Robbins Basic Pathology

Robbins Basic Pathology

8th edition

Vinay Kumar, MBBS, MD, FRCPath
Alice Hogge and Arthur Baer Professor
Chair, Department of Pathology
Vice Dean, Division of Biological Sciences and the Pritzker School of Medicine
University of Chicago
Chicago, Illinois

Abul K. Abbas, MBBS
Professor and Chair, Department of Pathology
University of California San Francisco
San Francisco, California

Nelson Fausto, MD
Chair, Department of Pathology
University of Washington School of Medicine
Seattle, Washington

Richard N. Mitchell, MD, PhD
Associate Professor
Department of Pathology and Health Sciences and Technology
Brigham and Women's Hospital and Harvard Medical School
Boston, Massachusetts

SAUNDERS
ELSEVIER

Robins Basic Pathology, 8e
Kumar, et al

Saunders
An imprint of Elsevier
1600 John F. Kennedy Blvd., Suite 1800
Philadelphia, Pennsylvania 19103-2899

Original ISBN: 978-1-4160-2973-1

This edition of Robins Basic Pathology, 8e by Vinay Kumar, MBBS, MD, FRCPath, et al is published by an arrangement with Elsevier Inc.

First Printed in India 2007
Reprinted 2008
Reprinted 2009

Indian Reprint ISBN: 978-81-312-1036-9

NOTICE

Knowledge and best practice in this field are constantly changing. As new research and experience broaden our knowledge, changes in practice, treatment and drug therapy may become necessary or appropriate. Readers are advised to check the most current information provided (i) on procedures featured or (ii) by the manufacturer of each product to be administered, to verify the recommended dose or formula, the method and duration of administration, and contraindications. It is the responsibility of the practitioner, relying on their own experience and knowledge of the patient, to make diagnoses, to determine dosages and the best treatment for each individual patient, and to take all appropriate safety precautions. To the fullest extent of the law, neither the Publisher nor the Authors assumes any liability for any injury and/or damage to persons or property arising out of or related to any use of the material contained in this book.

The Publisher

Published by Elsevier, a division of Reed Elsevier India Private Limited, Logix Park, First Floor, A-4 & A-5, Sector 16, Noida-201 301, U.P. (India).

Printed and bound at Solar Print Process, New Delhi

DEDICATION

In Memory of
Dr. Stanley L. Robbins (1915–2003)
and
Dr. Ramzi S. Cotran (1932–2000)

Dear friends, respected colleagues, and dedicated teachers

They leave a legacy of excellence that will enrich the lives of generations of future physicians.

Contributors

Charles E. Alpers, MD
Professor of Pathology and Adjunct Professor of Medicine
Department of Pathology
University of Washington Medical Center
Seattle, Washington

Jon C. Aster, MD, PhD
Associate Professor of Pathology
Department of Pathology
Brigham and Women's Hospital
Boston, Massachusetts

Agnes B. Fogo, MD
Professor of Pathology, Medicine, and Pediatrics
Director, Renal/EM Laboratory
Vanderbilt University Medical Center
Nashville, Tennessee

Matthew P. Frosch, MD, PhD
C.S. Kubik Laboratory for Neuropathology
Department of Pathology
Massachusetts General Hospital
Boston, Massachusetts

Alexander J.F. Lazar, MD, PhD
Assistant Professor of Pathology
Departments of Pathology and Dermatology
Sarcoma Research Center
University of Texas MD Anderson Cancer Center
Houston, Texas

Anirban Maitra, MBBS
Associate Professor of Pathology, Oncology, and Genetic Medicine
The Sol Goldman Pancreatic Cancer Research Center
Johns Hopkins University School of Medicine
Baltimore, Maryland

Anthony Montag, MD
Professor
Department of Pathology
University of Chicago
Chicago, Illinois

Frederick J. Schoen, MD, PhD
Professor of Pathology and Health Sciences and Technology
Harvard Medical School
Executive Vice-Chairman
Brigham and Women's Hospital
Boston, Massachusetts

Thomas P. Stricker, MD, PhD
Department of Pathology
University of Chicago
Chicago, Illinois

Preface

The remarkable advances made in the study of human disease mechanisms make this an exciting time for students of Pathology. We have attempted to capture this enthusiasm in Robbins Basic Pathology. As in the past, this edition has been extensively revised and in some areas completely rewritten. Cutting edge discoveries, such as the role of microRNAs in gene regulation and their impact on the unraveling of human diseases such as cancer, are included. Such advances in basic sciences ultimately help us in understanding diseases in the individual patient. Thus, we have strived to include the impact of scientific advances on diseases of organ systems described throughout the text. While many of the "breakthroughs" on the bench have not yet reached the bedside, we have included them in measured "doses" so that students can begin to experience the excitement that is ahead in their careers.

Realizing that the modern medical student feels inundated in trying to synthesize the essentials with the "state of the art," we have introduced a new feature in this edition. Scattered throughout the text are highlighted Summary Boxes designed to provide the students with key "take home" messages. We are keen to know from both students and instructors the utility of this feature.

Many new pieces of four-color art—schematics, flow charts, and diagrammatic representations of disease—have been added to facilitate the understanding of difficult concepts such as the molecular basis of cancer, interactions of HIV with its receptors, and the biochemical basis of apoptotic cell death. More illustrations have been added bringing the total to more than 1,000. Formatting and color palettes of the tables have been changed for greater clarity.

Despite the extensive changes and revisions, our goals remain substantially unaltered. As in previous editions, we have strived to provide a balanced, accurate, and up-to-date view of the central body of pathology. Gross and microscopic changes are highlighted for ready reference. The strong emphasis on clinicopathologic correlations is maintained, and wherever understood, the impact of molecular pathology on the practice of medicine is highlighted. We are pleased that all of this was accomplished without a "bulge" in the waistline of the text. The approximately 50 page increase is accounted for by the Summary boxes and new illustrations.

We continue to firmly believe that clarity of writing and proper usage of language enhance comprehension and facilitate the learning process. Generations of students have told us that they enjoy reading this book. We hope that this edition will be worthy of and possibly enhance the tradition of its forebears.

Acknowledgments

Any large endeavor of this type cannot be completed without the help of many individuals. First and foremost we thank the contributors of various chapters. Many are veterans of the older sib of this text, the so-called "Big Robbins". They are listed in the table of contents as well as in the chapters themselves. To each of them a special thanks.

Beverly Shackelford (UT Southwestern at Dallas), who has assisted one of us (VK) over the past 23 years, continued to be "the point person" who made sure that everyone did his or her job and served as a liaison with the publishers. No amount of "thank-yous" can fully capture our indebtedness to her. Vera Davis and Ruthie Cornelius deserve thanks for coordinating the tasks from Chicago, and Ana Narvaez from San Francisco. We are fortunate to continue our collaboration with Jim Perkins, whose illustrations bring to life abstract ideas and clarify difficult concepts.

Many colleagues have enhanced the text by providing helpful critiques in their areas of interest. These include Drs. Pedram Argani, Eugene Chang, Suzanne Conzen, Jennifer Cuthbert, Gerard Evan, Sandeep Gurbuxani, Aliya Husain, Ron McLawhon, Kay Macleod, Raminder Kumar, Tamara Lotan, Marcus Peter, Rish Pai, Peter Pytel, Paul Schumacker, Brad Stohr, Helen Te, Ken Thompson, and Rebecca Wilcox. Others have provided us with photographic gems from their personal collections. They are individually acknowledged in the credits to their contribution(s). For any unintended omissions we offer our apologies.

Many at Elsevier deserve recognition for their role in the production of this book. This text was fortunate to be in the hands of Jacquie McMahon and Rebecca Gruliow, our developmental editors. Others deserving of our thanks are Mary Stermel (Project Manager) and Ellen Zanolle (Design Manager).We were fortunate to be able work again with Ellen Sklar as our production editor. Few can match her dedication to quality and understanding of the complexities of textbook production. William Schmitt, Publishing Director of Medical Textbooks, continued to be our cheerleader and friend.

Ventures such as this exact a heavy toll from the families of the authors. We thank them for their tolerance of our absences, physically and emotionally. We are blessed and strengthened by their unconditional support and love, and for their sharing with us the belief that our efforts are worthwhile and useful. We are especially grateful to our wives Raminder Kumar, Ann Abbas, Ann DeLancey, and Diane Mitchell, who continue to provide silent but firm support.

And finally, Vinay Kumar welcomes three new colleagues to this edition, Abul Abbas, Nelson Fausto, and Rick Mitchell. While their names appear on the cover of this book for the first time, we have collaborated on many other texts of the Robbins family in the past. We are joined not only by coauthorship but also by a shared vision of excellence in teaching. Despite differences in opinions and individual styles, this partnership has increased our mutual respect, and our friendship grows stronger.

VK

AA

NF

RM

Contents*

*Chapters without any listed contributors have been written by the editors

Chapter 1

Cell Injury, Cell Death, and Adaptations

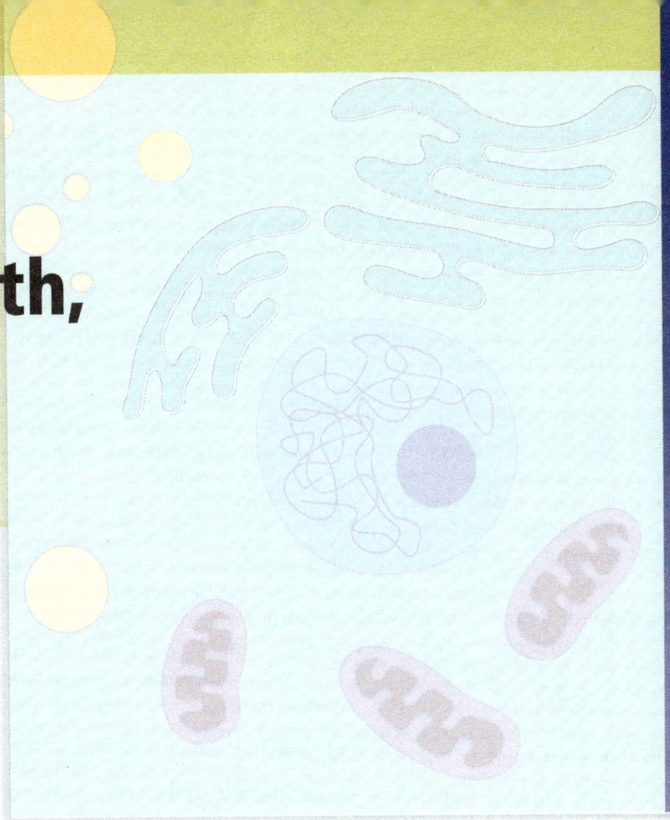

INTRODUCTION TO PATHOLOGY

Literally translated, *pathology* is the study (*logos*) of suffering (*pathos*). It is a discipline that bridges clinical practice and basic science, and it involves the investigation of the causes (*etiology*) of disease as well as the underlying mechanisms (*pathogenesis*) that result in the presenting signs and symptoms of the patient. Pathologists use a variety of molecular, microbiologic, and immunologic techniques to understand the biochemical, structural, and functional changes that occur in cells, tissues, and organs. To render diagnoses and guide therapy, pathologists identify changes in the gross or microscopic appearance (*morphology*) of cells and tissues, and biochemical alterations in body fluids (such as blood and urine). Traditionally, the discipline is divided into general pathology and systemic pathology; the former focuses on the fundamental cellular and tissue responses to pathologic stimuli, while the latter examines the particular responses of specialized organs. In this book we first cover the broad principles of general pathology and then progress to specific disease processes in individual organs.

OVERVIEW OF CELLULAR RESPONSES TO STRESS AND NOXIOUS STIMULI

Cells are active participants in their environment, constantly adjusting their structure and function to accommodate changing demands and extracellular stresses. Cells tend to maintain their intracellular milieu within a fairly narrow range of physiologic parameters; that is, they maintain normal *homeostasis*. As cells encounter physiologic stresses or pathologic stimuli, they can undergo adaptation, achieving a new steady state and preserving viability and function. The principal adaptive responses are *hypertrophy, hyperplasia, atrophy,* and *metaplasia.* If the adaptive capability is exceeded or if the external stress is inherently harmful, *cell injury* develops (Fig. 1–1). Within certain limits injury is *reversible,* and cells return to a stable baseline; however, severe or persistent stress results in *irreversible injury* and death of the affected cells. *Cell death* is one of the most crucial events in the evolution of disease in any tissue or organ. It results from diverse causes, including ischemia (lack of blood flow), infections, toxins, and immune reactions. Cell death is also a normal and essential process in embryogenesis, the development of organs, and the maintenance of homeostasis.

The relationships between normal, adapted, and reversibly and irreversibly injured cells are well illustrated by the responses of the heart to different types of stress (Fig. 1–2). Myocardium subjected to persistent increased load, as in hypertension or with a stenotic valve, adapts by undergoing *hypertrophy*—an increase in the size of the individual cells and ultimately the entire heart—to generate the required higher contractile force. If the increased demand is not relieved, or if the myocardium is subjected to reduced blood flow (*ischemia*) from an occluded coronary artery, the muscle cells may undergo injury. Myocardium may be reversibly injured if the stress

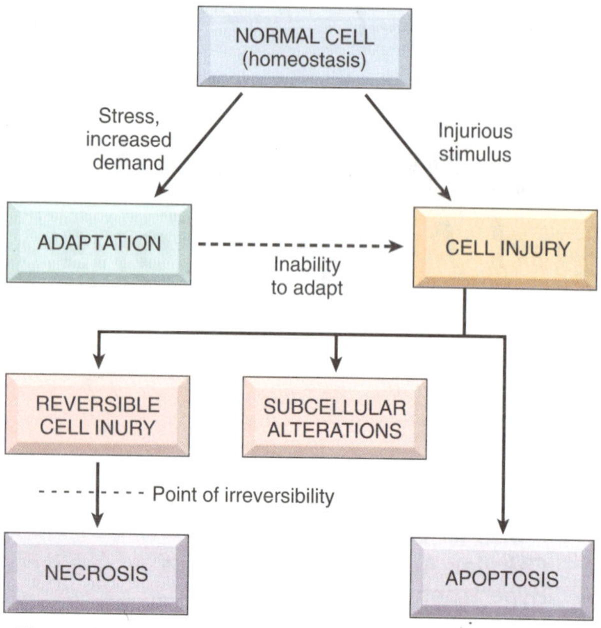

Figure 1–1

Stages in the cellular response to stress and injurious stimuli.

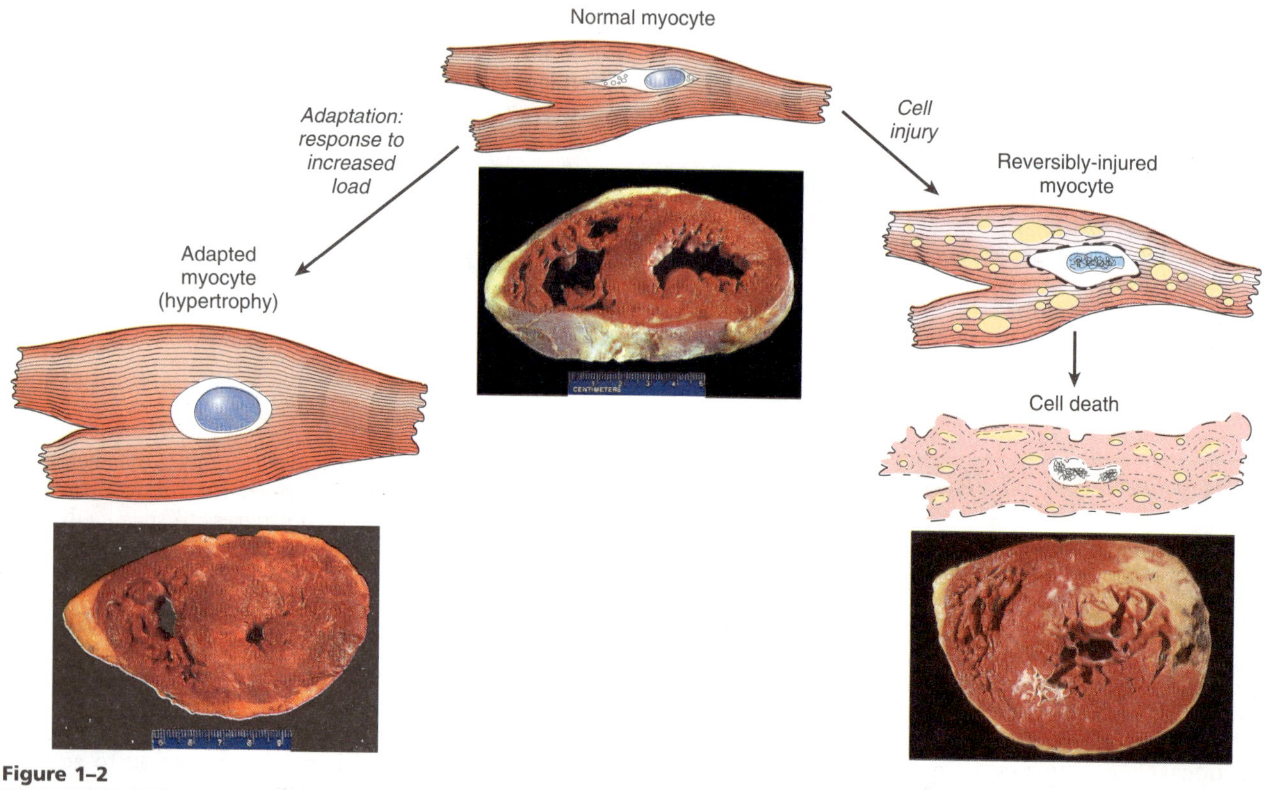

Figure 1–2

The relationship between normal, adapted, reversibly injured, and dead myocardial cells. The cellular adaptation depicted here is hypertrophy, the type of reversible injury is ischemia, and the irreversible injury is ischemic coagulative necrosis. In the example of myocardial hypertrophy (*lower left*), the left ventricular wall is thicker than 2 cm (normal, 1–1.5 cm). Reversibly injured myocardium shows functional effects without any gross or light microscopic changes, or reversible changes like cellular swelling and fatty change (shown here). In the specimen showing necrosis (*lower right*) the transmural light area in the posterolateral left ventricle represents an acute myocardial infarction. All three transverse sections of myocardium have been stained with triphenyltetrazolium chloride, an enzyme substrate that colors viable myocardium magenta. Failure to stain is due to enzyme loss after cell death.

is mild or the arterial occlusion is incomplete or sufficiently brief, or it may undergo irreversible injury (*infarction*) after complete or prolonged occlusion. Note, too, that stresses and injury affect not only the morphology but also the functional status of cells and tissues. Thus, reversibly injured myocytes are not dead and may resemble normal myocytes morphologically; however, they are transiently noncontractile, and therefore, even mild injury can have a lethal clinical impact. Whether a specific form of stress induces adaptation or causes reversible or irreversible injury depends not only on the nature and severity of the stress but also on several other variables, including cellular metabolism, blood supply, and nutritional status.

In this chapter we discuss first how cells adapt to stresses and then the causes, mechanisms, and consequences of the various forms of acute cell damage, including reversible cell injury, subcellular alterations, and cell death. We conclude with three other processes that affect cells and tissues: intracellular accumulations, pathologic calcification, and cell aging.

CELLULAR ADAPTATIONS TO STRESS

Adaptations are reversible changes in the number, size, phenotype, metabolic activity, or functions of cells in response to changes in their environment. *Physiologic adaptations* usually represent responses of cells to normal stimulation by hormones or endogenous chemical mediators (e.g., the hormone-induced enlargement of the breast and uterus during pregnancy). *Pathologic adaptations* are responses to stress that allow cells to modulate their structure and function and thus escape injury. Such adaptations can take several distinct forms.

Hypertrophy

Hypertrophy is an increase in the size of cells resulting in increase in the size of the organ. In contrast, hyperplasia (discussed next) is characterized by an increase in cell number. Stated another way, in pure hypertrophy there are no new cells, just bigger cells, enlarged by an increased amount of structural proteins and organelles. Hyperplasia is an adaptive response in cells capable of replication, whereas hypertrophy occurs when cells are incapable of dividing. *Hypertrophy can be physiologic or pathologic* and is caused either by increased functional demand or by specific hormonal stimulation. Hypertrophy and hyperplasia can also occur together, and obviously both result in an enlarged (*hypertrophic*) organ. Thus, the massive physiologic enlargement of the uterus during pregnancy occurs as a consequence of estrogen-stimulated smooth muscle hypertrophy and smooth muscle hyperplasia (Fig. 1–3). In contrast, the striated muscle cells in both the skeletal muscle and the heart can undergo only hypertrophy in response to increased demand because in the adult they have limited capacity to divide. Therefore, the avid weightlifter can develop a rippled physique only by hypertrophy of individual skeletal muscle cells induced by an increased workload. Examples of pathologic cellular hypertrophy include the cardiac enlargement that occurs with hypertension or aortic valve disease (see Fig. 1–2).

The mechanisms driving cardiac hypertrophy involve at least two types of signals: *mechanical triggers,* such as stretch, and *trophic triggers,* such as activation of α-adrenergic receptors. These stimuli turn on signal transduction pathways that lead to the induction of a number of genes, which in turn stimulate synthesis of numerous cellular proteins, including growth factors and structural proteins. The result is the synthesis of more proteins and

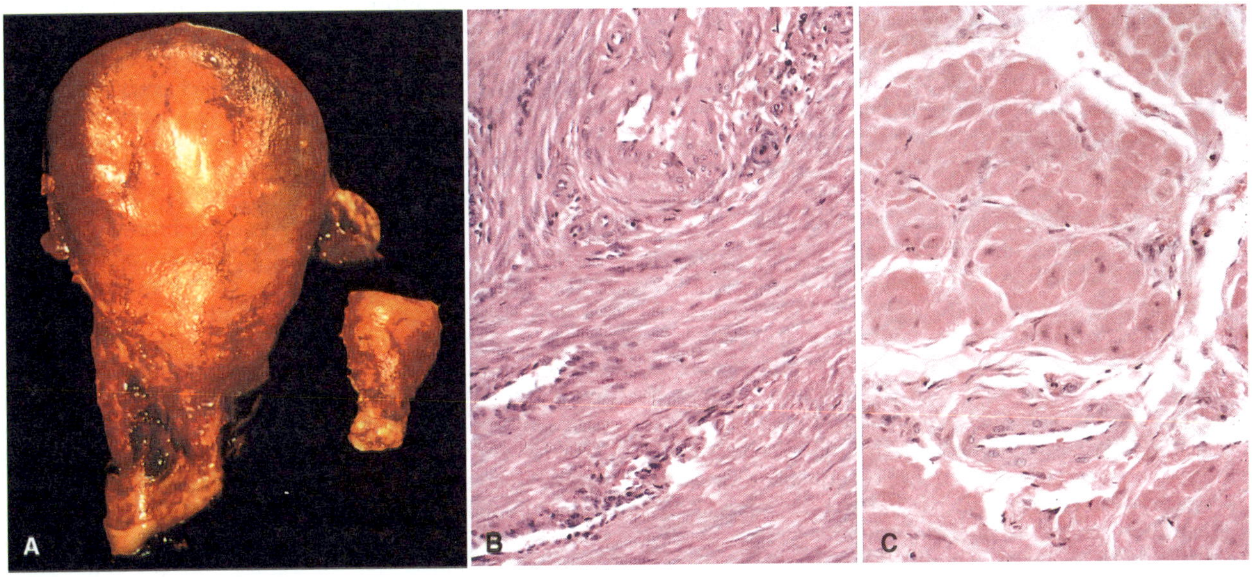

Figure 1–3

Physiologic hypertrophy of the uterus during pregnancy. **A,** Gross appearance of a normal uterus (*right*) and a gravid uterus (*left*) that was removed for postpartum bleeding. **B,** Small spindle-shaped uterine smooth muscle cells from a normal uterus. Compare this with (**C**) large, plump hypertrophied smooth muscle cells from a gravid uterus (**B** and **C,** same magnification).

myofilaments per cell, which achieves improved performance and thus a balance between the demand and the cell's functional capacity. There may also be a switch of contractile proteins from adult to fetal or neonatal forms. For example, during muscle hypertrophy, the α-myosin heavy chain is replaced by the β form of the myosin heavy chain, which has a slower, more energetically economical contraction. Whatever the exact mechanisms of hypertrophy, a limit is reached beyond which the enlargement of muscle mass can no longer compensate for the increased burden. When this happens in the heart, several "degenerative" changes occur in the myocardial fibers, of which the most important are fragmentation and loss of myofibrillar contractile elements. The variables that limit continued hypertrophy and cause the regressive changes are incompletely understood. There may be finite limits of the vasculature to adequately supply the enlarged fibers, of the mitochondria to supply adenosine triphosphate (ATP), or of the biosynthetic machinery to provide the contractile proteins or other cytoskeletal elements. The net result of these changes is ventricular dilation and ultimately cardiac failure, a sequence of events that illustrates how *an adaptation to stress can progress to functionally significant cell injury if the stress is not relieved.*

Hyperplasia

As discussed above, hyperplasia takes place if the cell population is capable of replication; it may occur with hypertrophy and often in response to the same stimuli.

Hyperplasia can be physiologic or pathologic.

- The two types of *physiologic hyperplasia* are (1) *hormonal hyperplasia,* exemplified by the proliferation of the glandular epithelium of the female breast at puberty and during pregnancy; and (2) *compensatory hyperplasia,* that is, hyperplasia that occurs when a portion of the tissue is removed or diseased. For example, when a liver is partially resected, mitotic activity in the remaining cells begins as early as 12 hours later, eventually restoring the liver to its normal weight. The stimuli for hyperplasia in this setting are polypeptide growth factors produced by remnant hepatocytes as well as nonparenchymal cells in the liver. After restoration of the liver mass, cell proliferation is "turned off" by various growth inhibitors (Chapter 3).
- Most forms of *pathologic hyperplasia* are caused by excessive hormonal or growth factor stimulation. For example, after a normal menstrual period there is a burst of uterine epithelial proliferation that is normally tightly regulated by stimulation through pituitary hormones and ovarian estrogen and by inhibition through progesterone. However, if the balance between estrogen and progesterone is disturbed, endometrial hyperplasia ensues, a common cause of abnormal menstrual bleeding. Hyperplasia is also an important response of connective tissue cells in wound healing, in which proliferating fibroblasts and blood vessels aid in repair (Chapter 3). In this process, growth factors are produced by white blood cells (leukocytes) responding to the injury and by cells in the extracellular matrix. Stimulation by growth factors is also involved in the hyperplasia that is associated with certain viral infections; for example, papillomaviruses cause skin warts and mucosal lesions composed of masses of hyperplastic epithelium. Here the growth factors may be produced by the virus or by infected cells. It is important to note that in all these situations, the hyperplastic process remains controlled; if hormonal or growth factor stimulation abates, the hyperplasia disappears. It is this sensitivity to normal regulatory control mechanisms that distinguishes benign pathologic hyperplasias from cancer, in which the growth control mechanisms become dysregulated or ineffective (Chapter 6). Nevertheless, pathologic hyperplasia constitutes a fertile soil in which cancerous proliferation may eventually arise. Thus, patients with hyperplasia of the endometrium are at increased risk of developing endometrial cancer, and certain papillomavirus infections predispose to cervical cancers (Chapter 19).

Atrophy

Shrinkage in the size of the cell by the loss of cell substance is known as atrophy. When a sufficient number of cells is involved, the entire tissue or organ diminishes in size, becoming atrophic (Fig. 1–4). It should be emphasized that *although atrophic cells may have diminished function, they are not dead.*

Causes of atrophy include a decreased workload (e.g., immobilization of a limb to permit healing of a fracture), loss of innervation, diminished blood supply, inadequate nutrition, loss of endocrine stimulation, and aging (senile atrophy). Although some of these stimuli are physiologic (e.g., the loss of hormone stimulation in menopause) and others pathologic (e.g., denervation), the fundamental cellular changes are identical. They represent a retreat by the cell to a smaller size at which survival is still possible; a new equilibrium is achieved between cell size and diminished blood supply, nutrition, or trophic stimulation.

Atrophy results from decreased protein synthesis and increased protein degradation in cells. Protein synthesis decreases because of reduced metabolic activity. The degradation of cellular proteins occurs mainly by the *ubiquitin-proteasome pathway.* Nutrient deficiency and disuse may activate ubiquitin ligases, which attach multiple copies of the small peptide ubiquitin to cellular proteins and target these proteins for degradation in proteasomes. This pathway is also thought to be responsible for the accelerated proteolysis seen in a variety of catabolic conditions, including cancer cachexia.

In many situations, atrophy is also accompanied by increased *autophagy,* with resulting increases in the number of *autophagic vacuoles.* Autophagy ("self-eating") is the process in which the starved cell eats its own components in an attempt to find nutrients and survive. We will describe this process later.

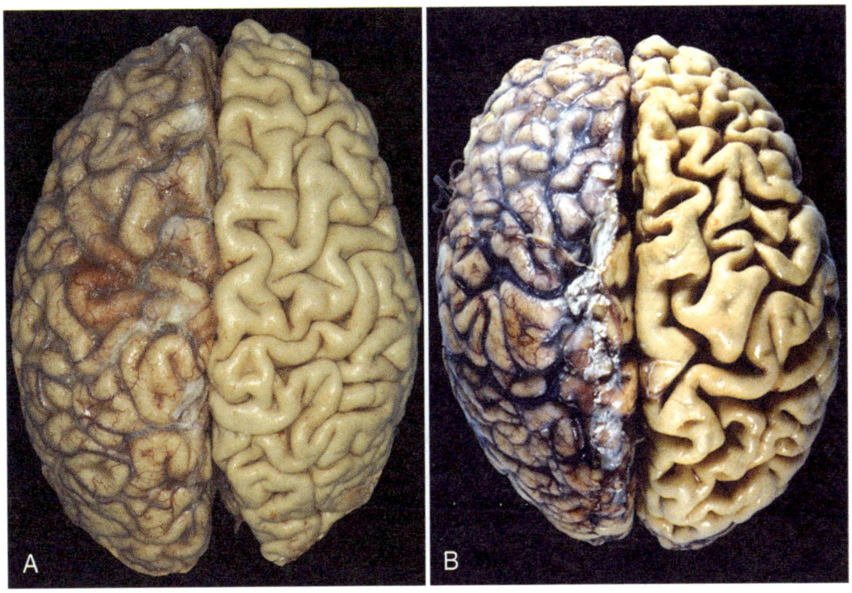

Figure 1–4

Atrophy. **A,** Normal brain of a young adult. **B,** Atrophy of the brain in an 82-year-old male with atherosclerotic disease. Atrophy of the brain is due to aging and reduced blood supply. Note that loss of brain substance narrows the gyri and widens the sulci. The meninges have been stripped from the right half of each specimen to reveal the surface of the brain.

Metaplasia

Metaplasia is a reversible change in which one adult cell type (epithelial or mesenchymal) is replaced by another adult cell type. In this type of cellular adaptation, cells sensitive to a particular stress are replaced by other cell types better able to withstand the adverse environment. Metaplasia is thought to arise by genetic "reprogramming" of stem cells rather than transdifferentiation of already differentiated cells.

Epithelial metaplasia is exemplified by the squamous change that occurs in the respiratory epithelium in habitual cigarette smokers (Fig. 1–5). The normal ciliated columnar epithelial cells of the trachea and bronchi are focally or widely replaced by stratified squamous epithelial cells. Vitamin A deficiency may also induce squamous metaplasia in the respiratory epithelium. The "rugged" stratified squamous epithelium may be able to survive under circumstances that the more fragile specialized epithelium would not tolerate. *Although the metaplastic squamous epithelium has survival advantages, important protective mechanisms are lost,* such as mucus secretion and ciliary clearance of particulate matter. Epithelial metaplasia is therefore a double-edged sword; moreover, *the influences that induce metaplastic transformation, if persistent, may predispose to malignant transformation of the epithelium.* In fact, in a common form of lung cancer, squamous metaplasia of the respiratory epithelium often coexists with cancers composed of malignant squamous cells. It is thought that cigarette smoking initially causes squamous metaplasia, and cancers arise later in some of these altered foci. Metaplasia need not always occur in the direction of columnar to squamous epithelium; in chronic gastric reflux, the normal stratified squamous epithelium of the lower esophagus may undergo metaplastic transformation to gastric or intestinal-type columnar epithelium. Metaplasia may also occur in mesenchymal cells but less clearly as an adaptive response. For example, bone is occasionally formed in soft tissues, particularly in foci of injury.

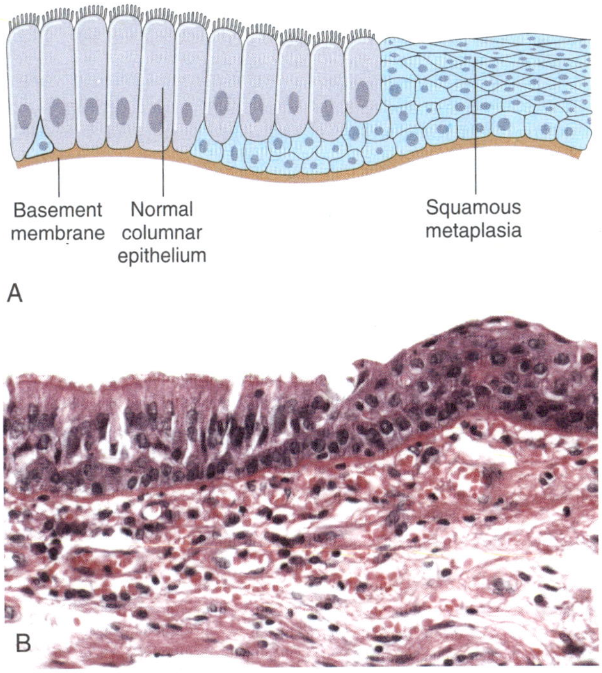

Figure 1–5

Metaplasia of normal columnar (*left*) to squamous epithelium (*right*) in a bronchus, shown **(A)** schematically and **(B)** histologically.

SUMMARY

Cellular Adaptations to Stress

- *Hypertrophy:* increased cell and organ size, often in response to increased workload; induced by mechanical stress and by growth factors; occurs in tissues incapable of cell division
- *Hyperplasia:* increased cell numbers in response to hormones and other growth factors; occurs in tissues whose cells are able to divide
- *Atrophy:* decreased cell and organ size, as a result of decreased nutrient supply or disuse; associated with decreased synthesis and increased proteolytic breakdown of cellular organelles
- *Metaplasia:* change in phenotype of differentiated cells, often a response to chronic irritation that makes cells better able to withstand the stress; usually induced by altered differentiation pathway of tissue stem cells; may result in reduced functions or increased propensity for malignant transformation.

OVERVIEW OF CELL INJURY AND CELL DEATH

As stated at the beginning of the chapter, cell injury results when cells are stressed so severely that they are no longer able to adapt or when cells are exposed to inherently damaging agents or suffer from intrinsic abnormalities. Different injurious stimuli affect many metabolic pathways and cellular organelles. Injury may progress through a reversible stage and culminate in cell death (see Fig. 1–1).

- *Reversible cell injury.* In early stages or mild forms of injury the functional and morphologic changes are reversible if the damaging stimulus is removed. At this stage, although there may be significant structural and functional abnormalities, the injury has typically not progressed to severe membrane damage and nuclear dissolution.
- *Cell death.* With continuing damage, the injury becomes irreversible, at which time the cell cannot recover and it dies. *There are two types of cell death—necrosis and apoptosis—which differ in their morphology, mechanisms, and roles in disease and physiology* (Fig. 1–6 and Table 1–1). When damage to membranes is severe, enzymes leak out of lysosomes, enter the cytoplasm, and digest the cell, resulting in *necrosis.* Cellular contents also leak out through the damaged plasma membrane and elicit a host reaction (inflammation). Necrosis is the major pathway of cell death in many commonly encountered injuries, such as those resulting from ischemia, exposure to toxins, various infections, and trauma. When a cell is deprived of growth factors or the cell's DNA or proteins are damaged beyond repair, the cell kills itself by another

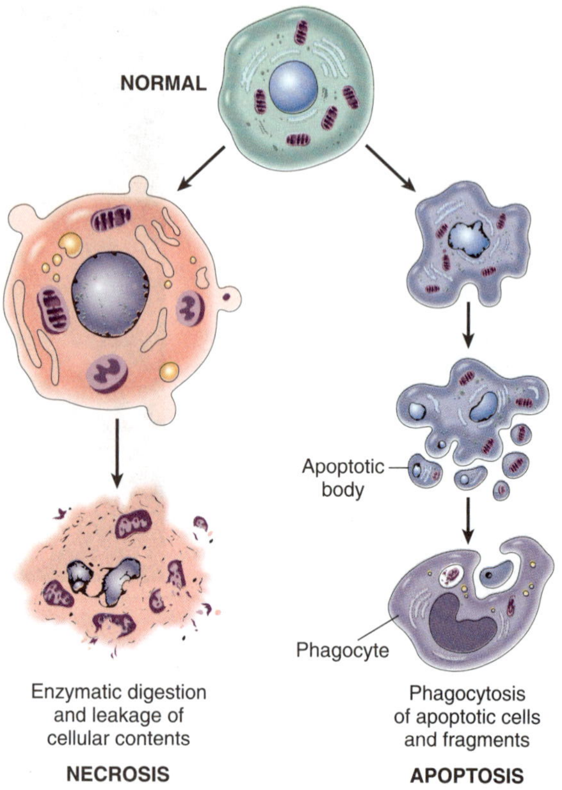

Figure 1–6

Cellular features of necrosis (*left*) and apoptosis (*right*). (Adapted from Walker NI, et al: Patterns of cell death. Methods Archiv Exp Pathol 13:18–32, 1988. With permission of S. Karger, Basel, Switzerland.)

Table 1–1 Features of Necrosis and Apoptosis

Feature	Necrosis	Apoptosis
Cell size	Enlarged (swelling)	Reduced (shrinkage)
Nucleus	Pyknosis → karyorrhexis → karyolysis	Fragmentation into nucleosome-size fragments
Plasma membrane	Disrupted	Intact; altered structure, especially orientation of lipids
Cellular contents	Enzymatic digestion; may leak out of cell	Intact; may be released in apoptotic bodies
Adjacent inflammation	Frequent	No
Physiologic or pathologic role	Invariably pathologic (culmination of irreversible cell injury)	Often physiologic, means of eliminating unwanted cells; may be pathologic after some forms of cell injury, especially DNA damage

type of death, called *apoptosis,* which is characterized by nuclear dissolution without complete loss of membrane integrity. Apoptosis is an active, energy-dependent, tightly regulated type of cell death that is seen in some specific situations. *Whereas necrosis is always a pathologic process, apoptosis serves many normal functions and is not necessarily associated with pathologic cell injury.* The morphologic features, mechanisms, and significance of these two death pathways are discussed in more detail later in the chapter.

CAUSES OF CELL INJURY

The causes of cell injury range from the gross physical trauma of a motor vehicle accident to the single gene defect that results in a defective enzyme underlying a specific metabolic disease. Most injurious stimuli can be grouped into the following categories.

Oxygen Deprivation. *Hypoxia,* or oxygen deficiency, interferes with aerobic oxidative respiration and is an extremely important and common cause of cell injury and death. Hypoxia should be distinguished from *ischemia,* which is a loss of blood supply in a tissue due to impeded arterial flow or reduced venous drainage. While ischemia is the most common cause of hypoxia, oxygen deficiency can also result from inadequate oxygenation of the blood, as in pneumonia, or reduction in the oxygen-carrying capacity of the blood, as in blood loss anemia or carbon monoxide (CO) poisoning. (CO forms a stable complex with hemoglobin that prevents oxygen binding.)

Chemical Agents. An enormous number of chemical substances can injure cells; even innocuous substances such as glucose or salt, if sufficiently concentrated, can so derange the osmotic environment that cell injury or death results. Oxygen at sufficiently high partial pressures is also toxic. Agents commonly known as poisons cause severe damage at the cellular level by altering membrane permeability, osmotic homeostasis, or the integrity of an enzyme or cofactor, and exposure to these poisons can culminate in the death of the whole organism. Other potentially toxic agents are encountered daily in our environment; these include air pollutants, insecticides, CO, asbestos, and social "stimuli" such as ethanol. Even therapeutic drugs can cause cell or tissue injury in a susceptible patient or if used excessively or inappropriately (Chapter 8).

Infectious Agents. These range from submicroscopic viruses to meter-long tapeworms; in between are the rickettsiae, bacteria, fungi, and protozoans. The diverse ways by which infectious pathogens cause injury are discussed in Chapter 9.

Immunologic Reactions. Although the immune system defends the body against pathogenic microbes, immune reactions can also result in cell and tissue injury. Examples include autoimmune reactions against one's own tissues and allergic reactions against environmental substances in genetically susceptible individuals (Chapter 5).

Genetic Defects. Genetic defects can result in pathologic changes as conspicuous as the congenital malformations associated with Down syndrome or as subtle as the single amino acid substitution in hemoglobin S giving rise to sickle cell anemia. Genetic defects may cause cell injury because of deficiency of functional proteins, such as enzymes in inborn errors of metabolism, or accumulation of damaged DNA or misfolded proteins, both of which trigger cell death when they are beyond repair. Variations in the genetic makeup can also influence the susceptibility of cells to injury by chemicals and other environmental insults.

Nutritional Imbalances. Even in the current era of burgeoning global affluence, nutritional deficiencies remain a major cause of cell injury. Protein-calorie insufficiency among underprivileged populations is only the most obvious example; specific vitamin deficiencies are not uncommon even in developed countries with high standards of living (Chapter 8). Ironically, excesses of nutrition are also important causes of morbidity and mortality; for example, obesity markedly increases the risk for type 2 diabetes mellitus. Moreover, diets rich in animal fat are strongly implicated in the development of atherosclerosis as well as in increased vulnerability to many disorders, including cancer.

Physical Agents. Trauma, extremes of temperatures, radiation, electric shock, and sudden changes in atmospheric pressure all have wide-ranging effects on cells (Chapter 8).

Aging. Cellular senescence leads to alterations in replicative and repair abilities of individual cells and tissues. All of these changes result in a diminished ability to respond to damage and, eventually, the death of cells and of the organism. The mechanisms underlying cellular aging are discussed at the end of this chapter.

THE MORPHOLOGY OF CELL AND TISSUE INJURY

It is useful to describe the basic alterations that occur in damaged cells before we discuss the biochemical mechanisms that bring about these changes. All stresses and noxious influences exert their effects first at the molecular or biochemical level. *Cellular function may be lost long before cell death occurs, and the morphologic changes of cell injury (or death) lag far behind both* (Fig. 1–7). For example, myocardial cells become noncontractile after 1 to 2 minutes of ischemia, although they do not die until 20 to 30 minutes of ischemia have elapsed. These myocytes do not appear dead by electron microscopy for 2 to 3 hours, and by light microscopy for 6 to 12 hours.

The cellular derangements of reversible injury can be repaired and, if the injurious stimulus abates, the cell will return to normalcy. Persistent or excessive injury, however, causes cells to pass the nebulous "point of no return" into *irreversible injury* and *cell death.* The events that determine when reversible injury becomes irreversible and progresses to cell death remain poorly understood. The clinical relevance of this question is obvious; if we can answer it we may be able to devise strategies for preventing cell injury from having permanent deleterious consequences. Although there are no definitive morphologic or biochemical correlates of irreversibility, *two phenomena*

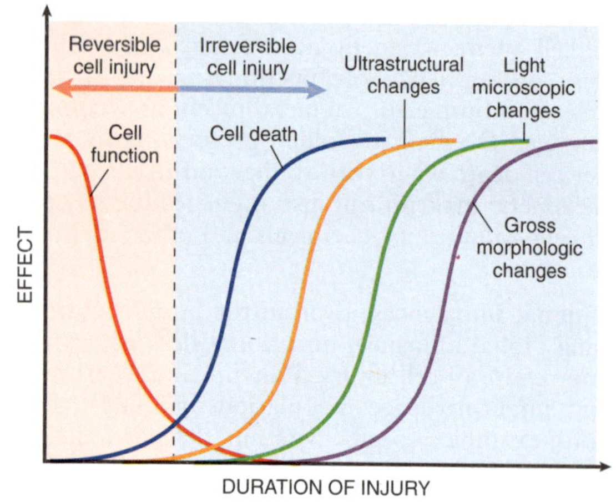

Figure 1–7

The relationship between cellular function, cell death, and the morphologic changes of cell injury. Note that cells may rapidly become nonfunctional after the onset of injury, although they are still viable, with potentially reversible damage; a longer duration of injury may eventually lead to irreversible injury and cell death. Note also that cell death typically precedes ultrastructural, light microscopic, and grossly visible morphologic changes.

consistently characterize irreversibility: the inability to reverse mitochondrial dysfunction (lack of oxidative phosphorylation and ATP generation) even after resolution of the original injury, and *profound disturbances in membrane function.* As mentioned earlier, injury to lysosomal membranes results in the enzymatic dissolution of the injured cell that is characteristic of necrosis.

Different injurious stimuli may induce death by necrosis or apoptosis (see Fig. 1–6 and Table 1–1). As mentioned above and detailed later, severe depletion of ATP and loss of membrane integrity are typically associated with necrosis. Apoptosis is an active and regulated process not associated with ATP depletion and it has many unique features, which we will describe separately later in the chapter.

Reversible Injury

The two main morphologic correlates of reversible cell injury are *cellular swelling* and *fatty change.* Cellular swelling is the result of failure of energy-dependent ion pumps in the plasma membrane, leading to an inability to maintain ionic and fluid homeostasis. Fatty change occurs in hypoxic injury and various forms of toxic or metabolic injury, and is manifested by the appearance of small or large lipid vacuoles in the cytoplasm. It occurs mainly in cells involved in and dependent on fat metabolism, such as hepatocytes and myocardial cells. The mechanisms of fatty change are discussed later in the chapter.

Morphology

Cellular swelling (Fig. 1–8B), the first manifestation of almost all forms of injury to cells, is difficult to appreciate with the light microscope; it may be more apparent at the level of the whole organ. When it affects many cells in an organ it causes some pallor, increased turgor, and increase in weight of the organ. Microscopic examination may reveal small, clear vacuoles within the cytoplasm; these represent distended and pinched-off segments of the ER. This pattern of nonlethal injury is sometimes called **hydropic change** or **vacuolar degeneration.** Swelling of cells is reversible. **Fatty change** is manifested by the appearance of lipid vacuoles in the cytoplasm. It is principally encountered in cells participating in fat metabolism (e.g., hepatocytes and myocardial cells) and is also reversible. Injured cells may also show increased eosinophilic staining, which becomes much more pronounced with progression to necrosis (described below).

The ultrastructural changes of reversible cell injury are illustrated schematically in Figure 1–9 and include (1) plasma membrane alterations such as blebbing, blunting or distortion of microvilli, and loosening of intercellular attachments; (2) mitochondrial changes such as swelling and the appearance of phospholipid-rich amorphous densities; (3) dilation of the ER with detachment of ribosomes and dissociation of polysomes; and (4) nuclear alterations, with clumping of chromatin.

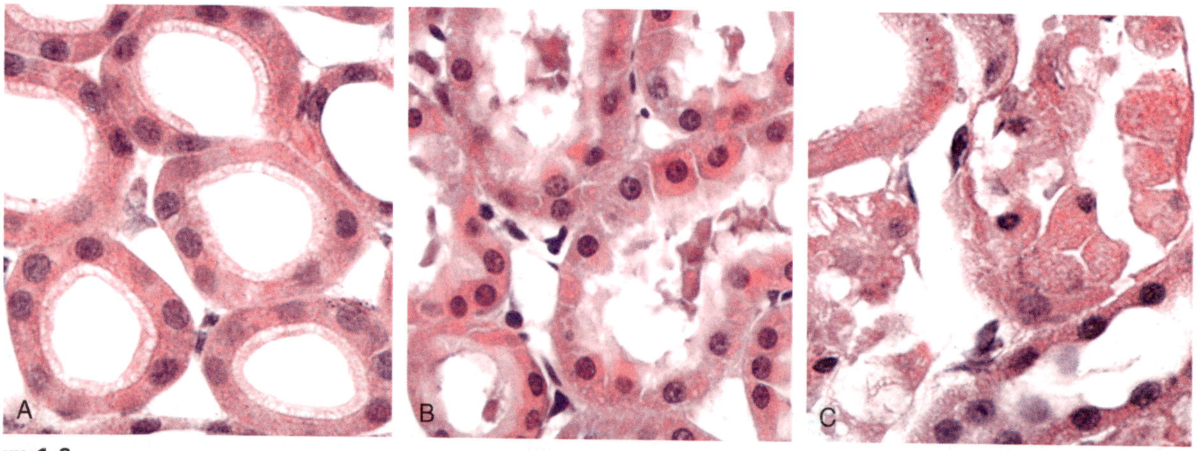

Figure 1–8

Morphologic changes in reversible and irreversible cell injury (necrosis). **A,** Normal kidney tubules with viable epithelial cells. **B,** Early (reversible) ischemic injury showing surface blebs, increased eosinophilia of cytoplasm, and swelling of occasional cells. **C,** Necrotic (irreversible) injury of epithelial cells, with loss of nuclei and fragmentation of cells and leakage of contents. The ultrastructural features of these stages of cell injury are shown in Fig. 1–9. (Courtesy of Drs. Neal Pinckard and M.A. Venkatachalam, University of Texas Health Sciences Center, San Antonio.)

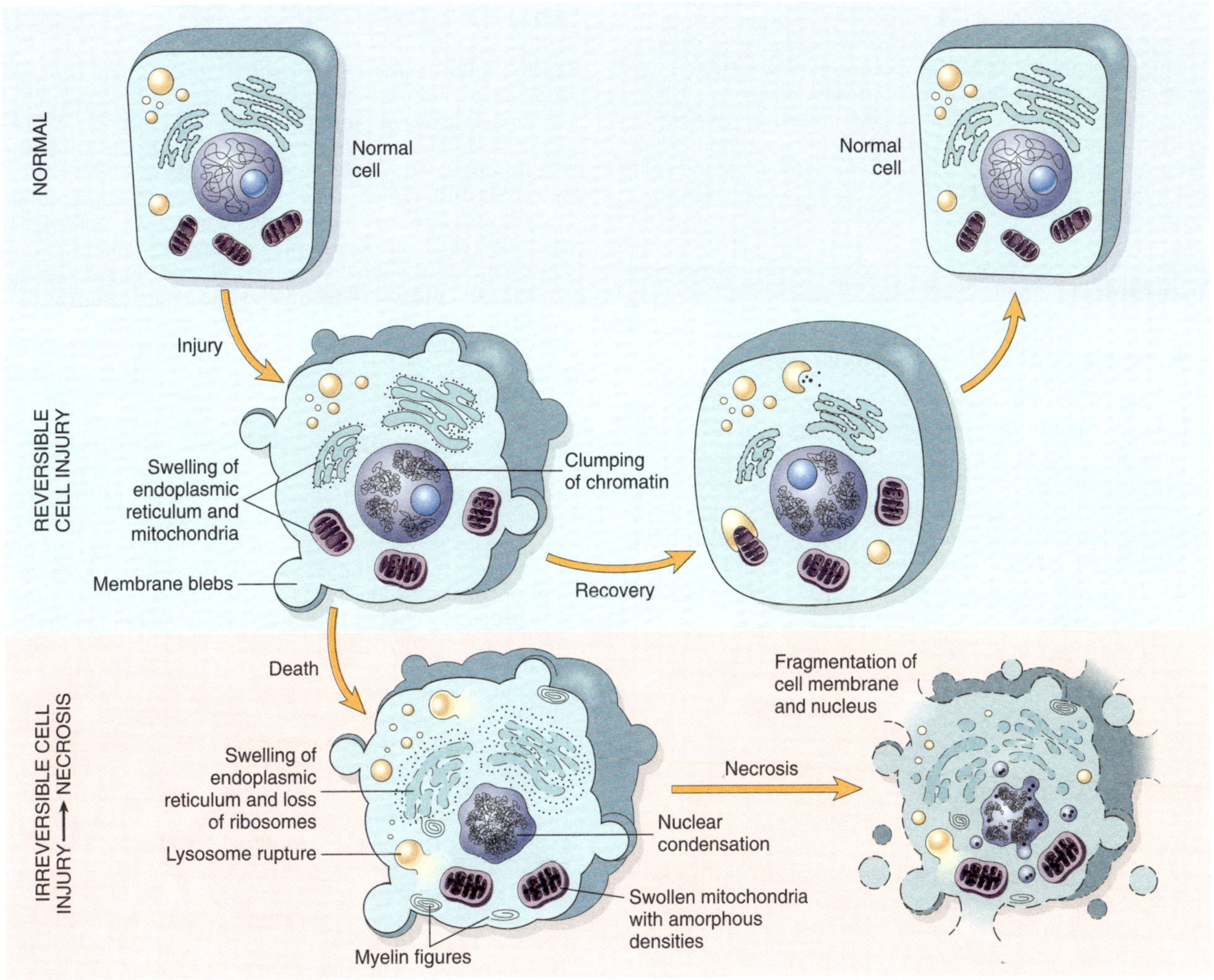

Figure 1–9

A normal cell and the changes in reversible and irreversible cell injury (necrosis).

Necrosis

The term *necrosis* was first used by morphologists to refer to a series of changes that accompany cell death, largely resulting from the degradative action of enzymes on lethally injured cells. Necrotic cells are unable to maintain membrane integrity, and their contents often leak out. The enzymes responsible for digestion of the cell are derived either from the lysosomes of the dying cells themselves or from the lysosomes of leukocytes that are recruited as part of the inflammatory reaction to the dead cells.

Morphology

In one common pattern of cell death resulting from lack of oxygen, the necrotic cells show **increased eosinophilia** (i.e., pink staining from the eosin dye, the "E" in "H&E"). This is attributable in part to increased binding of eosin to denatured cytoplasmic proteins and in part to loss of the basophilia that is normally imparted by the ribonucleic acid (RNA) in the cytoplasm (basophilia is the blue staining from the hematoxylin dye, the "H" in "H&E"). The cell may have a more glassy homogeneous appearance than viable cells, mostly because of the loss of glycogen particles. When enzymes have digested the cytoplasmic organelles, the cytoplasm becomes vacuolated and appears moth-eaten. Dead cells may be replaced by large, whorled phospholipid masses, called **myelin figures,** that are derived from damaged cellular membranes. They are thought to result from dissociation of lipoproteins with unmasking of phosphatide groups, promoting the uptake and intercalation of water between the lamellar stacks of membranes. These phospholipid precipitates are then either phagocytosed by other cells or further degraded into fatty acids; calcification of such fatty acid residues results in the generation of calcium soaps. Thus, the dead cells may ultimately become **calcified.** By electron microscopy (see Fig. 1–9), necrotic cells are characterized by discontinuities in plasma and organelle membranes, marked dilation of mitochondria with the appearance of large amorphous densities, disruption of lysosomes, intracytoplasmic myelin figures, and profound nuclear changes culminating in nuclear dissolution.

Nuclear changes assume one of three patterns, all due to breakdown of DNA and chromatin. The basophilia of the chromatin may fade (**karyolysis**), presumably secondary to deoxyribonuclease (DNase) activity. A second pattern is **pyknosis,** characterized by nuclear shrinkage and increased basophilia; the DNA condenses into a solid shrunken mass. In the third pattern, **karyorrhexis,** the pyknotic nucleus undergoes fragmentation. In 1 to 2 days, the nucleus in a dead cell completely disappears.

SUMMARY

Morphologic Alterations in Injured Cells

- *Reversible cell injury:* cell swelling, fatty change, plasma membrane blebbing and loss of microvilli, mitochondrial swelling, dilation of the ER, eosinophilia (due to decreased cytoplasmic RNA)
- *Necrosis:* increased eosinophilia; nuclear shrinkage, fragmentation, and dissolution; breakdown of plasma membrane and organellar membranes; myelin figures; leakage and enzymatic digestion of cellular contents
- *Apoptosis:* nuclear chromatin condensation; formation of apoptotic bodies (fragments of nuclei and cytoplasm)

Patterns of Tissue Necrosis

Necrosis of a collection of cells in a tissue or an organ, for instance in the ischemic myocardium, results in death of the entire tissue and sometimes an entire organ. There are several morphologically distinct patterns of tissue necrosis, which may provide clues about the underlying cause. Although the terms that describe these patterns do not reflect underlying mechanisms, the terms are used often and their implications are understood by both pathologists and clinicians.

Morphology

Coagulative necrosis is a form of tissue necrosis in which the component cells are dead but the basic tissue architecture is preserved for at least several days (Fig. 1–10). The affected tissues take on a firm texture. Presumably the injury denatures not only structural proteins but also enzymes and so blocks the proteolysis of the dead cells; as a result, eosinophilic, anucleate cells may persist for days or weeks. Ultimately, the necrotic cells are removed by phagocytosis of the cellular debris by infiltrating leukocytes and by digestion of the dead cells by the action of lysosomal enzymes of the leukocytes. Coagulative necrosis is characteristic of **infarcts** (areas of ischemic necrosis) in all solid organs except the brain.

Liquefactive necrosis is seen in focal bacterial or, occasionally, fungal infections, because microbes stimulate the accumulation of inflammatory cells and the enzymes of leukocytes digest ("liquefy") the tissue. For obscure reasons, hypoxic death of cells within the central nervous system often evokes liquefactive necrosis (Fig. 1–11). Whatever the pathogenesis, liquefaction completely digests the dead cells, resulting in transformation of the tissue into a liquid viscous mass. If the process was initiated by acute inflammation, the material is frequently creamy yellow and is called **pus** (Chapter 2).

Although **gangrenous necrosis** is not a distinctive pattern of cell death, the term is still commonly used in clinical practice. It is usually applied to a limb, generally the lower leg, that has lost its blood supply and has undergone coagulative necrosis involving multiple tissue layers. When bacterial infection is superimposed, coagulative necrosis is modified by the liquefactive action of the bacteria and the attracted leukocytes (so-called **wet gangrene**).

Caseous necrosis is encountered most often in foci of tuberculous infection. The term "caseous" (cheese-like) is derived from the friable yellow-white appearance of the area of necrosis (Fig. 1–12). On microscopic examination, the necrotic focus appears as a collection of fragmented or lysed cells with an amorphous granu-

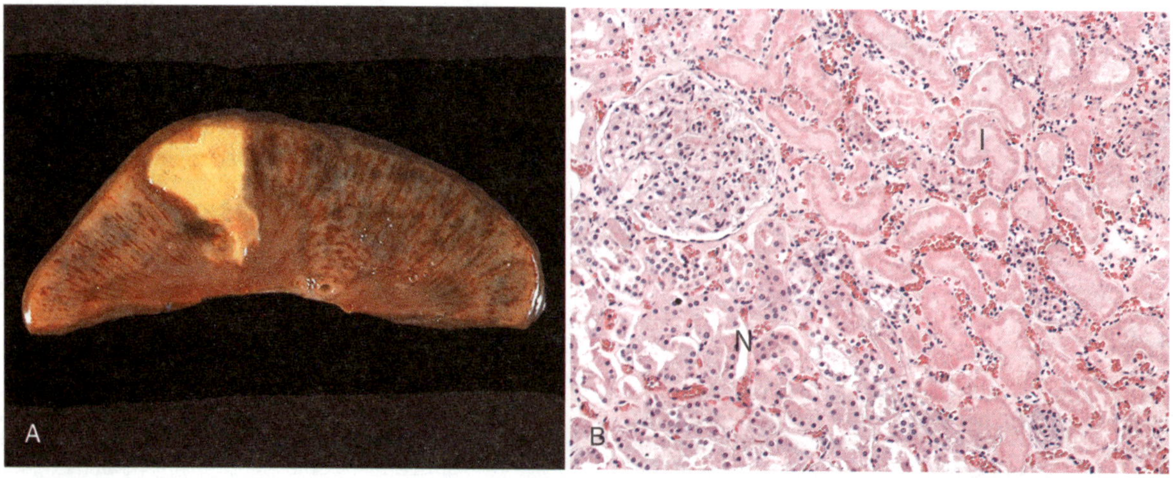

Figure 1–10

Coagulative necrosis. **A,** A wedge-shaped kidney infarct (yellow) with preservation of the outlines. **B,** Microscopic view of the edge of the infarct, with normal kidney (N) and necrotic cells in the infarct (I). The necrotic cells show preserved outlines with loss of nuclei, and an inflammatory infiltrate is present (difficult to discern at this magnification).

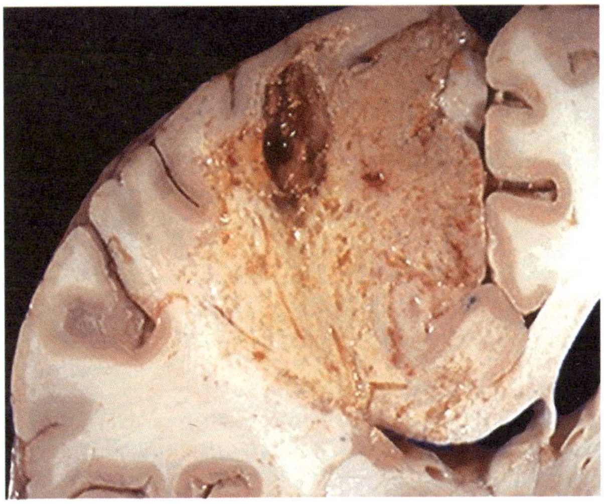

Figure 1–11

Liquefactive necrosis. An infarct in the brain, showing dissolution of the tissue.

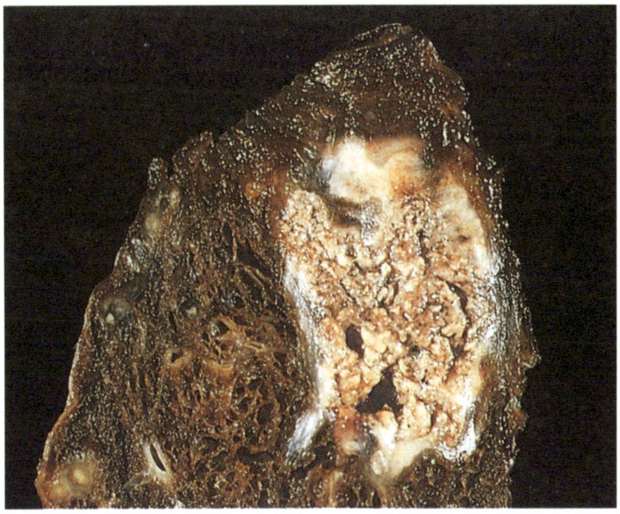

Figure 1–12

Caseous necrosis. A tuberculous lung with a large area of caseous necrosis containing yellow-white and cheesy debris.

lar appearance. Unlike coagulative necrosis, the tissue architecture is completely obliterated and cellular outlines cannot be discerned. Caseous necrosis is often enclosed within a distinctive inflammatory border; this appearance is characteristic of a focus of inflammation known as a **granuloma** (Chapter 2).

Fat necrosis, a term that is well fixed in medical parlance, refers to focal areas of fat destruction, typically resulting from release of activated pancreatic lipases into the substance of the pancreas and the peritoneal cavity. This occurs in the calamitous abdominal emergency known as acute pancreatitis (Chapter 17). In this disorder, pancreatic enzymes that have leaked out of acinar cells and ducts liquefy the membranes of fat cells in the peritoneum, and lipases split the triglyceride esters contained within fat cells. The released fatty acids combine with calcium to produce grossly visible chalky white areas (fat saponification), which enable the surgeon and the pathologist to identify the lesions (Fig. 1–13). On histologic examination, the foci of necrosis contain shadowy outlines of necrotic fat cells with basophilic calcium deposits, surrounded by an inflammatory reaction.

Fibrinoid necrosis is a special form of necrosis usually seen in immune reactions involving blood vessels. This pattern of necrosis is prominent when complexes of antigens and antibodies are deposited in the walls of arteries. Deposits of these "immune complexes," together with fibrin that has leaked out of vessels, result in a bright pink and amorphous appearance in H&E stains, called "fibrinoid" (fibrin-like) by pathologists (Fig. 1–14). The immunologically mediated diseases (e.g., polyarteritis nodosa) in which this type of necrosis is seen are described in Chapter 5.

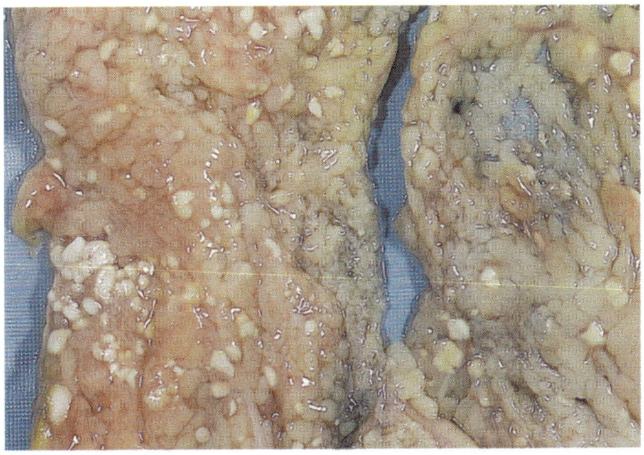

Figure 1–13

Fat necrosis in acute pancreatitis. The areas of white chalky deposits represent foci of fat necrosis with calcium soap formation (saponification) at sites of lipid breakdown in the mesentery.

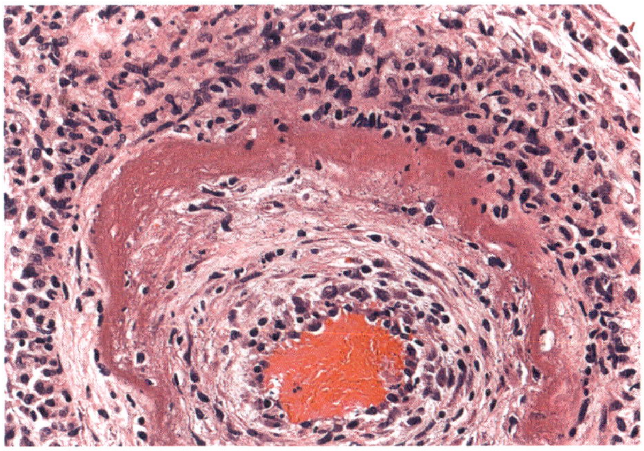

Figure 1–14

Fibrinoid necrosis in an artery in a patient with polyarteritis nodosa. The wall of the artery shows a circumferential bright pink area of necrosis with protein deposition and inflammation (dark nuclei of neutrophils).

Leakage of intracellular proteins through the damaged cell membrane and ultimately into the circulation provides a means of detecting tissue-specific necrosis using blood or serum samples. Cardiac muscle, for example, contains a unique isoform of the enzyme creatine kinase and of the contractile protein troponin, whereas hepatic bile duct epithelium contains a temperature-resistant isoform of the enzyme alkaline phosphatase, and hepatocytes contain transaminases. Irreversible injury and cell death in these tissues are reflected in increased serum levels of such proteins, and measurement of serum levels is used clinically to assess damage to these tissues.

Subcellular Responses to Injury

Thus far we have mainly focused on the whole tissue or the cell as a unit. However, certain agents and stresses induce distinctive alterations involving only subcellular organelles. Although some of these alterations occur in acute lethal injury, others are seen in chronic forms of cell injury, and still others are adaptive responses. In this section, some of the more common and interesting of these reactions are discussed.

Autophagy. Autophagy refers to lysosomal digestion of the cell's own components and is contrasted with *heterophagy,* in which a cell (usually a macrophage) ingests substances from the outside for intracellular destruction (Fig. 1–15). Autophagy is thought to be a survival mechanism in times of nutrient deprivation, such that the starved cell lives by eating its own contents. In this process, intracellular organelles and portions of cytosol are first sequestered from the cytoplasm in an *autophagic vacuole* formed from ribosome-free regions of the rough ER (RER). The vacuole fuses with lysosomes to form an *autophagolysosome,* and the cellular components are digested by lysosomal enzymes. Autophagy is initiated by several proteins that sense nutrient deprivation. If it is not corrected, autophagy may also signal cell death by apoptosis, a way of telling a stressed or starved cell that it can no longer cope by living on its own organelles.

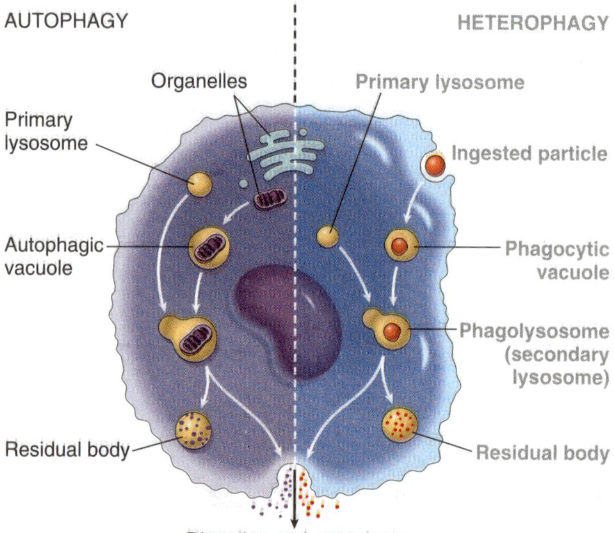

Figure 1–15

Autophagy (*right*) and heterophagy (*left*). (Redrawn from Fawcett DW: A Textbook of Histology, 11th ed. Philadelphia, WB Saunders, 1986, p 17.)

The enzymes in lysosomes can break down most proteins and carbohydrates, although some lipids remain undigested. Lysosomes with undigested debris may persist within cells as *residual bodies* or may be extruded. *Lipofuscin pigment* granules represent indigestible material resulting from free radical–mediated lipid peroxidation. Certain indigestible pigments, such as carbon particles inhaled from the atmosphere or inoculated pigment in tattoos, can persist in phagolysosomes of macrophages for decades (discussed later).

Lysosomes are also repositories wherein cells sequester materials that cannot be completely degraded. Hereditary *lysosomal storage disorders,* caused by deficiencies of enzymes that degrade various macromolecules, result in abnormal collections of intermediate metabolites in the lysosomes of cells all over the body; neurons are particularly susceptible to lethal injury from such accumulations (Chapter 7).

Induction (Hypertrophy) of Smooth ER. The smooth ER (SER) is involved in the metabolism of various chemicals, and cells exposed to these chemicals show hypertrophy of the ER as an adaptive response that may have important functional consequences. For instance, barbiturates are metabolized in the liver by the cytochrome P-450 mixed-function oxidase system found in the SER. Protracted use of barbiturates leads to a state of tolerance, with a decrease in the effects of the drug and the need to use increasing doses. This adaptation is due to increased volume (hypertrophy) of the SER of hepatocytes and increased P-450 enzymatic activity. Although P-450–mediated modification is often thought of as "detoxification," many compounds are rendered *more* injurious by this process; one example is carbon tetrachloride, discussed later. In addition, the products formed by this oxidative metabolism include reactive oxygen species (ROS), which can injure the cell. Cells adapted to one drug have increased capacity to metabolize other compounds handled by the same system. Thus, if patients taking phenobarbital for epilepsy increase their alcohol intake, they may have subtherapeutic levels of the antiseizure medication because of induction of SER in response to the alcohol.

Mitochondrial Alterations. As described later, mitochondrial dysfunction plays an important role in acute cell injury and death. In some nonlethal pathologic conditions, however, there may be alterations in the number, size, shape, and presumably function of mitochondria. For example, in cellular hypertrophy there is an increase in the number of mitochondria in cells; conversely, mitochondria decrease in number during cellular atrophy (probably via autophagy). Mitochondria may assume extremely large and abnormal shapes (*megamitochondria*), as seen in hepatocytes in various nutritional deficiencies and alcoholic liver disease. In certain inherited metabolic diseases of skeletal muscle, the *mitochondrial myopathies,* defects in mitochondrial metabolism are associated with increased numbers of unusually large mitochondria containing abnormal cristae.

Cytoskeletal Abnormalities. The cytoskeleton consists of actin and myosin filaments, microtubules, and various classes of intermediate filaments; several other nonpolymerized and nonfilamentous forms of contractile proteins also contribute to the cellular scaffold. The cytoskeleton is important for many cellular functions, including

- Intracellular transport of organelles and molecules
- Maintenance of basic cell architecture (e.g., cell polarity, distinguishing up and down)
- Transmission of cell-cell and cell–extracellular matrix signals to the nucleus
- Maintenance of mechanical strength for tissue integrity
- Cell mobility
- Phagocytosis

Cells and tissues respond to environmental stresses (e.g., shear stress in blood vessels or increased pressures in the heart) by constantly remodeling their intracellular scaffolding. Abnormalities of the cytoskeleton occur in a variety of pathologic states. These abnormalities may be manifested as an abnormal appearance and function of cells (hypertrophic cardiomyopathy; Chapter 11), aberrant movements of intracellular organelles, defective cell locomotion, or intracellular accumulations of fibrillar material as in alcoholic liver disease (Chapter 16). Perturbations in the organization of *microtubules* can cause sterility by inhibiting sperm motility, as well as defective mobility of cilia in the respiratory epithelium, resulting in chronic infections due to impaired clearance of inhaled bacteria (*Kartagener,* or the *immotile cilia, syndrome*). Microtubules are also essential for leukocyte migration and phagocytosis. Drugs that prevent microtubule polymerization (e.g., colchicine) are useful in treating gout, in which symptoms are due to movement of macrophages toward urate crystals with subsequent frustrated attempts at phagocytosis and inflammation. Since microtubules form the mitotic spindle, drugs that bind to microtubules (e.g., vinca alkaloids) are also antiproliferative and may therefore be useful as antitumor agents.

SUMMARY

Subcellular Alterations in Cell Injury: Effects of Injurious Agents on Organelles and Cellular Components

Some forms of cell injury affect particular organelles and have unique manifestations.

- *Autophagy:* In nutrient-deprived cells, organelles are enclosed in vacuoles that fuse with lysosomes. The organelles are digested but in some cases indigestible pigment (e.g. lipofuscin) remains.
- *Hypertrophy of SER:* Cells exposed to toxins that are metabolized in the SER show hypertrophy of the ER, a compensatory mechanism to maximize removal of the toxins.
- *Mitochondrial alterations:* Changes in the number, size, and shape of mitochondria are seen in diverse adaptations and responses to chronic injury.
- *Cytoskeletal alterations:* Some drugs and toxins interfere with the assembly and functions of cytoskeletal filaments or result in abnormal accumulations of filaments.

MECHANISMS OF CELL INJURY

Now that we have discussed the causes of cell injury and necrosis and their morphologic and functional correlates, we next consider in more detail the molecular basis of cell injury, and then illustrate the important principles with a few selected examples of common types of injury. The biochemical mechanisms linking any given injury with the resulting cellular and tissue manifestations are complex, interconnected, and tightly interwoven with many intracellular metabolic pathways. It is therefore often difficult to pinpoint specific molecular alterations caused by a particular insult. Nevertheless, several general principles are relevant to most forms of cell injury:

- *The cellular response to injurious stimuli depends on the type of injury, its duration, and its severity.* Thus, low doses of toxins or a brief duration of ischemia may lead to reversible cell injury, whereas larger toxin doses or longer ischemic intervals may result in irreversible injury and cell death.
- *The consequences of an injurious stimulus depend on the type, status, adaptability, and genetic makeup of the injured cell.* The same injury has vastly different outcomes depending on the cell type; thus, striated skeletal muscle in the leg accommodates complete ischemia for 2 to 3 hours without irreversible injury, whereas cardiac muscle dies after only 20 to 30 minutes. The nutritional (or hormonal) status can also be important; clearly, a glycogen-replete hepatocyte will tolerate ischemia much better than one that has just burned its last glucose molecule. Genetically determined diversity in metabolic pathways can also be important. For instance, when exposed to the same dose of a toxin, individuals who inherit variants in genes encoding cytochrome P-450 may catabolize the toxin at different rates, leading to different outcomes. Much effort is now directed toward understanding the role of genetic polymorphisms in responses to drugs and toxins and in disease susceptibility. The study of such interactions is called pharmacogenomics.
- *Cell injury results from functional and biochemical abnormalities in one or more of several essential cellular components* (Fig. 1–16). The most important targets of injurious stimuli are (1) mitochondria, the sites of ATP generation; (2) cell membranes, on which the ionic and osmotic homeostasis of the cell and its organelles depends; (3) protein synthesis; (4) the cytoskeleton; and (5) the genetic apparatus of the cell.

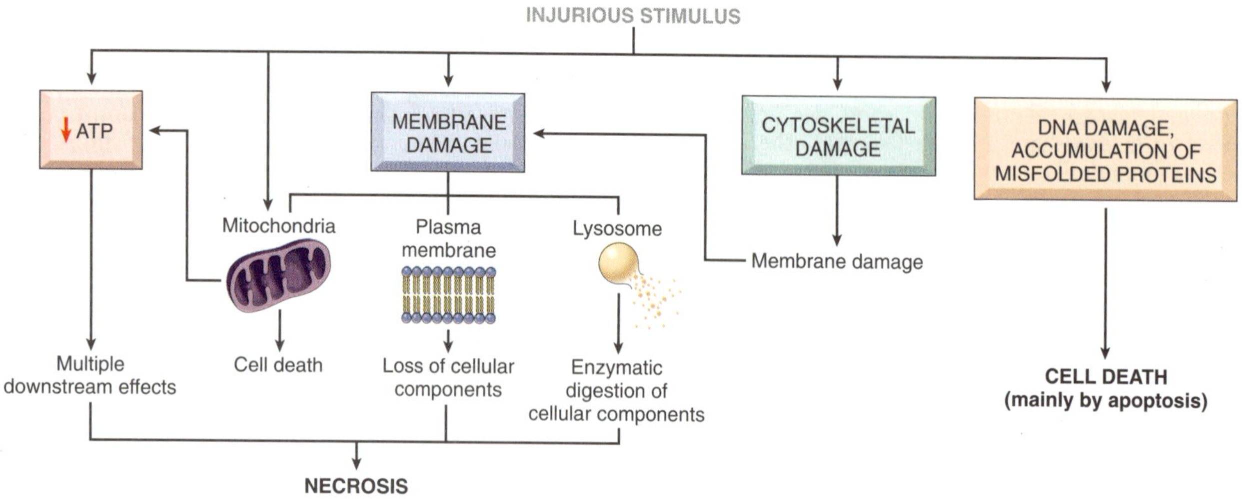

Figure 1–16

The principal cellular and biochemical sites of damage in cell injury. Note that loss of adenosine triphosphate (ATP) results first in reversible injury (not shown) and culminates in necrosis. Mitochondrial damage may lead to reversible injury and death by necrosis or apoptosis.

Depletion of ATP

ATP, the energy store of cells, is produced mainly by oxidative phosphorylation of adenosine diphosphate (ADP) during reduction of oxygen in the electron transport system of mitochondria. In addition, the glycolytic pathway can generate ATP in the absence of oxygen using glucose derived either from the circulation or from the hydrolysis of intracellular glycogen. The major causes of ATP depletion are reduced supply of oxygen and nutrients, mitochondrial damage, and the actions of some toxins (e.g., cyanide). Tissues with a greater glycolytic capacity (e.g., the liver) are able to survive loss of oxygen and decreased oxidative phosphorylation better than are tissues with limited capacity for glycolysis (e.g., the brain). High-energy phosphate in the form of ATP is required for virtually all synthetic and degradative processes within the cell, including membrane transport, protein synthesis, lipogenesis, and the deacylation-reacylation reactions necessary for phospholipid turnover. *Depletion of ATP to less than 5% to 10% of normal levels has widespread effects on many critical cellular systems* (Fig. 1–17).

- The activity of the *plasma membrane energy-dependent sodium pump* is reduced, resulting in intracellular accumulation of sodium and efflux of potassium. The net gain of solute is accompanied by iso-osmotic gain of water, causing *cell swelling* and dilation of the ER.
- There is a compensatory *increase in anaerobic glycolysis* in an attempt to maintain the cell's energy sources. As a consequence, intracellular glycogen stores are rapidly depleted, and lactic acid accumulates, leading to decreased intracellular pH and decreased activity of many cellular enzymes.
- *Failure of the Ca^{2+} pump* leads to influx of Ca^{2+}, with damaging effects on numerous cellular components, described below.
- Prolonged or worsening depletion of ATP causes *structural disruption of the protein synthetic apparatus,* manifested as detachment of ribosomes from the rough endoplastic reticulum (RER) and dissociation of polysomes into monosomes, with a consequent reduction in protein synthesis. Ultimately, there is irreversible damage to mitochondrial and lysosomal membranes, and the cell undergoes necrosis.

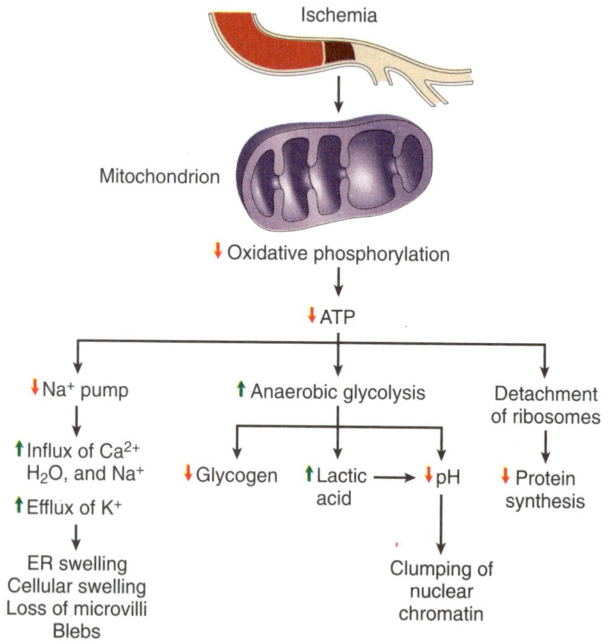

Figure 1–17

The initial functional and morphologic consequences of decreased intracellular adenosine triphosphate (ATP) during cell injury. ER, Endoplasmic reticulum.

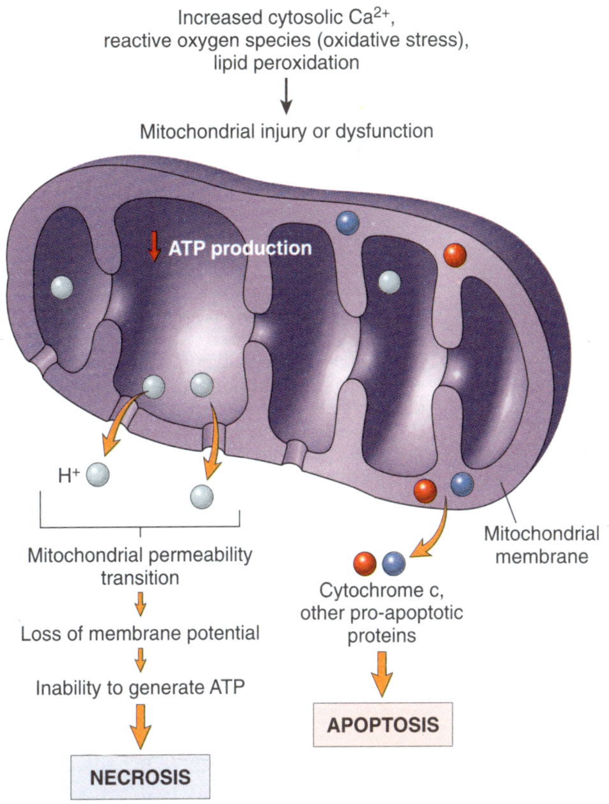

Figure 1–18

Consequences of mitochondrial dysfunction, culminating in cell death by necrosis or apoptosis. ATP, Adenosine triphosphate.

Damage to Mitochondria

Mitochondria are the cell's suppliers of life-sustaining energy in the form of ATP, but they are also critical players in cell injury and death. Mitochondria can be damaged by increases of cytosolic Ca^{2+}, reactive oxygen species (discussed below), and oxygen deprivation, and so they are sensitive to virtually all types of injurious stimuli, including hypoxia and toxins. There are two major consequences of mitochondrial damage (Fig. 1–18):

- Mitochondrial damage often results in the formation of a high-conductance channel in the mitochondrial membrane, called the mitochondrial permeability transition pore. The opening of this channel leads to the loss of mitochondrial membrane potential and pH changes, resulting in *failure of oxidative phosphorylation and progressive depletion of ATP*, culminating in necrosis of the cell.
- The mitochondria also contain several proteins that are capable of activating apoptotic pathways, including cytochrome *c* (the major protein involved in electron transport). Increased permeability of the mitochondrial membrane may result in leakage of these proteins into the cytosol and *death by apoptosis*. Thus, cytochrome *c* plays a key dual role in cell survival and death; in its normal location inside mitochondria, it is essential for energy generation and the life of the cell, but when mitochondria are damaged so severely that cytochrome *c* leaks out, it signals cells to die.

Influx of Calcium

Cytosolic free calcium is normally maintained by ATP-dependent calcium transporters at concentrations that are as much as 10,000 times lower than the concentration of extracellular calcium or of sequestered intracellular mitochondrial and ER calcium. Ischemia and certain toxins cause an increase in cytosolic calcium concentration, initially because of release of Ca^{2+} from the intracellular stores, and later resulting from increased influx across the plasma membrane. *Increased cytosolic Ca^{2+} activates a number of enzymes*, with potentially deleterious cellular effects (Fig. 1–19). These enzymes include phospholipases (which cause membrane damage), proteases (which break down both membrane and cytoskeletal proteins), endonucleases (which are responsible for DNA and chromatin fragmentation), and adenosine triphosphatases (ATPases; thereby hastening ATP depletion). Increased intracellular Ca^{2+} levels also result in the induction of apoptosis, by direct activation of caspases and by increasing mitochondrial permeability. The importance of Ca^{2+} in cell injury was established by the finding that depleting extracellular Ca^{2+} delays cell death after hypoxia and exposure to some toxins.

Accumulation of Oxygen-Derived Free Radicals (Oxidative Stress)

Free radicals are chemical species with a single unpaired electron in an outer orbital. Such chemical states are extremely unstable and readily react with inorganic and

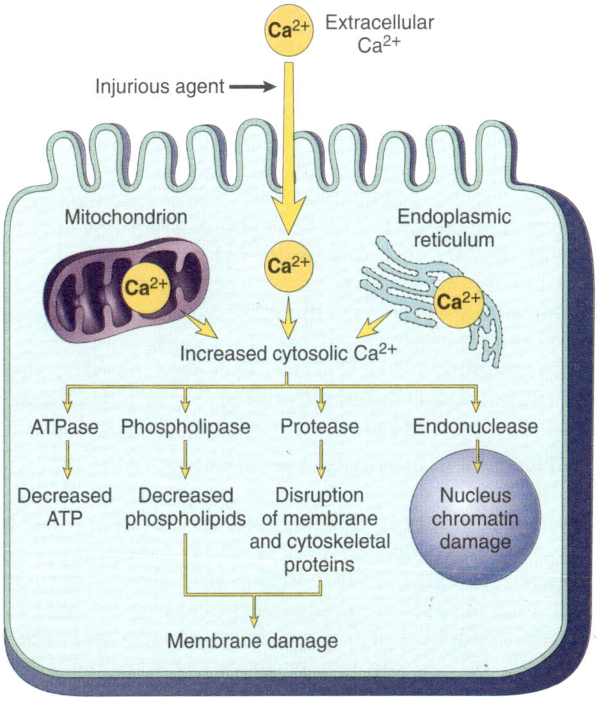

Figure 1–19

Sources and consequences of increased cytosolic calcium in cell injury. ATP, Adenosine triphosphate; ATPase, adenosine triphosphatase.

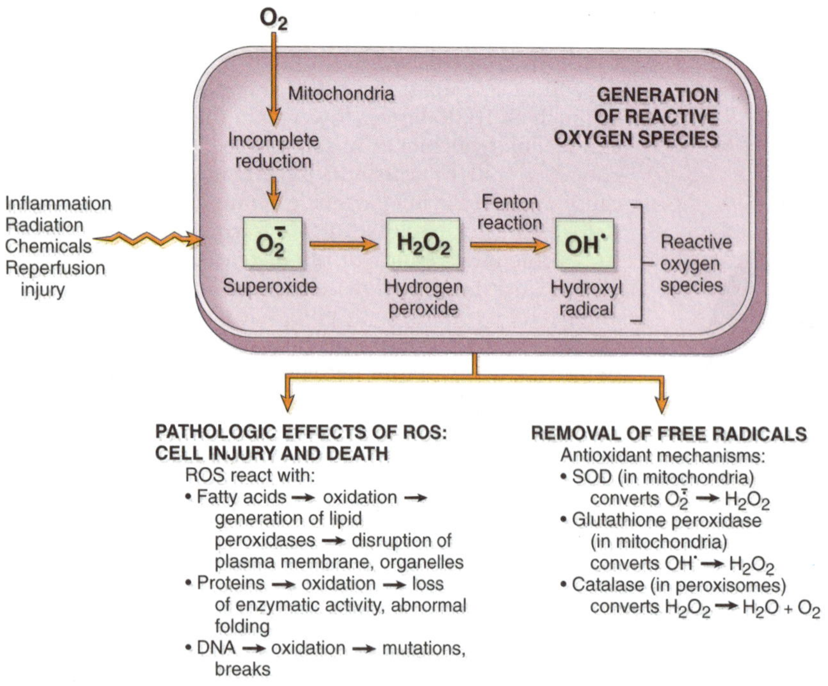

Figure 1–20

The role of reactive oxygen species (ROS) in cell injury. O_2 is converted to superoxide ($O_2^{\bar{\cdot}}$) by oxidative enzymes in the endoplasmic reticulum, mitochondria, plasma membrane, peroxisomes, and cytosol. $O_2^{\bar{\cdot}}$ is converted to H_2O_2 by dismutation and thence to $OH^{\bullet}$ by the Cu^{2+}/Fe^{2+}-catalyzed Fenton reaction. H_2O_2 is also derived directly from oxidases in peroxisomes (not shown). Also not shown is another potentially injurious free radical, singlet oxygen. Resultant free-radical damage to lipid (by peroxidation), proteins, and deoxyribonucleic acid (DNA) leads to various forms of cell injury. The major antioxidant enzymes are superoxide dismutase (SOD), catalase, and glutathione peroxidase.

organic chemicals; when generated in cells they avidly attack nucleic acids as well as a variety of cellular proteins and lipids. In addition, free radicals initiate autocatalytic reactions; molecules that react with free radicals are in turn converted into free radicals, thus propagating the chain of damage. *Reactive oxygen species (ROS)* are a type of oxygen-derived free radical whose role in cell injury is well established. They are produced normally in cells during mitochondrial respiration and energy generation, but they are degraded and removed by cellular defense systems. When the production of ROS increases or the scavenging systems are ineffective, the result is an excess of these free radicals, leading to a condition called *oxidative stress*. Cell injury in many circumstances involves damage by free radicals; these situations include ischemia-reperfusion (discussed below), chemical and radiation injury, toxicity from oxygen and other gases, cellular aging, microbial killing by phagocytic cells, and tissue injury caused by inflammatory cells.

The accumulation of free radicals is determined by their rates of production and removal (Fig. 1–20). Several reactions are responsible for the *generation of free radicals.*

- The reduction-oxidation (redox) reactions that occur during normal mitochondrial metabolism. During normal respiration, for example, molecular oxygen is sequentially reduced in mitochondria by the addition of four electrons to generate water. In the process, small amounts of toxic intermediate species are generated by partial reduction of oxygen; these include superoxide radicals ($O_2^{\bar{\cdot}}$), hydrogen peroxide (H_2O_2), and $OH^{\bullet}$. Transition metals such as copper and iron also accept or donate free electrons during certain intracellular reactions and thereby catalyze free-radical formation, as in the Fenton reaction ($Fe^{2+} + H_2O_2 \rightarrow Fe^{3+} + OH^{\bullet} + OH^{-}$).
- The absorption of radiant energy (e.g., ultraviolet light, x-rays). Ionizing radiation can hydrolyze water into hydroxyl ($OH^{\bullet}$) and hydrogen ($H^{\bullet}$) free radicals.
- The enzymatic metabolism of exogenous chemicals (e.g., carbon tetrachloride; see later)
- Inflammation, because free radicals are produced by leukocytes that enter tissues (see Chapter 2)
- Nitric oxide (NO), an important chemical mediator normally synthesized by a variety of cell types (Chapter 2), can act as a free radical or can be converted into highly reactive nitrite species

Cells have developed many *mechanisms to remove free radicals* and thereby minimize injury. Free radicals are inherently unstable and decay spontaneously. There are also several nonenzymatic and enzymatic systems that contribute to inactivation of free-radical reactions (see Fig. 1–20).

- The rate of spontaneous decay of superoxide is significantly increased by the action of superoxide dismutases (SODs) found in many cell types (catalyzing the reaction $2O_2^{\bar{\cdot}}\ 2H \rightarrow H_2O_2 + O_2$).
- Glutathione (GSH) peroxidase also protects against injury by catalyzing free-radical breakdown: $2OH^{\bullet} + 2GSH \rightarrow 2H_2O + GSSG$ (glutathione homodimer). The intracellular ratio of oxidized glutathione (GSSG) to reduced glutathione (GSH) is a reflection of the oxidative state of the cell and an important aspect of the cell's ability to catabolize free radicals.
- Catalase, present in peroxisomes, directs the degradation of hydrogen peroxide ($2H_2O_2 \rightarrow O_2 + 2H_2O$).
- Endogenous or exogenous antioxidants (e.g., vitamins E, A, and C, and β-carotene) may either block the formation of free radicals or scavenge them once they have formed.

- As mentioned above, *iron* and *copper* can catalyze the formation of ROS. The levels of these reactive metals are reduced by binding of the ions to storage and transport proteins (e.g., transferrin, ferritin, lactoferrin, and ceruloplasmin), thereby decreasing the formation of ROS.

ROS have many diverse effects on cells and have even been implicated in activation of cells by a variety of physiologic stimuli. However, three reactions are particularly relevant to *cell injury mediated by free radicals* (see Fig. 1–20):

- *Lipid peroxidation of membranes.* Double bonds in membrane polyunsaturated lipids are vulnerable to attack by oxygen-derived free radicals. The lipid-radical interactions yield peroxides, which are themselves unstable and reactive, and an autocatalytic chain reaction ensues.
- *Cross-linking of proteins.* Free radicals promote sulfhydryl-mediated protein cross-linking, resulting in enhanced degradation or loss of enzymatic activity. Free-radical reactions may also directly cause polypeptide fragmentation.
- *DNA fragmentation.* Free-radical reactions with thymine in nuclear and mitochondrial DNA produce single-strand breaks. Such DNA damage has been implicated in cell death, aging, and malignant transformation of cells.

Defects in Membrane Permeability

Early loss of selective membrane permeability leading ultimately to overt membrane damage is a consistent feature of most forms of cell injury (except apoptosis). The plasma membrane can be damaged by ischemia, various microbial toxins, lytic complement components, and a variety of physical and chemical agents. Several biochemical mechanisms may contribute to membrane damage (Fig. 1–21):

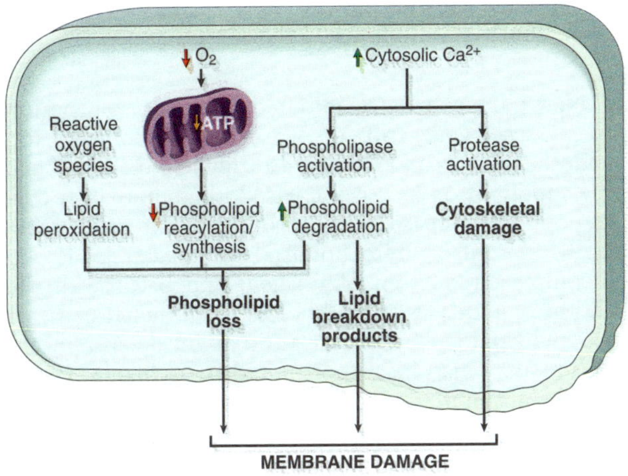

Figure 1–21

Mechanisms of membrane damage in cell injury. Decreased O_2 and increased cytosolic Ca^{2+} are typically seen in ischemia but may accompany other forms of cell injury. Reactive oxygen species, which are often produced on reperfusion of ischemic tissues, also cause membrane damage (not shown).

- *Decreased phospholipid synthesis.* The production of phospholipids in cells may be reduced whenever there is a fall in ATP levels, leading to decreased energy-dependent enzymatic activities. The reduced phospholipid synthesis may affect all cellular membranes including the mitochondria themselves, thus exacerbating the loss of ATP.
- *Increased phospholipid breakdown.* Severe cell injury is associated with increased degradation of membrane phospholipids, probably due to activation of endogenous phospholipases by increased levels of cytosolic Ca^{2+}.
- *ROS.* Oxygen free radicals cause injury to cell membranes by lipid peroxidation, discussed earlier.
- *Cytoskeletal abnormalities.* Cytoskeletal filaments serve as anchors connecting the plasma membrane to the cell interior. Activation of proteases by increased cytosolic Ca^{2+} may cause damage to elements of the cytoskeleton.
- *Lipid breakdown products.* These include unesterified free fatty acids, acyl carnitine, and lysophospholipids, catabolic products that are known to accumulate in injured cells as a result of phospholipid degradation. They have a detergent effect on membranes. They also either insert into the lipid bilayer of the membrane or exchange with membrane phospholipids, potentially causing changes in permeability and electrophysiologic alterations.

The most important sites of membrane damage during cell injury are the mitochondrial membrane, the plasma membrane, and membranes of lysosomes.

- *Mitochondrial membrane damage.* As discussed above, damage to mitochondrial membranes results in decreased production of ATP, culminating in necrosis, and release of proteins that trigger apoptotic death.
- *Plasma membrane damage.* Plasma membrane damage leads to loss of osmotic balance and influx of fluids and ions, as well as loss of cellular contents. The cells may also leak metabolites that are vital for the reconstitution of ATP, thus further depleting energy stores.
- *Injury to lysosomal membranes* results in leakage of their enzymes into the cytoplasm and activation of the acid hydrolases in the acidic intracellular pH of the injured (e.g., ischemic) cell. Lysosomes contain RNases, DNases, proteases, glucosidases, and other enzymes. Activation of these enzymes leads to enzymatic digestion of cell components, and the cells die by necrosis.

Damage to DNA and Proteins

Cells have mechanisms that repair damage to DNA, but if this damage is too severe to be corrected (e.g., after radiation injury or oxidative stress), the cell initiates its suicide program and dies by apoptosis. A similar reaction is triggered by improperly folded proteins, which may be the result of inherited mutations or external triggers such as free radicals. Since these mechanisms of cell injury typically cause apoptosis, they are discussed later in the chapter.

SUMMARY

Mechanisms of Cell Injury

- *ATP depletion:* failure of energy-dependent functions → reversible injury → necrosis
- *Mitochondrial damage:* ATP depletion → failure of energy-dependent cellular functions → ultimately, necrosis; under some conditions, leakage of proteins that cause apoptosis
- *Influx of calcium:* activation of enzymes that damage cellular components and may also trigger apoptosis
- *Accumulation of reactive oxygen species:* covalent modification of cellular proteins, lipids, nucleic acids
- *Increased permeability of cellular membranes:* may affect plasma membrane, lysosomal membranes, mitochondrial membranes; typically culminates in necrosis
- *Accumulation of damaged DNA and misfolded proteins:* triggers apoptosis

EXAMPLES OF CELL INJURY AND NECROSIS

To illustrate the evolution and biochemical mechanisms of cell injury, we conclude this section by discussing some commonly encountered examples of reversible cell injury and necrosis.

Ischemic and Hypoxic Injury

Ischemia, or diminished blood flow to a tissue, is the most common cause of cell injury in clinical medicine. In contrast to hypoxia, in which energy generation by anaerobic glycolysis can continue (albeit less efficiently than by oxidative pathways), ischemia also compromises the delivery of substrates for glycolysis. Consequently, anaerobic energy generation also ceases in ischemic tissues after potential substrates are exhausted or when glycolysis is inhibited by the accumulation of metabolites that would normally be removed by blood flow. Therefore, *ischemia injures tissues faster than does hypoxia.* The biochemical and structural changes in oxygen-deprived cells were discussed in detail earlier and the sequence of events is recapitulated below.

The fundamental biochemical abnormality in hypoxic cells that leads to cell injury is reduced intracellular generation of ATP, as a consequence of reduced supply of oxygen. As described above, loss of ATP leads to the *failure of many energy-dependent cellular systems, including* (1) *ion pumps* (leading to cell swelling, and influx of Ca^{2+}, with its deleterious consequences); (2) *depletion of glycogen stores,* apparent histologically by reduced staining for carbohydrates (e.g., by the periodic acid–Schiff stain), with accumulation of lactic acid, thus lowering the intracellular pH; and (3) *reduction in protein synthesis.*

The functional consequences may be severe at this stage. For instance, heart muscle ceases to contract within 60 seconds of coronary occlusion. However, loss of contractility does not mean cell death. If hypoxia continues, worsening ATP depletion causes further deterioration, with loss of microvilli and the formation of "blebs" (see Fig. 1–9). At this time, the entire cell and its organelles (mitochondria, ER) are markedly swollen, with increased concentrations of water, sodium, and chloride and a decreased concentration of potassium. *If oxygen is restored, all of these disturbances are reversible.*

If ischemia persists, irreversible injury and necrosis ensue. Irreversible injury is associated with severe swelling of mitochondria, extensive damage to plasma membranes, and swelling of lysosomes (see Fig. 1–9). Massive influx of calcium into the cell may occur. Death is mainly by necrosis, but apoptosis also contributes; the apoptotic pathway is activated probably by release of pro-apoptotic molecules from leaky mitochondria. The cell's components are progressively degraded, and there is widespread leakage of cellular enzymes into the extracellular space. Finally, the dead cells may become replaced by large masses composed of phospholipids in the form of myelin figures. These are then either phagocytosed by leukocytes or degraded further into fatty acids that may become calcified.

Ischemia-Reperfusion Injury

If cells are reversibly injured, the restoration of blood flow can result in cell recovery. However, under certain circumstances, the restoration of blood flow to ischemic but otherwise viable tissues results, paradoxically, in exacerbated and accelerated injury. As a result, tissues sustain the loss of cells *in addition to those that are irreversibly damaged at the end of the ischemic episode.* This so-called *ischemia-reperfusion injury* is a clinically important process that may contribute significantly to tissue damage in myocardial and cerebral infarctions.

Several mechanisms may account for the exacerbation of cell injury resulting from reperfusion into ischemic tissues:

- New damage may be initiated during reoxygenation by increased generation of *ROS* from parenchymal and endothelial cells and from infiltrating leukocytes. When the supply of oxygen is increased, there may be a corresponding increase in the production of ROS, especially because mitochondrial damage leads to incomplete reduction of oxygen, and because of the action of oxidases in leukocytes, endothelial cells, or parenchymal cells. Cellular antioxidant defense mechanisms may also be compromised by ischemia, favoring the accumulation of free radicals.
- Ischemic injury is associated with *inflammation,* which may increase with reperfusion because of increased influx of leukocytes and plasma proteins. The products of activated leukocytes may cause additional tissue injury (Chapter 2). Activation of the *complement system* may also contribute to ischemia-reperfusion injury. Some antibodies have a propensity to deposit in ischemic tissues for unknown reasons, and when blood

flow is resumed, complement proteins bind to the deposited antibodies, are activated, and exacerbate the cell injury and inflammation.

Chemical (Toxic) Injury

Chemicals induce cell injury by one of two general mechanisms.

- *Some chemicals act directly by combining with a critical molecular component or cellular organelle.* For example, in mercuric chloride poisoning, mercury binds to the sulfhydryl groups of various cell membrane proteins, causing inhibition of ATP-dependent transport and increased membrane permeability. Many antineoplastic chemotherapeutic agents also induce cell damage by direct cytotoxic effects. In such instances, the *greatest damage is sustained by the cells that use, absorb, excrete, or concentrate the compounds.*
- *Many other chemicals are not intrinsically biologically active but must be first converted to reactive toxic metabolites, which then act on target cells.* This modification is usually accomplished by the P-450 mixed-function oxidases in the smooth endoplasmic reticulum of the liver and other organs. Although the metabolites might cause membrane damage and cell injury by direct covalent binding to protein and lipids, the most important mechanism of cell injury involves the formation of free radicals. *Carbon tetrachloride* (CCl_4, which was used widely in the dry cleaning industry but is now banned) and the analgesic *acetaminophen* belong in this category. CCl_4, for example, is converted to the toxic free radical $CCl_3^{\bullet}$, principally in the liver. The free radicals cause autocatalytic membrane phospholipid peroxidation, with rapid breakdown of the ER. In less than 30 minutes after exposure to CCl_4, there is a decline in hepatic protein synthesis of enzymes and plasma proteins; within 2 hours, swelling of the smooth endoplasmic reticulum and dissociation of ribosomes from the smooth endoplasmic reticulum have occurred. There is reduced lipid export from the hepatocytes, as a result of their inability to synthesize apoprotein to form complexes with triglycerides and thereby facilitate lipoprotein secretion; the result is the "fatty liver" of CCl_4 poisoning. Mitochondrial injury follows, and subsequently diminished ATP stores result in defective ion transport and progressive cell swelling; the plasma membranes are further damaged by fatty aldehydes produced by lipid peroxidation in the ER. The end result can be calcium influx and eventually cell death.

APOPTOSIS

Apoptosis is a pathway of cell death that is induced by a tightly regulated suicide program in which cells destined to die activate enzymes capable of degrading the cells' own nuclear DNA and nuclear and cytoplasmic proteins. Fragments of the apoptotic cells then break off, giving the appearance that is responsible for the name (*apoptosis*, "falling off"). The plasma membrane of the apoptotic cell remains intact, but the membrane is altered in such a way that the cell and its fragments become avid targets for phagocytes. The dead cell is rapidly cleared before its contents have leaked out, and therefore cell death by this pathway does not elicit an inflammatory reaction in the host. Thus, apoptosis differs from necrosis, which is characterized by loss of membrane integrity, enzymatic digestion of cells, leakage of cellular contents, and frequently a host reaction (see Fig. 1–6 and Table 1–1). However, apoptosis and necrosis sometimes coexist, and apoptosis induced by some pathologic stimuli may progress to necrosis.

Causes of Apoptosis

Apoptosis occurs normally in many situations, and serves to eliminate potentially harmful cells and cells that have outlived their usefulness. It is also a pathologic event when cells are damaged beyond repair, especially when the damage affects the cell's DNA or proteins; in these situations, the irreparably damaged cell is eliminated.

Apoptosis in Physiologic Situations

Death by apoptosis is a normal phenomenon that serves to eliminate cells that are no longer needed and to maintain a steady number of various cell populations in tissues. It is important in the following physiologic situations:

- *The programmed destruction of cells during embryogenesis,* including implantation, organogenesis, developmental involution, and metamorphosis. The term "programmed cell death" was originally coined to denote death of specific cell types at defined times during the development of an organism. Apoptosis is a generic term for this pattern of cell death, regardless of the context, but it is often used interchangeably with "programmed cell death."
- *Involution of hormone-dependent tissues upon hormone deprivation,* such as endometrial cell breakdown during the menstrual cycle, and regression of the lactating breast after weaning
- *Cell loss in proliferating cell populations,* such as intestinal crypt epithelia, so as to maintain a constant number
- Death of cells that have served their useful purpose, such as neutrophils in an acute inflammatory response, and lymphocytes at the end of an immune response. In these situations, cells undergo apoptosis because they are deprived of necessary survival signals, such as growth factors.
- *Elimination of potentially harmful self-reactive lymphocytes,* either before or after they have completed their maturation, in order to prevent reactions against one's own tissues (Chapter 5)
- *Cell death induced by cytotoxic T lymphocytes,* a defense mechanism against viruses and tumors that serves to kill and eliminate virus-infected and neoplastic cells (Chapter 5)

Apoptosis in Pathologic Conditions

Apoptosis eliminates cells that are genetically altered or injured beyond repair without eliciting a severe host reaction, thus keeping the damage as contained as possible.

Death by apoptosis is responsible for loss of cells in a variety of pathologic states:

- *DNA damage.* Radiation, cytotoxic anticancer drugs, extremes of temperature, and even hypoxia can damage DNA, either directly or via production of free radicals. If repair mechanisms cannot cope with the injury, the cell triggers intrinsic mechanisms that induce apoptosis. In these situations, elimination of the cell may be a better alternative than risking mutations in the damaged DNA, which may progress to malignant transformation. These injurious stimuli cause apoptosis if the insult is mild, but larger doses of the same stimuli result in necrotic cell death. Inducing apoptosis of cancer cells is a desired effect of chemotherapeutic agents, many of which work by damaging DNA.
- *Accumulation of misfolded proteins.* Improperly folded proteins may arise because of mutations in the genes encoding these proteins or because of extrinsic factors, such as damage caused by free radicals. Excessive accumulation of these proteins in the ER leads to a condition called *ER stress,* which culminates in apoptotic death of cells.
- *Cell injury in certain infections,* particularly viral infections, in which loss of infected cells is largely due to apoptotic death that may be induced by the virus (as in adenovirus and human immunodeficiency virus infections) or by the host immune response (as in viral hepatitis)
- *Pathologic atrophy in parenchymal organs after duct obstruction,* such as occurs in the pancreas, parotid gland, and kidney

Mechanisms of Apoptosis

Apoptosis is an active enzymatic process in which nucleoproteins are broken down and then the cell is fragmented. Before discussing the molecular mechanisms, it is useful to review the morphology of this pathway of cell death.

Morphology

In H&E-stained tissue sections, apoptotic cells may appear as round or oval masses with intensely eosinophilic cytoplasm (Fig. 1–22). Nuclei show various stages of chromatin condensation and aggregation and, ultimately, karyorrhexis; at the molecular level this is reflected in fragmentation of DNA into nucleosome-sized pieces. The cells rapidly shrink, form cytoplasmic buds, and fragment into **apoptotic bodies** composed of membrane-bound vesicles of cytosol and organelles (see Fig. 1–6). Because these fragments are quickly extruded and phagocytosed without eliciting an inflammatory response, even substantial apoptosis may be histologically undetectable.

The fundamental event in apoptosis is the activation of enzymes called *caspases* (so named because they are *c*ysteine proteases that cleave proteins after *asp*artic residues). Activated caspases cleave numerous targets,

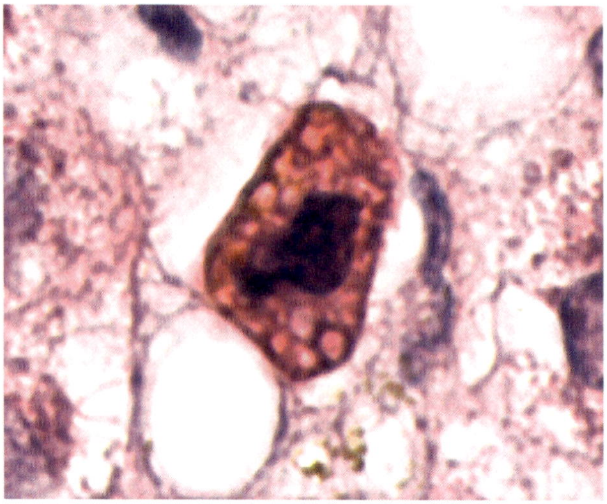

Figure 1–22

Apoptosis of a liver cell in viral hepatitis. The cell is reduced in size and contains brightly eosinophilic cytoplasm and a condensed nucleus.

culminating in activation of nucleases that degrade DNA and other enzymes that presumably destroy nucleoproteins and cytokeletal proteins. The activation of caspases depends on a finely tuned balance between pro- and anti-apoptotic molecular pathways. Two distinct pathways converge on caspase activation, called the *mitochondrial pathway* and the *death receptor pathway.* Although these pathways can interact, they are generally induced under different conditions, involve different molecules, and serve distinct roles in physiology and disease (Fig. 1–23).

The Mitochondrial (Intrinsic) Pathway of Apoptosis. Mitochondria contain several proteins that are capable of inducing apoptosis; these proteins include cytochrome *c* and antagonists of endogenous cytosolic inhibitors of apoptosis. The choice between cell survival and death is determined by the permeability of mitochondria, which is controlled by a family of more than 20 proteins, the prototype of which is Bcl-2. When cells are deprived of growth factors and trophic hormones, or are exposed to agents that damage DNA, or accumulate unacceptable amounts of misfolded proteins, a group of sensors is activated. Some of these sensors, which are members of the Bcl-2 family, in turn activate two pro-apoptotic members of the family called Bax and Bak, which dimerize, insert into the mitochondrial membrane, and form channels through which cytochrome *c* and other mitochondrial proteins escape into the cytosol. Other related sensors inhibit the anti-apoptotic molecules Bcl-2 and Bcl-x_L (see below), with the same end result—the leakage of mitochondrial proteins. Cytochrome *c*, together with some cofactors, activates caspase-9, while other proteins block the activities of caspase antagonists that function as physiologic inhibitors of apoptosis. The net result is the activation of the caspase cascade, ultimately leading to nuclear fragmentation. If cells are exposed to growth factors and other survival signals, they synthesize anti-apoptotic members of the Bcl-2 family, the two main ones of which are Bcl-2 itself and Bcl-x_L. These proteins antag-

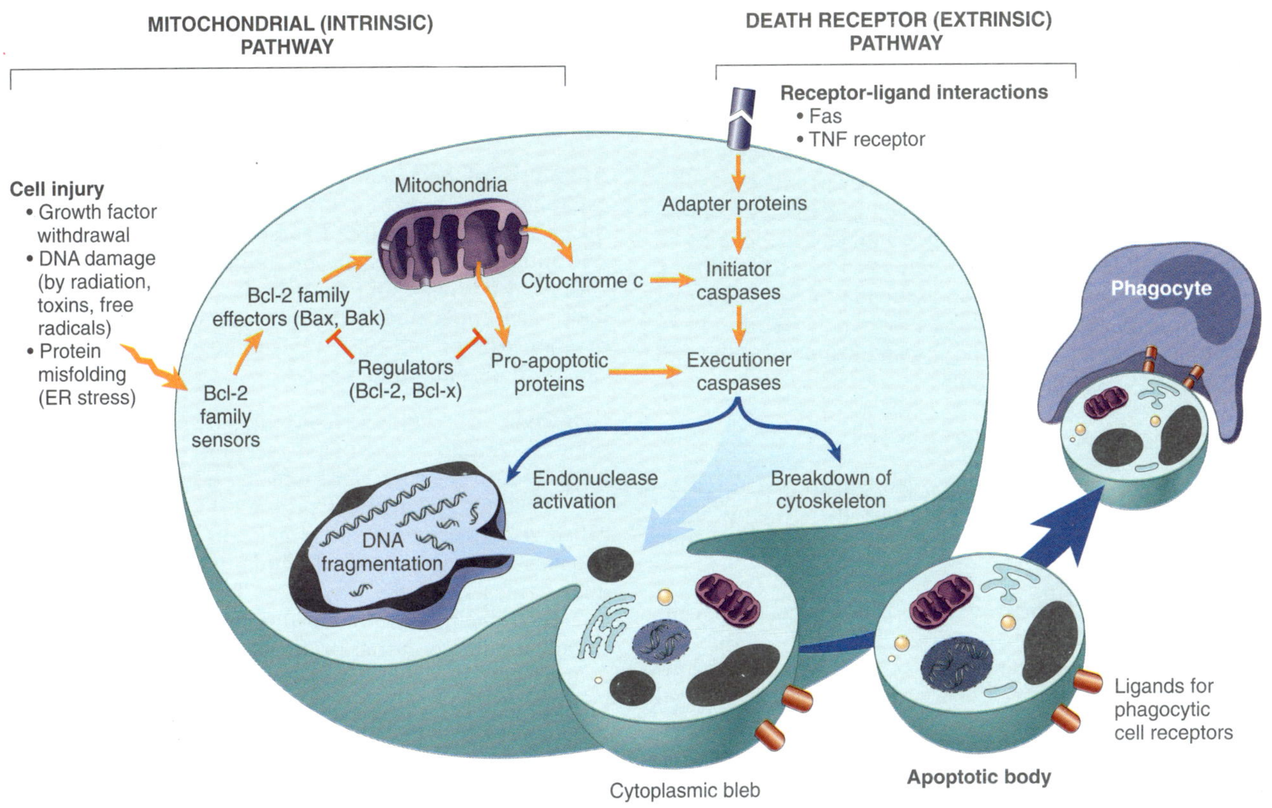

Figure 1–23

Mechanisms of apoptosis. The two pathways of apoptosis differ in their induction and regulation, and both culminate in the activation of "executioner" caspases. The induction of apoptosis is dependent on a balance between pro- and anti-apoptotic signals and intracellular proteins. The figure shows the pathways that induce apoptotic cell death, and the anti-apoptotic proteins that inhibit mitochondrial leakiness and cytochrome *c*–dependent caspase activation and thus function as regulators of mitochondrial apoptosis.

onize Bax and Bak, and thus limit the escape of mitochondrial pro-apoptotic proteins. Cells deprived of growth factors not only activate the pro-apoptotic proteins but also show reduced levels of Bcl-2 and Bcl-x_L, thus further tilting the balance toward death. The mitochondrial pathway seems to be the pathway that is responsible for most situations of apoptosis, as we shall discuss below.

The Death Receptor (Extrinsic) Pathway of Apoptosis. Many cells express surface molecules, called death receptors, that trigger apoptosis. Most of these are members of the tumor necrosis factor (TNF) receptor family that contain in their cytoplasmic regions a conserved "death domain," so named because it mediates interaction with other proteins. The prototypic death receptors are the type I TNF receptor and Fas (CD95). Fas-ligand (FasL) is a membrane protein expressed mainly on activated T lymphocytes. When these T cells recognize Fas-expressing targets, Fas molecules are cross-linked by the FasL and they bind adapter proteins, which in turn bind caspase-8. Clustering of many caspase molecules leads to their activation, thus initiating the caspase cascade. In many cell types caspase-8 may cleave and activate a pro-apoptotic member of the Bcl-2 family called Bid, thus feeding into the mitochondrial pathway. The combined activation of both pathways delivers a lethal blow to the cell. Cellular proteins, notably a caspase antagonist called FLIP, block activation of caspases downstream of death receptors. Interestingly, some viruses produce homologues of FLIP, and it is suggested that this is a mechanism that viruses use to keep infected cells alive. The death receptor pathway is involved in elimination of self-reactive lymphocytes and in killing of target cells by some cytotoxic T lymphocytes.

Clearance of Apoptotic Cells. Apoptotic cells undergo several changes in their membranes that promote their phagocytosis. In normal cells phosphatidylserine is present on the inner leaflet of the plasma membrane, but in apoptotic cells this phospholipid "flips" out and is expressed on the outer layer of the membrane, where it is recognized by macrophages. Cells that are dying by apoptosis also secrete soluble factors that recruit phagocytes. This facilitates prompt clearance of the dead cells before they undergo secondary membrane damage and release their cellular contents (which can result in inflammation). Some apoptotic bodies express adhesive glycoproteins that are recognized by phagocytes, and macrophages themselves may produce proteins that bind to apoptotic cells (but not to live cells) and target the dead cells for engulfment. Numerous macrophage receptors have been shown to be involved in the binding and engulfment of apoptotic cells. This process of phagocytosis of apoptotic cells is so efficient that dead cells disappear without leaving a trace, and inflammation is virtually absent.

Although we have emphasized the distinctions between necrosis and apoptosis, these two forms of cell death may coexist and be related mechanistically. For instance, DNA damage (seen in apoptosis) activates an enzyme called poly-ADP(ribose) polymerase, which depletes cellular supplies of nicotinamide adenine dinucleotide, leading to a fall in ATP levels and ultimately necrosis. In fact, even in common situations such as ischemia, it has been suggested that early cell death can be partly attributed to apoptosis, and necrosis is the dominant type of cell death late, with worsening ischemia.

Examples of Apoptosis

Cell death in many situations is known to be caused by apoptosis, and the selected examples listed below illustrate the role of this death pathway in normal physiology and in disease.

Growth Factor Deprivation. Hormone-sensitive cells deprived of the relevant hormone, lymphocytes that are not stimulated by antigens and cytokines, and neurons deprived of nerve growth factor die by apoptosis. In all these situations, apoptosis is triggered by the mitochondrial pathway and is attributable to activation of proapoptotic members of the Bcl-2 family and decreased synthesis of Bcl-2 and Bcl-x_L.

DNA Damage. Exposure of cells to radiation or chemotherapeutic agents induces DNA damage, and if this is too severe to be repaired it triggers apoptotic death. When DNA is damaged, the p53 protein accumulates in cells. It first arrests the cell cycle (at the G_1 phase) to allow time for repair (Chapter 6). However, if the damage is too great to be repaired successfully, p53 triggers apoptosis, mainly by activating sensors that ultimately activate Bax and Bak, and by stimulating synthesis of proapoptotic members of the Bcl-2 family. When p53 is mutated or absent (as it is in certain cancers), it is incapable of inducing apoptosis, so that cells with damaged DNA are allowed to survive. In such cells, the DNA damage may result in mutations or translocations that lead to neoplastic transformation (Chapter 6).

Accumulation of Misfolded Proteins. During normal protein synthesis, chaperones in the ER control the proper folding of newly synthesized proteins, and misfolded polypeptides are ubiquitinated and targeted for proteolysis. If, however, unfolded or misfolded proteins accumulate in the ER because of inherited mutations or stresses, they induce "ER stress" that triggers a number of cellular responses, collectively called the *unfolded protein response*. This response activates signaling pathways that increase the production of chaperones and retard protein translation, thus reducing the levels of misfolded proteins in the cell. However, if this response is unable to cope with the accumulation of misfolded proteins, the result is the activation of caspases that lead to apoptosis. Intracellular accumulation of abnormally folded proteins, caused by mutations, aging, or unknown environmental factors, is now recognized as a feature of a number of neurodegenerative diseases, including Alzheimer, Huntington, and Parkinson diseases, and possibly type II diabetes. Deprivation of glucose and oxygen, and stress such as heat, also result in protein misfolding, culminating in cell injury and death.

Apoptosis of Self-Reactive Lymphocytes. Lymphocytes capable of recognizing self antigens are normally produced in all individuals. If these lymphocytes encounter self antigens, the cells die by apoptosis. Both the mitochondrial pathway and the Fas death receptor pathway have been implicated in this process (Chapter 5). Failure of apoptosis of self-reactive lymphocytes is one of the causes of autoimmune diseases.

Cytotoxic T Lymphocyte–Mediated Apoptosis. Cytotoxic T lymphocytes (CTLs) recognize foreign antigens presented on the surface of infected host cells and tumor cells (Chapter 5). Upon activation, CTL granule proteases called *granzymes* enter the target cells. Granzymes cleave proteins at aspartate residues and are able to activate cellular caspases. In this way, the CTL kills target cells by directly inducing the effector phase of apoptosis, without engaging mitochondria or death receptors. CTLs also express FasL on their surface and may kill target cells by ligation of Fas receptors.

SUMMARY

Apoptosis

- Regulated mechanism of cell death that serves to eliminate unwanted and irreparably damaged cells, with the least possible host reaction
- Characterized by: enzymatic degradation of proteins and DNA, initiated by caspases; and recognition and removal of dead cells by phagocytes
- Initiated by two major pathways:
  - *Mitochondrial (intrinsic) pathway* is triggered by loss of survival signals, DNA damage and accumulation of misfolded proteins (ER stress); associated with leakage of pro-apoptotic proteins from mitochondrial membrane into the cytoplasm, where they trigger caspase activation; inhibited by anti-apoptotic members of the Bcl family, which are induced by survival signals including growth factors.
  - *Death receptor (extrinsic) pathway* is responsible for elimination of self-reactive lymphocytes and damage by cytotoxic T lymphocytes; is initiated by engagement of death receptors (members of the TNF receptor family) by ligands on adjacent cells.

This description of apoptosis concludes the discussion of cell injury and cell death. As we have seen, these processes are the root cause of many common diseases. We end this chapter with brief considerations of three other processes: intracellular accumulations of various substances and extracellular deposition of calcium, both of which are often associated with cell injury, and aging.

INTRACELLULAR ACCUMULATIONS

Under some circumstances cells may accumulate abnormal amounts of various substances, which may be harmless or associated with varying degrees of injury. The substance may be located in the cytoplasm, within organelles (typically lysosomes), or in the nucleus, and it may be synthesized by the affected cells or may be produced elsewhere.

There are three main pathways of abnormal intracellular accumulations (Fig. 1–24):

- A normal substance is produced at a normal or an increased rate, but the metabolic rate is inadequate to remove it. An example of this type of process is fatty change in the liver.
- A normal or an abnormal endogenous substance accumulates because of genetic or acquired defects in its folding, packaging, transport, or secretion. Mutations that cause defective folding and transport may lead to accumulation of proteins (e.g., α_1-antitrypsin deficiency).
- An inherited defect in an enzyme may result in failure to degrade a metabolite. The resulting disorders are called storage diseases (Chapter 7).
- An abnormal exogenous substance is deposited and accumulates because the cell has neither the enzymatic machinery to degrade the substance nor the ability to transport it to other sites. Accumulations of carbon or silica particles are examples of this type of alteration.

Fatty Change (Steatosis). *Fatty change* refers to any abnormal accumulation of triglycerides within parenchymal cells. It is most often seen in the liver, since this is the major organ involved in fat metabolism, but it may also occur in heart, skeletal muscle, kidney, and other organs. Steatosis may be caused by toxins, protein malnutrition, diabetes mellitus, obesity, and anoxia. *Alcohol abuse and diabetes associated with obesity are the most common causes of fatty change in the liver* (fatty liver) in industrialized nations.

Free fatty acids from adipose tissue or ingested food are normally transported into hepatocytes, where they are esterified to triglycerides, converted into cholesterol or phospholipids, or oxidized to ketone bodies (Fig. 1–25A). Some fatty acids are synthesized from acetate within the hepatocytes as well. Egress of the triglycerides from the hepatocytes requires the formation of complexes with apoproteins to form lipoproteins, which are able to enter the circulation (Chapter 7). Excess accumulation of triglycerides may result from defects at any step from fatty acid entry to lipoprotein exit, thus accounting for the occurrence of fatty liver after diverse hepatic insults. Hepatotoxins (e.g., alcohol) alter mitochondrial and SER function and thus inhibit fatty acid oxidation; CCl_4 and protein malnutrition decrease the synthesis of apoproteins; anoxia inhibits fatty acid oxidation; and starvation increases fatty acid mobilization from peripheral stores.

The significance of fatty change depends on the cause and severity of the accumulation. When mild it may have no effect on cellular function. More severe fatty change may transiently impair cellular function, but unless some vital intracellular process is irreversibly impaired (e.g., in

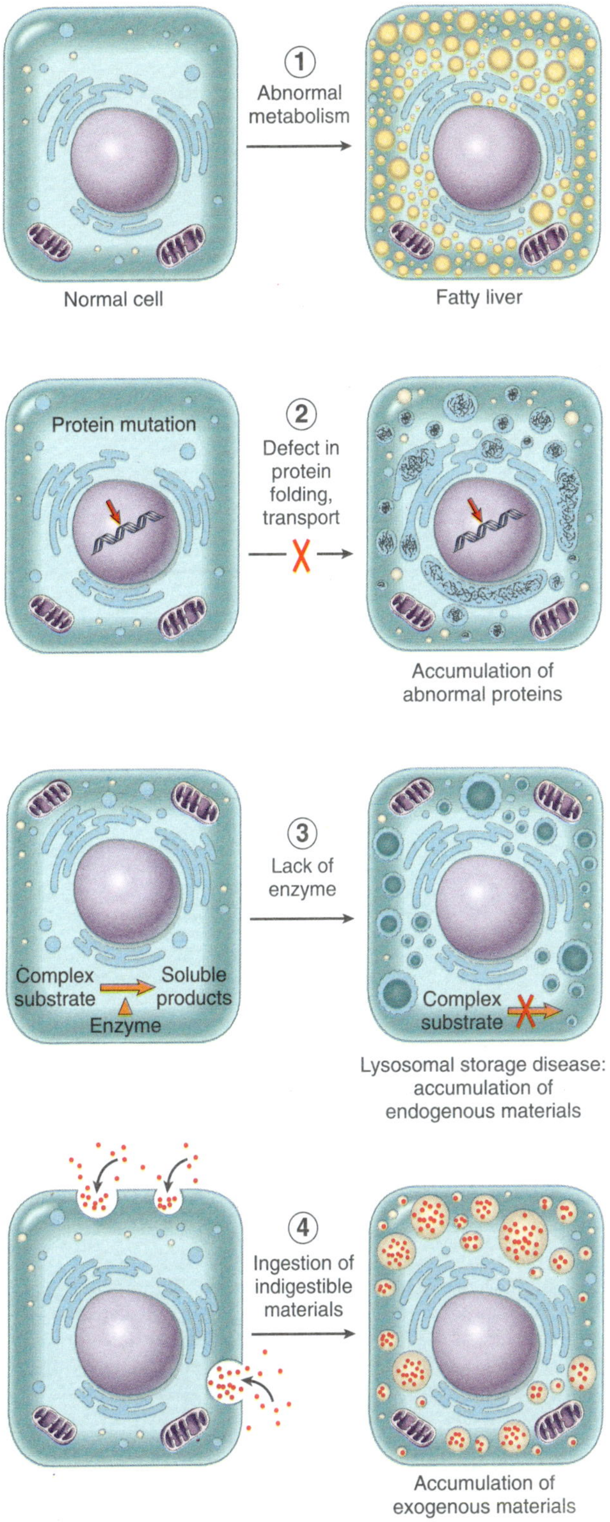

Figure 1–24

Mechanisms of intracellular accumulation. (1) Abnormal metabolism, as in fatty change in the liver. (2) Mutations causing alterations in protein folding and transport, so that defective molecules accumulate intracellularly. (3) A deficiency of critical enzymes responsible for breaking down certain compounds, causing substrates to accumulate in lysosomes, as in lysosomal storage diseases. (4) An inability to degrade phagocytosed particles, as in carbon pigment accumulation.

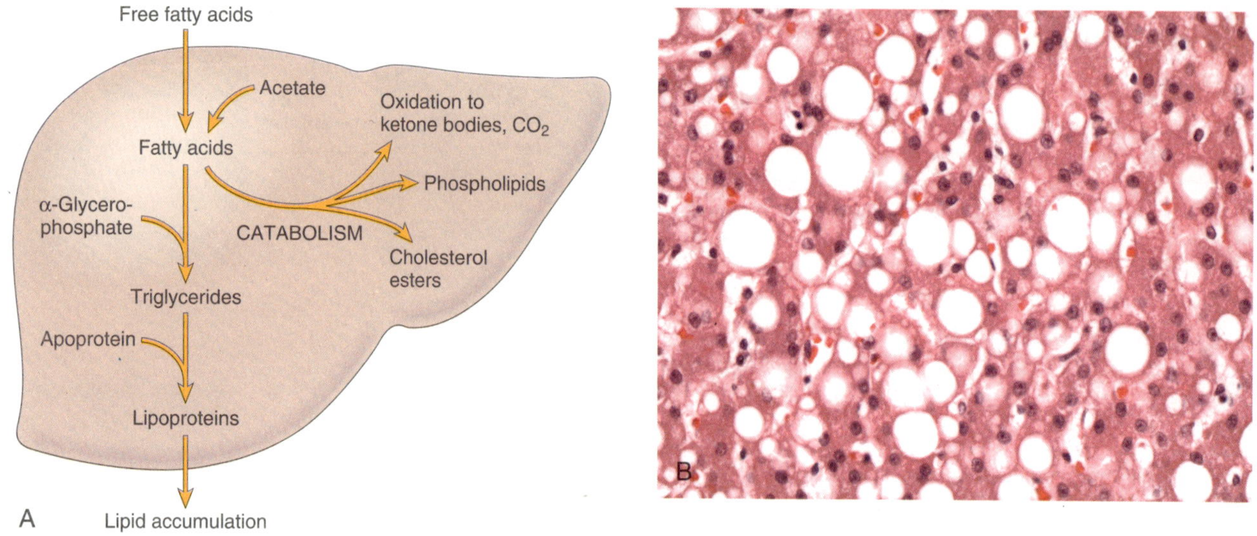

Figure 1–25

Fatty liver. **A,** The possible mechanisms leading to accumulation of triglycerides in fatty liver. Defects in any of the steps of uptake, catabolism, or secretion can lead to lipid accumulation. **B,** High-power detail of fatty change of the liver. In most cells the well-preserved nucleus is squeezed into the displaced rim of cytoplasm about the fat vacuole. (**B,** Courtesy of Dr. James Crawford, Department of Pathology, University of Florida School of Medicine, Gainesville, Florida.)

CCl_4 poisoning), fatty change is reversible. In the severe form, fatty change may precede cell death, and may be an early lesion in a serious liver disease called nonalcoholic steatohepatitis (Chapter 16).

Morphology

In any site, fatty accumulation appears as clear vacuoles within parenchymal cells. Special staining techniques are required to distinguish fat from intracellular water or glycogen, which can also produce clear vacuoles but have a different significance. To identify fat microscopically, tissues must be processed for sectioning without the organic solvents typically used in sample preparation. Usually, portions of tissue are therefore frozen to enable the cutting of thin sections for histologic examination; the fat is then identified by staining with Sudan IV or oil red O (these stain fat orange-red). Glycogen may be identified by staining for polysaccharides using the periodic acid–Schiff stain (which stains glycogen red-violet). If vacuoles do not stain for either fat or glycogen, they are presumed to be composed mostly of water.

Fatty change is most commonly seen in the liver and the heart. Mild fatty change in the **liver** may not affect the gross appearance. With increasing accumulation, the organ enlarges and becomes progressively yellow until, in extreme cases, it may weigh 3 to 6 kg (1.5–3 times the normal weight) and appear bright yellow, soft, and greasy. Early fatty change is seen by light microscopy as small fat vacuoles in the cytoplasm around the nucleus. In later stages, the vacuoles coalesce to create cleared spaces that displace the nucleus to the cell periphery (Fig. 1–25B). Occasionally contiguous cells rupture, and the enclosed fat globules unite to produce so-called fatty cysts.

In the **heart,** lipid is found in the form of small droplets, occurring in one of two patterns. Prolonged moderate hypoxia (as in profound anemia) results in focal intracellular fat deposits, creating grossly apparent bands of yellowed myocardium alternating with bands of darker, red-brown, uninvolved heart ("tigered effect"). The other pattern of fatty change is produced by more profound hypoxia or by some forms of toxic injury (e.g., diphtheria) and shows more uniformly affected myocytes.

Cholesterol and Cholesteryl Esters. Cellular cholesterol metabolism is tightly regulated to ensure normal cell membrane synthesis without significant intracellular accumulation. However, phagocytic cells may become overloaded with lipid (triglycerides, cholesterol, and cholesteryl esters) in several different pathologic processes.

Macrophages in contact with the lipid debris of necrotic cells or abnormal (e.g., oxidized) forms of lipoproteins may become stuffed with phagocytosed lipid. These macrophages may be filled with minute, membrane-bound vacuoles of lipid, imparting a foamy appearance to their cytoplasm (*foam cells*). In *atherosclerosis,* smooth muscle cells and macrophages are filled with lipid vacuoles composed of cholesterol and cholesteryl esters; these give atherosclerotic plaques their characteristic yellow color and contribute to the pathogenesis of the lesion (Chapter 10). In hereditary and acquired hyperlipidemic syndromes, macrophages accumulate intracellular cholesterol; when present in the subepithelial connective tissue of skin or in tendons, clusters of these foamy macrophages form masses called *xanthomas.*

Proteins. Morphologically visible protein accumulations are much less common than lipid accumulations; they may occur because excesses are presented to the cells or because the cells synthesize excessive amounts. In the kidney, for example, trace amounts of albumin filtered through the glomerulus are normally reabsorbed by pinocytosis in the proximal convoluted tubules. However, in disorders with heavy protein leakage across the glomerular filter (e.g.,

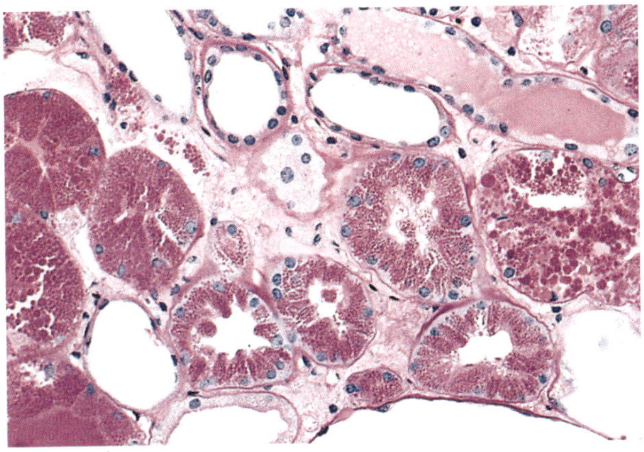

Figure 1–26

Protein reabsorption droplets in the renal tubular epithelium. (Courtesy of Dr. Helmut Rennke, Department of Pathology, Brigham and Women's Hospital, Boston, Massachusetts.)

nephrotic syndrome), there is a much larger reabsorption of the protein. Pinocytic vesicles containing this protein fuse with lysosomes, resulting in the histologic appearance of pink, hyaline cytoplasmic droplets (Fig. 1–26). The process is reversible; if the proteinuria abates, the protein droplets are metabolized and disappear. Another example is the marked accumulation of newly synthesized immunoglobulins that may occur in the RER of some plasma cells, forming rounded, eosinophilic *Russell bodies.*

Accumulations of intracellular proteins are also seen in certain types of cell injury. For example, the Mallory body, or "alcoholic hyalin," is an eosinophilic cytoplasmic inclusion in liver cells that is highly characteristic of alcoholic liver disease (Chapter 16). Such inclusions are composed predominantly of aggregated intermediate filaments that presumably resist degradation. The neurofibrillary tangle found in the brain in Alzheimer disease is an aggregated protein inclusion that contains microtubule-associated proteins and neurofilaments, a reflection of a disrupted neuronal cytoskeleton (Chapter 23).

Glycogen. Excessive intracellular deposits of glycogen are associated with abnormalities in the metabolism of either glucose or glycogen. In poorly controlled diabetes mellitus, the prime example of abnormal glucose metabolism, glycogen accumulates in renal tubular epithelium, cardiac myocytes, and β cells of the islets of Langerhans. Glycogen also accumulates within cells in a group of closely related genetic disorders collectively referred to as *glycogen storage diseases,* or *glycogenoses* (Chapter 7). In these diseases, enzymatic defects in the synthesis or breakdown of glycogen result in massive stockpiling, with secondary injury and cell death.

Pigments. Pigments are colored substances that are either exogenous, coming from outside the body, or endogenous, synthesized within the body itself.

- The most common exogenous pigment is *carbon* (an example is coal dust), a ubiquitous air pollutant of urban life. When inhaled, it is phagocytosed by alveolar macrophages and transported through lymphatic channels to the regional tracheobronchial lymph nodes. Aggregates of the pigment blacken the draining lymph nodes and pulmonary parenchyma (*anthracosis*).Heavy accumulations may induce emphysema or a fibroblastic reaction that can result in a serious lung disease called coal workers' pneumoconiosis (Chapter 13).
- Endogenous pigments include lipofuscin, melanin, and certain derivatives of hemoglobin. *Lipofuscin,* or "wear-and-tear pigment," is an insoluble brownish-yellow granular intracellular material that accumulates in a variety of tissues (particularly the heart, liver, and brain) as a function of age or atrophy. Lipofuscin represents complexes of lipid and protein that derive from the free radical–catalyzed peroxidation of polyunsaturated lipids of subcellular membranes. It is not injurious to the cell but is important as a marker of past free-radical injury. The brown pigment (Fig. 1–27), when present in large amounts, imparts an appearance to the tissue that is called *brown atrophy.* By electron microscopy, the pigment appears as perinuclear electron-dense granules (Fig. 1–27B).

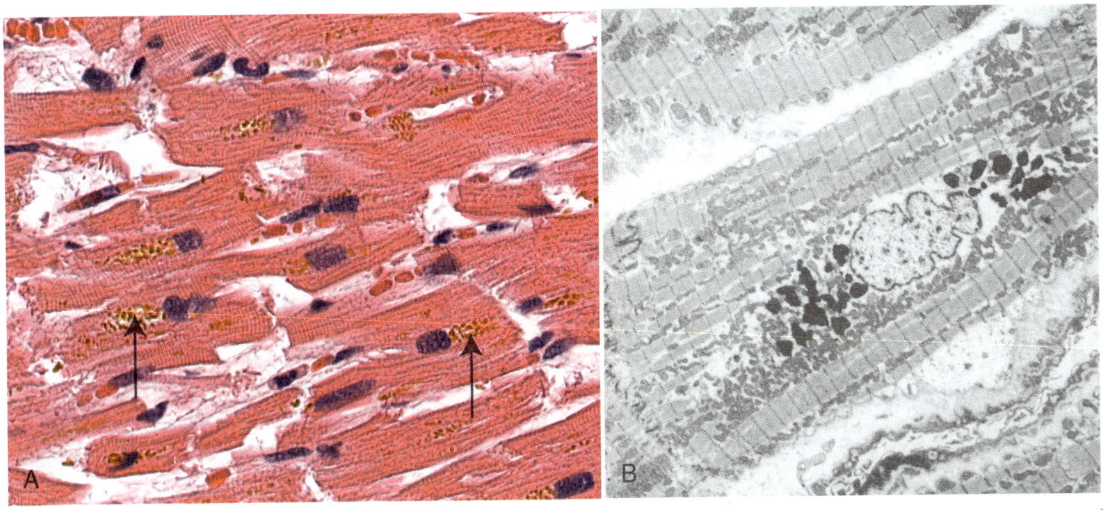

Figure 1–27

Lipofuscin granules in a cardiac myocyte. **A,** Light microscopy (deposits indicated by *arrows*). **B,** Electron microscopy. Note the perinuclear, intralysosomal location.

• *Melanin* is an endogenous, brown-black pigment produced in melanocytes following the tyrosinase-catalyzed oxidation of tyrosine to dihydroxyphenylalanine. It is synthesized exclusively by melanocytes located in the epidermis and acts as a screen against harmful ultraviolet radiation. Although melanocytes are the only source of melanin, adjacent basal keratinocytes in the skin can accumulate the pigment (e.g., in freckles), as can dermal macrophages.

• *Hemosiderin* is a hemoglobin-derived granular pigment that is golden yellow to brown and accumulates in tissues when there is a local or systemic excess of iron. Iron is normally stored within cells in association with the protein *apoferritin,* forming ferritin micelles. Hemosiderin pigment represents large aggregates of these ferritin micelles, readily visualized by light and electron microscopy; the iron can be unambiguously identified by the Prussian blue histochemical reaction (Fig. 1–28). Although hemosiderin accumulation is usually pathologic, small amounts of this pigment are normal in the mononuclear phagocytes of the bone marrow, spleen, and liver, where there is extensive red cell breakdown.

• Local excesses of iron, and consequently of hemosiderin, result from hemorrhage. The best example is the common bruise. After lysis of the erythrocytes at the site of hemorrhage, the red cell debris is phagocytosed by macrophages; the hemoglobin content is then catabolized by lysosomes with accumulation of the heme iron in hemosiderin. The array of colors through which the bruise passes reflects these transformations. The original red-blue color of hemoglobin is transformed to varying shades of green-blue by the local formation of biliverdin (green bile) and bilirubin (red bile) from the heme moiety; the iron ions of hemoglobin accumulate as golden-yellow hemosiderin.

• Whenever there is systemic overload of iron, hemosiderin is deposited in many organs and tissues, a condition called *hemosiderosis* (Chapter 12). It is found at first in the mononuclear phagocytes of the liver, bone marrow, spleen, and lymph nodes and in scattered macrophages throughout other organs. With progressive accumulation, parenchymal cells throughout the body (but principally the liver, pancreas, heart, and endocrine organs) become "bronzed" with accumulating pigment. Hemosiderosis occurs in the setting of (1) increased absorption of dietary iron, (2) impaired utilization of iron, (3) hemolytic anemias, and (4) transfusions (the transfused red cells constitute an exogenous load of iron). In most instances of systemic hemosiderosis, the iron pigment does not damage the parenchymal cells or impair organ function despite an impressive accumulation (Fig. 1–28). However, more extensive accumulations of iron are seen in *hereditary hemochromatosis* (Chapter 16), with tissue injury including liver fibrosis, heart failure, and diabetes mellitus.

PATHOLOGIC CALCIFICATION

Pathologic calcification is a common process in a wide variety of disease states; it implies the abnormal deposition of calcium salts, together with smaller amounts of iron, magnesium, and other minerals. When the deposition occurs in dead or dying tissues, it is called *dystrophic calcification; it occurs in the absence of calcium metabolic* derangements (i.e., with normal serum levels of calcium). In contrast, the deposition of calcium salts in normal tissues is known as *metastatic calcification and almost always reflects some derangement in calcium metabolism (hypercalcemia).* It should be noted that while hypercalcemia is not a prerequisite for dystrophic calcification, it can exacerbate it.

Dystrophic Calcification. Dystrophic calcification is encountered in areas of necrosis of any type. It is virtually inevitable in the *atheromas* of advanced atherosclerosis, associated with intimal injury in the aorta and large arteries and characterized by accumulation of lipids (Chapter 10). Although dystrophic calcification may be an incidental finding indicating insignificant past cell injury, it may also be a cause of organ dysfunction. For example, calcification can develop in aging or damaged heart valves, resulting in severely compromised valve

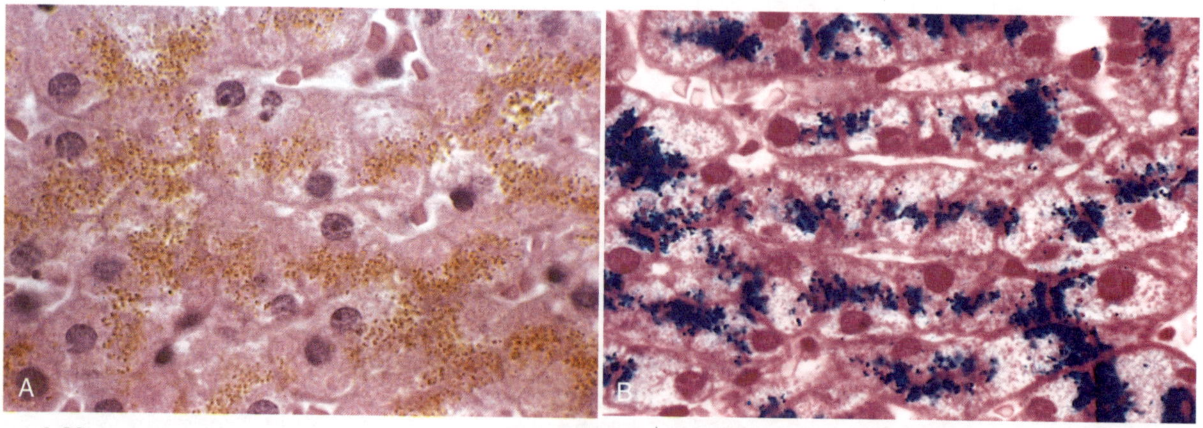

Figure 1–28

Hemosiderin granules in liver cells. **A,** H&E section showing golden-brown, finely granular pigment. **B,** Prussian blue reaction, specific for iron.

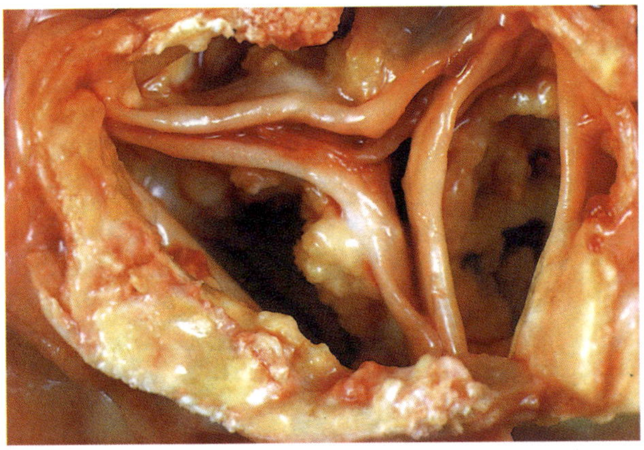

Figure 1–29

Calcification of the aortic valve. A view looking down onto the unopened aortic valve in a heart with calcific aortic stenosis. The semilunar cusps are thickened and fibrotic. Behind each cusp are large, irregular masses of dystrophic calcification that will prevent normal opening of the cusps.

motion. Dystrophic calcification of the aortic valves is an important cause of aortic stenosis in the elderly (Fig. 1–29).

Morphology

Regardless of the site, calcium salts are grossly seen as fine white granules or clumps, often felt as gritty deposits. Sometimes a tuberculous lymph node is essentially converted to radio-opaque stone. Histologically, calcification appears as intracellular and/or extracellular basophilic deposits. In time, heterotopic bone may be formed in the focus of calcification.

The pathogenesis of dystrophic calcification involves *initiation* (or nucleation) and *propagation,* both of which may be either intracellular or extracellular; the ultimate end product is the formation of crystalline *calcium phosphate.* Initiation in extracellular sites occurs in membrane-bound vesicles about 200 nm in diameter; in normal cartilage and bone they are known as *matrix vesicles,* and in pathologic calcification they derive from degenerating cells. It is thought that calcium is initially concentrated in these vesicles by its affinity for membrane phospholipids, while phosphates accumulate as a result of the action of membrane-bound phosphatases. Initiation of intracellular calcification occurs in the mitochondria of dead or dying cells that have lost their ability to regulate intracellular calcium. After initiation in either location, propagation of crystal formation occurs. This is dependent on the concentration of Ca^{2+} and PO_4^- in the extracellular spaces, the presence of mineral inhibitors, and the degree of collagenization, which enhances the rate of crystal growth.

Metastatic Calcification. Metastatic calcification can occur in normal tissues whenever there is hypercalcemia. The four major causes of hypercalcemia are (1) *increased secretion of parathyroid hormone,* due to either primary parathyroid tumors or production of parathyroid hormone-related protein by other malignant tumors; (2) *destruction of bone* due to the effects of accelerated turnover (e.g., *Paget disease*), immobilization, or tumors (increased bone catabolism associated with multiple myeloma, leukemia, or diffuse skeletal metastases); (3) *vitamin D–related disorders* including vitamin D intoxication and *sarcoidosis* (in which macrophages activate a vitamin D precursor); and (4) *renal failure,* in which phosphate retention leads to *secondary hyperparathyroidism.*

Morphology

Metastatic calcification can occur widely throughout the body but principally affects the interstitial tissues of the vasculature, kidneys, lungs, and gastric mucosa. The calcium deposits morphologically resemble those described in dystrophic calcification. Although they do not generally cause clinical dysfunction, extensive calcifications in the lungs may produce remarkable radiographs and respiratory deficits, and massive deposits in the kidney (**nephrocalcinosis**) can cause renal damage.

SUMMARY

Abnormal Intracellular Depositions and Calcifications

- Abnormal deposits of materials in cells and tissues are the result of excessive intake or defective transport or catabolism.
- Depositions of *lipids:*
  - *Fatty change:* accumulation of free triglycerides in cells, resulting from excessive intake or defective transport (often because of defects in synthesis of transport proteins); manifestation of reversible cell injury
  - *Cholesterol deposition:* result of defective catabolism and excessive intake; in macrophages and smooth muscle cells of vessel walls in atherosclerosis
- Deposition of *proteins:* reabsorbed proteins in kidney tubules; immunoglobulins in plasma cells
- Deposition of *glycogen:* in macrophages of patients with defects in lysosomal enzymes that break down glycogen (glycogen storage diseases)
- Deposition of *pigments:* typically indigestible pigments, such as carbon, lipofuscin (breakdown product of lipid peroxidation), iron (usually due to overload, as in hemosiderosis)
- Pathologic calcifications:
  - *Dystrophic calcification:* deposition of calcium at sites of cell injury and necrosis
  - *Metastatic calcification:* deposition of calcium in normal tissues, caused by hypercalcemia (usually a consequence of parathyroid hormone excess)

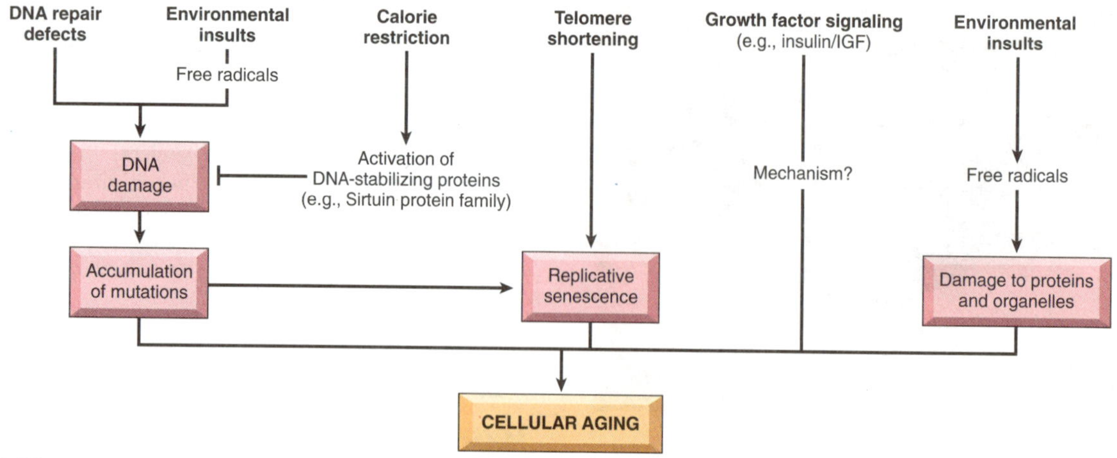

Figure 1–30

Mechanisms of cellular aging. Among the several pathways contributing to aging of cells and organisms, many have been defined in simple model organisms, and their relevance to aging in humans remains an area of active investigation. IGF, insulin-like growth factor.

CELLULAR AGING

Cellular aging is the result of a progressive decline in the proliferative capacity and life span of cells and the effects of continuous exposure to exogenous factors that cause accumulation of cellular and molecular damage (Fig. 1–30). The process of aging is conserved from yeast to humans, and—at least in simple model organisms—seems to be regulated by a limited number of genes. The idea that aging is controlled by particular genes has spurred enormous interest in defining its molecular pathways and in devising ways to manipulate a process that was once considered inexorable. Several mechanisms are known or suspected to be responsible for cellular aging.

- *DNA damage.* Cellular aging is associated with increasing DNA damage, which may happen during normal DNA replication and can be enhanced by free radicals. Although most DNA damage is repaired by DNA repair enzymes, some persists and accumulates as cells age. Some aging syndromes are associated with defects in DNA repair mechanisms, and the life span of model animals can be increased if responses to DNA damage are enhanced or proteins that stabilize DNA are introduced. In fact, the intervention that has most consistently prolonged life span in most species is *calorie restriction.* Recently, it has been proposed that calorie restriction imposes a level of stress that activates proteins of the Sirtuin family, such as Sir2, that function as histone deacetylases. These proteins may deacetylate and thereby activate DNA repair enzymes, thus stabilizing the DNA; in the absence of these proteins, DNA is prone to damage.
- *Decreased cellular replication.* All normal cells have a limited capacity for replication, and after a fixed number of divisions cells become arrested in a terminally nondividing state, known as *replicative senescence.* Aging is associated with progressive replicative senescence of cells. Cells from children have the capacity to undergo more rounds of replication than do cells from older people. In contrast, cells from patients with *Werner syndrome,* a rare disease characterized by premature aging, have a markedly reduced in vitro life span. In human cells, the mechanism of replicative senescence involves incomplete replication and progressive shortening of telomeres, which ultimately results in cell cycle arrest. *Telomeres* are short repeated sequences of DNA present at the linear ends of chromosomes that are important for ensuring the complete replication of chromosome ends and for protecting the ends from fusion and degradation. When somatic cells replicate, a small section of the telomere is not duplicated, and telomeres become progressively shortened. As the telomeres become shorter, the ends of chromosomes cannot be protected and are seen as broken DNA, which signals cell cycle arrest. The lengths of the telomeres are normally maintained by nucleotide addition mediated by an enzyme called *telomerase.* Telomerase is a specialized RNA-protein complex that uses its own RNA as a template for adding nucleotides to the ends of chromosomes. Telomerase activity is expressed in germ cells and is present at low levels in stem cells, but it is usually absent in most somatic tissues (Fig. 1–31). Therefore, as cells age their telomeres become shorter and they exit the cell cycle, resulting in an inability to generate new cells to replace damaged ones. Conversely, in immortal cancer cells, telomerase is reactivated and telomeres are not shortened, suggesting that telomere elongation might be an important—possibly essential—step in tumor formation. This is discussed more fully in Chapter 6. Despite such alluring observations, however, the relationship of telomerase activity and telomere length to aging and cancer has yet to be fully established.
- *Reduced regenerative capacity of tissue stem cells.* Recent studies suggest that with age, the p16

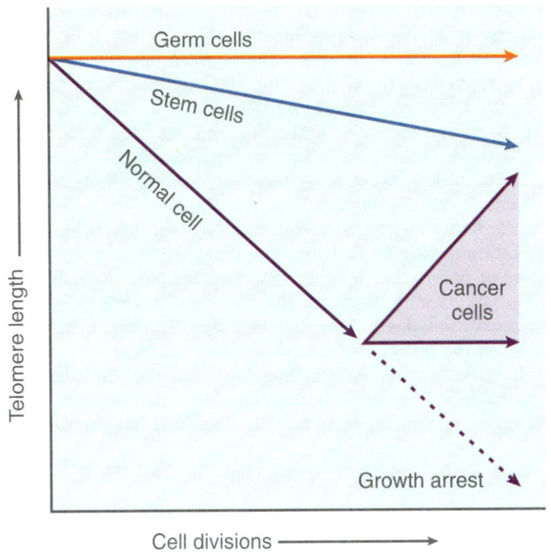

Figure 1–31

The role of telomeres and telomerase in replicative senescence of cells. Telomere length is plotted against the number of cell divisions. In normal somatic cells there is no telomerase activity, and telomeres progressively shorten with increasing cell divisions until growth arrest, or senescence, occurs. Germ cells and stem cells both contain active telomerase, but only the germ cells have sufficient levels of the enzyme to stabilize telomere length completely. In cancer cells, telomerase is often reactivated. (Modified by permission from Macmillan Publishers Ltd, from Holt SE, et al: Refining the telomer-telomerase hypothesis of aging and cancer. Nat Biotechnol 14:836, 1996.)

(CDKN2A) protein accumulates in stem cells, and they progressively lose their capacity to self-renew. p16 is a physiological inhibitor of cell cycle progression; as we discuss in Chapter 6, deletion or loss-of-function mutations of p16 are associated with cancer development.

- *Accumulation of metabolic damage.* Cellular life span is also determined by a balance between damage resulting from metabolic events occurring within the cell and counteracting molecular responses that can repair the damage. One group of potentially toxic products of normal metabolism is reactive oxygen species. As we have discussed earlier in the chapter, these byproducts of oxidative phosphorylation cause covalent modifications of proteins, lipids, and nucleic acids. Increased oxidative damage could result from repeated environmental exposure to such influences as ionizing radiation along with progressive reduction of antioxidant defense mechanisms. Damaged cellular organelles accumulate as cells age. This may also be the result of declining function of the proteasome, the proteolytic machine that serves to eliminate abnormal and unwanted intracellular proteins.
- Studies in model organisms, like the worm *Caenorhabditis elegans,* have shown that growth factors, such as insulin-like growth factor, and intracellular signaling pathways triggered by these hormones, tend to reduce life span. The underlying mechanisms are not fully understood, but these growth factors may attenuate Sir2 responses to cellular stress and thus reduce the stability of the DNA.

SUMMARY

Cellular Aging

- Results from combination of accumulating cellular damage (e.g., by free radicals), reduced capacity to divide (replicative senescence), and reduced ability to repair damaged DNA
- *Accumulation of DNA damage:* defective DNA repair mechanisms; DNA repair may be activated by calorie restriction (known to prolong aging in model organisms)
- *Replicative senescence:* reduced capacity of cells to divide because of decreasing amounts of telomerase and progressive shortening of chromosomal ends (telomeres)
- *Other factors:* progressive accumulation of metabolic damage; possible roles of growth factors that promote aging in simple model organisms

It should be apparent that the various forms of cellular derangements and adaptations described in this chapter cover a wide spectrum, ranging from adaptations in cell size, growth, and function; to the reversible and irreversible forms of acute cell injury; to the regulated type of cell death represented by apoptosis. Reference is made to all these alterations throughout this book because all organ injury and ultimately all clinical disease arise from derangements in cell structure and function.

BIBLIOGRAPHY

Balaban RS, Nemoto S, Finkel T: Mitochondria, oxidants, and aging. Cell 120:483, 2005. *[A good review of the role of free radicals in aging.]*

Blackburn EH: Switching and signaling at the telomere. Cell 106:661, 2001. *[This review describes the structure of telomeres and the molecular mechanisms of telomere function.]*

Danial NK, Korsmeyer SJ: Cell death: critical control points. Cell 116:205, 2004. *[Excellent review of the regulation of apoptosis, with emphasis on the Bcl-2 family of proteins.]*

Debnath J, Baehrecke EH, Kroemer G: Does autophagy contribute to cell death? Autophagy 1:66, 2005. *[Modern discussion of the possible links between autophagy and apoptosis.]*

Finkel T: Oxidant signals and oxidative stress. Curr Opin Cell Biol 15:247, 2003. *[Review of the physiologic and pathologic roles of oxygen-derived free radicals.]*

Frey N, Olson EN: Cardiac hypertrophy: the good, the bad, and the ugly. Annu Rev Physiol 65:45, 2003. *[Excellent discussion of the mechanisms of muscle hypertrophy, using the heart as the paradigm.]*

Fuchs E, Cleveland DW: A structural scaffolding of intermediate filaments in health and disease. Science 279:514, 1998. *[A succinct overview of the role of cytoskeleton in cell adaptation and disease.]*

Green DR, Kroemer G. The pathophysiology of mitochondrial cell death. Science 305:626, 2004. *[Overview of one of the two major pathways of apoptosis.]*

Guarente L, Picard F. Calorie restriction—the SIR2 connection. Cell 120:473, 2005. *[Current concepts of aging and how calorie restriction may retard the process.]*

Hathway DE: Toxic action/toxicity. Biol Rev Camb Philos Soc 75:95, 2000. *[A well-written overview of basic pathways of toxic injury and the intracellular responses to them.]*

Kaminski KA, et al: Oxidative stress and neutrophil activation—the two keystones of ischemia/reperfusion injury. Int J Cardiol 86:41,

2002. *[Discussion of the pathogenesis of ischemia-reperfusion injury.]*

Kaufman RJ: Orchestrating the unfolded protein response in health and disease. J Clin Invest 110:1389, 2002. *[Excellent discussion of how cells protect themselves from misfolded proteins, and how accumulation of these proteins can trigger cell death.]*

Lavrik I, Golks A, Krammer PH. Death receptor signaling. J Cell Sci 118:265, 2005. *[Review of the death receptor pathway of apoptosis.]*

Levine B. Eating oneself and uninvited guests: autophagy-related pathways in cellular defense. Cell 120:159, 2005. *[Modern review of the mechanisms and physiology of autophagy.]*

Lombard DB, et al: DNA repair, genome stability, and aging. Cell 120:497, 2005. *[The role of DNA damage in cellular aging.]*

McKinnell IW, Rudnicki MA: Molecular mechanisms of muscle atrophy. Cell 119:907, 2004. *[Discussion of the mechanisms of cellular atrophy.]*

Newmeyer DD, Ferguson-Miller S: Mitochondria: releasing power for life and unleashing the machineries of death. Cell 112:481, 2003. *[Excellent review of the many functions of mitochondria, with an emphasis on their role in cell death.]*

Ravichandran KS: "Recruitment signals" from apoptotic cells: invitation to a quiet meal. Cell 113:817, 2003. *[Discussion of how apoptotic cells are phagocytosed and cleared.]*

Szabo C: Mechanisms of cell necrosis. Crit Care Med 33:S530, 2005.

Tosh D, Slack JM: How cells change their phenotype. Nat Rev Mol Cell Biol 3:187, 2002. *[Review of metaplasia and the roles of stem cells and genetic reprogramming.]*

Toyokuni S: Reactive oxygen species-induced molecular damage and its application in pathology. Pathol Int 49:91, 1999. *[A review of mechanisms of free-radical injury and associated pathologies.]*

Zheng D, Saikumar P, Weinberg JM, Venkatachalam MA: Calcium in cell injury and death. Annu Rev Pathol 1:405, 2006. *[A recent review on the links between calcium and cell injury.]*

Ziegler U, Groscurth P: Morphological features of cell death. News Physiol Sci 19:124, 2004. *[Excellent, simple description of the morphology of cell death, and methods for detecting apoptotic cells.]*

Chapter 2

Acute and Chronic Inflammation

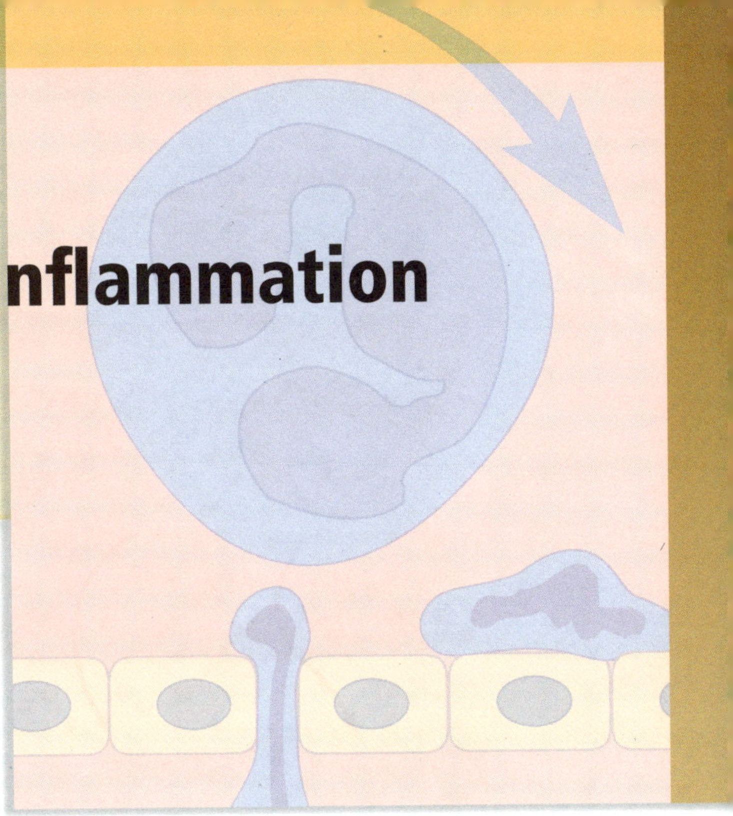

OVERVIEW OF INFLAMMATION

The survival of all organisms requires that they eliminate foreign invaders, such as infectious pathogens, and damaged tissues. These functions are mediated by a complex host response called *inflammation. Inflammation is a protective response intended to eliminate the initial cause of cell injury as well as the necrotic cells and tissues resulting from the original insult.* Inflammation accomplishes its protective mission by diluting, destroying, or otherwise neutralizing harmful agents (e.g., microbes and toxins). It then sets into motion the events that eventually heal and repair the sites of injury (Chapter 3). Without inflammation, infections would go unchecked and wounds would never heal. In the context of infections, inflammation is part of a broader protective response that immunologists refer to as *innate immunity* (Chapter 5).

Although inflammation helps clear infections and other noxious stimuli and initiates repair, the inflammatory reaction and the subsequent repair process can cause considerable harm. The components of the inflammatory reaction that destroy and eliminate microbes and dead tissues are capable of also injuring normal tissues. Therefore, injury may accompany entirely normal, beneficial inflammatory reactions, and the pathology may even become the dominant feature if the reaction is very strong (e.g., when the infection is severe), prolonged (e.g., when the eliciting agent resists eradication), or inappropriate (e.g., when it is directed against self-antigens in autoimmune diseases. or against usually harmless environmental antigens in allergic disorders). Some of the most vexing diseases of humans are disorders in which the pathophysiologic basis is inappropriate, often chronic, inflammation. This is why the process of inflammation is fundamental to virtually all of clinical medicine.

The cells and molecules of host defense normally circulate in the blood, and the goal of the inflammatory reaction is to bring them to the site of infection or tissue damage. Several types of cells and molecules play important roles in inflammation. These include blood leukocytes and plasma proteins, cells of vascular walls, and cells and extracellular matrix (ECM) of the surrounding connective tissue (Fig. 2–1).

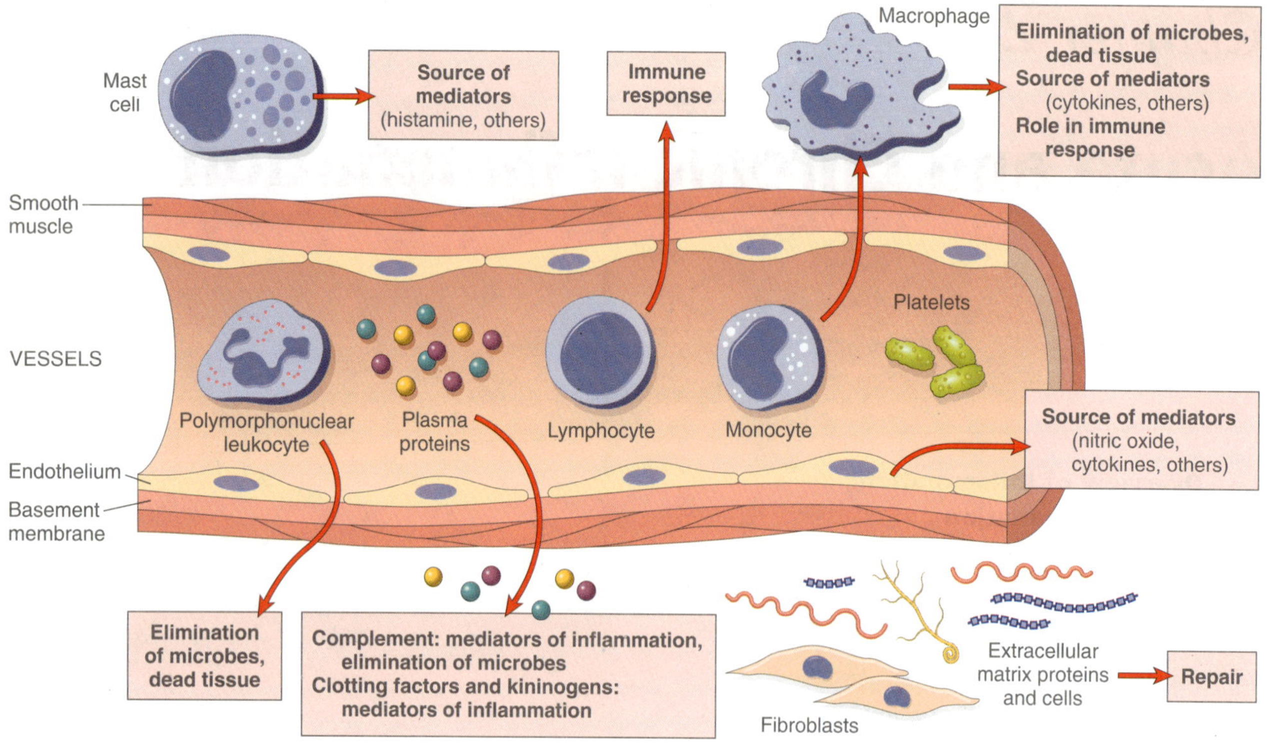

Figure 2–1

The components of acute and chronic inflammatory responses and their principal functions. The roles of these cells and molecules in inflammation will be described in this chapter.

Inflammation can be acute or chronic. Acute inflammation is rapid in onset and of short duration, lasting from a few minutes to as long as a few days, and is characterized by fluid and plasma protein exudation and a predominantly neutrophilic leukocyte accumulation. Chronic inflammation may be more insidious, is of longer duration (days to years), and is typified by influx of lymphocytes and macrophages with associated vascular proliferation and fibrosis (scarring). However, as we will see later, these basic forms of inflammation can overlap, and many variables modify their course and histologic appearance.

All acute inflammatory reactions follow a fairly stereotypical sequence in which blood vessels and leukocytes are the main participants. When a host encounters an injurious agent (e.g., a microbe) or dead cells, phagocytes that reside in tissues try to eliminate these agents. At the same time, phagocytes and other host cells react to the presence of the foreign or abnormal substance by liberating several protein and lipid molecules that function as chemical mediators of inflammation. Mediators are also produced from plasma proteins that react with the microbes or to injured tissues. Some of these mediators act on small blood vessels in the vicinity and promote the efflux of plasma and the recruitment of circulating leukocytes to the site where the offending agent is located. The recruited leukocytes are activated by the injurious agent and by locally produced mediators, and the activated leukocytes try to remove the offending agent by phagocytosis. An unfortunate side effect of the activation of leukocytes may be damage to normal host tissues.

The external manifestations of inflammation, often called its cardinal signs, result from the vascular changes and cell recruitment: heat (calor), redness (rubor), and swelling (tumor). The two additional cardinal features of acute inflammation, pain (dolor) and loss of function (functio laesa), occur as consequences of mediator elaboration and leukocyte-mediated damage. As the injurious agent is eliminated and anti-inflammatory mechanisms become active, the process subsides and the host returns to a normal state of health. If the injurious agent cannot be quickly eliminated, the result may be chronic inflammation.

SUMMARY

General Features of Inflammation

- Inflammation is a beneficial host response to foreign invaders and necrotic tissue, but it is itself capable of causing tissue damage.
- The main components of inflammation are a vascular reaction and a cellular response; both are activated by mediators that are derived from plasma proteins and various cells.
- The steps of the inflammatory response can be remembered as the five Rs: (1) Recognition of the

injurious agent, (2) Recruitment of leukocytes, (3) Removal of the agent, (4) Regulation (control) of the response, and (5) Resolution (repair).
• The outcome of acute inflammation is either elimination of the noxious stimulus followed by decline of the reaction and repair of the damaged tissue, or persistent injury resulting in chronic inflammation.

ACUTE INFLAMMATION

Acute inflammation is a rapid response to injury or microbes and other foreign substances that is designed to deliver leukocytes and plasma proteins to sites of injury. Once there, leukocytes clear the invaders and begin the process of digesting and getting rid of necrotic tissues.

Acute inflammation has two major components (Fig. 2–2):

- *Vascular changes:* alterations in vessel caliber resulting in increased blood flow (*vasodilation*) and structural changes that permit plasma proteins to leave the circulation (*increased vascular permeability*).
- *Cellular events:* emigration of the leukocytes from the microcirculation and accumulation in the focus of injury (*cellular recruitment and activation*). The principal leukocytes in acute inflammation are neutrophils (polymorphonuclear leukocytes).

Stimuli for Acute Inflammation

Acute inflammatory reactions may be triggered by a variety of stimuli.

- *Infections* (bacterial, viral, fungal, parasitic) are among the most common and medically important causes of inflammation.
- *Trauma* (blunt and penetrating) and *physical and chemical agents* (thermal injury, e.g., burns or frostbite; irradiation; some environmental chemicals) injure host cells and elicit inflammatory reactions.
- *Tissue necrosis* (from any cause), including ischemia (as in a myocardial infarct) and physical and chemical injury.
- *Foreign bodies* (splinters, dirt, sutures)
- *Immune reactions* (also called hypersensitivity reactions) against environmental substances or against self tissues. Because these stimuli for the inflammatory responses cannot be eliminated, such reactions tend to be persistent, often have features of chronic inflammation, and are important causes of morbidity and mortality. The term "immune-mediated inflammatory disease" is sometimes used to refer to this group of disorders.

Each of these stimuli may induce reactions with some distinctive characteristics, but all inflammatory reactions have the same basic features. We describe first the typical reactions of acute inflammation and its morphologic features, and then the chemical mediators responsible for these reactions.

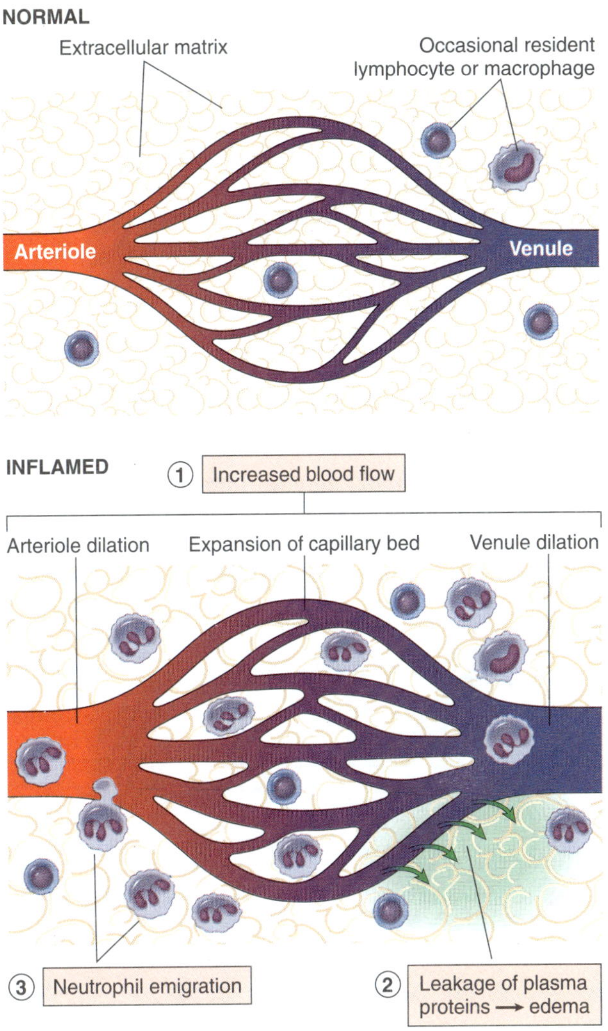

Figure 2–2

The major local manifestations of acute inflammation, compared to normal. (1) Vascular dilation and increased blood flow (causing erythema and warmth), (2) extravasation and deposition of plasma fluid and proteins (edema), and (3) leukocyte (mainly neutrophil) emigration and accumulation in the site of injury.

Vascular Changes

Changes in Vascular Caliber and Flow. Changes in blood vessels begin rapidly after infection or injury but may develop at variable rates, depending on the nature and severity of the original inflammatory stimulus.

- After transient vasoconstriction (lasting only for seconds), arteriolar *vasodilation* occurs, resulting in locally increased blood flow and engorgement of the down-stream capillary beds (see Fig. 2–2). This vascular expansion is the cause of the redness (*erythema*) and warmth characteristically seen in acute inflammation.
- As the microvasculature becomes more permeable, protein-rich fluid moves into the extravascular tissues. This causes the red blood cells to become more concentrated, thereby increasing blood viscosity and

slowing the circulation. These changes are reflected microscopically by numerous dilated small vessels packed with erythrocytes and slowly flowing blood, a process called *stasis.*

- As stasis develops, leukocytes (principally neutrophils) begin to accumulate along the vascular endothelial surface, a process called *margination.* This is the first step in the journey of the leukocytes through the vascular wall into the interstitial tissue (described later).

Increased Vascular Permeability. In the early phase of inflammation, arteriolar vasodilation and increased volume of blood flow lead to a rise in intravascular hydrostatic pressure, resulting in movement of fluid from capillaries into the tissues (Fig. 2–3). This fluid, called a *transudate,* is essentially an ultrafiltrate of blood plasma and contains little protein. However, transudation is soon eclipsed by increasing vascular permeability that allows the movement of protein-rich fluid and even cells (called an *exudate*) into the interstitium. The loss of protein-rich fluid into the perivascular space reduces the intravascular osmotic pressure and increases the osmotic pressure of the interstitial fluid. The net result is outflow of water and ions into the extravascular tissues. Fluid accumulation in extravascular spaces is called *edema;* the fluid may be a transudate or exudate. Whereas exudates are typical of inflammation, transudates accumulate in various noninflammatory conditions, which are mentioned in Figure 2–3 and described in more detail in Chapter 4.

Several mechanisms may contribute to increased vascular permeability in acute inflammatory reactions.

- *Endothelial cell contraction leading to intercellular gaps in postcapillary venules* is the most common cause of increased vascular permeability. It is a reversible process elicited by histamine, bradykinin, leukotrienes, and many other chemical mediators. Endothelial cell contraction occurs rapidly after binding of mediators to specific receptors, is usually short-lived (15–30 minutes), and is called the *immediate transient response.* A slower and more prolonged retraction of endothelial cells, resulting from changes in the cytoskeleton, may be induced by cytokines such as tumor necrosis factor (TNF) and interleukin-1 (IL-1). This reaction may take 4 to 6 hours to develop after the initial trigger and persist for 24 hours or more.
- *Endothelial injury* results in vascular leakage by causing endothelial cell necrosis and detachment. Direct injury to endothelial cells is usually seen after severe injuries (e.g., burns and some infections). In

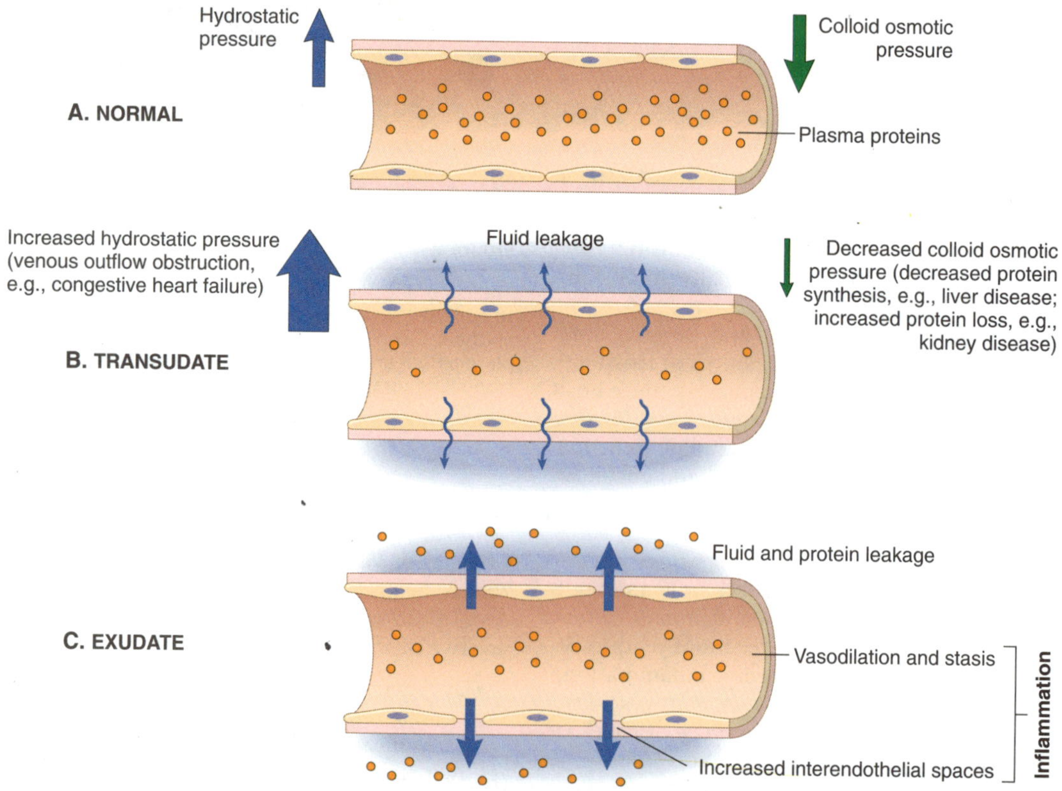

Figure 2–3

Formation of transudates and exudates. **A,** Normal hydrostatic pressure (*blue arrows*) is about 32 mm Hg at the arterial end of a capillary bed and 12 mm Hg at the venous end; the mean colloid osmotic pressure of tissues is approximately 25 mm Hg (*green arrows*), which is equal to the mean capillary pressure. Therefore, the net flow of fluid across the vascular bed is almost nil. **B,** A transudate is formed when fluid leaks out because of increased hydrostatic pressure or decreased osmotic pressure. **C,** An exudate is formed in inflammation because vascular permeability increases as a result of increased interendothelial spaces.

most cases leakage begins immediately after the injury and persists for several hours (or days) until the damaged vessels are thrombosed or repaired. Therefore, this reaction is known as the *immediate sustained response*. Venules, capillaries, and arterioles can all be affected, depending on the site of the injury. Direct injury to endothelial cells may also induce a *delayed prolonged leakage* that begins after a delay of 2 to 12 hours, lasts for several hours or even days, and involves venules and capillaries. Examples include mild to moderate thermal injury, certain bacterial toxins, and x- or ultraviolet irradiation (i.e., the sunburn that appears the evening after a day in the sun).

- *Leukocyte-mediated endothelial injury* may occur as a consequence of leukocyte accumulation along the vessel wall. As discussed later, activated leukocytes release many toxic mediators that may cause endothelial injury or detachment.
- *Increased transcytosis* of proteins via an intracellular vesicular pathway augments venular permeability, especially after exposure to certain mediators such as vascular endothelial growth factor (VEGF). Transcytosis occurs via channels formed by fusion of intracellular vesicles.
- *Leakage from new blood vessels.* As described in Chapter 3, tissue repair involves new blood vessel formation (*angiogenesis*). These vessel sprouts remain leaky until proliferating endothelial cells mature sufficiently to form intercellular junctions. New endothelial cells also have increased expression of receptors for vasoactive mediators, and some of the factors that induce angiogenesis (e.g., VEGF) directly induce increased vascular permeability via transcytosis.

Although these mechanisms are separable, all of them may participate in the response to a particular stimulus. For example, in a thermal burn, leakage results from chemically mediated endothelial contraction as well as from direct injury and leukocyte-mediated endothelial damage.

Responses of Lymphatic Vessels. Much of the emphasis in the discussion of inflammation is on the reactions of blood vessels, but lymphatics also participate in the response. As is well known, the small amount of interstitial fluid formed normally is removed by lymphatic drainage. In inflammation, lymph flow is increased and helps drain edema fluid from the extravascular space. Because the junctions of lymphatics are loose, lymphatic fluid eventually equilibrates with extravascular fluid. In addition to fluid, leukocytes and cell debris may also find their way into lymph. In severe inflammatory reactions, especially to microbes, the lymphatics may transport the offending agent. The lymphatics may become secondarily inflamed (*lymphangitis*), as may the draining lymph nodes (*lymphadenitis*). Inflamed lymph nodes are often enlarged, because of hyperplasia of the lymphoid follicles and increased numbers of lymphocytes and phagocytic cells lining the sinuses of the lymph nodes. This constellation of pathologic changes is termed reactive, or inflammatory, lymphadenitis (Chapter 12). For clinicians, the presence of red streaks near a skin wound is a telltale sign of an infection in the wound. This streaking follows the course of the lymphatic channels and is diagnostic of lymphangitis; it may be accompanied by painful enlargement of the draining lymph nodes, indicating lymphadenitis.

SUMMARY

Vascular Reactions in Acute Inflammation

- *Vasodilation* is induced by chemical mediators such as histamine (described later), and is the cause of erythema and stasis of blood flow.
- *Increased vascular permeability* is induced by histamine, kinins and other mediators that produce gaps between endothelial cells, by direct or leukocyte-induced endothelial injury, and by increased passage of fluids through the endothelium; increased vascular permeability allows plasma proteins and leukocytes to enter sites of infection or tissue damage; fluid leak through blood vessels results in edema.

Cellular Events: Leukocyte Recruitment and Activation

As mentioned above, an important function of the inflammatory response is to deliver leukocytes to the site of injury and to activate them. Leukocytes ingest offending agents, kill bacteria and other microbes, and eliminate necrotic tissue and foreign substances. A price that is paid for the defensive potency of leukocytes is that, once activated, they may induce tissue damage and prolong inflammation, since the leukocyte products that destroy microbes can also injure normal host tissues. Therefore, key to the normal function of leukocytes in host defense is to ensure that they are recruited and activated only when needed (i.e., in response to foreign invaders and dead tissues).

Leukocyte Recruitment

The sequence of events in the recruitment of leukocytes from the vascular lumen to the extravascular space consists of (1) margination, adhesion to endothelium, and rolling along the vessel wall; (2) firm adhesion to the endothelium; (3) transmigration between endothelial cells; and (4) migration in interstitial tissues toward a chemotactic stimulus (Fig. 2–4). Rolling, adhesion, and transmigration are mediated by the binding of complementary adhesion molecules on leukocytes and endothelial surfaces (see below). Chemical mediators—chemoattractants and certain cytokines—affect these processes by modulating the surface expression or avidity of the adhesion molecules and by stimulating directional movement of the leukocytes.

Margination and Rolling. As blood flows from capillaries into postcapillary venules, circulating cells are swept by laminar flow against the vessel wall. In addition, the smaller red cells tend to move faster than the larger white cells. As a result, leukocytes are pushed

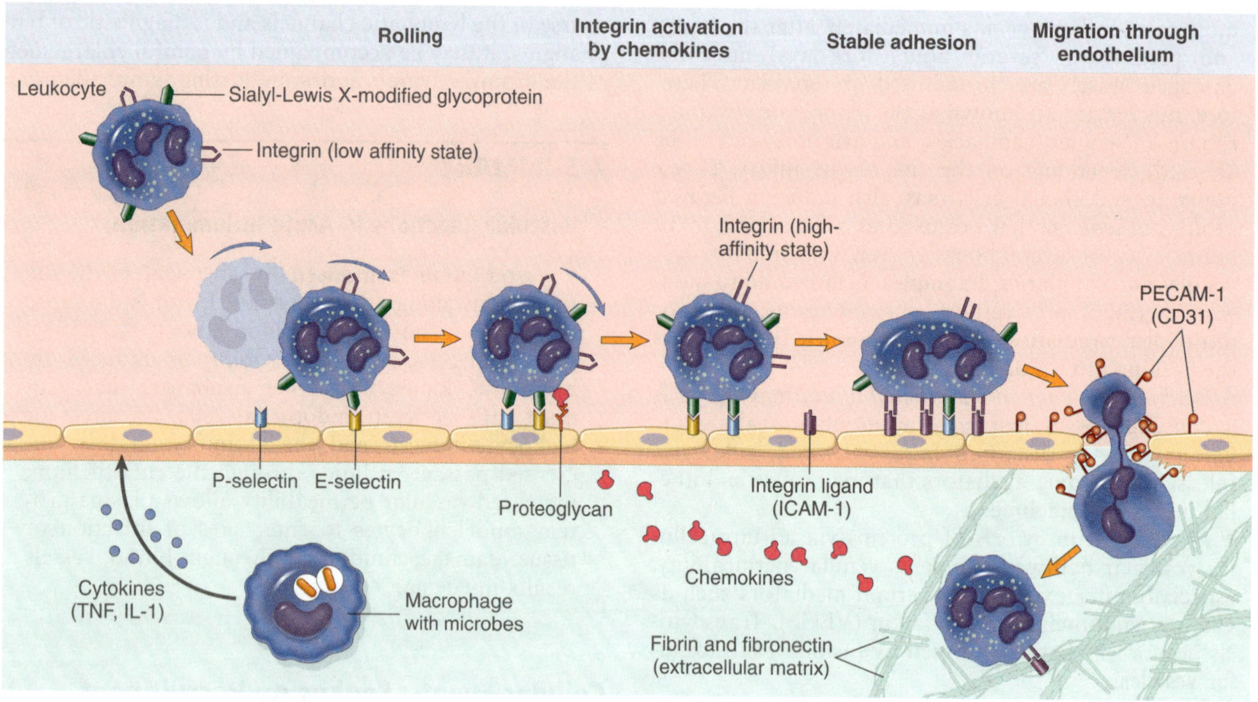

Figure 2–4

The complex process of leukocyte migration through blood vessels, shown here for neutrophils. The leukocytes first roll, then become activated and adhere to endothelium, then transmigrate across the endothelium, pierce the basement membrane, and migrate toward chemoattractants emanating from the source of injury. Different molecules play predominant roles in different steps of this process – selectins in rolling; chemokines (usually displayed bound to proteoglycans) in activating the neutrophils to increase avidity of integrins; integrins in firm adhesion; and CD31 (PECAM-1) in transmigration. ICAM-1, intercellular adhesion molecule 1; IL-1, interleukin 1; PECAM-1, platelet endothelial cell adhesion molecule 1; TNF, tumor necrosis factor.

out of the central axial column and thus have a better opportunity to interact with lining endothelial cells, especially as stasis sets in. This process of leukocyte accumulation at the periphery of vessels is called *margination.* Subsequently, leukocytes tumble on the endothelial surface, transiently sticking along the way, a process called *rolling.*

The weak and transient adhesions involved in rolling are mediated by the *selectin* family of adhesion molecules (Table 2–1). Selectins are receptors expressed on leukocytes and endothelium that contain an extracellular domain that binds sugars (hence the *lectin* part of the name). The three members of this family are E-selectin (also called CD62E), expressed on endothelial cells; P-selectin (CD62P), present on endothelium and platelets; and L-selectin (CD62L), on the surface of most leukocytes. Selectins bind sialylated oligosaccharides (e.g., sialyl–Lewis X on leukocytes) that are attached to mucin-like glycoproteins on various cells. The endothelial selectins are typically expressed at low levels or are not present at all on normal cells. They are upregulated after stimulation by specific mediators. Therefore, binding of leukocytes is largely restricted to endothelium at sites of infection or tissue injury (where the mediators are produced). For example, in nonactivated endothelial cells, P-selectin is found primarily in intracellular Weibel-Palade bodies; however, within minutes of exposure to mediators such as histamine or thrombin, P-selectin is distributed to the cell surface, where it can facilitate leukocyte binding. Similarly, E-selectin, which is not expressed on normal endothelium, is induced after stimulation by inflammatory mediators such as IL-1 and TNF.

Adhesion and Transmigration. The next step in the reaction of leukocytes is firm *adhesion* to endothelial surfaces. This adhesion is mediated by *integrins* expressed on leukocyte cell surfaces interacting with their ligands on endothelial cells (see Fig. 2–4 and Table 2–1). Integrins are transmembrane heterodimeric glycoproteins (composed of different α and β chains) that also function as cell receptors for extracellular matrix (Chapter 3). Integrins are normally expressed on leukocyte plasma membranes in a low-affinity form and do not adhere to their appropriate ligands until the leukocytes are activated by chemokines. Chemokines are chemoattractant cytokines that are secreted by many cells at sites of inflammation and are displayed bound to proteoglycans on the endothelial surface. (Cytokines are described later.) When the adherent leukocytes encounter the displayed chemokines, the cells are activated, and their integrins undergo conformational changes and cluster together, thus converting to a high-affinity form. At the same time, other cytokines, notably TNF and IL-1 (also secreted at sites of infection and injury), activate endothelial cells to increase their expression of ligands for integrins. These ligands include ICAM-1 (intercellular adhesion molecule 1), which binds to the integrins LFA-1 (CD11a/CD18) and Mac-1 (CD11b/CD18), and VCAM-1 (vascular cell adhesion

Table 2–1 Endothelial and Leukocyte Adhesion Molecules

Endothelial Molecule	Leukocyte Molecule	Major Role
P-selectin	Sialyl–Lewis X–modified proteins	Rolling (neutrophils, monocytes, lymphocytes)
E-selectin	Sialyl–Lewis X-modified proteins	Rolling and adhesion (neutrophils, monocytes, T lymphocytes)
GlyCam-1, CD34	L-selectin	Rolling (neutrophils, monocytes)*
ICAM-1 (immunoglobulin family)	CD11/CD18 integrins (LFA-1, Mac-1)	Adhesion, arrest, transmigration (neutrophils, monocytes, lymphocytes)
VCAM-1 (immunoglobulin family)	VLA-4 integrin	Adhesion (eosinophils, monocytes, lymphocytes)
CD31	CD31	Transmigration (all leukocytes)

*L-selectin–CD34 interactions are also involved in the "homing" of circulating lymphocytes to the high endotheilial venules in lymph nodes.
ICAM-1, Intercellular adhesion molecule 1; LFA-1, leukocyte function-associated antigen 1; VCAM-1, vascular cell adhesion molecule 1; VLA-4, very late antigen 4.

molecule 1), which binds to the integrin VLA-4 (see Table 2–1). The net result of cytokine-stimulated increased integrin affinity and increased expression of integrin ligands is stable attachment of leukocytes to endothelial cells at sites of inflammation.

After being arrested on the endothelial surface, leukocytes *migrate* through the vessel wall primarily by squeezing between cells at intercellular junctions (although intracellular movement through endothelial cell cytoplasm has also been described). This movement of leukocytes, called *diapedesis,* occurs mainly in the venules of the systemic vasculature; it has also been noted in capillaries in the pulmonary circulation. Migration of leukocytes is driven by chemokines produced in extravascular tissues, which stimulate movement of the leukocytes toward their chemical gradient. In addition, PECAM-1 (platelet endothelial cell adhesion molecule 1, also called CD31), a cellular adhesion molecule expressed on leukocytes and endothelial cells, mediates the binding events needed for leukocytes to traverse the endothelium. After passing through the endothelium, leukocytes cross vascular basement membranes by focally degrading them with secreted collagenases.

Chemotaxis. After extravasating from the blood, leukocytes migrate toward sites of infection or injury along a chemical gradient by a process called *chemotaxis.* Both exogenous and endogenous substances can be chemotactic for leukocytes, including (1) bacterial products, particularly peptides with *N*-formylmethionine termini; (2) cytokines, especially those of the *chemokine* family; (3) components of the complement system, particularly C5a; and (4) products of the lipoxygenase pathway of arachidonic acid (AA) metabolism, particularly leukotriene B_4 (LTB_4). These mediators, which are described in more detail later, are produced in response to infections and tissue damage and during immunologic reactions. Leukocyte infiltration in all these situations results from the actions of various combinations of mediators.

Chemotactic molecules bind to specific cell surface receptors, which are members of the seven-transmembrane G-protein coupled receptor family. Binding of the chemoattractants results in G-protein–mediated signal transduction events, some of which lead to increased cytosolic calcium, which triggers the assembly of cytoskeletal contractile elements necessary for movement. Leukocytes move by extending *pseudopods* that anchor to the ECM and then pull the cell in the direction of the extension. Thus, at the pseudopod's leading edge, actin monomers are polymerized into long filaments; at the same time, actin filaments elsewhere in the cell are disassembled to allow flow in the direction of the extending pseudopod. The direction of such movement is specified by a higher density of receptor–chemotactic ligand interactions at the leading edge of the cell.

The type of emigrating leukocyte varies with the age of the inflammatory response and with the type of stimulus. In most forms of acute inflammation, *neutrophils predominate in the inflammatory infiltrate during the first 6 to 24 hours and are replaced by monocytes in 24 to 48 hours* (Fig. 2–5). Several features of leukocytes account for this sequence: neutrophils are more numerous in the blood, they respond more rapidly to chemokines, and they may attach more firmly to the adhesion molecules that are rapidly induced on endothelial cells, such as P- and E-selectins. In addition, after entering tissues, neutrophils are short-lived—they die by apoptosis and disappear within 24 to 48 hours—while monocytes survive longer. There are exceptions to this pattern of cellular exudation, however. In certain infections (e.g., those caused by *Pseudomonas* organisms) the cellular infiltrate is dominated by continuously recruited neutrophils for several days; in viral infections lymphocytes may be the first cells to arrive; and in some hypersensitivity reactions eosinophilic granulocytes may be the main cell type.

SUMMARY

Leukocyte Recruitment to Sites of Inflammation

- Leukocytes are recruited from the blood into the extravascular tissue where infectious pathogens or damaged tissues may be located, migrate to the site of infection or tissue injury, and are activated to perform their functions.

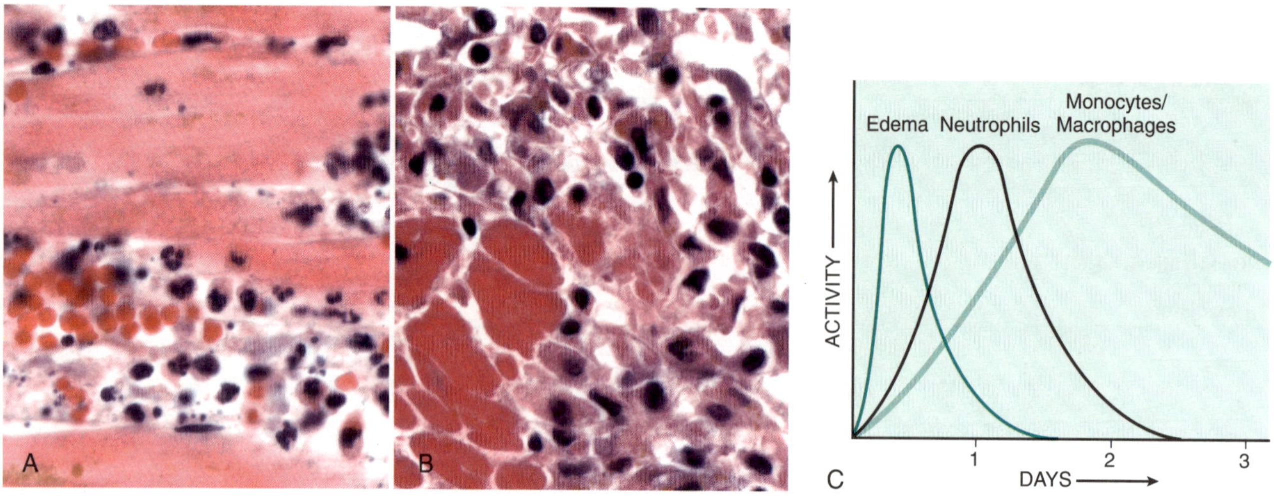

Figure 2–5

Nature of leukocyte infiltrates in inflammatory reactions. The photomicrographs show an inflammatory reaction in the myocardium after ischemic necrosis (infarction). **A,** Early (neutrophilic) infiltrates and congested blood vessels. **B,** Later (mononuclear) cellular infiltrates. **C,** The kinetics of edema and cellular infiltration are approximations. For sake of simplicity, edema is shown as an acute transient response, although secondary waves of delayed edema and neutrophil infiltration can also occur.

- Leukocyte recruitment is a multi-step process consisting of loose attachment to and rolling on endothelium (mediated by selectins); firm attachment to endothelium (mediated by integrins); and migration through inter-endothelial spaces.
- Various cytokines promote expression of selectins and integrin ligands on endothelium (TNF, IL-1), increase the avidity of integrins for their ligands (chemokines), and promote directional migration of leukocytes (also chemokines); many of these cytokines are produced by tissue macrophages and other cells responding to the pathogens or damaged tissues.
- Neutrophils predominate in the early inflammatory infiltrate and are later replaced by macrophages.

Leukocyte Activation

Once leukocytes have been recruited to the site of infection or tissue necrosis, they must be activated to perform their functions. Stimuli for activation include microbes, products of necrotic cells, and several mediators that are described later. Leukocytes express on their surface different kinds of receptors that sense the presence of microbes. These include Toll-like receptors (TLRs, named for their homology to *Drosophila* Toll protein), which recognize endotoxin (LPS) and many other bacterial and viral products; seven-transmembrane G-protein–coupled receptors, which recognize certain bacterial peptides and mediators produced in response to microbes; and other receptor families (Fig. 2–6). Engagement of these receptors by microbial products or by various mediators of inflammation induces a number of responses in leukocytes that are part of their normal defensive functions and are grouped under the generic term *leukocyte activation* (see Fig. 2–6). Leukocyte activation results in many enhanced functions:

- Phagocytosis of particles, an early step in the elimination of harmful substances.
- Production of substances that destroy phagocytosed microbes and remove dead tissues; these leukocyte products include lysosomal enzymes and reactive oxygen and nitrogen species.
- Production of mediators that amplify the inflammatory reaction, including arachidonic acid metabolites and cytokines.

Phagocytosis. Phagocytosis consists of three distinct but interrelated steps (Fig. 2–7): (1) recognition and attachment of the particle to the ingesting leukocyte; (2) engulfment, with subsequent formation of a phagocytic vacuole; and (3) killing and degradation of the ingested material.

Leukocytes bind and ingest most microorganisms and dead cells via specific surface receptors, which recognize either components of the microbes and dead cells, or host proteins, called *opsonins,* that coat microbes and target them for phagocytosis (a process called *opsonization*). The most important opsonins are antibodies of the immunoglobulin G (IgG) class that bind to microbial surface antigens, breakdown products of the complement protein C3 (described below), and plasma carbohydrate-binding lectins called *collectins,* which bind to microbial cell-wall sugar groups. These opsonins either are present in the blood ready to coat microbes or are produced in response to the microbes. Leukocytes express receptors for opsonins that facilitate rapid phagocytosis of the coated microbes. These receptors include the Fc receptor for IgG (called FcγRI), complement receptors 1 and 3 (CR1 and 3) for complement fragments, and C1q for the collectins.

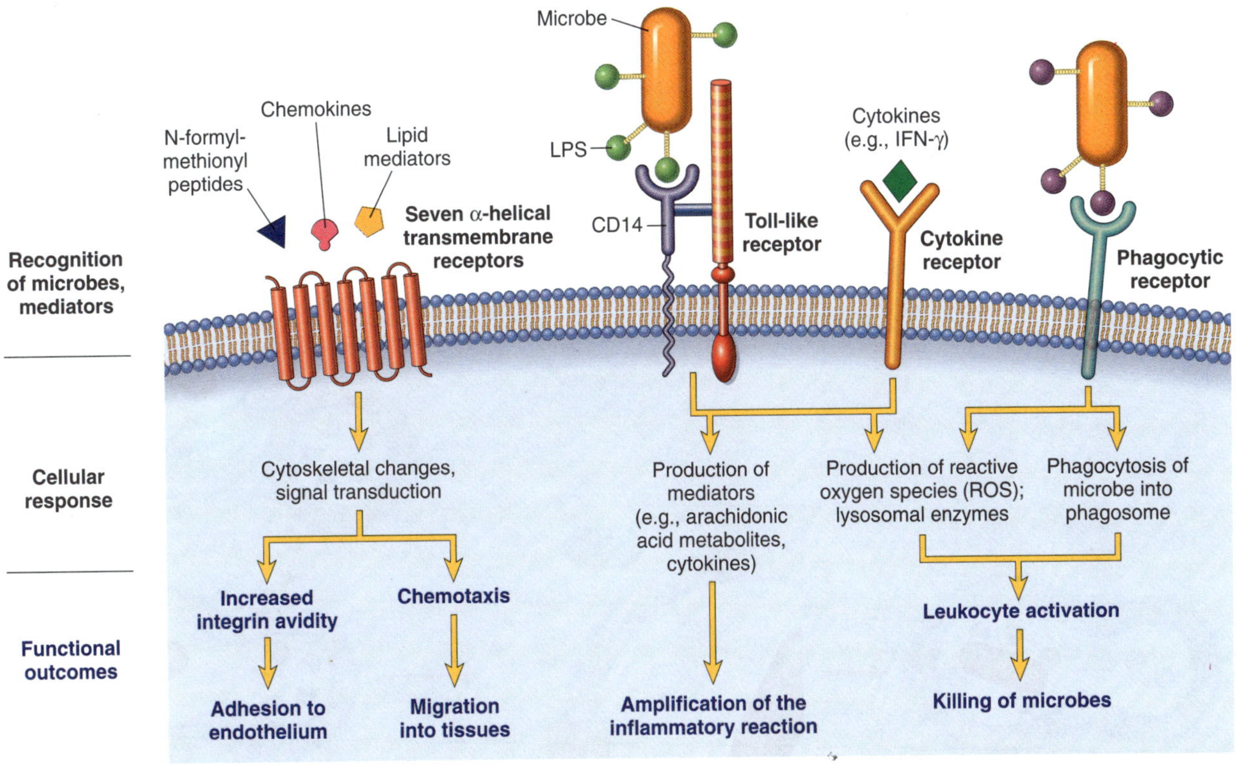

Figure 2–6

Leukocyte activation. Different classes of cell surface receptors of leukocytes recognize different stimuli. The receptors initiate responses that mediate the functions of the leukocytes. Only some receptors are depicted (see text for details). LPS first binds to a circulating LPS-binding protein (not shown). IFN-γ, interferon γ; LPS, lipopolysaccharide.

Binding of opsonized particles triggers *engulfment;* in addition, IgG binding to FcR and binding of complement products to C3 receptors induces cellular activation that enhances degradation of ingested microbes. In engulfment, pseudopods are extended around the object, eventually forming a phagocytic vacuole. The membrane of the vacuole then fuses with the membrane of a lysosomal granule, resulting in discharge of the granule's contents into the *phagolysosome.*

Killing and Degradation of Microbes. The culmination of the phagocytosis of microbes is killing and degradation of the ingested particles. The key steps in this reaction are the production of microbicidal substances within lysosomes and fusion of the lysosomes with phagosomes, thus selectively exposing the ingested particles to the destructive mechanisms of the leukocytes. The most important microbicidal substances are reactive oxygen species (ROS; see Fig. 2–7) and lysosomal enzymes. Phagocytosis stimulates an *oxidative burst* characterized by a sudden increase in oxygen consumption, glycogen catabolism (glycogenolysis), increased glucose oxidation, and production of ROS. The generation of the oxygen metabolites is due to rapid activation of a leukocyte NADPH oxidase, called the *phagocyte oxidase,* which oxidizes NADPH (reduced nicotinamide adenine dinucleotide phosphate) and, in the process, converts oxygen to superoxide ion ($O_2^{\bullet}$). Superoxide is then converted by spontaneous dismutation into hydrogen peroxide ($O_2^{\bullet} + 2H^+ \rightarrow H_2O_2$). These ROS act as free radicals and destroy microbes; the mechanisms of action of free radicals were described in Chapter 1. The quantities of H_2O_2 produced are generally insufficient to kill most bacteria (although superoxide and hydroxyl radical formation may be sufficient to do so). However, the lysosomes of neutrophils (called *azurophilic granules*) contain the enzyme myeloperoxidase (MPO), and in the presence of a halide such as Cl^-, MPO converts H_2O_2 to $HOCl^{\bullet}$ (hypochlorous radical). $HOCl^{\bullet}$ is a powerful oxidant and antimicrobial agent (NaOCl is the active ingredient in chlorine bleach) that kills bacteria by halogenation, or by protein and lipid peroxidation. Fortunately, the phagocyte oxidase is active only after its cytosolic subunit translocates to the membrane of the phagolysosome; thus, the reactive end products are generated mainly within the vesicles, and the phagocyte itself is not damaged. After the oxygen burst, H_2O_2 is eventually broken down to water and O_2 by the actions of catalase, and the other ROS are also degraded (Chapter 1). Reactive nitrogen species, particularly NO, act in the same way as ROS.

The dead microorganisms are then degraded by the action of lysosomal acid hydrolases. Perhaps the most important lysosomal enzyme involved in bacterial killing is elastase.

It is important to note that in addition to ROS and enzymes, several other constituents of leukocyte granules are capable of killing infectious pathogens. These include *bactericidal permeability-increasing protein* (causing phospholipase activation and membrane phospholipid

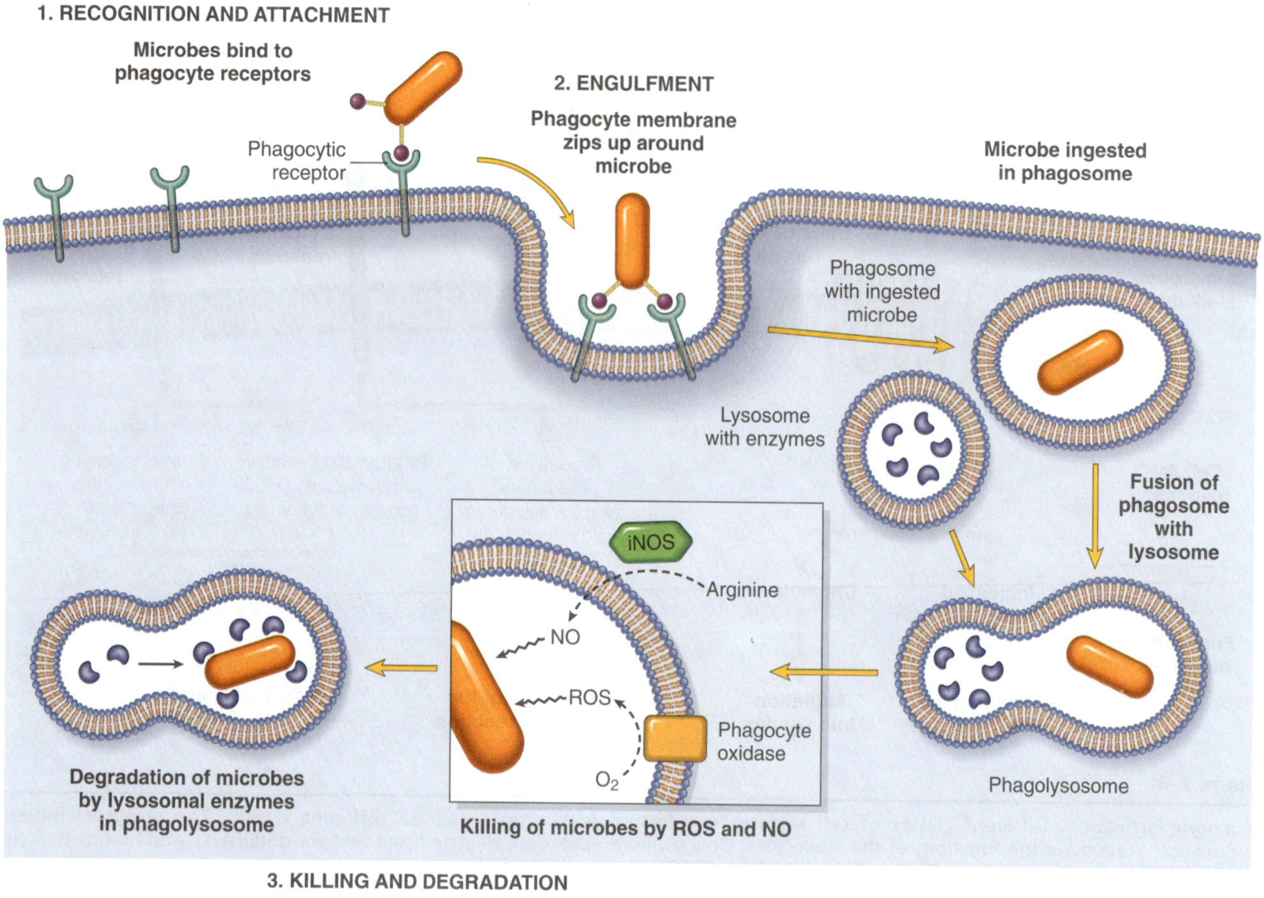

Figure 2–7

Phagocytosis of a particle (e.g., a bacterium) involves (1) attachment and binding of the particle to receptors on the leukocyte surface, (2) engulfment and fusion of the phagocytic vacuole with granules (lysosomes), and (3) destruction of the ingested particle. iNOS, Inducible nitric oxide synthase; NO, nitric oxide; ROS, reactive oxygen species.

degradation), *lysozyme* (causing degradation of bacterial coat oligosaccharides), *major basic protein* (an important eosinophil granule constituent that is cytotoxic for parasites), and *defensins* (peptides that kill microbes by creating holes in their membranes).

Leukocyte-Induced Tissue Injury

Leukocytes are important causes of injury to normal cells and tissues under several circumstances:

- As part of a normal defense reaction against infectious microbes, when "bystander" tissues are injured. In some infections that are difficult to eradicate, such as tuberculosis and certain viral diseases, the host response contributes more to the pathology than does the microbe itself.
- As a normal attempt to clear damaged and dead tissues (e.g., after a myocardial infarction). Inflammation may prolong and exacerbate the injurious consequences of the infarction, especially upon reperfusion (Chapter 1).
- When the inflammatory response is inappropriately directed against host tissues, as in certain autoimmune diseases, or when the host reacts excessively against non-toxic environmental substances, such as allergic diseases that induce asthma (discussed in Chapter 5).

In all these situations, the mechanisms by which leukocytes damage normal tissues are the same as the mechanisms involved in antimicrobial defense, because once the leukocytes are activated, their effector mechanisms do not distinguish between offender and host. During activation and phagocytosis, leukocytes may release toxic products not only within the phagolysosome but also into the extracellular space. The most important of these substances are *lysosomal enzymes,* present in the granules, and *reactive oxygen and nitrogen species.* In fact, if unchecked or inappropriately directed against host tissues, leukocytes themselves become offenders. Leukocyte-dependent tissue injury underlies many acute and chronic human diseases (Table 2–2), as will become evident in the discussion of specific disorders throughout this book.

The contents of lysosomal granules are secreted by leukocytes into the extracellular milieu by several mechanisms.

- If the phagocytic vacuole remains transiently open to the outside before complete closure of the phagolysosome (*regurgitation during feeding*).
- If cells encounter materials that cannot be easily ingested, such as immune complexes deposited on immovable flat surfaces (e.g., glomerular basement membrane), the attempt to phagocytose these sub-

stances (*frustrated phagocytosis*) triggers strong leukocyte activation, and lysosomal enzymes are released into the surrounding tissue or lumen.

- Following phagocytosis of potentially injurious substances, such as urate crystals, which damage the membrane of the phagolysosome.

Activated leukocytes, especially macrophages, also secrete many *cytokines,* which stimulate further inflammation and have important systemic effects, to be discussed later.

SUMMARY

Leukocyte Effector Mechanisms

- Leukocytes can eliminate microbes and dead cells by phagocytosis, followed by their destruction in phagolysosomes.
- Destruction is caused by free radicals (ROS, NO) generated in activated leukocytes and lysosomal enzymes.
- Enzymes and ROS may be released into the extracellular environment.
- The mechanisms that function to eliminate microbes and dead cells (the physiologic role of inflammation) are also capable of damaging normal tissues (the pathologic consequences of inflammation).

Table 2–2 Clinical Examples of Leukocyte-Induced Injury: Inflammatory Disorders*

Disorders	Cells and Molecules Involved in Injury
Acute	
Acute respiratory distress syndrome	Neutrophils
Acute transplant rejection	Lymphocytes; antibodies and complement
Asthma	Eosinophils; IgE antibodies
Glomerulonephritis	Antibodies and complement; neutrophils, monocytes
Septic shock	Cytokines
Vasculitis	Antibodies and complement; neutrophils
Chronic	
Arthritis	Lymphocytes, macrophages; antibodies
Asthma	Eosinophils, other leukocytes; IgE antibodies
Atherosclerosis	Macrophages; lymphocytes?
Chronic transplant rejection	Lymphocytes; cytokines
Pulmonary fibrosis	Macrophages; fibroblasts

*Listed are selected examples of diseases in which the host inflammatory response and accompanying tissue injury play a significant role in the disease. These disorders and their pathogenesis are discussed in much more detail in subsequent chapters.

Defects in Leukocyte Function

Since leukocytes play a central role in host defense, it is not surprising that defects in leukocyte function, both acquired and inherited, lead to increased susceptibility to infections, which may be recurrent and life-threatening (Table 2–3). The most common causes of defective inflammation are bone marrow suppression caused by tumors and chemotherapy or radiation (resulting in decreased leukocyte numbers), and metabolic diseases such as diabetes (causing abnormal leukocyte functions). These are described elsewhere in the book.

The genetic disorders, although individually rare, illustrate the importance of particular molecular pathways in the complex inflammatory response. Some of the better understood inherited diseases are the following:

- *Defects in leukocyte adhesion.* In *leukocyte adhesion deficiency type 1 (LAD-1),* defective synthesis of the CD18 β subunit of the leukocyte integrins LFA-1 and Mac-1 leads to impaired leukocyte adhesion to and migration through endothelium, and defective phagocytosis and generation of an oxidative burst. *Leukocyte adhesion deficiency type 2* (*LAD-2*) is caused by a defect in fucose metabolism resulting in the absence of sialyl–Lewis X, the oligosaccharide on leukocytes that binds to selectins on activated endothelium. Its clinical manifestations are similar to but milder than those of LAD-1.
- *Defects in microbicidal activity.* An example is *chronic granulomatous disease,* a genetic deficiency in one of the several components of the phagocyte oxidase responsible for generating ROS. In these patients, engulfment of bacteria does not result in activation of oxygen-dependent killing mechanisms. In an attempt to control these infections, the microbes are surrounded by activated macrophages, forming the "granulomas" (see later) that give the disease its distinctive pathology and its name.
- *Defects in phagolysosome formation.* One such disorder, *Chédiak-Higashi syndrome,* is an autosomal recessive disease that results from disordered intracellular trafficking of organelles, ultimately impairing the fusion of lysosomes with phagosomes. The secretion of lytic secretory granules by cytotoxic T lymphocytes is also affected, explaining the severe immunodeficiency seen in the disorder.
- Rare patients with defective host defenses have been shown to carry mutations in Toll-like receptor signaling pathways.

Outcomes of Acute Inflammation

Although the consequences of acute inflammation are modified by the nature and intensity of the injury, the site and tissue affected, and the ability of the host to mount

Table 2–3 Defects in Leukocyte Function

Disease	Defect
Acquired	
Bone marrow suppression: tumors, radiation, and chemotherapy	Production of leukocytes
Thermal injury, diabetes, malignancy, sepsis, immunodeficiencies	Chemotaxis
Hemodialysis, diabetes mellitus	Adhesion
Leukemia, anemia, sepsis, diabetes, neonates, malnutrition	Phagocytosis and microbicidal activity
Genetic	
Leukocyte adhesion deficiency 1	β chain of CD11/CD18 integrins
Leukocyte adhesion deficiency 2	Fucosyl transferase required for synthesis of sialylated oligosaccharide (receptor for selectins)
Chronic granulomatous disease	Decreased oxidative burst
X-linked	NADPH oxidase (membrane component)
Autosomal recessive	NADPH oxidase (cytoplasmic components)
Myeloperoxidase (MPO) deficiency	Absent MPO–H_2O_2 system
Chédiak-Higashi syndrome	Protein involved in organelle membrane docking and fusion

Modified from Gallin JI: Disorders of phagocytic cells. In Gallin JI, et al (eds): Inflammation: Basic Principles and Clinical Correlates, 2nd ed. New York, Raven Press, 1992, pp 860, 861.

a response, *acute inflammation* generally has one of three outcomes (Fig. 2–8):

- *Resolution.* When the injury is limited or short-lived, when there has been no or minimal tissue damage, and when the tissue is capable of replacing any irreversibly injured cells, the usual outcome is restoration to histologic and functional normalcy. *Termination of the acute inflammatory response* involves neutralization, decay or enzymatic degradation of the various chemical mediators, normalization of vascular permeability, and cessation of leukocyte emigration with subsequent death (by apoptosis) of extravasated neutrophils. Furthermore, leukocytes begin to produce mediators that inhibit inflammation and thus limit the reaction. Eventually, the combined efforts of lymphatic drainage and macrophage ingestion of necrotic debris lead to the clearance of the edema fluid, inflammatory cells, and detritus from the battlefield (Fig. 2–9).
- *Progression to chronic inflammation* may follow acute inflammation if the offending agent is not removed. In some instances, signs of chronic inflammation may be present at the onset of injury (e.g., in viral infections or immune responses to self-antigens). Depending on the extent of the initial and continuing tissue injury, as well as the capacity of the affected tissues to regrow, chronic inflammation may be followed by restoration of normal structure and function or may lead to scarring.
- *Scarring* or *fibrosis* (Chapter 3) results after substantial tissue destruction or when inflammation occurs in tissues that do not regenerate. In addition, extensive fibrinous exudates (due to increased vascular permeability) may not be completely absorbed and are *organized* by ingrowth of connective tissue, with resultant fibrosis. *Abscesses* may form in the setting of extensive neutrophilic infiltrates (see later) or in certain bacterial or fungal infections (these organisms are then said to be *pyogenic,* or "pus forming"). Because of the underlying tissue destruction (including damage to the ECM), the *usual outcome of abscess formation is scarring.*

SUMMARY

Sequence of Events in Acute Inflammation

- The vascular changes in acute inflammation are characterized by increased blood flow secondary to arteriolar and capillary bed dilation (erythema and warmth).
- Increased vascular permeability, either through widened interendothelial cell junctions of the venules or by direct endothelial cell injury, results in an exudate of protein-rich extravascular fluid (tissue edema).
- The leukocytes, initially predominantly neutrophils, adhere to the endothelium via adhesion molecules, then leave the microvasculature and migrate to the site of injury under the influence of chemotactic agents.
- Phagocytosis, killing, and degradation of the offending agent follow.
- Genetic or acquired defects in leukocyte functions give rise to recurrent infections.
- The outcome of acute inflammation may be removal of the exudate with restoration of normal tissue architecture (resolution); transition to chronic inflammation; or extensive destruction of the tissue resulting in scarring.

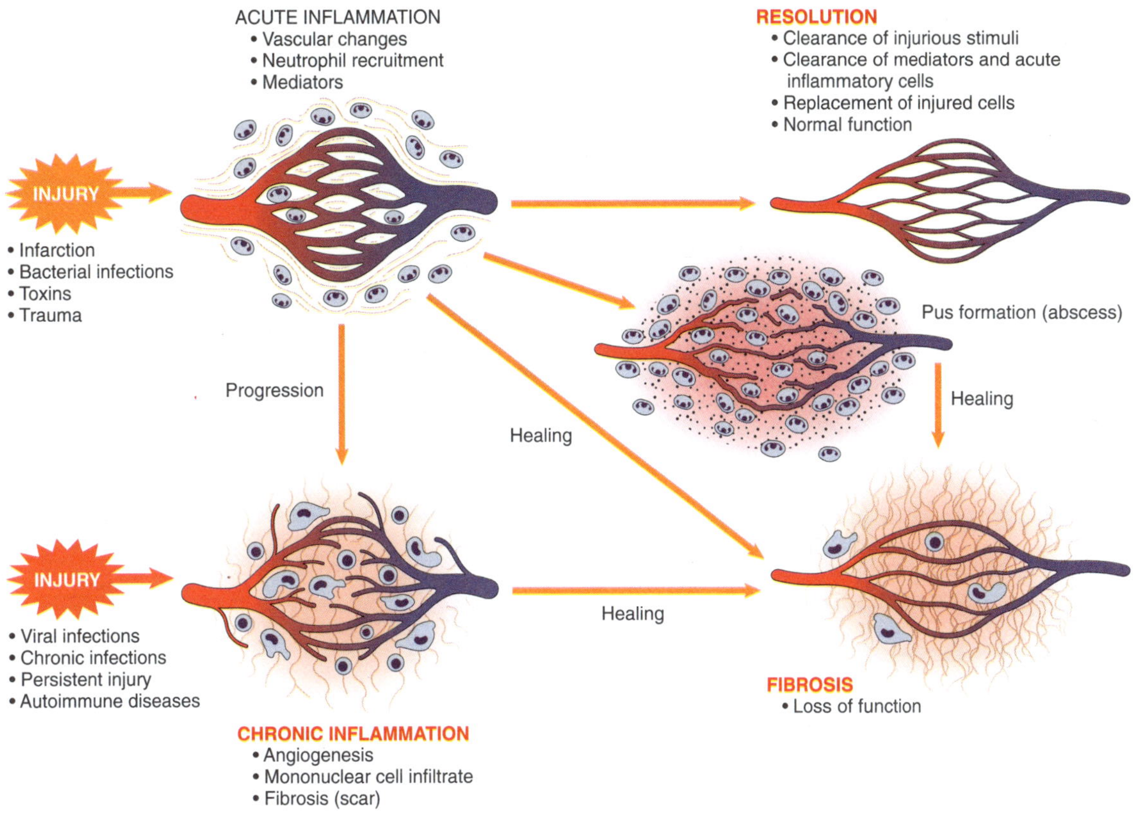

Figure 2–8

Outcomes of acute inflammation: resolution, healing by scarring (fibrosis), or chronic inflammation (see text).

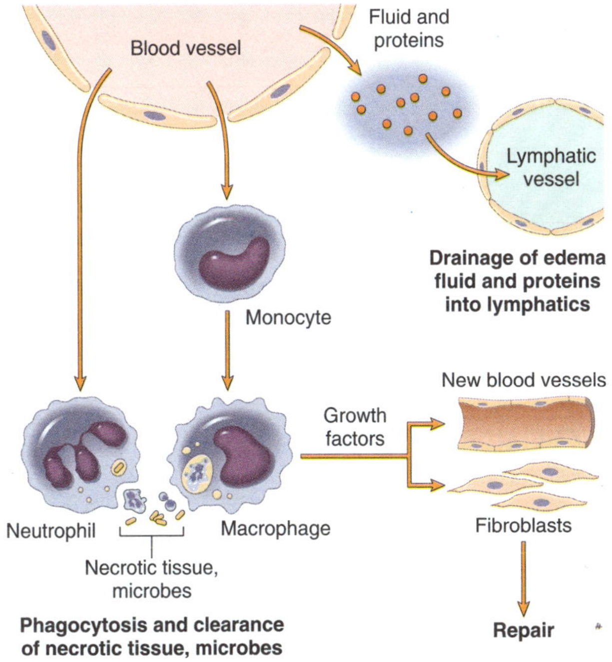

Figure 2–9

Events in the resolution of inflammation. Phagocytes clear the fluid, leukocytes and dead tissue, and fluid and proteins are removed by lymphatic drainage. (Modified from Haslett C, Henson PM: In Clark R, Henson PM [eds]: The Molecular and Cellular Biology of Wound Repair. New York, Plenum Press, 1996. With kind permission of Springer Science and Business Media.)

MORPHOLOGIC PATTERNS OF ACUTE INFLAMMATION

The vascular and cellular reactions that characterize acute inflammation are reflected in the morphologic appearance of the reaction. The severity of the inflammatory response, its specific cause, and the particular tissue involved can all modify the basic morphology of acute inflammation, producing distinctive appearances. The importance of recognizing these morphologic patterns is that they are often associated with different eliciting stimuli and clinical situations.

Morphology

Serous inflammation is characterized by the outpouring of a watery, relatively protein-poor fluid that, depending on the site of injury, derives either from the serum or from the secretions of mesothelial cells lining the peritoneal, pleural, and pericardial cavities. The skin blister resulting from a burn or viral infection is a good example of a serous effusion accumulated either within or immediately beneath the epidermis of the skin (Fig. 2–10). Fluid in a serous cavity is called an **effusion**.

Fibrinous inflammation occurs as a consequence of more severe injuries, resulting in greater vascular permeability that allows large molecules (such as fibrinogen) to pass the endothelial barrier. Histologically, the accumulated extravascular fibrin appears as an eosinophilic meshwork of threads or sometimes as an amorphous coagulum (Fig. 2–11). A fibrinous exudate is characteristic of inflammation in the lining of body cavities, such as the meninges, pericardium, and pleura. Such exudates may be degraded by fibrinolysis, and the accumulated debris may be removed by macrophages, resulting in restoration of the normal tissue structure **(resolution)**. However, failure to completely remove the fibrin results in the ingrowth of fibroblasts and blood vessels **(organization)**, leading ultimately to scarring that may have significant clinical consequences. For example, organization of a fibrinous pericardial exudate forms dense fibrous scar tissue that bridges or obliterates the pericardial space and restricts myocardial function.

Suppurative (purulent) inflammation is manifested by the presence of large amounts of purulent exudate (pus) consisting of neutrophils, necrotic cells, and edema fluid. Certain organisms (e.g., staphylococci) are more likely to induce such localized suppuration and are therefore referred to as pyogenic. **Abscesses** are focal collections of pus that may be caused by seeding of pyogenic organisms into a tissue or by secondary infections of necrotic foci. Abscesses typically have a central, largely necrotic region rimmed by a layer of preserved neutrophils (Fig. 2–12), with a surrounding zone of dilated vessels and fibroblastic proliferation indicative of early repair. As time passes the abscess may become completely walled off and eventually be replaced by connective tissue.

An **ulcer** is a local defect, or excavation, of the surface of an organ or tissue that is produced by necrosis of cells and sloughing (shedding) of inflammatory necrotic tissue (Fig. 2–13). Ulceration can occur only when tissue necrosis and resultant inflammation exist on or near a surface. It is most commonly encountered in (1) inflammatory necrosis of the mucosa of the mouth, stomach, intestines, or genitourinary tract; and (2) tissue necrosis and subcutaneous inflammation of the lower extremities in older persons who have circulatory disturbances that predispose to extensive necrosis. Ulcerations are best exemplified by peptic ulcer of the stomach or duodenum, in which acute and chronic inflammation coexist. During the acute stage there is intense polymorphonuclear infiltration and vascular dilation in the margins of the defect. With chronicity, the margins and base of the ulcer develop scarring with accumulation of lymphocytes, macrophages, and plasma cells.

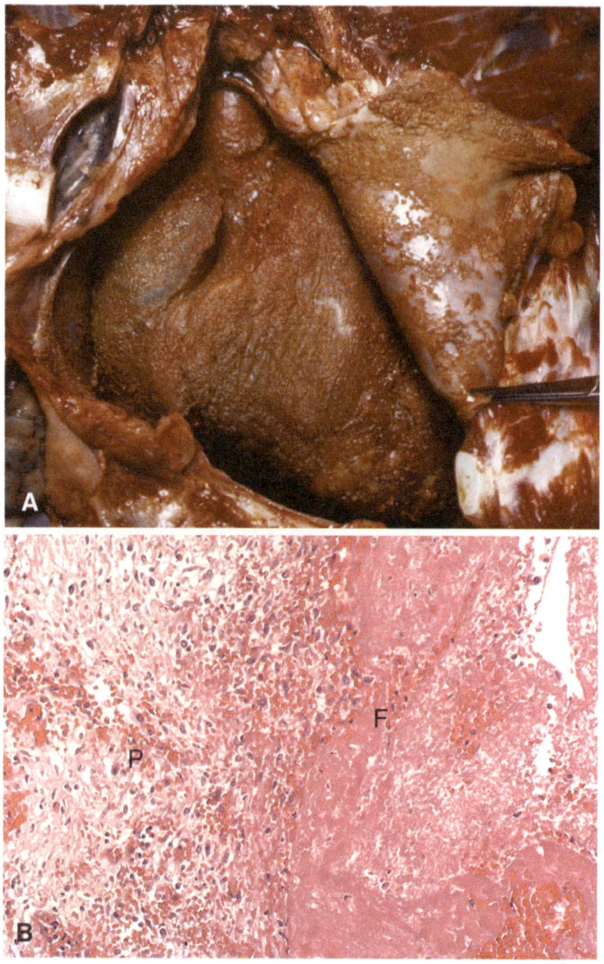

Figure 2–11

Fibrinous pericarditis. **A,** Deposits of fibrin on the pericardium. **B,** A pink meshwork of fibrin exudate (F) overlies the pericardial surface (P).

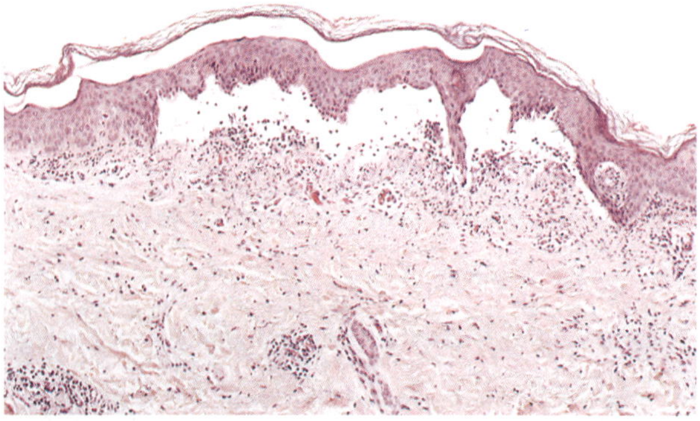

Figure 2–10

Serous inflammation. Low-power view of a cross-section of a skin blister showing the epidermis separated from the dermis by a focal collection of serous effusion.

CHEMICAL MEDIATORS OF INFLAMMATION

Having described the vascular and cellular events in acute inflammation, and the accompanying morphologic alterations, we will next describe the chemical mediators that are responsible for these events. Many mediators are known, and this knowledge has been used to design a large armamentarium of anti-inflammatory drugs, which are prominent on our pharmacy shelves. In this section, we will emphasize general properties of the mediators of inflammation and highlight only some of the more important molecules.

- *Mediators may be produced locally by cells at the site of inflammation, or they may be circulating in the*

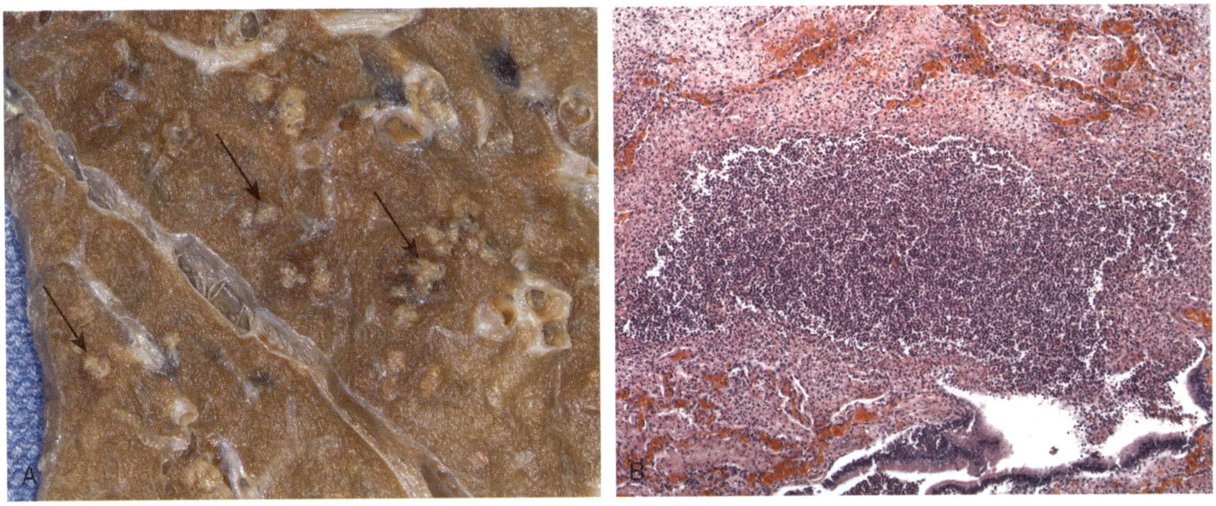

Figure 2–12

Purulent inflammation. **A,** Multiple bacterial abscesses in the lung (*arrows*) in a case of bronchopneumonia. **B,** The abscess contains neutrophils and cellular debris, and is surrounded by congested blood vessels.

plasma (typically synthesized by the liver) as inactive precursors that are activated at the site of inflammation (Fig. 2–14 and Table 2–4). Cell-derived mediators are normally sequestered in intracellular granules and are rapidly secreted upon cellular activation (e.g., histamine in mast cells) or are synthesized de novo in response to a stimulus (e.g., prostaglandins and cytokines). Plasma-protein–derived mediators (complement proteins, kinins) typically undergo proteolytic cleavage to acquire their biologic activities.

- *Most mediators induce their effects by binding to specific receptors on target cells.* Mediators may act on only one or a very few targets, or they may have widespread actions, with differing outcomes depending on which cell type they affect. Some mediators have direct enzymatic and/or toxic activities (e.g., lysosomal proteases and ROS).
- *Mediators may stimulate target cells to release secondary effector molecules.* Different mediators may have similar actions, in which case they may amplify a particular response, or they may have opposing effects, thus serving to control the response.
- *The actions of most mediators are tightly regulated.* Once activated and released from the cell, mediators quickly decay (e.g., arachidonic acid metabolites), are inactivated by enzymes (e.g., kininase inactivates bradykinin), are eliminated (e.g., antioxidants scavenge toxic oxygen metabolites), or are inhibited (complement-inhibitory proteins).

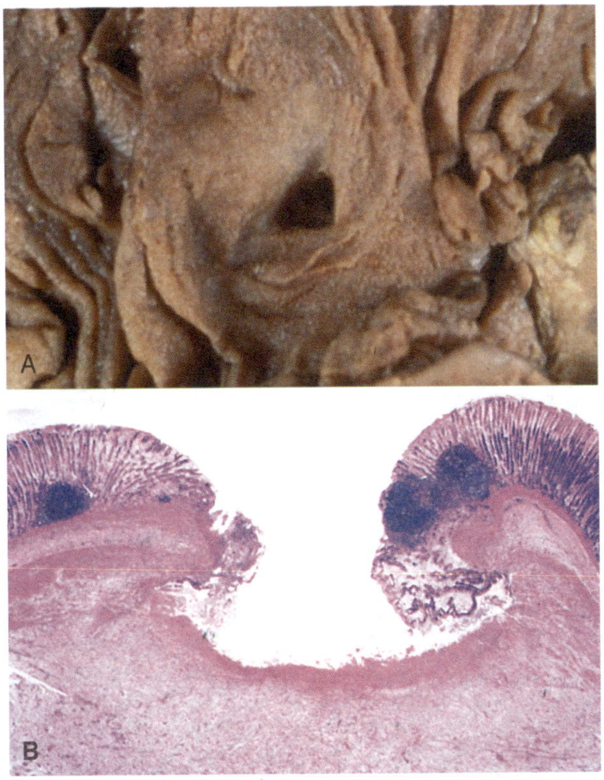

Figure 2–13

The morphology of an ulcer. **A,** A chronic duodenal ulcer. **B,** Low-power cross-section of a duodenal ulcer crater with an acute inflammatory exudate in the base.

Cell-Derived Mediators

Tissue macrophages, mast cells, and endothelial cells at the site of inflammation, as well as leukocytes that are recruited to the site from the blood, are all capable of producing different mediators of inflammation.

Vasoactive Amines. The two vasoactive amines histamine and serotonin are stored as preformed molecules in mast cells and other cells and are among the first mediators to be released in acute inflammatory reactions. *Histamine* is produced by many cell types, particularly mast cells adjacent to vessels, as well as circulating basophils and platelets. Preformed histamine is released from mast cell granules in response to a variety of stimuli: (1) physical injury such as trauma or heat; (2) immune reactions involving binding of IgE antibodies to Fc receptors on mast cells (Chapter 5); (3) C3a and C5a fragments of

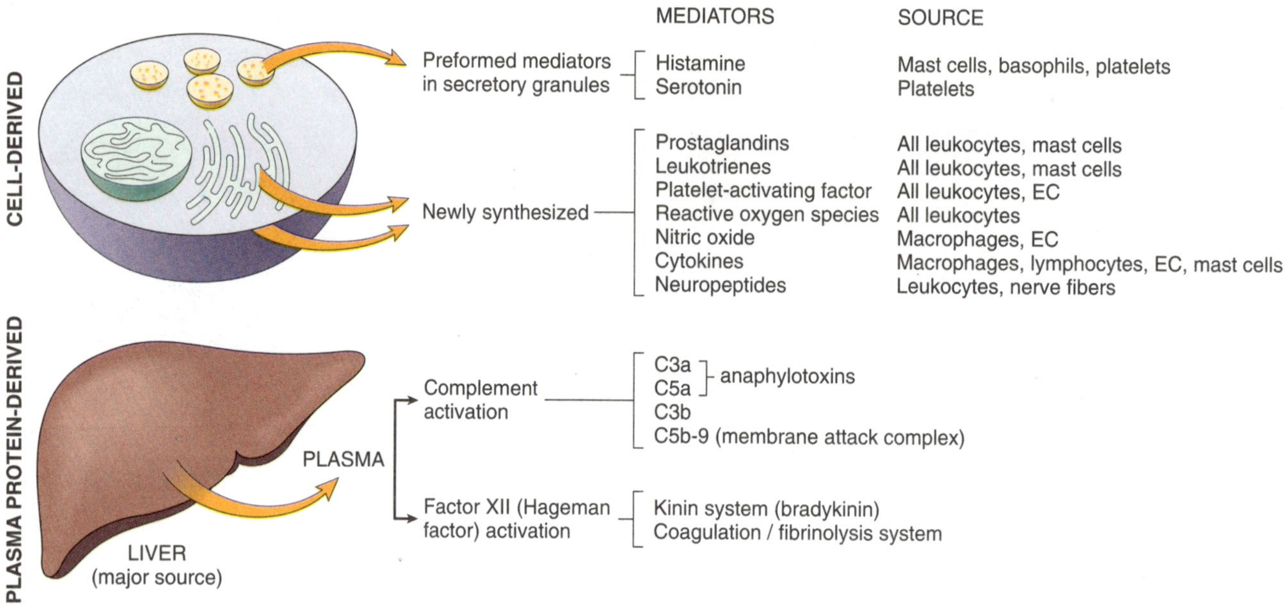

Figure 2–14

The principal chemical mediators of inflammation. EC, Endothelial cells.

complement, the so-called *anaphylatoxins* (see later); (4) leukocyte-derived histamine-releasing proteins; (5) neuropeptides (e.g., substance P); and (6) certain cytokines (e.g., IL-1 and IL-8). In humans, histamine causes arteriolar dilation and is the principal mediator of the immediate phase of increased vascular permeability, inducing venular endothelial contraction and interendothelial gaps. Soon after its release, histamine is inactivated by histaminase.

Serotonin (5-hydroxytryptamine) is also a preformed vasoactive mediator, with effects similar to those of histamine. It is found primarily within platelet dense body

Table 2–4 The Actions of the Principal Mediators of Inflammation

Mediator	Source	Principal Actions
Cell-Derived		
Histamine	Mast cells, basophils, platelets	Vasodilation, increased vascular permeability, endothelial activation
Serotonin	Platelets	Vasodilation, increased vascular permeability
Prostaglandins	Mast cells, leukocytes	Vasodilation, pain, fever
Leukotrienes	Mast cells, leukocytes	Increased vascular permeability, chemotaxis, leukocyte adhesion and activation
Platelet-activating factor	Leukocytes, endothelial cells	Vasodilation, increased vascular permeability, leukocyte adhesion, chemotaxis, degranulation, oxidative burst
Reactive oxygen species	Leukocytes	Killing of microbes, tissue damage
Nitric oxide	Endothelium, macrophages	Vascular smooth muscle relaxation; killing of microbes
Cytokines (e.g. TNF, IL-1)	Macrophages, lymphocytes, endothelial cells, mast cells	Local endothelial activation (expression of adhesion molecules), systemic acute-phase response; in severe infections, septic shock
Chemokines	Leukocytes, activated macrophages	Chemotaxis, leukocyte activation
Plasma Protein-Derived		
Complement	Plasma (produced in liver)	Leukocyte chemotaxis and activation, opsonization, vasodilation (mast cell stimulation)
Kinins	Plasma (produced in liver)	Increased vascular permeability, smooth muscle contraction, vasodilation, pain
Proteases activated during coagulation	Plasma (produced in liver)	Endothelial activation, leukocyte recruitment

IL-1, Interleukin-1; TNF, tumor necrosis factor.

granules (along with histamine, adenosine diphosphate, and calcium) and is released during platelet aggregation (Chapter 4).

Arachidonic Acid (AA) Metabolites: Prostaglandins, Leukotrienes, and Lipoxins. Products derived from the metabolism of AA affect a variety of biologic processes, including inflammation and hemostasis. AA metabolites (also called *eicosanoids*) can mediate virtually every step of inflammation (Table 2–5); their synthesis is increased at sites of inflammatory response, and agents that inhibit their synthesis also diminish inflammation. They can be thought of as short-range hormones that act locally at the site of generation and then decay spontaneously or are enzymatically destroyed. Leukocytes, mast cells, endothelial cells, and platelets are the major sources of AA metabolites in inflammation.

AA is a 20-carbon polyunsaturated fatty acid (with four double bonds) derived primarily from dietary linoleic acid and present in the body mainly in its esterified form as a component of cell membrane phospholipids. It is released from these phospholipids via cellular phospholipases that have been activated by mechanical, chemical, or physical stimuli, or by inflammatory mediators such as C5a. AA metabolism proceeds along one of two major enzymatic pathways: *Cyclooxygenase* stimulates the synthesis of *prostaglandins and thromboxanes*, and *lipoxygenase* is responsible for production of *leukotrienes* and *lipoxins* (Fig. 2–15).

- *Cyclooxygenase pathway.* Products of this pathway include prostaglandin E_2 (PGE_2), PGD_2, $PGF_2\alpha$, PGI_2 (prostacyclin), and thromboxane A_2 (TXA_2), each derived by the action of a specific enzyme on an intermediate. Some of these enzymes have a restricted tissue distribution. For example, platelets contain the enzyme thromboxane synthase, and hence TXA_2, a potent platelet-aggregating agent and vasoconstrictor, is the major PG produced in these cells. Endothelial cells, on the other hand, lack thromboxane synthase but contain prostacyclin synthase, which is responsible for the formation of PGI_2, a vasodilator and a potent inhibitor of platelet aggregation. The opposing roles of TXA_2 and PGI_2 in hemostasis are further discussed in Chapter 4. PGD_2 is the major metabolite of the cyclooxygenase pathway in mast cells; along with PGE_2 and $PGF_2\alpha$ (which are more widely distributed), it causes vasodilation and potentiates edema formation. The PGs are also involved in the pathogenesis of pain and fever in inflammation; PGE_2 augments pain sensitivity to a variety of other stimuli and interacts with cytokines to cause fever.
- *Lipoxygenase pathway.* 5-Lipoxygenase is the predominant AA-metabolizing enzyme in neutrophils. The 5-hydroperoxy derivative of AA, 5-HPETE (5-hydroperoxyeicosatetraenoic acid), is quite unstable and is either reduced to 5-HETE (5-hydroxyeicosatetraenoic acid) (which is chemotactic for neutrophils) or converted into a family of compounds collectively called *leukotrienes* (see Fig. 2–15). The first leukotriene generated from 5-HPETE is called *leukotriene A_4* (LTA_4), which in turn gives rise to LTB_4 or LTC_4. LTB_4 is produced by neutrophils and some macrophages and is a potent chemotactic agent for neutrophils. LTC_4 and its subsequent metabolites, LTD_4 and LTE_4, are produced mainly in mast cells and cause vasoconstriction, bronchospasm, and increased vascular permeability.

  Lipoxins function mainly as inhibitors of inflammation. Once leukocytes enter tissues, they gradually change their major lipoxygenase-derived AA products to lipoxins, which inhibit neutrophil chemotaxis and adhesion to endothelium, thus serving as endogenous antagonists of leukotrienes. Platelets that are activated and adherent to leukocytes are also important sources of lipoxins. Platelets alone cannot synthesize lipoxins A_4 and B_4 (LXA_4 and LXB_4), but they can form these mediators from an intermediate derived from adjacent neutrophils, by a transcellular biosynthetic pathway. By this mechanism AA products can pass from one cell to the other.

Table 2–5 Principal Inflammatory Actions of Arachidonic Acid Metabolites (Eicosanoids)

Action	Eicosanoid
Vasodilation	PGI_2 (prostacyclin), PGE_1, PGE_2, PGD_2
Vasoconstriction	Thromboxane A_2, leukotrienes C_4, D_4, E_4
Increased vascular permeability	Leukotrienes C_4, D_4, E_4
Chemotaxis, leukocyte adhesion	Leukotriene B_4

The central role of eicosanoids in inflammatory processes is emphasized by the clinical utility of agents that block eicosanoid synthesis. Aspirin and most nonsteroidal anti-inflammatory drugs (NSAIDs), such as ibuprofen, inhibit cyclooxygenase activity and thus all PG synthesis (hence their efficacy in treating pain and fever). There are two forms of the cyclooxygenase enzyme, called COX-1 and COX-2. COX-1 (but not COX-2) is expressed in the gastric mucosa, and the mucosal PGs generated by COX-1 are protective against acid-induced damage. Thus, inhibition of cyclooxygenases by aspirin and other nonsteroidal anti-inflammatory drugs (which inhibit both COX-1 and COX-2) predisposes to gastric ulceration. To preserve the anti-inflammatory effects of cyclooxygenase inhibition but prevent the harmful effects on gastric mucosa, highly selective COX-2 inhibitors are now available. However, recent clinical trials reveal that COX-2 inhibitors have their own problems. They seem to affect PGI_2 synthesis more than TXA_2 production and hence can induce a prothrombotic state. This can lead to a greater incidence of acute coronary artery disease. Glucocorticoids, which are powerful anti-inflammatory agents, act in part by inhibiting the activity of phospholipase A_2 and thus inhibiting the release of AA from membrane lipids.

Platelet-Activating Factor. Originally named for its ability to aggregate platelets and cause degranulation, platelet-activating factor (PAF) is another phospholipid-derived mediator with a broad spectrum of inflammatory effects. PAF is *acetyl glycerol ether phosphocholine;* it is gener-

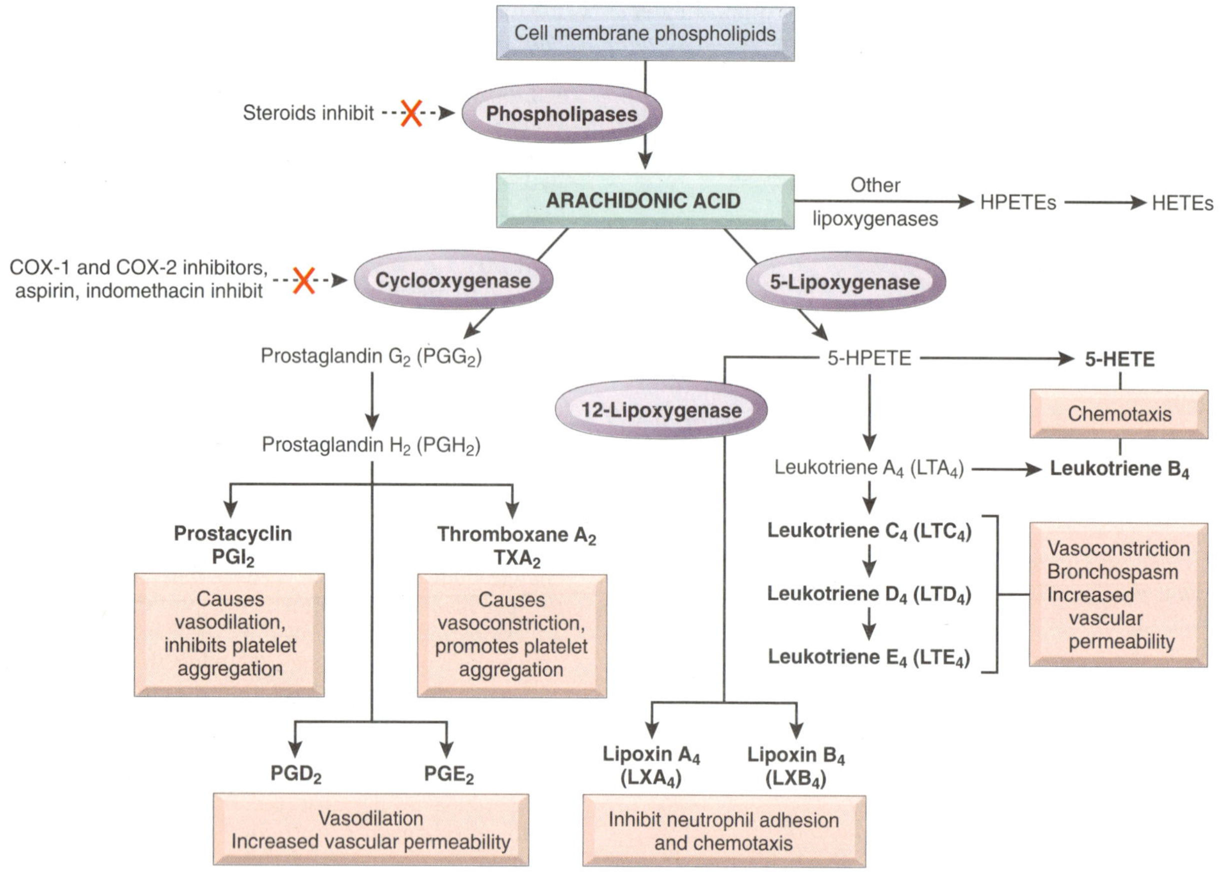

Figure 2–15

Generation of arachidonic acid metabolites and their roles in inflammation. Note the enzymatic activities whose inhibition through pharmacologic intervention blocks major pathways (denoted with a red X). COX-1, COX-2, Cyclooxygenase 1 and 2; HETE, hydroxyeicosatetraenoic acid; HPETE, hydroperoxyeicosatetraenoic acid.

ated from the membrane phospholipids of neutrophils, monocytes, basophils, endothelial cells, and platelets (and other cells) by the action of phospholipase A_2. PAF acts directly on target cells via a specific G-protein–coupled receptor. In addition to stimulating platelets, PAF causes vasoconstriction and bronchoconstriction and is 100 to 1,000 times more potent than is histamine in inducing vasodilation and increased vascular permeability. PAF can elicit most of the reactions of inflammation, including enhanced leukocyte adhesion, chemotaxis, leukocyte degranulation, and the oxidative burst; it also stimulates the synthesis of other mediators, particularly eicosanoids.

Cytokines. Cytokines are polypeptide products of many cell types that function as mediators of inflammation and immune responses (Chapter 5). Different cytokines are involved in the earliest immune and inflammatory reactions to noxious stimuli and in the later adaptive (specific) immune responses to microbes. Some cytokines stimulate bone marrow precursors to produce more leukocytes, thus replacing the ones that are consumed during inflammation and immune responses. Molecularly characterized cytokines are called *interleukins* (abbreviated IL and numbered), referring to their ability to mediate communications between leukocytes. However, many interleukins act on cells other than leukocytes, and many cytokines that do act on leukocytes are not called interleukins, for historical reasons.

The major cytokines in acute inflammation are TNF and IL-1, as well as a group of chemoattractant cytokines called *chemokines*. Other cytokines that are more important in chronic inflammation include interferon-γ (IFN-γ) and IL-12.

Tumor Necrosis Factor and Interleukin-1. TNF and IL-1 are produced by activated macrophages, as well as mast cells, endothelial cells, and some other cell types (Fig. 2–16). Their secretion is stimulated by microbial products, such as bacterial endotoxin, immune complexes, and products of T lymphocytes generated during adaptive immune responses. The principal role of these cytokines in inflammation is in *endothelial activation.* Both TNF and IL-1 stimulate the expression of adhesion molecules on endothelial cells, resulting in increased leukocyte binding and recruitment, and enhance the production of additional cytokines (notably chemokines) and eicosanoids. TNF also increases the thrombogenicity of endothelium and causes aggregation and activation of neutrophils, and IL-1 activates tissue fibroblasts, resulting in increased proliferation and production of ECM.

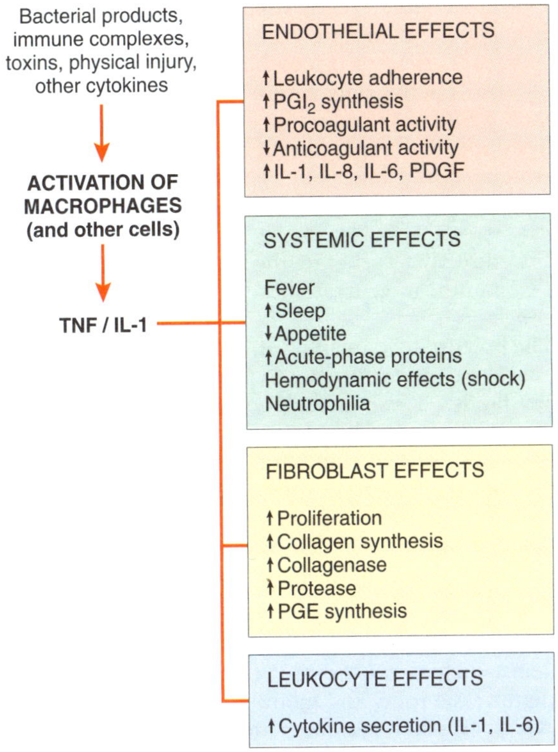

Figure 2–16

Major effects of tumor necrosis factor (TNF) and interleukin 1 (IL-1) in inflammation. PDGF, Platelet-derived growth factor; PGE, prostaglandin E; PGI, prostaglandin I.

Although TNF and IL-1 are secreted by macrophages and other cells at sites of inflammation, they may enter the circulation and act at distant sites to induce the *systemic acute-phase reaction* that is often associated with infection and inflammatory diseases. Components of this reaction include fever, lethargy, hepatic synthesis of various acute-phase proteins, metabolic wasting (*cachexia*), neutrophil release into the circulation, and release of adrenocorticotropic hormone (inducing corticosteroid synthesis and release). These systemic manifestations of inflammation are described later in the chapter.

Chemokines. The *chemokines* are a family of small (8–10 kD), structurally related proteins that act primarily as chemoattractants for different subsets of leukocytes. The two main functions of chemokines are in leukocyte recruitment in inflammation and in the normal anatomic organization of cells in lymphoid and other tissues. Combinations of chemokines that are produced transiently in response to inflammatory stimuli recruit particular cell populations (e.g., neutrophils, eosinophils, or lymphocytes) to sites of inflammation. Chemokines also activate leukocytes; one consequence of such activation, which was mentioned earlier, is increased affinity of leukocyte integrins for their ligands on endothelial cells. Some chemokines are produced constitutively in tissues and are responsible for the anatomic segregation of different cell populations in tissues (e.g., the segregation of T and B lymphocytes in different areas of lymph nodes and spleen). Many chemokines are displayed bound to proteoglycans on endothelial cells or in the ECM, providing high local concentration gradients where needed. Chemokines mediate their activities by binding to specific G-protein–coupled receptors on target cells; two of these chemokine receptors (called CXCR4 and CCR5) are important coreceptors for the binding and entry of the human immunodeficiency virus into lymphocytes (Chapter 5).

Chemokines are classified into four groups based on the arrangement of highly conserved cysteine residues. The two major groups are the CXC and CC chemokines:

- CXC chemokines have one amino acid separating the conserved cysteines and act primarily on neutrophils. IL-8 is typical of this group; it is produced by activated macrophages, endothelial cells, mast cells, and fibroblasts, mainly in response to microbial products and other cytokines such as IL-1 and TNF.
- CC chemokines have adjacent cysteine residues and include monocyte chemoattractant protein 1 (MCP-1) and macrophage inflammatory protein 1α (MIP-1α) (both chemotactic predominantly for monocytes), RANTES (regulated on activation normal T expressed and secreted) (chemotactic for memory CD4+ T cells and monocytes), and eotaxin (chemotactic for eosinophils).

Reactive Oxygen Species. ROS are synthesized via the NADPH oxidase (phagocyte oxidase) pathway and are released from neutrophils and macrophages that are activated by microbes, immune complexes, cytokines, and a variety of other inflammatory stimuli. The synthesis and regulation of these oxygen-derived free radicals were described in Chapter 1, in the context of cell injury. When the ROS are produced within lysosomes they function to destroy phagocytosed microbes and necrotic cells, much like NO. When secreted at low levels, ROS can increase chemokine, cytokine, and adhesion molecule expression, thus amplifying the cascade of inflammatory mediators. At higher levels, these mediators are responsible for tissue injury by several mechanisms, including (1) endothelial damage, with thrombosis and increased permeability; (2) protease activation and antiprotease inactivation, with a net increase in breakdown of the ECM; and (3) direct injury to other cell types (e.g., tumor cells, erythrocytes, parenchymal cells). Fortunately, various antioxidant protective mechanisms (e.g., catalase, superoxide dismutase, and glutathione) are present in tissues and blood to minimize the toxicity of the oxygen metabolites (Chapter 1).

Nitric Oxide. *NO* is a short-lived, soluble, free-radical gas produced by many cell types and capable of mediating a variety of functions (Fig. 2–17). In the central nervous system it regulates neurotransmitter release as well as blood flow. Macrophages use it as a cytotoxic metabolite for killing microbes and tumor cells. When produced by endothelial cells (where it was originally named *endothelium-derived relaxation factor*), it causes smooth muscle relaxation and vasodilation.

NO is synthesized de novo from L-arginine, molecular oxygen, and NADPH by the enzyme nitric oxide synthase (NOS). There are three isoforms of NOS, with different

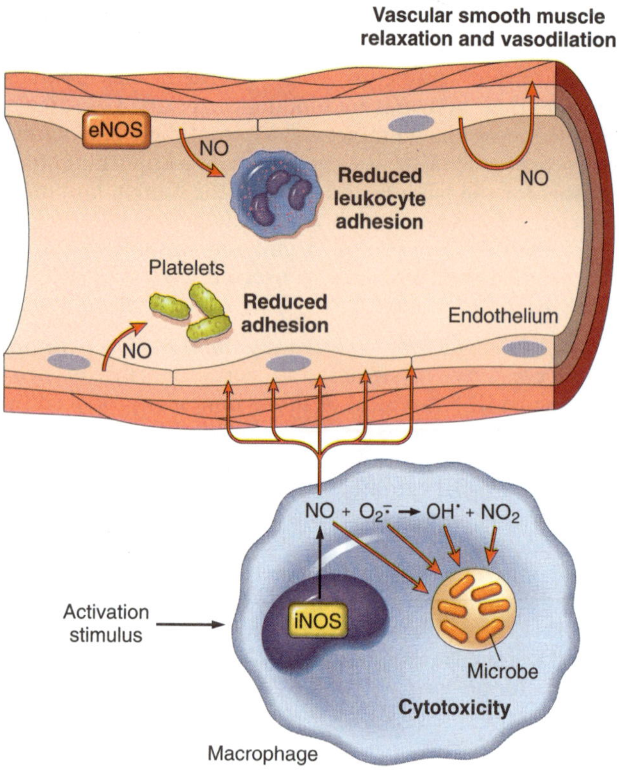

Figure 2–17

Sources and effects of nitric oxide (NO) in inflammation. NO synthesized by endothelial cells (mostly via endothelial cell [type III] NO synthase [eNOS]) and by macrophages (mostly via inducible [type II] NO synthase [iNOS]) causes vasodilation and reduces platelet and leukocyte adhesion; NO produced in phagocytes is also cytotoxic to microbes.

tissue distributions. Type I (nNOS) is a constitutively expressed neuronal NOS, which does not play a significant role in inflammation. Type II (iNOS) is an inducible enzyme present in macrophages and endothelial cells; it is induced by a number of inflammatory cytokines and mediators, most notably by IL-1, TNF, and IFN-γ, and by bacterial endotoxin, and is responsible for production of NO in inflammatory reactions. iNOS is also present in many other cell types, including hepatocytes, cardiac myocytes, and respiratory epithelium. Type III (eNOS) is a constitutively synthesized NOS found primarily (but not exclusively) within endothelium.

NO plays many roles in inflammation (see Fig. 2–17), including (1) relaxation of vascular smooth muscle (vasodilation), (2) antagonism of all stages of platelet activation (adhesion, aggregation, and degranulation), (3) reduction of leukocyte recruitment at inflammatory sites, and (4) action as a microbicidal (cytotoxic) agent (with or without superoxide radicals) in activated macrophages.

Lysosomal Enzymes of Leukocytes. The lysosomal granules of neutrophils and monocytes contain many molecules that can mediate acute inflammation. These may be released after cell death, by leakage during the formation of the phagocytic vacuole, or during futile attempts to phagocytose large, indigestible surfaces, as described earlier. The most important of these lysosomal molecules are enzymes. *Acid proteases* have acidic pH optima and are generally active only within phagolysosomes, whereas *neutral proteases,* including elastase, collagenase, and cathepsin, are active in the ECM and cause destructive, deforming tissue injury by degrading elastin, collagen, basement membrane, and other matrix proteins. Neutral proteases can also cleave the complement proteins C3 and C5 directly to generate the vasoactive mediators C3a and C5a and can generate bradykinin-like peptides from kininogen.

The potentially damaging effects of lysosomal enzymes are checked by *antiproteases* present in the serum and tissue fluids. These include α_1-antitrypsin, the major inhibitor of neutrophil elastase, and α_2-macroglobulin. Deficiencies of these inhibitors may result in sustained activation of leukocyte proteases, resulting in tissue destruction at sites of leukocyte accumulation. For instance, α_1-antitrypsin deficiency in the lung can cause a severe panacinar emphysema (Chapter 13).

Neuropeptides. Like the vasoactive amines, neuropeptides can initiate inflammatory responses; these are small proteins, such as *substance P,* that transmit pain signals, regulate vessel tone, and modulate vascular permeability. Nerve fibers that secrete neuropeptides are especially prominent in the lung and gastrointestinal tract.

SUMMARY

Major Cell-derived Mediators of Inflammation

- *Vasoactive amines*: histamine, serotonin; main effects are vasodilation and increased vascular permeability
- *Arachidonic acid metabolites*: *prostaglandins* and *leukotrienes*; several forms exist and are involved in vascular reactions, leukocyte chemotaxis, and other reactions of inflammation; antagonized by lipoxins
- *Cytokines*: proteins produced by many cell types; usually act at short range; mediate multiple effects, mainly in leukocyte recruitment and migration; principal ones in acute inflammation are TNF, IL-1, and chemokines
- *Reactive oxygen species*: role in microbial killing, tissue injury
- *Nitric oxide*: vasodilation, microbial killing
- *Lysosomal enzymes*: role in microbial killing, tissue injury

Plasma Protein-Derived Mediators

Circulating proteins of three interrelated systems—the complement, kinin, and coagulation systems—are involved in several aspects of the inflammatory reaction.

Complement. *The complement system* consists of plasma proteins that play an important role in host defense (immunity) and inflammation. Upon activation, different complement proteins coat (opsonize) particles, such as microbes, for phagocytosis and destruction, and contribute to the inflammatory response by increasing vascular permeability and leukocyte chemotaxis. Complement activation ultimately generates a porelike membrane attack complex (MAC) that punches holes in the membranes of invading microbes.

Complement components (numbered C1 to C9) are present in plasma in inactive forms, and many of them are activated by proteolysis to themselves acquire proteolytic activity, thus setting up an enzymatic cascade. The critical step in the generation of biologically active complement products is the activation of the third component, C3 (Fig. 2–18). C3 cleavage occurs (1) via the *classical pathway,* triggered by fixation of the first complement component C1 to antigen-antibody complexes; (2) through the *alternative pathway,* triggered by bacterial polysaccharides (e.g., endotoxin) and other microbial cell-wall components, and involving a distinct set of plasma proteins including *properdin* and *factors B* and *D;* and (3) by the *lectin pathway,* in which a plasma lectin binds to mannose residues on microbes and activates an early component of the classical pathway (but in the absence of antibodies). All three pathways lead to the formation of a *C3 convertase* that cleaves C3 to C3a and C3b. C3b deposits on the cell or microbial surface where complement was activated and then binds to the C3 convertase complex to form C5 convertase; this complex cleaves C5 to generate C5a and C5b and initiate the final stages of assembly of C6 to C9. There are many connections between the various circulating systems of inflammation and clotting. For instance, thrombin (generated during blood coagulation) may cleave C5, thus triggering the complement pathway. The complement-derived factors that are produced along the way affect a variety of phenomena in acute inflammation:

- *Vascular effects.* C3a and C5a increase vascular permeability and cause vasodilation by inducing mast cells to release histamine. These complement products are also called *anaphylatoxins* because their actions mimic those of mast cells, which are the main cellular effectors of the severe allergic reaction called anaphylaxis (Chapter 5). C5a also activates the lipoxygenase pathway of AA metabolism in neutrophils and macrophages, causing release of more inflammatory mediators.
- *Leukocyte activation, adhesion, and chemotaxis.* C5a activates leukocytes, increasing their adhesion to endothelium, and is a potent chemotactic agent for neutrophils, monocytes, eosinophils, and basophils.
- *Phagocytosis.* When fixed to a microbial surface, C3b and its inactive proteolytic product iC3b act as opsonins, augmenting phagocytosis by neutrophils and macrophages, which express receptors for these complement products.

The activation of complement is tightly controlled by cell-associated and circulating *regulatory proteins.* The presence of these inhibitors in host cell membranes protects normal cells from inappropriate damage during

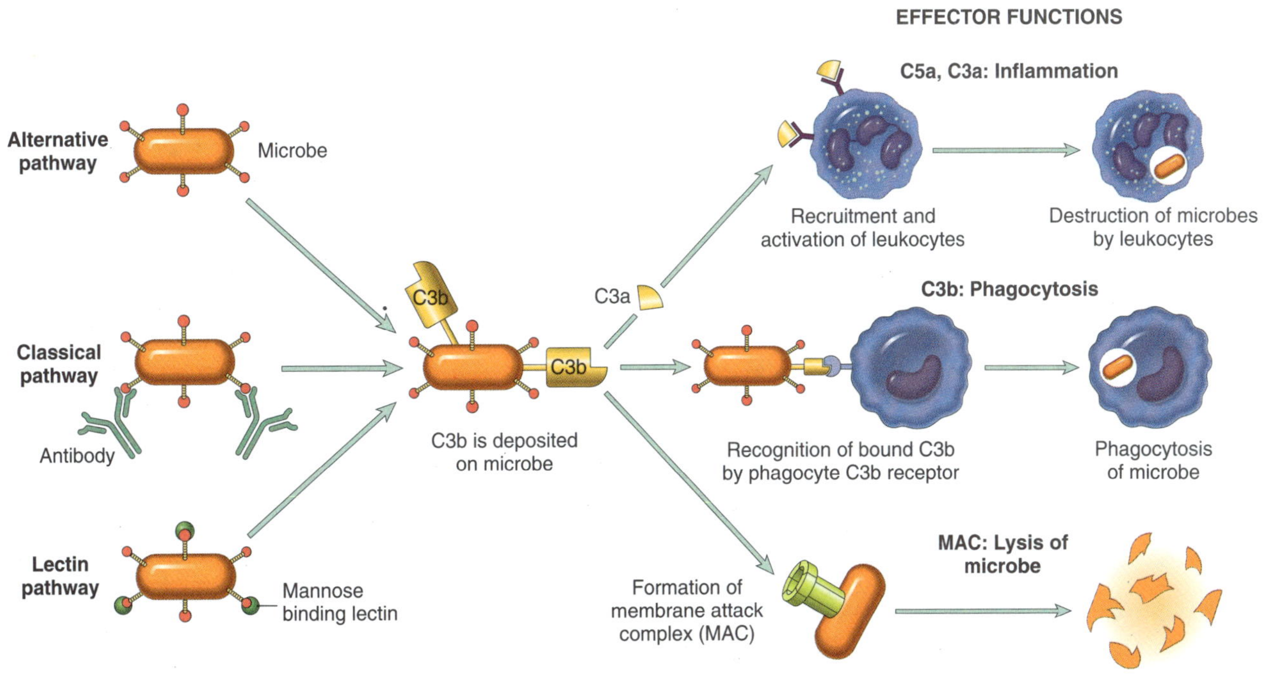

Figure 2–18

The activation and functions of the complement system. Activation of complement by different pathways leads to cleavage of C3. The functions of the complement system are mediated by breakdown products of C3 and other complement proteins, and by the membrane attack complex (MAC).

protective reactions against microbes. However, inappropriate or excessive complement activation (e.g., in antibody-mediated diseases) can overwhelm the regulatory systems, and this is why complement activation is responsible for serious tissue injury in a variety of immunologic disorders (Chapter 5).

Coagulation and Kinin Systems. A central event in the generation of several circulating mediators of inflammation is activation of *Hageman factor* (Fig. 2–19). Activated Hageman factor (factor XIIa) initiates four systems involved in the inflammatory response: (1) the kinin system, producing vasoactive kinins; (2) the clotting system, inducing the activation of thrombin, fibrinopeptides, and factor X, all with inflammatory properties; (3) the fibrinolytic system, producing plasmin and inactivating thrombin; and (4) the complement system, producing the anaphylatoxins C3a and C5a. Hageman factor (also known as *factor XII* of the *intrinsic coagulation cascade*) is a protein synthesized by the liver that circulates in an inactive form until it encounters collagen, basement membrane, or activated platelets (e.g., at a site of endothelial injury). With the assistance of a high-molecular-weight kininogen (HMWK) cofactor, factor XII then undergoes a conformational change (becoming factor XIIa), exposing an active serine center that can cleave several protein substrates of the kinin and coagulation systems.

In the *clotting system* (Chapter 4), the factor XIIa-driven proteolytic cascade leads to activation of *thrombin,* which then cleaves circulating soluble fibrinogen to generate an insoluble *fibrin clot. Factor Xa,* an intermediate in the clotting cascade, causes increased vascular permeability and leukocyte emigration. Thrombin participates in inflammation by binding to protease-activated receptors that are expressed on platelets, endothelial cells, and many other cell types. Binding of thrombin to these receptors on endothelial cells leads to their activation and enhanced leukocyte adhesion. In addition, thrombin generates *fibrinopeptides* (during fibrinogen cleavage) that increase vascular permeability and are chemotactic for leukocytes.

While activated Hageman factor is inducing clotting, it is concurrently activating the *fibrinolytic system.* This mechanism exists to limit clotting by cleaving fibrin, thereby solubilizing the fibrin clot. Without fibrinolysis and other regulatory mechanisms, initiation of the coagulation cascade, even by trivial injury, would culminate in continuous and irrevocable clotting of the entire vasculature (Chapter 4). *Plasminogen activator* (released from endothelium, leukocytes, and other tissues) and *kallikrein* cleave *plasminogen,* a plasma protein bound up

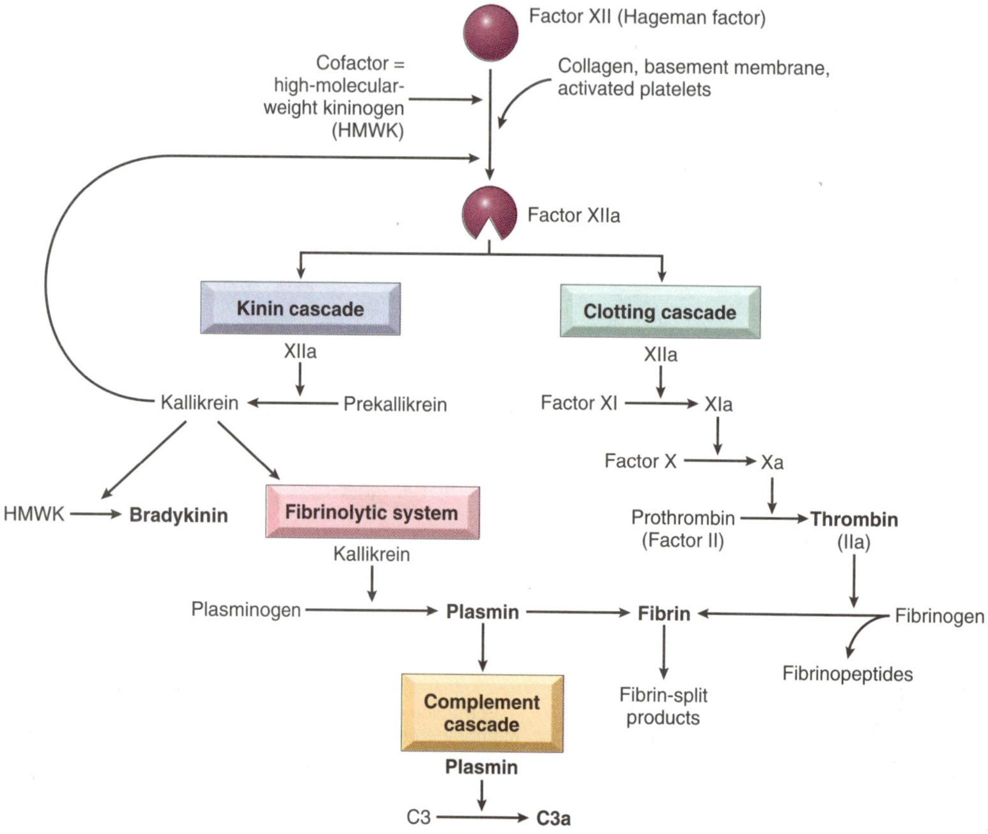

Figure 2–19

Interrelationships among the four plasma mediator systems triggered by activation of factor XII (Hageman factor). See text for details.

in the evolving fibrin clot. The resulting product, *plasmin*, is a multifunctional protease that cleaves fibrin and is therefore important in lysing clots. However, fibrinolysis also participates in multiple steps in the vascular phenomena of inflammation. For example, fibrin degradation products increase vascular permeability, while plasmin cleaves the C3 complement protein, resulting in production of C3a and vasodilation and increased vascular permeability. Plasmin can also activate Hageman factor, thereby amplifying the entire set of responses.

Kinin system activation leads ultimately to the formation of *bradykinin* from its circulating precursor, HMWK (see Fig. 2–19). Like histamine, bradykinin causes increased vascular permeability, arteriolar dilation, and bronchial smooth muscle contraction. It also causes pain when injected into the skin. The actions of bradykinin are short-lived because it is rapidly degraded by kininases present in plasma and tissues. It is important to note that *kallikrein,* an intermediate in the kinin cascade with chemotactic activity, is also a potent activator of Hageman factor and is thus another link between the kinin and clotting systems.

SUMMARY

Plasma Protein-Derived Mediators of Inflammation

- *Complement proteins:* Activation of the complement system by microbes or antibodies leads to the generation of multiple breakdown products, which are responsible for leukocyte chemotaxis, opsonization and phagocytosis of microbes and other particles, and cell killing
- *Coagulation proteins:* Activated factor XII triggers the clotting, kinin and complement cascades, and activates the fibrinolytic system
- *Kinins:* Produced by proteolytic cleavage of precursors; mediate vascular reaction, pain

It is evident from the preceding discussion that many molecules are involved in different aspects of the inflammatory reaction, and these molecules often interact with, amplify, and antagonize one another. From this almost bewildering potpourri of chemical mediators, it is possible to identify the major contributors to various components of acute inflammation (Table 2–6). Despite our quite sophisticated understanding of these mediators, we still do not fully understand why some stimuli elicit inflammatory reactions. For instance, we have mentioned from the outset that necrotic cells are a powerful stimulus for inflammation, but how dead cells trigger this reaction is not yet established. Hypoxia itself induces an inflammatory response, in part by stimulating the production of mediators, such as VEGF, that increase vascular permeability.

Table 2–6 Role of Mediators in Different Reactions of Inflammation

Vasodilation	Prostaglandins Nitric oxide Histamine
Increased vascular permeability	Histamine and serotonin C3a and C5a (by liberating vasoactive amines from mast cells, other cells) Bradykinin Leukotrienes C_4, D_4, E_4 PAF Substance P
Leukocyte recruitment and activation	TNF, IL-1 Chemokines C3a, C5a Leukotriene B_4 (Bacterial products, e.g., *N*-formyl methyl peptides)
Fever	IL-1, TNF Prostaglandins
Pain	Prostaglandins Bradykinin Neuropeptides
Tissue damage	Lysosomal enzymes of leukocytes Reactive oxygen species Nitric oxide

IL-1, Interleukin-1; PAF, platelet-activating factor; TNF, tumor necrosis factor.

CHRONIC INFLAMMATION

Chronic inflammation is inflammation of prolonged duration (weeks to months to years) in which *active inflammation, tissue injury, and healing proceed simultaneously.* In contrast to acute inflammation, which is distinguished by vascular changes, edema, and a predominantly neutrophilic infiltrate, chronic inflammation is characterized by (Fig. 2–20; also see Fig. 2–8)

- *Infiltration with mononuclear cells,* including macrophages, lymphocytes, and plasma cells
- *Tissue destruction,* largely induced by the products of the inflammatory cells
- *Repair, involving new vessel proliferation (angiogenesis) and fibrosis*

As indicated in Figure 2–8, acute inflammation may progress to chronic inflammation. This transition occurs when the acute response cannot be resolved, either because of the persistence of the injurious agent or because of interference with the normal process of healing. For example, a peptic ulcer of the duodenum initially shows acute inflammation followed by the beginning stages of resolution. However, recurrent bouts of duodenal epithelial injury interrupt this process and result in a lesion characterized by both acute and chronic inflammation (Chapter 15). Alternatively, some forms of injury (e.g., viral infections) engender a response that involves chronic inflammation from the onset.

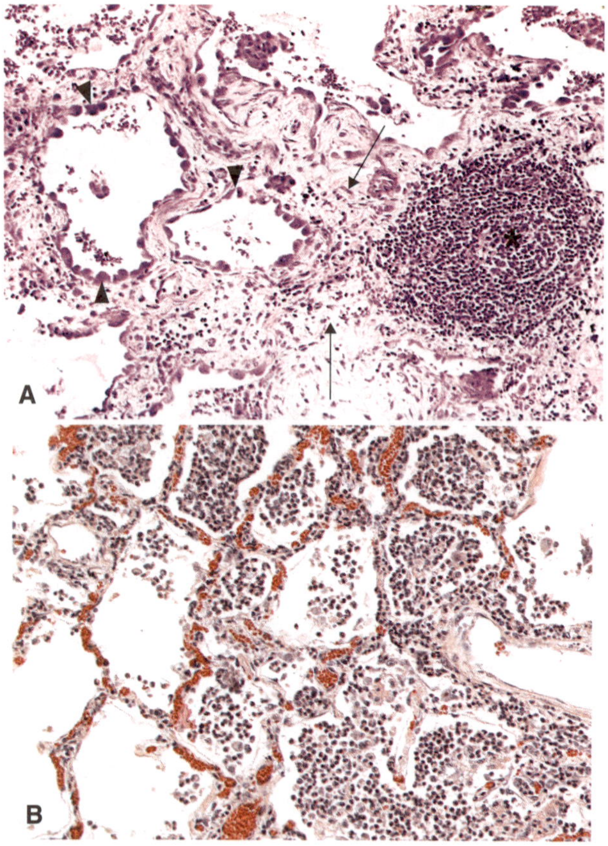

Figure 2–20

A, Chronic inflammation in the lung, showing the characteristic histologic features: collection of chronic inflammatory cells (*asterisk*), destruction of parenchyma (normal alveoli are replaced by spaces lined by cuboidal epithelium, *arrowheads*), and replacement by connective tissue (fibrosis, *arrows*). **B,** By contrast, in acute inflammation of the lung (acute bronchopneumonia), neutrophils fill the alveolar spaces and blood vessels are congested.

Chronic inflammation arises in the following settings:

- *Persistent infections* by microbes that are difficult to eradicate. These include mycobacteria, *Treponema pallidum* (causative organism of syphilis), and certain viruses and fungi, all of which tend to establish persistent infections and elicit a T lymphocyte–mediated immune response called *delayed-type hypersensitivity* (Chapter 5). In fact, most viral infections elicit chronic inflammatory reactions dominated by lymphocytes and macrophages.
- *Immune-mediated inflammatory diseases (hypersensitivity diseases)*. Diseases that are caused by excessive and inappropriate activation of the immune system are increasingly recognized as being important health problems (Chapter 5). Under certain conditions, immune reactions develop against the individual's own tissues, leading to *autoimmune diseases*. In these diseases, autoantigens evoke a self-perpetuating immune reaction that results in chronic tissue damage and inflammation. Inflammation secondary to autoimmunity plays an important role in several common and debilitating chronic diseases, such as rheumatoid arthritis and inflammatory bowel disease. Immune responses against common environmental substances are the cause of *allergic diseases,* such as bronchial asthma. Immune-mediated diseases may show morphologic patterns of mixed acute and chronic inflammation because they are characterized by repeated bouts of inflammation. Because the eliciting antigens cannot be eliminated, these disorders tend to be chronic and intractable.
- *Prolonged exposure to potentially toxic agents.* Examples include nondegradable exogenous materials such as inhaled particulate silica, which can induce a chronic inflammatory response in the lungs (*silicosis,* Chapter 13), and endogenous agents such as chronically elevated plasma lipid components, which may contribute to *atherosclerosis* (Chapter 10).

Chronic Inflammatory Cells and Mediators

A fundamental feature of chronic inflammation is its persistence, and this results from complex interactions between the cells that are recruited to the site of inflammation and are activated at this site. Understanding the pathogenesis of chronic inflammatory reactions requires an appreciation of these cells and their biologic responses and functions.

Macrophages. *Macrophages,* the dominant cells of chronic inflammation, are tissue cells derived from circulating blood *monocytes* after their emigration from the bloodstream. Macrophages are normally diffusely scattered in most connective tissues, and are also found in organs such as the liver (where they are called *Kupffer cells*), spleen and lymph nodes (called *sinus histiocytes*), central nervous system (*microglial cells*), and lungs (*alveolar macrophages*). Together these cells comprise the so-called *mononuclear phagocyte system,* also known by the older name of reticulo-endothelial system. In all tissues, macrophages act as filters for particulate matter, microbes, and senescent cells, as well as acting as sentinels to alert the specific components of the adaptive immune system (T and B lymphocytes) to injurious stimuli (Chapter 5).

The half-life of circulating monocytes is about 1 day; under the influence of adhesion molecules and chemotactic factors, they begin to migrate to a site of injury within 24 to 48 hours after the onset of acute inflammation, as described above. When monocytes reach the extravascular tissue, they undergo transformation into larger macrophages, which have longer half-lives and a greater capacity for phagocytosis than do blood monocytes. Macrophages may also become *activated,* resulting in increased cell size, increased content of lysosomal enzymes, more active metabolism, and greater ability to kill ingested organisms. By light microscopy, activated macrophages appear large, flat, and pink (in H&E stains); this appearance may be similar to that of squamous epithelial cells, and cells with such an appearance are therefore sometimes called *epithelioid cells.* Activation signals include bacterial *endotoxin* and other microbial products, cytokines secreted by sensitized T lymphocytes (in particular the cytokine IFN-γ) , various mediators produced during acute inflammation, and ECM proteins such as fibronectin. After activation, macrophages secrete a wide variety of biologically active products that, if unchecked, can result in the tissue injury and fibrosis that are characteristic of chronic inflammation (Fig. 2–21). These products include

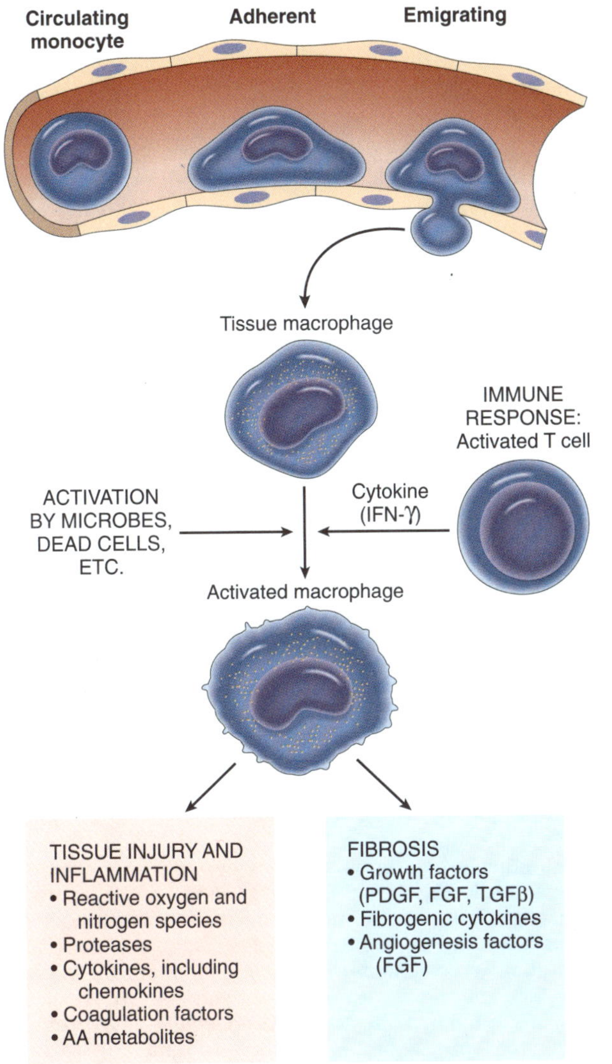

Figure 2–21

The roles of activated macrophages in chronic inflammation. Macrophages are activated by nonimmunologic stimuli such as bacterial endotoxin or by cytokines from immune-activated T cells, particularly interferon-γ (IFN-γ). The products made by activated macrophages that cause tissue injury and fibrosis are indicated. AA, Arachidonic acid; PDGF, platelet-derived growth factor; FGF, fibroblast growth factor; TGF-β, transforming growth factor β.

- *Acid and neutral proteases.* Recall that the latter were also implicated as mediators of tissue damage in acute inflammation. Other enzymes, such as *plasminogen activator,* greatly amplify the generation of proinflammatory substances.
- *ROS and NO*
- *AA metabolites* (*eicosanoids*)
- *Cytokines* such as IL-1 and TNF, as well as a variety of *growth factors* that influence the proliferation of smooth muscle cells and fibroblasts and the production of ECM

After the initiating stimulus is eliminated and the inflammatory reaction abates, macrophages eventually die or wander off into lymphatics. In chronic inflammatory sites, however, macrophage accumulation persists, and macrophages can proliferate. Steady release of lymphocyte-derived chemokines and other cytokines is an important mechanism by which macrophages are recruited to or immobilized in inflammatory sites. IFN-γ can also induce macrophages to fuse into large, multinucleated cells called *giant cells.*

Lymphocytes, Plasma Cells, Eosinophils, and Mast Cells. Lymphocytes are mobilized to the setting of any specific immune stimulus (i.e., infections) as well as non-immune-mediated inflammation (e.g., due to infarction or tissue trauma). Both T and B lymphocytes migrate into inflammatory sites using some of the same adhesion molecule pairs and chemokines that recruit other leukocytes. Lymphocytes and macrophages interact in a bidirectional way, and these interactions play an important role in chronic inflammation (Fig. 2–22). Macrophages display antigens to T cells, express membrane molecules (called *costimulators*), and produce cytokines (notably IL-12) that stimulate T-cell responses (Chapter 5). Activated T lymphocytes, in turn, produce cytokines, and one of these, IFN-γ, is a powerful activator of macrophages, promoting more antigen presentation and cytokine secretion. The result is a cycle of cellular reactions that fuel and sustain chronic inflammation. Plasma cells develop from activated B lymphocytes and produce antibodies directed either against persistent antigens in the inflammatory site or against altered tissue components. In some strong chronic inflammatory reactions, the accumulation of lymphocytes, antigen-presenting cells, and plasma cells may assume the morphologic features of lymphoid organs, and akin to lymph nodes, may even contain well-formed germinal centers. This pattern of lymphoid organogenesis is often seen in the synovium of patients with long-standing rheumatoid arthritis.

Eosinophils are characteristically found in inflammatory sites around parasitic infections or as part of immune reactions mediated by IgE, typically associated with *allergies.* Their recruitment is driven by adhesion molecules similar to those used by neutrophils, and by specific chemokines (e.g., eotaxin) derived from leukocytes or epithelial cells. Eosinophil granules contain major basic protein, a highly charged cationic protein that is toxic to parasites but also causes epithelial cell necrosis.

Mast cells are sentinel cells widely distributed in connective tissues throughout the body, and they can participate in both acute and chronic inflammatory responses. In atopic individuals (individuals prone to allergic reactions), mast cells are "armed" with IgE antibody specific for certain environmental antigens. When these antigens are subsequently encountered, the IgE-coated mast cells are triggered to release histamines and AA metabolites that elicit the early vascular changes of acute inflammation. IgE-armed mast cells are central players in *allergic reactions,* including *anaphylactic shock* (Chapter 5). Mast cells can also elaborate cytokines such as TNF and chemokines and may play a beneficial role in some infections.

An important final point: *although neutrophils are the classic hallmarks of acute inflammation, many forms of chronic inflammation may nevertheless continue to show extensive neutrophilic infiltrates,* as a result of either persistent microbes or necrotic cells, or mediators elaborated by macrophages.

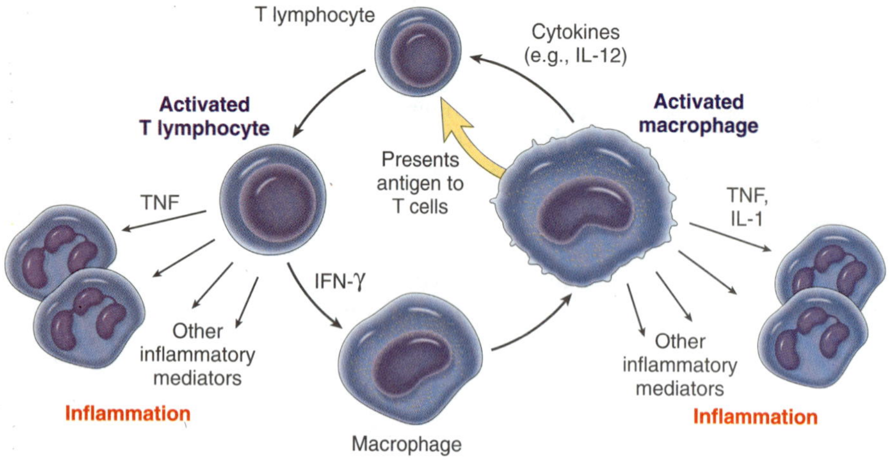

Figure 2–22

Macrophage–lymphocyte interactions in chronic inflammation. Activated lymphocytes and macrophages stimulate each other, and both cell types release inflammatory mediators that affect other cells. IFN-γ, interferon-γ; IL-1, interleukin 1; TNF, tumor necrosis factor.

Granulomatous Inflammation

Granulomatous inflammation is a distinctive pattern of chronic inflammation characterized by aggregates of activated macrophages that assume an epithelioid appearance. Granulomas are encountered in certain specific pathologic states; consequently, recognition of the granulomatous pattern is important because of the limited number of conditions (some life-threatening) that cause it (Table 2–7). Granulomas can form in the setting of persistent T-cell responses to certain microbes (such as *Mycobacterium tuberculosis, T. pallidum,* or fungi), where T-cell-derived cytokines are responsible for chronic macrophage activation. *Tuberculosis is the prototype of a granulomatous disease caused by infection and should always be excluded as the cause when granulomas are identified.* Granulomas may also develop in response to relatively inert foreign bodies (e.g., suture or splinter), forming so-called *foreign body granulomas.* The formation of a granuloma effectively "walls off" the offending agent and is therefore a useful defense mechanism. However, granuloma formation does not always lead to eradication of the causal agent, which is frequently resistant to killing or degradation, and granulomatous inflammation with subsequent fibrosis may even be the major cause of organ dysfunction in some diseases, such as tuberculosis.

Morphology

In the usual H&E preparations (Fig. 2–23), epithelioid cells in granulomas have pink, granular cytoplasm with indistinct cell boundaries. The aggregates of epithelioid macrophages are surrounded by a collar of lymphocytes secreting the cytokines responsible for continuing macrophage activation. Older granulomas may have a rim of fibroblasts and connective tissue. Frequently, but not invariably, multinucleated **giant cells** 40 to 50 μm in diameter are found in granulomas. They consist of a large mass of cytoplasm and many nuclei, and they derive from the fusion of 20 or more macrophages. In granulomas associated with certain infectious organisms (most classically the tubercle bacillus), a combination of hypoxia and free-radical injury leads to a central zone of necrosis. Grossly, this has a granular, cheesy appearance and is therefore called **caseous necrosis** (Chapters 1 and 13). Microscopically, this necrotic material appears as amorphous, structureless, granular debris, with complete loss of cellular details. Healing of granulomas is accompanied by fibrosis that may be quite extensive.

Table 2–7 Examples of Diseases with Granulomatous Inflammation

Disease	Cause	Tissue Reaction
Tuberculosis	*Mycobacterium tuberculosis*	Noncaseating tubercle (granuloma prototype): a focus of epithelioid cells, rimmed by fibroblasts, lymphocytes, histiocytes, occasional giant cells Caseating tubercle: central amorphous granular debris, loss of all cellular detail; acid-fast bacilli
Leprosy	*Mycobacterium leprae*	Acid-fast bacilli in macrophages; noncaseating granulomas
Syphilis	*Treponema pallidum*	Gumma: microscopic to grossly visible lesion, enclosing wall of histiocytes; plasma cell infiltrate; central cells are necrotic without loss of cellular outline
Cat-scratch disease	Gram-negative bacillus	Rounded or stellate granuloma containing central granular debris and recognizable neutrophils; giant cells uncommon
Sarcoidosis	Unknown etiology	Noncaseating granulomas with abundant activated macrophages
Crohn disease (inflammatory bowel disease)	Immune reaction against intestinal bacterial, self-antigens	Occasional noncaseating granulomas in wall of intestine, with dense chronic inflammatory infiltrate

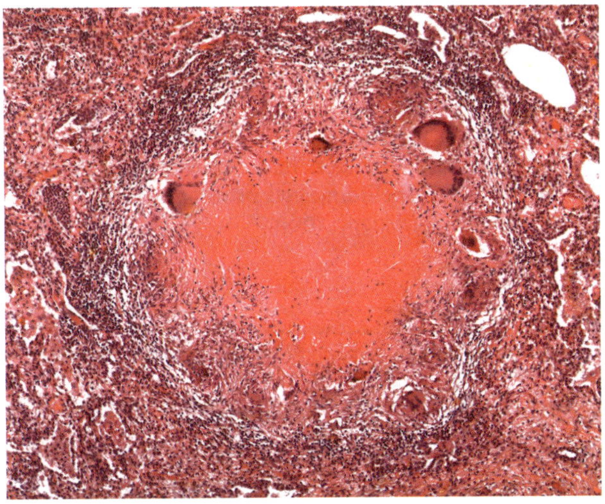

Figure 2–23

A typical granuloma resulting from infection with *Mycobacterium tuberculosis* showing central caseous necrosis, activated epithelioid macrophages, many giant cells, and a peripheral accumulation of lymphocytes.

SUMMARY

Features of Chronic Inflammation

- Prolonged host response to persistent stimulus
- Caused by microbes that resist elimination, immune responses against self and environmental antigens, and some toxic substances (e.g. silica); underlies many medically important diseases
- Characterized by coexisting inflammation, tissue injury, attempted repair by scarring, and immune response
- Cellular infiltrate consists of macrophages, lymphocytes, plasma cells; fibrosis is often prominent
- Mediated by cytokines produced by macrophages and lymphocytes (notably T lymphocytes); bidirectional interactions between these cells tend to amplify and prolong the inflammatory reaction

SYSTEMIC EFFECTS OF INFLAMMATION

Anyone who has suffered through a severe bout of a viral illness (such as influenza) has experienced the systemic effects of inflammation, collectively called the *acute-phase reaction,* or the systemic inflammatory response syndrome. *The cytokines TNF, IL-1, and IL-6* are the most important mediators of the acute-phase reaction. These cytokines are produced by leukocytes (and other cell types) in response to infection or in immune reactions and are released systemically. Often TNF induces the production of IL-1, which in turn stimulates the production of IL-6, forming a cascade of cytokines. TNF and IL-1 have similar biologic actions, although these may differ in subtle ways (see Fig. 2–16). IL-6 stimulates the hepatic synthesis of a number of plasma proteins, described below.

The acute-phase response consists of several clinical and pathologic changes.

- *Fever,* characterized by an elevation of body temperature, usually by 1° to 4°C, is one of the most prominent manifestations of the acute-phase response, especially when inflammation is caused by infection. Fever is produced in response to substances called *pyrogens* that act by stimulating prostaglandin (PG) synthesis in the vascular and perivascular cells of the hypothalamus. Bacterial products, such as lipopolysaccharide (LPS; called *exogenous pyrogens*), stimulate leukocytes to release cytokines such as IL-1 and TNF (called *endogenous pyrogens*) that increase the levels of cyclooxygenases that convert AA into prostaglandins. In the hypothalamus the PGs, especially PGE_2, stimulate the production of neurotransmitters, which function to reset the temperature set point at a higher level. NSAIDs, including aspirin, reduce fever by inhibiting cyclooxygenase and thus blocking PG synthesis. An elevated body temperature has been shown to help amphibians ward off microbial infections, and it is assumed that fever does the same for mammals, although the mechanism is unknown.
- *Elevated plasma levels of acute-phase proteins,* which are plasma proteins, mostly synthesized in the liver, whose concentrations may increase several 100-fold as part of the response to inflammatory stimuli. Three of the best-known of these proteins are C-reactive protein (CRP), fibrinogen, and serum amyloid A (SAA) protein. Synthesis of these molecules by hepatocytes is up-regulated by cytokines, especially IL-6. Many acute-phase proteins, such as CRP and SAA, bind to microbial cell walls, and they may act as opsonins and fix complement, thus promoting the elimination of the microbes. Fibrinogen binds to erythrocytes and causes them to form stacks (rouleaux) that sediment more rapidly at unit gravity than do individual erythrocytes. This is the basis for measuring the *erythrocyte sedimentation rate (ESR)* as a simple test for the systemic inflammatory response, caused by any number of stimuli, including LPS. Elevated serum levels of CRP are now used as a marker for increased risk of myocardial infarction or stroke in patients with atherosclerotic vascular disease. It is believed that inflammation is involved in the development of atherosclerosis (Chapter 10), and increased CRP is a measure of inflammation.
- *Leukocytosis* is a common feature of inflammatory reactions, especially those induced by bacterial infection. The leukocyte count usually climbs to 15,000 or 20,000 cells/μL, but sometimes it may reach extraordinarily high levels, as high as 40,000 to 100,000 cells/μL. These extreme elevations are referred to as *leukemoid reactions* because they are similar to the white cell counts obtained in leukemia. The leukocytosis occurs initially because of accelerated release of cells from the bone marrow postmitotic reserve pool

(caused by cytokines, including TNF and IL-1) and is therefore associated with a rise in the number of more immature neutrophils in the blood (*shift to the left*). Prolonged infection also stimulates production of colony-stimulating factors (CSFs), leading to increased bone marrow output of leukocytes, which compensates for the loss of these cells in the inflammatory reaction. Most bacterial infections induce an increase in the blood neutrophil count, called *neutrophilia*. Viral infections, such as infectious mononucleosis, mumps, and German measles, are associated with increased numbers of lymphocytes (*lymphocytosis*). Bronchial asthma, hay fever, and parasite infestations all involve an increase in the absolute number of eosinophils, creating an *eosinophilia*. Certain infections (typhoid fever and infections caused by some viruses, rickettsiae, and certain protozoa) are paradoxically associated with a decreased number of circulating white cells (*leukopenia*), likely because of cytokine-induced sequestration of lymphocytes in lymph nodes.

- Other manifestations of the acute-phase response include increased heart rate and blood pressure; decreased sweating, mainly because of redirection of blood flow from cutaneous to deep vascular beds, to minimize heat loss through the skin; and rigors (shivering), chills (perception of being cold as the hypothalamus resets the body temperature), anorexia, somnolence, and malaise, probably because of the actions of cytokines on brain cells. Chronic inflammation is associated with a wasting syndrome called *cachexia*, which is mainly the result of TNF-mediated appetite suppression and mobilization of fat stores.
- In severe bacterial infections (*sepsis*), the large amounts of organisms and LPS in the blood or extravascular tissue stimulate the production of enormous quantities of several cytokines, notably TNF, as well as IL-12 and IL-1. As a result, circulating levels of these cytokines increase, and the nature of the host response changes. High levels of TNF cause disseminated intravascular coagulation (DIC), hypoglycemia, and hypotensive shock. This clinical triad is described as *septic shock;* it is discussed in more detail in Chapter 4.

SUMMARY

Systemic Effects of Inflammation

- *Fever*: cytokines (TNF, IL-1) stimulate production of prostaglandins in hypothalamus
- Production of *acute-phase proteins*: C-reactive protein, others; synthesis stimulated by cytokines (IL-6, others) acting on liver cells
- *Leukocytosis*: cytokines (colony-stimulating factors) stimulate production of leukocytes from precursors in the bone marrow
- In some severe infections, *septic shock*: fall in blood pressure, disseminated intravascular coagulation, metabolic abnormalities; induced by high levels of TNF

Having concluded our discussion of the cellular and molecular events in acute and chronic inflammation, we must consider the changes induced by the body's attempts to heal the damage, the process of *repair.* As described next, in Chapter 3, the repair begins almost as soon as the inflammatory changes have started and involves several processes, including cell proliferation and differentiation, and ECM deposition.

BIBLIOGRAPHY

Cook-Mills JM, Deem TL: Active participation of endothelial cells in inflammation. J Leuk Biol 77:487, 2005. *[A review of endothelial adhesion molecules and their regulation.]*

Cotran RS, Mayadas TN: Endothelial adhesion molecules in health and disease. Pathol Biol 46:164, 1998. *[A well-written overview of the molecules mediating leukocyte adhesion and their mechanisms of regulation.]*

Coughlin SR: Thrombin signaling and protease-activated receptors. Nature 407:258, 2000. *[Excellent review of the role of protease-activated receptors in inflammation.]*

Funk CD: Prostaglandins and leukotrienes: advances in eicosanoid biology. Science 294:1871, 2001. *[An update on this family of mediators.]*

Gabay C, Kushner I: Acute-phase proteins and other systemic responses to inflammation. N Engl J Med 30:448, 1999. *[Description of the proteins of the acute-phase response.]*

Graham DJ: COX-2 inhibitors, other NSAIDs and cardiovascular risk. The seduction of common sense. JAMA 296: published online Sep. 12, 2006. *[A critical analysis of the untoward effects of COX-2 inhibitors.]*

Guo RF, Ward PA: Role of C5a in inflammatory responses. Annu Rev Immunol 23:821, 2005. *[Update on the role of this complement protein in inflammation.]*

Jaeschke H, Smith CW: Mechanisms of neutrophil-induced parenchymal injury. J Leukoc Biol 61:647, 1997. *[Review of the pathways and mediators of neutrophil-mediated injury.]*

Johnston B, Butcher EC: Chemokines in rapid leukocyte adhesion triggering and migration Semin Immunol 14:83, 2002. *[Good update on the role of chemokines in inflammation.]*

Laroux FS, et al: Role of nitric oxide in inflammation. Acta Physiol Scand 173:113, 2001. *[A review of the many actions of NO.]*

Lentsch AB, Ward PA: Regulation of inflammatory vascular damage. J Pathol 190:343, 2000. *[Discussion of the mechanisms of endothelial damage and increased vascular permeability.]*

Luster AD, Alon R, von Andrian UH: Immune cell migration in inflammation: present and future therapeutic targets. Nat Immunol 6:1182, 2005. *[Excellent review of the molecular basis of leukocyte recruitment in inflammation.]*

Muller WA: Leukocyte-endothelial cell interactions in the inflammatory response. Lab Invest 82:521, 2002. *[Review of the mechanisms of leukocyte migration through blood vessels.]*

Munford RS: Severe sepsis and septic shock: the role of Gram-negative bacteremia. Annual Review of Pathology: Mechanisms of Disease 1:467, 2006.

Saharinen P, et al: Lymphatic vasculature: development, molecular regulation, and role in tumor metastasis and inflammation. Trends Immunol 25:387, 2004. *[Excellent review on the biology of lymphatic vessels.]*

Sallusto F, Mackay CR: Chemokines and their receptors in homeostasis and inflammation. Curr Opin Immunol 16:724, 2004. *[An up-to-date review.]*

Segal AW: How neutrophils kill microbes. Annu Rev Immunol 23:197, 2005. *[Good review of microbicidal mechanisms of leukocytes.]*

Serhan CN, Savill J: Resolution of inflammation: the beginning programs the end. Nat Immunol 6:1191, 2005. *[Excellent discussion of the mechanisms involved in termination of the inflammatory response.]*

Underhill DM, Ozinsky A: Phagocytosis of microbes: complexity in action. Annu Rev Immunol 20:825, 2002. *[Excellent review of the biology and molecular mechanisms of phagocytosis.]*

Chapter 3

Tissue Repair: Regeneration, Healing, and Fibrosis

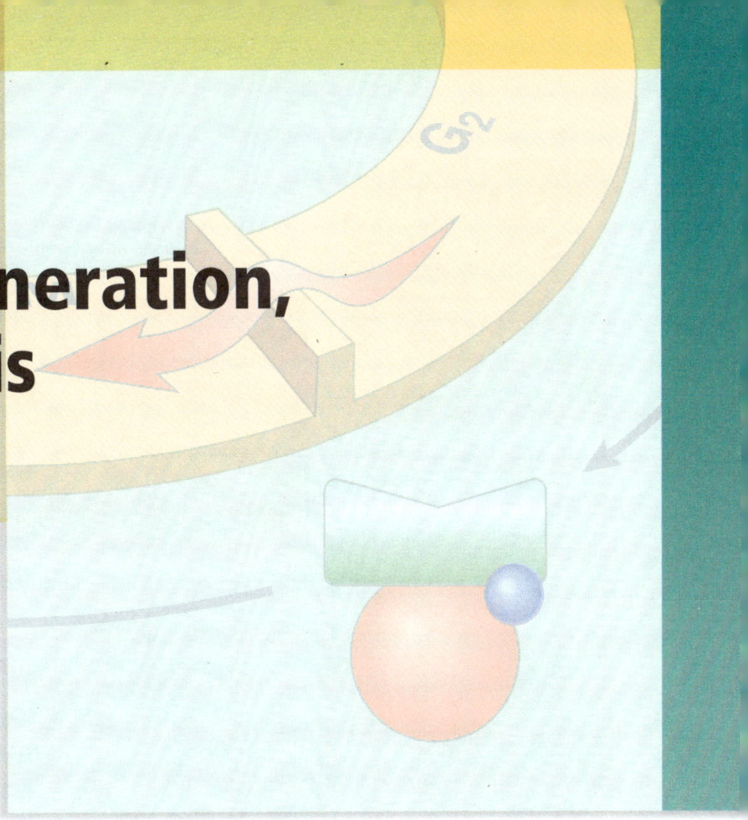

Critical to the survival of an organism is the ability to repair the damage caused by toxic insults and inflammation. The inflammatory response to microbes and injured tissues not only serves to eliminate these dangers but also sets into motion the process of repair. *Repair* refers to the restoration of tissue architecture and function after an injury. It occurs by two types of reactions (Fig. 3–1). Some tissues are able to replace the damaged components and essentially return to a normal state; this process is called *regeneration*. If the injured tissues are incapable of complete restitution, or if the supporting structures of the tissue are severely damaged, repair occurs by laying down of connective (fibrous) tissue, a process termed *healing* that results in *scar formation*. Although the fibrous scar is not normal, it provides enough structural stability that the injured tissue is usually able to function. After many common types of injury, both regeneration and scar formation contribute in varying degrees to the ultimate repair. The term *fibrosis* is most often used to describe the extensive deposition of collagen that occurs in the lungs, liver, kidney, and other organs as a consequence of chronic inflammation, or in the myocardium after extensive ischemic necrosis (infarction). If fibrosis develops in a tissue space occupied by an inflammatory exudate it is called *organization* (as in organizing pneumonia affecting the lung).

Repair involves the proliferation of various cells, and close interactions between cells and the extracellular matrix (ECM). Therefore, an understanding of the process of repair requires some knowledge of the control of cell proliferation and the functions of the ECM. In this chapter we first discuss the principles of cellular proliferation, the roles of stem cells in tissue homeostasis, and the roles of growth factors in the proliferation of different cell types involved in repair. This is followed by a discussion of some important properties of the ECM, and how it is involved in repair. These sections lay the foundation for a consideration of the salient features of regeneration and healing by scar formation, concluding with a description of cutaneous wound healing as an illustration of the repair process.

THE CONTROL OF CELL PROLIFERATION

As we will discuss later, several cell types proliferate during tissue repair. These include the remnants of the injured tissue (which attempt to restore normal structure),

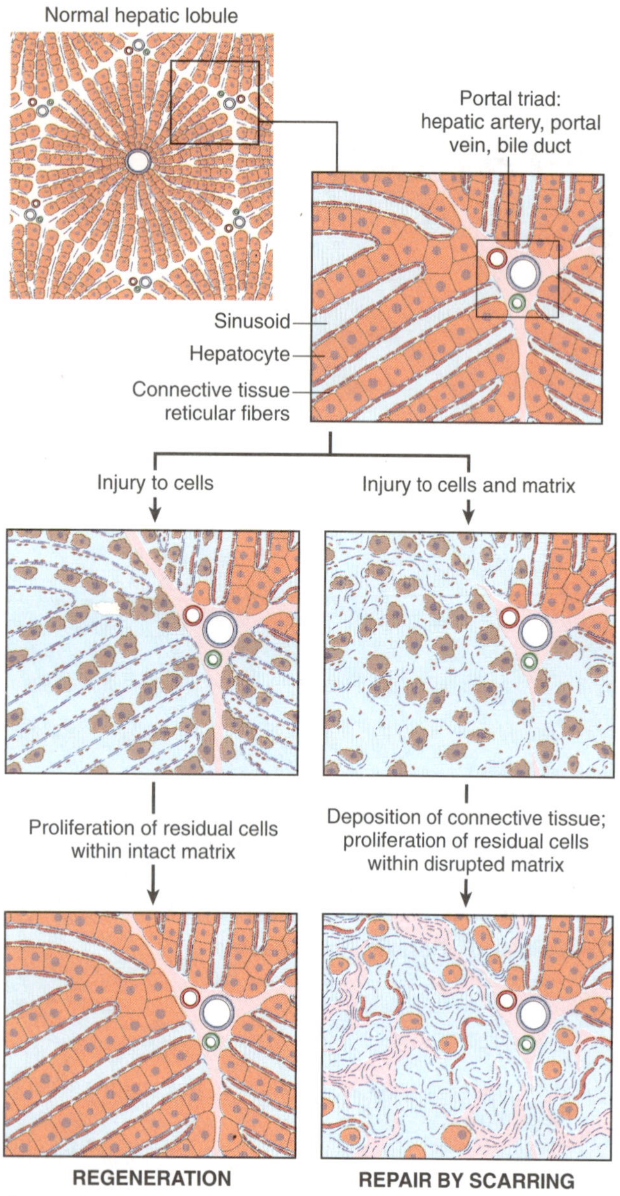

Figure 3–1

Mechanisms of tissue repair. In this example, injury to the liver is repaired by regeneration if only the hepatocytes are damaged, or by laying down of fibrous tissue if the matrix is also injured.

vascular endothelial cells (to create new vessels that provide the nutrients needed for the repair process), and fibroblasts (the source of the fibrous tissue that forms the scar to fill defects that cannot be corrected by regeneration) (Fig. 3–1). The proliferation of these cell types is driven by proteins that are collectively called *growth factors*. The production of polypeptide growth factors, responses of cells to these factors, and the ability of these cells to divide and expand in numbers are all important determinants of the adequacy of the repair process. In the following sections we describe the regulation of cell proliferation and the nature and activities of growth factors.

The normal size of cell populations is determined by a balance of cell proliferation, cell death by apoptosis, and emergence of new differentiated cells from stem cells (Fig. 3–2). Below we first discuss cell proliferation and stem cells, and then the capacities of different tissues to divide and self renew.

The Cell Cycle

To understand physiologic cell proliferation (as in repair) and pathologic proliferation (as in cancer), it is important to learn about the cell cycle and its regulation. Here we briefly summarize the main features of the cell cycle and its control mechanisms. A more detailed discussion of these topics is presented in Chapter 6, in the context of neoplasia.

The key processes in the proliferation of cells are DNA replication and mitosis. The sequence of events that control these two processes is known as the *cell cycle*. The cell cycle consists of a series of steps at which the cell checks for the accuracy of the process and instructs itself to proceed to the next step (Fig. 3–3). Because of its central role in growth regulation, *the cell cycle has multiple controls*, both positive and negative. The cycle consists of the presynthetic growth phase 1 *(G_1)*, the DNA synthesis phase *(S)*, the premitotic growth phase 2 *(G_2)*, and the mitotic phase *(M)*. Non-dividing cells are either in cell cycle arrest in G_1 or they exit the cycle to enter a phase called G_0. Any stimulus that initiates cell prolifer-

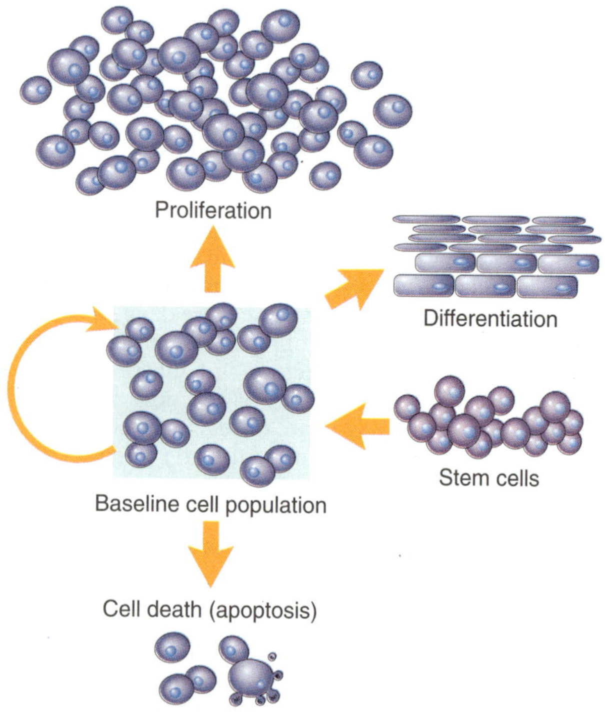

Figure 3–2

Mechanisms regulating cell populations. Cell numbers can be altered by increased or decreased rates of stem cell input, cell death via apoptosis, or changes in the rates of proliferation or differentiation. (Modified from McCarthy NJ, et al: Apoptosis in the development of the immune system: growth factors, clonal selection and *bcl-2*. Cancer Metastasis Rev 11:157, 1992.)

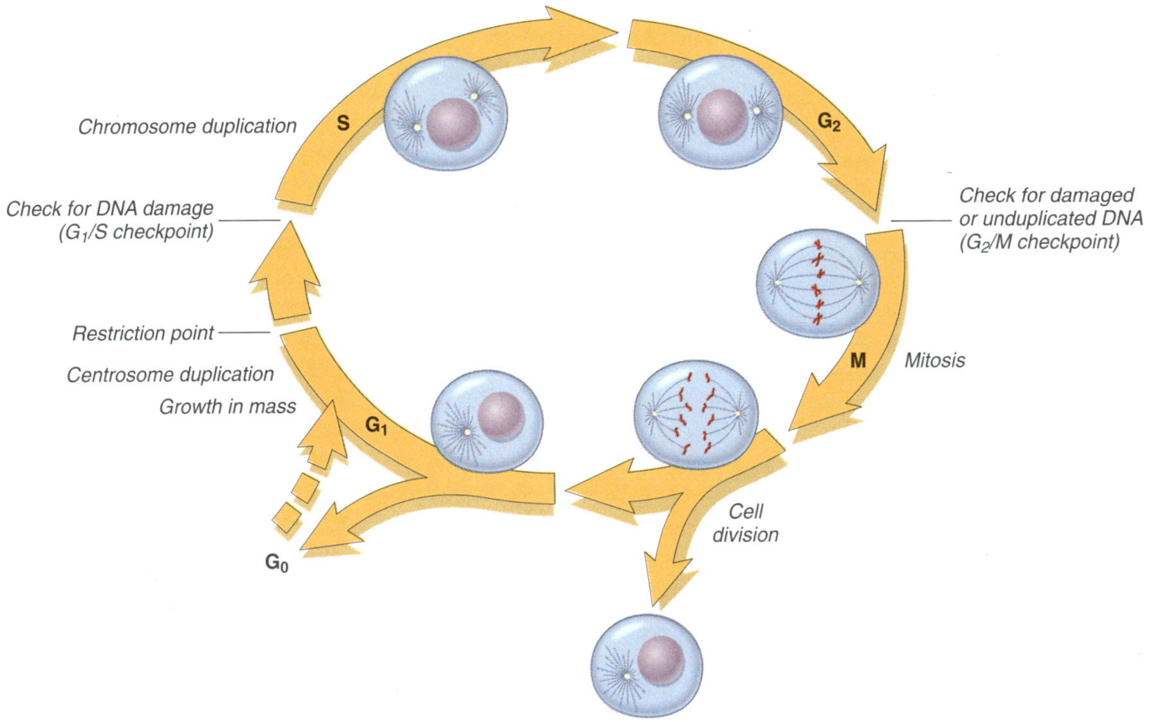

Figure 3–3

Cell populations and cycle landmarks. Note the cell cycle stages (G_0, G_1, S, G_2 and M), the G_1 restriction point, and the G_1/S and G_2/M checkpoints. While some cell populations continuously cycle and proliferate (e.g., epidermis, GI epithelium), others are quiescent (in G_0) but can enter the cell cycle (e.g., hepatocytes); permanent cells (e.g., neurons and cardiac myocytes) do not have the capacity to proliferate (see text). (Modified from Pollard TD, Earnshaw WC: Cell Biology. Philadelphia, WB Saunders, 2002.)

ation, such as exposure to growth factors, needs to promote the *G_0/G_1 transition* and the entry of cells into the first, i.e. G_1, phase of the cycle. Further progression is determined by the ability of the cell to traverse an intrinsic quality control mechanism for cell integrity, known as *checkpoint control*. Checkpoint controls prevent DNA replication or mitosis of damaged cells and either transiently stop the cell cycle to allow for DNA repair or eliminate irreversibly damaged cells by apoptosis. Progression through the cell cycle from G_1 is regulated by proteins called *cyclins*, which form complexes with enzymes called *cyclin-dependent kinases (CDKs)*. CDKs work by promoting DNA replication and various aspects of the mitotic process and are required for cell cycle progression; CDKs are suppressed during G_1 by multiple mechanisms (Chapter 6). As we shall see below, a major action of growth factors is to overcome these checkpoint controls by releasing the suppression of CDK activity. Once cells enter the S phase, the DNA is replicated and the cell progresses through G_2 and mitosis.

Proliferative Capacities of Tissues

The ability of tissues to repair themselves is critically influenced by their intrinsic proliferative capacity. Based on this criterion, the tissues of the body are divided into three groups.

Continuously Dividing Tissues. Cells of these tissues (also known as *labile tissues*) are continuously being lost and replaced by maturation from stem cells and by proliferation of mature cells. Labile cells include hematopoietic cells in the bone marrow and the majority of surface epithelia, such as the stratified squamous surfaces of the skin, oral cavity, vagina, and cervix; the cuboidal epithelia of the ducts draining exocrine organs (e.g., salivary glands, pancreas, biliary tract); the columnar epithelium of the gastrointestinal tract, uterus, and fallopian tubes; and the transitional epithelium of the urinary tract. These tissues can readily regenerate after injury as long as the pool of stem cells is preserved.

Stable Tissues. Cells of these tissues are quiescent (in the G_0 stage of the cell cycle) and have only minimal replicative activity in their normal state. However, these cells are capable of proliferating in response to injury or loss of tissue mass. Stable cells constitute the *parenchyma* of most solid tissues, such as liver, kidney, and pancreas. They also include endothelial cells, fibroblasts, and smooth muscle cells; the proliferation of these cells is particularly important in wound healing. With the exception of liver, stable tissues have a limited capacity to regenerate after injury.

Permanent Tissues. The cells of these tissues are considered to be terminally differentiated and nonproliferative in postnatal life. The majority of neurons and cardiac muscle cells belong to this category. Thus, injury to brain or heart is irreversible and results in a scar, because neurons and cardiac myocytes do not divide. Limited stem cell replication and differentiation occurs in some areas of the adult brain, and there is some evidence that heart muscle cells may proliferate after myocardial necrosis. Nevertheless, whatever proliferative capacity may exist in these tissues, it is insufficient to produce tissue regeneration after injury. Skeletal muscle is usually classified as a permanent tissue, but satellite cells attached to the endomysial sheath provide some regenerative capacity for this tissue. In permanent tissues, repair is typically dominated by scar formation.

With the exception of tissues composed primarily of nondividing permanent cells (e.g., cardiac muscle and nerve), most mature tissues contain variable proportions of three cell types: continuously dividing cells, quiescent cells that can return to the cell cycle, and nondividing cells.

Stem Cells

In most continuously dividing tissues the mature cells are terminally differentiated and short-lived. As mature cells die the tissue is replenished by the differentiation of cells generated from stem cells. Thus, in these tissues there is a homeostatic equilibrium between the replication and differentiation of stem cells and the death of the mature, fully differentiated cells. Such relationships are particularly evident in the multilayered epithelium of the skin and the gastrointestinal tract, in which stem cell niches have been identified near the basal layer of the epithelium. Cells differentiate progressively as they migrate to the upper layers of the epithelium; they ultimately die and are shed from the surface of the tissue.

Stem cells are characterized by two important properties: self-renewal capacity and asymmetric replication. Asymmetric replication of stem cells means that after each cell division, some progeny enter a differentiation pathway, while others remain undifferentiated, retaining their self-renewal capacity. Stem cells with the capacity to generate multiple cell lineages (*pluripotent stem cells*) can be isolated from embryos and are called *embryonic stem (ES) cells.* As mentioned above, stem cells are normally present in proliferative tissues and generate cell lineages specific for the tissue. However, it is now recognized that stem cells with the capacity to generate multiple lineages are present in the bone marrow and several other tissues of adult individuals. These cells are called *tissue stem cells* or *adult stem cells.* Whether tissue stem cells have similar differentiation capacity (referred to as *differentiation plasticity*) as ES cells remains the subject of active research and much dispute. *Bone marrow stem cells* have very broad differentiation capabilities, being able to generate fat, cartilage, bone, endothelium, and muscle. This developmental plasticity was first interpreted as being the consequence of *transdifferentiation,* that is, the change in the differentiation program of an already committed cell. Most likely, however, developmental plasticity involves the selection of a specific pathway from the many differentiation pathways available to uncommitted progenitor cells.

The new field of *regenerative medicine* has as its main goal the regeneration and repopulation of damaged organs using ES or adult stem cells. One of the most exciting prospects in this field is the type of stem cell therapy known as *therapeutic cloning.* The main steps of this procedure are illustrated in Figure 3–4. Other potential therapeutic strategies using stem cells involve transplanting stem cells into areas of injury, mobilization of stem cells from the bone marrow into injured tissue, and the use of stem cell culture systems to produce large amounts of differentiated cells for transplantation into injured tissue.

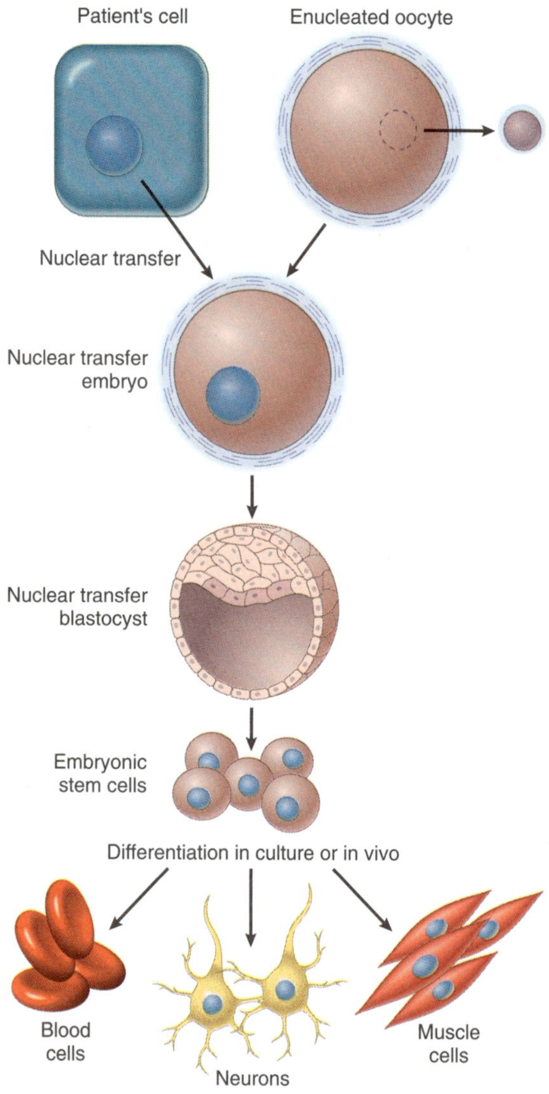

Figure 3–4

Steps involved in therapeutic cloning using embryonic stem (ES) cells for cell therapy. In this procedure the diploid nucleus of a cell from a patient is introduced into an enucleated oocyte. The oocyte is activated, and the zygote divides to become a blastocyst containing donor DNA. The blastocyst is dissociated to obtain ES cells; these cells are capable of differentiating into various tissues, either in culture or after transplantation into the donor. The goal of the procedure is to reconstitute or repopulate damaged organs from a patient using the cells of the patient, thus avoiding immunologic rejection. (Modified from Hochedlinger K, Jaenisch R: Nuclear transplantation, embryonic stem cells, and the potential for cell therapy. N Engl J Med 349:275, 2003. Copyright © 2003 Massachusetts Medical Society. Adapted with permission 2006. All rights reserved.)

SUMMARY

Cell Proliferation, the Cell Cycle, and Stem Cells

- Cell proliferation is regulated by cyclins that, when complexed with cyclin-dependent kinases (CDKs), regulate the phosphorylation of proteins involved in cell cycle progression leading to DNA replication and mitosis.
- The cell cycle is tightly regulated by stimulators and inhibitors, and contains intrinsic checkpoint controls to prevent replication of abnormal cells.
- Tissues are divided into labile, stable and permanent, according to the proliferative capacity of their cells.
- Continuously dividing tissues (labile tissues) contain stem cells that differentiate to replenish lost cells and maintain tissue homeostasis.
- Stem cells from embryos (ES cells) are pluripotent; adult tissues, particularly the bone marrow, contain adult stem cells capable of generating multiple cell lineages.

THE NATURE AND MECHANISMS OF ACTION OF GROWTH FACTORS

Cell proliferation can be triggered by many chemical mediators, such as growth factors, hormones, and cytokines. Although hormones and many cytokines are involved in the stimulation or inhibition of cell growth, they have many other functions and are traditionally discussed separately (they are alluded to in various sections of this book). Signals from the ECM are also important inducers of cell replication, and they will be discussed later. In this section, we focus on *polypeptide growth factors*, whose major role is to promote cell survival and proliferation and which are important in regeneration and healing.

Expansion of cell populations usually involves an increase in cell size (growth), cell division (mitosis), and protection from apoptotic death (survival). Strictly speaking, the term "growth factors" should be used for proteins that increase cell size, and "mitogens" and "survival factor" should be used for molecules with the other activities. However, many growth factors have all these activities, and by convention "growth factor" is used for a protein that expands cell populations by stimulating cell division (usually accompanied by increased cell size) and by promoting cell survival.

Most growth factors have pleiotropic effects; that is, in addition to stimulating cellular proliferation, they stimulate migration, differentiation and contractility, and enhance the synthesis of specialized proteins (such as collagen in fibroblasts). A growth factor may act on a specific cell type or on multiple cell types. They induce cell proliferation by binding to specific receptors and affecting the expression of genes whose products typically have several functions—they relieve blocks on cell cycle progression (thus promoting replication), they prevent apoptosis, and they enhance the synthesis of cellular proteins in preparation for mitosis. A major activity of growth factors is to stimulate the function of growth control genes, many of which are called *protooncogenes* because mutations in them lead to unrestrained cell proliferation characteristic of cancer (oncogenesis) (Chapter 6). Some growth factors stimulate proliferation of some cells and inhibit cycling of other cells. In fact, a growth factor can have opposite effects on the same cell depending on its concentration. An example of such a growth factor is transforming growth factor-β (TGF-β).

There is a huge (and ever-increasing) list of known growth factors. Rather than attempt an exhaustive cataloguing, we will highlight only selected molecules that contribute to tissue repair (Table 3–1). Many of the growth factors that are involved in repair are produced by leukocytes that are recruited to the site of injury or are activated at this site, as part of the inflammatory process. Other growth factors are produced by the parenchymal cells or the stromal (connective tissue) cells in response to cell injury or loss. Below we discuss general principles of how these growth factors work. We return to the roles of individual growth factors in the repair process later in the chapter.

Signaling Mechanisms of Growth Factor Receptors

The major intracellular signaling pathways induced by growth factor receptors are similar to those of many other cellular receptors that recognize extracellular ligands. The binding of a ligand to its receptor triggers a series of events by which extracellular signals are transduced into the cell, leading to the stimulation or repression of gene expression. Signaling may occur directly in the same cell, between adjacent cells, or over greater distances (Fig. 3–5).

- *Autocrine* signaling, in which a substance acts predominantly (or even exclusively) on the cell that secretes it. This pathway is important in the immune response (e.g. lymphocyte proliferation induced by some cytokines) and in compensatory epithelial hyperplasia (e.g., liver regeneration).
- *Paracrine* signaling, in which a substance affects cells in the immediate vicinity of the cell that released the agent. This pathway is important for recruiting inflammatory cells to the site of infection (Chapter 2), and for wound healing.
- *Endocrine* signaling, in which a regulatory substance, such as a hormone, is released into the bloodstream and acts on target cells at a distance.

Receptor proteins are generally located on the cell surface, but they may be intracellular; in the latter case, the ligands must be sufficiently hydrophobic to enter the cell (e.g., vitamin D, or steroid and thyroid hormones). *The binding of a ligand to its cell surface receptor leads to a cascade of secondary intracellular events that culminate in transcription factor activation or repression, leading to cellular responses.* For some intracellular receptors, ligand binding leads to the formation of receptor-ligand

Table 3–1 Growth Factors and Cytokines Involved in Regeneration and Wound Healing

Cytokine	Symbol	Source	Functions
Epidermal growth factor	EGF	Activated macrophages, salivary glands, keratinocytes, and many other cells	Mitogenic for keratinocytes and fibroblasts; stimulates keratinocyte migration and granulation tissue formation
Transforming growth factor α	TGF-α	Activated macrophages, T lymphocytes, keratinocytes, and many other cells	Similar to EGF; stimulates replication of hepatocytes and many epithelial cells
Hepatocyte growth factor (scatter factor)	HGF	Mesenchymal cells	Enhances proliferation of epithelial and endothelial cells, and of hepatocytes; increases cell motility
Vascular endothelial cell growth factor (isoforms A, B, C, D)	VEGF	Mesenchymal cells	Increases vascular permeability; mitogenic for endothelial cells (see text)
Platelet-derived growth factor (isoforms A, B, C, D)	PDGF	Platelets, macrophages, endothelial cells, keratinocytes, smooth muscle cells	Chemotactic for PMNs, macrophages, fibroblasts, and smooth muscle cells; activates PMNs, macrophages, and fibroblasts; mitogenic for fibroblasts, endothelial cells, and smooth muscles cells; stimulates production of MMPs, fibronectin, and HA; stimulates angiogenesis and wound remodeling; regulates integrin expression
Fibroblast growth factor 1 (acidic), -2 (basic), and family	FGF-1, -2	Macrophages, mast cells, T lymphocytes, endothelial cells, fibroblasts, and many tissues	Chemotactic for fibroblasts; mitogenic for fibroblasts and keratinocytes; stimulates keratinocyte migration, angiogenesis, wound contraction, and matrix deposition
Transforming growth factor β (isoforms 1, 2, 3)	TGF-β	Platelets, T lymphocytes, macrophages, endothelial cells, keratinocytes, smooth muscle cells, fibroblasts	Chemotactic for PMNs, macrophages, lymphocytes, fibroblasts, and smooth muscle cells; stimulates TIMP synthesis, angiogenesis, and fibroplasia; inhibits production of MMPs and keratinocyte proliferation; regulates integrin expression and other cytokines
Keratinocyte growth factor (FGF-7)	KGF	Fibroblasts	Stimulates keratinocyte migration, proliferation, and differentiation

HA, Hyaluronic acid; MMPs, matrix metalloproteinase; PMNs, polymorphonuclear cells; TIMP, tissue inhibitor of matrix metalloproteinase.
Modified from Schwartz SI: Principles of Surgery. McGraw Hill, New York, 1999.

complexes that directly associate with nuclear DNA and activate or turn off gene transcription. In some cases, cytoplasmic transcription factors called STATs (discussed later) migrate into the nucleus and bind to DNA directly. Regardless of their origin, transcription factors bind to gene promoters and enhancers to trigger or inhibit transcription.

Figure 3–6 presents an overview of signal transduction originating from three types of receptors: receptors with tyrosine kinase activity, G-protein–coupled receptors, and receptors without intrinsic enzymatic activity:

- *Receptors with intrinsic kinase activity.* These are usually dimeric transmembrane molecules with an extracellular ligand-binding domain; ligand binding causes stable dimerization with subsequent phosphorylation of the receptor subunits. Once phosphorylated, the receptors can activate other intracellular proteins (e.g., RAS, phosphatidylinositol 3-[PI3] kinase, phospholipase Cγ [PLC-γ]) and stimulate a cascade of events leading to entry into the cell cycle and cell cycle progression, or induction of other transcriptional programs. An especially important pathway stimulated by *RAS* activation is the *mitogen-activated protein (MAP) kinase cascade,* which is involved in the intracellular signaling of many growth factors, including *epidermal growth factor (EGF), vascular endothelial growth factor (VEGF), fibroblast growth factor (FGF),* and *hepatocyte growth factor (HGF).*
- *G-protein–coupled receptors.* These receptors contain seven transmembrane α-helix segments and are also known as *seven transmembrane G-protein–coupled receptors.* After ligand binding, the receptors associate with intracellular guanosine triphosphate (GTP)-binding proteins (G proteins) that contain guanosine diphosphate (GDP). Binding of the G proteins causes the exchange of GDP with GTP, resulting in activation of the proteins. Among the several transduction pathways activated through G-protein–coupled receptors are those involving *cyclic AMP (cAMP),* and the generation of *inositol-1,4,5,-triphosphate (IP_3), which releases calcium from the endoplasmic reticulum.* Receptors in this category constitute the largest family of plasma membrane receptors (more than 1500 members have been identified) and include those for epinephrine, vasopressin, serotonin, histamine, and glucagon, as well as the chemokines (Chapter 2).
- *Receptors without intrinsic enzymatic activity.* These are usually monomeric transmembrane molecules with an extracellular ligand-binding domain; ligand interaction induces an intracellular conformational change

that allows association with intracellular protein kinases called *Janus kinases (JAKs)*. Phosphorylation of JAKs activates cytoplasmic transcription factors called *STATs (signal transducers and activators of transcription)*, which shuttle directly into the nucleus. Ligands for these receptors include many cytokines, the interferons, colony-stimulating factors, growth hormone, and erythropoietin.

Note that not all ligands induce stimulatory signals; in fact, growth-inhibitory signals inducing direct inhibition or inhibition caused by cell-cell contact (*contact inhibition*) are equally important. For instance, the TGF-β receptor has intrinsic kinase activity, and when in complex with TGF-β it phosphorylates specific intracellular proteins, which in turn increase the synthesis of CDK inhibitors and block the activity of transcription factors and cell cycle progression.

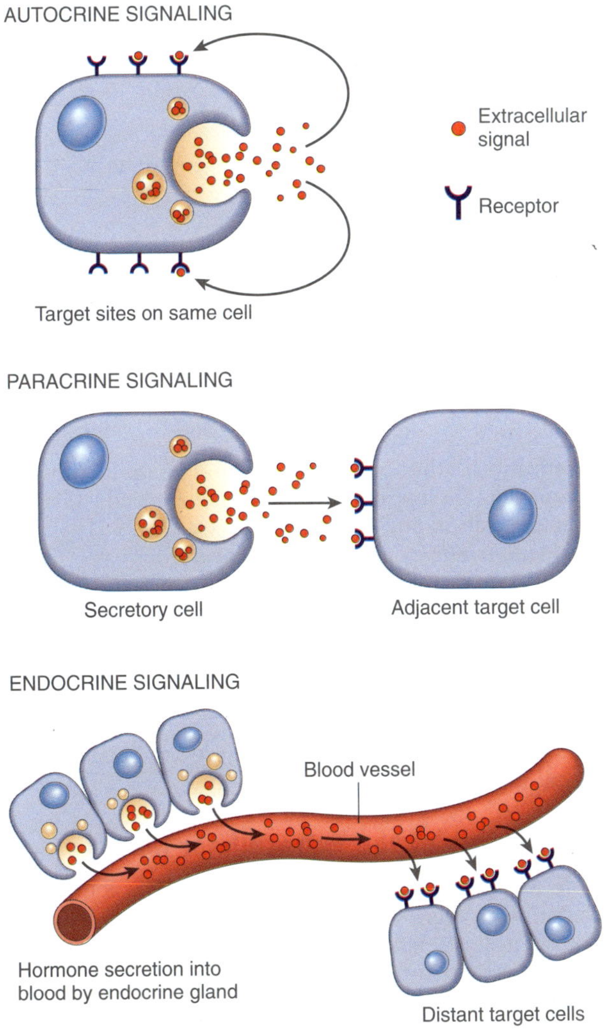

Figure 3–5

Patterns of extracellular signaling, demonstrating autocrine, paracrine, and endocrine signaling (see text). (Modified from Lodish, et al [eds]: Molecular Cell Biology, 3rd ed. New York, WH Freeman, 1995.)

SUMMARY

Growth Factors, Receptors and Signal Transduction

- Polypeptide growth factors act in autocrine, paracrine, or endocrine manner.
- Growth factors are produced transiently in response to an external stimulus and act by binding to cellular receptors. Different classes of growth factor receptors include receptors with intrinsic kinase activity, G-protein–coupled receptors and receptors without intrinsic kinase activity.
- Growth factors such as EGF and HGF bind to receptors with intrinsic kinase activity, and trigger a cascade of phosphorylating events through MAP kinases, which culminate in transcription factor activation and DNA replication.
- Cytokines generally bind to receptors without kinase activity; such receptors interact with cytoplasmic transcription factors that move into the nucleus.
- Most growth factors have multiple effects, such as cell migration, differentiation, stimulation of angiogenesis and fibrogenesis in addition to cell proliferation.

EXTRACELLULAR MATRIX (ECM) AND CELL-MATRIX INTERACTIONS

Tissue repair depends not only on growth factor activity but also on interactions between cells and ECM components. The ECM is a *dynamic, constantly remodeling* macromolecular complex synthesized locally, which assembles into a network that surrounds cells. It constitutes a significant proportion of any tissue. ECM sequesters water, providing turgor to soft tissues, and minerals, giving rigidity to bone. By supplying a substratum for cell adhesion and serving as a reservoir for growth factors, *ECM regulates the proliferation, movement, and differentiation of the cells living within it.* Synthesis and degradation of ECM accompanies morphogenesis, wound healing, chronic fibrotic processes, and tumor invasion and metastasis.

ECM occurs in two basic forms: *interstitial matrix* and *basement membrane* (Fig. 3–7).

Interstitial Matrix. This is present in the spaces between cells in connective tissue, and between epithelium and supportive vascular and smooth muscle structures; it is synthesized by mesenchymal cells (e.g., fibroblasts) and tends to form a three-dimensional, amorphous gel. Its major constituents are fibrillar and nonfibrillar collagens, as well as fibronectin, elastin, proteoglycans, hyaluronate, and other elements (described later).

Basement Membrane. The seemingly random array of interstitial matrix in connective tissues becomes highly organized around epithelial cells, endothelial cells, and smooth muscle cells, forming the specialized basement

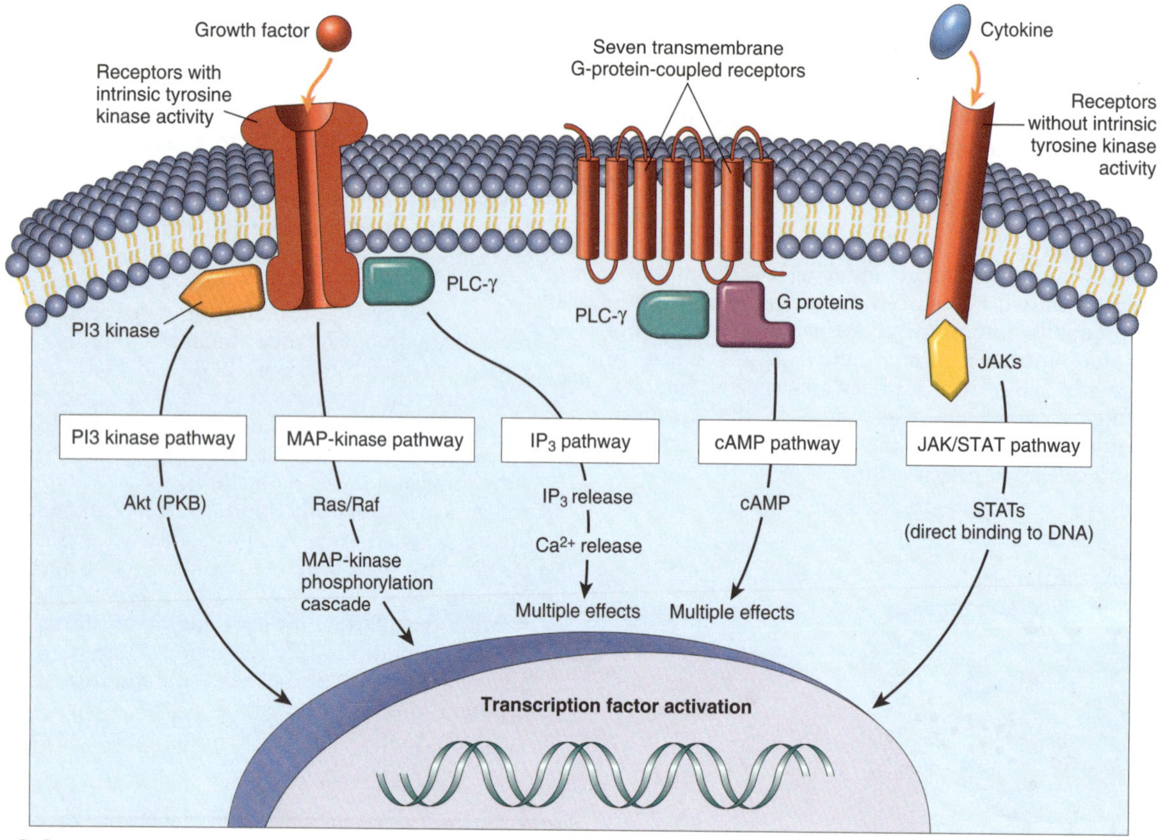

Figure 3–6

An overview of the major types of cell surface receptors and their principal signal transduction pathways leading to transcription factor activation (see text). Shown are receptors with intrinsic tyrosine kinase activity, seven transmembrane G-protein-coupled receptors, and receptors without intrinsic tyrosine kinase activity. cAMP, Cyclic adenosine monophosphate; IP_3, inositol triphosphate; JAK, Janus kinase; MAP kinase, mitogen-activated protein kinase; PI3 kinase, phosphatidylinositol 3-kinase; PKB, protein kinase B (also known as Akt); PLC-γ, phospholipase Cγ; STAT, signal transducers and activators of transcription.

membrane. The basement membrane lies beneath the epithelium and is synthesized by overlying epithelium and underlying mesenchymal cells; it tends to form a platelike "chicken wire" mesh. Its major constituents are amorphous nonfibrillar type IV collagen and laminin (see later).

Roles of the Extracellular Matrix

The ECM is much more than a space filler around cells. Its various functions include:

- *Mechanical support* for cell anchorage and cell migration, and maintenance of cell polarity
- *Control of cell growth.* ECM components can regulate cell proliferation by signaling through cellular receptors of the integrin family.
- *Maintenance of cell differentiation.* The type of ECM proteins can affect the degree of differentiation of the cells in the tissue, also acting largely via cell surface integrins.
- *Scaffolding for tissue renewal.* The maintenance of normal tissue structure requires a basement membrane or stromal scaffold. The integrity of the basement membrane or the stroma of the parenchymal cells is critical for the organized regeneration of tissues. It is particularly noteworthy that although labile and stable cells are capable of regeneration, injury to these tissues results in restitution of the normal structure only if the ECM is not damaged. Disruption of these structures leads to collagen deposition and scar formation (see Fig. 3–1).
- *Establishment of tissue microenvironments.* Basement membrane acts as a boundary between epithelium and underlying connective tissue and also forms part of the filtration apparatus in the kidney.
- *Storage and presentation of regulatory molecules.* For example, growth factors like FGF and HGF are excreted and stored in the ECM in some tissues. This allows the rapid deployment of growth factors after local injury, or during regeneration.

Components of the Extracellular Matrix

There are three basic components of ECM: (1) fibrous structural proteins such as collagens and elastins, which confer tensile strength and recoil; (2) water-hydrated gels such as proteoglycans and hyaluronan, which permit resilience and lubrication; and (3) adhesive glycoproteins that connect the matrix elements to one another and to cells (see Fig. 3–7).

Collagen. The collagens are fibrous structural proteins that confer tensile strength; without them human beings would be reduced to a clump of cells connected by neurons. Collagens are composed of three separate

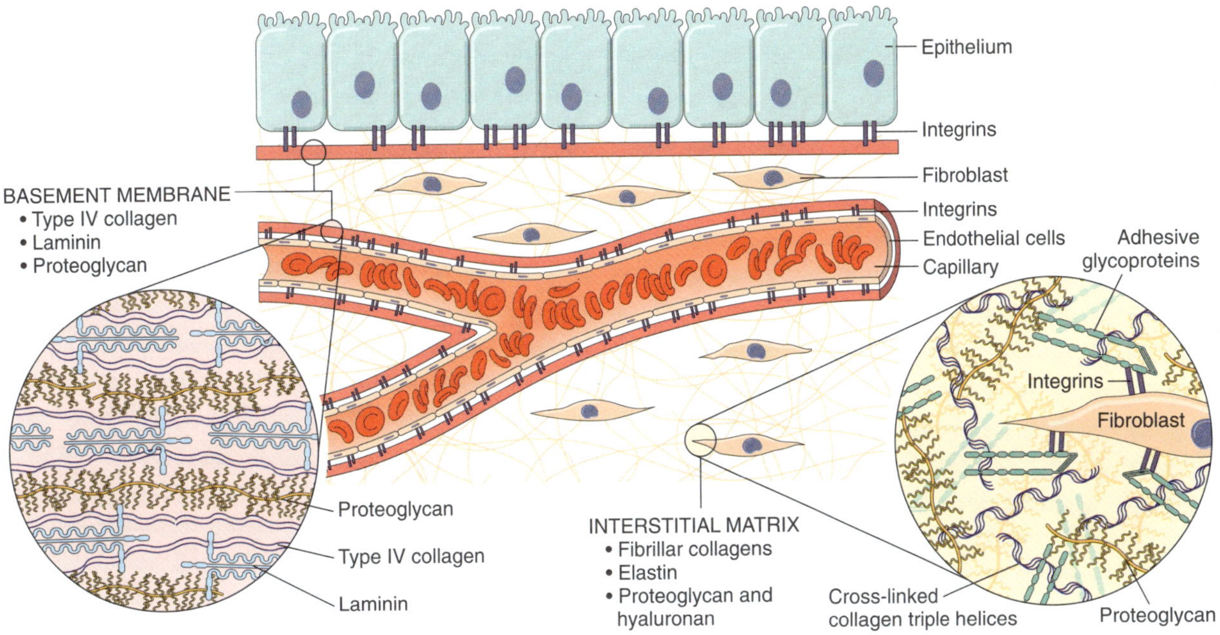

Figure 3–7

The major components of the extracellular matrix (ECM), including collagens, proteoglycans, and adhesive glycoproteins. Note that although there are some overlaps in their constituents, basement membrane and interstitial ECM have different general compositions and architecture. Both epithelial and mesenchymal cells (e.g., fibroblasts) interact with ECM via integrins. For the sake of simplification, many ECM components have been left out (e.g., elastin, fibrillin, hyaluronan, syndecan).

polypeptide chains braided into a ropelike triple helix. The collagen proteins are rich in hydroxyproline and hydroxylysine. About 30 collagen types have been identified, some of which are unique to specific cells and tissues. Some collagen types (e.g., types I, II, III, and V) form *fibrils* by virtue of lateral cross-linking of the triple helices. The fibrillar collagens form a major proportion of the connective tissue in healing wounds and particularly in scars. The tensile strength of the fibrillar collagens derives from their cross-linking, which is the result of covalent bonds catalyzed by the enzyme lysyl-oxidase. This process is dependent on vitamin C; therefore, children with ascorbate deficiency have skeletal deformities, bleed easily because of weak vascular wall basement membrane, and heal poorly. Genetic defects in these collagens cause diseases such as osteogenesis imperfecta and Ehlers-Danlos syndrome. Other collagens are nonfibrillar and may form basement membrane (type IV), or be components of other structures such as intervertebral discs (type IX) or dermal-epidermal junctions (type VII).

Elastin. Although tensile strength is derived from the fibrillar collagens, the ability of tissues to recoil and return to a baseline structure after physical stress is conferred by elastic tissue. This is especially important in the walls of large vessels (which must accommodate recurrent pulsatile flow), as well as in the uterus, skin, and ligaments. Morphologically, elastic fibers consist of a central core of *elastin* surrounded by a meshlike network of *fibrillin* glycoprotein. Like collagens, elastins require a glycine in every third position, but they differ from collagen by having fewer cross-links. The fibrillin meshwork serves as a scaffold for the deposition of elastin and assembly of elastic fibers; defects in fibrillin synthesis lead to skeletal abnormalities and weakened aortic walls (*Marfan syndrome;* Chapter 7).

Proteoglycans and Hyaluronan. Proteoglycans form highly hydrated compressible gels conferring resilience and lubrication (such as in the cartilage in joints). They consist of long polysaccharides called *glycosaminoglycans* (examples are *dermatan sulfate* and *heparan sulfate*) linked to a protein backbone. *Hyaluronan,* a huge molecule composed of many disaccharide repeats without a protein core, is also an important constituent of the ECM. Because of its ability to bind water, it forms a viscous, gelatin-like matrix. Besides providing compressibility to a tissue, proteoglycans also serve as reservoirs for growth factors secreted into the ECM (e.g., FGF and HGF). Proteoglycans can also be integral cell membrane proteins and have roles in cell proliferation, migration, and adhesion. For example, the transmembrane proteoglycan *syndecan* has attached hyaluronan chains that can bind such matrix growth factors as FGF, facilitating the interaction of FGF with cell surface receptors (Fig. 3–8). *Syndecan* also associates with the intracellular actin cytoskeleton and thereby helps to maintain normal epithelial sheet morphology.

Adhesive Glycoproteins and Adhesion Receptors. Adhesive glycoproteins and adhesion receptors are structurally diverse molecules involved in cell-to-cell adhesion, the linkage between cells and ECM, and binding between ECM components. The adhesive glycoproteins include fibronectin (major component of the interstitial ECM) and laminin (major constituent of basement membrane); they are described here as prototypical of the overall group. The adhesion receptors, also known as cell adhesion molecules (*CAMs*), are grouped into four families:

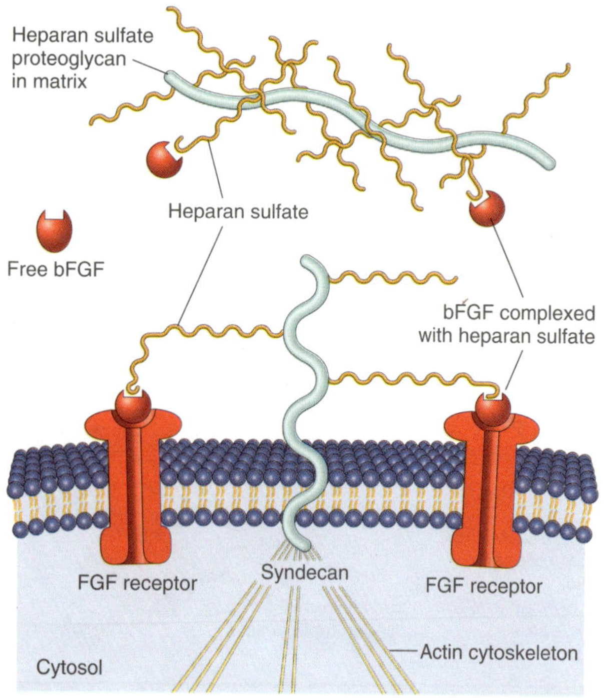

Figure 3–8

Proteoglycans in the ECM and on cells act as reservoirs for growth factors. Heparan sulfate binds basic fibroblast growth factor (FGF-2) secreted into the ECM. Any subsequent injury to the ECM can release FGF-2, which stimulates the recruitment of inflammatory cells, fibroblast activation, and new blood vessel formation. Syndecan is a cell surface proteoglycan with a transmembrane core protein and attached extracellular glycosaminoglycan side chains. The glycosaminoglycan chains can also bind free FGF-2 from the ECM and mediate interactions with cell surface FGF receptors. The cytoplasmic tail of syndecan attaches to the intracellular actin cytoskeleton and helps maintain the architecture of epithelial sheets. (Modified from Lodish H, et al [eds]: Molecular Cell Biology, 3rd ed. New York, WH Freeman, 1995.)

immunoglobulins, cadherins, selectins, and integrins. Only the integrins will be discussed here.

Fibronectin is a large (450-kD) disulfide-linked heterodimer synthesized by a variety of cells, including fibroblasts, monocytes, and endothelium. Fibronectin messenger RNA (mRNA) has two splice forms, which generate tissue and plasma fibronectin. Fibronectins have specific domains that bind to a wide spectrum of ECM components (e.g., collagen, fibrin, heparin, and proteoglycans) and can also attach to cell integrins via a tripeptide arginine–glycine–aspartic acid (abbreviated RGD) motif. Tissue fibronectin forms fibrillar aggregates at wound healing sites; plasma fibronectin binds to fibrin to form the provisional blood clot of a wound, which serves as substratum for ECM deposition and re-epithelialization.

Laminin is the most abundant glycoprotein in basement membrane. It is a 820-kD cross-shaped heterotrimer that connects cells to underlying ECM components such as type IV collagen and heparan sulfate. Besides mediating attachment to basement membrane, laminin can also modulate cell proliferation, differentiation, and motility.

Integrins are a family of transmembrane heterodimeric glycoproteins composed of α and β chains that are the main cellular receptors for ECM components, such as fibronectins and laminins. We discussed some of the integrins as leukocyte surface molecules that mediate firm adhesion and transmigration across endothelium at sites of inflammation, and we will meet them again when we discuss platelet aggregation in Chapter 4. Integrins are present in the plasma membrane of most animal cells, with the exception of red blood cells. They bind to many ECM components through RGD motifs, initiating signaling cascades that can affect cell locomotion, proliferation, and differentiation. Their intracellular domains link to actin filaments at focal adhesion complexes, through adaptor proteins such as talin and vinculin (Fig. 3–9). Integrin signal transduction utilizes the same intracellular signaling pathways used by growth factor receptors; for example, integrin-mediated adhesion to fibronectin can trigger elements of the MAP kinase, PI3 kinase, and protein kinase C pathways. In this manner, extracellular mechanical forces can be coupled to intracellular synthetic and transcriptional pathways (Fig. 3–9).

SUMMARY

Extracellular Matrix and Tissue Repair

- The ECM consists of: the interstitial matrix between cells, made up of collagens and several glycoproteins; and basement membranes underlying epithelia and surrounding vessels, made up of nonfibrillar collagen and laminin.
- The ECM serves several important functions:
  - It provides mechanical support to tissues; this is the role of collagens and elastin.
  - It acts as a substrate for cell growth and the formation of tissue microenvironments.
  - It regulates cell proliferation and differentiation; proteoglycans bind growth factors and display them at high concentration, and fibronectin and laminin stimulate cells via cellular integrin receptors.
- An intact ECM is required for tissue regeneration, and if the ECM is damaged, repair can only be accomplished by scar formation.

Having described the basic components of tissue repair, we now proceed to a discussion of repair by regeneration and by scar formation.

CELL AND TISSUE REGENERATION

As discussed above, cell renewal occurs continuously in labile tissues, such as the bone marrow, gut epithelium, and the skin. Damage to epithelia or an increased loss of blood cells can be corrected by the proliferation and differentiation of stem cells and, in the bone marrow, by proliferation of more differentiated progenitors. The renewal of hematopoietic cells is driven by growth factors

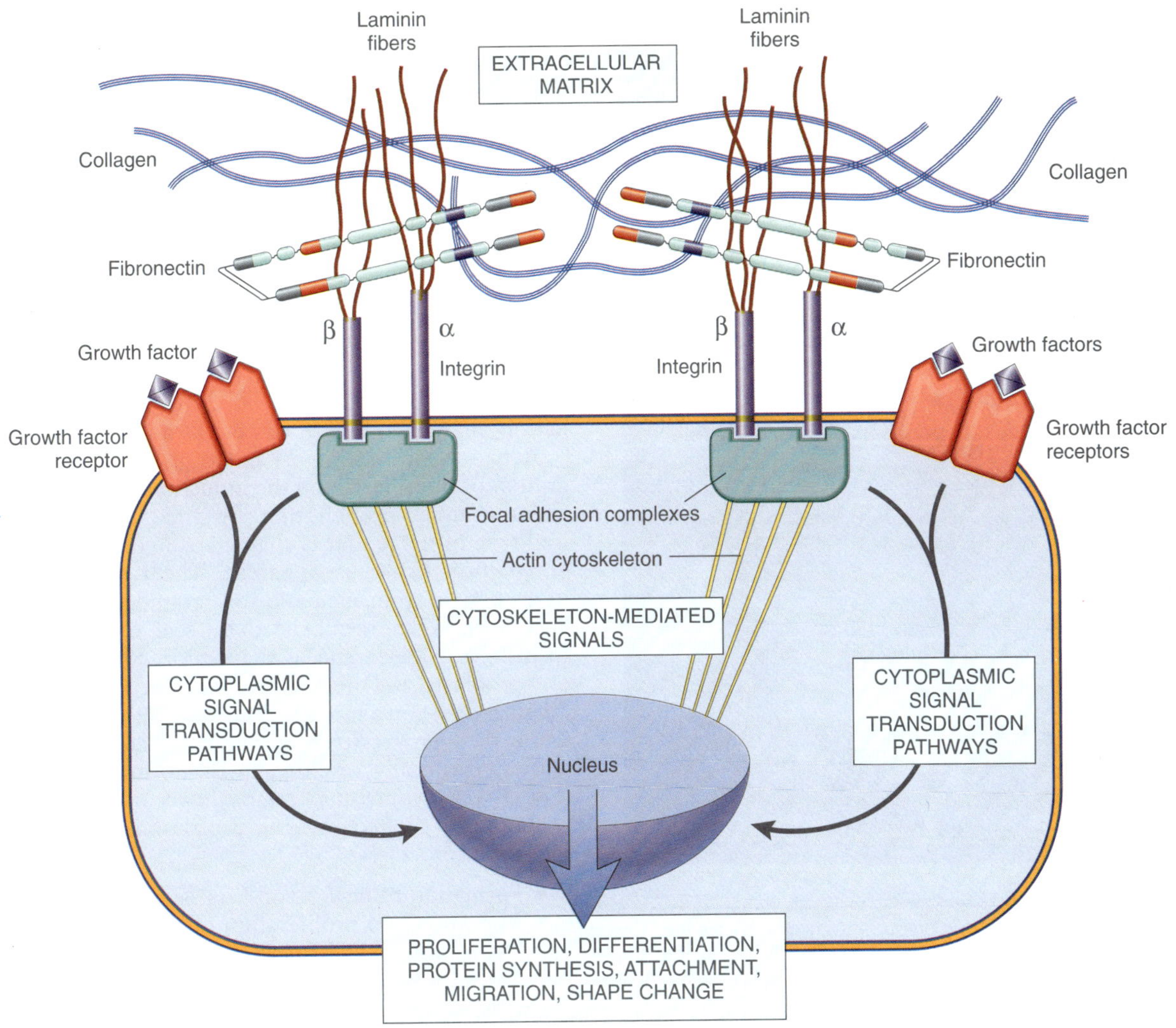

Figure 3–9

Mechanisms by which ECM components (e.g., fibronectin and laminin) and growth factors can influence cell proliferation, motility, differentiation, and protein synthesis. Integrins bind ECM and interact with the cytoskeleton at focal adhesion complexes (protein aggregates that include vinculin, α-actin, and talin). This can initiate the production of intracellular second messengers or can directly mediate nuclear signals. Cell surface receptors for growth factors activate signal transduction pathways that overlap with those activated by integrins. Signals received from growth factors and ECM components are integrated by the cell to yield various responses, including changes in cell proliferation, locomotion, and differentiation.

called *colony-stimulative factors (CSFs)*, which are produced in response to increased consumption or loss of blood cells. It is not known if growth factors play a role in the renewal of labile epithelia.

Tissue regeneration can occur in parenchymal organs with stable cell populations, but with the exception of the liver, this is usually a limited process. Pancreas, adrenal, thyroid, and lung tissues have some regenerative capacity. The surgical removal of a kidney elicits in the contralateral kidney a compensatory response that consists of both hypertrophy and hyperplasia of proximal duct cells. The mechanisms underlying this response are not understood. Much more dramatic, however, is the regenerative response of the liver that occurs after surgical removal of hepatic tissue. As much as 40% to 60% of the liver may be removed in a procedure called living-donor transplantation, in which a portion of the liver is resected from a normal individual and is transplanted into a recipient with end-stage liver disease (Fig. 3–10), or after partial hepatectomies performed for tumor removal. In all of these situations, the tissue resection triggers a proliferative response of the remaining hepatocytes (which are normally quiescent), and the subsequent replication of hepatic nonparenchymal cells. In experimental systems, hepatocyte replication after partial hepatectomy is initiated by cytokines (e.g., tumor necrosis factor [TNF] and interleukin 6 [IL-6]) that "prime" the cells for replication by stimulating the transition from G_0 to G_1 in the cell cycle. Progression through the cell cycle is dependent on the activity of growth factors such as *HGF and the EGF family of factors, which includes transforming growth factor α.*

- *HGF* is produced by fibroblasts, endothelial cells, and liver nonparenchymal cells. It induces proliferation

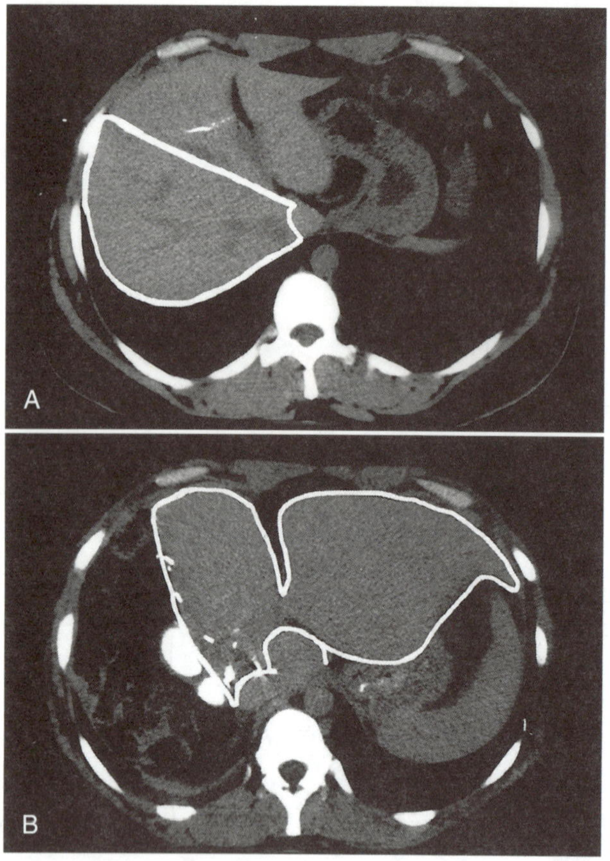

Figure 3–10

Regeneration of human liver. Computed tomography scans of the donor liver in living-donor liver transplantation. **A,** The liver of the donor before the operation. Note the right lobe *(outline),* which will be resected and used as a transplant. **B,** Scan of the same liver 1 week after resection of the right lobe; note the enlargement of the left lobe (outline) without regrowth of the right lobe. (Courtesy of R. Troisi, MD, Ghent University, Flanders, Belgium.)

of hepatocytes and most epithelial cells, including those in the skin, mammary gland, and lungs. HGF binds to a specific tyrosine kinase receptor (MET), which is frequently overexpressed in human cancers.

- *EGF and TGF-α* share a common receptor (epidermal growth factor receptor, or EGFR) with intrinsic tyrosine kinase activity. The "EGFR" is actually a family of receptors that respond to EGF, TGF-α, and other ligands of the EGF family. EGF/TGF-α is mitogenic for hepatocytes and most epithelial cells, including keratinocytes. In cutaneous wound healing EGF is produced by keratinocytes, macrophages, and other inflammatory cells. The main EGFR (referred to as EGFR1 or ERB B1) is frequently overexpressed in lung and some brain tumors and is an important therapeutic target for the treatment of these conditions. ERB B2 (also known as HER-2/NEU) has received great attention because of its overexpression in breast cancers, in which it is a target for effective cancer control (discussed in Chapter 6).

It should be emphasized that extensive regeneration or compensatory hyperplasia can occur only if the residual tissue is structurally and functionally intact, as after partial surgical resection. By contrast, if the tissue is damaged by infection or inflammation, regeneration is incomplete and is accompanied by scarring.

REPAIR BY CONNECTIVE TISSUE

If tissue injury is severe or chronic, and results in damage to parenchymal cells and epithelia as well as the stromal framework, or if nondividing cells are injured, repair cannot be accomplished by regeneration alone. Under these conditions, repair occurs by replacement of the nonregenerated cells with connective tissue, or by a combination of regeneration of some cells and scar formation.

Repair begins within 24 hours of injury by the emigration of fibroblasts and the induction of fibroblast and endothelial cell proliferation. By 3 to 5 days, a specialized type of tissue that is characteristic of healing, called *granulation tissue,* is apparent. The term granulation tissue derives from the pink, soft, granular gross appearance, such as that seen beneath the scab of a skin wound. Its histologic appearance is characterized by proliferation of fibroblasts and new thin-walled, delicate capillaries (angiogenesis), in a loose ECM (Fig. 3–11A). Granulation tissue then progressively accumulates connective tissue matrix, eventually resulting in the formation of a scar (Fig. 3–11B), which may remodel over time.

Repair by connective tissue deposition consists of four sequential processes:

- Formation of new blood vessels (*angiogenesis*)
- Migration and proliferation of fibroblasts
- Deposition of ECM (*scar formation*)
- Maturation and reorganization of the fibrous tissue (*remodeling*)

Angiogenesis

Blood vessels are assembled by two processes: *vasculogenesis,* in which the primitive vascular network is assembled from *angioblasts* (endothelial cell precursors) during embryonic development; and *angiogenesis,* or *neovascularization,* in which preexisting vessels send out capillary sprouts to produce new vessels (Fig. 3–12). Angiogenesis is a critical process in healing at sites of injury, in the development of collateral circulations at sites of ischemia, and in allowing tumors to increase in size beyond the constraints of their original blood supply. It has recently been found that endothelial precursor cells may migrate from the bone marrow to areas of injury and participate in angiogenesis at these sites. Much work has been done to understand the mechanisms underlying angiogenesis, and therapies to either augment the process (e.g., to improve blood flow to a heart ravaged by coronary atherosclerosis) or inhibit it (to frustrate tumor growth) are being developed.

The main steps that occur in angiogenesis from preexisting vessels are listed below.

- Vasodilation in response to nitric oxide and increased permeability of the preexisting vessel induced by vascular endothelial growth factor (VEGF)

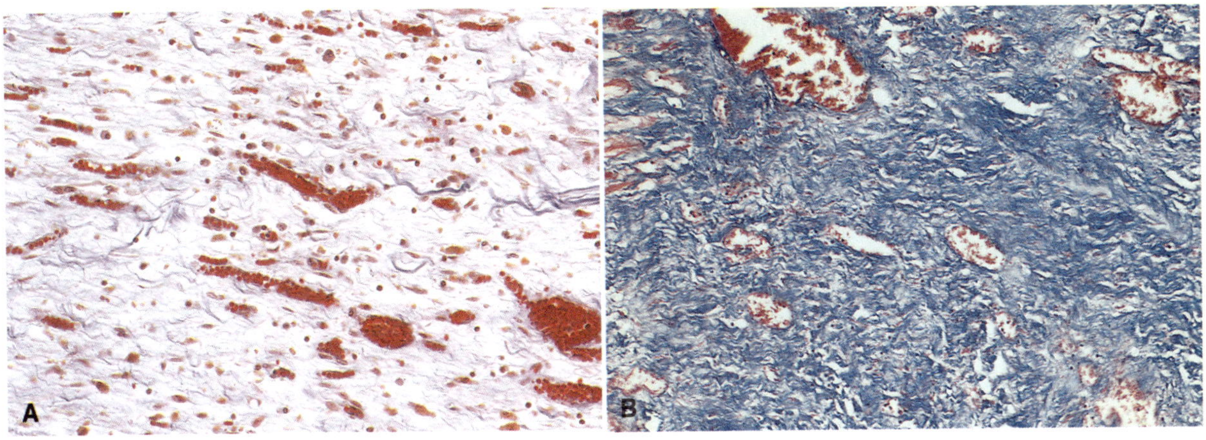

Figure 3–11

A, Granulation tissue showing numerous blood vessels, edema, and a loose ECM containing occasional inflammatory cells. Collagen is stained *blue* by the trichrome stain; minimal mature collagen can be seen at this point. **B,** Trichrome stain of mature scar, showing dense collagen with only scattered vascular channels.

- Migration of endothelial cells toward the area of tissue injury
- Proliferation of endothelial cells just behind the leading front of migrating cells
- Inhibition of endothelial cell proliferation and remodeling into capillary tubes
- Recruitment of periendothelial cells (pericytes for small capillaries and smooth muscle cells for larger vessels) to form the mature vessel

As mentioned, bone marrow endothelial precursor cells may also contribute to angiogenesis. The nature of

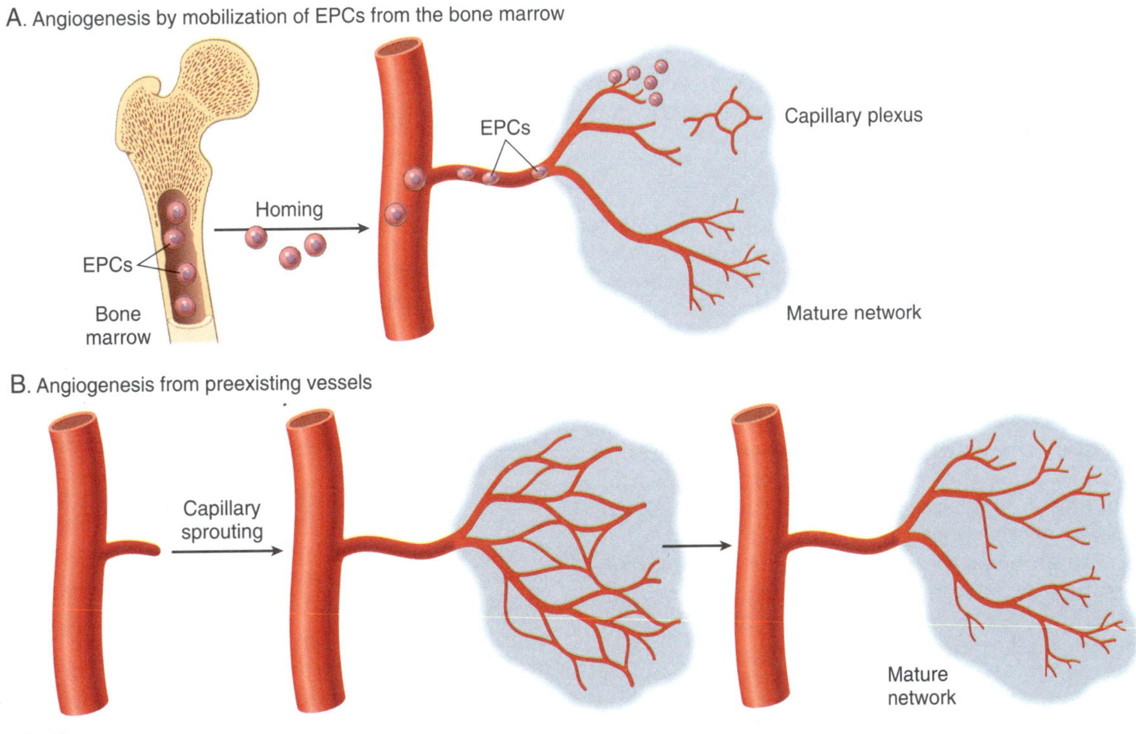

Figure 3–12

Angiogenesis resulting from, **A,** the mobilization of bone marrow endothelial precursor cells (EPCs), and, **B,** from preexisting vessels at the site of injury. EPCs can be mobilized from the bone marrow and migrate to a site of injury or tumor growth. At these sites EPCs differentiate and form a mature network by linking with preexisting vessels. In angiogenesis from preexisting vessels, endothelial cells from these vessels become motile and proliferate to form capillary sprouts. Regardless of the mechanism of angiogenesis, vessel maturation requires the recruitment of pericytes and smooth muscle cells to form the periendothelial layer. (Modified from Conway EM et al., Molecular mechanisms of blood vessel growth. Cardiovasc Res 49:507, 2001.)

the homing mechanism by which endothelial precursor cells located in the bone marrow migrate into sites of injury is unknown. These cells may participate in the replacement of lost endothelial cells, in the re-endothelialization of vascular implants, in the neovascularization of cutaneous wounds and ischemic tissues, and in tumor development.

New vessels formed during angiogenesis are leaky because of incompletely formed interendothelial junctions and because VEGF increases vessel permeability. This leakiness explains why granulation tissue is often edematous, and accounts in part for the edema that may persist in healing wounds long after the acute inflammatory response has resolved. Structural ECM proteins participate in the process of vessel sprouting in angiogenesis, largely through interactions with integrin receptors in endothelial cells. Nonstructural ECM proteins contribute to angiogenesis by destabilizing cell–ECM interactions to facilitate continued cell migration (e.g., *thrombospondin* and *tenascin* C) or degrade the ECM to permit remodeling and ingrowth of vessels (e.g., *plasminogen activator* and *matrix metalloproteinases [MMPs]*).

Growth Factors Involved in Angiogenesis. Several factors induce angiogenesis, but the most important are *VEGF* and *basic fibroblast growth factor (FGF-2)*.

VEGFs constitute a family of growth factors that include VEGF-A, -B, -C, and -D. VEGF-A is generally referred to as VEGF; VEGF-C selectively regulates lymphoid vasculature. VEGFs are dimeric glycoproteins with many isoforms. Listed below are some of the properties of VEGF:

- VEGFs are expressed at low levels in most tissues and are highly expressed in kidney podocytes and myocardial cells.
- VEGFs bind to a family of receptors (VEGFR-1, -2, and -3) with tyrosine kinase activity. The most important of these receptors for angiogenesis is VEGFR-2, which is restricted to endothelial cells. Targeted mutations in this receptor result in lack of vasculogenesis.
- Several agents can induce VEGFs, *the most important being hypoxia.* Other inducers are platelet-derived growth factor (PDGF), TGF-β, and TGF-α.

In angiogenesis originating from preexisting local vessels, VEGF stimulates both proliferation and motility of endothelial cells, thus initiating the process of capillary sprouting. In angiogenesis involving endothelial cell precursors from the bone marrow, VEGF acts through VEGFR-2 to mobilize these cells from the bone marrow and to induce proliferation and motility of these cells at the sites of angiogenesis. Regardless of the process that leads to capillary formation, new vessels need to be stabilized by the recruitment of pericytes and smooth muscle cells and by the deposition of connective tissue. *Angiopoietins 1* and *2 (Ang 1* and *Ang 2)* and the growth factors PDGF and TGF-β participate in the stabilization process. In particular, Ang1 interacts with a receptor on endothelial cells called Tie2 to recruit periendothelial cells. PDGF participates in the recruitment of smooth muscle cells; TGF-β enhances the production of ECM proteins.

FGFs constitute a family of factors with more than 20 members. The best characterized are *FGF-1 (acidic FGF)* and *FGF-2 (basic FGF)*. These growth factors are produced by many cell types and bind to a family of plasma membrane receptors that have tyrosine kinase activity. Released FGF can bind to heparan sulfate and be stored in the ECM. FGF-2 participates in angiogenesis mostly by stimulating the proliferation of endothelial cells. It also promotes the migration of macrophages and fibroblasts to the damaged area, and stimulates epithelial cell migration to cover epidermal wounds. *Keratinocyte growth factor (FGF-7)* may participate in cutaneous wound healing by enhancing the proliferation and migration of keratinocytes and may also protect the integrity of the epithelium of the oral cavity and gastrointestinal tract.

Migration of Fibroblasts and ECM Deposition (Scar Formation)

Scar formation builds on the granulation tissue framework of new vessels and loose ECM that develop early at the repair site. It occurs in two steps: *(1) migration and proliferation of fibroblasts into the site of injury and (2) deposition of ECM by these cells.* The recruitment and stimulation of fibroblasts is driven by many growth factors, *including PDGF, FGF-2 (described above), and TGF-β.* One source of these factors is the activated endothelium, but more importantly, growth factors are also elaborated by inflammatory cells. Macrophages, in particular, are important cellular constituents of granulation tissue, and besides clearing extracellular debris and fibrin at the site of injury, they elaborate a host of mediators that induce fibroblast proliferation and ECM production. Sites of inflammation are also rich in mast cells, and with the appropriate chemotactic milieu lymphocytes may also be present. Each of these can contribute directly or indirectly to fibroblast proliferation and activation.

As healing progresses, the number of proliferating fibroblasts and new vessels decreases; however, the fibroblasts progressively assume a more synthetic phenotype, and hence there is increased deposition of ECM. Collagen synthesis, in particular, is critical to the development of strength in a healing wound site. As described later, collagen synthesis by fibroblasts begins early in wound healing (days 3 to 5) and continues for several weeks, depending on the size of the wound. As described below, many of the same growth factors that regulate fibroblast proliferation also participate in stimulating ECM synthesis. *Net collagen accumulation, however, depends not only on increased synthesis but also on diminished collagen degradation* (discussed later). Ultimately, the granulation tissue scaffolding evolves into a scar composed of largely inactive, spindle-shaped fibroblasts, dense collagen, fragments of elastic tissue, and other ECM components (see Fig. 3–11B). As the scar matures, there is progressive vascular regression, which eventually transforms the highly vascularized granulation tissue into a pale, largely avascular scar.

Growth Factors Involved in ECM Deposition and Scar Formation. Many growth factors are involved in these processes, including TGF-β, PDGF, and FGF. Because FGF is also involved in angiogenesis, it was described earlier. Here we briefly describe some properties of TGF-β and PDGF.

TGF-β belongs to a family of homologous polypeptides (TGF-β1, -β2, and -β3) that includes other members such as bone morphogenetic proteins, activins, and inhibins. TGF-β1 has a widespread distribution and is usually referred to as TGF-β. The active factor binds to two cell surface receptors with serine/threonine kinase activity, triggering the phosphorylation of transcription factors called *smads*. TGF-β has many and often opposite effects, depending on the cell type and the metabolic state of the tissue. In the context of inflammation and repair, TGF-β has two main functions:

- *TGF-β is a potent fibrogenic agent.* It stimulates the production of collagen, fibronectin, and proteoglycans, and it inhibits collagen degradation by both decreasing proteinase activity and increasing the activity of tissue inhibitors of proteinases known as TIMPs (discussed below). TGF-β is involved not only in scar formation after injury but also in the development of fibrosis in lung, liver, and kidneys that follows chronic inflammation.
- *TGF-β inhibits lymphocyte proliferation and can have a strong anti-inflammatory effect.* Mice lacking TGF-β have widespread inflammation and abundant lymphocyte proliferation.

PDGF belongs to a family of closely related proteins, each consisting of two chains, designated A and B. There are five main PDGF isoforms, designated AA, AB, BB, CC, and DD. PDGFs bind to receptors designated as PDGFR α and PDGFR β. PDGF BB is the prototype for the family and is referred to as PDGF. It is stored in platelets and released on platelet activation, and produced by endothelial cells, activated macrophages, smooth muscle cells, and many tumor cells. PDGF causes migration and proliferation of fibroblasts, smooth muscle cells, and macrophages.

Cytokines (discussed in Chapter 2 as mediators of inflammation and in Chapter 5, in the context of immune responses) may also function as growth factors and participate in ECM deposition and scar formation. IL-1 and TNF, for example, induce fibroblast proliferation and can have a fibrogenic effect. They are also chemotactic for fibroblasts and stimulate the synthesis of collagen and collagenase by these cells.

ECM and Tissue Remodeling

The transition from granulation tissue to scar involves shifts in the composition of the ECM; even after its synthesis and deposition, scar ECM continues to be modified and remodeled. *The outcome of the repair process is, in part, a balance between ECM synthesis and degradation.* We have already discussed the cells and factors that regulate ECM synthesis. The *degradation* of collagens and other ECM components is accomplished by a family of matrix metalloproteinases (MMPs), which are dependent on *zinc ions* for their activity. MMPs should be distinguished from neutrophil elastase, cathepsin G, plasmin, and other *serine proteinases* that can also degrade ECM but are not metalloenzymes. MMPs include *interstitial collagenases,* which cleave fibrillar collagen (MMP-1,-2 and -3); *gelatinases* (MMP-2 and 9), which degrade amorphous collagen and fibronectin; and *stromelysins* (MMP-3, -10, and -11), which degrade a variety of ECM constituents, including proteoglycans, laminin, fibronectin, and amorphous collagen.

MMPs are produced by a variety of cell types (fibroblasts, macrophages, neutrophils, synovial cells, and some epithelial cells), and their synthesis and secretion are regulated by growth factors, cytokines, and other agents (Fig. 3–13). Their synthesis is inhibited by TGF-β and may be suppressed pharmacologically with steroids. Given the potential to wreak havoc in tissues, *the activity of the MMPs is tightly controlled.* Thus, they are typically elaborated as inactive (*zymogen*) precursors that must be first activated; this is accomplished by certain chemicals or proteases (e.g., plasmin) likely to be present only at sites of injury. In addition, activated collagenases

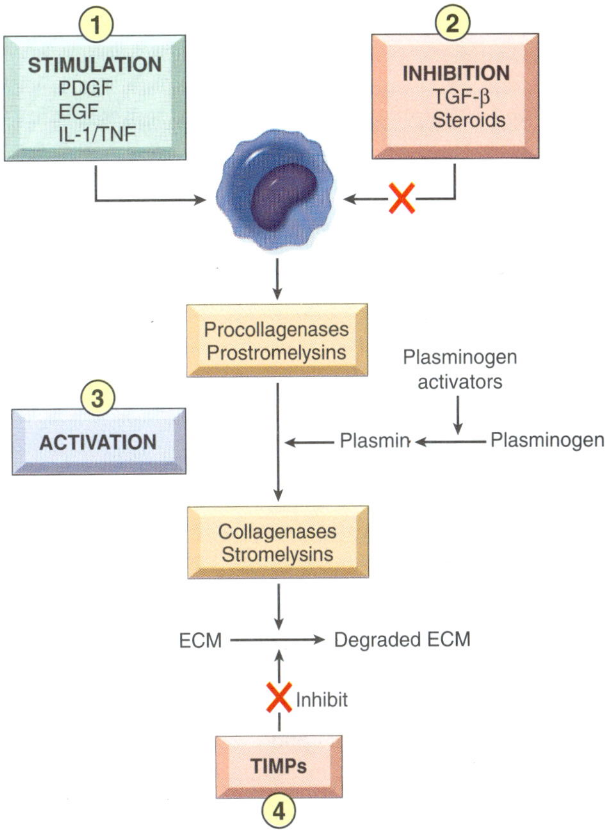

Figure 3–13

Matrix metalloproteinase regulation. The four mechanisms shown include (1) regulation of synthesis by a variety of growth factors or cytokines, (2) inhibition of synthesis by corticosteroids or transforming growth factor β (TGF-β), (3) regulation of the activation of the secreted but inactive precursors, and (4) blockade of the enzymes by specific tissue inhibitors of metalloproteinases (TIMPs). ECM, Extracellular matrix; EGF, epidermal growth factor; IL-1, interleukin 1; PDGF, platelet-derived growth factor; TNF, tumor necrosis factor. (Modified from Matrisian LM: Metalloproteinases and their inhibitors in matrix remodeling. Trends Genet 6:122, 1990.)

can be rapidly inhibited by specific tissue inhibitors of metalloproteinases (*TIMPs*), produced by most mesenchymal cells. MMPs and their inhibitors are spatially and temporally regulated in healing wounds. They are essential in the debridement of injured sites and in the remodeling of the ECM.

A large and important family of enzymes related to MMPs is called *ADAM* (a disintegrin and metalloproteinase). ADAMs are anchored to the plasma membrane and cleave and release extracellular domains of cell surface proteins, such as TNF, TGF-α, and other members of the EGF family.

SUMMARY

Regeneration and Repair by Connective Tissue

- Tissues can be repaired by regeneration with complete restoration of form and function, or by replacement with connective tissue and scar formation
- The main components of connective tissue repair are angiogenesis, migration and proliferation of fibroblasts, collagen synthesis, and connective tissue remodeling.
- Repair by connective tissue starts with the formation of granulation tissue and culminates in the laying down of fibrous tissue.
- Multiple growth factors stimulate the proliferation of the cell types involved in repair.
- TGF-β is a potent fibrogenic agent; ECM deposition depends on the balance between fibrogenic agents, metalloproteinases (MMPs) that digest ECM, and the tissue inhibitors of MMPs (TIMPs).

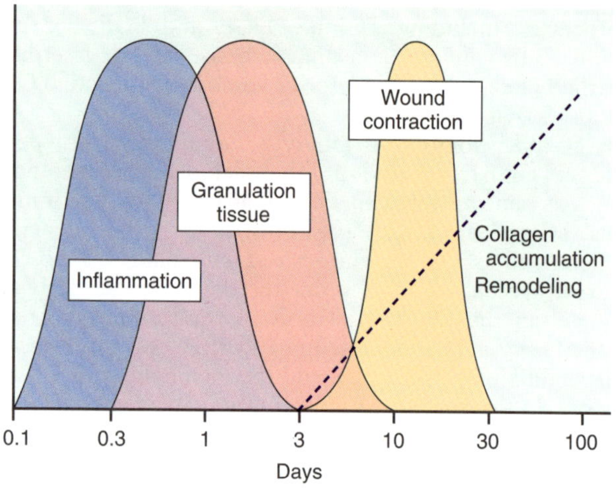

Figure 3–14

Phases of wound healing. Wound contraction occurs only in healing by second intention (see text). (Data from Clark RAF: Cutaneous wound repair. I. Basic biologic considerations. J Am Acad Dermatol 13:702, 1985.)

CUTANEOUS WOUND HEALING

So far, we have discussed general aspects of healing. In this section we specifically describe the healing of skin wounds (*cutaneous wound healing*). This is a process that involves both epithelial regeneration and the formation of connective tissue scar and is thus illustrative of the general principles that apply to wound healing in all tissues. Specialized cell types first clear the inciting injury and then progressively build the scaffolding to fill in any defect. Re-epithelialization of the wound surface takes place mostly by cell migration from the edges of the wound. The events are orchestrated by interplay of growth factors and ECM; physical conditions, including the forces generated by changes in cell shape, also contribute. The properties of various growth factors involved in repair have already been discussed; Table 3–2 lists the main factors that act at each wound healing step. However, one should be aware that different tissues in the body have specific cells and features that modify the basic scheme discussed here.

Cutaneous wound healing has three main phases: *(1) inflammation, (2) formation of granulation tissue, and (3) ECM deposition and remodeling* (Fig. 3–14). Larger wounds also *contract* during the healing process (discussed later). As we have already seen, events in wound healing overlap to a great extent and cannot be completely separated from each other. Based on the nature of the wound, *the healing of cutaneous wounds can occur by first or second intention.*

Table 3–2 Growth Factors and Cytokines Affecting Various Steps in Wound Healing

Epithelial proliferation	EGF, TGF-α, KGF, HGF
Monocyte chemotaxis	PDGF, FGF, TGF-β
Fibroblast migration	PDGF, FGF, TGF-β
Fibroblast proliferation	PDGF, EGF, FGF, TNF
Angiogenesis	VEGF, Ang, FGF
Collagen synthesis	TGF-β, PDGF
Collagenase secretion	PDGF, FGF, EGF, TNF; TGF-β inhibits

Ang, Angiopoietin; TNF, tumor necrosis factor. See Table 3–1 for other abbreviations.

Healing by First Intention

One of the simplest examples of wound repair is the healing of a clean, uninfected surgical incision approximated by surgical sutures (Fig. 3–15). This is referred to as *primary union*, or *healing by first intention.* The incision causes only focal disruption of epithelial basement membrane continuity and death of a relatively few epithelial and connective tissue cells. As a result, epithelial regeneration predominates over fibrosis. A small scar is formed, but there is minimal wound contraction. The narrow incisional space first fills with fibrin-clotted blood, which is rapidly invaded by granulation tissue and covered by new epithelium.

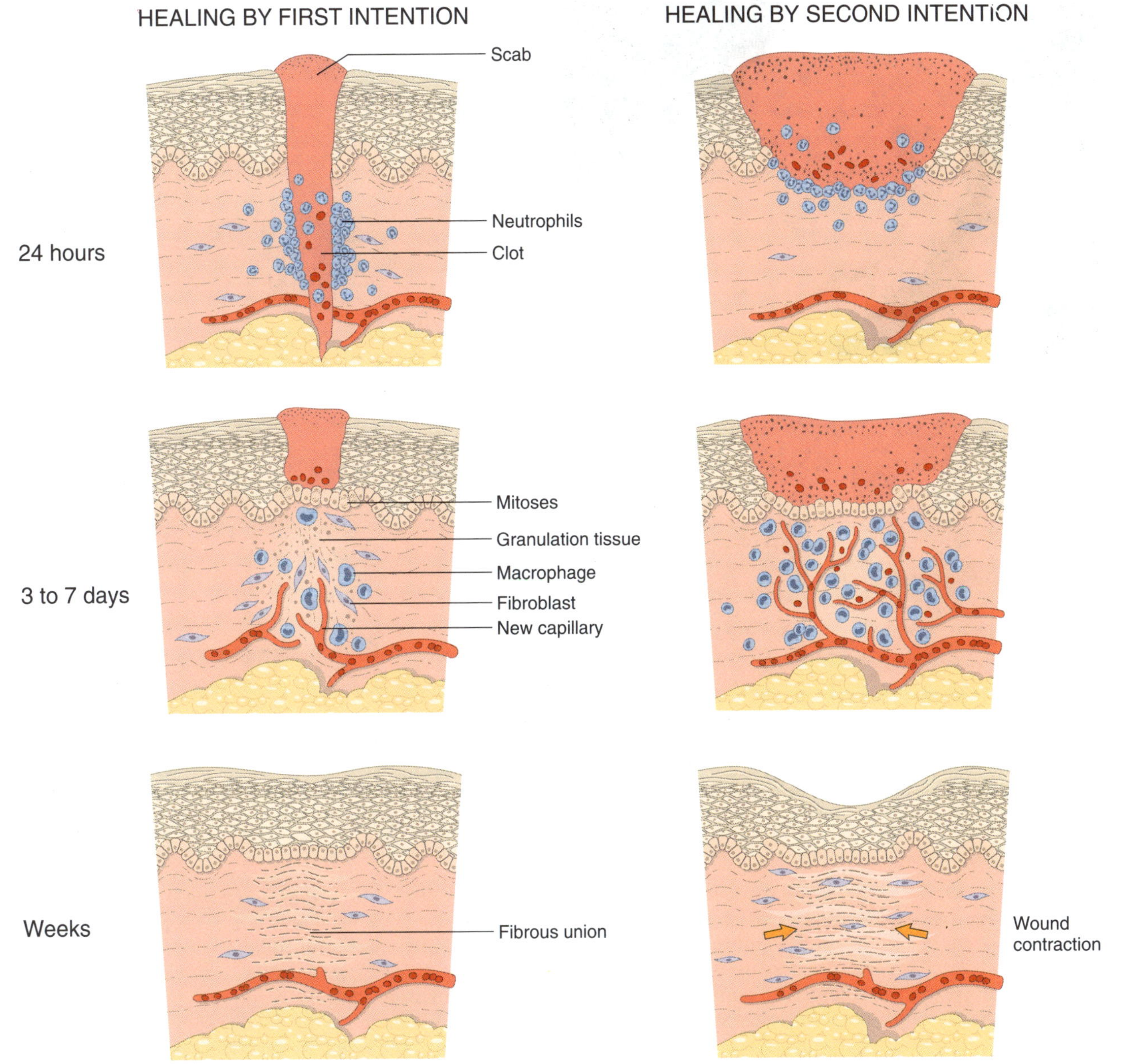

Figure 3–15

Steps in wound healing by first intention (*left*) and second intention (*right*). In the latter, note the large amount of granulation tissue and wound contraction.

Within 24 hours, neutrophils are seen at the incision margin, migrating toward the *fibrin clot.* Basal cells at the cut edge of the epidermis begin to show increased mitotic activity. Within 24 to 48 hours, epithelial cells from both edges have begun to migrate and proliferate along the dermis, depositing basement membrane components as they progress. The cells meet in the midline beneath the surface scab, yielding a thin but continuous epithelial layer.

By day 3, neutrophils have been largely replaced by macrophages, and granulation tissue progressively invades the incision space. Collagen fibers are now evident at the incision margins, but these are vertically oriented and do not bridge the incision. Epithelial cell proliferation continues, yielding a thickened epidermal covering layer.

By day 5, neovascularization reaches its peak as granulation tissue fills the incisional space. Collagen fibrils become more abundant and begin to bridge the incision. The epidermis recovers its normal thickness as differentiation of surface cells yields a mature epidermal architecture with surface keratinization.

During the second week, there is continued collagen accumulation and fibroblast proliferation. The leukocyte infiltrate, edema, and increased vascularity are substantially diminished. The long process of "blanching" begins, accomplished by increasing collagen deposition within the incisional scar and the regression of vascular channels.

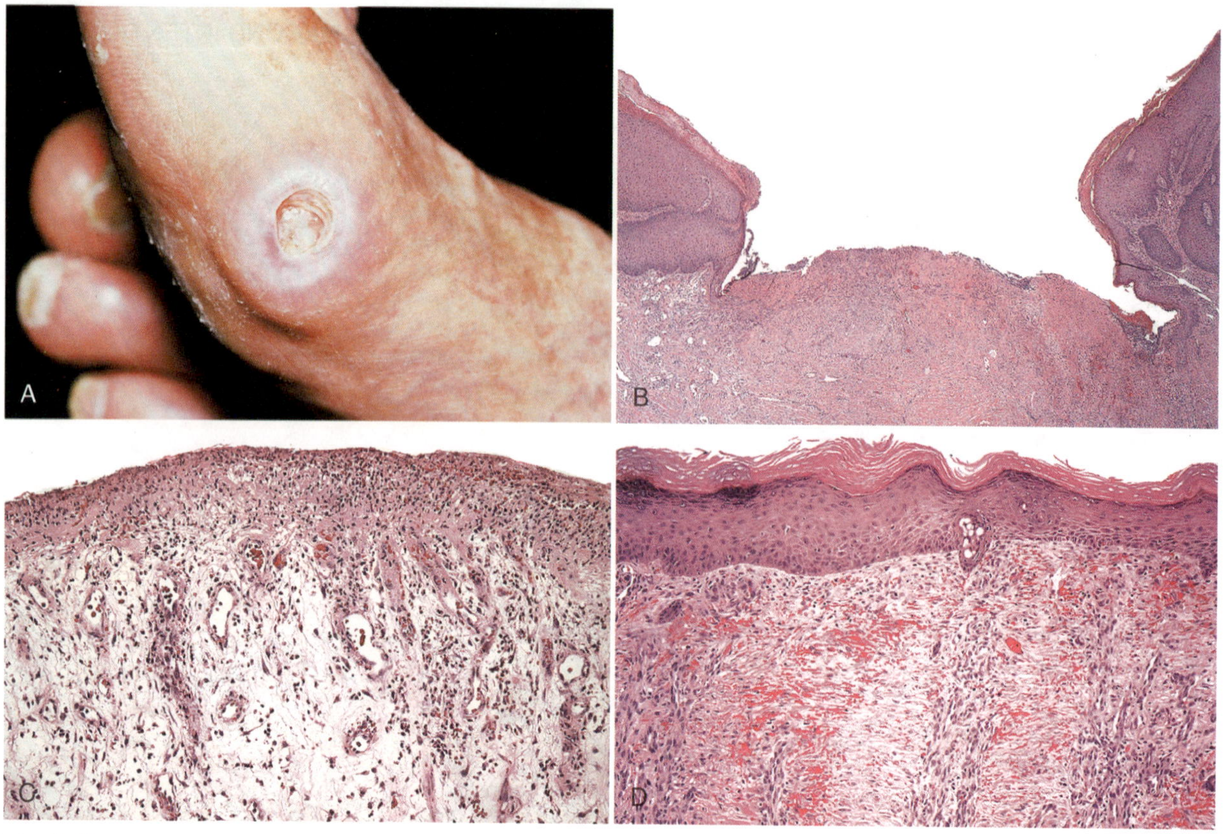

Figure 3–16

Healing of skin ulcers. **A,** Pressure ulcer of the skin, commonly found in diabetic patients. **B,** A skin ulcer with a large gap between the edges of the lesion. **C,** A thin layer of epidermal re-epithelialization, and extensive granulation tissue formation in the dermis. **D,** Continuing re-epithelialization of the epidermis and wound contraction. (Courtesy of Z. Argenyi, MD, University of Washington, Seattle.)

By the end of the first month, the scar comprises a cellular connective tissue largely devoid of inflammatory cells and covered by an essentially normal epidermis. However, the dermal appendages destroyed in the line of the incision are permanently lost. The tensile strength of the wound increases with time, as described later.

Healing by Second Intention

When cell or tissue loss is more extensive, such as in large wounds, abscess formation, and ulceration, the repair process is more complex, as is also the case after infarction in parenchymal organs. In second-intention healing, also known as *healing by secondary union* (Figs. 3–15 and 3–16), the inflammatory reaction is more intense, there is abundant development of granulation tissue, and the wound contracts by the action of *myofibroblasts.* This is followed by accumulation of ECM and formation of a large scar.

Secondary healing differs from primary healing in several respects:

- *A larger clot or scab* rich in fibrin and fibronectin forms at the surface of the wound.
- *Inflammation is more intense* because large tissue defects have a greater volume of necrotic debris, exudate, and fibrin that must be removed. Consequently, large defects have a greater potential for secondary, inflammation-mediated, injury (Chapter 2).
- *Much larger amounts of granulation tissue are formed.* Larger defects require a greater volume of granulation tissue to fill in the gaps and provide the underlying framework for the regrowth of tissue epithelium. A greater volume of granulation tissue generally results in a greater mass of scar tissue.
- *Secondary healing involves wound contraction.* Within 6 weeks, for example, large skin defects may be reduced to 5% to 10% of their original size, largely by contraction. This process has been ascribed to the presence of *myofibroblasts,* which are modified fibroblasts exhibiting many of the ultrastructural and functional features of contractile smooth muscle cells.

Wound Strength

Carefully sutured wounds have approximately 70% of the strength of unwounded skin, largely because of the placement of the sutures. When sutures are removed, usually at 1 week, wound strength is approximately 10% of that of unwounded skin, but this increases rapidly over the next 4 weeks. The recovery of tensile strength results from collagen synthesis exceeding degradation during the first 2 months, and from structural modifications of collagen (e.g., cross-linking and increased fiber size) when synthesis declines at later times. Wound strength reaches approximately 70% to 80% of normal by 3 months but usually does not substantially improve beyond that point.

PATHOLOGIC ASPECTS OF REPAIR

Wound healing may be altered by a variety of influences, frequently reducing the quality or adequacy of the reparative process. *Particularly important are infections and diabetes.* Variables that modify wound healing may be extrinsic (e.g., infection) or intrinsic to the injured tissue:

- *Infection* is the single most important cause of delay in healing; it prolongs the inflammation phase of the process and potentially increases the local tissue injury. *Nutrition* has profound effects on wound healing; protein deficiency, for example, and particularly vitamin C deficiency, inhibits collagen synthesis and retards healing. *Glucocorticoids* (steroids) have well-documented anti-inflammatory effects, and their administration may result in poor wound strength due to diminished fibrosis. In some instances, however, the anti-inflammatory effects of glucocorticoids are desirable. For example, in corneal infections, glucocorticoids are sometimes prescribed (along with antibiotics) to reduce the likelihood of opacity that may result from collagen deposition. *Mechanical variables* such as increased local pressure or torsion may cause wounds to pull apart, or *dehisce. Poor perfusion,* due either to arteriosclerosis and diabetes or to obstructed venous drainage (e.g. in varicose veins), also impairs healing. Finally, *foreign bodies* such as fragments of steel, glass, or even bone impede healing.
- *The type (and volume) of tissue injured* is critical. *Complete restoration can occur only in tissues composed of stable and labile cells;* even then, extensive injury will probably result in incomplete tissue regeneration and at least partial loss of function. *Injury to tissues composed of permanent cells must inevitably result in scarring* with, at most, attempts at functional compensation by the remaining viable elements. Such is the case with healing of a myocardial infarct.
- *The location of the injury* and the character of the tissue in which the injury occurs are also important. For example, *inflammation arising in tissue spaces (e.g., pleural, peritoneal, synovial cavities) develops extensive exudates.* Subsequent repair may occur by digestion of the exudate, initiated by the proteolytic enzymes of leukocytes and resorption of the liquefied exudate. This is called *resolution,* and in the absence of cellular necrosis, normal tissue architecture is generally restored. However, in the setting of larger accumulations, the exudate undergoes *organization:* granulation tissue grows into the exudate, and a fibrous scar ultimately forms.

Aberrations of cell growth and ECM production may occur even in what begins as normal wound healing. For example, the accumulation of exuberant amounts of collagen can give rise to prominent, raised scars known as *keloids* (Fig. 3–17). There appears to be a heritable predisposition to keloid formation, and the condition is more common in blacks. Healing wounds may also generate excessive granulation tissue that protrudes above the level of the surrounding skin and hinders re-epithelialization. This is called *exuberant granulation,* or *proud flesh,* and restoration of epithelial continuity requires cautery or surgical resection of the granulation tissue.

The mechanisms underlying the disabling *fibrosis* associated with chronic inflammatory diseases such as rheumatoid arthritis, pulmonary fibrosis, and cirrhosis have many similarities to those involved in normal wound healing. In these diseases, persistent stimulation of fibrogenesis results from chronic immune reactions that sustain the synthesis and secretion of growth factors, fibrogenic cytokines, and proteases. For example, collagen degradation by collagenases, normally important in wound remodeling, is responsible for much of the joint destruction seen in rheumatoid arthritis (Chapter 5).

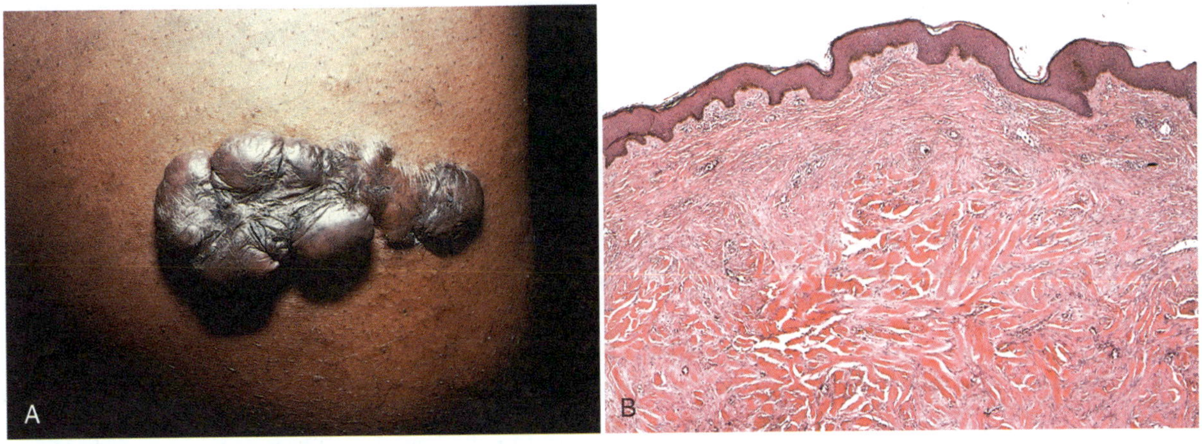

Figure 3–17

Keloid. **A,** Excess collagen deposition in the skin forming a raised scar known as a keloid. **B,** Thick connective tissue deposition in the dermis. (**A,** From Murphy GF, Herzberg AJ: Atlas of Dermatology. Philadelphia, WB Saunders, 1996. **B,** Courtesy of Z. Argenyi, MD, University of Washington, Seattle.)

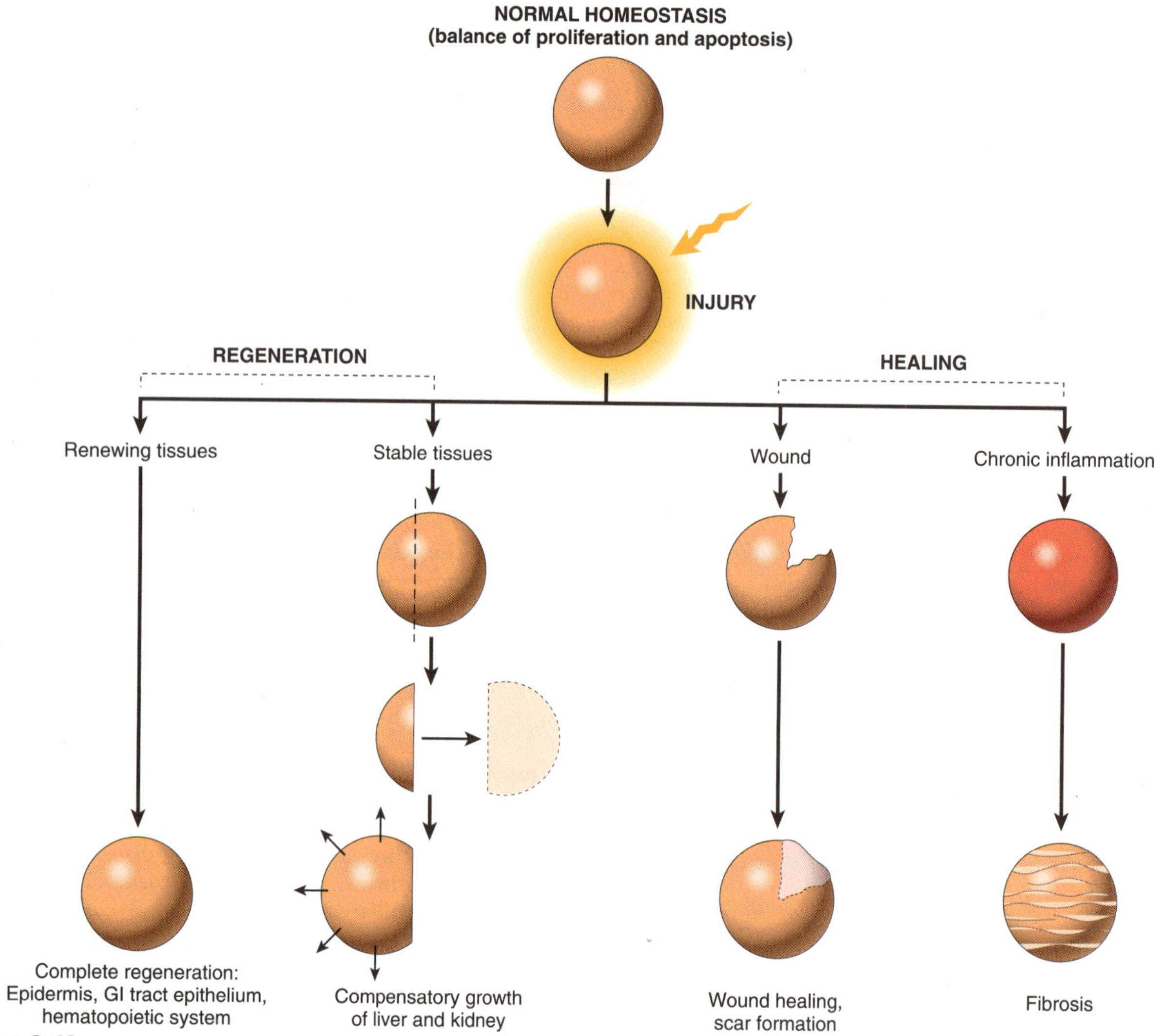

Figure 3–18

Overview of repair responses. Repair after injury can occur by regeneration of cells or tissues that restores normal tissue structure, or by healing, which leads to the formation of a scar. Chronic inflammation may cause massive fibrosis.

SUMMARY

Cutaneous Wound Healing and Pathologic Aspects of Repair

- The main phases of cutaneous wound healing are inflammation, formation of granulation tissue, and ECM remodeling.
- Cutaneous wounds can heal by primary union (first intention) or secondary union (secondary intention); secondary healing involves more extensive scarring and wound contraction.
- Wound healing can be altered by many conditions, particularly infection and diabetes; the type, volume and location of the injury are important factors for healing.
- Excessive production of ECM can cause keloids in the skin.
- Persistent stimulation of collagen synthesis in chronic inflammatory diseases leads to fibrosis of the tissue.

OVERVIEW OF REPAIR PROCESSES

In this chapter we discussed various processes of tissue repair and their molecular mechanisms. A general overview of these processes is presented in Figure 3–18. We have seen that not all injuries result in permanent damage, and that stable tissues such as the liver and tubular epithelium of the kidney can grow to compensate for tissue loss. Thus, some injuries can be resolved with almost perfect restoration of structure and function by cell and tissue regeneration. More often, though—depending on the type and extent of injury, the nature of the injured tissue, and persistence of inflammatory stimuli—injury results in some degree of residual scarring. Although it is functionally imperfect, a scar provides a resilient permanent patch that allows the remaining intact parenchyma to continue functioning. Occasionally, however, the scarring may be so large that it results in massive fibrosis, or so situated that it causes permanent dysfunction. In a healed myocardial infarct, for example, the fibrous tissue not only represents a loss of functioning muscle but by involving the conduction system may cause heart blocks or provide a surface for thrombus formation.

BIBLIOGRAPHY

Armulik L, et al: Endothelial/pericyte interactions. Circ Res 97:512, 2005. *[A review of the process of vessel maturation and its abnormalities.]*

Aicher A, et al: Mobilizing endothelial progenitor cells. Hypertension 45:321, 2005. *[A review of the data on the involvement of endothelial precursor cells from the bone marrow in angiogenesis.]*

Bartek J, et al: Checking on DNA damage in S phase. Nat Rev Mol Cell Biol 5:792, 2004. *[A discussion of cell cycle checkpoints.]*

Bjerknes M, Cheng H: Gastrointestinal stem cells. II Intestinal stem cells. Am J Physiol Gastrointest Liver Physiol 289:G381, 2005. *[An excellent review of cell population dynamics in intestinal epithelia, and the role of Notch and Wnt signaling.]*

Byrne AM, et al: Angiogenic and cell survival functions of vascular endothelial growth factor (VEGF). J Cell Mol Med 9:777, 2005. *[A comprehensive review of VEGF functions in various biological responses including wound healing, and the prospects of therapeutic strategies targeting VEGF receptors.]*

Carmeliet P: Angiogenesis in life, disease and medicine. Nature 438:932, 2005. *[A current review of the main aspects of normal and abnormal angiogenesis.]*

Carlson BM: Some principles of regeneration in mammalian systems. Anat Rec 287:4, 2005. *[A very thoughtful review of the evolutionary aspects and general mechanisms of limb and organ regeneration.]*

Eswarakumar VP, et al: Cellular signaling by fibroblast growth factor receptors. Cytokine Growth Factor Rev 16:139, 2005. *[A comprehensive review of the mechanisms of signal transduction and cellular responses induced by FGFs.]*

Evans M: Embryonic stem cells: a perspective. Novartis Found Symp 265:98, 2005. *[A very basic and well written review of the main properties of stem cells.]*

Falanga V (ed): *Cutaneous Wound Healing*. London, Martin Dunitz, 2001. *[A comprehensive book that contains chapters on basic and clinical aspects of wound healing.]*

Falanga V: Wound healing and its impairment in the diabetic foot. Lancet 366:1736, 2005. *[A review of the phases and mechanisms of cutaneous wound healing, and the impairment of the process in chronic wounds.]*

Fausto N: Liver regeneration and repair: hepatocytes, progenitor cells and stem cells. Hepatology 39:1477, 2004. *[A review of the cellular and molecular mechanisms of liver regeneration.]*

Feng XH, Derynck R: Specificity and versatility in TGF-β signaling through Smads. Annu Rev Cell Dev Biol 21:659, 2005. *[A review of the signal transduction pathways involving smads and the multiple biological responses elicited by TGF-β.]*

Finch PW, Rubin JS: Keratinocyte growth factor/fibroblast growth factor 7, a homeostatic factor with therapeutic potential for epithelial protection and repair. *[A review of the role of KGF in maintaining the integrity of surface epithelia, and of ongoing clinical trials.]*

Henry G, Garner WL: Inflammatory mediators in wound healing. Surg Clin North Am 83:483, 2003. *[A review of the interactions between inflammation and wound healing.]*

Holterman CE, Rudnicki MA: Molecular regulation of satellite cell function. Semin Cell Dev Biol 16:575, 2005. *[An interesting discussion of repair mechanisms in skeletal muscle.]*

Hynes RO: Integrins: bidirectional, allosteric signaling machines. Cell 110:673, 2002. *[An excellent review of the molecular mechanisms of integrin signaling, linking ECM components to intracellular signal transduction pathways.]*

Jones PF: Not just angiogenesis—wider role for the angiopoietins. J Pathol 201:515, 2003. *[A general review on the biological roles of angiopoietins.]*

Lee JW, Juliano R: Mitogenic signal transduction by integrin- and growth factor receptor—mediated pathways. Mol Cell 17:188, 2004. *[Another excellent review on integrin signaling.]*

Martin P, Leibovich SJ: Inflammatory cells during wound repair: the good, the bad, and the ugly. Trends Cell Biol 15:599, 2005. *[Good review on the multiple roles of inflammatory cells in repair.]*

Mott JD, Werb Z: Regulation of matrix biology by matrix metalloproteinases. Curr Opin Cell Biol 16:558, 2004. *[An interesting analysis of multiple effects of metalloproteinases on the ECM and cell surface-anchored molecules.]*

Nagy JA, Dvorak AM, Dvorak HF: VEGF-A and the induction of pathological angiogenesis. Annual Review of Pathology: Mechanisms of Disease, Vol. 2:251, 2007. *[A review of physiologic and pathologic angiogenesis.]*

Reed SI: Ratchets and clocks: the cell cycle, ubiquitylation and protein turnover. Nat Rev Mol Cell Biol 4:855, 2003. *[A review of regulatory mechanisms of cell cycle transitions, with emphasis on post-translational mechanisms.]*

Singer AJ, Clark RA: Cutaneous wound healing. N Engl J Med 341:738, 1999. *[An excellent and beautifully illustrated review on wound healing in the skin.]*

Singh AB, Harris RC: Autocrine, paracrine and juxtacrine signaling by EGFR ligands. Cell Signal 17:1183, 2005. *[A review of the mechanisms of cleavage of precursor molecules and signal transduction by members of the EGF family.]*

Tammela T, et al: The biology of vascular endothelial growth factors. Cardiovasc Res 65:550, 2005. *[A review of the angiogenic and lymphangiogenic effects of VEGFs.]*

Taub R: Liver regeneration: from myth to mechanism. Nat Rev Mol Cell Biol 5:836, 2004. *[A comprehensive review of the molecular mechanisms of liver regeneration.]*

Tomasek JJ, et al: Myofibroblasts and mechano-regulation of connective tissue remodeling. Nat Rev Mol Cell Biol 3:349, 2002. *[A review of myofibroblasts and wound contraction.]*

Vats A, et al: Stem cells. Lancet 366:592, 2005. *[A general discussion of therapeutic approaches using stem cells.]*

Wormald S, Hilton DJ: Inhibitors of cytokine signal transduction. J Biol Chem 279:821, 2004. *[A review of the JAK/STAT pathway and its inhibitors.]*

Chapter 4

Hemodynamic Disorders, Thrombosis, and Shock

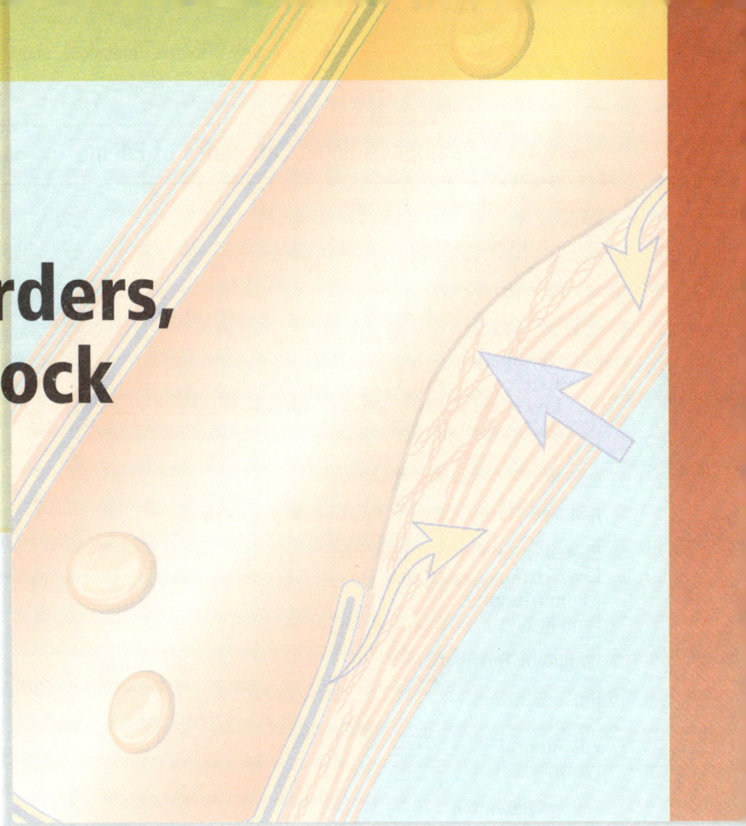

The health of cells and tissues depends not only on an *intact circulation* to deliver oxygen and remove wastes but also on *normal fluid homeostasis.* Normal fluid homeostasis requires vessel wall integrity as well as maintenance of intravascular pressure and osmolarity within certain physiologic ranges. Increases in vascular volume or pressure, decreases in plasma protein content, or alterations in endothelial function can result in a net outward movement of water across the vascular wall. Such water extravasation into interstitial spaces is called *edema;* depending on its location, edema may have minimal or profound effects. Thus, in the lower extremities edema fluid causes primarily swelling; however, in the lungs, edema fluid will fill alveoli and can result in life-threatening breathing difficulties.

Normal fluid homeostasis also means maintaining blood as a liquid until such time as injury necessitates formation of a clot. Absence of clotting after vascular injury results in *hemorrhage;* local bleeding can compromise regional tissue perfusion, while more extensive hemorrhage can result in hypotension (*shock*) and death. Conversely, inappropriate clotting (*thrombosis*) or migration of clots (*embolism*) can obstruct tissue blood supplies and cause cell death (*infarction*).

Abnormal fluid homeostasis (i.e., hemorrhage or thrombosis) underlies three of the most important causes of morbidity and mortality in Western society: myocardial infarction, pulmonary embolism, and cerebrovascular accident (stroke).

EDEMA

Approximately 60% of lean body weight is water, two-thirds of which is intracellular and the remainder is in extracellular compartments, mostly as interstitial fluid; only 5% of total body water is in blood plasma. The term *edema* signifies increased fluid in the interstitial tissue spaces; fluid collections in different body cavities are variously designated *hydrothorax, hydropericardium,* or *hydroperitoneum* (the last is more commonly called *ascites*). *Anasarca* is a severe and generalized edema with profound subcutaneous tissue swelling.

There are several pathophysiologic categories of edema (Table 4–1). The mechanism of inflammatory edema mostly involves increased vascular permeability and is discussed in Chapter 2; *noninflammatory causes of edema* are described below.

The movement of fluid between vascular and interstitial spaces is controlled mainly by the opposing effects of vascular hydrostatic pressure and plasma colloid osmotic pressure. Normally, the exit of fluid into the interstitium

Table 4–1 Pathophysiologic Categories of Edema

Increased Hydrostatic Pressure
Impaired venous return
Congestive heart failure
Constrictive pericarditis
Ascites (liver cirrhosis)
Venous obstruction or compression
Thrombosis
External pressure (e.g., mass)
Lower extremity inactivity with prolonged dependency
Arteriolar dilation
Heat
Neurohumoral dysregulation
Reduced Plasma Osmotic Pressure (Hypoproteinemia)
Protein-losing glomerulopathies (nephrotic syndrome)
Liver cirrhosis (ascites)
Malnutrition
Protein-losing gastroenteropathy
Lymphatic Obstruction
Inflammatory
Neoplastic
Postsurgical
Postirradiation
Sodium Retention
Excessive salt intake with renal insufficiency
Increased tubular reabsorption of sodium
Renal hypoperfusion
Increased renin-angiotensin-aldosterone secretion
Inflammation
Acute inflammation
Chronic inflammation
Angiogenesis

Modified from Leaf A, Cotran RS: Renal Pathophysiology, 3rd ed. New York, Oxford University Press, 1985, p 146.

from the arteriolar end of the microcirculation is nearly balanced by inflow at the venular end; the lymphatics drain a small residual amount of excess interstitial fluid. Either increased capillary pressure or diminished colloid osmotic pressure can result in increased interstitial fluid (Fig. 4–1). As extravascular fluid accumulates in either case, the increased tissue hydrostatic and plasma osmotic pressures eventually achieve a new equilibrium, and water re-enters the venules. Excess interstitial edema fluid is removed by lymphatic drainage, ultimately returning to the bloodstream via the thoracic duct (see Fig. 4–1); clearly, lymphatic obstruction (e.g., due to scarring or tumor) can also impair fluid drainage and cause edema. Finally, sodium retention (with its obligatory associated water) due to renal disease can also cause edema.

The edema fluid occurring with volume or pressure overload, or under conditions of reduced plasma protein, is typically a protein-poor *transudate;* it has a specific gravity less than 1.012. Conversely, because of the increased vascular permeability, inflammatory edema is a protein-rich *exudate* with a specific gravity that is usually greater than 1.020 (see Fig. 2–3, Chapter 2).

Increased Hydrostatic Pressure. *Localized* increases in intravascular pressure can result from impaired venous return; for example, lower extremity deep venous thrombosis can cause edema restricted to the distal portion of the affected leg. *Generalized* increases in venous pressure, with resultant systemic edema, occur most commonly in *congestive heart failure* (Chapter 11), affecting right ventricular cardiac function. Although increased venous hydrostatic pressure is contributory, the pathogenesis of cardiac edema is more complex (Fig. 4–2). In congestive heart failure, reduced cardiac output translates into reduced renal perfusion. Renal hypoperfusion in turn triggers the renin-angiotensin-aldosterone axis, inducing sodium and water retention by the kidneys (*secondary aldosteronism*). This mechanism normally functions to increase intravascular volume and thereby improve cardiac output to restore normal renal perfusion. However, if the failing heart cannot increase cardiac output, the extra fluid load causes increased venous pressure and, eventually, edema. Unless cardiac output is restored or renal water retention reduced (e.g., by salt restriction, diuretics, or aldosterone antagonists), a cycle of renal fluid retention and worsening edema ensues. Although salt restriction, diuretics, and aldosterone antagonists are discussed here in the context of edema in congestive heart failure, it should be understood that they are also of value in the management of generalized edema resulting from a variety of other causes.

Reduced Plasma Osmotic Pressure. Albumin is the serum protein most responsible for maintaining intravascular colloid osmotic pressure; reduced osmotic pressure

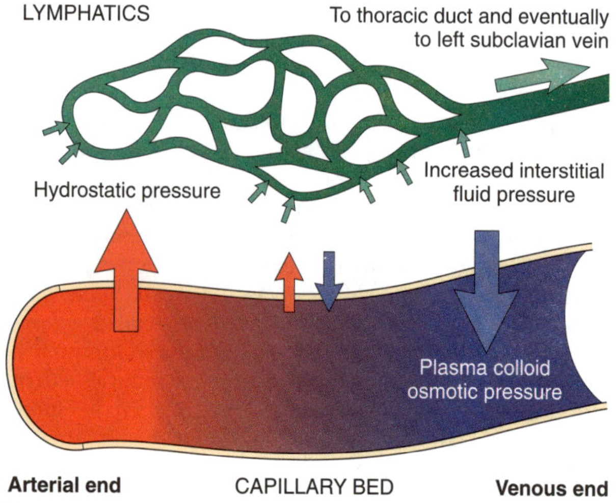

Figure 4–1

Variables affecting fluid transit across capillary walls. Capillary hydrostatic and osmotic forces are normally balanced so that there is no *net* loss or gain of fluid across the capillary bed. However, *increased* hydrostatic pressure or *diminished* plasma osmotic pressure leads to a net accumulation of extravascular fluid (edema). As the interstitial fluid pressure increases, tissue lymphatics remove much of the excess volume, eventually returning it to the circulation via the thoracic duct. If the ability of the lymphatics to drain tissue fluid is exceeded, persistent tissue edema results.

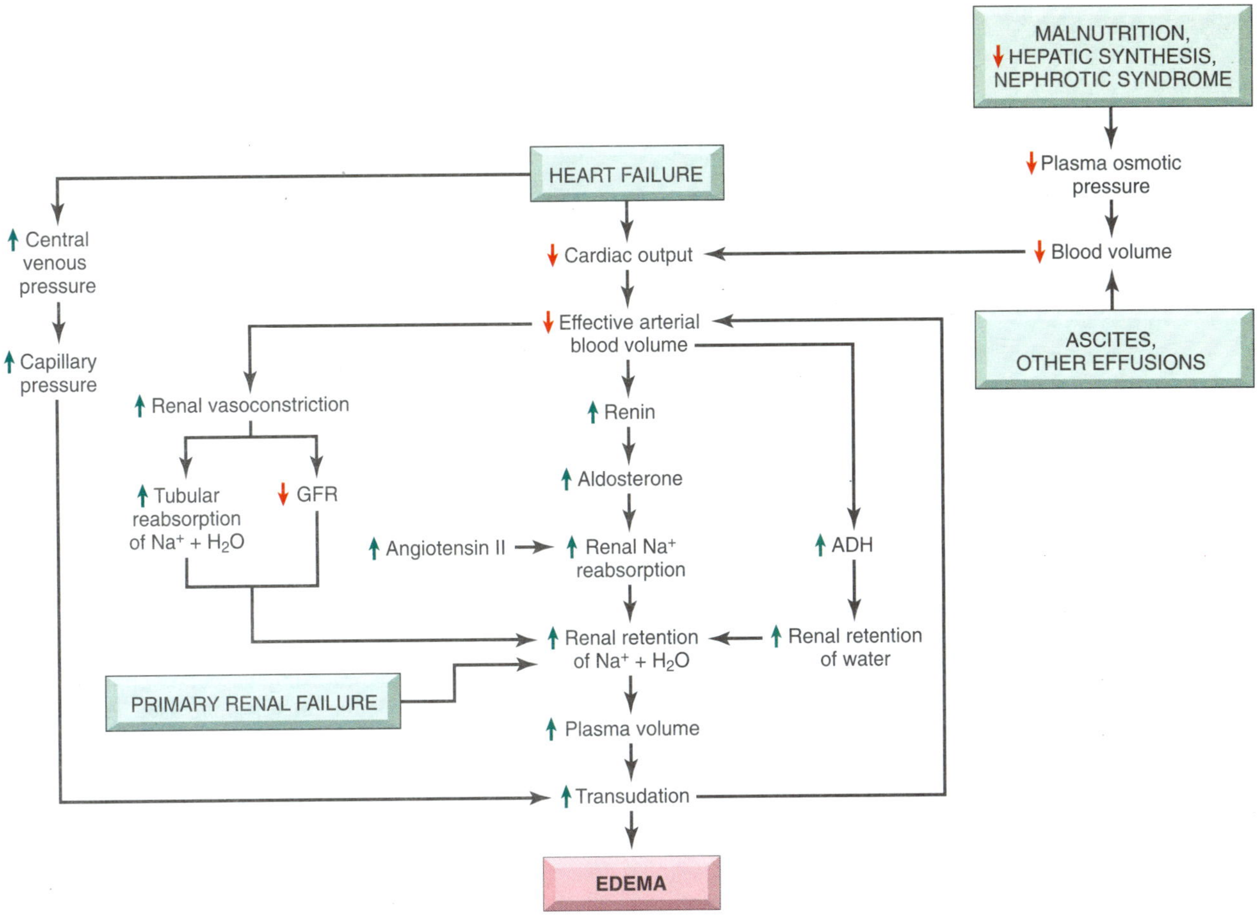

Figure 4–2

Pathways leading to systemic edema due to primary heart failure, primary renal failure, or reduced plasma osmotic pressure (e.g., from malnutrition, diminished hepatic synthesis, or protein loss due to the nephrotic syndrome). ADH, antidiuretic hormone; GFR, glomerular filtration rate.

occurs when albumin is inadequately synthesized or is lost from the circulation. An important cause of albumin loss is the *nephrotic syndrome* (Chapter 14), in which glomerular capillary walls become leaky; patients typically present with generalized edema. Reduced albumin synthesis occurs in the setting of diffuse liver diseases (e.g., cirrhosis; Chapter 16) or due to protein malnutrition (Chapter 8). In each case, reduced plasma osmotic pressure leads to a net movement of fluid into the interstitial tissues with subsequent plasma volume contraction. Predictably, reduced intravascular volume leads to renal hypoperfusion followed by secondary aldosteronism. Unfortunately, the retained salt and water cannot correct the plasma volume deficit since the primary defect of low serum proteins persists. As with congestive heart failure, edema precipitated by low protein is exacerbated by secondary salt and fluid retention.

Lymphatic Obstruction. Impaired lymphatic drainage and consequent *lymphedema* is usually localized; it can result from inflammatory or neoplastic obstruction. For example, the parasitic infection *filariasis* can cause extensive inguinal lymphatic and lymph node fibrosis. The resultant edema of the external genitalia and lower limbs can be so massive as to earn the appellation *elephantiasis*. Cancer of the breast can be treated by resection and/or irradiation of the associated axillary lymph nodes; the resultant scarring and loss of lymphatic drainage can cause severe upper extremity edema. In breast carcinoma infiltration and obstruction of superficial lymphatics can also cause edema of the overlying skin, the so-called *peau d'orange* (orange peel) appearance. Such a finely pitted surface results from an accentuation of depressions in the skin at the site of hair follicles.

Sodium and Water Retention. Salt retention can also be a primary cause of edema. Increased salt—with the obligate accompanying water—causes both increased hydrostatic pressure (due to expansion of the intravascular volume) and reduced vascular osmotic pressure. Salt retention can occur with any compromise of renal function, as in *poststreptococcal glomerulonephritis* and *acute renal failure* (Chapter 14).

SUMMARY

Edema

- Edema is extravasation of fluid from vessels into interstitial spaces; the fluid may be protein poor (transudate) or may be protein rich (exudate).
- Edema results from any of the following conditions:
  - Increased hydrostatic pressure, caused by a reduction in venous return (as in heart failure)
  - Decreased colloid osmotic pressure, caused by reduced concentration of plasma albumin (due to decreased synthesis, as in liver disease, or increased loss, as in kidney disease)
  - Lymphatic obstruction that impairs interstitial fluid clearance (as in scarring, tumors, or certain infections)
  - Primary renal sodium retention (in renal failure)
  - Increased vascular permeability (in inflammation)

Morphology

Edema is most easily recognized grossly; microscopically, edema fluid is reflected primarily as a clearing and separation of the extracellular matrix elements with subtle cell swelling. Although any organ or tissue in the body may be involved, edema is most commonly encountered in subcutaneous tissues, lungs, and brain.

Subcutaneous edema can be diffuse or more prominent in regions with high hydrostatic pressures; the ultimate distribution depends on the underlying etiology. Even diffuse edema is usually more prominent in certain body areas as a result of the effects of gravity; a gravity-dependent distribution is referred to as **dependent edema** (e.g., involving the legs when standing, or involving the sacrum when recumbent). **Dependent edema is a prominent feature of cardiac failure, particularly of the right ventricle.** Edema due to **renal dysfunction** or **nephrotic syndrome** is generally more severe than cardiac edema **and affects all parts of the body equally.** Nevertheless, severe edema early in the disease course can still manifest disproportionately in tissues with a loose connective tissue matrix (e.g., the eyelids, causing **periorbital edema**). Finger pressure over significantly edematous subcutaneous tissue displaces the interstitial fluid and leaves a finger-shaped depression, so-called **pitting edema.**

Pulmonary edema is a common clinical problem most frequently seen in the setting of left ventricular failure (with a dependent distribution in the lungs), but it also occurs in renal failure, acute respiratory distress syndrome (ARDS; Chapter 13), pulmonary infections, and hypersensitivity reactions. The lungs typically weigh two to three times their normal weight, and sectioning reveals frothy, sometimes blood-tinged fluid representing a mixture of air, edema fluid, and extravasated red cells.

Edema of the brain may be localized to sites of focal injury (e.g., infarct, abscesses or neoplasms) or may be generalized, as in encephalitis, hypertensive crises, or obstruction to the brain's venous outflow. Trauma may result in local or generalized edema, depending on the nature and extent of the injury. With generalized edema, the brain is grossly swollen with narrowed sulci and distended gyri showing signs of flattening against the unyielding skull (Chapter 23).

Clinical Correlation. The effects of edema may range from merely annoying to rapidly fatal. Subcutaneous tissue edema in cardiac or renal failure is important primarily because it indicates underlying disease; however, when significant it can also impair wound healing or the clearance of infection. In contrast, pulmonary edema can cause death by interfering with normal ventilatory function. Not only does fluid collect in the alveolar septa around capillaries and impede oxygen diffusion, but edema fluid in the alveolar spaces also creates a favorable environment for bacterial infection. Brain edema is serious and can be rapidly fatal. If severe, brain edema can cause *herniation* (extrusion of the brain) through the foramen magnum; the brainstem vascular supply can also be compressed by edema causing increased intracranial pressure. Either state can injure the medullary centers and can cause death (Chapter 23).

HYPEREMIA AND CONGESTION

The terms *hyperemia* and *congestion* both indicate a local increased volume of blood in a particular tissue. Hyperemia is an *active process* resulting from augmented blood flow due to arteriolar dilation (e.g., at sites of inflammation or in skeletal muscle during exercise). The affected tissue is redder than normal because of engorgement with oxygenated blood. Congestion is a *passive process* resulting from impaired venous return out of a tissue. It may occur systemically, as in cardiac failure, or it may be local, resulting from an isolated venous obstruction. The tissue has a blue-red color *(cyanosis)*, especially as worsening congestion leads to accumulation of deoxygenated hemoglobin in the affected tissues (Fig. 4–3).

Congestion of capillary beds is closely related to the development of edema, so that congestion and edema commonly occur together. In long-standing congestion, called *chronic passive congestion*, the stasis of poorly oxygenated blood causes chronic hypoxia, which in turn can result in degeneration or death of parenchymal cells and subsequent tissue fibrosis. Capillary rupture at such sites of chronic congestion can also cause small foci of hemorrhage; phagocytosis and catabolism of the erythrocyte debris can result in accumulations of hemosiderin-laden macrophages.

Morphology

Cut surfaces of hyperemic or congested tissues are hemorrhagic and wet. Microscopically, **acute pulmonary congestion** is characterized by alveolar capillaries engorged with blood; there may also be associated alveolar septal edema and/or focal minute intra-alveolar hemorrhage. In **chronic pulmonary congestion** the septa become thickened and fibrotic, and the alveolar spaces may contain numerous hemosiderin-laden macrophages ("heart failure cells"). In **acute hepatic congestion** the central vein and sinusoids are distended with blood, and there may even be central hepatocyte degeneration; the periportal hepatocytes, better oxygenated because of their proximity to hepatic arterioles, undergo less severe hypoxia and may develop only fatty change. In **chronic passive congestion** of the liver the central regions of the hepatic lobules are grossly red-brown and slightly depressed (because of a loss of cells) and are accentuated against the surrounding zones of uncongested tan, sometimes fatty, liver ("nutmeg liver"; Fig. 4–4A). Microscopically, there is centrilobular necrosis with hepatocyte drop-out, hemorrhage, and hemosiderin-laden macrophages (Fig. 4–4B). In long-standing, severe hepatic congestion (most commonly associated with heart failure), hepatic fibrosis ("cardiac cirrhosis") can develop. It is important to note that because the central portion of the hepatic lobule is the last to receive blood, centrilobular necrosis can also occur whenever there is reduced hepatic blood flow (including shock from any cause); there need not be previous hepatic congestion.

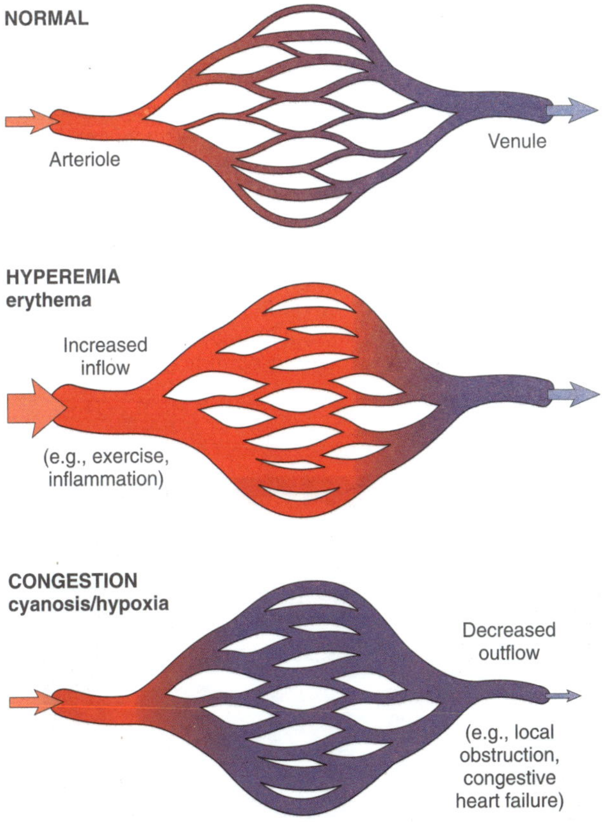

Figure 4–3

Hyperemia versus congestion. In both cases there is an increased volume and pressure of blood in a given tissue with associated capillary dilation and a potential for fluid extravasation. In hyperemia, increased inflow leads to engorgement with oxygenated blood, resulting in *erythema.* In congestion, diminished outflow leads to a capillary bed swollen with deoxygenated venous blood and resulting in *cyanosis.*

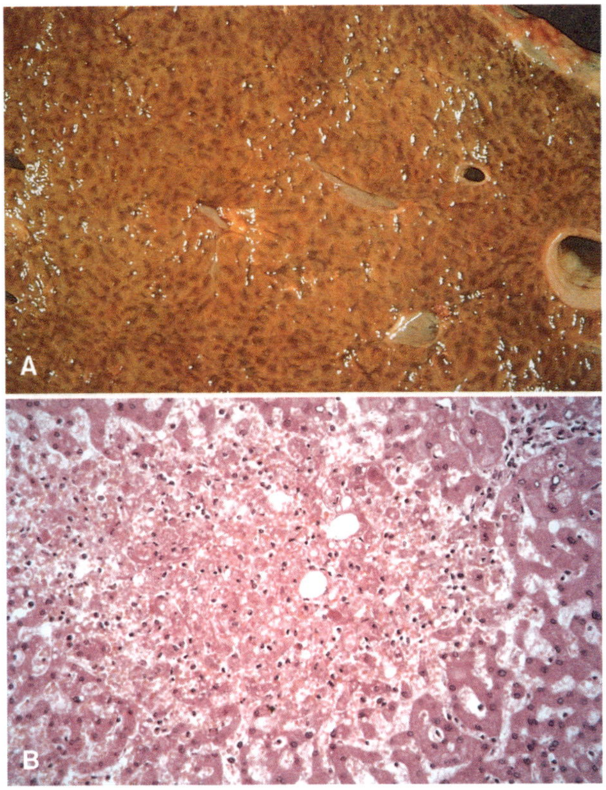

Figure 4–4

Liver with chronic passive congestion and hemorrhagic necrosis. **A,** Central areas are red and slightly depressed compared with the surrounding tan viable parenchyma, forming a "nutmeg liver" pattern (so called because it resembles the alternating pattern of light and dark seen when a whole nutmeg is cut). **B,** Centrilobular necrosis with degenerating hepatocytes and hemorrhage. (Courtesy of Dr. James Crawford, Department of Pathology, University of Florida, Gainesville, Florida.)

HEMORRHAGE

Hemorrhage is extravasation of blood from vessels into the extravascular space. As described above, capillary bleeding can occur under conditions of chronic congestion; an increased tendency to hemorrhage (usually with insignificant injury) occurs in a wide variety of clinical disorders collectively called *hemorrhagic diatheses.* Rupture of a large artery or vein results in severe hemorrhage, and is almost always due to vascular injury, including trauma, atherosclerosis, or inflammatory or neoplastic erosion of the vessel wall.

- Hemorrhage can be external or can be confined within a tissue; any accumulation is referred to as a *hematoma.* Hematomas can be relatively insignificant (e.g., a bruise) or can involve so much bleeding as to cause death (e.g., a massive retroperitoneal hematoma resulting from rupture of a dissecting aortic aneurysm; Chapter 10).

- Minute (1- to 2-mm) hemorrhages into skin, mucous membranes, or serosal surfaces are called *petechiae* (Fig. 4–5A) and are typically associated with locally increased intravascular pressure, low platelet counts (*thrombocytopenia*), defective platelet function, or clotting factor deficiencies.
- Slightly larger (3- to 5-mm) hemorrhages are called *purpura* and can be associated with many of the same disorders that cause petechiae; in addition, purpura can occur with trauma, vascular inflammation (*vasculitis*), or increased vascular fragility.
- Larger (1- to 2-cm) subcutaneous hematomas (bruises) are called *ecchymoses*. The erythrocytes in these local hemorrhages are phagocytosed and degraded by macrophages; the hemoglobin (red-blue color) is enzymatically converted into bilirubin (blue-green color) and eventually into hemosiderin (golden-brown), accounting for the characteristic color changes in a hematoma.
- Large accumulations of blood in one or another of the body cavities are called *hemothorax, hemopericardium, hemoperitoneum,* or *hemarthrosis* (in joints). Patients with extensive hemorrhages occasionally develop jaundice from the massive breakdown of red blood cells and systemic increases in bilirubin.

The clinical significance of hemorrhage depends on the volume and rate of blood loss. Rapid removal of as much as 20% of the blood volume or slow losses of even larger amounts may have little impact in healthy adults; greater losses, however, can cause *hemorrhagic (hypovolemic) shock* (discussed later). The site of hemorrhage is also important; bleeding that would be trivial in the subcutaneous tissues may cause death if located in the brain (Fig. 4–5B). Finally, chronic or recurrent external blood loss (e.g., a peptic ulcer or menstrual bleeding) causes a net loss of iron, frequently culminating in an iron deficiency anemia. In contrast, when red cells are retained (e.g., with hemorrhage into body cavities or tissues), the iron can be reutilized for hemoglobin synthesis.

HEMOSTASIS AND THROMBOSIS

Normal hemostasis is a consequence of tightly regulated processes that maintain blood in a fluid, clot-free state in normal vessels while inducing the rapid formation of a localized *hemostatic plug* at the site of vascular injury. The pathologic form of hemostasis is *thrombosis;* it involves blood clot (*thrombus*) formation in uninjured vessels or thrombotic occlusion of a vessel after relatively minor injury. Both hemostasis and thrombosis involve three components: the *vascular wall, platelets,* and the *coagulation cascade.* We begin our discussion with the process of normal hemostasis and a description of its regulation.

Normal Hemostasis

The sequence of events in hemostasis at a site of vascular injury is shown in Figure 4–6. After initial injury a brief period of *arteriolar vasoconstriction* occurs mostly as a result of reflex neurogenic mechanisms and is augmented by the local secretion of factors such as *endothelin* (a potent endothelium-derived vasoconstrictor; Fig. 4–6A). The effect is transient, and bleeding would resume were it not for activation of the platelet and coagulation systems.

Endothelial injury also exposes highly thrombogenic subendothelial extracellular matrix, allowing platelets to adhere and be activated. *Activation* of platelets results in a dramatic shape change (from small rounded disks to flat plates with markedly increased surface area) and release of secretory granules. Within minutes the secreted products have recruited additional platelets (*aggregation*) to form a hemostatic plug; this is the process of *primary hemostasis* (Fig. 4–6B).

Tissue factor is also exposed at the site of injury. Also known as *factor III* and *thromboplastin,* tissue factor is a membrane-bound procoagulant glycoprotein synthesized by endothelium. It acts in conjunction with factor

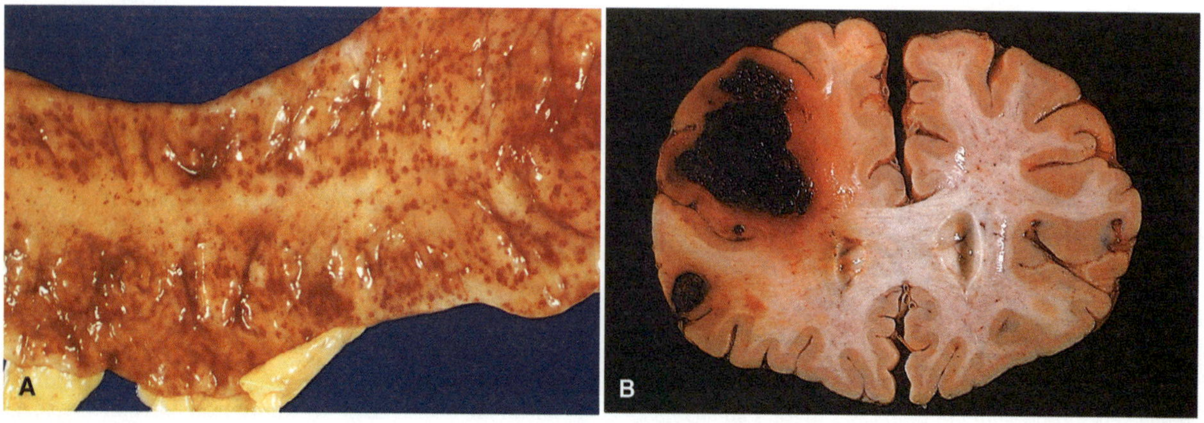

Figure 4–5

A, Punctate petechial hemorrhages of the colonic mucosa, a consequence of thrombocytopenia. **B,** Fatal intracerebral hemorrhage. Even relatively inconsequential volumes of hemorrhage in a critical location, or into a closed space (such as the cranium), can have fatal outcomes.

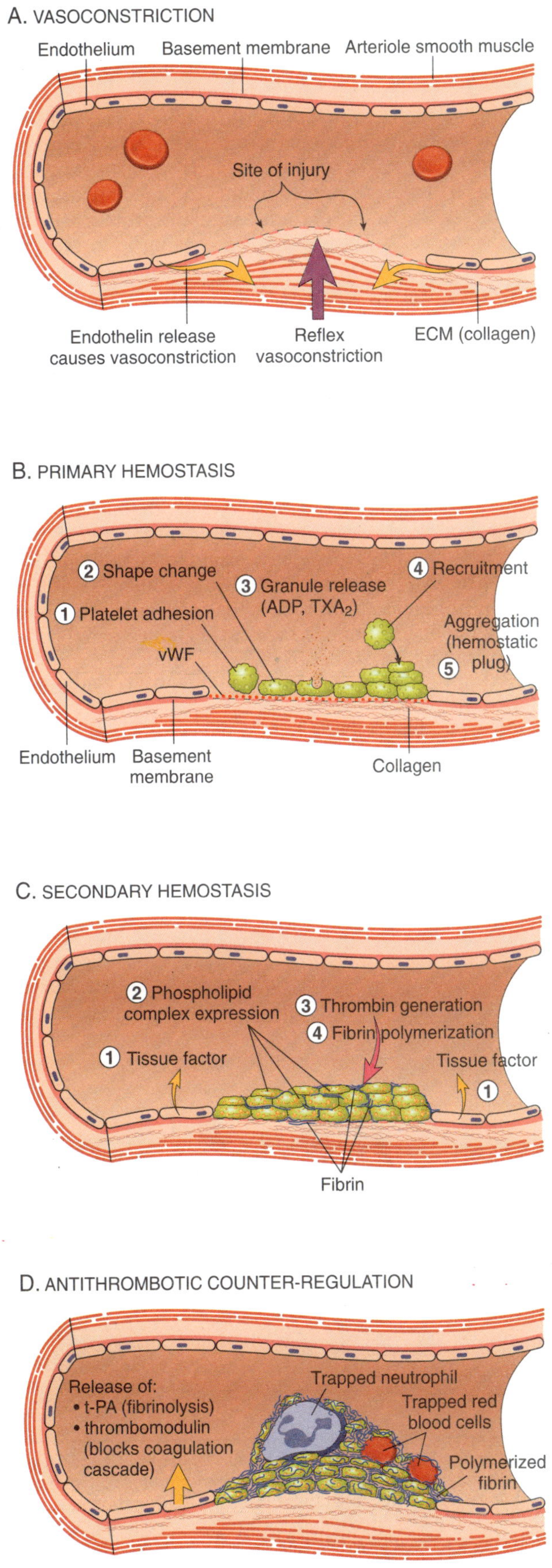

Figure 4–6

Normal hemostasis. **A,** After vascular injury, local neurohumoral factors induce a transient vasoconstriction. **B,** Platelets adhere (via GpIb receptors) to exposed extracellular matrix (ECM) by binding to von Willebrand factor (vWF) and are activated, undergoing a shape change and granule release. Released adenosine diphosphate (ADP) and thromboxane A_2 (TXA_2) lead to further platelet aggregation (via binding of fibrinogen to platelet GpIIb-IIIa receptors), to form the primary hemostatic plug. **C,** Local activation of the coagulation cascade (involving tissue factor and platelet phospholipids) results in fibrin polymerization, "cementing" the platelets into a definitive secondary hemostatic plug. **D,** Counter-regulatory mechanisms, such as release of t-PA (tissue plasminogen activator, a fibrinolytic product) and thrombomodulin (interfering with the coagulation cascade), limit the hemostatic process to the site of injury.

VII (see below) as the major in vivo pathway to activate the coagulation cascade, eventually culminating in *thrombin generation.* Thrombin cleaves circulating fibrinogen into insoluble *fibrin,* creating a fibrin meshwork deposition. Thrombin also induces further platelet recruitment and granule release. This *secondary hemostasis* sequence (Fig. 4–6C) lasts longer than the initial platelet plug.

Polymerized fibrin and platelet aggregates form a solid *permanent plug* to prevent any additional hemorrhage. At this stage counter-regulatory mechanisms (e.g., *tissue plasminogen activator, t-PA*) are set into motion to limit the hemostatic plug to the site of injury (see Fig. 4–6D).

The following sections discuss these events in greater detail.

Endothelium

Endothelial cells modulate several (and frequently opposing) aspects of normal hemostasis. The balance between endothelial anti- and prothrombotic activities determines whether thrombus formation, propagation, or dissolution occurs. At baseline, endothelial cells exhibit antiplatelet, anticoagulant, and fibrinolytic properties; however, they are capable (after injury or activation) of exhibiting numerous procoagulant activities (Fig. 4–7). It should also be remembered that endothelium can be activated by infectious agents, by hemodynamic factors, by plasma mediators, and (most significantly) by cytokines (Chapter 2).

Antithrombotic Properties

Under most circumstances, endothelial cells maintain an environment that promotes liquid blood flow by blocking platelet adhesion and aggregation, by inhibiting the coagulation cascade, and by lysing blood clots.

Antiplatelet Effects. An intact endothelium prevents platelets (and plasma coagulation factors) from interacting with the highly thrombogenic subendothelial ECM. Nonactivated platelets do not adhere to the endothelium, a property intrinsic to the plasma membrane of endothelium. Moreover, if platelets are activated (e.g., after focal endothelial injury), they are inhibited from adhering to the surrounding uninjured endothelium by endothelial prostacyclin (PGI_2) and nitric oxide (Chapter 2). Both mediators are potent vasodilators and inhibitors of

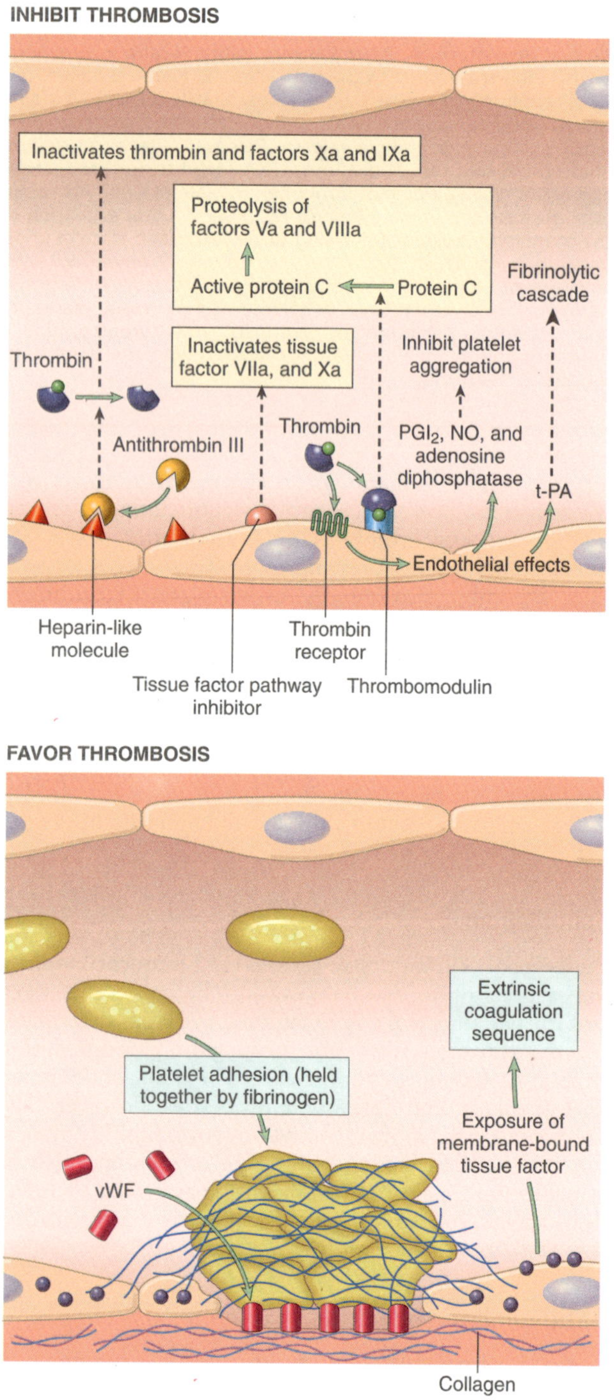

Figure 4–7

Pro- and anticoagulant activities of endothelium. Not shown are pro- and antifibrinolytic properties of endothelium (see text). NO, nitric oxide; PGI_2, prostacyclin; t-PA, tissue plasminogen activator; vWF, von Willebrand factor. The thrombin receptor is also called a protease-activated receptor (PAR; see text).

platelet aggregation; their synthesis by endothelial cells is stimulated by several factors (e.g., thrombin and cytokines) produced during coagulation. Endothelial cells also elaborate adenosine diphosphatase, which degrades adenosine diphosphate (ADP) and further inhibits platelet aggregation (see below).

Anticoagulant Effects. Anticoagulant effects are mediated by membrane-associated, heparin-like molecules and thrombomodulin (see Fig. 4–7). The *heparin-like molecules* act indirectly; they are cofactors that allow *antithrombin III* to inactivate thrombin, factor Xa, and several other coagulation factors (see later). *Thrombomodulin* also acts indirectly; it binds to thrombin, converting it from a procoagulant to an anticoagulant capable of activating the anticoagulant protein C. Activated protein C, in turn, inhibits clotting by proteolytic cleavage of factors Va and VIIIa; it requires protein S, synthesized by endothelial cells, as a cofactor.

Fibrinolytic Properties. Endothelial cells synthesize tissue plasminogen activator (*t-PA*), promoting fibrinolytic activity to clear fibrin deposits from endothelial surfaces (see Fig. 4–6D).

Prothrombotic Properties

While endothelial cells exhibit properties that usually limit blood clotting, they can also become prothrombotic, with activities that affect platelets, coagulation proteins, and the fibrinolytic system. Endothelial injury results in platelet adhesion to subendothelial collagen; this occurs through *von Willebrand factor (vWF),* an essential cofactor for binding platelets to collagen and other surfaces. vWF (both circulating and collagen bound) is synthesized largely by normal endothelium. Loss of endothelium exposes previously deposited vWF and allows circulating vWF to also bind to the basement membrane; in quick order, platelets adhere via their glycoprotein Ib (GpIb) receptors (Fig. 4–8).

Cytokines such as tumor necrosis factor (TNF) or interleukin-1 (IL-1) as well as bacterial endotoxin all induce endothelial cell production of *tissue factor;* as we will see

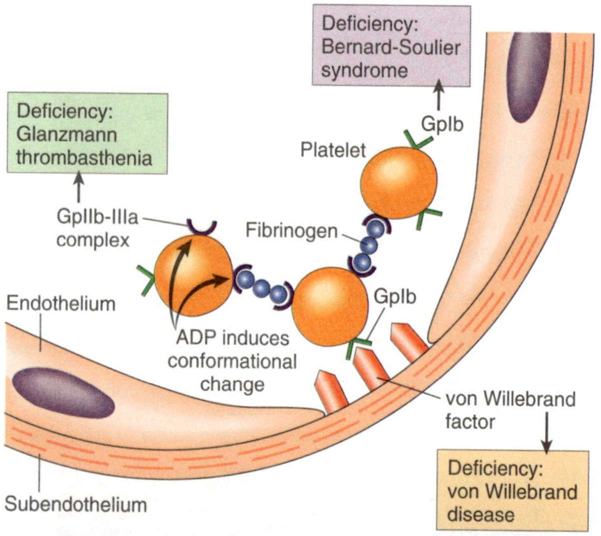

Figure 4–8

Platelet adhesion and aggregation. Von Willebrand factor functions as an adhesion bridge between subendothelial collagen and the glycoprotein Ib (GpIb) platelet receptor. Aggregation is accomplished by binding of fibrinogen to platelet GpIIb-IIIa receptors and bridging many platelets together. Congenital deficiencies in the various receptors or bridging molecules lead to the diseases indicated in the colored boxes. ADP, adenosine diphosphate.

below, tissue factor activates the extrinsic clotting pathway. By binding activated IXa and Xa (see below), endothelial cells augment the catalytic activities of these coagulation factors. Finally, endothelial cells also secrete *plasminogen activator inhibitors (PAIs)*, which depress fibrinolysis (not shown in Fig. 4–7).

SUMMARY

Contribution of Endothelial Cells to Coagulation

- Intact endothelial cells maintain liquid blood flow by actively inhibiting platelet adherence, preventing coagulation factor activation, and lysing blood clots that may form.
- Endothelial cells can be stimulated by direct injury or by various cytokines that are produced during inflammation. Such stimulation results in expression of procoagulant proteins (e.g., tissue factor and vWF) that contribute to local thrombus formation.
- Loss of endothelial integrity exposes underlying vWF and basement membrane collagen, both substrates for platelet aggregation and thrombus formation.

Platelets

Platelets play a critical role in normal hemostasis. When circulating and nonactivated they are membrane-bound smooth disks expressing several glycoprotein receptors of the integrin family and containing two types of granules:

- α-*Granules* express the adhesion molecule P-selectin on their membranes (Chapter 2) and contain fibrinogen, fibronectin, factors V and VIII, platelet factor 4 (a heparin-binding chemokine), platelet-derived growth factor (PDGF), and transforming growth factor α (TGF-α).
- *Dense* bodies, or δ granules, contain adenine nucleotides (ADP and ATP), ionized calcium, histamine, serotonin, and epinephrine.

After vascular injury, platelets encounter ECM constituents (of which collagen is the most important) and additional proteins (vWF being critical) that are normally not exposed when the endothelial layer is intact. Upon contact with these proteins, platelets undergo three reactions: (1) adhesion and shape change, (2) secretion (release reaction), and (3) aggregation (see Fig. 4–6B).

Platelet Adhesion. Adhesion to ECM is mediated largely via interactions with vWF acting as a bridge between platelet surface receptors (e.g., GpIb) and exposed collagen (see Fig. 4–8). Although platelets can adhere directly to ECM, vWF-GpIb associations are required to overcome the high shear forces of flowing blood. Genetic deficiencies of vWF (von Willebrand disease; Chapter 12) or its receptors result in bleeding disorders, highlighting the importance of these interactions. Conversely, failure of the normal proteolytic processing of vWF from high-molecular-weight multimers to smaller forms leads to aberrant platelet aggregation in the circulation; this defect in vWF processing causes *thrombotic thrombocytopenic purpura,* one of the so-called *thrombotic microangiopathies* (see Chapter 12).

Secretion (Release Reaction). Secretion of both granule types occurs soon after adhesion. Various agonists can bind specific platelet surface receptors and initiate an intracellular phosphorylation cascade that leads to degranulation. Release of dense body contents is especially important, since calcium is required in the coagulation cascade and ADP is a potent mediator of *platelet aggregation* (platelets adhering to other platelets—discussed next). ADP also begets additional platelet ADP release, amplifying the aggregation process. Finally, platelet activation increases surface expression of *phospholipid complexes,* which provide a critical nucleation and binding site for calcium and coagulation factors in the *intrinsic clotting pathway* (see later).

Platelet Aggregation. Aggregation follows platelet adhesion and granule release. In addition to ADP, platelet-synthesized thromboxane A_2 (TXA_2; Chapter 2) is also an important stimulus for platelet aggregation. ADP and TXA_2 together drive an autocatalytic process that promotes formation of an enlarging platelet aggregate, the *primary hemostatic plug.* This primary aggregation is reversible. However, with activation of the coagulation cascade, the generation of *thrombin* results in two processes that make an irreversible hemostatic plug. Thrombin binds to a platelet surface receptor (protease-activated receptor, or PAR, see below); in association with ADP and TXA_2, this interaction induces further platelet aggregation. *Platelet contraction* follows, creating an irreversibly fused mass of platelets ("viscous metamorphosis") constituting the definitive *secondary hemostatic plug.* Concurrently, thrombin converts fibrinogen to *fibrin* within and about the platelet plug, contributing to the overall stability of the clot (see below).

Both erythrocytes and leukocytes are also found in hemostatic plugs; leukocytes adhere to platelets and endothelium via adhesion molecules and contribute to the inflammatory response that accompanies thrombosis. Thrombin also contributes by directly stimulating neutrophil and monocyte adhesion and by generating chemotactic *fibrin split products* from the cleavage of fibrinogen.

Importance of Fibrinogen in Platelet Aggregation. The binding of ADP to its platelet receptor induces a conformational change of the GpIIb-IIIa receptors, allowing them to bind fibrinogen. Fibrinogen then acts to connect many platelets together to form large aggregates (see Fig. 4–8). The importance of these interactions is amply demonstrated by the bleeding disorders that occur in patients with congenitally deficient or inactive GpIIb-IIIa proteins. Moreover, the clinical recognition of the central role of these GpIIb-IIIa receptors in platelet cross-linking led to the development of antagonists that can potently block platelet aggregation—either by interfering with ADP binding, as with clopidogrel, or by binding to the GpIIb-IIIa receptors, as with monoclonal antibodies.

Interaction of Platelets and Endothelium. The interplay of platelets and endothelium has a profound impact on the formation of a clot. Prostaglandin PGI_2 (synthesized by endothelium) is a vasodilator and inhibits platelet aggregation, whereas TXA_2 is a platelet-derived prostaglandin that activates platelet aggregation and is a potent vasoconstrictor. Effects mediated by PGI_2 and TXA_2 constitute exquisitely balanced pathways for modulating human platelet function: in the normal state, intravascular platelet aggregation is prevented, whereas endothelial injury favors the formation of hemostatic plugs. The clinical use of aspirin (a cyclooxygenase inhibitor) in patients at risk for coronary thrombosis is related to its ability to inhibit the synthesis of TXA_2. In a manner similar to that of PGI_2, nitric oxide also acts as a vasodilator and inhibitor of platelet aggregation (see Fig. 4–7).

SUMMARY

Platelet Aggregation

- Endothelial injury exposes the underlying basement membrane ECM; platelets adhere to the ECM and become activated by binding to vWF through GpIb platelet receptors.
- Upon activation, platelets secrete granule products that include calcium (activates coagulation proteins) and ADP (mediates further platelet aggregation and degranulation). Activated platelets also synthesize TXA_2 (increases platelet activation and causes vasoconstriction).
- Activated platelets expose phospholipid complexes that provide an important surface for coagulation-protein activation (see below).
- Released ADP stimulates formation of a primary hemostatic plug by activating platelet GpIIb-IIIa receptors that in turn facilitate fibrinogen binding and cross-linking.
- The formation of the definitive secondary hemostatic plug requires the activation of thrombin to cleave fibrinogen and form polymerized fibrin via the coagulation cascade (see below).

Coagulation Cascade

The *coagulation cascade* constitutes the third component of the hemostatic process and is a major contributor to thrombosis. The pathways are schematically presented in Figure 4–9; only general principles are discussed here.

- The coagulation cascade is essentially an amplifying series of enzymatic conversions; each step in the process proteolytically cleaves an inactive proenzyme into an activated enzyme, eventually culminating in *thrombin* formation; thrombin is the most important enzyme regulating the coagulation process. Thrombin converts the soluble plasma protein *fibrinogen* into *fibrin* monomers that polymerize into an insoluble gel; this gel encases platelets and other circulating cells in the definitive secondary hemostatic plug. Fibrin polymers are stabilized by the transglutaminase cross-linking activity of factor XIIIa.
- Each reaction in the pathway results from the assembly of a complex composed of an *enzyme* (activated coagulation factor), a *substrate* (proenzyme form of coagulation factor), and a *cofactor* (reaction accelerator). These components are assembled on a *phospholipid complex* and held together by *calcium ions.* Thus, clotting tends to remain localized to phospholipid-rich sites where such an assembly can occur, for example, on the surface of activated platelets. Two such reactions are the sequential conversion of factor X to Xa and then factor II (prothrombin) to IIa (thrombin) are illustrated in Figure 4–10. Parenthetically, the ability of coagulation factors II, XII, IX, and X to bind to calcium requires that additional γ-carboxyl groups be enzymatically appended to certain glutamic acid residues on these proteins. This reaction requires vitamin K as a cofactor and is antagonized by drugs such as *coumadin,* which is therefore useful for patients who require anticoagulation on a chronic basis—or such as *warfarin,* which can be used as a rodenticide to cause exsanguination.
- The blood coagulation scheme has been traditionally classified into *extrinsic* and *intrinsic* pathways that converge with the activation of factor X (see Fig. 4–9). The extrinsic pathway was so designated because it required the addition of an exogenous trigger (originally provided by tissue extracts); the intrinsic pathway required only exposing factor XII (Hageman factor) to a thrombogenic surface (even glass would suffice). However, this classification, although useful for clinical testing (see below), is largely an artifact of in vitro testing, since several interconnections exist between the two pathways. The extrinsic pathway is the most physiologically relevant of the two in driving coagulation after vascular damage; it is activated by *tissue factor* (also known as *thromboplastin* or factor III), a membrane-bound lipoprotein expressed at sites of injury (see Fig. 4–9).
- The clinical pathology lab assesses the two pathways using two standard assays: *prothrombin time* (PT) and *partial thromboplastin time* (PPT).

The PT assay screens for the activity of the proteins in the extrinsic pathway (factors VII, X, II, V, and fibrinogen) by adding phospholipids and tissue factor to a patient's citrated plasma (sodium citrate chelates any calcium present and prevents spontaneous clotting). The clotting reaction is started by adding exogenous calcium, and the time to fibrin clot formation (usually 11–13 seconds) is recorded. Typically, this is expressed as ratio of the patient's PT to the mean PT for a group of normal patients, othewise known as the International Normalized Ratio (INR). In addition to its value as a screening assay for the normal activity of the extrinsic pathway factors, the PT is also sensitive to the effects of coumadin. It is therefore used to monitor the efficacy of coumadin anticoagulation

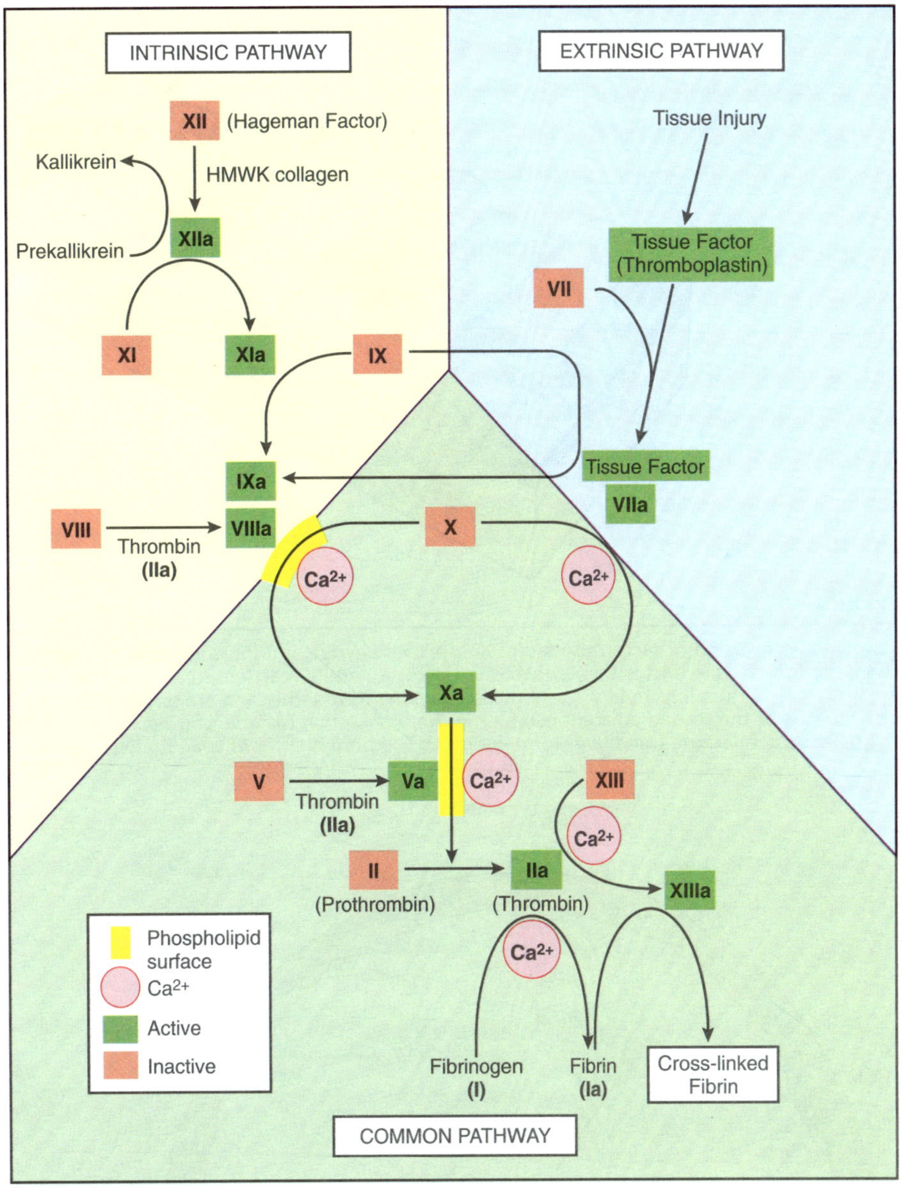

Figure 4–9

The classical coagulation cascade. Note the common link between the intrinsic and extrinsic pathways at the level of factor IX activation. Factors in red boxes represent inactive molecules; activated factors are indicated with a lower-case *a* and a green box. HMWK, high-molecular-weight kininogen. Not shown are the inhibitory anticoagulant pathways (see Figs. 4–7 and 4–12).

therapy; ideally, the INR is maintained between 2 and 3 in patients receiving coumadin.

The PTT assay screens for the activity of the proteins in the intrinsic pathway (factors XII, XI, IX, VIII, X, V, II, and fibrinogen) by adding first an appropriate surface (e.g., ground glass) and phospholipids to a patient's citrated plasma, and then exogenous calcium. The time to clot formation (usually 28–35 seconds) is recorded. In addition to its value in screening for the normal activity of intrinsic pathway factors, the PTT assay's sensitivity to the effects of heparin makes it useful to monitor the efficacy of heparin therapy for acute thrombosis or embolism.

• In addition to catalyzing the final steps in the coagulation cascade, thrombin exerts a wide variety of effects on the local vasculature and inflammatory milieu; it even actively participates in limiting the extent of the hemostatic process (Fig. 4–11). Most of these thrombin-mediated effects occur through protease activated receptors belonging to a family of seven transmembrane proteins coupled to G proteins (see Fig. 4-7).

• Once activated, the coagulation cascade must be restricted to the local site of vascular injury to prevent runaway clotting of the entire vascular tree. In addition to the restriction of factor activation to sites of exposed phospholipids, three categories of natural anticoagulants function to control clotting: *antithrombins, proteins C and S,* and *tissue factor pathway inhibitor* (TFPI).

- Antithrombins (e.g., antithrombin III) inhibit the activity of thrombin and other serine proteases, factors IXa, Xa, XIa, and XIIa. Antithrombin III is activated by binding to heparin-like molecules on endothelial cells—hence the usefulness of

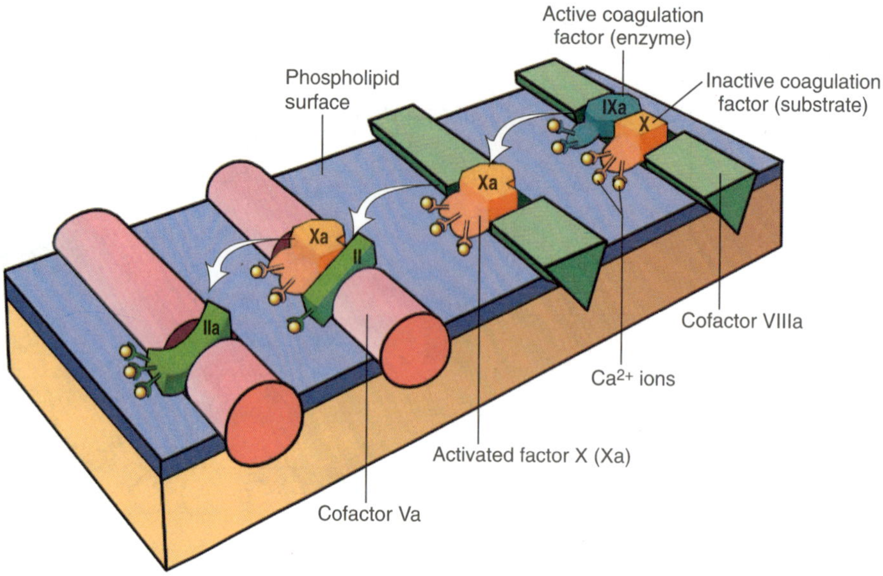

Figure 4–10

Sequential conversion of factor X to factor Xa, followed by factor II (prothrombin) to factor IIa (thrombin). The initial reaction complex consists of an enzyme (factor IXa), a substrate (factor X), and a reaction accelerator (factor VIIIa), all assembled on a platelet phospholipid surface. Calcium ions hold the assembled components together and are essential for the reaction. Activated factor Xa becomes the enzyme part of the second adjacent complex in the coagulation cascade, converting the prothrombin substrate to IIa using factor Va as the reaction accelerator. (Modified from Mann KG: The biochemistry of coagulation. Clin Lab Med 4:217, 1984.)

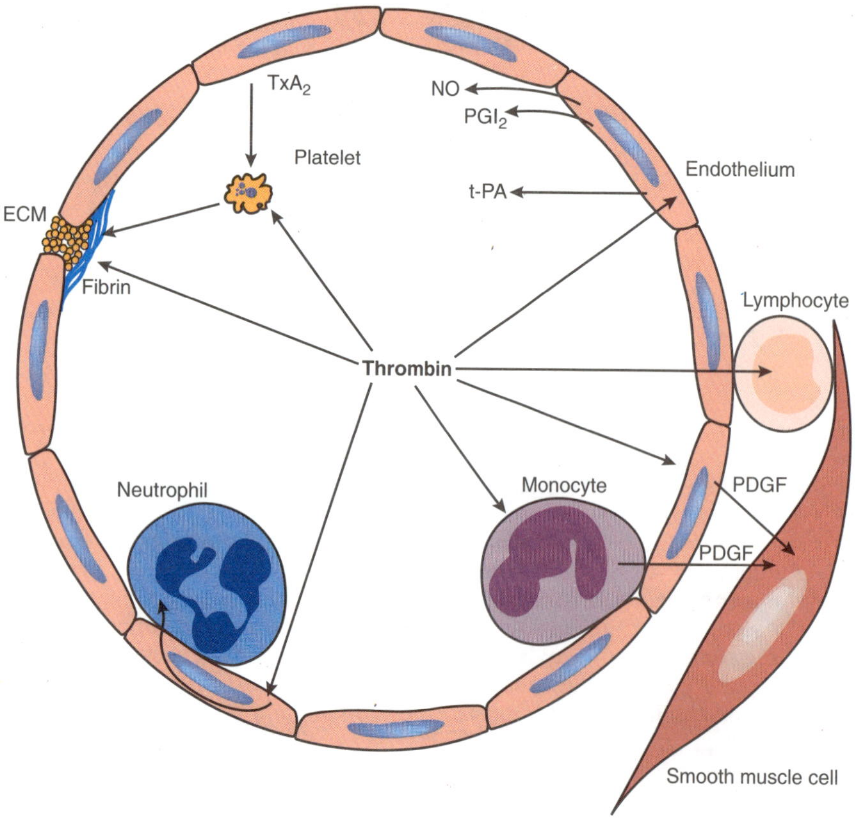

Figure 4–11

Role of thrombin in hemostasis and cellular activation. Thrombin plays a critical role in generating cross-linked fibrin via cleavage of fibrinogen to fibrin and activation of factor XIII. Through protease-activated receptors (PARs, see text), thrombin also modulates several cellular activities. It directly induces platelet aggregation and TXA_2 secretion and can activate endothelium to generate leukocyte adhesion molecule and a variety of fibrinolytic (t-PA), vasoactive (NO, PGI_2), and cytokine (PDGF) mediators. Thrombin also directly activates leukocytes. ECM, extracellular matrix; NO, nitric oxide; PDGF, platelet-derived growth factor; PGI_2, prostacyclin; TXA_2, thromboxane A_2; t-PA, tissue plasminogen activator. See Figure 4–7 for additional anticoagulant modulators of thrombin activity, such as antithrombin III and thrombomodulin. (Courtesy of Shaun Coughlin, MD, PhD, Cardiovascular Research Institute, University of California at San Francisco; modified with permission.)

administering heparin in clinical situations to reduce thrombotic activity (see Fig. 4–7).

- Proteins C and S are two vitamin K–dependent proteins that inactivate the cofactors Va and VIIIa. Protein C activation by thrombomodulin was described earlier; protein S is a cofactor for protein C activity (see Fig. 4–7).
- TFPI is a protein secreted by endothelium (and other cell types) that inactivates factor Xa and tissue factor–VIIa complexes (see Fig. 4–7).

• Activation of the clotting cascade also sets into motion a *fibrinolytic cascade* that moderates the size of the ultimate clot. Fibrinolysis is largely accomplished by the enzymatic activity of *plasmin,* which breaks down fibrin and interferes with its polymerization (Fig. 4–12). The resulting *fibrin split products* (FSPs, or *fibrin degradation products*) can also act as weak anticoagulants. As a clinical correlate, elevated levels of FSPs (clinical laboratories most frequently measure the fibrin *D-dimer*) are helpful in diagnosing abnormal thrombotic states including disseminated intravascular coagulation (DIC), deep venous thrombosis, or pulmonary thromboembolism (described in detail later).

Plasmin is generated by enzymatic degradation of the inactive circulating precursor *plasminogen* either by a factor XII–dependent pathway or by plasminogen activators (PAs; see Fig. 4–12). The most important of the PAs is *t-PA,* which is synthesized principally by endothelial cells and is most active when attached to fibrin. The affinity for fibrin makes t-PA a useful therapeutic agent, since it largely confines fibrinolytic activity to sites of recent thrombosis. *Urokinase-like PA (u-PA)* is another PA present in plasma and in various tissues; it can activate plasmin in the fluid phase. Finally, plasminogen can be cleaved to its active form by the bacterial product *streptokinase,* an activity that may be clinically significant in various bacterial infections. As with any potent regulatory component, the activity of plasmin is also tightly restricted. To prevent excess plasmin from lysing thrombi indiscriminately elsewhere in the body, free plasmin rapidly forms a complex with circulating α_2-antiplasmin and is inactivated (see Fig. 4–12).

• Endothelial cells further modulate the coagulation/anticoagulation balance by releasing PAIs, which block fibrinolysis and confer an overall procoagulation effect (see Fig. 4–12). The PAIs are increased by certain cytokines and probably play a role in the intravascular thrombosis accompanying severe inflammation.

SUMMARY

Coagulation Factors

• Coagulation occurs via the sequential enzymatic conversion of a cascade of circulating and locally synthesized proteins. Tissue factor elaborated at sites of injury is the most important initiator of the coagulation cascade; at the final stage of coagulation, thrombin converts fibrinogen into insoluble fibrin, which helps to form the definitive hemostatic plug.

• Coagulation is normally constrained to sites of vascular injury by:

- Limiting enzymatic activation to phospholipid complexes provided by activated platelets
- Natural anticoagulants elaborated at sites of endothelial injury or during activation of the coagulation cascade
- Induction of fibrinolytic pathways involving plasmin through the activities of various PAs

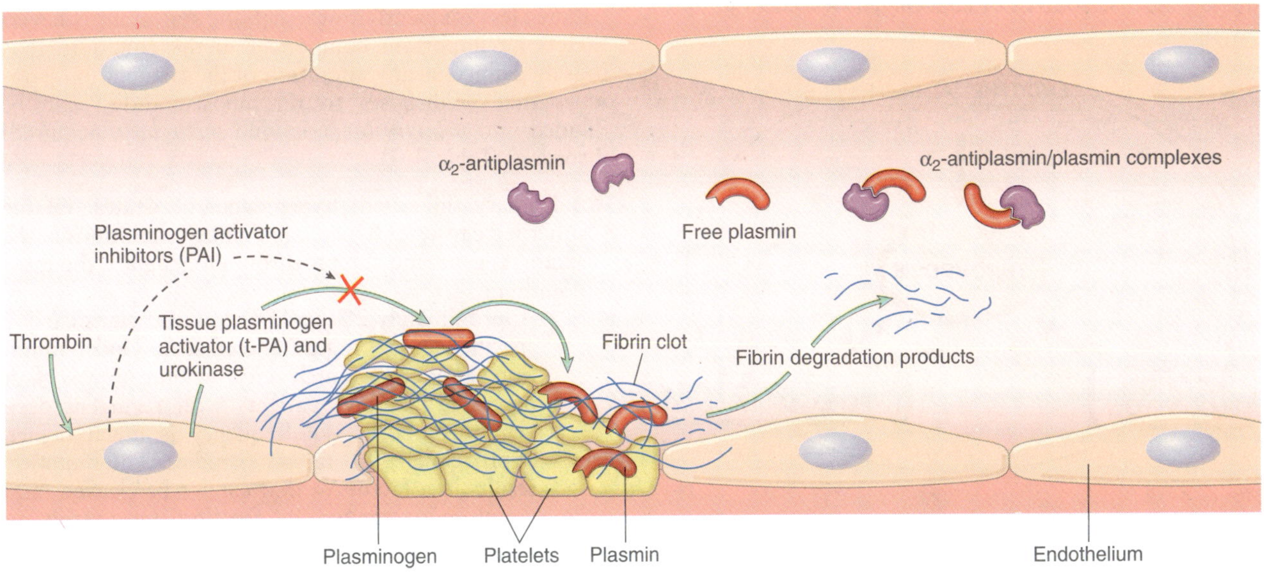

Figure 4–12

The fibrinolytic system, illustrating various plasminogen activators and inhibitors (see text).

Thrombosis

Having discussed the process of normal hemostasis, we can now turn our attention to the dysregulation that underlies thrombus formation.

Pathogenesis. There are three primary influences on thrombus formation (called *Virchow's triad*): (1) endothelial injury, (2) stasis *or* turbulence of blood flow, and (3) blood hypercoagulability (Fig. 4–13).

Endothelial Injury. This is a dominant influence, since endothelial loss by itself can lead to thrombosis. It is particularly important for thrombus formation occurring in the heart or in the arterial circulation, where the normally high flow rates might otherwise hamper clotting by preventing platelet adhesion or diluting coagulation factors. Thus, thrombus formation within the cardiac chambers (e.g., after endocardial injury due to myocardial infarction), over ulcerated plaques in atherosclerotic arteries, or at sites of traumatic or inflammatory vascular injury *(vasculitis)* is largely a function of endothelial injury. Clearly, physical loss of endothelium leads to exposure of subendothelial ECM, adhesion of platelets, release of tissue factor, and local depletion of PGI_2 and plasminogen activators. *However, it is important to note that endothelium need not be denuded or physically disrupted to contribute to the development of thrombosis; any perturbation in the dynamic balance of the prothrombotic and antithrombotic activities of endothelium can influence local clotting events* (see Fig. 4–7). Thus, dysfunctional endothelium may elaborate greater amounts of procoagulant factors (e.g., platelet adhesion molecules, tissue factor, plasminogen activator inhibitors) or may synthesize fewer anticoagulant effectors (e.g., thrombomodulin, PGI_2, t-PA). Significant endothelial dysfunction (in the absence of endothelial cell loss) may occur with hypertension, turbulent flow over scarred valves, or by the action of bacterial endotoxins. Even relatively subtle influences, such as homocystinuria, hypercholesterolemia, radiation, or products absorbed from cigarette smoke, may be sources of endothelial dysfunction.

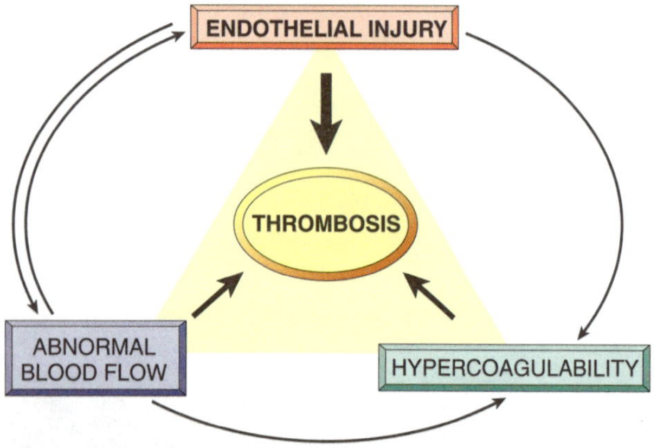

Figure 4–13

Virchow's triad in thrombosis. Integrity of endothelium is the most important factor. Injury to endothelial cells can also alter local blood flow and affect coagulability. Abnormal blood flow (stasis or turbulence), in turn, can cause endothelial injury. The factors may act independently or may combine to promote thrombus formation.

Alterations in Normal Blood Flow. *Turbulence* contributes to arterial and cardiac thrombosis by causing endothelial injury or dysfunction, as well as by forming countercurrents and local pockets of stasis; *stasis* is a major contributor to the development of venous thrombi. Normal blood flow is *laminar,* such that platelets flow centrally in the vessel lumen, separated from the endothelium by a slower moving clear zone of plasma. Stasis and turbulence therefore:

- Disrupt laminar flow and bring platelets into contact with the endothelium
- Prevent dilution of activated clotting factors by fresh-flowing blood
- Retard the inflow of clotting factor inhibitors and permit the buildup of thrombi
- Promote endothelial cell activation, resulting in local thrombosis, leukocyte adhesion, etc.

Turbulence and stasis contribute to thrombosis in several clinical settings. Ulcerated atherosclerotic plaques not only expose subendothelial ECM but also cause turbulence. Abnormal aortic and arterial dilations, called *aneurysms*, create local stasis and consequently a fertile site for thrombosis (Chapter 10). Acute myocardial infarction results in focally noncontractile myocardium; ventricular remodeling after more remote infarction can lead to aneurysm formation. In both cases cardiac mural thrombi form more easily because of the local blood stasis (Chapter 11). Mitral valve stenosis (e.g., after rheumatic heart disease) results in left atrial dilation. In conjunction with atrial fibrillation, a dilated atrium is a site of profound stasis and a prime location for development of thrombi. *Hyperviscosity syndromes* (such as *polycythemia;* Chapter 12) increase resistance to flow and cause small vessel stasis; the deformed red cells in sickle cell anemia (Chapter 12) cause vascular occlusions, with the resultant stasis also predisposing to thrombosis.

Hypercoagulability. Hypercoagulability generally contributes less frequently to thrombotic states but is nevertheless an important component in the equation. It is loosely defined as any alteration of the coagulation pathways that predisposes to thrombosis, and it can be divided into *primary* (genetic) and *secondary* (acquired) disorders (Table 4–2).

- Primary (inherited) hypercoagulable states. Of the inherited causes of hypercoagulability, mutations in the factor V gene and the prothrombin gene are the most common:
  - Approximately 2% to 15% of Caucasians carry a specific factor V mutation (called the Leiden mutation after the Dutch city where it was first described); among patients with recurrent deep vein thrombosis, the frequency is much higher, approaching 60% in some studies. The mutation results in a factor Va that cannot be cleaved (and therefore inactivated) by protein C; as a result, an important antithrombotic counter-regulatory pathway is lost (see Fig. 4–7).
  - A single-nucleotide substitution (G to A) in the 3′ untranslated region of the prothrombin gene is a fairly common allele (1% to 2% of the popula-

Table 4–2 Hypercoagulable States

Primary (Genetic)	
Common	
	Mutation in factor V gene (factor V Leiden)
	Mutation in prothrombin gene
	Mutation in methyltetrahydrofolate gene
Rare	
	Antithrombin III deficiency
	Protein C deficiency
	Protein S deficiency
Very rare	
	Fibrinolysis defects
Secondary (Acquired)	
High risk for thrombosis	
	Prolonged bedrest or immobilization
	Myocardial infarction
	Atrial fibrillation
	Tissue damage (surgery, fracture, burns)
	Cancer
	Prosthetic cardiac valves
	Disseminated intravascular coagulation
	Heparin-induced thrombocytopenia
	Antiphospholipid antibody syndrome (lupus anticoagulant syndrome)
Lower risk for thrombosis	
	Cardiomyopathy
	Nephrotic syndrome
	Hyperestrogenic states (pregnancy)
	Oral contraceptive use
	Sickle cell anemia
	Smoking

tion), resulting in increased prothrombin transcription, and a nearly threefold increased risk of venous thromboses.

Less common primary hypercoagulable states include inherited deficiencies of anticoagulants such as antithrombin III, protein C, or protein S; affected patients typically present with venous thrombosis and recurrent thromboembolism in adolescence or early adult life. Congenitally elevated levels of homocysteine contribute to arterial and venous thromboses (and to the development of atherosclerosis; Chapter 10); the prothrombotic effects of homocysteine are attributed to inhibition of antithrombin III and/or thrombomodulin. Point mutations in tetrahydrofolate reductase genes are associated with mild homocysteinemia in certain white and Asian populations, although the association of the mutations with thrombosis is not well established.

Although these inherited disorders are uncommon causes of significant hypercoagulable states on their own, collectively they are significant for two reasons. First, mutations can be co-inherited, and the resulting risk of a thrombotic diathesis is synergistic. Second, individuals with such mutations have a significantly increased frequency of venous thrombosis in the setting of other acquired risk factors (e.g., pregnancy or prolonged bedrest). Thus, factor V Leiden heterozygosity (which by itself may not be significant) can be sufficiently synergistic with the enforced inactivity during a cross-country plane flight to induce deep venous thromboses. Therefore, inherited causes of hypercoagulability should be considered in young patients (i.e., younger than 50 years), even when other acquired etiologies are present (see below).

- Secondary (acquired) hypercoagulable states. Unlike the hereditary disorders, the pathogenesis of *acquired thrombotic diatheses* is frequently multifactorial and is therefore more complicated (see Table 4–2). In some situations (e.g., cardiac failure or trauma), stasis or vascular injury may be most important. Hypercoagulability is associated with oral contraceptive use and the hyperestrogenic state of pregnancy, probably related to increased hepatic synthesis of coagulation factors and reduced synthesis of antithrombin III. In disseminated cancers, release of procoagulant tumor products predisposes to thrombosis. The hypercoagulability seen with advancing age has been attributed to increasing platelet aggregation and reduced endothelial PGI_2 release. Smoking and obesity promote hypercoagulability by unknown mechanisms.

Among the acquired causes of thrombotic diathesis, the *heparin-induced thrombocytopenia (HIT) syndrome* and *antiphospholipid antibody syndrome* (previously called the *lupus anticoagulant syndrome*) deserve special mention.

- Seen in as many as 5% of the population, the HIT syndrome occurs when administration of unfractionated heparin (for therapeutic anticoagulation) induces autoantibodies to complexes of heparin and a platelet membrane protein (platelet factor 4) (Chapter 12). This antibody binds to similar complexes present on platelet and endothelial surfaces, resulting in platelet activation and endothelial cell injury, and a net *prothrombotic state.* The occurrence of HIT syndrome can be reduced by using low-molecular-weight heparin preparations that retain anticoagulant activity but do not interact with platelets; these preparations have the additional advantage of a prolonged serum half-life.
- Antiphospholipid antibody syndrome has protean manifestations, including recurrent thrombosis, repeated miscarriages, cardiac valve vegetations, and thrombocytopenia; it is associated with autoantibodies directed against anionic phospholipids (e.g., cardiolipin) or—more accurately—plasma protein antigens that are unveiled by binding to such phospholipids (e.g., prothrombin). In vivo these antibodies induce a *hypercoagulable state,* by inducing direct platelet activation or by interfering with endothelial cell production of PGI_2. However, in vitro (in the absence of platelets and endothelium) the antibodies merely interfere with phospholipid complex assembly and thus inhibit coagulation (hence the designation *lupus anticoagulant*). Patients with antibodies to cardiolipins also have a false-positive serologic test for syphilis, because the antigen in the standard tests is embedded in cardiolipin.

There are two types of antiphospholipid antibody syndrome. Many patients have *secondary antiphospholipid syndrome* due to a well-defined autoimmune disease, such as systemic lupus erythematosus (Chapter

5). In contrast, those who exhibit only the manifestations of a hypercoagulable state without evidence of other autoimmune disorder are designated as having *primary antiphospholipid syndrome.* Patients with antiphospholipid antibody syndrome are at increased risk of a fatal event (as many as 7% in one series). Therapy involves anticoagulation, with immunosuppression in refractory cases. Although antiphospholipid antibodies are associated with thrombotic diatheses, they have also been identified in 5% to 15% of apparently normal individuals, implying that they may be necessary but not sufficient to cause full-blown antiphospholipid antibody syndrome.

Morphology

Thrombi can develop anywhere in the cardiovascular system (e.g., in cardiac chambers, on valves, or in arteries, veins, or capillaries). The size and shape of a thrombus depend on the site of origin and the cause. Arterial or cardiac thrombi typically begin at sites of endothelial injury or turbulence; venous thrombi characteristically occur at sites of stasis. Thrombi are focally attached to the underlying vascular surface; arterial thrombi tend to grow in a retrograde direction from the point of attachment, while venous thrombi extend in the direction of blood flow (thus both tend to propagate toward the heart). The propagating portion of a thrombus tends to be poorly attached and therefore prone to fragmentation, generating an **embolus**.

Thrombi can have grossly (and microscopically) apparent laminations called **lines of Zahn**; these represent pale platelet and fibrin layers alternating with darker erythrocyte-rich layers. Such lines are significant only in that they represent thrombosis in the setting of flowing blood; their presence can therefore potentially distinguish antemortem thrombosis from the bland nonlaminated clots that occur in the postmortem state (see also below). Although such lines are typically not as apparent in veins or smaller arteries (thrombi formed in sluggish venous flow usually resemble statically coagulated blood), careful evaluation generally reveals ill-defined laminations.

Thrombi occurring in heart chambers or in the aortic lumen are designated **mural thrombi.** Abnormal myocardial contraction (resulting from arrhythmias, dilated cardiomyopathy, or myocardial infarction) or endomyocardial injury (caused by myocarditis, catheter trauma) promotes cardiac mural thrombi (Fig. 4–14A), while ulcerated atherosclerotic plaques and aneurysmal dilation promote aortic thrombosis (Fig. 4–14B).

Arterial thrombi are frequently occlusive and are produced by platelet and coagulation activation; they are typically a friable meshwork of platelets, fibrin, erythrocytes, and degenerating leukocytes. Although arterial thrombi are usually superimposed on an atherosclerotic plaque, other vascular injury (vasculitis, trauma) can be involved.

Venous thrombosis (phlebothrombosis) is almost invariably occlusive, and the thrombus can create a long cast of the lumen; venous thrombosis is largely the result of activation of the coagulation cascade, and platelets play a secondary role. Because these thrombi form in the sluggish venous circulation, they also tend to contain more enmeshed erythrocytes and are therefore called red, or stasis, thrombi. The veins of the lower extremities are most commonly affected (90% of venous thromboses); however, venous thrombi can occur in the upper extremities, periprostatic plexus, or ovarian and periuterine veins; under special circumstances they may be found in the dural sinuses, portal vein, or hepatic vein.

Postmortem clots can sometimes be mistaken at autopsy for venous thrombi. However, postmortem "thrombi" are gelatinous, with a dark red dependent portion where red cells have settled by gravity, and a yellow "chicken fat" supernatant, and they are usually not attached to the underlying wall. In contrast, red thrombi are firmer and are focally attached, and sectioning reveals strands of gray fibrin.

Thrombi on heart valves are called **vegetations.** Bacterial or fungal blood-borne infections can cause valve damage, subsequently leading to large thrombotic masses (infective endocarditis, Chapter 11). Sterile vegetations can also develop on noninfected valves in hypercoagulable states, so-called **nonbacterial thrombotic endocarditis** (Chapter 11). Less commonly, sterile, verrucous endocarditis (Libman-Sacks endocarditis) can occur in the setting of systemic lupus erythematosus (Chapter 5).

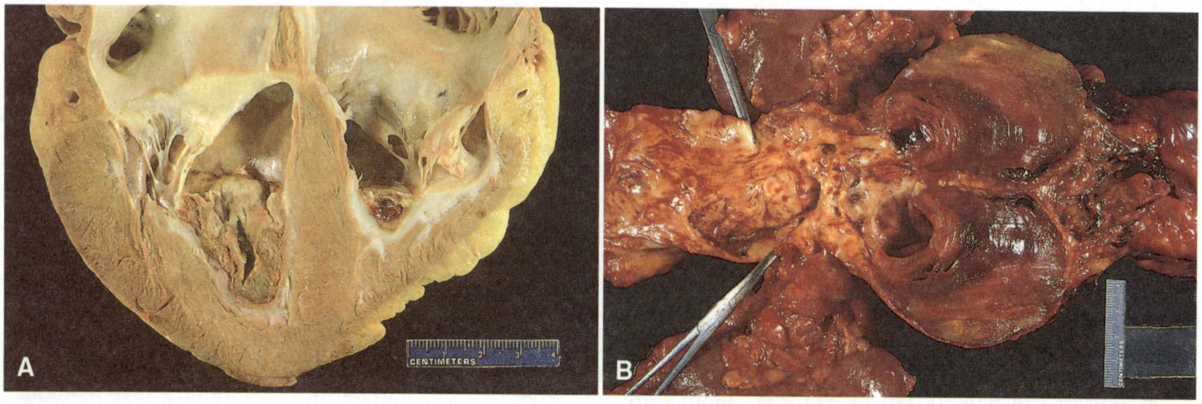

Figure 4–14

Mural thrombi. **A,** Thrombus in the left and right ventricular apices, overlying white fibrous scar. **B,** Laminated thrombus in a dilated abdominal aortic aneurysm. Numerous friable mural thrombi are also superimposed on advanced atherosclerotic lesions of the more proximal aorta (*left side of picture*).

Fate of the Thrombus. If a patient survives the initial thrombosis, in the ensuing days or weeks thrombi undergo some combination of the following four events:

- *Propagation.* Thrombi accumulate additional platelets and fibrin, eventually causing vessel obstruction.
- *Embolization.* Thrombi dislodge or fragment and are transported elsewhere in the vasculature.
- *Dissolution.* Thrombi are removed by fibrinolytic activity.
- *Organization and recanalization.* Thrombi induce inflammation and fibrosis *(organization).* These can eventually *recanalize* (re-establishing some degree of flow), or they can be incorporated into a thickened vessel wall.

Propagation was discussed above, and embolization is covered in greater detail below. Dissolution is the result of fibrinolytic activation, which leads to rapid shrinkage and even total lysis of *recent* thrombi. With older thrombi, extensive fibrin polymerization renders the thrombus substantially more resistant to proteolysis, and lysis is ineffectual. This is clinically significant because therapeutic administration of fibrinolytic agents (e.g., t-PA in the setting of acute coronary thrombosis) is generally effective only within a few hours of thrombus formation.

Older thrombi become *organized* by the ingrowth of endothelial cells, smooth muscle cells, and fibroblasts into the fibrin-rich clot (Fig. 4–15). Capillary channels are eventually formed that, to a limited extent, can create conduits along the length of the thrombus and thereby re-establish the continuity of the original lumen. Although the channels may not successfully restore significant flow to many obstructed vessels, recanalization can potentially convert a thrombus into a vascularized mass of connective tissue that is eventually incorporated into the vessel wall and remains as a subendothelial swelling. Eventually, with contraction of the mesenchymal cells only a fibrous lump may remain to mark the original thrombus site. Occasionally, instead of organizing, the center of a thrombus undergoes enzymatic digestion, presumably because of the release of lysosomal enzymes from trapped leukocytes and platelets.

Clinical Correlations: Venous versus Arterial Thrombosis. Thrombi are significant because *they cause obstruction of arteries and veins and are potential sources of emboli.* Which effect is most important depends on the site of thrombosis. Venous thrombi can cause congestion and edema in vascular beds distal to an obstruction, but they are most worrisome for their capacity to embolize to the lungs and cause death (see below). Conversely, while arterial thrombi can embolize and even cause downstream tissue infarction (see below), their role in vascular obstruction at critical sites (e.g., coronary and cerebral vessels) is much more significant clinically.

Venous Thrombosis (Phlebothrombosis). Most venous thrombi occur in the superficial or deep veins of the leg. Superficial venous thrombi usually occur in the saphenous system, particularly when there are varicosities. Such superficial thrombi can cause local congestion, swelling, pain, and tenderness along the course of the involved vein, but they rarely embolize. Nevertheless, the local edema and impaired venous drainage do predispose the overlying skin to infections from minor trauma and to the development of *varicose ulcers.* Deep thrombi in the larger leg veins at or above the knee joint (e.g., popliteal, femoral, and iliac veins) are more serious because they may embolize. Although they may cause local pain and edema, the venous obstruction may be rapidly offset by collateral bypass channels. Consequently, deep venous thromboses are entirely asymptomatic in approximately 50% of patients and are recognized in retrospect only after they have embolized.

Deep venous thrombosis can occur with stasis or in a variety of hypercoagulable states, as described earlier (see Table 4–2). Cardiac failure is an obvious reason for stasis in the venous circulation. Trauma, surgery, and burns usually result in reduced physical activity, injury to vessels, release of procoagulant substances from tissues, and/or reduced t-PA activity. There are many influences

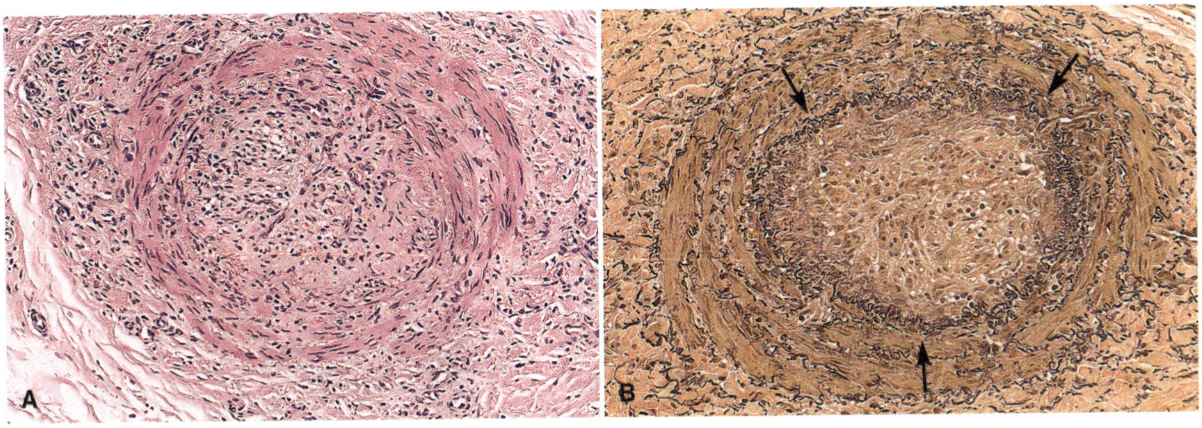

Figure 4–15

Low-power view of an artery with an old thrombus. **A,** H&E-stained section. **B,** Stain for elastic tissue. The original lumen is delineated by the internal elastic lamina (*arrows*) and is totally filled with organized thrombus, now punctuated by a number of recanalized channels (white spaces).

contributing to the thrombotic propensity of peripartum and postpartum states; in addition to the potential for amniotic fluid infusion into the circulation during parturition (see below), late pregnancy and the postpartum period are associated with hypercoagulability. Tumor-associated procoagulant release is largely responsible for the increased risk of thromboembolic phenomena seen in disseminated cancers (called *migratory thrombophlebitis*, or *Trousseau's syndrome*). Regardless of the specific clinical setting, advanced age, bedrest, and immobilization increase the risk of deep venous thrombosis because reduced physical activity diminishes the milking action of muscles in the lower leg and so slows venous return.

Cardiac and Arterial Thrombosis. *Atherosclerosis* is a major initiator of thromboses, because it is associated with loss of endothelial integrity and abnormal vascular flow (see Fig. 4–14B). Cardiac mural thrombi can occur in the setting of myocardial infarction related to dyskinetic myocardial contraction as well as damage to the adjacent endocardium (see Fig. 4–14A). *Rheumatic heart disease* (Chapter 11) can cause atrial mural thrombi due to mitral valve stenosis, followed by left atrial dilation and concurrent atrial fibrillation. In addition to the obstructive consequences, cardiac and aortic mural thrombi can also embolize peripherally. Virtually any tissue can be affected, but brain, kidneys, and spleen are prime targets because of their large volume of blood flow.

SUMMARY

Thrombosis

- Thrombus development depends on the relative contribution of the components of Virchow's triad:
  - Endothelial injury (e.g., by toxins, hypertension, inflammation, or metabolic products)
  - Abnormal blood flow – stasis or turbulence (e.g., due to aneurysms, atherosclerotic plaque)
  - Hypercoagulability, which can be either primary (e.g., factor V Leiden, increased prothrombin synthesis, antithrombin III deficiency) or secondary (e.g., bedrest, tissue damage, malignancy)
- Thrombi may propagate, resolve, become organized, or embolize.
- Thrombosis causes tissue injury by local vascular occlusion or by distal embolization.

EMBOLISM

An embolus is a detached intravascular solid, liquid, or gaseous mass that is carried by the blood to a site distant from its point of origin. Virtually 99% of all emboli represent some part of a dislodged thrombus, hence the term *thromboembolism*. Rare forms of emboli include fat droplets, bubbles of air or nitrogen, atherosclerotic debris (*cholesterol emboli*), tumor fragments, bits of bone marrow, or foreign bodies such as bullets. However, unless otherwise specified, an embolism should be considered to be thrombotic in origin. Inevitably, emboli lodge in vessels too small to permit further passage, resulting in partial or complete vascular occlusion. The consequences of thromboembolism include ischemic necrosis (*infarction*) of downstream tissue. Depending on the site of origin, emboli may lodge anywhere in the vascular tree; the clinical outcomes are best understood from the standpoint of whether emboli lodge in the pulmonary or systemic circulations.

Pulmonary Thromboembolism

Pulmonary embolism has an incidence of 20 to 25 per 100,000 hospitalized patients. Although the rate of fatal pulmonary emboli (as assessed at autopsy) has declined from 6% to 2% over the last quarter century, pulmonary embolism still causes about 200,000 deaths per year in the United States. In more than 95% of cases, venous emboli originate from deep leg vein thrombi above the level of the knee (described above). They are carried through progressively larger channels and pass through the right side of the heart before entering the pulmonary vasculature. Depending on the size of the embolus, it may occlude the main pulmonary artery, impact across the bifurcation (*saddle embolus*), or pass out into the smaller, branching arterioles (Fig. 4–16). Frequently, there are multiple emboli, perhaps sequentially, or as a shower of smaller emboli from a single large thrombus; in general, *the patient who has had one pulmonary embolus is at high risk of having more.* Rarely, an embolus can pass through an interatrial or interventricular defect, thereby entering the systemic circulation (*paradoxical embolism*). The following is an overview of pulmonary emboli; see Chapter 13 for a more complete discussion.

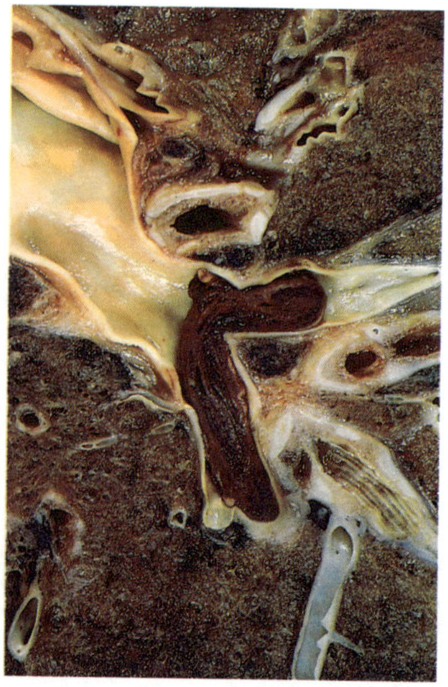

Figure 4–16

Embolus derived from a lower extremity deep venous thrombosis and now impacted in a pulmonary artery branch.

- Most pulmonary emboli (60% to 80%) are clinically silent because they are small. They eventually become organized and become incorporated into the vascular wall; in some cases, organization of the thromboembolus leaves behind a delicate, bridging fibrous *web*.
- Sudden death, right ventricular failure (*cor pulmonale*), or cardiovascular collapse occurs when 60% or more of the pulmonary circulation is obstructed with emboli.
- Embolic obstruction of medium-sized arteries can cause pulmonary hemorrhage but usually not pulmonary infarction because the lung has a dual blood supply and the intact bronchial arterial circulation continues to supply blood to the area. However, a similar embolus in the setting of left-sided cardiac failure (and resultant sluggish bronchial artery blood flow) may result in a large infarct.
- Embolic obstruction of small end-arteriolar pulmonary branches usually does result in associated infarction.
- Many emboli occurring over a period of time may cause pulmonary hypertension with right ventricular failure.

Systemic Thromboembolism

Systemic thromboembolism refers to emboli in the arterial circulation. Most (80%) arise from intracardiac mural thrombi, two-thirds of which are associated with left ventricular wall infarcts and another quarter with dilated left atria (e.g., secondary to mitral valve disease). The remainder originate from aortic aneurysms, thrombi on ulcerated atherosclerotic plaques, or fragmentation of valvular vegetations (Chapter 11). A very small fraction of systemic emboli appear to arise in veins but end up in the arterial circulation, through interventricular defects. These are called *paradoxical emboli.* In contrast to venous emboli, which tend to lodge primarily in one vascular bed (the lung), arterial emboli can travel to a wide variety of sites; the site of arrest depends on the point of origin of the thromboembolus and the relative blood flow through the downstream tissues. The major sites for arteriolar embolization are the lower extremities (75%) and the brain (10%), with the intestines, kidneys, and spleen affected to a lesser extent. The consequences of embolization in a tissue depend on vulnerability to ischemia, caliber of the occluded vessel, and the collateral blood supply; in general, arterial embolization causes infarction of the affected tissues.

Fat Embolism

Microscopic fat globules can be found in the circulation after fractures of long bones (which contain fatty marrow) or after soft-tissue trauma. Fat enters the circulation by rupture of the marrow vascular sinusoids or rupture of venules in injured tissues. Although fat and marrow embolism occurs in some 90% of individuals with severe skeletal injuries (Fig. 4–17), fewer than 10% of such patients show any clinical findings. *Fat embolism syndrome is characterized by pulmonary insufficiency, neurologic symptoms, anemia, and thrombocytopenia; it is fatal in about 10% of cases.* Typically, the symptoms appear 1 to 3 days after injury, with sudden onset of tachypnea, dyspnea, and tachycardia. Neurologic symptoms include irritability and restlessness, with progression to delirium or coma.

The pathogenesis of fat emboli syndrome probably involves both mechanical obstruction and biochemical injury. Fat microemboli occlude pulmonary and cerebral microvasculature; vascular occlusion is aggravated by local platelet and erythrocyte aggregation. This pathology is further exacerbated by free fatty acid release from the fat globules, causing local toxic injury to endothelium. Platelet activation and recruitment of granulocytes (with free radical, protease, and eicosanoid release; Chapter 2) complete the vascular assault. Because lipids are dissolved out of tissue preparations by the solvents routinely used in paraffin embedding, the microscopic demonstration of fat microglobules (i.e., in the absence of accompanying marrow) typically requires specialized techniques, including frozen sections and fat stains.

Air Embolism

Gas bubbles within the circulation can obstruct vascular flow (and cause distal ischemic injury) almost as readily as thrombotic masses can. Air may enter the circulation during obstetric procedures or as a consequence of chest wall injury. Generally, more than 100 mL of air are required to produce a clinical effect; bubbles can coalesce to form frothy masses sufficiently large to occlude major vessels.

A particular form of gas embolism, called *decompression sickness,* occurs when individuals are exposed to sudden changes in atmospheric pressure. Scuba and deep-sea divers, and underwater construction workers are at risk. When air is breathed at high pressure (e.g., during a deep-sea dive), increased amounts of gas (particularly nitrogen) become dissolved in the blood and tissues. If the diver then ascends (depressurizes) too rapidly, the nitrogen expands in the tissues and bubbles out of solution in the blood to form gas emboli that can induce focal ischemia in a number of tissues, including brain and heart.

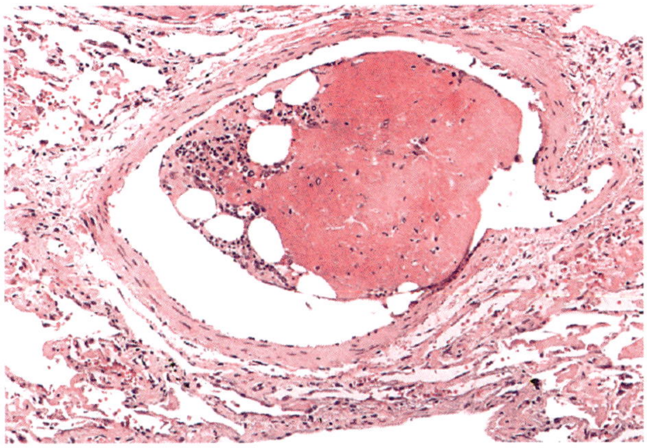

Figure 4–17

Bone marrow embolus in the pulmonary circulation. The cellular elements on the left side of the embolus are hematopoietic precursors, while the cleared vacuoles represent marrow fat. The relatively uniform red area on the right of the embolus is an early organizing thrombus.

The rapid formation of gas bubbles within skeletal muscles and supporting tissues in and about joints is responsible for the painful condition called *the bends* (so named in the 1880s because afflicted individuals characteristically arched their backs in a manner reminiscent of a then-popular women's fashion called the *Grecian Bend*). In the lungs, gas bubbles in the vasculature cause edema, hemorrhages, and focal atelectasis or emphysema, leading to respiratory distress, called the *chokes*. A more chronic form of decompression sickness is called *caisson disease,* where persistence of gas emboli in the bones leads to multiple foci of ischemic necrosis; the heads of the femurs, tibias, and humeri are most commonly affected.

Treating acute decompression sickness requires placing the affected individual in a compression chamber to increase barometric pressure and force the gas bubbles back into solution. Subsequent slow decompression theoretically permits gradual resorption and exhalation of the gases so that obstructive bubbles do not re-form.

Amniotic Fluid Embolism

Amniotic fluid embolism is a grave but fortunately uncommon complication of labor and the immediate postpartum period (1 in 50,000 deliveries). It has a mortality rate in excess of 20% to 40%. The onset is characterized by sudden severe dyspnea, cyanosis, and hypotensive shock, followed by seizures and coma. If the patient survives the initial crisis, pulmonary edema typically develops, along with (in half the patients) disseminated intravascular coagulation (DIC), due to release of thrombogenic substances from amniotic fluid.

The underlying cause is entry of amniotic fluid (and its contents) into the maternal circulation via a tear in the placental membranes and rupture of uterine veins. Classically, there is marked pulmonary edema and diffuse alveolar damage (Chapter 13), with the pulmonary microcirculation containing squamous cells shed from fetal skin, lanugo hair, fat from vernix caseosa, and mucin derived from the fetal respiratory or gastrointestinal tracts. Systemic fibrin thrombi indicate the onset of DIC.

SUMMARY

Embolism

- An embolus is any detached solid, liquid, or gaseous mass carried by the blood to a site distant from its origin; the vast majority are part of a dislodged thrombus.
- Pulmonary emboli derive primarily from lower extremity deep vein thrombosis; their effect (sudden death, right heart failure, pulmonary hemorrhage, or infarction) depends on the size of the embolus.
- Systemic emboli derive primarily from cardiac mural or valvular thrombi, aortic aneurysms, or atherosclerotic plaque; whether an embolus causes tissue infarction depends on the site of embolization and collateral circulation.

INFARCTION

An infarct is an area of ischemic necrosis caused by occlusion of either the arterial supply or the venous drainage in a particular tissue. Tissue infarction is a common and extremely important cause of clinical illness. More than half of all deaths in the United States are caused by cardiovascular disease, and most of these are attributable to myocardial or cerebral infarction. Pulmonary infarction is a common complication in several clinical settings, bowel infarction is frequently fatal, and ischemic necrosis of the extremities (gangrene) is a serious problem in the diabetic population.

Nearly 99% of all infarcts result from thrombotic or embolic events, and almost all result from arterial occlusion. Occasionally, infarction may also be caused by other mechanisms, such as local vasospasm, expansion of an atheroma secondary to intraplaque hemorrhage, or extrinsic compression of a vessel (e.g., by tumor). Uncommon causes include vessel twisting (e.g., in testicular torsion or bowel volvulus), vascular compression by edema or entrapment in a hernia sac, or traumatic vessel rupture. Although venous thrombosis can cause infarction, it more often merely induces venous obstruction and congestion. Usually, bypass channels open rapidly after the occlusion forms, providing some outflow from the area that, in turn, improves the arterial inflow. Infarcts caused by venous thrombosis are more likely in organs with a single venous outflow channel (e.g., testis and ovary).

Morphology

Infarcts are classified on the basis of their color (reflecting the amount of hemorrhage) and the presence or absence of microbial infection. Therefore, infarcts may be either red (hemorrhagic) or white (anemic) and may be either septic or bland.

Red infarcts (Fig. 4–18A) occur (1) with venous occlusions (such as in ovarian torsion); (2) in loose tissues (such as lung) that allow blood to collect in the infarcted zone; (3) in tissues with dual circulations such as lung and small intestine, permitting flow of blood from an unobstructed parallel supply into a necrotic area (such perfusion not being sufficient to rescue the ischemic tissues); (4) in tissues that were previously congested because of sluggish venous outflow; (5) when flow is re-established to a site of previous arterial occlusion and necrosis (e.g., fragmentation of an occlusive embolus or angioplasty of a thrombotic lesion).

White infarcts occur with arterial occlusions or in solid organs (such as heart, spleen, and kidney), where the solidity of the tissue limits the amount of hemorrhage that can seep into the area of ischemic necrosis from adjoining capillary beds (Fig. 4–18B).

All infarcts tend to be wedge shaped, with the occluded vessel at the apex and the periphery of the organ forming the base (see Fig. 4–18); when the base is a serosal surface there can be an overlying fibrinous exudate. At the outset, all infarcts are poorly defined and slightly hemorrhagic. The margins of both types of infarcts tend to become better defined with time by a narrow rim of congestion attributable to inflammation at the edge of the lesion.

In solid organs, the relatively few extravasated red cells are lysed, with the released hemoglobin remaining in the form of hemosiderin. Thus, infarcts resulting from arterial occlusions typically become progressively more pale and sharply defined with time (see Fig. 4–18B). In spongy organs, by comparison, the hemorrhage is too extensive to permit the lesion ever to become pale (see Fig. 4–18A). Over the course of a few days, however, it does become firmer and browner, reflecting the accumulation of hemosiderin pigment.

The dominant histologic characteristic of infarction is **ischemic coagulative necrosis** (Chapter 1). An inflammatory response begins to develop along the margins of infarcts within a few hours and is usually well defined within 1 to 2 days. Eventually the inflammatory response is followed by a reparative response beginning in the preserved margins (Chapter 3). In stable or labile tissues, parenchymal regeneration can occur at the periphery, where underlying stromal architecture is spared. However, most infarcts are ultimately replaced by scar (Fig. 4–19). The brain is an exception to these generalizations; ischemic tissue injury in the central nervous system results in liquefactive necrosis (Chapter 1).

Septic infarctions occur when bacterial vegetations from a heart valve embolize or when microbes seed an area of necrotic tissue. In these cases the infarct is converted into an abscess, with a correspondingly greater inflammatory response (Chapter 2). The eventual sequence of organization, however, follows the pattern previously described.

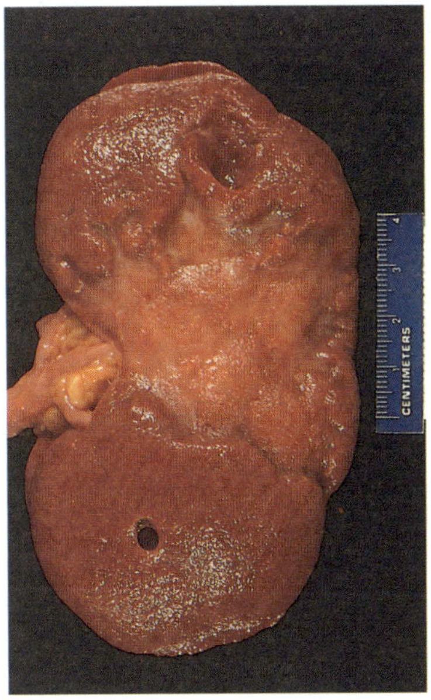

Figure 4–19

Remote kidney infarct, now replaced by a large fibrotic scar.

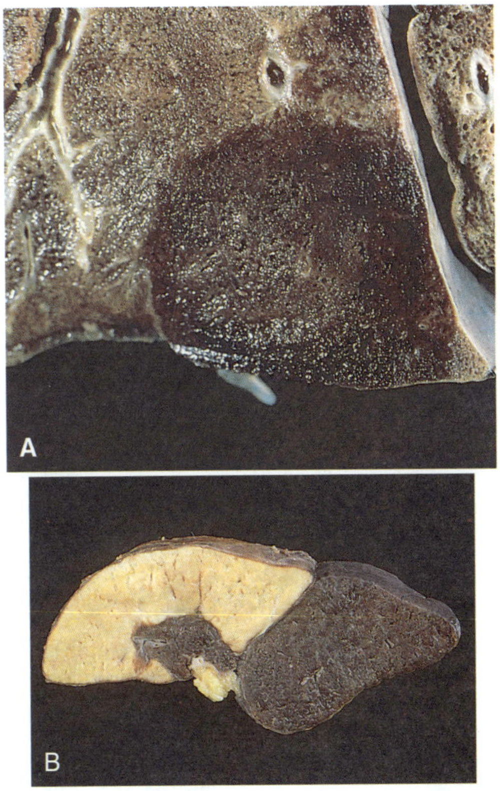

Figure 4–18

Red and white infarcts. **A**, Hemorrhagic, roughly wedge-shaped pulmonary infarct (*red infarct*). **B**, Sharply demarcated pale infarct in the spleen (*white infarct*).

Factors That Influence Development of an Infarct. Vascular occlusion can have no or minimal effect, or can cause death of a tissue or even the individual. *The major determinants of the eventual outcome include the nature of the vascular supply, the rate of development of the occlusion, vulnerability to hypoxia, and the oxygen content of blood.*

Nature of the Vascular Supply. The availability of an alternative blood supply is the most important determinant of whether occlusion of a vessel will cause damage. For example, as mentioned above, lungs have a dual pulmonary and bronchial artery blood supply; thus, obstruction of small pulmonary arterioles does not cause infarction in an otherwise healthy individual with an intact bronchial circulation. Similarly, the liver, with its dual hepatic artery and portal vein circulation, and the hand and forearm, with their dual radial and ulnar arterial supply, are all relatively resistant to infarction. In contrast, renal and splenic circulations are end-arterial, and obstruction of such vessels generally causes infarction.

Rate of Development of Occlusion. Slowly developing occlusions are less likely to cause infarction because they provide time for the development of alternative perfusion pathways. For example, small interarteriolar anastomoses—normally with minimal functional flow—interconnect the three major coronary arteries in the heart. If one of the coronaries is slowly occluded (e.g., by an encroaching atherosclerotic plaque), flow within this collateral circulation may increase sufficiently to prevent infarction, even though the major coronary artery is eventually occluded.

Vulnerability to Hypoxia. The susceptibility of a tissue to hypoxia influences the likelihood of infarction. Neurons undergo irreversible damage when deprived of their blood supply for only 3 to 4 minutes. Myocardial cells, though hardier than neurons, are also quite sensitive and die after only 20 to 30 minutes of ischemia. In contrast, fibroblasts within myocardium remain viable after many hours of ischemia.

Oxygen Content of Blood. The partial pressure of oxygen in blood also determines the outcome of vascular occlusion. Partial flow obstruction of a small vessel in an anemic or cyanotic patient might lead to tissue infarction, whereas it would be without effect under conditions of normal oxygen tension. In this way congestive heart failure, with compromised flow and ventilation, could cause infarction in the setting of an otherwise inconsequential blockage.

SUMMARY

Infarction

- Infarcts are areas of ischemic, usually coagulative, necrosis caused by occlusion of arterial supply or less commonly venous drainage.
- Infarcts are most commonly caused by formation of occlusive arterial thrombi, or embolization of arterial or venous thrombi.
- Infarcts caused by venous occlusion, or in loose tissues with dual blood supply, are typically hemorrhagic (red) whereas those caused by arterial occlusion in compact tissues are pale (white) in color.

SHOCK

Shock is the final common pathway for a number of potentially lethal clinical events, including severe hemorrhage, extensive trauma or burns, large myocardial infarction, massive pulmonary embolism, and microbial sepsis. Regardless of the underlying pathology, *shock gives rise to systemic hypoperfusion; it can be caused either by reduced cardiac output or by reduced effective circulating blood volume. The end results are hypotension, impaired tissue perfusion, and cellular hypoxia.* Although the hypoxic and metabolic effects of hypoperfusion initially cause only reversible cellular injury, persistence of shock eventually causes irreversible tissue injury and can culminate in the death of the patient.

There are three general categories of shock: cardiogenic, hypovolemic, and septic (Table 4–3). The mechanisms underlying cardiogenic and hypovolemic shock are fairly straightforward; septic shock is substantially more complicated and is discussed in further detail below.

- *Cardiogenic shock* results from failure of the cardiac pump. This may be caused by myocardial damage (infarction), ventricular arrhythmias, extrinsic compression (cardiac tamponade, Chapter 11), or outflow obstruction (e.g., pulmonary embolism).
- *Hypovolemic shock* results from loss of blood or plasma volume. This may be caused by hemorrhage, fluid loss from severe burns, or trauma.

Table 4–3 Three Major Types of Shock

Type of Shock	Clinical Examples	Principal Mechanisms
Cardiogenic		
	Myocardial infarction Ventricular rupture Arrhythmia Cardiac tamponade Pulmonary embolism	Failure of myocardial pump resulting from intrinsic myocardial damage, extrinsic pressure, or obstruction to outflow
Hypovolemic		
	Hemorrhage Fluid loss (e.g., vomiting, diarrhea, burns, or trauma)	Inadequate blood or plasma volume
Septic		
	Overwhelming microbial infections Endotoxic shock Gram-positive septicemia Fungal sepsis Superantigens (e.g. toxic shock syndrome)	Peripheral vasodilation and pooling of blood; endothelial activation/injury; leukocyte-induced damage; disseminated intravascular coagulation; activation of cytokine cascades

- *Septic shock* is caused by microbial infection. Most commonly this occurs in the setting of gram-negative infections (*endotoxic shock*), but it can also occur with gram-positive and fungal infections. Notably, there need not be systemic bacteremia to induce septic shock; host inflammatory responses to local extravascular infections may be sufficient (see below).

Less commonly, shock may occur in the setting of an anesthetic accident or a spinal cord injury (*neurogenic shock*), as a result of loss of vascular tone and peripheral pooling of blood. *Anaphylactic shock* represents systemic vasodilation and increased vascular permeability caused by an immunoglobulin E hypersensitivity reaction (Chapter 5). In these situations, acute severe widespread vasodilation results in tissue hypoperfusion and cellular anoxia.

Pathogenesis of Septic Shock

With a 25% to 50% mortality rate, septic shock ranks first among the causes of death in intensive care units and accounts for more than 200,000 deaths annually in the United States. Moreover, the continuing increase in the incidence of sepsis syndromes is attributable to improved life support for high-risk patients, an increase in invasive procedures, and the growing numbers of immunocompromised hosts (secondary to chemotherapy, immunosuppression, or infection with the human immunodeficiency virus). Septic shock results from the host innate immune response to infectious organisms that may be blood borne or localized to a particular site.

Most cases of septic shock (approximately 70%) are caused by endotoxin-producing gram-negative bacilli (Chapter 9)—hence the term *endotoxic shock*. Endotoxins are bacterial wall lipopolysaccharides (LPS) consisting of a toxic fatty acid (*lipid A*) core common to all gram-negative bacteria, and a complex polysaccharide coat (including O *antigen*) unique for each species. Analogous molecules in the walls of gram-positive bacteria and fungi can also elicit septic shock.

All of the cellular and hemodynamic effects of septic shock can be reproduced by LPS injection alone. Free LPS attaches to a circulating LPS-binding protein, and the complex then binds to a specific receptor (CD14) on monocytes, macrophages, and neutrophils. Engagement of CD14 (even at doses as minute as *10 pg/mL*) results in intracellular signaling via an associated "Toll-like receptor" protein 4 (TLR-4), resulting in profound activation of mononuclear cells and production of potent effector cytokines such as IL-1 and TNF (Chapter 2). These cytokines act on endothelial cells and have a variety of effects including reduced synthesis of anticoagulation factors such as tissue factor pathway inhibitor and thrombomodulin (see Fig. 4–7). The effects of the cytokines may be amplified by TLR-4 engagement on endothelial cells.

TLR–mediated activation helps to trigger the innate immune system to efficiently eradicate invading microbes (Chapter 5). Unfortunately, depending on the dosage and the extent of immune and vascular activation, the secondary effects of LPS release can also cause severe pathologic changes, including fatal shock.

At low doses, LPS predominantly activates monocytes, macrophages, and neutrophils; it can also directly activate complement, thereby contributing to local eradication of bacteria. Mononuclear phagocytes respond to LPS by producing TNF, which in turn induces IL-1 synthesis. Both TNF and IL-1 act on endothelial cells (and other cell types) to produce additional cytokines (e.g., IL-6 and IL-8) and induce adhesion molecules (Chapter 2). Thus, the initial release of LPS results in a circumscribed cytokine cascade (Fig. 4–20 and Fig. 4–21) that enhances the *local* acute inflammatory response and improves clearance of the infection.

With moderately severe infections, and therefore with higher levels of LPS (and a consequent augmentation of the cytokine cascade), cytokine-induced secondary effectors (e.g., nitric oxide and platelet-activating factor; Chapter 2) become significant. In addition, systemic effects of TNF and IL-1 may begin to be seen, including fever, increased synthesis of acute-phase reactants, and increased production of circulating neutrophils (see Fig. 4–21). Higher LPS levels tip the endothelium toward a net procoagulant phenotype.

Finally, at still higher levels of LPS, the syndrome of septic shock supervenes (see Fig. 4–21); the same cytokine and secondary mediators, now at high levels, result in

- Systemic vasodilation (hypotension)
- Diminished myocardial contractility
- Widespread endothelial injury and activation, causing systemic leukocyte adhesion and diffuse alveolar capillary damage in the lung (Chapter 13)

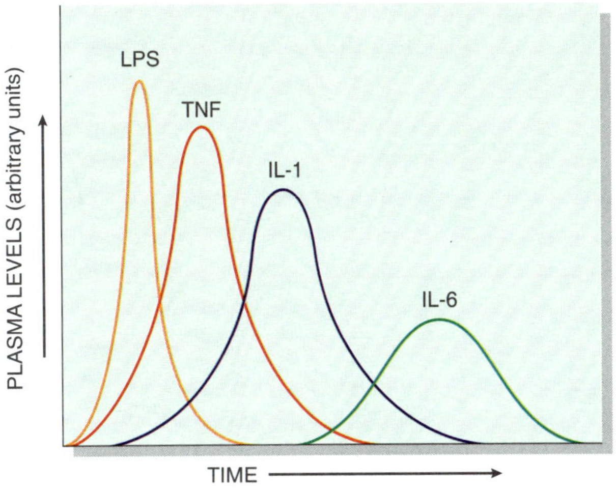

Figure 4–20

Cytokine cascade in sepsis. After lipopolysaccharide (LPS) release there are successive waves of tumor necrosis factor (TNF), interleukin 1 (IL-1), and IL-6 secretion. (Modified from Abbas AK, et al: Cellular and Molecular Immunology, 4th ed. Philadelphia, WB Saunders, 2000.)

- Activation of the coagulation system, culminating in disseminated intravascular coagulation (DIC) (Chapter 12)

The hypoperfusion resulting from the combined effects of widespread vasodilation, myocardial pump failure, and DIC causes *multiorgan system failure* that affects the liver, kidneys, and central nervous system, among others. Unless the underlying infection (and LPS overload) is rapidly brought under control, the patient usually dies. In some experimental animal models, soluble CD14, antibodies to LPS-binding proteins, or pharmacologic inhibitors of the secondary mediators (e.g., nitric oxide synthesis) have demonstrated some efficacy in protecting against septic shock. Unfortunately, these interventions have not yet proved of significant clinical benefit in patients, perhaps because many different pathways and mediators are activated by LPS.

An interesting group of bacterial proteins called *superantigens* also causes a syndrome similar to septic shock (e.g., *toxic shock syndrome toxin 1*, responsible for the *toxic shock syndrome*). Superantigens are polyclonal T-lymphocyte activators that induce systemic inflammatory cytokine cascades similar to those that occur in response to LPS. Their actions can result in a variety of clinical manifestations ranging from a diffuse rash to vasodilation, hypotension, and death.

Stages of Shock

Shock is a progressive disorder that if uncorrected leads to death. Unless the insult is massive and rapidly lethal (e.g., a massive hemorrhage from a ruptured aortic aneurysm), shock tends to evolve through three general (albeit somewhat artificial) stages. These stages have been documented most clearly in hypovolemic shock but are common to other forms as well:

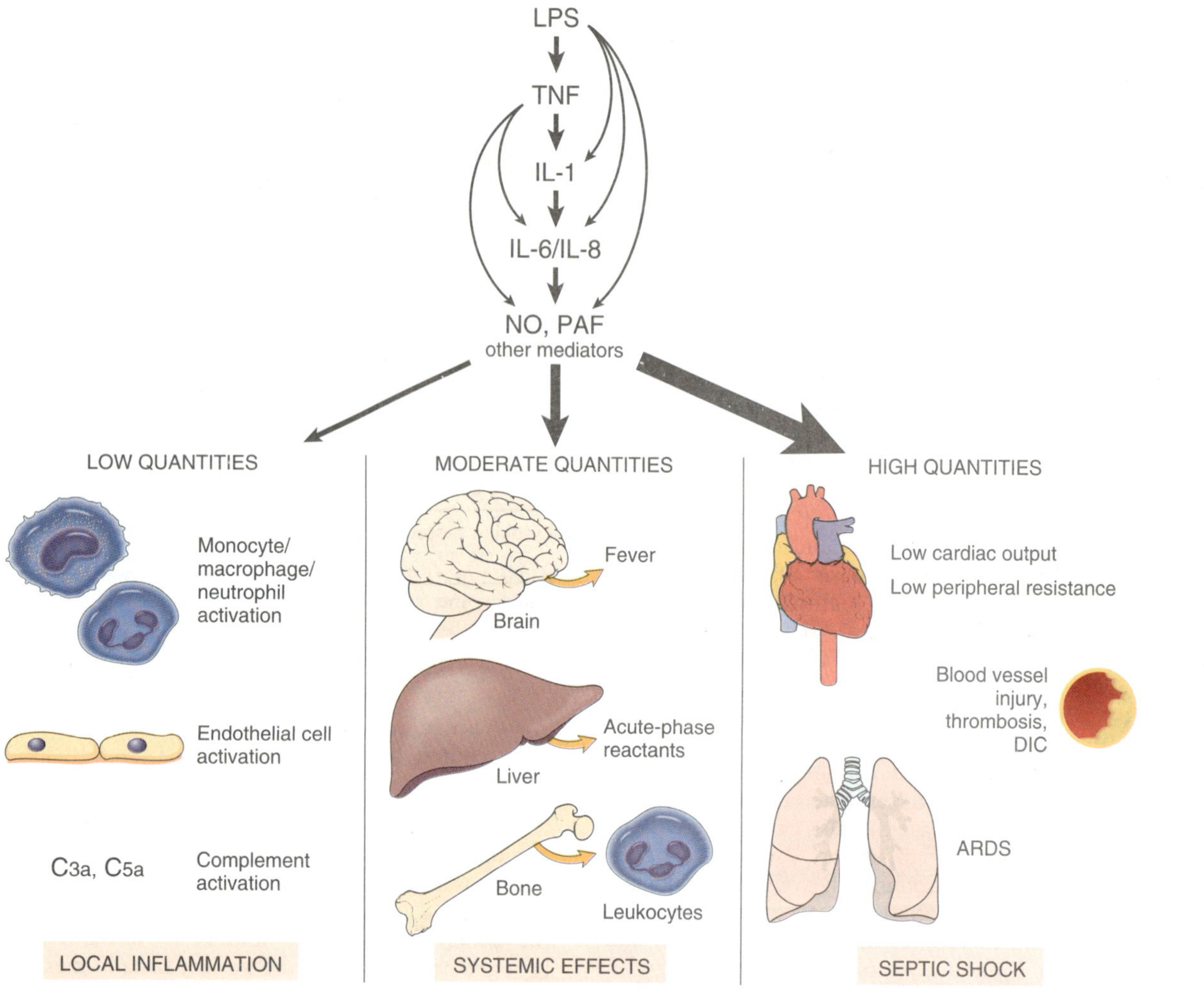

Figure 4–21

Effects of lipopolysaccharide (LPS) and secondarily induced effector molecules. LPS initiates the cytokine cascade described in Fig. 4–21. In addition, LPS and the secondary mediators can also directly stimulate downstream cytokine production, as indicated. Secondary effectors that become important include nitric oxide (NO) and platelet-activating factor (PAF). At low levels, only local inflammatory effects are seen. With moderate levels, more systemic events occur in addition to the local vascular effects. At high concentrations, the syndrome of septic shock supervenes. ARDS, adult respiratory distress syndrome; DIC, disseminated intravascular coagulation; IL-1, interleukin 1; IL-6, interleukin 6; IL-8, interleukin 8; TNF, tumor necrosis factor. (Modified from Abbas AK, et al: Cellular and Molecular Immunology, 4th ed. Philadelphia, WB Saunders, 2000.)

- An initial *nonprogressive stage* during which reflex compensatory mechanisms are activated and perfusion of vital organs is maintained
- A *progressive stage* characterized by tissue hypoperfusion and onset of worsening circulatory and metabolic imbalances
- An *irreversible stage* that sets in after the body has incurred cellular and tissue injury so severe that even if the hemodynamic defects are corrected, survival is not possible

In the early, nonprogressive phase of shock, various *neurohumoral mechanisms* help maintain cardiac output and blood pressure. These include baroreceptor reflexes, release of catecholamines, activation of the renin-angiotensin axis, antidiuretic hormone release, and generalized sympathetic stimulation. The net effect is *tachycardia, peripheral vasoconstriction,* and *renal conservation of fluid.* Cutaneous vasoconstriction, for example, is responsible for the characteristic coolness and pallor of skin in shock (although septic shock may initially cause cutaneous *vasodilation* and thus present with *warm, flushed skin*). Coronary and cerebral vessels are less sensitive to the sympathetic response and thus maintain relatively normal caliber, blood flow, and oxygen delivery to their respective vital organs.

If the underlying causes are not corrected, shock passes imperceptibly to the progressive phase, during which there is widespread tissue hypoxia. In the setting of persistent oxygen deficit, intracellular aerobic respiration is replaced by anaerobic glycolysis, with excessive production of lactic acid. The resultant metabolic *lactic acidosis lowers the tissue pH and blunts the vasomotor response;* arterioles dilate, and blood begins to pool in the microcirculation. Peripheral pooling not only worsens the cardiac output but also puts endothelial cells at risk of developing anoxic injury with subsequent DIC. With widespread tissue hypoxia, vital organs are affected and begin to fail.

Unless there is intervention, the process eventually enters an irreversible stage. Widespread cell injury is reflected in lysosomal enzyme leakage, further aggravating the shock state. Myocardial contractile function worsens, in part because of nitric oxide synthesis. If ischemic bowel allows intestinal flora to enter the circulation, endotoxic shock may also be superimposed. At this point, the patient has complete renal shutdown due to ischemic acute tubular necrosis (Chapter 14), and, despite heroic measures, the downward clinical spiral almost inevitably culminates in death.

Morphology

The cellular and tissue changes induced by shock are essentially those of hypoxic injury (Chapter 1), due to some combination of hypoperfusion and microvascular thrombosis. Since shock is characterized by **failure of many organ systems**, the cellular changes may appear in any tissue. Nevertheless, they are particularly evident in the brain, heart, kidneys, adrenal glands, and gastrointestinal tract. Fibrin thrombi may be identified in virtually any tissue, although they are usually most readily visualized in kidney glomeruli. The **adrenal changes** in shock are those seen in all forms of stress; essentially there is cortical cell lipid depletion. This reflects not adrenal exhaustion but instead conversion of the relatively inactive vacuolated cells to metabolically active cells that use stored lipids for the synthesis of steroids. The **kidneys** typically reveal acute tubular necrosis (Chapter 14) so that oliguria, anuria, and electrolyte disturbances dominate the clinical picture. The **gastrointestinal tract** may mainfest focal mucosal hemorrhage and necrosis. The **lungs** are seldom affected in pure hypovolemic shock, because they are somewhat resistant to hypoxic injury. However, when shock is caused by bacterial sepsis or trauma, changes of **diffuse alveolar damage** (Chapter 13) may develop, the so-called shock lung.

With the exception of neuronal and myocyte ischemic loss, virtually all tissues may revert to normal if the patient survives. Unfortunately, most patients with irreversible changes due to severe shock die before the tissues can recover.

Clinical Course. The clinical manifestations of shock depend on the precipitating insult. In hypovolemic and cardiogenic shock, the patient presents with *hypotension;* a weak, rapid pulse; tachypnea; and cool, clammy, cyanotic skin. In septic shock, however, the skin may be warm and flushed as a result of peripheral vasodilation. The initial threat to life stems from the underlying catastrophe that precipitated the shock state (e.g., a myocardial infarct, severe hemorrhage, or bacterial infection). Rapidly, however, the cardiac, cerebral, and pulmonary changes that occur secondary to the shock state materially worsen the problem. If patients survive the initial complications, they enter a second phase, dominated by renal insufficiency and marked by a progressive fall in urine output as well as acidosis, and severe fluid and electrolyte imbalances.

The prognosis varies with the origin of shock and its duration. Thus, 80% to 90% of young, otherwise healthy patients with hypovolemic shock survive with appropriate management, whereas cardiogenic shock associated with extensive myocardial infarction, or gram-negative sepsis carries a mortality rate of 75%, even with care that is state of the art.

SUMMARY

Shock

- Shock causes systemic hypoperfusion due to either reduced cardiac output or reduced circulating blood volume.
- The most common causes of shock are cardiogenic (cardiac pump failure due, for example, to myocardial infarction), hypovolemic (due, for example, to blood loss), and sepsis (due to infections).
- Septic shock results from the host innate immune response to bacterial or fungal cell molecules (most commonly endotoxin), with systemic production of cytokines, such as TNF and IL-1, that affect endothelial and inflammatory cell activation.
- Hypotension, DIC, and metabolic disturbances constitute the clinical triad of septic shock.
- Shock of any form causes pathology by inducing prolonged tissue hypoxic injury.

BIBLIOGRAPHY

Aird WC: The role of the endothelium in severe sepsis and multiple organ dysfunction syndrome. Blood 101:3765, 2003 *[Mechanisms by which endothelial injury and dysfunction contribute to septic shock.]*

Andrews RK, Berndt MC: Platelet physiology and thrombosis. Thromb Res 114:447, 2004 *[Good review of normal platelet function in hemostasis.]*

Baker MD, Acharya KR: Superantigens: structure-function relationships. Int J Med Microbiol 293:529, 2004. *[Although the article is primarily about superantigen structure, there is a good overview of the pathogeneis of superantigen-mediated disease.]*

Caine GJ, et al: The hypercoagulable state of malignancy: pathogenesis and current debate. Neoplasia 4:465, 2002 *[Good discussion of the pathways by which cancer predisposes to thrombosis.]*

Cesarman-Maus G, Hajjar KA: Molecular mechanisms of fibrinolysis. Br J Haematol 129:307, 2005. *[Long and detailed summary of fibrinolytic pathways, including therapeutic interventions.]*

Coughlin SR, Camerer E: PARticipation in inflammation. J Clin Invest 111:25, 2003. *[Review of the roles played by thrombin-cleaved protease-activated receptors in inflammation.]*

Dahlback B: Blood coagulation and its regulation by anticoagulant pathways: genetic pathogenesis of bleeding and thrombotic diseases. J Intern Med 257:209, 2005. *[Good review for one-stop reading on normal and abnormal hemostasis.]*

Eilertsen KE, Osterud B: Tissue factor: pathophysiology and cellular biology. Blood Coagul Fibrinolysis 15:521, 2004. *[Concise overview of tissue factor physiology as well as the increasing recognition of its role in disease states.]*

Feero WG: Genetic thrombophilia. Prim Care 31: 685, 2004. *[Readable summary of hereditary forms of hypercoagulable states, with emphasis on diagnosis and treatment.]*

Galley HF, Webster NR: Physiology of the endothelium. Br J Anaesth 93:105, 2004. *[Excellent overview of endothelial function in health and disease; in addition to hemostasis and thrombosis, the role of endothelium in inflammatory processes is also described.]*

Gallus AS: Travel, venous thromboembolism, and thrombophilia. Semin Thromb Hemost 31:90, 2005. *[Review of the roles of acute immobilization and concurrent hereditary hypercoagulable risk factors in deep venous thrombosis.]*

Goldhaber SZ: Pulmonary embolism. N Engl J Med 339:93, 1998. *[An excellent and thorough review of the pathophysiologic and clinical issues regarding pulmonary embolism; even though this is an "older" reference, it is still quite good and relevant.]*

Hotchkiss RS, Karl IE: Medical progress: the pathophysiology and treatment of sepsis. N Engl J Med 348:138, 2003. *[Well written and reasonably up-to-date overview of the pathogenesis and therapy for septic shock.]*

Johnson CM, et al: Hypercoagulable states: a review. Vasc Endovascular Surg 39:123, 2005. *[A basic, practical summary of the major hypercoagulable states, including diagnosis, and therapeutic goals.]*

Kottke-Marchant K: Genetic polymorphisms associated with venous and arterial thrombosis: an overview. Arch Pathol Lab Med 126:295, 2002. *[Excellent summary of the known genetic loci that contribute to hypercoagulable states.]*

Levi M, et al: New treatment strategies for disseminated intravascular coagulation based on current understanding of the pathophysiology. Ann Med 36:41, 2004. *[Superb overview of the pathophysiology and potential therapeutic interventions in DIC.]*

Lopez JA, et al: Deep venous thrombosis. Hematology (Am Soc Hematol Educ Program). 439–456, 2004. *[Good review at a medical student/house officer level; part of a larger offering with multiple additional hemostasis/thrombosis topics.]*

Michiels C: Endothelial cell functions. J Cell Physiol 196:430, 2003. *[A complete and readable overview of endothelial cell biology.]*

Munford RS: Severe sepsis and septic shock: the role of gram-negative bacteremia. Annu Rev Pathol 1:467–496, 2006. *[An interesting and somewhat provocative view regarding the pathogenesis of septic shock.]*

Murugappan S, et al: Platelet receptors for adenine nucleotides and thromboxane A_2. Semin Thromb Hemost 30:411, 2004. *[A thorough, albeit dry, review of platelet-activating receptors and their therapeutic ligands.]*

Parisi DM, et al: Fat embolism syndrome. Am J Orthop 31:507, 2002. *[Decent overview of pathogenesis and clinical issues.]*

Perozzi KJ, Englert NC: Amniotic fluid embolism: an obstetric emergency. Crit Care Nurse 24:54, 2004. *[Review of the mechanisms of pathology, with an emphasis on diagnosis and intervention.]*

Pierangeli SS, et al: Intracellular signaling triggered by antiphospholipid antibodies in platelets and endothelial cells: a pathway to targeted therapies. Thromb Res 114:467, 2004. *[Good summary of the antiphospholipid syndrome, with emphasis on diagnosis and therapeutics.]*

Rahimtoola A, Bergin JD: Acute pulmonary embolism: an update on diagnosis and management. Curr Probl Cardiol 30:61, 2005. *[A thorough, exhaustive, and well-referenced discussion of pulmonary embolism.]*

Rand JH: The antiphospholipid syndrome. Ann Rev Med 54:409, 2003. *[Review of the pathogenesis, diagnosis, and treatment of the entity.]*

Rumbaut RE, et al: Microvascular thrombosis models in venules and arterioles in vivo. Microcirculation 12:259, 2005. *[Good overview of the experimental evidence for the mechanisms underlying thrombosis, in an issue with several other excellent summaries related to hemostasis.]*

Van Amersfoortes ES, et al: Receptors, mediators, and mechanisms involved in bacterial sepsis and septic shock. Clin Microbiol Rev 16:379, 2003. *[Reasonably complete overview of the molecular pathways involved in septic shock.]*

Warkentin TE: An overview of the heparin-induced thrombocytopenia syndrome. Semin Thromb Hemost 30:273, 2004. *[Excellent summary of the pathophysiology, diagnosis, and therapy of HIT.]*

Wu KK, Matijevic-Aleksic N: Molecular aspects of thrombosis and antithrombotic drugs. Crit Rev Clin Lab Sci. 42:249, 2005. *[Lengthy, thorough overview of the mechanisms of thrombus formation with emphasis on targets for therapeutic intervention.]*

Chapter 5

Diseases of the Immune System

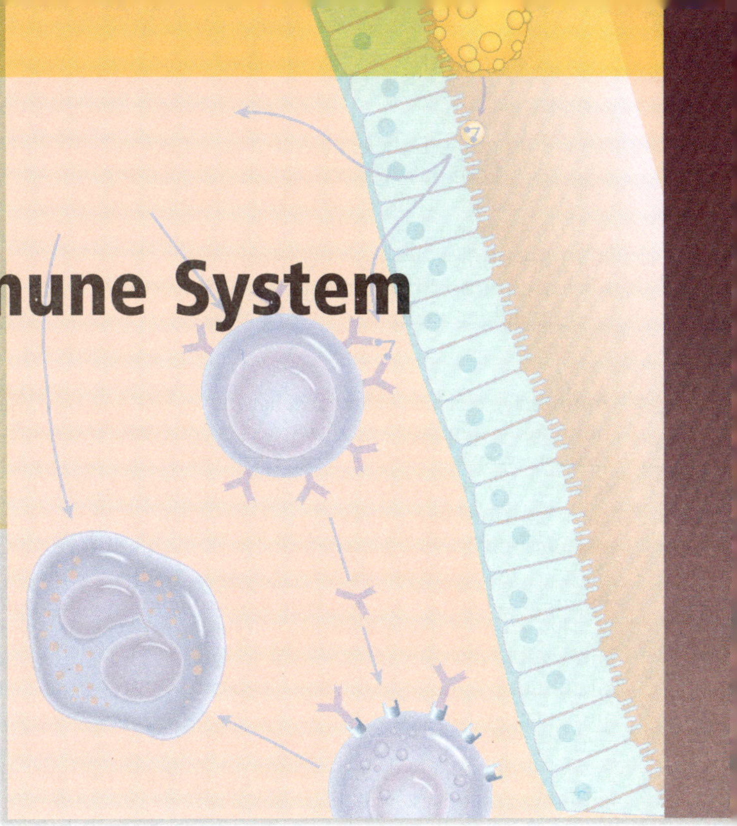

Immunity refers to protection against infections, and the immune system is the collection of cells and molecules that are responsible for defending us against the countless pathogenic microbes in our environment. Deficiencies in immune defenses result in an increased susceptibility to infections, which can be life-threatening if the deficits are not corrected. On the other hand, the immune system is itself capable of causing great harm and is the root cause of some of the most vexing and intractable diseases of the modern world. Thus, diseases of immunity range from those caused by "too little" to those caused by "too much or inappropriate" immune activity. This chapter starts with a brief review of some of the basic concepts of lymphocyte biology and normal immune responses, which establishes the foundation for our discussion of transplant rejection and diseases caused by defective or inappropriate immune responses. The chapter concludes with a discussion of *amyloidosis,* a disease characterized by the abnormal extracellular deposition of certain proteins (some of which are produced in the setting of immune responses).

INNATE AND ADAPTIVE IMMUNITY

Defense against microbes consists of two types of reactions (Fig. 5–1). *Innate immunity* (also called natural, or native, immunity) is mediated by cells and proteins that are always present and poised to fight against microbes and are called into action immediately in response to infection. The major components of innate immunity are epithelial barriers of the skin, gastrointestinal tract, and respiratory tract, which prevent microbe entry (and have to be breached for a microbe to establish infection); phagocytic leukocytes (neutrophils and macrophages); a specialized cell type called the natural killer (NK) cell; and several circulating plasma proteins, the most important of which are the proteins of the complement system.

The innate immune response is able to prevent and control many infections. However, many pathogenic microbes have evolved to overcome innate immune defenses, and protection against these infections requires the more powerful mechanisms of *adaptive immunity* (also called acquired, or specific, immunity). Adaptive immunity is normally silent and responds (or "adapts") to the presence of infectious microbes by becoming active, expanding, and generating potent mechanisms for neutralizing and eliminating the microbes. The components of the adaptive immune system are lymphocytes and their products. By convention, the terms "immune system" and "immune response" refer to adaptive immunity.

There are two types of adaptive immune responses: *humoral immunity,* mediated by soluble antibody proteins that are produced by B lymphocytes (also called B cells), and *cell-mediated (or cellular) immunity,* mediated by T lymphocytes (also called T cells) (Fig. 5–2). Anti-

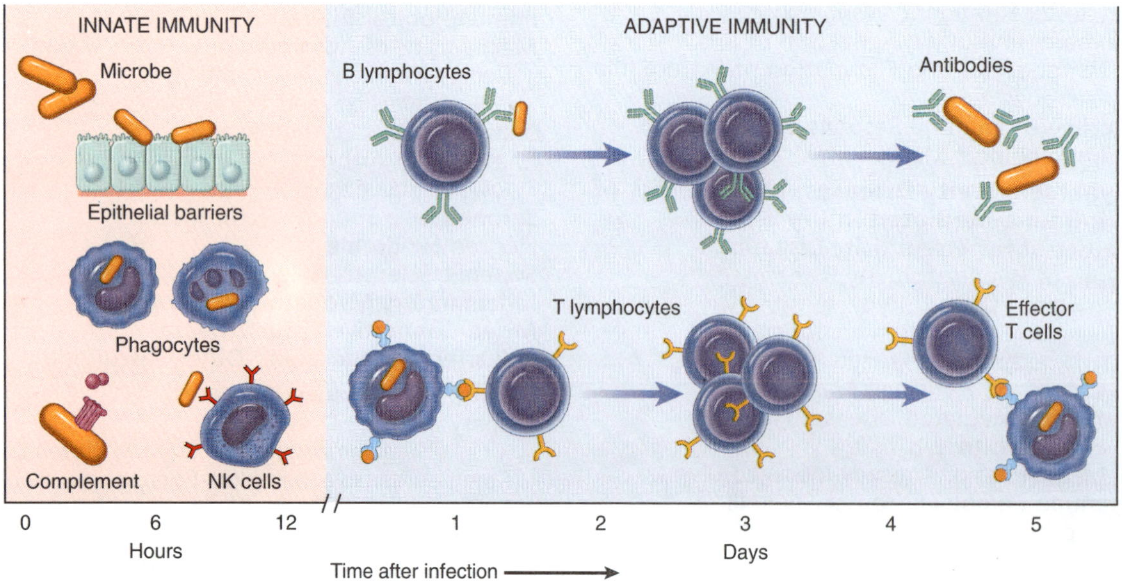

Figure 5–1

The principal mechanisms of innate immunity and adaptive immunity. NK cells, natural killer cells.

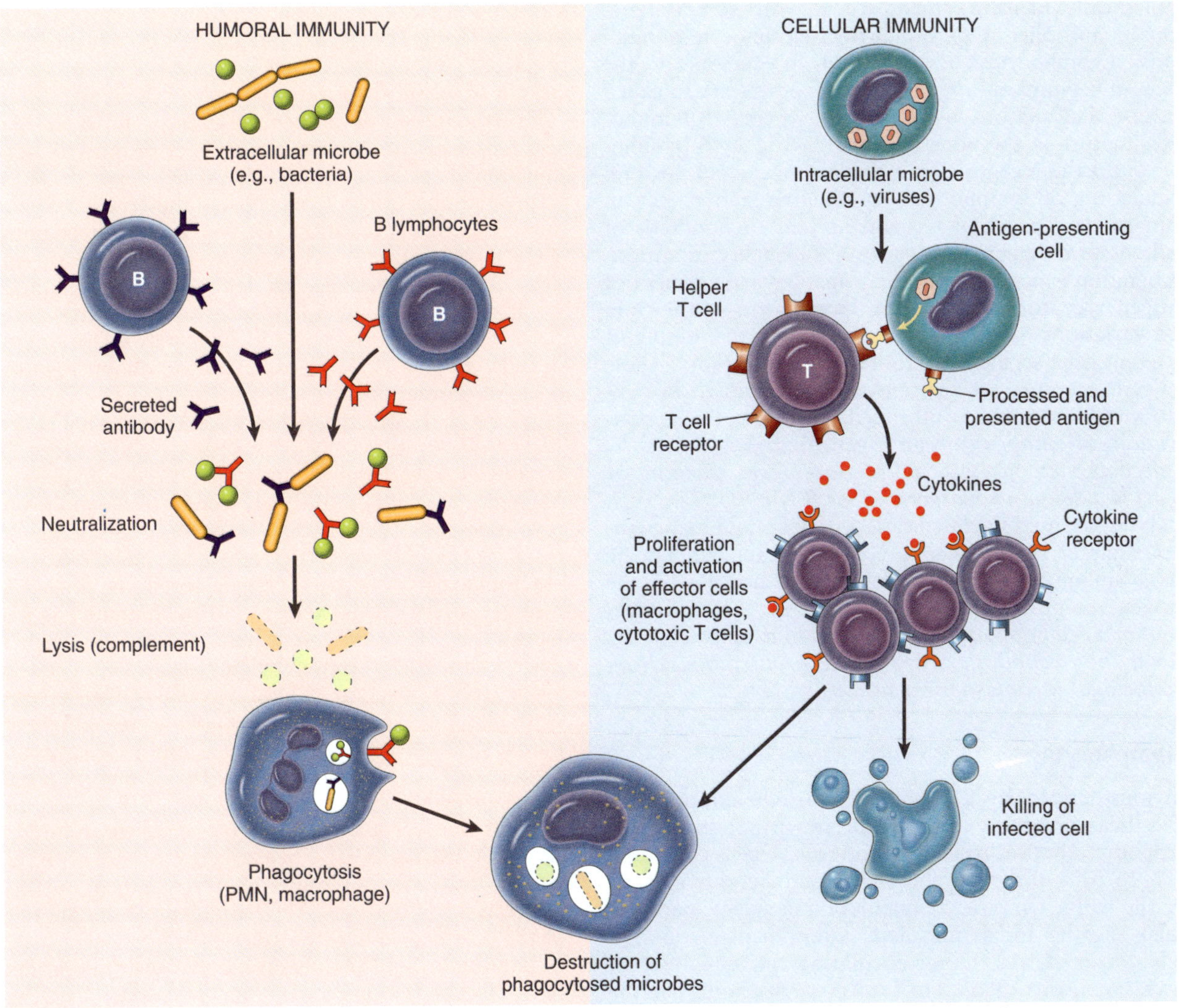

Figure 5–2

Humoral and cell-mediated immunity. In humoral immunity, B lymphocytes secrete antibodies that eliminate extracellular microbes. In cell-mediated immunity, T lymphocytes either activate macrophages to destroy phagocytosed microbes or kill infected cells. PMN, polymorphonuclear leukocyte.

bodies provide protection against extracellular microbes in the blood, mucosal secretions, and tissues. T lymphocytes are important in defense against intracellular microbes. They work by either directly killing infected cells (accomplished by cytotoxic T lymphocytes) or by activating phagocytes to kill ingested microbes, via the production of soluble protein mediators called cytokines (made by helper T cells). The main properties and functions of the cells of the immune system are described below.

When the immune system is inappropriately triggered or not properly controlled, the same mechanisms that are involved in host defense cause tissue injury and disease. The reaction of the cells of innate and adaptive immunity may be manifested as *inflammation*. As we discussed in Chapter 2, inflammation is a beneficial process, but it is also the basis of many human diseases. Later in this chapter we will discuss the ways by which the immune response triggers pathologic inflammatory reactions.

CELLS AND TISSUES OF THE IMMUNE SYSTEM

The cells of the immune system consist of lymphocytes, which are the mediators of adaptive immunity; specialized antigen-presenting cells (APCs), which capture and display microbial and other antigens to the lymphocytes; and various effector cells, which perform the task of eliminating the antigens (typically, microbes), the ultimate "effect" of the immune response. A remarkable feature of the immune system is how intricately and efficiently the responses of these different cell types are orchestrated and regulated.

Lymphocytes

Lymphocytes are present in the circulation and in various lymphoid organs. Although all lymphocytes appear morphologically identical, there are actually several functionally and phenotypically distinct lymphocyte populations. Lymphocytes develop from precursors in the generative lymphoid organs; T lymphocytes are so called because they mature in the thymus, whereas B lymphocytes mature in the bone marrow. Each T or B lymphocyte expresses receptors for a single antigen, and the total population of lymphocytes (numbering about 10^{12} in humans) is capable of recognizing tens or hundreds of millions of antigens. This enormous diversity of antigen recognition is generated by the somatic rearrangement of antigen receptor genes during lymphocyte maturation, and variations that are introduced during the joining of different gene segments to form antigen receptors. These antigen receptors are rearranged and expressed in lymphocytes but not in any other cell. Therefore, the *demonstration of antigen receptor gene rearrangements by molecular methods (e.g., polymerase chain reaction, or PCR) is a definitive marker of T or B lymphocytes.* Such analyses are used in classification of lymphoid malignancies (Chapter 12). Furthermore, because each lymphocyte has a unique DNA rearrangement (and hence a unique antigen receptor), *molecular analysis of the rearrangement in a cell population can be used to distinguish polyclonal (non-neoplastic) lymphocyte proliferations from monoclonal (neoplastic) expansions.*

T Lymphocytes

Thymus-derived, or T, lymphocytes are the effector cells of cellular immunity and provide important stimuli for antibody responses to protein antigens. T cells constitute 60% to 70% of the lymphocytes in peripheral blood and are the major lymphocyte population in splenic periarteriolar sheaths and lymph node interfollicular zones. T cells do not detect free or circulating antigens. Instead, the vast majority (>95%) of T cells recognize only peptide fragments of protein antigens that are displayed on other cells bound to proteins of the major histocompatibility complex (MHC; or in humans, human leukocyte antigen [HLA] complex). The MHC was discovered on the basis of studies of graft rejection or acceptance (tissue, or "histo," compatibility). It is now known that the normal function of MHC molecules is to display peptides for recognition by T lymphocytes. By forcing T cells to see MHC-bound peptides, the system ensures that T cells can recognize antigens in other cells and thus perform their function of killing infected cells or activating phagocytes or B lymphocytes that have ingested protein antigens. In every individual, T cells recognize only peptides displayed by that individual's MHC molecules, which, of course, are the only MHC molecules that the T cells will encounter normally. This phenomenon is called *MHC restriction.* In MHC-restricted T cells, the T-cell receptor (TCR) is a heterodimer composed of disulfide-linked α and β protein chains (Fig. 5–3A); each chain has a variable region that participates in binding a particular peptide antigen and a constant region that interacts with associated signaling molecules. MHC molecules are described below.

TCRs are noncovalently linked to a cluster of five invariant polypeptide chains, the γ, δ, and ε proteins of the CD3 molecular complex and two ζ chains (see Fig. 5–3A). The CD3 proteins and ζ chains do not themselves bind antigens; instead, they interact with the constant region of the TCR to transduce intracellular signals after TCR recognition of antigen. In addition to these signaling proteins, T cells express a number of other invariant function–associated molecules. CD4 and CD8 are expressed on distinct T-cell subsets and serve as coreceptors for T-cell activation. During antigen recognition, CD4 molecules on T cells bind to invariant portions of class II MHC molecules (see later) on selected APCs; in an analogous fashion, CD8 binds to class I MHC molecules. CD4 is expressed on approximately 60% of mature T cells, whereas CD8 is expressed on about 30% of T cells; in normal healthy individuals, the CD4/CD8 ratio is about 2:1. The CD4- and CD8-expressing T cells (called CD4+ and CD8+ cells, respectively) perform different but overlapping functions. CD4+ T cells are "helper" T cells because they secrete soluble molecules (*cytokines*) that help B cells to produce antibodies (the origin of the name "helper" cells) and also help macrophages to destroy phagocytosed microbes. The central role of CD4+ helper cells in immunity is highlighted by the severe compromise that results from the destruction of this subset by human immunodeficiency virus (HIV) infection. CD8+ T cells can also secrete cytokines, but they play a more important role in directly killing virus-infected or tumor cells, and hence are called "cytotoxic" T lymphocytes (CTLs). Other important invariant proteins on T cells include CD28, which functions as the receptor for molecules that are induced on APCs by microbes (and are called costimulators), and various adhesion molecules that strengthen the bond between the T cells and APCs and control the migration of the T cells to different tissues.

In a minority of peripheral blood T cells and in many of the T cells associated with mucosal surfaces (e.g., lung and gastrointestinal tract), the TCRs are heterodimers of γ and δ chains, which are similar but not identical to the α and β chains of most TCRs. Such *γδ T cells* do not express CD4 or CD8 and recognize nonprotein molecules (e.g., bacterial lipoglycans), but their functional roles are not well understood. Another small population of T cells expresses markers of T cells and NK cells. These *NKT cells* recognize microbial glycolipids, but their importance in host defense is also not established. The antigen receptors of γδ T cells and NKT cells are much less diverse than the receptors of "conventional" T cells, suggesting that the former recognize conserved microbial structures. In this respect, γδ T cells and NKT cells resemble cells of innate immunity.

Another population of T cells that is receiving great attention is called *regulatory T lymphocytes.* This cell type is described later, in context of tolerance of self antigens.

MHC Molecules: the Peptide Display System of Adaptive Immunity

Because MHC molecules are fundamental to T-cell recognition of antigens, and variations in MHC molecules are associated with immunologic diseases, it is important to review the structure and function of these molecules. The

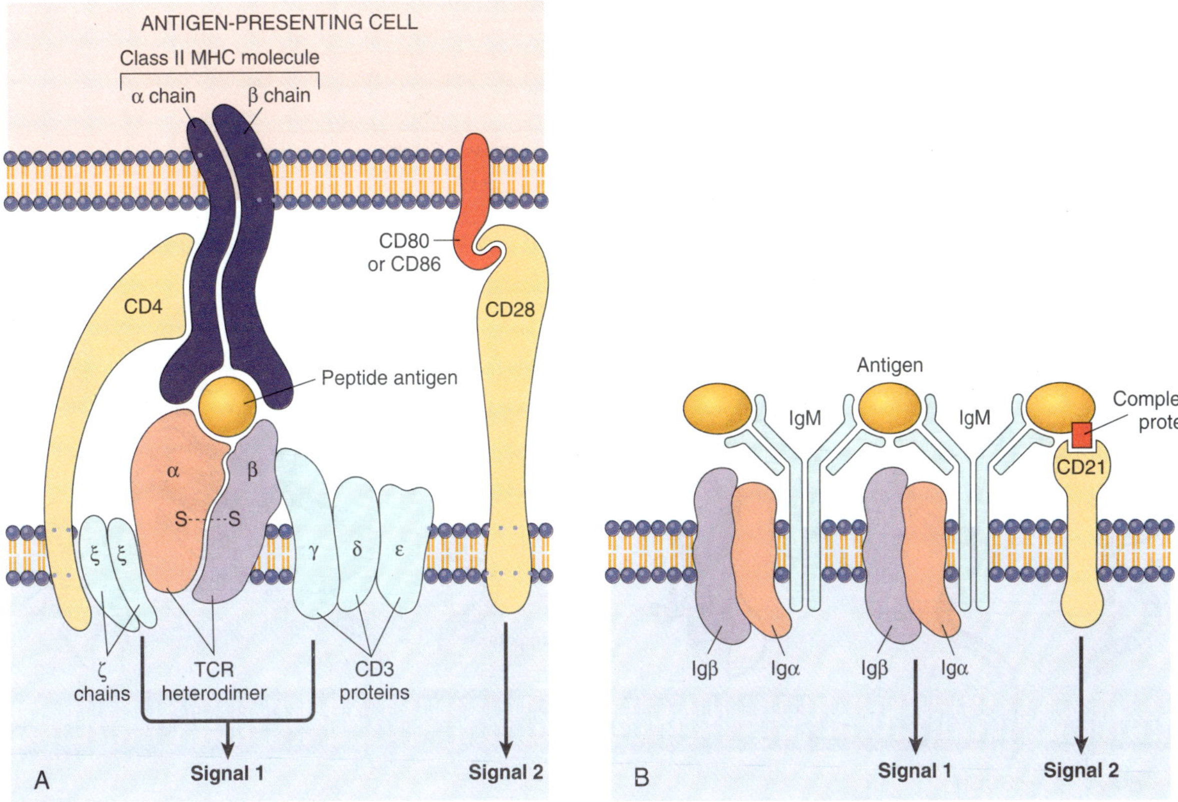

Figure 5–3

Lymphocyte antigen receptors. **A,** The T-cell receptor (TCR) complex and other molecules involved in T-cell activation. The TCRα and TCRβ chains recognize antigen (in the form of peptide–MHC complexes expressed on antigen-presenting cells), and the linked CD3 complex initiates activating signals. CD4 and CD28 are also involved in T-cell activation. (Note that some T cells express CD8 and not CD4; these molecules serve analogous roles.) **B,** The B-cell receptor complex is composed of membrane IgM (or IgD, not shown) and the associated signaling proteins Igα and Igβ. CD21 is a receptor for a complement component that promotes B-cell activation.

human MHC, known as the *human leukocyte antigen (HLA) complex,* consists of a cluster of genes on chromosome 6 (Fig. 5–4). The HLA system is highly polymorphic; that is, there are several alternative forms (*alleles*) of a gene at each locus (e.g., >400 different HLA-B alleles have been described). Such diversity provides a system whereby a vast array of peptides can be displayed by MHC molecules for recognition by T cells. As we shall see, this polymorphism also constitutes a formidable barrier to organ transplantation.

On the basis of their chemical structure, tissue distribution, and function, MHC gene products fall into three categories:

- *Class I MHC molecules* are encoded by three closely linked loci, designated *HLA-A, HLA-B,* and *HLA-C* (see Fig. 5–4). Each of these molecules is a heterodimer, consisting of a polymorphic 44-kD α chain noncovalently associated with a 12-kD nonpolymorphic β_2-microglobulin (encoded by a separate gene on chromosome 15). The extracellular portion of the α chain contains a cleft where foreign peptides bind to MHC molecules for presentation to CD8+ T cells. In general, class I MHC molecules bind to peptides derived from proteins synthesized within the cell (e.g., viral antigens). Because class I MHC molecules are present on all nucleated cells, all virus-infected cells can be detected and eliminated by CTLs.
- *Class II MHC molecules* are encoded by genes in the *HLA-D* region, which contains at least three subregions: *DP, DQ,* and *DR.* Class II MHC molecules are heterodimers of noncovalently linked polymorphic α and β subunits (see Fig. 5–4). As in class I, the extracellular portion of the class II MHC heterodimer contains a cleft for the binding of antigenic peptides. Unlike in class I, the tissue distribution of class II MHC–expressing cells is quite restricted; they are constitutively expressed mainly on APCs (notably, dendritic cells), and macrophages, and B cells. In general, class II MHC molecules bind to peptides derived from proteins synthesized outside the cell (e.g., those derived from extracellular bacteria). This allows CD4+ T cells to recognize the presence of extracellular pathogens and to orchestrate a protective response.
- Class III proteins include some of the complement components (C2, C3, and Bf); genes encoding tumor necrosis factor (TNF) and lymphotoxin (LT, or TNF-β) are also located within the MHC. Although genetically linked to class I and II molecules, class III molecules and the cytokine genes do not form a part of the peptide display system and will not be discussed further.

Every individual inherits one HLA allele from each parent and thus typically expresses two different molecules for every locus. Cells of a heterozygous individual

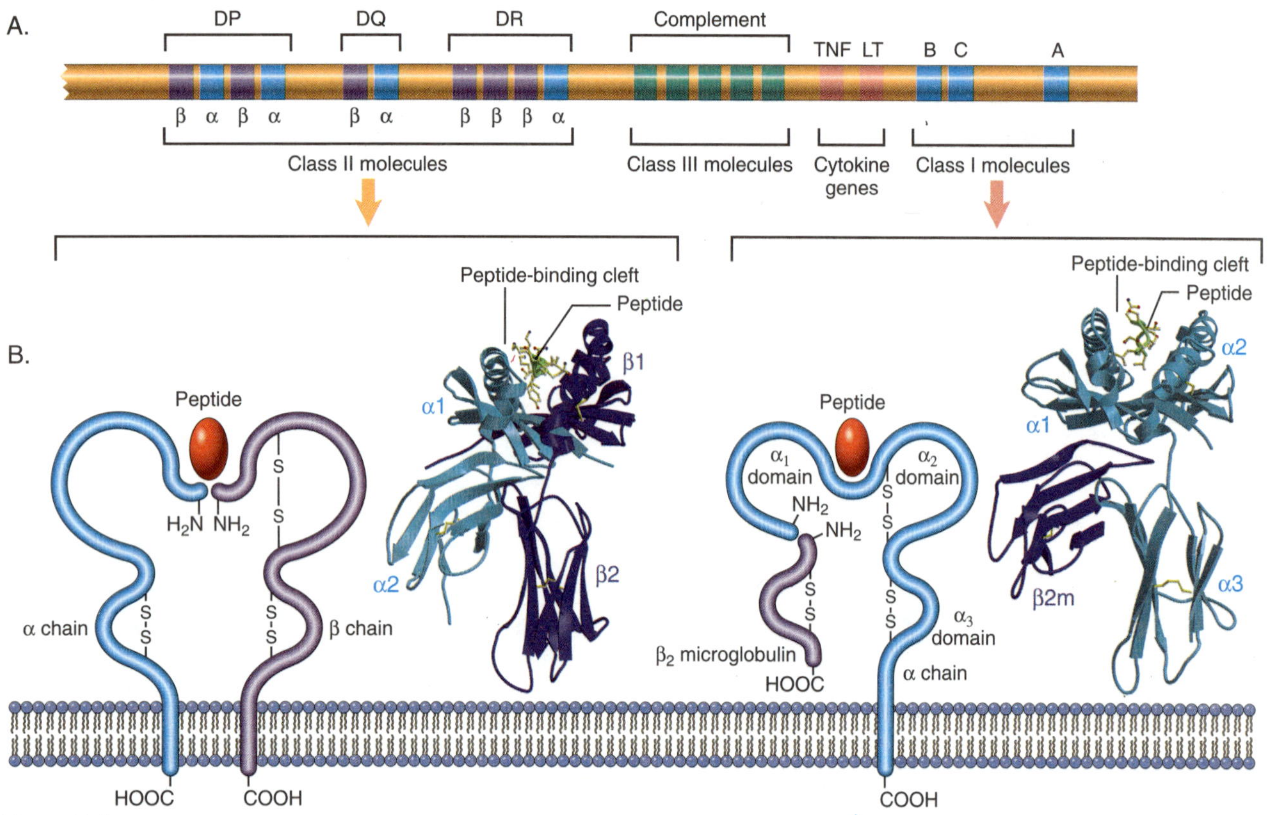

Figure 5–4

The HLA complex and the structure of HLA molecules. **A,** The location of genes in the HLA complex. The sizes and distances between genes are not to scale. The class II region also contains genes that encode several proteins involved in antigen processing (not shown). **B,** Schematic diagrams and crystal structures of class I and class II HLA molecules. LT, leukotriene; TNF, tumor necrosis factor. (Crystal structures are courtesy of Dr. P. Bjorkman, California Institute of Technology, Pasadena, California.)

can therefore express six different class I HLA molecules: three of maternal origin and three of paternal origin. Similarly, a given individual expresses maternal and paternal alleles of the class II MHC loci; because some HLA-D α and β chains can mix and match with each other, each class II–expressing cell can have as many as 20 different class II MHC molecules. *Different MHC alleles bind to different peptide fragments depending on the particular amino acid sequence of a given peptide;* the expression of many different MHC molecules allows each cell to present a wide array of peptide antigens.

As a result of the polymorphism at the major HLA loci in the population, a virtually infinite number of combinations of molecules exist, and each individual expresses a unique MHC antigenic profile on his or her cells. The combination of HLA alleles in each individual is called the *HLA haplotype*. The implications of HLA polymorphism are obvious in the context of transplantation—because every individual has HLA alleles that differ to some extent from every other individual, grafts from any person will evoke immune responses in any other person and be rejected (except, of course, for identical twins). In fact, HLA molecules were discovered in the course of early attempts at tissue transplantation. HLA molecules of the graft evoke both humoral and cell-mediated responses, eventually leading to graft destruction (discussed later in this chapter). This ability of MHC molecules to trigger immune responses is the reason these molecules are often called "antigens." It is believed that the polymorphism of MHC genes arose to enable the population to display and respond to any conceivable microbial peptide.

The role of the MHC in T-cell stimulation also has important implications for the genetic control of immune responses. The ability of any given MHC allele to bind the peptide antigens generated from a particular pathogen will determine whether an individual's T cells can actually "see" and respond to that pathogen. In other words, an individual will recognize and mount an immune response against a given antigen only if he or she inherits MHC molecules that can bind the antigenic peptide and present it to T cells. The inheritance of particular alleles influences both protective and harmful immune responses. For example, if the antigen is ragweed pollen and the response is an allergic reaction, inheritance of some HLA genes may make individuals susceptible to this disease. On the other hand, good responsiveness to a viral antigen, determined by inheritance of certain HLA alleles, may be beneficial for the host.

Finally, many diseases are associated with particular HLA alleles. These HLA-linked diseases can be broadly grouped into the following categories: (1) *inflammatory diseases,* including ankylosing spondylitis and several postinfectious arthropathies, all associated with *HLA-B27;* and (2) *autoimmune diseases,* including autoimmune endocrinopathies, associated with certain

DR alleles. The mechanisms underlying all these associations are not understood at present. The best known association is between ankylosing spondylitis and the *HLA-B27* allele; individuals who possess this allele have a 90-fold greater chance (relative risk) of developing the disease than do those who are negative for *HLA-B27*. We will return to a discussion of HLA linkage when we consider autoimmune diseases.

B Lymphocytes

Bone marrow–derived, or B, lymphocytes comprise 10% to 20% of the circulating peripheral lymphocyte population. They are also present in bone marrow and in the follicles of peripheral lymphoid tissues (lymph nodes, spleen, tonsils, and other mucosal tissues). Stimulation of follicular B cells leads to the formation of a central zone of large, activated B cells in follicles, called a *germinal center.* B cells are the only cell lineage that synthesize antibodies, also called immunoglobulins (Ig).

B cells recognize antigen via monomeric membrane-bound antibody of the immunoglobulin M (IgM) class, associated with signaling molecules to form the B-cell receptor (BCR) complex (see Fig. 5–3B). Whereas T cells can recognize only MHC-associated peptides, B cells can recognize and respond to many more chemical structures, including proteins, lipids, polysaccharides, nucleic acids, and small chemicals; furthermore, B cells (and antibodies) recognize native (conformational) forms of these antigens. As with TCRs, each antibody has a unique antigen specificity. The diversity of antibodies is generated during somatic rearrangements of Ig genes. B cells express several invariant molecules that are responsible for signal transduction and for activation of the cells (see Fig. 5–3B). These molecules include the CD40 receptor, which binds to its ligand expressed on helper T cells, and CD21 (also known as the CR2 complement receptor), which recognizes a complement breakdown product that is frequently deposited on microbes.

After stimulation, B cells differentiate into *plasma cells,* which secrete large amounts of antibodies, the mediators of humoral immunity. There are five classes, or isotypes, of immunoglobulins: IgG, IgM, and IgA constitute more than 95% of circulating antibodies. IgA is the major isotype in mucosal secretions, IgE is present in the circulation at very low concentrations and is also found attached to the surfaces of tissue mast cells, and IgD is expressed on the surfaces of B cells but is not secreted. As outlined below, each isotype has characteristic abilities to activate complement or recruit inflammatory cells and thus plays a different role in host defense and disease states.

Natural Killer Cells

Natural killer (NK) cells are lymphocytes that arise from the common lymphoid progenitor that gives rise to T and B lymphocytes. However, NK cells are cells of innate immunity and do not express highly variable and clonally distributed receptors for antigens. Therefore, they do not have specificities as diverse as do T cells or B cells. NK cells use a limited set of activating receptors to recognize molecules expressed on stressed or infected cells or cells with DNA damage, and then kill these cells, thus eliminating irreparably damaged cells and potential reservoirs of infection. NK cells have another unique specificity. To avoid attacking normal host cells, NK cells express inhibitory receptors that recognize self class I MHC molecules, which are expressed on all healthy cells; engagement of these inhibitory receptors typically overrides the activating receptors and thus prevents activation of the NK cells. Infections (especially viral infections) and stress are associated with loss of expression of class I MHC molecules. When this happens, the NK cells are released from their inhibition and are able to respond to the activating ligands that were induced by the stress and ultimately destroy the unhealthy host cells.

Antigen-Presenting Cells

The immune system contains several cell types that are specialized to capture microbial antigens and display these to lymphocytes. Foremost among these APCs are dendritic cells (DCs), the major cells for displaying protein antigens to naive T cells to initiate immune responses. Several other cell types present antigens to different lymphocytes at various stages of immune responses.

Dendritic Cells

Cells with dendritic morphology (i.e., with fine dendritic cytoplasmic processes) occur as two functionally distinct types. Interdigitating DCs, or more simply, DCs, are nonphagocytic cells that express high levels of class II MHC and T-cell costimulatory molecules. Immature DCs reside in epithelia, where they are strategically located to capture entering microbes; an example is the Langerhans cell of the epidermis. Mature DCs are present in the T-cell zones of lymphoid tissues, where they present antigens to T cells circulating through these tissues. DCs are also present in the interstitium of many nonlymphoid organs, such as the heart and lungs, where they can capture the antigens of microbes that have invaded the tissues.

The second type of DCs is called *follicular dendritic cells (FDCs).* They are located in the germinal centers of lymphoid follicles in the spleen and lymph nodes. These cells bear receptors for the Fc tails of IgG and for complement proteins, and hence efficiently trap antigen bound to antibodies and complement. These cells display antigens to activated B lymphocytes in lymphoid follicles and promote secondary antibody responses.

Other APCs

Macrophages ingest microbes and other particulate antigens and display peptides for recognition by T lymphocytes. These T cells in turn activate the macrophages to kill the microbes, the central reaction of cell-mediated immunity. B cells present peptides to helper T cells and receive signals that stimulate antibody responses to protein antigens.

Effector Cells

Many different types of leukocytes perform the ultimate task of the adaptive immune response, which is to eliminate infections. NK cells are frontline effector cells because of their ability to rapidly react against "stressed" cells. Antibody-secreting plasma cells are effector cells of humoral immunity. T lymphocytes, both CD4+ helper T cells and CD8+ CTLs, are effector cells of cell-mediated immunity. These lymphocytes often function in host defense together with other cells. Macrophages, which were described in Chapter 2, bind microbes that are coated with antibodies or complement, and phagocytose and destroy these microbes, thus serving as effector cells of humoral immunity. Macrophages also respond to signals from helper T cells and improve their ability to destroy phagocytosed microbes, thus serving as effector cells of cellular immunity. T lymphocytes secrete cytokines that recruit and activate other leukocytes, such as neutrophils and eosinophils, and all these cell types function in defense against various pathogens. The same effector cells are responsible for tissue injury in inflammatory diseases caused by abnormal immune responses.

Lymphoid Tissues

The lymphoid tissues of the body are divided into generative (primary) organs, where lymphocytes express antigen receptors and mature, and peripheral (secondary) lymphoid organs, where adaptive immune responses develop. The generative organs are the thymus and bone marrow, and the peripheral organs are the lymph nodes, spleen, and mucosal and cutaneous lymphoid tissues. Mature lymphocytes recirculate through the peripheral organs, searching for microbial antigens to which they can recognize and respond. An important characteristic of these organs is that T and B lymphocytes are anatomically segregated until they are needed (i.e., until they are activated by antigens). This process is described below.

SUMMARY

Cells and Tissues of the Immune System

- Lymphocytes are the mediators of adaptive immunity and the only cells that produce specific and diverse receptors for antigens.
- *T (thymus-derived) lymphocytes* express antigen receptors called T cell receptors (TCRs) that recognize peptide fragments of protein antigens that are displayed by MHC molecules on the surface of antigen-presenting cells.
- *B (bone marrow-derived) lymphocytes* express membrane-bound antibodies that recognize a wide variety of antigens. B cells are activated to become plasma cells, which secrete antibodies.
- *Natural killer (NK) cells* kill cells that are infected by some microbes, or are stressed and damaged beyond repair. NK cells express inhibitory receptors that recognize MHC molecules that are normally expressed on healthy cells, and are thus prevented from killing normal cells.
- *Antigen-presenting cells (APCs)* capture microbes and other antigens, transport them to lymphoid organs, and display them for recognition by lymphocytes. The most efficient APCs are *dendritic cells,* which live in epithelia and most tissues.
- The cells of the immune system are organized in tissues, some of which are the sites of production of mature lymphocytes (the generative lymphoid organs, the bone marrow and thymus), and others are the sites of immune responses (the peripheral lymphoid organs, including lymph nodes, spleen, and mucosal lymphoid tissues).

OVERVIEW OF NORMAL IMMUNE RESPONSES

Now that we have described the major components of the immune system, it is useful to summarize the key features of normal immune responses. This will serve as the foundation for the subsequent discussion of diseases caused by deficient or uncontrolled immune responses.

The Early Innate Immune Response to Microbes

The principal barriers between hosts and their environment are the epithelia of the skin and the gastrointestinal and respiratory tracts. Infectious microbes usually enter through these routes and attempt to colonize the hosts. Epithelia serve as physical and functional barriers to infections, simultaneously impeding the entry of microbes and interfering with their growth through production of natural antimicrobial agents. If microbes are able to traverse these epithelia, they encounter the defense mechanisms of innate immunity, which are designed to react rapidly against microbes and their products. Phagocytes, including neutrophils and macrophages, ingest microbes into vesicles and destroy them by producing microbicidal substances in these vesicles; macrophages also secrete cytokines, which stimulate inflammation and lymphocyte responses. Phagocytes, dendritic cells, and many other cell types also turn on a variety of antimicrobial mechanisms, including secreted proteins called cytokines (described later), in response to recognition of microbes. Cells use several receptors to sense microbes; foremost among these are proteins called *Toll-like receptors,* so named because of homology with the *Drosophila* Toll protein, that recognize bacterial and viral components. NK cells kill virus-infected cells and produce the macrophage-activating cytokine, IFN-γ. Many plasma proteins are involved in host defense, including the proteins of the complement system, which are activated by microbes by the "alternative" pathway and whose products kill microbes and coat (opsonize) them for phagocytosis. In addition to combating infections, innate immune responses stimulate subsequent adaptive immunity, providing signals that are essential for initiating the responses of antigen-specific T and B lymphocytes.

The Capture and Display of Microbial Antigens

Microbes that enter through epithelia, and their protein antigens, are captured by DCs that are resident in these epithelia, and the cell-bound antigens are transported to draining lymph nodes (see Fig. 5–6). Protein antigens are processed in the APCs to generate peptides that are displayed on the surface of the APCs bound to MHC molecules. Antigens in different cellular compartments are displayed by different MHC molecules and are recognized by different subsets of T cells. Antigens that are ingested from the extracellular environment are processed in endosomal and lysosomal vesicles, and displayed bound to class II MHC molecules. Because CD4 binds to class II MHC molecules, CD4+ helper T cells recognize class II-associated peptides, which are usually derived from ingested proteins. In contrast, antigens in the cytoplasm are displayed by class I MHC molecules and are recognized by CD8+ cytotoxic T cells, because CD8 binds to class I MHC. This segregation of different antigens is key to the specialized functions of CD4+ and CD8+ T cells; as we discuss below, the two classes of T cells are designed to combat microbes that are located in different cellular compartments. Protein antigens, as well as polysaccharides and other nonprotein antigens, are also recognized by B lymphocytes in the lymphoid follicles of the peripheral lymphoid organs.

At the same time as the antigens of a microbe are recognized by B and T lymphocytes, the microbe elicits an innate immune response; in the case of immunization with a protein antigen, this innate response is induced by the adjuvant administered with the antigen. The innate immune response activates APCs to express costimulatory molecules and secrete cytokines that stimulate the proliferation and differentiation of T lymphocytes. The principal costimulators for T cells are the B7 molecules (CD80 and CD86) that are expressed on professional APCs and recognized by the CD28 receptor on naive T cells. The innate immune response to some microbes and polysaccharides also results in the activation of complement, generating cleavage products that enhance the proliferation and differentiation of B lymphocytes. Thus, antigen (signal 1 in Fig. 5–3) and molecules produced during innate immune responses (signal 2 in Fig. 5–3) function cooperatively to activate antigen-specific lymphocytes. The requirement for microbe-triggered signal 2 ensures that the adaptive immune response is induced by microbes and not by harmless substances.

Antigen recognition and costimulation together trigger the functional responses of the antigen-specific lymphocytes. These cellular responses proceed in steps, which are also reflected in the sequence of events in adaptive immune responses (Fig. 5–5). Although these phases are similar in all immune responses, the reactions of T and B lymphocytes differ in important ways and are best considered separately.

Cell-Mediated Immunity: Activation of T Lymphocytes and Elimination of Cell-Associated Microbes

Naive T lymphocytes are activated by antigen and costimulators in peripheral lymphoid organs, and proliferate and differentiate into effector cells that migrate to any site where the antigen (microbe) is present (Fig. 5–6). Upon activation, T lymphocytes secrete soluble proteins

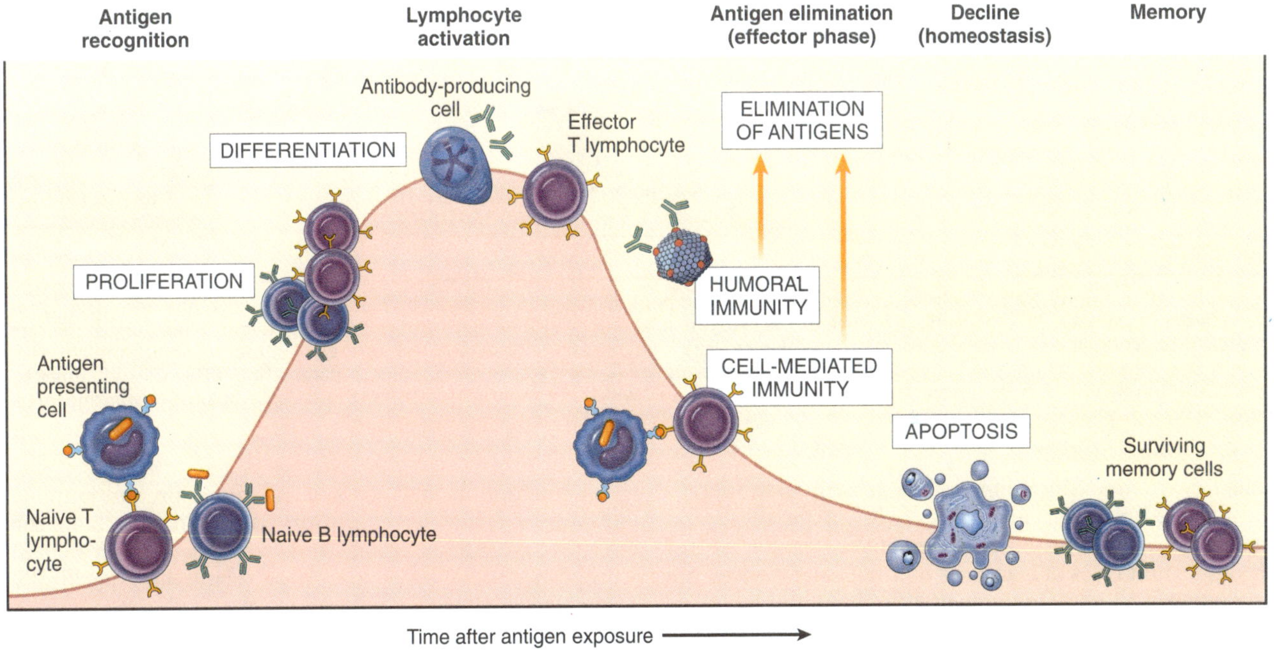

Figure 5–5

Adaptive immune responses consist of sequential phases: recognition of antigen by specific lymphocytes, activation of lymphocytes (consisting of their proliferation and differentiation into effector cells), and the effector phase (elimination of antigen). The response declines as antigen is eliminated, and most of the antigen-stimulated lymphocytes die by apoptosis. The antigen-specific cells that survive are responsible for memory. The duration of each phase may vary in different immune responses. The *y*-axis represents an arbitrary measure of the magnitude of the response. These principles apply to humoral immunity (mediated by B lymphocytes) and cell-mediated immunity (mediated by T lymphocytes).

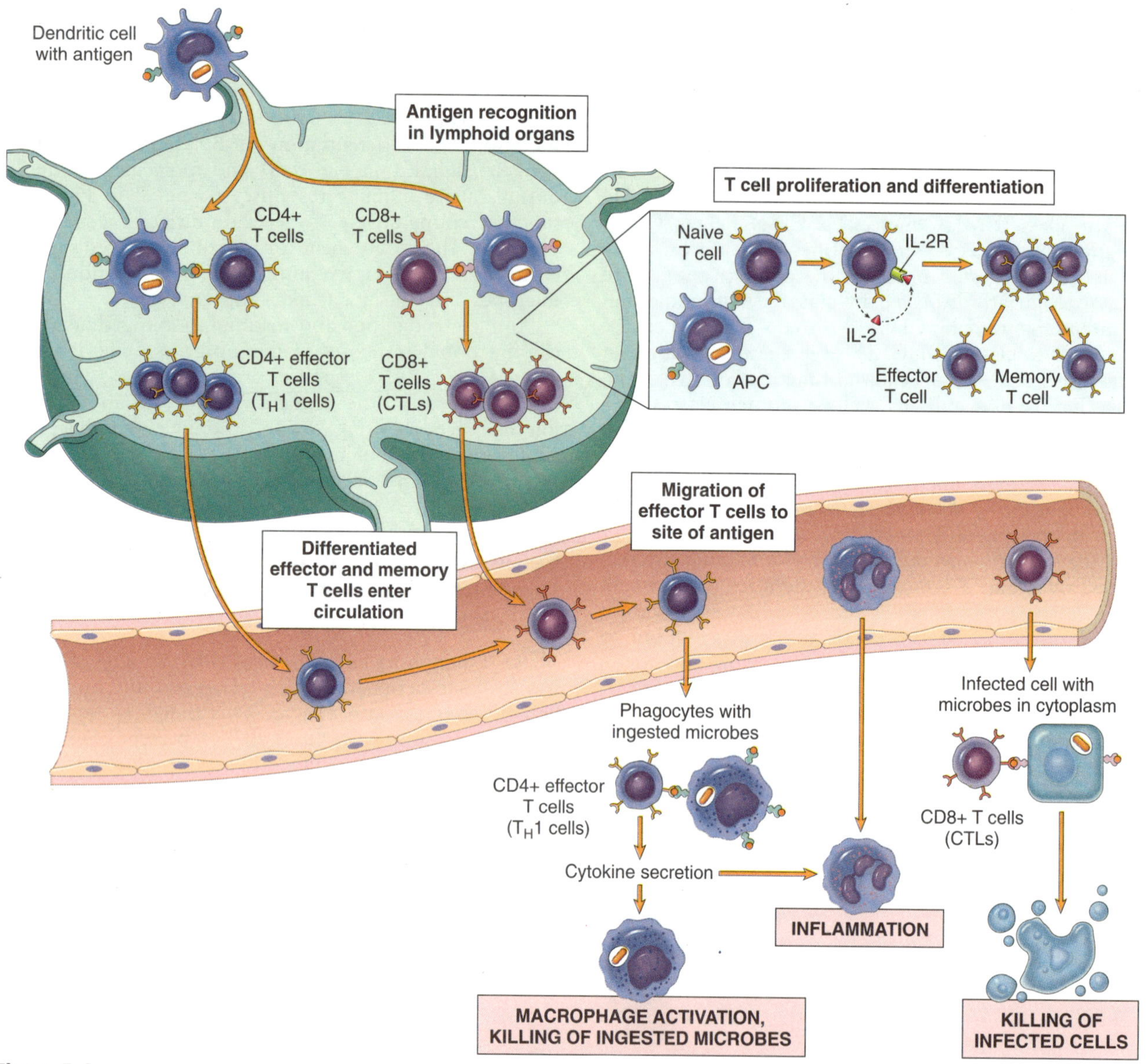

Figure 5–6

Cell-mediated immunity. Naive T cells recognize MHC-associated peptide antigens displayed on dendritic cells in lymph nodes. The T cells are activated to proliferate (under the influence of the cytokine IL-2) and to differentiate into effector and memory cells, which migrate to sites of infection and serve various functions in cell-mediated immunity. Effector CD4+ T cells of the T_H1 subset recognize the antigens of microbes ingested by phagocytes and activate the phagocytes to kill the microbes and induce inflammation. CD8+ CTLs kill infected cells harboring microbes in the cytoplasm. Not shown are T_H2 cells, which are especially important in defense against helminthic infections. Some activated T cells differentiate into long-lived memory cells. APC, antigen-presenting cell.

called *cytokines,* which function as growth and differentiation factors for lymphocytes and other cells, and mediate communications between leukocytes. Because of the important roles of cytokines in immune responses and inflammation, and in inflammatory and immunologic diseases, it is important to understand their properties and actions.

Cytokines: Messenger Molecules of the Immune System

Cytokines are polypeptide products of many cell types (but principally activated lymphocytes and macrophages) that function as mediators of inflammation and immune responses. They were introduced in Chapter 2 in the context of inflammation; here we review their general properties and focus on those cytokines specifically involved in adaptive immunity.

Although different cytokines have diverse actions and functions, they all share some common features. Cytokines are synthesized and secreted in response to external stimuli, which may be microbial products, antigen recognition, and other cytokines. Their secretion is typically transient and is controlled by transcription and post-translational mechanisms. The actions of cytokines may be *autocrine* (on the cell that produces the cytokine), *paracrine* (on adjacent cells), and, less commonly, endocrine (at a distance from the site of production). The effects of cytokines tend to be *pleiotropic* (one cytokine has effects on many cell types) and *redundant* (the same activity may be induced by many proteins).

Cytokines may be grouped into several classes based on their biologic activities and functions.

- *Cytokines involved in innate immunity and inflammation,* the earliest host response to microbes and dead cells. The major cytokines in this group are TNF and interleukin-1 (IL-1), a group of chemoattractant cytokines called chemokines, IL-12, and IFN-γ. Major sources of these cytokines are activated macrophages and DCs, as well as endothelial cells, lymphocytes, mast cells, and other cell types. These were described in Chapter 2.
- *Cytokines that regulate lymphocyte responses and effector functions in adaptive immunity.* Different cytokines are involved in the proliferation and differentiation of lymphocytes (e.g., IL-2 and IL-4), and in the activation of various effector cells (e.g., IFN-γ, which activates macrophages, and IL-5, which activates eosinophils). The major sources of these cytokines are CD4+ helper T lymphocytes stimulated by antigens and costimulators. These cytokines are key participants in the induction and effector phases of adaptive cell-mediated immune responses (see below).
- *Cytokines that stimulate hematopoiesis.* Many of these are called *colony-stimulating factors.* They function to increase the output of leukocytes from the bone marrow and to thus replenish leukocytes that are consumed during immune and inflammatory reactions.

Effector Functions of T Lymphocytes

One of the earliest responses of CD4+ helper T cells is secretion of the cytokine IL-2 and expression of high-affinity receptors for IL-2. IL-2 is a growth factor that acts on these T lymphocytes and stimulates their proliferation, leading to an increase in the number of antigen-specific lymphocytes. Some of the progeny of the expanded pool of T cells differentiate into effector cells that can secrete different sets of cytokines and thus perform different functions. *The best defined subsets of CD4+ helper cells are the T_H1 and T_H2 subsets.* T_H1 cells produce the cytokine IFN-γ, which activates macrophages and stimulates B cells to produce antibodies that activate complement and coat microbes for phagocytosis. T_H2 cells produce IL-4, which stimulates B cells to differentiate into IgE-secreting plasma cells; IL-5, which activates eosinophils; and IL-13, which activates mucosal epithelial cells to secrete mucus and expel microbes. A third subset, called T_H17, has been described recently that produces the cytokine IL-17, which promotes inflammation, and is believed to play an important role in some T cell–mediated inflammatory disorders. These effector cells migrate to sites of infection and accompanying tissue damage. When the differentiated effectors again encounter cell-associated microbes, they are activated to perform the functions that are responsible for elimination of the microbes. The key mediators of the functions of helper T cells are the surface molecule called CD40 ligand (CD40L), which binds to its receptor, CD40, on B cells and macrophages, and various cytokines. Differentiated CD4+ effector T cells of the T_H1 subset recognize microbial peptides on macrophages that have ingested the microbes. The T cells express CD40L, which engages CD40 on the macrophages, and the T cells secrete the cytokine, IFN-γ, which is a potent macrophage activator. The combination of CD40- and IFN-γ–mediated activation results in the induction of potent microbicidal substances in the macrophages, including reactive oxygen species and nitric oxide, leading to the destruction of ingested microbes. T_H2 cells elicit cellular defense reactions that are dominated by eosinophils and not macrophages. As we discuss below, CD4+ helper T cells also stimulate B-cell responses by CD40L and cytokines.

Activated CD8+ lymphocytes differentiate into CTLs that kill cells harboring microbes in the cytoplasm. These microbes may be viruses that infect many cell types, or bacteria that are ingested by macrophages but have learned to escape from phagocytic vesicles into the cytoplasm (where they are inaccessible to the killing machinery of phagocytes, which is largely confined to vesicles). By destroying the infected cells, CTLs eliminate the reservoirs of infection.

Humoral Immunity: Activation of B Lymphocytes and Elimination of Extracellular Microbes

Upon activation, B lymphocytes proliferate and then differentiate into plasma cells that secrete different classes of antibodies with distinct functions (Fig. 5–7). Many polysaccharide and lipid antigens have multiple identical antigenic determinants (epitopes) that are able to engage several antigen receptor molecules on each B cell and initiate the process of B-cell activation. Typical globular protein antigens are not able to bind to many antigen receptors, and the full response of B cells to protein antigens requires help from CD4+ T cells. B cells can also act as APCs, i.e. ingest protein antigens, degrade them, and display peptides bound to class II MHC molecules for recognition by helper T cells. The helper T cells express CD40L and secrete cytokines, which work together to activate the B cells.

Some of the progeny of the expanded B-cell clones differentiate into antibody-secreting plasma cells. Each plasma cell secretes antibodies that have the same antigen binding site as the cell surface antibodies (B-cell receptors) that first recognized the antigen. Polysaccharides and lipids stimulate secretion mainly of IgM antibody. Protein antigens, by virtue of CD40L- and cytokine-mediated helper T-cell actions, induce the production of antibodies of different classes (IgG, IgA, IgE). This production of functionally different antibodies, all with the same specificity, is called *heavy-chain class (isotype) switching;* it provides plasticity in the antibody response, allowing antibodies to serve many functions. Helper T cells also stimulate the production of antibodies with higher and higher affinity for the antigen. This process, called *affin-*

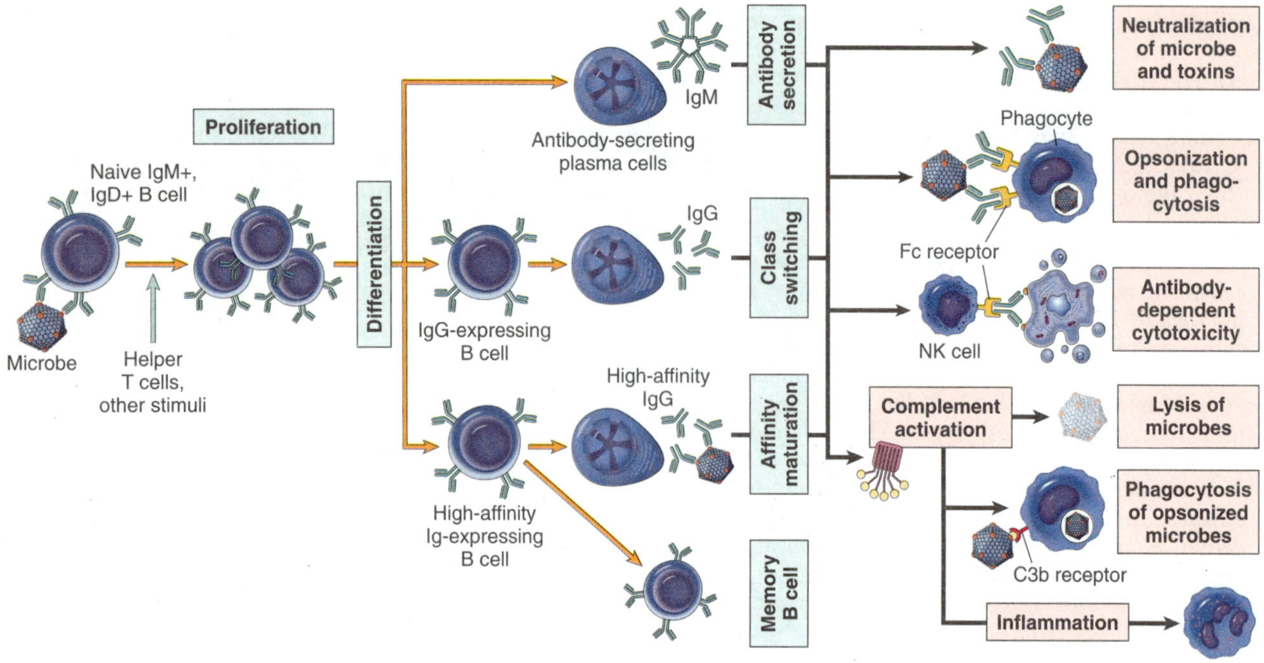

Figure 5–7

Humoral immunity. Naive B lymphocytes recognize antigens, and under the influence of helper T cells and other stimuli (not shown), the B cells are activated to proliferate and to differentiate into antibody-secreting plasma cells. Some of the activated B cells undergo heavy-chain class switching and affinity maturation, and some become long-lived memory cells. Antibodies of different heavy-chain isotypes (classes) perform different effector functions, shown on the right.

ity maturation, improves the quality of the humoral immune response.

The humoral immune response combats microbes in numerous ways (see Fig. 5–7).

- Antibodies bind to microbes and prevent them from infecting cells, thus "neutralizing" the microbes.
- IgG antibodies coat ("opsonize") microbes and target them for phagocytosis, since phagocytes (neutrophils and macrophages) express receptors for the Fc tails of IgG.
- IgG and IgM activate the complement system by the classical pathway, and complement products promote phagocytosis and destruction of microbes. Most opsonizing and complement-fixing IgG antibodies are stimulated by T_H1 helper cells, which respond to many bacteria and viruses, and IgG antibodies are important mechanisms of defense against these microbes.
- IgA is secreted in mucosal tissues and neutralizes microbes in the lumens of the respiratory and gastrointestinal tracts (and other mucosal tissues).
- IgG is actively transported across the placenta and protects the newborn until the immune system becomes mature.
- IgE coats helminthic parasites, and functions with mast cells and eosinophils to kill the parasites. As mentioned above, T_H2 helper cells secrete cytokines that stimulate the production of IgE and activate eosinophils, and thus the response to helminths is orchestrated by T_H2 cells.

Most circulating antibodies have half-lives of about 3 weeks. Some antibody-secreting plasma cells migrate to the bone marrow and live for years, continuing to produce low levels of antibodies.

Decline of Immune Responses and Immunologic Memory

The majority of effector lymphocytes induced by an infectious pathogen die by apoptosis after the microbe is eliminated, thus returning the immune system to its basal resting state. This return to a stable or steady state is called homeostasis. It occurs because microbes provide essential stimuli for lymphocyte survival and activation and effector cells are short-lived. Therefore, as the stimuli are eliminated, the activated lymphocytes are no longer kept alive.

The initial activation of lymphocytes also generates long-lived memory cells, which may survive for years after the infection. Memory cells are an expanded pool of antigen-specific lymphocytes (more numerous than the naive cells specific for any antigen that are present before encounter with that antigen), and memory cells respond faster and more effectively against the antigen than do naive cells. This is why the generation of memory cells is an important goal of vaccination.

This brief discussion of the normal immune response sets the stage for a consideration of the situations in which immune responses become abnormal, and how these abnormalities lead to tissue injury and disease.

SUMMARY

Overview of Normal Immune Responses

- The physiologic function of the immune system is defense against infectious microbes.
- The early reaction to microbes is mediated by the mechanisms of *innate immunity,* which are ready to respond to microbes. These mechanisms include epithelial barriers, phagocytes, NK cells, and plasma proteins, e.g., of the complement system. The reaction of innate immunity is often manifested as *inflammation.*
- The defense reactions of *adaptive immunity* develop slowly, but are more potent and specialized.
- Microbes and other foreign antigens are captured by dendritic cells and transported to lymph nodes, where the antigens are recognized by naïve lymphocytes. The lymphocytes are activated to proliferate and differentiate into effector and memory cells.
- *Cell-mediated immunity* is the reaction of T lymphocytes, designed to combat cell-associated microbes (e.g., phagocytosed microbes and microbes in the cytoplasm of infected cells). *Humoral immunity* is mediated by antibodies and is effective against extracellular microbes (in the circulation and mucosal lumens).
- CD4+ helper T cells help B cells to make antibodies, activate macrophages to destroy ingested microbes, and regulate all immune responses to protein antigens. The functions of CD4+ T cells are mediated by secreted proteins called *cytokines.* CD8+ cytotoxic T lymphocytes kill cells that express antigens in the cytoplasm that are seen as foreign (e.g. virus-infected and tumor cells).
- Antibodies secreted by plasma cells neutralize microbes and block their infectivity, and promote the phagocytosis and destruction of pathogens. Antibodies also confer passive immunity to neonates.

HYPERSENSITIVITY DISEASES: MECHANISMS OF IMMUNE-MEDIATED INJURY

Immune responses are capable of causing tissue injury and diseases that are called *hypersensitivity diseases.* This term originated from the idea that individuals who mount immune responses against an antigen are said to be "sensitized" to that antigen, and therefore, pathologic or excessive reactions are manifestations of "hypersensitivity." Normally, an exquisite system of checks and balances optimizes the eradication of infecting organisms without serious injury to host tissues. However, immune responses may be inadequately controlled or inappropriately targeted to host tissues, and in these situations, the normally beneficial response is the cause of disease. In the following sections, we will describe the causes and general mechanisms of hypersensitivity diseases, and then specific situations in which the immune response is responsible for the disease.

Causes of Hypersensitivity Diseases

Pathologic immune responses may be directed against different types of antigens, and may result from various underlying abnormalities.

- *Autoimmunity.* Normally, the immune system does not react against an individual's own antigens. This phenomenon is called *self-tolerance,* implying that all of us "tolerate" our own antigens. Sometimes, self-tolerance fails, resulting in reactions against one's own cells and tissues that are called *autoimmunity.* The diseases caused by autoimmunity are referred to as *autoimmune diseases.* We will return to the mechanisms of self-tolerance and autoimmunity later in this chapter.
- *Reactions against microbes.* There are many types of reactions against microbial antigens that may cause disease. In some cases, the reaction appears to be excessive or the microbial antigen is unusually persistent. If antibodies are produced against such antigens, the antibodies may bind to the microbial antigens to produce immune complexes, which deposit in tissues and trigger inflammation; this is the underlying mechanism of *poststreptococcal glomerulonephritis* (Chapter 14). T-cell responses against persistent microbes may give rise to severe inflammation, sometimes with the formation of granulomas (Chapter 2); this is the cause of tissue injury in tuberculosis and other infections. Rarely, antibodies or T cells reactive with a microbe cross-react with a host tissue; this is believed to be the basis of *rheumatic heart disease* (Chapter 11). Sometimes the disease-causing immune response may be entirely normal, but in the process of eradicating the infection host tissues are injured. In *viral hepatitis,* the virus that infects liver cells is not cytopathic, but it is recognized as foreign by the immune system. Cytotoxic T cells try to eliminate infected cells, and this normal immune response damages liver cells.
- *Reactions against environmental antigens.* Most healthy individuals do not react strongly against common environmental substances (e.g., pollens, animal danders, or dust mites), but almost 20% of the population is "allergic" to these substances. Allergies are diseases caused by unusual immune responses to a variety of noninfectious, and otherwise harmless, antigens to which all individuals are exposed but against which only some react.

In all these conditions, tissue injury is caused by the same mechanisms that normally function to eliminate infectious pathogens, namely antibodies, effector T lymphocytes, and various other effector cells. The problem in these diseases is that the response is triggered and maintained inappropriately. Because the stimuli for these abnormal immune responses are difficult or impossible to eliminate (e.g., self antigens, persistent microbes, or environmental antigens), and the immune system has many intrinsic positive feedback loops (amplification mechanisms), once a pathologic immune response starts it is difficult to control or terminate it. Therefore, these hypersensitivity diseases tend to be chronic, often debilitating, and are therapeutic challenges. Since inflammation, typically chronic inflammation, is a major component of the pathology of these disorders, they are sometimes grouped under the rubric *immune-mediated inflammatory diseases.*

Types of Hypersensitivity Diseases

Hypersensitivity reactions are traditionally subdivided into four types; three are variations on antibody-mediated injury, whereas the fourth is cell mediated (Table 5–1). The rationale for this classification is that the mechanism of immune injury is often a good predictor of the clinical manifestations and may even help to guide the therapy. However, this classification of immune-mediated disease is not perfect, because several immune reactions may coexist in one disease.

- *Immediate (type I) hypersensitivity* results from the activation of the T_H2 subset of CD4+ helper T cells by environmental antigens, leading to the production of IgE antibodies, which become attached to mast cells. When these IgE molecules bind the antigen (allergen), the mast cells are triggered to release mediators that transiently affect vascular permeability and induce smooth muscle contraction in various organs, and may stimulate more prolonged inflammation (the late phase reaction). These diseases are commonly called *allergies.*
- *Antibody-mediated (type II) hypersensitivity* disorders are caused by antibodies that bind to fixed tissue or cell surface antigens and promote phagocytosis and destruction of the coated cells or trigger pathologic inflammation in tissues.
- *Immune complex–mediated (type III) hypersensitivity* disorders are caused by antibodies binding to antigens to form complexes that circulate and may deposit in vascular beds and stimulate inflammation, typically secondary to complement activation. Tissue injury in these diseases is the result of the inflammation.
- *T-cell–mediated (type IV) hypersensitivity* disorders are cell-mediated immune responses in which T lymphocytes cause tissue injury, either by producing cytokines that induce inflammation and activate macrophages, or by directly killing host cells.

Immediate (Type I) Hypersensitivity

Immediate hypersensitivity is a tissue reaction that occurs rapidly (typically within minutes) after the interaction of antigen with IgE antibody that is bound to the surface of mast cells in a sensitized host. The reaction is initiated by entry of an antigen, which is called an allergen because it triggers allergy. Many allergens are environmental substances that are harmless for most individuals. Some individuals apparently inherit genes that make them susceptible to allergies. This susceptibility is manifested by the propensity of these individuals to make strong T_H2 responses and, subsequently, IgE antibody against the allergens. The IgE is central to the activation of the mast cells and release of mediators that are responsible for the clinical and pathologic manifestations of the reaction. Immediate hypersensitivity may occur as a local reaction that is merely annoying (e.g., seasonal rhinitis, or hay fever) or severely debilitating (asthma) or may culminate in a fatal systemic disorder (anaphylaxis).

Sequence of Events in Immediate Hypersensitivity Reactions

Most hypersensitivity reactions follow the same sequence of cellular responses (Fig. 5–8).

- *Activation of T_H2 cells and production of IgE antibody.* Allergens may be introduced by inhalation, ingestion, or injection. Variables that probably contribute to the strong T_H2 responses to allergens include

Table 5–1 Mechanisms of Immunologically Mediated Diseases

Type	Prototype Disorder	Immune Mechanisms	Pathologic Lesions
Immediate (type I) hypersensitivity	Anaphylaxis, allergies, bronchial asthma (atopic forms)	Production of IgE antibody → immediate release of vasoactive amines and other mediators from mast cells; recruitment of inflammatory cells (late-phase reaction)	Vascular dilation, edema, smooth muscle contraction, mucus production, inflammation
Antibody-mediated (type II) hypersensitivity	Autoimmune hemolytic anemia; Goodpasture syndrome	Production of IgG, IgM → binds to antigen on target cell or tissue → phagocytosis or lysis of target cell by activated complement or Fc receptors; recruitment of leukocytes	Phagocytosis and lysis of cells; inflammation; in some diseases, functional derangements without cell or tissue injury
Immune complex–mediated (type III) hypersensitivity	Systemic lupus erythematosus; some forms of glomerulonephritis; serum sickness; Arthus reaction	Deposition of antigen–antibody complexes → complement activation → recruitment of leukocytes by complement products and Fc receptors → release of enzymes and other toxic molecules	Inflammation, necrotizing vasculitis (fibrinoid necrosis)
T-cell–mediated (type IV) hypersensitivity	Contact dermatitis; multiple sclerosis; type I diabetes; transplant rejection; tuberculosis	Activated T lymphocytes → (i) release of cytokines and macrophage activation; (ii) T-cell–mediated cytotoxicity	Perivascular cellular infiltrates, edema, cell destruction, granuloma formation

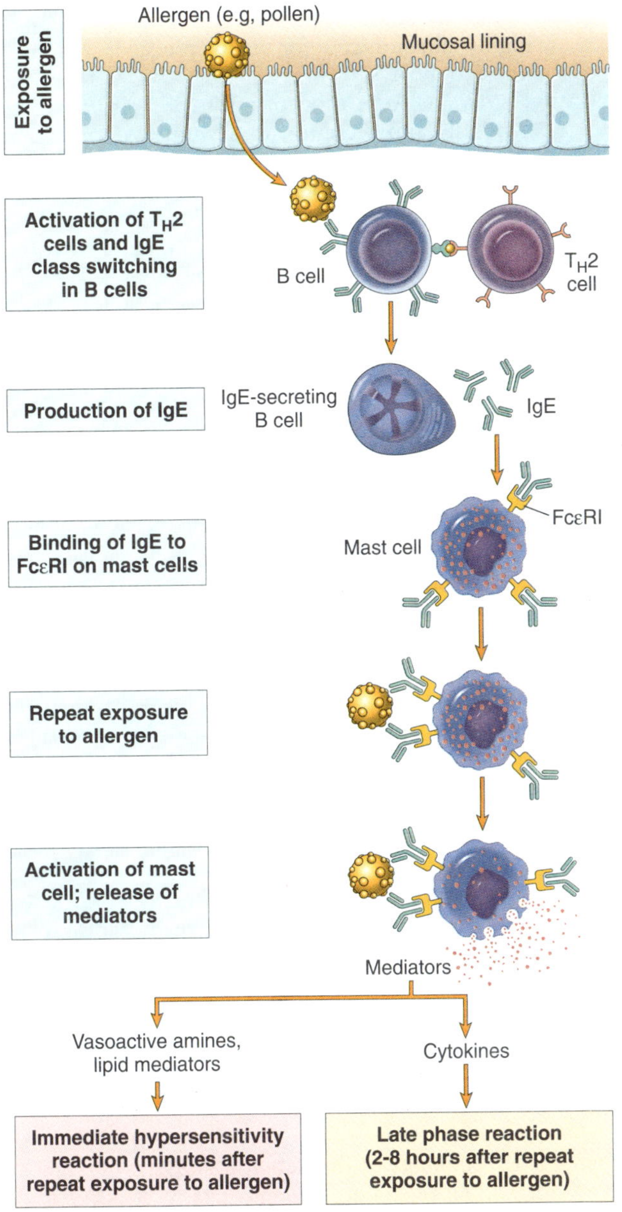

Figure 5–8

Sequence of events in immediate (type 1) hypersensitivity. Immediate hypersensitivity reactions are initiated by the introduction of an allergen, which stimulates T_H2 responses and IgE production. IgE binds to Fc receptors (FcεRI) on mast cells, and subsequent exposure to the allergen activates the mast cells to secrete the mediators that are responsible for the pathologic manifestations of immediate hypersensitivity.

the route of entry, dose, and chronicity of antigen exposure; the absence of inflammation and innate immunity at the time of allergen recognition; and the genetic makeup of the host. It is not clear if allergenic substances also have unique structural properties that endow them with the ability to elicit T_H2 responses. The T_H2 cells that are induced secrete several cytokines that are responsible for essentially all the reactions of immediate hypersensitivity. IL-4 stimulates B cells specific for the allergen to undergo heavy-chain class switching to IgE and to secrete this isotype. IL-5 activates eosinophils that are recruited to the reaction, and IL-13 acts on epithelial cells and stimulates mucus secretion. T_H2 cells are often recruited to the site of allergic reactions in response to chemokines that are produced locally; among these chemokines is eotaxin, which also recruits eosinophils to the same site.

The central role of T_H2 cells and IgE antibody in immediate hypersensitivity reactions is well established from clinical observations and experimental studies. Levels of serum IgE (and, in some studies, the numbers of T_H2 cells in the blood) are increased in individuals who suffer from allergies, and reducing IgE levels is of therapeutic benefit.

- *Sensitization of mast cells by IgE antibody.* Mast cells are derived from bone marrow, are widely distributed in tissues, and often reside near blood vessels and nerves and in subepithelial locations. Mast cells express a high-affinity receptor for the Fc portion of the ε heavy chain of IgE, called FcεRI. Even though the serum concentration of IgE is very low (in the range of 1–100 μg/mL), the affinity of the mast cell FcεRI receptor is so high that it is always occupied by IgE. These antibody-bearing mast cells are "sensitized" to react if the antigen binds to the antibody molecules. Basophils are the circulating counterparts of mast cells. They also express FcεRI, but their role in most immediate hypersensitivity reactions is not established (since these reactions occur in tissues and not in the circulation). The third cell type that expresses FcεRI are eosinophils, which are often present in these reactions and also have a role in IgE-mediated host defense against helminth infections, described below.
- *Activation of mast cells and release of mediators.* When individuals who were sensitized by exposure to an allergen are re-exposed to the allergen, it binds to multiple specific IgE molecules on mast cells, usually at or near the site of allergen entry. When these IgE molecules are cross-linked, a series of biochemical signals is triggered in the mast cells. The signals culminate in the secretion of various mediators from the mast cells. Three groups of mediators are the most important in different immediate hypersensitivity reactions (Fig. 5–9):
    - *Vasoactive amines released from granule stores.* The granules of mast cells contain histamine, which is released within seconds or minutes of activation. Histamine causes vasodilation, increased vascular permeability, smooth muscle contraction, and increased secretion of mucus. Other rapidly released mediators include adenosine (which causes bronchoconstriction and inhibits platelet aggregation) and chemotactic factors for neutrophils and eosinophils. Other mast cell granule contents that may be secreted include several neutral proteases (e.g., tryptase), which may damage tissues and also generate kinins and cleave complement components to produce additional chemotactic and inflammatory

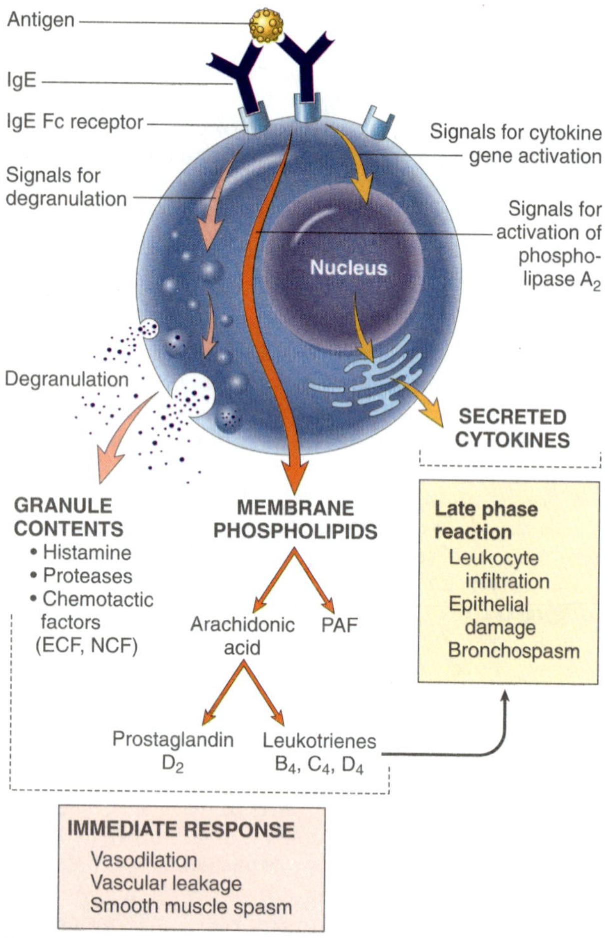

Figure 5–9

Mast cell mediators. Upon activation, mast cells release various classes of mediators that are responsible for the immediate and late-phase reactions. ECF, eosinophil chemotactic factor; NCF, neutrophil chemotactic factor (neither of these has been biochemically defined); PAF, platelet-activating factor.

factors (e.g., C3a; Chapter 2). The granules also contain acidic proteoglycans (heparin, chondroitin sulfate), the main function of which seems to be as a storage matrix for the amines.

- *Newly synthesized lipid mediators.* Mast cells synthesize and secrete prostaglandins and leukotrienes, by the same pathways as do other leukocytes (Chapter 2). These lipid mediators have several actions that are important in immediate hypersensitivity reactions. *Prostaglandin D_2 (PGD_2)* is the most abundant mediator generated by the cyclooxygenase pathway in mast cells. It causes intense bronchospasm as well as increased mucus secretion. *Leukotrienes C_4 and D_4 (LTC_4, LTD_4)* are the most potent vasoactive and spasmogenic agents known; on a molar basis, they are several thousand times more active than histamine in increasing vascular permeability and causing bronchial smooth muscle contraction. *LTB_4* is highly chemotactic for neutrophils, eosinophils, and monocytes.
- *Cytokines.* Activation of mast cells results in the synthesis and secretion of several cytokines that are important for the late-phase reaction. These include TNF and chemokines, which recruit and activate leukocytes (Chapter 2), IL-4 and IL-5, which amplify the T_H2-initiated immune reaction, and IL-13, which stimulates epithelial cell mucus secretion.

In summary, a variety of compounds that act on blood vessels, smooth muscle, and leukocytes mediate type I hypersensitivity reactions (Table 5–2). Some of these compounds are released rapidly from sensitized mast cells and are responsible for the intense immediate reactions associated with conditions such as systemic anaphylaxis. Others, such as cytokines, are responsible for the inflammation seen in late-phase reactions.

- *Late-phase reactions.* Often, the IgE-triggered reaction has two well-defined phases (Fig. 5–10): (1) the immediate response, characterized by vasodilation, vascular leakage, and smooth muscle spasm, usually evident within 5 to 30 minutes after exposure to an allergen and subsiding by 60 minutes; and (2) a second, late-phase reaction that usually sets in 2 to 8 hours later and may last for several days and is characterized by inflammation as well as tissue destruction, such as mucosal epithelial cell damage. The dominant inflammatory cells in the late-phase reaction are neutrophils, eosinophils, and lymphocytes, especially T_H2 cells. *Neutrophils* are recruited by various chemokines; their roles in inflammation were described in Chapter 2. *Eosinophils* are recruited by eotaxin and other chemokines released from TNF-activated epithelium

Table 5–2 Summary of the Action of Mast Cell Mediators in Immediate (Type I) Hypersensitivity

Action	Mediator
Vasodilation, increased vascular permeability	Histamine PAF Leukotrienes C_4, D_4, E_4 Neutral proteases that activate complement and kinins Prostaglandin D_2
Smooth muscle spasm	Leukotrienes C_4, D_4, E_4 Histamine Prostaglandins PAF
Cellular infiltration	Cytokines (e.g., chemokines, TNF) Leukotriene B_4 Eosinophil and neutrophil chemotactic factors (not defined biochemically)

PAF, platelet-activating factor; TNF, tumor necrosis factor.

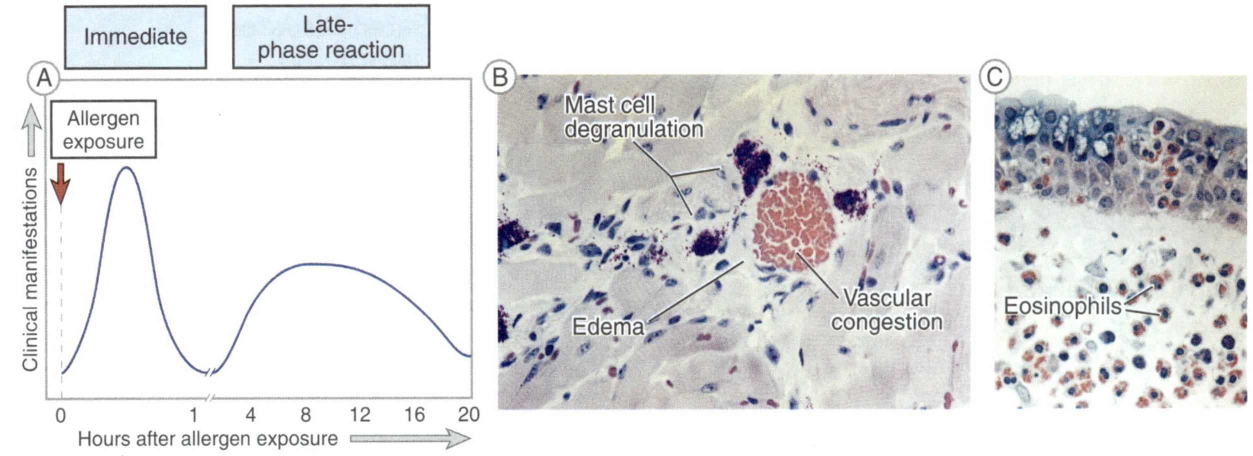

Figure 5–10

Immediate hypersensitivity. **A,** Kinetics of the immediate and late-phase reactions. The immediate vascular and smooth muscle reaction to allergen develops within minutes after challenge (allergen exposure in a previously sensitized individual), and the late-phase reaction develops 2 to 24 hours later. **B–C,** Morphology: The immediate reaction (**B**) is characterized by vasodilation, congestion, and edema, and the late-phase reaction (**C**) is characterized by an inflammatory infiltrate rich in eosinophils, neutrophils, and T cells. (Micrographs courtesy of Dr. Daniel Friend, Department of Pathology, Brigham and Women's Hospital, Boston, Massachusetts.)

and are important effectors of tissue injury in the late-phase response. Eosinophils produce major basic protein and eosinophil cationic protein, which are toxic to epithelial cells, and LTC_4 and platelet-activating factor, which promote inflammation. Cytokines produced by *T_H2 cells* have multiple actions, which are described above. The recruited leukocytes can amplify and sustain the inflammatory response even in the absence of continuous allergen exposure. In addition, inflammatory leukocytes are responsible for much of the epithelial cell injury in immediate hypersensitivity. Because inflammation is a major component of many allergic diseases, notably asthma and atopic dermatitis, therapy usually includes anti-inflammatory drugs such as corticosteroids.

Clinical and Pathologic Manifestations

An immediate hypersensitivity reaction may occur as a systemic disorder or as a local reaction. The nature of the reaction is often determined by the route of antigen exposure. Systemic (parenteral) administration of protein antigens (e.g., in bee venom) or drugs (e.g., penicillin) may result in *systemic anaphylaxis.* Within minutes of an exposure in a sensitized host, itching, *urticaria* (hives), and skin erythema appear, followed in short order by profound respiratory difficulty caused by pulmonary bronchoconstriction and accentuated by hypersecretion of mucus. Laryngeal edema may exacerbate matters by causing upper airway obstruction. In addition, the musculature of the entire gastrointestinal tract may be affected, with resultant vomiting, abdominal cramps, and diarrhea. Without immediate intervention, there may be systemic vasodilation with fall in blood pressure *(anaphylactic shock),* and the patient may progress to circulatory collapse and death within minutes.

Local reactions generally occur when the antigen is confined to a particular site, such as skin (contact, causing urticaria), gastrointestinal tract (ingestion, causing diarrhea), or lung (inhalation, causing bronchoconstriction). The common forms of skin and food allergies, hay fever, and certain forms of asthma are examples of localized allergic reactions.

Susceptibility to localized type I reactions is genetically controlled, and the term *atopy* is used to imply familial predisposition to such localized reactions. Patients who suffer from nasobronchial allergy (including hay fever and some forms of asthma) often have a family history of similar conditions. Linkage studies have identified several chromosomal regions that are associated with susceptibility to asthma and other allergic diseases. Among the candidate genes that are present close to these chromosomal loci are genes that encode HLA molecules (which may confer immune responsiveness to particular allergens), cytokines (which may control T_H2 responses), a component of the FcεRI, and ADAM33, a metalloproteinase that may be involved in tissue remodeling in the airways.

Before this discussion of immediate hypersensitivity is closed, it is worth noting that these reactions clearly did not evolve to engender human discomfort and disease. The immune response dependent on T_H2 cells and IgE, in particular the late-phase inflammatory reaction, plays an important protective role in parasitic infections. IgE antibodies are produced in response to many helminthic infections, and their physiologic function is to target helminths for destruction by eosinophils and mast cells. Mast cells are also involved in defense against bacterial infections. And snake aficionados will be relieved to hear that their mast cells may protect them from some snake venoms by releasing granule proteases that degrade the toxins. Why these beneficial responses are inappropriately activated by harmless environmental antigens, giving rise to allergies, remains a puzzle.

SUMMARY

Immediate (Type I) Hypersensitivity

- Also called allergic reactions, or allergies
- Induced by environmental antigens (allergens) that stimulate strong T_H2 responses and IgE production in genetically susceptible individuals
- IgE coats mast cells by binding to Fcε receptors; re-exposure to the allergen leads to cross-linking of the IgE and FcεRI, activation of mast cells, and release of mediators.
- Principal mediators are histamine, proteases and other granule contents; prostaglandins and leukotrienes; cytokines.
- Mediators are responsible for the immediate vascular and smooth muscle reactions and the late-phase reaction (inflammation).
- The clinical manifestations may be local or systemic, and range from mildly annoying rhinitis to fatal anaphylaxis.

Antibody-Mediated Diseases (Type II Hypersensitivity)

Antibody-mediated (type II) hypersensitivity disorders are caused by antibodies directed against target antigens on the surface of cells or other tissue components. The antigens may be normal molecules intrinsic to cell membranes or extracellular matrix, or they may be adsorbed exogenous antigens (e.g., a drug metabolite). Antibody-mediated abnormalities are the underlying cause of many human diseases; examples of these are listed in Table 5–3. In all these disorders the tissue damage or functional abnormalities result from a limited number of mechanisms.

Mechanisms of Antibody-Mediated Diseases

Antibodies cause disease by targeting cells for phagocytosis, by activating the complement system, and by interfering with normal cellular functions (Fig. 5–11). The antibodies that are responsible are typically high-affinity antibodies capable of activating complement and binding to the Fc receptors of phagocytes.

- *Opsonization and phagocytosis.* When circulating cells, such as erythrocytes or platelets, are coated (opsonized) with autoantibodies, with or without complement proteins, the cells become targets for phagocytosis by neutrophils and macrophages (see Fig. 5–11A). These phagocytes express receptors for the Fc

Table 5–3 Examples of Antibody-Mediated Diseases (Type II Hypersensitivity)

Disease	Target Antigen	Mechanisms of Disease	Clinicopathologic Manifestations
Autoimmune hemolytic anemia	Erythrocyte membrane proteins (Rh blood group antigens, I antigen)	Opsonization and phagocytosis of erythrocytes	Hemolysis, anemia
Autoimmune thrombocytopenic purpura	Platelet membrane proteins (gpllb:Illa integrin)	Opsonization and phagocytosis of platelets	Bleeding
Pemphigus vulgaris	Proteins in intercellular junctions of epidermal cells (epidermal cadherin)	Antibody-mediated activation of proteases, disruption of intercellular adhesions	Skin vesicles (bullae)
Vasculitis caused by ANCA	Neutrophil granule proteins, presumably released from activated neutrophils	Neutrophil degranulation and inflammation	Vasculitis
Goodpasture syndrome	Noncollagenous protein in basement membranes of kidney glomeruli and lung alveoli	Complement- and Fc receptor–mediated inflammation	Nephritis, lung hemorrhage
Acute rheumatic fever	Streptococcal cell wall antigen; antibody cross-reacts with myocardial antigen	Inflammation, macrophage activation	Myocarditis, arthritis
Myasthenia gravis	Acetylcholine receptor	Antibody inhibits acetylcholine binding, down-modulates receptors	Muscle weakness, paralysis
Graves disease (hyperthyroidism)	TSH receptor	Antibody-mediated stimulation of TSH receptors	Hyperthyroidism
Insulin-resistant diabetes	Insulin receptor	Antibody inhibits binding of insulin	Hyperglycemia, ketoacidosis
Pernicious anemia	Intrinsic factor of gastric parietal cells	Neutralization of intrinsic factor, decreased absorption of vitamin B_{12}	Abnormal erythropoiesis, anemia

ANCA, antineutrophil cytoplasmic antibodies; TSH, thyroid-stimulating hormone.

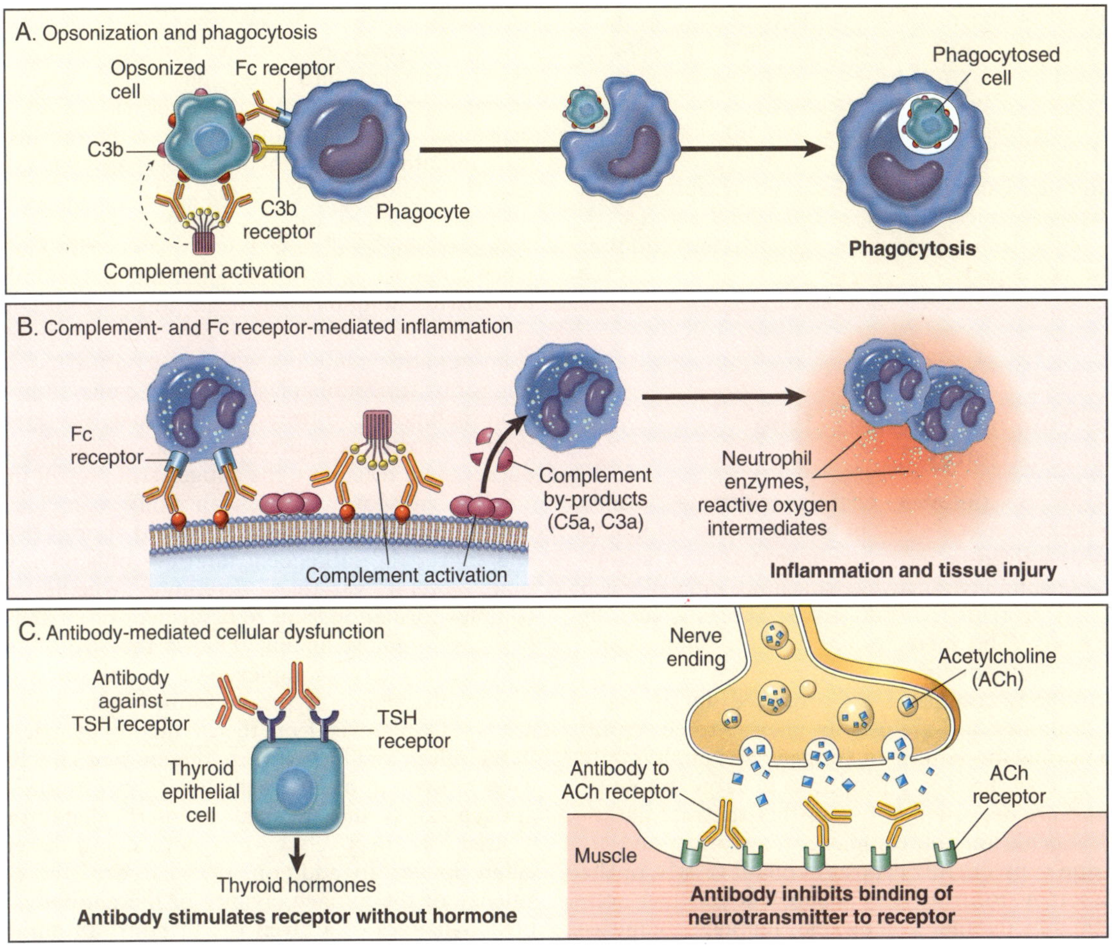

Figure 5–11

Effector mechanisms of antibody-mediated injury. **A,** Opsonization of cells by antibodies and complement components, and ingestion of opsonized cells by phagocytes. **B,** Inflammation induced by antibody binding to Fc receptors of leukocytes and by complement breakdown products. **C,** Antireceptor antibodies disturb the normal function of receptors. In these examples, antibodies against the thyroid-stimulating hormone (TSH) receptor activate thyroid cells in Graves disease, and acetylcholine (ACh) receptor antibodies impair neuromuscular transmission in myasthenia gravis.

tails of IgG antibodies and for breakdown products of the C3 complement protein, and use these receptors to bind and ingest opsonized particles. Opsonized cells are usually eliminated in the spleen, and this is why splenectomy is of some benefit in autoimmune thrombocytopenia and hemolytic anemia.

• *Inflammation.* Antibodies bound to cellular or tissue antigens activate the complement system by the "classical" pathway (Fig. 5–11B). Products of complement activation recruit neutrophils and monocytes, triggering inflammation in tissues, opsonize cells for phagocytosis, and lyse cells, especially erythrocytes. Leukocytes may also be activated by engagement of Fc receptors, which recognize the bound antibodies.

• *Antibody-mediated cellular dysfunction.* In some cases, antibodies directed against cell surface receptors impair or dysregulate cellular function without causing cell injury or inflammation (Fig. 5–11C). In myasthenia gravis, antibodies against acetylcholine receptors in the motor end plates of skeletal muscles inhibit neuromuscular transmission, with resultant muscle weakness. Antibodies can also stimulate cell function inappropriately. In Graves' disease, antibodies against the thyroid-stimulating hormone receptor stimulate thyroid epithelial cells to secrete thyroid hormones, resulting in hyperthyroidism. Antibodies against hormones and other essential proteins can neutralize and block the actions of these molecules, causing functional derangements.

SUMMARY

Pathogenesis of Diseases Caused by Antibodies and Immune Complexes

• Antibodies can coat (opsonize) cells, with or without complement proteins, and target these cells for *phagocytosis* by phagocytes (macrophages), which express receptors for the Fc tails of IgG and for complement proteins. The result is depletion of the opsonized cells.

- Antibodies and immune complexes may deposit in tissues or blood vessels, and elicit an *acute inflammatory reaction* by activating complement, with release of breakdown products, or by engaging Fc receptors of leukocytes. The inflammatory reaction causes tissue injury.
- Antibodies can bind to cell surface receptors or essential molecules, and cause *functional derangements* (either inhibition or unregulated activation) without cell injury.

Immune Complex Diseases (Type III Hypersensitivity)

Antigen–antibody (immune) complexes that are formed in the circulation may deposit in blood vessels, leading to complement activation and acute inflammation. The antigens in these complexes may be exogenous antigens, such as microbial proteins, or endogenous antigens, such as nucleoproteins. The mere formation of immune complexes does not equate with hypersensitivity disease; antigen–antibody complexes are produced during many immune responses and are usually phagocytosed, representing a normal mechanism of antigen removal. It is only when these complexes are produced in large amounts, persist, and are deposited in tissues that they are pathogenic. Pathogenic immune complexes may form in the circulation and subsequently deposit in blood vessels, or the complexes may form at sites where antigen has been planted (in situ immune complexes). Immune complex–mediated injury is systemic when complexes are formed in the circulation and are deposited in several organs, or localized to particular organs (e.g., kidneys, joints, or skin) if the complexes are formed and deposited in a specific site. The mechanism of tissue injury is the same regardless of the pattern of distribution; however, the sequence of events and the conditions leading to the formation of systemic and local immune complexes are different and will be considered separately. Immune complex diseases are some of the most common immunologic diseases (Table 5–4).

Systemic Immune Complex Disease

The pathogenesis of systemic immune complex disease can be divided into three phases: (1) formation of antigen–antibody complexes in the circulation and (2) deposition of the immune complexes in various tissues, thus initiating (3) an inflammatory reaction in various sites throughout the body (Fig. 5–12).

Acute serum sickness is the prototype of a systemic immune complex disease. It was first described in humans when large amounts of foreign serum were administered for passive immunization (e.g., horse serum containing antidiphtheria antibody); it is now seen only infrequently (e.g., in patients injected with horse antithymocyte globulin for treatment of aplastic anemia, a mercifully uncommon therapeutic strategy). Approximately 5 days after a foreign protein is injected, specific antibodies are produced; these react with the antigen still present in the circulation to form antigen–antibody complexes. The complexes deposit in blood vessels in various tissue beds and trigger the subsequent injurious inflammatory reaction. Several variables determine whether immune complex formation leads to tissue deposition and disease. Perhaps foremost among these is the size of the complexes. Very large complexes or complexes with many free IgG Fc regions (typically formed in antibody excess) are rapidly removed from the circulation by macrophages in the spleen and liver and are therefore usually harmless. The most pathogenic complexes are formed during antigen excess and are small or intermediate in size, are cleared less effectively by phagocytes, and therefore circulate longer. In addition, the charge of the complex, valency of the antigen, avidity of the antibody, and the hemodynamics of a given vascular bed all influence the tendency to develop disease. The favored sites of deposition are kidneys, joints, and small blood vessels in many tissues. Localization in the kidney and joints is explained in part by the high hemodynamic pressures associated with the filtration function of the glomerulus and the synovium. If complexes are to leave the circulation and deposit within or outside the vessel wall, an increase in vascular permeability must also occur. This is probably triggered when immune complexes bind to leukocytes and mast cells via Fc and C3b receptors and stimulate release of mediators that increase vascular permeability.

Table 5–4 Examples of Immune Complex–Mediated Diseases

Disease	Antigen Involved	Clinicopathologic Manifestations
Systemic lupus erythematosus	Nuclear antigens	Nephritis, skin lesions, arthritis, others
Poststreptococcal glomerulonephritis	Streptococcal cell wall antigen(s); may be "planted" in glomerular basement membrane	Nephritis
Polyarteritis nodosa	Hepatitis B virus antigen	Systemic vasculitis
Reactive arthritis	Bacterial antigens (*Yersinia*)	Acute arthritis
Serum sickness	Various proteins, such as foreign serum protein (horse anti-thymocyte globulin)	Arthritis, vasculitis, nephritis
Arthus reaction (experimental)	Various foreign proteins	Cutaneous vasculitis

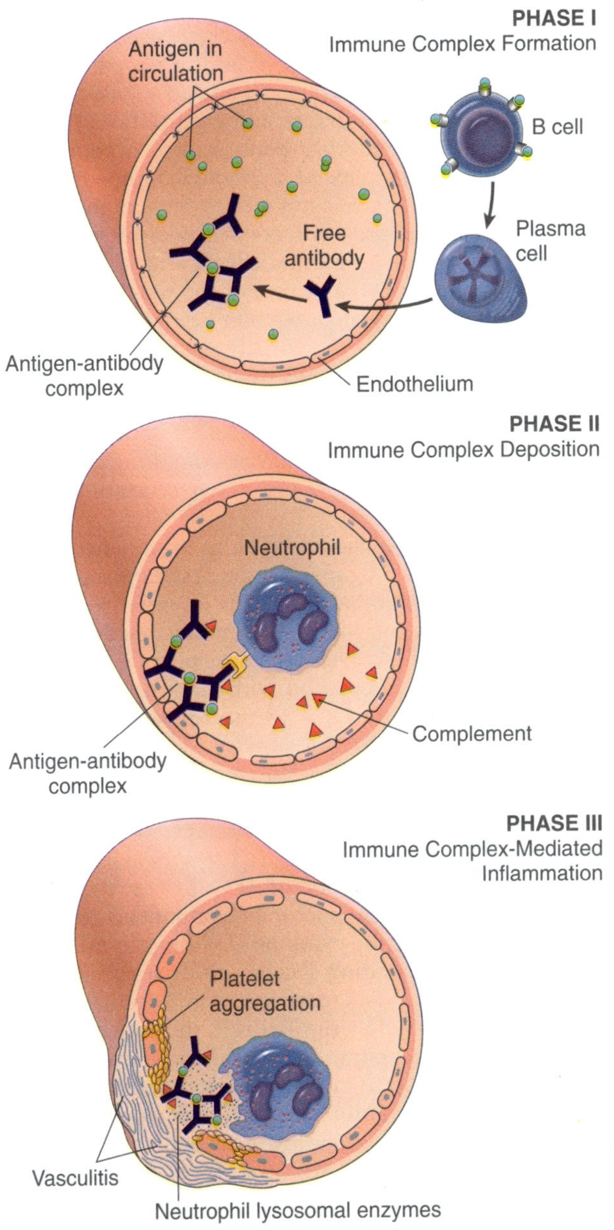

Figure 5–12

Immune complex disease. The sequential phases in the induction of systemic immune complex–mediated diseases (type III hypersensitivity).

Once complexes are deposited in the tissue, the third phase, the inflammatory reaction, ensues. During this phase (approximately 10 days after antigen administration), clinical features such as fever, urticaria, arthralgias, lymph node enlargement, and proteinuria appear. Wherever immune complexes deposit, the tissue damage is similar. The immune complexes activate the complement system, leading to the release of biologically active fragments such as the anaphylatoxins (C3a and C5a), which increase vascular permeability and are chemotactic for neutrophils and monocytes (Chapter 2). The complexes also bind to Fcγ receptors on neutrophils and monocytes and activate these cells. Attempted phagocytosis of immune complexes by the leukocytes results in the secretion of a variety of additional proinflammatory substances, including prostaglandins, vasodilator peptides, and chemotactic substances, as well as lysosomal enzymes capable of digesting basement membrane, collagen, elastin, and cartilage, and reactive-oxygen species that damage tissues. Immune complexes can also cause platelet aggregation and activate Hageman factor; both of these reactions augment the inflammatory process and initiate formation of microthrombi, which contribute to the tissue injury by producing local ischemia (see Fig. 5–12). The resultant pathologic lesion is termed *vasculitis* if it occurs in blood vessels, *glomerulonephritis* if it occurs in renal glomeruli, *arthritis* if it occurs in the joints, and so on.

Predictably, the antibody classes that induce such lesions are complement-fixing antibodies (i.e., IgG and IgM) and antibodies that bind to phagocyte Fc receptors (IgG). Because IgA can activate complement by the alternative pathway, IgA-containing complexes may also induce tissue injury. During the active phase of the disease, consumption of complement may result in decreased serum complement levels. The role of complement- and Fc receptor–dependent inflammation in the pathogenesis of the tissue injury is supported by the observations that experimental depletion of serum complement levels or knockout of Fc receptors in mice greatly reduces the severity of lesions, as does depletion of neutrophils.

Morphology

The morphologic appearance of immune complex injury is dominated by acute **necrotizing vasculitis,** microthrombi, and superimposed ischemic necrosis accompanied by acute inflammation of the affected organs. The necrotic vessel wall takes on a smudgy eosinophilic appearance called **fibrinoid necrosis,** caused by protein deposition (see Fig. 1–14, Chapter 1). Immune complexes can be visualized in the tissues, usually in the vascular wall; examples of such deposits in the kidney lupus are shown in Figure 5–21E. In due course the lesions tend to resolve, especially when they were brought about by a single exposure to antigen (e.g., acute serum sickness and acute poststreptococcal glomerulonephritis [Chapter 14]). However, chronic immune complex disease develops when there is persistent antigenemia or repeated exposure to an antigen. This occurs in some human diseases, such as systemic lupus erythematosus (SLE). Most often, even though the morphologic changes and other findings strongly implicate immune complex disease, the inciting antigens are unknown.

Local Immune Complex Disease

A model of local immune complex diseases is the *Arthus reaction,* an area of tissue necrosis resulting from acute immune complex vasculitis. The reaction is produced experimentally by injecting an antigen into the skin of a previously immunized animal (i.e., preformed antibodies against the antigen are already present in the circulation). Because of the initial antibody excess, immune complexes are formed as the antigen diffuses into the vascular wall; these are precipitated at the site of injection and trigger the same inflammatory reaction and histologic appearance as in systemic immune complex disease. Arthus lesions evolve over a few hours and reach a peak 4 to 10 hours after injection, when the injection site develops visible edema with severe hemorrhage, occasionally followed by ulceration.

T-Cell–Mediated (Type IV) Hypersensitivity

The occurrence and significance of T-lymphocyte–mediated tissue injury have been increasingly appreciated as the methods for detecting and purifying T cells from patients' circulation and lesions have improved. This group of diseases has received great interest because many of the new, rationally designed biologic therapies for immune-mediated inflammatory diseases have been developed to target abnormal T-cell reactions. Several autoimmune disorders, as well as pathologic reactions to environmental chemicals and persistent microbes, are now known to be caused by T cells (Table 5–5). Two types of T-cell reactions are capable of causing tissue injury and disease: (1) *delayed-type hypersensitivity (DTH), initiated by CD4+ T cells,* and (2) *direct cell* cytotoxicity, *mediated by CD8+ T cells* (Fig. 5–13). In DTH, T_H1-type CD4+ T cells secrete cytokines, leading to recruitment of other cells, especially macrophages, which are the major effector cells of injury. In cell-mediated cytotoxicity, cytotoxic CD8+ T cells are responsible for tissue damage.

Delayed-Type Hypersensitivity

A classic example of DTH is the *tuberculin reaction,* elicited by antigen challenge in an individual already sensitized to the tubercle bacillus by a previous infection (Chapter 13). Between 8 and 12 hours after intracutaneous injection of tuberculin (a protein extract of the tubercle bacillus), a local area of erythema and induration appears, reaching a peak (typically 1–2 cm in diameter) in 24 to 72 hours (hence the adjective, *delayed*) and thereafter slowly subsiding. Histologically, the DTH reaction is characterized by perivascular accumulation ("cuffing") of CD4+ helper T cells and macrophages (Fig. 5–14). Local secretion of cytokines by these mononuclear inflammatory cells leads to increased microvascular permeability, giving rise to dermal edema and fibrin deposition; the latter is the main cause of the tissue induration in these responses. The tuberculin response is used to screen populations for individuals who have had prior exposure to tuberculosis and therefore have circulating memory T cells specific for mycobacterial proteins. Notably, immunosuppression or loss of CD4+ T cells (e.g., resulting from HIV infection) may lead to a negative tuberculin response even in the presence of a severe infection.

The sequence of events in DTH, as exemplified by the tuberculin reaction, begins with the first exposure of the individual to tubercle bacilli, and is essentially the same as the reactions of cell-mediated immunity (see Fig. 5–6). Naive CD4+ T lymphocytes recognize peptide antigens of tubercle bacilli in association with class II MHC molecules on the surface of DCs (or macrophages) that have processed the mycobacterial antigens. This process leads to the generation of effector and memory CD4+ cells of the T_H1 type, some of which may remain in the circulation or tissues for years. Many variables may determine why some stimuli induce a T_H1 response. Foremost among these is the activation of APCs by the engagement of Toll-like receptors by microbial components, resulting in the production of the cytokine *IL-12* by the APCs. IL-12 acts on the responding T cells and drives their differentiation along the T_H1 pathway. The cytokine IFN-γ, made by NK cells and by the T_H1 cells themselves, further promotes T_H1 differentiation, providing a powerful positive feedback loop. On subsequent exposure to the antigen (e.g., tuberculin), the previously generated T_H1 effector and memory cells are recruited to the site of

Table 5–5 Examples of T-Cell-Mediated (Type IV) Hypersensitivity

Disease	Specificity of Pathogenic T cells	Clinicopathologic Manifestations
Type 1 diabetes mellitus	Antigens of pancreatic islet β cells (insulin, glutamic acid decarboxylase, others)	Insulitis (chronic inflammation in islets), destruction of β cells; diabetes
Multiple sclerosis	Protein antigens in CNS myelin (myelin basic protein, proteolipid protein)	Demyelination in CNS with perivascular inflammation; paralysis, ocular lesions
Rheumatoid arthritis	Unknown antigen in joint synovium (type II collagen?); role of antibodies?	Chronic arthritis with inflammation, destruction of articular cartilage and bone
Peripheral neuropathy; Guillain-Barré syndrome?	Protein antigens of peripheral nerve myelin	Neuritis, paralysis
Inflammatory bowel disease (Crohn's disease)	Unknown antigen; may be derived from intestinal microbes	Chronic inflammation of ileum and colon, often with granulomas; fibrosis, stricture
Contact dermatitis	Environmental chemicals, e.g., poison ivy (pentadecylcatechol)	Dermatitis, with itching; usually short-lived, may be chronic with persistent exposure

CNS, central nervous system.

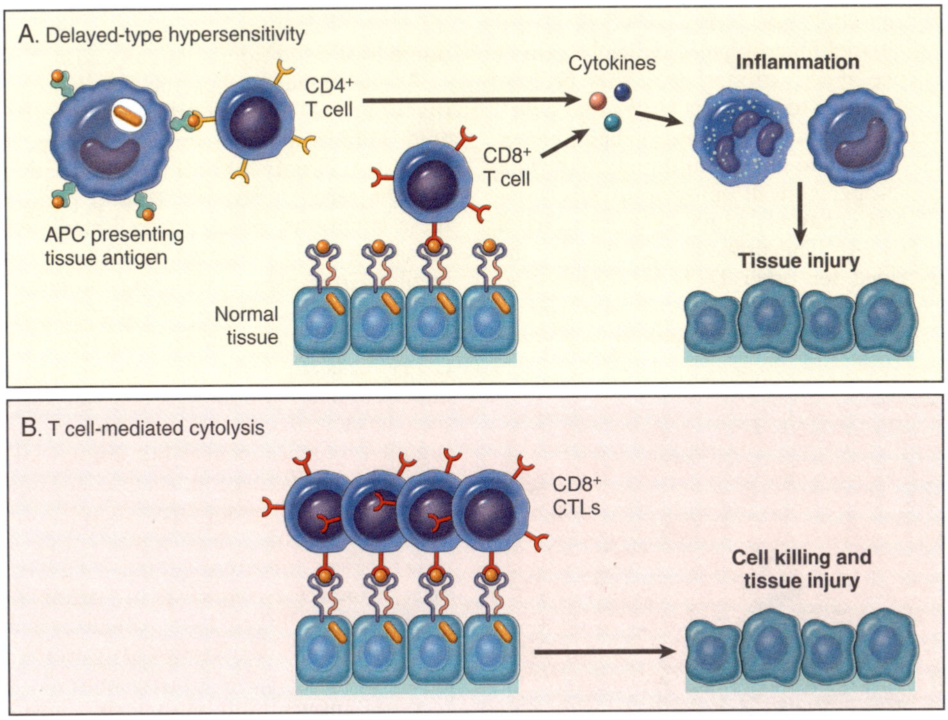

Figure 5–13

Mechanisms of T-cell-mediated (type IV) hypersensitivity reactions. **A,** In delayed-type hypersensitivity reactions, CD4+ T cells (and sometimes CD8+ cells) respond to tissue antigens by secreting cytokines that stimulate inflammation and activate phagocytes, leading to tissue injury. **B,** In some diseases, CD8+ CTLs directly kill tissue cells. APC, antigen-presenting cell.

antigen exposure and are activated by the antigen presented by local APCs. The T_H1 cells secrete *IFN-γ,* which is the most potent macrophage-activating cytokine known and the major mediator of the DTH reaction.

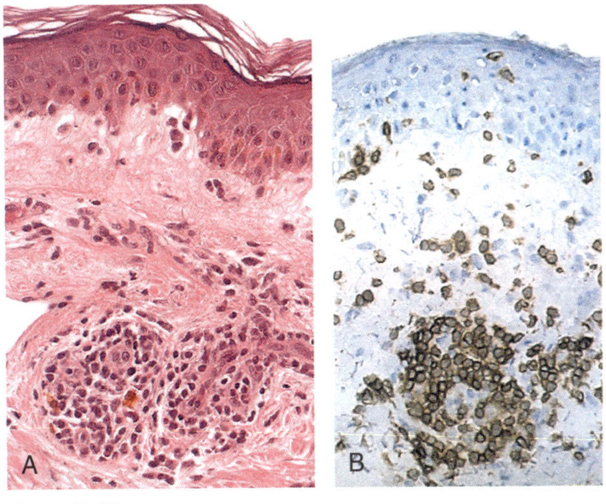

Figure 5–14

Delayed-type hypersensitivity reaction in the skin. **A,** Perivascular accumulation ("cuffing") of mononuclear inflammatory cells (lymphocytes and macrophages), with associated dermal edema and fibrin deposition. **B,** Immunoperoxidase staining reveals a predominantly perivascular cellular infiltrate that marks positively with anti-CD4 antibodies. (**B,** Courtesy of Dr. Louis Picker, Department of Pathology, Oregon Health Sciences University, Portland, Oregon.)

Activated macrophages have increased phagocytic and microbicidal activity. They also secrete several polypeptide growth factors, including platelet-derived growth factor (PDGF) and transforming growth factor β (TGF-β), which stimulate fibroblast proliferation and augment collagen synthesis. Thus, activation by IFN-γ enhances the ability of macrophages to eliminate offending agents; if the activation is sustained, fibrosis ensues. Activated macrophages also express more class II MHC molecules and costimulators, leading to augmented antigen presentation capacity, and the cells secrete more IL-12, thus stimulating more T_H1 responses. Because of these multiple feedback loops, DTH reactions become chronic unless the offending agent is eliminated or the cycle is interrupted therapeutically.

Other cytokines produced by T_H1 cells also play significant roles in the DTH reaction. *IL-2* causes the proliferation of the T cells that have accumulated at sites of DTH. *TNF* and *lymphotoxin* are cytokines that exert important effects on endothelial cells: (1) increased secretion of nitric oxide and prostacyclin, causing local vasodilation and increased blood flow; (2) increased expression of selectins and ligands for integrins (Chapter 2), adhesion molecules that promote leukocyte attachment; and (3) secretion of chemokines such as IL-8. Together, these changes facilitate the recruitment of lymphocytes and monocytes to the site of DTH responses.

Prolonged DTH reactions against persistent microbes or other stimuli may result in a special morphologic pattern of reaction called *granulomatous inflammation.* The initial perivascular CD4+ T-cell infiltrate is progressively replaced by macrophages over a period of 2 to 3 weeks; these accumulated macrophages typically exhibit morphologic evidence of activation, that is, they become large, flat, and eosinophilic (denoted as *epithelioid cells*). The epithelioid cells occasionally fuse under the influence of cytokines (e.g., IFN-γ) to form multinucleated *giant cells*. A microscopic aggregate of epithelioid cells, typically surrounded by a collar of lymphocytes, is called a *granuloma* (Fig. 5–15A). The process is essentially the same as that described for other DTH responses (Fig. 5–15B). Older granulomas develop an enclosing rim of fibroblasts and connective tissue. Recognition of a granuloma is of diagnostic importance because of the limited number of conditions that can cause it (Chapter 2).

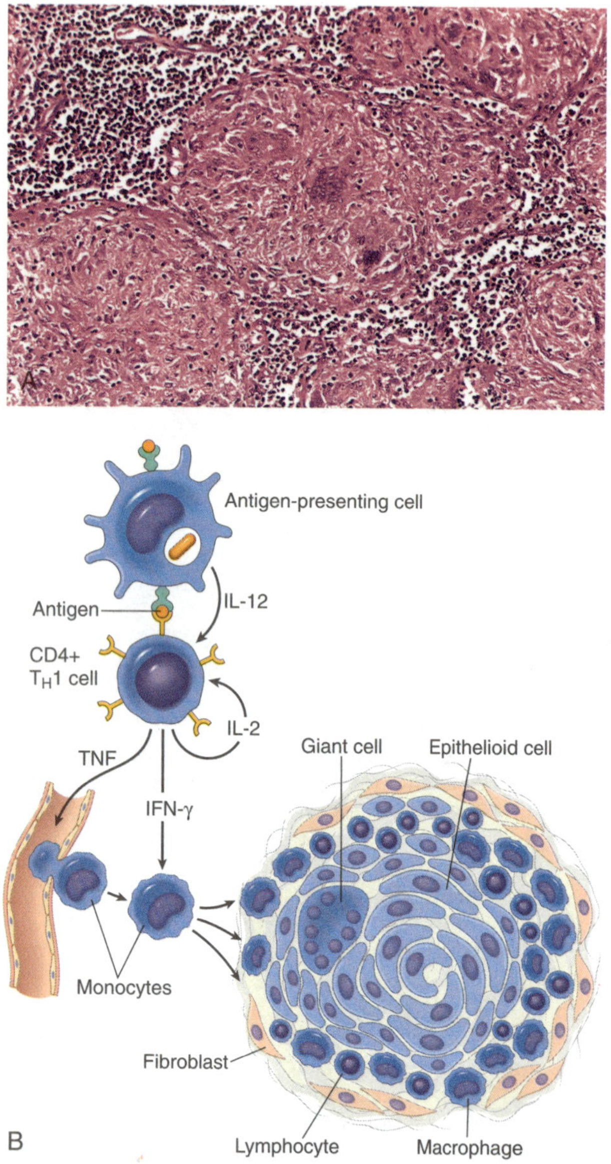

Figure 5–15

Granulomatous inflammation. **A,** A section of a lymph node shows several granulomas, each made up of an aggregate of epithelioid cells and surrounded by lymphocytes. The granuloma in the center shows several multinucleate giant cells. **B,** The events that give rise to the formation of granulomas in type IV hypersensitivity reactions. Note the role played by T-cell-derived cytokines. (**A,** Courtesy of Dr. Trace Worrell, Department of Pathology, University of Texas Southwestern Medical School, Dallas, Texas.)

As mentioned earlier, the T cell–macrophage reaction that typifies DTH is also the central reaction of cell-mediated immunity, a major mechanism of host defense against a variety of intracellular pathogens, including mycobacteria, fungi, and certain parasites. In many of these situations, protective cell-mediated immunity and damaging DTH may coexist. The same reaction may be involved in transplant rejection and tumor immunity. The critical role of CD4+ T cells in protective, cell-mediated immunity is evident in patients with AIDS. The loss of CD4+ cells in these patients results in a markedly impaired host response against intracellular pathogens such as *Mycobacterium tuberculosis*. The bacteria are engulfed by macrophages but are not killed, and instead of granuloma formation, there is accumulation of unactivated macrophages poorly adapted to deal with the invading microbe.

DTH reactions are the underlying basis of several diseases. *Contact dermatitis* is an example of tissue injury resulting from DTH. It is evoked by contact with pentadecylcatechol (also known as urushiol, the active component of poison ivy and poison oak, which probably becomes antigenic by binding to a host protein). Exposure of a sensitized host elicits the reaction, typically manifested as a vesicular dermatitis. The basic mechanism is similar to that described for tuberculin sensitivity. On reexposure to the plants, sensitized T_H1 CD4+ cells accumulate in the dermis and migrate toward the antigen within the epidermis. Here they release cytokines that damage keratinocytes, causing separation of these cells and formation of an intraepidermal vesicle. It has long been thought that several systemic diseases, such as type 1 diabetes, multiple sclerosis, and Crohn disease, are caused by T_H1 reactions against self-antigens. However, recent studies, mostly in mice, have implicated another CD4+ T-cell subset, the "T_H17" cells, in immune reactions. The signature cytokine of this subset is IL-17, which is a potent inducer of inflammation. It may be that T_H17 cells are important contributors to inflammatory diseases, such as Crohn disease and multiple sclerosis.

T-Cell–Mediated Cytotoxicity

In this form of T-cell–mediated hypersensitivity, CD8+ CTLs kill antigen-bearing target cells. As discussed earlier, class I MHC molecules bind to intracellular peptide antigens and present the peptides to CD8+ T lymphocytes, stimulating the differentiation of these T cells into effector cells called CTLs. CTLs play a critical role in resistance to virus infections and some tumors. The principal mechanism of killing by CTLs is dependent on the perforin-granzyme system. Perforin and granzymes are stored in the granules of CTLs and are rapidly released when CTLs engage their targets (cells bearing the appropriate class I MHC–bound peptides). Perforin binds to the plasma membrane of the target cells and promotes the entry of granzymes, which are proteases that specifically cleave and thereby activate cellular caspases. These enzymes induce apoptotic death of the target cells (Chapter 1). CTLs play an important role in the rejection of solid-organ transplants and may contribute to many

SUMMARY

Mechanisms of T-Cell-Mediated Hypersensitivity Reactions

- *Delayed-type hypersensitivity (DTH):* CD4+ T cells are activated by exposure to a protein antigen and differentiate into T_H1 effector cells. Subsequent exposure to the antigen results in the secretion of cytokines. IFN-γ activates macrophages to produce substances that cause tissue damage and promote fibrosis, and TNF promotes inflammation.
- *T-cell–mediated cytotoxicity:* CD8+ cytotoxic T lymphocytes (CTLs) specific for an antigen recognize cells expressing the target antigen and kill these cells. CD8+ T cells also secrete IFN-γ.

immunologic diseases, such as type 1 diabetes (in which insulin-producing β cells in pancreatic islets are destroyed by an autoimmune T-cell reaction).

Having described the basic mechanisms of pathologic immune reactions, we proceed to a discussion of two categories of reactions that are of great clinical importance: transplant rejection and autoimmunity.

REJECTION OF TRANSPLANTS

The major barrier to transplantation of organs from one individual to another of the same species (called *allografts*) is immunologic rejection of the transplanted tissue. Rejection is a complex phenomenon involving both cell- and antibody-mediated hypersensitivity reactions directed against histocompatibility molecules on the foreign graft. The key to successful transplantation has been the development of therapies that prevent or minimize rejection. Below we discuss how grafts are recognized as foreign and how they are rejected.

Immune Recognition of Allografts

Rejection of allografts is a response to MHC molecules, which are so polymorphic that no two individuals in an outbred population are likely to express exactly the same set of MHC molecules (except, of course, for identical twins). There are two main mechanisms by which the host immune system recognizes and responds to the MHC molecules on the graft (Fig. 5–16).

- *Direct recognition.* Host T cells directly recognize the allogeneic (foreign) MHC molecules that are expressed on graft cells. Direct recognition of foreign MHC seems to violate the rule of MHC restriction, which states that in every individual, all the T cells are educated to recognize foreign antigens displayed by only that individual's MHC molecules. It is suggested that allogeneic MHC molecules (with any bound peptides) structurally mimic self-MHC and foreign peptide, and so direct recognition of the allogeneic MHC is essentially an immunologic cross-reaction. Because DCs in the graft express high levels of MHC as well as important costimulatory molecules, they are the most likely APCs in direct recognition. Host CD4+ helper T cells are triggered into proliferation and cytokine production by recognition of donor class II MHC (HLA-D) molecules and drive the DTH response. CD8+ T cells recognize class I MHC (HLA-A, -B) and differentiate into CTLs, which kill the cells in the graft.
- *Indirect recognition.* In this instance, host CD4+ T cells recognize donor MHC molecules after these molecules are picked up, processed, and presented by the *host's* own APCs. This is similar to the physiologic processing and presentation of other foreign (e.g., microbial) antigens. This form of recognition mainly activates DTH pathways; CTLs that develop by indirect recognition cannot directly recognize and kill graft cells. The indirect pathway is also involved in the production of antibodies against graft alloantigens; if these antigens are proteins, they are picked up by host B cells, and peptides are presented to helper T cells, which then stimulate antibody responses.

Effector Mechanisms of Graft Rejection

Both T cells and antibodies reactive with the graft are involved in the rejection of most solid-organ allografts (see Fig. 5–16).

T-Cell–Mediated Rejection

CTLs kill cells in the grafted tissue, causing parenchymal and, perhaps more importantly, endothelial cell death (resulting in thrombosis and graft ischemia). Cytokine-secreting CD4+ T cells trigger DTH reactions, with increased vascular permeability and local accumulation of mononuclear cells (lymphocytes and macrophages). Activated microphages can injure graft cells and vasculature. The microvascular injury also results in tissue ischemia, which contributes to graft destruction.

Antibody-Mediated Rejection

Although T cells are of paramount importance in allograft rejection, antibodies also mediate some forms of rejection. Alloantibodies directed against graft MHC molecules and other alloantigens bind to the graft endothelium and cause injury (and secondary thrombosis) via complement activation and recruitment of leukocytes. Superimposed on the immunologic vascular damage are platelet aggregation and coagulation (caused by complement activation), adding further ischemic insult to the injury. Histologically, this form of rejection resembles the vasculitis of antibody-mediated hypersensitivity, described earlier. Local deposition of complement breakdown products (specifically C4d) is now widely used to detect humoral (antibody-mediated) rejection of kidney allografts.

Hyperacute rejection is a special form of rejection occurring in the setting where *preformed antidonor antibodies* are present in the circulation of the host before transplant. This may occur in multiparous women who have anti-HLA antibodies against paternal antigens encountered during pregnancy, or in individuals exposed

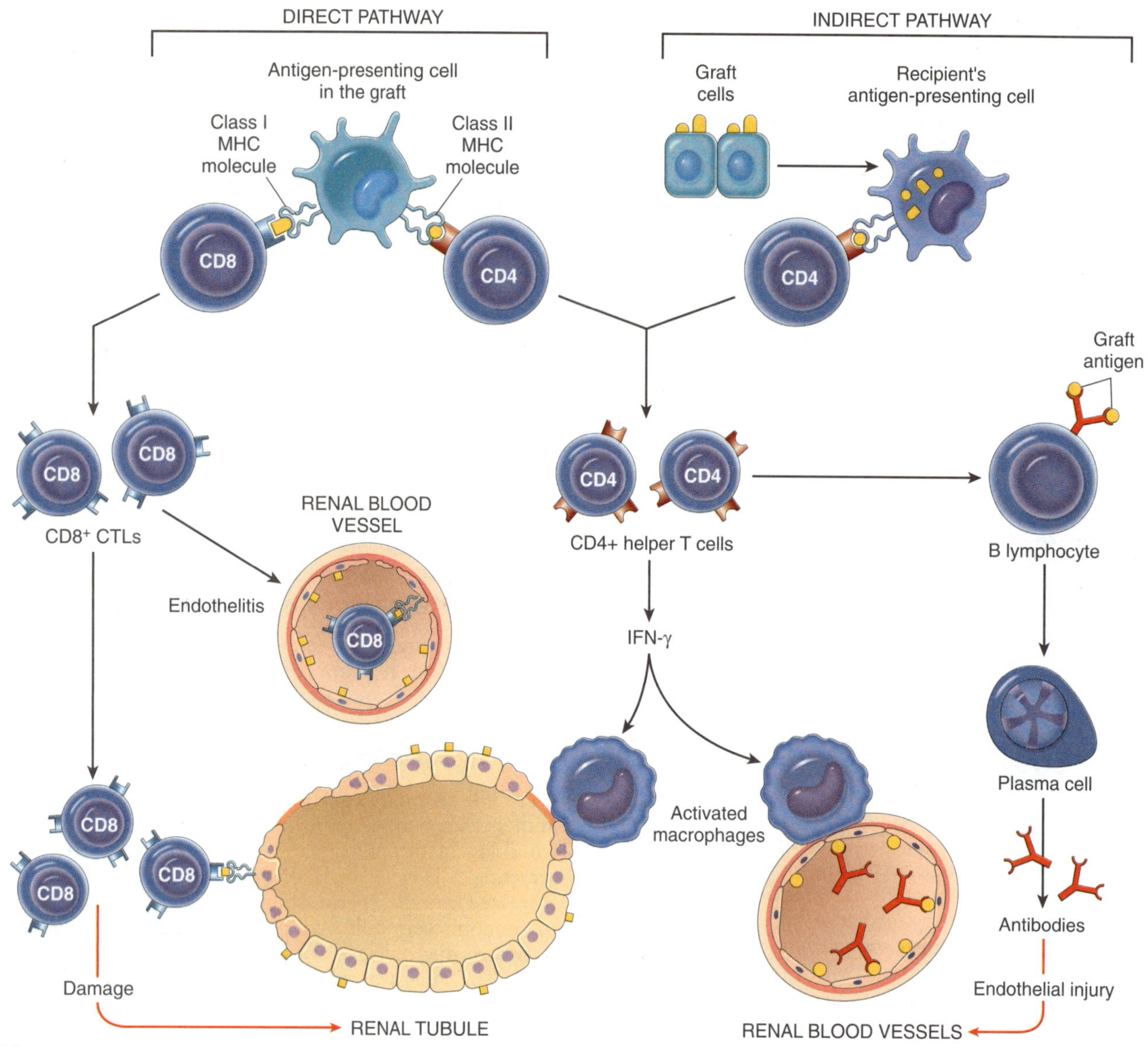

Figure 5–16

Recognition and rejection of organ allografts. In the direct pathway, donor class I and class II MHC antigens on antigen-presenting cells (APCs) in the graft (along with costimulators, not shown) are recognized by host CD8+ cytotoxic T cells and CD4+ helper T cells, respectively. CD4+ cells proliferate and produce cytokines (e.g., IFN-γ), which induce tissue damage by a local delayed-hypersensitivity reaction. CD8+ T cells responding to graft antigens differentiate into CTLs that kill graft cells. In the indirect pathway, graft antigens are displayed by host APCs and activate CD4+ T cells, which damage the graft by a local delayed-hypersensitivity reaction and stimulate B lymphocytes to produce antibodies.

to foreign HLA (on platelets or leukocytes) from prior blood transfusions. Obviously, such antibodies may also be present in a host who has previously rejected an organ transplant. Transplantation in this setting results in immediate rejection (within minutes to hours) because the circulating antibodies rapidly bind to the endothelium of the grafted organ, with subsequent complement activation and vascular thrombosis. Note that with the current practice of screening potential recipients for preformed anti-HLA antibodies and cross-matching (testing recipients for the presence of antibodies directed against a specific donor's lymphocytes), hyperacute rejection occurs in less than 0.4% of transplants.

Morphology

On the basis of the mechanisms involved, the resulting morphology, and the tempo of the various processes, rejection reactions have been classified as hyperacute, acute, and chronic (Fig. 5–17). The morphology of these patterns is described in the context of renal transplants; however, similar changes are encountered in any other vascularized organ transplant.

Hyperacute Rejection. Hyperacute rejection occurs within minutes to a few hours after transplantation in a presensitized host and is typically recognized by the

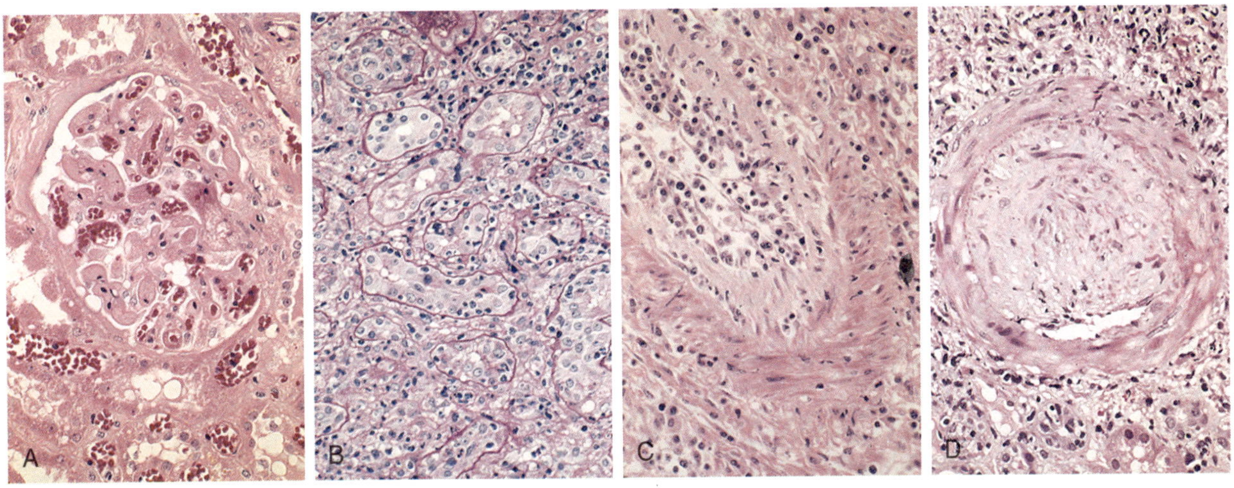

Figure 5–17

Morphologic patterns of graft rejection. **A,** Hyperacute rejection of a kidney allograft showing endothelial damage, platelet and thrombin thrombi in a glomerulus. **B,** Acute cellular rejection of a kidney allograft with inflammatory cells in the interstitium and between epithelial cells of the tubules. **C,** Acute humoral rejection of a kidney allograft (rejection vasculitis) with inflammatory cells and proliferating smooth muscle cells in the intima. **D,** Chronic rejection in a kidney allograft with graft arteriosclerosis. The arterial lumen is replaced by an accumulation of smooth muscle cells and connective tissue in the intima. (Courtesy of Dr. Helmut Rennke, Department of Pathology, Brigham and Women's Hospital and Harvard Medical School, Boston, Massachusetts.)

surgeon just after the vascular anastomosis is completed. In contrast to a nonrejecting kidney graft that regains a normal pink color and tissue turgor and promptly excretes urine, a hyperacutely rejecting kidney rapidly becomes cyanotic, mottled, and flaccid and may excrete only a few drops of bloody fluid. The histology is characterized by widespread acute arteritis and arteriolitis, vessel thrombosis, and ischemic necrosis, all resulting from the binding of preformed antibodies to graft endothelium. Virtually all arterioles and arteries exhibit characteristic acute fibrinoid necrosis of their walls, with narrowing or complete occlusion of the lumens by precipitated fibrin and cellular debris (see Fig. 5–17A).

Acute Rejection. Acute rejection may occur within days to weeks of transplantation in a nonimmunosuppressed host or may appear months or even years later, even in the presence of adequate immunosuppression. Acute rejection is caused by both cellular and humoral immune mechanisms, and in any one patient one or the other may predominate. Histologically, cellular rejection is marked by an interstitial mononuclear cell infiltrate with associated edema and parenchymal injury, whereas humoral rejection is associated with vasculitis.

Acute cellular rejection is most commonly seen within the first months after transplantation and is typically accompanied by clinical signs of renal failure. Histologically, there is usually extensive interstitial CD4+ and CD8+ T-cell infiltration with edema and mild interstitial hemorrhage (see Fig. 5–17B). Glomerular and peritubular capillaries contain large numbers of mononuclear cells, which may also invade the tubules and cause focal tubular necrosis. In addition to tubular injury, CD8+ T cells may also injure the endothelium, causing an endotheliitis. Cyclosporine (a widely used immunosuppressive agent) is also nephrotoxic and causes so-called arteriolar hyaline deposits. Renal biopsy is used to distinguish rejection from drug toxicity. Accurate recognition of cellular rejection is important, because in the absence of an accompanying arteritis patients typically respond promptly to increased immunosuppressive therapy.

Acute humoral rejection (rejection vasculitis) caused by antidonor antibodies may also be present in acute graft rejection. The histologic lesions may take the form of necrotizing vasculitis with endothelial cell necrosis; neutrophilic infiltration; deposition of antibody, complement, and fibrin; and thrombosis. Such lesions may be associated with ischemic necrosis of the renal parenchyma. In many cases, the vasculitis is less acute and is characterized by marked thickening of the intima by proliferating fibroblasts, myocytes, and foamy macrophages (see Fig. 5–17C). The resultant narrowing of the arterioles may cause infarction or renal cortical atrophy. The proliferative vascular lesions mimic arteriosclerotic thickening and are believed to be caused by cytokines that stimulate proliferation of vascular smooth muscle cells.

Chronic Rejection. Patients with chronic rejection present clinically late after transplantation (months to years) with a progressive rise in serum creatinine levels (an index of renal dysfunction) over a period of 4 to 6 months. Chronic rejection is dominated by vascular changes, interstitial fibrosis, and loss of renal parenchyma; there are typically only mild or even no ongoing cellular parenchymal infiltrates. The vascular changes occur predominantly in the arteries and arterioles, which exhibit intimal smooth muscle cell proliferation and extracellular matrix synthesis (Fig. 5–20D). These lesions ultimately compromise vascular perfusion and result in renal ischemia manifested by loss or hyalinization of glomeruli, interstitial fibrosis, and tubular atrophy. The vascular lesion may be caused by cytokines released by activated T cells that act on the cells of the vascular wall, and it may be the end stage of the proliferative arteritis described earlier. Chronic rejection does not respond to standard immunosuppression regimens.

SUMMARY

Recognition and Rejection of Organ Transplants (Allografts)

- The graft rejection response is initiated mainly by host T cells that recognize the foreign HLA antigens of the graft, either directly (on APCs in the graft) or indirectly (after uptake and presentation by host APCs).
- Types and mechanisms of rejection:
  1. *Hyperacute rejection.* Preformed antidonor antibodies bind to graft endothelium immediately after transplantation, leading to thrombosis, ischemic damage, and rapid graft failure.
  2. *Acute cellular rejection.* T cells destroy graft parenchyma by cytotoxicity and DTH reaction.
  3. *Acute vascular rejection.* T cells and antibodies damage graft vasculature.
  4. *Chronic rejection.* Dominated by arteriosclerosis, this type is probably caused by T-cell reaction and secretion of cytokines that induce proliferation of vascular smooth muscle cells, associated with parenchymal fibrosis.

Methods of Improving Graft Survival

Because HLA molecules are the major targets in transplant rejection, better matching of the donor and the recipient improves graft survival. The benefits of HLA matching are most dramatic in living related donor kidney transplants, and survival improves with increasing number of loci matched. However, as drugs for immunosuppression have improved, HLA matching is not even attempted in some situations, such as heart, lung, and liver transplantation; in these cases, the recipient often needs a transplant urgently and other considerations, such as anatomic compatibility, are of greater practical importance.

Immunosuppression of the recipient is a practical necessity in all organ transplantation except in the case of identical twins. At present, drugs such as cyclosporine, the related FK506, mofetil mycophenolate (MMF), rapamycin, azathioprine, corticosteroids, antilymphocyte globulins, and monoclonal antibodies (e.g., monoclonal anti-CD3) are used. Cyclosporine and FK506 suppress T-cell-mediated immunity by inhibiting transcription of cytokine genes, in particular, the gene for IL-2. Although immunosuppression has made transplantation of many organs feasible, there is still a price to be paid. Global immunosuppression results in increased susceptibility to opportunistic fungal, viral, and other infections. These patients are also at increased risk for developing Epstein-Barr virus (EBV)–induced lymphomas, human papillomavirus–induced squamous cell carcinomas, and Kaposi sarcoma (KS). To circumvent the untoward effects of immunosuppression, much effort is devoted to inducing donor-specific tolerance in host T cells. One strategy being pursued is to prevent host T cells from receiving costimulatory signals from donor DCs during the initial phase of sensitization. This can be accomplished by administration of agents to interrupt the interaction between the B7 molecules on the DCs of the graft with the CD28 receptors on host T cells. This will interrupt the second signal for T-cell activation and either induce apoptosis or render the T cells functionally unresponsive.

Transplantation of Hematopoietic Cells

Bone marrow transplantation is increasingly used as therapy for hematopoietic and some nonhematopoietic malignancies, aplastic anemias, and certain immune deficiency states. Hematopoietic stem cells are usually obtained from donor bone marrow but may also be harvested from peripheral blood after mobilization by administration of hematopoietic growth factors. The recipient receives chemotherapy and/or irradiation to destroy malignant cells (e.g., in leukemia) and to create a graft bed; then, stem cells are infused. *Rejection of allogeneic bone marrow transplants* seems to be mediated by some combination of host T cells and NK cells that are resistant to radiation therapy and chemotherapy. *Two major problems complicate this form of transplantation: graft-versus-host disease (GVHD) and immune deficiency.*

- *GVHD* occurs when immunologically competent T cells (or their precursors) are transplanted into recipients who are immunologically compromised. Although GVHD happens most commonly in the setting of allogeneic bone marrow transplantation (usually involving minor histocompatibility mismatches between donor and recipient), it may also occur after transplantation of solid organs rich in lymphoid cells (e.g., the liver) or after transfusion of nonirradiated blood. When an immunologically compromised host receives allogeneic bone marrow cells, the host cannot reject the graft, but T cells present in the donor marrow recognize the recipient's tissue as "foreign" and react against it. This results in the activation of both CD4+ and CD8+ T cells, ultimately generating DTH and CTL responses.

Acute GVHD (occurring days to weeks after transplant) *causes epithelial cell necrosis in three principal target organs: liver, skin, and gut.* Destruction of small bile ducts gives rise to jaundice, and mucosal ulceration of the gut results in bloody diarrhea. Cutaneous involvement is manifested by a generalized rash. *Chronic GVHD* may follow the acute syndrome or may occur insidiously. These patients develop skin lesions resembling those of systemic sclerosis (discussed later) and manifestations mimicking other autoimmune disorders.

GVHD is a potentially lethal complication that can be minimized but not eliminated by HLA matching. As another potential solution, donor T cells can be depleted before marrow transplant. This protocol has proved to be a mixed blessing: the risk of GVHD is reduced, but the incidence of graft failure and the recurrence of leukemia increase. It seems that the multifunctional T cells not only mediate GVHD but also are required for the efficient engraftment of the transplanted bone marrow stem cells and elimination of leukemia cells (so-called *graft-versus-leukemia* effect).

- *Immune deficiencies*, often of prolonged duration, occur in recipients of bone marrow transplants. Among the many reasons for this are the slow reconstitution of the host immune system, which is often destroyed or suppressed to allow the graft to take, and an inability to fully regenerate all the necessary immune cells. The consequence of the immune deficiency is that recipients are susceptible to a variety of infections, mostly viral, such as cytomegalovirus (CMV) and EBV infections.

AUTOIMMUNE DISEASES

The evidence is compelling that an immune reaction to *self-antigens* (i.e., *autoimmunity*) is the cause of certain human diseases; a growing number of entities have been attributed to this process (Table 5–6). However, in many of these disorders the proof is not definitive, and an important caveat is that the simple presence of autoreactive antibodies or T cells does *not* equate to autoimmune disease. For example, low-affinity antibodies and T cells reactive with self-antigens can be readily demonstrated in most otherwise healthy individuals; presumably, these antibodies and T cells are not pathogenic and are of little consequence. Moreover, similar innocuous autoantibodies to self-antigens are frequently generated following other forms of injury (e.g., ischemia) and may even serve a physiologic role in the removal of products of tissue breakdown. The evidence that the diseases listed in Table 5–6 are indeed the result of autoimmune reactions is more persuasive for some than for others. Thus, the presence of a multiplicity of autoantibodies accounts for many of the clinical and pathologic manifestations of SLE. Moreover, these autoantibodies can be identified within lesions by immunofluorescence and electron-microscopic techniques. In many other disorders, an autoimmune etiology is suspected but is unproven. Indeed, in some cases of apparent autoimmunity the response may be directed against an exogenous antigen, such as a microbial protein; such is the probable pathogenesis of the vasculitis in many cases of polyarteritis nodosa.

Presumed autoimmune diseases range from those in which specific immune responses are directed against one particular organ or cell type and result in localized tissue damage, to multisystem diseases characterized by lesions in many organs and associated with multiple autoantibodies or cell-mediated reactions against numerous self-antigens. In the systemic diseases, the lesions affect principally the connective tissue and blood vessels of the various organs involved. Thus, even though the systemic reactions are not specifically directed against constituents of connective tissue or blood vessels, the diseases are often referred to as "collagen vascular" or "connective tissue" disorders.

It is obvious that autoimmunity implies loss of self-tolerance, and the question arises as to how this happens. To understand the pathogenesis of autoimmunity, it is important to first familiarize ourselves with the mechanisms of normal immunologic tolerance.

Table 5–6 Autoimmune Diseases

Organ-Specific	Systemic
Hashimoto thyroiditis	Systemic lupus erythematosus
Autoimmune hemolytic anemia	Rheumatoid arthritis
Autoimmune atrophic gastritis of pernicious anemia	Sjögren syndrome
Multiple sclerosis	Reiter syndrome
Autoimmune orchitis	Inflammatory myopathies*
Goodpasture syndrome	Systemic sclerosis (scleroderma)*
Autoimmune thrombocytopenia	Polyarteritis nodosa*
Insulin-dependent diabetes mellitus	
Myasthenia gravis	
Graves' disease	
Primary biliary cirrhosis*	
Autoimmune (chronic active) hepatitis*	
Ulcerative colitis	

*The evidence supporting an autoimmune basis of these disorders is not strong.

Immunological Tolerance

Immunological tolerance is unresponsiveness to an antigen that is induced by exposure of specific lymphocytes to that antigen. Self-tolerance refers to a lack of immune responsiveness to one's own tissue antigens. During the generation of billions of antigen receptors in developing T and B lymphocytes, it is not surprising that receptors are produced that can recognize self-antigens. Since these antigens cannot all be concealed from the immune system, there must be means of eliminating or controlling self-reactive lymphocytes. Several mechanisms work in concert to select against self-reactivity and to thus prevent immune reactions against one's own antigens. These mechanisms are broadly divided into two groups: central tolerance and peripheral tolerance (Fig. 5–18).

- *Central tolerance.* This refers to deletion of self-reactive T and B lymphocytes during their maturation in central lymphoid organs (i.e., in the thymus for T cells and in the bone marrow for B cells). Many autologous (self) protein antigens are processed and presented by thymic APCs in association with self-MHC. Any developing T cell that expresses a receptor for such a self-antigen is negatively selected (deleted by apoptosis), and the resulting peripheral T-cell pool is thereby depleted of self-reactive cells (see Fig. 5–18). An exciting recent advance has been the identification of putative transcription factors that induce the expression of apparently peripheral tissue antigens in the thymus. One such factor is called the autoimmune regulator (AIRE); mutations in the *AIRE* gene are responsible for an autoimmune polyendocrine syndrome in which T

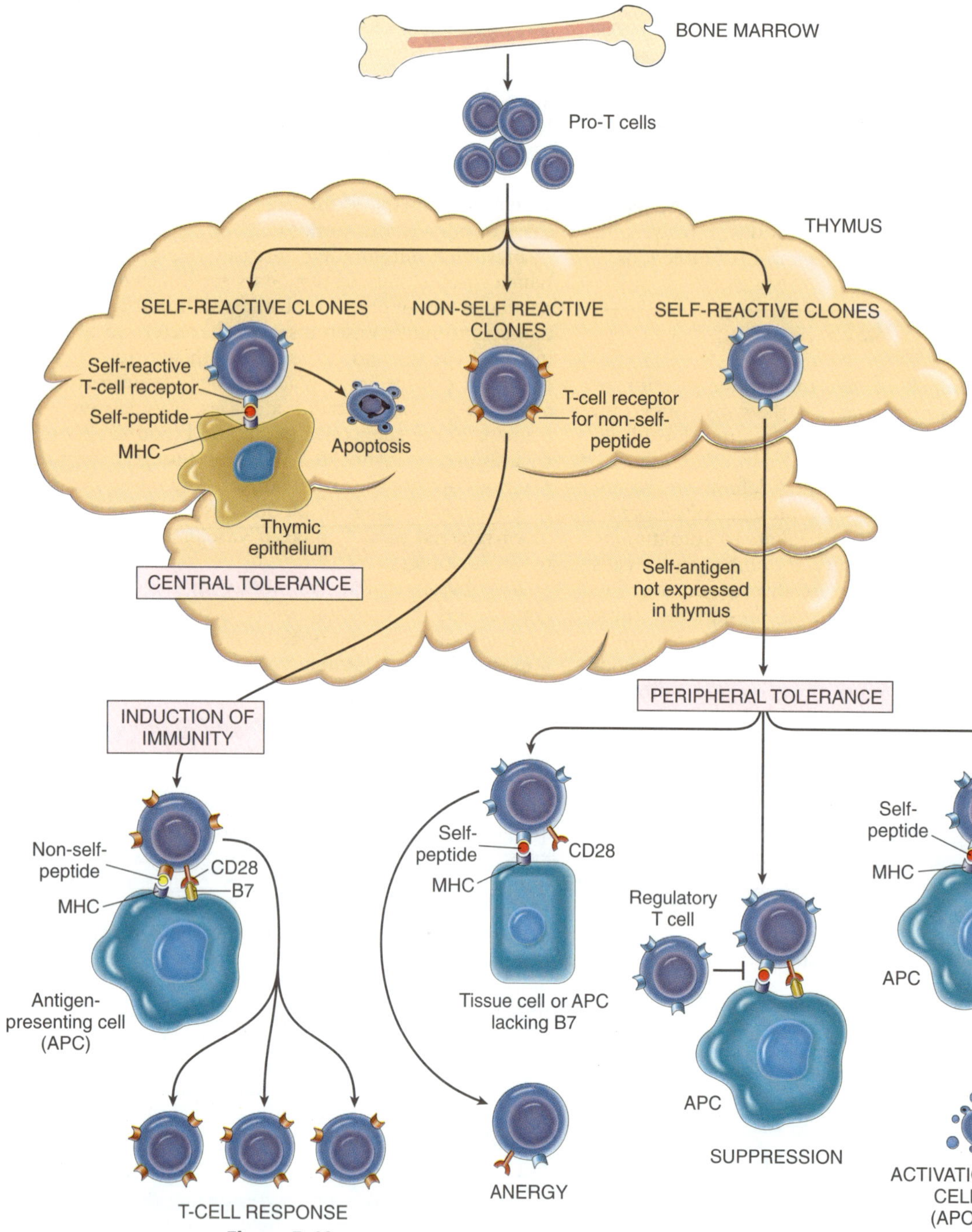

Figure 5–18

The principal mechanisms of central and peripheral self-tolerance in CD4+ T cells.

cells specific for multiple self-antigens escape deletion, presumably because these self-antigens are not expressed in the thymus. Some T cells that encounter self-antigens in the thymus are not killed but differentiate into regulatory T cells, which are described below.

Immature B cells that recognize, with high affinity, self-antigens in the bone marrow may also die by apoptosis. Some self-reactive B cells may not be deleted but may undergo a second round of rearrangement of antigen receptor genes and express new receptors that are no longer self-reactive (a process called "receptor editing").

Unfortunately, the process of deletion of self-reactive lymphocytes is far from perfect. Many self-antigens may not be present in the thymus, and hence T cells bearing receptors for such autoantigens escape into the periphery. There is similar "slippage" in the B-cell system as well, and B cells that bear receptors for a variety of self-antigens, including thyroglobulin, collagen, and DNA, can be found in healthy individuals.

- *Peripheral tolerance.* Self-reactive T cells that escape negative selection in the thymus can potentially wreak havoc unless they are deleted or effectively muzzled. Several mechanisms in the *peripheral* tissues that silence such potentially autoreactive T cells have been identified:
  - *Anergy:* This refers to functional inactivation (rather than death) of lymphocytes induced by encounter with antigens under certain conditions. Recall that activation of T cells requires two signals: recognition of peptide antigen in association with self-MHC molecules on APCs, and a set of second costimulatory signals (e.g., via B7 molecules) provided by the APCs. If the second costimulatory signals are not delivered, or if an inhibitory receptor on the T cell (rather than the costimulatory receptor) is engaged when the cell encounters self-antigen, the T cell becomes anergic and cannot respond to the antigen (see Fig. 5–21). Because costimulatory molecules are not strongly expressed on most normal tissues, the encounter between autoreactive T cells and self-antigens in tissues may result in anergy. B cells can also become anergic if they encounter antigen in the absence of specific helper T cells.
  - *Suppression by regulatory T cells:* The responses of T lymphocytes to self-antigens may be actively suppressed by *regulatory T cells.* The best-defined populations of regulatory T cells express CD25, one of the chains of the receptor for IL-2, and require IL-2 for their generation and survival. These cells also express a unique transcription factor called FoxP3, and this one protein seems to be both necessary and sufficient for the development of regulatory cells. Mutations in the *FOXP3* gene are responsible for a systemic autoimmune disease called IPEX (immune dysregulation, polyendocrinopathy, enteropathy, X-linked syndrome), which is associated with deficiency of regulatory T cells. The probable mechanism by which regulatory T cells control immune responses is by secreting immunosuppressive cytokines (e.g., IL-10 and TGF-β), which can dampen a variety of T-cell responses.
  - *Activation-induced cell death:* Another mechanism of peripheral tolerance involves apoptosis of mature lymphocytes as a result of self-antigen recognition. T cells that are repeatedly stimulated by antigens in vitro undergo apoptosis. One mechanism of apoptosis is the death receptor Fas (a member of the TNF receptor family) being engaged by its ligand coexpressed on the same cells. The same pathway is important for the deletion of self-reactive B cells by Fas ligand expressed on helper T cells. The importance of this pathway of self-tolerance is illustrated by the discovery that mutations in the *FAS* gene are responsible for an autoimmune disease called the autoimmune lymphoproliferative syndrome, characterized by lymphadenopathy and multiple autoantibodies including anti-DNA. Defects in Fas and Fas ligand are also the cause of similar autoimmune diseases in mice.

Mechanisms of Autoimmunity

Now that we have summarized the principal mechanisms of self-tolerance, we can ask how these mechanisms might break down to give rise to pathologic autoimmunity. Unfortunately, there are no simple answers to this question, and we still do not understand the underlying causes of most human autoimmune diseases. We referred above to mutations that compromise one or another pathway of self-tolerance and cause pathologic autoimmunity. These single-gene mutations are extremely informative, and they help to establish the biologic significance of the various pathways of self-tolerance. The diseases caused by such mutations are rare, however, and most autoimmune diseases cannot be explained by defects in single genes.

The breakdown of self-tolerance and the development of autoimmunity are probably related to the inheritance of various susceptibility genes and changes in tissues, often induced by infections or injury, that alter the display and recognition of self-antigens (Fig. 5–19).

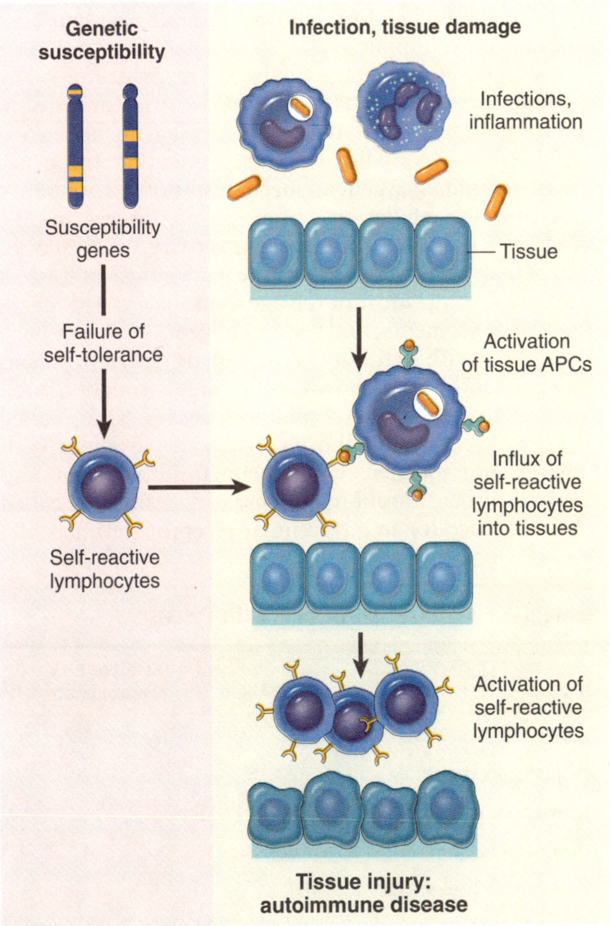

Figure 5–19

Pathogenesis of autoimmunity. Autoimmunity arises from many causes, including the inheritance of susceptibility genes that may interfere with self-tolerance, and environmental triggers (inflammation, other inflammatory stimuli) that promote lymphocyte entry into tissues, activation of self-reactive lymphocytes, and tissue injury.

Genetic Factors in Autoimmunity

There is abundant evidence that susceptibility genes play an important role in the development of autoimmune diseases.

- Autoimmune diseases have a tendency to run in families, and there is a greater incidence of the same disease in monozygotic than in dizygotic twins.
- Several autoimmune diseases are linked with the *HLA locus,* especially class II alleles *(HLA-DR, -DQ).* The frequency of a disease in an individual with a particular HLA allele, compared to individuals who do not inherit that allele, is called the *relative risk* (Table 5–7). The relative risk ranges from 3–4 for rheumatoid arthritis and *HLA-DR4* to as high as 90–100 for ankylosing spondylitis and *HLA-B27.* However, the role of MHC genes in autoimmunity is still not clear, especially because MHC molecules do not distinguish between self and foreign peptide antigens. It should also be noted that most individuals with a susceptibility-related MHC allele never develop any disease, and, conversely, individuals without the relevant MHC gene can develop the disease. Expression of a particular MHC gene is therefore but one variable that can contribute to autoimmunity.
- Genome-wide linkage analyses are revealing many genetic loci that are associated with different autoimmune diseases. Some of these loci seem to be associated with several diseases, suggesting that the genes involved influence general mechanisms of self-tolerance and immune regulation. Other loci are disease specific and may influence end-organ sensitivity or display of particular self-antigens. Despite enormous interest in this area, so far most of the associations are with chromosomal segments, and the actual genes have not been identified with certainty. Two genetic polymorphisms have recently been shown to be quite strongly associated with certain autoimmune diseases. One, called *PTPN22,* encodes a phosphatase, and particular variants are associated with rheumatoid arthritis and several other autoimmune diseases. Another, called *NOD2,* encodes an intracellular receptor for microbial peptides, and certain variants or mutants of this gene are present in as many as 25% of patients with Crohn's disease in some populations. How these genes contribute to autoimmunity is not established.

Table 5–7 Association of HLA with Disease

Disease	HLA Allele	Relative Risk (approximate %)
Ankylosing spondylitis	*B27*	90–100
Postgonococcal arthritis	*B27*	14
Acute anterior uveitis	*B27*	15
Rheumatoid arthritis	*DR4*	4
Autoimmune hepatitis	*DR3*	14
Primary Sjögren syndrome	*DR3*	10
Type 1 diabetes mellitus	*DR3* *DR4* *DR3/DR4*	5 6 15
21-Hydroxylase deficiency	*Bw47*	15

Role of Infections and Tissue Injury

A variety of microbes, including bacteria, mycoplasmas, and viruses, have been implicated as triggers for autoimmunity. Microbes may induce autoimmune reactions by several mechanisms:

- Viruses and other microbes, particularly certain bacteria such as streptococci and *Klebsiella* organisms, may share cross-reacting epitopes with self-antigens, such that responses to the microbial antigen may attack self-tissues. This phenomenon is called *molecular mimicry.* It is the probable cause of a few diseases, the best example being rheumatic heart disease, in which an immune response against streptococci cross-reacts with cardiac antigens. It is not known if more subtle mimicry plays a role in other autoimmune diseases.
- Microbial infections with resultant tissue necrosis and inflammation can cause up-regulation of costimulatory molecules on resting APCs in tissue, thus favoring a breakdown of T-cell anergy and subsequent T-cell activation.
- The display of tissue antigens may be altered by infections and other triggers. Local tissue injury for any reason may lead to the release of self-antigens and autoimmune responses.

Clearly, there is no lack of possible mechanisms to explain how infectious agents might participate in the pathogenesis of autoimmunity. At present, however, there is no evidence that clearly implicates any microbe in the causation of human autoimmune diseases. Adding to the complexity are recent suggestions (based largely on epidemiologic data) that infections may paradoxically protect individuals from some autoimmune diseases, notably type 1 diabetes and multiple sclerosis. The possible mechanisms underlying this effect are not understood.

An autoimmune response may itself promote further autoimmune attack by a process that has been called *epitope spreading.* Each self-protein has relatively few antigenic determinants (epitopes) that are effectively processed and presented to T cells. Most T cells capable of reacting to such dominant epitopes are either deleted in the thymus or rendered unresponsive in the periphery. By contrast, a large number of self-determinants are not processed and therefore are not recognized by the immune system; thus, T cells specific for such "cryptic" self-epitopes are not deleted. Tissue injury caused by an autoimmune response or any other cause may lead to exposure of cryptic epitopes that are subsequently presented to T cells in an immunogenic form. The activation of such autoreactive T cells is called "epitope spreading" because the immune response "spreads" to epitopes that were not recognized initially. The progression and chronicity of the autoimmune response may be maintained by recruitment of autoreactive T cells that recognize these normally cryptic self-determinants.

SUMMARY

Immunological Tolerance and Autoimmunity

- Tolerance (unresponsiveness) to self-antigens is a fundamental property of the immune system, and breakdown of tolerance is the basis of autoimmune diseases.
- *Central tolerance:* immature lymphocytes that recognize self-antigens in the central (generative) lymphoid organs are killed by apoptosis; in the B-cell lineage, some of the self-reactive lymphocytes switch to new antigen receptors that are not self-reactive.
- *Peripheral tolerance:* mature lymphocytes that recognize self-antigens in peripheral tissues become functionally inactive (anergic), or are suppressed by regulatory T lymphocytes, or die by apoptosis.
- The variables that lead to a failure of self-tolerance and the development of autoimmunity include (1) inheritance of susceptibility genes that may disrupt different tolerance pathways, and (2) infections and tissue alterations that may expose self-antigens and activate APCs and lymphocytes in the tissues.

Against this general background, the individual systemic autoimmune diseases will be discussed. Although each disease is discussed separately, it will be apparent that there is considerable overlap in their clinical, serologic, and morphologic features. Only the systemic autoimmune diseases are considered in this chapter; the autoimmune diseases that affect single organ systems are more appropriately discussed in the chapters that deal with the relevant organs.

Systemic Lupus Erythematosus

Systemic lupus erythematosus (SLE) is a multisystem autoimmune disease of protean manifestations and variable behavior. Clinically, it is an unpredictable, remitting and relapsing disease of acute or insidious onset that may involve virtually any organ in the body; however, it affects principally the skin, kidneys, serosal membranes, joints, and heart. Immunologically, the disease is associated with an enormous array of autoantibodies, classically including *antinuclear antibodies (ANAs).* The clinical presentation of SLE is so variable and it has so many overlaps with other autoimmune diseases (rheumatoid arthritis, polymyositis, and others) that it has been necessary to develop diagnostic criteria for SLE (Table 5–8). The diagnosis is established if a patient demonstrates four or more of the criteria during any interval of observation.

SLE is a fairly common disease; its prevalence may be as high as 1 case per 2500 persons in certain populations. Like many autoimmune diseases, there is a strong (approximately 9 : 1) female preponderance, affecting 1 in 700 women of childbearing age. The disease is more common and severe in black Americans, affecting 1 in

in…

Etiolo… *SLE is a* … a large nu… damage tissu… complex depo… antibodies is im… standing the patho…

Spectrum of Auto… been identified against a… components of the cell th… nor species. Another grou… against surface antigens of bl… …ther is reactive with proteins in com… …olipids (antiphospholipid antibodies; Cha…

Antinuclear Antibodies. ANAs a… …cted against several nuclear antigens and can be gro… …d into four categories: (1) antibodies to DNA, (2) antibodies to histones, (3) antibodies to nonhistone proteins bound to RNA, and (4) antibodies to nucleolar antigens. Table 5–9 lists several ANAs and their association with SLE as well as with other autoimmune diseases to be discussed later. Several techniques are used to detect ANAs. Clinically, the most commonly used method is indirect immunofluorescence, which detects antibodies reactive with a variety of nuclear antigens, including DNA, RNA, and proteins *(generic ANAs).* The pattern of nuclear fluorescence suggests the type of antibody present in the patient's serum, and four basic patterns are recognized:

- Homogeneous or diffuse staining usually reflects antibodies to chromatin, histones, and double-stranded DNA (dsDNA).
- Rim or peripheral staining patterns are most commonly indicative of antibodies to dsDNA.
- Speckled pattern is the most common pattern and refers to the presence of uniform or variable-sized speckles. It reflects the presence of antibodies to non-DNA nuclear constituents such as histones and ribonucleoproteins (RNPs).
- Nucleolar pattern refers to the presence of a few discrete spots of fluorescence within the nucleus that represent antibodies to nucleolar RNA. This pattern is reported most often in patients with systemic sclerosis.

The immunofluorescence test for ANAs is positive in virtually every patient with SLE, so that the test is quite *sensitive.* However, it is *not specific,* because patients with other autoimmune diseases (and 5% to 15% of normal persons) also score positive (see Table 5–9). Moreover, the fluorescence patterns are not absolutely specific for the type of antibody, and because of the plethora of antibodies, many combinations frequently exist. It should be noted that the presence of antibodies to dsDNA, or to the so-called Smith (Sm) antigen, is virtually diagnostic of SLE.

Other Autoantibodies. Antibodies against blood cells, including red cells, platelets, and lymphocytes, are found in many patients. Antiphospholipid antibodies are

...ssification of Systemic Lupus Erythematosus*

	...tion
	Fixed erythema, flat or raised, over the malar eminences, tending to spare the nasolabial folds
	Erythematous raised patches with adherent keratotic scaling and follicular plugging; atrophic scarring may occur in older lesions
.. Photosensitivity	Rash as a result of unusual reaction to sunlight, by patient history or physician observation
4. Oral ulcers	Oral or nasopharyngeal ulceration, usually painless, observed by a physician
5. Arthritis	Nonerosive arthritis involving two or more peripheral joints, characterized by tenderness, swelling, or effusion
6. Serositis	Pleuritis—convincing history of pleuritic pain or rub heard by a physician or evidence of pleural effusion, or Pericarditis—documented by electrocardiogram or rub or evidence of pericardial effusion
7. Renal disorder	Persistent proteinuria >0.5 gm/dL or >3+ if quantitation not performed or Cellular casts—may be red blood cell, hemoglobin, granular, tubular, or mixed
8. Neurologic disorder	Seizures: in the absence of offending drugs or known metabolic derangements (e.g., uremia, ketoacidosis, or electrolyte imbalance) or Psychosis: in the absence of offending drugs or known metabolic derangements (e.g., uremia, ketoacidosis, or electrolyte imbalance)
9. Hematologic disorder	Hemolytic anemia: with reticulocytosis, or Leukopenia: $<4.0 \times 10^9$ cells per liter (4000 cells per mm^3) total on two or more occasions or Lymphopenia: $<1.5 \times 10^9$ cells per liter (1500 cells per mm^3) on two or more occasions or Thrombocytopenia: $<100 \times 10^9$ cells per liter (100×10^3 cells per mm^3) in the absence of offending drugs
10. Immunologic disorder	Anti-DNA antibody to native DNA in abnormal titer or Anti-Sm: presence of antibody to Sm nuclear antigen or Positive finding of antiphospholipid antibodies based on (1) an abnormal serum level of IgG or IgM anticardiolipin antibodies, (2) a positive test for lupus anticoagulant using a standard test, or (3) a false-positive serologic test for syphilis known to be positive for at least 6 months and confirmed by negative *Treponema pallidum* immobilization or fluorescent treponemal antibody absorption test
11. Antinuclear antibody	An abnormal titer of antinuclear antibody by immunofluorescence or an equivalent assay at any point in time and in the absence of drugs known to be associated with drug-induced lupus syndrome

*The proposed classification is based on 11 criteria. For the purpose of identifying patients in clinical studies, a person is said to have systemic lupus erythematosus if any 4 or more of the 11 criteria are present, serially or simultaneously, during any interval of observation.

Data from Tan EM, et al.: The revised criteria for the classification of systemic lupus erythematosus. Arthritis Rheum 25:1271, 1982; and Hochberg MC: Updating the American College of Rheumatology revised criteria for the classification of systemic lupus erythematosus. Arthritis Rheum 40:1725, 1997.

present in 40% to 50% of lupus patients and react with a wide variety of proteins in complex with phospholipids. Some bind to cardiolipin antigen, used in serologic tests for syphilis, and therefore lupus patients may have a false-positive test result for syphilis. Because phospholipids are required for blood clotting, patients with antiphospholipid antibodies may also display prolongation of in vitro clotting tests, such as the partial thromboplastin time. Therefore, these antibodies are referred to as "lupus anticoagulants" even though the patients who have them actually have a prothrombotic state (the *antiphospholipid antibody syndrome;* Chapter 4). They tend to have venous and arterial thromboses, thrombocytopenia, and recurrent spontaneous miscarriages.

Immunologic Factors. All the immunologic findings in SLE patients clearly suggest that some fundamental derangement of the immune system is at work in its pathogenesis. *One model for the pathogenesis of the disease proposes a combination of increased generation or defective clearance of nuclear antigens released from apoptotic cells, and a failure of T- and B-cell tolerance to these self-antigens* (Fig. 5–20). However, despite a variety of reported T- and B-cell immunologic abnormalities in SLE patients, it has not been possible to establish any of them as causal. For years, intrinsic B-cell hyperactivity was considered a central feature of SLE pathogenesis. However, molecular analyses of anti-dsDNA antibodies indicate that they are high-affinity, isotype-switched antibodies whose production requires T-cell help. Therefore, it is now thought that tolerance has failed in both CD4+ helper T cells and B cells specific for nuclear (and other) self-antigens. The molecular mechanisms for failure of tolerance remain unknown. Recent studies indicate that the peripheral blood cells of SLE patients show evidence of overproduction of the cytokine IFN-α and of increased responses to this cytokine. IFN-α is an antiviral cytokine

Table 5-9 Antinuclear Antibodies in Various Autoimmune Diseases*

Nature of Antigen	Antibody System	Disease, % Positive: SLE	Drug-Induced LE	Systemic Sclerosis – Diffuse	Limited Scleroderma (CREST)	Sjögren Syndrome	Inflammatory Myopathies
Many nuclear antigens (DNA, RNA, proteins)	Generic ANAs (indirect IF)	>95	>95	70–90	70–90	50–80	40–60
Native DNA	Anti-dsDNA	40–60	<5	<5	<5	<5	<5
Histones	Antihistone	50–70	>95	<5	<5	<5	<5
Core proteins of small nuclear ribonucleoprotein particles (Smith antigen)	Anti-Sm	20–30	<5	<5	<5	<5	<5
Ribonucleoprotein (U1RNP)	Nuclear RNP	30–40	<5	15	10	<5	<5
RNP	SS-A (Ro)	30–50	<5	<5	<5	70–95	10
RNP	SS-B (La)	10–15	<5	<5	<5	60–90	<5
DNA topoisomerase I	Scl-70	<5	<5	28–70	10–18	<5	<5
Centromeric proteins	Anticentromere	<5	<5	22–36	90	<5	<5
Histidyl-tRNA synthetase	Jo-1	<5	<5	<5	<5	<5	25

ANA, antinuclear antibodies; dsDNA, double-stranded DNA; IF, immunofluorescence; LE, lupus erythematosus; RNP, ribonucleoprotein; SLE, systemic lupus erythematosus.
*Boxed entries indicate high correlation.

produced during the early innate immune response to many viruses. The relevance of the "interferon signature" to the development of SLE is intriguing but remains unexplained. Persistent activation of B cells by self nucleoproteins engaging Toll-like receptors has also been invoked as a mechanism of autoantibody production.

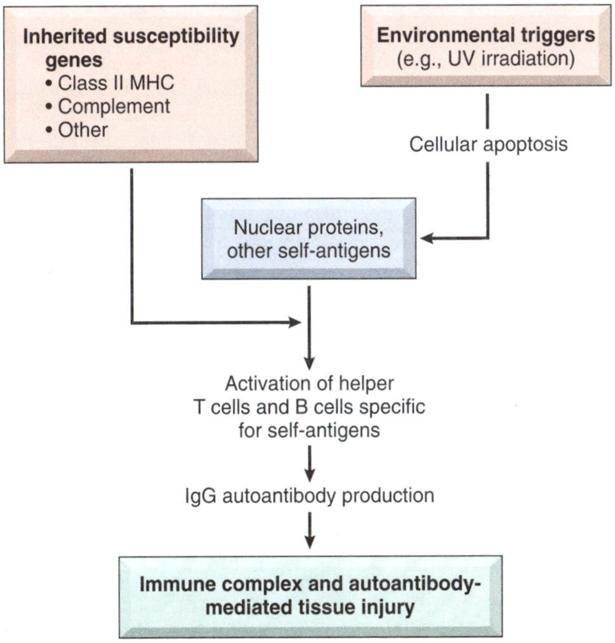

Figure 5–20

Model for the pathogenesis of systemic lupus erythematosus (SLE). The importance of apoptotic cells as the source of self-antigens is speculative. How susceptibility genes promote activation of self-reactive lymphocytes is unknown. (Modified from Kotzin BL: Systemic lupus erythematosus. Cell 65:303, copyright 1996, with permission from Elsevier.)

Genetic Variables. Many lines of evidence support a genetic predisposition to SLE.

- There is a high rate of concordance in monozygotic twins (25%) versus dizygotic twins (1% to 3%).
- Family members have an increased risk of developing SLE, and up to 20% of clinically unaffected first-degree relatives may reveal autoantibodies.
- In North American white populations there is a positive association between SLE and class II HLA genes, particularly at the *HLA-DQ* locus.
- Some lupus patients (about 6%) have inherited deficiencies of complement components. Lack of complement presumably impairs removal of immune complexes from the circulation and favors tissue deposition, giving rise to tissue injury. The C1q component of complement is involved in phagocytosis of apoptotic cells, and its deficiency may lead to persistence of these cells and, hence, of nuclear antigens.
- In mouse models of SLE, different genes are believed to influence B-cell hyperactivity, production of specific anti-DNA antibodies, and end-organ damage to the kidneys. The homologous genes in humans have not been identified.

Nongenetic Variables. *Ultraviolet (UV) radiation* (sun exposure) exacerbates the lesions of SLE. A postulated mechanism of this is that UV radiation causes apoptosis of host cells, leading to an increased burden of nuclear fragments (see Fig. 5–20). An example of nongenetic (e.g., environmental) variables in initiating SLE is the occurrence of a lupus-like syndrome in patients receiving certain drugs, including procainamide and hydralazine.

Most patients treated with procainamide for more than 6 months develop ANAs, with clinical features of SLE appearing in 15% to 20% of them. *Sex hormones* also seem to exert an important influence on the occurrence of SLE; witness the overwhelming female preponderance of the disease. The mechanism of this hormonal effect is not known.

Mechanisms of Tissue Injury. Regardless of the exact sequence by which autoantibodies are formed, they are clearly the mediators of tissue injury. Most of the systemic lesions are mediated by immune complexes (type III hypersensitivity). DNA/anti-DNA complexes can be detected in the glomeruli, and low serum levels of complement coupled with granular complement deposits in the glomeruli further support the role of immune complexes in the disease. In addition, autoantibodies against red cells, white cells, and platelets promote destruction and phagocytosis of these cells (type II hypersensitivity). There is no evidence that the ANAs involved in immune complex formation can permeate intact cells. However, if cell nuclei are exposed, the ANAs can bind to them. In tissues, nuclei of damaged cells react with ANAs, lose their chromatin pattern, and become homogeneous, to produce so-called *LE bodies* or *hematoxylin bodies*. An in vitro correlate of this is the *LE cell,* a neutrophil or macrophage that has engulfed the denatured nucleus of another injured cell. When blood is withdrawn and agitated, a number of leukocytes are sufficiently damaged to expose their nuclei to ANAs, with secondary complement activation; these antibody- and complement-opsonized nuclei are then readily phagocytosed. Although the LE cell test is positive in as many as 70% of patients with SLE, it is now largely of historical interest.

Morphology

SLE is a systemic disease with protean manifestations (see Table 5–8). The morphologic changes in SLE are therefore extremely variable and depend on the nature of the autoantibodies, the tissue in which immune complexes deposit, and the course and duration of disease. The most characteristic morphologic changes result from the deposition of immune complexes in a variety of tissues.

An **acute necrotizing vasculitis** affecting small arteries and arterioles may be present in any tissue. The arteritis is characterized by necrosis and by fibrinoid deposits within vessel walls containing antibody, DNA, complement fragments, and fibrinogen; a transmural and perivascular leukocytic infiltrate is also frequently present. In chronic stages, vessels show fibrous thickening with luminal narrowing.

Kidney involvement is one of the most important clinical features of SLE, with renal failure being the most common cause of death. The focus here is on glomerular pathology, although interstitial and tubular lesions are also seen in SLE.

The pathogenesis of all forms of **glomerulonephritis** in SLE involves deposition of DNA/anti-DNA complexes within the glomeruli. These evoke an inflammatory response that may cause proliferation of the endothelial, mesangial, and/or epithelial cells and, in severe cases, necrosis of the glomeruli. Although the kidney appears normal by light microscopy in 25% to 30% of cases, almost all cases of SLE show some renal abnormality if examined by immunofluorescence and electron microscopy. According to the World Health Organization morphologic classification, there are five patterns of glomerular disease in SLE (none of which is specific to the disease): **class I,** normal by light, electron, and immunofluorescence microscopy (less than 5% of SLE patients); **class II,** mesangial lupus glomerulonephritis; **class III,** focal proliferative glomerulonephritis; **class IV,** diffuse proliferative glomerulonephritis; and **class V,** membranous glomerulonephritis.

Mesangial lupus glomerulonephritis (class II) is seen in 10% to 25% of cases and is associated with mild clinical symptoms. Immune complexes deposit in the mesangium, with a slight increase in the mesangial matrix and cellularity.

Focal proliferative glomerulonephritis (class III) is seen in 20% to 35% of cases, and, as the name suggests, lesions are visualized in only portions of fewer than half the glomeruli. Typically, one or two foci within an otherwise normal glomerulus show swelling and proliferation of endothelial and mesangial cells, infiltration by neutrophils, and/or fibrinoid deposits with capillary thrombi (Fig. 5–21A). Focal glomerulonephritis is usually associated with only mild microscopic hematuria and proteinuria; a transition to a more diffuse form of renal involvement is associated with more severe disease.

Diffuse proliferative glomerulonephritis (class IV) is the most serious form of renal lesions in SLE and is also the most common, occurring in 35% to 60% of patients. Most of the glomeruli show endothelial and mesangial proliferation affecting the entire glomerulus, leading to diffuse hypercellularity of the glomeruli (Fig. 5–21B), producing in some cases epithelial crescents that fill Bowman's space. When extensive, immune complexes create an overall thickening of the capillary wall, resembling rigid "wire loops" on routine light microscopy (Fig. 5–21C). Electron microscopy reveals electron-dense subendothelial immune complexes (between endothelium and basement membrane; Fig. 5–21D). Immune complexes can be visualized by staining with fluorescent antibodies directed against immunoglobulins or complement, resulting in a granular fluorescent staining pattern (Fig. 5–21E). In due course, glomerular injury gives rise to scarring (glomerulosclerosis). Most of these patients have hematuria with moderate to severe proteinuria, hypertension, and renal insufficiency.

Membranous glomerulonephritis (class V) occurs in 10% to 15% of cases and is the designation for glomerular disease characterized by widespread thickening of the capillary wall. Membranous glomerulonephritis associated with SLE is very similar to that encountered in idiopathic membranous nephropathy (Chapter 14). Thickening of capillary walls is caused by increased deposition of basement membrane–like material, as well as accumulation of immune complexes. Patients with this histologic change almost always have severe proteinuria with overt nephrotic syndrome (Chapter 14).

The **skin** is involved in the majority of patients; a characteristic erythematous or maculopapular eruption over the malar eminences and bridge of the nose ("butterfly pattern") is observed in about half. Exposure to sunlight (UV light) exacerbates the erythema (so-called **photosensitivity**), and a similar rash may be present

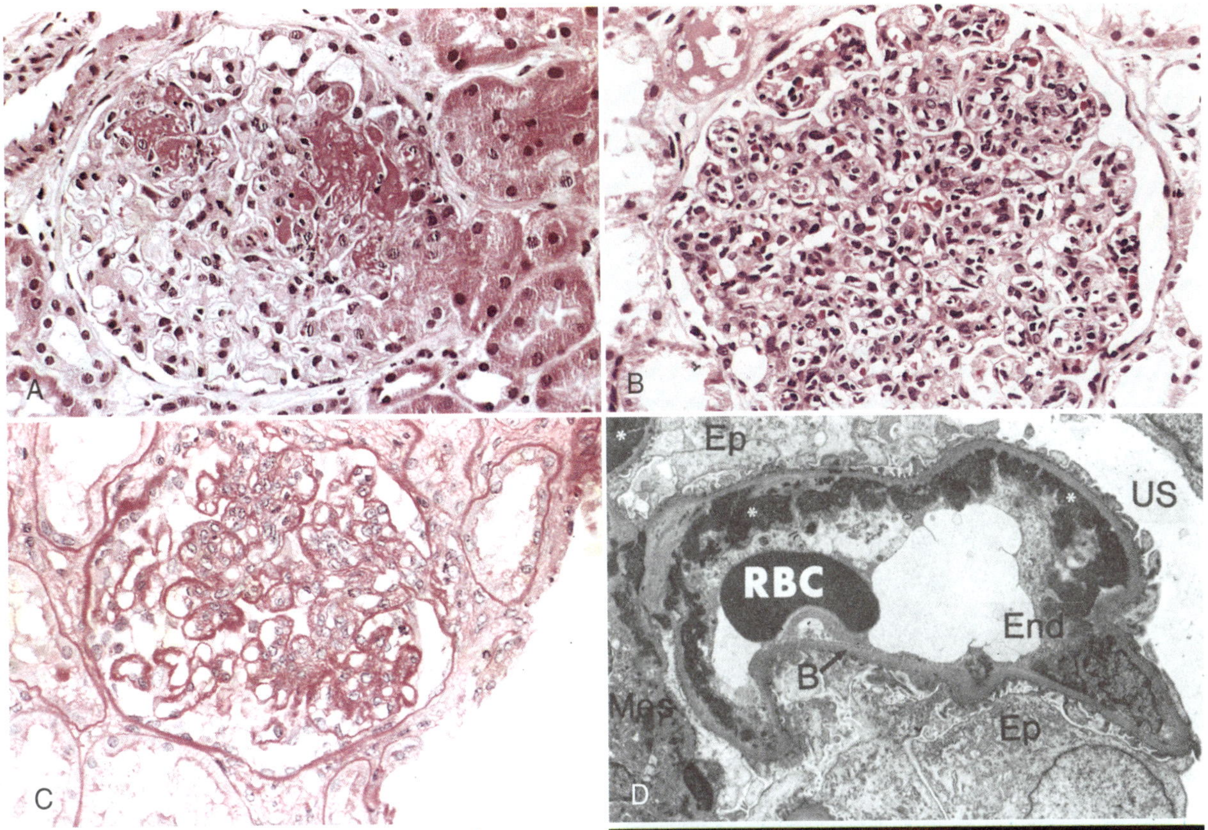

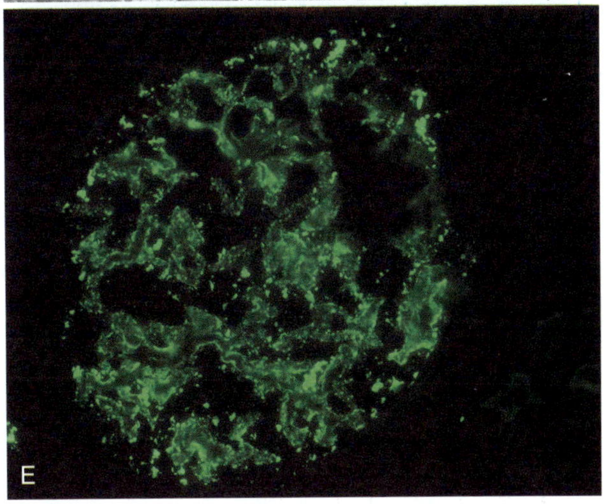

Figure 5–21

Lupus nephritis. **A,** Focal proliferative glomerulonephritis, with two focal necrotizing lesions at the 11 o'clock and 2 o'clock positions (H&E stain). **B,** Diffuse proliferative glomerulonephritis. Note the marked increase in cellularity throughout the glomerulus (H&E stain). **C,** Lupus nephritis showing a glomerulus with several "wire loop" lesions representing extensive subendothelial deposits of immune complexes (periodic acid–Schiff stain). **D,** Electron micrograph of a renal glomerular capillary loop from a patient with SLE nephritis. Subendothelial dense deposits correspond to "wire loops" seen by light microscopy. **E,** Deposition of IgG antibody in a granular pattern, detected by immunofluorescence. B, basement membrane; End, endothelium; Ep, epithelial cell with foot processes; Mes, mesangium; RBC, red blood cell in capillary lumen; US, urinary space; *, electron-dense deposits in subendothelial location. (**A–C,** courtesy of Dr. Helmut Rennke, Department of Pathology, Brigham and Women's Hospital, Boston, Massachusetts. **D,** Courtesy of Dr. Edwin Eigenbrodt, Department of Pathology, University of Texas, Southwestern Medical School, Dallas. **E,** Courtesy of Dr. Jean Olson, Department of Pathology, University of California, San Francisco, California.)

elsewhere on the extremities and trunk, frequently in sun-exposed areas. Histologically, there is liquefactive degeneration of the basal layer of the epidermis, edema at the dermoepidermal junction, and mononuclear infiltrates around blood vessels and skin appendages (Fig. 5–22A). Immunofluorescence microscopy reveals deposition of Ig and complement at the dermoepidermal junction (Fig. 5–22B); similar Ig and complement deposits may also be present in apparently uninvolved skin.

Joint involvement is frequent but is usually not associated with striking anatomic changes nor with joint deformity. When present, it consists of swelling and a nonspecific mononuclear cell infiltration in the synovial membranes. Erosion of the membranes and destruction of articular cartilage, such as occurs with rheumatoid arthritis, is exceedingly rare.

Central nervous system (CNS) involvement is also very common, with focal neurologic deficits and/or neuropsychiatric symptoms. CNS disease is often ascribed to vascular lesions causing ischemia or multifocal cerebral microinfarcts. Small vessel angiopathy with noninflammatory intimal proliferation is the most frequent pathological lesion; frank vasculitis is uncommon. The angiopathy may result from thrombosis caused by antiphospholipid antibodies. Premature ath-

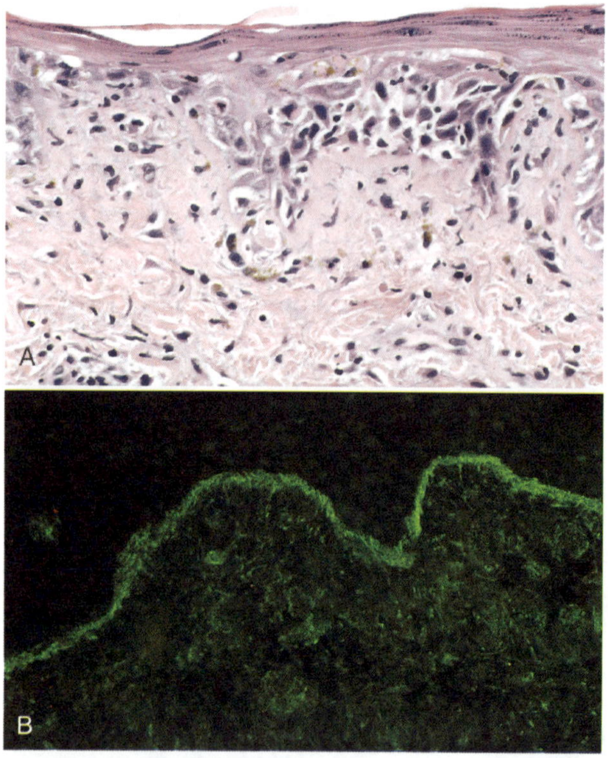

Figure 5–22

SLE involving the skin. **A,** An H&E-stained section shows liquefactive degeneration of the basal layer of the epidermis and edema at the dermoepidermal junction. **B,** An immunofluorescence micrograph stained for IgG reveals deposits of Ig along the dermoepidermal junction. (**A,** Courtesy of Dr. Jag Bhawan, Boston University School of Medicine, Boston, Massachusetts. **B,** Courtesy of Dr. Richard Sontheimer, Department of Dermatology, University of Texas Southwestern Medical School, Dallas, Texas.)

erosclerosis occurs, and may contribute to CNS ischemia. It has also been postulated that anti-neuronal antibodies cause neuronal dysfunction, but this hypothesis remains unproved.

The **spleen** may be moderately enlarged. Capsular fibrous thickening is common, as is follicular hyperplasia with numerous plasma cells in the red pulp. Central penicilliary arteries characteristically show thickening and perivascular fibrosis, producing **onion-skin lesions**.

Pericardium and pleura, in particular, are **serosal membranes** that show a variety of inflammatory changes in SLE ranging (in the acute phase) from serous effusions to fibrinous exudates and progressing to fibrous opacification in the chronic stage.

Involvement of the heart is manifested primarily in the form of pericarditis. Myocarditis, in the form of a nonspecific mononuclear cell infiltrate, and valvular lesions, called **Libman-Sacks endocarditis**, also occur but are less common in the current era of aggressive corticosteroid therapy. The valvular **nonbacterial verrucous endocarditis** takes the form of irregular, 1- to 3-mm warty deposits, distinctively on either surface of the leaflets (i.e., on the surface exposed to the forward flow of the blood or on the underside of the leaflet) (see Chapter 11). An increasing number of patients also show clinical and anatomic manifestations of coronary artery disease. The basis of accelerated atherosclerosis is not fully understood, but it seems to be multifactorial; certainly, immune complexes can deposit in the coronary vasculature and lead to endothelial damage by that pathway. Moreover, glucocorticoid treatment causes alterations in lipid metabolism, and renal disease (common in SLE) causes hypertension; both of these are risk factors for atherosclerosis (Chapter 10).

Many **other organs and tissues** may be involved. The changes consist essentially of acute vasculitis of the small vessels, foci of mononuclear infiltrations, and fibrinoid deposits. In addition, lungs may reveal interstitial fibrosis, along with pleural inflammation; the liver shows nonspecific inflammation of the portal tracts.

Clinical Manifestations. The diagnosis of SLE may be obvious in a young woman with a classic butterfly rash over the face, fever, arthritis, pleuritic chest pain, and photosensitivity. However, in many patients the presentation of SLE is subtle and puzzling, taking forms such as a febrile illness of unknown origin, abnormal urinary findings, or neuropsychiatric manifestations, including psychosis. A variety of clinical findings may point toward renal involvement, including hematuria, red cell casts, proteinuria, and, in some cases, the classic nephrotic syndrome (Chapter 14). Renal failure may occur, especially in patients with diffuse proliferative or membranous glomerulonephritis, or both. The hematologic derangements mentioned (see Table 5–8) may in some cases be the presenting manifestation as well as the dominant clinical problem. ANAs can be found in virtually 100% of patients, but they can also be found in patients with other autoimmune disorders; nevertheless, anti-dsDNA antibodies and antibodies to the so-called Smith (Sm) antigen are considered highly diagnostic of SLE. Serum complement levels are low, typically as a result of deposition of immune complexes.

The course of SLE is extremely variable. Even without therapy, some patients follow a relatively benign course with only skin manifestations and/or mild hematuria. Rare cases rapidly progress to death within months. Most often the disease is characterized by remissions and relapses spanning years to decades. Acute flare-ups are usually controlled by steroids or other immunosuppressive drugs. Overall, with current therapies, 90% five-year and 80% ten-year survivals can be expected. Renal failure, intercurrent infections, and diffuse CNS involvement are the major causes of death.

SUMMARY

Systemic Lupus Erythematosus

- SLE is a systemic autoimmune disease caused by autoantibodies produced against numerous self-antigens and the formation of immune complexes.
- The major autoantibodies, and the ones responsible for the formation of circulating immune com-

plexes, are directed against nuclear antigens. Other autoantibodies react with erythrocytes, platelets, and various complexes of phospholipids with proteins.

- Disease manifestations include nephritis, skin lesions and arthritis (caused by the deposition of immune complexes), and hematologic and neurologic abnormalities.
- The underlying cause of the breakdown in self-tolerance in SLE is unknown; it may include excess or persistence of nuclear antigens, multiple inherited susceptibility genes, and environmental triggers (e.g., UV irradiation, which results in cellular apoptosis and release of nuclear proteins).

Rheumatoid Arthritis

Rheumatoid arthritis (RA) is a systemic, chronic inflammatory disease affecting many tissues but principally attacking the joints to produce a *nonsuppurative proliferative synovitis that frequently progresses to destroy articular cartilage and underlying bone with resulting disabling arthritis*. When extra-articular involvement develops—for example, of the skin, heart, blood vessels, muscles, and lungs—RA may resemble SLE or scleroderma.

RA is a very common condition, with a prevalence of approximately 1%; it is three to five times more common in women than in men. The peak incidence is in the second to fourth decades of life, but no age is immune. Morphology will be considered first, as a background to a discussion of pathogenesis.

Morphology

A broad spectrum of morphologic alterations is seen in RA; the most severe occur in the joints. RA typically presents as **symmetric arthritis, principally affecting the small joints** of the hands and feet, ankles, knees, wrists, elbows, and shoulders. Typically, the proximal interphalangeal and metacarpophalangeal joints are affected, but distal interphalangeal joints are spared. Axial involvement, when it occurs, is limited to the upper cervical spine; similarly, hip joint involvement is extremely uncommon. Histologically, the affected joints show **chronic synovitis,** characterized by (1) synovial cell hyperplasia and proliferation; (2) dense perivascular inflammatory cell infiltrates (frequently forming lymphoid follicles) in the synovium composed of CD4+ T cells, plasma cells, and macrophages; (3) increased vascularity due to angiogenesis; (4) neutrophils and aggregates of organizing fibrin on the synovial surface and in the joint space; and (5) increased osteoclast activity in the underlying bone, leading to synovial penetration and bone erosion. The classic appearance is that of a **pannus,** formed by proliferating synovial-lining cells admixed with inflammatory cells, granulation tissue, and fibrous connective tissue; the overgrowth of this tissue is so exuberant that the usually thin, smooth synovial membrane is transformed into lush, edematous, frondlike (villous) projections (Fig. 5–23). With full-blown inflammatory joint involvement, periarticular soft tissue edema usually develops, classically manifested first by fusiform swelling of the proximal interphalangeal joints. With progression of the disease, the articular cartilage subjacent to the pannus is eroded and, in time, virtually destroyed. The subarticular bone may also be attacked and eroded. Eventually the pannus fills the joint space, and subsequent **fibrosis and calcification** may cause

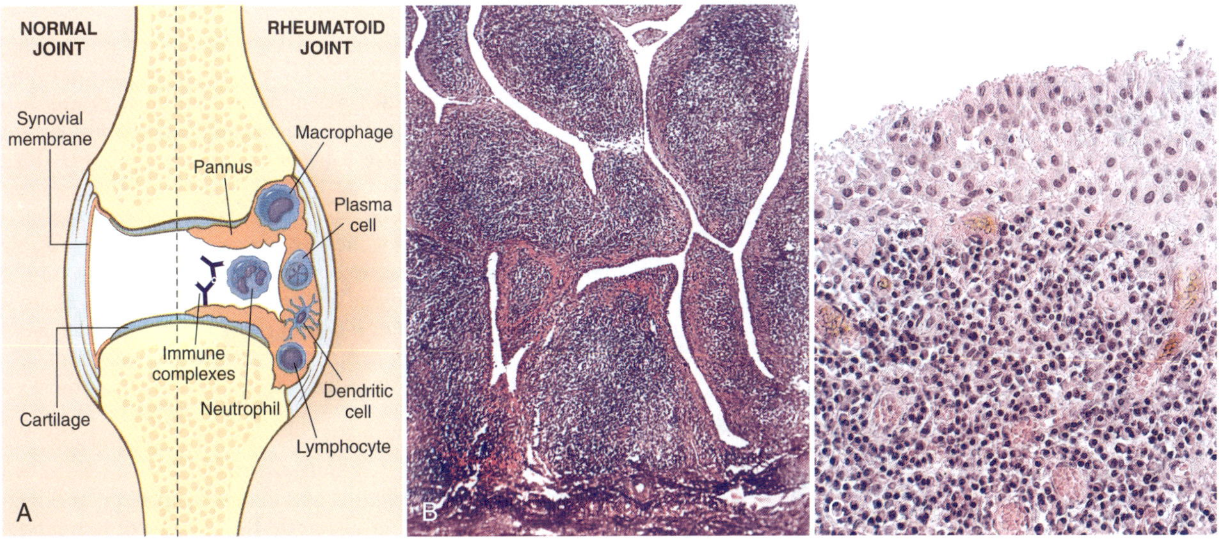

Figure 5–23

Rheumatoid arthritis. **A,** A joint lesion. **B,** Low magnification reveals marked synovial hypertrophy with formation of villi. **C,** At higher magnification, dense lymphoid aggregates are seen in the synovium. (**A,** Modified with permission from Feldmann M: Development of anti-TNF therapy for rheumatoid arthritis. Nat Rev Immunol 2:364, 2002.)

permanent **ankylosis.** The radiographic hallmarks are joint effusions and juxta-articular osteopenia with erosions and narrowing of the joint space and loss of articular cartilage. Destruction of tendons, ligaments, and joint capsules produces the characteristic deformities, including radial deviation of the wrist, ulnar deviation of the fingers, and flexion-hyperextension abnormalities of the fingers (swan-neck deformity, boutonnière deformity).

Rheumatoid subcutaneous nodules develop in about one-fourth of patients, occurring along the extensor surface of the forearm or other areas subjected to mechanical pressure; rarely they can form in the lungs, spleen, heart, aorta, and other viscera. Rheumatoid nodules are firm, nontender, oval or rounded masses as large as 2 cm in diameter. Microscopically, they are characterized by a central focus of fibrinoid necrosis surrounded by a palisade of macrophages, which in turn is rimmed by granulation tissue (Fig. 5–24).

Patients with severe erosive disease, rheumatoid nodules, and high titers of **rheumatoid factor** (circulating IgM that binds IgG; see later) are at risk of developing vasculitic syndromes; acute necrotizing vasculitis may involve small or large arteries. Serosal involvement may manifest as fibrinous pleuritis or pericarditis or both. Lung parenchyma may be damaged by progressive interstitial fibrosis. Ocular changes such as uveitis and keratoconjunctivitis (similar to those seen in Sjögren syndrome; see later) may be prominent in some cases.

Pathogenesis. The joint inflammation in RA is immunologically mediated, and there is a clear genetic predisposition to the disease, but the initiating agent or agents and the precise interplay between genetic and environmental variables are not yet understood. It is proposed that the disease is initiated, in a genetically predisposed individual, by activation of *CD4+ helper T cells* responding to some arthritogenic agent, possibly microbial, or to some self-antigen (Fig. 5–25). The activated T cells produce *cytokines* that (1) activate macrophages and other cells in the joint space, releasing degradative enzymes and other factors that perpetuate inflammation, and (2) activate B cells, resulting in the production of antibodies, some of which are directed against self-antigens in the joint. The rheumatoid synovium is rich in both lymphocyte- and macrophage-derived cytokines. The activity of these cytokines accounts for many features of rheumatoid synovitis; some, such as TNF, promote leukocyte recruitment, others activate macrophages, and yet others, such as IL-1, cause proliferation of synovial cells and fibroblasts. The cytokines also stimulate secretion by synovial cells and chondrocytes of proteolytic and matrix-degrading enzymes. Activated T cells in RA lesions have also been shown to express impressive amounts of a cytokine called RANK ligand, which induces osteoclast differentiation and activation and may play a key role in the bone resorption seen in destructive joint lesions (Chapter 21). Despite the plethora of cytokines produced in the joint in RA, TNF appears to play a pivotal role. This is demonstrated by the remarkable effectiveness of TNF antagonists in the disease, even in patients who are resistant to other therapies.

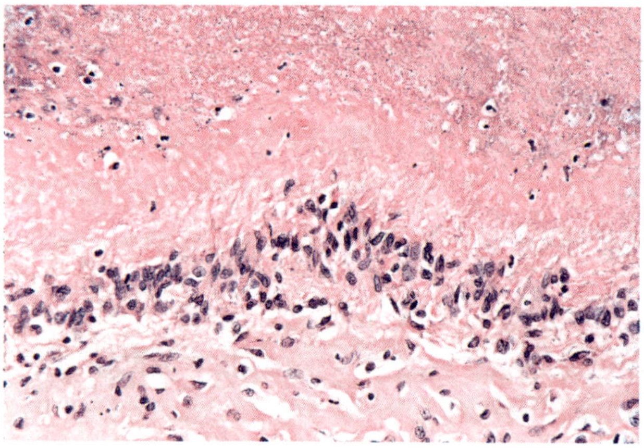

Figure 5–24

Rheumatoid nodule. Subcutaneous nodule with an area of necrosis (*top*) surrounded by a palisade of macrophages and scattered chronic inflammatory cells.

The role of *antibodies* in the disease is suspected from a variety of experimental and clinical observations. About 80% of patients have serum IgM (and, less frequently, IgG) autoantibodies that bind to the Fc portions of their own (self) IgG. These autoantibodies are called *rheumatoid factor (RF)*. They may form immune complexes with self-IgG that deposit in joints and other tissues, leading to inflammation and tissue damage. However, the role of RF in the pathogenesis of the joint or extra-articular lesions has not been established, and about 20% of patients do not have RF, suggesting that these autoantibodies are not essential for tissue injury in RA.

Genetic variables in the pathogenesis of RA are suggested by the increased frequency of this disease among first-degree relatives and a high concordance rate in monozygotic twins; there are also associations of *HLA-DR4* and polymorphisms in the *PTPN22* gene with RA.

Finally, there are the elusive *infectious agents* whose antigens may activate T or B cells. Many candidates have been considered, but none has been conclusively proved. Suspects include EBV, *Borrelia* species, *Mycoplasma* species, parvoviruses, and mycobacteria.

Clinical Course. Although RA is basically a symmetric polyarticular arthritis, there may also be constitutional symptoms such as weakness, malaise, and low-grade fever. Many of the systemic manifestations result from the same mediators that cause joint inflammation (e.g., IL-1 and TNF). The arthritis first appears insidiously, with aching and stiffness of the joints, particularly in the morning. As the disease advances, the joints become enlarged, motion is limited, and in time complete ankylosis may appear. Vasculitic involvement of the extremities may give rise to *Raynaud phenomenon* and chronic leg ulcers. Such multisystem involvement must be distinguished from SLE, scleroderma, polymyositis, dermatomyositis, and Lyme disease, as well as other forms of arthritis. Helpful in making the correct diagnosis are (1) characteristic radiographic findings; (2) sterile, turbid synovial fluid with decreased viscosity, poor mucin clot formation, and inclusion-bearing neutrophils; and (3) RF (80% of patients).

The clinical course of RA is highly variable. In a minority of patients the disease may become stabilized or may even regress; most of the remainder pursues a chronic, remitting-relapsing course. The natural history of the disease has been one of progressive joint destruction

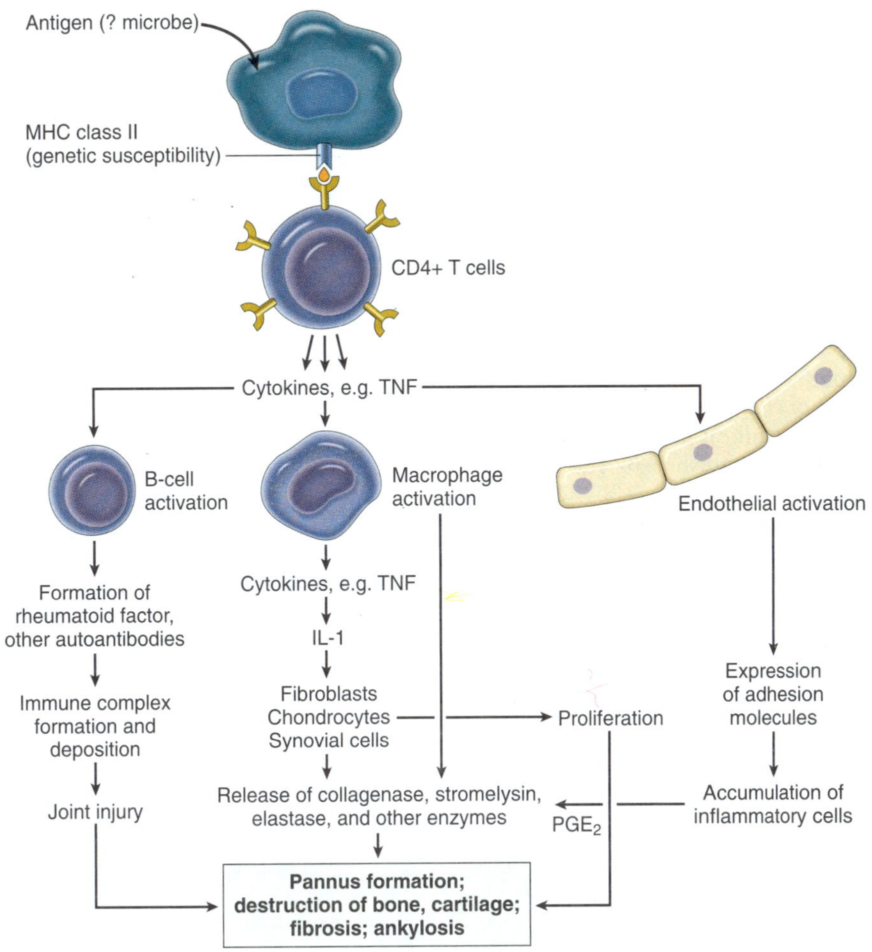

Figure 5–25

Model for the pathogenesis of rheumatoid arthritis. CD4+ T cells reacting against an unknown arthritogenic antigen are believed to stimulate autoantibody production and to activate macrophages and other cells in the joint synovium. PGE_2, prostaglandin E_2.

leading to disability after 10–15 years. However, the outcome has been dramatically improved by recent advances in therapy, including aggressive treatment of early RA and the introduction of highly ineffective biologic agents that antagonize TNF. RA is an important cause of reactive amyloidosis (discussed later), which develops in 5% to 10% of these patients, particularly those with long-standing severe disease.

SUMMARY

Rheumatoid Arthritis

- RA is a chronic inflammatory disease that affects mainly the joints, especially small joints, but can affect multiple tissues.
- The disease is caused by an autoimmune response against an unknown self antigen(s), which leads to T-cell reactions in the joint with production of cytokines that activate phagocytes that damage tissues and stimulate proliferation of synovial cells (synovitis). The cytokine TNF plays a central role, and antagonists against TNF are of great benefit. Antibodies may also contribute to the disease.

Juvenile Rheumatoid Arthritis

Juvenile RA (JRA) refers to chronic idiopathic arthritis that occurs in children. It is not a single disease but a heterogeneous group of disorders, most of which differ significantly from the adult form of RA except for the destructive nature of the arthritis. RF is typically absent, as are rheumatoid nodules. Extra-articular inflammatory manifestations such as uveitis may be present. Some variants involve relatively few larger joints such as knees, elbows, and ankles and are thus called *pauciarticular.* Some cases of JRA are associated with *HLA-B27,* and their clinical features overlap with the spondyloarthropathies described next. One variant, previously called Still disease, has an acute febrile onset and systemic manifestations, including leukocytosis (white blood cell counts of 15,000–25,000 cells/μL), hepatosplenomegaly, lymphadenopathy, and rash.

Seronegative Spondyloarthropathies

For years, several entities in this group of disorders were considered variants of RA; however, careful clinical, morphologic, and genetic studies have distinguished these disorders from RA. The spondyloarthropathies are characterized by the following features:

- Pathologic changes that begin in the ligamentous attachments to bone rather than in the synovium
- Involvement of the sacroiliac joints, with or without arthritis in other peripheral joints
- Absence of RFs (hence the name "seronegative" spondyloarthropathies)
- Association with *HLA-B27*

This group of disorders includes several clinical entities, of which *ankylosing spondylitis* is the prototype. Others include Reiter syndrome, psoriatic arthritis, spondylitis associated with inflammatory bowel diseases, and reactive arthropathies after infections (e.g., with *Yersinia, Shigella, Salmonella, Helicobacter,* or *Campylobacter*). Sacroiliitis is a common manifestation in all of these disorders; they are distinguished by the particular peripheral joints involved, as well as by associated extraskeletal manifestations (for example, urethritis, conjunctivitis, and uveitis are characteristic of Reiter syndrome). Although a triggering infection and immune mechanisms are thought to underlie most of the seronegative spondyloarthropathies, their pathogenesis remains obscure.

Sjögren Syndrome

Sjögren syndrome is a clinicopathologic entity characterized by dry eyes (*keratoconjunctivitis sicca*) and dry mouth (*xerostomia*), resulting from immune-mediated destruction of the lacrimal and salivary glands. It occurs as an isolated disorder (primary form), also known as the *sicca syndrome,* or more often in association with another autoimmune disease (secondary form). Among the associated disorders, RA is the most common, but some patients have SLE, polymyositis, systemic sclerosis, vasculitis, or thyroiditis.

Etiology and Pathogenesis. Several lines of evidence suggest that Sjögren syndrome is an autoimmune disease in which the ductal epithelial cells of the exocrine glands are the primary target. Nevertheless, there is also systemic B-cell hyperactivity, as evidenced by the presence of ANAs and RF (even in the absence of associated RA). Most patients with primary Sjögren syndrome have autoantibodies to the RNP antigens SS-A (Ro) and SS-B (La); note that these antibodies are also present in some SLE patients and are therefore not diagnostic for Sjögren syndrome (see Table 5–9). Although patients with high-titer anti-SS-A antibodies are more likely to have systemic (extraglandular) manifestations, there is no evidence that the autoantibodies cause primary tissue injury. Analogous to SLE as well, the disease is probably initiated by a loss of tolerance in the CD4+ T-cell population, although the nature of the target autoantigen is unknown. A viral trigger has also been suggested, but no causative virus has been identified conclusively. *Genetic variables* play a role in the pathogenesis of Sjögren syndrome. As with SLE, inheritance of certain class II MHC alleles predisposes to the development of specific RNP autoantibodies.

Morphology

Lacrimal and salivary glands are the primary targets, but other secretory glands, including those in the nasopharynx, upper airway, and vagina, may also be involved. Involved tissues show an intense lymphocyte (primarily activated CD4+ T cells) and plasma-cell infiltrate, occasionally forming lymphoid follicles with germinal centers. There is associated destruction of the native architecture (Fig. 5–26).

Lacrimal gland destruction results in a lack of tears, leading to drying of the corneal epithelium, with subsequent inflammation, erosion, and ulceration (**keratoconjunctivitis**). Similar changes may occur in the oral mucosa as a result of loss of salivary gland output, giving rise to mucosal atrophy, with inflammatory fissuring and ulceration (**xerostomia**). Dryness and crusting of the nose may lead to ulcerations and even perforation of the nasal septum. When the respiratory passages are involved, secondary laryngitis, bronchitis, and pneumonitis may appear. Approximately 25% of the patients (especially those with anti-SS-A antibodies) develop extraglandular disease affecting the CNS, skin, kidneys, and muscles. Renal lesions take the form of mild interstitial nephritis associated with tubular transport defects; unlike in SLE, glomerulonephritis is rare.

Clinical Course. Approximately 90% of Sjögren syndrome cases occur in women between the ages of 35 and 45 years. Patients present with dry mouth, lack of tears, and the resultant complications just described. Salivary glands are often enlarged as a result of lymphocytic infiltrates (see Fig. 5–26). Extraglandular manifestations include synovitis, pulmonary fibrosis, and peripheral neuropathy. About 60% of Sjögren patients have an accompanying autoimmune disorder such as RA. Notably, there is a 40-fold increased risk of developing a non-Hodgkin B-cell lymphoma, arising in the setting of the initial robust polyclonal B-cell proliferation. These so-called marginal zone lymphomas are discussed in Chapter 12.

SUMMARY

Sjögren Syndrome

- Sjögren syndrome is an inflammatory disease that affects primarily the salivary and lacrimal glands, causing dryness of the mouth and eyes.
- The disease is believed to be caused by an autoimmune T-cell reaction against an unknown self antigen(s) expressed in these glands, or immune reactions against the antigens of a virus that infects the tissues.

Systemic Sclerosis (Scleroderma)

Although commonly called *scleroderma,* this disorder is better labeled systemic sclerosis (SS), because it is characterized by excessive fibrosis throughout the body and

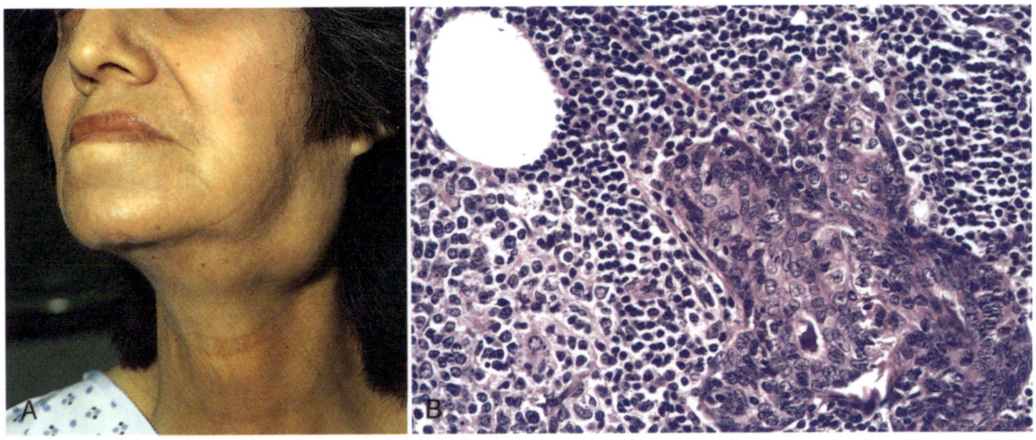

Figure 5–26

Sjögren syndrome. **A,** Enlargement of the salivary gland. **B,** The histologic view shows intense lymphocytic and plasma cell infiltration with ductal epithelial hyperplasia. (**A,** Courtesy of Dr. Richard Sontheimer, Department of Dermatology, University of Texas Southwestern Medical School, Dallas, Texas. **B,** Courtesy of Dr. Dennis Burns, Department of Pathology, University of Texas Southwestern Medical School, Dallas, Texas.)

not just the skin. Cutaneous involvement is the usual presenting symptom and eventually appears in approximately 95% of cases, but it is the visceral involvement—of the gastrointestinal tract, lungs, kidneys, heart, and skeletal muscles—that produces the major morbidity and mortality.

SS can be classified into two groups based on its clinical course:

- *Diffuse scleroderma,* characterized by initial widespread skin involvement, with rapid progression and early visceral involvement
- *Limited scleroderma,* with relatively mild skin involvement, often confined to the fingers and face. Involvement of the viscera occurs late, and hence the disease in these patients generally has a fairly benign course. This is also called the CREST syndrome because of its frequent features of calcinosis, Raynaud phenomenon, esophageal dysmotility, sclerodactyly, and telangiectasia.

Etiology and Pathogenesis. *Fibroblast activation with excessive fibrosis is the hallmark of systemic sclerosis.* The cause is unknown, although it is attributed to abnormal activation of the immune system and microvascular injury and not to any intrinsic defect in fibroblasts or in collagen synthesis. It is proposed that CD4+ cells responding to an as yet unidentified antigen accumulate in the skin and release cytokines that activate mast cells and macrophages; in turn, these cells release fibrogenic cytokines such as IL-1, PDGF, TGF-β, and fibroblast growth factors. The possibility that activated T cells play a role in the pathogenesis of SS is supported by the observation that several features of this disease (including the cutaneous sclerosis) are seen in chronic GVHD, a disorder resulting from sustained activation of T cells in recipients of allogeneic bone marrow transplants. B-cell activation also occurs, as indicated by the presence of hypergammaglobulinemia and ANAs. Although humoral immunity does not play any significant role in the pathogenesis of SS, two of the ANAs are virtually unique to this disease and are therefore useful in diagnosis (see Table 5–9). One of these, directed against *DNA topoisomerase I (anti-Scl 70),* is highly specific; it is present in as many as 70% of patients with diffuse scleroderma (and in less than 1% of patients with other connective tissue diseases) and is a marker for patients likely to develop more aggressive disease with pulmonary fibrosis and peripheral vascular pathology. The other ANA is an *anti-centromere antibody,* found in as many as 90% of patients with limited scleroderma (i.e., the CREST syndrome); it indicates a relatively benign course.

Microvascular disease is also consistently present early in the course of SS, although the mechanisms of endothelial injury remain mysterious. It is possible that endothelial cells are activated and subsequently injured by the local T-cell reaction. Repeated cycles of endothelial damage followed by platelet aggregation lead to release of platelet factors (e.g., PDGF) that trigger periadventitial fibrosis and narrowing of the microvasculature, with eventual ischemic injury.

Morphology

Virtually any organ may be affected in SS, but the most prominent changes are found in the skin, musculoskeletal system, gastrointestinal tract, lungs, kidneys, and heart.

Skin. The vast majority of patients have diffuse, sclerotic atrophy of the skin, usually beginning in the fingers and distal regions of the upper extremities and extending proximally to involve the upper arms, shoulders, neck, and face. In the early stages, affected skin areas are somewhat edematous and have a doughy consistency. Histologically, there are edema and perivascular infiltrates containing CD4+ T cells. Capillaries and small arteries (as large as 500 μm in diameter) may show thickening of the basal lamina, endothelial cell damage, and partial occlusion. With progression, the edematous phase is replaced by progressive fibrosis of the dermis, which becomes tightly bound to the subcutaneous structures. There is marked increase of compact collagen in the dermis along with thinning of the epidermis, atrophy of the dermal appendages, and hyaline thickening of the walls of dermal arterioles and capillaries (Fig. 5–27A, B). Focal and sometimes diffuse subcutaneous calcifications may develop, especially in patients with the CREST syndrome. In advanced stages the fingers take on a tapered, clawlike appearance with limitation of motion in the joints (Fig. 5–27C), and the face becomes a drawn mask. Loss of blood supply may lead to cutaneous ulcerations and to atrophic changes in the terminal phalanges, including autoamputation.

Gastrointestinal Tract. The gastrointestinal tract is affected in approximately 90% of patients. Progressive atrophy and collagenous fibrous replacement of the muscularis may develop at any level of the gut but are most severe in the esophagus, with the lower two-thirds often developing an inflexibility not unlike a rubber hose. The associated dysfunction of the lower esophageal sphincter gives rise to gastroesophageal reflux and its complications, including Barrett metaplasia (Chapter 15) and strictures. The mucosa is thinned and may be ulcerated, and there is excessive collagenization of the lamina propria and submucosa. Loss of villi and microvilli in the small bowel is the anatomic basis for the malabsorption syndrome sometimes encountered.

bacterial overgrowth due to dysmotility is also an issue

Musculoskeletal System. Synovial hyperplasia and inflammation is common in the early stages; fibrosis later ensues. Although these changes are reminiscent of RA, joint destruction is not common in SS. In a small subset of patients (approximately 10%), inflammatory myositis indistinguishable from polymyositis may develop.

Lungs. The lungs are affected in more than 50% of patients; this may manifest as pulmonary hypertension and/or interstitial fibrosis. Pulmonary vasospasm from pulmonary vascular endothelial dysfunction is considered important in the pathogenesis of pulmonary hypertension. Pulmonary fibrosis, when present, is indistinguishable from that seen in idiopathic pulmonary fibrosis (Chapter 13).

Kidneys. Renal abnormalities occur in two-thirds of patients with SS, most typically associated with thickening of the vessel walls of interlobular arteries (150–500 μm in diameter). These show intimal-cell proliferation with deposition of various glycoproteins and acid mucopolysaccharides. Although similar to the changes seen in malignant hypertension, the alterations in SS are restricted to vessels 150 to 500 μm in diameter and are not always associated with hypertension. Hypertension does occur in 30% of patients and in 20% of those patients takes an ominously malignant course (malignant hypertension). In hypertensive patients, vascular alterations are more pronounced and are often associated with fibrinoid necrosis involving the arterioles together with thrombosis and infarction. Such patients often die of renal failure, accounting for about half the deaths in patients with SS. There are no specific glomerular changes.

Heart. Patchy myocardial fibrosis, along with thickening of intramyocardial arterioles, occurs in one-third of the patients; this is putatively caused by microvascular injury and resultant ischemia (so-called cardiac Raynaud). Because of the changes in the lung, right ventricular hypertrophy and failure (cor pulmonale) are frequent.

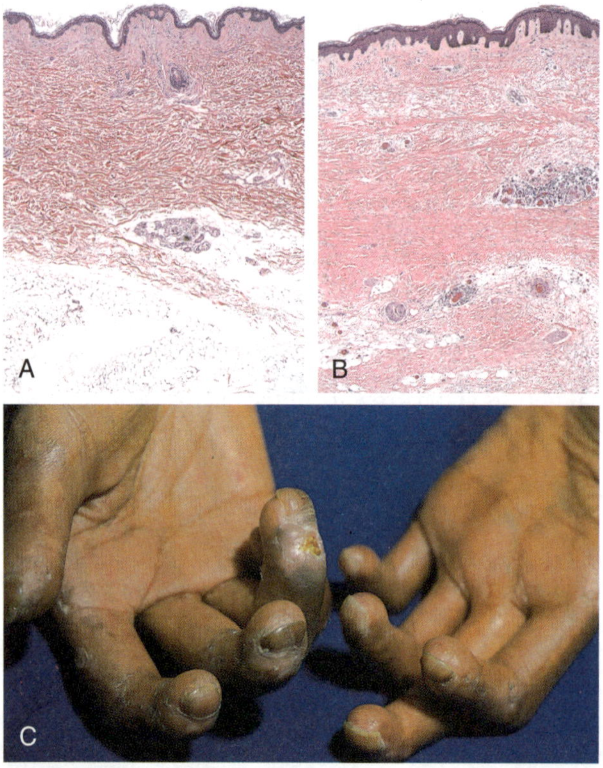

Figure 5–27

Systemic sclerosis. **A,** Normal skin. **B,** Extensive deposition of dense collagen in the dermis. **C,** The extensive subcutaneous fibrosis has virtually immobilized the fingers, creating a clawlike flexion deformity. Loss of blood supply has led to cutaneous ulcerations. (Courtesy of Dr. Richard Sontheimer. Department of Dermatology, University of Texas Southwestern Medical School, Dallas, Texas.)

Clinical Course. SS affects women three times more often than men, with a peak incidence in the 50- to 60-year age group. There is a substantial overlap in presentation between SS and RA, SLE, and dermatomyositis (see later); the distinctive feature of SS is the striking cutaneous involvement. Almost all patients develop *Raynaud phenomenon,* a vascular disorder characterized by reversible vasospasm of the arteries. Typically the hands turn white on exposure to cold, reflecting vasospasm, followed by a blue color as ischemia and cyanosis supervene. Finally, the color changes to red as reactive vasodilation occurs. Progressive collagenization of the skin leads to atrophy of the hands, with increasing stiffness and eventually complete immobilization of the joints. Difficulty in swallowing results from esophageal fibrosis and resultant hypomotility. Eventually, destruction of the esophageal wall leads to atony and dilation. Malabsorption may appear if the submucosal and muscular atrophy and fibrosis involve the small intestine. Dyspnea and chronic cough reflect the pulmonary changes; with advanced lung involvement, secondary pulmonary hypertension may develop, leading to right-sided cardiac failure. Renal functional impairment secondary to both the advance of SS and the concomitant malignant hypertension is frequently marked.

The course of diffuse SS is difficult to predict. In most patients the disease pursues a steady, slow, downhill course over the span of many years, although in the absence of renal involvement, life span may be normal. The overall 10-year survival rate ranges from 35% to 70%. The chances of survival are significantly better for patients with localized scleroderma than for those with the usual diffuse progressive disease. *Limited scleroderma,* or CREST syndrome, frequently has Raynaud phenomenon as its presenting feature. It is associated with limited skin involvement confined to the fingers and face, and these two features may be present for decades before the appearance of visceral lesions.

SUMMARY

Systemic Sclerosis

- Systemic sclerosis (commonly called *scleroderma*) is characterized by progressive fibrosis involving the skin, gastrointestinal tract, and other tissues.
- Fibrosis may be the result of activation of fibroblasts by cytokines produced by T cells, but what triggers T-cell responses is unknown.
- Endothelial injury and microvascular disease are commonly present in the lesions of systemic sclerosis, perhaps causing chronic ischemia, but the pathogenesis of vascular injury is not known.

Inflammatory Myopathies

Inflammatory myopathies make up a heterogeneous group of rare disorders characterized by immune-mediated muscle injury and inflammation. Based on the clinical, morphologic, and immunologic features, three disorders—*polymyositis, dermatomyositis,* and *inclusion body myositis*—have been described. These may occur alone or in conjunction with other autoimmune diseases, such as SS. Women with dermatomyositis have a slightly increased risk of developing visceral cancers (of the lung, ovary, stomach).

Clinically, these diseases are characterized by usually symmetric muscle weakness initially affecting large muscles of the trunk, neck, and limbs. Thus, tasks such as getting up from a chair or climbing steps become increasingly difficult. In dermatomyositis an associated rash (classically described as a *lilac* or *heliotrope* discoloration) affects the upper eyelids and causes periorbital edema. Histologically, there is infiltration by lymphocytes, and both degenerating and regenerating muscle fibers are seen (Fig. 5–28). The pattern of muscle injury and the location of the inflammatory infiltrates are fairly distinctive for each subtype.

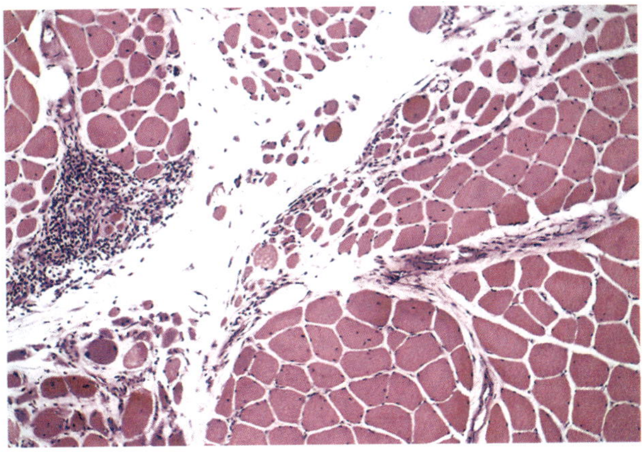

Figure 5–28

Dermatomyositis. Perifascicular inflammation and atrophy in a skeletal muscle. (Courtesy of Dr. Dennis Burns, Department of Pathology, University of Texas Southwestern Medical School, Dallas, Texas.)

The immunologic evidence supports antibody-mediated tissue injury in dermatomyositis, whereas polymyositis and inclusion body myositis seem to be mediated by CTLs. ANAs are present in most patients. Of these, only Jo-1 antibodies, directed against transfer RNA synthetase, are specific for this group of disorders (see Table 5–9).

The diagnosis of these myopathies is based on clinical features, laboratory evidence of muscle injury (e.g., increased blood levels of creatine kinase), electromyography, and biopsy.

Mixed Connective Tissue Disease

The term *mixed connective tissue disease* refers to a spectrum of pathologic processes in patients who clinically present with several features suggestive of SLE, polymyositis, and SS; they also have *high titers of antibodies to an RNP antigen called U1RNP.* Two other features of mixed connective tissue disease are the paucity of renal disease and an extremely good response to corticosteroids, both of which suggest a favorable long-term prognosis.

Mixed connective tissue disease may present as arthritis, swelling of the hands, Raynaud phenomenon, esophageal dysmotility, myositis, leukopenia and anemia, fever, lymphadenopathy, and/or hypergammaglobulinemia. Because of these overlapping features, it is not entirely clear whether mixed connective tissue disease constitutes a distinct disease or represents heterogeneous subsets of SLE, systemic sclerosis, and polymyositis; most authorities do not consider it a specific entity.

Polyarteritis Nodosa and Other Vasculitides

Polyarteritis nodosa belongs to a group of diseases characterized by necrotizing inflammation of the walls of blood vessels, most likely of an immune pathogenesis. The general term *noninfectious necrotizing vasculitis* differentiates these conditions from those attributable to direct vessel infection (e.g., an abscess) and serves to emphasize that any type of vessel may be involved—arteries, arterioles, veins, or capillaries. A detailed classification and description of vasculitides is presented in Chapter 10.

IMMUNE DEFICIENCY DISEASES

Immune deficiency diseases may be caused by inherited defects affecting immune system development, or they may result from secondary effects of other diseases (e.g., infection, malnutrition, aging, immunosuppression, autoimmunity, or chemotherapy). Clinically, patients with immune deficiency present with increased susceptibility to infections as well as to certain forms of cancer. The type of infections in a given patient depends largely on the component of the immune system that is affected. Patients with defects in Ig, complement, or phagocytic cells typically suffer from recurrent infections with pyogenic bacteria, whereas those with defects in cell-mediated immunity are prone to infections caused by viruses, fungi, and intracellular bacteria. Here we describe some of the more important primary immune deficiencies, followed by a detailed description of the acquired immunodeficiency syndrome (AIDS), the most devastating example of secondary immune deficiency.

Primary Immune Deficiencies

Primary immune deficiency states are (fortunately) rare but have nevertheless contributed greatly to our understanding of the development and function of the immune system. Most primary immune deficiency diseases are genetically determined and affect either adaptive immunity (i.e., humoral or cellular) or innate host defense mechanisms, including complement proteins and cells such as phagocytes and NK cells. Defects in adaptive immunity are often subclassified on the basis of the primary component involved (i.e., B cells or T cells, or both); however, because of the interactions between T and B lymphocytes, these distinctions are not clear-cut. For instance, T-cell defects frequently lead to impaired antibody synthesis, and hence isolated deficiencies of T cells may be indistinguishable from combined deficiencies of T and B cells. Most primary immune deficiencies come to attention early in life (between 6 months and 2 years of age), usually because the affected infants are susceptible to recurrent infections. One of the most impressive accomplishments of modern molecular biology has been the identification of the genetic basis of many primary immune deficiencies (Fig. 5–29), laying the foundation for future gene replacement therapy.

X-Linked Agammaglobulinemia (XLA, Bruton Disease)

X-Linked agammaglobulinemia (XLA), or Bruton disease, is one of the more common forms of primary immune deficiency. It is *characterized by the failure of pre-B cells to differentiate into B cells;* as a consequence, and as the name implies, there is a resultant absence of gamma globulin in the blood. During normal B-cell maturation, Ig heavy-chain genes are rearranged first, followed by light-chain rearrangement. At each stage, signals are received from the expressed components of the antigen receptor that drive maturation to the next stage; these signals act as quality controls, to ensure that the correct receptor proteins are being produced. In XLA, B-cell maturation stops after the initial heavy-chain gene rearrangement because of mutations in a tyrosine kinase that is associated with the pre-B-cell receptor and is involved in pre-B-cell signal transduction. This kinase is called *Bruton tyrosine kinase* or *B-cell tyrosine kinase (BTK).* When it is nonfunctional the pre-B-cell receptor cannot signal the cells to proceed along the maturation pathway. As a result, Ig light chains are not produced, and the complete Ig molecule containing heavy and light chains cannot be assembled and transported to the cell membrane, although free heavy chains can be found in the cytoplasm. Because *BTK* maps to the X chromosome, the disorder is seen in males.

Classically, this disease is characterized by

- Absent or markedly decreased numbers of B cells in the circulation, with depressed serum levels of all classes of immunoglobulins. The numbers of pre-B cells in the bone marrow may be normal or reduced.
- Underdeveloped or rudimentary germinal centers in peripheral lymphoid tissues, including lymph nodes, Peyer patches, the appendix, and tonsils
- Absence of plasma cells throughout the body
- Normal T-cell–mediated responses

XLA does not become apparent until approximately 6 months of age, when maternal immunoglobulins are depleted. In most cases, recurrent bacterial infections such as acute and chronic pharyngitis, sinusitis, otitis media, bronchitis, and pneumonia suggest an underlying immune defect. The causal organisms are typically those bacterial pathogens that are cleared by antibody-mediated opsonization and phagocytosis (e.g., *Haemophilus influenzae, Streptococcus pneumoniae,* or *Staphylococcus aureus*). Because antibodies are important for neutralizing viruses, these patients are also susceptible to certain viral infections, especially those caused by enteroviruses. Similarly, *Giardia lamblia,* an intestinal protozoan usually neutralized by secreted IgA, cannot be efficiently cleared and causes persistent infections. Fortunately, replacement therapy with intravenous Ig from pooled human serum allows the majority of patients to adequately combat bacterial infections. Patients with XLA clear most viral, fungal, and protozoal infections, because their T-cell-mediated immunity is intact. For unclear reasons, autoimmune diseases (such as RA and dermatomyositis) occur in as many as 20% of patients with this disease.

Common Variable Immunodeficiency

This is a heterogeneous group of disorders characterized by hypogammaglobulinemia, impaired antibody responses to infection (or vaccination), and increased susceptibility to infections. The clinical manifestations are

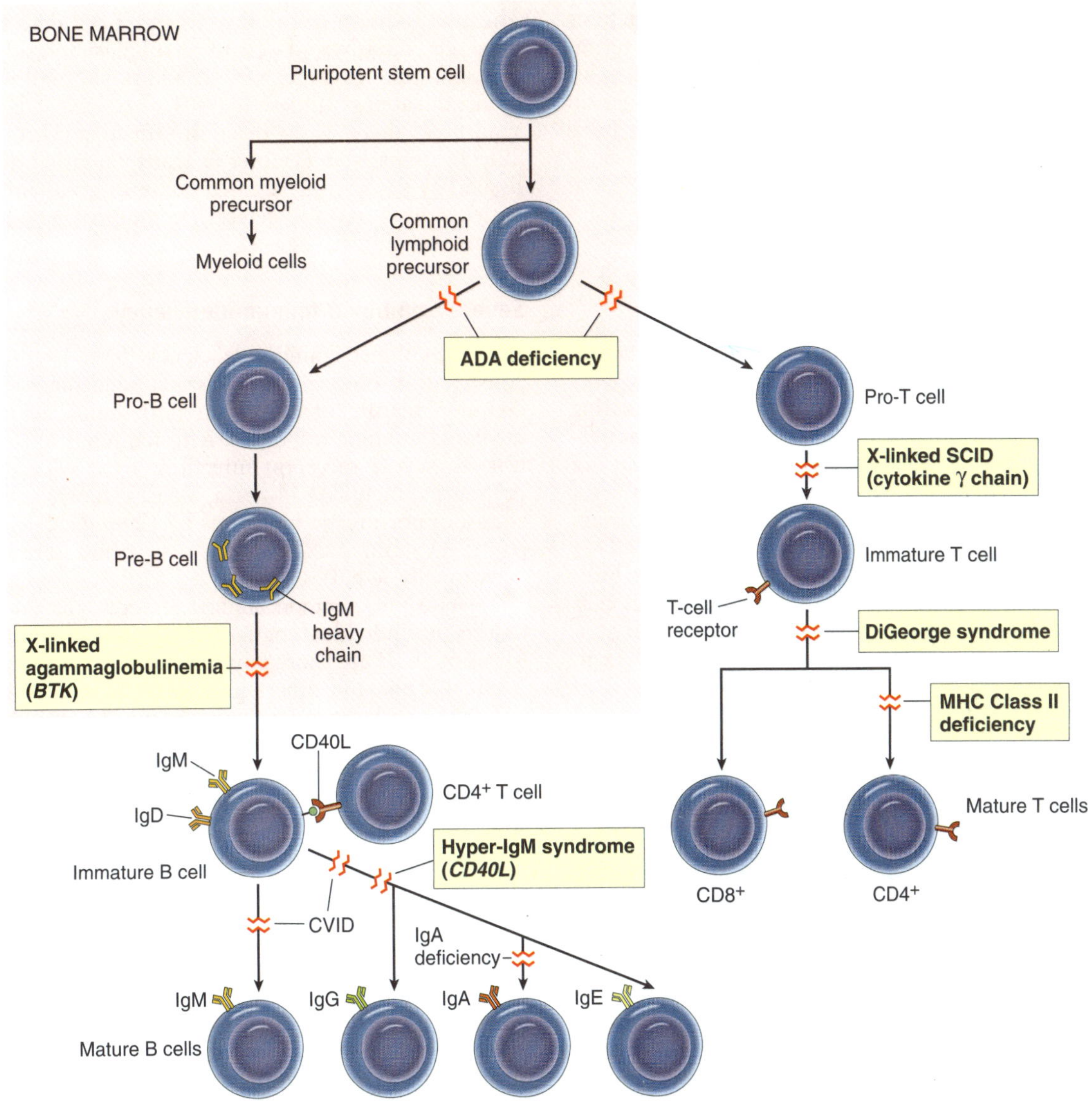

Figure 5–29

Primary immune deficiency diseases. Lymphocyte development and sites of block in primary immune deficiency diseases. The affected genes are indicated in parentheses for some of the disorders. ADA, adenosine deaminase; CD40L, CD40 ligand (also known as CD154); CVID, common variable immunodeficiency; SCID, severe combined immunodeficiency.

superficially similar to those of XLA, but in common variable immunodeficiency the sexes are affected equally and the onset of symptoms is much later, in the second or third decade of life. The diagnosis is usually one of exclusion (after other causes of immune deficiency are ruled out); the basis of the Ig deficiency is variable (hence the name). Although most patients have normal numbers of mature B cells, plasma cells are absent, suggesting a block in antigen-stimulated B-cell differentiation. The defective antibody production has been variably attributed to intrinsic B-cell defects, deficient T-cell help, or excessive T-cell suppressor activity. Paradoxically, these patients are prone to develop a variety of autoimmune disorders (hemolytic anemia, pernicious anemia), as well as lymphoid tumors. Some patients with this disease have mutations in B-cell receptors for certain growth factors, or in molecules involved in T cell–B cell interactions. However, the genetic basis of most cases of the disease is not known.

Isolated IgA Deficiency

The most common of all the primary immune deficiency diseases, IgA deficiency affects about 1 in 700 white individuals. Recall that IgA is the major Ig in mucosal secretions and is thus involved in airway and gastrointestinal defense. Although most individuals with this condition are asymptomatic, weakened mucosal defenses predispose patients to recurrent sinopulmonary infections and diarrhea. There is also a significant (but unexplained) association with autoimmune diseases. The pathogenesis of IgA deficiency seems to involve a block in the terminal differentiation of IgA-secreting B cells to plasma cells; IgM and IgG subclasses of antibodies are present in normal or even supranormal levels. The molecular basis of this defect is not understood.

Hyper-IgM Syndrome

In a normal immune response to protein antigen, IgM antibodies are produced first, followed by the sequential elaboration of IgG, IgA, and IgE antibodies. As we discussed earlier in this chapter, the orderly appearance of different antibody types is called *heavy-chain class (isotype) switching* and is important for generating classes of antibody that can effectively activate complement and/or opsonize bacterial pathogens. The ability of IgM-producing B cells to turn on the transcription of genes that encode other Ig isotypes depends on certain cytokines, as well as contact-mediated signals from CD4+ helper T cells. The contact-dependent signals are provided by interaction between CD40 molecules on B cells and CD40L (also known as CD154), expressed on activated helper T cells. Patients with the hyper-IgM syndrome produce normal (or even supranormal) levels of IgM antibodies to antigens but lack the ability to produce the IgG, IgA, or IgE isotypes; the underlying defect is an inability of T cells to induce B-cell isotype switching. The most common genetic abnormality is mutation of the gene encoding CD40L. This gene is located on the X chromosome; consequently, in approximately 70% of the cases, hyper-IgM syndrome is X-linked. In the remaining patients, the mutations affect CD40 or other molecules involved in class switching, notably an enzyme called *activation-induced deaminase*.

Although the disease is diagnosed and named because of the antibody abnormality, there is also a defect in cell-mediated immunity because the CD40–CD40L interaction is critical for helper T cell–mediated activation of macrophages, the central reaction of cell-mediated immunity. Male patients with the X-linked form of hyper-IgM syndrome present with recurrent pyogenic infections due to low levels of opsonizing IgG antibodies. These patients are also susceptible to a variety of intracellular pathogens that are normally combated by cell-mediated immunity, including *Pneumocystis jiroveci* (formerly called *P. carinii*).

Thymic Hypoplasia: DiGeorge Syndrome

DiGeorge syndrome results from a congenital defect in thymic development with deficient T-cell maturation. T cells are absent in the lymph nodes, spleen, and peripheral blood, and infants with this defect are extremely vulnerable to viral, fungal, and protozoal infections. Patients are also susceptible to infection with intracellular bacteria, because of defective T-cell–mediated immunity. B cells and serum immunoglobulins are generally unaffected.

The disorder is a consequence of a developmental malformation affecting the third and fourth pharyngeal pouches—structures that give rise to the thymus, parathyroid glands, and portions of the face and aortic arch. Thus, in addition to the thymic and T-cell defects, there may be parathyroid gland hypoplasia resulting in hypocalcemic tetany, as well as additional midline developmental abnormalities. In 90% of cases of DiGeorge syndrome there is a deletion affecting chromosome 22q11, discussed in Chapter 7. Transplantation of thymic tissue has successfully treated some of these infants. In patients with partial defects, immunity may improve spontaneously with age.

Severe Combined Immunodeficiency

Severe combined immunodeficiency (SCID) represents a constellation of genetically distinct syndromes with the common feature of defects in both humoral and cell-mediated immune responses. Affected infants are susceptible to severe recurrent infections by a wide array of pathogens, including bacteria, viruses, fungi, and protozoans; opportunistic infections by *Candida, Pneumocystis,* CMV, and *Pseudomonas* also cause serious (and occasionally lethal) disease.

Despite the common clinical features, the underlying defects in individual patients are quite diverse. Some forms of SCID are caused by a single defect affecting both T and B cells, and others may result from a primary T-cell deficit with secondary impairment of humoral immunity. Approximately half of the cases are X-linked; these are caused by mutations in the gene encoding the common γ chain shared by the receptors for the cytokines IL-2, IL-4, IL-7, IL-9, and IL-15. Of these cytokines, IL-7 is the most important in this disease because it is the growth factor responsible for stimulating the survival and expansion of immature B- and T-cell precursors in the generative lymphoid organs. Another 40% to 50% of SCID cases are inherited in an autosomal recessive fashion, with approximately half of these caused by mutations in *adenosine deaminase (ADA),* an enzyme involved in purine metabolism. ADA deficiency results in accumulation of adenosine and deoxyadenosine triphosphate metabolites, which inhibit DNA synthesis and are toxic to lymphocytes. The other autosomal recessive cases of SCID are attributed to defects in another purine metabolic pathway, primary failure of class II MHC expression, or mutations in genes encoding the recombinase responsible for the rearrangement of lymphocyte antigen-receptor genes.

In the two most common forms of SCID (cytokine receptor common γ chain mutation and ADA deficiency), the thymus is hypoplastic. Lymph nodes and lymphoid tissues (e.g., in the tonsils, gut, and appendix) are atrophic and lack B-cell germinal centers as well as paracortical T cells. Affected patients may have marked lymphopenia, with both T- and B-cell deficiency; others may have increased numbers of immature T cells and/or large numbers of B cells that are nonfunctional because of a lack of T-cell help. Patients with SCID are currently treated by bone marrow transplantation. X-SCID is the first disease in which gene therapy has been used to successfully replace the mutated gene, but the approach is being re-evaluated because some of the treated patients have developed T-cell leukemias, presumably because the introduced gene inserted close to a cellular oncogene.

Immune Deficiency with Thrombocytopenia and Eczema: Wiskott-Aldrich Syndrome

Wiskott-Aldrich syndrome is an X-linked recessive disease characterized by thrombocytopenia, eczema, and a marked vulnerability to recurrent infection, ending in early death; the only treatment is bone marrow transplantation. This is a curious syndrome, in that the clinical presentation and immunologic deficits are difficult to explain on the basis of the known underlying genetic defect. The thymus is initially normal, but there is progressive age-related depletion of T lymphocytes in the peripheral blood and lymph nodes, with concurrent loss of cellular immunity. Additionally, patients do not effectively synthesize antibodies to polysaccharide antigens, and are therefore particularly susceptible to encapsulated, pyogenic bacteria. (However, B-cell responses to polysaccharide antigens do not require T-cell help!) Affected patients are also prone to developing malignant lymphomas. The responsible gene maps to the X chromosome and encodes a protein *(Wiskott-Aldrich syndrome protein)* that links several membrane receptors to the cytoskeleton. Although the mechanism is not known, a defect in this protein could result in abnormal cellular morphology (including platelet shape changes?) or defective cytoskeleton-dependent activation signals in lymphocytes and other leukocytes, with abnormal cell-cell adhesions and leukocyte migration.

Genetic Deficiencies of Components of Innate Immunity

Several genetic defects have been shown to affect molecules or cells that are important in the early innate immune response to microbes.

Complement Proteins. As discussed earlier in this chapter and in Chapter 2, complement components play important roles in inflammatory and immunologic responses. Consequently, hereditary deficiency of complement components, especially C3 (critical for both the classical and alternative pathways), results in an increased susceptibility to infection with pyogenic bacteria. Inherited deficiencies of C1q, C2, and C4 do not make individuals susceptible to infections, but they do increase the risk of immune complex–mediated disease (e.g., SLE), possibly by impairing the clearance of apoptotic cells or of antigen-antibody complexes from the circulation. Deficiencies of the late components of the classical complement pathway (C5–C8) result in recurrent infections by *Neisseria* (gonococci, meningococci) but, curiously, not by other microbes. Lack of the regulatory protein C1 inhibitor allows unfettered C1 activation, with the generation of down-stream vasoactive complement mediators; the result is *hereditary angioedema,* characterized by recurrent episodes of localized edema affecting the skin and/or mucous membranes.

Phagocytes. Several congenital defects in phagocytes are known. These include defects in the phagocyte oxidase enzyme, the cause of *chronic granulomatous disease,* and defects in integrins and selectin ligands, causing the *leukocyte adhesion deficiencies.* These disorders were described in Chapter 2.

SUMMARY

Primary (Congenital) Immune Deficiency Diseases

- Caused by mutations in genes involved in lymphocyte maturation or function, or in innate immunity
- Some of the common disorders are
  - *XLA:* failure of B-cell maturation, absence of antibodies; mutations in *BTK* gene, which encodes B-cell tyrosine kinase, required for maturation signals from the pre-B cell and B-cell receptors
  - *Common variable immunodeficiency:* defects in antibody production; cause unknown in most cases
  - *Selective IgA deficiency:* failure of IgA production; cause unknown
  - *X- SCID:* failure of T-cell and B-cell maturation; mutation in the common γ chain of a cytokine receptor, leading to failure of IL-7 signaling and defective lymphopoiesis
  - *Autosomal SCID:* failure of T-cell development, secondary defect in antibody responses; approximately 50% of cases caused by mutation in the gene encoding ADA, leading to accumulation of toxic metabolites during lymphocyte maturation and proliferation
  - *X-linked hyper-IgM syndrome:* failure to produce isotype-switched high-affinity antibodies (IgG, IgA, IgE); mutation in gene encoding CD40L
- Clinical presentation: increased susceptibility to infections in early life

Secondary Immune Deficiencies

Immune deficiencies secondary to other diseases or therapies are much more common than the primary (inherited) disorders. Secondary immune deficiencies may be encountered in patients with malnutrition, infection, cancer, renal disease, or sarcoidosis. However, the most common cases of immune deficiency are therapy-induced suppression of the bone marrow and of lymphocyte function.

In the following section, we describe AIDS, an immune deficiency that has become one of the great scourges of mankind.

Acquired Immunodeficiency Syndrome

AIDS is a retroviral disease caused by the human immunodeficiency virus (HIV). It is characterized by infection and depletion of CD4+ T lymphocytes, and by profound immunosuppression leading to opportunistic infections, secondary neoplasms, and neurologic manifestations. Although AIDS was first described in the United States, it has now been reported in virtually every country in the world. Worldwide, more than 22 million people have died of AIDS since the epidemic was recognized in 1981;

about 42 million people are living with the disease, and there are an estimated 5 million infections each year. Worldwide, 95% of HIV infections are in developing countries, with Africa alone carrying more than 50% of the HIV burden. Although the largest number of infections is in Africa, the most rapid increases in HIV infection in the past decade are in Southeast Asian countries, including Thailand, India, and Indonesia. The statistics are only slightly better in the industrialized nations; for example, approximately 1 million US citizens are infected (roughly 1 in 300). Moreover, more Americans (more than 500,000) have died of AIDS than died in both world wars combined. Although AIDS-related death rates continue to decline from a 1995 peak, AIDS still represents the fifth most common cause of death in adults between the ages of 25 and 44.

Because of the combined work of many scientists and clinicians, there has been an explosion of new knowledge about this modern plague. So rapid is the pace of research on the biology of HIV that any text covering the topic will probably be out of date by the time it goes to press. Nevertheless, the following will attempt to summarize the currently available information on HIV epidemiology, etiology, pathogenesis, and clinical features.

Epidemiology

Epidemiologic studies in the United States have identified five groups at risk for developing AIDS, and these are similar in other countries, except as noted below. Transmission of HIV occurs under conditions that facilitate the exchange of blood or body fluids that contain the virus or virus-infected cells. Thus, *the major routes of HIV infection are sexual contact, parenteral inoculation,* and *passage of the virus from infected mothers to their newborns.* The case distributions listed below are in the United States; in about 10% of cases the risk factors are unknown or not reported.

- Homosexual or bisexual males constitute the largest group of infected individuals, accounting for 48% of reported cases in the period 2001–2004 and 56% of infected men (approximately 4% of these also inject drugs). However, transmission of AIDS in this category is declining, with less than 50% of new cases attributable to male homosexual contacts.
- Heterosexual contacts of members of other high-risk groups constituted about 34% of infections in 2001–2004. In Africa and Asia, this is by far the largest group of new infections, and the majority of new cases are in women infected by male partners.
- Intravenous drug abusers with no history of homosexuality compose the next largest group, representing about 17% of all patients.
- Recipients of blood and blood components (but not hemophiliacs) who received transfusions of HIV-infected whole blood or components (e.g., platelets, plasma) account for <1% of patients.
- Hemophiliacs, especially those who received large amounts of factor VIII or IX concentrates before 1985, make up less than <1% of all cases.
- The epidemiology of HIV infection and AIDS is quite different in children (diagnosed when younger than 13 years of age). About 1% of all AIDS cases occur in this population, and the vast majority (about 90%) results from vertical transmission of virus from infected mother to the fetus or newborn.

Sexual Transmission. *Sexual transmission* is by far the major mode of infection worldwide, accounting for more than 75% of all cases of HIV transmission. Although most sexually transmitted cases in the United States are still due to homosexual or bisexual male contacts, *the vast majority of sexually transmitted HIV infections globally are due to heterosexual activity.* Even in the United States, the rate of increase of heterosexual transmission has outpaced transmission by other means; such spread accounts for the dramatic increase in HIV infection in female sex partners of male intravenous drug abusers.

The virus is present in semen, both extracellularly and within mononuclear inflammatory cells, and it enters the recipient's body through lacerations or abrasions in mucosa. Viral transmission can occur either by direct entry of virus or infected cells into blood vessels breached by trauma or by uptake into mucosal DCs. Clearly, all forms of sexual transmission are aided and abetted by the concomitant presence of other sexually transmitted diseases that cause genital ulcerations, including syphilis, chancroid, and herpes simplex virus. Gonorrhea and *Chlamydia* also act as cofactors for HIV transmission, primarily by increasing the seminal fluid content of inflammatory cells (presumably carrying HIV). In addition to male-to-male and male-to-female transmission, HIV is present in the vaginal and cervical cells of infected women and can also be spread from females to males, albeit about eightfold less efficiently.

Parenteral Transmission. *Parenteral transmission* of HIV is well documented in three different groups: intravenous drug abusers (the largest group), hemophiliacs receiving factor VIII or IX concentrates, and random recipients of blood transfusion. Among intravenous drug abusers, transmission occurs through shared needles, syringes, or other paraphernalia contaminated with HIV-containing blood.

Transmission of HIV by transfusion of blood or blood products such as lyophilized factor VIII concentrates has been virtually eliminated since 1985. Four public health measures are responsible: screening of donated blood and plasma for antibody to HIV, screening for HIV-associated p24 antigen (detectable before the development of antibodies), heat treatment of clotting factor concentrates, and screening of donors on the basis of history. With all these measures, the risk of transfusion-associated HIV infection in the United States has been reduced to roughly 1 in 676,000 donations. This translates into approximately 18 out of 12 million donations that may transmit HIV. With the advent of nucleic acid testing, this already small risk will show further decline.

Mother-to-Infant Transmission. As noted earlier, mother-to-infant *vertical transmission* is the major cause of pediatric AIDS. Three routes are involved: in utero, by transplacental spread; intrapartum, during delivery; and via ingestion of HIV-contaminated breast milk. Of these, the transplacental and intrapartum routes account for most cases. Vertical transmission rates worldwide vary from 25% to 35%, with a 15% to 25% rate reported in the United States; higher rates of infection occur with high maternal viral load and/or the presence of chorioamnionitis, presumably by increasing placental accumulation of inflammatory cells.

Because of the dismal outcome of AIDS, the lay public is justifiably concerned about the spread of HIV infection outside recognized high-risk groups. Many of these anxieties can be laid to rest, as extensive studies indicate that *HIV infection cannot be transmitted by casual personal contact in the home, workplace, or school, and no convincing evidence for spread by insect bites has been obtained.* There is an extremely small but definite risk for transmission of HIV infection to health care workers. Seroconversion has been documented after accidental needle-stick injury or exposure of nonintact skin to infected blood in laboratory accidents, with a rate about 0.3% per accidental exposure. By comparison, the rate of seroconversion after accidental exposure to hepatitis B–infected blood is about 6% to 30%. Transmission of HIV from an infected health care worker to a patient is extremely rare.

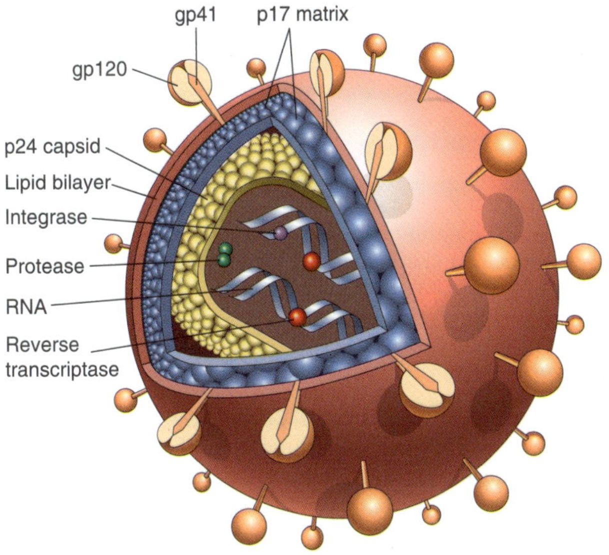

Figure 5–30

The structure of HIV. The human immune deficiency virus (HIV)-1 virion. The viral particle is covered by a lipid bilayer derived from the host cell and studded with viral glycoproteins gp41 and gp120.

Etiology

AIDS is caused by HIV, a human retrovirus belonging to the lentivirus family (which also includes feline immunodeficiency virus, simian immunodeficiency virus, visna virus of sheep, and the equine infectious anemia virus). Two genetically different but antigenically related forms of HIV, called *HIV-1* and *HIV-2,* have been isolated from patients with AIDS. HIV-1 is the more common type associated with AIDS in the United States, Europe, and Central Africa, whereas HIV-2 causes a similar disease principally in West Africa. Specific tests for HIV-2 are now available, and blood collected for transfusion is also routinely screened for HIV-2 seropositivity. The ensuing discussion relates primarily to HIV-1 and diseases caused by it, but it is generally applicable to HIV-2 as well.

Structure of HIV

Like most retroviruses, the HIV-1 virion is spherical and contains an electron-dense, cone-shaped core surrounded by a lipid envelope derived from the host cell membrane (Fig. 5–30). The virus core contains: (1) major capsid protein p24, (2) nucleocapsid protein p7/p9, (3) two copies of genomic RNA, and (4) three viral enzymes (protease, reverse transcriptase, and integrase). p24 is the most readily detected viral antigen and is therefore the target for the antibodies used to diagnose HIV infection in blood screening. The viral core is surrounded by a matrix protein called *p17,* lying beneath the virion envelope. The viral envelope itself is studded by two viral glycoproteins (gp120 and gp41), critical for HIV infection of cells. The HIV-1 proviral genome contains the *gag, pol,* and *env* genes, which code for various viral proteins. The products of the *gag* and *pol* genes are translated initially into large precursor proteins that must be cleaved by the viral protease to yield the mature proteins. The highly effective anti-HIV-1 protease inhibitor drugs thus prevent viral assembly by inhibiting the formation of mature viral proteins.

In addition to these three standard retroviral genes, HIV contains several other genes (given three-letter names such as *tat, rev, vif, nef, vpr,* and *vpu*) that regulate the synthesis and assembly of infectious viral particles. The product of the *tat* (transactivator) gene, for example, is critical for virus replication, causing a 1000-fold increase in the transcription of viral genes. The nef protein activates intracellular kinase activity (affecting T-cell activation, viral replication, and viral infectivity) and reduces surface expression of CD4 and MHC molecules on infected cells. The progression of HIV infection in vivo is dependent on *nef;* strains of simian immunodeficiency virus with mutated *nef* genes cause AIDS in monkeys at a markedly decreased rate, and humans infected with a *nef*-defective HIV-1 strain display low viral burden, with AIDS onset at a substantially slower pace than for nonmutant strains. The products of various regulatory genes are important for HIV pathogenicity, and several therapeutic approaches are being developed to block their actions.

Molecular analysis of different viral isolates reveals considerable variability in many parts of the HIV genome. This variability is due to the relatively low fidelity of the viral polymerase, with estimates of one mistake for each 10^5 replicated nucleotides. Most variations cluster in certain regions of the envelope glycoproteins. Because the immune response against HIV-1 is targeted against its envelope, such extreme variability in antigen structure poses a formidable barrier for vaccine development.

On the basis of the molecular analysis, HIV-1 can be divided into two groups, designated *M* (major) and *O* (outlier). Group M viruses, the more common form worldwide, are further divided into subtypes (also called *clades*), designated A through J. The clades differ in their geographic distribution, with B being the most common form in Western Europe and the United States and E being the most common in Thailand. Beyond molecular homologies, the clades also show differences in modes of transmission. Thus, E clade is spread predominantly by heterosexual contact (male-to-female), presumably because of its ability to infect vaginal subepithelial DCs. By contrast, B clade virus grows poorly in DCs and may be transmitted by monocytes and lymphocytes.

Pathogenesis

The two major targets of HIV infection are the immune system and the CNS. The life cycle of the virus is best understood in terms of its interactions with the immune system.

Life Cycle of HIV. *The entry of HIV into cells requires the CD4 molecule, which acts as a high-affinity receptor for the virus* (Fig. 5–31). This explains the tropism of the virus for CD4+ T cells and its ability to infect other CD4+ cells, particularly macrophages and DCs. However, binding to CD4 is not sufficient for infection; the HIV envelope gp120 must also bind to other cell surface molecules (*coreceptors*) to facilitate cell entry. Two cell surface chemokine receptors, CCR5 and CXCR4, serve this role. HIV envelope gp120 (noncovalently attached to transmembrane gp41) binds initially to CD4 molecules (see Fig. 5–31). This binding leads to a conformational change that exposes a new recognition site on gp120 for the CXCR4 (mostly on T cells) or CCR5 (mostly on macrophages) coreceptors. The gp41 then undergoes a conformational change that allows it to insert into the target membrane, and this process facilitates fusion of the virus with the cell. After fusion, the virus core containing the HIV genome enters the cytoplasm of the cell.

The coreceptors are critical components of the HIV infection process, and their discovery resolved some previously unexplained observations regarding HIV tropism. It had been known that HIV strains could be classified according to their relative ability to infect macrophages and/or CD4+ T cells. Macrophage-tropic (R5 virus) strains infect both monocytes/macrophages and freshly isolated peripheral blood T cells, whereas T-cell tropic (X4 virus) strains infect only activated T cell lines. This selectivity is now explained by selective coreceptor usage. R5 strains use CCR5 as their coreceptor, and, because CCR5 is expressed on both monocytes and T cells, these cells succumb to infection by R5 strains. Conversely, X4 strains bind to CXCR4, which is expressed on T cell lines (and not on monocytes/macrophages), so that only activated T cells are susceptible. Interestingly, approximately 90% of HIV infections are initially transmitted by R5 strains. However, over the course of infection, X4 viruses gradually accumulate; these are especially virulent and are responsible for T-cell depletion in the final rapid phase of disease progression. It is thought that during the course of HIV infection, R5 strains evolve into X4 strains, as a result of mutations in genes that encode gp120. Individuals with defective CCR5 receptors (in US whites, 20% are heterozygous and 1% are homozygous for the mutant CCR5) are relatively resistant to developing AIDS, despite repeated HIV exposure in vivo. Because of the significance of HIV-coreceptor interaction in the pathogenesis of AIDS, preventing this interaction may be of significant therapeutic importance.

Once internalized, the viral genome undergoes reverse transcription, leading to formation of complementary DNA (cDNA). In quiescent T cells, HIV proviral cDNA may remain in the cytoplasm in a linear episomal form. However, in dividing T cells, the cDNA enters the nucleus and becomes integrated into the host genome. After integration, the provirus may remain nontranscribed for months or years, and the infection becomes *latent;* alter-

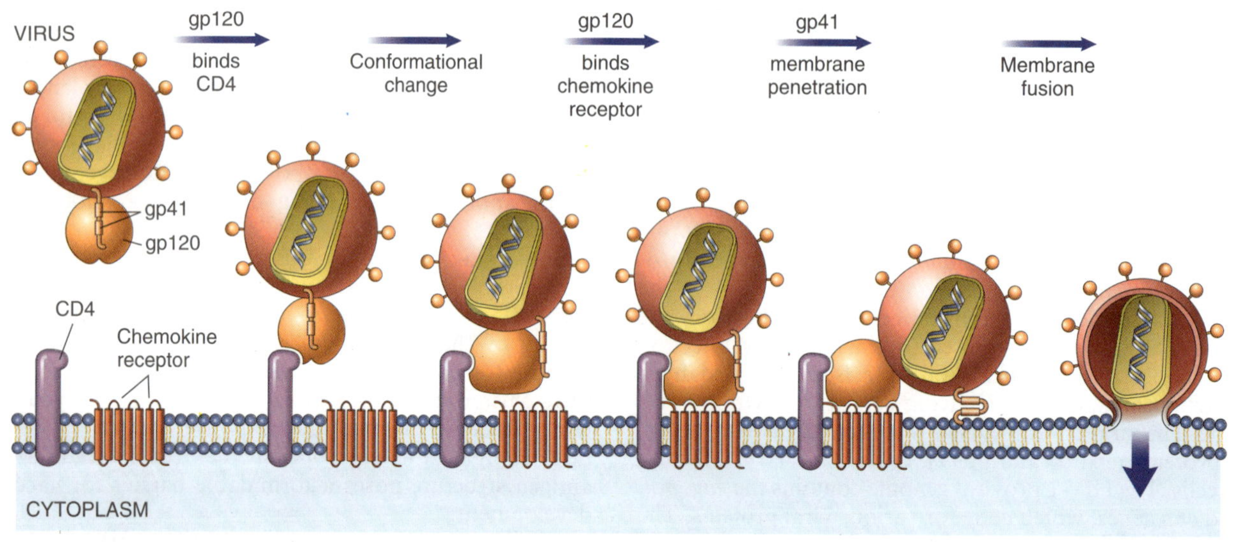

Figure 5–31

Molecular basis of HIV entry into host cells. Interactions with CD4 and a chemokine receptor ("coreceptor"). (Adapted by permission from Macmillan Publishers Ltd, from Wain-Hobson S: HIV. One on one meets two. Nature 384:117, copyright 1996.)

natively, proviral DNA may be transcribed to form complete viral particles that bud from the cell membrane. Such productive infections, associated with extensive viral budding, lead to cell death. It is important to note that although HIV-1 can infect resting T cells, the initiation of proviral DNA transcription (and hence productive infection) occurs only when the infected cell is activated by exposure to antigens or cytokines. Thus, in a cruel twist, physiologic responses to infections and other stimuli promote the death of HIV-infected T cells.

Progression of HIV Infection. *HIV disease begins with acute infection, which is only partly controlled by the host immune response, and advances to chronic progressive infection of peripheral lymphoid tissues* (Fig. 5–32). The first cell types to be infected may be memory CD4+ T cells (which express CCR5) in mucosal lymphoid tissues. Because the mucosal tissues are the largest reservoir of T cells in the body and a major site of residence of memory T cells, the death of these cells results in considerable depletion of lymphocytes.

The transition from the acute phase to a chronic phase of infection is characterized by dissemination of the virus, viremia, and the development of host immune responses. Dendritic cells in epithelia at sites of virus entry capture the virus and then migrate into the lymph nodes. Once in lymphoid tissues, dendritic cells may pass HIV on to CD4+ T cells through direct cell-cell contact. Within days after the first exposure to HIV, viral replication can be detected in the lymph nodes. This replication leads to viremia, during which high numbers of HIV particles are present in the patient's blood, accompanied by an acute HIV syndrome that includes a variety of nonspecific signs and symptoms typical of many viral diseases. The virus disseminates throughout the body and infects helper T cells, macrophages, and dendritic cells in peripheral lymphoid tissues. As the infection spreads, the immune system mounts both humoral and cell-mediated immune responses directed at viral antigens. These immune responses partially control the infection and viral production, and such control is reflected by a drop in viremia to low but detectable levels by about 12 weeks after the primary exposure.

In the next, chronic phase of the disease, lymph nodes and the spleen are sites of continuous HIV replication and cell destruction (see Fig. 5–32). During this period of the disease, the immune system remains competent at handling most infections with opportunistic microbes, and few or no clinical manifestations of the HIV infection are present. Therefore, this phase of HIV disease is called the *clinical latency period.* Although the majority of peripheral blood T cells do not harbor the virus, destruction of CD4+ T cells within lymphoid tissues steadily progresses during the latent period, and the number of circulating blood CD4+ T cells steadily declines. More than 90% of the body's approximately 10^{12} T cells are normally found in lymphoid tissues, and it is estimated that HIV destroys up to 1 to 2 × 10^9 CD4+ T cells every day. Early in the course of the disease, the body may continue to make new CD4+ T cells, and therefore CD4+ T cells can be replaced almost as quickly as they are destroyed. At this stage, up to 10% of CD4+ T cells in lymphoid organs may be infected, but the number of circulating CD4+ T cells that are infected at any one time may be less than 0.1% of the total CD4+ T cells in an individual. Eventually, over a period of years, the continuous cycle of virus infection and T cell death leads to

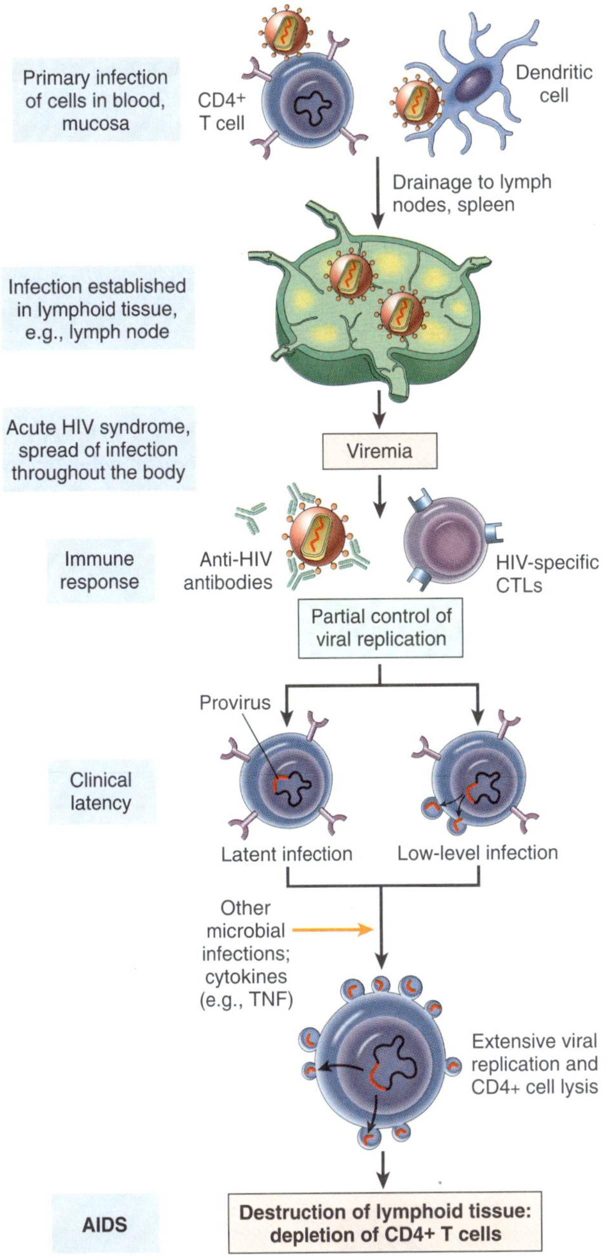

Figure 5–32

Pathogenesis of HIV infection. Initially, HIV infects T cells and macrophages directly or is carried to these cells by Langerhans cells. Viral replication in the regional lymph nodes leads to viremia and widespread seeding of lymphoid tissue. The viremia is controlled by the host immune response (not shown), and the patient then enters a phase of clinical latency. During this phase, viral replication in both T cells and macrophages continues unabated, but there is some immune containment of virus (not illustrated). There continues a gradual erosion of CD4+ cells by productive infection (or other mechanisms, not shown). Ultimately, CD4+ cell numbers decline and the patient develops clinical symptoms of full-blown AIDS. Macrophages are also parasitized by the virus early; they are not lysed by HIV and they transport the virus to tissues, particularly the brain.

a steady decline in the number of CD4+ T cells in the lymphoid tissues and the circulation.

In addition to T-cell depletion, abnormalities have been described in many components of the immune system (summarized in Table 5–10). Below we describe the major defects in immune cells during the course of HIV infection.

Mechanisms of T-cell Depletion in HIV Infection. *The major mechanism of loss of CD4+ T cells is lytic HIV infection of the cells, and cell death during viral replication and production of virions* (Fig. 5–33). Like other cytopathic viruses, HIV disrupts cellular functions sufficiently to cause death of infected cells. In addition to direct cell lysis, other mechanisms may cause T-cell loss:

- Loss of immature precursors of CD4+ T cells, either by direct infection of thymic progenitor cells or by infection of accessory cells that secrete cytokines essential for CD4+ T-cell maturation. The result is decreased production of mature CD4+ T cells.
- Chronic activation of uninfected cells by HIV antigens or by other concurrent infectious microbes may lead to apoptosis of the T cells. Because of this "activation-induced death" of uninfected cells, the numbers of T cells that die may be much greater than the number of HIV-infected cells.
- Infection of various cells in lymphoid tissues may disrupt the normal architecture, leading to impaired immune responses.
- Fusion of infected and uninfected cells causes formation of syncytia (giant cells). In tissue culture, the

Table 5–10 Major Abnormalities of Immune Function in AIDS

Lymphopenia
Predominantly caused by selective loss of the CD4 helper T-cell subset; inversion of CD4:CD8 ratio
Decreased T-Cell Function in Vivo
Preferential loss of activated and memory T cells Decreased delayed-type hypersensitivity Susceptibility to opportunistic infections Susceptibility to neoplasms
Altered T-Cell Function in Vitro
Decreased proliferative response to mitogens, alloantigens, and soluble antigens Decreased cytotoxicity Decreased helper function for B-cell antibody production Decreased IL-2 AND IFN-γ production
Altered Monocyte or Macrophage Functions
Decreased chemotaxis and phagocytosis Decreased HLA class II antigen expression Diminished capacity to present antigen to T cells Increased spontaneous secretion of IL-1, TNF, IL-6
Polyclonal B-Cell Activation
Hypergammaglobulinemia and circulating immune complexes Inability to mount de novo antibody response to a new antigen Poor responses to normal signals for B-cell activation in vitro

IFN-γ, interferon-γ; IL-1, interleukin-1; TNF, tumor necrosis factor.

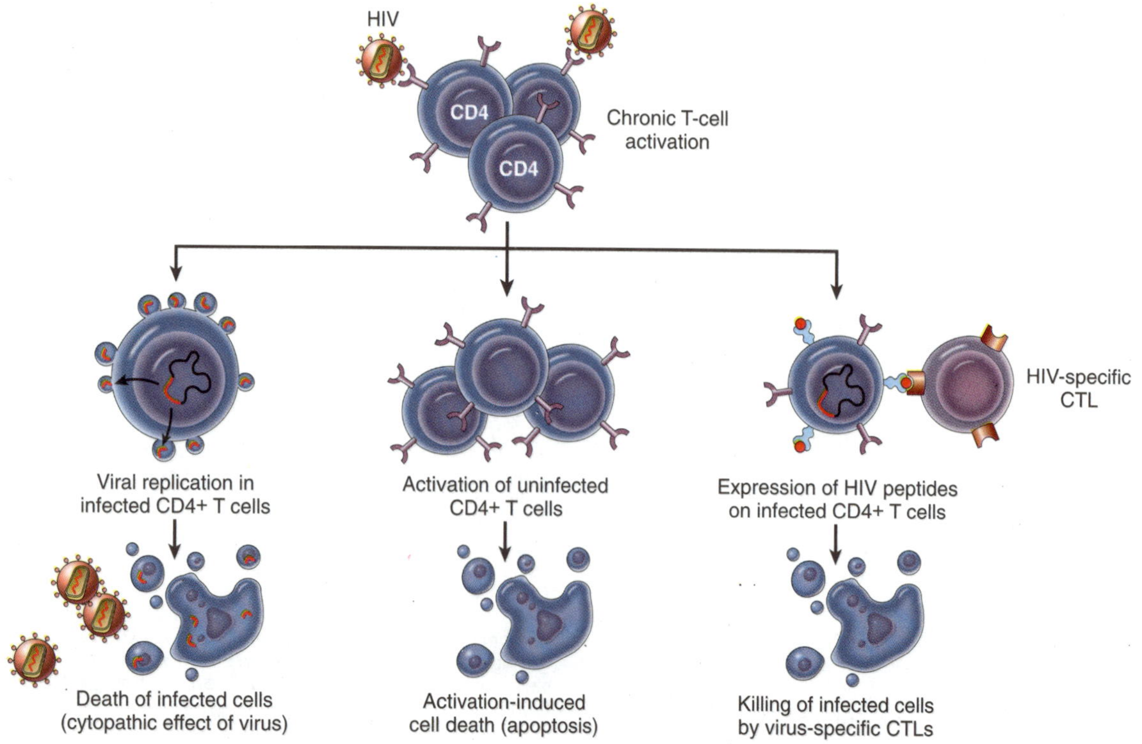

Figure 5–33

Mechanisms of CD4 cell loss in HIV infection. Some of the principal known and postulated mechanisms of T-cell depletion after HIV infection are shown.

gp120 expressed on productively infected cells binds to CD4 molecules on uninfected T cells, followed by cell fusion, ballooning, and death within a few hours. This property of syncytia formation is confined to the X4 strain of HIV.

- Uninfected CD4+ T cells may bind soluble gp120 to the CD4 molecule, leading to aberrant signaling and apoptosis.
- Infected CD4+ T cells may be killed by HIV-specific CD8+ CTLs.

The loss of CD4+ cells leads to an inversion of the CD4:CD8 ratio in the peripheral blood. Thus, while the normal CD4:CD8 ratio is close to 2, patients with AIDS have a ratio of 0.5. Such inversion is a common finding in AIDS, but it may also occur in other viral infections and is therefore not diagnostic.

Although marked reduction in CD4+ T cells is a hallmark of AIDS and can account for much of the immune deficiency late in the course of HIV infection, there is also compelling evidence for *qualitative defects in T-cell function that can be detected even in asymptomatic HIV-infected persons.* Such defects include reduced antigen-induced T-cell proliferation, impaired T_H1 cytokine production, and abnormal intracellular signaling. There is also a selective loss of memory CD4+ T cells early in the course of the disease, possibly related to the higher level of CCR5 expression in this T-cell subset.

Low-level chronic or latent infection of T cells (and macrophages) is an important feature of HIV infection. Although only rare CD4+ T cells express infectious virus early in the course of infection, up to 30% of lymph node T cells can be demonstrated to actually harbor the HIV genome. It is widely believed that integrated provirus, without virus production (*latent infection*), can persist within cells for months or years. Even with highly active antiretroviral therapy (which can eliminate most of the virus in the blood), latent virus lurks in lymph node CD4+ cells (as many as 0.05% of resting, long-lived CD4+ T cells are infected). *Completion of the viral life cycle in latently infected cells requires cell activation.* Thus, if latently infected CD4+ cells are activated by environmental antigens, an unfortunate consequence is increased HIV proviral DNA transcription. This leads to virion production and, in the case of T cells, also results in cell lysis. In addition, TNF, IL-1, and IL-6 produced by activated macrophages during normal immune responses can also lead to increased HIV gene transcription (see Fig. 5–32). Thus, it seems that HIV thrives when the host macrophages and T cells are physiologically activated (e.g., via intercurrent infection by other microbial agents). The life styles of most HIV-infected patients in the United States place them at increased risk for recurrent exposure to other sexually transmitted diseases; in Africa, socioeconomic conditions probably impose a higher burden of chronic microbial infections. It is easy to understand how AIDS patients develop a vicious cycle of T-cell destruction: infections to which these patients are prone because of diminished helper T-cell function lead to increased production of proinflammatory cytokines, which, in turn, stimulate more HIV production, followed by infection and loss of additional CD4+ T cells.

Monocytes/Macrophages in HIV Infection. In addition to infection of CD4+ T cells, infection of monocytes and macrophages is also extremely important in the pathogenesis of HIV disease. Similar to T cells, most of the HIV-infected macrophages are found in the tissues and not in peripheral blood. As many as 10% to 50% of macrophages in certain tissues, such as brain and lungs, may be infected. Several additional aspects of macrophage HIV infection warrant emphasis:

- Although cell division is required for integration and subsequent replication of most retroviruses, HIV-1 can infect and multiply in terminally differentiated nondividing macrophages, a property conferred by the HIV-1 *vpr* gene.
- Infected macrophages bud relatively small amounts of virus from the cell surface but contain large numbers of virus particles located in intracellular vesicles.
- In contrast to CD4+ T cells, macrophages are quite resistant to the cytopathic effects of HIV and can, therefore, harbor the virus for long periods.
- In more than 90% of cases, HIV infection is transmitted by R5 strains. The more virulent X4 strains that evolve later in the course of HIV infection are inefficient in transmitting HIV. This suggests that the initial infection of macrophages (or DCs) is critical for HIV transmission.

Thus, in all likelihood, macrophages are the gatekeepers of HIV infection. Besides providing a portal for initial transmission, monocytes and macrophages are viral reservoirs and factories, whose output remains largely protected from host defenses. Circulating monocytes also provide a vehicle for HIV transport to various parts of the body, particularly the nervous system. In late stages of HIV infection, when the CD4+ T-cell numbers are massively depleted, macrophages remain a major site of continued viral replication. Although the number of HIV-infected monocytes in the circulation is low, their functional deficits (e.g., impaired microbicidal activity, decreased chemotaxis, abnormal cytokine production, and diminished antigen presentation capacity) have important bearing on host defenses.

DCs in HIV Infection. In addition to macrophages, two types of DCs are also important targets for the initiation and maintenance of HIV infection: mucosal and follicular DCs. As discussed earlier, DCs in mucosal epithelia capture the virus and transport it to regional lymph nodes, where CD4+ T cells are infected. Follicular DCs in the germinal centers of lymph nodes are important reservoirs of HIV. Although some follicular DCs are infected by HIV, most virus particles are found on the surface of their dendritic processes, including bound to Fc receptors via HIV/anti-HIV antibody complexes. The antibody-coated virions localized to follicular DCs retain the ability to infect CD4+ T cells. HIV infection of macrophages and DCs may also impair the functions of these cell populations, with secondary effects on T-cell responsiveness.

B Cells and Other Lymphocytes in HIV Infection. Although much attention has been focused on T cells and macrophages, patients with AIDS also display profound abnormalities of B-cell function. Paradoxically, these patients have hypergammaglobulinemia and circulating immune complexes as a result of polyclonal B-cell activation. This may result from multiple factors, including infection with CMV or EBV, both of which are polyclonal B-cell activators. The HIV gp41 itself can promote B-cell growth and differentiation, and HIV-infected macrophages produce increased amounts of IL-6, which drives B-cell activation. Despite the presence of spontaneously activated B cells, patients with AIDS are unable to mount antibody responses to newly encountered antigens. Not only is this attributable to deficient T-cell help, but antibody responses against T-independent antigens are also suppressed, suggesting additional B-cell defects. Impaired humoral immunity renders these patients susceptible to encapsulated bacteria (e.g., *S. pneumoniae* and *H. influenzae*) that require antibodies for effective opsonization and clearance.

CD4+ T cells play a pivotal role in regulating the immune response: they produce a plethora of cytokines, chemotactic factors, and hematopoietic growth factors (e.g., granulocyte-macrophage colony-stimulating factor). Therefore, loss of this "master cell" has ripple effects on virtually every other cell of the immune system, as summarized in Table 5–10.

Pathogenesis of CNS Involvement. The pathogenesis of the neurologic manifestations in AIDS deserves special mention because, in addition to the lymphoid system, the nervous system is a major target of HIV infection. Macrophages and cells belonging to the monocyte and macrophage lineage (microglia) are the predominant cell types in the brain that are infected with HIV. The virus is most likely carried into the brain by infected monocytes (thus, brain HIV isolates are almost exclusively of the R5 type). The mechanism of HIV-induced damage of the brain, however, remains obscure. Because neurons are not infected by HIV, and the extent of neuropathologic changes is often less than might be expected from the severity of neurologic symptoms, most experts believe that the neurologic deficit is caused indirectly by viral products and soluble factors (e.g., cytokines such as TNF) produced by macrophages/microglia. In addition, nitric oxide induced in neuronal cells by gp41 and direct damage of neurons by soluble HIV gp120 have been postulated.

SUMMARY

HIV Life Cycle and the Pathogenesis of AIDS

- *Virus entry into cells:* requires CD4 and co-receptors, which are receptors for chemokines; involves binding of viral gp120 and fusion with the cell mediated by viral gp41 protein; main cellular targets are CD4+ helper T cells, macrophages, and DCs
- *Viral replication:* provirus genome integrates into host cell DNA; viral gene expression is triggered by stimuli that activate infected cells (e.g., infectious microbes, cytokines produced during normal immune responses)
- *Progression of infection:* acute infection of mucosal T cells and DCs; viremia with dissemination of virus; latent infection of cells in lymphoid tissue; continuing viral replication and progressive loss of CD4+ T cells.
- *Mechanisms of immune deficiency:*
  - Loss of CD4+ T cells: T-cell death during viral replication and budding (similar to other cytopathic infections); apoptosis as a result of chronic stimulation; decreased thymic output; functional defects
  - Defective macrophage and DC functions
  - Destruction of architecture of lymphoid tissues (late)

Natural History of HIV Infection

The clinical course of HIV infection can best be understood in terms of an interplay between HIV and the immune system. Three phases reflecting the dynamics of virus–host interaction can be recognized: (1) an early *acute phase,* (2) a middle *chronic phase,* and (3) a final *crisis phase* (Fig. 5–34).

- The *acute phase* represents the initial response of an immunocompetent adult to HIV infection. Clinically, this is typically a self-limited illness that develops in 50% to 70% of adults 3 to 6 weeks after infection; it is characterized by nonspecific symptoms including sore throat, myalgia, fever, rash, and sometimes aseptic meningitis. This phase is also characterized by high levels of virus production, viremia, and widespread seeding of the peripheral lymphoid tissues, typically with a modest reduction in CD4+ T cells. Soon, however, a virus-specific immune response develops, evidenced by seroconversion (usually within 3 to 17 weeks of exposure) and by the development of virus-specific CD8+ CTLs. As viremia abates, CD4+ T cells return to nearly normal numbers. However, the reduction in plasma virus does not signal the end of viral replication, which continues within CD4+ T cells and macrophages in the tissues (particularly lymphoid organs).
- The middle, *chronic phase* represents a stage of relative containment of the virus. The immune system is largely intact at this point, but there is *continued HIV replication that may last for several years.* Patients either are asymptomatic or develop persistent lymphadenopathy, and many patients have "minor" opportunistic infections such as thrush (*Candida*) or herpes zoster. During this phase, viral replication in the lymphoid tissues continues unabated. The extensive viral turnover is associated with continued loss of CD4+ cells, but a large proportion of the CD4+ cells is replenished and the decline of CD4+ cells in the peripheral blood is modest. After an extended and variable period, the number of CD4+ cells begins to decline, the proportion of the surviving CD4+ cells

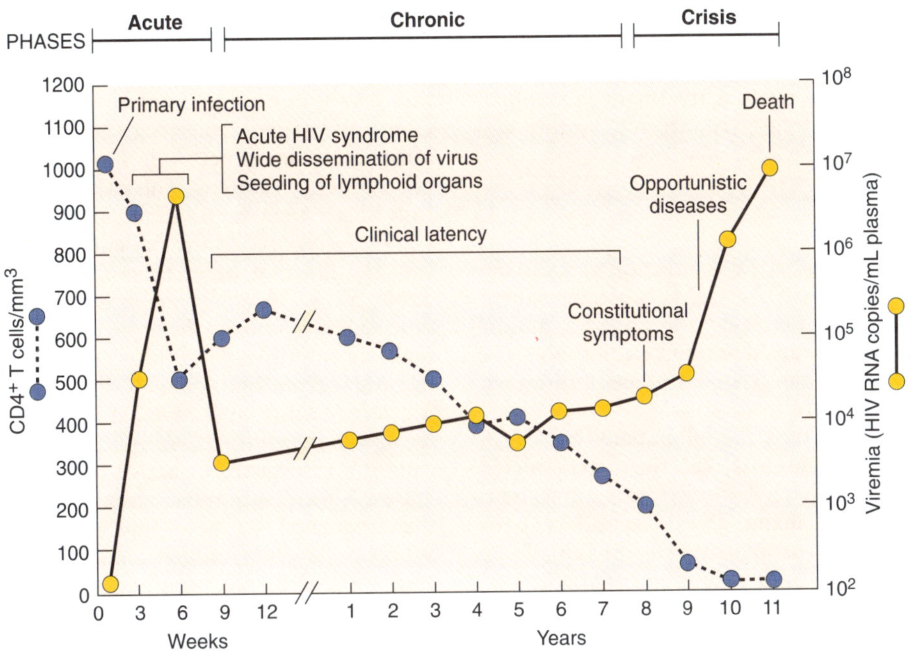

Figure 5–34

Clinical course of HIV infection. During the early period after primary infection, there is widespread dissemination of virus and a sharp decrease in the number of CD4+ T cells in peripheral blood. An immune response to HIV ensues, with a decrease in viremia followed by a prolonged period of clinical latency. During this period, viral replication continues. The CD4+ T-cell count gradually decreases during the subsequent years, until it reaches a critical level below which there is a substantial risk of opportunistic diseases. (Redrawn from Fauci AS, Lane I-IC: Human immunodeficiency virus disease: AIDS and related conditions. In Fauci AS, et al (eds): Harrison's Principles of Internal Medicine, 14th ed. New York, McGraw-Hill, 1997, p 1791. Reproduced with permission of The McGraw-Hill Companies.)

infected with HIV increases, and host defenses begin to wane. Persistent lymphadenopathy with significant constitutional symptoms (fever, rash, fatigue) reflects the onset of immune system decompensation, escalation of viral replication, and the onset of the "crisis" phase.

- The final, *crisis phase* is characterized by a catastrophic breakdown of host defenses, a marked increase in viremia, and clinical disease. Typically, patients present with fever of more than 1 month's duration, fatigue, weight loss, and diarrhea; the CD4+ cell count is reduced below 500 cells/μL. After a variable interval, patients develop serious opportunistic infections, secondary neoplasms, and/or neurologic manifestations (so-called *AIDS-defining conditions*), and the patient is said to have full-blown AIDS. Even if the usual AIDS-defining conditions are not manifest, Centers for Disease Control (CDC) guidelines define any HIV-infected individual with CD4+ cell counts less than or equal to 200 per microliter as having AIDS.

In the absence of treatment, most patients with HIV infection develop AIDS after a chronic phase lasting 7 to 10 years. Exceptions to this include *rapid progressors* and long-term *nonprogressors*. In rapid progressors, the middle, chronic phase is telescoped to 2 to 3 years after primary infection. Nonprogressors (fewer than 5% of infected persons) are defined as HIV-infected individuals who remain asymptomatic for 10 years or more, with stable CD4+ counts and low levels of plasma viremia; notably, AIDS eventually develops in the majority of these patients, albeit after a much prolonged clinical latency. Despite much study, the reason for nonprogression is not known.

Because the loss of immune containment is associated with declining CD4+ T-cell counts, the CDC classification of HIV infection stratifies patients into three categories on the basis of CD4+ T-cell counts: more than 500 cells/μL, between 200 and 500 cells/μL, and less than 200 cells/μL. Patients in the first group are generally asymptomatic; counts below 500 cells/μL are associated with early symptoms, and a decline of CD4+ T-cell levels below 200 cells/μL is associated with severe immunosuppression. For clinical management, CD4+ cell counts are an important adjunct to HIV viral load measurements. The significance of these two measurements, however, is slightly different: whereas CD4+ cell counts indicate the status of the patient's disease at the time of measurement, the viral load provides information about the direction in which the disease is progressing.

It should be evident from our discussion that in each of the three phases of HIV infection viral replication continues to occur at a fairly brisk rate. Even in the middle, chronic phase, before the severe decline in the CD4+ cell count, there is extensive viral production. In other words, *HIV infection lacks a phase of true microbiologic latency,* that is, a phase during which *all* the HIV is in the form of proviral DNA and no cell is productively infected. Multiple-drug antiretroviral therapy has dramatically slowed the progression of the disease and the frequency of opportunistic infections and other complications. However, the available therapy does not eliminate all the virus, and the disease can recur if treatment is stopped. It is also not known if drug-resistant viral strains will become widespread.

Clinical Features

The clinical manifestations of HIV infection range from a mild acute illness to severe disease. Because the salient clinical features of the acute, early and chronic, middle phases of HIV infection were described earlier, only the clinical manifestations of the terminal phase, full-blown AIDS, are summarized here.

In the United States the typical adult patient with AIDS presents with fever, weight loss, diarrhea, generalized lymphadenopathy, multiple opportunistic infections, neurologic disease, and (in many cases) secondary neoplasms. The infections and neoplasms listed in Table 5–11 are included in the surveillance definition of AIDS.

Opportunistic Infections. Opportunistic infections have accounted for approximately 80% of deaths in patients with AIDS. Their spectrum is constantly changing, and their incidence is decreasing markedly as a result of more effective highly active antiretroviral therapy. A brief summary of selected opportunistic infections is provided here.

Pneumonia caused by the opportunistic fungus *Pneumocystis jiroveci* (representing reactivation of a previous latent infection) is the presenting feature in many cases, although its incidence is declining as a result of effective prophylactic regimens. The risk of developing this infection is extremely high in individuals with fewer than 200 CD4+ T cells/μL. Many patients present with an opportunistic infection other than *P. jiroveci* pneumonia (see Table 5–11). Among the most common are recurrent mucosal candidiasis, disseminated CMV infection (particularly enteritis and retinitis), severe ulcerating oral and perianal herpes simplex, and disseminated infection with *M. tuberculosis* and atypical mycobacteria *(Mycobacterium avium-intracellulare)*. The AIDS epidemic has caused a resurgence of active tuberculosis in the United States. Although in most cases it represents reactivation, the frequency of new infections is also increasing. Whereas *M. tuberculosis* manifests itself early in the course of AIDS, infections with atypical mycobacteria are seen late in the course of HIV disease, usually occurring in patients with fewer than 100 CD4+ cells/μL. Toxoplasmosis is the most common secondary infection of the CNS. Cryptococcal meningitis is also quite frequent. Persistent diarrhea, which is common in patients with AIDS, is often caused by *Cryptosporidium* or *Isospora belli* infections, but bacterial pathogens such as *Salmonella* species and *Shigella* species may also be involved. Because of depressed humoral immunity, AIDS patients are susceptible to infections with *S. pneumoniae* and *H. influenzae.*

Table 5–11 AIDS-Defining Opportunistic Infections and Neoplasms Found in Patients with HIV Infection

Infections
PROTOZOAL AND HELMINTHIC INFECTIONS
Cryptosporidiosis or isosporidiosis (enteritis)
Pneumocystosis (pneumonia or disseminated infection)
Toxoplasmosis (pneumonia or CNS infection)
FUNGAL INFECTIONS
Candidiasis (esophageal, tracheal, or pulmonary)
Cryptococcosis (CNS infection)
Coccidioidomycosis (disseminated)
Histoplasmosis (disseminated)
BACTERIAL INFECTIONS
Mycobacteriosis ("atypical," e.g., *Mycobacterium avium-intracellulare,* disseminated or extrapulmonary; *M. tuberculosis,*pulmonary or extrapulmonary)
Nocardiosis (pneumonia, meningitis, disseminated)
Salmonella infections, disseminated
VIRAL INFECTIONS
Cytogegalovirus (pulmonary, intestinal, retinitis, or CNS infections)
Herpes simplex virus (localized or disseminated)
Varicella-zoster virus (localized or disseminated)
Progressive multifocal leukoencephalopathy
Neoplasms
Kaposi sacroma
Non-Hodgkin lymphomas (Burkitt, immunoblastic)
Primary lymphoma of brain
Invasive cancer of uterine cervix

CNS, central nervous system.

Neoplasms. Patients with AIDS have a high incidence of certain tumors, particularly Kaposi sarcoma (KS), non-Hodgkin lymphomas, and cervical cancer in women. The basis of the increased risk of malignancy is multifactorial: profound defects in T-cell immunity, dysregulated B-cell and monocyte functions, and multiple infections with known (e.g., human herpesvirus type 8, EBV, human papillomavirus) and unknown viruses.

KS, a vascular tumor that is otherwise rare in the United States (Chapter 10), is the most common neoplasm in AIDS patients (although its incidence has decreased significantly with anti-retroviral therapy). The tumor is far more common among homosexual or bisexual males than in intravenous drug abusers or patients belonging to other risk groups. The lesions can arise early, before the immune system is compromised, or in advanced stages of HIV infection. Unlike the lesions in sporadic cases of KS, those that occur in AIDS patients are multicentric and tend to be more aggressive; they can affect the skin, mucous membranes, gastrointestinal tract, lymph nodes, and lungs. The lesions contain spindle cells that share features with endothelial cells and smooth muscle cells and are believed to be lymphatic endothelial cells or mesenchymal cells that can form vascular channels. In different patients, the lesions are monoclonal or oligoclonal or even polyclonal, indicating that KS is not always a typical tumor.

KS is caused by a herpesvirus called Kaposi sarcoma herpesvirus (KSHV) or human herpesvirus-8 (HHV-8).

The mechanisms linking infection with this virus to the vascular lesions are unknown. One hypothesis is that KSHV infects lymphatic endothelial or other cells, and in concert with cytokines produced by HIV-infected immune cells, stimulates proliferation of the vascular cells. The KSHV genome contains homologues of several human genes known to affect cellular survival and proliferation. Why the proliferating cells develop some features of tumors is unclear.

Non-Hodgkin lymphomas constitute the second most common type of AIDS-associated tumors. These tumors are highly aggressive, occur most frequently in severely immunosuppressed patients, and involve many extranodal sites. The brain is the most common extranodal site, and hence primary lymphoma of the brain is considered an AIDS-defining condition. In keeping with their aggressive clinical course, most such lymphomas have a diffuse large-cell histologic picture (Chapter 12). As with the majority of other diffuse large-cell lymphomas, those that occur in the setting of AIDS are primarily of B-cell origin. At least in some cases (30% to 40%), these lymphomas are associated with EBV and progress from polyclonal to monoclonal B-cell lesions. Another less common AIDS-related lymphoma is the body cavity lymphoma that is also associated with KSHV infection; it grows exclusively in body cavities in the form of pleural, peritoneal, and pericardial effusions.

Cervical carcinoma is also increased in patients with AIDS. This is attributable to a high prevalence of human papillomavirus infection in patients with AIDS whose immune systems are compromised. This virus is believed to be intimately associated with squamous cell carcinoma of the cervix and its precursor lesions, cervical dysplasia and carcinoma in situ (Chapter 19). Hence, gynecologic examination should be part of the routine evaluation of HIV-infected women.

CNS Involvement. Involvement of the CNS is a common and important manifestation of AIDS. At autopsy 90% of patients show some form of neurologic involvement, and 40% to 60% have clinically evident neurologic dysfunction. Significantly, in some patients neurologic manifestations may be the sole or earliest presenting feature of HIV infection. In addition to opportunistic infections and neoplasms, several virally determined neuropathologic changes occur. These include an aseptic meningitis occurring at the time of seroconversion, vacuolar myelopathy, peripheral neuropathies, and (most commonly) a progressive encephalopathy clinically designated the *AIDS-dementia complex* (Chapter 23).

Morphology

The anatomic changes in the tissues (with the exception of lesions in the brain) are neither specific nor diagnostic. In general, the pathologic features of AIDS are those of widespread opportunistic infections, KS, and lymphoid tumors. Most of these lesions are discussed elsewhere, because they also occur in patients who do not have HIV infection. To appreciate the distinctive nature of lesions in the CNS, they are discussed in the context of other disorders affecting the brain (Chapter 23). Here the focus is on changes in the lymphoid organs.

Biopsy specimens from enlarged lymph nodes in the early stages of HIV infection reveal a **marked follicular hyperplasia** (Chapter 12). The medulla contains abundant **plasma cells**. These changes, affecting primarily the B-cell areas of the node, are the morphologic counterparts of the polyclonal B-cell activation and hypergammaglobulinemia seen in AIDS patients. In addition to changes in the follicles, the sinuses show increased cellularity, due primarily to increased numbers of macrophages but also contributed to by B-cell lymphoblasts and plasma cells. HIV particles can be demonstrated within the germinal centers, concentrated on the villous processes of the follicular DCs. Viral DNA can also be detected in macrophages and CD4+ T cells.

With disease progression, the frenzy of B-cell proliferation gives way to a pattern of severe follicular involution and generalized lymphocyte depletion. The organized network of follicular DCs is disrupted, and the follicles may even become hyalinized. These "burnt-out" lymph nodes are atrophic and small and may harbor numerous opportunistic pathogens. Because of profound immunosuppression, the inflammatory response to infections both in the lymph nodes and at extranodal sites may be sparse or atypical. For example, with severe immunosuppression, mycobacteria do not evoke granuloma formation, because CD4+ T cells are lacking. In the empty-looking lymph nodes and in other organs, the presence of infectious agents may not be readily apparent without the application of special stains. As might be expected, lymphoid depletion is not confined to the nodes; in the later stages of AIDS, the spleen and thymus also appear to be "wastelands."

Non-Hodgkin lymphomas, involving the nodes as well as extranodal sites such as liver, gastrointestinal tract, and bone marrow, are primarily high-grade diffuse B-cell neoplasms (Chapter 12).

Since the emergence of AIDS in 1981, the concerted efforts of epidemiologists, immunologists, and molecular biologists have resulted in spectacular advances in our understanding of this disorder. Despite all this progress, however, the prognosis of patients with AIDS remains poor. Although the mortality rate has begun to decline in the United States as a result of the use of potent combinations of antiretroviral drugs, all treated patients still carry viral DNA in their lymphoid tissues. Can there be a cure with persistent virus? Although a considerable effort has been mounted to develop a vaccine, many hurdles remain to be crossed before vaccine-based prophylaxis or treatment becomes a reality. Molecular analyses have revealed an alarming degree of variation in viral isolates from different patients, rendering vaccine development even more difficult. A further complication to this task is that the nature of the protective immune response is not yet fully understood. Consequently, at present, prevention and effective public health measures, combined with antiretroviral therapy, are the mainstays in the fight against AIDS.

AMYLOIDOSIS

Amyloidosis is a condition associated with a number of inherited and inflammatory disorders in which extracellular deposits of fibrillar proteins are responsible for tissue damage and functional compromise. These abnormal fibrils are produced by the aggregation of misfolded proteins (which are soluble in their normal folded configuration). The fibrillar deposits bind a wide variety of proteoglycans and glycosaminoglycans, including heparan sulfate and dermatan sulfate, and plasma proteins, notably serum amyloid P component (SAP). The presence of abundant charged sugar groups in these adsorbed proteins give the deposits staining characteristics that were thought to resemble starch (amylose). Therefore, the deposits were called *amyloid,* a name that is firmly entrenched despite the realization that the deposits are unrelated to "starch."

Pathogenesis of Amyloid Deposition. *Amyloidosis is fundamentally a disorder of protein misfolding.* Amyloid is not a structurally homogeneous protein, although it always has the same morphologic appearance. In fact, more than 20 (at last count, 23) different proteins can aggregate and form fibrils with the appearance of amyloid. Regardless of their derivation, all amyloid deposits are composed of nonbranching fibrils, 7.5 to 10 nm in diameter, each formed of β-sheet polypeptide chains that are wound together (Fig. 5–35). The dye Congo red binds to these fibrils and produces a red–green dichroism (birefringence), which is commonly used to identify amyloid desposits in tissues.

Several factors may contribute to the aggregation of certain proteins and the formation of fibrils that deposit in extracellular tissues (Fig. 5–36).

- The protein may have a tendency to form aggregates of misfolded forms but does so only when its concentration reaches abnormally high levels. This may happen as an individual ages (senile amyloidosis), or when its production is increased (e.g., in chronic inflammatory states), or if excretion of the protein is impaired (amyloidosis associated with long-term dialysis).
- A mutation may give rise to a form of a protein that has a tendency to fold improperly and form aggregates (hereditary amyloidosis).
- Limited proteolysis may generate a protein that forms amyloid fibrils (amyloidosis associated with Alzheimer disease).

Of the more than 20 biochemically distinct forms of amyloid proteins that have been identified, three are most common:

- The *AL (amyloid light chain) protein* is produced by plasma cells and is made up of complete immunoglobulin (Ig) light chains, the amino-terminal fragments of light chains, or both. Only a few types of Ig light chains are prone to forming aggregates, probably because they contain amino acid residues that destabilize the domain structure. As expected, the deposition of amyloid fibril protein of the AL type is associated with some form of monoclonal B-cell proliferation.
- The *AA (amyloid-associated) fibril* is a unique nonimmunoglobulin protein derived from a larger (12-kD) serum precursor called *SAA (serum amyloid-associated) protein* that is synthesized in the liver. The production of this protein is increased in inflammatory states as part of the "acute phase response"; therefore this form of amyloidosis is associated with chronic inflammatory disorders. Increased production of SAA is probably not sufficient to generate amyloid deposits. It is believed that SAA is normally degraded to soluble end products by macrophage-derived enzymes. Defective proteolysis may produce misfolded, incompletely degraded SAA, leading to aggregation and deposition as AA fibrils. Although this is a plausible hypothesis, specific enzymatic defects have not been identified in any patient.
- *Aβ amyloid* is found in the cerebral lesions of *Alzheimer disease.* Aβ is a 4-kD peptide that constitutes the core of cerebral plaques and the amyloid deposits in cerebral blood vessels in this disease. The Aβ protein is derived from a much larger transmembrane glycoprotein called *amyloid precursor protein* (APP) (Chapter 23).

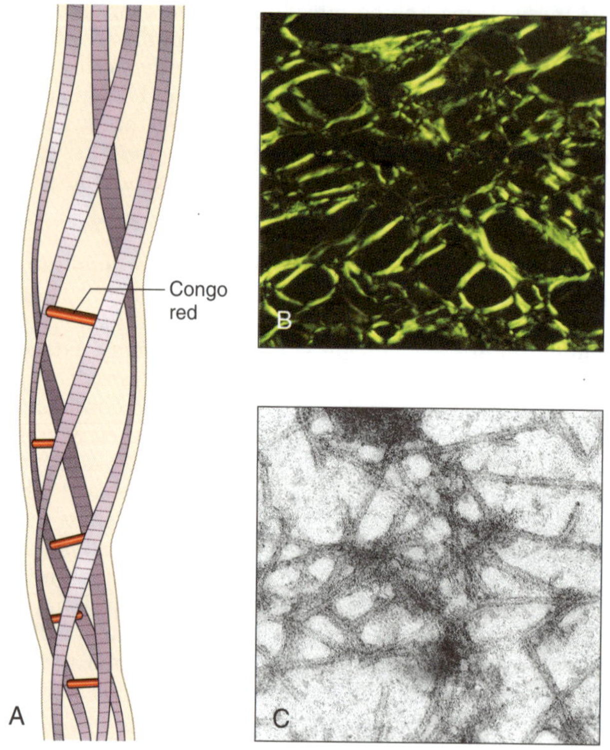

Figure 5–35

Structure of amyloid. **A,** Schematic diagram of an amyloid fiber showing fibrils (4 shown, may be up to 6) wound around one another with regularly spaced binding of the Congo red dye. **B,** Congo red staining shows an apple-green birefringence under polarized light, a diagnostic feature of amyloid. **C,** Electron micrograph of 7.5–10 nm amyloid fibrils. (Reproduced from Merlini, G. and Bellotti, V. Molecular mechanisms of amyloidosis. New Engl J Med 349:583–596, 2003. Copyright 2003 Massachusetts Medical Society. All rights reserved.)

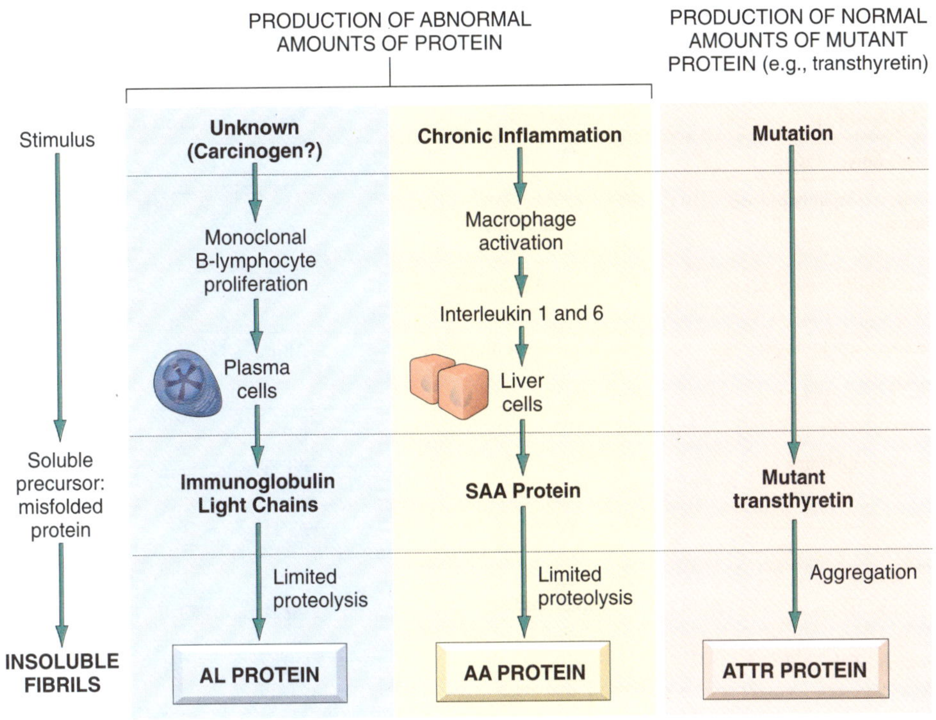

Figure 5–36

Pathogenesis of amyloidosis. The proposed mechanisms underlying deposition of the major forms of amyloid fibrils.

Several other proteins have been found in amyloid deposits in a variety of clinical settings:

- *Transthyretin* (TTR) is a normal serum protein that binds and transports thyroxine and retinol, hence the name. Mutations in the gene encoding transthyretin result in the production of a protein (and its fragments) that aggregate and form amyloid deposits. The resultant diseases are called *familial amyloid polyneuropathies*. Transthyretin is also deposited in the heart of aged individuals (senile systemic amyloidosis); in such cases the protein is structurally normal, but it accumulates at high concentrations. Some cases of familial amyloidosis are associated with deposits of mutant *lysozyme*.
- *β2-microglobulin,* a component of the MHC class I molecules and a normal serum protein, has been identified as the amyloid fibril subunit (Aβ2m) in amyloidosis that complicates the course of patients on *long-term hemodialysis*. Aβ2m fibers are structurally similar to normal β2m protein. This protein is present in high concentrations in the serum of patients with renal disease and is retained in the circulation because it is not efficiently filtered through dialysis membranes. In some series, as many as 60% to 80% of patients on long-term dialysis developed amyloid deposits in the synovium, joints, and tendon sheaths.
- Amyloid deposits derived from diverse precursors such as hormones (procalcitonin) and keratin have also been reported.

Classification of Amyloidosis. Because a given biochemical form of amyloid (e.g., AA) may be associated with amyloid deposition in diverse clinical settings, a combined biochemical and clinical classification is followed for this discussion (Table 5–12). Amyloid may be *systemic* (generalized), involving several organ systems, or it may be *localized,* when deposits are limited to a single organ, such as the heart. On clinical grounds, the systemic, or generalized, pattern is subclassified into *primary amyloidosis* when associated with some immunocyte dyscrasia, or *secondary amyloidosis* when it occurs as a complication of an underlying chronic inflammatory or tissue destructive process. *Hereditary* or *familial amyloidosis* constitutes a separate, albeit heterogeneous group, with several distinctive patterns of organ involvement.

Immunocyte Dyscrasias with Amyloidosis (Primary Amyloidosis). Amyloid in this category is usually systemic in distribution and is of the AL type. With approximately 3000 new cases each year in the United States, this is the most common form of amyloidosis. The best example in this category is amyloidosis associated with *multiple myeloma,* a malignant neoplasm of plasma cells (Chapter 12). The malignant B cells characteristically synthesize abnormal amounts of a single specific Ig (monoclonal gammopathy), producing an M (myeloma) protein spike on serum electrophoresis. In addition to the synthesis of whole Ig molecules, plasma cells may also synthesize and secrete either the γ or κ light chain, also known as *Bence Jones proteins* (by virtue of the small molecular size of the Bence Jones proteins, they are also frequently excreted in the urine). These are present in the serum of as many as 70% of patients with multiple myeloma, and almost all patients with myeloma who develop amyloidosis have Bence Jones proteins in the

Table 5–12 Classification of Amyloidosis

Clinicopathologic Category	Associated Diseases	Major Fibril Protein	Chemically Related Precursor Protein
Systemic (Generalized) Amyloidosis			
Immunocyte dyscrasias with amyloidosis (primary amyloidosis)	Multiple myeloma and other monoclonal B-cell proliferations	AL	Immunoglobulin light chains, chiefly γ type
Reactive systemic amyloidosis (secondary amyloidosis)	Chronic inflammatory conditions	AA	SAA
Hemodialysis-associated amyloidosis	Chronic renal failure	$A\beta_2m$	β_2-microglobulin
Hereditary Amyloidosis			
Familial Mediterranean fever		AA	SAA
Familial amyloidotic neuropathies (several types)		ATTR	Transthyretin
Senile Amyloidosis		ATTR	Transthyretin
Localized Amyloidosis			
Senile cerebral	Alzheimer disease	Aβ	APP
Endocrine			
Medullary carcinoma of thyroid		A Cal	Calcitonin
Islets of Langerhans	Type 2 diabetes	AIAPP	Islet amyloid peptide
Isolated atrial amyloidosis		AANF	Atrial natriuretic factor

serum or urine, or both. However, only 6% to 15% of myeloma patients who have free light chains develop amyloidosis. Clearly, the presence of Bence Jones proteins, though necessary, is by itself not sufficient to produce amyloidosis. Other variables, such as the type of light chain produced and its catabolism, contribute to the "amyloidogenic potential" and influence the deposition of Bence Jones proteins.

The great majority of patients with AL amyloid do not have classic multiple myeloma or any other overt B-cell neoplasm; such cases are nevertheless classified as primary amyloidosis because their clinical features derive from the effects of amyloid deposition without any other associated disease. In virtually all such cases, patients have a modest increase in the number of plasma cells in the bone marrow, and monoclonal immunoglobulins or free light chains can be found in the serum or urine. Clearly, these patients have an underlying B-cell dyscrasia in which production of an abnormal protein, rather than production of tumor masses, is the predominant manifestation.

Reactive Systemic Amyloidosis. The amyloid deposits in this pattern are systemic in distribution and are composed of AA protein. This category was previously referred to as *secondary amyloidosis,* because it is secondary to an associated inflammatory condition. The feature common to most cases of reactive systemic amyloidosis is protracted cell injury occurring in a spectrum of infectious and noninfectious chronic inflammatory conditions. Classically, tuberculosis, bronchiectasis, and chronic osteomyelitis were the most common causes; with the advent of effective antimicrobial therapies, reactive systemic amyloidosis is seen most frequently in the setting of chronic inflammation caused by autoimmune states (e.g., RA, ankylosing spondylitis, and inflammatory bowel disease). RA is particularly prone to develop amyloidosis, with amyloid deposition seen in as many as 3% of such patients. Chronic skin infections caused by "skin-popping" of narcotics are also associated with amyloid deposition. Finally, reactive systemic amyloidosis may also occur in association with tumors not derived from immune cells, the two most common being renal cell carcinoma and Hodgkin lymphoma.

Familial (Hereditary) Amyloidosis. A variety of familial forms of amyloidosis have been described; most are rare and occur in limited geographic areas. The best characterized is an autosomal recessive condition called *familial Mediterranean fever.* This is a febrile disorder characterized by attacks of fever accompanied by inflammation of serosal surfaces, including peritoneum, pleura, and synovial membrane. This disorder is encountered largely in individuals of Armenian, Sephardic Jewish, and Arabic origins. It is associated with widespread tissue involvement indistinguishable from reactive systemic amyloidosis. The amyloid fibril proteins are made up of AA proteins, suggesting that this form of amyloidosis is related to the recurrent bouts of inflammation that characterize this disease. The gene for familial Mediterranean fever has been cloned, and its product is called *pyrin;* although its exact function is not known, it has been suggested that pyrin is responsible for regulating acute inflammation, presumably by inhibiting the function of neutrophils. With a mutation in this gene, minor traumas unleash a vigorous, tissue-damaging inflammatory response.

In contrast to familial Mediterranean fever, a group of autosomal dominant familial disorders is characterized by deposition of amyloid predominantly in the peripheral and autonomic nerves. These familial amyloidotic polyneuropathies have been described in kindreds in different parts of the world, for example, in Portugal, Japan, Sweden, and the United States. As mentioned previously, the fibrils in these familial polyneuropathies are made up of mutant ATTRs.

Localized Amyloidosis. Sometimes amyloid deposits are limited to a single organ or tissue without involvement of any other site in the body. The deposits may produce grossly detectable nodular masses or be evident only on microscopic examination. Nodular (tumor-forming) deposits of amyloid are most often encountered in the lung, larynx, skin, urinary bladder, tongue, and the region about the eye. Frequently, there are infiltrates of lymphocytes and plasma cells in the periphery of these amyloid masses, raising the question of whether the mononuclear infiltrate is a response to the deposition of amyloid or instead is responsible for it. At least in some cases, the amyloid consists of AL protein and may therefore represent a localized form of immunocyte-derived amyloid.

Endocrine Amyloid. Microscopic deposits of localized amyloid may be found in certain endocrine tumors, such as medullary carcinoma of the thyroid gland, islet tumors of the pancreas, pheochromocytomas, and undifferentiated carcinomas of the stomach, as well as in the islets of Langerhans in patients with type 2 diabetes mellitus. In these settings, the amyloidogenic proteins seem to be derived either from polypeptide hormones (medullary carcinoma) or from unique proteins (e.g., islet amyloid polypeptide).

Amyloid of Aging. Several well-documented forms of amyloid deposition occur with aging. *Senile systemic amyloidosis* refers to the systemic deposition of amyloid in elderly patients (usually in their 70s and 80s). Because of the dominant involvement and related dysfunction of the heart (typically presenting as a restrictive cardiomyopathy and arrhythmias), this form is also called *senile cardiac amyloidosis.* The amyloid in this form is composed of the normal TTR molecule. In addition, another form predominantly affecting only the heart results from the deposition of *a mutant form of TTR.* Approximately 4% of the black population in the United States is a carrier of the mutant allele, and cardiomyopathy has been identified in both homozygous and heterozygous patients.

Morphology

There are no consistent or distinctive patterns of organ or tissue distribution of amyloid deposits in any of the categories cited. Nonetheless, a few generalizations can be made. In amyloidosis secondary to chronic inflammatory disorders, kidneys, liver, spleen, lymph nodes, adrenals, and thyroid, as well as many other tissues, are typically affected. Although immunocyte-associated amyloidosis cannot reliably be distinguished from the secondary form by its organ distribution, it more often involves the heart, gastrointestinal tract, respiratory tract, peripheral nerves, skin, and tongue. However, the same organs affected by reactive systemic amyloidosis (secondary amyloidosis), including kidneys, liver, and spleen, may also contain deposits in the immunocyte-associated form of the disease. The localization of amyloid deposits in the hereditary syndromes is varied. In familial Mediterranean fever the amyloidosis may be widespread, involving the kidneys, blood vessels, spleen, respiratory tract, and (rarely) liver. The localization of amyloid in the remaining hereditary syndromes can be inferred from the designation of these entities.

Whatever the clinical disorder, the amyloidosis may or may not be apparent on macroscopic examination. Often small amounts are not recognized until the surface of the cut organ is painted with iodine and sulfuric acid. This yields mahogany brown staining of the amyloid deposits. When amyloid accumulates in larger amounts, the organ is frequently enlarged and the tissue appears gray with a waxy, firm consistency. **Histologically, the amyloid deposition is always extracellular and begins between cells,** often closely adjacent to basement membranes. As the amyloid accumulates, it encroaches on the cells, in time surrounding and destroying them. In the immunocyte-associated form, perivascular and vascular localizations are common.

The histologic diagnosis of amyloid is based almost entirely on its staining characteristics. The most commonly used staining technique uses the dye Congo red, which under ordinary light imparts a pink or red color to amyloid deposits. Under polarized light the Congo red–stained amyloid shows so-called apple-green birefringence (Fig. 5–37). This reaction is shared by all forms of amyloid and is caused by the crossed β-pleated configuration of amyloid fibrils. Confirmation can be obtained by electron microscopy, which reveals amorphous nonoriented thin fibrils. AA, AL, and ATTR types of amyloid can also be distinguished by specific immunohistochemical staining.

Because the pattern of organ involvement in different clinical forms of amyloidosis is variable, each of the major organ involvements is described separately.

Kidney. Amyloidosis of the kidney is the most common and most serious involvement in the disease. Grossly, the kidney may appear unchanged, or it may be abnormally large, pale, gray, and firm; in long-standing cases, the kidney may be reduced in size. Microscopically, the **amyloid deposits are found principally in the glomeruli,** but they are also present in the interstitial peritubular tissue as well as in the walls of the blood vessels. The glomerulus first develops focal deposits within the mesangial matrix and diffuse or nodular thickenings of the basement membranes of the capillary loops. With progression, the deposition encroaches on the capillary lumina and eventually leads to total obliteration of the vascular tuft (Fig. 5–38A). The interstitial peritubular deposits are frequently associated with the appearance of amorphous pink casts within the tubular lumens, presumably of a proteinaceous nature. Amyloid deposits may develop in the walls of blood vessels of all sizes, often causing marked vascular narrowing.

Spleen. Amyloidosis of the spleen often causes moderate or even marked enlargement (200–800 gm). For obscure reasons, one of two patterns may develop. The deposits may be virtually limited to the splenic follicles, producing tapioca-like granules on gross examination ("sago spleen"), or the involvement may affect principally the splenic sinuses and eventually extend to the splenic pulp, forming large, sheetlike deposits ("larda-

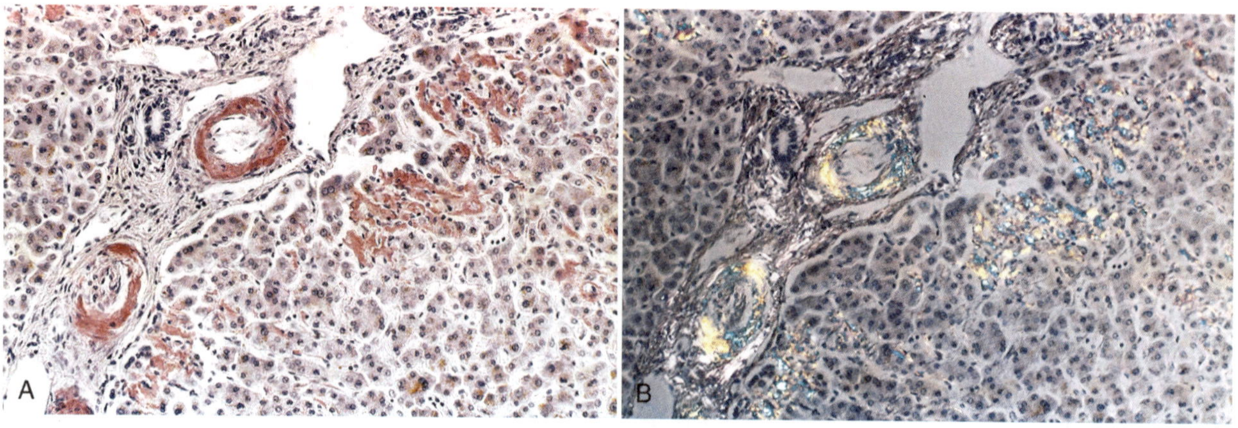

Figure 5–37

Amyloidosis. **A,** A section of the liver stained with Congo red reveals pink-red deposits of amyloid in the walls of blood vessels and along sinusoids. **B,** Note the yellow-green birefringence of the deposits when observed by polarizing microscope. (Courtesy of Dr. Trace Worrell and Sandy Hinton, Department of Pathology, University of Texas Southwestern Medical School, Dallas, Texas.)

ceous spleen"). In both patterns the spleen is firm in consistency, and cut surfaces reveal pale gray, waxy deposits.

Liver. Amyloidosis of the liver may cause massive enlargement (as much as 9000 gm). In such advanced cases the liver is extremely pale, grayish, and waxy on both the external surface and the cut section. Histologically, **amyloid deposits first appear in the space of Disse** and then progressively enlarge to encroach on the adjacent hepatic parenchyma and sinusoids (see Fig. 5–37). The trapped liver cells undergo compression atrophy and are eventually replaced by sheets of amyloid; remarkably, normal liver function may be preserved even in the setting of severe involvement.

Heart. Amyloidosis of the heart may occur either as isolated organ involvement or as part of a systemic distribution. When accompanied by systemic involvement, it is usually associated with immunocyte dyscrasias. The isolated form (senile amyloidosis) is usually confined to older individuals. The deposits may not be evident on gross examination, or they may cause minimal to moderate cardiac enlargement. The most characteristic gross findings are gray-pink, dewdrop-like subendocardial elevations, particularly evident in the atrial chambers. On histologic examination, deposits are typically found throughout the myocardium, beginning **between myocardial fibers** and eventually causing their pressure atrophy (Fig. 5–38B).

Other Organs. Amyloidosis of other organs is generally encountered in systemic disease. The adrenals, thyroid, and pituitary are common sites of involvement. In this case also the amyloid deposition begins in relation to stromal and endothelial cells and progressively encroaches on the parenchymal cells. Surprisingly, large amounts of amyloid may be present in any of these endocrine glands without apparent disturbance of function. In the gastrointestinal tract, a relatively favored site, amyloid may be found at all levels, sometimes producing tumorous masses that must be distin-

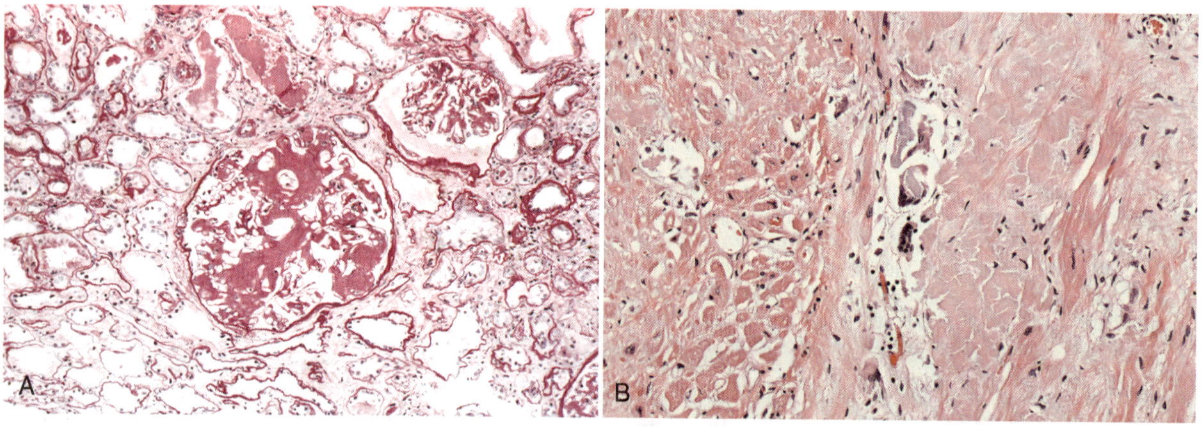

Figure 5–38

Amyloidosis. **A,** Amyloidosis of the kidney. The glomerular architecture is almost totally obliterated by the massive accumulation of amyloid. **B,** Cardiac amyloidosis. The atrophic myocardial fibers are separated by structureless, pink-staining amyloid.

guished from neoplasms. Nodular depositions in the tongue may produce **macroglossia**. On the basis of the frequent involvement of the gastrointestinal tract in systemic cases, gingival, intestinal, and rectal biopsies serve in the diagnosis of suspected cases. Deposition of β_2-microglobulin amyloid in patients receiving long-term dialysis occurs most commonly in the **carpal ligaments of the wrist**, resulting in compression of the median nerve (carpal tunnel syndrome).

Clinical Correlation. Amyloidosis may be an unsuspected finding at autopsy in a patient who has no apparent related clinical manifestations, or it may be responsible for serious clinical dysfunction and even death. All depends on the particular sites or organs affected and the severity of the involvement. Nonspecific complaints such as weakness, fatigue, and weight loss are the most common initial symptoms. Later in the course, amyloidosis tends to manifest in one of several ways: by *renal disease, hepatomegaly, splenomegaly, or cardiac abnormalities*. Renal involvement giving rise to severe proteinuria (*nephrotic syndrome;* Chapter 14) is often the major cause of symptoms in reactive systemic amyloidosis. Progression of the renal disease may lead to renal failure, which is an important cause of death in amyloidosis. The hepatosplenomegaly rarely causes significant clinical dysfunction, but it may be the presenting finding. Cardiac amyloidosis may manifest as conduction disturbances or as restrictive cardiomyopathy (Chapter 11). Cardiac arrhythmias are an important cause of death in cardiac amyloidosis. In one large series, 40% of the patients with AL amyloid died of cardiac disease.

The diagnosis of amyloidosis may be suspected from the clinical signs and symptoms and from some of the findings mentioned; however, more specific tests must often be done for definitive diagnosis. *Biopsy and subsequent Congo red staining is the most important tool in the diagnosis of amyloidosis.* In general, biopsy is taken from the organ suspected to be involved. For example, renal biopsy is useful in the presence of urinary abnormalities. Rectal and gingival biopsy specimens contain amyloid in as many as 75% of cases with generalized amyloidosis. Examination of abdominal fat aspirates stained with Congo red is a simple, low-risk method. In suspected cases of AL amyloidosis, serum and urinary protein electrophoresis and immunoelectrophoresis should be performed. Bone marrow aspirate in such cases usually shows plasmacytosis, even if skeletal lesions of multiple myeloma are not present.

The outlook for patients with generalized amyloidosis is poor, with the mean survival time after diagnosis ranging from 1 to 3 years. In AA amyloidosis, the prognosis depends to some extent on the control of the underlying condition. Patients with myeloma-associated amyloidosis have a poorer prognosis, although they may respond to cytotoxic drugs used to treat the underlying disorder. Resorption of amyloid after treatment of the associated condition has been reported, but this is a rare occurrence.

SUMMARY

Amyloidosis

- Amyloidosis is a disorder characterized by the extracellular deposits of misfolded proteins that aggregate to form insoluble fibrils.
- The deposition of these proteins may result from: excessive production of proteins that are prone to misfolding and aggregation; mutations that produce proteins that cannot fold properly and tend to aggregate; defective or incomplete proteolytic degradation of extracellular proteins.
- Amyloidosis may be localized or systemic. It is seen in association with a variety of primary disorders, including monoclonal B-cell proliferations (in which the amyloid deposits consist of immunologlobulin light chains); chronic inflammatory diseases such as rheumatoid arthritis (deposits of amyloid A protein, derived from an acute-phase protein produced in inflammation); Alzheimer disease (amyloid β protein); familial conditions in which the amyloid deposits consist of mutants of normal proteins (e.g. transthyretin in familial amyloid polyneuropathies); amyloidosis associated with dialysis (deposits of β2-microglobulin, whose clearance is defective).
- Amyloid deposits cause tissue injury and impair normal function by causing pressure on cells and tissues. They do not evoke an inflammatory response.

BIBLIOGRAPHY

Buckley RH: Primary immunodeficiency diseases: dissectors of the immune system. Immunol Rev 185:206, 2002. *[Excellent review of the molecular basis and therapy of the major primary immunodeficiency diseases.]*

Cookson W: The immunogenetics of asthma and eczema: a new focus on the epithelium. Nat Rev Immunol 4:978, 2004. *[Review of genes associated with asthma, and a discussion of new ideas about the role of abnormalities in epithelia in the pathogenesis of asthma and allergic dermatitis.]*

Crow MK, Kirou KA: Interferon-alpha in systemic lupus erythematosus. Curr Opin Rheumatol 16:541, 2004. *[Discussion of new findings suggesting a role for the cytokine IFN-α in SLE.]*

Cunningham-Rundles C, Ponda PP: Molecular defects in T-ad B-cell primary immunodeficiency diseases. Nat Rev Immunol 5:880, 2006. *[Excellent, up-to-date review of primary imunodeficiencies.]*

Dalakas MC, Hohlfeld R: Polymyositis and dermatomyositis. Lancet 362:971, 2003. *[Excellent comprehensive review of the two major inflammatory myopathies.]*

Davidson A, Diamond B: Autoimmune diseases. N Engl J Med 345:340, 2001. *[A readable overview of the etiology, pathogenesis, and therapy for autoimmune diseases.]*

Frankel AD, Young JA: HIV-1: fifteen proteins and an RNA. Annu Rev Biochem 67:1, 1998. *[Excellent review of the biochemistry of the major proteins of HIV.]*

Gaffney PM, et al.: Recent advances in the genetics of systemic lupus erythematosus. Rheum Dis Clin North Am 28:111, 2002. *[Review of the genes associated with SLE in humans and in mouse models.]*

Galli SJ, et al.: Mast cells as "tunable" effector and immunoregulatory cells: recent advances. Annu Rev Immunol 23:749, 2005. *[Modern discussion of the activation and regulation of mast cells, and their roles in allergic diseases.]*

Ganem D: KSHV infection and the pathogenesis of Kaposi's sarcoma. Annu Rev Pathol 1:273, 2006. *[Excellent and thoughtful discussion of the current understanding of Kaposi sarcoma.]*

Gonzalez-Scarano F, Martin-Garcia J: The neuropathogenesis of AIDS. Nat Rev Immunol 5:69, 2005. *[Excellent discussion of the pathogenesis of HIV-associated dementia.]*

Goodnow CC, et al.: Cellular and genetic mechanisms of self tolerance and autoimmunity. Nature 435:590, 2005. *[Excellent modern review of the molecular mechanisms of self-tolerance and how they may break down to give rise to autoimmune disease.]*

Greene WC, Peterlin BM: Charting HIV's remarkable voyage through the cell: basic science as a passport to future therapy. Nat Med 8:673, 2002. *[Excellent review of the molecular mechanisms of HIV entry into cells and viral gene expression and replication.]*

Grossman Z, et al.: CD4+ T-cell depletion in HIV infection: are we closer to understanding the cause? Nat Med 8:319, 2002. *[Thoughtful discussion of the possible mechanisms of T-cell depletion in HIV infection, and the controversies in the field.]*

Hansen A, et al.: New concepts in the pathogenesis of Sjögren syndrome: many questions, fewer answers. Curr Opin Rheumatol 15:563, 2003. *[Discussion of what is known and uncertain about this clinically important disease.]*

Heeger PS: T-cell allorecognition and transplant rejection: a summary and update. Am J Transplant 3:525, 2003. *[Good review of the mechanisms of recognition and rejection of allografts.]*

Hoffman RW, Greidinger EL: Mixed connective tissue disease. Curr Opin Rheumatol 12:386, 2000. *[A good discussion of this puzzling clinical entity.]*

Kay AB: Allergy and allergic diseases. First of two parts. N Engl J Med 344:30, 109, 2001. *[Superb two-part review of the mechanisms and manifestations of type I hypersensitivity.]*

Lanier LL: NK cell recognition. Annu Rev Immunol 23:225, 2005. *[Excellent review of the activating and inhibitory receptors of NK cells and their biologic roles.]*

Lee DM, Weinblatt ME: Rheumatoid arthritis. Lancet 358:903, 2001. *[An authoritative article summarizing clinical aspects of rheumatoid arthritis.]*

Letvin NL, Walker BD: Immunopathogenesis and immunotherapy in AIDS virus infections. Nat Med 9:861, 2003. *[Excellent discussion of the immune responses to HIV, viral escape mechanisms, mechanisms of immunodeficiency, and how this knowledge may help to guide therapeutic approaches.]*

Levine JS, et al.: The antiphospholipid syndrome. N Engl J Med 346:752, 2002. *[An excellent discussion of this not uncommon syndrome.]*

Libby P, Pober JS: Chronic rejection. Immunity 14:387, 2001. *[Well-written summary of the mechanisms of allograft arteriopathy.]*

Marrack P, et al.: Autoimmune disease: why and where it occurs. Nat Med 7:899, 2001. *[Excellent discussion of the interplay of environmental and genetic factors in the development of autoimmune diseases.]*

McCune JM: The dynamics of CD4+ T-cell depletion in HIV disease. Nature 410:974, 2001. *[An excellent discussion of factors that cause loss of CD4+ T cells.]*

Merlini G, Bellotti V: Molecular mechanisms of amyloidosis. N Engl J Med 349:583, 2003. *[Good review of the general pathogenic mechanisms in various forms of systemic amyloidosis.]*

Pascual M, et al.: Strategies to improve long-term outcomes after renal transplantation. N Engl J Med 346:580, 2002. *[Review of the current treatment of graft rejection and prospects for the future.]*

Pepys MB: Amyloidosis. Ann Rev Med 57:223, 2006. *[An excellent review of the pathogenesis, clinical features and therapeutic approaches in amyloidosis.]*

Rioux JD, Abbas AK: Paths to understanding the genetic basis of autoimmune disease. Nature 435:584, 2005. *[Discussion of the current understanding of the genetics of autoimmunity, with illustrative examples of informative genes that are known to be associated with different autoimmune diseases.]*

Ruiz-Irastorza G, et al.: Systemic lupus erythematosus. Lancet 357:1027, 2001. *[Update on clinical issues related to the pathogenesis and therapy of SLE.]*

Sakaguchi S: Naturally arising Foxp3-expressing CD25+CD4+ regulatory T cells in immunological tolerance to self and non-self. Nat Immunol 6:345, 2005. *[Up-to-date discussion of the properties and functions of this fascinating population of T cells.]*

Schwartz RH: T cell anergy. Ann Rev Immunol 21:305, 2003. *[Excellent review of one of the important mechanisms of T-cell tolerance.]*

Sepkowitz KA: AIDS—the first 20 years. N Engl J Med 344:1764, 2001. *[Excellent historical review of the AIDS epidemic and insights gleaned from the long-term perspective.]*

Stevenson M: HIV-1 pathogenesis. Nat Med 9:853, 2003. *[Thoughtful discussion of the pathogenesis of AIDS, what is not known, and how non-human primate models may provide new insights.]*

VanderBorght A, et al.: The autoimmune pathogenesis of rheumatoid arthritis: role of autoreactive T cells and new immunotherapies. Semin Arthritis Rheum 31:160, 2001. *[An up-to-date summary of the role for autoimmunity in the pathogenesis of rheumatoid arthritis.]*

Walker LS, Abbas AK: The enemy within: keeping self-reactive T cells at bay in the periphery. Nat Rev Immunol 2:11, 2002. *[Review of the known molecular mechanisms of peripheral T-cell tolerance.]*

Walsh NC, Gravallese EM: Bone loss in inflammatory arthritis: mechanisms and treatment strategies. Curr Opin Rheumatol 16:419, 2004. *[A concise and authoritative review of the mechanisms underlying the destructive bone lesions in rheumatoid arthritis.]*

Chapter 6

Neoplasia

THOMAS P. STRICKER, MD, PhD
VINAY KUMAR, MD

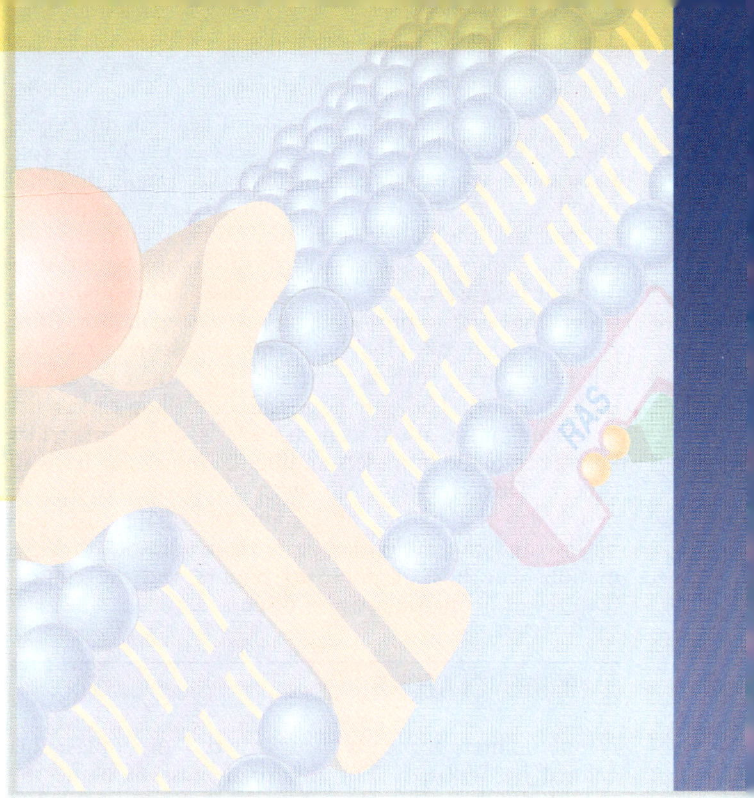

Cancer is the second leading cause of death in the United States; only cardiovascular diseases exact a higher toll. Even more agonizing than the mortality rate is the emotional and physical suffering inflicted by neoplasms. Patients and the public often ask, "When will there be a cure for cancer?" The answer to this simple question is difficult because cancer is not one disease but many disorders that share a profound growth dysregulation. Some cancers, such as Hodgkin lymphomas, are curable, whereas others, such as cancer of the pancreas, have a high mortality. The only hope for controlling cancer lies in learning more about its pathogenesis, and great strides have been made in understanding the molecular basis of cancer. This chapter deals with the basic biology of neoplasia—the nature of benign and malignant neoplasms and the molecular basis of neoplastic transformation. The host response to tumors and the clinical features of neoplasia are also discussed.

NOMENCLATURE

Neoplasia literally means "new growth." A neoplasm, as defined by Willis, is "an abnormal mass of tissue the growth of which exceeds and is uncoordinated with that of the normal tissues and persists in the same excessive manner after the cessation of the stimuli which evoked the change." *Fundamental to the origin of all neoplasms are heritable (genetic) changes that allow excessive and unregulated proliferation that is independent of physiologic growth-regulatory stimuli.* Neoplastic cells are said to be transformed because they continue to replicate, apparently oblivious to the regulatory influences that control normal cell growth. Neoplasms therefore enjoy a certain degree of autonomy and more or less steadily increase in size regardless of their local environment and the nutritional status of the host. Their autonomy is by no means complete, however. Some neoplasms require endocrine support, and such dependencies sometimes can be exploited to the disadvantage of the neoplasm. All neoplasms depend on the host for their nutrition and blood supply.

In common medical usage, a neoplasm is often referred to as a *tumor,* and the study of tumors is called *oncology* (from *oncos,* "tumor," and *logos,* "study of"). In oncology, the division of neoplasms into benign and malignant categories is important. This categorization is based on a judgment of a neoplasm's potential clinical behavior.

A tumor is said to be *benign* when its microscopic and gross characteristics are considered to be relatively innocent, implying that it will remain localized, it cannot spread to other sites, and is amenable to local surgical removal; the patient generally survives. It should be noted, however, that benign tumors can produce more than localized lumps, and sometimes they are responsible for serious disease, as pointed out later.

Malignant tumors are collectively referred to as *cancers,* derived from the Latin word for *crab*—that is, they adhere to any part that they seize in an obstinate manner, similar to a crab's behavior. *Malignant,* as applied to a neoplasm, implies that the lesion can invade and destroy adjacent structures and spread to distant sites (metastasize) to cause death. Not all cancers pursue so deadly a course. Some are less aggressive and are treated successfully, but the designation *malignant* constitutes a red flag.

All tumors, benign and malignant, have two basic components: (1) the *parenchyma,* made up of transformed or neoplastic cells, and (2) the supporting, host-derived, non-neoplastic *stroma,* made up of connective tissue, blood vessels, and host-derived inflammatory cells. The parenchyma of the neoplasm largely determines its biologic behavior, and it is this component from which the tumor derives its name. The stroma is crucial to the growth of the neoplasm, since it carries the blood supply and provides support for the growth of parenchymal cells. As will be discussed later, stromal cells and neoplastic cells carry on a two-way conversation that influences the growth of the tumor.

Benign Tumors. In general, benign tumors are designated by attaching the suffix *-oma* to the cell type from which the tumor arises. A benign tumor arising in fibrous tissue is a *fibroma;* a benign cartilaginous tumor is a *chondroma.* The nomenclature of benign epithelial tumors is more complex. They are classified sometimes on the basis of their microscopic pattern and sometimes on the basis of their macroscopic pattern. Others are classified by their cells of origin.

For instance, the term *adenoma* is applied to benign epithelial neoplasms producing gland patterns and to neoplasms derived from glands but not necessarily exhibiting gland patterns. A benign epithelial neoplasm arising from renal tubule cells and growing in glandlike patterns would be termed an adenoma, as would a mass of benign epithelial cells that produces no glandular patterns but has its origin in the adrenal cortex. *Papillomas* are benign epithelial neoplasms, growing on any surface, that produce microscopic or macroscopic finger-like fronds. A *polyp* is a mass that projects above a mucosal surface, as in the gut, to form a macroscopically visible structure (Fig. 6–1). Although this term is commonly used for benign tumors, some malignant tumors also may appear as polyps. *Cystadenomas* are hollow cystic masses; typically they are seen in the ovary.

Malignant Tumors. The nomenclature of malignant tumors essentially follows that of benign tumors, with certain additions and exceptions.

Malignant neoplasms arising in mesenchymal tissue or its derivatives are called *sarcomas.* A cancer of fibrous tissue origin is a *fibro*sarcoma, and a malignant neoplasm composed of chondrocytes is a *chondro*sarcoma. Sarcomas are designated by their histogenesis (i.e., the cell type of which they are composed). Malignant neoplasms of epithelial cell origin are called *carcinomas.* It must be remembered that the epithelia of the body are derived from all three germ-cell layers; a malignant neoplasm arising in the renal tubular epithelium (mesoderm) is a carcinoma, as are the cancers arising in the skin (ectoderm) and lining epithelium of the gut (endoderm). It is evident that mesoderm may give rise to carcinomas (epithelial) and sarcomas (mesenchymal). Carcinomas may be qualified further. Carcinomas that grow in a glandular pattern are called *adenocarcinomas,* and those that

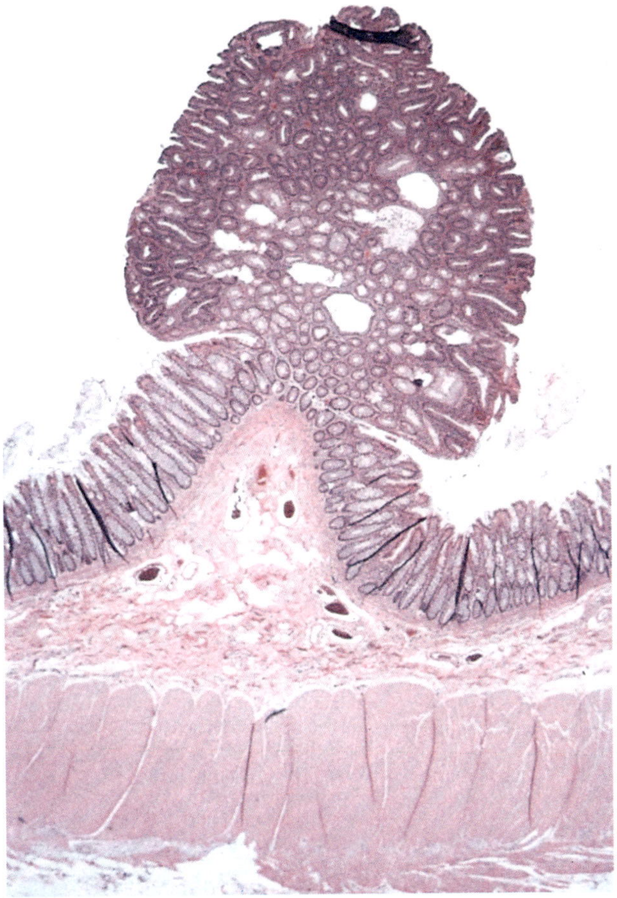

Figure 6–1

Colonic polyp. This benign glandular tumor (adenoma) is projecting into the colonic lumen and is attached to the mucosa by a distinct stalk.

produce squamous cells are called *squamous cell carcinomas*. Sometimes the tissue or organ of origin can be identified, as in the designation of renal cell adenocarcinoma or cholangiocarcinoma, which implies an origin from bile ducts. Sometimes the tumor shows little or no differentiation and must be called *poorly differentiated or undifferentiated carcinoma*.

The parenchymal cells in a neoplasm, whether benign or malignant, resemble each other, as though all had been derived from a single progenitor. Indeed, neoplasms are of monoclonal origin, as is discussed later. In some instances, however, the tumor cells may undergo *divergent differentiation*, creating so-called *mixed tumors*. The best example is mixed tumor of salivary gland. These tumors have obvious epithelial components dispersed throughout a fibromyxoid stroma, sometimes harboring islands of cartilage or bone (Fig. 6–2). All of these diverse elements are thought to derive from epithelial cells, myoepithelial cells, or both in the salivary glands, and the preferred designation of these neoplasms is *pleomorphic adenoma*. Fibroadenoma of the female breast is another common mixed tumor. This benign tumor contains a mixture of proliferated ductal elements (adenoma) embedded in a loose fibrous tissue (fibroma). Although studies suggest that only the fibrous component is neoplastic, the term *fibroadenoma* remains in common usage.

The multifaceted mixed tumors should not be confused with a *teratoma*, which contains recognizable mature or immature cells or tissues representative of more than one germ-cell layer and sometimes all three. Teratomas originate from totipotential stem cells such as those normally present in the ovary and testis and sometimes abnormally present in sequestered midline embryonic rests. Such cells have the capacity to differentiate into any of the cell types found in the adult body and so, not surprisingly, may give rise to neoplasms that mimic, in a helter-skelter fashion, bits of bone, epithelium, muscle, fat, nerve, and other tissues.

The specific names of the more common forms of neoplasms are presented in Table 6–1. Some glaring inconsistencies may be noted. For example, the terms *lymphoma, mesothelioma, melanoma,* and *seminoma* are used for malignant neoplasms. These inappropriate usages are firmly entrenched in medical terminology.

There are other instances of confusing terminology. *Hamartoma* is a malformation that presents as a mass of disorganized tissue indigenous to the particular site. One may see a mass of mature but disorganized hepatic cells, blood vessels, and possibly bile ducts within the liver, or there may be a hamartomatous nodule in the lung containing islands of cartilage, bronchi, and blood vessels. Another misnomer is the term *choristoma*. This congenital anomaly is better described as a *heterotopic rest* of cells. For example, a small nodule of well-developed and normally organized pancreatic tissue may be found in the submucosa of the stomach, duodenum, or small intestine. This heterotopic rest may be replete with islets of Langerhans and exocrine glands. The term *choristoma*, connoting a neoplasm, imparts to the heterotopic rest a gravity far beyond its usual trivial significance. Although the terminology of neoplasms is regrettably not simple, it is important because it is the language by which the nature and significance of tumors are categorized.

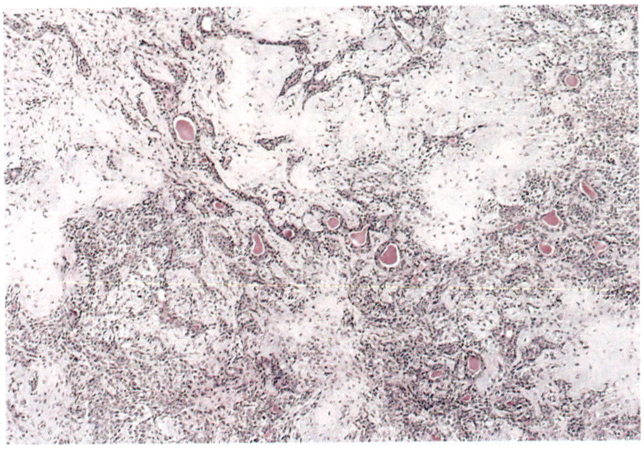

Figure 6–2

Mixed tumor of the parotid gland contains epithelial cells forming ducts and myxoid stroma that resembles cartilage. (Courtesy of Dr. Trace Worrell, Department of Pathology, University of Texas Southwestern Medical School, Dallas, Texas.)

Table 6–1 Nomenclature of Tumors

Tissue of Origin	Benign	Malignant
Composed of One Parenchymal Cell Type		
Connective tissue and derivatives	Fibroma	Fibrosarcoma
	Lipoma	Liposarcoma
	Chondroma	Chondrosarcoma
	Osteoma	Osteogenic sarcoma
Endothelial and related tissues		
Blood vessels	Hemangioma	Angiosarcoma
Lymph vessels	Lymphangioma	Lymphangiosarcoma
Synovium		Synovial sarcoma
Mesothelium		Mesothelioma
Brain coverings	Meningioma	Invasive meningioma
Blood cells and related cells		
Hematopoietic cells		Leukemias
Lymphoid tissue		Lymphomas
Muscle		
Smooth	Leiomyoma	Leiomyosarcoma
Striated	Rhabdomyoma	Rhabdomyosarcoma
Tumors of epithelial origin		
Stratified squamous	Squamous cell papilloma	Squamous cell or epidermoid carcinoma
Basal cells of skin or adnexa		Basal cell carcinoma
Epithelial lining of glands or ducts	Adenoma	Adenocarcinoma
	Papilloma	Papillary carcinomas
	Cystadenoma	Cystadenocarcinoma
Respiratory passages	Bronchial adenoma	Bronchogenic carcinoma
Renal epithelium	Renal tubular adenoma	Renal cell carcinoma
Liver cells	Liver cell adenoma	Hepatocellular carcinoma
Urinary tract epithelium (transitional)	Urothelial papilloma	Urothelial carcinoma
Placental epithelium	Hydatidiform mole	Choriocarcinoma
Testicular epithelium (germ cells)		Seminoma
		Embryonal carcinoma
Tumors of melanocytes	Nevus	Malignant melanoma
More Than One Neoplastic Cell Type—Mixed Tumors, Usually Derived from One Germ Cell Layer		
Salivary glands	Pleomorphic adenoma (mixed tumor of salivary gland)	Malignant mixed tumor of salivary gland
Renal anlage		Wilms tumor
More Than One Neoplastic Cell Type Derived from More Than One Germ Cell Layer—Teratogenous		
Totipotential cells in gonads or in embryonic rests	Mature teratoma, dermoid cyst	Immature teratoma, teratocarcinoma

CHARACTERISTICS OF BENIGN AND MALIGNANT NEOPLASMS

Nothing is more important to the patient with a tumor than being told "It is benign." In most instances such a prediction can be made with remarkable accuracy based on long-established clinical and anatomic criteria, but some neoplasms defy easy characterization. Certain features may indicate innocence, and others may indicate malignancy. These problems are not the rule, however, and there are four fundamental features by which benign and malignant tumors can be distinguished. These are differentiation and anaplasia, rate of growth, local invasion, and metastasis.

Differentiation and Anaplasia

Differentiation and anaplasia refer only to the parenchymal cells that constitute the transformed elements of neoplasms. The differentiation of parenchymal cells refers to the extent to which they resemble their normal forebears morphologically and functionally. The stroma carrying the blood supply is crucial to the growth of tumors but does not aid in the separation of benign from malignant ones. The amount of stromal connective tissue does determine, however, the consistency of a neoplasm. Certain cancers induce a dense, abundant fibrous stroma (desmoplasia), making them hard, so-called scirrhous tumors.

Benign neoplasms are composed of well-differentiated cells that closely resemble their normal counterparts. A lipoma is made up of mature fat cells laden with cytoplasmic lipid vacuoles, and a chondroma is made up of mature cartilage cells that synthesize their usual cartilaginous matrix—evidence of morphologic and functional differentiation. In well-differentiated benign tumors, mitoses are extremely scant in number and are of normal configuration.

Malignant neoplasms are characterized by a wide range of parenchymal cell differentiation, from surprisingly well differentiated (Fig. 6–3) to completely undifferentiated. For example, well-differentiated adenocarcinomas of the thyroid may contain normal-appearing follicles. Such tumors sometimes may be difficult to distinguish from benign proliferations. Between the two extremes lie tumors loosely referred to as *moderately well differentiated.*

The better the differentiation of the cell, the more completely it retains the functional capabilities found in its normal counterparts. Benign neoplasms and even well-differentiated cancers of endocrine glands frequently elaborate the hormones characteristic of their origin. Well-differentiated squamous cell carcinomas elaborate keratin (see Fig. 6–3), just as well-differentiated hepatocellular carcinomas elaborate bile. In other instances unanticipated functions emerge. Some cancers may elaborate fetal proteins not produced by comparable cells in the adult. Cancers of nonendocrine origin may produce so-called ectopic hormones. For example, certain lung carcinomas may produce adrenocorticotropic hormone (ACTH), parathyroid-like hormone, insulin, glucagon, and others. More is said about these phenomena later. Despite exceptions, *the more rapidly growing and the more anaplastic a tumor, the less likely it is to have specialized functional activity.*

Malignant neoplasms that are composed of undifferentiated cells are said to be *anaplastic.* Lack of differentiation, or anaplasia, is considered a hallmark of malignancy. The term *anaplasia* literally means "to form backward." It implies dedifferentiation, or loss of the structural and functional differentiation of normal cells. It is now known, however, that at least some cancers arise from stem cells in tissues; in these tumors failure of differentiation, rather than dedifferentiation of specialized cells, accounts for undifferentiated tumors. Recent studies also indicate that, in some cases dedifferentiation of apparently mature cells does occur during carcinogenesis.

Anaplastic cells display marked *pleomorphism* (i.e., marked variation in size and shape) (Fig. 6–4). Characteristically the *nuclei are extremely hyperchromatic* (darkly stained) and large. The nuclear-to-cytoplasmic ratio may approach 1:1 instead of the normal 1:4 or 1:6. *Giant cells* that are considerably larger than their neighbors may be formed and possess either one enormous nucleus or several nuclei. *Anaplastic nuclei are variable and bizarre in size and shape.* The chromatin is coarse and clumped, and nucleoli may be of astounding size. More important, *mitoses are often numerous and distinctly atypical;* anarchic multiple spindles may be seen and sometimes appear as tripolar or quadripolar forms (Fig. 6–5). Also, anaplastic cells usually fail to develop recognizable patterns of orientation to one another (i.e., they lose normal polarity). They may grow in sheets, with total loss of communal structures, such as gland formations or stratified squamous architecture. Anaplasia is the most extreme disturbance in cell growth encountered in the spectrum of cellular proliferations.

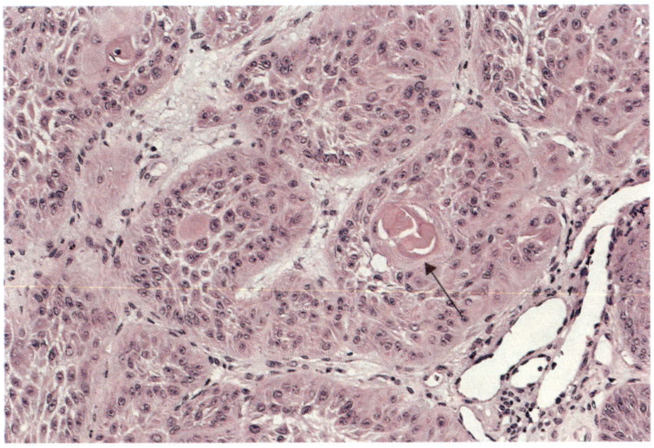

Figure 6–3

Well-differentiated squamous cell carcinoma of the skin. The tumor cells are strikingly similar to normal squamous epithelial cells, with intercellular bridges and nests of keratin pearls *(arrow).* (Courtesy of Dr. Trace Worrell, Department of Pathology University of Texas, Southwestern Medical School, Dallas, Texas.)

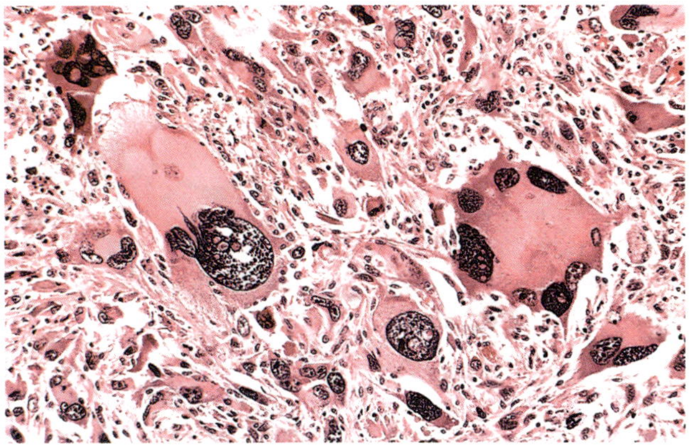

Figure 6–4

Anaplastic tumor of the skeletal muscle (rhabdomyosarcoma). Note the marked cellular and nuclear pleomorphism, hyperchromatic nuclei, and tumor giant cells. (Courtesy of Dr. Trace Worrell, Department of Pathology, University of Texas Southwestern Medical School, Dallas, Texas.)

Before we leave the subject of differentiation and anaplasia, we should discuss *dysplasia,* a term used to describe disorderly but non-neoplastic proliferation. Dysplasia is encountered principally in the epithelia. It is a *loss in the uniformity of individual cells and in their architectural orientation.* Dysplastic cells exhibit considerable pleomorphism and often possess hyperchromatic nuclei that are abnormally large for the size of the cell. Mitotic figures are more abundant than usual. Frequently the mitoses appear in abnormal locations within the epithelium. In dysplastic stratified squamous epithelium, mitoses are not confined to the basal layers, where they normally occur, but may appear at all levels and even in surface cells. There is considerable architectural anarchy. For example, the usual progressive maturation of tall cells in the basal layer to flattened squames on the surface may be lost and replaced by a disordered scrambling of dark basal-appearing cells (Fig. 6–6). When dysplastic changes are marked and involve the entire thickness of the epithelium, the lesion is referred to as *carcinoma in situ,* a pre-invasive stage of cancer (Chapter 19). Although

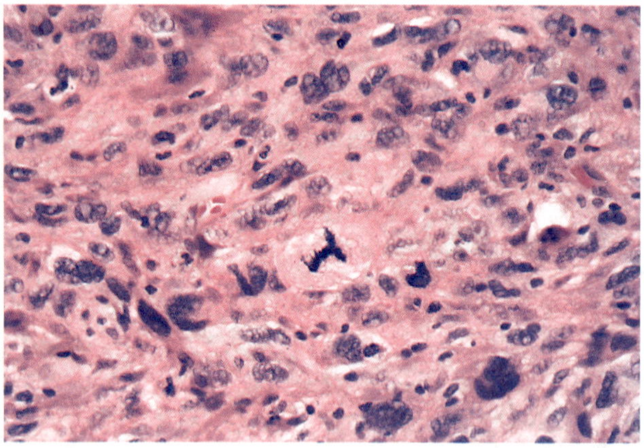

Figure 6–5

High-power detail view of anaplastic tumor cells shows cellular and nuclear variation in size and shape. The prominent cell in the center field has an abnormal tripolar spindle.

dysplastic changes are often found adjacent to foci of malignant transformation, and long-term studies of cigarette smokers show that epithelial dysplasia almost invariably antedates the appearance of cancer, *the term dysplasia without qualifications does not indicate cancer, and dysplasias do not necessarily progress to cancer.* Mild-to-moderate changes that do not involve the entire thickness of epithelium may be reversible, and with removal of the putative inciting causes, the epithelium may revert to normal.

Rate of Growth

Most benign tumors grow slowly, and most cancers grow much faster, eventually spreading locally and to distant sites (metastasizing) and causing death. There are many exceptions to this generalization, however, and some benign tumors grow more rapidly than some cancers. For example, the rate of growth of leiomyomas (benign smooth muscle tumors) of the uterus is influenced by the circulating levels of estrogens. They may increase rapidly in size during pregnancy then cease growing, becoming largely fibrocalcific, after menopause. Other influences, such as adequacy of blood supply or pressure constraints, also may affect the growth rate of benign tumors. Adenomas of the pituitary gland locked into the sella turcica have been observed to shrink suddenly. Presumably, they undergo a wave of necrosis as progressive enlargement compresses their blood supply. Despite these caveats and the variation in growth rate from one neoplasm to another, it is generally true that most benign tumors increase in size slowly over the span of months to years.

The rate of growth of malignant tumors correlates in general with their level of differentiation. In other words, rapidly growing tumors tend to be poorly differentiated. However, there is wide variation in the rate of growth. Some grow slowly for years, then enter a phase of rapid growth, signifying the emergence of an aggressive subclone of transformed cells. Others grow relatively slowly and steadily, and there are exceptional instances when growth comes almost to a standstill. Even more exceptionally, some cancers (particularly choriocarcinomas) have disappeared spontaneously as they have become totally necrotic, leaving only secondary metastatic implants. Despite these rarities, most cancers progressively enlarge over time, some slowly, others rapidly, but the notion that they "emerge out of the blue" is not true. Many lines of experimental and clinical evidence document that most if not all cancers take years and sometimes decades to evolve into clinically overt lesions. Rapidly growing malignant tumors often contain central areas of ischemic necrosis because the tumor blood supply, derived from the host, fails to keep pace with the oxygen needs of the expanding mass of cells.

Cancer Stem Cells and Lineages. A clinically detectable tumor contains a heterogeneous population of cells, which originated from the clonal growth of a single cell. It has been hypothesized that this population contains

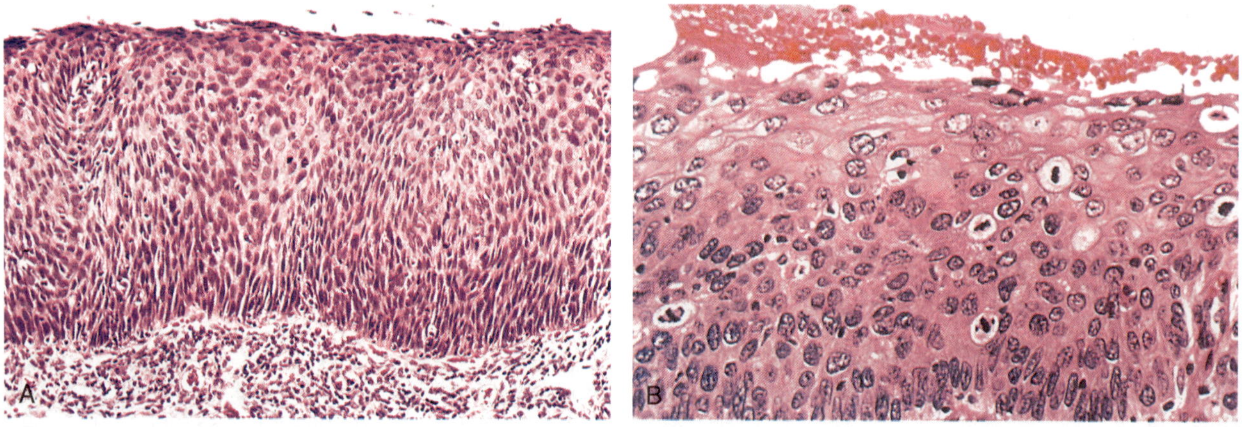

Figure 6–6

A, Carcinoma in situ. Low-power view shows the entire thickness of the epithelium is replaced by atypical dysplastic cells. There is no orderly differentiation of squamous cells. The basement membrane is intact, and there is no tumor in the subepithelial stroma. **B,** High-power view of another region shows failure of normal differentiation, marked nuclear and cellular pleomorphism, and numerous mitotic figures extending toward the surface. The intact basement membrane (below) is not seen in this section.

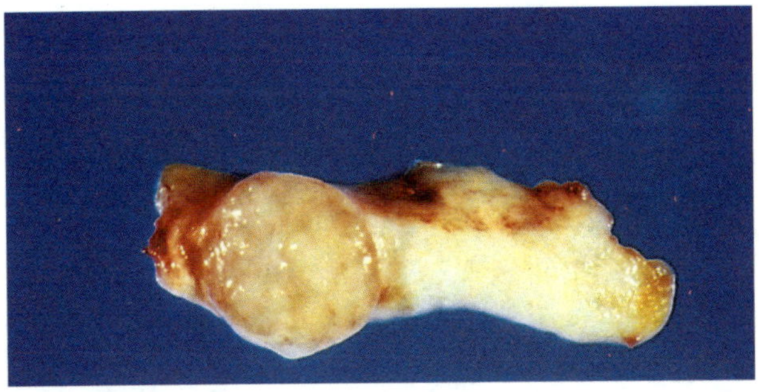

Figure 6–7

Fibroadenoma of the breast. The tan-colored, encapsulated small tumor is sharply demarcated from the whiter breast tissue.

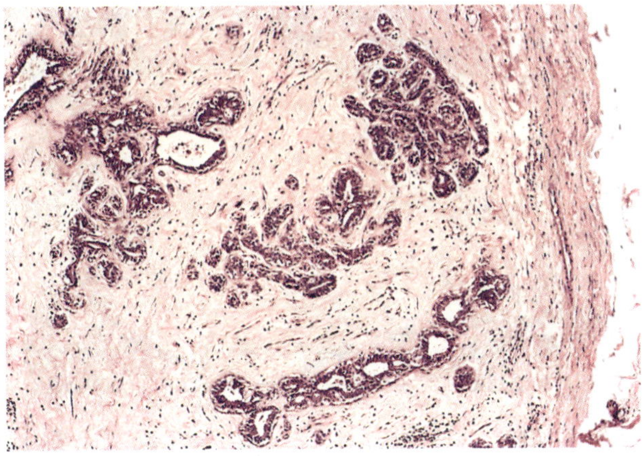

Figure 6–8

Microscopic view of fibroadenoma of the breast seen in Figure 6–7. The fibrous capsule *(right)* sharply delimits the tumor from the surrounding tissue. (Courtesy of Dr. Trace Worrell, Department of Pathology, University of Texas Southwestern Medical School, Dallas, Texas.)

cancer stem cells, which, in analogy to tissue stem cells, have the capacity to initiate and sustain the tumor. Recently, cancer stem cells, sometimes called tumor-initiating cells, were identified in breast cancer, glioblastoma multiforme (a brain tumor), and acute myeloid leukemia. Cancer stem cells constitute fewer than 2% of the cells in breast tumors and 0.1% to 1.0% of cells in acute myeloid leukemia. These findings have important implications for cancer treatment. Therapies that may efficiently kill the progeny of cancer stem cells would leave in place the cells capable of regenerating the tumor. Whether cancer stem cells exist in all tumors is not yet clear.

Local Invasion

A benign neoplasm remains localized at its site of origin. It does not have the capacity to infiltrate, invade, or metastasize to distant sites, as do malignant neoplasms. For example, as fibromas and adenomas slowly expand, most develop an enclosing fibrous capsule that separates them from the host tissue. This capsule probably is derived from the stroma of the host tissue as the parenchymal cells atrophy under the pressure of the expanding tumor. The stroma of the tumor itself also may contribute to the capsule (Figs. 6–7 and 6–8). It should be emphasized, however, that *not all benign neoplasms are encapsulated.* For example, the leiomyoma of the uterus is discretely demarcated from the surrounding smooth muscle by a zone of compressed and attenuated normal myometrium, but there is no well-developed capsule. Nonetheless, a well-defined cleavage plane exists around these lesions. A few benign tumors are neither encapsulated nor discretely defined; this is particularly true of some vascular benign neoplasms of the dermis. These exceptions are pointed out only to emphasize that although encapsulation is the rule in benign tumors, the lack of a capsule does not imply that a tumor is malignant.

Cancers grow by progressive infiltration, invasion, destruction, and penetration of the surrounding tissue (Figs. 6–9 and 6–10). They do not develop well-defined capsules. There are, however, occasional instances in which a slowly growing malignant tumor deceptively appears to be encased by the stroma of the surrounding host tissue, but microscopic examination usually reveals tiny crablike feet penetrating the margin and infiltrating adjacent structures. The infiltrative mode of growth makes it necessary to remove a wide margin of surrounding normal tissue when surgical excision of a malignant tumor is attempted. Surgical pathologists carefully examine the margins of resected tumors to ensure that they are devoid of cancer cells *(clean margins). Next to the development of metastases, local invasiveness is the most reliable feature that distinguishes malignant from benign tumors.*

Metastasis

The term *metastasis* connotes the development of secondary implants (metastases) discontinuous with the primary tumor, in remote tissues (Fig. 6–11). *The properties of invasiveness and, even more so, metastasis, more unequivocally identify a neoplasm as malignant than any of the other attributes of a tumor.* Not all cancers have equivalent ability to metastasize, however. At one extreme are basal cell carcinomas of the skin and most primary tumors of the central nervous system that are highly invasive in their primary sites of origin but rarely metastasize. At the other extreme are osteogenic (bone) sarcomas, which usually have metastasized to the lungs at the time of initial discovery.

Approximately 30% of newly diagnosed patients with solid tumors (excluding skin cancers other than melanomas) present with clinically evident metastases. An additional 20% have occult (hidden) metastases at the time of diagnosis.

In general, the more anaplastic and the larger the primary neoplasm, the more likely is metastatic spread; however, exceptions abound. Extremely small cancers have been known to metastasize, and, conversely, some large and ominous-looking lesions may not spread. Dissemination strongly prejudices, if it does not preclude, the possibility of cure of the disease, so it is obvious that,

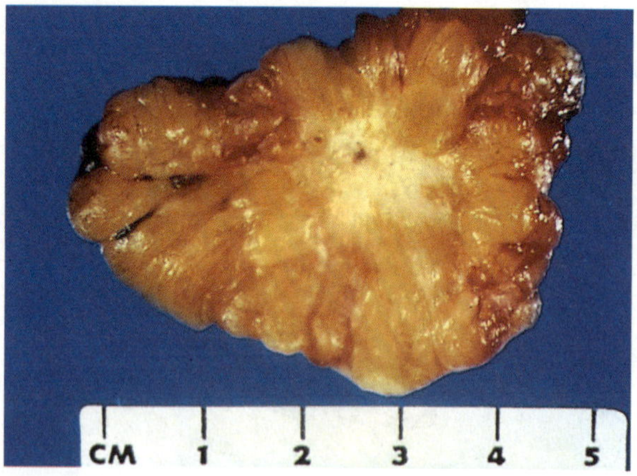

Figure 6–9

Cut section of invasive ductal carcinoma of the breast. The lesion is retracted, infiltrating the surrounding breast substance, and would be stony-hard on palpation.

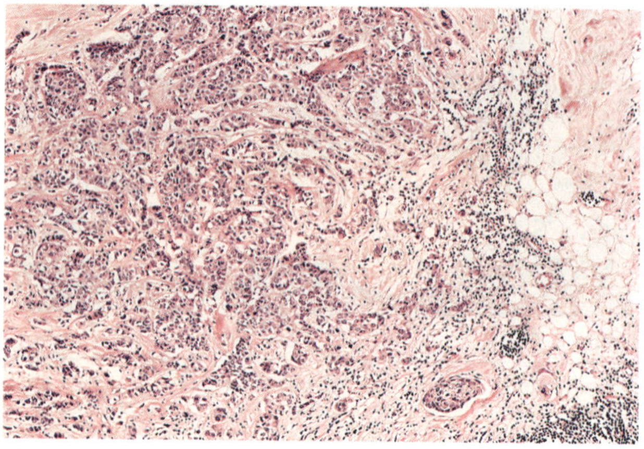

Figure 6–10

Microscopic view of breast carcinoma seen in Figure 6–9 illustrates the invasion of breast stroma and fat by nests and cords of tumor cells (compare with Fig. 6–8). Note the absence of a well-defined capsule. (Courtesy of Dr. Trace Worrell, Department of Pathology, University of Texas Southwestern Medical School, Dallas, Texas.)

short of prevention of cancer, no achievement would confer greater benefit on patients than methods to prevent metastasis.

Malignant neoplasms disseminate by one of three pathways: (1) seeding within body cavities, (2) lymphatic spread, or (3) hematogenous spread.

Spread by seeding occurs when neoplasms invade a natural body cavity. This mode of dissemination is particularly characteristic of cancers of the ovary, which often cover the peritoneal surfaces widely. The implants literally may glaze all peritoneal surfaces and yet not invade the underlying parenchyma of the abdominal organs. Here is an instance of the ability to reimplant elsewhere that seems to be separable from the capacity to invade. Neoplasms of the central nervous system, such as a medulloblastoma or ependymoma, may penetrate the cerebral ventricles and be carried by the cerebrospinal fluid to reimplant on the meningeal surfaces, either within the brain or in the spinal cord.

Lymphatic spread is more typical of carcinomas, whereas *hematogenous spread* is favored by sarcomas. There are numerous interconnections, however, between the lymphatic and vascular systems, and so all forms of cancer may disseminate through either or both systems. The pattern of lymph node involvement depends principally on the site of the primary neoplasm and the natural pathways of lymphatic drainage of the site. Lung carcinomas arising in the respiratory passages metastasize first to the regional bronchial lymph nodes, then to the tracheobronchial and hilar nodes. Carcinoma of the breast usually arises in the upper outer quadrant and first spreads to the axillary nodes. However, medial breast lesions may drain through the chest wall to the nodes along the internal mammary artery. Thereafter, in both instances, the supraclavicular and infraclavicular nodes may be seeded. In some cases, the cancer cells seem to traverse the lymphatic channels within the immediately proximate nodes to be trapped in subsequent lymph nodes, producing so-called *skip metastases*. The cells may traverse all of the lymph nodes ultimately to reach the vascular compartment via the thoracic duct.

A "sentinal lymph node" is defined as the first lymph node in a regional lymphatic basin that receives lymph flow from a primary tumor. It can be delineated by injection of blue dyes or radiolabelled tracers. Biopsy of sentinal lymph nodes allows determination of the extent of spread of tumor, and can be used to plan treatment.

It should be noted that although enlargement of nodes near a primary neoplasm should arouse strong suspicions of metastatic spread, it does not always imply cancerous involvement. The necrotic products of the neoplasm and tumor antigens often evoke reactive changes in the nodes, such as enlargement and hyperplasia of the follicles (lymphadenitis) and proliferation of macrophages in the subcapsular sinuses (sinus histiocytosis).

Hematogenous spread is the most feared consequence of a cancer. It is the favored pathway for sarcomas, but carcinomas use it as well. As might be expected, arteries are penetrated less readily than are veins. With venous invasion, the blood-borne cells follow the venous flow draining the site of the neoplasm, with tumor cells often

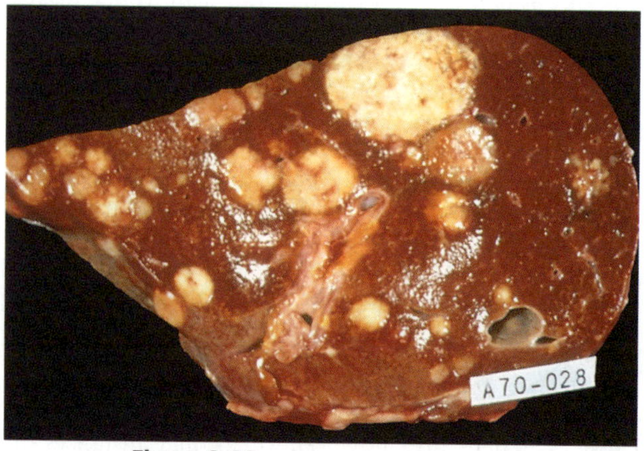

Figure 6–11

A liver studded with metastatic cancer.

stopping in the first capillary bed they encounter. Since all portal area drainage flows to the liver, and all caval blood flows to the lungs, *the liver and lungs are the most frequently involved secondary sites in hematogenous dissemination.* Cancers arising near the vertebral column often embolize through the paravertebral plexus; this pathway probably is involved in the frequent vertebral metastases of carcinomas of the thyroid and prostate.

Certain carcinomas have a propensity to invade veins. Renal cell carcinoma often invades the renal vein to grow in a snakelike fashion up the inferior vena cava, sometimes reaching the right side of the heart. Hepatocellular carcinomas often penetrate portal and hepatic radicles to grow within them into the main venous channels. Remarkably, such intravenous growth may not be accompanied by widespread dissemination.

Many observations suggest that mere anatomic localization of the neoplasm and natural pathways of venous drainage do not wholly explain the systemic distributions of metastases. For example, prostatic carcinoma preferentially spreads to bone, bronchogenic carcinomas tend to involve the adrenals and the brain, and neuroblastomas spread to the liver and bones. Conversely, skeletal muscles, although rich in capillaries, are rarely the site of secondary deposits. The molecular basis of such tissue-specific homing of tumor cells is discussed later.

In conclusion, the various features discussed in the preceding sections, as summarized below and in Figure 6–12, usually permit the differentiation of benign and malignant neoplasms. Against this background of the structure and behavior of neoplasms, we can turn to some considerations of their nature and origins.

SUMMARY

Characteristics of Benign and Malignant Tumors

- Benign and malignant tumors can be distinguished on the basis of the degree of differentiation, rate of growth, local invasiveness, and distant spread.
- Benign tumors resemble the tissue of origin and are well differentiated; malignant tumors are poorly or completely undifferentiated (anaplastic).
- Benign tumors are slow growing, whereas malignant tumors generally grow faster.
- Benign tumors are well circumscribed and have a capsule; malignant tumors are poorly circumscribed and invade the surrounding normal tissues.
- Benign tumors remain localized to the site of origin, whereas malignant tumors are locally invasive and they metastasize to distant sites.

EPIDEMIOLOGY

Because cancer is a disorder of cell growth and behavior, its ultimate cause must be defined at the cellular and molecular levels. Cancer epidemiology can contribute substantially to knowledge about the origin of cancer. The now well-established concept that cigarette smoking is causally associated with lung cancer arose primarily from epidemiologic studies. A comparison of the incidence of colon cancer and dietary patterns in the western world

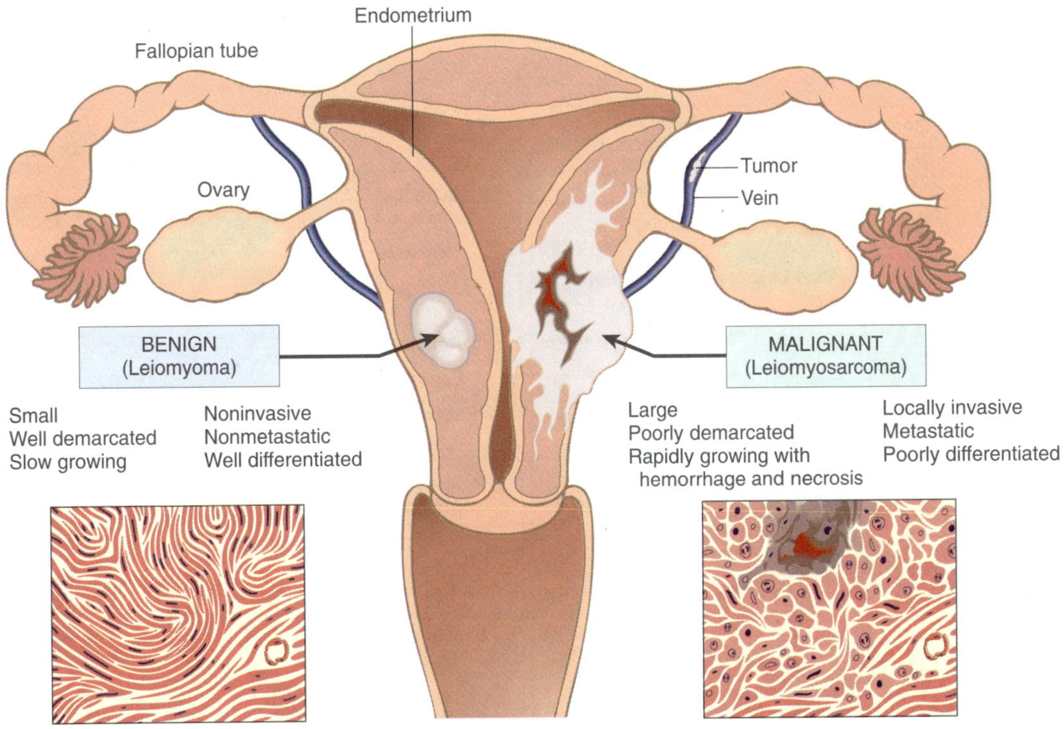

Figure 6–12

Comparison between a benign tumor of the myometrium (leiomyoma) and a malignant tumor of similar origin (leiomyosarcoma).

and Africa led to the recognition that dietary fat and fiber content may figure importantly in the causation of this cancer. Major insights into the causes of cancer can be obtained by epidemiologic studies that relate particular environmental, racial (possibly hereditary), and cultural influences to the occurrence of specific neoplasms. Certain diseases associated with an increased risk of developing cancer (preneoplastic disorders) also provide clues to the pathogenesis of cancer. In the following discussion we first summarize the overall incidence of cancer to gain an insight into the magnitude of the cancer problem, then we review some issues relating to the patient and environment that influence the predisposition to cancer.

Cancer Incidence

Some perspective on the likelihood of developing a specific form of cancer can be gained from national incidence and mortality data. Overall, it is estimated that about *1.4 million* new cancer cases will occur in 2006, and 565,000 people will die of cancer in the United States. The incidence of the most common forms of cancer and the major killers is presented in Figure 6–13.

Over several decades, the death rates of many forms of malignant neoplasia have changed. Particularly notable is the significant increase in the overall cancer death rate among men that was attributable largely to lung cancer, but this has finally begun to drop. In contrast, the overall death rate among women has fallen slightly, mostly as a result of the decline in death rates from cancers of the uterine cervix, stomach, and large bowel. These welcome trends have more than counterbalanced the striking climb in the rate of lung cancer among women, which not long ago was a relatively uncommon form of neoplasia in this sex. The declining death rate from cervical cancer is directly related to widespread use of cytologic smear studies for early detection of this tumor while it is still curable. The causes of decline in death rates for cancers of the stomach are obscure; however, there have been speculations about decreasing exposure to dietary carcinogens.

Geographic and Environmental Variables

Although many impressive advances in understanding the molecular pathogenesis of cancer have been made by analyzing hereditary cancers, it is fair to state that environmental factors that give rise to somatic mutations are the predominant cause of the most common sporadic cancers. This notion is supported by the geographic differences in death rates from specific forms of cancer. For example, death rates from breast cancer are about fourfold to fivefold higher in the United States and Europe compared with Japan. Conversely, the death rate for stomach carcinoma in men and women is about seven times higher in Japan than in the United States. Liver cell carcinoma is relatively infrequent in the United States but is the most lethal cancer among many African populations. Nearly all the evidence indicates that these geographic differences are environmental rather than genetic in origin. Nisei (second-generation Japanese living in the United States) have mortality rates for certain forms of cancer that are intermediate between those of natives of Japan and of Americans who have lived in the United States for many generations. The two rates come closer with each passing generation.

There is no paucity of environmental carcinogens. They lurk in the ambient environment, in the workplace, in food, and in personal practices. They can be as uni-

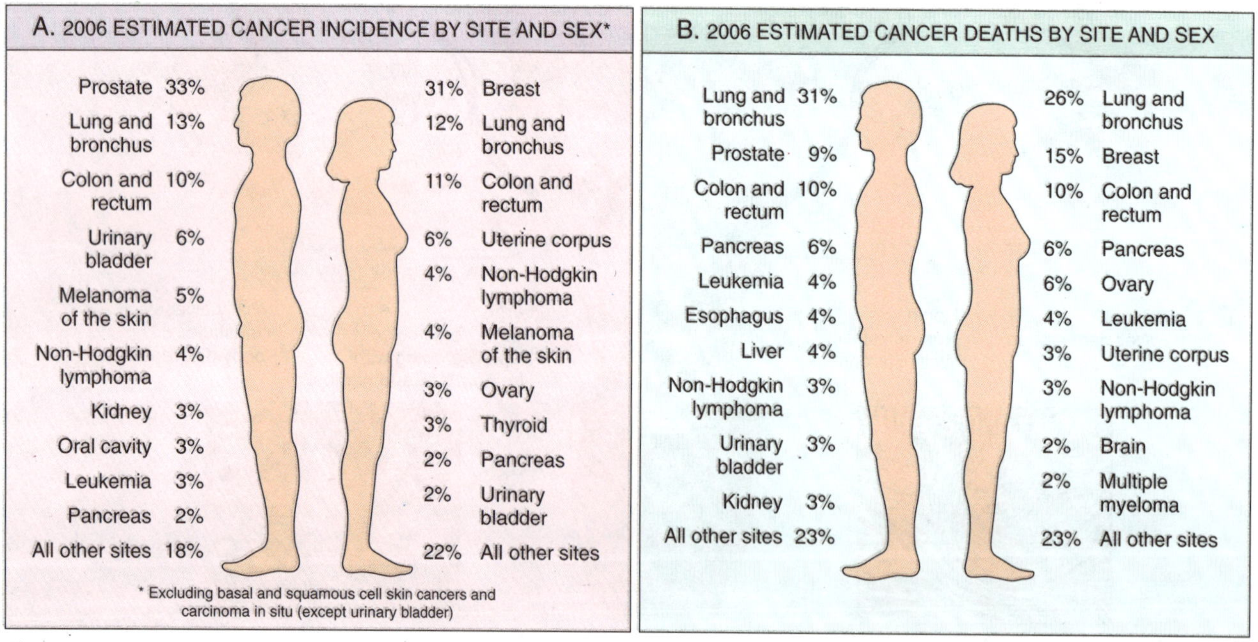

Figure 6–13

Cancer incidence and mortality by site and sex. (Adapted from Jemal A, et al.: Cancer statistics, 2006. CA Cancer J Clin 56:106, 2006.)

Table 6–2 Occupational Cancers

Agents or Groups of Agents	Human Cancer Site and Type for Which Reasonable Evidence Is Available	Typical Use or Occurrence
Arsenic and arsenic compounds	Lung, skin, hemangiosarcoma	Byproduct of metal smelting. Component of alloys, electrical and semiconductor devices, medications and herbicides, fungicides, and animal dips
Asbestos	Lung, mesothelioma; gastrointestinal tract (esophagus, stomach, large intestine)	Formerly used for many applications because of fire, heat, and friction resistance; still found in existing construction as well as fire-resistant textiles, friction materials (i.e., brake linings), underlayment and roofing papers, and floor tiles
Benzene	Leukemia, Hodgkin lymphoma	Principal component of light oil. Although use as solvent is discouraged, many applications exist in printing and lithography, paint, rubber, dry cleaning, adhesives and coatings, and detergents. Formerly widely used as solvent and fumigant
Beryllium and beryllium compounds	Lung	Missile fuel and space vehicles. Hardener for lightweight metal alloys, particularly in aerospace applications and nuclear reactors
Cadmium and cadmium compounds	Prostate	Uses include yellow pigments and phosphors. Found in solders. Used in batteries and as alloy and in metal platings and coatings
Chromium compounds	Lung	Component of metal alloys, paints, pigments, and preservatives
Ethylene oxide	Leukemia	Ripening agent for fruits and nuts. Used in rocket propellant and chemical synthesis, in fumigants for foodstuffs and textiles, and in sterilants for hospital equipment
Nickel compounds	Nose, lung	Nickel plating. Component of ferrous alloys, ceramics, and batteries. Byproduct of stainless-steel arc welding
Radon and its decay products	Lung	From decay of minerals containing uranium. Can be serious hazard in quarries and mines
Vinyl chloride	Angiosarcoma, liver	Refrigerant. Monomer for vinyl polymers. Adhesive for plastics. Formerly inert aerosol propellant in pressurized containers

Modified from Stellman JM, Stellman SD: Cancer and workplace. CA Cancer J Clin 46:70–92, 1996 with permission from Lippincott Williams & Wilkins.

versal as sunlight, can be found particularly in urban settings (e.g., asbestos), or can be limited to a certain occupation (Table 6–2). Certain features of diet have been implicated as possible predisposing influences. Among the possible environmental influences, the most distressing are those incurred in personal practices, notably cigarette smoking and chronic alcohol consumption. The risk of cervical cancer is linked to age at first intercourse and the number of sex partners (pointing to a causal role for venereal transmission of an oncogenic virus). There is no escape: It seems that everything one does to earn a livelihood, to subsist, or to enjoy life turns out to be illegal, immoral, or fattening, or—most disturbing—possibly carcinogenic.

Age

In general, the frequency of cancer increases with age. Most cancer mortality occurs between ages 55 and 75; the rate declines, along with the population base, after age 75. The rising incidence with age may be explained by the accumulation of somatic mutations associated with the emergence of malignant neoplasms (discussed later). The decline in immune competence that accompanies aging also may be a factor.

Cancer causes slightly more than 10% of all deaths among children younger than 15 years (Chapter 7). The major lethal cancers in children are leukemia, tumors of the central nervous system, lymphomas, soft tissue sarcomas, and bone sarcomas. As discussed later, study of several childhood tumors, particularly retinoblastoma and Wilms tumor, has provided novel insights into the pathogenesis of malignant transformation.

Heredity

The evidence now indicates that for many types of cancer, including the most common forms, there exist not only environmental influences but also hereditary predispositions. Hereditary forms of cancer can be divided into three categories (Table 6–3).

Inherited Cancer Syndromes. Inherited cancer syndromes include several well-defined cancers in which inheritance

Table 6–3 Inherited Predisposition to Cancer

Gene	Inherited Predisposition
Inherited Cancer Syndromes (Autosomal Dominant)	
RB	Retinoblastoma
p53	Li-Fraumeni syndrome (various tumors)
p16INK4A	Melanoma
APC	Familial adenomatous polyposis/colon cancer
NF1, NF2	Neurofibromatosis 1 and 2
BRCA1, BRCA2	Breast and ovarian tumors
MEN1, RET	Multiple endocrine neoplasia 1 and 2
MSH2, MLH1, MSH6	Hereditary nonpolyposis colon cancer
PATCH	Nevoid basal cell carcinoma syndrome
Familial Cancers	
Familial clustering of cases, but role of inherited predisposition not clear for each individual	
Breast cancer (not linked to BRCA1 or BRCA2)	
Ovarian cancer	
Pancreatic cancer	
Inherited Autosomal Recessive Syndromes of Defective DNA Repair	
Xeroderma pigmentosum	
Ataxia-telangiectasia	
Bloom syndrome	
Fanconi anemia	

of a single mutant gene greatly increases the risk of developing a tumor. The predisposition to these tumors shows an autosomal dominant pattern of inheritance. Childhood retinoblastoma is the most striking example of this category. Approximately 40% of retinoblastomas are familial. As is discussed later, a *tumor suppressor gene* has been implicated in the pathogenesis of this tumor. Carriers of this gene have a 10,000-fold increased risk of developing retinoblastoma, usually bilaterally. They also have a greatly increased risk of developing a second cancer, particularly osteogenic sarcoma. Familial adenomatous polyposis is another hereditary disorder marked by an extraordinarily high risk of cancer. Individuals who inherit the autosomal dominant mutation have, at birth or soon thereafter, innumerable polypoid adenomas of the colon, and virtually 100% of patients develop a carcinoma of the colon by age 50 (see Table 6–3).

Tumors within this group often are associated with a specific marker phenotype. There may be multiple benign tumors in the affected tissue, as occurs in familial polyposis of the colon and in multiple endocrine neoplasia. Sometimes, there are abnormalities in tissue that are not the target of transformation (e.g., Lisch nodules and café-au-lait spots in neurofibromatosis type 1; Chapter 23).

Familial Cancers. Virtually all the common types of cancers that occur sporadically have been reported to occur in familial forms. Examples include carcinomas of colon, breast, ovary, and brain. *Features that characterize familial cancers include early age at onset, tumors arising in two or more close relatives of the index case, and sometimes multiple or bilateral tumors.* Familial cancers are not associated with specific marker phenotypes. For example, in contrast to the familial adenomatous polyposis syndrome, familial colonic cancers do not arise in preexisting benign polyps. The transmission pattern of familial cancers is not clear. In general, siblings have a relative risk between 2 and 3. Segregation analysis of large families usually reveals that predisposition to the tumors is dominant, but multifactorial inheritance cannot be easily ruled out. As discussed later, certain familial cancers can be linked to the inheritance of mutant genes.

Autosomal Recessive Syndromes of Defective DNA Repair. Besides the dominantly inherited precancerous conditions, a small group of autosomal recessive disorders is collectively characterized by chromosomal or DNA instability. One of the best-studied examples is xeroderma pigmentosum, in which DNA repair is defective. This and other familial disorders of DNA instability are described later.

In summary, no more than 5% to 10% of all human cancers fall into one of the three aforementioned categories. What can be said about the influence of heredity in the large preponderance of malignant tumors? There is emerging evidence that the influence of hereditary factors is subtle and indirect. The genotype may influence the likelihood of one's developing environmentally induced cancers. For example, polymorphisms in drug-metabolizing enzymes confer genetic predisposition to lung cancers in cigarette smokers. A striking genetic predisposition to developing mesotheliomas (an asbestos-associated tumor) also has been noted, but the relevant gene is not yet known.

Acquired Preneoplastic Disorders

In addition to the genetic influences described earlier, certain clinical conditions are well-recognized predispositions to the development of malignant neoplasia and are referred to as *preneoplastic disorders.* This designation is unfortunate because it implies a certain inevitability, but in fact, although such conditions may increase the likelihood, in most instances cancer does not develop. A brief listing of the chief conditions follows:

- Persistent regenerative cell replication (e.g., squamous cell carcinoma in the margins of a chronic skin fistula or in a long-unhealed skin wound; hepatocellular carcinoma in cirrhosis of the liver)
- Hyperplastic and dysplastic proliferations (e.g., endometrial carcinoma in atypical endometrial hyperplasia; bronchogenic carcinoma in the dysplastic bronchial mucosa of habitual cigarette smokers)
- Chronic atrophic gastritis (e.g., gastric carcinoma in pernicious anemia or following long-standing *Helicobacter pylori* infection)
- Chronic ulcerative colitis (e.g., an increased incidence of colorectal carcinoma in long-standing disease)

- Leukoplakia of the oral cavity, vulva, or penis (e.g., increased risk of squamous cell carcinoma)
- Villous adenomas of the colon (e.g., high risk of transformation to colorectal carcinoma)

In this context it may be asked, "What is the risk of malignant change in a benign neoplasm?" or, stated differently, "Are benign tumors precancerous?" In general the answer is no, but inevitably there are exceptions, and perhaps it is better to say that each type of benign tumor is associated with a particular level of risk, ranging from high to virtually nonexistent. For example, adenomas of the colon as they enlarge can undergo malignant transformation in 50% of cases; in contrast, malignant change is extremely rare in leiomyomas of the uterus.

SUMMARY

Epidemiology of Cancer

- The incidence of cancer varies with age, race, geographic factors, and genetic backgrounds. Cancers are most common at the two extremes of age. The geographic variation results mostly from different environmental exposures.
- Most cancers are sporadic, but some are familial. Predisposition to hereditary cancers may be autosomal dominant or autosomal recessive. The former are usually linked to inheritance of a germ-line mutation of cancer suppressor genes, whereas the latter are typically associated with inherited defects in DNA repair.
- Familial cancers tend to be bilateral and arise earlier in life than their sporadic counterparts.

CARCINOGENESIS: THE MOLECULAR BASIS OF CANCER

It could be argued that the proliferation of literature on the molecular basis of cancer has outpaced the growth of even the most malignant of tumors. It is easy to get lost in the growing forest of information. First, we list some fundamental principles before delving into the details of the genetic basis of cancer.

Nonlethal genetic damage lies at the heart of carcinogenesis. Such genetic damage (or mutation) may be acquired by the action of environmental agents, such as chemicals, radiation, or viruses, or it may be inherited in the germ line. The genetic hypothesis of cancer implies that a tumor mass results from the clonal expansion of a single progenitor cell that has incurred genetic damage (i.e., tumors are monoclonal). This expectation has been realized in most tumors that have been analyzed. Clonality of tumors is assessed readily in women who are heterozygous for polymorphic X-linked markers, such as the enzyme glucose-6-phosphate dehydrogenase or X-linked restriction-fragment-length polymorphisms. The principle underlying such an analysis is illustrated in Figure 6–14.

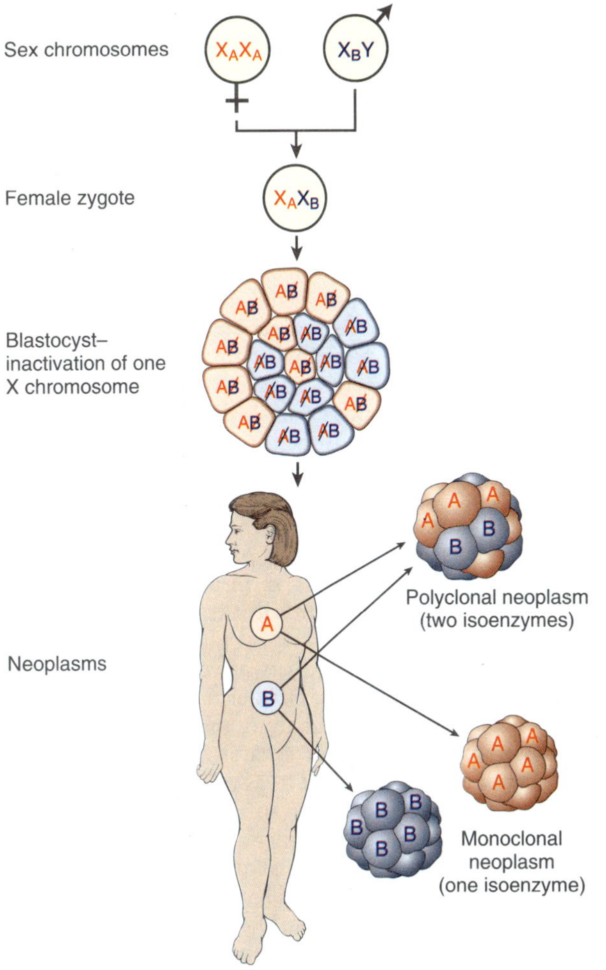

Figure 6–14

Diagram depicting the use of X-linked isoenzyme cell markers as evidence of the monoclonality of neoplasms. Because of random X inactivation, all females are mosaics with two cell populations (with glucose-6-phosphate dehydrogenase isoenzyme A or B in this case). When neoplasms that arise in women who are heterozygous for X-linked markers are analyzed, they are made up of cells that contain the active maternal (X_A) or the paternal (X_B) X chromosome, but not both. Currently, X-linked molecular markers are used more commonly than isoenzyme variants.

Four classes of normal regulatory genes—growth-promoting proto-oncogenes, growth-inhibiting tumor suppressor genes, genes that regulate programmed cell death (i.e., apoptosis), and genes involved in DNA repair—are the principal targets of genetic damage. Collectively the genetic alterations in tumor cells confer upon them growth and survival advantages over normal cells, as will be evident from the discussion that follows.

Mutant alleles of proto-oncogenes are called oncogenes. They are considered dominant because mutation of a single allele can lead to cellular transformation. In contrast, typically both normal alleles of tumor suppressor genes must be damaged for transformation to occur, so this family of genes is sometimes referred to as recessive oncogenes. However, recent work has clearly shown that, in some cases, loss of a single allele of a tumor suppressor gene can promote transformation (haploinsufficiency). Genes that regulate apoptosis may be dominant, as are proto-oncogenes, or they may behave as tumor suppressor genes. Tumor suppressor genes are usefully placed into two general groups, promoters and caretakers. Promoters are the traditional tumor suppressor genes, such as *RB* or *p53*, where mutation of the gene leads to transformation by releasing the brakes on cellular proliferation. Caretaker genes are responsible for processes that ensure the integrity of the genome, such as DNA repair. Mutation of caretaker genes does not directly transform cells by affecting proliferation or apoptosis. Instead, DNA repair genes affect cell proliferation or survival indirectly by influencing the ability of the organism to repair nonlethal damage in other genes, including proto-oncogenes, tumor suppressor genes, and genes that regulate apoptosis. A disability in the DNA repair genes can predispose cells to widespread mutations in the genome and thus to neoplastic transformation. Cells with mutations in caretaker genes are said to have developed a *mutator phenotype*.

Carcinogenesis is a multistep process at both the phenotypic and the genetic levels, resulting from the accumulation of multiple mutations. As discussed earlier, malignant neoplasms have several phenotypic attributes, such as excessive growth, local invasiveness, and the ability to form distant metastases. Furthermore, it is well established that over a period of time, many tumors become more aggressive and acquire greater malignant potential. This phenomenon is referred to as tumor progression and is not simply represented by an increase in tumor size. Careful clinical and experimental studies reveal that increasing malignancy is often acquired in an incremental fashion. At the molecular level, tumor progression and associated heterogeneity most likely result from multiple mutations that accumulate independently in different cells, generating subclones with different characteristics (Fig. 6–15) such as ability to invade, rate of growth, metastatic ability, karyotype, hormonal responsiveness, and susceptibility to anti-neoplastic drugs. Some of the mutations may be lethal; others may spur cell growth by affecting proto-oncogenes or cancer suppressor genes. *Even though most malignant tumors are monoclonal in origin, by the time they become clinically evident, their constituent cells are extremely heterogeneous.* During progression, tumor cells are subjected to immune and nonimmune selection pressures. For example, cells that are highly antigenic are destroyed by host defenses, whereas those with reduced growth factor requirements are positively selected. A growing tumor, therefore, tends to be enriched for subclones that "beat the odds" and are adept at survival, growth, invasion, and metastasis.

SUMMARY

Overview of Carcinogenesis

- Tumors arise from clonal growth of cells that have incurred mutations in four classes of genes. These include genes that regulate cell growth (proto-oncogenes and tumor suppressor genes) and those that regulate apoptosis and DNA repair.
- Mutation in no single gene is sufficient to cause cancer. Typically, the phenotypic attributes characteristic of malignancy develop when multiple mutations involving multiple genes accumulate. The stepwise accumulation of mutations and increasing malignancy is referred to as tumor progression.

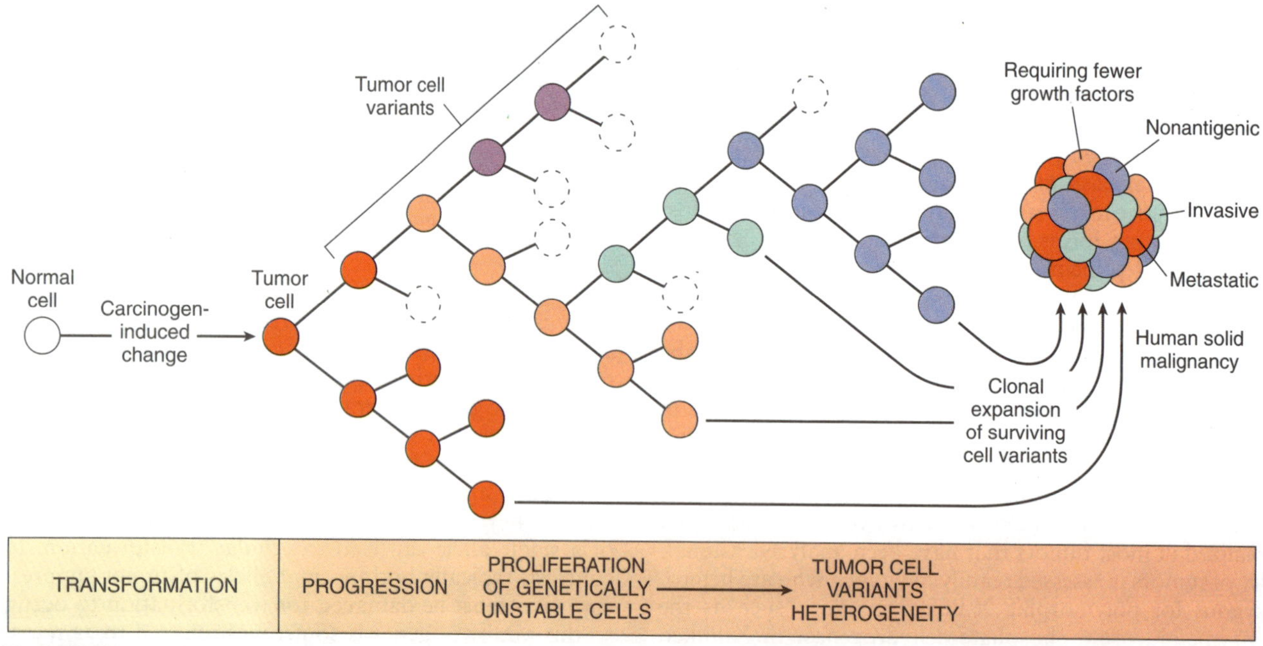

Figure 6–15

Tumor progression and generation of heterogeneity. New subclones arise from the descendants of the original transformed cell by multiple mutations. With progression the tumor mass becomes enriched for variants that are more adept at evading host defenses and are likely to be more aggressive.

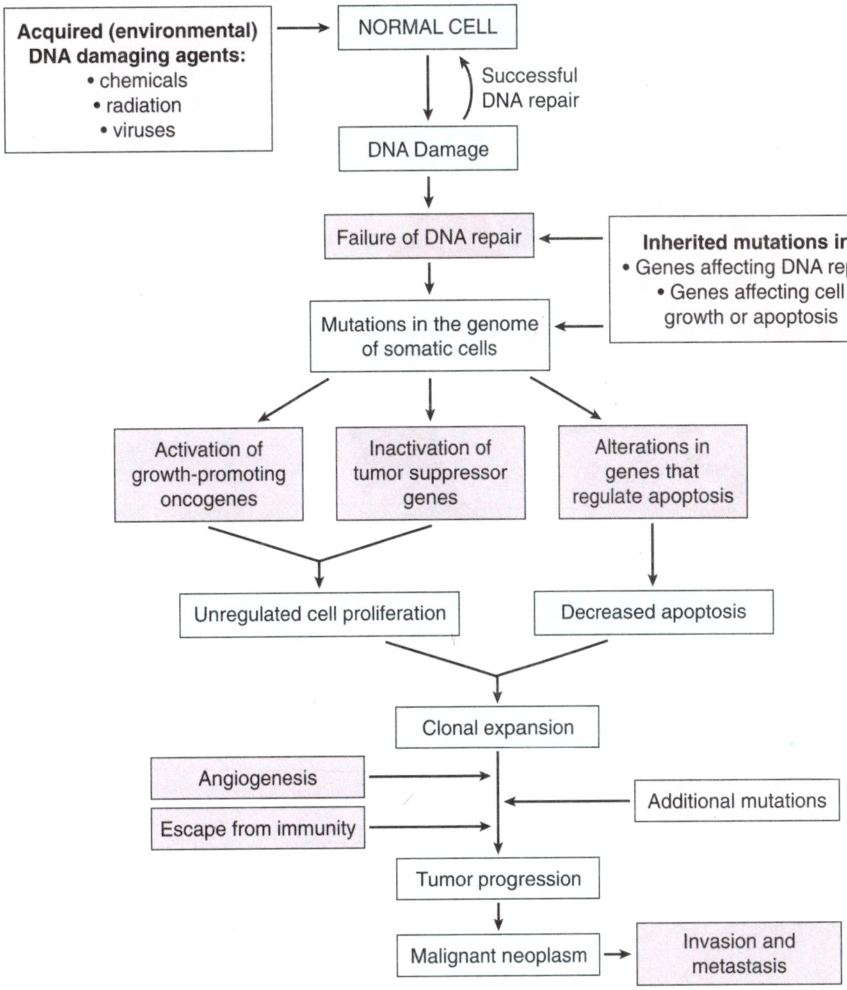

Figure 6–16

Flow chart depicting a simplified scheme of the molecular basis of cancer.

With this overview (Fig. 6–16), we can now address in detail the molecular pathogenesis of cancer and discuss the carcinogenic agents that inflict genetic damage. In the past 20 years hundreds of cancer-associated genes have been discovered. Some, such as *p53,* are commonly mutated; others, such as *c-ABL,* are affected only in certain leukemias. Each cancer gene has a specific function, the dysregulation of which contributes to the origin or progression of malignancy. It is best therefore to consider cancer-related genes in the context of seven fundamental changes in cell physiology that together dictate the malignant phenotype. All except the mutator phenotype are illustrated in Figure 6–17:

1. Self-sufficiency in growth signals
2. Insensitivity to growth-inhibitory signals
3. Evasion of apoptosis
4. Limitless replicative potential (i.e., overcoming cellular senescence and avoiding mitotic catastrophe)
5. Development of sustained angiogenesis
6. Ability to invade and metastasize
7. Genomic instability resulting from defects in DNA repair

Mutations in genes that regulate some or all of these cellular traits are seen in every cancer, and hence these will form the basis of our discussion of the molecular origins of cancer. In the ensuing discussion it should be noted that gene symbols are italicized but their protein products are not (e.g., *RB* gene and RB protein).

Self-Sufficiency in Growth Signals

Genes that promote autonomous cell growth in cancer cells are called *oncogenes.* They are derived by mutations in proto-oncogenes and are characterized by the ability to promote cell growth in the absence of normal growth-promoting signals. Their products, called *oncoproteins,* resemble the normal products of proto-oncogenes except that oncoproteins are devoid of important regulatory elements, and their production in the transformed cells does not depend on growth factors or other external signals. To aid in the understanding of the nature and functions of oncoproteins, it is necessary to review briefly the sequence of events that characterize normal cell proliferation; these were introduced in Chapter 3. Under physiologic conditions, cell proliferation can be readily resolved into the following steps:

- The binding of a growth factor to its specific receptor on the cell membrane

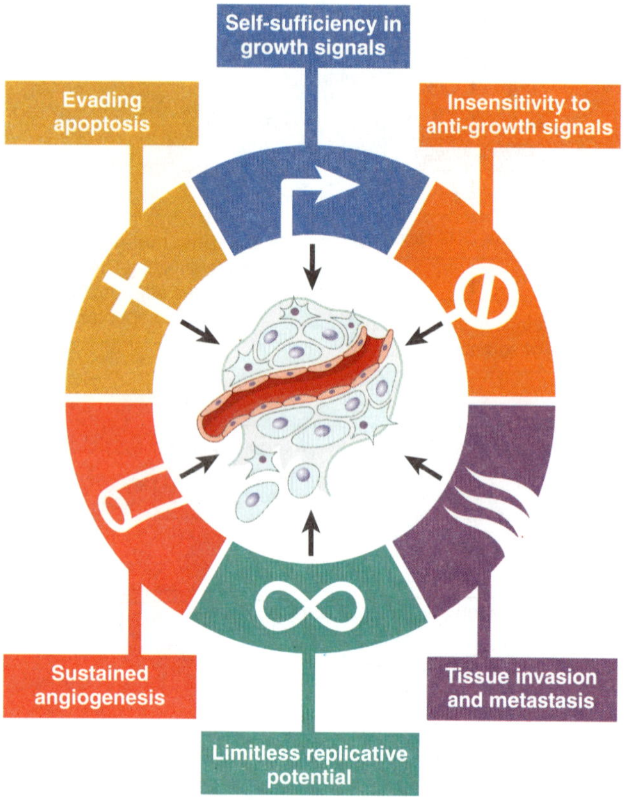

Figure 6–17

Six hallmarks of cancer. Most cancer cells acquire these properties during their development, typically by mutations in the relevant genes. (From Hanahan D, Weinberg RA: The hallmarks of cancer. Cell 100:57, 2000.)

- Transient and limited activation of the growth factor receptor, which in turn activates several signal-transducing proteins on the inner leaflet of the plasma membrane
- Transmission of the transduced signal across the cytosol to the nucleus via second messengers or a cascade of signal transduction molecules
- Induction and activation of nuclear regulatory factors that initiate DNA transcription
- Entry and progression of the cell into the cell cycle, resulting ultimately in cell division

With this background we can identify the strategies used by cancer cells to acquire self-sufficiency in growth signals. They can be grouped on the basis of their role in the signal transduction cascade and cell cycle regulation. Indeed, each one of the steps above is susceptible to corruption by cancer cells.

Growth Factors

All normal cells require stimulation by growth factors to undergo proliferation. Most soluble growth factors are made by one cell type and act on a neighboring cell to stimulate proliferation (paracrine action). Many cancer cells acquire growth self-sufficiency, however, by acquiring the ability to synthesize the same growth factors to which they are responsive. For example, many glioblastomas secrete platelet-derived growth factor (PDGF) and express the PDGF receptor, and many sarcomas make both transforming growth factor-α (TGF-α) and its receptor. Similar autocrine loops are fairly common in many types of cancer. Genes that encode homologues of fibroblast growth factors (e.g., *hst-1* and *FGF3*) have been detected in several gastrointestinal and breast tumors; FGF-2 is expressed in human melanomas but not normal melanocytes. Hepatocyte growth factor (HGF) and its receptor c-Met are both overexpressed in follicular carcinomas of the thyroid. In many instances the growth factor gene itself is not altered or mutated, but the products of other oncogenes (e.g., *RAS*) stimulate overexpression of growth factor genes and the subsequent development of an autocrine loop.

Growth Factor Receptors

The next group in the sequence of signal transduction is growth factor receptors, and several oncogenes that result from the overexpression or mutation of growth factor receptors have been identified. Mutant receptor proteins deliver continuous mitogenic signals to cells, even in the absence of the growth factor in the environment. More common than mutations is overexpression of growth factor receptors, which can render cancer cells hyper-responsive to levels of the growth factor that would not normally trigger proliferation. The best-documented examples of overexpression involve the epidermal growth factor (EGF) receptor family. *ERBB1,* the EGF receptor, is overexpressed in 80% of squamous cell carcinomas of the lung, 50% or more of glioblastomas, and 80 to 100% of epithelial tumors of the head and neck. A related receptor, called *HER2/NEU (ERBB2),* is amplified in 25% to 30% of breast cancers and adenocarcinomas of the lung, ovary, and salivary glands. These tumors are exquisitely sensitive to the mitogenic effects of small amounts of growth factors, and a high level of HER2/NEU protein in breast cancer cells is a harbinger of poor prognosis. The significance of *HER2/NEU* in the pathogenesis of breast cancers is illustrated dramatically by the clinical benefit derived from blocking the extracellular domain of this receptor with anti-*HER2/NEU* antibodies. Treatment of breast cancer with anti-HER2/NEU antibody is an elegant example of "bench to bedside" medicine.

Signal-Transducing Proteins

A relatively common mechanism by which cancer cells acquire growth autonomy is mutations in genes that encode various components of the signaling pathways downstream of growth factor receptors. These signaling molecules couple growth factor receptors to their nuclear targets. Many such signaling proteins are associated with the inner leaflet of the plasma membrane, where they receive signals from activated growth factor receptors and transmit them to the nucleus, either through second messengers or through a cascade of phosphorylation and activation of signal transduction molecules. Two important members in this category are *RAS* and *ABL.* Each of these is discussed briefly.

RAS is the most commonly mutated proto-oncogene in human tumors. Indeed, approximately 30% of all human tumors contain mutated versions of the *RAS* gene, and the incidence is even higher in some specific cancers (e.g., colon and pancreatic adenocarcinomas). RAS is a member of a family of small G proteins that bind guanosine nucleotides (guanosine triphosphate [GTP] and guanosine diphosphate [GDP]), similar to the larger trimolecular G proteins. Normal RAS proteins flip back and forth between an excited signal-transmitting state and a quiescent state. RAS proteins are inactive when bound to GDP; stimulation of cells by growth factors leads to exchange of GDP for GTP and subsequent conformational changes that generates active RAS (Fig. 6–18). The activated RAS in turn stimulates down-stream regulators of proliferation, such as the *RAF–mitogen-activated protein (MAP) kinase mitogenic cascade,* which floods the nucleus with signals for cell proliferation. The excited signal-emitting stage of the normal RAS protein is short-lived, however, because its intrinsic guanosine triphosphatase (GTPase) activity hydrolyzes GTP to GDP, releasing a phosphate group and returning the protein to its quiescent inactive state. The GTPase activity of activated RAS protein is magnified dramatically by a family of GTPase-activating proteins (GAPs), which act as molecular brakes that prevent uncontrolled RAS activation by favoring hydrolysis of GTP to GDP.

The *RAS* gene is most commonly activated by point mutations. Molecular analyses of *RAS* mutations have revealed three hot spots, which encode residues either within the GTP-binding pocket or the enzymatic region essential for GTP hydrolysis. Mutations at these locations interfere with GTP hydrolysis that is essential to convert RAS into an inactive form. RAS is thus trapped in its activated GTP-bound form, and the cell is forced into a continuously proliferating state. It follows from this scenario that the consequences of mutations in RAS protein would be mimicked by mutations in the GAPs that fail to restrain normal RAS proteins. Indeed, disabling mutation of neurofibromin 1, a GAP, is associated with familial neurofibromatosis type 1 (Chapter 23).

In addition to *RAS,* several non–receptor-associated tyrosine kinases function as signal transduction molecules. In this group, *ABL* is the most well defined with respect to carcinogenesis. The *ABL* proto-oncogene has tyrosine kinase activity that is dampened by internal negative regulatory domains. In chronic myeloid leukemia and certain acute leukemias, this activity is unleashed

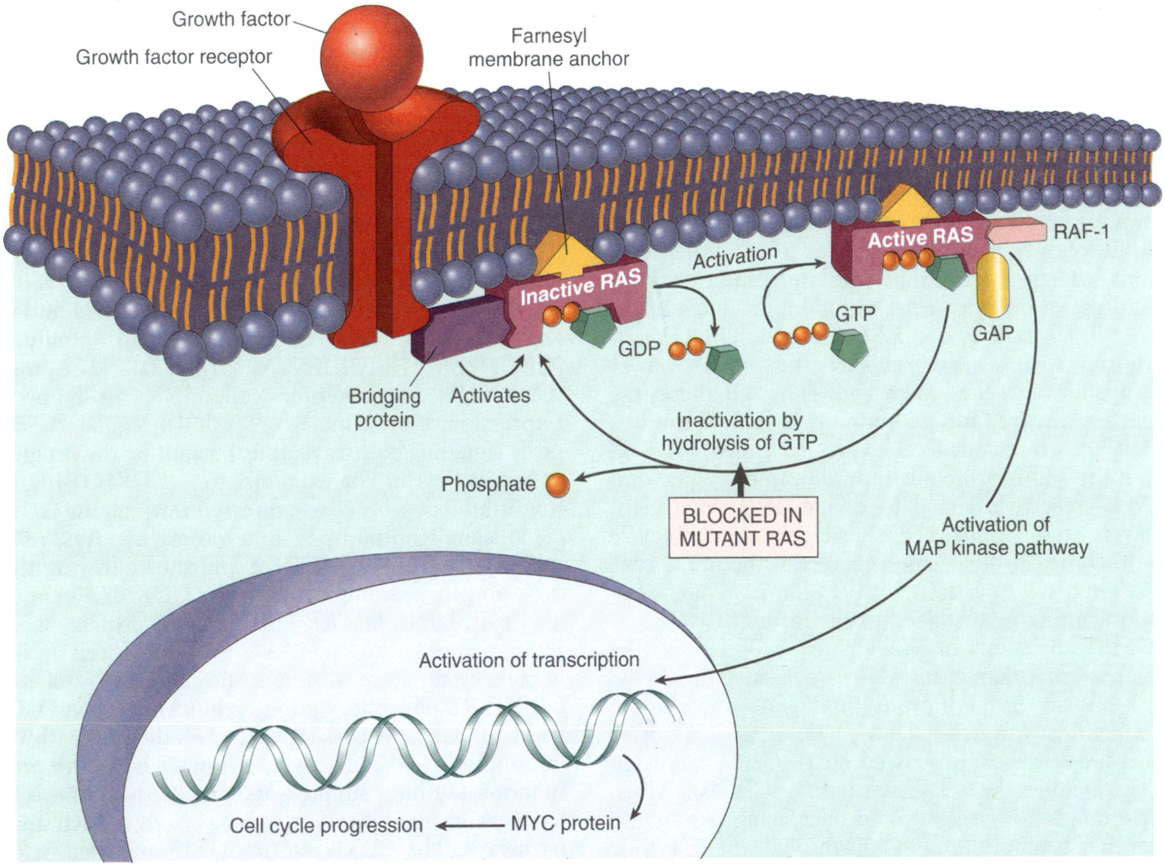

Figure 6–18

Model for action of *RAS* genes. When a normal cell is stimulated through a growth factor receptor, inactive (GDP-bound) RAS is activated to a GTP-bound state. Activated RAS recruits RAF-1 and stimulates the MAP-kinase pathway to transmit growth-promoting signals to the nucleus. *MYC* gene is one of several targets of the activated RAS pathway. The mutant RAS protein is permanently activated because of inability to hydrolyze GTP, leading to continuous stimulation of cells without any external trigger. The anchoring of RAS to the cell membrane by the farnesyl moiety is essential for its action, and drugs that inhibit farnesylation can inhibit RAS action.

because the *ABL* gene is translocated from its normal abode on chromosome 9 to chromosome 22, where it fuses with part of the breakpoint cluster region *(BCR)* gene. The BCR-ABL hybrid protein has potent, unregulated tyrosine kinase activity, which activates several pathways, including the *RAS-RAF* cascade. Other studies have revealed a completely novel function of *ABL* in oncogenesis. Normal ABL protein localizes in the nucleus, where its role is to promote apoptosis of cells that suffer DNA damage. This is analogous to the role of the *p53* gene (discussed later). The *BCR-ABL* gene cannot perform this function, because it is retained in the cytoplasm as a result of abnormal tyrosine kinase activity. Thus, a cell with *BCR-ABL* fusion gene is dysregulated in two ways: inappropriate tyrosine kinase activity leads to growth autonomy, while simultaneously apoptosis is impaired.

The crucial role of *BCR-ABL* in transformation has been confirmed by the dramatic clinical response of patients with chronic myeloid leukemia after therapy with an inhibitor of the BCR-ABL fusion kinase called imatinib mesylate (Gleevec); this is another example of rational drug design emerging from an understanding of the molecular basis of cancer.

Nuclear Transcription Factors

Ultimately, all signal transduction pathways enter the nucleus and have an impact on a large bank of responder genes that orchestrate the cells' orderly advance through the mitotic cycle. Indeed, the ultimate consequence of signaling through oncogenes like *RAS* or *ABL* is inappropriate and continuous stimulation of nuclear transcription factors that drive growth-promoting genes. Growth autonomy may thus occur as a consequence of mutations affecting genes that regulate transcription of DNA. A host of oncoproteins, including products of the *MYC, MYB, JUN, FOS,* and *REL* oncogenes, function as transcription factors that regulate the expression of growth-promoting genes, such as cyclins. Of these, the *MYC* gene is involved most commonly in human tumors. The *MYC* proto-oncogene is expressed in virtually all cells, and the MYC protein is induced rapidly when quiescent cells receive a signal to divide. In normal cells, MYC levels decline to near basal level when the cell cycle begins. In contrast, oncogenic versions of the *MYC* gene are associated with persistent expression or overexpression, contributing to sustained proliferation.

The MYC protein can either activate or repress the transcription of other genes. Those activated by MYC include several growth-promoting genes, including cyclin-dependent kinases (CDKs), whose products drive cells into the cell cycle (discussed next). Genes repressed by MYC include the CDK inhibitors (CDKIs). Thus, MYC promotes tumorigenesis by increasing expression of genes that promote progression through the cell cycle and repressing genes that slow or prevent progression through the cell cycle. Dysregulation of the *MYC* gene resulting from a t(8;14) translocation occurs in Burkitt lymphoma, a B-cell tumor. *MYC* is also amplified in breast, colon, lung, and many other cancers; the related *N-MYC* and *L-MYC* genes are amplified in neuroblastomas and small-cell cancers of lung.

Cyclins and Cyclin-Dependent Kinases (CDKs)

The ultimate outcome of all growth-promoting stimuli is the entry of quiescent cells into the cell cycle. Cancers may become autonomous if the genes that drive the cell cycle become dysregulated by mutations or amplification. As alluded to in Chapter 3, the orderly progression of cells through the various phases of the cell cycle is orchestrated by CDKs, which are activated by binding to *cyclins,* so called because of the cyclic nature of their production and degradation. The CDK-cyclin complexes phosphorylate crucial target proteins that drive the cell through the cell cycle. On completion of this task, cyclin levels decline rapidly. More than 15 cyclins have been identified; cyclins D, E, A, and B appear sequentially during the cell cycle and bind to one or more CDK. The cell cycle may thus be seen as a relay race in which each lap is regulated by a distinct set of cyclins, and as one set of cyclins leaves the track, the next set takes over (Fig. 6–19).

With this background it is easy to appreciate that mutations that dysregulate the activity of cyclins and CDKs would favor cell proliferation. Mishaps affecting the expression of cyclin D or CDK4 seem to be a common event in neoplastic transformation. The cyclin D genes are overexpressed in many cancers, including those affecting the breast, esophagus, liver, and a subset of lymphomas. Amplification of the *CDK4* gene occurs in melanomas, sarcomas, and glioblastomas. Mutations affecting cyclin B and cyclin E and other CDKs also occur, but they are much less frequent than those affecting cyclin D/CDK4.

While cyclins arouse the CDKs, their inhibitors (CDKIs), of which there are many, silence the CDKs and exert negative control over the cell cycle. One family of CDKIs, composed of three proteins, called p21 [CDKN1A], p27 [CDKN1B], and p57 [CDKN1C], inhibits the CDKs broadly, whereas the other family of CDKIs has selective effects on cyclin D/CDK4 and cyclin D/CDK6. The four members of this family (p15 [CDKN2B], p16 [CDKN2A], p18 [CDKN2C], and p19 [CDKN2D]) are sometimes called INK4 (A–D) proteins. Expression of these inhibitors is down-regulated by mitogenic signaling pathways, thus promoting the progression of the cell cycle. For example, p27 [CDKN1B], a CDKI that inhibits cyclin E, is expressed throughout G_1. Mitogenic signals obtund p27 in a variety of ways, relieving inhibition of cyclin E–CDK2 and thus allowing the cell cycle to proceed. Interestingly, the *CDKN2A* gene locus, also called *INK4a/ARF,* encodes two protein products: the p16 INK4A and p14ARF. Both block cell cycle progression but have different targets. p16 [CDKN2A] inhibits RB phosphorylation by blocking cyclin D–CDK4 complex, whereas p14ARF activates the p53 pathway by inhibiting MDM2 (discussed below). Thus, both proteins function as tumor suppressors, and deletion of this locus, frequent in many tumors, impacts both the RB and p53 pathways. The CDKIs are frequently mutated or otherwise silenced in many human malignancies. Germ-line mutations of *CDKN2A* are associated with 25% of melanoma-prone kindreds. Somatically acquired deletion or inactivation of *CDKN2A* is seen in 75% of pancreatic carcinomas, 40% to 70% of glioblastomas, 50% of esophageal cancers, and 20% of non-small-cell lung carcinomas, soft tissue sarcomas, and bladder cancers.

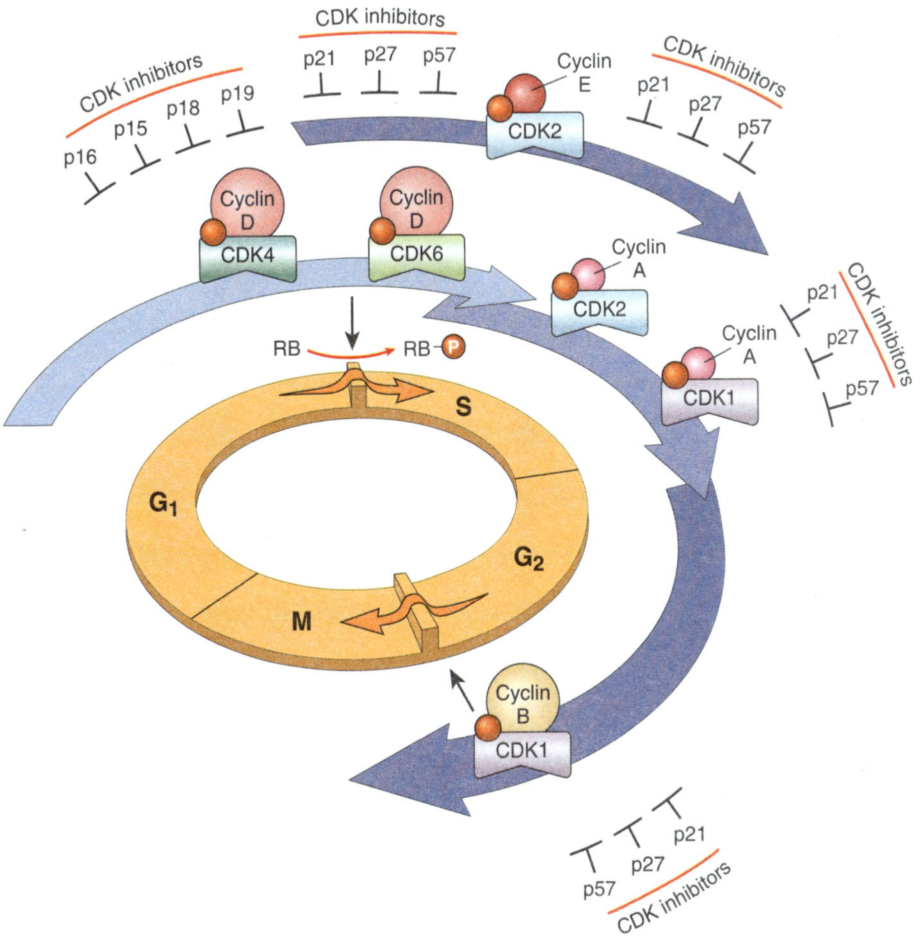

Figure 6–19

Schematic illustration of the role of cyclins, CDKs, and CDKIs in regulating the cell cycle. The shaded arrows represent the phases of the cell cycle during which specific cyclin-CDK complexes are active. As illustrated, cyclin D–CDK4, cyclin D–CDK6, and cyclin E–CDK2 regulate the G_1-to-S transition by phosphorylation of the RB protein (pRB). Cyclin A–CDK2 and cyclin A–CDK1 are active in the S phase. Cyclin B–CDK1 is essential for the G_2-to-M transition. Two families of CDK inhibitors can block activity of CDKs and progression through the cell cycle. The so-called INK4 inhibitors composed of p16, p15, p18, and p19, act on cyclin D–CDK4 and cyclin D–CDK6. The other family of three inhibitors, p21, p27, and p57, can inhibit all CDKs.

SUMMARY

Oncogenes that Promote Unregulated Proliferation (Self-sufficiency in Growth Signals)

Proto-oncogenes: normal cellular genes whose products promote cell proliferation
Oncogenes: mutant versions of proto-oncogenes that function autonomously without a requirement for normal growth-promoting signals

Oncogenes can promote uncontrolled cell proliferation by several mechanisms:

- Stimulus-independent expression of growth factor and its receptor, setting up an autocrine loop of cell proliferation
  - PDGF-PDGF-receptor in brain tumors
- Mutations in genes encoding growth factor receptors, leading to overexpression or constitutive signaling by the receptor (e.g., EGF receptors)
  - EGF-receptor family members, including HER2/NEU (breast, lung, and other tumors)
- Mutations in genes encoding signaling molecules
  - RAS is commonly mutated in human cancers; normally flips between resting GDP-bound state and active GTP-bound state; mutations block hydrolysis of GTP to GDP, leading to unchecked signaling
  - Fusion of ABL tyrosine kinase with BCR protein in certain leukemias generates a hybrid protein with constitutive kinase activity
- Overproduction or unregulated activity of transcription factors
  - Translocation of MYC in some lymphomas leads to overexpression and unregulated expression of its target genes controlling cell cycling and survival
- Mutations that activate cyclin genes or inactivate normal regulators of cyclins and cyclin-dependent kinases

- Complexes of cyclins with cyclin-dependent kinases (CDKs) drive the cell cycle by phosphorylating various substrates; CDKs are controlled by inhibitors; mutations in genes encoding cyclins, CDKs, and CDK inhibitors result in uncontrolled cell cycle progression. Such mutations are found in wide variety of cancers including melanomas, brain, lung, and pancreatic cancer.

Insensitivity to Growth-Inhibitory Signals

Isaac Newton predicted that every action has an equal and opposite reaction. Although Newton was not a cancer biologist, his formulation holds true for cell growth. Whereas oncogenes encode proteins that promote cell growth, the products of tumor suppressor genes apply brakes to cell proliferation. Disruption of such genes renders cells refractory to growth inhibition and mimics the growth-promoting effects of oncogenes. In this section we describe tumor suppressor genes, their products, and possible mechanisms by which loss of their function contributes to unregulated cell growth.

We begin our discussion with the retinoblastoma *(RB)* gene, the first and prototypic cancer suppressor gene to be discovered. Similar to many advances in medicine, the discovery of cancer suppressor genes was accomplished by the study of a rare disease, in this case retinoblastoma, an uncommon childhood tumor. Approximately 60% of retinoblastomas are sporadic, and the remaining ones are familial, the predisposition to develop the tumor being transmitted as an autosomal dominant trait. To account for the sporadic and familial occurrence of an identical tumor, Knudson, in 1974, proposed his now famous *two-hit* hypothesis, which in molecular terms can be stated as follows:

- Two mutations *(hits)* are required to produce retinoblastoma. These involve the *RB* gene, located on chromosome 13q14. Both of the normal alleles of the *RB* locus must be inactivated (two hits) for the development of retinoblastoma (Fig. 6–20).
- In familial cases, children inherit one defective copy of the *RB* gene in the germ line; the other copy is normal. Retinoblastoma develops when the normal *RB* gene is lost in retinoblasts as a result of somatic mutation. Because in retinoblastoma families only a single somatic mutation is required for expression of the disease, the familial transmission follows an autosomal dominant inheritance pattern.
- In sporadic cases, both normal *RB* alleles are lost by somatic mutation in one of the retinoblasts. The end result is the same: a retinal cell that has lost both of the normal copies of the *RB* gene becomes cancerous.

Although the loss of normal *RB* genes was discovered initially in retinoblastomas, it is now evident that homozygous loss of this gene is a fairly common event in several tumors, including breast cancer, small-cell cancer of the lung, and bladder cancer. Patients with familial retinoblastoma also are at greatly increased risk of developing osteosarcomas and some soft tissue sarcomas.

At this point, we should clarify some terminology. A cell heterozygous at the *RB* locus is not neoplastic. Tumors develop when the cell becomes *homozygous* for the mutant allele or, in other words, *loses heterozygosity* of the normal *RB* gene.

The signals and signal-transducing pathways for growth inhibition are much less well understood than are those for growth promotion. Nevertheless, it is reasonable to assume that, similar to mitogenic signals, growth-inhibitory signals may originate outside the cell and use receptors, signal transducers, and nuclear transcription regulators to accomplish their effects. The tumor suppressor genes seem to encode various components of this growth-inhibitory pathway.

In principle, antigrowth signals can prevent cell proliferation by two complementary mechanisms. The signal may cause dividing cells to go into G_0 (quiescence), where they remain until external cues prod their reentry into the proliferative pool. Alternatively the cells may enter a post-mitotic, differentiated pool and lose replicative potential. It is useful to begin our discussion of growth-inhibitory mechanisms and their evasion by focusing initially on the *RB* gene, the prototypic tumor suppressor gene.

SUMMARY

Insensitivity to Growth-Inhibitory Signals

- Tumor suppressor genes encode proteins that inhibit cellular proliferation by regulating the cell cycle. Unlike oncogenes, both copies of the gene must be lost for tumor development, leading to loss of heterozygosity at the gene locus.
- In cases with familial predisposition to develop tumors, the affected individuals inherit one defective (nonfunctional) copy of a tumor suppressor gene and lose the second one through somatic mutation. In sporadic cases both copies are lost through somatic mutations.

RB Gene and Cell Cycle

Much is known about the *RB* gene, because this was the first tumor suppressor gene discovered. The *RB* gene product is a DNA-binding protein that is expressed in every cell type examined, where it exists in an *active hypophosphorylated* and an *inactive hyperphosphorylated state.* The importance of RB lies in its enforcement of G_1, or the gap between mitosis (M) and DNA replication (S). In embryos, cell divisions proceed at an amazing clip, with DNA replication beginning immediately after mitosis ends. However, as development proceeds, two gaps are incorporated into the cell cycle: Gap 1 (G_1) between mitosis (M) and DNA replication (S), and Gap 2 (G_2) between DNA replication (S) and mitosis (M) (see Fig. 6–19). Although each phase of the cell cycle circuitry is monitored carefully, the transition from G_1 to S is believed to be an extremely important checkpoint in the

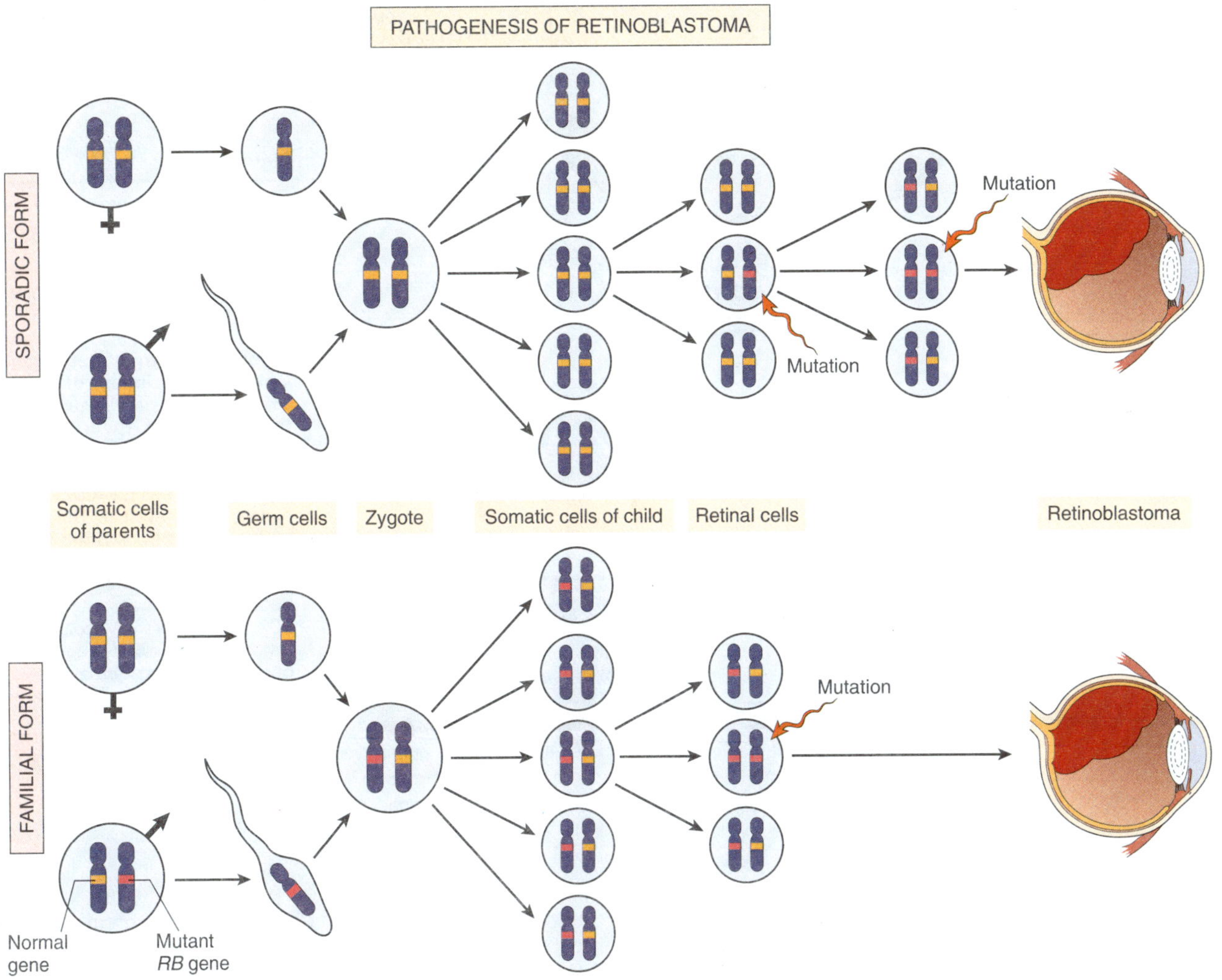

Figure 6–20

Pathogenesis of retinoblastoma. Two mutations of the *RB* locus on chromosome 13q14 lead to neoplastic proliferation of the retinal cells. In the familial form, all somatic cells inherit one mutant *RB* gene from a carrier parent. The second mutation affects the *RB* locus in one of the retinal cells after birth. In the sporadic form, both mutations at the *RB* locus are acquired by the retinal cells after birth.

cell cycle clock. Once cells cross the G_1 checkpoint they can pause the cell cycle for a time, but they are obligated to complete mitosis. In G_1, however, cells can exit the cell cycle, either temporarily, called quiescence, or permanently, called senescence. In G_1, therefore, diverse signals are integrated to determine whether the cell should enter the cell cycle, exit the cell cycle and differentiate, or die. RB is a key node in this decision process. To understand why RB is such a crucial player, we must review the mechanisms that enforce the G_1 phase.

The initiation of DNA replication requires the activity of cyclin E/CDK2 complexes, and expression of cyclin E is dependent on the E2F family of transcription factors. Early in G_1, RB is in its hypophosphorylated active form, and it binds to and inhibits the E2F family of transcription factors, preventing transcription of cyclin E. Hypophosphorylated RB blocks E2F-mediated transcription in at least two ways (Fig. 6–21). First, it sequesters E2F, preventing it from interacting with other transcriptional activators. Second, RB recruits chromatin remodeling proteins, such as histone deacetylases and histone methyltransferases, which bind to the promoters of E2F-responsive genes such as cyclin E. These enzymes modify chromatin at the promoters to make DNA insensitive to transcription factors. This situation is changed upon mitogenic signaling. Growth factor signaling leads to cyclin D expression and activation of cyclin D–CDK4/6 complexes. These complexes phosphorylate RB, inactivating the protein and releasing E2F to induce target genes such as cyclin E. Expression of cyclin E then stimulates DNA replication and progression through the cell cycle. When the cells enter S phase, they are committed to divide without additional growth factor stimulation. During the ensuing M phase, the phosphate groups are removed from RB by cellular phosphatases, regenerating the hypophosphorylated form of RB.

E2F is not the sole target of RB. The versatile RB protein has been shown to bind to a variety of other transcription factors that regulate cell differentiation. For example, RB stimulates myocyte-, adipocyte-,

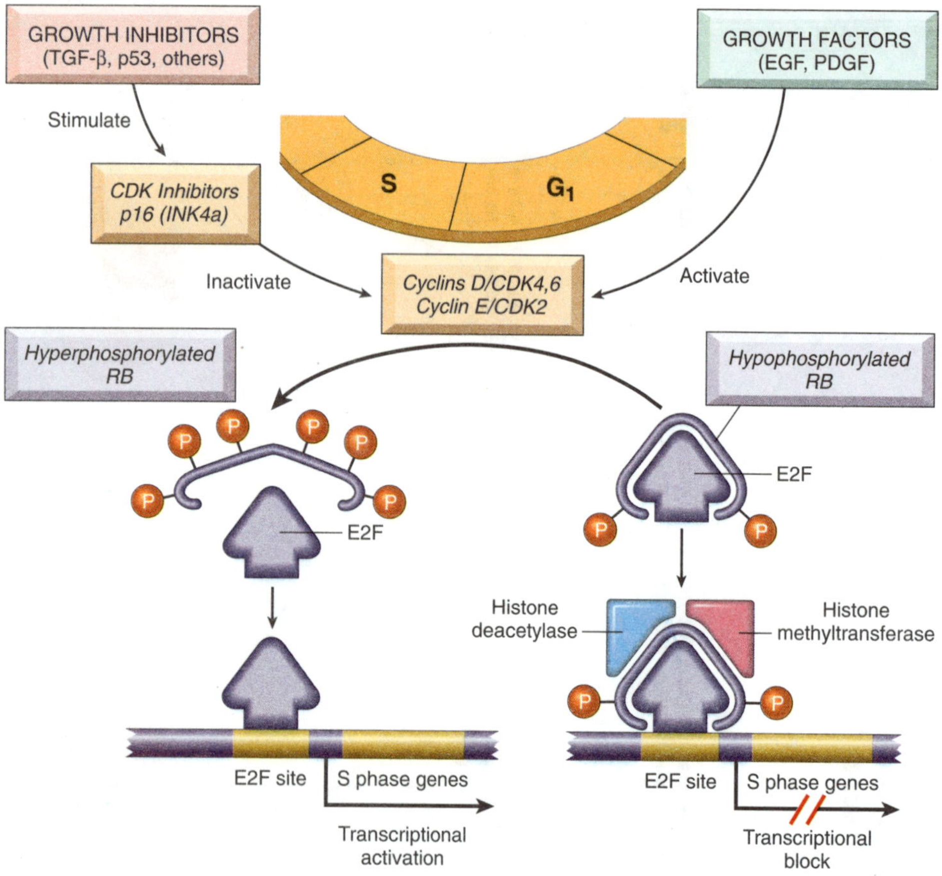

Figure 6–21

The role of RB in regulating the G_1–S checkpoint of the cell cycle. Hypophosphorylated RB in complex with the E2F transcription factors binds to DNA, recruits chromatin remodeling factors (histone deacetylases and histone methyltransferases), and inhibits transcription of genes whose products are required for the S phase of the cell cycle. When RB is phosphorylated by the cyclin D–CDK4, cyclin D–CDK6, and cyclin E–CDK2 complexes, it releases E2F. The latter then activates transcription of S-phase genes. The phosphorylation of RB is inhibited by CDKIs, because they inactivate cyclin-CDK complexes. Virtually all cancer cells show dysregulation of the G_1–S checkpoint as a result of mutation in one of four genes that regulate the phosphorylation of RB; these genes are *RB, CDK4, cyclin D,* and *CDKN2A [p16]*. EGF, epidermal growth factor; PDGF, platelet-derived growth factor.

melanocyte-, and macrophage-specific transcription factors. Thus, the RB pathway couples control of cell cycle progression at G_1 with differentiation, which may explain how differentiation is associated with exit from the cell cycle. In addition to these dual activities, RB can also induce senescence, discussed below.

Given that RB is central to the control of the cell cycle, one may ask why *RB* is not mutated in every cancer. Mutations in other genes that control RB phosphorylation can mimic the effect of *RB* loss; such genes are mutated in many cancers that seem to have normal *RB* genes. For example, mutational activation of CDK4 or overexpression of cyclin D would favor cell proliferation by facilitating RB phosphorylation and inactivation. Indeed, cyclin D is overexpressed in many tumors because of gene amplification or translocation. Mutational inactivation of CDKIs also would drive the cell cycle by unregulated activation of cyclins and CDKs. As mentioned above, the *CDKN2A* gene is an extremely common target of deletion or mutational inactivation in human tumors.

The emerging paradigm is that loss of normal cell cycle control is central to malignant transformation and that at least one of the four key regulators of the cell cycle (CDKN2A, cyclin D, CDK4, RB) is mutated in most human cancers. Furthermore, the transforming proteins of several oncogenic animal and human DNA viruses seem to act, in part, by neutralizing the growth-inhibitory activities of RB. Simian virus 40 and polyomavirus large-T antigens, adenovirus EIA protein, and human papillomavirus (HPV) E7 protein all bind to the hypophosphorylated form of RB. The RB protein, unable to bind to the E2F transcription factors, is functionally deleted, and the cells lose the ability to be inhibited by antigrowth signals that funnel through the RB nexus.

SUMMARY

RB Gene and Cell Cycle

- RB exerts antiproliferative effects by controlling the G_1-to-S transition of the cell cycle. In its active form RB is hypophosphorylated and binds to E2F transcription factor. This interaction prevents transcription of genes like cyclin E that are needed for DNA replication, and so the cells are arrested in G_1.
- Growth factor signaling leads to cyclin D expression, activation of the cyclin D–CDK4/6 complexes, inactivation of RB by phosphorylation, and thus release of E2F.
- Loss of cell cycle control is fundamental to malignant transformation. Almost all cancers will have disabled the G_1 checkpoint, by mutation of either *RB* or genes that affect RB function, like cyclin D, CDK4, and CDKIs.
- Many oncogenic DNA viruses, like HPV, encode proteins (e.g., E7) that bind to RB and render it nonfunctional.

p53 Gene: Guardian of the Genome

The *p53* tumor suppressor gene is one of the most commonly mutated genes in human cancers. *p53 thwarts neoplastic transformation by three interlocking mechanisms: activation of temporary cell cycle arrest (termed quiescence), induction of permanent cell cycle arrest (termed senescence), or triggering of programmed cell death (termed apoptosis).* Fundamentally, *p53* can be viewed as a central monitor of stress, directing the stressed cells toward an appropriate response. A variety of stresses can trigger the *p53* response pathways, including anoxia, inappropriate oncogene expression (e.g., *MYC* or *RAS*), and damage to the integrity of DNA. By managing the DNA-damage response, *p53* plays a central role in maintaining the integrity of the genome, as will be evident from the following discussion.

In nonstressed, healthy cells, p53 has a short half-life (20 minutes) because of its association with MDM2, a protein that targets it for destruction. When the cell is stressed, for example by an assault on its DNA, p53 undergoes post-transcriptional modifications that release it from MDM2 and increase its half-life. During the process of being unshackled from MDM2, p53 also becomes activated as a transcription factor. Dozens of genes whose transcription is triggered by p53 have been found. They can be grouped into two broad categories: those that cause cell cycle arrest and those that cause apoptosis. If DNA damage can be repaired during cell cycle arrest, the cell reverts to a normal state; if the repair fails, p53 induces apoptosis or senescence. These actions are discussed next.

The manner in which p53 senses DNA damage and determines the adequacy of DNA repair are not completely understood. The key initiators of the DNA-damage pathway are two related protein kinases: *ataxia-telangiectasia mutated (ATM) and ataxia-telangiectasia mutated related (ATR).* As the name implies, the *ATM* gene was originally identified as the germ-line mutation in patients with ataxia-telangiectasia. Patients with this disease, which is characterized by an inability to repair certain kinds of DNA damage, suffer from an increased incidence of cancer. The types of damage sensed by ATM and ATR are different, but the down-stream pathways they activate are similar. Once triggered, both ATM and ATR phosphorylate a variety of targets, including p53 and DNA repair proteins. Phosphorylation of these two targets leads to a pause in the cell cycle and stimulation of DNA repair pathways respectively.

p53-*mediated cell cycle arrest may be considered the primordial response to DNA damage* (Fig. 6–22). It occurs late in the G_1 phase and is caused mainly by *p53*-dependent transcription of the CDKI *CDKN1A (p21).* The *CDKN1A* gene, as described earlier, inhibits cyclin-CDK complexes and prevents phosphorylation of RB essential for cells to enter G_1 phase. Such a pause in cell cycling is welcome, because it gives the cells "breathing time" to repair DNA damage. p53 also helps the process by inducing certain proteins, such as GADD45 (growth arrest and DNA damage), that help in DNA repair. p53 can stimulate DNA repair pathways by transcription-independent mechanisms as well. If DNA damage is repaired successfully, p53 up-regulates transcription of MDM2, leading to destruction of p53 and relief of the cell cycle block. If the damage cannot be repaired, the cell may enter p53-induced senescence or undergo p53-directed apoptosis.

p53-*induced senescence is a permanent cell cycle arrest* characterized by specific changes in morphology and gene expression that differentiate it from quiescence or reversible cell cycle arrest. Senescence requires activation of p53 and/or RB and expression of their mediators, such as the CDKIs. Such cell cycle arrest is generally irreversible, although it may require the continued expression of p53. The mechanisms of senescence are unclear but seem to involve global chromatin changes, which drastically and permanently alter gene expression.

p53-induced apoptosis of cells with irreversible DNA damage is the ultimate protective mechanism against neoplastic transformation. It is mediated by several pro-apoptotic genes such as *BAX* and *PUMA* (described later).

To summarize, p53 *senses DNA damage and assists in DNA repair by causing* G_1 *arrest and inducing DNA repair genes.* A cell with damaged DNA that cannot be repaired is directed by p53 *to either enter senescence or undergo apoptosis (see Fig. 6–22). In view of these activities,* p53 *has been rightfully called a "guardian of the genome."* With homozygous loss of *p53*, DNA damage goes unrepaired, mutations become fixed in dividing cells, and the cell turns onto a one-way street leading to malignant transformation.

Confirming the importance of *p53* in controlling carcinogenesis, more than 70% of human cancers have a defect in this gene, and the remaining malignant neoplasms have defects in genes up-stream or down-stream of *p53*. Homozygous loss of the *p53* gene is found in virtually every type of cancer, including carcinomas of the lung, colon, and breast—the three leading causes of cancer deaths. In most cases, inactivating mutations affecting both *p53* alleles are acquired in somatic cells. Less commonly, some individuals inherit a mutant *p53* allele; this disease is called the *Li-Fraumeni syndrome.* As with the *RB* gene, inheritance of one mutant allele predisposes individuals to develop malignant tumors because only one additional hit is needed to inactivate the second, normal allele. Patients with the *Li-Fraumeni syndrome* have a 25-fold greater chance of developing a malignant tumor by age 50 compared with the general population. In contrast to patients who inherit a mutant *RB* allele, the spectrum of tumors that develop in patients with the Li-Fraumeni syndrome is varied; the most common types of tumors are sarcomas, breast cancer, leukemia, brain tumors, and carcinomas of the adrenal cortex. Compared with sporadic tumors, patients with Li-Fraumeni syndrome develop tumors at a younger age and may develop multiple primary tumors.

As with RB protein, normal p53 also can be rendered nonfunctional by certain DNA viruses. Proteins encoded by oncogenic HPVs, hepatitis B virus (HBV), and possibly Epstein-Barr virus (EBV) can bind to normal p53 and nullify its protective function. Thus, DNA viruses can subvert two of the best-understood tumor suppressor genes, *RB* and *p53*.

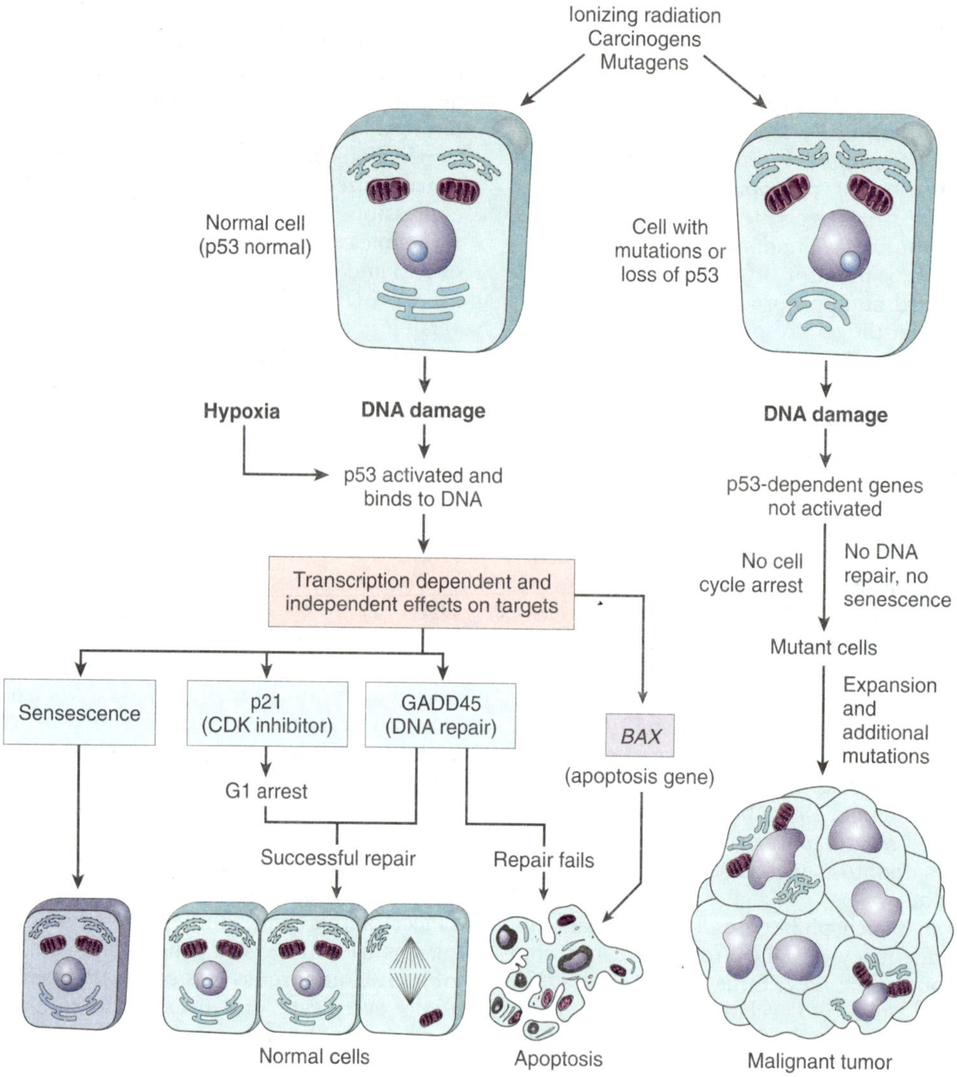

Figure 6–22

The role of *p53* in maintaining the integrity of the genome. Activation of normal *p53* by DNA-damaging agents or by hypoxia leads to cell cycle arrest in G_1 and induction of DNA repair, by transcriptional up-regulation of the cyclin-dependent kinase inhibitor *CDKN1A* (p21) and the *GADD45* genes. Successful repair of DNA allows cells to proceed with the cell cycle; if DNA repair fails, *p53* triggers either apoptosis or senescence. In cells with loss or mutations of *p53,* DNA damage does not induce cell cycle arrest or DNA repair, and genetically damaged cells proliferate, giving rise eventually to malignant neoplasms.

SUMMARY

p53 Gene: Guardian of the Genome

- p53 is the central monitor of stress in the cell and can be activated by anoxia, inappropriate oncogene signaling, or DNA damage. Activated p53 controls the expression and activity of genes involved in cell cycle arrest, DNA repair, cellular senescence, and apoptosis.
- DNA damage leads to activation of p53 by phosphorylation. Activated p53 drives transcription of *CDKN1A (p21)* that prevents RB phosphorylation and therefore causes a G_1-S block in the cell cycle. This pause allows the cells to repair DNA damage.
- If DNA damage cannot be repaired, p53 induces cellular senescence or apoptosis.
- Of human tumors, 70% have homozygous loss of *p53*. Patients with the rare Li-Fraumeni syndrome inherit one defective copy in the germ line and lose the second one in somatic tissues; such individuals develop a variety of tumors.
- As with RB, p53 can be incapacitated by binding to proteins encoded by oncogenic DNA viruses like HPV, and possibly EBV and HBV.

Transforming Growth Factor-β Pathway

Although much is known about the circuitry that applies brakes to the cell cycle, the molecules that transmit antiproliferative signals to cells are less well characterized. Best known is TGF-β, a member of a family of dimeric growth factors that includes bone morphogenetic proteins and activins. In most normal epithelial, endothelial, and hematopoietic cells, TGF-β is a potent inhibitor of proliferation. It regulates cellular processes by binding to a complex composed of TGF-β receptors I and II. Dimerization of the receptor upon ligand binding leads to a cascade of events that result in the transcriptional activation of CDKIs with growth-suppressing activity, as well as repression of growth-promoting genes such as *c-MYC, CDK2, CDK4,* and cyclins A and E.

In many forms of cancer, the growth-inhibiting effects of TGF-β pathways are impaired by mutations in the TGF-β signaling pathway. These mutations may affect the type II TGF-β receptor or SMAD molecules that serve to transduce antiproliferative signals from the receptor to the nucleus. Mutations affecting the type II receptor are seen in cancers of the colon, stomach, and endometrium. Mutational inactivation of SMAD4, one of 10 proteins involved in TGF-β signaling, is common in pancreatic cancers. *In 100% of pancreatic cancers and 83% of colon cancers, at least one component of the TGF-β pathway is mutated.*

Adenomatous Polyposis Coli–β-Catenin Pathway

In the rare hereditary disease called adenomatous polyposis coli (APC), patients develop numerous adenomatous polyps in the colon that have a very high incidence of transformation into colonic cancers. These patients consistently show loss of a tumor suppressor gene called *APC* (named for the disease). The *APC* gene exerts antiproliferative effects in an unusual manner. It is a cytoplasmic protein whose dominant function is to regulate the intracellular levels of β-catenin, a protein with many functions. On the one hand, β-catenin binds to the cytoplasmic portion of E-cadherin, a cell surface protein that mediates intercellular interactions; on the other hand, it can translocate to the nucleus and activate cell proliferation. Here the focus is on the latter function of this protein. β-catenin is an important component of the so-called WNT signaling pathway that regulates cell proliferation (illustrated in Fig. 6–23). WNT is a soluble factor that can induce cellular proliferation. It does so by binding to its receptor and transmitting signals that prevent the degradation of β-catenin, allowing it to translocate to the nucleus, where it acts as a transcriptional activator in conjunction with another molecule, called TcF (see Fig. 6–23B). In quiescent cells, which are not exposed to WNT, cytoplasmic β-catenin is degraded by a *destruction complex,* of which APC is an integral

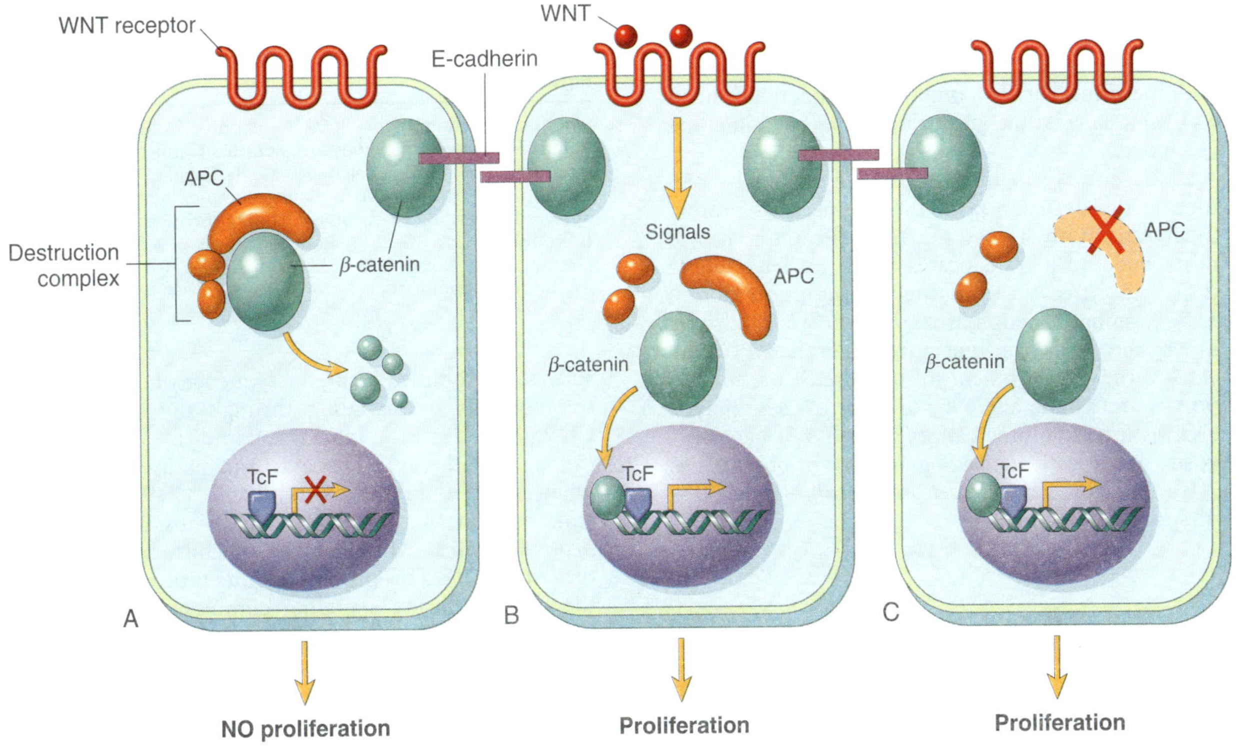

Figure 6–23

A–C, The role of APC in regulating the stability and function of β-catenin. APC and β-catenin are components of the WNT signaling pathway. In resting cells (not exposed to WNT), β-catenin forms a macromolecular complex containing the APC protein. This complex leads to the destruction of β-catenin, and intracellular levels of β-catenin are low. When cells are stimulated by secreted WNT molecules, the *destruction complex* is deactivated, β-catenin degradation does not occur, and cytoplasmic levels increase. β-catenin translocates to the nucleus, where it binds to TcF, a transcription factor that activates several genes involved in the cell cycle. When APC is mutated or absent, the destruction of β-catenin cannot occur. β-catenin translocates to the nucleus and coactivates genes that promote the cell cycle, and cells behave as if they are under constant stimulation by the WNT pathway.

part (see Fig. 6–23A). With loss of APC (in malignant cells), β-catenin degradation is prevented, and the WNT signaling response is inappropriately activated in the absence of WNT (see Fig. 6–23C). This leads to transcription of growth-promoting genes, such as cyclin D1 and *MYC*.

APC behaves as a typical tumor suppressor gene. Individuals born with one mutant allele develop hundreds to thousands of adenomatous polyps in the colon during their teens or 20s, which show loss of the other *APC* allele. Almost invariably, one or more polyps undergo malignant transformation upon accumulation of other mutations in the cells within the polyp, as discussed later. *APC* mutations are seen in 70% to 80% of sporadic colon cancers. Colonic cancers that have normal *APC* genes show activating mutations of β-catenin that render them refractory to the degrading action of APC.

SUMMARY

Transforming Growth Factor-β and Adenomatous Polyposis Coli–β-Catenin Pathways

- TGF-β inhibits proliferation of many cell types by activation of growth-inhibiting genes like CDKIs and suppression of growth-promoting genes like *MYC* and cyclins.
- TGF-β function is compromised in many tumors by mutations in its receptors (colon, stomach, endometrium) or by mutational inactivation of *SMAD* genes that transduce TGF-β signaling (pancreas).
- *APC* gene exerts antiproliferative actions by regulating the destruction of the cytoplasmic protein β-catenin. With a loss of *APC*, β-catenin is not destroyed and it translocates to the nucleus, where it acts as a growth-promoting transcription factor.
- In familial adenomatous polyposis syndrome inheritance of a germ-line mutation in the *APC* gene causes the development of hundreds of colonic polyps at a young age. One or more of these polyps evolves into a colonic cancer with loss of heterozygosity at the *APC* locus. Somatic loss of both alleles of the of *APC* gene is seen in approximately 70% of sporadic colon cancers.

Evasion of Apoptosis

Accumulation of neoplastic cells may result not only from activation of growth-promoting oncogenes or inactivation of growth-suppressing tumor suppressor genes, but also from mutations in the genes that regulate apoptosis. A large family of genes that regulate apoptosis has been identified. Before we can understand how tumor cells evade apoptosis, it is essential to review briefly the biochemical pathways to apoptosis. As discussed in Chapter 1, there are two distinct programs that activate apoptosis, the extrinsic and intrinsic pathways. Figure 6–24

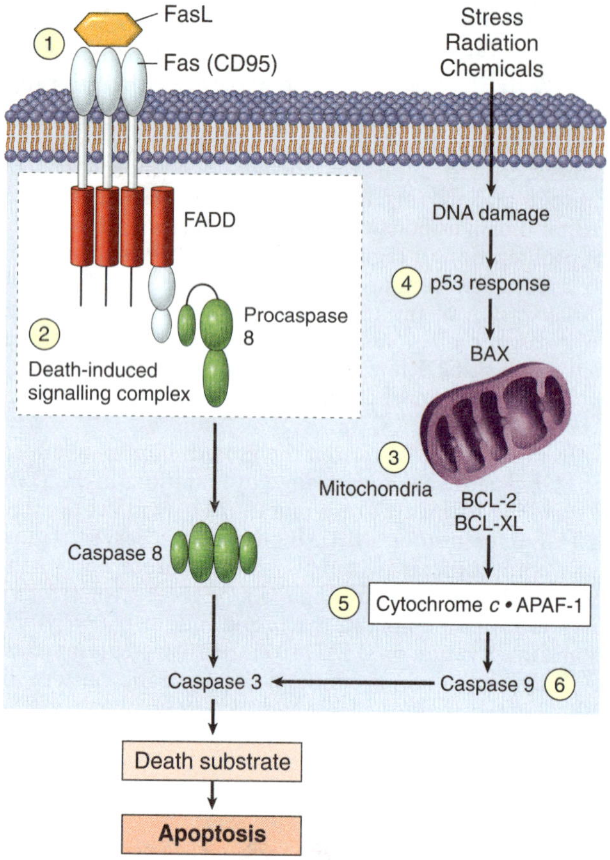

Figure 6–24

Simplified schema of CD95 receptor–induced and DNA damage–triggered pathways of apoptosis and mechanisms used by tumor cells to evade cell death. (1) Reduced CD95 level. (2) Inactivation of death-induced signaling complex by FLICE protein. (3) Reduced egress of cytochrome c from mitochondrion as a result of up-regulation of BCL2. (4) Reduced levels of pro-apoptotic BAX resulting from loss of p53. (5) Loss of APAF-1. (6) Up-regulation of inhibitors of apoptosis.

shows, in simplified form, the sequence of events that lead to apoptosis by signaling through the death receptor CD95/Fas (extrinsic pathway) and by DNA damage (intrinsic pathway). The extrinsic pathway is initiated when CD95 is bound to its ligand, CD95L, leading to trimerization of the receptor and thus its cytoplasmic *death domains*, which attract the intracellular adaptor protein FADD. This protein recruits procaspase 8 to form the death-inducing signaling complex. Procaspase 8 is activated by cleavage into smaller subunits, generating caspase 8. Caspase 8 then activates down-stream caspases such as caspase 3, a typical *executioner caspase* that cleaves DNA and other substrates to cause cell death. The intrinsic pathway of apoptosis is triggered by a variety of stimuli, including withdrawal of survival factors, stress, and injury. Activation of this pathway leads to permeabilization of mitochondrial outer membrane, with resultant release of molecules, such as cytochrome *c*, that initiate apoptosis. The integrity of the mitochondrial outer membrane is regulated by pro-apoptotic and anti-apoptotic members of the BCL2 family of proteins. The pro-apoptotic proteins, BAX and BAK, are required for apoptosis and directly promote mitochondrial permeabilization. Their action is inhibited by the anti-apoptotic members of this family exemplified by BCL2 and BCL-XL. A third set of proteins (so-called BH3-only proteins) including BAD, BID, and PUMA, regulate the balance between the pro- and anti-apoptotic members of the BCL2 family. The BH3-only proteins promote apoptosis by neutralizing the actions of anti-apoptotic proteins like BCL2 and BCL-XL. When the sum total of all BH3 proteins expressed "overwhelms" the anti-apoptotic BCL2/BCLXl protein barrier, BAX and BAK are activated and form pores in the mitochondrial membrane. Cytochrome *c* leaks into the cytosol, where it binds to APAF-1, activating caspase 9. Like caspase 8 of the extrinsic pathway, caspase 9 can cleave and activate the executioner caspases. Because of the pro-apoptotic effect of BH3 only proteins, efforts are underway to develop of BH3 mimetic drugs.

Within this framework, it is possible to illustrate the multiple sites at which apoptosis is frustrated by cancer cells (see Fig. 6–24). Starting from the surface, reduced levels of CD95 may render the tumor cells less susceptible to apoptosis by Fas ligand (FasL). Some tumors have high levels of FLIP, a protein that can bind death-inducing signaling complex and prevent activation of caspase 8. Of all these genes, perhaps *best established is the role of BCL2 in protecting tumor cells from apoptosis.* As discussed later, approximately 85% of B-cell lymphomas of the follicular type (Chapter 12) carry a characteristic t(14;18) (q32;q21) translocation. Recall that 14q32, the site where immunoglobulin heavy-chain genes are found, is also involved in the pathogenesis of Burkitt lymphoma. Juxtaposition of this transcriptionally active locus with *BCL2* (located at 18q21) causes overexpression of the BCL2 protein. This in turn increases the BCL2/BCL-XL buffer, protecting lymphocytes from apoptosis and allowing them to survive for long periods; there is therefore a steady accumulation of B lymphocytes, resulting in lymphadenopathy and marrow infiltration. Because BCL2-overexpressing lymphomas arise in large part from reduced cell death rather than explosive cell proliferation, they tend to be indolent (slow growing) compared with many other lymphomas.

As mentioned before, *p53 is an important pro-apoptotic gene that induces apoptosis in cells that are unable to repair DNA damage.* The actions of *p53* are mediated in part by transcriptional activation of *BAX*, but there are other connections as well between p53 and the apoptotic machinery.

SUMMARY

Evasion of Apoptosis

- Apoptosis can be initiated through the extrinsic or intrinsic pathways.
- Both pathways result in the activation of a proteolytic cascade of caspases that destroys the cell.
- Mitochondrial outer membrane permeabilization is regulated by the balance between pro-apoptotic (e.g., BAX, BAK) and anti-apoptotic molecules (BCL2, BCL-XL). BH-3-only molecules activate apoptosis by tilting the balance in favor of the pro-apoptotic molecules.
- In 85% of follicular B-cell lymphomas the anti-apoptotic gene *BCL2* is activated by the t(8;14) translocation.

Limitless Replicative Potential

As was discussed in the section on cellular aging (Chapter 1), most normal human cells have a capacity of 60 to 70 doublings. After this, the cells lose the capacity to divide and enter senescence. This phenomenon has been ascribed to progressive shortening of *telomeres* at the ends of chromosomes. Indeed, short telomeres seem to be recognized by the DNA repair machinery as double-stranded DNA breaks, and this leads to cell cycle arrest mediated by *p53* and *RB*. Cells in which the checkpoints are disabled by *p53* or *RB* mutations, the nonhomologous end-joining pathway is activated as a last-ditch effort to save the cell, joining the shortened ends of two chromosomes. This inappropriately activated repair system results in dicentric chromosomes that are pulled apart at anaphase, resulting in new double-stranded DNA breaks. The resulting genomic instability from the repeated bridge-fusion-breakage cycles eventually produces mitotic catastrophe, characterized by massive cell death. *It follows that for tumors to grow indefinitely, as they often do, loss of growth restraints is not enough. Tumor cells must also develop ways to avoid both cellular senescence and mitotic catastrophe* (Fig. 6–25). If during crisis a cell manages to reactivate telomerase, the bridge-fusion-breakage cycles cease and the cell is able to avoid death. However, during this period of genomic instability that precedes telomerase activation, numerous mutations could accumulate, helping the cell march toward malignancy. Passage through a period of genomic instability probably explains the complex karyotypes frequently seen in human carcinomas. Telomerase, active in normal stem cells, is normally absent from, or at very low levels in, most somatic cells. By contrast, telomere maintenance is seen in virtually all types of cancers. In 85% to 95% of cancers, this is due to up-regulation of the enzyme telomerase. A few tumors use other mechanisms, termed alternative lengthening of telomeres, which probably depend on DNA recombination. Interestingly, in the progression from colonic adenoma to colonic adenocarcinoma, early lesions had a high degree of genomic instability with low telomerase expression, whereas malignant lesions had complex karyotypes with high levels of telomerase activity, consistent with a model of telomere-driven tumorigenesis in human cancer. Several other mechanisms of genomic instability are discussed later.

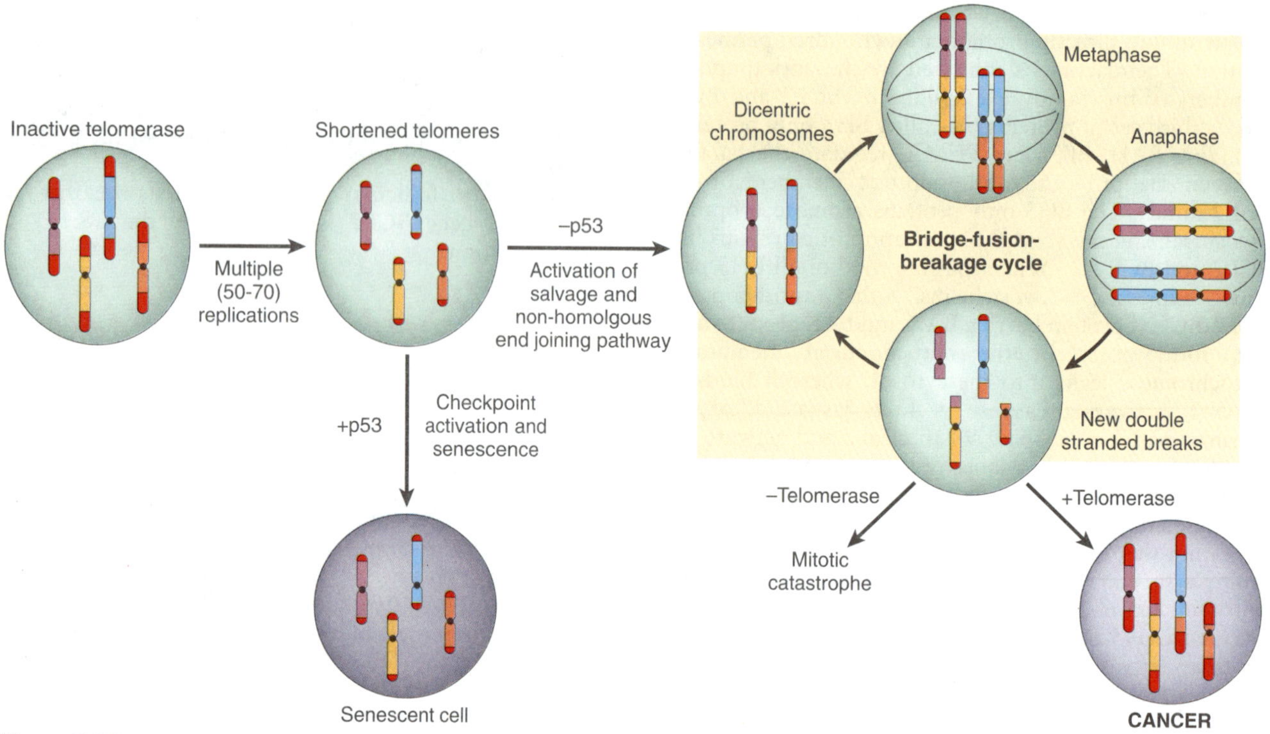

Figure 6–25

Schematic illustration of the sequence of events in the development of limitless replicative potential. Replication of somatic cells, which do not express telomerase, leads to shortened telomeres. In the presence of competent checkpoints, cells undergo arrest and enter nonreplicative senescence. In the absence of checkpoints, DNA repair pathways are inappropriately activated, leading to the formation of dicentric chromosomes. At mitosis, the dicentric chromosomes are pulled apart, generating random double-stranded breaks, which then activate DNA repair pathways, leading to the random association of double-stranded ends and the formation, again, of dicentric chromosomes. Cells undergo numerous rounds of this bridge-fusion-breakage cycle, which generates massive chromosomal instability and numerous mutations. If cells fail to re-express telomerase, they eventually undergo mitotic catastrophe and death. Re-expression of telomerase allows the cells to escape the bridge-fusion-breakage cycle, thus promoting their survival and tumorigenesis.

SUMMARY

Limitless Replicative Potential

- In normal cells, which lack expression of telomerase, the shortened telomeres generated by cell division eventually activate cell cycle checkpoints, leading to senescence and placing a limit on the number of divisions a cell may undergo.
- In cells that have disabled checkpoints, DNA repair pathways are inappropriately activated by shortened telomeres, leading to massive chromosomal instability and mitotic crisis.
- Tumor cells reactivate telomerase, thus staving off mitotic catastrophe and achieving immortality.

Development of Sustained Angiogenesis

Even with all the genetic abnormalities discussed above, tumors cannot enlarge beyond 1 to 2 mm in diameter unless they are vascularized. Like normal tissues, tumors require delivery of oxygen and nutrients and removal of waste products; presumably the 1- to 2-mm zone represents the maximal distance across which oxygen, nutrients, and waste can diffuse from blood vessels. Cancer cells can stimulate neo-angiogenesis, during which new vessels sprout from previously existing capillaries, or, in some cases, vasculogenesis, in which endothelial cells are recruited from the bone marrow (Chapter 3). Tumor vasculature is abnormal, however. The vessels are leaky, dilated, and have a haphazard pattern of connection. Neovascularization has a dual effect on tumor growth: Perfusion supplies needed nutrients and oxygen, and newly formed endothelial cells stimulate the growth of adjacent tumor cells by secreting growth factors, such as insulin-like growth factors, PDGF, and granulocyte-macrophage colony-stimulating factor. Angiogenesis is required not only for continued tumor growth but also for access to the vasculature and hence for metastasis. *Angiogenesis is thus a necessary biologic correlate of malignancy.*

How do growing tumors develop a blood supply? The emerging paradigm is that tumor angiogenesis is controlled by the balance between angiogenic factors and factors that inhibit angiogenesis. Early in their growth, most human tumors do not induce angiogenesis. They remain small or in situ for years until the angiogenic switch terminates this stage of vascular quiescence. The molecular basis of the angiogenic switch involves increased production of angiogenic factors and/or loss of angiogenesis inhibitors. These factors may be produced directly by the tumor cells themselves or by inflammatory cells (e.g., macrophages) or other stromal cells associated with the tumors. The angiogenic switch is controlled by several physiologic stimuli, such as hypoxia. Relative lack of oxygen stimulates production of a variety of pro-angiogenic cytokines, such as vascular endothelial growth factor (VEGF), through activation of hypoxia-induced factor-1α (HIF1α), an oxygen-sensitive transcription factor. HIF1α is continuously produced, but in normoxic settings the von Hippel–Lindau protein (VHL) binds to HIF1α, leading to ubiquitination and destruction of HIF1α. In hypoxic conditions, such as a tumor that has reached a critical size, the lack of oxygen prevents HIF1α recognition by VHL, and it is not destroyed. HIF1α translocates to the nucleus and activates transcription of its target genes, such as VEGF. Because of these activities, VHL acts as a tumor suppressor gene, and germ-line mutations of the *VHL* gene are associated with hereditary renal cell cancers, pheochromocytomas, hemangiomas of the central nervous system, retinal angiomas, and renal cysts (*VHL syndrome*). Both pro- and anti-angiogenic factors are regulated by many other genes frequently mutated in cancer. For example, in normal cells, *p53* can stimulate expression of anti-angiogenic molecules, such as thrombospondin-1, and repress expression of pro-angiogenic molecules, such as VEGF. Thus, loss of *p53* in tumor cells not only removes the cell cycle checkpoints listed above, but also provides a more permissive environment for angiogenesis. The transcription of VEGF is also influenced by signals from the RAS-MAP kinase pathway, and mutations of *RAS* or *MYC* up-regulate the production of VEGF.

Proteases, either elaborated by the tumor cells directly or from stromal cells in response to the tumor, are also involved in regulating the balance between angiogenic and anti-angiogenic factors. Many proteases can release the angiogenic basic FGF stored in the extracellular matrix (ECM); conversely, three potent angiogenesis inhibitors—angiostatin, endostatin, and vasculostatin—are produced by proteolytic cleavage of plasminogen, collagen, and transthyretin, respectively. Because of the crucial role of angiogenesis in tumor growth, much interest is focused on anti-angiogenesis therapy. Indeed, anti-VEGF antibody is now approved for the treatment of several types of cancers.

SUMMARY

Development of Sustained Angiogenesis

- Vascularization of tumors is essential for their growth and is controlled by the balance between angiogenic and anti-angiogenic factors that are produced by tumor and stromal cells.
- Hypoxia triggers angiogenesis through the actions of HIF1α. Because of its ability to degrade HIF1α and thus prevent angiogenesis, VHL acts as a tumor suppressor gene. Inheritance of germ-line mutations of this gene causes VHL syndrome, characterized by the development of a variety of tumors.
- Many other factors regulate angiogenesis; for example, p53 induces synthesis of the angiogenesis inhibitor thrombospondin-1.

Ability to Invade and Metastasize

The spread of tumors is a complex process involving a series of sequential steps, diagrammed in Figure 6–26. Predictably, this sequence of steps may be interrupted at any stage by either host-related or tumor-related factors. For the purpose of discussion, the metastatic cascade can be subdivided into two phases: invasion of ECM and vascular dissemination, and homing of tumor cells.

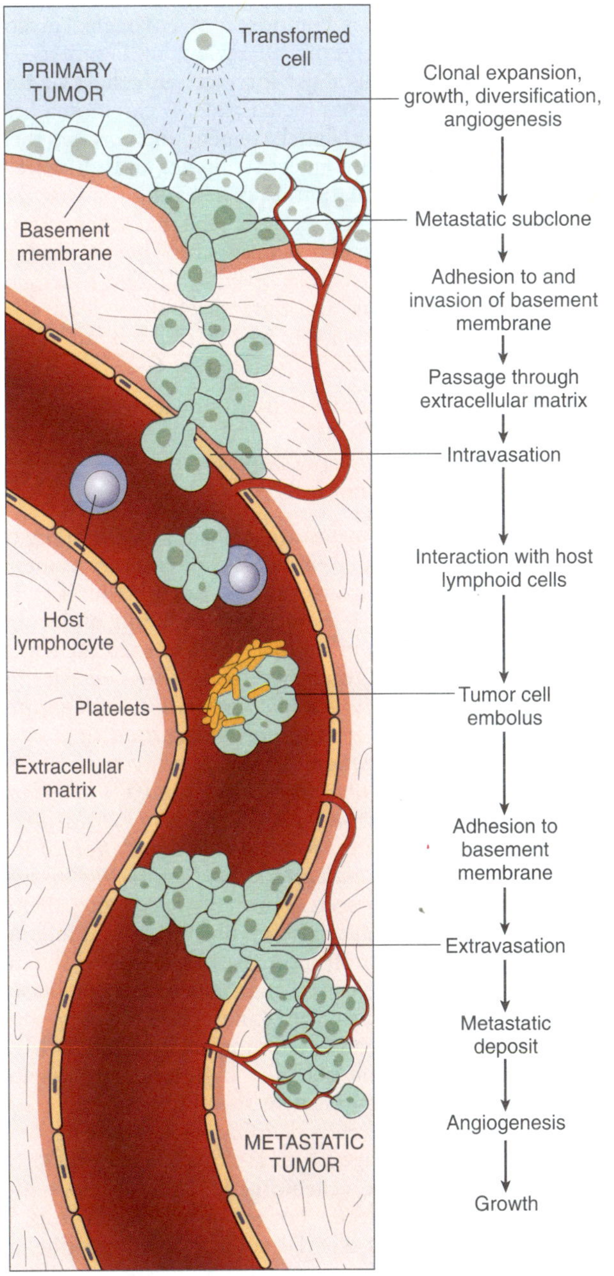

Figure 6–26

The metastatic cascade. Schematic illustration of the sequential steps involved in the hematogenous spread of a tumor.

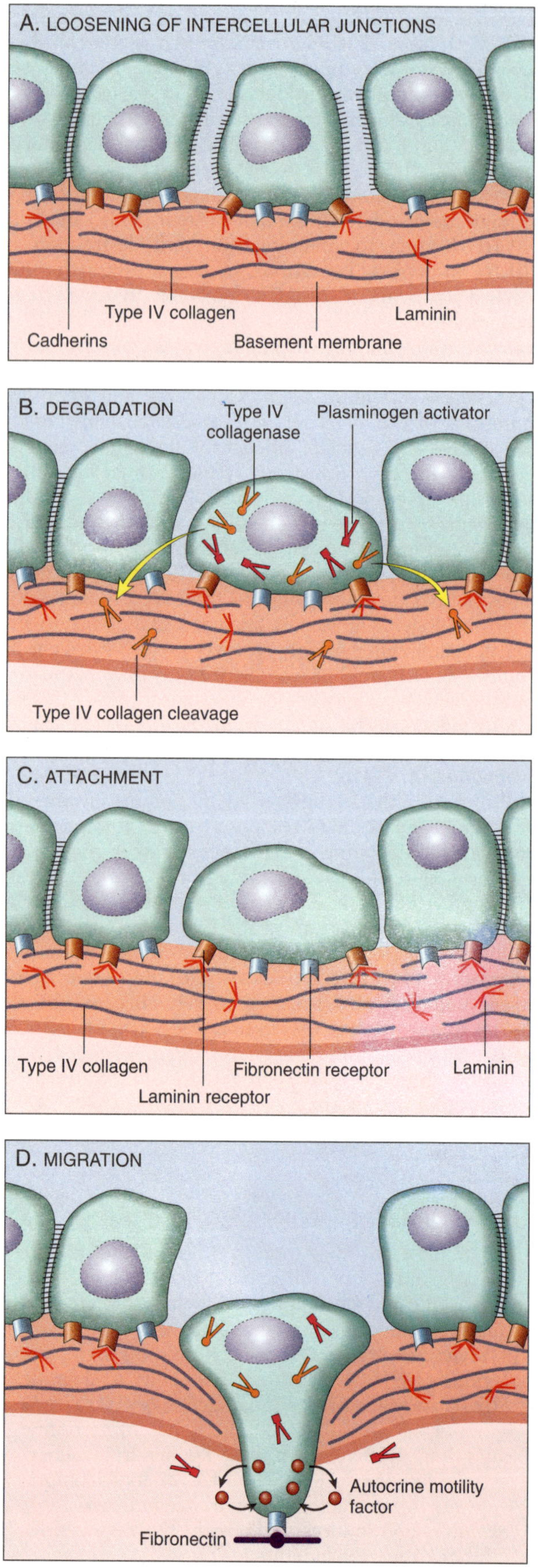

Figure 6–27

A–D, Schematic illustration of the sequence of events in the invasion of epithelial basement membranes by tumor cells. Tumor cells detach from each other because of reduced adhesiveness, then secrete proteolytic enzymes, degrading the basement membrane. Binding to proteolytically generated binding sites and tumor cell migration follow.

Invasion of Extracellular Matrix (ECM)

As is well known, human tissues are organized into a series of compartments separated from each other by two types of ECM: basement membranes and interstitial connective tissue. Though organized differently, each of these components of ECM is composed of collagens, glycoproteins, and proteoglycans. A review of Figure 6–26 reveals that tumor cells must interact with the ECM at several stages in the metastatic cascade. A carcinoma first must breach the underlying basement membrane, then traverse the interstitial connective tissue, and ultimately gain access to the circulation by penetrating the vascular basement membrane. This cycle is repeated when tumor cell emboli extravasate at a distant site. Thus, to metastasize, a tumor cell must cross several different basement membranes, as well as negotiate through at least two interstitial matrices. Invasion of the ECM is an active process that requires four steps (see Fig. 6–27):

1. Detachment of tumor cells from each other
2. Degradation of ECM
3. Attachment to novel ECM components
4. Migration of tumor cells

The first step in the metastatic cascade is a *loosening* of tumor cells. As mentioned earlier, E-cadherins act as intercellular glues, and their cytoplasmic portions bind to β-catenin (see Fig. 6–23). Adjacent E-cadherin molecules keep the cells together; in addition, as discussed earlier, E-cadherin can transmit antigrowth signals by sequestering β-catenin. *E-cadherin function is lost in almost all epithelial cancers, either by mutational inactivation of E-cadherin genes, by activation of β-catenin genes, or by inappropriate expression of the SNAIL and TWIST transcription factors, which suppress E-cadherin expression.*

The second step in invasion is local *degradation of the basement membrane and interstitial connective tissue.* Tumor cells may either secrete proteolytic enzymes themselves or induce stromal cells (e.g., fibroblasts and inflammatory cells) to elaborate proteases. Multiple different families of proteases, such as matrix metalloproteinases (MMPs), cathepsin D, and urokinase plasminogen activator, have been implicated in tumor cell invasion. MMPs regulate tumor invasion not only by remodeling insoluble components of the basement membrane and interstitial matrix but also by releasing ECM-sequestered growth factors. Indeed, cleavage products of collagen and proteoglycans also have chemotactic, angiogenic, and growth-promoting effects. For example, MMP-9 is a gelatinase that cleaves type IV collagen of the epithelial and vascular basement membrane and also stimulates release of VEGF from ECM-sequestered pools. Benign tumors of the breast, colon, and stomach show little type

IV collagenase activity, whereas their malignant counterparts overexpress this enzyme. Concurrently, the levels of metalloproteinase inhibitors are reduced so that the balance is tilted greatly toward tissue degradation. Indeed, overexpression of MMPs and other proteases have been reported for many tumors. Because of these observations, attempts are being made to use protease inhibitors as therapeutic agents.

The third step in invasion involves *changes in attachment of tumor cells to ECM proteins*. Normal epithelial cells have receptors, such as integrins, for basement membrane laminin and collagens that are polarized at their basal surface; these receptors help to maintain the cells in a resting, differentiated state. Loss of adhesion in normal cells leads to induction of apoptosis, while, not surprisingly, tumor cells are resistant to this form of cell death. Additionally, the matrix itself is modified in ways that promote invasion and metastasis. For example, cleavage of the basement membrane proteins collagen IV and laminin by MMP-2 or MMP-9 generates novel sites that bind to receptors on tumor cells and stimulate migration.

Locomotion is the final step of invasion, propelling tumor cells through the degraded basement membranes and zones of matrix proteolysis. Migration is a complex, multistep process that involves many families of receptors and signaling proteins that eventually impinge on the actin cytoskeleton. Such movement seems to be potentiated and directed by tumor cell–derived cytokines, such as autocrine motility factors. In addition, cleavage products of matrix components (e.g., collagen, laminin) and some growth factors (e.g., insulin-like growth factors I and II) have chemotactic activity for tumor cells. Stromal cells also produce paracrine effectors of cell motility, such as hepatocyte growth factor/scatter factor (HGF/SCF), which bind to receptors on tumor cells. Concentrations of HGF/SCF are elevated at the advancing edges of the highly invasive brain tumor glioblastoma multiforme, supporting their role in motility.

It has become clear in recent years, however, that the ECM and stromal cells surrounding tumor cells do not merely represent a static barrier for tumor cells to traverse but rather represent a variable environment in which reciprocal signaling between tumor cells and stromal cells may either promote or prevent tumorigenesis and/or tumor progression. Stromal cells that interact with tumors include innate and adaptive immune cells (discussed later), as well as fibroblasts. A variety of studies have demonstrated that tumor-associated fibroblasts exhibit altered expression of genes that encode ECM molecules, proteases, protease inhibitors, and various growth factors. Thus, tumor cells live in a complex and ever-changing milieu composed of ECM, growth factors, fibroblasts, and immune cells, with significant cross-talk among all the components. The most successful tumors may be those that can co-opt and adapt this environment to their own nefarious ends.

Vascular Dissemination and Homing of Tumor Cells

When in the circulation, tumor cells are vulnerable to destruction by host immune cells (discussed later). In the bloodstream, some tumor cells form emboli by aggregating and adhering to circulating leukocytes, particularly platelets; aggregated tumor cells are thus afforded some protection from the antitumor host effector cells. Most tumor cells, however, circulate as single cells. Extravasation of free tumor cells or tumor emboli involves adhesion to the vascular endothelium, followed by egress through the basement membrane into the organ parenchyma by mechanisms similar to those involved in invasion.

The site of extravasation and the organ distribution of metastases generally can be predicted by the location of the primary tumor and its vascular or lymphatic drainage. Many tumors metastasize to the organ that represents the first capillary bed they encounter after entering the circulation. However, in many cases the natural pathways of drainage do not readily explain the distribution of metastases. As pointed out earlier, some tumors (e.g., lung cancers) tend to involve the adrenals with some regularity but almost never spread to skeletal muscle. Such organ tropism may be related to the expression of adhesion molecules by tumor cells whose ligands are expressed preferentially on the endothelium of target organs. Another mechanism of site-specific homing involves chemokines and their receptors. As discussed in Chapter 2, chemokines participate in directed movement (chemotaxis) of leukocytes, and it seems that cancer cells use similar tricks to home in on specific tissues. Human breast cancer cells express high levels of the chemokine receptors *CXCR4* and *CCR7*. The ligands for these receptors (i.e., chemokines CXCL12 and CCL21) are highly expressed only in those organs where breast cancer cells metastasize. On the basis of this observation, it is speculated that blockade of chemokine receptors may limit metastases. After extravasation, tumor cells are dependent on a receptive stroma for growth. Thus, tumors may fail to metastasize to certain target tissues because they present a nonpermissive growth environment. Despite the foregoing considerations, the precise localization of metastases cannot be predicted with any form of cancer. Evidently many tumors have not read the relevant chapters of the pathology textbooks!

Molecular Genetics of Metastasis

A long-held theory of tumor progression suggests that, as tumors grow, individual cells randomly accumulate mutations, creating subclones with distinct combinations of mutations. According to this hypothesis only a small subpopulation of the tumor cells contains all the mutations necessary for metastasis. However, recent experiments, in which gene profiling of primary tumors and metastatic deposits has been compared, challenge this hypothesis. For example, a subset of breast cancers has a gene expression signature similar to that found in metastases, although no clinical evidence for metastasis is apparent. In these tumors it seems that most if not all cells develop a predilection for metastatic spread early, during primary carcinogenesis. Metastases, according to this view, are not dependent on the stochastic generation of metastatic subclones postulated above. It should be noted, however, that gene expression analyses like those described above would not detect a small subset of metastatic subclones within a large tumor. Perhaps both mechanisms are operative, with aggressive tumors acquiring a metastases-permissive gene expression pattern early in tumorigenesis that requires some additional random mutations to complete the metastatic phenotype.

One open question in the field is, are there genes whose principal or sole contribution to tumorigenesis is to control metastases? This question is of more than academic interest, because if altered forms of certain genes promote or suppress the metastatic phenotype, their detection in a primary tumor would have both prognostic and therapeutic implications. Metastasis is a complex phenomenon involving a variety of steps and pathways described above. It is thought therefore that, unlike transformation, in which a subset of proteins like p53 and RB seem to play a key role, genes that function as "metastasis oncogenes" or "metastatic suppressors" are rare. Among candidates for such metastasis oncogenes are SNAIL and TWIST, which encode transcription factors whose primary function is to promote a process called epithelial-to-mesenchymal transition (EMT). In EMT, carcinoma cells down-regulate certain epithelial markers (e.g., E-cadherin) and up-regulate certain mesenchymal markers (e.g., vimentin and smooth muscle actin). These changes are believed to favor the development of a promigratory phenotype that is essential for metastasis. Loss of E-cadherin expression seems to be a key event in EMT, and SNAIL and TWIST are transcriptional repressors that promote EMT by down-regulating E-cadherin expression. EMT has been documented mainly in breast cancers; whether this is a general phenomenon remains to be established.

SUMMARY

Invasion and Metastasis

- Ability to invade tissues, a hallmark of malignancy, occurs in four steps: loosening of cell-cell contacts, degradation of ECM, attachment to novel ECM components, and migration of tumor cells.
- Cell-cell contacts are lost by the inactivation of E-cadherin through a variety of pathways.
- Basement membranes and interstitial matrix degradation is mediated by proteolytic enzymes secreted by tumor cells and stromal cells, such as MMPs and cathepsins.
- Proteolytic enzymes also release growth factors sequestered in the ECM and generate chemotactic and angiogenic fragments from cleavage of ECM glycoproteins.
- The metastatic site of many tumors can be predicted by the location of the primary tumor. Many tumors arrest in the first capillary bed they encounter (lung and liver, most commonly).
- Some tumors show organ tropism, probably due to expression of adhesion or chemokine receptors whose ligands are expressed by the metastatic site.

Genomic Instability—Enabler of Malignancy

In the preceding section we discussed six defining features of malignancy and the genetic alterations that are responsible for the phenotypic attributes of cancer cells. How do these mutations arise? Although humans literally swim in environmental agents that are mutagenic (e.g., chemicals, radiation, sunlight), cancers are relatively rare outcomes of these encounters. This state of affairs results from the ability of normal cells to repair DNA damage. The importance of DNA repair in maintaining the integrity of the genome is highlighted by several inherited disorders in which genes that encode proteins involved in DNA repair are defective. *Individuals born with such inherited defects in DNA repair proteins are at a greatly increased risk of developing cancer.* Typically, genomic instability occurs when both copies of the gene are lost; however, recent work has suggested that at least a subset of these genes may promote cancer in a haploinsufficient manner. Defects in three types of DNA repair systems—mismatch repair, nucleotide excision repair, and recombination repair—are presented next.

Hereditary Nonpolyposis Colon Cancer Syndrome. The role of DNA repair genes in predisposition to cancer is illustrated dramatically by hereditary nonpolyposis colon carcinoma (HNPCC) syndrome. This disorder, characterized by familial carcinomas of the colon affecting predominantly the cecum and proximal colon (Chapter 15), results from defects in genes involved in DNA mismatch repair. When a strand of DNA is being repaired, these genes act as "spell checkers." For example, if there is an erroneous pairing of G with T rather than the normal A with T, the mismatch repair genes correct the defect. Without these "proofreaders," errors gradually accumulate in several genes, including proto-oncogenes and cancer suppressor genes. Mutations in at least four mismatch repair genes have been found to underlie HNPCC (Chapter 15). Each affected individual inherits one defective copy of one of several DNA mismatch repair genes and acquires the second hit in colonic epithelial cells. Thus, DNA repair genes behave like tumor suppressor genes in their mode of inheritance, but in contrast to tumor suppressor genes (and oncogenes), they affect cell growth only indirectly—by allowing mutations in other genes during the process of normal cell division. One of the hallmarks of patients with mismatch repair defects is microsatellite instability (MSI). Microsatellites are tandem repeats of one to six nucleotides found throughout the genome. In normal people, the length of these microsatellites remains constant. However, in patients with HNPCC, these satellites are unstable and increase or decrease in length. Although HNPCC accounts only for 2% to 4% of all colonic cancers, MSI can be detected in about 15% of sporadic cancers. The growth-regulating genes that are mutated in HNPCC patients have not yet been fully characterized.

Xeroderma Pigmentosum. Patients with another inherited disorder, xeroderma pigmentosum, are at increased risk for the development of cancers of the skin exposed to the ultraviolet (UV) light contained in sun rays. The basis of this disorder is defective DNA repair. UV light causes cross-linking of pyrimidine residues, preventing normal DNA replication. Such DNA damage is repaired by the nucleotide excision repair system. Several proteins are involved in nucleotide excision repair, and an inherited loss of any one can give rise to xeroderma pigmentosum.

Diseases with Defects in DNA Repair by Homologous Recombination. A group of autosomal recessive disorders comprising Bloom syndrome, ataxia-telangiectasia, and Fanconi anemia is characterized by hypersensitivity to other DNA-damaging agents, such as ionizing radiation (Bloom syndrome and ataxia-telangiectasia), or DNA cross-linking agents, such as nitrogen mustard (Fanconi anemia). Their phenotype is complex and includes, in addition to predisposition to cancer, features such as neural symptoms (ataxia-telangiectasia), anemia (Fanconi anemia), and developmental defects (Bloom syndrome). As mentioned earlier, the gene mutated in ataxia-telangiectasia is *ATM,* which seems to be important in recognizing and responding to DNA damage caused by ionizing radiation. Evidence for the role of DNA repair genes in the origin of cancer also comes from the study of hereditary breast cancer. Mutations in two genes, *BRCA1* and *BRCA2,* account for 80% of cases of familial breast cancer. In addition to breast cancer, women with *BRCA1* mutations have a substantially higher risk of epithelial ovarian cancers, and men have a slightly higher risk of prostate cancer. Likewise, mutations in the *BRCA2* gene increase the risk of breast cancer in both men and women as well as cancer of the ovary, prostate, pancreas, bile ducts, stomach, and melanocytes. Although the functions of these genes have not been elucidated fully, cells that lack these genes develop chromosomal breaks and severe aneuploidy. Indeed, both genes seem to function, at least in part, in the homologous recombination DNA repair pathway. For example, BRCA1 forms a complex with other proteins in the homologous recombination pathway and is also linked to the ATM checkpoint pathway. *BRCA2* was identified as one of several genes mutated in Fanconi anemia and the BRCA2 protein has been shown to bind to RAD51, a protein required for catalysis of the primary reaction of homologous recombination. Similar to other tumor suppressor genes, both copies of *BRCA1* and *BRCA2* must be inactivated for cancer to develop. Although linkage of *BRCA1* and *BRCA2* to familial breast cancers is established, these genes are rarely inactivated in sporadic cases of breast cancer. In this regard, *BRCA1* and *BRCA2* are different from other tumor suppressor genes, such as *APC* and *p53,* which are inactivated in both familial and sporadic cancers.

SUMMARY

Genomic Instability—Enabler of Malignancy

- Individuals with inherited mutations of genes involved in DNA repair systems are at a greatly increased risk of developing cancer.
- Patients with HNPCC syndrome have defects in the mismatch repair system and develop carcinomas of the colon. These patients show microsatellite instability (MSI), in which short repeats throughout the genome change in length.
- Patients with xeroderma pigmentosum have a defect in the nucleotide excision repair pathway and are at increased risk for the development of cancers of the skin exposed to UV light, because of an inability to repair pyrimidine dimers.
- Syndromes involving defects in the homologous recombination DNA repair system compose a group of disorders (Bloom syndrome, ataxia-telangiectasia, and Fanconi anemia) that are characterized by hypersensitivity to DNA-damaging agents, such as ionizing radiation. *BRCA1* and *BRCA2,* which are mutated in familial breast cancers, are involved in DNA repair.

MicroRNAs (MiRNAs) and Cancer

As discussed in Chapter 7, miRNAs are non-coding, single-stranded RNAs, approximately 22 nucleotides in length, that function as negative regulators of genes. They inhibit gene expression post-transcriptionally by repressing translation, or in some cases, by mRNA cleavage. Given that miRNAs control cell growth, differentiation, and cell survival, it is not surprising that there is accumulating evidence to support their role in carcinogenesis. As illustrated by Figure 6–28, miRNAs can participate in neoplastic transformation either by increasing the expression of oncogenes or reducing the expression of tumor suppressor genes. If an miRNA inhibits the translation of an oncogene, a reduction in the quantity or function of that miRNA will lead to overproduction of the oncogene product. Conversely, if the target of an miRNA is a tumor suppressor gene, then overactivity of the miRNA can reduce the tumor suppressor protein. Such relationships have already been established by miRNA profiling of several human tumors. For example, downregulation or deletion of certain miRNAs in some leukemias and lymphomas results in increased expression of BCL2, the anti-apoptotic gene. Thus, by negatively regulating BCL2, such miRNAs behave as tumor suppressor genes. Similar miRNA-mediated upregulation of RAS, and MYC oncogenes has also been detected in lung tumors and in certain B cell leukemias respectively. In some brain and breast tumors there is 5–100 fold greater expression of certain miRNAs. Although the targets of these miRNAs have not been identified, presumably they are unidentified tumor suppressor genes, whose activities are reduced by the overexpressed miRNA.

These findings not only provide novel insights into carcinogenesis, they also have practical implications. For instance, drugs that inhibit or augment the functions of miRNAs could be useful in chemotherapy. Since miRNAs regulate normal cellular differentiation, the patterns of miRNA expression ("miRNA profiling") can provide

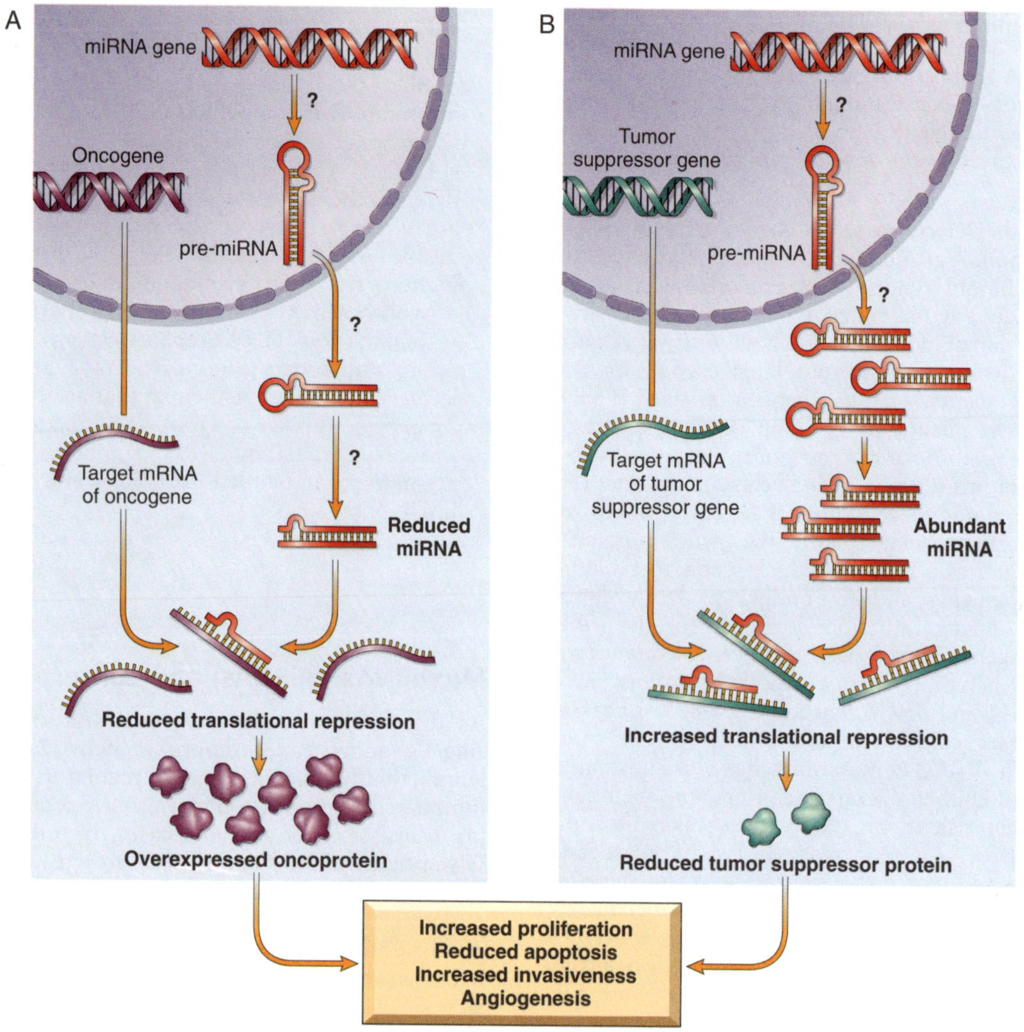

Figure 6–28

Role of miRNAs in tumorigenesis. **A**. Reduced activity of a miRNA that inhibits translation of an oncogene gives rise to an excess of oncoproteins. **B**. Overactivity of a miRNA that targets a tumor suppression gene reduces the production of the tumor suppressor protein. Question marks in A and B are meant to indicate that the mechanisms by which changes in the level or activity of miRNA are not entirely known.

clues to the cell of origin and classification of tumors. Much remains to be learned about these oncogenic miRNAs, or so called "oncomirs."

Molecular Basis of Multistep Carcinogenesis

Given that malignant tumors must develop several fundamental abnormalities, discussed above, it follows that *each cancer must result from accumulation of multiple mutations*. Indeed, recently completed genome-wide analysis of breast and colon cancers has revealed that individual tumors accumulate an average of 90 mutant genes. A much smaller subset of these (≈11/tumor) were mutated at significant frequency. Included among these are some known oncogenes and tumor suppressor genes, while others were not previously known to be tumor-associated. Each of these alterations represents crucial steps in the progression from a normal cell to a malignant tumor. Furthermore, *it seems that evolution has installed a variety of "intrinsic tumor-suppressive mechanisms" such as apoptosis and senescence that thwart the actions of growth-promoting mutations*. Indeed, in cells with competent checkpoints, oncogenic signaling through genes like *RAS* leads not to transformation, but to senescence or apoptosis. Thus, emergence of malignant tumors requires mutational loss of many genes including those that regulate apoptosis and senescence. A dramatic example of incremental acquisition of the malignant phenotype is documented by the study of colon carcinoma. These lesions are believed to evolve through a series of morphologically identifiable stages: colon epithelial hyperplasia followed by formation of adenomas that progressively enlarge and ultimately undergo malignant transformation (Chapter 15). The proposed molecular correlates of this adenoma-carcinoma sequence are illustrated in Figure 6–29. According to this scheme, inactivation of the *APC* tumor suppressor gene occurs first, followed by activation of *RAS* and, ultimately, loss of a tumor suppressor gene on 18q and loss of *p53*. The precise temporal sequence of mutations may be different in each organ and tumor type.

Karyotypic Changes in Tumors

The genetic damage that activates oncogenes or inactivates tumor suppressor genes may be subtle (e.g., point mutations) or large enough to be detected in a karyotype. As previously discussed, the *RAS* oncogene represents the best example of activation by point mutation. In certain neoplasms, karyotypic abnormalities are nonrandom and common. Specific abnormalities have been identified in most leukemias and lymphomas, and in an increasing number of nonhematopoietic tumors. The common types of nonrandom structural abnormalities in tumor cells are (1) balanced translocations, (2) deletions, and (3) cytogenetic manifestations of gene amplification. In addition, whole chromosomes may be gained or lost, termed aneuploidy.

Balanced Translocations. Balanced translocations are extremely common, especially in hematopoietic neoplasms. Translocations can activate proto-oncogenes in two ways. First, specific translocations can result in overexpression of proto-oncogenes by removing them from their normal regulatory elements and placing them under control of an inappropriate promoter. Second, translocations can result in fusion genes, combining the DNA sequence of two unrelated genes in new ways. This results in the expression of growth-promoting chimeric proteins. Most notable is the Philadelphia (Ph) chromosome in chronic myeloid leukemia, comprising a reciprocal and balanced translocation between chromosomes 22 and, usually, 9 (Fig. 6–30). As a consequence, chromosome 22 appears abbreviated. *This cytogenetic change, seen in more than 90% of cases of chronic myeloid leukemia, is a reliable marker of the disease. The few Ph chromosome–negative cases of chronic myeloid leukemia show molecular evidence of the BCR-ABL rearrangement, the crucial consequence of Ph translocation.* As mentioned earlier, such changes give rise to the *BCR-ABL* fusion gene with potent tyrosine kinase activity. In more than 90% of cases of Burkitt lymphoma the cells have a translocation, usually between chromosomes 8 and 14. This leads to overexpression of *MYC* gene on chromosome 8 by juxtaposition with immunoglobulin heavy chain gene on chromosome 14. In follicular B-cell lymphomas, a reciprocal translocation between chromosomes 14 and 18 leads to overexpression of the *BCL2* gene on chromosome 18.

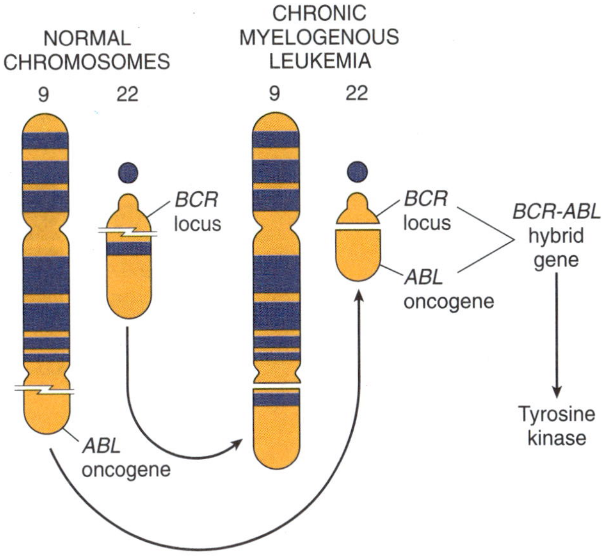

Figure 6–30

The chromosomal translocation and associated oncogene in chronic myeloid leukemia.

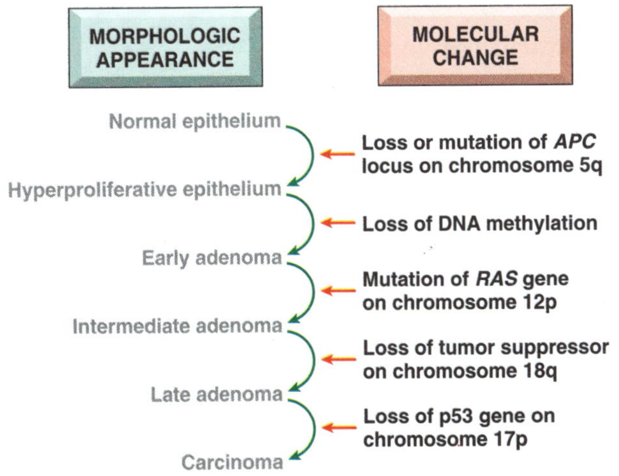

Figure 6–29

Molecular model for the evolution of colorectal cancers through the adenoma-carcinoma sequence. (Based on studies of Fearon ER, Vogelstein B: A genetic model of colorectal carcinogenesis. Cell 61:759, 1990.)

Hematopoietic cells are most commonly the targets of such translocations, probably because these cells purposefully make DNA breaks during the processes of antibody or T-cell receptor recombination. However, several solid tumors have also been shown to possess a recurrent translocation, such as the t(11;22)(q24;12) translocation in Ewing sarcoma that results in fusion of the EWS transcription factor with Fli-1. Recently, a subset of prostate cancers has been shown to possess a fusion protein between a prostate-expressed protein and members of the ETS family of transcription factors.

Deletions. Chromosomal deletions are the second most prevalent structural abnormality in tumor cells. *Compared with translocations, deletions are more common in nonhematopoietic solid tumors.* As discussed, deletions of chromosome 13q band 14 are associated with retinoblastoma. Deletions of 17p, 5q, and 18q have all been noted in colorectal cancers; these regions harbor three tumor suppressor genes. Deletion of 3p, noted in several tumors, is extremely common in small-cell lung carcinomas, and the hunt is on for one or more cancer suppressor genes at this locale.

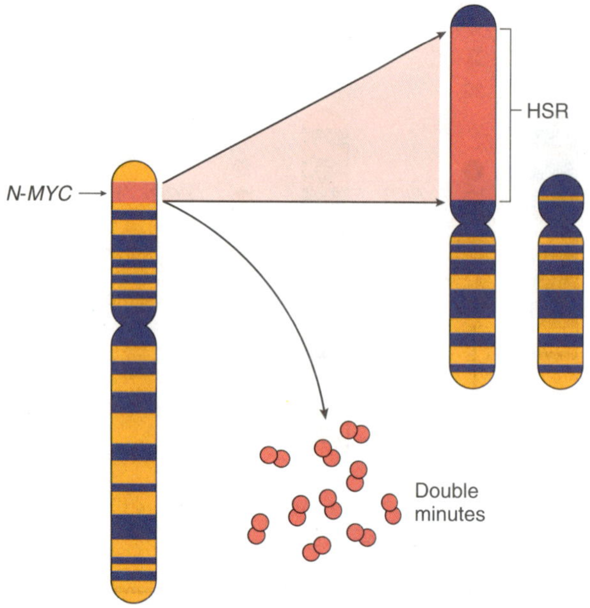

Figure 6–31

Amplification of the *N-MYC* gene in human neuroblastoma. The *N-MYC* gene, present normally on chromosome 2p, becomes amplified and is seen either as extra chromosomal double minutes or as a chromosomally integrated homogeneous-staining region (HSR). The integration involves other autosomes, such as 4, 9, or 13. (Modified from Brodeur GM, et al.: Clinical implication of oncogene activation in human neuroblastomas. Cancer 58:541, 1986. Reprinted by permission of Wiley-Liss, Inc, a subsidiary of John Wiley & Sons, Inc.)

Gene Amplifications. There are two karyotypic manifestations of gene amplification: homogeneously staining regions on single chromosomes and double minutes (Fig. 6–31), which are seen as small paired fragments of chromatin. Neuroblastomas and breast cancers are the best-studied examples of gene amplification involving the *N-MYC* and *HER-2/NEU* genes respectively.

Epigenetic Changes

Epigenetics concerns reversible, heritable changes in gene expression that occur without mutation. It has become evident during the past few years that certain tumor suppressor genes may be inactivated, not because of structural changes, but because the gene is silenced by hypermethylation of promoter sequences. For example, *p14ARF* is silenced in colon and stomach cancers, and *p16INK4a* is silenced in various types of cancers. Furthermore, *BRCA1* in breast cancer, *VHL* in renal cell cancer, and the *MLH1* mismatch repair gene in colorectal cancer are frequently silenced by methylation of the promoter. Interestingly, although the promoters of some tumor suppressor genes are hypermethylated in tumor cells, the entire genome seems to be hypomethylated compared with normal cells. Genome-wide hypomethylation has been shown to cause chromosomal instability and can induce tumors in mice. Thus epigenetic changes may influence carcinogenesis in many ways.

SUMMARY

Karyotypic Changes in Tumors

- Tumor cells may develop a variety of nonrandom chromosomal abnormalities that contribute to malignancy; these include balanced translocations, deletions, and cytogenetic manifestations of gene amplification.
- Balanced translocations contribute to carcinogenesis by overexpression of oncogenes or generation of novel fusion proteins with altered signaling capacity. Deletions frequently affect tumor suppressor genes, whereas gene amplification increases the expression of oncogenes.
- Tumor suppressor genes and DNA repair genes may also be silenced by epigenetic changes, which involve reversible, heritable changes in gene expression that occur, not by mutation, but by methylation of the promoter.

ETIOLOGY OF CANCER: CARCINOGENIC AGENTS

Genetic damage lies at the heart of carcinogenesis. What agents inflict such damage? Three classes of carcinogenic agents can be identified: (1) chemicals, (2) radiant energy, and (3) microbial agents. Chemicals and radiant energy are documented causes of cancer in humans, and oncogenic viruses are involved in the pathogenesis of tumors in several animal models and at least in some human tumors. In the following discussion, each class of agents is considered separately, but it is important to note that several may act in concert or sequentially to produce the multiple genetic abnormalities characteristic of neoplastic cells.

Chemical Carcinogens

More than 200 years ago, the London surgeon Sir Percival Pott correctly attributed scrotal skin cancer in chimney sweeps to chronic exposure to soot. Based on this observation, the Danish Chimney Sweeps Guild ruled that its members must bathe daily. No public health measure since that time has achieved so much in the control of a form of cancer. Subsequently, hundreds of chemicals have been shown to be carcinogenic in animals.

Some of the major agents are presented in Table 6–4. A few comments are offered on a handful of these.

Direct-Acting Agents

Direct-acting agents require no metabolic conversion to become carcinogenic. They are in general weak carcinogens but are important because some of them are cancer chemotherapeutic drugs (e.g., alkylating agents) that have successfully cured, controlled, or delayed recurrence of

Table 6–4 Major Chemical Carcinogens

Direct-Acting Carcinogens
ALKYLATING AGENTS
β-Propiolactone
Dimethyl sulfate
Diepoxybutane
Anticancer drugs (cyclophosphamide, chlorambucil, nitrosoureas, and others)
ACYLATING AGENTS
1-Acetyl-imidazole
Dimethylcarbamyl chloride
Procarcinogens That Require Metabolic Activation
POLYCYCLIC AND HETEROCYCLIC AROMATIC HYDROCARBONS
Benz(*a*)anthracene
Benzo(*a*)pyrene
Dibenz(*a*, *h*)anthracene
3-Methylcholanthrene
7, 12-Dimethylbenz(*a*)anthracene
AROMATIC AMINES, AMIDES, AZO DYES
2-Naphthylamine (β-naphthylamine)
Benzidine
2-Acetylaminofluorene
Dimethylaminoazobenzene (butter yellow)
Natural Plant and Microbial Products
Aflatoxin B_1
Griseofulvin
Cycasin
Safrole
Betel nuts
OTHERS
Nitrosamine and amides
Vinyl chloride, nickel, chromium
Insecticides, fungicides
Polychlorinated biphenyls

certain types of cancer (e.g., leukemia, lymphoma, Hodgkin lymphoma, and ovarian carcinoma), only to evoke later a second form of cancer, usually leukemia. This situation is even more tragic when their initial use has been for non-neoplastic disorders, such as rheumatoid arthritis or Wegener granulomatosis. The risk of induced cancer is low, but its existence dictates judicious use of such agents.

Indirect-Acting Agents

The designation *indirect-acting agent* refers to chemicals that require metabolic conversion to an *ultimate carcinogen* before they become active. Some of the most potent indirect chemical carcinogens—the polycyclic hydrocarbons—are present in fossil fuels. For example, benzo*[a]*pyrene and other carcinogens are formed in the high-temperature combustion of tobacco in cigarette smoking. *These products are implicated in the causation of lung cancer in cigarette smokers.* Polycyclic hydrocarbons may also be produced from animal fats during the process of broiling meats and are present in smoked meats and fish. The principal active products in many hydrocarbons are epoxides, which form covalent adducts (addition products) with molecules in the cell, principally DNA, but also with RNA and proteins.

The aromatic amines and azo dyes are another class of indirect-acting carcinogens. Before its carcinogenicity was recognized, β-naphthylamine was responsible for a 50-fold increased incidence of bladder cancers in heavily exposed workers in the aniline dye and rubber industries. Many other occupational carcinogens were listed in Table 6–2. Because indirect-acting carcinogens require metabolic activation for their conversion to DNA-damaging agents, much interest is focused on the enzymatic pathways that are involved, such as the cytochrome P-450–dependent monooxygenases. The genes that encode these enzymes are polymorphic, and enzyme activity varies among different individuals. It is widely believed that the susceptibility to chemical carcinogenesis depends at least in part on the specific allelic form of the enzyme inherited. Thus, it may be possible in the future to assess cancer risk in a given individual by genetic analysis of such enzyme polymorphisms.

A few other agents merit brief mention. Aflatoxin B_1 is of interest because it is a naturally occurring agent produced by some strains of *Aspergillus,* a mold that grows on improperly stored grains and nuts. There is a *strong correlation between the dietary level of this food contaminant and the incidence of hepatocellular carcinoma in some parts of Africa and the Far East.* Additionally, vinyl chloride, arsenic, nickel, chromium, insecticides, fungicides, and polychlorinated biphenyls are potential carcinogens in the workplace and about the house. Finally, nitrites used as food preservatives have caused concern, since they cause nitrosylation of amines contained in the food. The nitrosoamines so formed are suspected to be carcinogenic.

Mechanisms of Action of Chemical Carcinogens

Because malignant transformation results from mutations, it should come as no surprise that most chemical carcinogens are mutagenic. Indeed, all direct and ultimate carcinogens contain highly reactive electrophile groups that form chemical adducts with DNA, as well as with proteins and RNA. Although any gene may be the target of chemical carcinogens, the commonly mutated oncogenes and tumor suppressors, such as *RAS* and *p53,* are important targets of chemical carcinogens. Indeed, specific chemical carcinogens, such as aflatoxin B_1, produce characteristic mutations in the *p53* gene, such that detection of the "*signature mutation*" within the *p53* gene establishes aflatoxin as the causative agent. These associations are proving useful tools in epidemiologic studies of chemical carcinogenesis.

Carcinogenicity of some chemicals is augmented by subsequent administration of *promoters* (e.g., phorbol esters, hormones, phenols, and drugs) that by themselves are nontumorigenic. To be effective, repeated or sustained exposure to the promoter must *follow* the application of the mutagenic chemical, or *initiator.* The initiation-promotion sequence of chemical carcinogenesis raises an important question: Since promoters are not mutagenic, how do they contribute to tumorigenesis? Although the effects of tumor promoters are pleiotropic, *induction of cell proliferation is a sine qua non of tumor promotion.* It seems most likely that while the application of an initiator may cause the mutational activation of an oncogene such as *RAS,* subsequent application of promoters leads to clonal expansion of initiated (mutated) cells. Forced to proliferate, the initiated clone of cells accumulates additional mutations, developing eventually into a malignant tumor. Indeed, the concept that sustained cell proliferation increases the risk of mutagenesis, and hence neoplastic transformation, is also applicable to human carcinogenesis. For example, pathologic hyperplasia of the endometrium (Chapter 19) and increased regenerative activity that accompanies chronic liver cell injury are associated with the development of cancer in these organs. Were it not for the DNA repair mechanisms discussed earlier, the incidence of chemically induced cancers in all likelihood would be much higher. As mentioned above, the rare hereditary disorders of DNA repair, including xeroderma pigmentosum, are associated with greatly increased risk of cancers induced by UV light and certain chemicals.

SUMMARY

Chemical Carcinogens

- Chemical carcinogens have highly reactive eletrophile groups that directly damage DNA, leading to mutations and eventually cancer.
- Direct-acting agents do not require metabolic conversion to become carcinogenic, while indirect-acting agents are not active until converted to an ultimate carcinogen by endogenous metabolic pathways. Hence polymorphisms of endogenous enzymes like cytochrome P-450 may influence carcinogenesis.
- Following exposure of a cell to a mutagen or an initiator, tumorigenesis can be enhanced by exposure to promoters, which stimulate proliferation of the mutated cells.
- Examples of human carcinogens include direct-acting (e.g., alkylating agents used for chemotherapy), indirect-acting (e.g., benzopyrene, azo dyes, and aflatoxin), and promoters/agents that cause pathologic hyperplasias of liver, endometrium.

Radiation Carcinogenesis

Radiation, whatever its source (UV rays of sunlight, x-rays, nuclear fission, radionuclides) is an established carcinogen. Unprotected miners of radioactive elements have a 10-fold increased incidence of lung cancers. Follow-up of survivors of the atomic bombs dropped on Hiroshima and Nagasaki disclosed a markedly increased incidence of leukemia—principally acute and chronic myeloid leukemia—after an average latent period of about 7 years, as well as an increased mortality rate from thyroid, breast, colon, and lung carcinomas. The nuclear power accident at Chernobyl in the former Soviet Union continues to exact its toll in the form of high cancer incidence in the surrounding areas. Therapeutic irradiation of the head and neck can give rise to papillary thyroid cancers years later. The oncogenic properties of ionizing radiation are related to its mutagenic effects; it causes chromosome breakage, translocations, and, less frequently, point mutations. Biologically, double-stranded DNA breaks seem to be the most important form of DNA damage caused by radiation. There is also some evidence that nonlethal doses of radiation may induce genomic instability, favoring carcinogenesis.

The oncogenic effect of UV rays merits special mention because it highlights the importance of DNA repair in carcinogenesis. Natural UV radiation derived from the sun can cause skin cancers (melanomas, squamous cell carcinomas, and basal cell carcinomas). At greatest risk are fair-skinned people who live in locales such as Australia and New Zealand that receive a great deal of sunlight. Nonmelanoma skin cancers are associated with total cumulative exposure to UV radiation, whereas melanomas are associated with intense intermittent exposure—as occurs with sunbathing. UV light has several biologic effects on cells. Of particular relevance to carcinogenesis is the ability to damage DNA by forming pyrimidine dimers. This type of DNA damage is repaired by the nucleotide excision repair pathway. With extensive exposure to UV light, the repair systems may be overwhelmed, and skin cancer results. As mentioned above, patients with the inherited disease *xeroderma pigmentosum* have a defect in the nucleotide excision repair pathway. As expected, there is a greatly increased predisposition to skin cancers in this disorder.

SUMMARY

Radiation Carcinogenesis

- Ionizing radiation causes chromosome breakage, translocations, and, less frequently, point mutations, leading to genetic damage and carcinogenesis.
- UV rays induce the formation of pyrimidine dimers within DNA, leading to mutations. Therefore UV rays can give rise to squamous cell carcinomas and melanomas of the skin.

Viral and Microbial Oncogenesis

Many DNA and RNA viruses have proved to be oncogenic in animals as disparate as frogs and primates. Despite intense scrutiny, however, only a few viruses have been linked with human cancer. Our discussion focuses on human oncogenic viruses. Also discussed is the emerging role of the bacterium *H. pylori* in gastric cancer.

Oncogenic RNA Viruses

The study of oncogenic retroviruses in animals has provided spectacular insights into the genetic basis of cancer. However, human T-cell leukemia virus-1 (HTLV-1) is the only retrovirus that has been demonstrated to cause cancer in humans. HTLV-1 is associated with a form of T-cell leukemia/lymphoma that is endemic in certain parts of Japan and the Caribbean basin but is found sporadically elsewhere, including the United States. Similar to the human immunodeficiency virus (HIV), HTLV-1 has tropism for CD4+ T cells, and this subset of T cells is the major target for neoplastic transformation. Human infection requires transmission of infected T cells via sexual intercourse, blood products, or breastfeeding. Leukemia develops only in about 3% to 5% of infected individuals after a long latent period of 20 to 50 years.

There is little doubt that HTLV-1 infection of T lymphocytes is necessary for leukemogenesis, but the molecular mechanisms of transformation are not clear. HTLV-1 does not contain a *viral oncogene,* and in contrast to certain animal retroviruses, no consistent integration site next to a cellular oncogene has been discovered. Indeed, the long latency period between initial infection and development of disease suggests a multistep process, during which many oncogenic mutations are accumulated.

The genome of HTLV-1 contains, in addition to the usual retroviral genes, a unique region called *pX*. This region encodes several genes, including one called *TAX*. The TAX protein has been shown to be necessary and sufficient for cellular transformation. By interacting with several transcription factors, such as NF-κB, the TAX protein can transactivate the expression of genes that encode cytokines, cytokine receptors, and costimulatory molecules. This inappropriate gene expression leads to autocrine signaling loops and increased activation of pro-mitogenic signaling cascades. Furthermore, TAX can drive progression through the cell cycle by directly binding to and activating cyclins. In addition, TAX can repress the function of several tumor suppressor genes that control the cell cycle, including *CDKN2A/p16* and *p53*. From these and other observations the following scenario is emerging (Fig. 6–32): The *TAX* gene turns on several cytokine genes and their receptors (IL-2 and IL-2R, IL-15, and IL-15R), setting up an autocrine system that drives T-cell proliferation. Of these cytokines, IL-15 seems to be more important, but much remains to be defined. Additionally, a parallel paracrine pathway is activated by increased production of granulocyte-macrophage colony-stimulating factor, which stimulates neighboring macrophages to produce other T-cell mitogens. Initially the T-cell proliferation is polyclonal because the virus infects many cells, but, because of TAX-based inactivation of tumor suppressor genes such as *p53,* the proliferating T cells are at increased risk of secondary transforming events (mutations), which lead ultimately to the outgrowth of a monoclonal neoplastic T-cell population.

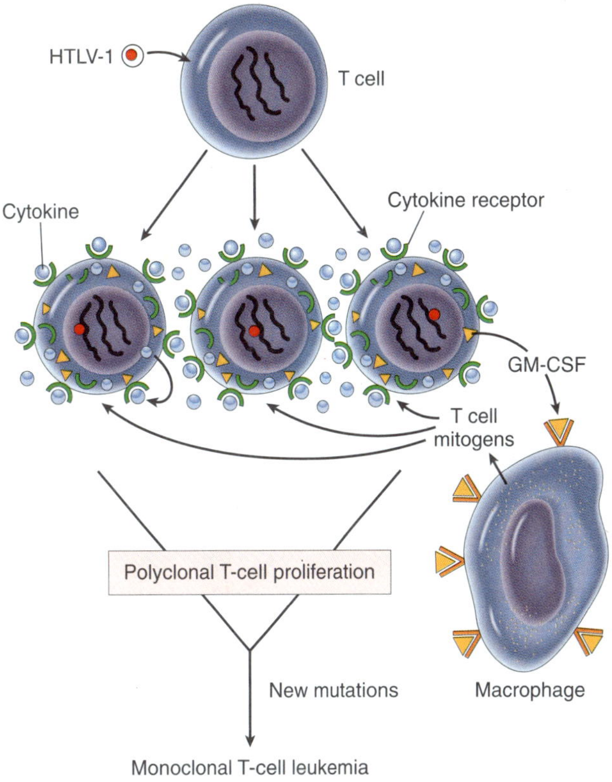

Figure 6–32

Pathogenesis of human T-cell lymphotropic virus (HTLV-1)–induced T-cell leukemia/lymphoma. HTLV-1 infects many T cells and initially causes polyclonal proliferation by autocrine and paracrine pathways triggered by the *TAX* gene. Simultaneously, TAX neutralizes growth-inhibitory signals by affecting *p53* and *CDKN2A/p16* genes. Ultimately, a monoclonal T-cell leukemia/lymphoma results when one proliferating T cell suffers additional mutations.

SUMMARY

Oncogenic RNA Viruses

- HTLV-1 causes a T-cell leukemia that is endemic in Japan and the Caribbean.
- HTLV-1 encodes a viral TAX protein, which turns on genes for cytokines and their receptors in infected T cells. This sets up autocrine and paracrine signaling loops that stimulate T-cell proliferation. Although this proliferation is initially polyclonal, the proliferating T cells are at increased risk of secondary mutations that lead to the outgrowth of a monoclonal leukemia.

Oncogenic DNA Viruses

As with RNA viruses, several oncogenic DNA viruses that cause tumors in animals have been identified. Four DNA viruses—human papillomavirus (HPV), Epstein-Barr virus (EBV), Kaposi sarcoma herpesvirus (KSHV, also called human herpesvirus 8), and hepatitis B virus (HBV)—are of special interest, because they are strongly associated with human cancer. KSHV and Kaposi sarcoma were discussed in Chapter 5. The others are presented here.

Human Papillomavirus

Scores of genetically distinct types of HPV have been identified. Some types (e.g., 1, 2, 4, and 7) definitely cause benign squamous papillomas (warts) in humans (Chapters 19 and 22). By contrast, high-risk HPVs (e.g., 16 and 18) have been implicated in the genesis of several cancers, particularly squamous cell carcinoma of the cervix and anogenital region. In addition, at least 20% of oropharyngeal cancers are associated with HPV. In contrast to cervical cancers, genital warts have low malignant potential and are associated with low-risk HPVs predominantly HPV-6 and HPV-11.

The oncogenic potential of HPV can be related to products of two early viral genes, E6 and E7. Together, they interact with a variety of growth-regulating proteins encoded by protooncogenes and tumor suppressor genes. The E7 protein binds to the retinoblastoma protein and displaces the E2F transcription factors that are normally sequestered by RB, promoting progression through the cell cycle. Interestingly, E7 protein from high-risk HPV types has a higher affinity for RB than does E7 from low-risk HPV types. E7 also inactivates the CDKIs CDKN1A/p21 and CDNK1B/p27. E7 proteins from high-risk HPV types (types 16, 18, and 31) also bind and presumably activate cyclins E and A. The E6 protein has complementary effects. It binds to and mediates the degradation of p53 and BAX, a pro-apoptotic member of the BCL2 family, and it activates telomerase. In analogy with E7, E6 from high-risk HPV types has a higher affinity for p53 than E6 from low-risk HPV types. Interestingly, in benign warts the HPV genome is maintained in a nonintegrated episomal form, while in cancers the HPV genome is randomly integrated into the host genome. Integration interrupts the viral DNA, resulting in overexpression of the oncoproteins E6 and E7. Furthermore, cells in which the viral genome has integrated show significantly more genomic instability.

To summarize, *infection with high-risk HPV types simulates the loss of tumor suppressor genes, activates cyclins, inhibits apoptosis, and combats cellular senescence.* Thus, it is evident that many of the hallmarks of cancer discussed earlier are driven by HPV proteins. However, infection with HPV itself is not sufficient for carcinogenesis. For example, when human keratinocytes are transfected with DNA from HPV 16, 18, or 31 in vitro, they are immortalized, but they do not form tumors in experimental animals. Cotransfection with a mutated *RAS* gene results in full malignant transformation. These data strongly suggest that HPV, in all likelihood, acts in concert with other environmental factors (Chapter 19). However, the primacy of HPV infection in the causation of cervical cancer is attested to by the near complete protection from this cancer by anti-HPV vaccines.

Epstein-Barr Virus

EBV has been implicated in the pathogenesis of several human tumors: Burkitt lymphoma, B-cell lymphomas in patients with acquired immunodeficiency syndrome and other causes of immunosuppression, a subset of Hodgkin lymphoma, and nasopharyngeal carcinoma. Except for nasopharyngeal carcinoma, all others are B-cell tumors. A subset of T-cell lymphomas and the rare NK-cell lymphomas may also be related to EBV.

Burkitt lymphoma is endemic in certain parts of Africa and is sporadic elsewhere. In endemic areas, tumor cells in virtually all patients carry the EBV genome. The molecular basis of B-cell proliferations induced by EBV is complex. EBV uses the complement receptor, CD21, to attach to and infect B cells. In vitro such infection leads to polyclonal B-cell proliferation and generation of B-lymphoblastoid cell lines. One of the EBV-encoded genes, called *LMP-1,* acts as an oncogene, and its expression in transgenic mice induces B-cell lymphomas. *LMP-1* promotes B-cell proliferation by activating signaling pathways, such as NF-κB and JAK/STAT, which mimic B-cell activation via the B-cell surface molecule CD40. Concurrently, *LMP-1* prevents apoptosis by activating BCL2. Thus, the virus "borrows" a normal B-cell activation pathway to promote its own replication by expanding the pool of cells susceptible to infection. Another EBV-encoded gene, *EBNA-2,* transactivates several host genes, including cyclin D and the *src* family genes. In addition, the EBV genome contains a viral cytokine, vIL-10, that was pirated from the host genome. This viral cytokine can prevent macrophages and monocytes from activating T cells and is required for EBV-dependent transformation of B cells.

In immunologically normal individuals, EBV-driven polyclonal B-cell proliferation in vivo is readily controlled, and the individual either remains asymptomatic or develops a self-limited episode of infectious mononucleosis (Chapter 12). Evasion of the immune system seems to be a key step in EBV-related oncogenesis. In regions of the world where Burkitt lymphoma is endemic, concomitant (endemic) malaria (or other infections) impair immune competence, allowing sustained B-cell proliferation. Interestingly, although *LMP-1* is the primary transforming oncogene in the EBV genome, it is not expressed in EBV-derived Burkitt lymphoma, because it is also one of the major viral antigens recognized by the immune system. Presumably, infected cells expressing viral antigens such as LMP-1 are kept in check by the immune system. Lymphoma cells emerge only when additional mutations, such as the t(8;14) translocation, a consistent feature of this tumor, activate the *MYC* oncogene. *MYC* activation may substitute for *LMP-1* signaling, allowing the tumor cells to down-regulate *LMP-1* and evade the immune system. In keeping with this scenario, EBV-derived B-cell lymphomas from immunocompromised patients, discussed below, retain expression of LMP-1. It should be noted that in nonendemic areas, 80% of tumors do not harbor the EBV genome, but all tumors possess the specific t(8;14) translocation. This observation suggests that, although non-African Burkitt lymphomas are triggered by mechanisms other than EBV, they develop cancer by similar pathways.

In immunosuppressed patients, including those with HIV disease and organ transplant recipients, EBV-infected B cells undergo polyclonal expansion, producing lymphoblastoid-like cells. In contrast to Burkitt lymphoma, the B lymphoblasts in immunosuppressed patients do express viral antigens, such as LMP-1, that are recognized by T cells. These potentially lethal proliferations can be subdued if the immunologic status of the host improves, as may occur with withdrawal of immunosuppressive drugs in transplant recipients.

Nasopharyngeal carcinoma is endemic in southern China and some other locales, and the EBV genome is found in all tumors. LMP-1 is expressed in epithelial cells as well. In these cells, as in B cells, *LMP-1* activates the NF-κB pathway. Furthermore, *LMP-1* induces the expression of pro-angiogenic factors such as VEGF, FGF-2, MMP-9, and COX2, which may contribute to oncogenesis. As in Burkitt lymphoma, EBV acts in concert with other, unidentified, factors (Chapter 13).

SUMMARY

Oncogenic DNA Viruses

- HPV has been associated with benign warts, as well as cervical cancer.
- The oncogenic ability of HPV is related to the expression of two viral oncoproteins, E6 and E7; they bind to RB and p53, respectively, neutralizing their function; they also activate cyclins.
- E6 and E7 from high-risk HPV (that give rise to cancers) have higher affinity for their targets than E6 and E7 from low-risk HPV (that give rise to low-grade tumors).
- EBV has been implicated in the pathogenesis of Burkitt lymphomas, lymphomas in immunosuppressed individuals with HIV infection or organ transplantation, some forms of Hodgkin lymphoma, and nasopharyngeal carcinoma. All except the nasopharyngeal cancers are B-cell tumors.
- Certain EBV gene products contribute to oncogenesis by stimulating a normal B-cell proliferation pathway. Concomitant compromise of immune competence allows sustained B-cell proliferation and eventually development of lymphoma with occurrence of additional mutations such as t(8;14), leading to activation of the *MYC* gene.

Hepatitis B and Hepatitis C Viruses

The epidemiologic evidence linking chronic HBV and hepatitis C virus (HCV) infection with hepatocellular carcinoma is strong (Chapter 16). It is estimated that 70% to 85% of hepatocellular carcinomas worldwide are due to infection with HBV or HCV. However, the mode of action of these viruses in tumorigenesis is not fully elucidated. The HBV and HCV genomes do not encode any viral oncoproteins, and although the HBV DNA is integrated within the human genome, there is no consistent pattern of integration in liver cells. Indeed, the oncogenic effects of HBV and HCV are multifactorial, but the dominant effect seems to be immunologically mediated chronic inflammation with hepatocyte death leading to regeneration, and genomic damage. Although the immune system is generally thought to be protective, recent work has demonstrated that in the setting of unresolved chronic inflammation, as occurs in viral hepatitis or chronic gastritis cause by *H. pylori* (see below), the immune response may become maladaptive, promoting tumorigenesis.

As with any cause of hepatocellular injury, chronic viral infection leads to the compensatory proliferation of hepatocytes. This regenerative process is aided and abetted by a plethora of growth factors, cytokines, chemokines, and other bioactive substances produced by activated immune cells that promote cell survival, tissue remodeling, and angiogenesis. The activated immune cells also produce other mediators, such as reactive oxygen species, that are genotoxic and mutagenic. One key molecular step seems to be activation of the NF-κB pathway in hepatocytes caused by mediators derived from the activated immune cells. Activation of the NF-κB pathway within hepatocytes blocks apoptosis, allowing the dividing hepatocytes to incur genotoxic stress and to accumulate mutations. Although this seems to be the dominant mechanism in the pathogenesis of viral-induced hepatocellular carcinoma, both HBV and HCV also contain proteins within their genomes that may more directly promote the development of cancer. The HBV genome contains a gene known as *HBx*, and mice transgenic for this gene develop hepatocellular cancers. *HBx* can directly or indirectly activate a variety of transcription factors and several signal transduction pathways. In addition, viral integration can cause secondary rearrangements of chromosomes, including multiple deletions that may harbor unknown tumor suppressor genes.

Though not a DNA virus, HCV is also strongly linked to the pathogenesis of liver cancer. The molecular mechanisms used by HCV are less well defined than are those of HBV. In addition to chronic liver cell injury and compensatory regeneration, components of the HCV genome, such as the HCV core protein may have a direct effect on tumorigenesis, possibly by activating a variety of growth-promoting signal transduction pathways.

SUMMARY

Hepatitis B and Hepatitis C Viruses

- Between 70% and 85% of hepatocellular carcinomas worldwide are due to infection with HBV or HCV.
- The oncogenic effects of HBV and HCV are multifactorial, but the dominant effect seems to be immunologically mediated chronic inflammation, hepatocellular injury, stimulation of hepatocyte proliferation, and production of reactive oxygen species that can damage DNA.
- The HBx protein of HBV and the HCV core protein can activate a variety of signal transduction pathways that may also contribute to carcinogenesis.

Helicobacter pylori

First incriminated as a cause of peptic ulcers, *H. pylori* now has acquired the dubious distinction of being the first bacterium classified as a carcinogen. Indeed, *H. pylori* infection is implicated in the genesis of both gastric adenocarcinomas and gastric lymphomas.

The scenario for the development of gastric adenocarcinoma is similar to that of HBV- and HCV-induced liver cancer. It involves increased epithelial cell proliferation in a background of chronic inflammation. As in viral hepatitis, the inflammatory milieu contains numerous genotoxic agents, such as reactive oxygen species. There is an initial development of chronic inflammation/gastritis, followed by gastric atrophy, intestinal metaplasia of the lining cells, dysplasia, and cancer. This sequence takes decades to complete and occurs in only 3% of infected patients. Like HBV and HCV, the *H. pylori* genome also contains genes directly implicated in oncogenesis. Strains associated with gastric adenocarcinoma have been shown to contain a "pathogenicity island" that contains cytotoxin-associated A *(CagA)* gene. Although *H. pylori* is noninvasive, *CagA* is injected into gastric epithelial cells, where it has a variety of effects, including the initiation of a signaling cascade that mimics unregulated growth factor stimulation.

As mentioned above, *H. pylori* is associated with an increased risk for the development of gastric lymphomas as well. The gastric lymphomas are of B-cell origin, and because the transformed B cells normally reside in the marginal zones of lymphoid follicles, these tumors are also called MALT lymphomas (marginal zone–associated lymphomas; Chapter 12). Their molecular pathogenesis is incompletely understood but seems to involve strain-specific *H. pylori* factors, as well as host genetic factors, such as polymorphisms in the promoters of inflammatory cytokines such as IL-1β and tumor necrosis factor (TNF). It is thought that *H. pylori* infection leads to the formation of *H. pylori*–reactive T cells, which in turn cause polyclonal B-cell proliferations. In time, a monoclonal B-cell tumor emerges in the proliferating B cells, perhaps as a result of accumulation of mutations in growth-regulatory genes. In keeping with this, early in the course of disease, eradication of *H. pylori* "cures" the lymphoma by removing antigenic stimulus for T cells.

SUMMARY

Helicobacter pylori

- *H. pylori* infection has been implicated in both gastric adenocarcinoma and MALT lymphoma.
- The mechanism of *H. pylori*–induced gastric cancers is multifactorial, including immunologically mediated chronic inflammation, stimulation of gastric cell proliferation, and production of reactive oxygen species that damage DNA. *H. pylori* pathogenicity genes, such as *CagA,* may also contribute by stimulating growth factor pathways.
- It is thought that *H. pylori* infection leads to polyclonal B-cell proliferations and that eventually a monoclonal B-cell tumor (MALT lymphoma) emerges as a result of accumulation of mutations.

HOST DEFENSE AGAINST TUMORS: TUMOR IMMUNITY

The idea that tumors are not entirely self was conceived by Ehrlich, who proposed that immune-mediated recognition of autologous tumor cells may be a "positive mechanism" capable of eliminating transformed cells. Subsequently, Lewis Thomas and McFarlane Burnet formalized this concept by coining the term *immune surveillance* to refer to recognition and destruction of non-self tumor cells on their appearance. That cancers occur implies that immune surveillance is imperfect; however, that some tumors escape such policing does not preclude the possibility that others may have been aborted. Here we address certain questions about tumor immunity: What is the nature of tumor antigens? What host effector systems may recognize tumor cells? Is tumor immunity effective against spontaneous neoplasms?

Tumor Antigens

Antigens that elicit an immune response have been demonstrated in many experimentally induced tumors and in some human cancers. Initially, they were broadly classified into two categories based on their patterns of expression: *tumor-specific antigens,* which are present only on tumor cells and not on any normal cells, and *tumor-associated antigens,* which are present on tumor cells and also on some normal cells. This classification, however, is imperfect, because many antigens thought to be tumor specific turned out to be expressed by some normal cells as well. The modern classification of tumor antigens is based on their molecular structure and source. An important advance in the field of tumor immunology was the development of techniques for identifying tumor antigens that were recognized by cytotoxic T lymphocytes (CTLs), because CTLs are the major immune defense mechanism against tumors. Recall that CTLs recognize peptides derived from cytoplasmic proteins that are displayed bound to class I major histocompatibility complex (MHC) molecules (Chapter 5). Below we describe the main classes of tumor antigens (Fig. 6–33).

Products of Mutated Oncogenes and Tumor Suppressor Genes. Neoplastic transformation, as we have discussed, results from genetic alterations, some of which may result in the expression of cell surface antigens that are seen as non-self by the immune system. Antigens in this category are derived from mutant oncoproteins and cancer suppressor proteins. Unique tumor antigens arise from products of *β-catenin, RAS, p53,* and *CDK4* genes, which frequently are mutated in tumors. Because the mutant

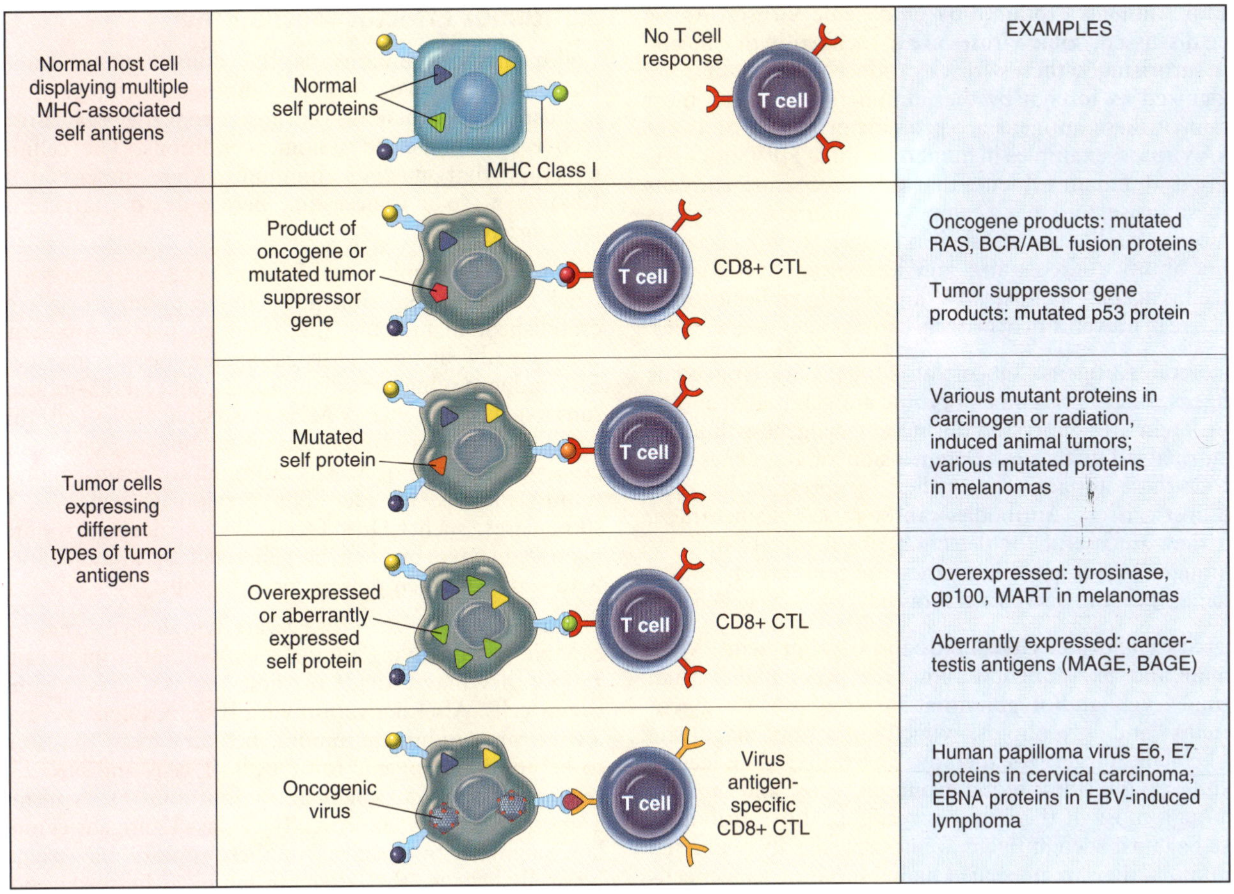

Figure 6–33

Tumor antigens recognized by CD8+ T cells. (Modified from Abbas AK, Lichtman AH: Cellular and Molecular Immunology, 5th ed. Philadelphia, WB Saunders, 2003.)

proteins are present only in tumors, their peptides are expressed only in tumor cells. Since many tumors may carry the same mutation, such antigens are shared by different tumors. Although CTLs can be induced against such antigens, they do not appear to elicit protective responses in vivo.

Products of Other Mutated Genes. Because of the genetic instability of tumor cells, many genes are mutated in these cells, including genes whose products are not related to the transformed phenotype and have no known function. Products of these mutated genes are potential tumor antigens. These antigens are extremely diverse, because the carcinogens that induce the tumors may randomly mutagenize virtually any host gene. Mutated cellular proteins are found more frequently in chemical carcinogen- or radiation-induced animal tumors than in spontaneous human cancers. They can be targeted by the immune system, since there is no self-tolerance against them.

Overexpressed or Aberrantly Expressed Cellular Proteins. Tumor antigens may be normal cellular proteins that are abnormally expressed in tumor cells and elicit immune responses. In a subset of human melanomas some tumor antigens are structurally normal proteins that are produced at low levels in normal cells and overexpressed in tumor cells. One such antigen is tyrosinase, an enzyme involved in melanin biosynthesis that is expressed only in normal melanocytes and melanomas. T cells from melanoma patients recognize peptides derived from tyrosinase, raising the possibility that tyrosinase vaccines may stimulate such responses to melanomas; clinical trials with these vaccines are ongoing. It may be surprising that these patients are able to respond to a normal self-antigen. The probable explanation is that tyrosinase is normally produced in such small amounts and in so few cells that it is not recognized by the immune system and fails to induce tolerance.

Another group, the so called "cancer-testis" antigens, are encoded by genes that are silent in all adult tissues except the testis—hence their name. Although the protein is present in the testis it is not expressed on the cell surface in an antigenic form, because sperm do not express MHC class I antigens. Thus, for all practical purposes, these antigens are tumor specific. Prototypic of this group is the MAGE family of genes. Although they are tumor specific, MAGE antigens are not unique for individual tumors. MAGE-1 is expressed on 37% of melanomas and a variable number of lung, liver, stomach, and esophageal carcinomas. Similar antigens called GAGE, BAGE, and RAGE have been detected in other tumors.

Tumor Antigens Produced by Oncogenic Viruses. As we have discussed, some viruses are associated with cancers. Not surprisingly, these viruses produce proteins that are recognized as foreign by the immune system. The most potent of these antigens are proteins produced by latent DNA viruses; examples in humans include HPV and EBV. There is abundant evidence that CTLs recognize antigens of these viruses and that a competent immune system plays a role in surveillance against virus-induced tumors because of its ability to recognize and kill virus-infected cells. Indeed, vaccines against HPV antigens have been found effective in prevention of cervical cancers in young females.

Oncofetal Antigens. Oncofetal antigens or embryonic antigens, such as carcinoembryonic antigen (CEA) and α-fetoprotein, are expressed during embryogenesis but not in normal adult tissues. Derepression of the genes that encode these antigens causes their reexpression in colon and liver cancers. Antibodies can be raised against these, and they are useful for detection of oncofetal antigens. Although, as discussed later, they are not entirely tumor specific, they can serve as serum markers for cancer.

Altered Cell Surface Glycolipids and Glycoproteins. Most human and experimental tumors express higher than normal levels and/or abnormal forms of surface glycoproteins and glycolipids, which may be diagnostic markers and targets for therapy. These altered molecules include gangliosides, blood group antigens, and mucins. Although most of the epitopes recognized by antibodies raised against such antigens are not specifically expressed on tumors, they are present at higher levels on cancer cells than on normal cells. This class of antigens is a target for cancer therapy with specific antibodies.

Several mucins are of special interest and have been the focus of diagnostic and therapeutic studies. These include CA-125 and CA-19-9, expressed on ovarian carcinomas, and MUC-1, expressed on breast carcinomas. Unlike many other types of mucins, MUC-1 is an integral membrane protein that is normally expressed only on the apical surface of breast ductal epithelium, a site that is relatively sequestered from the immune system. In ductal carcinomas of the breast, however, the molecule is expressed in an unpolarized fashion and contains new, tumor-specific carbohydrate and peptide epitopes. These epitopes induce both antibody and T-cell responses in cancer patients and are therefore being considered as candidates for tumor vaccines.

Cell Type–Specific Differentiation Antigens. Tumors express molecules that are normally present on the cells of origin. These antigens are called *differentiation antigens,* because they are specific for particular lineages or differentiation stages of various cell types. Their importance is as potential targets for immunotherapy and for identifying the tissue of origin of tumors. For example, lymphomas may be diagnosed as B-cell–derived tumors by the detection of surface markers characteristic of this lineage, such as CD10 and CD20. Antibodies against these molecules are also used for tumor immunotherapy. These differentiation antigens are typically normal self-antigens, and therefore they do not induce immune responses in tumor-bearing hosts.

Antitumor Effector Mechanisms

Cell-mediated immunity is the dominant anti-tumor mechanism in vivo. Although antibodies can be made against tumors, there is no evidence that they play a protective role under physiologic conditions. The cellular effectors that mediate immunity were described in Chapter 5, so it is necessary here only to characterize them briefly.

Cytotoxic T Lymphocytes. The role of specifically sensitized CTLs in experimentally induced tumors is well established. In humans, they seem to play a protective role, chiefly against virus-associated neoplasms (e.g., EBV-induced Burkitt lymphoma and HPV-induced tumors). The presence of MHC-restricted CD8+ cells that can kill autologous tumor cells within human tumors suggests that the role of T cells in immunity against human tumors may be broader than previously suspected. In some cases, such CD8+ T cells do not develop spontaneously in vivo but can be generated by immunization with tumor antigen-pulsed dendritic cells.

Natural Killer Cells. NK cells are lymphocytes that are capable of destroying tumor cells without prior sensitization; they may provide the first line of defense against tumor cells. After activation with IL-2, NK cells can lyse a wide range of human tumors, including many that seem to be nonimmunogenic for T cells. T cells and NK cells seem to provide complementary antitumor mechanisms. Tumors that fail to express MHC class I antigens cannot be recognized by T cells, but these tumors may trigger NK cells because the latter are inhibited by recognition of normal autologous class I molecules (Chapter 5). The triggering receptors on NK cells are extremely diverse and belong to several gene families. NKG2D proteins expressed on NK cells and some T cells are important activating receptors. They recognize stress-induced antigens that are expressed on tumor cells and cells that have incurred DNA damage and are at risk for neoplastic transformation.

Macrophages. Activated macrophages exhibit cytotoxicity against tumor cells in vitro. T cells, NK cells, and macrophages may collaborate in antitumor reactivity, because interferon-γ, a cytokine secreted by T cells and NK cells, is a potent activator of macrophages. Activated macrophages may kill tumors by mechanisms similar to those used to kill microbes (e.g., production of reactive oxygen metabolites; Chapter 2) or by secretion of tumor necrosis factor (TNF).

Humoral Mechanisms. Although there is no evidence for the protective effects of anti-tumor antibodies against spontaneous tumors, administration of monoclonal antibodies against tumor cells can be therapeutically effective. A monoclonal antibody against CD20, a B cell surface antigen, is widely used for treatment of certain non-Hodgkin lymphomas.

Immune Surveillance

Given the host of possible and potential antitumor mechanisms, is there any evidence that they operate in vivo to prevent the emergence of neoplasms? The strongest argument for the existence of immune surveillance is the increased frequency of cancers in immunodeficient hosts. About 5% of individuals with congenital immunodeficiencies develop cancers, a rate that is about 200 times that for individuals without such immunodeficiencies. Analogously, immunosuppressed transplant recipients and patients with acquired immunodeficiency syndrome have increased numbers of malignancies. It should be noted that most (but not all) of these neoplasms are lymphomas, often lymphomas of activated B cells. Particularly illustrative is X-linked lymphoproliferative disorder. When affected boys develop an EBV infection, such infection does not take the usual self-limited form of infectious mononucleosis but instead evolves into a chronic or sometimes fatal form of infectious mononucleosis or, even worse, malignant lymphoma.

Most cancers occur in individuals who do not suffer from any overt immunodeficiency. If immune surveillance exists, how do cancers evade the immune system in immunocompetent hosts? Several escape mechanisms have been proposed:

- *Selective outgrowth of antigen-negative variants.* During tumor progression, strongly immunogenic subclones may be eliminated.
- *Loss or reduced expression of histocompatibility molecules.* Tumor cells may fail to express normal levels of HLA class I, escaping attack by CTLs. Such cells, however, may trigger NK cells.
- *Immunosuppression.* Many oncogenic agents (e.g., chemicals and ionizing radiation) suppress host immune responses. Tumors or tumor products also may be immunosuppressive. For example, TGF-β, secreted in large quantities by many tumors, is a potent immunosuppressant. In some cases, the immune response induced by the tumor may inhibit tumor immunity. Several mechanisms of such inhibition have been described. For instance, recognition of tumor cells may lead to engagement of the T-cell inhibitory receptor, CTLA-4, or activation of regulatory T cells that suppress immune responses.

It is worth mentioning that although much of the focus in the field of tumor immunity has been on the mechanisms by which the host immune system defends against tumors, there is some recent evidence that, paradoxically, the immune system may promote the growth of tumors. It is possible that activated lymphocytes and macrophages produce growth factors for tumor cells. Enzymes, such as MMPs, that enhance tumor invasion, may also be produced. Harnessing the protective actions of the immune system and abolishing its ability to increase tumor growth is obviously an important goal of immunologists and oncologists.

SUMMARY

Immune Surveillance

- Tumor cells can be recognized by the immune system as non-self and destroyed.
- Antitumor activity is mediated by predominantly cell-mediated mechanisms. Tumor antigens are presented on the cell surface by MHC class I molecules and are recognized by CD8+ CTLs.
- The different classes of tumor antigens include products of mutated proto-oncogenes, tumor suppressor genes, overexpressed or aberrantly expressed proteins, tumor antigens produced by oncogenic viruses, oncofetal antigens, altered glycolipids and glycoproteins, and cell type–specific differentiation antigens.
- Immunosuppressed patients have an increased risk of cancer.
- In immunocompetent patients, tumors may avoid the immune system by several mechanisms, including selective outgrowth of antigen-negative variants, loss or reduced expression of histocompatibility antigens, and immunosuppression mediated by secretion of factors (e.g., TGF-β) from the tumor.

CLINICAL ASPECTS OF NEOPLASIA

Ultimately the importance of neoplasms lies in their effects on patients. Although malignant tumors are of course more threatening than benign tumors, any tumor, even a benign one, may cause morbidity and mortality. Indeed, both malignant and benign tumors may cause problems because of (1) location and impingement on adjacent structures, (2) functional activity such as hormone synthesis or the development of paraneoplastic syndromes, (3) bleeding and infections when the tumor ulcerates through adjacent surfaces, (4) symptoms that result from rupture or infarction, and (5) cachexia or wasting. The following discussion considers the effects of a tumor on the host, the grading and clinical staging of cancer, and the laboratory diagnosis of neoplasms.

Effects of Tumor on Host

Location is crucial in both benign and malignant tumors. A small (1-cm) pituitary adenoma can compress and destroy the surrounding normal gland and give rise to hypopituitarism. A 0.5-cm leiomyoma in the wall of the renal artery may lead to renal ischemia and serious hypertension. A comparably small carcinoma within the common bile duct may induce fatal biliary tract obstruction.

Hormone production is seen with benign and malignant neoplasms arising in endocrine glands. Adenomas and carcinomas arising in the β-cells of the islets of the pancreas can produce hyperinsulinism, sometimes fatal. Analogously, some adenomas and carcinomas of the adrenal cortex elaborate corticosteroids that affect the patient (e.g., aldosterone, which induces sodium retention, hypertension, and hypokalemia). Such hormonal activity is more likely with a well-differentiated benign tumor than with a corresponding carcinoma.

A tumor may ulcerate through a surface, with consequent bleeding or secondary infection. Benign or malignant neoplasms that protrude into the gut lumen may become caught in the peristaltic pull of the gut, causing intussusception (Chapter 15) and intestinal obstruction or infarction.

Cancer Cachexia

Many cancer patients suffer progressive loss of body fat and lean body mass, accompanied by profound weakness, anorexia, and anemia, referred to as *cachexia.* There is some correlation between the size and extent of spread of the cancer and the severity of the cachexia. However, cachexia is not caused by the nutritional demands of the tumor. Although patients with cancer are often anorexic, current evidence indicates that cachexia results from the action of soluble factors such as cytokines produced by the tumor and the host rather than reduced food intake. In patients with cancer, calorie expenditure remains high, and basal metabolic rate is increased, despite reduced food intake. This is in contrast to the lower metabolic rate that occurs as an adaptational response in starvation. The basis of these metabolic abnormalities is not fully understood. It is suspected that TNF produced by macrophages in response to tumor cells or by the tumor cells themselves mediates cachexia. TNF suppresses appetite and inhibits the action of lipoprotein lipase, inhibiting the release of free fatty acids from lipoproteins. Additionally, a protein-mobilizing factor called proteolysis-inducing factor, which causes breakdown of skeletal muscle proteins by the ubiquitin-proteosome pathway, has been detected in the serum of cancer patients. Other molecules with lipolytic action also have been found. There is no satisfactory treatment for cancer cachexia other than removal of the underlying cause, the tumor.

Paraneoplastic Syndromes

Symptom complexes that occur in patients with cancer and that cannot be readily explained by local or distant spread of the tumor or by the elaboration of hormones indigenous to the tissue of origin of the tumor are referred to as *paraneoplastic syndromes.* They appear in 10% to 15% of patients with cancer, and it is important to recognize them for several reasons:

- They may represent the earliest manifestation of an occult neoplasm.
- In affected patients, they may represent significant clinical problems and may even be lethal.
- They may mimic metastatic disease and confound treatment.

The paraneoplastic syndromes are diverse and are associated with many different tumors (Table 6–5). *The most common syndromes are hypercalcemia, Cushing syndrome, and nonbacterial thrombotic endocarditis;* the neoplasms most often associated with these and other syndromes are lung and breast cancers and hematologic malignancies. Hypercalcemia in cancer patients is multifactorial, but the most important mechanism is the synthesis of a parathyroid hormone–related protein (PTHrP) by tumor cells. Also implicated are other tumor-derived factors, such as TGF-α, a polypeptide factor that activates osteoclasts, and the active form of vitamin D. Another possible mechanism for hypercalcemia is widespread osteolytic metastatic disease of bone, but *it should be noted that hypercalcemia resulting from skeletal metastases is not a paraneoplastic syndrome.* Cushing syndrome as a paraneoplastic phenomenon is usually related to ectopic production of ACTH or ACTH-like polypeptides by cancer cells, as occurs in small-cell cancers of the lung. Sometimes one tumor induces several syndromes concurrently. For example, bronchogenic carcinomas may elaborate products identical to or having the effects of ACTH, antidiuretic hormone, parathyroid hormone, serotonin, human chorionic gonadotropin, and other bioactive substances.

Paraneoplastic syndromes may also manifest as hypercoagulability leading to venous thrombosis and nonbacterial thrombotic endocarditis (Chapter 11). Other manifestations are clubbing of the fingers and hypertrophic osteoarthropathy in patients with lung carcinomas (Chapter 13). Still others are discussed in the consideration of cancers of the various organs of the body.

Grading and Staging of Cancer

Methods to quantify the probable clinical aggressiveness of a given neoplasm and its apparent extent and spread in the individual patient are necessary for making accurate prognosis and for comparing end results of various treatment protocols. For instance, the results of treating extremely small, highly differentiated thyroid adenocarcinomas that are localized to the thyroid gland are likely to be different from those obtained from treating highly anaplastic thyroid cancers that have invaded the neck organs.

The *grading* of a cancer attempts to establish some estimate of its aggressiveness or level of malignancy based on the cytologic differentiation of tumor cells and the number of mitoses within the tumor. The cancer may be classified as grade I, II, III, or IV, in order of increasing anaplasia. Criteria for the individual grades vary with each form of neoplasia and so are not detailed here. Difficulties in establishing clear-cut criteria have led in some instances to descriptive characterizations (e.g., "well-differentiated adenocarcinoma with no evidence of vascular or lymphatic invasion" or "highly anaplastic sarcoma with extensive vascular invasion").

Staging of cancers is based on the size of the primary lesion, its extent of spread to regional lymph nodes, and the presence or absence of metastases. This assessment is usually based on clinical and radiographic examination (computed tomography and magnetic resonance imaging) and in some cases surgical exploration. Two methods of staging are currently in use: the TNM system (*T,* primary tumor; *N,* regional lymph node involvement; *M,* metastases) and the AJC (American Joint Committee) system. In the TNM system, T1, T2, T3, and T4 describe the increasing size of the primary lesion; N0, N1, N2, and

Table 6–5 Paraneoplastic Syndromes

Clinical Syndromes	Major Forms of Underlying Cancer	Causal Mechanism
Endocrinopathies		
Cushing syndrome	Small-cell carcinoma of lung Pancreatic carcinoma Neural tumors	ACTH or ACTH-like substance
Syndrome of inappropriate antidiuretic hormone secretion	Small-cell carcinoma of lung; intracranial neoplasms	Antidiuretic hormone or atrial natriuretic hormones
Hypercalcemia	Squamous cell carcinoma of lung Breast carcinoma Renal carcinoma Adult T-cell leukemia/lymphoma Ovarian carcinoma	Parathyroid hormone-related protein, TGF-α, TNF, IL-1
Hypoglycemia	Fibrosarcoma Other mesenchymal sarcomas Hepatocellular carcinoma	Insulin or insulin-like substance
Carcinoid syndrome	Bronchial adenoma (carcinoid) Pancreatic carcinoma Gastric carcinoma	Serotonin, bradykinin
Polycythemia	Renal carcinoma Cerebellar hemangioma Hepatocellular carcinoma	Erythropoietin
Nerve and Muscle Syndrome		
Myasthenia	Bronchogenic carcinoma	Immunologic
Disorders of the central and peripheral nervous systems	Breast carcinoma	
Dermatologic Disorders		
Acanthosis nigricans	Gastric carcinoma Lung carcinoma Uterine carcinoma	Immunologic; secretion of epidermal growth factor
Dermatomyositis	Bronchogenic, breast carcinoma	Immunologic
Osseous, Articular, and Soft-Tissue Changes		
Hypertrophic osteoarthropathy and clubbing of the fingers	Bronchogenic carcinoma	Unknown
Vascular and Hematologic Changes		
Venous thrombosis (Trousseau phenomenon)	Pancreatic carcinoma Bronchogenic carcinoma Other cancers	Tumor products (mucins that activate clotting)
Nonbacterial thrombotic endocarditis	Advanced cancers	Hypercoagulability
Anemia	Thymic neoplasms	Unkown
Others		
Nephrotic syndrome	Various cancers	Tumor antigens, immune complexes

ACTH, adrenocorticotropic hormone; TGF, transforming growth factor; TNF, tumor necrosis factor; IL, interleukin.

N3 indicate progressively advancing node involvement; and M0 and M1 reflect the absence or presence of distant metastases. In the AJC method, the cancers are divided into stages 0 to IV, incorporating the size of primary lesions and the presence of nodal spread and of distant metastases. Examples of the application of these two staging systems are cited in subsequent chapters. It is worth noting that *when compared with grading, staging has proved to be of greater clinical value.*

SUMMARY

Clinical Aspects of Tumors

- Cachexia, defined by progressive loss of body fat and lean body mass, accompanied by profound weakness, anorexia, and anemia, is caused by release of cytokines by the tumor or host.

• Paraneoplastic syndromes, defined by systemic symptoms that cannot be explained by tumor spread or by hormones appropriate to the tissue, are caused by the ectopic production and secretion of bioactive substances, such as ACTH, PTHrP, or TGF-α.
• Grading of tumors is determined by cytologic appearance and is based on the idea that behavior and differentiation are related, with poorly differentiated tumors having more aggressive behavior.
• Staging, determined by surgical exploration or imaging, is based on size, local and regional lymph node spread, and distant metastases. Staging has greater clinical value than grading.

Laboratory Diagnosis of Cancer

Morphologic Methods

In most instances, the laboratory diagnosis of cancer is not difficult. The two ends of the benign–malignant spectrum pose no problems; however, in the middle lies a "no man's land" where the wise tread cautiously. Clinicians tend to underestimate the contributions they make to the diagnosis of a neoplasm. Clinical data are invaluable for optimal pathologic diagnosis. Radiation-induced changes in the skin or mucosa can be similar to those of cancer. Sections taken from a healing fracture can mimic an osteosarcoma. The laboratory evaluation of a lesion can be only as good as the specimen submitted for examination. The specimen must be adequate, representative, and properly preserved.

Several sampling approaches are available, including excision or biopsy, fine-needle aspiration, and cytologic smears. When excision of a lesion is not possible, selection of an appropriate site for biopsy of a large mass requires awareness that the margins may not be representative and the center may be largely necrotic. Analogously with disseminated lymphoma (i.e., involving many nodes), nodes in the inguinal region that drain large areas of the body often undergo reactive changes that may mask neoplastic involvement. Requesting *frozen-section* diagnosis is sometimes desirable, as, for example, in determining the nature of a mass lesion or in evaluating the regional lymph nodes in a patient with cancer for metastasis. This method, in which a sample is quick-frozen and sectioned, permits histologic evaluation within minutes. In experienced, competent hands, frozen-section diagnosis is accurate, but there are particular instances in which the better histologic detail provided by the more time-consuming routine methods is needed. In such instances, it is better to wait a few days, despite the drawbacks, than to perform inadequate or unnecessary surgery.

Fine-needle aspiration of tumors is another approach that is widely used. It involves aspiration of cells from a mass, followed by cytologic examination of the smear. This procedure is used most commonly with readily palpable lesions affecting the breast, thyroid, lymph nodes, and salivary glands. Modern imaging techniques permit extension of the method to deeper structures, such as the liver, pancreas, and pelvic lymph nodes. It obviates surgery and its attendant risks. Although it entails some difficulties, such as small sample size and sampling errors, in experienced hands it can be extremely reliable, rapid, and useful.

Cytologic (Papanicolaou) smears provide another method for the detection of cancer. Historically, this approach has been used widely for the discovery of carcinoma of the cervix, often at an in situ stage, but now it is used with many other forms of suspected malignancy, such as endometrial carcinoma, bronchogenic carcinoma, bladder and prostate tumors, and gastric carcinomas; for the identification of tumor cells in abdominal, pleural, joint, and cerebrospinal fluids; and, less commonly, with other forms of neoplasia. Neoplastic cells are less cohesive than others and so are shed into fluids or secretions (Fig. 6–34). The shed cells are evaluated for features of anaplasia indicative of their origin from a tumor. The gratifying control of cervical cancer is the best testament to the value of the cytologic method.

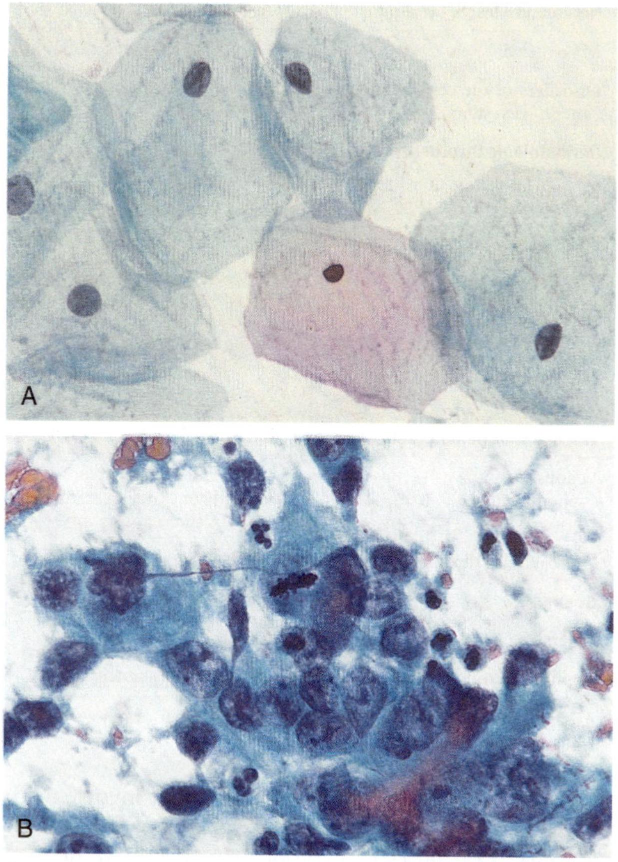

Figure 6–34

A, Normal Papanicolaou smear from the uterine cervix. Large, flat cells with small nuclei. **B,** Abnormal smear containing a sheet of malignant cells with large hyperchromatic nuclei. There is nuclear pleomorphism, and one cell is in mitosis. There are few interspersed neutrophils with compact lobated nuclei and much smaller size. (Courtesy of Dr. Richard M. DeMay, Department of Pathology, University of Chicago, Chicago, Illinois.)

Immunocytochemistry offers a powerful adjunct to routine histology. Detection of cytokeratin by specific monoclonal antibodies labeled with peroxidase points to a diagnosis of undifferentiated carcinoma rather than large-cell lymphoma. Similarly, detection of prostate-specific antigen (PSA) in metastatic deposits by immunohistochemistry allows definitive diagnosis of a primary tumor in the prostate. Immunocytochemical detection of estrogen receptors allows prognostication and directs therapeutic intervention in breast cancers.

Flow cytometry is used routinely in the classification of leukemias and lymphomas. In this method, fluorescent antibodies against cell surface molecules and differentiation antigens are used to obtain the phenotype of malignant cells.

Tumor Markers

Biochemical assays for tumor-associated enzymes, hormones, and other tumor markers in the blood cannot be utilized for definitive diagnosis of cancer; however, they contribute to finding cases and in some instances are useful in determining the effectiveness of therapy or the appearance of a recurrence. The application of these assays is considered with many of the specific forms of neoplasia discussed in other chapters, so only a few examples suffice here. PSA, used to screen for prostatic adenocarcinoma, may be one of the most used, and most successful, tumor markers in clinical practice. Prostatic carcinoma can be suspected when elevated levels of PSA are found in the blood. However, PSA screening also highlights problems encountered by virtually every tumor marker. Although PSA levels are often elevated in cancer, PSA levels also may be elevated in benign prostatic hyperplasia (Chapter 18). Furthermore, there is no PSA level that ensures that a patient does not have prostate cancer. *Thus, the PSA test suffers from both low sensitivity and low specificity*. Other tumor markers occasionally used in clinical practice include carcinoembryonic antigen (CEA), which is elaborated by carcinomas of the colon, pancreas, stomach, and breast, and α-fetoprotein, which is produced by hepatocellular carcinomas, yolk sac remnants in the gonads, and occasionally teratocarcinomas and embryonal cell carcinomas. Unfortunately, like PSA, both of these markers can be produced by a variety of non-neoplastic conditions as well. Thus, CEA and α-fetoprotein assays lack both specificity and sensitivity required for the early detection of cancers. They are still particularly useful in the detection of recurrences after excision. With successful resection of the tumor, these markers disappear from the serum; their reappearance almost always signifies the beginning of the end. CEA is further discussed in Chapter 15 and α-fetoprotein in Chapter 16.

Molecular Diagnosis

An increasing number of molecular techniques are being used for the diagnosis of tumors and for predicting their behavior.

1. *Diagnosis of malignancy.* Because each T and B cell has unique rearrangement of its antigen receptor genes, polymerase chain reaction (PCR)–based detection of T-cell receptor or immunoglobulin genes allows distinction between monoclonal (neoplastic) and polyclonal (reactive) proliferations. Many hematopoietic neoplasms, and a few solid tumors, are defined by particular translocations, and thus the diagnosis can be made by detection of such translocations. For example, fluorescence in situ hybridization (FISH) or PCR (Chapter 7) can be used to detect translocations characteristic of Ewing sarcoma and several leukemias and lymphomas. PCR-based detection of *BCR-ABL* transcripts provides the molecular diagnosis of chronic myeloid leukemia.
2. *Prognosis and behavior.* Certain genetic alterations are associated with a poor prognosis, and thus the presence of these alterations determines the patient's subsequent therapy. FISH and PCR methods can be used to detect amplification of oncogenes such as *HER-2/NEU* and *N-MYC*, which provide prognostic and therapeutic information for breast cancers and neuroblastomas.
3. *Detection of minimal residual disease.* Another emerging use of molecular techniques is detection of minimal residual disease after treatment. For example, detection of *BCR-ABL* transcripts by PCR gives a measure of residual disease, in patients treated for chronic myeloid leukemia.
4. *Diagnosis of hereditary predisposition to cancer.* Germ-line mutation of several tumor suppressor genes, such as *BRCA1*, increases a patient's risk of developing certain types of cancer. Thus, detection of these mutated alleles may allow the patient and physician to devise an aggressive screening protocol, as well as to consider prophylactic surgery. In addition, such detection allows genetic counseling of relatives at risk.

Molecular Profiling of Tumors

One of the most exciting advances in the molecular analysis of tumors has been made possible by DNA-microarray analysis. This technique allows simultaneous measurements of the expression levels of several thousand genes. The principle of this so-called gene chip technology is illustrated in Figure 6–35 and described briefly here.

As can be seen, the process begins by extraction of mRNA from any two sources (e.g., normal and malignant, normal and preneoplastic, or two tumors of the same histologic type). cDNA copies of the mRNA are synthesized in vitro with fluorescently labeled nucleotides. The fluorescence-labeled cDNA strands are hybridized to sequence-specific DNA probes linked to a solid support, such as a silicon chip. A 1-cm^2 chip can contain thousands of probes arranged in an array of columns and rows. After hybridization, high-resolution laser scanning detects fluorescent signals from each of the spots. The fluorescence intensity of each spot is proportional to the level of expression of the original mRNA used to synthesize the cDNA hybridized to that spot. For each sample, therefore, the expression level of thousands of genes is obtained, and by using bioinformatic tools,

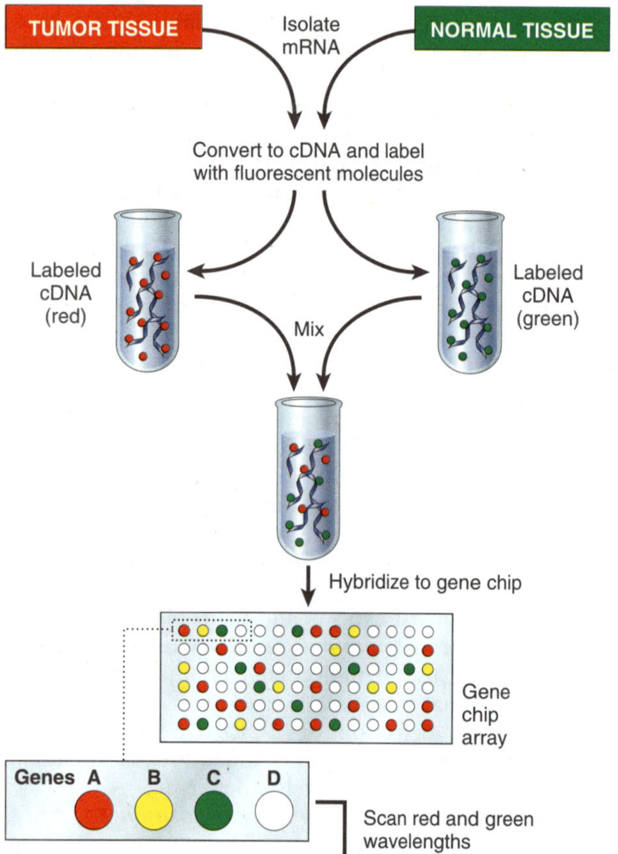

Results:

Fluorescence intensity Red	Fluorescence intensity Green		Conclusion
Gene A	+++	+	Up-regulated in neoplastic tissue
Gene B	++	++	Unchanged in neoplastic tissue
Gene C	+	+++	Down-regulated in neoplastic tissue
Gene D	–	–	Not expressed in either tissue

Figure 6–35

Schematic illustration of cDNA microarray analysis. mRNA is extracted from the samples, reverse transcribed to cDNA, and labeled with fluorescent molecules. In the case illustrated, *red* fluorescent molecules were used for normal cDNA, and *green* molecules were used for tumor cDNA. The labeled cDNAs are mixed and applied to a gene chip, which contains thousands of DNA probes representing known genes. The labeled cDNAs hybridize to spots that contain complementary sequences. The hybridization is detected by laser scanning of the chip, and the results are read in units of red or green fluorescence intensity. In the example shown, spot A has high red fluorescence, indicating that a greater number of cDNAs from neoplastic cells hybridized to gene A. Thus, gene A seems to be up-regulated in tumor cells. (Courtesy of Dr. Robert Anders, Department of Pathology, University of Chicago, Chicago, Illinois.)

the relative levels of gene expression in different samples can be compared. In essence, a molecular profile is generated for each tissue analyzed.

Such analysis has revealed that phenotypically identical large B-cell lymphomas (Chapter 12) from different patients are heterogeneous with respect to their gene expression. Nevertheless, clusters of gene expression patterns can be detected that allow segregation of phenotypically similar tumors into distinct subcategories with dramatically different survival rates. This type of molecular profiling indicates that the currently available morphologic and molecular tools are insufficient for stratification of tumors into prognostically different subgroups. Similar analyses have been performed on breast cancers and melanomas. Although the data currently available have to be validated by prospective analysis of a larger cohort of patients, the proof of principle has been obtained. It is likely that, in the near future, molecular profiling will become an adjunct in the diagnosis, classification, and management of cancer. This type of analysis may also reveal novel gene targets for development of new drugs. Thus, therapy may be tailored to the specific genes dysregulated in a given tumor. Who knows, advertisements for "designer genes" may appear side by side with ads for "designer jeans"!

SUMMARY

Laboratory Diagnosis of Cancer

- Several sampling approaches exist for the diagnosis of tumors, including excision, biopsy, fine-needle aspiration, and cytologic smears.
- Immunohistochemistry and flow cytometry help in the diagnosis and classification of tumors, because distinct protein expression patterns define different entities.
- Proteins released by tumors into the serum, such as PSA, can be used to screen populations for cancer and to monitor recurrence following treatment.
- Molecular analyses are used to determine diagnosis, prognosis, the detection of minimal residual disease, and the diagnosis of hereditary predisposition to cancer.
- Molecular profiling of tumors by cDNA arrays can determine expression of large segments of the genome at once and can be useful in molecular stratification of otherwise identical tumors for the purpose of treatment and prognostication.

BIBLIOGRAPHY

Bergers G, Benjamin LE: Tumorigenesis and the angiogenic switch. Nat Rev Cancer 3:401, 2003. *[Review discussing the molecular mechanisms involved in the angiogenic switch.]*

Blume-Jensen P, Hunter T: Oncogenic kinase signaling. Nature 411:355, 2001. *[Authoritative review of the role that kinase signaling plays in tumorigenesis.]*

Damania B: Oncogenic gamma-herpesviruses: comparison of viral proteins involved in tumorigenesis. Nat Rev Microbiol 2:656, 2004. *[Excellent summary of the molecular mechanisms underlying EBV, KSHV, and HVS tumorigenesis.]*

Farazi PA, De Pinho RA: Hepatocellular carcinoma pathogenesis; from genes to environment. Nat Rev Cancer 6:674, 2006. *[Excellent review of the role of HBV and HCV in liver cancer.]*

Grassman R, et al: Molecular mechanisms of cellular transformation by HTLV-1 Tax. Oncogene 24:5976, 2005. *[Excellent summary of the many effects of Tax gene function in transformation by HTLV-1.]*

Green DR, Kroemer G: The pathophysiology of mitochondrial cell death. Science 305:626, 2004. *[Recent review on the central role of the mitochondria in apoptosis.]*

Hanahan D, Weinberg RA: The hallmarks of cancer. Cell 100:57, 2000. *[An excellent, brief account of the fundamental properties of cancer and their molecular basis. The organization of genetic changes in cancer is based on this article.]*

Jordan CT, Guzman ML, Noble M: Cancer stem cells. New Engl J Med 355:1253, 2006. *[Excellent summary of current knowledge of cancer stem cells.]*

Kastan MB, Bartek J: Cell-cycle checkpoints and cancer. Nature 432:316, 2004. *[A detailed review on the mechanisms of cell-cycle checkpoints and how they must be disrupted in cancer.]*

Kustok JL, Wang F: The spectrum of Epstein-Barr associated disease. Annu Rev Pathol Mech Dis 1:375, 2006. *[Good discussion of EBV-induced tumors.]*

Liang TJ, Heller T: Pathogenesis of hepatitis C–associated hepatocellular carcinoma. Gastroenterology 127:S62, 2004. *[A discussion summarizing the pathogenesis of hepatitis C–induced hepatocellular carcinoma.]*

Lichtenstein P, et al.: Environmental and heritable factors in causation of cancers. N Engl J Med 343:78, 2000. *[A large study of twins and cancer risk from Sweden.]*

Little JB: Radiation carcinogenesis. Carcinogenesis 21:397, 2000. *[An update written by a pioneer in the field of radiation injury.]*

Lowe SW, et al.: Intrinsic tumour suppression. Nature 432:307, 2004. *[Excellent review of the innate networks that signal to suppress tumorigenesis and the way in which these pathways are disrupted in cancer.]*

Massague J: G1 cell-cycle control and cancer. Nature 432:298, 2004. *[A scholarly review of the G1 checkpoint, its central role in preventing tumorigenesis, and how it may be corrupted by cancers.]*

Nagy JA, Dvorak AM, Dvorak HF: VEGF-A and the induction of pathological angiogenesis. Annual Review of Pathology: Mechanisms of Disease, Vol. 2:251, 2007. *[A review of physiologic and pathologic angiogenesis.]*

O'Shaughnessy JA: Molecular signatures predict outcomes of breast cancer. New Engl J Med 355:615, 2006. *[Discussion of gene expression profiling in management of breast cancer.]*

Peek RM Jr, Crabtree JE: *Helicobacter* infection and gastric neoplasia. J Pathol 208:233, 2006. *[Recent review discussing H. pylori and both gastric adenocarcinoma and MALToma.]*

Sancar A, et al.: Molecular mechanisms of mammalian DNA repair and the DNA damage checkpoints. Annu Rev Biochem 73:39, 2004. *[Review of the molecular pathways involved in both DNA checkpoints and repair of DNA damage.]*

Sharpless NE, DePinho RA: Telomeres, stem cells, senescence, and cancer. J Clin Invest 113(2):160, 2004. *[Summary of the telomere hypothesis.]*

Sjöblom T, et al: The consensus coding sequences of human breast and colorectal cancers. Science 314:268, 2006. *[A tour de force of cancer genomics, describes the complete genetic sequence of 11 breast and 11 colon cancers.]*

Thiery JP, Sleeman JP: Complex networks orchestrate epithelial-mesenchymal transitions. Nat Rev Mol Cell Biol 7:131, 2006. *[Excellent review of the molecular mechanisms underlying epithelial-to-mesenchymal transition.]*

Tlsty T, Coussens LM: Tumor stroma and regulation of cancer development. Annu Rev Pathol Mech Dis 1:119, 2006. *[An exhaustive discussion of the interplay between tumor cells and tumor stroma.]*

Ward RJ, Dirks PB: Cancer stem cells: at the headwaters of tumor development. Annual Review of Pathology: Mechanisms of Disease, Vol. 2:175, 2007. *[A discussion of the role of cancer stem cells in carcinogenesis.]*

Williams GM: Mechanisms of chemical carcinogenesis and application to human cancer risk assessment. Toxicology 166:3, 2001. *[A brief overview of chemical carcinogenesis.]*

Willis SN, Adams JM: Life in the balance: how BH 3-only proteins induce apoptosis. Curr Opin Cell Biol 17:617, 2005. *[A summary of how BH3 proteins regulate the BCL2 family members.]*

Yee KS, Vousden KH: Complicating the complexity of p53. Carcinogenesis. 26:1317, 2005. *[Roundup of recent discoveries of p53 biology.]*

Zlotnik A: Chemokines and cancer. Int J Cancer 119:2026, 2006. *[Role of chemokines in metastases.]*

Chapter 7

Genetic and Pediatric Diseases

VINAY KUMAR, MD
ANIRBAN MAITRA, MBBS

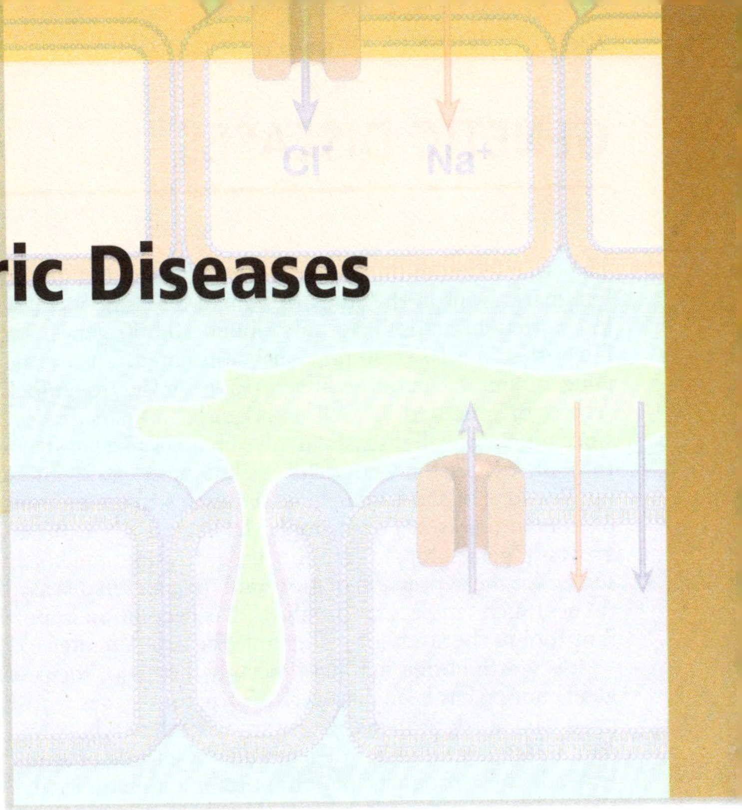

GENETIC DISEASES

The completion of the human genome project has been a landmark event in the study of human diseases. We now know that humans have only about 30,000 genes, far fewer than the 100,000 previously estimated. The unraveling of our "genetic architecture" promises to unlock secrets of inherited as well as acquired human disease, since ultimately all diseases involve changes in gene structure or expression. Powerful technologies now allow applications of the human gene sequences to the analysis of human diseases. For example, DNA and RNA microarrays ("gene chips") can be used to simultaneously screen for the expression of thousands of genes in diseased tissues. Such "molecular profiling" has become an important tool in the study of malignant diseases (Chapter 6).

It is worth noting that until recently the major focus of gene hunting has been discovery of structural genes whose products encode proteins. Recent studies indicate, however, that a very large number of genes do not encode proteins. Instead, their products play important regulatory functions. The most recent among this class are genes that encode small RNA molecules, so-called microRNAs (miRNAs). miRNAs, unlike other RNAs, do not encode proteins but instead inhibit gene expression. Silencing of gene expression by miRNA is preserved in all living forms from plants to humans and therefore must be a fundamental mechanism of gene regulation. Because of their profound influence on gene regulation, miRNAs are assuming central importance in understanding normal developmental pathways, as well as pathologic conditions, such as cancer. Such is the importance of the discovery of gene silencing by miRNAs that Andrew Fire and Craig Mello were awarded the Nobel prize in physiology or medicine in 2006, a mere eight years after they published their work in 1998.

By current estimates, there are approximately 1000 genes in humans that encode miRNAs, accounting for about 3% of the human genome. Transcription of miRNA genes produces primary microRNA transcript (pri-miRNA), which is processed within the nucleus to form another structure, called pre-miRNA (Fig. 7–1). With the help of specific transporter proteins, pre-miRNA is exported to the cytoplasm. Additional "cutting" by an enzyme, appropriately called Dicer, generates mature miRNAs that are about 21 to 30 nucleotides in length (hence the name "micro"). At this stage the miRNA is still double-stranded. Next, the miRNA unwinds, and single strands of this duplex are incorporated into a multiprotein complex called RNA-induced silencing complex (RISC). Base pairing between the miRNA strand and its target mRNA directs the RISC to either cause mRNA cleavage or repress its translation. In this way, the gene from which the target mRNA was derived is silenced (at a post-transcriptional state). Given that the numbers of miRNA genes are far fewer than those that encode proteins, it follows that a given miRNA can silence many target genes. The precise mechanism by which the target specificity of miRNA is determined remains to be fully elucidated.

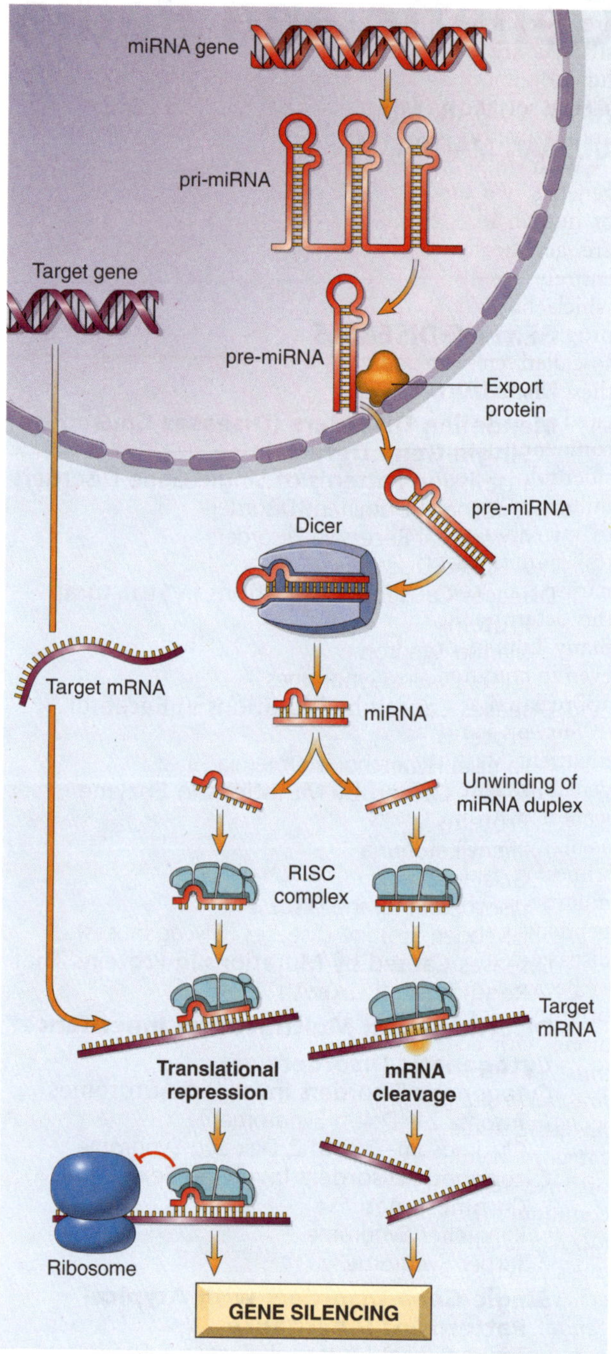

Figure 7–1

Generation of micro RNAs and their mode of action in regulating gene function. Pri-miRNA, primary microRNA transcript; Pre-miRNA, precursor microRNA; RISC, RNA-induced silencing complex.

Another species of gene-silencing RNA, called small interfering RNAs (siRNAs), works in a manner quite similar to that of miRNA. Unlike miRNA, however, siRNA precursors are introduced by investigators into the cell. Their processing by Dicer and functioning via RISC are essentially similar to that described for miRNA. siRNAs are becoming powerful tools for studying gene function and may in the future be used therapeutically to silence specific genes, such as oncogenes, whose products are involved in neoplastic transformation.

With this background of developments in human genetics, we can turn to the time-honored classification of human diseases into three categories: (1) those that are genetically determined, (2) those that are almost entirely environmentally determined, and (3) those to which both nature and nurture contribute. However, progress in understanding the molecular basis of many so-called environmental disorders has tended to blur these distinctions. At one time, microbial infections were cited as examples of disorders arising wholly from environmental influences, but it is now clear that to a considerable extent, an individual's genetic makeup influences his or her immune response and susceptibility to microbiologic infections. Despite the complexities of this nature-nurture interplay, there is little doubt that nature (i.e., the genetic component) plays a major, if not the determining, role in the occurrence and severity of many human diseases. In fact, the genetic contribution even in common diseases is far greater than is commonly appreciated.

Surveys indicate that as many as 20% of the pediatric inpatients in university hospitals suffer from disorders of genetic origin. These data describe only the tip of the iceberg. Chromosomal aberrations have been identified in as many as 50% of spontaneous abortuses during the first trimester, and many more abortuses probably had gene mutations. Only those mutations compatible with independent existence constitute the reservoir of genetic disease in the population at large.

Because several pediatric disorders are of genetic origin, we discuss developmental and pediatric diseases along with genetic diseases in this chapter. However, *it must be borne in mind that not all genetic disorders present in infancy and childhood, and conversely, many pediatric diseases are not of genetic origin.* To the latter category belong diseases resulting from immaturity of organ systems. In this context it is helpful to clarify three commonly used terms: hereditary, familial, and congenital. *Hereditary* disorders, by definition, are derived from one's parents, are transmitted in the gametes through the generations, and therefore are *familial.* The term *congenital* simply implies "present at birth." It should be noted that some congenital diseases are not genetic (e.g., congenital syphilis). On the other hand, not all genetic diseases are congenital; the expression of Huntington disease, for example, begins only after the third or fourth decade of life.

It is beyond the scope of this book to review normal human genetics, but it is beneficial to recall some fundamental concepts that have a bearing on the understanding of genetic diseases.

MUTATIONS

As is well known, the term *mutation* refers to permanent changes in the DNA. Those that affect germ cells are transmitted to the progeny and may give rise to inherited diseases. Mutations in somatic cells are not transmitted to the progeny but are important in the causation of cancers and some congenital malformations.

Details of specific mutations and their effects are discussed along with the relevant disorders throughout this text. Here we cite only some common examples of gene mutations and their effects.

Point mutations result from the substitution of a single nucleotide base by a different base, resulting in the replacement of one amino acid by another in the protein product. The mutation giving rise to sickle cell anemia is an excellent example of a point mutation that alters the meaning of the genetic code. Such mutations are sometimes called *missense mutations.*

In contrast, certain point mutations may change an amino acid codon to a chain termination codon, or *stop codon.* Such "nonsense" mutations interrupt translation, and the resultant truncated proteins are rapidly degraded.

Frameshift mutations occur when the insertion or deletion of one or two base pairs alters the reading frame of the DNA strand.

Trinucleotide repeat mutations belong to a special category, because these mutations are characterized by amplification of a sequence of 3 nucleotides. Although the specific nucleotide sequence that undergoes amplification differs in various disorders, all affected sequences share the nucleotides guanine (G) and cytosine (C). For example, in fragile X syndrome, prototypical of this category of disorders, there are 200 to 4000 tandem repeats of the sequence CGG within a gene called *FMR1.* In normal populations, the number of repeats is small, averaging 29. The expansions of the trinucleotide sequences prevent normal expression of the *FMR1* gene, thus giving rise to mental retardation. Another distinguishing feature of trinucleotide repeat mutations is that they are dynamic (i.e., the degree of amplification increases during gametogenesis). These features, discussed in greater detail later in this chapter, influence the pattern of inheritance and the phenotypic manifestations of the diseases caused by this class of mutations.

With this brief review of the nature of mutations, we can turn our attention to the three major categories of genetic disorders: (1) those related to mutant genes of large effect, (2) diseases with multifactorial (polygenic) inheritance, and (3) those arising from chromosomal aberrations. The first category, sometimes referred to as *mendelian disorders,* includes many uncommon conditions, such as the storage diseases and inborn errors of metabolism, all resulting from single-gene mutations of large effect. Most of these conditions are hereditary and familial. The second category includes some of the most common disorders of humans, such as hypertension and diabetes mellitus. Multifactorial, or polygenic, inheritance implies that both genetic and environmental influences condition the expression of a phenotypic characteristic or disease. The third category includes disorders that are the consequence of numeric or structural abnormalities in the chromosomes.

To these well-known categories, it is necessary to add a heterogeneous group of genetic disorders that, like mendelian disorders, involve single genes but do not follow simple mendelian rules of inheritance. These single-gene disorders with nonclassic inheritance include those resulting from triplet repeat mutations, those arising from mutations in mitochondrial DNA, and those in which the transmission is influenced by an epigenetic phenomenon called *genomic imprinting.*

Each of these four categories is discussed separately.

MENDELIAN DISORDERS (DISEASES CAUSED BY SINGLE-GENE DEFECTS)

Single-gene defects (mutations) follow the well-known mendelian patterns of inheritance. Thus, the conditions they produce are often called *mendelian disorders* (Table 7–1). Although individually each is rare, altogether they account for approximately 1% of all adult admissions to hospitals and about 6% to 8% of all pediatric hospital admissions.

Mutations involving single genes follow one of three patterns of inheritance: autosomal dominant, autosomal recessive, or X-linked. Although gene expression is usually described as dominant or recessive, it should be remembered that in some cases both alleles of a gene pair may be fully expressed in the heterozygote, a condition called *codominance.* Histocompatibility and blood group antigens are good examples of codominant inheritance, as well as of *polymorphism* (i.e., the presence of many allelic forms of a single gene).

A single-gene mutation may lead to many phenotypic effects (*pleiotropy*), and conversely, mutations at several genetic loci may produce the same trait (*genetic heterogeneity*). For example, Marfan syndrome, which results from a basic defect in connective tissue, is associated with widespread effects involving the skeleton, eye, and cardiovascular system, all of which stem from a mutation in the gene encoding fibrillin, a component of connective tissues. On the other hand, retinitis pigmentosa, an inherited cause of abnormal retinal pigmentation and consequent visual impairment, can be caused by several different types of mutations. Recognition of genetic heterogeneity not only is important in genetic counseling but also facilitates the understanding of the pathogenesis of common disorders such as diabetes mellitus (Chapter 20).

Table 7–1 Prevalence of Selected Monogenic Disorders Among Liveborn Infants

Disorder	Estimated Prevalence
Autosomal Dominant	
Familial hypercholesterolemia	1 in 500
Polycystic kidney disease	1 in 1250
Huntington disease	1 in 2500
Hereditary spherocytosis	1 in 5000
Marfan syndrome	1 in 20,000
Autosomal Recessive	
Sickle cell anemia	1 in 625 (US blacks)
Cystic fibrosis	1 in 2000 (Caucasians)
Tay-Sachs disease	1 in 3000 (US Jews)
Phenylketonuria	1 in 12,000
Mucopolysaccharidoses (all types)	1 in 25,000
Glycogen storage diseases (all types)	1 in 50,000
Galactosemia	1 in 57,000
X-Linked	
Duchenne muscular dystrophy	1 in 7000
Hemophilia	1 in 10,000

Table 7–2 Common Autosomal Dominant Disorders

System	Disorder
Nervous	Huntington disease Neurofibromatosis Myotonic dystrophy Tuberous sclerosis
Urinary	Polycystic kidney disease
Gastrointestinal	Familial polyposis coli
Hematopoietic	Hereditary spherocytosis Von Willebrand disease
Skeletal	Marfan syndrome* Ehlers-Danlos syndrome (some variants)* Osteogenesis imperfecta Achondroplasia
Metabolic	Familial hypercholesterolemia* Acute intermittent porphyria

*Discussed in this chapter. Other disorders listed are discussed in appropriate chapters of this book.

Transmission Patterns of Single-Gene Disorders

Autosomal Dominant Disorders

Autosomal dominant disorders are manifested in the heterozygous state, so at least one parent of an index case is usually affected; both males and females are affected, and both can transmit the condition. When an affected person marries an unaffected one, every child has one chance in two of having the disease. The following features also pertain to autosomal dominant diseases (Table 7–2):

- With any autosomal dominant disorder, some patients do not have affected parents. Such patients owe their disorder to new mutations involving either the egg or the sperm from which they were derived. Their siblings are neither affected nor at increased risk of developing the disease.
- Clinical features can be modified by reduced penetrance and variable expressivity. Some individuals inherit the mutant gene but are phenotypically normal. This is referred to as reduced penetrance. The variables that affect penetrance are not clearly understood. In contrast to penetrance, if a trait is seen in all individuals carrying the mutant gene but is expressed differ-

ently among individuals, the phenomenon is called variable expressivity. For example, manifestations of neurofibromatosis 1 range from brownish spots on the skin to multiple tumors and skeletal deformities.

- In many conditions the age at onset is delayed and symptoms and signs do not appear until adulthood (as in Huntington disease).
- In autosomal dominant disorders, a 50% reduction in the normal gene product is associated with clinical symptoms. Because a 50% loss of enzyme activity can usually be compensated for, involved genes usually do not encode enzyme proteins. Two major categories of nonenzyme proteins are usually affected in autosomal dominant disorders:
  - Those involved in regulation of complex metabolic pathways, often subject to feedback control (examples are membrane receptors and transport proteins). One example of this is familial hypercholesterolemia, which results from mutation in the low-density lipoprotein (LDL) receptor gene (discussed later).
  - Key structural proteins, such as collagen and cytoskeletal components of the red cell membrane (e.g., spectrin)

The biochemical mechanisms by which a 50% reduction in the levels of such proteins results in an abnormal phenotype are not fully understood. In some cases, especially when the gene encodes one subunit of a multimeric protein, the product of the mutant allele can interfere with the assembly of a functionally normal multimer. For example, the collagen molecule is a trimer in which the three collagen chains are arranged in a helical configuration. Even with a single mutant collagen chain, normal collagen trimers cannot be formed, and hence there is a marked deficiency of collagen. In this instance the mutant allele is called *dominant negative,* because it impairs the function of a normal allele. This effect is illustrated by some forms of osteogenesis imperfecta (Chapter 21).

Autosomal Recessive Disorders

Autosomal recessive diseases make up the largest group of mendelian disorders. They occur when both of the alleles at a given gene locus are mutants; therefore, such disorders are characterized by the following features: (1) The trait does not usually affect the parents, but siblings may show the disease; (2) siblings have one chance in four of being affected (i.e., the recurrence risk is 25% for each birth); and (3) if the mutant gene occurs with a low frequency in the population, there is a strong likelihood that the proband is the product of a consanguineous marriage.

In contrast to the features of autosomal dominant diseases, the following features generally apply to most autosomal recessive disorders (Table 7–3):

- The expression of the defect tends to be more uniform than in autosomal dominant disorders.
- Complete penetrance is common.
- Onset is frequently early in life.
- Although new mutations for recessive disorders do occur, they are rarely detected clinically. Because the affected individual is an asymptomatic heterozygote, several generations may pass before the descendants of such a person mate with other heterozygotes and produce affected offspring.
- In many cases, enzyme proteins are affected by the mutation. In heterozygotes, equal amounts of normal and defective enzyme are synthesized. Usually the natural "margin of safety" ensures that cells with half of their complement of the enzyme function normally.

Table 7–3 Autosomal Recessive Disorders

System	Disorder
Metabolic*	Cystic fibrosis* Phenylketonuria* Galactosemia* Homocystinuria Lysosomal storage diseases* α_1-Antitrypsin deficiency Wilson disease Hemochromatosis Glycogen storage diseases*
Hematopoietic	Sickle cell anemia Thalassemias
Endocrine	Congenital adrenal hyperplasia
Skeletal	Ehlers-Danlos syndrome (some variants)* Alkaptonuria
Nervous atrophies	Neurogenic muscular Friedreich ataxia Spinal muscular atrophy

*Discussed in this chapter. Many others are discussed elsewhere in the book.

X-Linked Disorders

All sex-linked disorders are X-linked. No Y-linked diseases are as yet known. Save for determinants that dictate male differentiation, the only characteristic that may be located on the Y chromosome is the attribute of hairy ears, which is not altogether devastating. Most X-linked disorders are X-linked recessive and are characterized by the following features (Table 7–4):

- They are transmitted by heterozygous female carriers only to sons, who of course are hemizygous for the X chromosome.
- Heterozygous females rarely express the full phenotypic change, because they have the paired normal allele; however, because of the inactivation of one of the X chromosomes in females (discussed later), it is remotely possible for the normal allele to be inactivated in most cells, permitting full expression of the disease in heterozygous females.
- An affected male does not transmit the disorder to sons, but all daughters are carriers. Sons of heterozygous women have one chance in two of receiving the mutant gene.

There are a very few X-linked dominant diseases and they are much less common than disorders arising from autosomal mutations. Their inheritance pattern is characterized by transmission of the disease to 50% of the

Table 7–4 X-Linked Recessive Disorders

System	Disease
Musculoskeletal	Duchenne muscular dystrophy
Blood	Hemophilias A and B Chronic granulomatous disease Glucose-6-phosphate dehydrogenase deficiency
Immune	Agammaglobulinemia X-linked severe combined immunodeficiency (SCID) Wiskott-Aldrich syndrome
Metabolic	Diabetes insipidus Lesch-Nyhan syndrome
Nervous	Fragile X syndrome*

*Discussed in this chapter.

sons and daughters of an affected heterozygous female. An affected male cannot transmit the disease to his sons, but all daughters are affected.

Although mendelian disorders are often grouped according to their patterns of transmission, it is perhaps more appropriate to categorize them on the basis of the nature of the protein that is affected, because in large part the type of protein affected determines the pattern of inheritance. Hence, in Table 7–5, selected single-gene disorders are classified into broad groupings on the basis of the protein abnormality.

SUMMARY

Transmission Patterns of Single-Gene Disorders

- Autosomal dominant disorders are characterized by expression in heterozygous state; they affect males and females equally, and both sexes can transmit the disorder.
- Enzyme proteins are not affected in autosomal dominant disorders; instead, receptors and structural proteins are involved.
- Autosomal recessive diseases occur when both copies of a gene are mutated and frequently involve enzyme proteins. Male and females are affected equally.
- X-linked disorders are transmitted by heterozygous females to their sons who manifest the disease. Female carriers are usually protected because of random inactivation of one X chromosome.

Diseases Caused by Mutations in Structural Proteins

Marfan Syndrome

In this autosomal dominant disorder of connective tissues, the basic biochemical abnormality affects *fibrillin 1*. This glycoprotein, secreted by fibroblasts, is the major component of microfibrils found in the extracellular matrix. Microfibrils serve as scaffolding for the deposition of elastin and are considered integral components of elastic fibers. Fibrillin 1 is encoded by the *FBN1* gene, which maps to chromosome 15q21. Mutations in the *FBN1* gene are found in all patients with Marfan syndrome. However, molecular diagnosis of Marfan syndrome is not feasible, because more than 500 distinct mutations affecting the *FBN1* gene have been found. Since heterozygotes have clinical symptoms, it follows that the mutant fibrillin 1 protein must act as a dominant negative by preventing the assembly of normal microfibrils.

While many of the abnormalities in Marfan syndrome can be explained on the basis of structural failure of connective tissues, some, such as overgrowth of bones and myxomatous changes in mitral valves, are difficult to relate to simple loss of fibrillin. Recent studies in mouse models of Marfan syndrome suggest an additional dysregulation of transforming growth factor β (TGF-β) production. It seems that with deficiency of fibrillin-1 there is increased TGF-β production. This cytokine secondarily regulates connective tissue growth and architecture. In support of this hypothesis, mutations in the TGF-β type II receptor give rise to a related syndrome, called Marfan syndrome, type II. The prevalence of Marfan syndrome is estimated to be 1 per 20,000. Approximately 75% of cases are familial, and the rest are sporadic, arising from new mutations in the germ cells of parents.

Although connective tissue throughout the body is affected, the principal clinical manifestations relate to three systems: the skeleton, the eyes, and the cardiovascular system.

Morphology

Skeletal abnormalities are the most obvious feature of Marfan syndrome. Patients have a slender, elongated habitus with abnormally long legs, arms, and fingers (arachnodactyly); a high-arched palate; and hyperextensibility of joints. A variety of spinal deformities, such as severe kyphoscoliosis, may appear. The chest is deformed, exhibiting either pectus excavatum (i.e., deeply depressed sternum) or a pigeon-breast deformity. President Lincoln is thought to have had features suggestive of Marfan syndrome. The most characteristic **ocular change** is bilateral dislocation, or subluxation, of the lens owing to weakness of its suspensory ligaments. It should be noted that the ciliary zonules that support the lens are devoid of elastin and are made up exclusively of fibrillin. Most serious, however, is the involvement of the **cardiovascular system**. Fragmentation of the elastic fibers in the tunica media of the aorta predisposes to aneurysmal dilation and aortic dissection (Chapter 10). These changes are not specific for Marfan syndrome. Similar lesions occur in patients with hypertension and in aging. Loss of medial support causes dilation of the aortic valve ring, giving rise to aortic incompetence. The cardiac valves, especially the mitral and, less commonly, the tricuspid valve, may be excessively distensible and regurgitant (floppy valve syndrome), giving rise to congestive cardiac failure (Chapter 11). Death from aortic rupture may occur at

Table 7–5 Biochemical Basis and Inheritance Pattern of Some Mendelian Disorders

Protein Type/Function	Examples	Pattern of Inheritance	Diseases
Enzymes	Phenylalanine hydroxylase Hexosaminidase Adenosine deaminase	Autosomal recessive	Phenylketonuria Tay-Sachs disease Severe combined immunodeficiency
Enzyme inhibitor	α_1-Antitrypsin	Autosomal recessive	Emphysema and liver disease
Receptor transport	Low-density lipoprotein receptor	Autosomal dominant	Familial hypercholesterolemia
Oxygen transport	Hemoglobin	Autosomal codominant*	α-Thalassemia β-Thalassemia Sickle cell anemia
Ion transport	Cystic fibrosis transmembrane conductance regulator	Autosomal recessive	Cystic fibrosis
Structural support			
Extracellular	Collagen	Autosomal dominant	Osteogenesis imperfecta; Ehlers-Danlos syndromes†
	Fibrillin	Autosomal dominant	Marfan syndrome
Cell membrane	Dystrophin	X-linked recessive	Duchenne/Becker muscular dystrophy
	Spectrin, ankyrin, or protein 4.1	Autosomal dominant	Hereditary spherocytosis
Hemostasis	Factor VIII	X-linked recessive	Hemophilia A
Growth regulation	RB protein NF-1 protein	Autosomal dominant Autosomal dominant	Hereditary retinoblastoma Neurofibromatosis type 1

* Heterozygotes either are asymptomatic or have mild disease.
† Some variants of Ehlers-Danlos syndrome are autosomal recessive or X-linked recessive.

any age and is the most common cause of death. Less commonly, cardiac failure is the terminal event.

Although the lesions described are typical of Marfan syndrome, they are not seen in all cases. There is much variation in clinical expression, and some patients may exhibit predominantly cardiovascular lesions with minimal skeletal and ocular changes. The variable expressivity is believed to be related to different allelic mutations in the fibrillin gene.

Ehlers-Danlos Syndromes

Ehlers-Danlos syndromes (EDSs) are characterized by defects in collagen synthesis or structure. All are single-gene disorders, but the mode of inheritance encompasses all three of the mendelian patterns. It should be recalled that there are approximately 30 distinct types of collagen, and all of them have characteristic tissue distributions and are the products of different genes. To some extent, the clinical heterogeneity of EDS can be explained by mutations in different collagen genes.

At least six clinical and genetic variants of EDS are recognized. Because defective collagen is present in all the variants, certain clinical features are common to all.

As might be expected, tissues rich in collagen, such as skin, ligaments, and joints, are frequently involved in most variants of EDS. Because the abnormal collagen fibers lack adequate tensile strength, *skin is hyperextensible and joints are hypermobile.* These features permit grotesque contortions, such as bending the thumb backward to touch the forearm and bending the knee upward to create almost a right angle. Indeed, it is believed that most contortionists have one of the EDSs; however, a predisposition to joint dislocation is one of the prices paid for this virtuosity. *The skin is extraordinarily stretchable, extremely fragile,* and *vulnerable to trauma.* Minor injuries produce gaping defects, and surgical repair or any surgical intervention is accomplished only with great difficulty because of the lack of normal tensile strength. The basic defect in connective tissue may lead to serious internal complications, including rupture of the colon and large arteries (vascular EDS); ocular fragility, with rupture of the cornea and retinal detachment (kyphoscoliosis EDS); and diaphragmatic hernias (classic EDS), among others.

The molecular bases of EDS are varied and include the following:

- *Deficiency of the enzyme lysyl hydroxylase.* Decreased hydroxylation of lysyl residues in types I and III collagen interferes with the normal cross-links among collagen molecules. As might be expected, this variant (kyphoscoliosis EDS), resulting from an enzyme deficiency, is inherited as an autosomal recessive disorder.
- *Deficient synthesis of type III collagen resulting from mutations affecting the COL3A1* gene. This variant (vascular type) is inherited as an autosomal dominant disorder and is characterized by weakness of tissues rich in type III collagen (e.g., blood vessels, bowel wall).
- *Defective conversion of procollagen type I to collagen,* resulting from a mutation in two type I collagen genes (*COL1A1* and *COL1A2*) in arthrochalasia-type EDS.

SUMMARY

Marfan Syndrome

- Marfan syndrome is caused by a mutation in the gene encoding fibrillin, which is required for structural integrity of connective tissues.
- The major tissues affected are the skeleton, eyes, and cardiovascular system.
- Clinical features include tall stature, long fingers, bilateral subluxation of lens, floppy mitral valve, aortic aneurysm, and aortic dissection.

Ehlers-Danlos Syndromes

- There are six variants of Ehlers-Danlos syndromes, all caused by defects in collagen synthesis or assembly. Each of the variants is caused by a distinct mutation.
- Clinical features are fragile, hyperextensible skin vulnerable to trauma, hypermobile joints, and rupture of internal organs like colon, cornea, and large arteries. Wound healing is poor.

Diseases Caused by Mutations in Receptor Proteins

Familial Hypercholesterolemia

Familial hypercholesterolemia is among the most common mendelian disorders; the frequency of heterozygotes is one in 500 in the general population. It is caused by a mutation in the gene that specifies the receptor for LDL, the form in which 70% of total plasma cholesterol is transported. As you know, cholesterol may be derived from the diet or from endogenous synthesis. Dietary triglycerides and cholesterol are incorporated into chylomicrons in the intestinal mucosa, which drain via the gut lymphatics into the blood. These chylomicrons are hydrolyzed by an endothelial lipoprotein lipase in the capillaries of muscle and fat. The chylomicron remnants, rich in cholesterol, are then delivered to the liver. Some of the cholesterol enters the metabolic pool (to be described), and some is excreted as free cholesterol or bile acids into the biliary tract. The endogenous synthesis of cholesterol and LDL begins in the liver (Fig. 7–2). The first step in the synthesis of LDL is the secretion of triglyceride-rich very-low-density lipoprotein (VLDL) by the liver into the blood. In the capillaries of adipose tissue and muscle, the VLDL particle undergoes lipolysis and is converted to intermediate-density lipoprotein (IDL). Compared with VLDL, the content of triglyceride is reduced and that of cholesteryl esters enriched in IDL, but IDL retains on its surface two of the three VLDL-associated apolipoproteins, B-100 and E. Further metabolism of IDL occurs along two pathways: Most of the IDL particles are taken up by the liver through the LDL receptor described later; others are converted to cholesterol-rich LDL by a further loss of triglycerides and apolipoprotein E. In the liver cells, IDL is recycled to generate VLDL.

Two-thirds of the resultant LDL particles are metabolized by the LDL receptor pathway, and the rest is metabolized by a receptor for oxidized LDL (scavenger receptor), to be described later. The LDL receptor binds to apolipoproteins B-100 and E and hence is involved in the transport of both LDL and IDL. Although the LDL receptors are widely distributed, approximately 75% are located on hepatocytes, so the liver plays an extremely important role in LDL metabolism. The first step in the receptor-mediated transport of LDL involves binding to the cell surface receptor, followed by endocytotic internalization (Fig. 7–3). Within the cell, the endocytic vesicles fuse with the lysosomes, and the LDL molecule is enzymatically degraded, resulting ultimately in the release of free cholesterol into the cytoplasm. The cholesterol not only is used by the cell for membrane synthesis but also takes part in intracellular cholesterol homeostasis by a sophisticated system of feedback control:

- It suppresses cholesterol synthesis by inhibiting the activity of the enzyme 3-hydroxy-3-methylglutaryl (3-HMG) coenzyme A reductase (HMG-CoA reductase), which is the rate-limiting enzyme in the synthetic pathway.
- It activates the enzyme acyl-CoA: cholesterol acyltransferase (ACAT), which favors esterification and storage of excess cholesterol.
- It down-regulates the synthesis of cell surface LDL receptors, thus protecting cells from excessive accumulation of cholesterol.

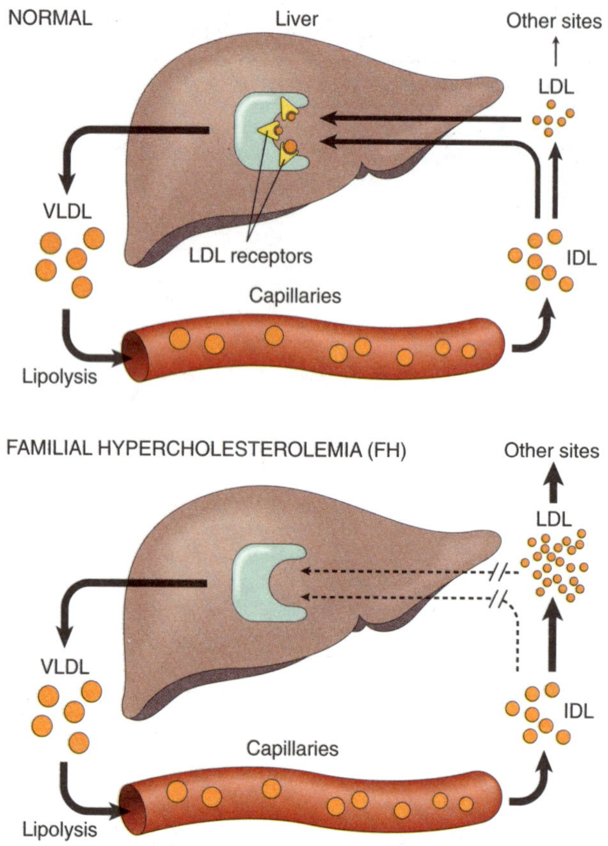

Figure 7–2

Low-density lipoprotein (LDL) metabolism and the role of the liver in its synthesis and catabolism, in normal persons and those with familial hypercholesterolemia. IDL, intermediate-density lipoprotein; VLDL, very-low-density lipoprotein.

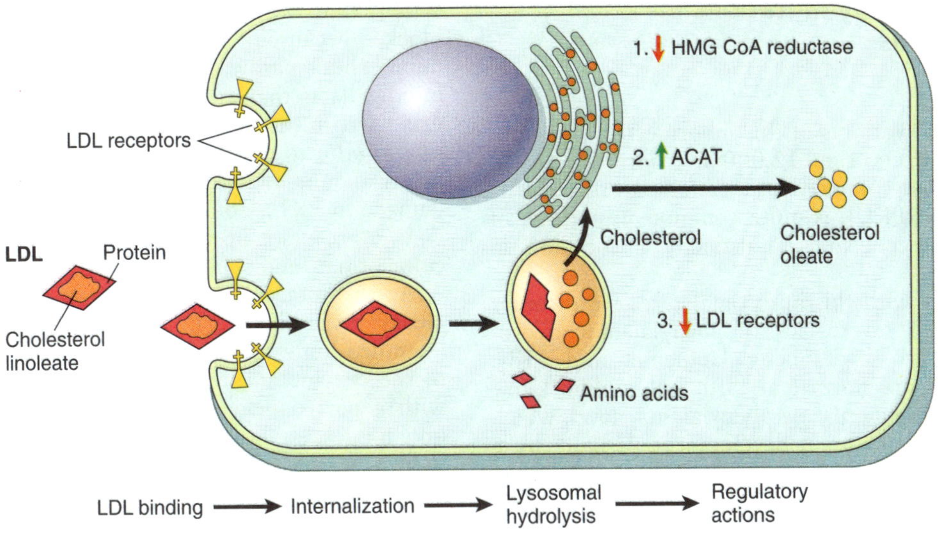

Figure 7–3

Sequential steps in low-density lipoprotein (LDL) pathway in mammalian cells. The arrows show three regulatory functions of free cholesterol: (1) Suppression of cholesterol synthesis by inhibition of HMGCoA reductase, (2) storage of excess cholesterol by activation of ACAT, and (3) reduced synthesis of LDL receptors. ACAT, acyl-CoA:cholesterol acyltransferase; HMG-CoA reductase, 3-hydroxy-3-methylglutaryl coenzyme A reductase. (Modified from Goldstein JL, Brown MS: The LDL receptor defect in familial hypercholesterolemia. Implications for pathogenesis and therapy. Med Clin North Am 66:335, 1982.)

The transport of LDL by the scavenger receptors, alluded to earlier, seems to take place in cells of the mononuclear phagocyte system and possibly in other cells as well. Monocytes and macrophages have receptors for chemically modified (e.g., acetylated or oxidized) LDLs. The amount catabolized by this "scavenger receptor" pathway is directly related to the plasma cholesterol level.

In familial hypercholesterolemia, mutations in the LDL receptor gene impair the intracellular transport and catabolism of LDL, resulting in accumulation of LDL cholesterol in the plasma. In addition, the absence of LDL receptors on liver cells also impairs the transport of IDL into the liver, and hence a greater proportion of plasma IDL is converted into LDL. Thus, patients with familial hypercholesterolemia develop excessive levels of serum cholesterol as a result of the combined effects of reduced catabolism and excessive biosynthesis (see Fig. 7–2). In the presence of such hypercholesterolemia, there is a marked increase of cholesterol traffic into the monocyte macrophages and vascular walls via the scavenger receptor. This accounts for the appearance of skin xanthomas and premature atherosclerosis.

Familial hypercholesterolemia is an autosomal dominant disease. Heterozygotes have a two- to threefold elevation of plasma cholesterol levels, whereas homozygotes may have in excess of a fivefold elevation. Although their cholesterol levels are elevated from birth, heterozygotes remain asymptomatic until adult life, when they develop cholesterol deposits (xanthomas) along tendon sheaths and premature atherosclerosis resulting in coronary artery disease. Homozygous persons are much more severely affected, developing cutaneous xanthomas in childhood and often dying of myocardial infarction by the age of 15 years.

Analysis of the cloned LDL receptor gene has revealed that more than 900 different mutations can give rise to familial hypercholesterolemia. These can be grouped in five categories. Class I mutations are uncommon, and they are associated with loss of receptor synthesis. With class II mutations, the most prevalent form, the receptor protein is synthesized, but its transport from the endoplasmic reticulum to the Golgi apparatus is impaired. Class III mutations produce receptors that are transported to the cell surface but fail to bind LDL normally. Class IV mutations give rise to receptors that fail to internalize after binding to LDL, while class V mutations encode receptors that can bind LDL and are internalized but are trapped in endosomes because dissociation of receptor and bound LDL does not occur.

The discovery of the critical role of LDL receptors in cholesterol homeostasis has led to the rational design of the statin family of drugs that are now widely used to lower plasma cholesterol. They inhibit the activity of HMG-CoA reductase and thus promote greater synthesis of LDL receptor (see Fig. 7–3).

SUMMARY

Familial Hypercholesterolemia

- Familial hypercholesterolemia is an autosomal dominant disorder caused by mutations in the LDL receptor gene.
- Patients develop hypercholesterolemia due to impaired transport of LDL into the cells.
- In heterozygotes, elevated serum cholesterol greatly increases the risk of atherosclerosis and resultant coronary artery disease; homozygotes have an even greater increase in serum cholesterol and occurrence of ischemic heart disease. Cholesterol also deposits along tendon sheaths to produce xanthomas.

Diseases Caused by Mutations in Enzyme Proteins

Phenylketonuria

There are several variants of this inborn error of metabolism, which affects 1 in 12,000 live-born Caucasian infants. The most common form, referred to as *classic phenylketonuria* (PKU), is quite common in persons of Scandinavian descent and is distinctly uncommon in blacks and Jews.

Homozygotes with this autosomal recessive disorder classically have a severe lack of phenylalanine hydroxylase, leading to hyperphenylalaninemia and PKU. Affected infants are normal at birth but within a few weeks develop a rising plasma phenylalanine level, which in some way impairs brain development. Usually by 6 months of life *severe mental retardation* becomes all too evident; fewer than 4% of untreated phenylketonuric children have IQs greater than 50 or 60. About one-third of these children are never able to walk, and two-thirds cannot talk. *Seizures,* other neurologic abnormalities, *decreased pigmentation of hair and skin,* and *eczema* often accompany the *mental retardation* in untreated children. Hyperphenylalaninemia and the resultant mental retardation can be avoided by restriction of phenylalanine intake early in life. Hence, several screening procedures are routinely performed to detect PKU in the immediate postnatal period.

Many female PKU patients, treated with diet early in life, reach childbearing age and are clinically normal. Most of them have marked hyperphenylalaninemia, because dietary treatment is discontinued after they reach adulthood. Children born to such women are profoundly mentally retarded and have multiple congenital anomalies, even though the infants themselves are heterozygotes. This syndrome, termed *maternal PKU,* results from the teratogenic effects of phenylalanine that crosses the placenta and affects the developing fetus. Hence, it is imperative that maternal phenylalanine levels be lowered by dietary means before conception. Maternal hyperphenylalaninemia also increases the risk of spontaneous abortions.

The biochemical abnormality in PKU is an inability to convert phenylalanine into tyrosine. In normal children, less than 50% of the dietary intake of phenylalanine is necessary for protein synthesis. The remainder is converted to tyrosine by the phenylalanine hydroxylase system (Fig. 7–4). When phenylalanine metabolism is blocked because of a lack of phenylalanine hydroxylase, minor shunt pathways come into play, yielding several intermediates that are excreted in large amounts in the urine and in the sweat. These impart a *strong musty or mousy odor* to affected infants. It is believed that excess phenylalanine or its metabolites contribute to the brain damage in PKU. Concomitant lack of tyrosine (see Fig. 7–4), a precursor of melanin, is responsible for the light color of hair and skin.

At the molecular level, approximately 400 mutant alleles of the phenylalanine hydroxylase gene have been identified, only some of which cause a severe deficiency of the enzyme and thus result in classic PKU. In those with a partial deficiency of phenylalanine hydroxylase only modest elevations of phenylalanine levels occur, and there is no neurologic damage. This condition, referred to as non-PKU hyperphenylalaninemia, is important to recognize because affected individuals may test positive in screening tests but do not develop the stigmata of classic PKU. Measurement of serum phenylalanine levels is necessary to differentiate non-PKU hyperphenylalaninemia from PKU. Because of the numerous disease-causing alleles of the phenylalanine hydroxylase gene, molecular diagnosis is not feasible. Once a biochemical diagnosis is established, the specific mutation causing PKU can be determined. With this information, carrier testing of at-risk family members can be performed.

As alluded to earlier, several variant forms of PKU have been identified. These account for 2% to 3% of all cases of PKU and result from deficiencies of enzymes other than phenylalanine hydroxylase, such as dihydropteridine reductase (see Fig. 7–4). *It is clinically important to recognize these variant forms of PKU, because they cannot be treated by dietary restriction of phenylalanine.*

Galactosemia

Galactosemia is an autosomal recessive disorder of galactose metabolism that affects one in 30,000 live-born infants. Normally, lactase splits lactose, the major carbohydrate of mammalian milk, into glucose and galactose in the intestinal microvilli. Galactose is then converted to glucose in several steps, in one of which the enzyme galactose-1-phosphate uridyltransferase is required. Lack of this enzyme is responsible for galactosemia. As a result

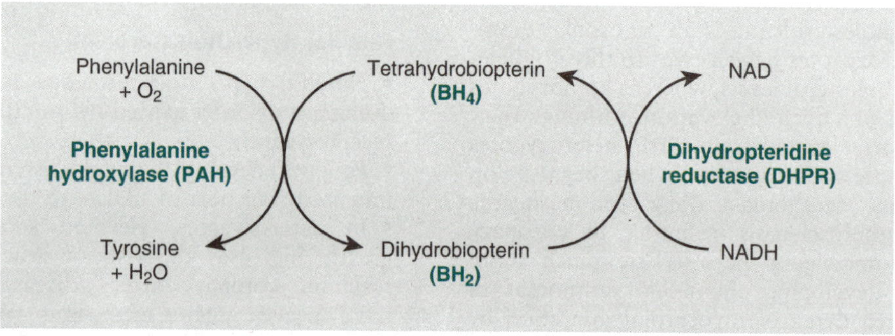

Figure 7–4

The phenylalanine hydroxylase system. NAD(H), Nicotinamide adenine dinucleotide (reduced form).

of this lack of transferase, galactose 1-phosphate and other metabolites, including galactitol, accumulate in many tissues, including the liver, spleen, lens of the eye, kidney, and cerebral cortex.

The liver, eyes, and brain bear the brunt of the damage. The early-developing hepatomegaly is due largely to fatty change, but in time widespread scarring that closely resembles the cirrhosis of alcohol abuse may supervene (Chapter 16). Opacification of the lens (cataracts) develops, probably because the lens absorbs water and swells as galactitol, produced by alternative metabolic pathways, accumulates and increases its tonicity. Nonspecific alterations appear in the central nervous system (CNS), including loss of nerve cells, gliosis, and edema. There is still no clear understanding of the mechanism of injury to the liver and brain.

Almost from birth, these infants fail to thrive. *Vomiting and diarrhea* appear within a few days of milk ingestion. *Jaundice* and *hepatomegaly* usually become evident during the first week of life. Accumulation of galactose and galactose 1-phosphate in the kidney impairs amino acid transport, resulting in aminoaciduria. There is an increased frequency of fulminant *Escherichia coli* septicemia. Without appropriate dietary therapy, long-term complications such as cataracts, speech defects, neurologic deficits, and ovarian failure may occur in older children and adults.

Most of the clinical and morphologic changes can be prevented by early removal of galactose from the diet for at least the first 2 years of life. The diagnosis is established by assay of the transferase in leukocytes and erythrocytes. Antenatal diagnosis is possible by enzyme assays or DNA-based testing of cultured amniocytes or chorionic villi.

SUMMARY

Phenylketonuria

- Phenylketonuria is an autosomal recessive disorder caused by a lack of the enzyme phenylalanine hydroxylase and consequent inability to metabolize phenylalanine.
- Clinical features include severe mental retardation, seizures, and decreased pigmentation of skin that can be avoided by restricting the intake of phenylalanine in the diet.
- Female PKU patients who discontinue dietary treatment can give birth to mentally retarded children with malformations due to transplacental passage of phenylalanine metabolites.

Galactosemia

- Galactosemia is caused by an inherited lack of galactose-1-phosphate uridyltransferase causing accumulation of galactose 1-phosphate and its metabolites in tissues.
- Clinical features include jaundice, liver damage, cataracts, neural damage, vomiting and diarrhea, and *E. coli* sepsis. Dietary restriction of galactose can prevent these.

Lysosomal Storage Diseases

Lysosomes, as is well known, contain a variety of hydrolytic enzymes that are involved in the breakdown of complex substrates, such as sphingolipids and mucopolysaccharides, into soluble end products. These large molecules may be derived from the turnover of intracellular organelles that enter the lysosomes by autophagocytosis, or they may be acquired from outside the cells by phagocytosis. With an inherited lack of a lysosomal enzyme, catabolism of its substrate remains incomplete, leading to accumulation of the partially degraded insoluble metabolites within the lysosomes (Fig. 7–5). Approximately 40 lysosomal storage diseases have been identified, each resulting from the functional absence of a specific lysosomal enzyme or proteins involved in their function. Traditionally, lysosomal storage disorders are divided into broad categories based on the biochemical nature of the substrates and the accumulated metabolites, but a more mechanistic classification is based on the underlying molecular defect (Table 7–6). Within each group are several entities, each resulting from the deficiency of a specific enzyme. Despite this complexity, certain features are common to most diseases in this group:

- Autosomal recessive transmission
- Commonly affect infants and young children
- Storage of insoluble intermediates in the mononuclear phagocyte system, giving rise to hepatosplenomegaly
- Frequent CNS involvement with associated neuronal damage
- Cellular dysfunctions, caused not only by storage of undigested material but also by a cascade of secondary events triggered, for example, by macrophage activation and release of cytokines.

Fortunately for both medical students and the potential victims of the diseases, most of these conditions are very rare, and their detailed description is better relegated to specialized texts and reviews. Only a few of the more common conditions are considered here. Type II glycogen storage disease (Pompe disease), also a lysosomal disorder, is discussed later.

Tay-Sachs Disease (G_{M2} Gangliosidosis: Deficiency in Hexosaminidase α Subunit). Gangliosidoses are characterized by accumulation of gangliosides, principally in the brain, as a result of a deficiency of a catabolic lysosomal enzyme. Depending on the ganglioside involved, these disorders are subclassified into G_{M1} and G_{M2} categories. Tay-Sachs disease, by far the most common of all gangliosidoses, is characterized by a mutation in and consequent deficiency of the α subunit of the enzyme hexosaminidase A, which is necessary for the degradation of G_{M2}. More than 90 mutations have been described; most affect protein folding or intracellular transport. The brain is principally affected, because it is most involved in ganglioside metabolism. *The storage of G_{M2}* occurs within neurons, axon cylinders of nerves, and glial cells throughout the CNS. Affected cells appear swollen, possibly foamy (Fig. 7–6A). Electron microscopy reveals a whorled configuration within lysosomes (Fig. 7–6B). These

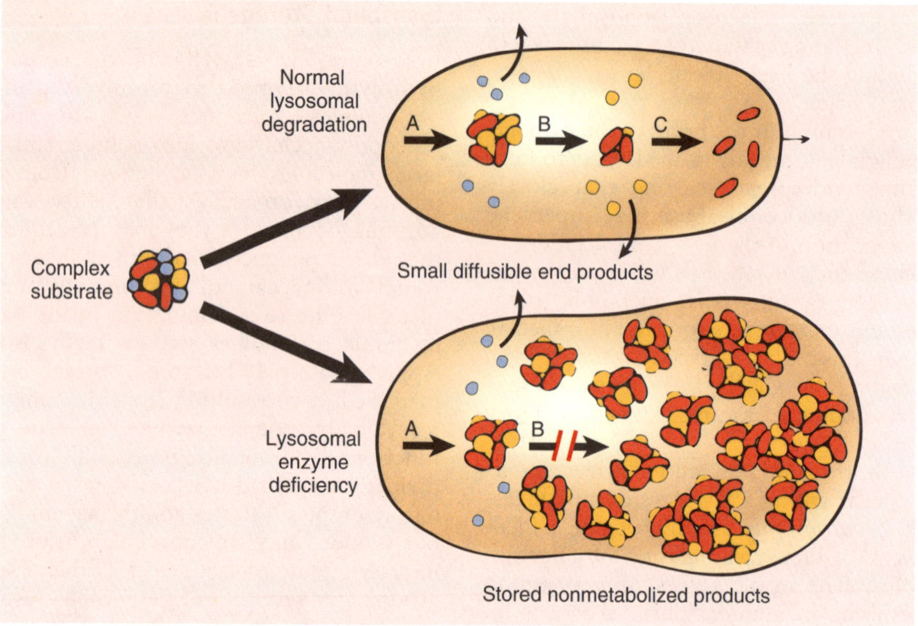

Figure 7–5

Pathogenesis of lysosomal storage diseases. In this example, a complex substrate is normally degraded by a series of lysosomal enzymes (**A**, **B**, and **C**) into soluble end products. If there is a deficiency or malfunction of one of the enzymes (e.g., **B**), catabolism is incomplete, and insoluble intermediates accumulate in the lysosomes.

anatomic changes are found throughout the CNS (including the spinal cord), peripheral nerves, and autonomic nervous system. The retina is usually involved as well.

The molecular bases of neuronal injury are not fully understood. Because in many cases the mutant protein is misfolded, it induces the so-called "unfolded protein" response (Chapter 1). If such misfolded proteins are not stabilized by chaperones, they trigger apoptosis. These findings have given rise to the possibility of chaperone therapy for this and similar lysosomal storage diseases.

Tay-Sachs disease, like other lipidoses, is most common among Ashkenazi Jews, among whom the frequency of heterozygous carriers is estimated to be one in 30. Heterozygotes can be reliably detected by estimating the level of hexosaminidase in the serum or by DNA analysis. In the most common acute infantile variant of Tay-Sachs disease, infants appear normal at birth, but

Table 7–6 Lysosomal Storage Disorders

Disease category	Disease	Deficiency
Primary lysosomal hydrolase defect	Gaucher disease GM1 gangliosidosis Tay-Sachs disease Sandhoff disease Fabry disease Krabbe disease Niemann-Pick disease types A and B	Glucosylceramidase G_{M1}-β-galactosidase β-Hexosaminidase A β-Hexosaminidase A and B α-Galactosidase A β-Galactosyl ceramidase Sphingomyelinase
Post-translational processing defect of lysosomal enzymes	Mucosulfatidosis	Multiple sulfatases
Trafficking defect for lysosomal enzymes	Mucolipidosis types II and IIIA	*N*-acetyl glucosamine phosphoryl transferase
Defect in lysosomal enzyme protection	Galactosialidosis	Protective protein cathepsin A (β-galactosidase and neuraminidase)
Defect in soluble nonenzymatic lysosomal proteins	GM2 activator protein deficiency, variant AB	GM2 activator protein
Transmembrane (nonenzymic) protein	Sphingolipid activator protein deficiency Niemann-Pick disease type C (NPC) Salia disease (free sialic acid storage)	Sphingolipid activator protein *NPC1* and *NPC2* Sialin

Modified from Jeyakumar M, et al: Storage solutions: treating lysosomal disorders of the brain. Nature Rev Neurosci 6:1, 2005.

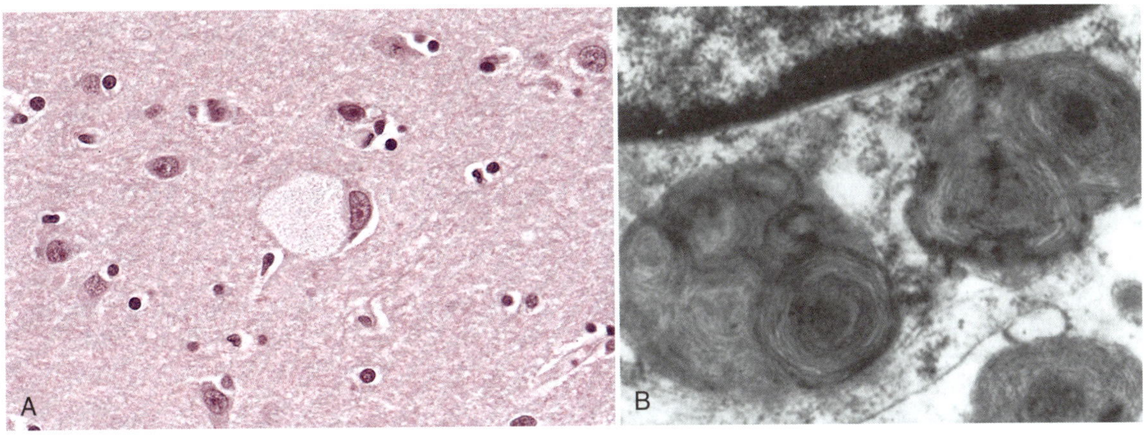

Figure 7–6

A, Ganglion cells in Tay-Sachs disease. Under the light microscope, a large neuron has obvious lipid vacuolation. **B,** Tay-Sachs disease. A portion of a neuron under the electron microscope shows prominent lysosomes with whorled configurations. Part of the nucleus is shown above. (**A** Courtesy of Dr. Arthur Weinberg, Department of Pathology, University of Texas Southwestern Medical Center, Dallas, Texas. **B** Courtesy of Dr. Joe Rutledge, Children's Regional Medical Center, Seattle, Washington.)

motor weakness begins at 3 to 6 months of age, followed by mental retardation, blindness, and severe neurologic dysfunctions. Death occurs within 2 or 3 years.

Niemann-Pick Disease, Types A and B. These two related entities are characterized by a primary deficiency of acid sphingomyelinase and the resultant accumulation of sphingomyelin. In type A, characterized by a severe deficiency of sphingomyelinase, the breakdown of sphingomyelin into ceramide and phosphorylcholine is impaired, and excess sphingomyelin accumulates in all phagocytic cells and in the neurons. The macrophages become stuffed with droplets or particles of the complex lipid, imparting a fine vacuolation or foaminess to the cytoplasm (Fig. 7–7). Because of their high content of phagocytic cells, *the organs most severely* affected are the *spleen, liver, bone marrow, lymph nodes, and lungs.* The splenic enlargement may be striking. In addition, the entire CNS, including the spinal cord and ganglia, is involved in this tragic, inexorable process. The affected neurons are enlarged and vacuolated as a result of the storage of lipids. This variant manifests itself in infancy with *massive visceromegaly and severe neurologic deterioration.* Death usually occurs within the first 3 years of life. By comparison, patients with the type B variant have organomegaly but no neurologic symptoms. Estimation of sphingomyelinase activity in the leukocytes or cultured fibroblasts can be used for diagnosis of suspected cases, as well as for detection of carriers. Antenatal diagnosis is possible by enzyme assays or DNA probe analysis.

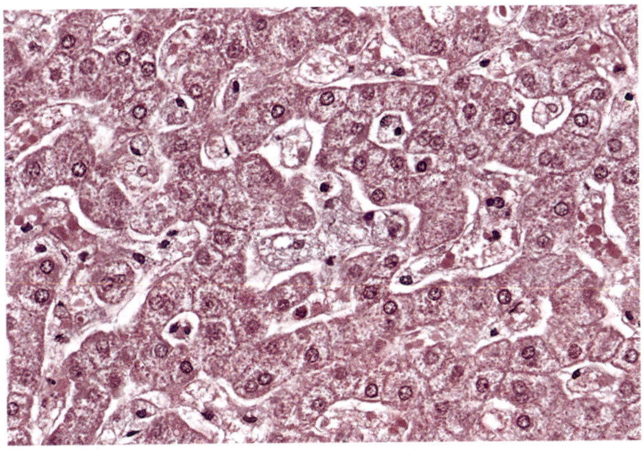

Figure 7–7

Niemann-Pick disease in liver. The hepatocytes and Kupffer cells have a foamy, vacuolated appearance resulting from deposition of lipids. (Courtesy of Dr. Arthur Weinberg, Department of Pathology, University of Texas Southwestern Medical Center, Dallas, Texas.)

Niemann-Pick Disease Type C. Although previously considered to be related to types A and B Niemann-Pick disease, type C (NPC) is quite distinct at the biochemical and molecular levels and is more common than types A and B combined. Mutations in two related genes, *NPC1* and *NPC2,* can give rise to it, with *NPC1* being responsible for the majority of cases. Unlike most other lysosomal storage diseases, NPC is due to a primary defect in lipid transport. Affected cells accumulate cholesterol as well as gangliosides such as G_{M1} and G_{M2}. The precise biochemical step affected by the *NPC1* gene is still not clear. NPC is clinically heterogeneous: the most common form presents in childhood and is marked by ataxia, vertical supranuclear gaze palsy, dystonia, dysarthria, and psychomotor regression.

Gaucher Disease. This disease results from mutation in the gene that encodes glucosylceramidase. There are five autosomal recessive variants of Gaucher disease resulting from distinct allelic mutations. Common to all is variably deficient activity of a glucosylceramidase that normally cleaves the glucose residue from ceramide. This leads to an accumulation of glucosylceramide in the mononuclear phagocytic cells and their transformation into so-called Gaucher cells. Normally the glycolipids derived from the breakdown of senescent blood cells, particularly erythrocytes, are sequentially degraded. In Gaucher disease, the degradation stops at the level of glucosylceramides, which, in transit through the blood as macromolecules, are engulfed by the phagocytic cells of the body, especially in the liver, spleen, and bone marrow. These phagocytes (Gaucher cells) become enlarged, with some becoming as large as 100 μm, because of the accumulation of distended lysosomes, and develop a pathognomonic cytoplasmic appearance characterized as "wrinkled tissue paper" (Fig. 7–8). No distinct vacuolation is present. It is evident now that Gaucher disease is caused not just by the burden of storage material but also by activation of the macrophages. High levels of macrophage-derived cytokines, such as interleukins (IL-2, IL-6) and tumor necrosis factor (TNF) are found in affected tissues.

One variant, type I, also called the *chronic non-neuronopathic form,* accounts for 99% of cases of Gaucher disease. It is characterized by clinical or radiographic bone involvement (osteopenia, focal lytic lesions, and osteonecrosis) in 70% to 100% of cases. Additional features are hepatosplenomegaly and the absence of CNS involvement. The spleen often enlarges massively, filling the entire abdomen. Gaucher cells are found in the liver, spleen, lymph nodes, and bone marrow. Marrow replacement and cortical erosion may produce radiographically visible skeletal lesions, as well as a reduction in the formed elements of blood. Bone changes are believed to be caused by macrophage-derived cytokines, listed above. Type I is most common in Ashkenazi Jews and, unlike other variants, it is compatible with long life. Types II and III variants are characterized by neurologic signs and symptoms. In type II, the symptoms start before 2 years of age and are more severe, whereas in type III, the symptoms appear later and are milder. Although the liver and spleen are also involved, the clinical features are dominated by neurologic disturbances. In addition to these, there is a perinatal-lethal form characterized by hepatosplenomegaly, skin lesions, and non-immune hydrops (see later). In the so-called cardiovascular form, there is involvement and calcification of mitral and aortic valves.

The level of glucosylceramidase in leukocytes or cultured fibroblasts is helpful in diagnosis and in the detection of heterozygotes. Current therapy is aimed at enzyme replacement by infusion of purified enzyme. A newer form of therapy involves reducing the substrate (glucosylceramide) by administration of drugs that inhibit glucosylceramide synthetase. Since glucosylceramide is reduced, its accumulation is also reduced. On the horizon is glucosylceramidase gene therapy involving infusion of autologous hematopoietic stem cells transfected with the normal gene.

Mucopolysaccharidoses. Mucopolysaccharidoses (MPSs) are characterized by defective degradation (and therefore excessive storage) of mucopolysaccharides in various tissues. Recall that mucopolysaccharides form a part of ground substance and are synthesized by connective tissue fibroblasts. Most of the mucopolysaccharide is secreted into the ground substance, but a certain fraction is degraded within lysosomes. Several enzymes are involved in this catabolic pathway; it is the lack of these enzymes that leads to accumulation of mucopolysaccharides within the lysosomes. Several clinical variants of MPS, classified numerically from MPS I to MPS VII, have been described, each resulting from the deficiency of one specific enzyme. The mucopolysaccharides that accumulate within the tissues include dermatan sulfate, heparan sulfate, keratan sulfate, and (in some cases) chondroitin sulfate.

In general, the MPSs are progressive disorders characterized by involvement of many organs, including the liver, spleen, heart, and blood vessels. Most are associated with *coarse facial features, clouding of the cornea, joint stiffness, and mental retardation.* Urinary excretion of the accumulated mucopolysaccharides is often increased. All of these disorders except one are inherited as autosomal recessive conditions; the exception, Hunter syndrome, is an X-linked recessive disease. Of the seven recognized variants, only two well-characterized syndromes are discussed briefly here.

Mucopolysaccharidosis type I refers to a spectrum of three disorders varying from mild to severe, all caused by a deficiency of α-L-iduronidase. At the two ends of the spectrum are Hurler syndrome and Scheie syndrome,

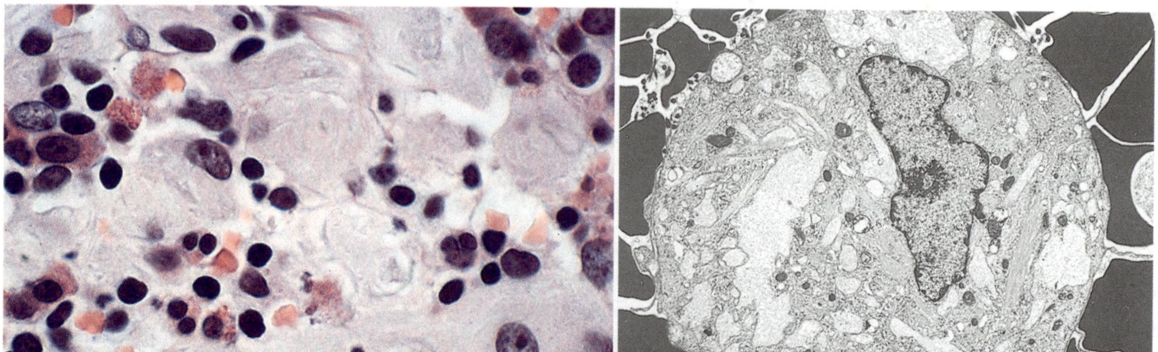

Figure 7–8

Gaucher disease involving the bone marrow. **A,** Gaucher cells with abundant lipid-laden granular cytoplasm. **B,** Electron micrograph of Gaucher cells with elongated distended lysosomes. (Courtesy of Dr. Mathew Fries, Department of Pathology, University of Texas Southwestern Medical Center, Dallas, Texas.)

with the Hurler-Scheie syndrome occupying the middle position. In Hurler syndrome, affected children have a life expectancy of 6 to 10 years. Like patients with most other forms of MPS, they develop coarse facial features associated with skeletal deformities. Death is often due to cardiac complications resulting from the formation of raised endothelial and endocardial lesions by the deposition of mucopolysaccharides in the coronary arteries and heart valves. Accumulation of dermatan sulfate and heparan sulfate is seen in cells of the mononuclear phagocyte system, in fibroblasts, and within endothelium and smooth muscle cells of the vascular wall. The affected cells are swollen and have clear cytoplasm, resulting from the accumulation of material positive for periodic acid–Schiff stain within engorged, vacuolated lysosomes. Lysosomal inclusions are also found in neurons, accounting for the mental retardation.

The other variant of MPS, called type II, or *Hunter syndrome,* differs from Hurler syndrome in its mode of inheritance (X-linked), the absence of corneal clouding, and often its milder clinical course. As in Hurler syndrome, the accumulated mucopolysaccharides in Hunter syndrome are heparan sulfate and dermatan sulfate, but this results from a deficiency of L-iduronate sulfatase. Despite the difference in enzyme deficiency, an accumulation of identical substrates occurs because breakdown of heparan sulfate and dermatan sulfate requires both α-L-iduronidase and the sulfatase; if either one is missing, further degradation is blocked.

SUMMARY

Lysosomal Storage Diseases

- *Tay-Sachs disease* is caused by an inability to metabolize G_{M2} gangliosides due to lack of lysosomal hexosaminidase A. G_{M2} gangliosides accumulate in the CNS and cause severe mental retardation, blindness, motor weakness, and death by 2–3 years of age.
- *Niemann-Pick disease types A and B* are caused by a deficiency of sphingomeylinase. In the more severe type A variant, accumulation of sphingomyelin in the nervous system results in neuronal damage. Lipid is also stored in phagocytes within the liver, spleen, bone marrow, and lymph nodes, causing their enlargement. In type B, neuronal damage is not present.
- *Niemann-Pick type C* disease is caused by a defect in cholesterol transport and resultant accumulation of cholesterol and gangliosides in the nervous system. Affected children have ataxia, dysarthria, and psychomotor regression.
- *Gaucher disease* results from lack of the lysosomal enzyme glucosylceramidase and accumulation of glucosylceramide in mononuclear phagocytic cells. In the most common, type I variant, affected phagocytes become enlarged (Gaucher cells) and accumulate in liver, spleen, and bone marrow, causing hepatosplenomegaly and bone erosion. Type II and III have variable neuronal involvement.
- *Mucopolysaccharidoses* result from accumulation of mucopolysaccharides in many tissues including liver, spleen, heart, blood vessels, brain, cornea, and joints. Affected patients in all forms have coarse facial features. In Hurler syndrome there is corneal clouding, coronary arterial and valvular depositions, and death in childhood. Hunter syndrome has a milder course.

Glycogen Storage Diseases (Glycogenoses)

An inherited deficiency of any one of the enzymes involved in glycogen synthesis or degradation can result in excessive accumulation of glycogen or some abnormal form of glycogen in various tissues. The type of glycogen stored, its intracellular location, and the tissue distribution of the affected cells vary depending on the specific enzyme deficiency. Regardless of the tissue or cells affected, the glycogen is most often stored within the cytoplasm, or sometimes within nuclei. One variant, Pompe disease, is a form of lysosomal storage disease, because the missing enzyme is localized to lysosomes. Most glycogenoses are inherited as autosomal recessive diseases, as is common with "missing enzyme" syndromes.

Approximately a dozen forms of glycogenoses have been described on the basis of specific enzyme deficiencies. On the basis of pathophysiology, they can be grouped into three categories (Table 7–7):

- *Hepatic type.* Liver contains several enzymes that synthesize glycogen for storage and also break it down into free glucose. Hence, a deficiency of the hepatic enzymes involved in glycogen metabolism is associated with two major clinical effects: *enlargement of the liver due to storage of glycogen* and *hypoglycemia due to a failure of glucose production* (Fig. 7–9). Von Gierke disease (type I glycogenosis), resulting from a lack of glucose-6-phosphatase, is the most important example of the hepatic form of glycogenosis (see Table 7–7).
- *Myopathic type.* In striated muscle, glycogen is an important source of energy. Not surprisingly, most forms of glycogen storage disease affect muscles. When enzymes that are involved in glycolysis are deficient, glycogen storage occurs in muscles and there is an associated muscle weakness due to impaired energy production. Typically, *the myopathic forms of glycogen storage diseases are marked by muscle cramps after exercise, myoglobinuria, and failure of exercise to induce an elevation in blood lactate levels because of a block in glycolysis.* McArdle disease (type V glycogenosis), resulting from a deficiency of muscle phosphorylase, is the prototype of myopathic glycogenoses.
- Two other forms of glycogenoses do not fit into either of the two categories described. Type II glycogenosis (*Pompe disease*) is caused by a deficiency

Table 7–7 Principal Subgroups of Glycogenoses

Clinicopathologic Category	Specific Type	Enzyme Deficiency	Morphologic Changes	Clinical Features
Hepatic type	Hepatorenal (von Gierke disease, type I)	Glucose-6-phosphatase	Hepatomegaly: intracytoplasmic accumulations of glycogen and small amounts of lipid; intranuclear glycogen Renomegaly: intracytoplasmic accumulations of glycogen in cortical tubular epithelial cells	In untreated patients, failure to thrive, stunted growth, hepatomegaly, and renomegaly Hypoglycemia due to failure of glucose mobilization, often leading to convulsions Hyperlipidemia and hyperuricemia resulting from deranged glucose metabolism; many patients develop gout and skin xanthomas. Bleeding tendency due to platelet dysfunction With treatment (providing continuous source of glucose), most patients survive and develop late complications (e.g., hepatic adenomas).
Myopathic type	McArdle syndrome (type V)	Muscle phosphorylase	Sketetal muscle only—accumulations of glycogen predominant in subsarcolemmal location	Painful cramps associated with strenuous exercise Myoglobinuria occurs in 50% of cases. Onset in adulthood (>20 yr) Muscular exercise fails to raise lactate level in venous blood. Compatible with normal longevity
Miscellaneous type	Generalized glycogenosis (Pompe disease, type II)	Lysosomal glucosidase (acid maltase)	Mild hepatomegaly: ballooning of lysosomes with glycogen creating lacy cytoplasmic pattern Cardiomegaly: glycogen within sarcoplasm as well as membrane-bound Skeletal muscle: similar to heart (see cardiomegaly)	Massive cardiomegaly, muscle hypotonia, and cardiorespiratory failure within 2 yr Milder adult form with only skeletal muscle involvement presents with chronic myopathy.

of lysosomal acid maltase and so is associated with deposition of glycogen in virtually every organ, but cardiomegaly is most prominent. Brancher glycogenosis (type IV) is caused by deposition of an abnormal form of glycogen, with detrimental effects on the liver, heart, and muscles.

SUMMARY

Glycogen Storage Diseases

- Inherited deficiency of enzymes involved in glycogen metabolism can result in storage of normal or abnormal forms of glycogen, predominantly in liver or muscles or in all tissues.
- In the *hepatic form* (von Gierke disease), liver cells store glycogen because of a lack of hepatic glucose-6-phosphatase. There are several *myopathic forms,* including McArdle disease, in which muscle phosphorylase lack gives rise to storage in skeletal muscles and cramps after exercise. In *Pompe disease* there is lack of lysosomal acid maltase, and all organs are affected but heart involvement is predominant.

Diseases Caused by Mutations in Proteins That Regulate Cell Growth

As was detailed in Chapter 6, two classes of genes, proto-oncogenes and tumor suppressor genes, regulate normal cell growth and differentiation. Mutations affecting these genes, most often in somatic cells, are involved in the pathogenesis of tumors. In approximately 5% of all cancers, however, mutations affecting certain tumor suppressor genes are present in all cells of the body, including germ cells, and hence can be transmitted to the offspring. These mutant genes predispose the offspring to hereditary tumors, a topic discussed in greater detail in Chapter 6.

DISORDERS WITH MULTIFACTORIAL INHERITANCE

Multifactorial (also called *polygenic*) inheritance is involved in many of the physiologic characteristics of humans (e.g., height, weight, blood pressure, hair color). A multifactorial physiologic or pathologic trait may be defined as one governed by the additive effect of two or more genes of small effect, conditioned by environmental, nongenetic influences. Even monozygous twins reared separately may achieve different heights because of nutritional or other environmental influences. When surveyed in a large population, phenotypic attributes governed by multifactorial inheritance fall on a continuous Gaussian distribution (Fig. 7–10). Presumably, there is some threshold effect, so that a disorder becomes manifest only when a certain number of effector genes, as well as conditioning environmental influences, are involved. The threshold effect also explains why parents of a child with a polygenic disorder may themselves be normal. Once the threshold value is exceeded, the severity of the disease is directly proportional to the number and the degree of influence of the pathologic genes.

The following features characterize multifactorial inheritance. These have been established for the multifactorial inheritance of congenital malformations and, in all likelihood, obtain for other multifactorial diseases.

- The risk of expressing a multifactorial disorder is conditioned by the number of mutant genes inherited. Thus, the risk is greater in siblings of patients having severe expressions of the disorder.
- The rate of recurrence of the disorder (2% to 7%) is the same for all first-degree relatives (i.e., parents, siblings, and offspring) of the affected individual. Thus, if parents have had one affected child, the risk that the next child will be affected is between 2% and 7%. Similarly, there is the same chance that one of the parents will be affected.

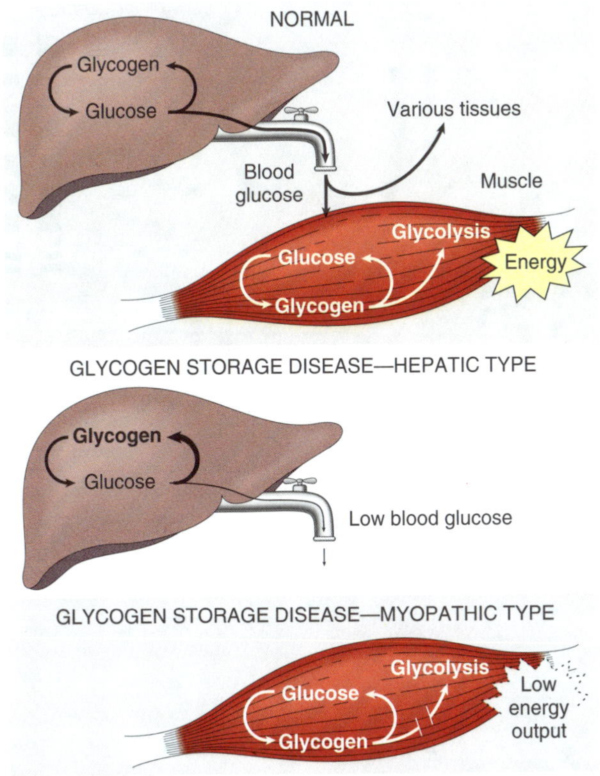

Figure 7–9

Top, A simplified scheme of normal glycogen metabolism in the liver and skeletal muscles. **Middle,** The effects of an inherited deficiency of hepatic enzymes involved in glycogen metabolism. **Bottom,** The consequences of a genetic deficiency in the enzymes that metabolize glycogen in skeletal muscles.

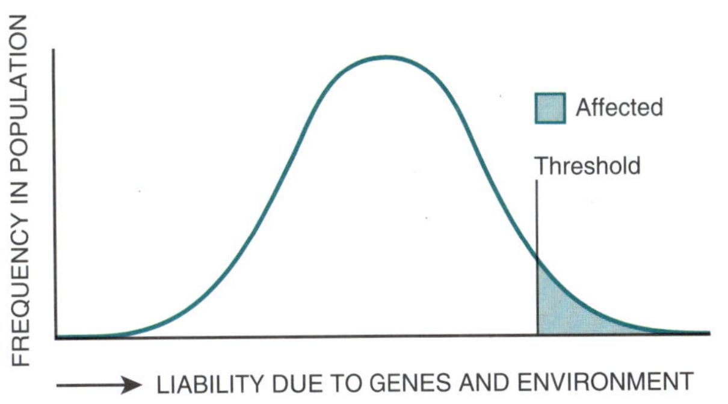

Figure 7–10

Multifactorial inheritance. The continuous distribution of the liability to develop a multifactorial disease is determined by many genes and the environment. A threshold of liability indicates the limit beyond which disease is expressed. (Adapted from Elsas LJ II, Priest JH: Medical genetics. In Sodeman WA, Sodeman TM [eds]: Pathologic Physiology: Mechanisms of Disease, 7th ed. Philadelphia, WB Saunders, 1985, p 59.)

- The likelihood that both identical twins will be affected is significantly less than 100% but is much greater than the chance that both nonidentical twins will be affected. Experience has proved, for example, that the frequency of concordance for identical twins is in the range of 20% to 40%.
- The risk of recurrence of the phenotypic abnormality in subsequent pregnancies depends on the outcome in previous pregnancies. When one child is affected, there is as high as a 7% chance that the next child will be affected, but after two affected siblings, the risk rises to about 9%.

This form of inheritance is believed to underlie such common diseases as diabetes mellitus, hypertension, gout, schizophrenia, bipolar disorder, and certain forms of congenital heart disease, as well as some skeletal abnormalities. Hypertension provides an excellent example of multifactorial inheritance. There is good evidence that the level of blood pressure of an individual, at least in some part, is under genetic control, apparently governed by many genes of small effect. The pressure levels of the population at large fall along a continuous Gaussian curve of distribution. At some arbitrary level of blood pressure, hypertension is said to exist, because pressures above this level are associated with a significant disadvantage to the individual. (Chapter 10.)

CYTOGENETIC DISORDERS

Chromosomal abnormalities occur much more frequently than is generally appreciated. It is estimated that approximately one of 200 newborn infants has some form of chromosomal abnormality. The figure is much higher in fetuses that do not survive to term. It is estimated that in 50% of first-trimester abortions, the fetus has a chromosomal abnormality. Cytogenetic disorders may result from alterations in the number or structure of chromosomes and may affect autosomes or sex chromosomes.

Before we embark on a discussion of chromosomal aberrations, it should be recalled that karyotyping is the basic tool of the cytogeneticist. A karyotype is a photographic representation of a stained metaphase spread in which the chromosomes are arranged in order of decreasing length. A variety of techniques for staining chromosomes have been developed. With the widely used Giemsa stain (G banding) technique, each chromosome set can be seen to possess a distinctive pattern of alternating light and dark bands of variable widths (Fig. 7–11). The use of banding techniques allows certain identification of each chromosome, as well as precise localization of structural changes in the chromosomes (described later).

Numeric Abnormalities. In humans, the normal chromosome count is 46 (i.e., $2n=46$). Any exact multiple of the haploid number (n) is called *euploid.* Chromosome numbers such as $3n$ and $4n$ are called *polyploid.* Polyploidy generally results in a spontaneous abortion. Any number that is not an exact multiple of n is called *aneuploid.* The chief cause of aneuploidy is nondisjunction of a homologous pair of chromosomes at the first meiotic division or a failure of sister chromatids to separate during the second meiotic division. The latter may also occur during somatic cell division, leading to the production of two aneuploid cells. Failure of pairing of homologous chromosomes followed by random assortment (anaphase lag) can also lead to aneuploidy. When nondisjunction occurs at the time of meiosis, the gametes formed have either an extra chromosome ($n+1$) or one less chromosome ($n-1$). Fertilization of such gametes by normal gametes would result in two types of zygotes: trisomic, with an extra chromosome ($2n+1$), or monosomic ($2n-1$). Monosomy involving an autosome is incompatible with life, whereas trisomies of certain autosomes and monosomy involving sex chromosomes are compatible with life. These, as we shall see, are associated with variable degrees of phenotypic abnormality. *Mosaicism* is a term used to describe the presence of two or more populations of cells in the same individual. In the context of chromosome numbers, postzygotic mitotic nondisjunction would result in the production of a trisomic and a monosomic daughter cell; the descendants of these cells would then produce a mosaic. As discussed later, mosaicism affecting sex chromosomes is common, whereas autosomal mosaicism is not.

Structural Abnormalities. Structural changes in the chromosomes usually result from chromosomal breakage followed by loss or rearrangement of material. Such changes are usually designated using a cytogenetic shorthand in which p (petit) denotes the short arm of a chromosome, and q, the long arm. Each arm is then divided into numbered regions (1, 2, 3, and so on) from centromere

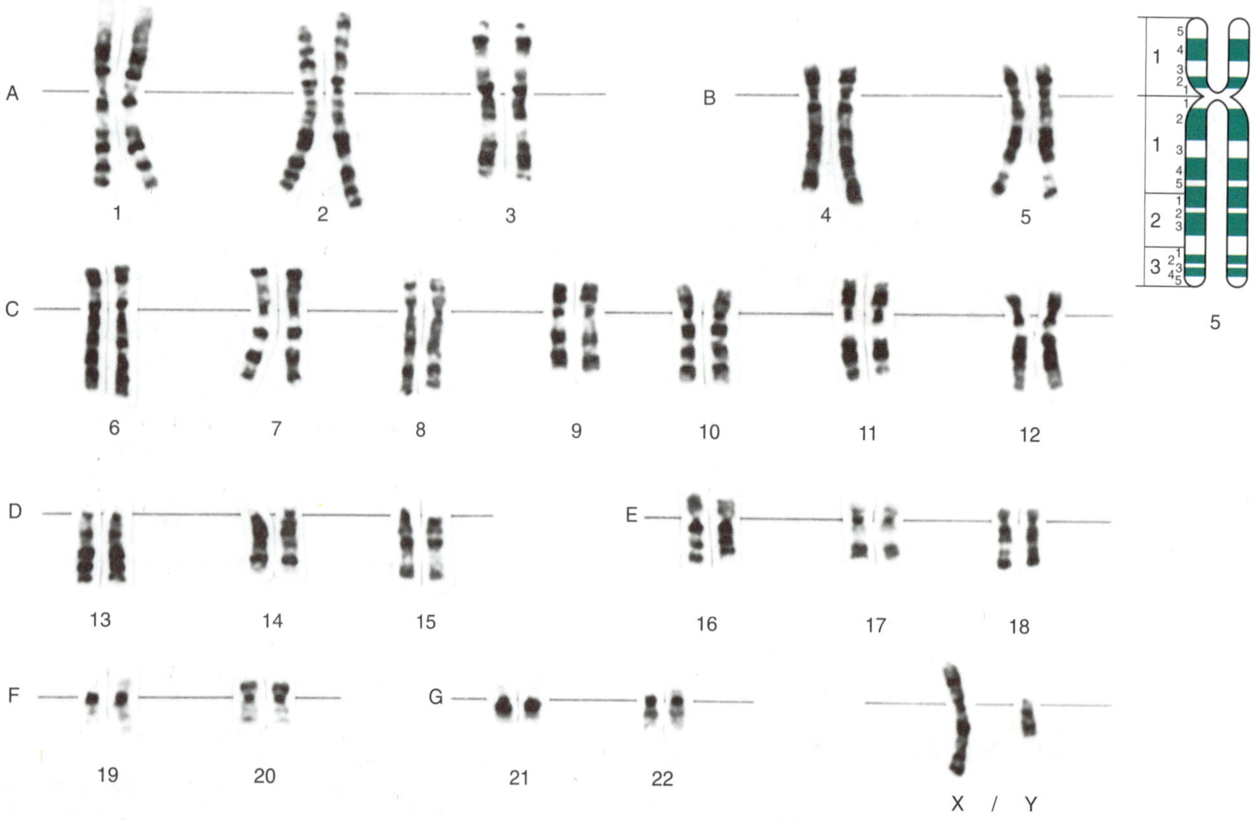

Figure 7–11

Normal male karyotype with G banding. (Courtesy of Dr. Nancy R. Schneider, Department of Pathology, University of Texas Southwestern Medical School, Dallas, Texas.) Also shown is chromosome 5 in mid-metaphase with G banding to indicate the nomenclature of arms, regions, and bands. Clear areas are negative or pale-staining, G bands, and green areas are positive G bands.

outward, and within each region the bands are numerically ordered (see Fig. 7–11). Thus, 2q34 indicates chromosome 2, long arm, region 3, band 4. The patterns of chromosomal rearrangement after breakage (Fig. 7–12) are as follows:

- *Translocation* implies transfer of a part of one chromosome to another chromosome. The process is usually reciprocal (i.e., fragments are exchanged between two chromosomes). In genetic shorthand, translocations are indicated by *t* followed by the involved chromosomes in numeric order, for example, *46,XX,t(2;5)(q31;p14)*. This would indicate a reciprocal translocation involving the long arm (q) of chromosome 2 at region 3, band 1, and the short arm of chromosome 5, region 1, band 4. When the entire broken fragments are exchanged, the resulting balanced reciprocal translocation (Fig. 7–12) is not harmful to the carrier, who has the normal number of chromosomes and the full complement of genetic material. However, during gametogenesis, abnormal (unbalanced) gametes are formed, resulting in abnormal zygotes. A special pattern of translocation involving two acrocentric chromosomes is called *centric fusion type,* or *robertsonian,* translocation. Typically, the breaks occur close to the centromere, affecting the short arms of both chromosomes. Transfer of the segments leads to one very large chromosome and one extremely small one (see Fig. 7–12). The short fragments are lost, and the carrier has 45 chromosomes. Because the short arms of all acrocentric chromosomes carry highly redundant genes (e.g., ribosomal RNA genes), such loss is compatible with survival. However, difficulties arise during gametogenesis, resulting in the formation of unbalanced gametes that could lead to abnormal offspring.
- *Isochromosomes* result when the centromere divides horizontally rather than vertically. One of the two arms of the chromosome is then lost, and the remaining arm is duplicated, resulting in a chromosome with two short arms only or two long arms only. The most common isochromosome present in live births involves the long arm of the X chromosome and is designated *i(Xq)*. When fertilization occurs by a gamete that contains a normal X chromosome, there is monosomy for genes on Xp and trisomy for genes on Xq.
- *Deletion* involves loss of a portion of a chromosome. A single break may delete a terminal segment. Two interstitial breaks, with reunion of the proximal and distal segments, may result in loss of an intermediate segment. The isolated fragment, which lacks a centromere, almost never survives, and thus many genes are lost.
- *Inversions* occur when there are two interstitial breaks in a chromosome, and the segment reunites after a complete turnaround.
- A *ring chromosome* is a variant of a deletion. After loss of segments from each end of the chromosome, the arms unite to form a ring.

Against this background, we can turn first to some general features of chromosomal disorders, followed by some specific examples of diseases involving changes in the karyotype.

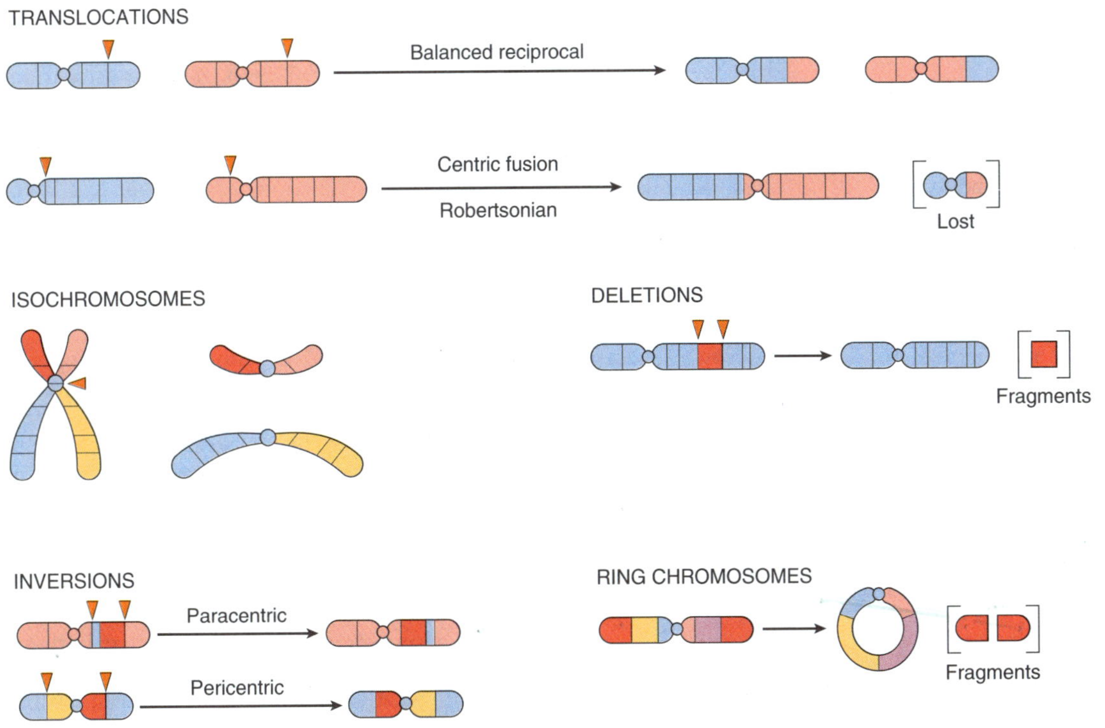

Figure 7–12

Types of chromosomal rearrangements.

- Chromosomal disorders may be associated with absence (deletion, monosomy), excess (trisomy), or abnormal rearrangements (translocations) of chromosomes.
- In general, loss of chromosomal material produces more severe defects than does gain of chromosomal material.
- Excess chromosomal material may result from a complete chromosome (as in trisomy) or from part of a chromosome (as in robertsonian translocation).
- Imbalances of sex chromosomes (excess or loss) are tolerated much better than are similar imbalances of autosomes.
- Sex chromosomal disorders often produce subtle abnormalities, sometimes not detected at birth. Infertility, a common manifestation, cannot be diagnosed until adolescence.
- In most cases, chromosomal disorders result from de novo changes (i.e., parents are normal, and risk of recurrence in siblings is low). An uncommon but important exception to this principle is exhibited by the translocation form of Down syndrome.

Cytogenetic Disorders Involving Autosomes

Three autosomal trisomies (21, 18, and 13) and one deletion syndrome (cri du chat syndrome), which results from partial deletion of the short arm of chromosome 5, were the first chromosomal abnormalities identified. More recently, several additional trisomies and deletion syndromes (such as that affecting 22q) have been described. Most of these disorders are quite uncommon, but their clinical features should permit ready recognition (Fig. 7–13).

Only trisomy 21 and 22q11.2 deletion occur with sufficient frequency to merit further consideration.

Trisomy 21 (Down Syndrome)

Down syndrome is the most common of the chromosomal disorders. About 95% of affected persons have trisomy 21, so their chromosome count is 47. As mentioned earlier, the most common cause of trisomy, and therefore of Down syndrome, is meiotic nondisjunction. The parents of such children have a normal karyotype and are normal in all respects. *Maternal age has a strong influence* on the incidence of Down syndrome. It occurs in 1 in 1550 live births in women younger than 20 years, in contrast to 1 in 25 live births in women older than 45 years. The correlation with maternal age suggests that in most cases the meiotic nondisjunction of chromosome 21 occurs in the ovum. Indeed, in 95% of cases the extra chromosome is of maternal origin. The reason for the increased susceptibility of the ovum to nondisjunction is not fully understood. No effect of paternal age has been found in those cases in which the extra chromosome is derived from the father.

In about 4% of all patients with trisomy 21, the extra chromosomal material is present not as an extra chromosome but as a translocation of the long arm of chromosome 21 to chromosome 22 or 14. Such cases are frequently (but not always) familial, and the translocated chromosome is inherited from one of the parents, who is most frequently a carrier of a robertsonian translocation. Approximately 1% of trisomy 21 patients are mosaics, usually having a mixture of 46- and 47-chromosome cells. These result from mitotic nondisjunction of chromosome 21 during an early stage of embryogenesis. Symptoms in such cases are variable and milder, depending on the proportion of abnormal cells.

Characteristic clinical features of Down syndrome include *epicanthic folds* and *flat facial profile* (see Fig. 7–13). Trisomy 21 is a leading cause of *mental retardation.* The degree of mental retardation is severe: IQ varies from 25 to 50. Congenital malformations are common and quite disabling. Approximately 40% of patients with trisomy 21 have *cardiac malformations,* which are responsible for most of the deaths in early childhood. *Serious infections* are another important cause of morbidity and mortality. As with most other clinical features, the basis of increased susceptibility to infection is not clearly understood. The chromosomal imbalance, in some undefined manner, also *increases the person's risk of developing acute leukemias,* particularly acute megakaryocytic leukemia.

The overall prognosis for individuals with Down syndrome has improved remarkably in the recent past as a result of better control of infections. Currently, the median age at death is 47 years. Most of those who survive into middle age develop histologic, metabolic, and neurochemical changes of Alzheimer disease (Chapter 24). Many develop frank dementia. The basis of this association is being actively investigated, with the hope of finding clues to the pathogenesis of Alzheimer disease.

Although the karyotype of Down syndrome has been known for decades, the molecular basis of this disease remains elusive. Data from the human genome project indicate that chromosome 21 carries approximately 300 genes. By molecular analysis of the translocation variants of Down syndrome, a 5-megabase region has been identified as the Down Syndrome Critical Region. Recent studies point a finger toward two genes within this region that regulate the function of NFAT (nuclear factor of activated T cells), a pleiotropic transcription factor that regulates many target genes in the developmental pathways.

Chromosome 22q11.2 Deletion Syndrome

Chromosome 22q11.2 syndrome encompasses a spectrum of disorders that result from a small interstitial deletion of band 11 on the long arm of chromosome 22. The clinical features of this deletion include congenital heart disease affecting the outflow tracts, abnormalities of the palate, facial dysmorphism, developmental delay, thymic hypoplasia with impaired T-cell immunity, and parathyroid hypoplasia causing hypocalcemia. Previously, these clinical features were believed to represent two different disorders: *DiGeorge syndrome* and *velocardiofacial syndrome.* However, it is now known that both are caused by 22q11.2 deletion. It is thought that variations in the size and position of the deletion is responsible for the variable clinical manifestations. When T-cell immunodeficiency and hypocalcemia are the dominant features, the patients are said to have *DiGeorge syndrome,* whereas

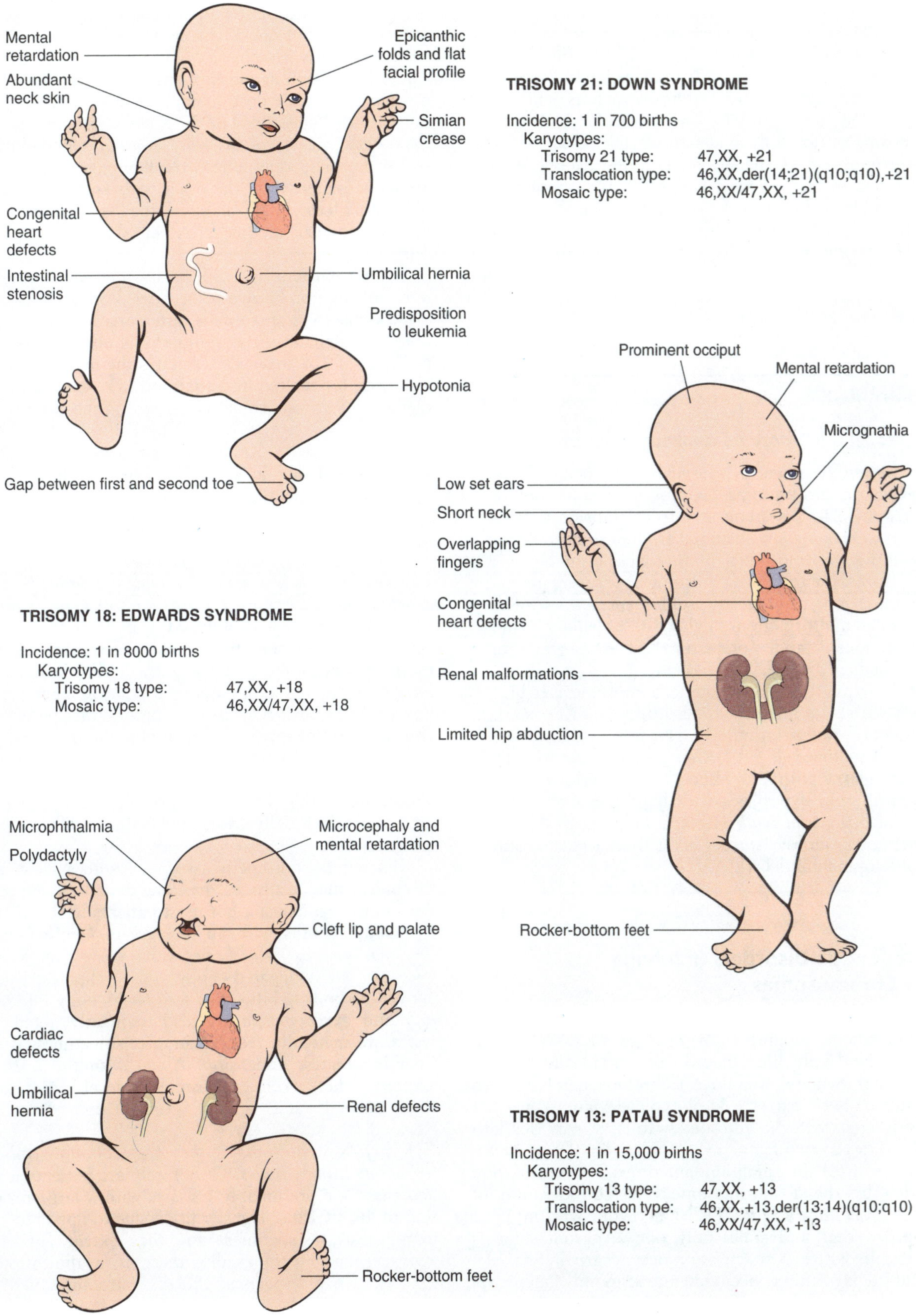

Figure 7–13

Clinical features and karyotypes of the three most common autosomal trisomies.

patients with the so-called *velocardiofacial syndrome* have mild immunodeficiency with pronounced dysmorphology and cardiac defects. In addition to these malformations, patients with 22q11.2 deletion are at a particularly high risk for psychoses such as schizophrenia and bipolar disorders. The molecular basis of this syndrome is not fully understood. The affected region of chromosome 11 encodes many genes. Among these, a transcription factor gene called *TBX1* is suspected to be responsible, since its loss seems to correlate with the occurrence of DiGeorge syndrome.

The diagnosis of this condition may be suspected on clinical grounds but can be established only by detection of the deletion by fluorescence in situ hybridization (FISH) (see Fig. 7–38B).

SUMMARY

Cytogenetic Disorders Involving Autosomes

- *Down syndrome* is caused by an extra copy of genes on chromosome 21, most commonly due to trisomy 21, less frequently from translocation of extra chromosomal material from chromosome 21 to other chromosomes or from mosaicism.
- Patients with Down syndrome have severe mental retardation, flat facial profile, epicanthic folds, cardiac malformations, higher risk of leukemia and infections, and premature development of Alzheimer disease.
- Deletion of genes from chromosome 22q11.2 gives rise to malformations affecting face, heart, thymus, and parathyroids. The resulting disorders are recognized as (1) *DiGeorge syndrome* (thymic hypoplasia with diminished T-cell immunity and parathyroid hypoplasia with hypocalcemia) or (2) *velocardiofacial syndrome* (congenital heart disease affecting outflow tracts, facial dysmorphism, and developmental delay).

Cytogenetic Disorders Involving Sex Chromosomes

A number of abnormal karyotypes involving the sex chromosomes, ranging from 45,X to 49,XXXXY, are compatible with life. Indeed, phenotypically normal males with two and even three Y chromosomes have been identified. Such extreme karyotypic deviations are not encountered with the autosomes. In large part this latitude relates to two factors: (1) lyonization of X chromosomes and (2) the small amount of genetic information carried by the Y chromosome. The consideration of lyonization must begin with Mary Lyon, who in 1962 proposed that in females only one X chromosome is genetically active. X inactivation occurs early in fetal life, about 16 days after conception, and randomly inactivates either the paternal or the maternal X chromosome in each of the primitive cells representing the developing embryo. Once inactivated, the same X chromosome remains genetically neutralized in all of the progeny of these cells. Moreover, all but one X chromosome is inactivated, and so a 48,XXXX female has only one active X chromosome. This phenomenon explains why normal females do not have a double dose (compared with males) of phenotypic attributes coded by the X chromosome. The Lyon hypothesis also explains why normal females are in reality mosaics, containing two cell populations: one with an active maternal X, the other with an active paternal X. Although essentially accurate, the Lyon hypothesis has been somewhat modified, as we shall discuss under Turner syndrome.

Extra Y chromosomes are readily tolerated because the only information known to be carried on the Y chromosome seems to relate to male differentiation. It should be noted that whatever the number of X chromosomes, the presence of a Y invariably dictates the male phenotype. The gene for male differentiation (*SRY*, sex-determining region of Y chromosome) is located on the short arm of the Y.

Two disorders—Klinefelter syndrome and Turner syndrome—arising in aberrations of sex chromosomes are described briefly.

Klinefelter Syndrome

This syndrome is best defined as male hypogonadism that develops when there are at least two X chromosomes and one or more Y chromosomes. Most patients are 47,XXY. This karyotype results from nondisjunction of sex chromosomes during meiosis. The extra X chromosome may be of either maternal or paternal origin. Advanced maternal age and a history of irradiation of either parent may contribute to the meiotic error resulting in this condition. Approximately 15% of patients show mosaic patterns, including 46,XY/47,XXY, 47,XXY/48,XXXY, and variations on this theme. The presence of a 46,XY line in mosaics is usually associated with a milder clinical condition.

Klinefelter syndrome is associated with a wide range of clinical manifestations. In some it may be expressed only as hypogonadism, but most patients have a distinctive body habitus with an *increase in length between the soles and the pubic bone,* which creates the appearance of an elongated body. Also characteristic is eunuchoid body habitus. *Reduced facial, body, and pubic hair* and *gynecomastia* are also frequently noted. The testes are markedly reduced in size, sometimes to only 2 cm in greatest dimension. Along with the *testicular atrophy,* the serum testosterone levels are lower than normal, and urinary gonadotropin levels are elevated.

Klinefelter syndrome is the most common cause of hypogonadism in males. Only rarely are patients fertile, and these are presumably mosaics with a large proportion of 46,XY cells. The sterility is due to impaired spermatogenesis, sometimes to the extent of total azoospermia. Histologically, there is hyalinization of tubules, which appear as ghostlike structures in tissue section. By contrast, Leydig cells are prominent, as a result of either hyperplasia or an apparent increase related to loss of tubules. Although Klinefelter syndrome

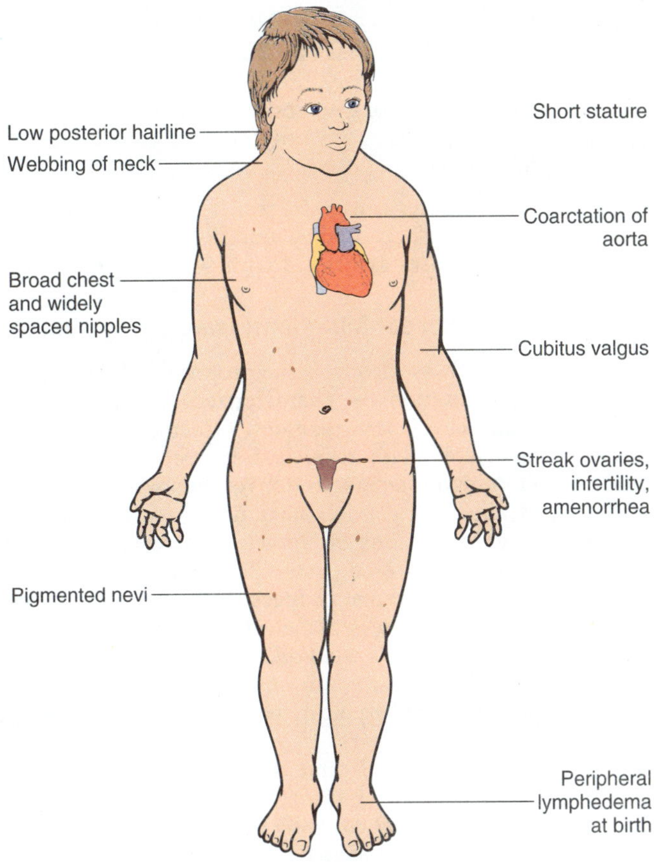

TURNER SYNDROME

Incidence: 1 in 3000 female births

Karyotypes:	
Classic:	45,X
Defective second X chromosome:	46,X,i(Xq)
	46,XXq–
	46,XXp–
	46,X, r(X)
Mosaic type:	45,X/46,XX

Figure 7–14

Clinical features and karyotypes of Turner syndrome.

may be associated with mental retardation, the degree of intellectual impairment is typically mild and in some cases is undetectable. The reduction in intelligence is correlated with the number of extra X chromosomes. Patients with Klinefelter syndrome have several associated disorders, such as breast cancer (20 times more common than in normal males), extragonadal germ cell tumors, and autoimmune diseases such as systemic lupus erythematosus.

Turner Syndrome

Turner syndrome, characterized by primary hypogonadism in phenotypic females, results from partial or complete monosomy of the short arm of the X chromosome. With routine cytogenetic methods, the entire X chromosome is missing in 57% of patients, resulting in a 45,X karyotype. These patients are the most severely affected, and the diagnosis can often be made at birth or early in childhood. Typical clinical features associated with 45,X Turner syndrome include significant growth retardation, leading to abnormally short stature (below third percentile); swelling of the nape of the neck due to distended lymphatic channels (in infancy) that is seen as webbing of the neck in older children; low posterior hairline; cubitus valgus (an increase in the carrying angle of the arms); shieldlike chest with widely spaced nipples; high-arched palate; lymphedema of the hands and feet; and a variety of congenital malformations such as horseshoe kidney, bicuspid aortic valve, and coarctation of the aorta (Fig. 7–14). Cardiovascular abnormalities are the most common cause of death in childhood. In adolescence, affected girls fail to develop normal secondary sex characteristics; the genitalia remain infantile, breast development is minimal, and little pubic hair appears. Most have primary amenorrhea, and morphologic examination reveals transformation of the ovaries into white streaks of fibrous stroma devoid of follicles. The mental status of these patients is usually normal, but subtle defects in nonverbal, visual-spatial information processing have been noted. Curiously, hypothyroidism caused by autoantibodies occurs especially in women with isochromosome Xp. As many as 50% of these develop clinical hypothyroidism. In adult patients, *a combination of short stature and primary amenorrhea should prompt strong suspicion of Turner syndrome*. The diagnosis is established by karyotyping.

Approximately 43% of patients with Turner syndrome either are mosaics (one of the cell lines being 45,X) or have structural abnormalities of the X chromosome. The most common is deletion of the small arm, resulting in the formation of an isochromosome of the long arm,

46,X,i(X)(q10). The net effect of the associated structural abnormalities is to produce partial monosomy of the X chromosome. Combinations of deletions and mosaicism are reported. It is important to appreciate the karyotypic heterogeneity associated with Turner syndrome because it is responsible for significant variations in the phenotype. In contrast to the patients with monosomy X, *those who are mosaics or have deletion variants may have an almost normal appearance and may present only with primary amenorrhea.*

It is pertinent to recall the Lyon hypothesis in the context of Turner syndrome. If only one active X chromosome were necessary for the development of normal females (as proposed in the Lyon hypothesis), patients with partial or complete loss of one X chromosome would not be expected to display the stigmata of Turner syndrome. In view of this inconsistency and other observations, the Lyon hypothesis has been modified. It is now known that although one X chromosome is inactivated in all cells during embryogenesis, it is selectively reactivated in germ cells before the first meiotic division. Furthermore, it seems that certain X chromosome genes remain active on both X chromosomes in many somatic cells of normal females. Thus, it seems that two copies of some X-linked genes are essential for normal gametogenesis and somatic development. Some of these genes are beginning to be identified. For example, a homeobox gene aptly called short-stature homeobox (*SHOX*), located on Xp22.33, seems to be involved in vertical growth. This is one of the genes that remain active on both copies of the X chromosome. Homologues of the *SHOX* gene are also found on the Y chromosome, ensuring that males with only one copy of the X chromosome develop normally.

SUMMARY

Cytogenetic Disorders Involving Sex Chromosomes

- In females one X chromosome, maternal or paternal, is randomly inactivated during development (Lyon hypothesis), and hence women carry two populations of cells (mosaics).
- In *Klinefelter syndrome* there are two or more X chromosomes with one Y chromosome as a result of nondisjunction of sex chromosomes. Patients have testicular atrophy, sterility, reduced body hair, gynecomastia, and eunuchoid body habitus. It is the most common cause of male sterility.
- In *Turner syndrome* there is partial or complete monosomy of genes on the short arm of the X chromosome, most commonly due to absence of one X chromosome (45X) and less commonly from mosaicism, or from deletions involving the short arm of the X chromosome. Short stature, webbing of the neck, cubitus valgus, cardiovascular malformations, amenorrhea, lack of secondary sex characteristics, and fibrotic ovaries are typical clinical features.

SINGLE-GENE DISORDERS WITH ATYPICAL PATTERNS OF INHERITANCE

Three groups of diseases resulting from mutations affecting single genes do not follow the mendelian rules of inheritance:

- Diseases caused by triplet-repeat mutations
- Diseases caused by mutations in mitochondrial genes
- Diseases associated with genomic imprinting.

Triplet-Repeat Mutations: Fragile X Syndrome

Fragile X syndrome is the prototype of diseases in which the mutation is characterized by a long repeating sequence of 3 nucleotides. Other examples of diseases associated with trinucleotide repeat mutations include Huntington disease and myotonic dystrophy. The origins of about 40 diseases have now been assigned to pathologic expansions of trinucleotide repeats, and all disorders discovered so far are associated with neurodegenerative changes. In each of these conditions, *amplification of specific sets of 3 nucleotides within the gene disrupts its function.* Certain unique features of trinucleotide-repeat mutations, described later, are responsible for the atypical pattern of inheritance of the associated diseases.

Fragile X syndrome is characterized by mental retardation and an abnormality in the X chromosome. *It is one of the most common causes of familial mental retardation.* The cytogenetic alteration, referred to as Fragile X, is induced by certain culture conditions and is seen as a *discontinuity of staining or constriction in the long arm of the X chromosome.* Clinically affected males have moderate to severe mental retardation. They express a characteristic physical phenotype that includes a long face with a large mandible, large everted ears, and large testicles (*macro-orchidism*). Although characteristic of fragile X syndrome, these abnormalities are not always present or may be quite subtle. The only distinctive physical abnormality that can be detected in at least 90% of postpubertal males with fragile X syndrome is macro-orchidism.

Fragile X syndrome results from a mutation in the *FMR1* gene, which maps to Xq27.3. Like all X-linked recessive disorders, this disease affects males. However, unlike patients with other X-linked recessive disorders, approximately 20% of males who are known to carry the fragile X mutation may be clinically and cytogenetically normal. These "carrier males" can transmit the disease to their grandsons through their phenotypically normal daughters. Another peculiarity is the presence of mental retardation in 50% of carrier females. These unusual features have been related to the dynamic nature of the mutation (Fig. 7–15). In the normal population, the number of CGG repeats in the *FMR1* gene is small, averaging around 29, whereas affected individuals have 200 to 4000 repeats. These so-called full mutations are believed to arise through an intermediate stage of *premutations* characterized by 52 to 200 CGG repeats. Carrier males and females have premutations. During oogenesis (but not spermatogenesis) the premutations can

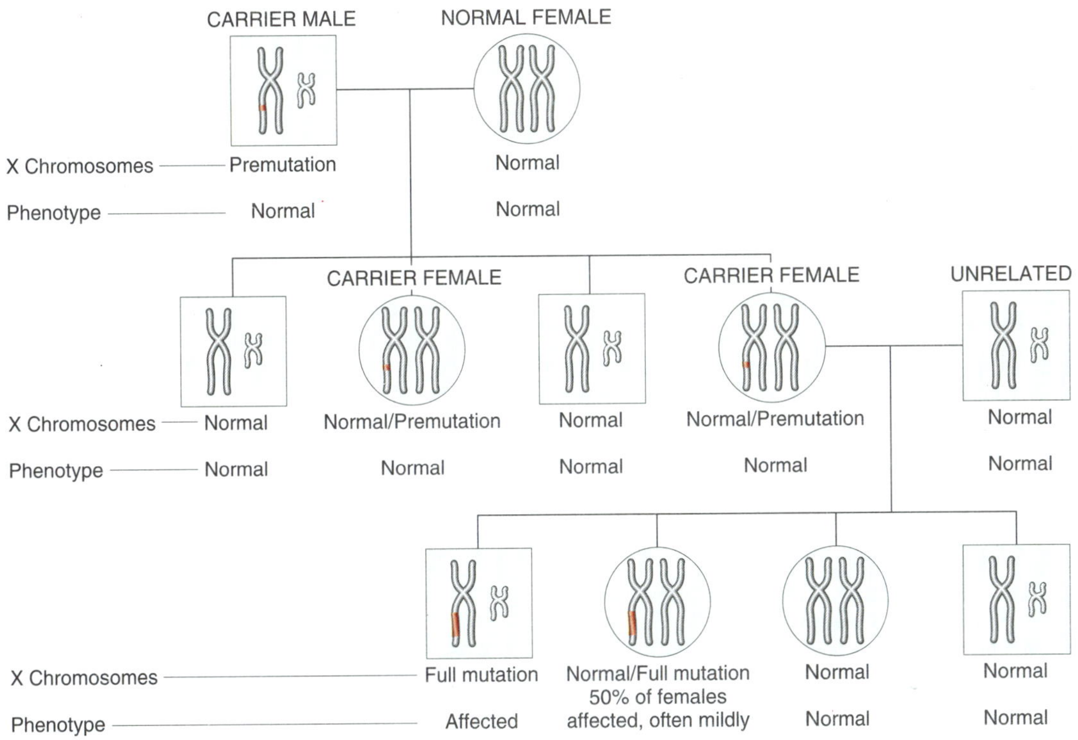

Figure 7–15

Fragile X pedigree. Note that in the first generation, all sons are normal and all females are carriers. During oogenesis in the carrier female, premutation expands to full mutation; hence, in the next generation, all males who inherit the X with full mutation are affected. However, only 50% of females who inherit the full mutation are affected, and often only mildly. (Based on an original sketch courtesy of Dr. Nancy Schneider, Department of Pathology, University of Texas Southwestern Medical School, Dallas, Texas.)

be converted to full mutations by further amplification of the CGG repeats, which can then be transmitted to both the sons and the daughters of the carrier female. These observations provide an explanation for why some carrier males are unaffected (they have premutations), and certain carrier females are affected (they inherit full mutations). Recent studies indicate that premutations are not so benign after all. *Approximately 30% of females carrying the premutation have premature ovarian failure (before the age of 40 years), and about one-third of premutation-carrying males exhibit a progressive neurodegenerative syndrome starting in their sixth decade.* This syndrome, referred to as fragile X–associated tremor/ataxia, is characterized by intention tremors and cerebellar ataxia and may progress to parkinsonism. However it is clear that the abnormalities in permutation carriers are milder and occur later in life.

The molecular basis of fragile X syndrome is beginning to be understood. The CGG repeats are located in the 5′ untranslated region of the *FMR1* gene (Fig. 7–16). In patients with this disease, the expanded CGG repeats are hypermethylated. Methylation then extends upstream into the promoter region, resulting in transcriptional silencing of the *FMR1* gene. The product of the *FMR1* gene, called FMR protein (FMRP), is widely expressed in normal tissues, but higher levels of tran-

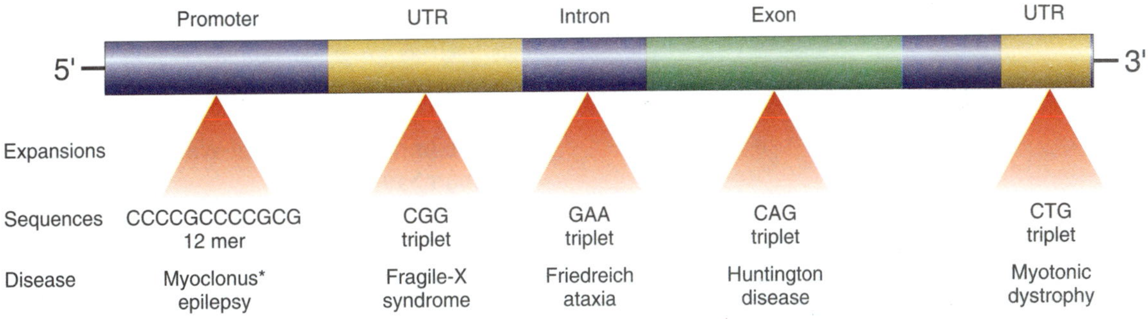

Figure 7–16

Sites of expansion and the affected sequence in selected diseases caused by nucleotide repeat mutations. UTR, untranslated region.

scripts are found in the brain and the testis. Current evidence suggests that FMRP is an RNA-binding protein that is transported from the cytoplasm to the nucleus, where it binds specific mRNAs and transports them to the axons and dendrites (Fig. 7–17). It is in the synapses that FMRP-mRNA complexes perform critical roles in regulating the translation of specific mRNAs. The absence of this finely coordinated "shuttle" function seems to underlie the causation of fragile X syndrome.

Before closing this discussion, it is appropriate to offer some general comments on other neurodegenerative diseases related to trinucleotide-repeat expansions.

- In all cases, gene functions are altered by an expansion of the repeats, but the precise threshold at which premutations are converted to full mutations differs with each disorder.
- While the expansion in fragile X syndrome occurs during oogenesis, in other disorders such as Huntington disease, premutations are converted to full mutations during spermatogenesis.
- The expansion may involve any part of the gene and can be grouped into two broad categories, those that affect untranslated regions (as in fragile X syndrome) or coding regions (as in Huntington disease). When mutations affect noncoding regions, there is "loss of function," since protein synthesis is suppressed (e.g., FMRP). By contrast, mutations involving translated parts of the gene give rise to abnormal proteins that interfere with function of normal proteins (e.g., Huntington disease). Many of these so-called gain-of-function mutations involve CAG repeats that encode polyglutamine tracts, and the resultant diseases are sometimes referred to as "polyglutamine diseases," affecting primarily the nervous system. Accumulation of mutant proteins in aggregates within the cytoplasm is a common feature of these diseases.

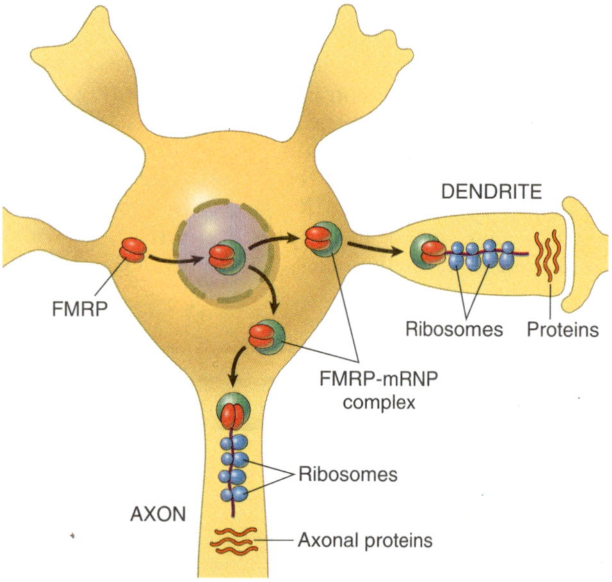

Figure 7–17

A model for the action of familial mental retardation protein (FMRP) in neurons. (Adapted from Hin P, Warren ST: New insights into fragile X syndrome: from molecules to neurobehavior. Trends Biochem Sci 28:152, 2003.)

SUMMARY

Fragile X Syndrome

- Pathologic amplification of trinucleotide repeats causes loss-of-function (fragile X syndrome) or gain-of-function mutations (Huntington disease). Most such mutations produce neurodegenerative disorders.
- Fragile X syndrome results from loss of *FMR1* gene function and is characterized by mental retardation, macro-orchidism, and abnormal facial features.
- In the normal population there are about 29 CGG repeats in the *FMR1* gene. Carrier males and females carry permutations with 52 to 200 CGG repeats that can expand to 4000 repeats (full mutations) during oogenesis. When full mutations are transmitted to progeny, fragile X syndrome occurs.

Diseases Caused By Mutations in Mitochondrial Genes

Mitochondria contain several genes that encode enzymes involved in oxidative phosphorylation. Inheritance of mitochondrial DNA differs from that of nuclear DNA in that the former is associated with *maternal inheritance.* The reason for this peculiarity is that ova contain mitochondria within their abundant cytoplasm, whereas spermatozoa contain few, if any, mitochondria. Hence, the mitochondrial DNA complement of the zygote is derived entirely from the ovum. Thus, mothers transmit mitochondrial genes to all of their offspring, both male and female; however, daughters but not sons transmit the DNA further to their progeny.

Diseases caused by mutations in mitochondrial genes are rare. Because mitochondrial DNA encodes enzymes involved in oxidative phosphorylation, diseases caused by mutations in such genes affect organs most dependent on oxidative phosphorylation (skeletal muscle, heart, brain). Leber hereditary optic neuropathy is the prototypical disorder in this group. This neurodegenerative disease manifests itself as progressive bilateral loss of central vision that leads in due course to blindness.

Genomic Imprinting: Prader-Willi and Angelman Syndromes

All humans inherit two copies of each gene, carried on homologous maternal and paternal chromosomes. It has usually been assumed that there is no difference between normal homologous genes derived from the mother or the father. Indeed, this is true for many genes. However, it has now been established that with respect to some genes, functional differences exist between the paternal and the maternal genes. These differences arise from an epigenetic process called *genomic imprinting,* whereby certain genes are differentially "inactivated" during paternal and maternal gametogenesis. Thus, *maternal imprinting* refers to transcriptional silencing of the maternal allele, whereas *paternal imprinting* implies that the paternal allele is inactivated. Imprinting occurs in ovum or sperm and is then stably transmitted to all somatic cells derived from the zygote.

Genomic imprinting is best illustrated by considering two uncommon genetic disorders: Prader-Willi syndrome and Angelman syndrome.

Prader-Willi syndrome is characterized by mental retardation, short stature, hypotonia, obesity, small hands and feet, and hypogonadism. In 60% to 75% of cases, an interstitial deletion of band q12 in the long arm of chromosome 15 [i.e., del(15)(q11;q13)] can be detected. In many patients without a detectable cytogenetic abnormality, FISH analysis reveals smaller deletions within the same region. *It is striking that in all cases the deletion affects the paternally derived chromosome 15.* In contrast with Prader-Willi syndrome, patients with the phenotypically distinct *Angelman syndrome* are born with a deletion of the same chromosomal region derived from their mothers. Patients with Angelman syndrome are also mentally retarded, but in addition they present with ataxic gait, seizures, and inappropriate laughter. Because of the laughter and ataxia, this syndrome is also called the *happy puppet syndrome.* A comparison of these two syndromes clearly demonstrates the "parent-of-origin" effects on gene function. If all the paternal and maternal genes contained within chromosome 15 were expressed in an identical fashion, clinical features resulting from these deletions would be expected to be identical regardless of the parental origin of chromosome 15.

The molecular basis of these two syndromes can be understood in the context of imprinting (Fig. 7–18). It is believed that a set of genes on maternal chromosome 15q12 is imprinted (and hence silenced), and thus the only functional alleles are provided by the paternal chromosome. When these are lost as a result of a deletion (in the paternal chromosome), the patient develops Prader-Willi syndrome. Conversely, a distinct gene that also maps to the same region of chromosome 15 is imprinted on the paternal chromosome. Only the maternally derived allele of the gene is normally active. Deletion of this maternal gene on chromosome 15 gives rise to the Angelman syndrome. Molecular studies of cytogenetically normal patients with Prader-Willi syndrome have revealed that in some cases both of the structurally normal chromosome 15s are derived from the mother. Inheritance of both chromosomes of a pair from one parent is called uniparental disomy. The net effect is the same (i.e., the patient does not have a functional set of genes from the [nonimprinted] paternal chromosome 15). Angelman syndrome, as might be expected, can also result from uniparental disomy of parental chromosome 15.

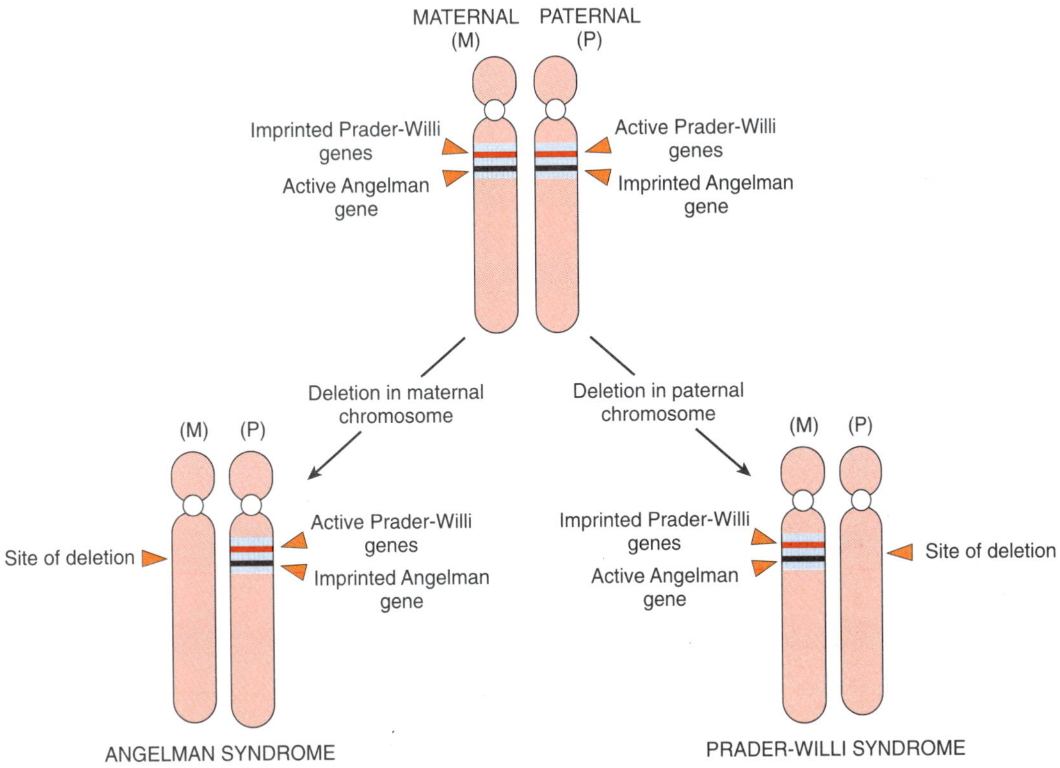

Figure 7–18

Genetics of Angelman and Prader-Willi syndromes.

The Angelman syndrome gene (imprinted on paternal chromosome) is now known to encode a ligase that has a role in the ubiquitin-proteasome proteolytic pathway (Chapter 1). This gene, called, somewhat laboriously, *UBE3A*, is expressed primarily from the maternal allele in specific regions of the normal brain. In Angelman syndrome, *UBE3A* is not expressed in these areas of the brain—hence the neurologic disorder. Prader-Willi syndrome, unlike Angelman syndrome, is most likely caused by the loss of several genes located between 15q11 and q13. These genes are still being fully characterized.

SUMMARY

Genomic Imprinting

- Imprinting involves transcriptional silencing of the paternal or maternal copies of certain genes during gametogenesis. For such genes only one functional copy exists in the individual. Loss of the functional allele (not imprinted) by deletions gives rise to diseases.
- *Prader-Willi syndrome* results from deletion of paternal chromosome 15q12 and is characterized by mental retardation, short stature, hypotonia, obesity, and hypogonadism.
- *Angelman syndrome* results from deletion of maternal chromosome 15q12 and is characterized by mental retardation, ataxia, seizures, and inappropriate laughter.

PEDIATRIC DISEASES

As mentioned earlier and illustrated by several examples, many diseases of infancy and childhood are of genetic origin. Others, though not genetic, either are unique to children or take distinctive forms in this stage of life and so merit the designation *pediatric diseases*. During each stage of development, infants and children are prey to a somewhat different group of diseases (Table 7–8). Clearly, diseases of infancy (i.e., the first year of life) pose the highest risk of mortality. During this phase, the neonatal period (the first 4 weeks of life) is unquestionably the most hazardous time.

Once the infant survives the first year of life, the outlook brightens considerably. However, it is sobering to note that between 1 year and 15 years of age, injuries

Table 7–8 Causes of Death by Age

Causes*	Rate†
Under 1 Year: All Causes	**727.4**
Congenital malformations, deformations, and chromosomal anomalies	
Disorders related to short gestation and low birth weight	
Sudden infant death syndrome (SIDS)	
Newborn affected by maternal complications of pregnancy	
Newborn affected by complications of placenta, cord, and membranes	
Respiratory distress of newborn	
Accidents (unintentional injuries)	
Bacterial sepsis of newborn	
Intrauterine hypoxia and birth asphyxia	
Diseases of the circulatory system	
All other causes	
1–4 Years: All Causes	**32.6**
Accidents and adverse effects	
Congenital malformations, deformations, chromosomal abnormalities	
Malignant neoplasms	
Homicide and legal intervention	
Disease of the heart‡	
Influenza and pneumonia	
5–14 Years: All Causes	**18.5**
Accidents and adverse effects	
Malignant neoplasms	
Homicide and legal intervention	
Congenital malformations, deformations, chromosomal abnormalities	
Suicide	
Diseases of the heart	
15–24 Years: All Causes	**80.7**
Accident and adverse effects	
Homicide	
Suicide	
Malignant neoplasms	
Diseases of the heart	

*Causes are listed in decreasing order of frequency.
†Rates are expressed per 100,000 population.
‡Excludes congenital heart disease. All causes and rates are preliminary 2000 statistics.
From Minino AM, Smith BL: Deaths: Preliminary data for 2000. National Vital Statistics Report, 49:12, 2001.

resulting from accidents are the leading cause of death. Not all conditions listed in Table 7–8 are described in this chapter, but only a select few that are most common. Although general principles of neoplastic disease and specific tumors are discussed elsewhere, a few tumors of children are described here to highlight the differences between pediatric and adult neoplasms.

CONGENITAL ANOMALIES

Congenital anomalies are structural defects that are present at birth, although some, such as cardiac defects and renal anomalies, may not become clinically apparent until years later. As will be evident from the ensuing discussion, the term *congenital* does not imply or exclude a genetic basis for birth defects. It is estimated that about 3% of newborns have a major anomaly, defined as a birth defect having either cosmetic or functional significance. As indicated in Table 7–8, congenital anomalies are an important cause of infant mortality. Moreover, they continue to be a significant cause of illness, disability, and death throughout the early years of life.

Before the etiology and pathogenesis of congenital anomalies are described, it is essential to define some of the terms used to describe errors in morphogenesis.

- *Malformations* represent primary errors of morphogenesis. In other words, there is an *intrinsically abnormal developmental process*. Malformations are usually multifactorial rather than the result of a single gene or chromosomal defect. They may present in several patterns. In some, such as congenital heart diseases, single body systems may be involved, whereas in other cases, multiple malformations involving many organs and tissues may coexist (Fig. 7–19).
- *Disruptions* result from secondary destruction of an organ or body region that was previously normal in development; thus, in contrast to malformations, disruptions arise from an *extrinsic disturbance in morphogenesis. Amniotic bands,* denoting rupture of amnion with resultant formation of "bands" that encircle, compress, or attach to parts of the developing fetus, are the classic example of a disruption (Fig. 7–20). A variety of environmental agents may cause disruptions (see later). Understandably, disruptions are not heritable and hence are not associated with risk of recurrence in subsequent pregnancies.
- *Deformations,* like disruptions, also represent an *extrinsic disturbance of development* rather than an intrinsic error of morphogenesis. Deformations are common problems, affecting approximately 2% of newborn infants to various degrees. Fundamental to the pathogenesis of deformations is localized or generalized compression of the growing fetus by abnormal biomechanical forces, leading eventually to a variety of structural abnormalities. The most common cause of such deformations is uterine constraint. Between the 35th and 38th weeks of gestation, rapid increase in the size of the fetus outpaces the growth of the uterus, and the relative amount of amniotic fluid (which normally acts as a cushion) also decreases. Thus, even the normal fetus is subjected to some form of uterine constraint. However, several variables increase the likelihood of excessive compression of the fetus, including maternal conditions such as first pregnancy, small uterus, mal-

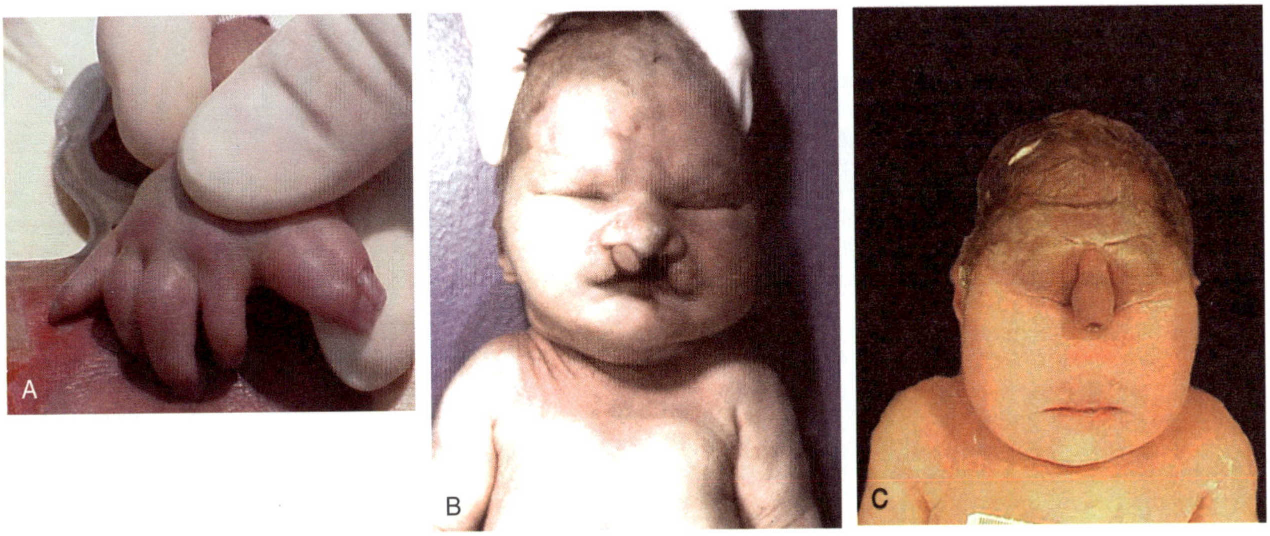

Figure 7–19

Human malformations can range in severity from the incidental to the lethal. **A,** *Polydactyly* (one or more extra digits) and *syndactyly* (fusion of digits), have little functional consequence when they occur in isolation. **B,** Similarly, *cleft lip,* with or without associated *cleft palate,* is compatible with life when it occurs as an isolated anomaly; in this case, however, the child had an underlying *malformation syndrome* (trisomy 13) and expired because of severe cardiac defects. **C,** Stillbirth representing a severe and essentially lethal malformation, in which the midface structures are fused or ill-formed; in almost all cases, this degree of external dysmorphogenesis is associated with severe internal anomalies such as maldevelopment of the brain and cardiac defects. (**A** and **C,** Courtesy of Dr. Reade Quinton. **B,** Courtesy of Dr. Beverly Rogers, Department of Pathology, University of Texas Southwestern Medical Center, Dallas, Texas.)

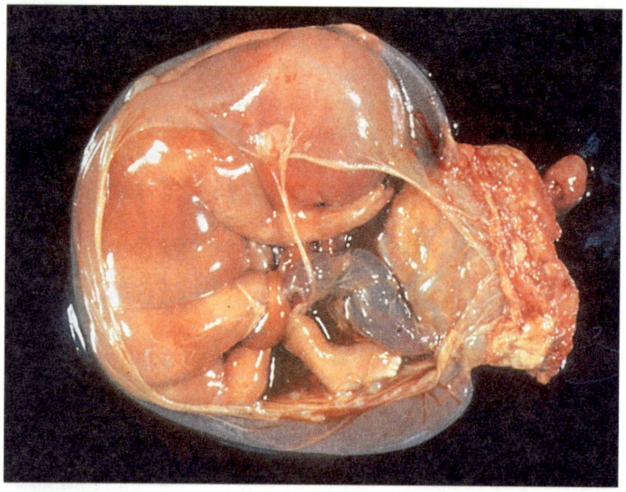

Figure 7–20

Disruptions occur in a normally developing organ because of an extrinsic abnormality that interferes with normal morphogenesis. *Amniotic bands* are a frequent cause of disruptions. In the illustrated example, note the placenta at the right of the diagram and the band of amnion extending from the top portion of the amniotic sac to encircle the leg of the fetus. (Courtesy of Dr. Theonia Boyd, Children's Hospital of Boston, Boston, Massachusetts.)

formed (bicornuate) uterus, and leiomyomas. Causes relating to the fetus, such as multiple fetuses, oligohydramnios, and abnormal fetal presentation, may also be involved.

- *Sequence* refers to multiple congenital anomalies that result from *secondary effects of a single localized aberration in organogenesis.* The initiating event may be a malformation, deformation, or disruption. An excellent example is the oligohydramnios (or Potter) sequence (Fig. 7–21A). Oligohydramnios, denoting decreased amniotic fluid, may be caused by a variety of unrelated maternal, placental, or fetal abnormalities. Chronic leakage of amniotic fluid due to rupture of the amnion, uteroplacental insufficiency resulting from maternal hypertension or severe toxemia, and renal agenesis in the fetus (because fetal urine is a major constituent of amniotic fluid) are all causes of oligohydramnios. The fetal compression associated with significant oligohydramnios in turn results in a classic phenotype in the newborn infant, including flattened facies and positional abnormalities of the hands and feet (Fig. 7–21B). The hips may be dislocated. Growth of the chest wall and the contained lungs is also compromised, sometimes to such an extent that survival is not possible. If the embryologic connection between these defects and the initiating event is not recognized, a sequence may be mistaken for a malformation syndrome.
- *Malformation syndrome* refers to the presence of several defects that cannot be explained on the basis of a single localizing initiating error in morphogenesis. Syndromes most often arise from a single causative condition (e.g., viral infection or a specific chromosomal abnormality) that simultaneously affects several tissues.

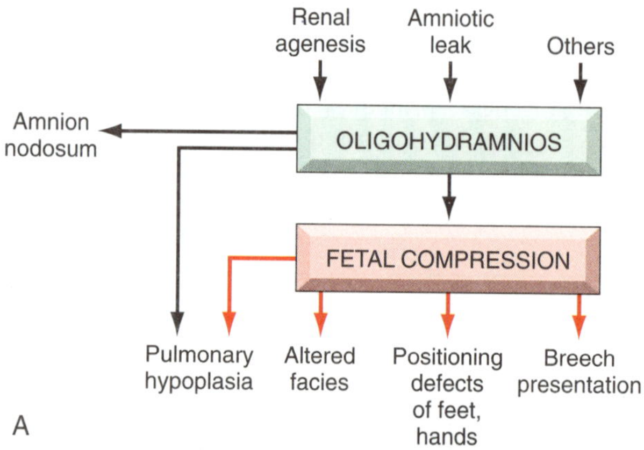

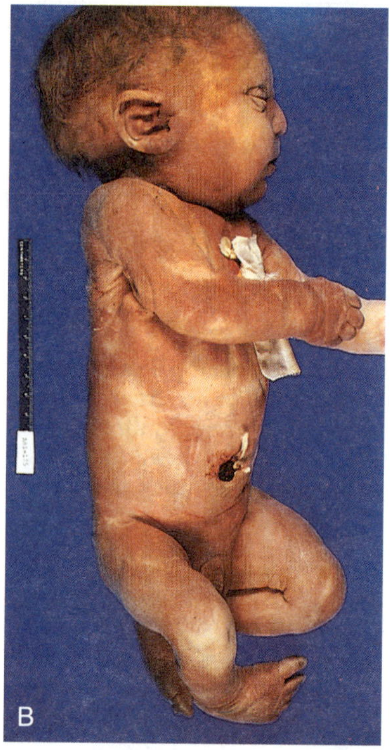

Figure 7–21

A, Pathogenesis of the oligohydramnios (Potter) sequence. **B,** Infant with oligohydramnios (Potter) sequence. Note flattened facial features and deformed foot (talipes equinovarus).

In addition to the global definitions listed previously, some general terms are applied to organ-specific malformations. *Agenesis* refers to the complete absence of an organ or its anlage, whereas *aplasia* and *hypoplasia* are used to indicate incomplete development or underdevelopment of an organ. *Atresia* describes the absence of an opening, usually of a hollow visceral organ or duct such as intestines and bile ducts.

Etiology. Known causes of errors in human malformations can be grouped into three major categories: *genetic, environmental,* and *multifactorial* (Table 7–9). *Almost half have no recognized cause.*

Genetic causes of malformations include all of the previously discussed mechanisms of genetic disease. Virtually all chromosomal syndromes are associated with congeni-

Table 7–9 Causes of Congenital Malformations in Humans

Cause	Malformed Live Births (%)
Genetic	
Chromosomal aberrations	10–15
Mendelian inheritance	2–10
Environmental	
Maternal/placental infections Rubella Toxoplasmosis Syphilis Cytomegalovirus infection Human immunodeficiency virus infection	2–3
Maternal disease states Diabetes Phenylketonuria Endocrinopathies	6–8
Drugs and chemicals Alcohol Folic acid antagonists Androgens Phenytoin Thalidomide Warfarin 13-*cis*-Retinoic acid Others	~1
Irradiation	~1
Multifactorial	**20–25**
Unknown	**40–60**

Adapted from Stevenson RE, et al. (eds): Human Malformations and Related Anomalies. New York, Oxford University Press, 1993, p 115.

tal malformations. Examples include Down syndrome and other trisomies, Turner syndrome, and Klinefelter syndrome. Most chromosomal disorders arise during gametogenesis and hence are not familial. Single-gene mutations, characterized by mendelian inheritance, may underlie major malformations. For example, holoprosencephaly is the most common developmental defect of the forebrain and midface in humans (see Chapter 23); mutations of *sonic hedgehog,* a gene involved in morphogenesis, have been reported in a subset of holoprosencephaly patients. Similarly, mutations of a downstream target of sonic hedgehog signaling, *GLI3,* have been reported in patients with anomalies of digits, either conjoined digits (*syndactyly*) or supernumerary digits (*polydactyly*).

Environmental influences, such as viral infections, drugs, and irradiation to which the mother was exposed during pregnancy, may cause fetal malformations (the appellation of "malformation" is loosely used in this context, since technically, these anomalies represent *disruptions*). Among the viral infections listed in Table 7–9, rubella was a major scourge of the 19th and early 20th centuries. Fortunately, maternal rubella and the resultant *rubella embryopathy* have been virtually eliminated in developed countries as a result of vaccination. A variety of drugs and chemicals have been suspected to be teratogenic, but perhaps less than 1% of congenital malformations are caused by these agents. The list includes thalidomide, alcohol, anticonvulsants, warfarin (oral anticoagulant), and 13-*cis*-retinoic acid, which is used in the treatment of severe acne. For example, *thalidomide,* once used as a tranquilizer in Europe and currently being considered for its anti-angiogenic properties, causes an extremely high incidence (50% to 80%) of limb malformations. *Alcohol,* perhaps the most widely used agent today, is an important environmental teratogen. Affected infants show prenatal and postnatal growth retardation, facial anomalies (microcephaly, short palpebral fissures, maxillary hypoplasia), and psychomotor disturbances. These in combination are labeled the *fetal alcohol syndrome.* While cigarette smoke-derived nicotine has not been convincingly demonstrated to be a teratogen, there is a high incidence of spontaneous abortions, premature labor, and placental abnormalities in pregnant smokers; babies born to mothers who smoke often have a low birth weight and may be prone to the sudden infant death syndrome. *In light of these findings, it is best to avoid nicotine exposure altogether during pregnancy.* Among maternal conditions listed in Table 7–9, *diabetes mellitus* is a common entity, and despite advances in antenatal obstetric monitoring and glucose control, the incidence of major malformations in infants of diabetic mothers stands between 6% and 10% in most series. Maternal hyperglycemia-induced fetal hyperinsulinemia results in fetal macrosomia (organomegaly and increased body fat and muscle mass); cardiac anomalies, neural tube defects, and other CNS malformations are some of the major anomalies seen in *diabetic embryopathy.*

Multifactorial inheritance, which implies the interaction of environmental influences with two or more genes of small effect, is the most common genetic cause of congenital malformations. Included in this category are some relatively common malformations such as cleft lip and palate and neural tube defects. The importance of environmental contributions to multifactorial inheritance is underscored by the dramatic reduction of the incidence of neural tube defects by periconceptional intake of folic acid in the diet. The recurrence risks and mode of transmission of multifactorial disorders were described earlier in this chapter.

Pathogenesis. The pathogenesis of congenital malformations is complex and still poorly understood, but two important general principles of developmental pathology are relevant regardless of the etiologic agent:

- *The timing of the prenatal insult has an important impact on both the occurrence and the type of malformation produced.* The intrauterine development of humans can be divided into two phases: the embryonic period, occupying the first 9 weeks of pregnancy, and the fetal period, which terminates at birth. In the early embryonic period (the first 3 weeks after fertilization), an injurious agent damages either enough cells to cause death and abortion, or only a few cells, presumably allowing the embryo to recover without developing defects. Between the 3rd and 9th weeks, the embryo is extremely susceptible to teratogenesis; the peak sensitivity during this period is between the fourth and fifth weeks. It is during this period that organs are being crafted out of the germ cell layers. The fetal period that follows organogenesis is marked chiefly by further growth and maturation of the organs, with greatly reduced susceptibility to teratogenic agents. Instead, the fetus is susceptible to growth retardation or injury to already-formed organs. It is therefore possible for the same teratogenic agent to produce different effects if exposure occurs at different times of gestation. For example, viral infections such as rubella produce disruption of the developmental program in the first trimester, but later during pregnancy, the result of viral infection is usually tissue injury accompanied by inflammation (see Perinatal Infections section below). The approximate timing of the insult can be gauged from the pattern of disruption that is present at birth or in the abortus. Thus, a ventricular septal defect resulting from exposure to a teratogen must have occurred before 6 weeks of gestation, because the ventricular septum closes at this time.

• *Genes that regulate morphogenesis may be the target of teratogens.* The role of single-gene mutations in causing human malformations is becoming increasingly evident. It is not surprising, therefore, that the function of genes controlling developmental events is likely to be affected by teratogens as well. One such class of genes, called homeobox (*HOX*) genes, regulates transcription of several other genes, and in experimental animals, agents that alter *HOX* gene expression are known to produce malformations. For example, infants born to mothers treated with retinoic acid for severe acne develop *retinoic acid embryopathy,* including CNS, cardiac, and craniofacial defects. In animals, retinoic acid exposure produces reproducible changes in *HOX* gene expression and causes a wide range of structural congenital malformations, mirroring those seen in retinoic acid embryopathy. A variety of other teratogens (e.g., the anticonvulsant sodium valproate) also mediate their effects through disruption of *HOX* gene expression.

SUMMARY

Congenital Anomalies

• Congenital anomalies result from intrinsic abnormalities (malformations) as well as extrinsic disturbances (deformations, disruptions).

• Congenital anomalies can result from genetic (chromosomal abnormalities, gene mutations), environmental (infections, drugs, alcohol), and multifactorial causes.

• The timing of the in utero insult has profound influence on the extent of congenital anomalies, with earlier events usually demonstrating greater impact.

PERINATAL INFECTIONS

Infections of the fetus and neonate may be acquired transcervically (ascending infections) or transplacentally (hematologic infections).

• Transcervical, or *ascending, infections* involve spread of infection from the cervicovaginal canal and may be acquired in utero or during birth. Most bacterial infections (e.g., α-hemolytic streptococcal infection) and a few viral infections (e.g., herpes simplex) are acquired in this manner. In general, the fetus acquires the infection by "inhaling" infected amniotic fluid into the lungs or by passing through an infected birth canal during delivery. Fetal infection is usually associated with inflammation of the placental membranes (chorioamnionitis) and inflammation of the umbilical cord (funisitis). This mode of spread usually gives rise to pneumonia and, in severe cases, to sepsis and meningitis.

• Transplacental infections gain access to the fetal bloodstream by crossing the placenta via the chorionic villi, and may occur at any time during gestation or occasionally, as may be the case with hepatitis B and human immunodeficiency virus, at the time of delivery via maternal-to-fetal transfusion. Most parasitic (e.g., toxoplasma, malaria) and viral infections, and a few bacterial infections (i.e., *Listeria, Treponema*) demonstrate this mode of hematogenous transmission. The clinical manifestations of these infections are highly variable, depending largely on the gestational timing and microorganism involved. The most important transplacental infections can be conveniently remembered by the acronym *TORCH.* The elements of the TORCH complex are the following: *Toxoplasma* (T), rubella virus (R), cytomegalovirus (C), herpesvirus (H), and any of a number of other (O) microbes such as *Treponema pallidum.* These agents are grouped together because they may evoke similar clinical and pathologic manifestations. TORCH infections occurring early in gestation may cause chronic sequela in the child, including growth restriction, mental retardation, cataracts, and congenital cardiac anomalies, while infections later in pregnancy result primarily in tissue injury accompanied by inflammation (encephalitis, chorioretinitis, hepatosplenomegaly, pneumonia, and myocarditis).

PREMATURITY AND FETAL GROWTH RESTRICTION

Prematurity is the second most common cause of neonatal mortality (second only to congenital anomalies), and is defined by a gestational age less than 37 weeks. As might be expected, infants born before completion of gestation also weigh less than normal (<2500 gm). The major risk factors for prematurity include premature rupture of membranes; intrauterine infection leading to inflammation of the placental membranes (chorioamnionitis); structural abnormalities of the uterus, cervix, and placenta; and multiple gestation (e.g., twin pregnancy). It is well established that children born before completion of the full period of gestation are subject to a higher incidence of morbidity and mortality than are full-term infants. The immaturity of organ systems in preterm infants makes them especially vulnerable to several complications discussed below, including:

• Hyaline membrane disease (respiratory distress syndrome).

• Necrotizing enterocolitis.

- Intraventricular and germinal matrix hemorrhage (Chapter 23).

Although preterm infants have low birth weights, it is usually appropriate once adjusted for their gestational age. In contrast, as many as one-third of infants who weigh less than 2500 gm are born at term and are therefore undergrown rather than immature. These small-for-gestational-age (SGA) infants suffer from fetal growth restriction. Fetal growth restriction may result from fetal, maternal, or placental abnormalities, although in many cases the specific cause is unknown.

- *Fetal factors* are those that intrinsically reduce growth potential of the fetus despite an adequate supply of nutrients from the mother. Prominent among such fetal conditions are *chromosomal disorders, congenital anomalies*, and *congenital infections*. Chromosomal abnormalities may be detected in as many as 17% of fetuses sampled for fetal growth restriction and in as many as 66% of fetuses with documented ultrasonographic malformations. *Fetal infection* should be considered in all growth-restricted neonates, with the TORCH group of infections (*see above*) being a common cause. When the causation is intrinsic to the fetus, growth retardation is *symmetric* (i.e., affects all organ systems equally).
- *Placental causes* include any factor that compromises the uteroplacental supply line. This may result from placenta previa (low implantation of the placenta), placental abruption (separation of placenta from the decidua by a retroplacental clot), or placental infarction. With placental (and maternal) causes of growth restriction, the growth retardation is *asymmetric* (i.e., the brain is spared relative to visceral organs such as the liver).
- *Maternal factors* are by far the most common cause of the growth deficit in SGA infants. These include vascular diseases such as preeclampsia ("toxemia of pregnancy") (Chapter 19) and chronic hypertension. The list of other maternal conditions associated with growth-restricted infants is long, but some of the avoidable influences are maternal narcotic abuse, alcohol intake, and heavy cigarette smoking (recall that many of these same causes are also involved in the pathogenesis of congenital anomalies). Drugs causing fetal growth restriction similarly include teratogens, such as the commonly administered anticonvulsant phenytoin (Dilantin), as well as nonteratogenic agents. Maternal malnutrition (in particular, prolonged hypoglycemia) may also affect fetal growth, but the association between growth-restricted infants and the nutritional status of the mother is complex.

The growth-restricted infant is handicapped not only in the perinatal period but also in childhood and adult life. These individuals are at increased risk for cerebral dysfunction, learning disabilities, and sensory (i.e., visual, hearing) impairment.

RESPIRATORY DISTRESS SYNDROME OF THE NEWBORN

There are many causes of respiratory distress in the newborn, including excessive sedation of the mother, fetal head injury during delivery, aspiration of blood or amniotic fluid, and intrauterine hypoxia brought about by coiling of the umbilical cord about the neck. However, the most common cause is respiratory distress syndrome (RDS), also known as *hyaline membrane disease* because of the formation of "membranes" in the peripheral air spaces of infants who succumb to this condition. Approximately 24,000 infants are affected by RDS each year, and in 2002, a little more than 1000 deaths were ascribed to this disease. The tremendous strides made in the prevention and management of RDS can be estimated by recalling that in the 1960s there were more than 25,000 deaths each year from this disorder.

Pathogenesis. *RDS is basically a disease of premature infants.* It occurs in about 60% of infants born at less than 28 weeks of gestation, 15% to 20% of those born between 32 and 36 weeks of gestation, and fewer than 5% of those born after 37 weeks of gestation. Other contributing influences are *maternal diabetes, cesarean section* before the onset of labor, and *twin gestation.*

The fundamental defect in RDS is the inability of the immature lung to synthesize sufficient surfactant. Surfactant is a complex of surface-active phospholipids, principally dipalmitoylphosphatidylcholine (lecithin), and at least two groups of surfactant-associated proteins. Surfactant is synthesized by type II pneumocytes and, with the healthy newborn's first breath, rapidly coats the surface of alveoli, reducing surface tension and thus decreasing the pressure required to keep alveoli open. In a lung deficient in surfactant, alveoli tend to collapse, and a relatively greater inspiratory effort is required with each breath to open the alveoli. The infant rapidly tires from breathing, and generalized atelectasis sets in. The resulting hypoxia sets into motion a sequence of events that lead to epithelial and endothelial damage and eventually to the formation of hyaline membranes (Fig. 7–22). As discussed later, this classical picture of surfactant deficiency is greatly modified by surfactant treatment.

Surfactant synthesis is regulated by hormones. Corticosteroids stimulate the formation of surfactant lipids and associated proteins. Therefore, conditions associated with intrauterine stress and fetal growth restriction that increase corticosteroid release lower the risk of developing RDS. Surfactant synthesis can be suppressed by the compensatory high blood levels of insulin in infants of diabetic mothers, which counteracts the effects of steroids. This may explain, in part, why infants of diabetic mothers have a higher risk of developing RDS. Labor is known to increase surfactant synthesis; hence, cesarean section before the onset of labor may increase the risk of RDS.

Morphology

The lungs in RDS infants are of normal size but are heavy and relatively airless. They have a mottled purple color, and microscopically the tissue appears solid, with poorly developed, generally collapsed (atelectatic) alveoli. If the infant dies within the first several hours of life, only necrotic cellular debris is present in the terminal bronchioles and alveolar ducts. Later in the course, characteristic **eosinophilic hyaline membranes** line the respiratory bronchioles, alveolar ducts, and random

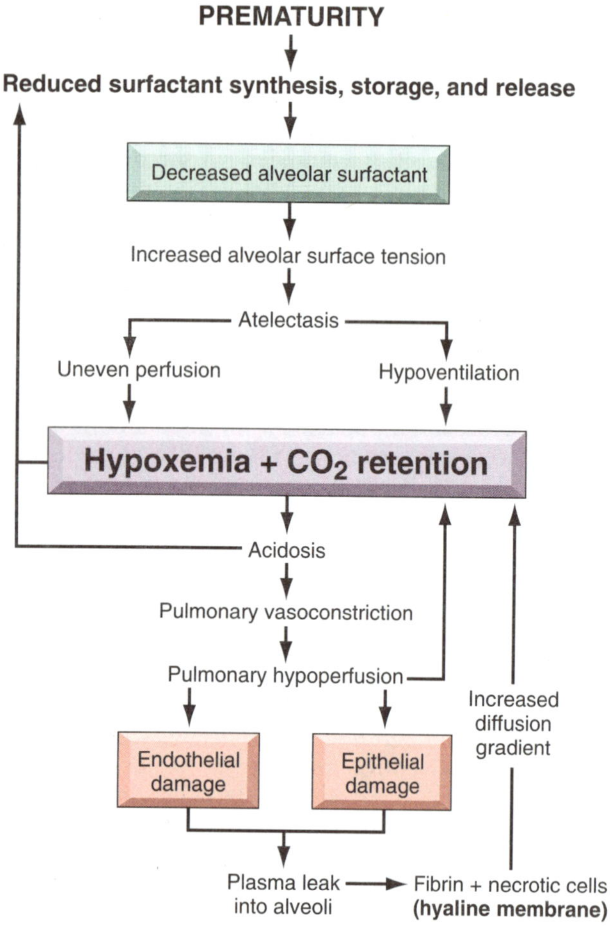

Figure 7–22

Pathophysiology of respiratory distress syndrome (see text).

alveoli (Fig. 7–23). These "membranes" contain necrotic epithelial cells admixed with extravasated plasma proteins. There is a remarkable paucity of neutrophilic inflammatory reaction associated with these membranes. The lesions of hyaline membrane disease are never seen in stillborn infants or in live-born infants who die within a few hours of birth. If the infant dies after several days, evidence of reparative changes, including proliferation of type II pneumocytes and interstitial fibrosis, is seen.

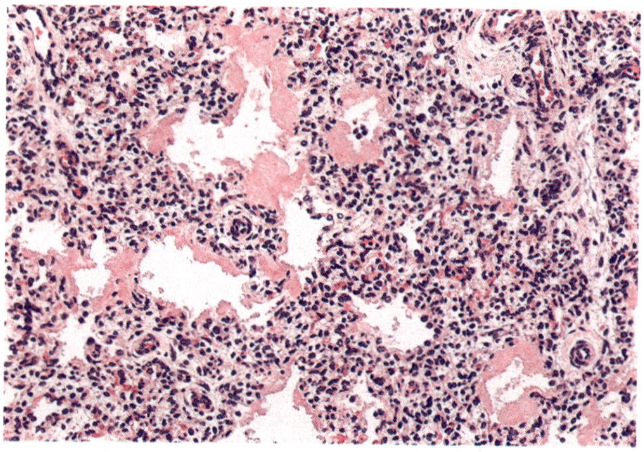

Figure 7–23

Hyaline membrane disease (H&E stain). There is alternating atelectasis and dilation of the alveoli. Note the eosinophilic thick hyaline membranes lining the dilated alveoli.

Clinical Features. The classic clinical presentation before the era of treatment with exogenous surfactant was described earlier. Currently, the actual clinical course and prognosis for neonatal RDS vary, dependent on the maturity and birth weight of the infant and the promptness of institution of therapy. A major thrust in the control of RDS focuses on prevention, either by delaying labor until the fetal lung reaches maturity or by inducing maturation of the lung in the fetus at risk. Critical to these objectives is the ability to assess fetal lung maturity accurately. Because pulmonary secretions are discharged into the amniotic fluid, analysis of amniotic fluid phospholipids provides a good estimate of the level of surfactant in the alveolar lining. Prophylactic administration of exogenous surfactant at birth to extremely premature infants (gestational age <28 weeks) has been shown to be very beneficial, such that it is now uncommon for infants to die of acute RDS.

In uncomplicated cases, recovery begins to occur within 3 or 4 days. In affected infants oxygen is required. However, high concentration of ventilator-administered oxygen for prolonged periods is associated with two well-known complications: *retrolental fibroplasia* (also called *retinopathy of prematurity*) in the eyes, and *bronchopulmonary dysplasia (BPD)*. Fortunately, both complications are now significantly less common as a result of gentler ventilation techniques, antenatal glucocorticoid therapy, and prophylactic surfactant treatments.

- Retinopathy of prematurity has a two-phase pathogenesis. During the *hyperoxic* phase of RDS therapy (phase I), expression of the pro-angiogenic vascular endothelial growth factor (VEGF) is markedly decreased, causing endothelial cell apoptosis; VEGF levels rebound after return to relatively hypoxic room air ventilation (phase II), inducing retinal vessel proliferation (*neovascularization*) characteristic of the lesions in the retina.
- *The major abnormality in BPD is a decrease in the number of mature alveoli, referred to as alveolar hypoplasia.* Thus, the current view is that BPD is most likely caused by an arrested development of alveolar septation at the so-called saccular stage of development. The levels of a variety of proinflammatory cytokines (TNF, macrophage inflammatory protein-1 and IL-8) are increased in the alveoli of infants who develop BPD, suggesting a role for these cytokines in arresting pulmonary development.

Infants who recover from RDS are also at increased risk for developing a variety of other complications associated with preterm birth; most important among these are *patent ductus arteriosus, intraventricular hemorrhage,* and *necrotizing enterocolitis.* Thus, although technologic advances help save the lives of many infants with

RDS, it also brings to the surface the exquisite fragility of the immature neonate.

SUMMARY

Neonatal Respiratory Distress Syndrome

- Neonatal RDS ("hyaline membrane disease") is a disease of prematurity (most cases occur in neonates <28 weeks gestational age).
- The fundamental abnormality in RDS is insufficient pulmonary surfactant, which results in failure of lungs to inflate after birth.
- The characteristic morphology in RDS is the presence of hyaline membranes (consisting of necrotic epithelial cells and plasma proteins) lining the airways.
- RDS can be ameliorated by prophylactic administration of steroids, surfactant therapy, and by improved ventilation techniques.
- Long-term sequela associated with RDS therapy include retinopathy of prematurity and bronchopulmonary dysplasia; the incidence of both complications has decreased with improvements in management of RDS.

NECROTIZING ENTEROCOLITIS

Necrotizing enterocolitis (NEC) most commonly occurs in premature infants, with the incidence of the disease being inversely proportional to the gestational age. It occurs in approximately one out of 10 very-low-birth-weight infants (<1500 gm). The cause of NEC is controversial, but in all likelihood it is multifactorial. *Intestinal ischemia* is a prerequisite and may result from either generalized hypoperfusion or selective reduction of blood flow to the intestines to divert oxygen to vital organs such as the brain. Other predisposing conditions include *bacterial colonization* of the gut and administration of *formula feeds,* both of which aggravate mucosal injury in the immature bowel.

NEC typically involves the terminal ileum, cecum, and right colon, although any part of the small or large intestine may be involved. The involved segment is distended, friable, and congested (Fig. 7–24), or it can be frankly gangrenous; intestinal perforation with accompanying peritonitis may be seen. Microscopically, mucosal or transmural coagulative necrosis, ulceration, bacterial colonization, and submucosal gas bubbles are all features associated with NEC. Reparative changes, such as granulation tissue and fibrosis, may be seen shortly after the acute episode.

The clinical course is fairly typical, with the onset of bloody stools, abdominal distention, and development of circulatory collapse. Abdominal radiographs often demonstrate gas within the intestinal wall (*pneumatosis intestinalis*). When detected early NEC can be often managed conservatively, but many cases (20% to 60%) require operative intervention and resection of the necrotic segments of bowel. NEC is associated with high perinatal mortality; infants who survive often develop *post-NEC strictures* from fibrosis caused by the healing process.

SUDDEN INFANT DEATH SYNDROME

Sudden infant death syndrome (SIDS) is a disease of unknown cause. The National Institute of Child Health

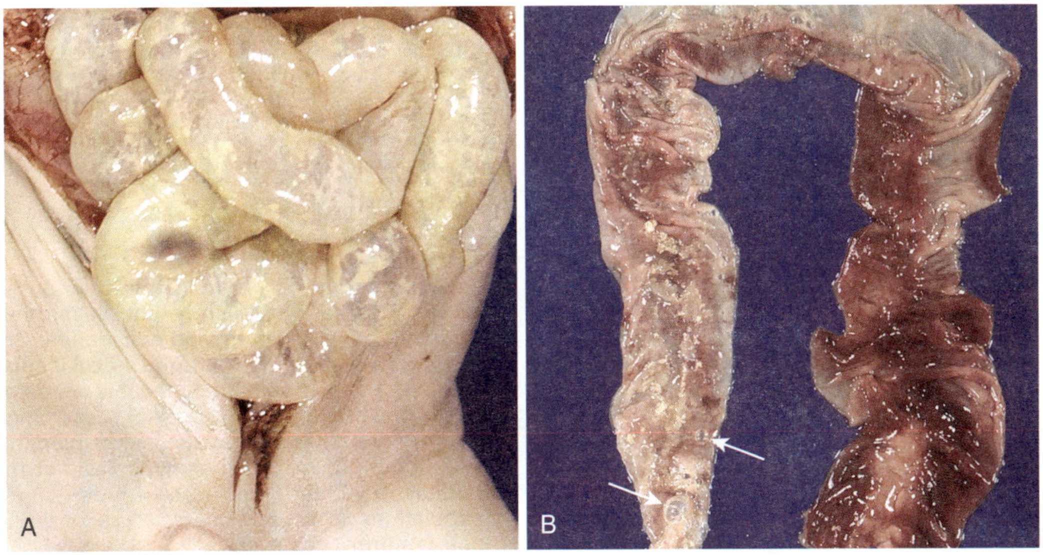

Figure 7–24

Necrotizing enterocolitis. **A,** Postmortem examination in a severe case shows that the entire small bowel is markedly distended with a perilously thin wall (usually this implies impending perforation). **B,** The congested portion of the ileum corresponds to areas of hemorrhagic infarction and transmural necrosis seen on microscopy. Submucosal gas bubbles (*pneumatosis intestinalis*) can be seen in several areas (*arrows*).

and Human Development defines *SIDS* as "the sudden death of an infant under 1 year of age which remains unexplained after a thorough case investigation, *including performance of a complete autopsy, examination of the death scene, and review of the clinical history.*" An aspect of SIDS that is not stressed in the definition is that the infant usually dies while asleep, hence the pseudonyms of *crib death* or *cot death*. SIDS is the leading cause of death between 1 month and 1 year of age in this country, and the third leading cause of death overall in infancy, after congenital anomalies and diseases of prematurity and low birth weight. In 90% of cases, the infant is younger than 6 months; most are between the ages of 2 and 4 months.

Pathogenesis. The circumstances surrounding SIDS have been explored in great detail, and it is generally accepted that it is a *multifactorial condition,* with a variable mixture of contributing causes in a given case. A "triple-risk" model of SIDS has been proposed, which postulates the intersection of three overlapping variables: (1) *a vulnerable infant,* (2) *a critical developmental period in homeostatic control,* and (3) *an exogenous stressor*(s). According to this model, several factors make the infant vulnerable to sudden death during the critical developmental period (i.e., 1 month to 1 year). These vulnerability factors may be attributable to the parents or the infant, while the exogenous stressor(s) is attributable to the environment (Table 7–10). Although numerous factors have been proposed to account for a vulnerable infant, *the most compelling hypothesis is that SIDS reflects a delayed development of arousal and cardiorespiratory control.* Regions of the brain stem, particularly the *arcuate nucleus* located in the ventral medullary surface, play a critical role in the body's "arousal" response to noxious stimuli such as hypercarbia, hypoxia, and thermal stress encountered during sleep. In addition, these areas regulate breathing, heart rate, and body temperature. In certain infants, for yet inexplicable reasons, there may be a maldevelopment or delay in maturation of this region, compromising the arousal response to noxious stimuli. Among the potential environmental causes, prone sleeping position, sleeping on soft surfaces, and thermal stress are possibly the most important modifiable risk factors for SIDS. The prone position predisposes an infant to one or more recognized noxious stimuli (hypoxia, hypercarbia, and thermal stress) during sleep. In addition, the prone position is also associated with decreased arousal responsiveness compared with the supine position. Results of studies from Europe, Australia, New Zealand, and the United States showed clearly increased risk for SIDS in infants who sleep in a prone position, prompting the American Academy of Pediatrics to recommend placing *healthy infants on their back* when laying them down to sleep. This "Back to Sleep" campaign has resulted in substantial decreases in SIDS-related deaths since its inception in 1994.

Table 7–10 Factors Associated with Sudden Infant Death Syndrome

Parental
Young maternal age (<20 years of age)
Maternal smoking during pregnancy
Drug abuse in *either* parent, specifically paternal marijuana and maternal opiate, cocaine use
Short intergestational intervals
Late or no prenatal care
Low socioeconomic group
African American and American Indian ethnicity (? socioeconomic factors)
Infant
Brain stem abnormalities associated defective arousal and cardiorespiratory control
Prematurity and/or low birth weight
Male sex
Product of a multiple birth
SIDS in an earlier sibling
Antecedent respiratory infections
?Gastroesophageal reflux
Environment
Prone sleep position
Sleeping on a soft surface
Hyperthermia
Postnatal passive smoking
Postmortem Abnormalities Detected in Cases of Sudden Unexpected Infant Death*
Infections
Viral myocarditis
Bronchopneumonia
Unsuspected congenital anomaly
Congenital aortic stenosis
Anomalous origin of the left coronary artery from the pulmonary artery
Traumatic child abuse
Intentional suffocation (filicide)
Genetic and metabolic defects
Cardiac sodium and potassium ion channel mutations
Fatty acid oxidation disorders (MCAD mutations)
Cardiomyopathy secondary to mitochondrial DNA mutations

*SIDS is not the only cause of sudden unexpected death in infancy; instead, it is *a diagnosis of exclusion*. Therefore, performance of an autopsy may reveal findings that would explain the cause of sudden unexpected death. These cases should *not*, strictly speaking, be labeled as "SIDS."

MCAD, medium-chain acyl-coenzyme A dehydrogenase.

Morphology

Anatomic studies of victims have yielded inconsistent histologic findings. **Multiple petechiae** are the most common finding in the typical SIDS autopsy (~80% of cases); these are usually present on the thymus, visceral and parietal pleura, and epicardium. Grossly, the lungs are usually congested, and **vascular engorgement** with or without **pulmonary edema** is demonstrable microscopically in the majority of cases. Sophisticated morphometric studies have revealed quantitative brain stem abnormalities such as **hypoplasia of the arcuate nucleus** or a subtle decrease in brain stem neuronal populations in several cases; these observations are not uniform, however, and not amenable to most "routine" autopsy procedures.

It should be noted that SIDS is not the only cause of sudden unexpected deaths in infancy. In fact, SIDS is a diagnosis of exclusion, requiring careful examination of the death scene and a complete postmortem examination. The latter can reveal an unsuspected cause of sudden death in as many as 20% or more of "SIDS" babies (see Table 7–10). Infections (e.g., viral myocarditis or bronchopneumonia) are the most common causes of sudden "unexpected" death, followed by an unsuspected congenital anomaly. As a result of advancements in molecular diagnostics, several genetic causes of sudden "unexpected" infant death have emerged. For example, fatty acid oxidation disorders, characterized by defects in mitochondrial fatty acid oxidative enzymes, may be responsible for as many as 5% of sudden deaths in infancy; of these, a deficiency in medium-chain acyl-coenzyme A dehydrogenase is the most common. Retrospective analyses of "SIDS" cases have also revealed mutations of cardiac sodium and potassium channels, which result in a form of cardiac arrhythmia characterized by prolonged QT intervals; these account for no more than 1% of SIDS deaths. SIDS in an earlier sibling is associated with a fivefold relative risk of recurrence; traumatic child abuse must be carefully excluded under these circumstances.

SUMMARY

Sudden Infant Death Syndrome

- SIDS is a disease of *unknown cause,* defined as the sudden death of an infant younger than 1 year of age, which remains unexplained after a thorough case investigation including performance of an autopsy. Most cases occur between 2 and 4 months of age.
- The most likely basis for SIDS is a delayed development in arousal reflexes and cardiorespiratory control.
- Numerous risk factors have been proposed, of which the prone sleeping position is best recognized; hence the success of the "Back to Sleep" program in reducing SIDS.

FETAL HYDROPS

Fetal hydrops refers to the accumulation of edema fluid in the fetus during intrauterine growth. The causes of fetal hydrops are manifold; the most important are listed in Table 7–11. Until recently, hemolytic anemia caused by Rh blood group incompatibility between mother and fetus (immune hydrops) was the most common cause, but with the successful prophylaxis of this disorder during pregnancy, causes of nonimmune hydrops have emerged as the principal culprits. Notably, the intrauterine fluid accumulation can be quite variable, from progressive, generalized edema of the fetus (*hydrops fetalis*), a usually lethal condition, to more localized degrees of edema, such as isolated pleural and peritoneal effusions, or postnuchal fluid accumulation (*cystic hygroma*) that are often compatible with life (Fig. 7–25). The mechanism of immune hydrops will be discussed first, followed by other important causes of fetal hydrops.

Table 7–11 Major Causes of Fetal Hydrops*

Cardiovascular
Malformations Tachyarrhythmia High-output failure
Chromosomal
Turner syndrome Trisomy 21, Trisomy 18
Fetal Anemia
Homozygous α-thalassemia Parvovirus B19 Immune hydrops (Rh and ABO incompatibility)
Twin Gestation
Twin-twin transfusion
Infection (excluding parvovirus)
Cytomegalovirus Syphilis Toxoplasmosis
Major Malformations
Tumors
Metabolic Disorders

*The cause of fetal hydrops may be undetermined ("idiopathic") in as many as 20% of cases.

Modified from Machin GA: Hydrops, cystic hygroma, hydrothorax, pericardial effusions, and fetal ascites. In Gilbert-Barnes (ed): Potter's Pathology of Fetus and Infant. St. Louis, Mosby, 1997.

Immune Hydrops

Immune hydrops results from an antibody-induced *hemolytic disease in the newborn* that is caused by blood group incompatibility between mother and fetus. Such an incompatibility occurs only when the fetus inherits red cell antigenic determinants from the father that are foreign to the mother. The most common antigens to result in clinically significant hemolysis are the Rh and ABO blood group antigens. Of the numerous antigens included in the Rh system, only the D antigen is a major cause of Rh incompatibility. Fetal red cells may reach the maternal circulation during the last trimester of pregnancy, when the cytotrophoblast is no longer present as a barrier, or during childbirth itself (fetomaternal bleed). The mother thus becomes sensitized to the foreign antigen and develops antibodies that can freely traverse the placenta to the fetus and cause red cell destruction. Once immune hemolysis is initiated, there is progressive anemia in the fetus, with resultant tissue ischemia, intrauterine cardiac failure, and peripheral pooling of fluid (edema). As discussed later, cardiac failure may be the final pathway by which edema occurs in many cases of nonimmune hydrops as well.

Several factors influence the immune response to Rh-positive fetal red cells that reach the maternal circulation.

- Concurrent ABO incompatibility protects the mother against Rh immunization, because the fetal red cells are promptly coated by isohemagglutinins and removed from the maternal circulation.

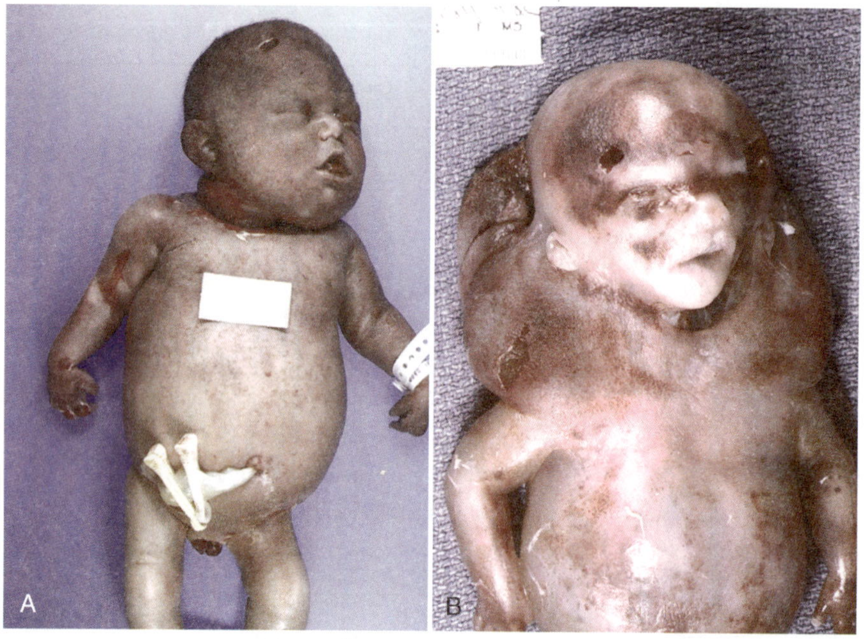

Figure 7–25

Hydrops fetalis. **A,** Generalized accumulation of fluid in the fetus. **B,** Fluid accumulation particularly prominent in the soft tissues of the neck. This condition has been termed *cystic hygroma*. Cystic hygromas are characteristically seen with, but not limited to, constitutional chromosomal anomalies such as 45,X karyotypes. (Courtesy of Dr. Beverly Rogers, Department of Pathology, University of Texas Southwestern Medical Center, Dallas, Texas.)

- The antibody response depends on the dose of immunizing antigen; hence, hemolytic disease develops only when the mother has experienced a significant transplacental bleed (>1 mL of Rh-positive red cells).
- The isotype of the antibody is important, because immunoglobulin G (IgG) (but not IgM) antibodies can cross the placenta. The initial exposure to Rh antigen evokes the formation of IgM antibodies, *so Rh disease is very uncommon with the first pregnancy*. Subsequent exposure during the second or third pregnancy generally leads to a brisk IgG antibody response.

Appreciation of the role of prior sensitization in the pathogenesis of Rh-hemolytic disease of the newborn has led to its remarkable control. Currently, Rh-negative mothers are given anti-D globulin soon after the delivery of an Rh-positive baby. The anti-D antibodies mask the antigenic sites on the fetal red cells that may have leaked into the maternal circulation during childbirth, thus preventing long-lasting sensitization to Rh antigens.

As a result of the remarkable success achieved in prevention of Rh hemolysis, fetomaternal ABO incompatibility is currently the most common cause of immune hemolytic disease of the newborn. Although ABO incompatibility occurs in approximately 20% to 25% of pregnancies, only a small fraction of infants subsequently born develop hemolysis, and in general the disease is much milder than is Rh incompatibility. ABO hemolytic disease occurs almost exclusively in infants of group A or B who are born to group O mothers. The normal anti-A and anti-B isohemagglutinins in group O mothers are usually of the IgM type and so do not cross the placenta. However, for reasons not well understood, certain group O women possess IgG antibodies directed against group A or B antigens (or both) even without prior sensitization. Therefore, the firstborn may be affected. Fortunately, even with transplacentally acquired antibodies, lysis of the infant's red cells is minimal. There is no effective method of preventing hemolytic disease resulting from ABO incompatibility.

Nonimmune Hydrops

The major causes of nonimmune hydrops include those associated with *cardiovascular defects, chromosomal anomalies,* and *fetal anemia.* Both structural cardiovascular defects and functional abnormalities (i.e., arrhythmias) may result in intrauterine cardiac failure and hydrops. Among the chromosomal anomalies, 45,X karyotype (Turner syndrome) and trisomies 21 and 18 are associated with fetal hydrops; usually the basis for this is the presence of underlying structural cardiac anomalies, although in Turner syndrome there may be an abnormality of lymphatic drainage from the neck leading to postnuchal fluid accumulation (*cystic hygromas*). Fetal anemias due to causes other than Rh or ABO incompatibility also result in hydrops. In fact, in some parts of the world (e.g., Southeast Asia), severe fetal anemia caused by homozygous α-thalassemia is probably the most common cause of fetal hydrops. Transplacental infection by parvovirus B19 is increasingly recognized as an important cause of fetal hydrops. The virus gains entry into erythroid precursors (normoblasts), where it replicates. This leads to erythrocyte maturation arrest and aplastic anemia. Parvoviral intranuclear inclusions can be seen within circulating and marrow erythroid precursors (Fig. 7–26). The basis for fetal hydrops in fetal anemia of both immune and nonimmune cause is tissue ischemia with secondary myocardial dysfunction and circulatory failure. Additionally, secondary liver failure may ensue,

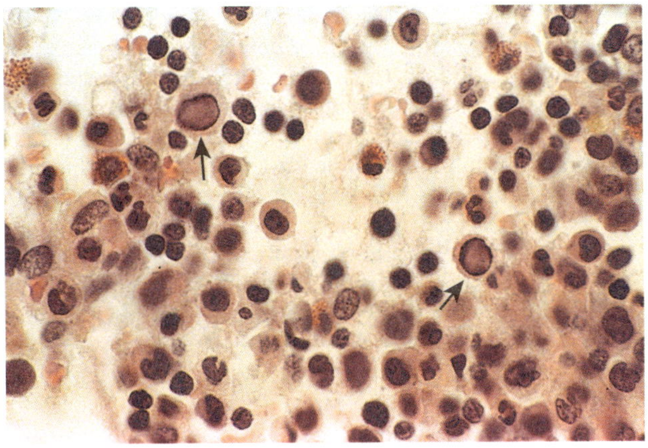

Figure 7–26

Bone marrow from an infant infected with parvovirus B19. The arrows point to two erythroid precursors with large homogeneous intranuclear inclusions and a surrounding peripheral rim of residual chromatin.

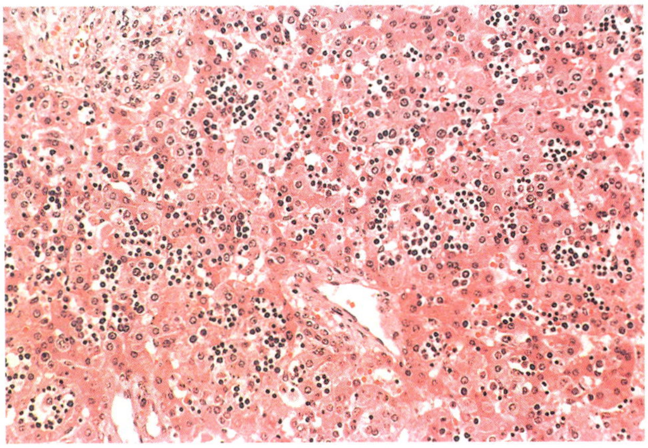

Figure 7–27

Numerous islands of extramedullary hematopoiesis (small *blue* cells) are scattered among mature hepatocytes in this infant with nonimmune hydrops fetalis.

with loss of synthetic function contributing to hypoalbuminemia, reduced plasma osmotic pressure, and edema.

Morphology

The anatomic findings in fetuses with intrauterine fluid accumulation vary with both the severity of the disease and the underlying etiology. As previously noted, **hydrops fetalis** represents the most severe and generalized manifestation (see Fig. 7–25), and lesser degrees of edema such as isolated pleural, peritoneal, or postnuchal fluid collections can occur. Accordingly, infants may be stillborn, die within the first few days, or recover completely. The presence of dysmorphic features suggests underlying constitutional chromosomal abnormalities; postmortem examination may reveal a cardiac anomaly. In hydrops associated with fetal anemia, both fetus and placenta are characteristically pale; in most cases, the liver and spleen are enlarged from **cardiac failure** and congestion. Additionally, the bone marrow shows compensatory hyperplasia of erythroid precursors (parvovirus-associated aplastic anemia being a notable exception), and **extramedullary hematopoiesis** is present in the liver, the spleen, and possibly other tissues such as the kidneys, the lungs, and even the heart. The increased hematopoietic activity accounts for the presence in the peripheral circulation of large numbers of immature red cells, including reticulocytes, normoblasts, and erythroblasts (**erythroblastosis fetalis**) (Fig. 7–27).

The presence of hemolysis in Rh or ABO incompatibility is associated with the added complication of increased circulating bilirubin from the red cell breakdown. The CNS may be damaged when hyperbilirubinemia is marked (usually above 20 mg/dL in full-term infants, often less in premature infants). The circulating unconjugated bilirubin is taken up by the brain tissue, on which it apparently exerts a toxic effect. The basal ganglia and brain stem are particularly prone to deposition of bilirubin pigment, which imparts a characteristic yellow hue to the parenchyma (**kernicterus**; Fig. 7–28).

Clinical Course. Early recognition of intrauterine fluid accumulation is imperative, since even severe cases can sometimes be salvaged with currently available therapy. Fetal hydrops that results from Rh incompatibility may be more or less accurately predicted, because it correlates well with rapidly rising Rh antibody titers in the mother during pregnancy. Amniotic fluid obtained by amniocentesis may show high levels of bilirubin. The human antiglobulin test (Coombs test, Chapter 12) is positive on fetal cord blood if the red cells have been coated by maternal antibody. Antenatal exchange transfusion is an effective form of therapy. Postnatally, phototherapy is helpful because visible light converts bilirubin to readily excreted dipyrroles. As already discussed, in an overwhelming majority of cases, administration of anti-D globulins to the mother can prevent the occurrence of

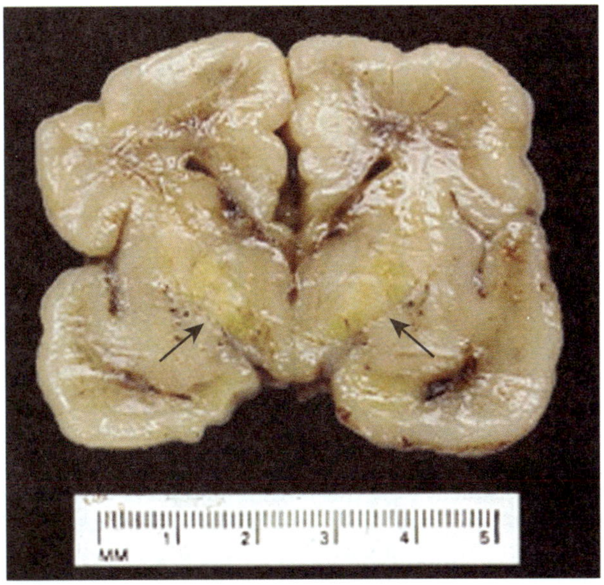

Figure 7–28

Kernicterus. Severe hyperbilirubinemia in the neonatal period—for example, secondary to immune hydrolysis—results in deposition of bilirubin pigment (*arrows*) in the brain parenchyma. This occurs because the blood-brain barrier is less well developed in the neonatal period than it is in adulthood. Infants who survive develop long-term neurologic sequelae.

immune hydrops in subsequent pregnancies. Group ABO hemolytic disease is more difficult to predict but is readily anticipated by awareness of the blood incompatibility between mother and father and by hemoglobin and bilirubin determinations in the vulnerable newborn infant. Needless to say, in fatal instances of fetal hydrops, a thorough postmortem examination is imperative to determine the cause and to exclude a potentially recurring cause such as a chromosomal abnormality.

SUMMARY

Fetal Hydrops

- Fetal hydrops refers to the accumulation of edema fluid in the fetus during intrauterine growth.
- The degree of fluid accumulation is variable, from generalized hydrops fetalis to localized cystic hygromas.
- The most common causes of fetal hydrops are *nonimmune* (chromosomal abnormalities, cardiovascular defects, and fetal anemia), while immune hydrops has become less frequent due to Rh antibody prophylaxis.
- Erythroblastosis fetalis (circulating immature erythroid precursors) is a characteristic finding of fetal anemia-associated hydrops.
- Hemolysis-induced hyperbilirubinemia can result in kernicterus in the basal ganglia and brain stem, particularly in premature infants.

CYSTIC FIBROSIS

With an incidence of 1 in 3200 live births in the United States, *cystic fibrosis (CF) is the most common lethal genetic disease that affects Caucasian populations.* It is uncommon among Asians (1 in 31,000 live births) and African Americans (1 in 15,000 live births). CF follows simple *autosomal recessive* transmission, and does not affect heterozygote carriers. There is, however, a bewildering compendium of phenotypic variation that results from diverse mutations in the CF-associated gene, the tissue-specific effects of loss of this gene's function, and the influence of newly recognized disease modifiers. It is fundamentally a *widespread disorder of epithelial transport affecting fluid secretion in exocrine glands and the epithelial lining of the respiratory, gastrointestinal (GI), and reproductive tracts.* Indeed, abnormally viscid mucus secretions that block the airways and the pancreatic ducts are responsible for the two most important clinical manifestations: recurrent and chronic pulmonary infections and pancreatic insufficiency. In addition, although the exocrine sweat glands are structurally normal (and remain so throughout the course of this disease), *a high level of sodium chloride in the sweat is a consistent and characteristic biochemical abnormality in CF.*

Pathogenesis. The primary defect in CF is abnormal function of an epithelial chloride channel protein encoded by the CF transmembrane conductance regulator (*CFTR*) gene on chromosome 7q31.2. The changes in mucus are considered secondary to the disturbance in transport of chloride ions. In normal epithelia the transport of chloride ions across the cell membrane occurs through transmembrane proteins such as CFTR that form chloride channels. Mutations in the *CFTR* gene render the epithelial membranes relatively impermeable to chloride ions (Fig. 7–29). However, the impact of this defect on transport function is tissue-specific. The major function of the CFTR protein in the sweat gland ducts is to reabsorb luminal chloride ions and augment sodium reabsorption. Therefore, in the sweat ducts, loss of CFTR function leads to decreased reabsorption of sodium chloride and production of hypertonic sweat (see Fig. 7–29, top). In contrast to the sweat glands, CFTR in the respiratory and intestinal epithelium forms one of the most important avenues for active luminal secretion of chloride. At these sites, *CFTR* mutations result in loss or reduction of chloride secretion into the lumen (see Fig. 7–29, bottom). Active luminal sodium absorption is also increased, and both of these ion changes increase passive water reabsorption from the lumen, lowering the water content of the surface fluid layer coating mucosal cells. Thus, unlike the sweat ducts, there is no difference in the salt concentration of the surface fluid layer coating the respiratory and intestinal mucosal cells in normal versus individuals with CF. Instead, the pathogenesis of respiratory and intestinal complications in CF seems to stem from an isotonic but low-volume surface fluid layer. In the lungs, this dehydration leads to defective mucociliary action and the accumulation of concentrated, viscid secretions that obstruct the air passages and predispose to recurrent pulmonary infections.

Since the *CFTR* gene was cloned in 1989, more than 800 disease-causing mutations have been identified. They can be classified as "severe" or "mild" depending on the location of the mutation in the gene sequence; "severe" mutations are associated with complete loss of CFTR protein function, while the product of a "mild" mutation retains residual function. The most common *CFTR* gene mutation leads to a deletion of 3 nucleotides coding for phenylalanine at amino acid position 508 (*ΔF508*). This is an example of a "severe" mutation. Worldwide, *ΔF508* mutation can be found in approximately 70% of CF patients. Since CF is an autosomal recessive disease, affected individuals harbor mutations on both alleles. As discussed later, the combination of mutations on the two alleles influences the overall phenotype, as well as organ-specific manifestations. Although CF remains one of the best known examples of the "one gene, one disease" axiom, there is increasing evidence that *genetic modifiers* besides *CFTR* modulate the frequency and severity of organ-specific manifestations. One example of a candidate genetic modifier is *mannose-binding lectin,* a key effector of innate immunity involved in phagocytosis of microorganisms. Polymorphisms in one or both mannose-binding lectin alleles that produce lower circulating levels of the protein are associated with a threefold higher risk of end-stage lung disease, and reduced survival subsequent to chronic bacterial infection in the setting of CF.

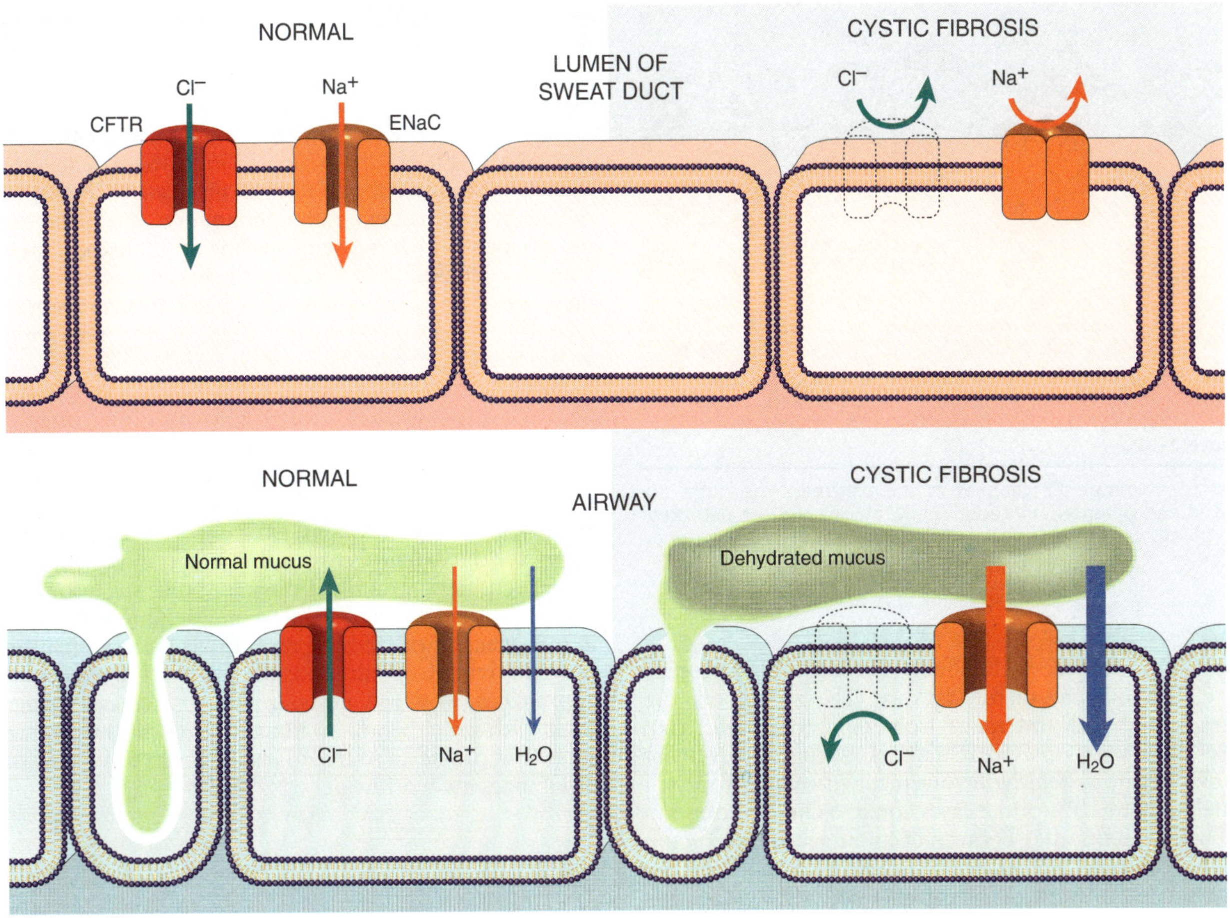

Figure 7–29

Chloride channel defect in the sweat duct (*top*) causes increased chloride and sodium concentration in sweat. In the airway (*bottom*), CF patients have decreased chloride secretion and increased sodium and water reabsorption leading to dehydration of the mucous layer coating epithelial cells, defective mucociliary action, and mucous plugging of airways. CFTR, cystic fibrosis transmembrane conductance regulator; ENaC, epithelial sodium channel responsible for intracellular sodium conduction.

Morphology

The anatomic changes are highly variable and depend on which glands are affected and on the severity of this involvement. **Pancreatic abnormalities** are present in 85% to 90% of patients with CF. In the milder cases, there may be only accumulations of mucus in the small ducts with some dilation of the exocrine glands. In more advanced cases, usually seen in older children or adolescents, the ducts are totally plugged, causing atrophy of the exocrine glands and progressive fibrosis (Fig. 7–30). The total loss of pancreatic exocrine secretion impairs fat absorption, and so avitaminosis A may contribute to squamous metaplasia of the lining epithelium of the ducts in the pancreas, which are already injured by the inspissated mucus secretions. Thick viscid plugs of mucus may also be found in the small intestine of infants. Sometimes these cause small-bowel obstruction, known as **meconium ileus.**

The **pulmonary changes** are the most serious complications of this disease (Fig. 7–31). These stem from the viscous mucus secretions of the submucosal glands of the respiratory tree with secondary obstruction and infection of the air passages. The bronchioles are often distended with thick mucus associated with marked hyperplasia and hypertrophy of the mucus-secreting cells. Superimposed infections give rise to severe chronic bronchitis and bronchiectasis. In many instances, lung abscesses develop. *Staphylococcus aureus, Haemophilus influenzae,* and *Pseudomonas aeruginosa* are the three most common organisms responsible for lung infections. Even more sinister is the increasing frequency of infection with another pseudomonad, *Burkholderia cepacia.* This opportunistic bacterium is particularly hardy, and infection with this organism has been associated with fulminant illness. The **liver involvement** follows the same basic pattern. Bile canaliculi are plugged by mucinous material, accompanied by ductular proliferation and portal inflammation. Hepatic **steatosis** is a common finding in liver biopsies. Over time, **cirrhosis** develops, resulting in diffuse hepatic nodularity. Such severe hepatic involvement is encountered in only approximately 5% of patients. **Azoospermia and infertility** are found in 95% of the males who survive to adulthood; **bilateral absence of the vas deferens** is a frequent finding in these patients. In some males, this may be the only feature suggesting an underlying *CFTR* mutation.

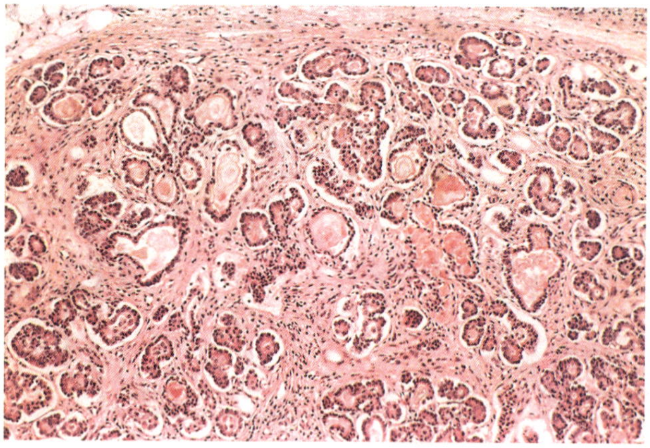

Figure 7–30

Mild to moderate CF changes in the pancreas. The ducts are dilated and plugged with eosinophilic mucin, and the parenchymal glands are atrophic and replaced by fibrous tissue.

Clinical Course. Few childhood diseases are as protean as CF in clinical manifestations. The symptoms are extremely varied and range from mild to severe, from onset at birth to onset years later, and from involvement of one organ system to involvement of many. Approximately 5% to 10% of the cases come to clinical attention at birth or soon after because of an attack of *meconium ileus. Exocrine pancreatic insufficiency* occurs in the majority (85% to 90%) of patients with CF and is associated with "severe" *CFTR* mutations on *both* alleles (e.g., *ΔF508/ΔF508*), whereas 10% to 15% of patients with one "severe" and one "mild" *CFTR* mutation, or two "mild" *CFTR* mutations, retain sufficient pancreatic exocrine function so as not to require enzyme supplementation (*pancreas-sufficient* phenotype). Pancreatic insufficiency is associated with malabsorption of protein and fat and increased fecal loss. Manifestations of malabsorption (e.g., large, foul stools; abdominal distention; and poor weight gain) appear during the first year of life. The faulty fat absorption may induce deficiency states of the fat-soluble vitamins, resulting in manifestations of avitaminosis A, D, or K. Hypoproteinemia may be severe enough to cause generalized edema. Persistent diarrhea may result in rectal prolapse in as many as 10% of children with CF. The *pancreas-sufficient* phenotype is usually not associated with other GI complications, and in general, these individuals demonstrate excellent growth and development. *"Idiopathic" chronic pancreatitis* occurs in a subset of patients with pancreas-sufficient CF and is associated with recurrent abdominal pain with life-threatening complications.

Cardiorespiratory complications, such as chronic cough, persistent lung infections, obstructive pulmonary disease, and cor pulmonale, are the most common cause of death (~80%) in patients followed by most CF centers in the United States. By 18 years of age, 80% of patients with classic CF harbor *P. aeruginosa*, and 3.5% harbor *B. cepacia*. With the indiscriminate use of antibiotic prophylaxis against *Staphylococcus*, there has been an unfortunate resurgence of resistant strains of *Pseudomonas* in many patients. *Recurrent sinonasal polyps* can occur in as many as 10% to 25% of patients with CF, and hence, children who present with this finding should be tested for abnormalities of sweat chloride. Significant *liver disease* occurs late in the natural history of CF and was formerly foreshadowed by pulmonary and pancreatic involvement; however, with increasing life expectancies, liver disease has also received increasing attention. In fact, next to cardiopulmonary and transplantation-related complications, liver disease is the third most common of death in CF.

In most cases, the diagnosis of CF is based on persistently elevated sweat electrolyte concentrations (often the mother makes the diagnosis because her infant tastes salty), characteristic clinical findings (sinopulmonary disease and GI manifestations), or a family history. Sequencing the *CFTR* gene is of course the "gold standard" for the diagnosis of CF. Therefore, in patients with clinical findings or family history (or both) suggesting this diagnosis, genetic analysis may be warranted. Advances in management of CF have meant that more patients are now surviving to adulthood; the median life expectancy approaches 30 years and continues to increase. Clinical trials with gene therapy in humans are still in their early stages but provide a source of encouragement for millions of CF patients worldwide.

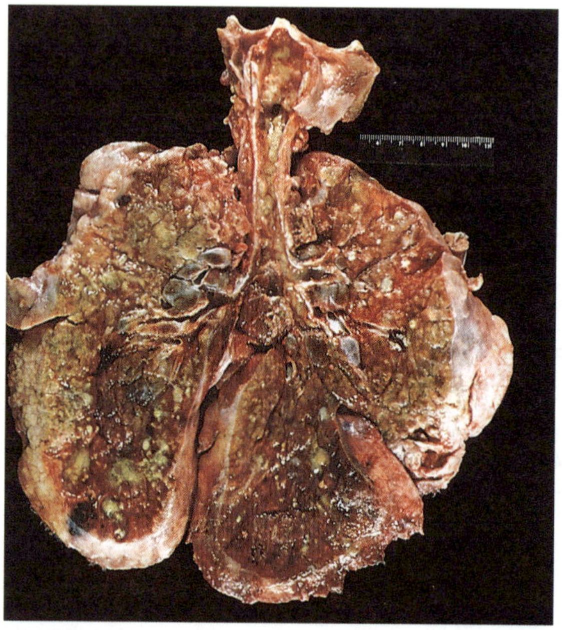

Figure 7–31

Lungs of a patient dying of CF. There is extensive mucous plugging and dilation of the tracheobronchial tree. The pulmonary parenchyma is consolidated by a combination of both secretions and pneumonia—the green color associated with *Pseudomonas* infections. (Courtesy of Dr. Eduardo Yunis, Children's Hospital of Pittsburgh, Pittsburgh, Pennsylvania.)

SUMMARY

Cystic Fibrosis

- CF is an autosomal recessive disease caused by mutations in the *CFTR* gene encoding the CF transmembrane regulator.
- The principal defect is of chloride ion transport, resulting in high salt concentrations in sweat, and viscous luminal secretions in respiratory and GI tracts.
- *CFTR* mutations can be severe (*ΔF508*), resulting in multisystem disease, or mild with limited disease extent and severity.
- Cardiopulmonary manifestations are the most common cause of mortality; pulmonary infections, especially with resistant pseudomonads, are frequent. Bronchiectasis and right-sided heart failure are long-term sequela.
- Pancreatic insufficiency is extremely common; infertility caused by congenital bilateral absence of vas deferens is a characteristic finding in adult CF patients.

TUMORS AND TUMOR-LIKE LESIONS OF INFANCY AND CHILDHOOD

Malignant neoplasms are the second most common cause of death in children between the ages of 4 and 14 years; only accidents exact a higher toll. Benign tumors are even more common than are cancers.

It is difficult to segregate, on morphologic grounds, true tumors from tumor-like lesions in the infant and child. In this context, two special categories of tumor-like lesions should be recognized.

Heterotopia or *choristoma* refers to microscopically normal cells or tissues that are present in abnormal locations. Examples include a pancreatic tissue "rest" found in the wall of the stomach or small intestine, or a small mass of adrenal cells found in the kidney, lungs, ovaries, or elsewhere. Heterotopic rests are usually of little significance, but they can be confused clinically with neoplasms.

Hamartoma refers to an excessive but focal overgrowth of cells and tissues native to the organ in which it occurs. Although the cellular elements are mature and identical to those found in the remainder of the organ, they do not reproduce the normal architecture of the surrounding tissue. Hamartomas can be thought of as the linkage between malformations and neoplasms. The line of demarcation between a hamartoma and a benign neoplasm is frequently tenuous and is variously interpreted. Hemangiomas, lymphangiomas, rhabdomyomas of the heart, and adenomas of the liver are considered by some to be hamartomas and by others to be true neoplasms.

Benign Tumors

Virtually any tumor may be encountered in the pediatric age group, but three—hemangiomas, lymphangiomas, and sacrococcygeal teratomas—deserve special mention here because they occur commonly in childhood.

Hemangiomas are the most common tumors of infancy. Both cavernous and capillary hemangiomas may be encountered (Chapter 10), although the latter are often more cellular than in adults, and hence are deceptively worrisome. In children most hemangiomas are located in the skin, particularly on the face and scalp, where they produce flat to elevated, irregular, red-blue masses; the flat, larger lesions are referred to as *port wine stains*. Hemangiomas may enlarge as the child gets older, but in many instances they spontaneously regress (Fig. 7–32). The vast majority of superficial hemangiomas have no more than a cosmetic significance; rarely, they may be the manifestation of a hereditary disorder associated with disease within internal organs, such as the von Hippel-Lindau and Sturge-Weber syndromes (Chapter 23).

Lymphangiomas represent the lymphatic counterpart of hemangiomas. They are characterized by cystic and cavernous spaces lined by endothelial cells and surrounded by lymphoid aggregates; the spaces usually contain pale fluid. They may occur on the skin but, more

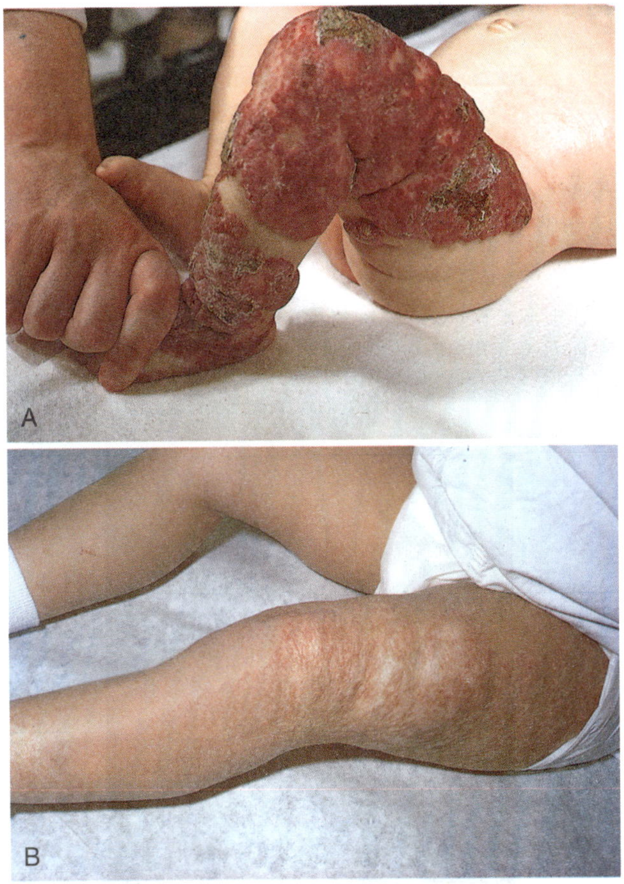

Figure 7–32

Congenital capillary hemangioma at birth (**A**) and at 2 years of age (**B**) after the lesion had undergone spontaneous regression. (Courtesy of Dr. Eduardo Yunis, Children's Hospital of Pittsburgh, Pittsburgh, Pennsylvania.)

importantly, are also encountered in the deeper regions of the neck, axilla, mediastinum, and retroperitoneum. Though histologically benign, they tend to increase in size after birth and may encroach on mediastinal structures or nerve trunks in axilla.

Sacrococcygeal teratomas are the most common germ cell tumors of childhood, accounting for 40% or more of cases (Fig. 7–33). In view of the overlap in the mechanisms underlying teratogenesis and oncogenesis, it is interesting that approximately 10% of sacrococcygeal teratomas are associated with congenital anomalies, primarily defects of the hindgut and cloacal region and other midline defects (e.g., meningocele, spina bifida) not believed to result from local effects of the tumor. Approximately 75% of these tumors are histologically mature with a benign course, and about 12% are unmistakably malignant and lethal (Chapter 18). The remainder is designated immature teratomas, and their malignant potential correlates with the amount of immature tissue elements present. Most of the benign teratomas are encountered in younger infants (<4 months), whereas children with malignant lesions tend to be somewhat older.

Malignant Tumors

The organ systems involved most commonly by malignant neoplasms in infancy and childhood include the hematopoietic system, neural tissue, and soft tissues (Table 7–12). This is in sharp contrast to adults, in whom tumors of the lung, heart, prostate, and colon are the most common forms. Malignant tumors of infancy and childhood differ biologically and histologically from those in adults. The main differences are as follows:

- Relatively frequent demonstration of a close relationship between abnormal development (teratogenesis) and tumor induction (oncogenesis)
- Prevalence of constitutional genetic abnormalities or syndromes that predispose to cancer

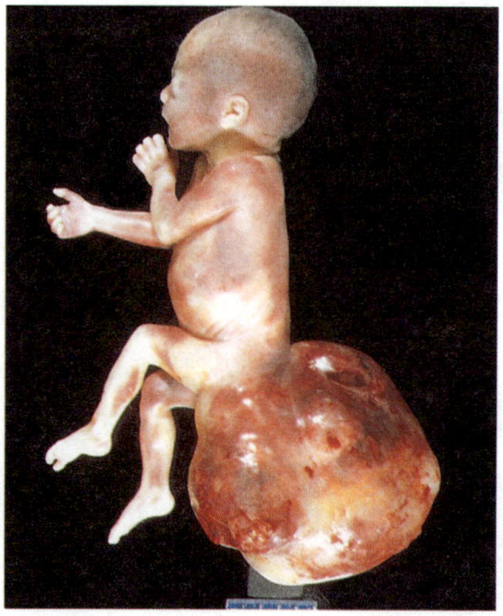

Figure 7–33

Sacrococcygeal teratoma. Note the size of the lesion compared with that of the infant.

Table 7–12 Common Malignant Neoplasms of Infancy and Childhood

0–4 Age yr	5–9 Age yr	10–14 Age yr
Leukemia	Leukemia	Hepatocellular carcinoma
Retinoblastoma	Retinoblastoma	Soft tissue sarcoma
Neuroblastoma	Neuroblastoma	Osteogenic sarcoma
Wilms' tumor	Hepatocellular carcinoma	Thyroid carcinoma
Hepatoblastoma	Soft tissue sarcoma	Hodgkin disease
Soft tissue sarcoma (especially rhabdomyosarcoma)	CNS tumors	
	Ewing tumor	
Teratomas	Lymphoma	
CNS tumors		

CNS, central nervous system.

- Tendency of fetal and neonatal malignancies to spontaneously regress or undergo "differentiation" into mature elements
- Improved survival or cure of many childhood tumors, so that more attention is now being paid to minimizing the adverse delayed effects of chemotherapy and radiotherapy in survivors, including the development of second malignancies

Histologically, many malignant pediatric neoplasms are unique. In general, they tend to have a primitive (*embryonal*) rather than pleomorphic-anaplastic microscopic appearance, and frequently they exhibit features of organogenesis specific to the site of tumor origin. Because of their primitive histologic appearance, many childhood tumors have been collectively referred to as *small, round, blue cell tumors*. These are characterized by sheets of cells with small, round nuclei. The tumors in this category include neuroblastoma, lymphoma, rhabdomyosarcoma, Ewing sarcoma (peripheral neuroectodermal tumor), and some cases of Wilms' tumor. There are usually sufficient distinctive features to render a definitive diagnosis on the basis of histologic examination alone, but when necessary, clinical and radiographic findings, combined with ancillary studies (e.g., chromosome analysis, immunoperoxidase stains, and electron microscopy) are used. Three common tumors—neuroblastoma, retinoblastoma, and Wilms' tumor—are described here to highlight the differences between pediatric tumors and those in adults.

Neuroblastoma

The term "neuroblastic tumor" includes tumors of the sympathetic ganglia and adrenal medulla that are derived from primordial neural crest cells populating these sites; neuroblastoma is the most important member of this family. It is the second most common solid malignancy of childhood after brain tumors, accounting for 7% to 10% of all pediatric neoplasms, and as many as 50% of malignancies diagnosed in infancy. Neuroblastomas demonstrate several unique features in their natural history, including *spontaneous regression* and *spontaneous- or therapy-induced maturation.* Most occur sporadically, but a few are familial with autosomal dominant transmission, and in such cases the neoplasms may involve both of the adrenals or multiple primary autonomic sites.

Morphology

In childhood, about 40% of neuroblastomas arise in the **adrenal medulla.** The remainder occur anywhere along the sympathetic chain, with the most common locations being the paravertebral region of the abdomen (25%) and posterior mediastinum (15%). Macroscopically, neuroblastomas range in size from minute nodules (the in situ lesions) to large masses weighing more than 1 kg. In situ neuroblastomas are reported to be 40 times more frequent than overt tumors. The great preponderance of these silent lesions spontaneously regress, leaving only a focus of fibrosis or calcification in the adult. Some neuroblastomas are often sharply demarcated with a fibrous pseudo-capsule, but others are far more infiltrative and invade surrounding structures, including the kidneys, renal vein, and vena cava, and envelop the aorta. On transection, they are composed of soft, gray-tan, brainlike tissue. Larger tumors have areas of necrosis, cystic softening, and hemorrhage.

Histologically, classic neuroblastomas are composed of small, primitive-appearing cells with dark nuclei, scant cytoplasm, and poorly defined cell borders growing in solid sheets (Fig. 7–34A). Mitotic activity, nuclear breakdown ("karyorrhexis"), and pleomorphism may be prominent. The background often demonstrates a faintly eosinophilic fibrillary material (neuropil) that corresponds to neuritic processes of the primitive neuroblasts. Typically, **rosettes** (Homer-Wright pseudo-rosettes) can be found in which the tumor cells are concentrically arranged about a central space filled with neuropil. Other helpful features include immunochemical detection of **neuron-specific enolase** and ultrastructural demonstration of small, membrane-bound, cytoplasmic catecholamine-containing secretory granules.

Some neoplasms show signs of **maturation**, either spontaneous or therapy-induced. Larger cells having more abundant cytoplasm with large vesicular nuclei and a prominent nucleolus, representing **ganglion cells** in various stages of maturation, may be found in tumors admixed with primitive neuroblasts (**ganglioneuroblastoma**). Even better differentiated lesions contain many more large cells resembling mature ganglion cells in the absence of residual neuroblasts; such neoplasms merit the designation **ganglioneuroma** (Fig. 7–34B). Maturation of neuroblasts into ganglion cells is usually accompanied by the appearance of Schwann cells. In fact, the presence of a "schwannian stroma" composed of organized fascicles of neuritic processes, mature **Schwann cells,** and fibroblasts is a histologic prerequisite for the designation of ganglioneuroblastoma and ganglioneuroma; ganglion cells in and of themselves do not fulfill the criteria for maturation.

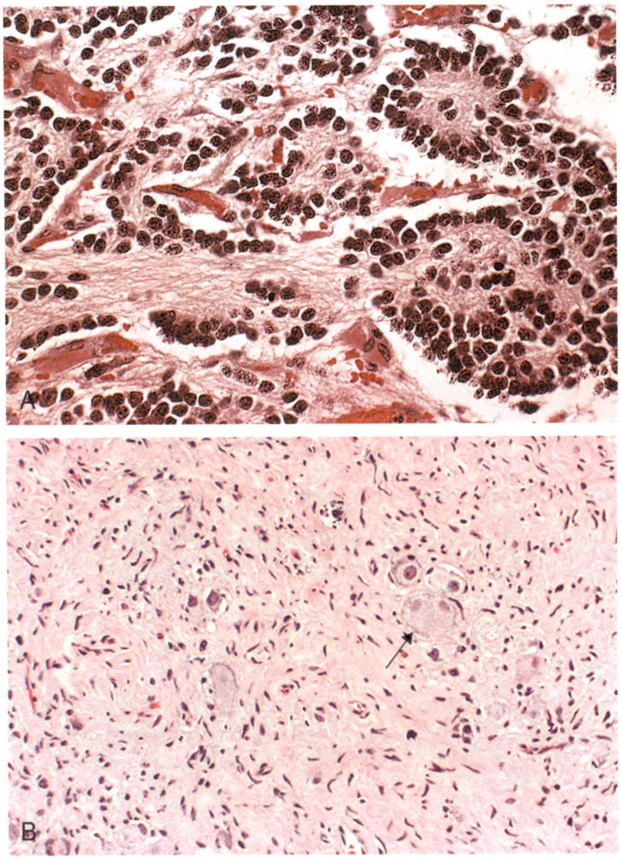

Figure 7–34

A, Neuroblastoma. This tumor is composed of small cells embedded in a finely fibrillar matrix (neuropil). A Homer-Wright pseudorosette (tumor cells arranged concentrically around a central core of neuropil) is seen in the upper right corner. **B,** Ganglioneuromas, arising from spontaneous or therapy-induced maturation of neuroblastomas, are characterized by clusters of large cells with vesicular nuclei and abundant eosinophilic cytoplasm (*arrow*), representing neoplastic ganglion cells. Spindle-shaped Schwann cells are present in the background stroma.

Prognosis. *Many factors influence prognosis, but the most important are the stage of the tumor and the age of the patient.* Staging of neuroblastomas (Table 7–13) assumes great importance in establishing a prognosis. Special note should be taken of stage 4S (S means special), because the outlook for these patients is excellent, despite the spread of disease. As noted in Table 7–13, the primary tumor would be classified as stages 1 or 2 but for the presence of metastases, which are limited to liver, skin, and bone marrow, without bone involvement. Such infants have an excellent prognosis with minimal therapy, and it is not uncommon for the primary or metastatic tumors to undergo spontaneous regression. The biologic basis of this welcome behavior is not clear. *Age is the other important determinant of outcome,* and children younger than 1 year have a much more favorable outlook than do older children at a comparable stage of disease. Most neoplasms in the infant years are stage 1 or 2, or stage 4S. *Morphology* is an independent prognostic variable in neuroblastic tumors; evidence of schwannian stroma and

Table 7-13 Staging of Neuroblastomas

Stage 1	Localized tumor with complete gross excision, with or without microscopic residual disease; representative ipsilateral nonadherent lymph nodes negative for tumor (nodes adherent to the primary tumor may be positive for tumor).
Stage 2A	Localized tumor with incomplete gross resection; representative ipsilateral nonadherent lymph nodes negative for tumor microscopically.
Stage 2B	Localized tumor with or without complete gross excision, ipsilateral nonadherent lymph nodes positive for tumor; enlarged contralateral lymph nodes, which are negative for tumor microscopically.
Stage 3	Unresectable unilateral tumor infiltrating across the midline with or without regional lymph node involvement; or localized unilateral tumor with contralateral regional lymph node involvement.
Stage 4	Any primary tumor with dissemination to distant lymph nodes, bone, bone marrow, liver, skin, and/or other organs (*except as defined for stage 4S*).
Stage 4S*	Localized primary tumor (as defined for stages 1, 2A, or 2B) with dissemination limited to skin, liver, and/or bone marrow (<10% of nucleated cells are constituted by neoplastic cells; >10% involvement of bone marrow is considered as stage 4); *stage 4S limited to infants <1 yr.*

*S = special.
Adapted from Brodeur GM, et al: The international neuroblastoma staging system. J Clinical Oncol 11:1466, 1993.

gangliocytic differentiation is indicative of a "favorable" histology. *Amplification of the MYCN oncogene* in neuroblastomas is a molecular event that has profound impact on prognosis. *MYCN* amplification is present in about 25% to 30% of primary tumors, most in advanced-stage disease; the greater the number of copies, the worse the prognosis. *MYCN* amplification is currently the most important genetic abnormality used in risk stratification of neuroblastic tumors. Deletion of the distal short arm of chromosome 1, gain of the distal long arm of chromosome 17, and overexpression of telomerase are all adverse prognostic factors, while expression of TrkA, a high-affinity receptor for nerve growth factor that is indicative of differentiation toward sympathetic ganglia lineage, is associated with favorable prognosis.

Clinical Course. Children younger than 2 years with neuroblastomas generally present with protuberant abdomen resulting from an abdominal mass, fever, and weight loss. In older children the neuroblastomas may remain unnoticed until metastases cause hepatomegaly, ascites, and bone pain. Neuroblastomas may metastasize widely through the hematogenous and lymphatic systems, particularly to liver, lungs, and bones, in addition to the bone marrow. In neonates, disseminated neuroblastomas may present with multiple cutaneous metastases with deep blue discoloration to the skin (earning the rather unfortunate moniker of "*blueberry muffin baby*"). As stated, above, there are many variables that influence the prognosis of neuroblastomas, but as a rule of thumb, stage and age are the paramount determinants. Tumors of all stages that occur in infants, as well as low-stage tumors in older children, are usually associated with favorable prognosis, while high-stage tumors in children >1 year of age have the poorest outcome. About 90% of neuroblastomas, regardless of location, produce catecholamines (similar to the catecholamines associated with pheochromocytomas), which are an important diagnostic feature (i.e., elevated blood levels of catecholamines and elevated urine levels of catecholamine metabolites such as vanillylmandelic acid [VMA] and homovanillic acid [HVA]). Despite the elaboration of catecholamines, hypertension is much less frequent with these neoplasms than with pheochromocytomas (Chapter 20).

SUMMARY

Neuroblastoma

- Neuroblastomas and related tumors arise from neural crest–derived cells in the sympathetic ganglia and adrenal medulla.
- Neuroblastomas are undifferentiated neoplasms, whereas ganglioneuroblastomas and ganglioneuromas demonstrate evidence of differentiation (Schwannian stroma and ganglion cells). Homer-Wright pseudo-rosettes are characteristic of neuroblastomas.
- Age and stage are the most important prognostic features; infants usually have a better prognosis than older children, while children with higher stage tumors fare worse.
- Neuroblastomas secrete catecholamines, whose metabolites (VMA/HVA) can be used for screening patients.

Retinoblastoma

Retinoblastoma is the most common malignant eye tumor of childhood. From a pathologic as well as a clinical standpoint, retinoblastoma is unusual in several aspects when compared with most other solid tumors. Retinoblastoma frequently occurs as a *congenital tumor,* it can be *multifocal* and *bilateral,* it undergoes *spontaneous regression,* and patients have a high incidence of *second primary tumors*. The incidence decreases with age, most cases being diagnosed before the age of 4 years.

Retinoblastomas occur in both familial and sporadic patterns. *Familial cases typically develop multiple tumors that are bilateral,* although they may be unifocal and unilateral. All of the sporadic nonheritable tumors are unilateral and unifocal. Patients with familial retinoblastoma are also at increased risk for developing *osteosarcoma* and other soft tissue tumors.

Approximately 60% to 70% of the tumors are associated with a germline mutation in the *RB1* gene and are hence heritable. The remaining 30% to 40% of the tumors develop sporadically, and these have somatic *RB1* gene mutations.

Morphology

Retinoblastoma is believed to arise from a cell of neuroepithelial origin, usually in the posterior retina (Fig. 7–35A). The tumors tend to be nodular masses, often with satellite seedings. On light microscopic examination, undifferentiated areas of these tumors are found to be composed of small, round cells with large hyperchromatic nuclei and scant cytoplasm, resembling undifferentiated retinoblasts.

Differentiated structures are found within many retinoblastomas, the most characteristic of these being the rosettes described by Flexner and Wintersteiner **(Flexner-Wintersteiner rosettes;** Fig. 7–35B). These structures consist of clusters of cuboidal or short columnar cells arranged around a central lumen (contrast with the **pseudo-rosettes** of neuroblastoma, which lack a central lumen). The nuclei are displaced away from the lumen, which by light microscopy appears to have a limiting membrane resembling the external limiting membrane of the retina.

Tumor cells may disseminate beyond the eye through the optic nerve or subarachnoid space. The most common sites of distant metastases are the CNS, skull, distal bones, and lymph nodes.

Clinical Features. The median age at presentation is 2 years, although the tumor may be present at birth. The presenting findings include poor vision, strabismus, a whitish hue to the pupil ("cat's eye reflex"), and pain and tenderness in the eye. Untreated, the tumors are usually fatal, but after early treatment with enucleation, chemotherapy, and radiotherapy, survival is the rule. As noted earlier, some tumors spontaneously regress, and patients with familial retinoblastoma are at increased risk for developing osteosarcoma and other soft tissue tumors.

Wilms' Tumor

Wilms' tumor, or *nephroblastoma,* is the most common primary tumor of the kidney in children. Most cases occur in children between 2 and 5 years of age. This tumor illustrates several important concepts of childhood tumors: the relationship between congenital malformation and increased risk of tumors, the histologic similarity between tumor and developing organ, and finally, the remarkable success in the treatment of childhood tumors. Each of these will be evident from the following discussion.

Three groups of congenital malformations are associated with an increased risk of developing Wilms' tumor. Patients with the *WAGR syndrome,* characterized by aniridia, genital abnormalities, and mental retardation, have a 33% chance of developing Wilms' tumor. Another group of patients, those with the so-called *Denys-Drash syndrome* (DDS) also has an extremely high risk (~90%) of developing Wilms' tumor. This syndrome is characterized by gonadal dysgenesis and renal abnormalities. Both of these conditions are associated with abnormalities of the Wilms' tumor 1 (*WT1*) gene, located on chromosome 11p13. The nature of genetic aberration differs, however. Patients with WAGR syndrome demonstrate loss of

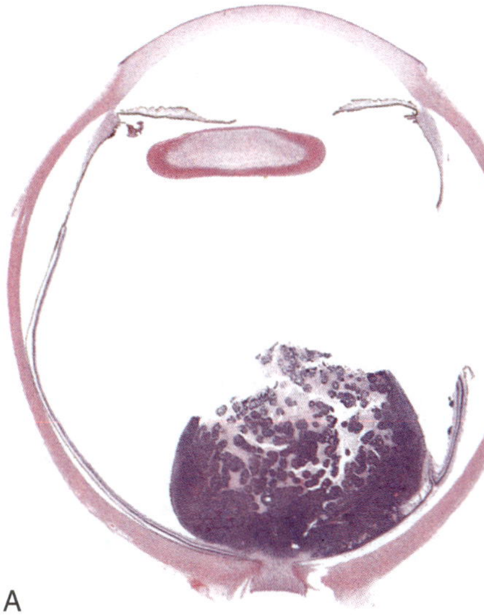

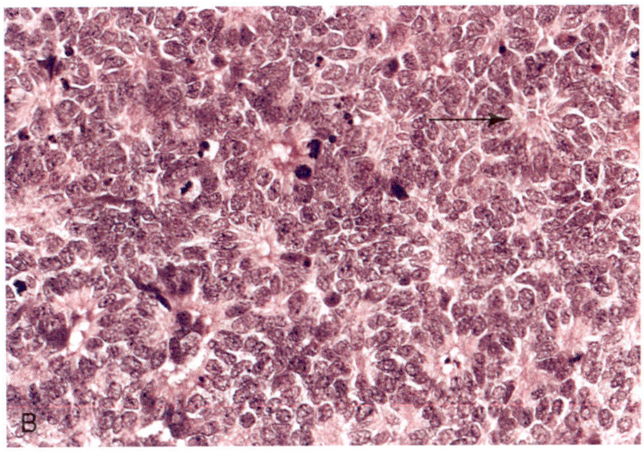

Figure 7–35

Retinoblastoma. **A,** Note poorly cohesive tumor in retina abutting optic nerve. **B,** Higher power view showing Flexner-Wintersteiner rosettes (*arrows*) and numerous mitotic figures.

genetic material (i.e., deletions) of *WT1*, and individuals with DDS harbor a dominant negative inactivating mutation in a critical region of the gene. (A dominant negative mutation interferes with the function of the remaining wild-type allele.) The *WT1* gene is critical to normal renal and gonadal development; it is not surprising therefore that constitutional inactivation of one copy of this gene results in genitourinary abnormalities in humans. A third group of patients, those with the *Beckwith-Wiedemann syndrome* (BWS), also has an increased risk of developing Wilms' tumor. These patients have enlargement of individual body organs (e.g., tongue, kidneys, or liver) or entire body segments (hemihypertrophy); enlargement of adrenal cortical cells (adrenal cytomegaly) is a characteristic microscopic feature. *BWS is an example of a disorder of genomic imprinting* (see earlier). The genetic locus that is involved in these patients is in band p15.5 of chromosome 11 distal to the *WT1* locus. Although this locus is called "*WT2*" for the second Wilms' tumor locus, the gene involved has not been identified. This region contains at least 10 genes that are normally expressed from only *one* of the two parental alleles, with transcriptional silencing of the other parental homologue by *methylation of the promoter region,* located up-stream of the transcription start site. One of the candidate genes in this region—insulin-like growth factor-2 (*IGF2*) is normally expressed solely from the *paternal allele,* while the maternal allele is imprinted (i.e., silenced) by methylation. In some Wilms' tumors, *loss of imprinting* (i.e., re-expression of *IGF2* by the maternal allele) can be demonstrated, leading to overexpression of the IGF2 protein, which is postulated to result in both organ enlargement and tumorigenesis. Thus, these associations suggest that in some cases congenital malformations and tumors represent related manifestations of genetic damage affecting a single gene or closely linked genes. In addition to Wilms' tumors, patients with BWS are also at increased risk for developing hepatoblastoma, adrenocortical tumors, rhabdomyosarcomas, and pancreatic tumors.

Morphology

Grossly, Wilms' tumor tends to present as a large, solitary, well-circumscribed mass, although 10% are either bilateral or multicentric at the time of diagnosis. On cut section, the tumor is soft, homogeneous, and tan to gray, with occasional foci of hemorrhage, cystic degeneration, and necrosis (Fig. 7–36).

Microscopically, Wilms' tumors are characterized by recognizable attempts to recapitulate different stages of nephrogenesis. The classic **triphasic combination** of blastemal, stromal, and epithelial cell types is observed in most lesions, although the percentage of each component is variable (Fig. 7–37). Sheets of small blue cells, with few distinctive features, characterize the blastemal component. Epithelial "differentiation" usually takes the form of **abortive tubules or glomeruli.** Stromal cells are usually fibrocytic or myxoid in nature, although skeletal muscle "differentiation" is not uncommon. Rarely, other heterologous elements are identified, including squamous or mucinous epithelium, smooth muscle, adipose tissue, cartilage, and osteoid and neurogenic tissue. Approximately 5% of tumors contain foci of **anaplasia** (cells with large, hyperchromatic, pleomorphic nuclei and abnormal mitoses) (see *inset,* Fig. 7–37). The presence of anaplasia correlates with underlying *p53* mutations, and the emergence of resistance to chemotherapy. The pattern of distribution of anaplastic cells within the primary tumor (focal versus diffuse) has important implications for prognosis (see later).

Nephrogenic rests are putative precursor lesions of Wilms' tumors and are sometimes present in the renal parenchyma adjacent to the tumor. Nephrogenic rests have a spectrum of histologic appearances, from expansile masses that resemble Wilms' tumors (hyperplastic rests) to sclerotic rests consisting predominantly of fibrous tissue with occasional admixed immature tubules or glomeruli. It is important to document the presence of nephrogenic rests in the resected specimen, since these patients are at an increased risk of developing Wilms' tumors in the **contralateral** kidney.

Clinical Course. Patients' complaints are usually referable to the tumor's enormous size. Commonly, there is a readily palpable abdominal mass, which may extend across the midline and down into the pelvis. Less often, the patient presents with fever and abdominal pain, with hematuria, or, occasionally, with intestinal obstruction as a result of pressure from the tumor. The prognosis for Wilms' tumor is generally very good, and excellent results are obtained with a combination of nephrectomy and chemotherapy. Anaplasia is a harbinger of adverse prognosis, but careful analyses by the National Wilms' Tumor Study group in the United States have shown that as long as the anaplasia is *focal* and confined within the resected nephrectomy specimen, the outcome is no different from tumors without evidence of anaplasia. In contrast, Wilms' tumors with *diffuse anaplasia,* especially those with extra-renal spread, have the least favorable outcome, underscoring the need for correctly identifying this histologic pattern.

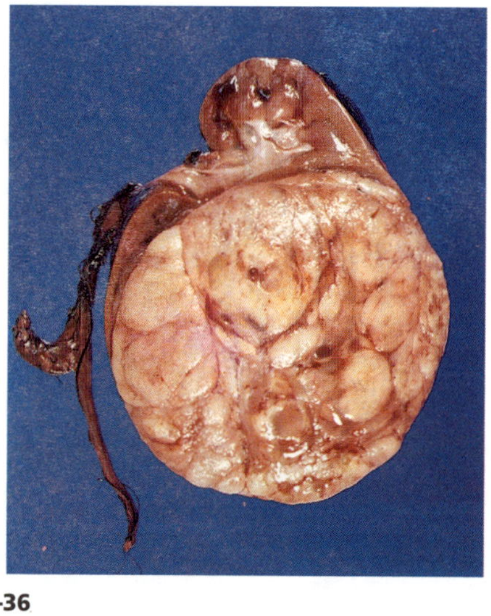

Figure 7–36

Wilms' tumor in the lower pole of the kidney with the characteristic tan to gray color and well-circumscribed margins.

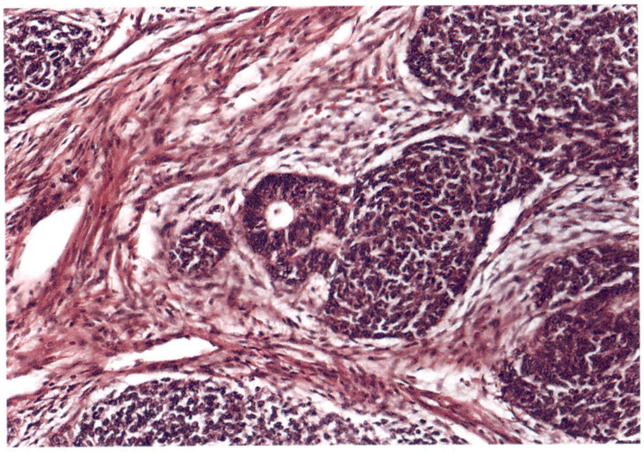

Figure 7–37

Triphasic histology of Wilms' tumor: the stromal component is composed of spindle-shaped cells in the less cellular area on the left; the immature tubule in the center is an example of the epithelial component, and the tightly packed blue cells the blastemal elements. (Courtesy of Dr. Charles Timmons, Department of Pathology, University of Texas Southwestern Medical School, Dallas, Texas.)

SUMMARY

Wilms' Tumor

- Wilms' tumor is the most common renal neoplasm of childhood.
- Patients with three syndromes are at increased risk for Wilms' tumors: WAGR, DDS, and BWS.
- WAGR and DDS are associated with *WT1* inactivation, while BWS arises through imprinting abnormalities at the *WT2* locus.
- The morphologic components of Wilms' tumor include blastema (small, round blue cells) and epithelial and stromal elements.
- Nephrogenic rests are precursor lesions of Wilms' tumors.

DIAGNOSIS OF GENETIC DISEASES

By definition, diseases with a genetic component should have an aberration in the genetic material of the individual. This aberration may be in the germline (i.e., present in each and every cell of the individual, as with the *CFTR* mutation in a CF patient) or be somatic (i.e., restricted to specific tissue types or lesions, as with the *MYCN* amplification in neuroblastoma cells). The sequencing of the human genome and the deposition of this sequence in publicly available databases on the Internet has greatly accelerated the hunt for disease-causing genes. In this section we will briefly outline some of the traditional and emerging technologies for unraveling the genetic bases of human diseases. Karyotype analysis of chromosomes by G-banding remains the classic approach for identifying changes at the chromosomal level; however, as one can imagine, the resolution of this technique is fairly low. In addition, a major limitation of karyotyping is that it is applicable only to cells that are dividing or can be induced to divide in vitro. To bypass these hurdles, both focused analysis of chromosomal regions by FISH and global genomic approaches such as comparative genomic hybridization (CGH) have become popular.

Fluorescence in Situ Hybridization

FISH utilizes DNA probes that recognize sequences specific to chromosomal regions. The usual size of a FISH probe is in the order of ~1 megabase (1×10^6 nt), and this defines the limit of resolution of this technique for identifying chromosomal changes. Such probes are labeled with fluorescent dyes and applied to metaphase spreads or interphase nuclei. The probe binds to its complementary sequence on the chromosome and thus labels the specific chromosomal region that can be visualized under a fluorescent microscope. The ability of FISH to circumvent the need for dividing cells is invaluable when a rapid diagnosis is warranted (e.g., in a critically ill infant suspected of having an underlying genetic disorder). Such analysis can be performed on prenatal samples (e.g., cells obtained by amniocentesis, chorionic villus biopsy, or umbilical cord blood), peripheral blood lymphocytes, and even archival tissue sections. FISH has been used for detection of numeric abnormalities of chromosomes (aneuploidy) (Fig. 7–38A); for the demonstration of subtle microdeletions (Fig. 7–38B) or complex translocations not detectable by routine karyotyping; for analysis of gene amplification (e.g., *MYCN* amplification in neuroblastomas); and for mapping newly isolated genes of interest to their chromosomal loci.

Comparative Genomic Hybridization (CGH)

It is obvious from the preceding discussion that FISH requires prior knowledge of the one or few specific chromosomal regions suspected of being altered in the test sample. However, chromosomal abnormalities can also be detected without prior knowledge of what these aberrations may be, using a global strategy like CGH. In CGH, the test DNA and a reference (normal) DNA are labeled with two different fluorescent dyes (most commonly, Cy5 and Cy3, which fluoresce red and green, respectively). The differentially labeled samples are then hybridized to each other. If the contributions of both samples are equal for a given chromosomal region (i.e., the test sample is diploid), then all regions of the genome will fluoresce yellow (due to an equal admixture of green and red dyes). In contrast, if the test sample shows an excess of DNA at any given chromosomal region (such as resulting from an amplification), there will be a corresponding excess of signal from the dye with which this sample was labeled. The reverse will be true in the event of a deletion, with an excess of the signal used for label-

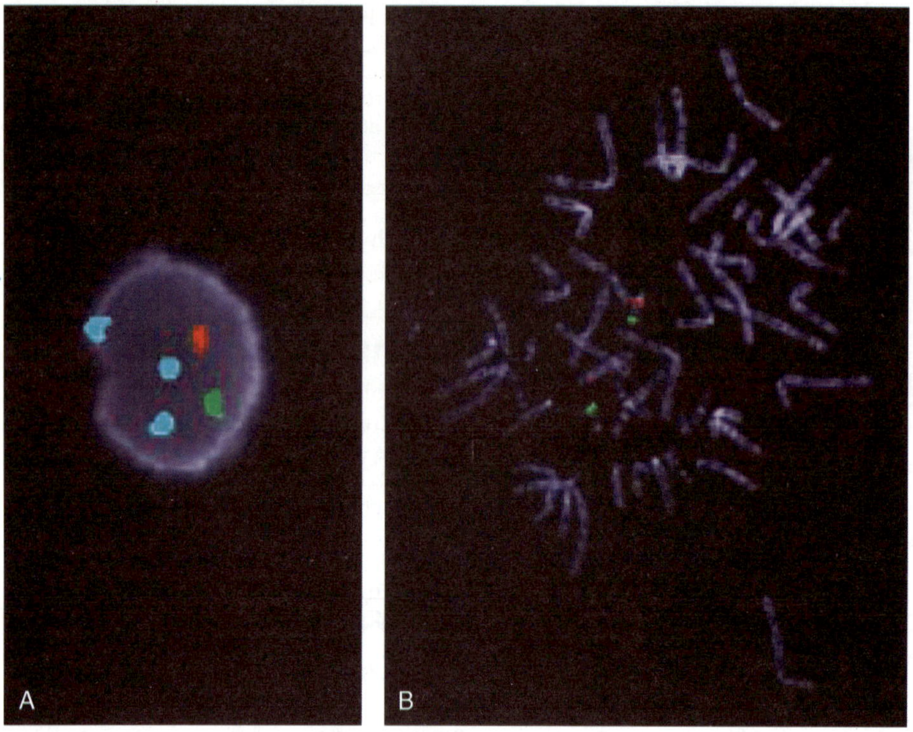

Figure 7–38

Fluorescence in situ hybridization (FISH). **A,** Interphase nucleus from a male patient with suspected trisomy 18. Three different fluorescent probes have been used in a "FISH cocktail"; the green probe hybridizes to the X chromosome centromere (one copy), the red probe to the Y chromosome centromere (one copy), and the aqua probe to the chromosome 18 centromere (three copies). **B,** A metaphase spread in which two fluorescent probes have been used, one hybridizing to chromosome 22q13 region (*green*) and the other hybridizing to chromosome 22q11.2 region (*red*). There are two 22q13 signals. One of the two chromosomes does not stain with the probe for 22q11.2, indicating a microdeletion in this region. This deletion gives rise to the 22q11.2 deletion syndrome (DiGeorge syndrome). (Courtesy of Dr. Nancy R. Schneider and Jeff Doolittle, Cytogenetics Laboratory, University of Texas Southwestern Medical Center, Dallas, Texas.)

ing the reference sample. Despite having a higher resolution than conventional cytogenetics, CGH still lacks the ability to detect submicroscopic alterations. Therefore, in recent years, an approach known as *array-based CGH* has been developed, wherein short segments of genomic DNA are "spotted" on a solid matrix, usually a glass slide. These segments of DNA are representations of the human genome at regularly spaced intervals, and usually cover all 22 autosomes and the X chromosome. Thereafter, the steps are similar to conventional CGH, except that hybridization of the two differentially labeled samples occurs on the glass slide (Fig. 7–39A). Amplifications and deletions in the test sample can now be significantly better localized, often up to a 200-kilobase (kb) resolution (Fig. 7–39B). Newer generations of microarrays using single-nucleotide polymorphisms (SNPs, see below) provide even higher resolution, and are currently being used to uncover copy number abnormalities in a variety of diseases, from cancer to autism.

Molecular Diagnosis of Genetic Disorders

Many genetic diseases are caused by alterations at the nucleotide level (i.e., mutations) that cannot be detected by FISH or even high-resolution array-based CGH. In the era predating the ready availability of molecular diagnostic assays, assays for single-gene ("mendelian") disorders depended on the identification of abnormal gene products (e.g., mutant hemoglobin or abnormal metabolites) or their clinical effects, such as mental retardation (e.g., in phenylketonuria). Now, it is possible to identify mutations at the DNA level and offer diagnostic tests for an increasing number of genetic disorders. The molecular diagnosis of inherited diseases has distinct advantages over other surrogate techniques:

- It is remarkably sensitive. The use of polymerase chain reaction (PCR) allows several million-fold amplification of DNA or RNA, making it possible to utilize as few as 1 or 100 cells for analysis. A few drops of blood or a piece of biopsy tissue can supply sufficient DNA for PCR amplification.
- DNA-based tests are not dependent on a gene product that may be produced only in certain specialized cells (e.g., brain) or expression of a gene that may occur late in life. Because the defective gene responsible for inherited genetic disorders is present in germline samples, every postzygotic cell carries the mutation.

These two features have profound implications for the *prenatal diagnosis* of genetic diseases, because a sufficient number of cells can be obtained from a few milliliters of amniotic fluid or from a biopsy of chorionic villus that can be performed as early as the first trimester. There are two distinct approaches to the molecular diagnosis of single-gene diseases: direct detection of DNA mutations and indirect detection based on linkage of the disease gene with surrogate markers in the genome. These two methods are described in the following sections.

Direct Detection of DNA Mutations by PCR Analysis

PCR analysis, which involves exponential amplification of DNA, is now widely used in molecular diagnosis. If RNA is used as the substrate, it is first reverse transcribed to obtain cDNA and then amplified by PCR. This method is often abbreviated as RT-PCR. One prerequisite for

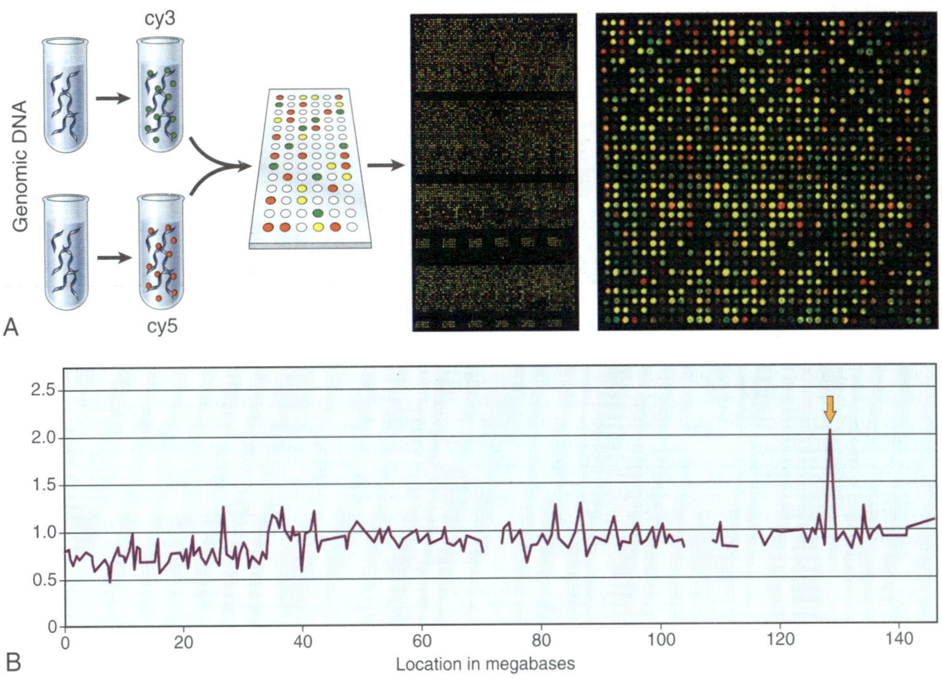

Figure 7–39

A, Array CGH is performed by hybridization of fluorescently labeled "test" DNA and "control" DNA on a slide that contains thousands of probes corresponding to defined chromosomal regions across the human genome. The resolution of most currently available array CGH is in the order of ~200 to 500 kb. Higher power view of the array demonstrates copy number aberrations in the "test" sample (Cy5, red), including regions of amplification (spots with excess of red signal) and deletion (spots with excess of green signal); yellow spots correspond to regions of normal (diploid) copy number. **B,** The hybridization signals are digitized resulting in a virtual karyotype of the genome of the "test" sample. In the illustrated example, array CGH of a cancer cell line identifies an amplification on the distal long arm of chromosome 8, which corresponds to increased copy number of the oncogene *MYC*. (**A,** From Snijders AM, et al.: Assembly of microarrays for genome-wide measurement of DNA copy number. Nat Genet 29:263, Web Figure A, Copyright 2001. Reprinted by permission from Macmillan Publishers Ltd.)

direct detection is that the sequence of the normal gene must be known. To detect the mutant gene, two primers that bind to the 3' and 5' ends of the normal sequence are designed. By utilizing appropriate DNA polymerases and thermal cycling, the target DNA is greatly amplified, producing millions of copies of the DNA sequence between the two primer sites. The subsequent identification of an abnormal sequence can then be performed in several ways:

- The DNA can be sequenced to obtain a readout of the order of nucleotides, and by comparison with a normal (wild-type) sequence, mutations can be identified. The ready availability of automated sequencers has made the previously laborious task of manual sequencing obsolete, and thousands of base pairs of genomic DNA can now be sequenced in a matter of hours. More recently, gene chips (microarrays) have become available that can be used for sequencing genes or portions of genes. Short sequences of DNA (oligonucleotides) that are complementary to the wild-type sequence and to known mutations are "tiled" adjacent to each other on the gene chip, and the DNA sample to be tested is hybridized to the array (Fig. 7–40). Before hybridization the sample is labeled with fluorescent dyes. The hybridization (and consequently, the fluorescent signal emitted) will be strongest at the oligonucleotide that is complementary to wild-type sequence if no mutations are present, while the presence of a mutation will cause hybridization to occur at the complementary mutant oligonucleotide. Computerized algorithms can then rapidly "decode" the DNA sequence for hundreds of thousands of base pairs of sequence from the fluorescent hybridization pattern on the chip, and identify potential mutations.
- Alternatively, the DNA can be digested with enzymes known as restriction enzymes that recognize, and then cut, DNA at specific sequences. If the specific mutation is known to affect a restriction site, then the amplified DNA can be digested. Because the mutation affects a restriction site, the mutant and normal alleles give rise to products of different sizes. These would appear as different bands on agarose gel electrophoresis. Needless to say, this approach is considerably lower in its throughput than automated or array-based sequencing, but remains useful for molecular diagnostics in instances when the causal mutation always occurs at an invariant nucleotide position.
- Another approach for identifying mutations at a specific nucleotide position (say, a codon 12 mutation in the *KRAS* oncogene that converts glycine [GGT] to aspartic acid [GAT]) would be to add fluorescently labeled nucleotides C and T to the PCR mixture, which are complementary to either the wild-type (G) or mutant (A) sequence, respectively. Since these two nucleotides are labeled with different fluorophores, the

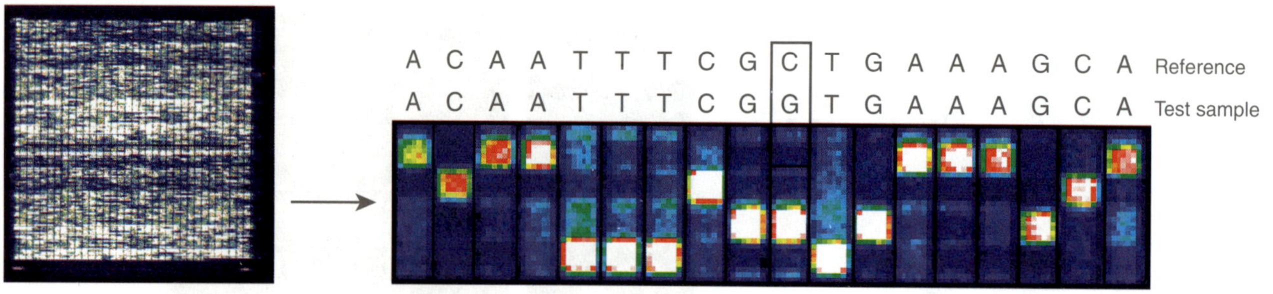

Figure 7–40

Microarray-based DNA sequencing. **Left panel,** A low-power digitized scan of a "gene chip" that is no larger than a nickel in size but is capable of sequencing thousands of base pairs of DNA. High-throughput microarrays have been used for sequencing whole organisms (such as viruses), organelles (such as the mitochondria), and entire human chromosomes. **Right panel,** A high-resolution view of the gene chip illustrates hybridization patterns corresponding to a stretch of DNA sequence. Typically, a computerized algorithm is available that can convert the individual hybridization patterns across the entire chip into actual sequence data within a matter of minutes ("conventional" sequencing technologies would required days to weeks for such analysis). Here, the sequence on top is the reference (wild-type) sequence, while the lower one correspond to the test sample sequence. As shown, the computerized algorithm has identified a C→G mutation in the test sample. (Adapted from Maitra A, et al.: The Human MitoChip: a high-throughput sequencing microarray for mitochondrial mutation detection. Genome Res 14:812, 2004.)

fluorescence emitted by the resulting PCR product can be of one or another color, depending on whether a "C" or a "T" becomes incorporated in the process of primer extension (Fig. 7–41). The advantage of this "allele-specific extension" strategy is that it can detect the presence of mutant DNA even in heterogeneous mixtures of normal and abnormal cells (for example, in clinical specimens obtained from patients suspected of harboring a malignancy). Many variations on this theme have been developed and are being currently used for mutation detection in the laboratory and clinical settings.

• PCR analysis is also very useful when a mutation is associated with deletions or expansions (Fig. 7–42). As discussed earlier, several diseases, such as the fragile X syndrome, are associated with trinucleotide repeats. Two primers that bind to a sequence at the 5' end of the *FMR1* gene, which is affected by trinucleotide repeats, are used to amplify the intervening sequences. Because there are large differences in the number of repeats, the size of the PCR products obtained from the DNA of normal individuals and those with premutation is quite different. These size differences are revealed by differential migration of the amplified DNA products on a gel.

Linkage Analysis

Direct diagnosis of mutations is possible only if the gene responsible for a genetic disorder is known and its sequence has been identified. In several diseases that have a genetic basis, including some common disorders, direct genetic diagnosis is not possible, either because the causal gene has not been identified or because the disease is multifactorial (polygenic) and no single gene is involved. In such cases, surrogate markers in the genome, also known as marker loci, must be used to localize the chromosomal regions of interest, based on their linkage to one or more putative disease-causing genes. *Linkage analysis* deals with assessing these marker loci in family members exhibiting the disease or trait of interest, with the assumption that marker loci very close to the disease allele, are transmitted through pedigrees. With time it becomes possible to define a "disease haplotype" based on a panel of marker loci all of which co-segregate with the putative disease allele. Eventually, linkage analysis facilitates localization and cloning of the disease allele. The marker loci utilized in linkage studies are naturally occurring variations in DNA sequences known as *poly-*

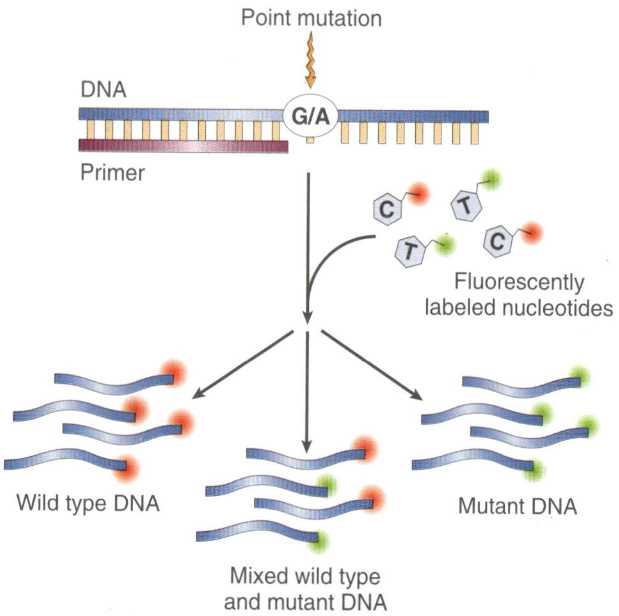

Figure 7–41

Allele-specific PCR for mutation detection in a heterogeneous sample containing an admixture of normal and mutant DNA. Nucleotides complementary to the mutant and wild-type nucleotides at the queried base position are labeled with different fluorophores, such that incorporation into the resulting PCR product yields fluorescent signals of varying intensity based on the ratio of mutant to wild-type DNA present.

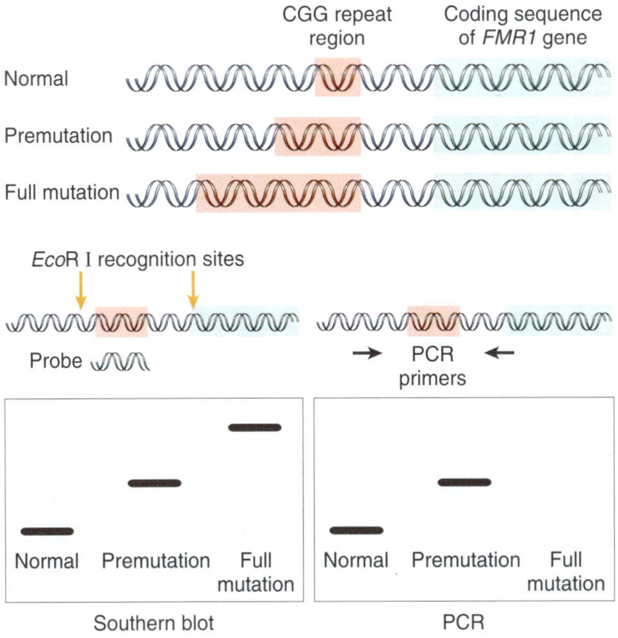

Figure 7–42

Molecular diagnosis of triplet-repeat expansion in fragile X syndrome. With PCR, the differences in the size of CGG repeat between normal and premutation give rise to products of different sizes and mobility. With a full mutation the region between the primers is too large to be amplified by conventional PCR. In Southern blot analysis, the DNA is cut by enzymes that flank the CGG repeat region and is then probed with a DNA that binds to the affected part of the gene. A single small band is seen in normal males, a band of higher molecular weight in males with premutation, and a very large (usually diffuse) band in those with the full mutation.

morphisms. DNA polymorphisms occur at a frequency of approximately one nucleotide in every ~1000–base pair stretch. These single nucleotide polymorphisms (SNPs) are found throughout the genome (e.g., in exons and introns and in regulatory sequences). SNPs serve both as a physical landmark within the genome and as a genetic marker whose transmission can be followed from parent to child. Because of their prevalence throughout the genome and relative stability, SNPs can be used in linkage analysis for identifying haplotypes associated with disease, leading to gene discovery and mapping. In the last decade, SNPs have become the genetic marker of choice for the study of complex genetic traits. Population studies have found some associations between specific SNPs and multifactorial diseases such as hypertension, heart disease, and diabetes. "SNP chips" that contain as many as half a million SNPs across the human genome are now available and provide an unprecedented opportunity to perform linkage analysis at a resolution previously inconceivable. Recently, an international consortium to generate genome-wide SNP haplotypes in different ethnic backgrounds (the "HapMap" project) completed its task; the public availability of this data will permit rapid generation of disease-associated haplotypes and subsequent localization of genes responsible for a host of diseases that have a genetic basis.

Indications for Genetic Analysis

In the preceding discussion we described some of the many techniques available today for the diagnosis of genetic diseases. To judiciously utilize these methods it is important to recognize which individuals require genetic testing. In general, genetic testing can be divided into prenatal and postnatal analysis. It may involve conventional cytogenetics, FISH, molecular diagnostics, or a combination of these techniques.

Prenatal genetic analysis should be offered to all patients who are at risk of having cytogenetically abnormal progeny. It can be performed on cells obtained by amniocentesis, on chorionic villus biopsy material, or on umbilical cord blood. Some important indications are the following:

- A mother of advanced age (>34 years), because of greater risk of trisomies
- A parent who is a carrier of a balanced reciprocal translocation, Robertsonian translocation, or inversion (in these cases the gametes may be unbalanced, and hence the progeny would be at risk for chromosomal disorders)
- A parent with a previous child with a chromosomal abnormality
- A parent who is a carrier of an X-linked genetic disorder (to determine fetal sex).

Postnatal genetic analysis is usually performed on peripheral blood lymphocytes. Indications are as follows:

- Multiple congenital anomalies
- Unexplained mental retardation and/or developmental delay
- Suspected aneuploidy (e.g., features of Down syndrome)
- Suspected unbalanced autosome (e.g., Prader-Willi syndrome)
- Suspected sex chromosomal abnormality (e.g., Turner syndrome)
- Suspected fragile X syndrome
- Infertility (to rule out sex chromosomal abnormality)
- Multiple spontaneous abortions (to rule out the parents as carriers of balanced translocation; both partners should be evaluated).

In closing, it should be pointed out that the progress in unraveling the genetic basis of human disease is likely to be breathtaking in the coming years. We all wait in anticipation.

BIBLIOGRAPHY

Altshuler D, et al: The International HapMap Consortium: a haplotype map of the human genome. Nature 437:1299, 2005. *[A seminal paper describing the completion of a haplotype map of the human genome.]*

Antonarakis SE, et al: Chromosome 21 and Down syndrome: from genomics to pathophysiology. Nat Rev Genet 5:725, 2004. *[An in-depth review of the molecular pathogenesis of Down syndrome—for the brave of heart!]*

Antshel KM, et al: 22q11.2 deletion syndrome: genetics, neuroanatomy, and cognitive behavioral features. Child Neuropsychol 11:5, 2005. *[A focus on the genetics and psychological problems in 22q11.2 syndrome.]*

Barkin RM, Gausche-Hill JA: Sudden infant death syndrome. In Marx (ed): Rosen's Emergency Medicine: Concepts and Clinical Practice, 5th ed. Baltimore, CV Mosby, 2002, p 2392. *[An up-to-date discussion of the pathogenesis and prevention of SIDS.]*

Carlson CS, et al: Mapping complex disease loci in whole genome association studies. Nature 429:446; 2004. *[A review on genetic approaches to mapping susceptibility genes for some of the most common human diseases that bear a genetic component.]*

Doull IJM: Recent advances in cystic fibrosis. Arch Dis Child 85:62, 2001. *[An excellent article addressing the complexity of pathogenesis, and genotype-phenotype correlations.]*

Epstein CJ: Critical genes in critical region. Nature 441:582, 2006. *[A succinct commentary on the role of NFAT transcription factor in Down syndrome.]*

Feinberg AP: The epigenetics of cancer etiology. Semin Cancer Biol 14:427, 2004. *[An outstanding review from the world expert on imprinting, highlighting the role of epigenetic abnormalities in the pathogenesis of cancers such as Wilms' tumors.]*

Goldstone AP: Prader-Willi syndrome: advances in genetics, pathophysiology and treatment. Trends Endocrinol Metab 15:12, 2004. *[A good discussion of this complex disorder.]*

Jeyakumar M, et al: Storage solutions: treating lysosomal disorders of the brain. Nat Rev Neurosci 6:1, 2005. *[A review that presents the current understanding of lysosomal storage diseases, with special emphasis on neuronal involvement.]*

Judge DP, Dietz HC: Marfan syndrome. Lancet 366:1965, 2005. *[An excellent summary of current thinking on pathogenesis of this disease.]*

Mitchell JJ, Scriver CR: Phenylalanine hydroxylase deficiency. Gene Reviews. Available at http://www.genetests.org. *[A comprehensive database that is regularly updated.]*

Patterson M: Niemann-Pick disease type C. Gene Reviews. Available at http://www.genetests.org. *[A detailed discussion of this newly discovered disease.]*

Person CE, et al: Repeat instability: mechanisms of dynamic mutations. Nat Rev Genet 6:729, 2005. *[A detailed discussion of the molecular basis of trinucleotide repeat mutations.]*

Pillai, RS: MicroRNA function: multiple mechanisms for a tiny RNA? RNA 11:1753, 2005. *[A detailed review.]*

Ranke MB, Saenger P: Turner syndrome. Lancet 358:309, 2001. *[An excellent basic and clinical review of Turner syndrome.]*

Rivera MN, Haber DA: Wilms tumor: Connecting tumorigenesis and organ development in the kidney. Nat Rev Cancer 5:699, 2005. *[An outstanding review on how Wilms' tumor epitomizes the connection between development and neoplasia.]*

Schwab M, et al: Neuroblastoma: biology and molecular and chromosomal pathology. Lancet Oncol 4:472, 2003. *[A comprehensive review of the major molecular alterations in neuroblastomas, and the use of genetics for prognostication.]*

Smyth CM, Bremmer WJ: Kleinfelter syndrome. Arch Intern Med 158:1309, 1998. *[An excellent clinical review.]*

Spitzer AR: Current controversies in the pathophysiology and prevention of sudden infant death syndrome. Curr Opin Pediatr 17:181, 2005. *[An update on research into causes of SIDS, particularly genetics and failure of arousal with discussion of approaches for SIDS prevention.]*

Stevenson M: Therapeutic potential of RNA interference. N Engl J Med 351:17, 2004. *[A glimpse into the future of miRNA applications.]*

Treszl A, et al: Genetic basis for necrotizing enterocolitis—risk factors and their relations to genetic polymorphisms. Front Biosci 11:570, 2006. *[A discussion on the potential etiologic factors contributing to NEC, and their relationship to the underlying genetic makeup of the individual.]*

Turcios NL: Cystic fibrosis—an overview. J Clin Gastroenterol 39:307, 2005. *[A concise update on the pathophysiology and clinical ramifications of cystic fibrosis.]*

Wattendorf DJ, et al: Diagnosis and management of fragile X syndrome. Am Fam Physician 72:111, 2005. *[An excellent and concise review of clinical features.]*

Chapter 8

Environmental and Nutritional Diseases

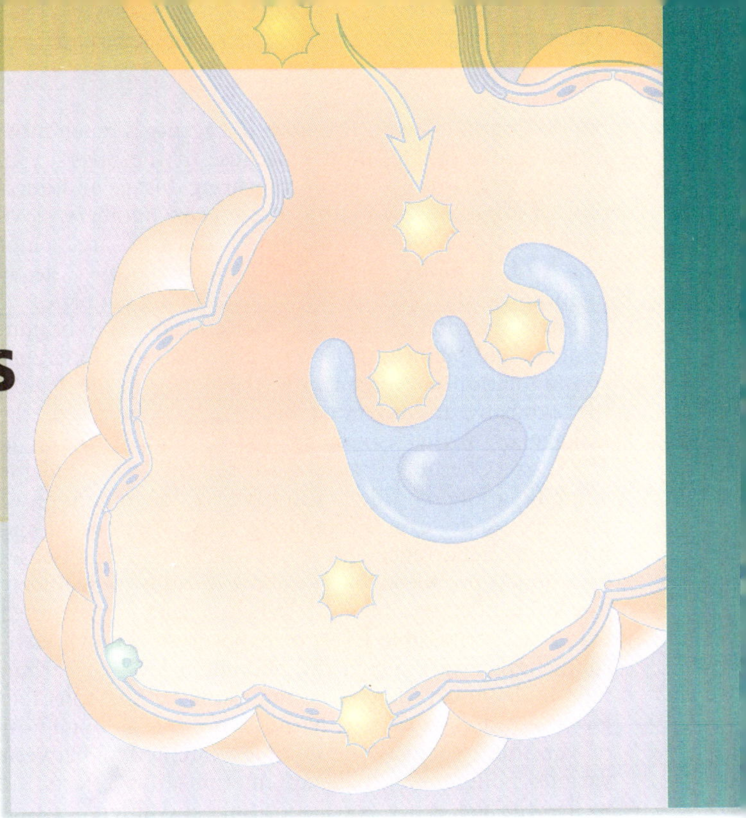

Many diseases can be caused or influenced by environmental factors. Broadly defined, the term "environment" encompasses the outdoor, indoor, and occupational environments in which we live. In each of these environments the air we breathe, the food and water we consume, and the direct exposure to toxic agents are major determinants of the health of the population. Another type of environment pertains more particularly to the individual ("personal environment") and is greatly influenced by the use of tobacco, alcohol ingestion, therapeutic and nontherapeutic drug consumption, diet, and the like. Factors in the personal environment generally have a larger effect on human health than does the ambient environment. The term *environmental diseases* refers to lesions and diseases caused by exposure to chemical or physical agents in the ambient, workplace, and personal environments, including diseases of nutritional origin. Environmental diseases are surprisingly common. The International Labor Organization has estimated that work-related injuries and illnesses kill 1.1 million people per year globally—more deaths than are caused by road accidents and wars combined. Most of these work-related problems are caused by illnesses rather than accidents. The burden of disease in the general population created by nonoccupational exposures to toxic agents is much more difficult to estimate, mostly because of the diversity of agents and the difficulties in measuring dosage and duration of exposures. Whatever the precise numbers, environmental (including nutritional) diseases are major causes of disability and suffering and constitute a heavy financial burden, particularly in developing countries.

Environmental diseases are often considered to be consequences of major disasters, such as the methyl mercury contamination of Minamata Bay in Japan in the 1960s, the exposure to dioxin in Seveso, Italy in 1976, the leakage of methyl isocyanate gas in Bhopal, India, in 1984, the Chernobyl nuclear accident in 1986, and the contamination of Tokyo subways by the organophosphate pesticide sarin. Fortunately, these are unusual and infrequent occurrences. Of major concern are the diseases and injury produced by chronic exposure to relatively low levels of contaminants. Several agencies in the United States set permissible levels of exposure to known environmental hazards (e.g., the maximum level of carbon monoxide in air that is noninjurious or the tolerable levels of radiation that are harmless or "safe"). But a host of variables, such as the complex interaction between various pollutants producing multiplicative effects, as well as the age, genetic predisposition, and different tissue sensitivities of exposed persons, create wide variations in individual sensitivity, limiting the value of establishing rigid "safe levels" for entire populations. Nevertheless, such levels are useful for comparative studies of the effects of harmful agents between specific populations, and for estimating risk of disease in heavily exposed individuals. With this brief overview of the nature and magnitude of the problem, we start by presenting some general comments about mechanisms of toxicity and then consider some of the more important environmental hazards.

GENERAL MECHANISMS OF TOXICITY

The number of chemicals available in the United States increases continuously, as the chemical industry markets almost 1000 new synthetic compounds per year. Of approximately 80,000 chemicals in use in the United States, only 600 have been tested experimentally for health effects. In Europe the number of available chemicals is less than one-half of that in the United States, but even these numbers are very high, since many of these chemicals are released in the environment as industrial products or discharged as human and animal wastes. *Toxicology* is defined as the science of poisons. It studies the distribution, effects, and mechanisms of action of toxic agents. More broadly, it also includes the study of the effects of physical agents such as radiation and heat. We now consider some basic principles regarding the toxicity of exogenous chemicals and drugs.

- The *definition of a poison* is not straightforward. It is basically a quantitative concept strictly dependent on *dosage*. The quote from Paracelsus in the 16th century that "all substances are poisons; the right dosage differentiates a poison from a remedy" is perhaps even more valid today, given the proliferation of therapeutic drugs with potentially harmful effects.
- Exogenous chemicals commonly referred to as *xenobiotics* may be present in air, water, food, and soil and are absorbed by the body through inhalation, ingestion, and skin contact (Fig. 8–1). Therapeutic drugs and drugs of abuse may be introduced intravenously or injected by other routes.
- Chemicals may be excreted in urine or feces or eliminated in expired air, or they may accumulate in bone, fat, brain, or other tissues.
- Chemicals may act at the site of entry, or they may be transported to other sites. Some agents are not modified

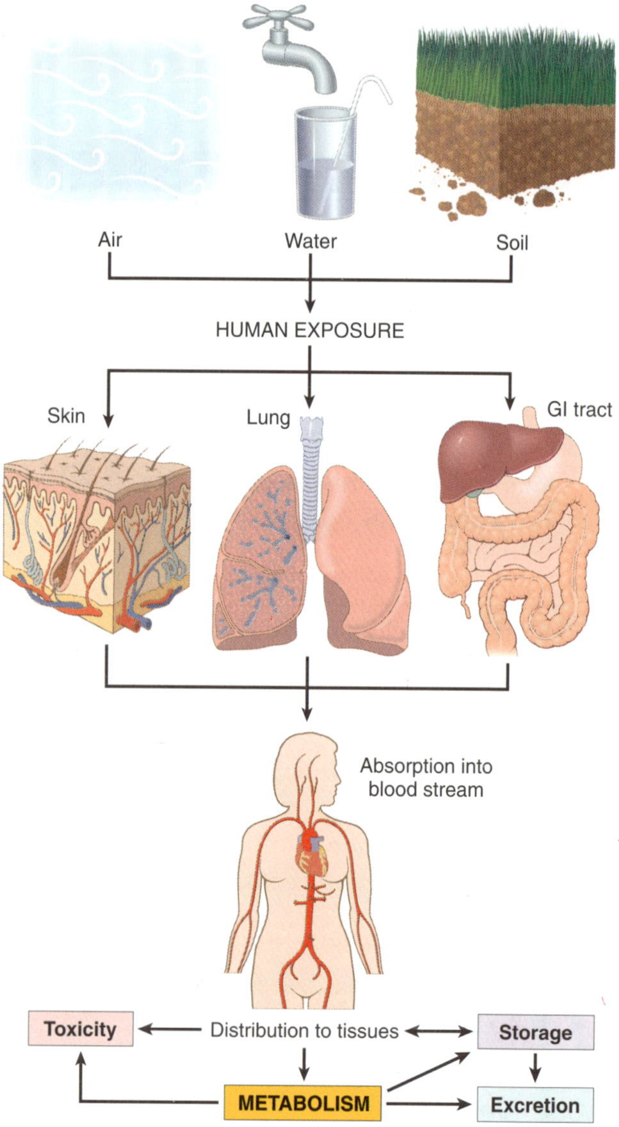

Figure 8–1

Human exposure to pollutants. Pollutants contained in air, water, and soil are absorbed through the lungs, GI tract, and skin. In the body they may act at the site of absorption but are generally transported through the bloodstream to various organs, where they may be stored or metabolized. Metabolism of xenobiotics may result in the formation of water-soluble compounds that are excreted or in activation of the agent, creating a toxic metabolite.

upon entry in the body, but most solvents and drugs are metabolized to form water-soluble products (*detoxification*) or are *activated to form toxic metabolites*.

- Most solvents and drugs are lipophilic, which facilitates their transport in the blood by lipoproteins and penetration through lipid components of cell membranes.
- The reactions that metabolize xenobiotics into nontoxic products, or activate xenobiotics to generate toxic compounds (Figs. 8–1 and 8–2), occur in two phases. In *phase I* reactions chemicals can undergo hydrolysis, oxidation, or reduction. Products of phase I reactions are often metabolized into water-soluble compounds through *phase II* reactions of glucuronidation, sulfation, methylation, and conjugation with glutathione (GSH). Water-soluble compounds are readily excreted.
- The most important component of phase I reactions is the *cytochrome P-450* system, primarily located in the endoplasmic reticulum (ER) of the liver but also present in skin, lungs, and gastrointestinal (GI) mucosa, and practically every organ. The system catalyzes reactions that either *detoxify xenobiotics or activate xenobiotics into active compounds that cause cellular injury*. Both types of reactions may produce, as a byproduct, *reactive oxygen species (ROS)*, which can cause cellular damage, as discussed in Chapter 1. Examples of metabolic activation of chemicals through the P-450 system are the production in the liver of the toxic trichloromethyl free radical from carbon tetrachloride, and the generation of a DNA-binding metabolite from benzo[*a*]pyrene (BaP), a carcinogen present in cigarette smoke. The cytochrome P-450 system also participates in the metabolism of a large number of common therapeutic drugs such as acetaminophen, barbiturates, and anticonvulsants, and in alcohol metabolism (discussed later in this chapter).
- There is great variation in the activity of P-450 enzymes among individuals. The variation may be a consequence of *genetic polymorphisms* in cytochrome P-450 enzymes, or it may result from the presence of other drugs that are also metabolized through the system. The activity of the enzymes may also be modified by diet (decreased by fasting or starvation), and induced by alcohol consumption and smoking.

ENVIRONMENTAL POLLUTION

Air Pollution

Precious as air is—especially to those deprived of it—it is often laden with many potential causes of disease. Airborne microorganisms have long been major causes of morbidity and mortality. More widespread are the chemical and particulate pollutants found in the air, especially in industrialized nations. Here, we consider these hazards in outdoor and indoor air.

Outdoor Air Pollution

The ambient air in industrialized nations is contaminated with an unsavory mixture of gaseous and particulate pollutants, more heavily in cities and in proximity to heavy industry. In the United States, the Environmental Protection Agency (EPA) monitors and sets allowable upper limits for six pollutants: sulfur dioxide, carbon monoxide, ozone, nitrogen dioxide, lead, and particulate matter. Together, some of these agents produce the well-known smog that sometimes stifles large cities such as Cairo, Los Angeles, Houston, Mexico City, and São Paulo. It may seem that air pollution is a modern phenomenon. This is not so, since Seneca wrote in AD 61 that he felt an alteration of his disposition as soon as he left the "pestilential vapors, soot and heavy air of Rome." The first environmental control law was proclaimed by Edward I in 1306 and was straightforward in its simplicity: "whoever should be found guilty of burning coal shall suffer the loss of his head." What has changed in modern times is the nature and sources of air pollutants, and the types of regulations that control their emission.

The lungs bear the brunt of the adverse consequences of air pollution, although air pollutants can affect many organ systems (see, for instance, the discussion of lead poisoning and carbon monoxide effects below). Except for some comments here on smoking, pollutant-caused

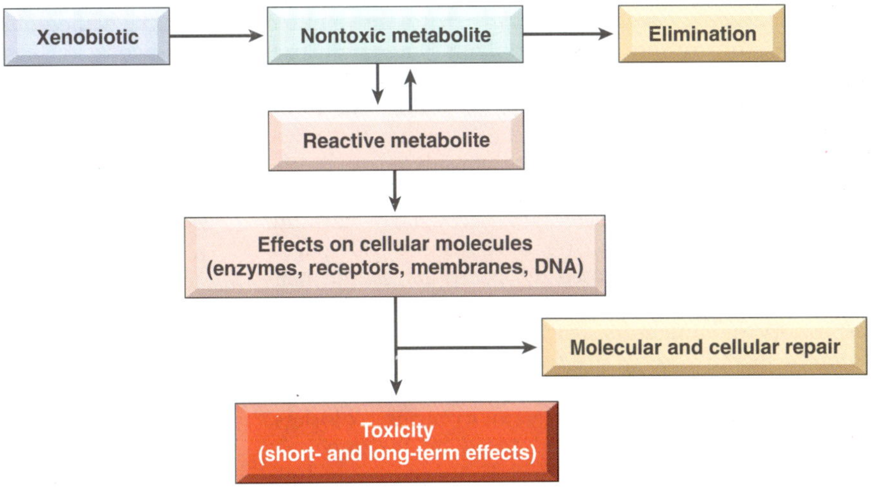

Figure 8–2

Xenobiotic metabolism. Xenobiotics can be metabolized to nontoxic metabolites and eliminated from the body (detoxification). However, their metabolism may also result in activation of the chemical leading to formation of a reactive metabolite that is toxic to cellular components. If repair is not effective, short- and long-term effects develop. (Based on Hodgson E: A Textbook of Modern Toxicology, 3rd ed. Fig. 1–1. Hoboken, New Jersey, John Wiley & Sons, 2004.)

Table 8–1 Health Effects of Outdoor Air Pollutants

Pollutant	Populations at Risk	Effects
Ozone	Healthy adults and children Athletes, outdoor workers Asthmatics	Decreased lung function Increased airway reactivity Lung inflammation Decreased exercise capacity Increased hospitalizations
Nitrogen dioxide	Healthy adults Asthmatics Children	Increased airway reactivity Decreased lung function Increased respiratory infections
Sulfur dioxide	Healthy adults Patients with chronic lung disease Asthmatics	Increased respiratory symptoms Increased mortality Increased hospitalization Decreased lung function
Acid aerosols	Healthy adults Children Asthmatics	Altered mucociliary clearance Increased respiratory infections Decreased lung function Increased hospitalizations
Particulates	Children Patients with chronic lung or heart disease Asthmatics	Increased respiratory infections Decreased lung function Excess mortality Increased attacks

Data from Bascom R, et al.: Health effects of outdoor air pollution. Am J Respir Crit Care Med 153(3):477, 1996.

lung diseases are discussed in Chapter 13. Here we comment on the major health effects of ozone, sulfur dioxide, particulates, and carbon monoxide (Table 8–1).

Ozone is one of the most intractable air pollutants, in that levels in many cities exceed the EPA standards. It is a gas formed by sunlight-driven reactions involving nitrogen oxides, which are released mostly by automobile exhaust. Together with oxides and *fine particulate matter,* it forms the familiar *"smog"* (named for a mixture of smoke and fog). Its toxicity relates to production of free radicals, which injure epithelial cells along the respiratory tract and type I alveolar cells. Low levels of ozone may be well tolerated by healthy individuals but are detrimental to lung function, especially in individuals with asthma or emphysema, and when combined with particulate pollution. Unfortunately, pollutants rarely occur singly but combine to create a veritable "witches' brew."

Sulfur dioxide, particles, and acid aerosols are emitted by coal- and oil-fired power plants and industrial processes burning these fuels. Particles are the most important harmful components of these mixtures. Although such particles have not been well characterized chemically or physically, they are considered to be the main cause of morbidity and mortality. Particles that are less than 10 µm in diameter are particularly harmful, since they remain in the airstream to reach the airspaces, where they are phagocytosed by macrophages and neutrophils, causing the release of mediators and inciting a respiratory inflammatory reaction. Larger particles are removed in the nose or are trapped by the mucociliary "escalator."

Carbon monoxide (CO) is a nonirritating, colorless, tasteless, odorless gas. It is produced by the imperfect oxidation of carbonaceous materials. Its sources include automotive engines, industries using fossil fuels, home heating with oil (not natural gas), and cigarette smoke. The low levels often found in ambient air may contribute to impaired respiratory function, but by themselves they are not life-threatening. However, individuals working in confined environments with high exposure to fumes, such as tunnel and underground garage workers, may develop chronic poisoning. CO is included here as an air pollutant, but it is also an important cause of accidental and suicidal death. In a small, closed garage, the average car exhaust can induce lethal coma within 5 minutes. CO is a systemic asphyxiant that kills by inducing central nervous system (CNS) depression, which appears so insidiously that victims may not even be aware of their plight and indeed may be unable to help themselves. Hemoglobin has a 200-fold greater affinity for CO than for oxygen. The resultant carboxyhemoglobin is incapable of carrying oxygen. Systemic hypoxia appears when the hemoglobin is 20% to 30% saturated with CO, and unconsciousness and death are probable with 60% to 70% saturation.

Morphology

Chronic poisoning by CO may develop because carboxyhemoglobin, once formed, is remarkably stable and, with low-level persistent exposure to CO, may accumulate to a life-threatening concentration in the blood. The slowly developing hypoxia can insidiously evoke widespread ischemic changes in the CNS; these are particularly marked in the basal ganglia and lenticular nuclei. With cessation of exposure to CO the patient usually recovers, but often there are permanent neurologic sequelae. The diagnosis of CO poisoning is critically dependent on the identification of significant levels of carboxyhemoglobin in the blood.

Acute poisoning by CO is generally a consequence of accidental exposure or suicide attempt. In light-skinned individuals, acute poisoning is marked by a characteristic **generalized cherry-red color of the skin and mucous membranes,** resulting from carboxyhemoglobin. If death occurs, depending on the rapidity of onset, morphologic changes may not be present; with longer survival, the brain may be slightly edematous, with punctate hemorrhages and hypoxia-induced neuronal changes. The morphologic changes are not specific; they simply imply systemic hypoxia. When exposure has not been prolonged, complete recovery is possible; however, sometimes impairments of memory, vision, hearing, and speech remain.

Indoor Air Pollution

As we increasingly "button up" our homes to exclude the environment, the potential for pollution of the indoor air increases. The commonest pollutant is tobacco smoke (discussed separately later), but additional offenders are CO, nitrogen dioxide (already mentioned as outdoor pollutants), and asbestos (discussed in Chapter 13). Only a few comments about some other agents will be made here.

Wood smoke, containing various oxides of nitrogen and carbon particulates, is an irritant that predisposes to lung infections and may contain carcinogenic polycyclic hydrocarbons. *Radon,* a radioactive gas derived from uranium, is widely present in soil and in homes. Although radon exposure is an occupational hazard that can cause lung cancer in uranium miners, it does not appear that low-level chronic exposures in the home increase lung cancer risk, at least for nonsmokers. *Bioaerosols* include microbiologic agents capable of causing infectious diseases such as Legionnaires' disease, viral pneumonia, and the common cold, as well as less threatening but nonetheless distressing allergens derived from pet dander, dust mites, and fungi and molds that can cause rhinitis, eye irritation, and even asthma.

SUMMARY

Environmental Diseases and Environmental Pollution

- Environmental diseases are conditions caused by exposure to chemical or physical agents in the ambient, workplace, and personal environments.
- Exogenous chemicals known as xenobiotics are absorbed by the body through inhalation, ingestion, and skin contact, and can either be eliminated from the body or accumulate in fat, bone, brain, and other tissues.
- Xenobiotics can be converted into non-toxic products, or be activated to generate toxic compounds, through a two-phase reaction process that involves the cytochrome P-450 system.
- The most common air pollutants are ozone, which in combination with oxides and particulate matter forms smog; sulfur dioxide; acid aerosols; and particles of less than 10 μm in diameter.
- Carbon monoxide is an air pollutant and important cause of death from accidents and suicide; it binds hemoglobin with high affinity and causes systemic asphyxiation with CNS depression.

Metals as Environmental Pollutants

Lead, mercury, arsenic, and cadmium are the heavy metals most commonly associated with harmful effects in human populations and are considered here.

Lead

Lead exposure occurs through contaminated air and food. For most of the twentieth century the major sources of lead in the environment were lead-containing house paints and gasoline. Although the use of lead-based paints and leaded gas has greatly diminished, lead contamination remains an important health hazard, particularly for children. There are many sources of lead in the environment, such as mines, foundries, batteries, and spray paints, all of which constitute occupational hazards. However, *flaking lead paint* in older houses and soil contamination pose major hazards to youngsters, and ingestion of as much as 200 μg/day may occur. Indeed, a single chip of lead paint the size of a thumbnail may contain 500,000 μg of lead, enough to produce highly toxic levels if completely absorbed. According to the 2005 report from the Centers for Disease Control (CDC), 1.6% of American children had blood lead levels in excess of 10 μg/dL (the maximal allowable level). This percentage has decreased from 4.4% in the early 1990s, but lead blood levels in children living in homes containing lead-based paint or lead-contaminated dust generally exceed the maximal allowed levels. Children absorb more than 50% of lead from food, while adults may absorb approximately 15%. A more permeable blood-brain barrier in children creates a high susceptibility to brain damage. The main clinical features of lead poisoning are shown in Figure 8–3.

Most of the absorbed lead (80% to 85%) is taken up by bone and developing teeth; lead competes with calcium, binds phosphates, and has a half-life in bone of 20 to 30 years. About 5% to 10% of the absorbed lead remains in the blood, and the remainder is distributed throughout soft tissues. *Excess lead causes neurologic effects in adults and children; peripheral neuropathies* predominate in adults, while central effects are more common in children. The effects of chronic lead exposure in children include a lower intellectual capacity manifested by low IQs, as well as behavioral problems such as hyperactivity and poor organizational skills. Lead-induced peripheral neuropathies in adults are generally reversible with elimination of lead exposure, but both peripheral and CNS abnormalities in children are gener-

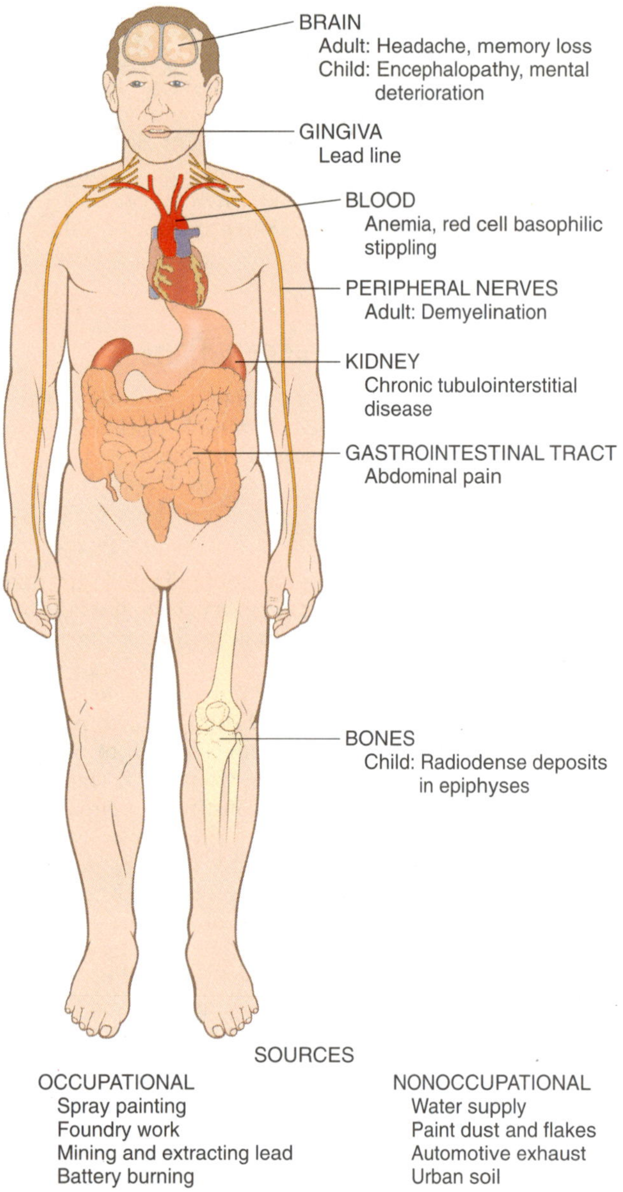

Figure 8–3

Pathologic features of lead poisoning.

ally irreversible. *Excess lead interferes with the normal remodeling of calcified cartilage* and primary bone trabeculae in the epiphyses in children, causing increased bone density, which is detected as radiodense "lead lines" on radiographs (Fig. 8–4). Lead lines of a different sort may also occur in the gums, where excess lead stimulates hyperpigmentation of the gum tissue adjacent to the teeth. Lead inhibits the healing of fractures by increasing chondrogenesis and delaying cartilage mineralization. Excretion of lead occurs via the kidneys, and acute exposures may cause damage to proximal tubules.

Lead has a high affinity for sulfhydryl groups and interferes with enzymes involved in heme synthesis (aminolevulinic acid dehydratase and delta ferrochelatase). Iron incorporation into heme is impaired, leading to *a microcytic, hypochromic anemia*. A characteristic finding is *basophilic stippling* of erythrocytes. Lead also inhibits the activity of sodium- and potassium-dependent adenosine triphosphatases in cell membranes, an effect that may increase the fragility of red blood cells, causing *hemolytic anemia*. The diagnosis of lead poisoning requires constant awareness of its prevalence. It may be suspected on the basis of neurologic changes in children or unexplained anemia with basophilic stippling in red cells. Elevated blood lead and free erythrocyte protoporphyrin levels (>50 µg/dL) or, alternatively, zinc-protoporphyrin levels are required for definitive diagnosis. In milder cases of lead exposure, anemia may be the most obvious abnormality detected.

Morphology

The major anatomic targets of lead toxicity are the blood, nervous system, GI tract, and kidneys (see Fig. 8–3).

Blood changes resulting from lead accumulation occur fairly early and are characteristic. Lead interferes with normal heme biosynthesis. As a consequence, zinc-protoporphyrin is formed instead of heme. Thus, the elevated blood levels of zinc-protoporphyrin or its product, free erythrocyte protoporphyrin, are important indicators of lead poisoning. Typically, a microcytic, hypochromic, hemolytic anemia appears. Even more distinctive is a punctate **basophilic stippling** of the erythrocytes.

Brain damage is prone to occur in children. It may be very subtle, producing mild dysfunction, or it may

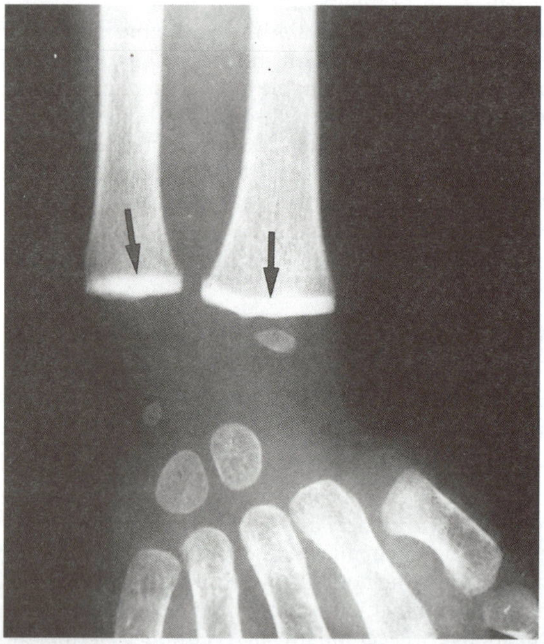

Figure 8–4

Lead poisoning. Impaired remodeling of calcified cartilage in the epiphyses (*arrows*) of the wrist has caused a marked increase in their radiodensity, so that they are as radiopaque as the cortical bone. (Courtesy of Dr. G.W. Dietz, Department of Radiology, University of Texas Southwestern Medical School, Dallas, Texas.)

be massive and lethal. In young children, sensory, motor, intellectual, and psychological impairments have been described, including reduced IQ; learning disabilities; retarded psychomotor development; blindness; and, in more severe cases, psychoses, seizures, and coma. Lead toxicity in the mother may impair brain development in the prenatal infant. The anatomic changes underlying the more subtle functional deficits are ill defined, but there is concern that some of the defects may be permanent. At the more severe end of the spectrum are marked brain edema, demyelination of the cerebral and cerebellar white matter, and necrosis of cortical neurons accompanied by diffuse astrocytic proliferation. In adults, the CNS is less often affected, but frequently a **peripheral demyelinating neuropathy** appears, typically involving the motor innervation of the most commonly used muscles. Thus, the extensor muscles of the wrist and fingers are often the first to be affected, followed by paralysis of the peroneal muscles (**wristdrop** and **footdrop**).

The GI tract is also a major source of clinical manifestations. Lead "colic" is characterized by extremely severe, poorly localized abdominal pain.

Kidneys may develop proximal tubular damage with intranuclear lead inclusions. Chronic renal damage leads eventually to interstitial fibrosis and possibly renal failure and findings suggestive of gout ("saturnine gout"). Other features of lead poisoning are shown in Figure 8–3.

Mercury

Humans have found many ways to use mercury throughout history, including as a pigment in cave paintings, a cosmetic, a remedy for syphilis, and a component of diuretics. Poisoning from inhalation of mercury vapors has long been recognized and is associated with tremor, gingivitis, and bizarre behavior, such as the "Mad Hatter" in Lewis Carroll's *Alice in Wonderland*. Today, the main sources of exposure to mercury are contaminated fish and dental amalgams, which release mercury vapors. In some areas of the world, mercury used in gold mining has contaminated rivers and streams. Inorganic mercury from the natural degassing of the earth's crust or from industrial contamination is converted to organic compounds such as methyl mercury by bacteria. Methyl mercury enters the food chain, and in carnivorous fish such as swordfish, shark, and blue fish, mercury levels may be a million-fold higher than in the surrounding water. The consumption of contaminated fish from the release of methyl mercury in Minamata Bay and the Agano River in Japan, and the consumption of bread containing grain treated with a methyl mercury–based fungicide in Iraq, caused widespread mortality and morbidity. The medical disorders associated with the Minamata episode became known as *"Minamata disease,"* and include cerebral palsy, deafness, blindness, and major CNS defects in children exposed in the uterus. *The developing brain is extremely sensitive to methyl mercury;* for this reason, the CDC has recommended that pregnant women reduce to a minimum their consumption of fish known to contain mercury. There has been much publicity about a possible relationship between thimerosal (a compound that contains ethyl mercury, until recently used as a preservative in some vaccines) and the development of autism, but there is little evidence for a relationship between thimerosal and autism.

Arsenic

Arsenic was the favorite poison in renaissance Italy and had some skilled practitioners among the Borgias and Medicis. Deliberate poisoning by arsenic is exceedingly rare today, but exposure to arsenic is an important health problem in many areas of the world. Arsenic is found naturally in soil and water and is used in wood preservatives, herbicides, and other agricultural products. It may be released in the environment from mines and smelting industries. Large concentrations of inorganic arsenic are present in ground water used for drinking in countries such as Bangladesh, Chile, and China. As many as 20 million people in Bangladesh drink water contaminated by arsenic. According to the World Health Organization, this constitutes the highest environmental cancer risk ever found.

The most toxic forms of arsenic are the trivalent compounds arsenic trioxide, sodium arsenite, and arsenic trichloride. If ingested in large quantities, arsenic causes acute toxicity consisting of severe disturbances of the gastrointestinal, cardiovascular and central nervous systems, often progressing to death. These effects may be attributed to the interference with mitochondrial oxidative phosphorylation. Chronic exposure to arsenic causes skin changes consisting of hyperpigmentation and hyperkeratosis. These alterations may be followed by the development of basal and squamous cell carcinomas (but not melanomas). The development of arsenic-induced skin tumors differs from those induced by sunlight by appearing on palms and soles, and by occurring as multiple lesions. Arsenic exposure is also associated with increased risk of the development of lung carcinomas, but the mechanisms of arsenic carcinogenesis in skin and lung have not been elucidated.

Cadmium

By contrast to other metals discussed in this section, cadmium is a relatively modern toxic agent. It is used mainly in nickel-cadmium batteries and is generally disposed of as household waste. It can contaminate soil and plants directly or through fertilizers and irrigation water. Food is the most important source of cadmium exposure for the general population. The health effects of excess cadmium consist of obstructive lung disease and kidney damage, which initially involves tubular damage that may progress to end-stage renal disease. Cadmium exposure can also cause skeletal abnormalities associated with calcium loss. Cadmium-containing water used to irrigate rice fields in Japan caused a disease in postmenopausal women known as "itai-itai" (ouch-ouch), which is a combination of osteoporosis and osteomalacia, associated with renal disease. A recent survey showed that 5% of the US population aged 20 years and older has urinary cadmium levels that, according to research data, may produce subtle kidney injury and increased calcium loss.

SUMMARY

Toxic Effects of Heavy Metals

- Lead, mercury, arsenic, and cadmium are the heavy metals most commonly associated with toxic effects in humans.
- Children absorb more ingested lead than adults; the main source of exposure for children is lead-containing paint.
- Excess lead causes CNS defects in children and peripheral neuropathy in adults. Excess lead competes with calcium in bones and interferes with the remodeling of cartilage; it also causes anemia.
- The major source of exposure to mercury is contaminated fish. The developing brain is highly sensitive to methyl mercury, which accumulates in the brain and blocks ion channels.
- Minamata disease resulting from exposure to high levels of mercury may include cerebral palsy, deafness, and blindness.
- Arsenic is naturally found in soil and water and is a component of some wood preservatives and herbicides. Excess arsenic interferes with mitochondrial oxidative phosphorylation and causes toxic effects in the GI tract, CNS, and cardiovascular system; long-term exposure causes skin lesions and carcinomas.
- Cadmium from nickel-cadmium batteries and chemical fertilizers can contaminate soil. Excess cadmium causes obstructive lung disease and kidney damage.

Industrial and Agricultural Exposures

More than 10 million occupational injuries per year occur in the United States, and about 65,000 people die as a consequence of occupational injuries and illnesses. Industrial exposures to toxic agents are as varied as the industries themselves. They range from mere irritation of the mucosa of the airways caused by fumes of formaldehyde or ammonia, to lung cancer secondary to exposure to asbestos, arsenic, or uranium mining, to leukemia after prolonged exposure to benzene. Human diseases associated with occupational exposures are listed in Table 8–2. Here are a few examples of important agents that contribute to environmental diseases. Toxicity caused by metals has already been discussed in this chapter.

- *Organic solvents* are widely used in huge quantities worldwide. Some, such as *chloroform and carbon tetrachloride,* are found in degreasing and dry cleaning agents and paint removers. Acute exposure to high levels of vapors from these agents can cause dizziness and confusion, leading to CNS depression and even coma. Lower levels have toxicity for the liver and kidneys. Occupational exposure of rubber workers to *benzene* and *1,3-butadiene* increases the risk of leukemia. Benzene is oxidized to an epoxide through hepatic CYP2E1, a component of the P-450 enzyme system already mentioned. The epoxide and other metabolites disrupt cell differentiation in the bone marrow, causing bone marrow aplasia and acute myeloblastic leukemia.
- *Polycyclic hydrocarbons* may be released from the combustion of fossil fuels, particularly at the high-

Table 8–2 Human Diseases Associated With Occupational Exposures

Organ/System	Effect	Toxicant
Cardiovascular system	Heart disease	Carbon monoxide, lead, solvents, cobalt, cadmium
Respiratory system	Nasal cancer	Isopropyl alcohol, wood dust
	Lung cancer	Radon, asbestos, silica, bis(chloromethyl)ether, nickel, arsenic, chromium, mustard gas
	Chronic obstructive lung disease	Grain dust, coal dust, cadmium
	Hypersensitivity	Beryllium, isocyanates
	Irritation	Ammonia, sulfur oxides, formaldehyde
	Fibrosis	Silica, asbestos, cobalt
Nervous system	Peripheral neuropathies	Solvents, acrylamide, methyl chloride, mercury, lead, arsenic, DDT
	Ataxic gait	Chlordane, toluene, acrylamide, mercury
	Central nervous system depression	Alcohols, ketones, aldehydes, solvents
	Cataracts	Ultraviolet radiation
Urinary system	Toxicity	Mercury, lead, glycol ethers, solvents
	Bladder cancer	Naphthylamines, 4-aminobiphenyl, benzidine, rubber products
Reproductive system	Male infertility	Lead, phthalate plasticizers
	Female infertility	Cadmium, lead
	Teratogenesis	Mercury, polychlorinated biphenyls
Hematopoietic system	Leukemia	Benzene, radon, uranium
Skin	Folliculitis and acneiform dermatosis	Polychlorinated biphenyls, dioxins, herbicides
	Cancer	Ultraviolet radiation
Gastrointestinal tract	Liver angiosarcoma	Vinyl chloride

Data from Leigh JP, et al.: Occupational injury and illness in the United States. Estimates of costs, morbidity, and mortality. Arch Intern Med 157:1557, 1997; Mitchell FL: Hazardous waste. In Rom WN (ed): Environmental and Occupational Medicine, 2nd ed. Boston, Little, Brown, 1992, p 1275; and Levi PE: Classes of toxic chemicals. In Hodgson E, Levi PE (eds): A Textbook of Modern Toxicology. Stamford, CT, Appleton & Lange, 1997, p 229.

temperature burning of coal and gas in steel foundries, and are also present in tar and soot. (Pott identified soot as the cause of scrotal cancers in chimney sweeps in 1775, as was mentioned in Chapter 6.) Polycyclic hydrocarbons are among the most potent carcinogens, and industrial exposures have been implicated in the causation of lung and bladder cancer.

- *Organochlorines.* Organochlorines (and halogenated organic compounds in general) are synthetic products that resist degradation and are lipophilic. Important organochlorines used as pesticides are *DDT (dichlorodiphenyltrichloroethane) and its metabolites,* and agents such as Lindane, Aldrin, and Dieldrin. Nonpesticide organochlorines include *polychlorinated byphenyls (PCBs) and dioxin* (*TCDD;* 2,3,7,8-tetrachlorodibenzo-*p*-dioxin). DDT was banned in the United States in 1973, but more than half of the United States population have detectable serum levels of *p,p'*-DDE, a long-lasting DDT metabolite. This substance is found in people 12 through 19 years old who were born after the ban on DDT. PCB and TCDD are also present in the blood of the majority of the population. *Most organochlorines are endocrine disruptors* and have anti-estrogenic or anti-androgenic activity (in experimental work, *p,p'*-DDE blocked androgen binding to its receptor). DDT poisoning in humans causes acute neurologic toxicity. Other health effects for humans have not been firmly established.
- *Dioxins, PCBs.* These can cause skin disorders such as folliculitis and acneiform dermatosis known as *chloracne,* which consists of acne, cyst formation, hyperpigmentation, and hyperkeratosis, generally around the face and behind the ears. It can be accompanied by abnormalities in the liver and CNS. Because PCBs induce the P-450 enzyme system, workers exposed to these substances may show abnormal drug metabolism. Environmental disasters in Japan and China in the late 1960s caused by the consumption of rice oil contaminated by PCBs during its production, poisoned about 2000 people in each episode. The primary manifestation of the disease (Yusho in Japan; Yu-Cheng in China) was chloracne and hyperpigmentation of the skin and nails. A bizarre case of intentional dioxin poisoning, which made international headlines and was a front-page illustration of chloracne, involved a candidate for office in the Ukraine who developed extensive chloracne and systemic symptoms as a consequence of eating a meal spiked with dioxin, offered by one of his "friends."
- Exposure to *phthalates* in laboratory animals causes endocrine disruption and a testicular dysgenesis syndrome manifested as hypospadias, cryptorchidism, and testicular cell abnormalities that are similar to conditions of unknown origin found in humans. Phthalates are plasticizers that are widely used in flexible plastics (as in food wraps), and medical containers, such as blood and serum bags. A matter of concern is that critically ill infants might receive large doses of phthalates from such bags, although effects in humans have not been firmly established.
- Exposure to *vinyl chloride,* used in the synthesis of polyvinyl resins, was found to cause (in rare individuals) angiosarcoma of the liver, an unusual type of liver tumor.
- Inhalation of mineral dusts causes chronic, non-neoplastic lung diseases called *pneumoconioses.* This term includes diseases induced by organic and inorganic particulates as well as chemical fume- and vapor-induced non-neoplastic lung diseases. The most common pneumoconioses are caused by exposures to mineral dust: *coal dust* (mining of hard coal), *silica* (sandblasting, stone cutting), *asbestos* (mining, fabrication, insulation work), and *beryllium* (mining, fabrication). Exposure to these agents nearly always occurs in the workplace. However, the increased risk of cancer as a result of asbestos exposure extends to family members of asbestos workers and to other individuals exposed outside the workplace. Pneumoconioses and their pathogenesis are discussed in Chapter 13.

EFFECTS OF TOBACCO

Tobacco is the most common exogenous cause of human cancers, being responsible for 90% of lung cancers. The main culprit is cigarette smoking, but smokeless tobacco (snuff, chewing tobacco) is also harmful to health and is an important cause of oral cancer. The use of tobacco products not only creates personal risks, but passive tobacco inhalation from the environment ("second-hand smoke") can cause lung cancer in nonsmokers. Cigarette smoking causes, worldwide, more than 4 million deaths annually, mostly from cardiovascular disease, various types of cancers, and chronic respiratory problems. It is expected that there will be 8 million tobacco-related deaths yearly by 2020, the major increase occurring in developing countries. It has been estimated that of the people alive today, approximately 500 million will die from tobacco-related illnesses. In the United States alone, tobacco is responsible for more than 400,000 deaths per year, one-third of these attributable to lung cancer.

Smoking is the most preventable cause of human death. It reduces overall survival, and the impact is dose dependent. For instance, while 80% of a population of nonsmokers are alive at age 70, only about 50% of smokers survive to that age (Fig. 8–5). *Cessation of smoking greatly reduces the risk of death from lung cancer,* and it even has an effect, albeit reduced, on individuals who stop smoking at age 60. Unfortunately, the prevalence of smoking is increasing in young people, particularly women. Recent surveys estimate that 12% of middle-school and 28% of high-school students had used tobacco products during the month before the survey. In the following section we discuss some of the agents contained in tobacco and diseases associated with tobacco consumption. Adverse effects of smoking in various organ systems are shown in Figure 8–6.

The number of potentially noxious chemicals in tobacco smoke is vast (tobacco contains between 2000 and 4000 substances). Table 8–3 provides only a partial list and includes the type of injury produced by these agents. *Nicotine,* an alkaloid present in tobacco leaves, is not a direct cause of tobacco-related diseases, but it is

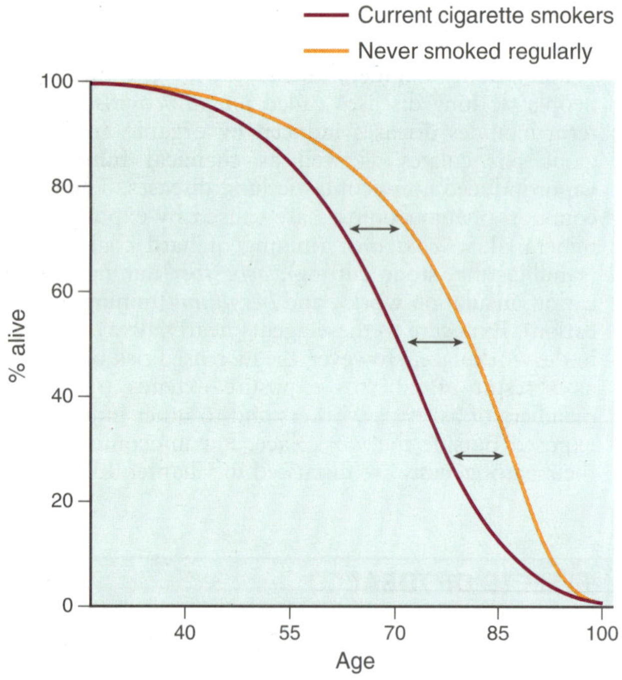

Figure 8–5

The effects of smoking on survival. The study compared age-specific death rates for current cigarette smokers with that of individuals who never smoke regularly (British Doctors Study). Measured at age 75, the difference in survival between smokers and nonsmokers is 7.5 years. (Modified from Stewart BW, Kleihues P [eds]: World Cancer Report, Lyon, IARC Press, 2003.)

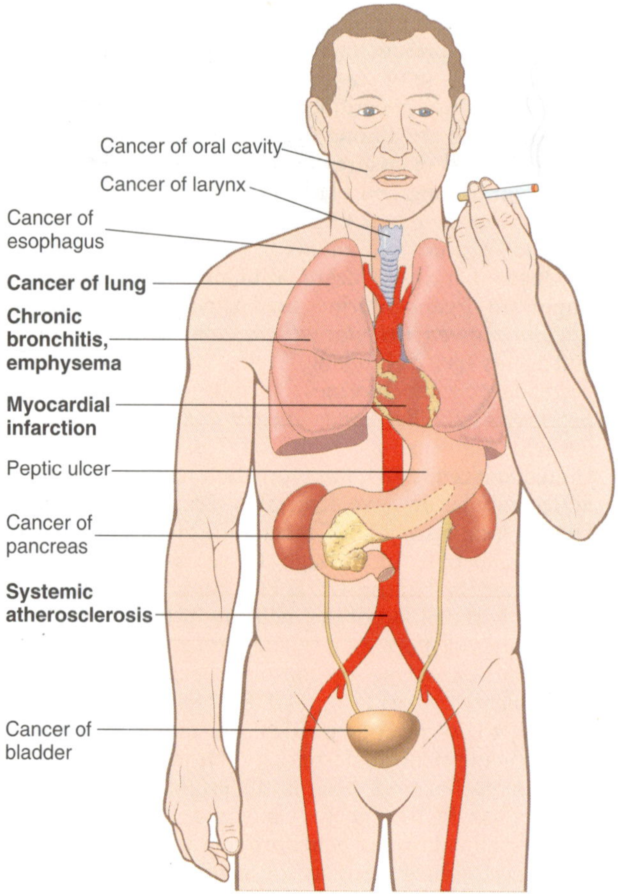

Figure 8–6

Adverse effects of smoking: the more common are in bold face.

addictive. Without it, it would be easy for smokers to stop the habit. Nicotine binds to receptors in the brain and, through the release of catecholamines, is responsible for the acute effects of smoking, such as the increase in heart rate and blood pressure, and the increase in cardiac contractility and output. The *most common diseases caused by cigarette smoking involve the lung and include emphysema, chronic bronchitis, and lung cancer,* all discussed in Chapter 13. Here we briefly mention the mechanisms responsible for some tobacco-induced diseases.

Agents in smoke have a direct irritant effect on the tracheobronchial mucosa, producing *inflammation and increased mucus production (bronchitis).* Cigarette smoke also causes the recruitment of leukocytes to the lung, with increased local elastase production and subsequent injury to lung tissue, leading to *emphysema. Components of cigarette smoke, particularly polycyclic hydrocarbons and nitrosamines* (Table 8–4), *are potent carcinogens in animals and are most likely involved in the causation of lung carcinomas in humans* (see Chapter 13). The risk of development of lung cancer is related to the intensity of exposure, frequently expressed in terms of "pack years" (e.g., one pack daily for 20 years equals 20 pack years) or in cigarettes smoked per day (Fig. 8–7). Moreover, smoking multiplies the risk of other carcinogenic influences; witness the 10-fold higher incidence of lung carcinomas in asbestos workers and uranium miners who smoke over those who do not smoke, and the interaction between tobacco consumption and alcohol in the development of oral cancers mentioned below.

Atherosclerosis and its major complication, myocardial infarction, are strongly linked to cigarette smoking. The causal mechanisms probably relate to several

Table 8–3 Effects of Selected Tobacco Smoke Constituents

Substance	Effect
Tar	Carcinogenesis
Polycyclic aromatic hydrocarbons	Carcinogenesis
Nicotine	Ganglionic stimulation and depression, tumor promotion
Phenol	Tumor promotion; mucosal irritation
Benzopyrene	Carcinogenesis
Carbon monoxide	Impaired oxygen transport and utilization
Formaldehyde	Toxicity to cilia; mucosal irritation
Oxides of nitrogen	Toxicity to cilia; mucosal irritation
Nitrosamine	Carcinogenesis

Table 8–4 Organ-Specific Carcinogens in Tobacco Smoke

Organ	Carcinogen
Lung, larynx	Polycyclic aromatic hydrocarbons 4-(Methylnitrosoamino)-1-(3-pyridyl)-1-buta-none (NNK) Polonium 210
Esophagus	*N'*-Nitrosonornicotine (NNN)
Pancreas	NNK (?)
Bladder	4-Aminobiphenyl, 2-naphthylamine
Oral cavity (smoking)	Polycyclic aromatic hydrocarbons, NNK, NNN
Oral cavity (snuff)	NNK, NNN, polonium 210

Data from Szczesny LB, Holbrook JH: Cigarette smoking. In Rom WH (ed): Environmental and Occupational Medicine, 2nd ed. Boston, Little, Brown, 1992, p 1211.

changes, including increased platelet aggregation, decreased myocardial oxygen supply (because of significant lung disease coupled with the hypoxia related to the CO content of cigarette smoke) accompanied by an increased oxygen demand, and a decreased threshold for ventricular fibrillation. Almost one-third of all heart attacks are associated with cigarette smoking. Smoking has a multiplicative effect when combined with hypertension and hypercholesterolemia.

In addition to lung cancers, *tobacco smoke contributes to the development of cancers of the oral cavity, esophagus, pancreas, and bladder.* Table 8–4 lists organ-specific carcinogens contained in tobacco smoke. Smoke and smokeless tobacco interact with alcohol in the development of laryngeal cancer. The combination of these agents has a multiplicative effect on the risk of developing this tumor (Fig. 8–8).

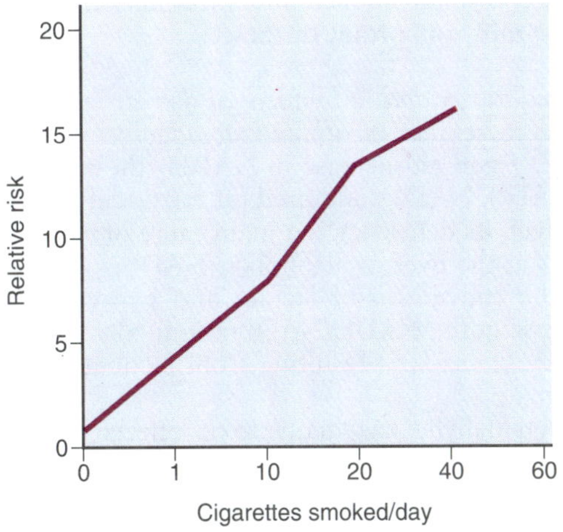

Figure 8–7

The risk of lung cancer is determined by the number of cigarettes smoked. (Modified from Stewart BW, Kleihues P [eds]: World Cancer Report, Lyon, IARC Press, 2003.)

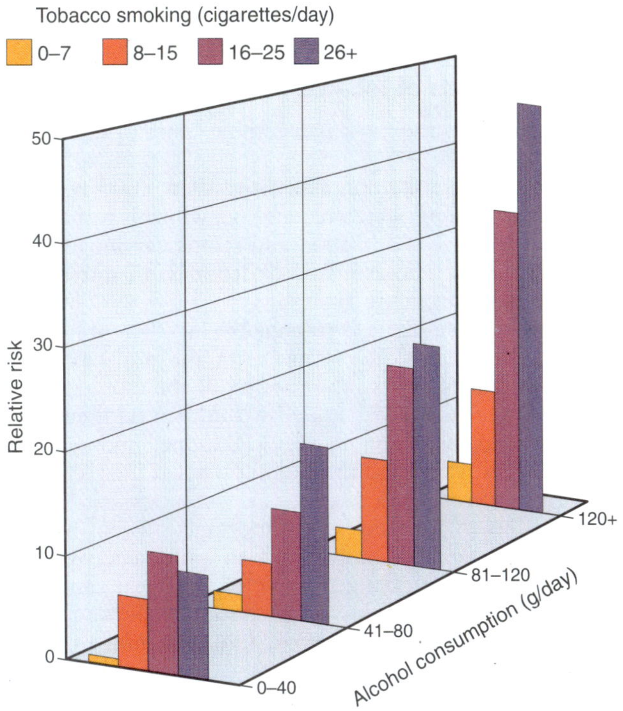

Figure 8–8

Multiplicative increase in the risk of laryngeal cancer from the interaction between cigarette smoking and alcohol consumption. (Redrawn from Stewart BW, Kleihues P (eds): World Cancer Report, Lyon, IARC Press, 2003.)

Maternal smoking increases the risk of spontaneous abortions and preterm births and results in intrauterine growth retardation (Chapter 7); however, birth weights of infants born to mothers who stopped smoking before pregnancy are normal.

Exposure to *environmental tobacco smoke (passive smoke inhalation)* is also associated with detrimental effects that result from active smoking. It is estimated that the relative risk of lung cancer in nonsmokers exposed to environmental smoke is about 1.3 times that of nonsmokers who are not exposed to smoke. In the United States, approximately 3000 lung cancer deaths in nonsmokers over the age of 35 years can be attributed each year to environmental tobacco smoke. Even more striking is the increased risk of coronary atherosclerosis and fatal myocardial infarction. Studies report that every year 30,000 to 60,000 cardiac deaths in the United States are associated with exposure to passive smoke. Children living in a household with an adult who smokes have an increased incidence of respiratory illnesses and asthma. Passive smoke inhalation in nonsmokers can be estimated by measuring the blood levels of *cotinine,* a metabolite of nicotine. Median cotinine levels in nonsmokers have decreased by more than 60% during the last 10 years, but exposure to environmental tobacco smoke in the home remains a major public health concern, particularly for children. It is clear that the transient pleasure a puff may give comes with a heavy long-term price.

SUMMARY

Health Effects of Tobacco

- Smoking is the most preventable cause of human death.
- Tobacco smoke contains more than 2000 compounds. Among these are nicotine, which is responsible for tobacco addiction and strong carcinogens, mainly polycyclic aromatic hydrocarbons, nitrosamines, and aromatic amines.
- Cigarette smoking is responsible for 90% of lung cancers. It also causes cancers of the oral cavity, larynx and pharynx, and cancers of the esophagus and stomach. It is associated with the development of carcinomas of the bladder and kidney and some leukemias. Cessation of smoking reduces the risk of lung cancer.
- Smokeless tobacco is an important cause of oral cancers. Tobacco consumption interacts with alcohol in multiplying the risk of laryngeal cancer and increases the risk of lung cancers from occupational exposures to asbestos, uranium, and other agents.
- Tobacco consumption is an important risk factor for atherosclerosis and myocardial infarction, peripheral vascular disease, and cerebrovascular disease. In the lungs, in addition to cancer, it causes emphysema, chronic bronchitis, and chronic obstructive disease.
- Maternal smoking increases the risk of abortion, premature birth, and intrauterine growth retardation.

EFFECTS OF ALCOHOL

Ethanol is consumed, at least partly, for its mood-altering properties, but when used in moderation it is socially acceptable and not injurious. When excessive amounts are used, alcohol can cause marked physical and psychological damage. Our purpose here is to describe the lesions directly associated with the abuse of alcohol.

Despite all the attention given to cocaine and heroin addiction, alcohol abuse is a more widespread hazard and claims many more lives. Fifty percent of adults in the western world drink alcohol, and about 5% to 10% have chronic alcoholism. It is estimated that *there are more than 10 million chronic alcoholics in the United States and that alcohol consumption is responsible for more than 100,000 deaths annually*. Almost 50% of these deaths result from accidents caused by drunken driving and alcohol-related homicides and suicides, and about 25% are a consequence of cirrhosis of the liver. After consumption, ethanol is absorbed unaltered in the stomach and small intestine. It is then distributed to all the tissues and fluids of the body in direct proportion to the blood level. Less than 10% is excreted unchanged in the urine, sweat, and breath. The amount exhaled is proportional to the blood level and forms the basis of the breath test used by law enforcement agencies. A concentration of 80 mg/dL in the blood constitutes the legal definition of drunk driving in most states. For an average individual, this alcohol concentration may be reached after consumption of about eight bottles of beer (6 to 16 gm of alcohol per bottle), 12 ounces of wine (9 to 18 gm of alcohol per glass) or 6 ounces of whiskey (about 11 gm of alcohol per ounce). Drowsiness occurs at 200 mg/dL, stupor at 300 mg/dL, and coma, with possible respiratory arrest, at higher levels. The rate of metabolism affects the blood alcohol level. Persons with chronic alcoholism can tolerate levels as high as 700 mg/dL, such tolerance is partially explained by accelerated ethanol metabolism caused by a 5- to 10-fold induction of cytochrome P-450 enzymes in the liver (see discussion below).

Most of the alcohol in the blood is biotransformed to acetaldehyde in the liver by three enzyme systems consisting of alcohol dehydrogenase, cytochrome P-450 isoenzymes, and catalase (Fig. 8–9). Catalase activity, which utilizes hydrogen peroxide as substrate, is of minor importance, because it metabolizes no more than 5% of ethanol in the liver. Acetaldehyde produced by alcohol metabolism through these systems is converted to acetate by acetaldehyde dehydrogenase, which is then utilized in the mitochondrial respiratory chain. *The main enzyme system involved in alcohol metabolism is alcohol dehydrogenase*, located in the cytosol of hepatocytes. At high blood alcohol levels, the microsomal ethanol-oxidizing system participates in the metabolism. This system involves cytochrome P-450 enzymes, particularly the CYP2E1 isoform, located in the smooth ER. Induction of P-450 enzymes by alcohol explains the increased susceptibility of alcoholics to other compounds metabolized by the same enzyme system, which include drugs (acetaminophen, cocaine), anesthetics, carcinogens, and industrial solvents. Note, however, that when alcohol is present in the blood at high concentrations, it competes with other CYP2E1 substrates and may delay the catabolism of other drugs, thus potentiating their effects. Several toxic effects result from ethanol metabolism. We mention only the most important of these.

- *Alcohol oxidation by alcohol dehydrogenase causes a decrease in nicotinamide adenine dinucleotide (NAD^+)* and an increase in NADH (the reduced form of NAD^+). NAD^+ is required for fatty acid oxidation in the liver. Its deficiency is a main cause of *accumulation of fat* in the liver of alcoholics. NAD^+ is also required for the conversion of lactate into pyruvate, and the increase in the $NADH/NAD^+$ ratio in alcoholics causes *metabolic acidosis* resulting from lactic acid accumulation.
- Acetaldehyde has many toxic effects and may be responsible for some of the acute effects of alcohol. The efficiency of alcohol metabolism varies between populations, depending on the composition of acetaldehyde dehydrogenase isozymes, and of mutations that decrease enzyme activity. About 50% of individuals of Asian background have deficiencies in acetaldehyde

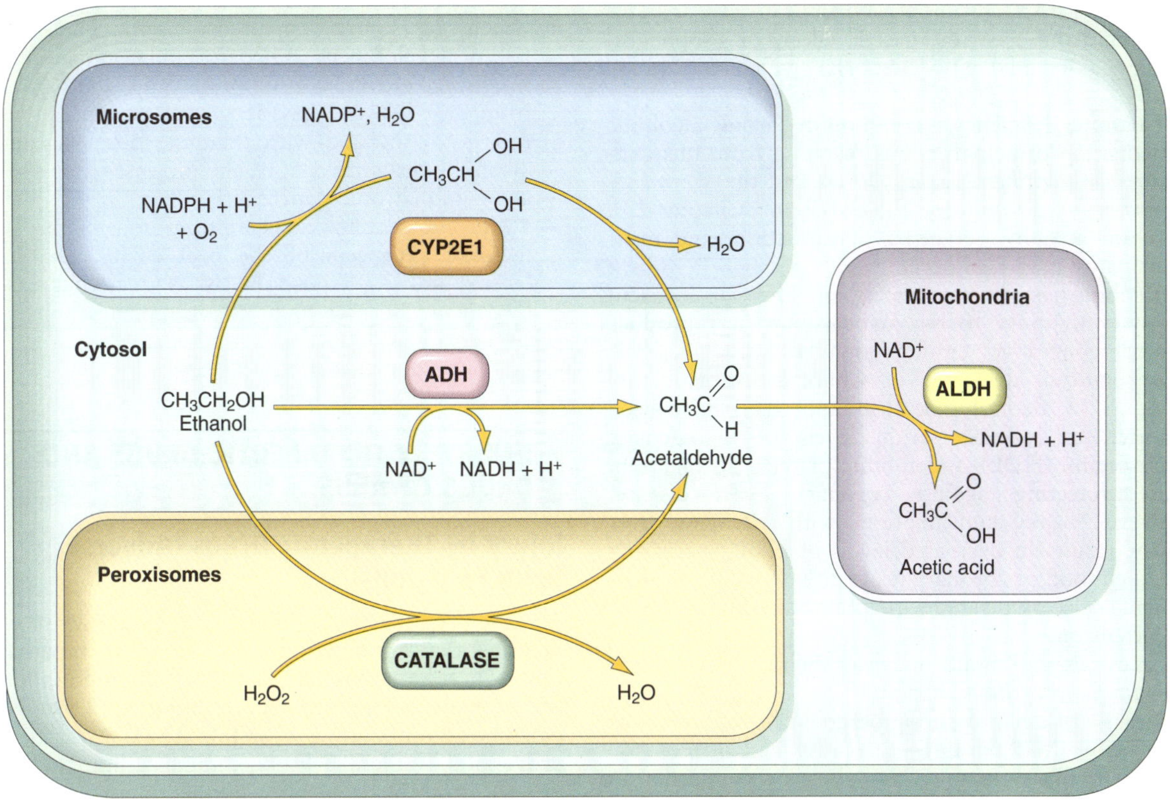

Figure 8–9

Metabolism of ethanol: oxidation of ethanol to acetaldehyde by three different routes, and the generation of acetic acid. Note that oxidation by alcohol dehydrogenase (ADH) takes place in the cytosol; the cytochrome P-450 system and its CYP2E1 isoform are located in the ER (microsomes), and catalase is located in peroxisomes. Oxidation of acetaldehyde by aldehyde dehydrogenase (ALDH) occurs in mitochondria. (From Parkinson A: Biotransformation of xenobiotics. In Klassen CD [ed]: Casarett and Doull's Toxicology: The Basic Science of Poisons, 6th ed. New York, McGraw-Hill, 2001, p 133.)

dehydrogenase activity. These individuals experience flushing, tachychardia, and hyperventilation after alcohol ingestion.

- *Metabolism of ethanol in the liver by CYP2E1 produces reactive oxygen species and causes lipid peroxidation of cell membranes.* Nevertheless, the precise mechanisms that account for alcohol-induced cellular injury have not been well defined.
- Alcohol may cause the release of endotoxin (lipopolysaccharide), a product of gram-negative bacteria from the intestinal flora. Endotoxin stimulates the release of tumor necrosis factor (TNF) and other cytokines from circulating macrophages and from Kupffer cells in the liver, causing cell injury.

The adverse effects of ethanol can be categorized into its acute effects and the consequences of chronic alcoholism.

Acute alcoholism exerts its effects mainly on the CNS, but it may induce hepatic and gastric changes that are reversible in the absence of continued alcohol consumption. Even with moderate intake of alcohol, multiple fat droplets accumulate in the cytoplasm of hepatocytes (*fatty change or hepatic steatosis*). The gastric changes are acute *gastritis and ulceration*. In the CNS, alcohol is a depressant, first affecting subcortical structures (probably the high brain stem reticular formation) that modulate cerebral cortical activity. Consequently there is stimulation and disordered cortical, motor, and intellectual behavior. At progressively higher blood levels, cortical neurons and then lower medullary centers are depressed, including those that regulate respiration. Respiratory arrest may follow.

Chronic alcoholism is responsible for morphologic alterations, primarily in the liver and stomach, but they may occur in virtually all organs and tissues. Chronic alcoholics suffer significant morbidity and have a shortened life span, related principally to damage to the liver, GI tract, CNS, cardiovascular system, and pancreas.

- The *liver* is the main site of chronic injury. In addition to fatty change, mentioned above, chronic alcoholism causes alcoholic hepatitis and cirrhosis, as described in Chapter 16. Cirrhosis is associated with portal hypertension and an increased risk for the development of hepatocellular carcinoma.

• In the *GI tract,* chronic alcoholism can cause massive bleeding from gastritis, gastric ulcer, or esophageal varices (associated with cirrhosis), which may prove fatal.
• Thiamine deficiency is common in chronic alcoholic patients; the principal lesions resulting from this deficiency are *peripheral neuropathies* and the *Wernicke-Korsakoff syndrome* (see Table 8–9 and Chapter 23). Cerebral atrophy, cerebellar degeneration, and optic neuropathy may also occur.
• Alcohol has diverse effects on the cardiovascular system. Injury to the myocardium may produce dilated congestive cardiomyopathy (*alcoholic cardiomyopathy*), discussed in Chapter 11. Moderate amounts of alcohol (one drink per day) have been reported to increase serum levels of high-density lipoproteins (HDL) and inhibit platelet aggregation, thus protecting against coronary heart disease. However, heavy consumption, with attendant liver injury, results in decreased levels of HDL, increasing the likelihood of coronary heart disease. Chronic alcoholism is also associated with an increased incidence of hypertension.
• Excess alcohol intake increases the risk of *acute and chronic pancreatitis* (Chapter 17).
• The use of ethanol during pregnancy—reportedly as little as one drink per day—can cause *fetal alcohol syndrome*. It consists of microcephaly, growth retardation and facial abnormalities in the newborn and reduction in mental functions in older children. It is difficult to establish the amount of alcohol consumption that can cause fetal alcohol syndrome, but consumption during the first trimester of pregnancy is particularly harmful.
• Chronic alcohol consumption is associated with an *increased incidence of cancer* of the oral cavity, esophagus, liver, and, possibly, breast in females. The mechanisms of the carcinogenic effect are uncertain.
• Ethanol is a substantial source of energy (empty calories). Chronic alcoholism leads to malnutrition and deficiencies, particularly of the B vitamins.

SUMMARY

Alcohol—Metabolism and Health Effects

• Acute alcohol abuse causes drowsiness at blood levels of approximately 200 mg/dL. Stupor and coma develop at higher levels.
• Alcohol is oxidized to acetaldehyde in the liver by alcohol dehydrogenase, by the cytochrome P-450 system, and by catalase, which is of minor importance. Acetaldehyde is converted to acetate in mitochondria and utilized in the respiratory chain.
• Alcohol oxidation by alcohol dehydrogenase depletes NAD, leading to accumulation of fat in the liver and metabolic acidosis.
• The main effects of chronic alcohol consumption are fatty liver, alcoholic hepatitis, and cirrhosis, which causes portal hypertension and increases the risk of development of hepatocellular carcinoma.
• Chronic alcohol consumption can cause bleeding from gastritis and gastric ulcers, peripheral neuropathy associated with thiamine deficiency, and alcoholic cardiomyopathy, and increases the risk for acute and chronic pancreatitis.
• Chronic alcohol consumption is a major risk factor for cancers of the oral cavity, pharynx, larynx, and esophagus. The risk is greatly increased by concurrent smoking or use of smokeless tobacco.

INJURY BY THERAPEUTIC DRUGS AND DRUGS OF ABUSE

Injury by Therapeutic Drugs (Adverse Drug Reactions)

Adverse drug reactions (ADRs) refer to untoward effects of drugs that are given in conventional therapeutic settings. These reactions are extremely common in the practice of medicine and are believed to affect 7% to 8% of patients admitted to a hospital. About 10% of these prove fatal. Table 8–5 lists common pathologic findings in ADRs and the drugs most frequently involved. As can be seen in the table, many of the drugs involved in ADRs, such as the antineoplastic agents, are highly potent, and the ADR is a calculated risk of the dosage assumed to achieve the maximal therapeutic effect. Commonly used drugs such as long-acting tetracyclines, which are used to treat diverse conditions, including acne, may produce localized or systemic reactions (Fig. 8–10). Because they are widely used, estrogens and oral contraceptives are discussed next in more detail. In addition, acetaminophen and aspirin, which are nonprescription drugs but are important causes of accidental or intentional overdose, merit special comment.

Exogenous Estrogens and Oral Contraceptives (OCs)

Exogenous Estrogens. Estrogen therapy, once used primarily for distressing menopausal symptoms (e.g., hot flashes), has been widely used in postmenopausal women, with or without added progestins, to prevent or slow the progression of osteoporosis (Chapter 21) and to reduce the likelihood of myocardial infarction. Such therapy is referred to as *hormone replacement therapy* (HRT). Given the fact that endogenous hyperestrinism increases the risk of developing ovarian carcinoma and, probably, breast carcinoma, there is understandable concern about the use of HRT. The main focus of controversy is the potential benefit of HRT as protection against ischemic myocardial disease. *Recent data has confirmed the adverse effects of HRT on endometrial and breast cancers but does not support the view that HRT offers protection against ischemic heart disease.* Here is a summary of the main adverse effects of HRT.

Table 8–5 Some Common Adverse Drug Reactions and Their Agents

Reaction	Major Offenders
Blood Dyscrasias*	
Granulocytopenia, aplastic anemia, pancytopenia	Antineoplastic agents, immunosuppressives, and chloramphenicol
Hemolytic anemia, thrombocytopenia	Penicillin, methyldopa, quinidine
Cutaneous	
Urticaria, macules, papules, vesicles, petechiae, exfoliative dermatitis, fixed drug eruptions, abnormal pigmentation	Antineoplastic agents, sulfonamides, hydantoins, some antibiotics, and many other agents
Cardiac	
Arrhythmias	Theophylline, hydantoins
Cardiomyopathy	Doxorubicin, daunorubicin
Renal	
Glomerulonephritis	Penicillamine
Acute tubular necrosis	Aminoglycoside antibiotics, cyclosporin, amphotericin B
Tubulointerstitial disease with papillary necrosis	Phenacetin, salicylates
Pulmonary	
Asthma	Salicylates
Acute pneumonitis	Nitrofurantoin
Interstitial fibrosis	Busulfan, nitrofurantoin, bleomycin
Hepatic	
Fatty change	Tetracycline
Diffuse hepatocellular damage	Halothane, isoniazid, acetominophen
Cholestasis	Chlorpromazine, estrogens, contraceptive agents
Systemic	
Anaphylaxis	Penicillin
Lupus erythematosus syndrome (drug-induced lupus)	Hydralazine, procainamide
Central Nervous System	
Tinnitus and dizziness	Salicylates
Acute dystonic reactions and parkinsonian syndrome	Phenothiazine antipsychotics
Respiratory depression	Sedatives

*Feature of almost half of all drug-related deaths.

• Results from randomized control trials show that *HRT increases the risk of ovarian cancer*. Unopposed estrogen therapy increases the risk of *endometrial carcinoma* three- to sixfold after 5 years of use and more than 10-fold after 10 years, but the risk is drastically reduced or eliminated when progestins are added to the therapeutic regimen. Therefore, estrogen in combination with a progestin is most commonly in use today for postmenopausal women. HRT causes a small increase in the risk of *breast cancers*. The risk of breast cancer is *not* eliminated by the combination of estrogen and progestins; quite the contrary, the combination therapy *increases* the risk over that for women taking estrogen alone.

• HRT increases risk of *venous thromboembolism*, including deep vein thrombosis, pulmonary embolism, and stroke, by about twofold. The increase is more pronounced during the first 2 years of treatment and in women who have other risk factors such as immobilization or factor V or prothrombin mutations.

• Estrogens and progestins increase blood levels of high-density lipoprotein and decrease levels of low-density lipoprotein. It was thought that these effects would be beneficial in protecting against atherosclerosis and ischemic heart disease. Indeed, several epidemiologic studies had suggested in the past that HRT beginning at or near the onset of menopause protected against ischemic heart disease. However, recently published large and well-controlled studies did not demonstrate a protective effect of HRT on the risk of myocardial infarction.

Oral Contraceptives. Although OCs have been in use for over 30 years, and despite innumerable analyses of their

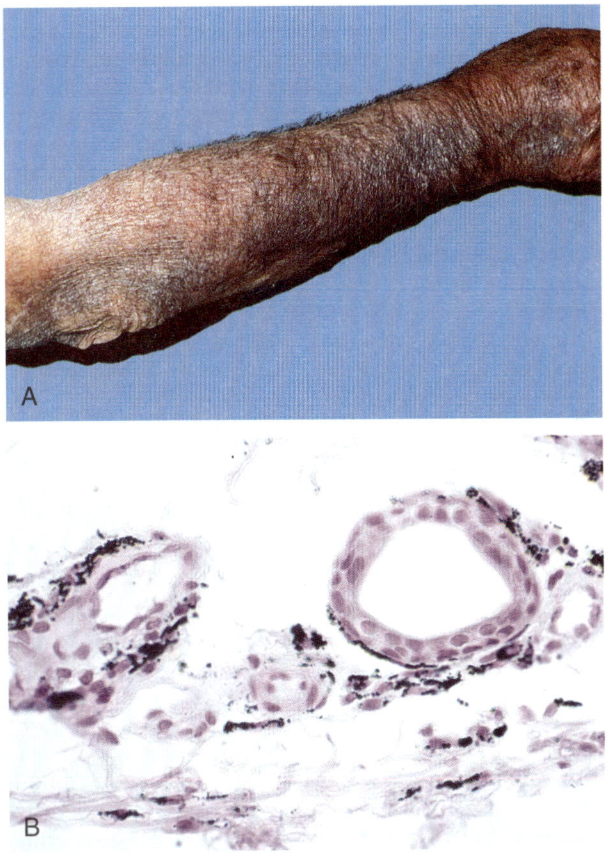

Figure 8–10

Adverse reaction to minocycline, a long-acting tetracycline derivative. **A,** Diffuse blue-gray pigmentation of the forearm, secondary to minocycline administration. **B,** Deposition of drug metabolite/iron/melanin pigment particles in the dermis. (Courtesy of Dr. Zsolt Argenyi, Department of Pathology, University of Washington, Seattle, Washington.)

risks and benefits, disagreement continues about their safety and adverse effects. They nearly always contain a synthetic estradiol and a variable amount of a progestin (combined OCs), but a few preparations contain only progestins. Currently prescribed OCs contain a smaller amount of estrogens (<50 μg/day) and are clearly associated with fewer side effects than were earlier formulations. Hence, the results of epidemiologic studies must be interpreted in the context of the dosage. Nevertheless, there is reasonable evidence to support the following conclusions:

- *Breast carcinoma.* Despite the disagreements, the prevailing opinion is that OCs do not cause an increase in breast cancer risk.
- *Endometrial cancer and ovarian cancers.* OCs have a protective effect against these tumors.
- *Cervical cancer.* OCs may increase risk of cervical carcinomas in women infected with human papilloma virus, although it is unclear whether the increased risk results from sexual activity.
- *Thromboembolism.* Most studies indicate that OCs, including the newer low-dose (<50 μg of estrogen) preparations, are clearly associated with a three- to sixfold increased risk of venous thrombosis and pulmonary thromboembolism because of increased hepatic synthesis of coagulation factors. This risk may be even higher with newer "third-generation" OCs that contain synthetic progestins, particularly in women who are carriers of the factor V Leiden mutation. The increased thrombotic risk from these agents seems to be a consequence of the generation of an acute-phase response, with increases in C-reactive protein and plasma viscosity.
- *Cardiovascular disease.* There is considerable uncertainty about the risk of atherosclerosis and myocardial infarction in users of OCs. It seems that OCs do not increase the risk of coronary artery disease in women younger than 30 years or in older women who are nonsmokers, but the risk does increase by about twofold in women older than 35 years who smoke.
- *Hepatic adenoma.* There is a well-defined association between the use of OCs and this rare benign hepatic tumor, especially in older women who have used OCs for prolonged periods. The tumor appears as a large, solitary, and well-encapsulated mass.

Obviously, the pros and cons of OCs must be viewed in the context of their wide applicability and acceptance as a form of contraception that protects against unwanted pregnancies.

Acetaminophen

At therapeutic doses, acetaminophen, a widely used nonprescription analgesic and antipyretic, is mostly conjugated in the liver with glucuronide or sulfate. About 5% or less is metabolized to NAPQI (*N*-acetyl-*p*-benzoquinoneimine) through the P-450 system. However, when taken in very large doses, *NAPQI accumulates, leading to hepatic necrosis* localized in the centrilobular areas of the hepatic lobules. The mechanisms of injury produced by NAPQI include (1) covalent binding to hepatic proteins and (2) depletion of glutathione (GSH). The depletion of GSH makes the hepatocytes more susceptible to cell death caused by reactive oxygen species. The window between the usual therapeutic dose (0.5 gm) and the toxic dose (15–25 gm) is large, and the drug is ordinarily very safe. Nevertheless accidental overdosage occurs in children, and suicide attempts using acetaminophen are not uncommon in adults, particularly in the United Kingdom. Toxicity begins with nausea, vomiting, diarrhea, and sometimes shock, followed in a few days by jaundice. Overdoses of acetaminophen can be treated at its early stages by administration of N-acetylcysteine, which restores GSH. With serious overdose, liver failure ensues. There is centrilobular necrosis that may extend to entire lobules, requiring liver transplantation for survival. Some patients show evidence of concurrent renal damage.

Aspirin (Acetylsalicylic Acid)

Overdose may result from accidental ingestion of a large number of 325 mg tablets by young children; in adults, overdose is frequently suicidal. The major untoward consequences are metabolic, with few morphologic changes. At first, respiratory alkalosis develops, followed by a metabolic acidosis that often proves fatal before anatomic changes can appear. Ingestion of as little as 2 to 4 gm by children or 10 to 30 gm by adults may be fatal, but survival has been reported after doses five times larger.

Chronic aspirin toxicity (salicylism) may develop in persons who take 3 gm or more daily (the dose required to treat chronic inflammatory conditions). Chronic salicylism is manifested by headache, dizziness, ringing in the ears (tinnitus), difficulty in hearing, mental confusion, drowsiness, nausea, vomiting, and diarrhea. The CNS changes may progress to convulsions and coma. The morphologic consequences of chronic salicylism are varied. Most often, there is an acute erosive gastritis (Chapter 15), which may produce overt or covert GI bleeding and lead to gastric ulceration. A bleeding tendency may appear concurrently with chronic toxicity, because aspirin acetylates platelet cyclooxygenase and blocks the ability to make thromboxane A_2, an activator of platelet aggregation. Petechial hemorrhages may appear in the skin and internal viscera, and bleeding from gastric ulcerations may be exaggerated.

Proprietary analgesic mixtures of aspirin and phenacetin or its active metabolite, acetaminophen, when taken over several years, can cause tubulointerstitial nephritis with renal papillary necrosis, referred to as *analgesic nephropathy* (Chapter 14).

Injury by Nontherapeutic Toxic Agents (Drug Abuse)

Drug abuse generally involves the use of mind-altering substances, beyond therapeutic or social norms. Drug addiction and overdose are serious public health problems. Common drugs of abuse are listed in Table 8–6. Here we consider cocaine, heroin, and marijuana, and briefly mention a few other drugs.

Table 8–6 Common Drugs of Abuse

Class	Molecular Target	Example
Opioid narcotics	Mu opioid receptor (agonist)	Heroin, hydromorphone (Dilaudid) Oxycodone (Percodan, Percocet, Oxycontin) Methadone (Dolophine) Meperidine (Demerol)
Sedative-hypnotics	$GABA_A$ receptor (agonist)	Barbiturates Ethanol Methaqualone (Quaalude) Glutethimide (Doriden) Ethchlorvynol (Placidyl)
Psychomotor stimulants	Dopamine transporter (antagonist) Serotonin receptors (toxicity)	Cocaine Amphetamine 3,4-methylenedioxymethamphetamine (MDMA, ecstasy)
Phencyclidine-like drugs	NMDA glutamate receptor channel (antagonist)	Phencyclidine (PCP, angel dust) Ketamine
Cannabinoids	CBI cannabinoid receptors (agonist)	Marijuana Hashish
Nicotine	Nicotine acetylcholine receptor (agonist)	Tobacco products
Hallucinogens	Serotonin $5\text{-}HT_2$ receptors (agonist)	Lysergic acid diethylamide (LSD) Mescaline Psilocybin

Data from Hyman SE: A 28-year-old man addicted to cocaine. JAMA 286:2586, 2001. GABA, γ-aminobutyric acid; $5\text{-}HT_2$, 5-hydroxytryptamine; NMDA, *N*-methy D-aspartate.

Cocaine

There has been a major escalation in the use of cocaine, along with its derivative "crack"; currently, there are an estimated 2 to 6 million cocaine users in the United States. Approximately 1.1% of middle-school and 2.3% of high-school students reported the use of cocaine in the month preceding a survey. Extracted from the leaves of the coca plant, cocaine is usually prepared as a water-soluble powder, cocaine hydrochloride, but when sold on the street it is liberally diluted with talcum powder, lactose, or other look-alikes. Crystallization of the pure alkaloid from cocaine hydrochloride yields nuggets of crack (so called because of the cracking or popping sound it makes when heated). The pharmacologic actions of cocaine and crack are identical, but crack is far more potent. Both forms of the drug are absorbed from all sites and so can be snorted, smoked after mixing with tobacco, ingested, or injected subcutaneously or intravenously.

Cocaine produces an intense euphoria and stimulation, making it one of the most addictive of all drugs. Experimental animals will press a lever more than 1000 times and forgo food and drink to obtain the drug. In the cocaine user, although physical dependence seems not to occur, the psychological withdrawal is profound and can be extremely difficult to treat. Intense cravings are particularly severe in the first several months after abstinence and can recur for years. Acute overdose produces seizures, cardiac arrhythmias, and respiratory arrest. The following are the important manifestations of cocaine toxicity.

Cardiovascular effects. The most serious physical effects of cocaine relate to its acute action on the cardiovascular system, where it behaves as a sympathomimetic agent (Fig. 8–11). It facilitates neurotransmission both in the CNS, where it blocks the reuptake of dopamine, and at adrenergic nerve endings, where it blocks the reuptake of both epinephrine and norepinephrine while stimulating the presynaptic release of norepinephrine. The net effect is the accumulation of these two neurotransmitters in synapses, resulting in excess stimulation, manifested by *tachycardia, hypertension,* and *peripheral vasoconstriction.* Cocaine also induces *myocardial ischemia,* the basis for which is multifactorial. It causes *coronary artery vasoconstriction* and promotes thrombus formation by facilitating platelet aggregation. Cigarette smoking potentiates cocaine-induced coronary vasospasm. Thus, the dual effect of cocaine, causing increased myocardial oxygen demand by its sympathomimetic action and, at the same time, reducing coronary blood flow, sets the stage for myocardial ischemia that may lead to myocardial infarction. Cocaine can also precipitate *lethal arrhythmias* by enhanced sympathetic activity as well as by disrupting normal ion (K^+, Ca^{2+}, Na^+) transport in the myocardium. These toxic effects are not necessarily dose related, and a fatal event may occur in a first-time user with what is a typical mood-altering dose.

CNS effects. The most common CNS findings are hyperpyrexia (thought to be caused by aberrations of the dopaminergic pathways that control body temperature) and seizures.

Effects on the fetus. In pregnant women, cocaine may cause decreased blood flow to the placenta, resulting in fetal hypoxia and spontaneous abortion. Neurologic development may be impaired in the fetus of pregnant women who are chronic drug users.

Chronic cocaine use. Chronic use may cause (1) perforation of the nasal septum in snorters, (2) decrease in

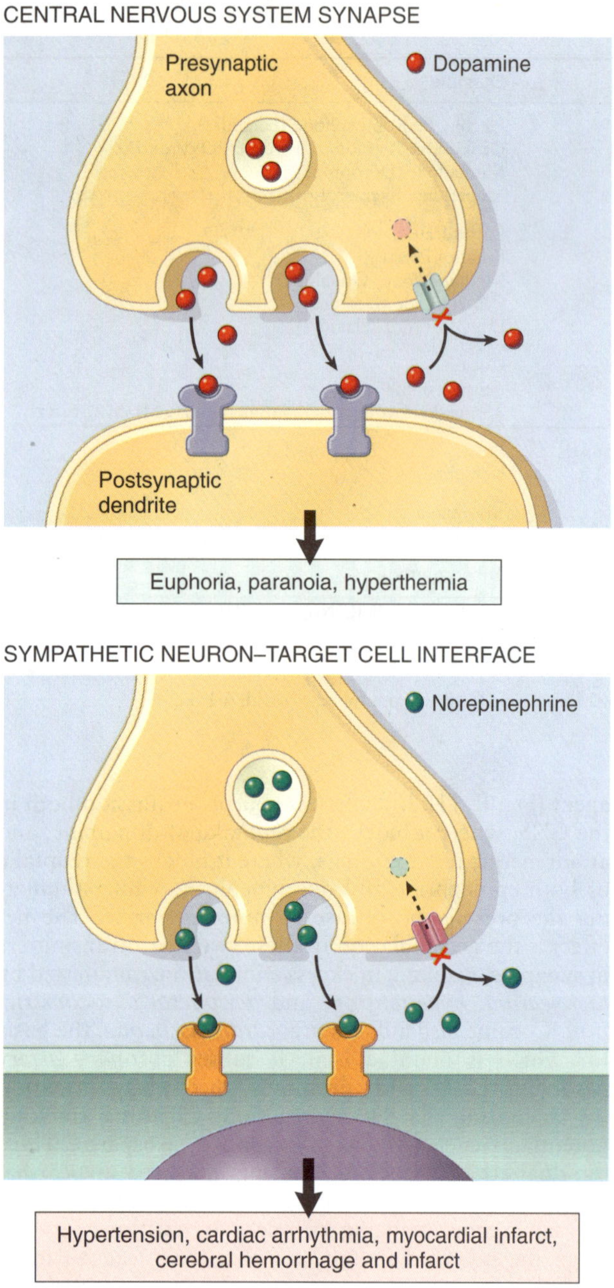

Figure 8–11

The effect of cocaine on neurotransmission. The drug inhibits reuptake of the neurotransmitters dopamine and norepinephrine in the central and peripheral nervous systems.

lung diffusing capacity in those who inhale the smoke, and (3) the development of dilated cardiomyopathy.

Heroin

Heroin is an addictive opioid derived from the poppy plant and is closely related to morphine. Its effects are even more harmful than those of cocaine. As sold on the street, it is cut (diluted) with an agent (often talc or quinine); thus, the size of the dose is not only variable but also usually unknown to the buyer. The heroin, along with any contaminating substances, is usually self-administered intravenously or subcutaneously. Effects are varied and include euphoria, hallucinations, somnolence, and sedation. Heroin has a wide range of adverse physical effects related to (1) the pharmacologic action of the agent, (2) reactions to the cutting agents or contaminants, (3) hypersensitivity reactions to the drug or its adulterants (quinine itself has neurologic, renal, and auditory toxicity), and (4) diseases contracted incident to the use of the needle. Some of the most important adverse effects of heroin are the following:

- *Sudden death.* Sudden death, usually related to overdose, is an ever-present risk because drug purity is generally unknown and may range from 2% to 90%. The yearly mortality in the United States is estimated to be between 1% and 3%. Sudden death can also occur if tolerance for the drug, built up over time, is lost (as during a period of incarceration). The mechanisms of death include profound respiratory depression, arrhythmia and cardiac arrest, and severe pulmonary edema.
- *Pulmonary problems.* Pulmonary complications include moderate to severe edema, septic embolism, lung abscess, opportunistic infections, and foreign body granulomas from talc and other adulterants. Although granulomas occur principally in the lung, they are sometimes found in the mononuclear phagocyte system, particularly in the spleen, liver, and lymph nodes that drain the upper extremities. Examination under polarized light often highlights trapped talc crystals, sometimes enclosed within foreign body giant cells.
- *Infections.* Infectious complications are common. The four sites most commonly affected are the skin and subcutaneous tissue, heart valves, liver, and lungs. In a series of addicted patients admitted to the hospital, more than 10% had endocarditis, which often takes a distinctive form involving right-sided heart valves, particularly the tricuspid. Most cases are caused by *Staphylococcus aureus,* but fungi and a multitude of other organisms have also been implicated. Viral hepatitis is the most common infection among addicted persons and is acquired by the sharing of dirty needles. In the United States, this practice has also led to a very high incidence of acquired immunodeficiency syndrome in intravenous drug abusers.
- *Skin.* Cutaneous lesions are probably the most frequent telltale sign of heroin addiction. Acute changes include abscesses, cellulitis, and ulcerations due to subcutaneous injections. Scarring at injection sites, hyperpigmentation over commonly used veins, and thrombosed veins are the usual sequelae of repeated intravenous inoculations.
- *Renal problems.* Kidney disease is a relatively common hazard. The two forms most frequently encountered are amyloidosis (generally secondary to skin infections) and focal glomerulosclerosis; both induce heavy proteinuria and the nephrotic syndrome.

Marijuana

Marijuana or "pot" is the most widely used illegal drug. It is made from the leaves of the *Cannabis sativa* plant, which contain the psychoactive substance Δ^9-tetrahydrocannabinol (THC). When it is smoked about 5% to 10%

is absorbed. Despite numerous studies, the central question of whether the drug has persistent adverse physical and functional effects remains unresolved. Some of the untoward anecdotal effects may be allergic or idiosyncratic reactions or may possibly be related to contaminants in the preparations rather than to marijuana's pharmacologic effects. On the other hand, two beneficial effects of THC are its capacity to decrease intraocular pressure in glaucoma and to combat intractable nausea secondary to cancer chemotherapy.

The functional and organic CNS consequences of marijuana have received great scrutiny. Clearly, its use distorts sensory perception and impairs motor coordination, but these acute effects generally clear in 4 to 5 hours. With continued use these changes may progress to cognitive and psychomotor impairments, such as inability to judge time, speed, and distance. Among adolescents, such changes often lead to automobile accidents. Marijuana increases the heart rate and sometimes blood pressure, and it may cause angina in a person with coronary artery disease.

The lungs are affected by chronic marijuana smoking; laryngitis, pharyngitis, bronchitis, cough and hoarseness, and asthma-like symptoms have all been described, along with mild but significant airway obstruction. Smoking a marijuana cigarette, compared with a tobacco cigarette, is associated with a threefold increase in the amount of tar inhaled and retained in the lungs. Presumably, the larger puff volume, deeper inhalation, and longer breath holding are responsible.

Other Illicit Drugs

The variety of drugs that have been tried by those seeking "new experiences" (highs, lows, "out-of-body experiences") defies belief. They include various stimulants, depressants, analgesics, and hallucinogens. Among these are PCP (phenylcyclidine, an anesthetic agent), LSD (lysergic acid diethylamide, the most potent hallucinogen known), "ecstasy" (MDMA, 3,4-methylenedioxymethamphetamine), oxycodone (an analgesic), and ketamine (an anesthetic agent used in animal surgery). Because they are used haphazardly and in various combinations, not much is known about their long-time deleterious effects, but LSD and ecstasy can cause serious health effects. Regarding their acute effects, this much is clear: they cause bizarre and often aggressive behavior that leads to violence, or depressive moods that may verge on suicide. Consumed in combination with alcohol, they are deadly agents of driving accidents.

SUMMARY

Drug Injury

- Drug injury may be caused by therapeutic drugs (adverse drug reactions) or non-therapeutic agents (drug abuse).
- Antineoplastic agents, long-acting tetracyclines and other antibiotics, hormone replacement therapy (HRT) and oral contraceptives (OC), acetaminophen, and aspirin are the drugs most frequently involved.
- HRT increases the risk of ovarian and breast cancers, and thromboembolism, but does not appear to protect against ischemic heart disease. OCs have a protective effect on endometrial and ovarian cancers, but increase the risk of thromboembolism and hepatic adenomas.
- Overdose of acetaminophen may cause centrilobular liver necrosis leading to liver failure. Early toxicity may be prevented by agents that restore GSH levels. Aspirin blocks the production of thromboxane A_2 and may produce gastric ulceration and bleeding.
- The common drugs of abuse include psychomotor stimulants (cocaine, amphetamine, ecstasy), opioid narcotics (heroin, methadone, oxycodone), hallucinogens (LSD, mescalin), cannabinoids (marijuana, hashish) and sedative hypnotics (barbiturates, ethanol).

INJURY BY PHYSICAL AGENTS

Injury induced by physical agents is divided into the following categories: mechanical trauma, thermal injury, electrical injury, and injury produced by ionizing radiation. Each type is considered separately.

Mechanical Trauma

Mechanical forces may inflict a variety of forms of damage. The type of injury depends on the shape of the colliding object, the amount of energy discharged at impact, and the tissues or organs that bear the impact. Bone and head injuries result in unique damage and are discussed elsewhere (Chapter 23). All soft tissues react similarly to mechanical forces, and the patterns of injury can be divided into abrasions, contusions, lacerations, incised wounds, and puncture wounds (Fig. 8–12).

Morphology

An **abrasion** is a wound produced by scraping or rubbing, resulting in removal of the superficial layer. Skin abrasions may remove only the epidermal layer. A **contusion,** or bruise, is a wound usually produced by a blunt object and is characterized by damage to blood vessels and extravasation of blood into tissues. A **laceration** is a tear or disruptive stretching of tissue caused by the application of force by a blunt object. In contrast to an incision, most lacerations have intact bridging blood vessels and jagged, irregular edges. An **incised wound** is one inflicted by a sharp instrument. The bridging blood vessels are severed. A **puncture wound** is caused by a long, narrow instrument and is termed penetrating when the instrument pierces the tissue and perforating when it traverses a tissue to also

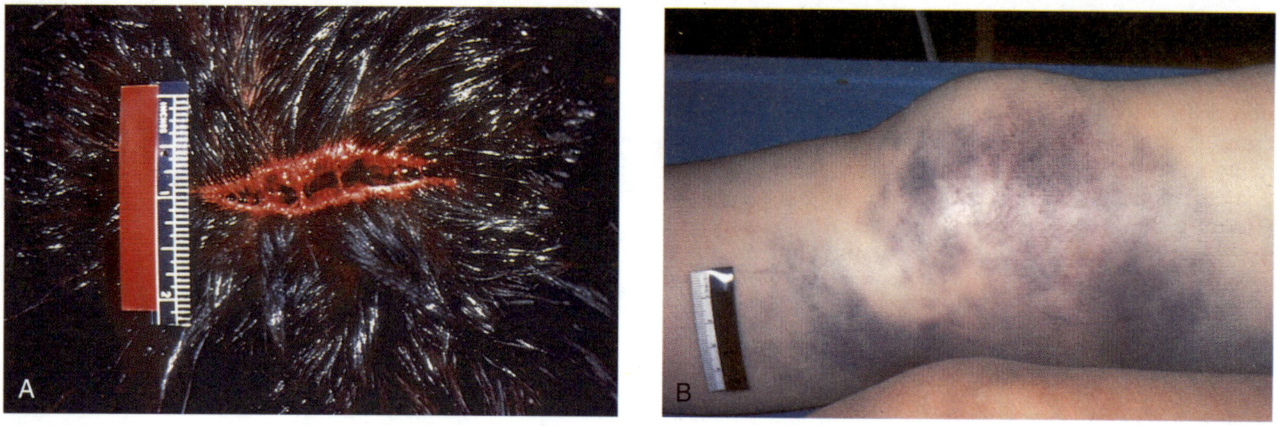

Figure 8–12

A, Laceration of the scalp: the bridging strands of fibrous tissues are evident. **B,** Contusion resulting from blunt trauma. The skin is intact but there is hemorrhage of subcutaneous vessels, producing extensive discoloration. (From the teaching collection of the Department of Pathology, University of Texas Southwestern Medical School, Dallas, Texas.)

create an exit wound. Gunshot wounds are special forms of puncture wounds that demonstrate distinctive features important to the forensic pathologist. For example, a wound from a bullet fired at close range leaves powder burns, whereas one fired from more than 4 or 5 feet away does not.

One of the most common causes of mechanical injury is **vehicular accident.** Injuries typically sustained result from (1) hitting a part of the interior of the vehicle or being hit by objects that enter the passenger compartment during the crash, such as engine parts; (2) being thrown from the vehicle; or (3) being trapped in a burning vehicle. The pattern of injury relates to whether one or all three of these mechanisms are operative. For example, in a head-on collision, a common pattern of injury sustained by a driver who is not wearing a seat belt includes trauma to the head (windshield impact), chest (steering column impact), and knees (dashboard impact). Under these conditions, common chest injuries include sternal and rib fractures, heart contusions, aortic lacerations, and (less commonly) lacerations of the spleen and liver. Thus, in caring for an automobile injury victim, it is essential to remember that internal wounds often accompany superficial abrasions, contusions, and lacerations. Indeed, in many cases, external evidence of serious internal damage is completely absent.

Thermal Injury

Both excess heat and excess cold are important causes of injury. Burns are all too common and are discussed first; a brief discussion of hyperthermia and hypothermia follows.

Thermal Burns

In the United States, burns cause 5000 deaths per year and result in the hospitalization of more than 10 times that many persons. Many victims are children, who are often scalded by hot liquids. Fortunately, since the 1970s marked decreases have been seen in both mortality rates and the length of hospitalizations. These improvements have been achieved by a better understanding of the systemic effects of massive burns and discoveries of better ways to prevent wound infection and facilitate the healing of skin surfaces.

The clinical significance of burns depends on the following important variables:

- Depth of the burn
- Percentage of body surface involved
- Possible presence of internal injuries from inhalation of hot and toxic fumes
- Promptness and efficacy of therapy, especially fluid and electrolyte management and prevention or control of wound infections

A *full-thickness* burn involves total destruction of the epidermis and dermis, with loss of the dermal appendages that would have provided cells for epithelial regeneration. Both third- and fourth-degree burns are in this category. In *partial-thickness* burns at least the deeper portions of the dermal appendages are spared. Partial-thickness burns include first-degree burns (epithelial involvement only) and second-degree burns (involving both epidermis and superficial dermis).

Morphology

Grossly, full-thickness burns are white or charred, dry, and anesthetic (because of nerve ending destruction), whereas, depending on the depth, partial-thickness burns are pink or mottled with blisters and are painful. Histologically, devitalized tissue reveals coagulative necrosis, adjacent to vital tissue that quickly accumulates inflammatory cells and marked exudation.

Despite continuous improvement in therapy, any burn exceeding 50% of the total body surface, whether superficial or deep, is grave and potentially fatal. With burns of more than 20% of the body surface, there is a rapid shift of body fluids into the interstitial compartments, both at the burn site and systemically, which can result in hypovolemic shock (Chapter 4). Because protein from the blood is lost into interstitial tissue, generalized edema, including pulmonary edema, may become severe.

Another important consideration in patients with burns is the degree of injury to the airways and lungs. Inhalation injury is frequent in persons trapped in burning buildings and may result from the direct effect of heat on the mouth, nose, and upper airways or from the inhalation of heated air and gases in the smoke. Water-soluble gases, such as chlorine, sulfur oxides, and ammonia, may react with water to form acids or alkalis, particularly in the upper airways, and so produce inflammation and swelling, which may lead to partial or complete airway obstruction. Lipid-soluble gases, such as nitrous oxide and products of burning plastics, are more likely to reach deeper airways, producing pneumonitis. Unlike shock, which develops within hours, pulmonary manifestations may not develop for 24 to 48 hours.

Organ system failure resulting from burn sepsis continues to be the leading cause of death in burned patients. The burn site is ideal for growth of microorganisms; the serum and debris provide nutrients, and the burn injury compromises blood flow, blocking effective inflammatory responses. The most common offender is the opportunist *Pseudomonas aeruginosa,* but antibiotic-resistant strains of other common hospital-acquired bacteria, such as *S. aureus,* and fungi, particularly *Candida* species, may also be involved. Furthermore, cellular and humoral defenses against infections are compromised, and both lymphocyte and phagocyte functions are impaired. Direct bacteremic spread and release of toxic substances such as endotoxin from the local site have dire consequences. Pneumonia or septic shock with renal failure and/or the acute respiratory distress syndrome (ARDS) (Chapter 13) are the most common serious sequelae.

Another very important pathophysiologic effect of burns is the development of a hypermetabolic state, with excess heat loss and an increased need for nutritional support. It is estimated that when more than 40% of the body surface is burned, the resting metabolic rate may approach twice normal.

Hyperthermia

Prolonged exposure to elevated ambient temperatures can result in heat cramps, heat exhaustion, and heat stroke.

- *Heat cramps* result from loss of electrolytes via sweating. Cramping of voluntary muscles, usually in association with vigorous exercise, is the hallmark. Heat-dissipating mechanisms are able to maintain normal core body temperature.
- *Heat exhaustion* is probably the most common hyperthermic syndrome. Its onset is sudden, with prostration and collapse, and it results from a failure of the cardiovascular system to compensate for hypovolemia, secondary to water depletion. After a period of collapse, which is usually brief, equilibrium is spontaneously re-established.
- *Heat stroke* is associated with high ambient temperatures and high humidity. Thermoregulatory mechanisms fail, sweating ceases, and core body temperature rises. Body temperatures of 112° to 113°F have been recorded in some terminal cases. Clinically, a rectal temperature of 106°F or higher is considered a grave prognostic sign, and the mortality rate for such patients exceeds 50%. The underlying mechanism is marked generalized peripheral vasodilation with peripheral pooling of blood and a decreased effective circulating blood volume. Necrosis of the muscles and myocardium may occur. Arrhythmias, disseminated intravascular coagulation, and other systemic effects are common. Elderly persons, individuals undergoing intense physical stress (including young athletes and military recruits), and persons with cardiovascular disease are prime candidates for heat stroke.

Hypothermia

Prolonged exposure to low ambient temperature leads to hypothermia, a condition seen all too frequently in homeless persons. High humidity, wet clothing, and dilation of superficial blood vessels occurring as a result of the ingestion of alcohol hasten the lowering of body temperature. At about 90°F, loss of consciousness occurs, followed by bradycardia and atrial fibrillation at lower core temperatures.

Local Reactions. Chilling or freezing of cells and tissues causes injury by two mechanisms:

Direct effects are probably mediated by physical disruptions within cells and high salt concentrations incident to the crystallization of the intra- and extracellular water.

Indirect effects are the result of circulatory changes. Depending on the rate at which the temperature drops and the duration of the drop, slowly developing chilling may induce vasoconstriction and increased permeability, leading to edema. Such changes are typical of "trench foot." Atrophy and fibrosis may follow. Alternatively, with sudden sharp drops in temperature that are persistent, the vasoconstriction and increased viscosity of the blood in the local area may cause ischemic injury and degenerative changes in peripheral nerves. In this situation, only after the temperature begins to return to normal do the vascular injury and increased permeability with exudation become evident. However, during the period of ischemia hypoxic changes and infarction of the affected tissues may develop (e.g., gangrene of toes or feet).

Electrical Injury

Electrical injuries, which may result in death, can arise from low-voltage currents (i.e., in the home and workplace) or from high-voltage currents from high-power lines or lightning. Injuries are of two types: (1) burns and (2) ventricular fibrillation or cardiac and respiratory center failure, resulting from disruption of normal electrical impulses. The type of injury and the severity and extent of burning depend on the amperage and path of the electric current within the body.

Voltage in the household and workplace (120 or 220 V) is high enough that with low resistance at the site of contact (as when the skin is wet), sufficient current can pass through the body to cause serious injury, including ventricular fibrillation. If current flow continues long enough, it generates enough heat to produce burns at the site of entry and exit as well as in internal organs. An important characteristic of alternating current, the type available in most homes, is that it induces tetanic muscle spasm, so that when a live wire or switch is grasped, irreversible clutching is likely to occur, prolonging the period of current flow. This results in a greater likelihood of developing extensive electrical burns and, in some cases, spasm of the chest wall muscles, producing death from asphyxia. Currents generated from high-voltage sources cause similar damage; however, because of the large current flows generated, these are more likely to produce paralysis of medullary centers and extensive burns. Lightning is a classic cause of high-voltage electrical injury.

Before leaving the subject of electrical injury, we should briefly mention the health risks of exposure to electromagnetic fields (EMFs), particularly those generated by transmission lines. Earlier studies linked exposure to EMFs to an increased risk of cancer, mainly leukemias, among electrical workers who worked on high-power lines and among children living near power transmission lines. However, *further analyses failed to confirm these findings*. EMF and microwave radiation, when sufficiently intense, may produce burns, usually of the skin and subjacent connective tissue, and both forms of radiation can interfere with cardiac pacemakers.

Injury Produced by Ionizing Radiation

Radiation is energy that travels in the form of waves or high-speed particles. Radiation has a wide range of energies that span the electromagnetic spectrum; it can be divided into nonionizing and ionizing radiation. The energy of nonionizing radiation, such as ultraviolet (UV) and infrared light, microwaves, and sound waves, can move atoms in a molecule or cause them to vibrate, but is not sufficient to displace bound electrons from atoms. By contrast, *ionizing radiation has sufficient energy to remove tightly bound electrons*. Collision of electrons with other molecules releases electrons in a reaction cascade referred to as ionization. The main sources of ionizing radiation are (1) *x-rays and γ rays,* which are electromagnetic waves of very high frequencies, and (2) high-energy neutrons, *alpha particles* (composed of two protons and two neutrons), and *beta particles,* which are essentially electrons. About 18% of the total dose of ionizing radiation received by the US population is human made, originating for the most part in medical devices and radioisotopes.

Ionizing radiation is indispensable in medical practice, but it is a two-edged sword. It is used in the treatment of cancer, in diagnostic imaging, and as therapeutic or diagnostic radioisotopes. However, it is also *mutagenic, carcinogenic, and teratogenic*. The following terms are used to express exposure, absorption, and dose of ionizing radiation:

- *Roentgen* (R), introduced in 1928, was the first unit of radiation measurement. It measures radiation exposure, but it is rarely used today. It represents the quantity of electrical charge produced in air by X- or γ radiation (1 R of exposure produces 2 billion ion pairs per cubic centimeter of air).
- *Gray* (Gy) is a unit that expresses the energy absorbed by a target tissue. It corresponds to the absorption of 10^4 ergs/gm of tissue. The centigray (cGy), which is the absorption of 100 ergs of energy per gram of tissue, is equivalent to the exposure of tissue to 100 R.
- *Sievert* (Sv) is a unit of equivalent dose that depends on the biologic rather than the physical effects of radiation. For the same absorbed dose, various types of radiation differ in the extent of damage they produce. The equivalent dose equalizes this variation and provides a uniform measuring unit. *The equivalent dose is expressed in sieverts and corresponds to the absorbed dose (expressed in Grays) × the relative biological effectiveness (RBE) of the radiation.* The RBE depends on the type of radiation, the type and volume of tissue exposed to radiation, the duration of the exposure, and some other biologic factors (discussed below). For instance, if equivalent amounts of energy enter the body in the form of α and γ radiation, the alpha particles would cause heavy damage in a restricted area, whereas γ rays would dissipate energy over a longer, deeper course and produce considerably less damage per unit of tissue. The effective dose of x-rays, computed tomography (CT), and other imaging and nuclear medicine procedures are commonly expressed in millisieverts (mSv). As examples, the effective radiation dosage of a single-film chest x-ray is approximately 0.01 mSv, while that of a CT scan of the chest is 6 to 8 mSv.
- *Curie* (Ci) represents the disintegrations per second of a spontaneously disintegrating radionuclide (radioisotope). One Ci is equal to 3.7×10^{10} disintegrations per second.

In addition to the physical properties of the radiation, its biologic effects depend heavily on the following variables:

- *Sensitivity of proliferating tissues.* Because ionizing radiation damages DNA, rapidly dividing cells are more vulnerable to injury than are quiescent cells. Except at extremely high doses that impair DNA transcription, DNA damage is compatible with survival in nondividing cells; however, during mitosis cells that have incurred irreparable DNA damage die, because chromosome abnormalities prevent normal division. Understandably, therefore, *tissues with a high rate of cell turnover, such as gonads, bone marrow, lymphoid tissue, and the mucosa of the GI tract, are extremely vulnerable to radiation,* and the injury is manifested early after exposure. Tissues with nondividing cells, such as brain and myocardium, do not suffer cell death, except at doses that are so high that transcription of vital molecules is affected.
- *Vascular damage.* Because tissues are made up of many cell types, the effects of radiation are complex.

Damage to endothelial cells, which are moderately sensitive to radiation, may cause narrowing or occlusion of blood vessels, leading to impaired healing, fibrosis, and chronic ischemic atrophy. These changes may appear months or years after exposure. Despite the low sensitivity of brain cells to radiation, vascular damage after irradiation can lead to late manifestations of radiation injury in this tissue.

- *Rate of delivery.* The rate of delivery significantly modifies the biologic effect. Although the effect of radiant energy is cumulative, delivery in divided doses may allow cells to repair some of the damage in the intervals. Thus, fractional doses of radiant energy have a cumulative effect only to the extent that repair during the intervals is incomplete. Radiotherapy of tumors exploits the capability of normal cells to self-repair and recover more rapidly than tumor cells avoiding much cumulative radiation damage.
- *Hypoxia.* Ionizing radiation may directly damage DNA (direct-target theory), but more often it does so indirectly, by producing free radicals from the radiolysis of water or interaction with molecular oxygen (indirect-target theory). Therefore, hypoxic tissues are relatively resistant to radiation injury. This *oxygen effect* is significant in the radiotherapy of neoplasms. The center of rapidly growing tumors may be poorly vascularized and therefore somewhat hypoxic, making radiotherapy less effective.
- *Field size.* The size of the field exposed to radiation has a great influence on its consequences. The body can sustain relatively high doses of radiation when they are delivered to small, carefully shielded fields, whereas smaller doses delivered to larger fields may be lethal.

DNA Damage and Carcinogenesis. Because its most important target is DNA, ionizing radiation kills dividing cells, and, as a consequence of mutations and chromosomal abnormalities, it can have delayed effects that are manifested years or decades later. Ionizing radiation can cause many types of damage in DNA, including base damage, single- and double-strand breaks, and cross-links between DNA and protein (Fig. 8–13). In surviving cells, simple defects may be reparable by various enzyme repair systems contained in mammalian cells (see Chapter 6). These repair systems are linked to cell cycle regulation through the activity of genes such as *ATM* that initiate signal transduction after the damage, and *p53*, which can transiently slow down the cell cycle to allow for DNA repair or trigger apoptosis of cells that are irreparable. However, double-strand breaks may persist without repair, or the repair of the lesion may be defective, creating mutations. If cell cycle checkpoints are not functioning (for instance, because of a mutation in *p53*), cells with abnormal and unstable genomes survive, and may expand as abnormal clones to eventually form tumors.

Fibrosis. A common consequence of radiation therapy for cancer is the development of fibrosis in the tissues included in the irradiated field (Fig. 8–14). Fibrosis may occur weeks or months after irradiation, leading to the replacement of dead parenchymal cells by connective tissue and the formation of scars and adhesions (see Chapter 3). As already mentioned, ionizing radiation causes vascular damage and consequent tissue ischemia. Vascular damage, the killing of tissue stem cells by ionizing radiation, and the release of cytokines and chemokines that promote an inflammatory reaction and fibroblast activation are the main contributors to the development of radiation-induced fibrosis.

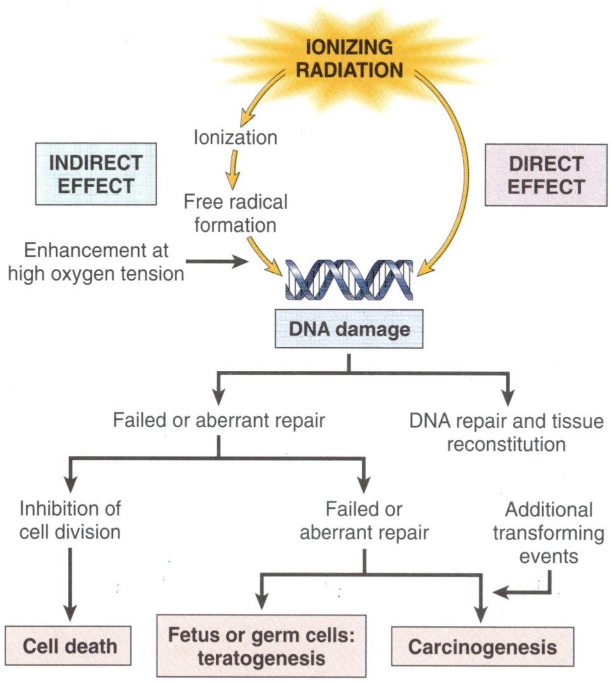

Figure 8–13

Effects of ionizing radiation on DNA and their consequences. The effects on DNA can be direct or, most importantly, indirect, through free-radical formation.

Morphology

Cells surviving radiant energy damage show a wide range of structural **changes in chromosomes**, including deletions, breaks, translocations, and fragmentation. The mitotic spindle often becomes disorderly, and polyploidy and aneuploidy may be encountered. **Nuclear swelling** and condensation and clumping of chromatin may appear; sometimes the nuclear membrane breaks. **Apoptosis** may occur. All forms of abnormal nuclear morphology may be produced. Giant cells with pleomorphic nuclei or more than one nucleus may appear and persist for years after exposure. At extremely high dose levels of radiant energy, nuclear pyknosis or lysis appears quickly as a marker of cell death.

In addition to affecting DNA and nuclei, radiant energy may induce a variety of **cytoplasmic changes**, including cytoplasmic swelling, mitochondrial distortion, and degeneration of the ER. Plasma membrane breaks and focal defects may appear. The histologic constellation of cellular pleomorphism, giant cell formation, changes in nuclei, and mitotic figures creates a more than passing similarity between radiation-

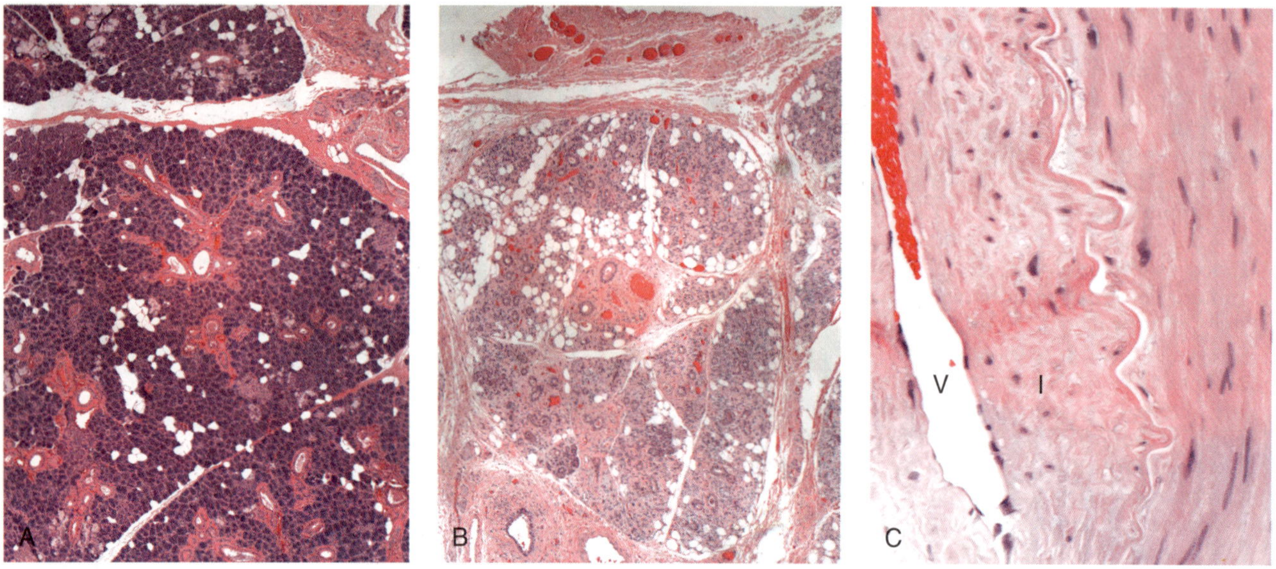

Figure 8–14

Vascular changes and fibrosis of salivary glands produced by radiation therapy of the neck region. **A,** Normal salivary gland; **B,** fibrosis caused by radiation; **C,** fibrosis and vascular changes consisting of fibrointimal thickening and arteriolar sclerosis. L, Vessel lumen; I, thickened intima. (Courtesy of Dr. Melissa Upton, Department of Pathology, University of Washington, Seattle, Washington.)

injured cells and cancer cells, a problem that plagues the pathologist when evaluating post-irradiation tissues for the possible persistence of tumor cells.

At the light microscopic level, vascular changes and interstitial fibrosis are prominent in irradiated tissues (Fig. 8–14). During the immediate post-irradiation period, vessels may show only dilation. Later, or with higher doses, a variety of degenerative changes appear, including endothelial cell swelling and vacuolation, or even dissolution with total necrosis of the walls of small vessels such as capillaries and venules. Affected vessels may rupture or thrombose. Still later, endothelial cell proliferation and collagenous hyalinization with thickening of the media are seen in irradiated vessels, resulting in marked narrowing or even obliteration of the vascular lumina. At this time, an increase in interstitial collagen in the irradiated field usually becomes evident, leading to scarring and contractions.

Effects on Organ Systems. Figure 8–15 depicts the main consequences of radiation injury. As already mentioned, *the most sensitive organs are the gonads, the hematopoietic and lymphoid systems, and the lining of the GI tract.* Estimated threshold doses for the effects of acute exposure to radiation in various organs are shown in Table 8–7. Here we briefly discuss the changes in the hematopoietic and lymphoid systems, as well as cancers induced by environmental or occupational exposure to ionizing radiation.

- *Hematopoietic and lymphoid systems.* The hematopoietic and lymphoid systems are extremely susceptible to radiation injury and deserve special mention. With high dose levels and large exposure fields, severe lymphopenia may appear within hours of irradiation, along with shrinkage of the lymph nodes and spleen. Radiation directly destroys lymphocytes, both in the circulating blood and in tissues (nodes, spleen, thymus, gut). With sublethal doses of radiation, regeneration from viable precursors is prompt, leading to restoration of a normal lymphocyte count in the blood within weeks to months. The circulating *granulocyte count* may first rise but begins to fall toward the end of the first week. Levels near zero may be reached during the second week. If the patient survives, recovery of the normal granulocyte count may require 2 to 3 months. *Platelets* are similarly affected, with the nadir of the count occurring somewhat later than that of granulocytes; recovery is similarly delayed. *Hematopoietic cells in the bone marrow,* including red cell precursors, are also quite sensitive to radiant energy. Erythrocytes are radioresistant, but anemia may nonetheless appear after 2 to 3 weeks and persist for months because of marrow damage.
- *Environmental exposure and cancer development.* Any cell capable of division that has sustained a mutation has the potential to become cancerous. Thus, an increased incidence of neoplasms may occur in any organ after exposure to ionizing radiation. The level of radiation required to increase the risk of cancer development is difficult to determine; sublethal but relatively high doses are clearly associated with an increased risk. This is documented by the increased incidence of leukemias and tumors at various sites (such as thyroid, breast, and lung) in survivors of the atomic bombings of Hiroshima and Nagasaki, in the increase in thyroid cancers in survivors of the Chernobyl accident, and also in residents of Pacific islands exposed to nuclear fallout.
- *Occupational exposure and cancer development. Radon* is a ubiquitous product of the spontaneous

decay of uranium. The carcinogenic agents are two radon decay byproducts (polonium-214 and -218 or "radon daughters"), which emit alpha particles and have a short half-life. These particulates are deposited in the lung, and chronic exposure in uranium miners may give rise to lung carcinomas. Risks are also present in homes in which the levels of radon are very high, comparable to those found in mines. However, there is little or no evidence to suggest that radon may be a contributor to the risk of lung cancer in the average household.

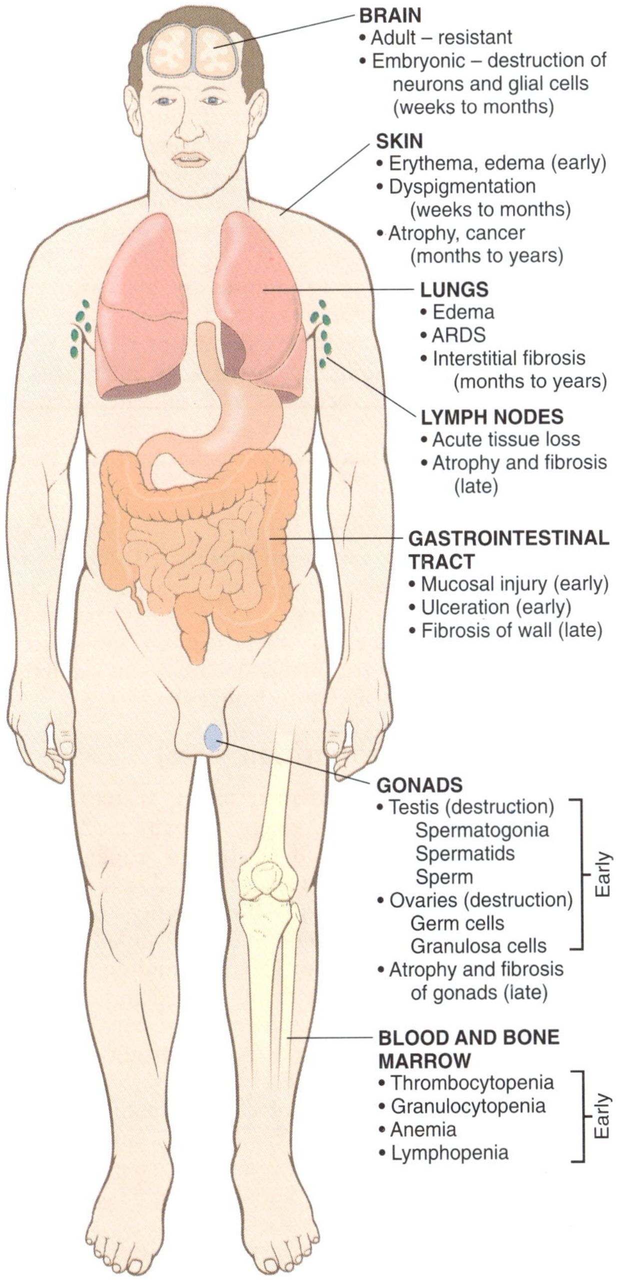

Figure 8–15

Overview of the major morphologic consequences of radiation injury. Early changes occur in hours to weeks; late changes occur in months to years. ARDS, acute respiratory distress syndrome.

Table 8–7 Estimated Threshold Doses for Acute Radiation Effects on Specific Organs

Health Effect	Organ	Dose (Sv)
Temporary sterility	Testes	0.15
Depression of hematopoiesis	Bone marrow	0.50
Reversible skin effects (e.g., erythema)	Skin	1.0–2.0
Permanent sterility	Ovaries	2.5–6.0
Temporary hair loss	Skin	3.0–5.0
Permanent sterility	Testis	3.5
Cataract	Lens of eye	5.0

Total-Body Irradiation. Exposure of large areas of the body to even very small doses of radiation may have devastating effects. Dosages below 1 Sv produce minimal or no symptoms. However, higher levels of exposure cause health effects known as acute radiation syndromes, which at progressively higher doses involve the hematopoietic system, GI system, and CNS. The syndromes associated with total-body exposure to ionizing radiation are presented in Table 8–8.

SUMMARY

Radiation Injury

- Ionizing radiation may injure the cells directly or indirectly by generating free radicals from water or molecular oxygen.
- Ionizing radiations damage DNA and therefore rapidly dividing cells such as germ cells, bone marrow and gastrointestinal tract are very sensitive to radiation injury.
- DNA damage that is not adequately repaired may result in mutations that predispose the cells to neoplastic transformation.
- Ionizing radiation may cause vascular damage and sclerosis, resulting in ischemic necrosis of parenchymal cells and their replacement by fibrous tissue.

NUTRITIONAL DISEASES

Millions of people in undeveloped or developing nations starve or live on the cruel edge of starvation, while those in the industrial world struggle to avoid calories and the attendant obesity or fear that what they eat may contribute to atherosclerosis and hypertension. So both the lack of nutrition and overnutrition continue to be major health concerns.

Table 8–8 Effects of Whole-Body Ionizing Radiation

	0–1 Sv	1–2 Sv	2–10 Sv	10–20 Sv	>50 Sv
Main site of injury	None	Lymphocytes	Bone marrow	Small bowel	Brain
Main signs and symptoms	–	Moderate leukopenia	Leukopenia, hemorrhage, epilation, vomiting	Diarrhea, fever, electrolyte imbalance, vomiting	Ataxia, coma, convulsions, vomiting
Timing	–	1 day to 1 week	4–6 weeks	5–14 days	1–4 hours
Lethality	–	None	Variable (0% to 80%)	100%	100%

Malnutrition

An appropriate diet should provide (1) sufficient energy, in the form of carbohydrates, fats, and proteins, for the body's daily metabolic needs; (2) essential (as well as nonessential) amino acids and fatty acids to be used as building blocks for synthesis of structural and functional proteins and lipids; and (3) vitamins and minerals, which function as coenzymes or hormones in vital metabolic pathways or, as in the case of calcium and phosphate, as important structural components. In *primary malnutrition,* one or all of these components are missing from the diet. By contrast, in *secondary, or conditioned, malnutrition,* the supply of nutrients is adequate, but malnutrition results from nutrient malabsorption, impaired nutrient utilization or storage, excess nutrient losses, or increased need for nutrients. The causes of secondary malnutrition can be grouped into three general but overlapping categories: (1) GI diseases, (2) chronic wasting diseases, and (3) acute critical illness.

Malnutrition is widespread and may be gross or subtle. Some common causes of dietary insufficiencies are listed here.

- *Poverty.* Homeless persons, aged individuals, and children of the poor often suffer from protein-energy malnutrition (PEM) as well as trace nutrient deficiencies. In poor countries, poverty, together with droughts, crop failure, and livestock deaths, creates the setting for malnourishment of children and adults.
- *Ignorance.* Even the affluent may fail to recognize that infants, adolescents, and pregnant women have increased nutritional needs. Ignorance about the nutritional content of various foods also contributes. A few examples are: (1) iron deficiency often develops in infants fed exclusively artificial milk diets, (2) polished rice used as the mainstay of a diet may lack adequate amounts of thiamine, and (3) iodine is often lacking from food and water in regions removed from the oceans, unless supplementation is provided.
- *Chronic alcoholism.* Alcoholic persons may sometimes suffer from PEM but are more frequently lacking in several vitamins, especially thiamine, pyridoxine, folate, and vitamin A, as a result of a combination of dietary deficiency, defective GI absorption, abnormal nutrient utilization and storage, increased metabolic needs, and an increased rate of loss. A failure to recognize the likelihood of thiamine deficiency in patients with chronic alcoholism may result in irreversible brain damage (e.g., Korsakoff psychosis, discussed in Chapter 23).
- *Acute and chronic illnesses.* The basal metabolic rate becomes accelerated in many illnesses (in patients with extensive burns, it may double), resulting in increased daily requirements for all nutrients. Failure to recognize these nutritional needs may delay recovery. PEM is often present in patients with metastatic cancers (see below).
- *Self-imposed dietary restriction.* Anorexia nervosa, bulimia, and less overt eating disorders affect a large population of individuals who are concerned about body image or suffer from an unreasonable fear of cardiovascular disease (anorexia and bulimia are discussed in a separate section in this chapter).
- *Other causes.* Additional causes of malnutrition include GI diseases, acquired and inherited malabsorption syndromes, specific drug therapies (which block uptake or utilization of particular nutrients), and total parenteral nutrition.

The sections that follow barely skim the surface of nutritional disorders. Particular attention is devoted to PEM, anorexia nervosa and bulimia, deficiencies of vitamins and trace minerals, obesity, and a brief overview of the relationships of diet to atherosclerosis and cancer. Other nutrients and nutritional issues are discussed in the context of specific diseases throughout the text.

Protein-Energy Malnutrition (PEM)

Severe PEM is a serious, often lethal, disease. It is common in poor countries, where as many as 25% of children may be affected and where it is a major contributor to the high death rates among children younger than 5 years. In the western Africa country of Niger, which suffered a severe famine in 2005, United Nation reports estimate that there are 150,000 children younger than 5 years who are severely malnourished and 650,000 who are moderately malnourished. In that country malnutrition is a direct or indirect cause of mortality in 60% of children younger than age 5.

PEM presents as a range of clinical syndromes, all characterized by a dietary intake of protein and calories inadequate to meet the body's needs. The two ends of the spectrum of syndromes are known as *marasmus* and *kwashiorkor*. In considering these conditions, it is important to remember that from a functional standpoint, there are two protein compartments in the body: the somatic compartment, represented by proteins in skeletal muscles, and the visceral compartment, represented by protein stores in the visceral organs, primarily the liver. These two compartments are regulated differently, and, as we shall see, the somatic compartment is affected more severely in marasmus, and the visceral compartment is depleted more severely in kwashiorkor. We first make brief comments on the clinical assessment of undernutrition and then discuss the clinical presentations of marasmus and kwashiorkor.

The most common victims of PEM worldwide are children. A child whose weight falls to less than 80% of normal is considered malnourished. The diagnosis of PEM is obvious in its most severe forms; in mild to moderate forms the usual approach is to compare the body weight for a given height with standard tables; other helpful parameters are the evaluation of fat stores, muscle mass, and serum proteins. With a loss of fat, the thickness of skinfolds (which includes skin and subcutaneous tissue) is reduced. If the somatic protein compartment is catabolized, the resultant reduction in muscle mass is reflected by reduced circumference of the midarm. Measurement of levels of serum proteins (albumin, transferrin, and others) provides a measure of the adequacy of the visceral protein compartment.

A child is considered to have *marasmus* when weight level falls to 60% of normal for sex, height, and age. A marasmic child suffers growth retardation and loss of muscle. The loss of muscle mass results from catabolism and depletion of the somatic protein compartment. This seems to be an adaptive response that provides the body with amino acids as a source of energy. Interestingly, the visceral protein compartment, which is presumably more precious and critical for survival, is depleted only marginally, and hence *serum albumin levels are either normal or only slightly reduced*. In addition to muscle proteins, subcutaneous fat is also mobilized and used as fuel. Leptin (discussed in the section on Obesity) production is low, which may stimulate the hypothalamic-pituitary-adrenal axis to produce high levels of cortisol that contribute to lipolysis. With such losses of muscle and subcutaneous fat, the *extremities are emaciated;* by comparison, the head appears too large for the body. Anemia and manifestations of multivitamin deficiencies are present, and there is evidence of *immune deficiency,* particularly T-cell–mediated immunity. Hence, concurrent infections are usually present, and they impose an additional stress on an already weakened body.

Kwashiorkor occurs when protein deprivation is relatively greater than the reduction in total calories (Fig. 8–16). This is the most common form of PEM seen in African children who have been weaned too early and subsequently fed, almost exclusively, a carbohydrate diet (the name kwashiorkor is from the Ga language in Ghana describing a disease of a baby due to the arrival of another child). The prevalence of kwashiorkor is also high in impoverished countries of Southeast Asia. Less severe forms may occur worldwide in persons with chronic diarrheal states in which protein is not absorbed or in those with chronic protein loss (e.g., protein-losing enteropathies, the nephrotic syndrome, or the aftermath of extensive burns). Cases of kwashiorkor resulting from fad diets or replacement of milk by rice-based beverages have been reported in the United States.

In kwashiorkor (unlike in marasmus), marked protein deprivation is associated with severe loss of the visceral protein compartment, and the resultant hypoalbuminemia gives rise to *generalized or dependent edema* (see Fig. 8–16). The weight of children with severe kwashiorkor is typically 60% to 80% of normal. However, the true loss of weight is masked by the increased fluid retention (edema). In further contrast to marasmus, there is relative sparing of subcutaneous fat and muscle mass. The modest loss of these compartments may also be masked by edema. Children with kwashiorkor have characteristic *skin lesions,* with alternating zones of hyperpigmentation, areas of desquamation, and hypopigmentation, giving a "flaky paint" appearance. *Hair changes* include overall loss of color or alternating bands of pale and darker hair, straightening, fine texture. and loss of firm attachment to the scalp. Other features that distinguish kwashiorkor from marasmus include an enlarged, *fatty liver* (resulting from reduced synthesis of the carrier protein component of lipoproteins) and the development of apathy, listlessness, and loss of appetite. As in marasmus, vitamin deficiencies are likely to be present, as are *defects in immunity* and *secondary infections*. In kwashiorkor, the physiologic stress brought about by infection is considered to be crucial to set in motion a catabolic state that aggravates the malnutrition. It should be emphasized that marasmus and kwashiorkor are two ends of a spectrum, and considerable overlap exists.

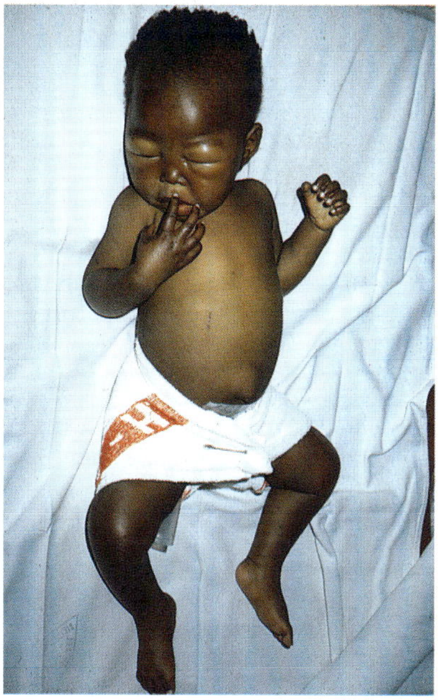

Figure 8–16

Kwashiorkor. The infant shows generalized edema, seen in the form of puffiness of the face, arms, and legs.

Secondary PEM is not uncommon in chronically ill or hospitalized patients. A particularly severe form of secondary PEM, called *cachexia,* commonly develops in patients with advanced cancer (Chapter 6). The wasting is all too apparent and often presages death. Although loss of appetite may partly explain it, cachexia may appear before a decrease in appetite. A number of explanations have been offered, including an elevated resting metabolic rate and the production of cytokines such as TNF in response to tumors, which stimulate fat mobilization from lipid stores.

Morphology

The central anatomic changes in PEM are (1) growth failure, (2) peripheral edema in kwashiorkor, and (3) loss of body fat and atrophy of muscle, more marked in marasmus.

The **liver** in kwashiorkor, but not in marasmus, is enlarged and fatty; superimposed cirrhosis is rare.

In kwashiorkor (rarely in marasmus) the **small bowel** shows a decrease in the mitotic index in the crypts of the glands, associated with mucosal atrophy and loss of villi and microvilli. In such cases concurrent loss of small intestinal enzymes occurs, most often manifested as disaccharidase deficiency. Hence, infants with kwashiorkor initially may not respond well to full-strength, milk-based diets. With treatment, the mucosal changes are reversible.

The **bone marrow** in both kwashiorkor and marasmus may be hypoplastic, mainly as a result of decreased numbers of red cell precursors. How much of this derangement is due to a deficiency of protein and folates and how much to reduced synthesis of transferrin and ceruloplasmin is uncertain. Thus, anemia is usually present, most often hypochromic microcytic anemia, but a concurrent deficiency of folates may lead to a mixed microcytic-macrocytic anemia.

The **brain** in infants who are born to malnourished mothers and who suffer from PEM during the first 1 or 2 years of life has been reported by some to show cerebral atrophy, a reduced number of neurons, and impaired myelinization of white matter.

Many other changes may be present, including (1) thymic and lymphoid atrophy (more marked in kwashiorkor than in marasmus), (2) anatomic alterations induced by intercurrent infections, particularly with all manner of endemic worms and other parasites, and (3) deficiencies of other required nutrients such as iodine and vitamins.

Anorexia Nervosa and Bulimia

Anorexia nervosa is self-induced starvation, resulting in marked weight loss; *bulimia* is a condition in which the patient binges on food and then induces vomiting. Bulimia is more common than anorexia nervosa and generally has a better prognosis. It is estimated to occur in 1% to 2% of women and 0.1% of men, with an average onset at 20 years of age. These eating disorders occur primarily in previously healthy young women who have developed an obsession with attaining thinness.

The clinical findings in anorexia nervosa are generally similar to those in severe PEM. In addition, effects on the endocrine system are prominent. *Amenorrhea,* resulting from decreased secretion of gonadotropin-releasing hormone (and subsequent decreased secretion of luteinizing and follicle-stimulating hormones), is so common that its presence is a diagnostic feature for the disorder. Other common findings, related to decreased thyroid hormone release, include cold intolerance, bradycardia, constipation, and changes in the skin and hair. In addition, dehydration and electrolyte abnormalities are frequently present. The skin becomes dry and scaly and may be yellow as a result of excess carotene in the blood. Body hair may be increased but is usually fine and pale (lanugo). Bone density is decreased, most likely because of low estrogen levels, which mimics the postmenopausal acceleration of osteoporosis. As expected with severe PEM, anemia, lymphopenia, and hypoalbuminemia may be present. A major complication of anorexia nervosa is an increased susceptibility to cardiac arrhythmia and sudden death, resulting in all likelihood from hypokalemia.

In bulimia, binge eating is the norm. Huge amounts of food, principally carbohydrates, are ingested, only to be followed by induced vomiting. Although menstrual irregularities are common, amenorrhea occurs in fewer than 50% of bulimic patients, probably because weight and gonadotropin levels are maintained near normal. The major medical complications are due to continual induced vomiting and chronic use of laxatives and diuretics. These include (1) electrolyte imbalances (hypokalemia), which predispose the patient to cardiac arrhythmias; (2) pulmonary aspiration of gastric contents; and (3) esophageal and stomach rupture. Nevertheless, there are no specific signs and symptoms for this syndrome, and the diagnosis must rely on a comprehensive psychologic assessment of the patient.

Vitamin Deficiencies

Thirteen vitamins are necessary for health; four (A, D, E, and K) are fat-soluble, and the remainder are water-soluble. The distinction between fat- and water-soluble vitamins is important; although the former are more readily stored in the body, they may be poorly absorbed in fat malabsorption disorders, caused by disturbances of digestive functions (discussed in Chapter 15). Certain vitamins can be synthesized endogenously—vitamin D from precursor steroids, vitamin K and biotin by the intestinal microflora, and niacin from tryptophan, an essential amino acid. Notwithstanding this endogenous synthesis, a dietary supply of all vitamins is essential for health.

A deficiency of vitamins may be primary (dietary in origin) or secondary (because of disturbances in intestinal absorption, transport in the blood, tissue storage, or metabolic conversion). In the following sections, vitamins A, D, and C are presented in some detail because of their wide-ranging functions and the morphologic changes of deficient states. This is followed by a summary in tabular form of the main consequences of deficiencies of the remaining vitamins (E, K, and the B complex) and some essential minerals. However, it should be emphasized that deficiency of a single vitamin is uncommon and that single- or multiple-vitamin deficiencies may be submerged in concurrent PEM.

Vitamin A

The fat-soluble vitamin A is a generic name for a group of related compounds that include *retinol, retinal, and retinoic acid,* which have similar biologic activities. Retinol is the chemical name given to vitamin A. It is the transport form and, as retinol ester, also the storage form. A widely used term, *retinoids,* refers to both natural and synthetic chemicals that are structurally related to vitamin A but may not necessarily have vitamin A activity. Animal-derived foods such as liver, fish, eggs, milk, and butter are important dietary sources of preformed vitamin A. Yellow and leafy green vegetables such as carrots, squash, and spinach supply large amounts of carotenoids, many of which are provitamins that can be metabolized to active vitamin A in the body. Carotenoids contribute approximately 30% of the vitamin A in human diets; the most important of these is β-carotene, which is efficiently converted to vitamin A. The recommended dietary allowance for vitamin A is expressed in retinol equivalents, to take into account both preformed vitamin A and β-carotene

As with all fats, the digestion and absorption of carotenes and retinoids require bile, pancreatic enzymes, and some level of antioxidant activity in the food. Retinol (generally ingested as retinol ester) and β-carotene are absorbed through the intestinal wall, where β-carotene is converted to retinol (Fig. 8–17). Retinol is then transported in chylomicrons to the liver for esterification and storage. Uptake in liver cells takes place through the apolipoprotein E receptor. More than 90% of the body's vitamin A reserves are stored in the liver, predominantly in the perisinusoidal stellate (Ito) cells. In healthy persons who consume an adequate diet, these reserves are sufficient for at least 6 months of vitamin A deprivation. Retinol esters stored in the liver can mobilized; before release, retinol binds to a specific retinol-binding protein (RBP), synthesized in the liver. The uptake of retinol/RBP in peripheral tissues is dependent on cell surface receptors that are specific for RBP rather than for retinol. After uptake by these cells, retinol binds to a cellular RBP, and the RBP is released back into the blood. Retinol may be stored in peripheral tissues as retinyl ester or be oxidized to form retinoic acid.

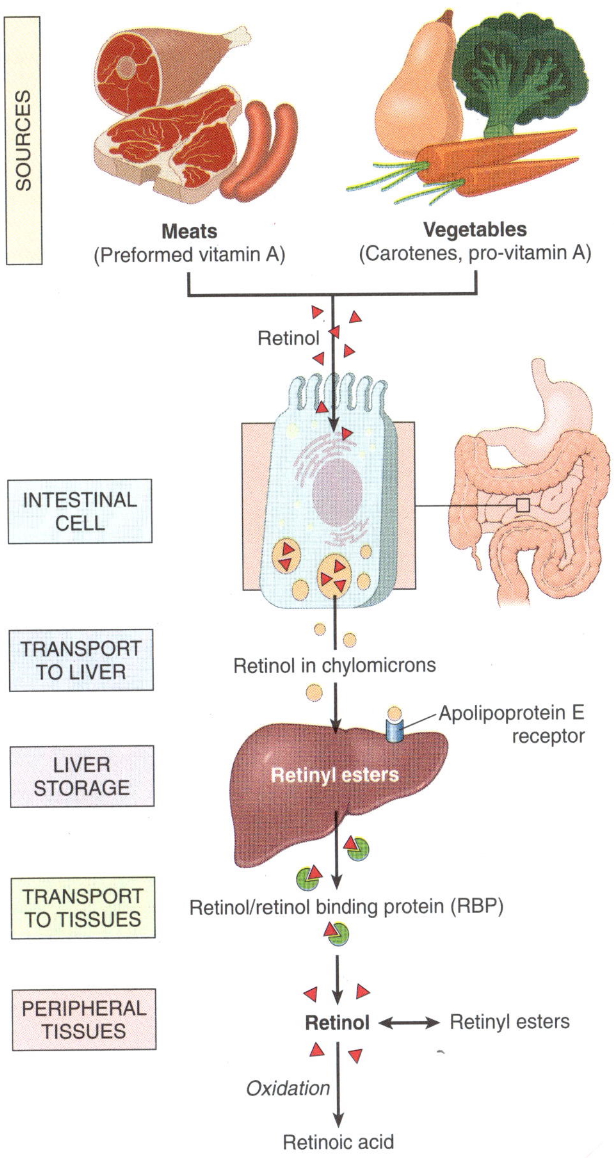

Figure 8–17

Vitamin A metabolism.

Function. In humans, the best-defined functions of vitamin A are

- Maintaining normal vision in reduced light
- Potentiating the differentiation of specialized epithelial cells, mainly mucus-secreting cells
- Enhancing immunity to infections, particularly in children with measles.

In addition, the retinoids, β-carotene, and some related carotenoids can function as photoprotective and antioxidant agents. Retinoids have broad biologic effects, including effects on embryonic development, cellular differentiation and proliferation, and lipid metabolism.

The *visual process* involves four forms of vitamin A–containing pigments: rhodopsin in the rods, which is the most light-sensitive pigment and therefore important in reduced light; and three iodopsins in cone cells, each responsive to a specific color in bright light. The synthesis of rhodopsin from retinol involves (1) oxidation to all-*trans*-retinal, (2) isomerization to 11-*cis*-retinal, and (3) interaction with the rod protein, opsin, to form rhodopsin. A photon of light causes the isomerization of 11-*cis*-retinal to all-*trans*-retinal, and a sequence of configuration changes in rhodopsin, which produce a visual signal. In the process, a nerve impulse is generated (by changes in membrane potential), and transmitted via neurons from the retina to the brain. During dark adaptation, some of the all-*trans*-retinal is reconverted to 11-*cis*-retinal but most is reduced to retinol and lost to the retina, dictating the need for continuous supply of retinol.

Vitamin A and retinoids play an important role in the orderly *differentiation of mucus-secreting epithelium;* when a deficiency state exists, the epithelium undergoes squamous metaplasia and differentiation to a keratinizing epithelium. All-*trans*-retinoic acid (ATRA), a potent acid derivative of vitamin A, exerts its effects by binding to retinoic acid receptors (RARs). These receptors are obligatory partners of nuclear receptors for 9-*cis*-retinoic acid (RXR), forming RAR/RXR heterodimers. The RAR/RXR heterodimer binds to retinoic acid response elements present in the promoter region of multiple genes that encode cell receptors and secreted proteins, including receptors for growth factors, and tumor suppressor genes. ATRA induces temporary remission of promyelocytic leukemia (PML). In this leukemia the t(15:17) translocation (Chapter 12) results in the fusion of a truncated *RAR-α* gene on chromosome 17 with the *PML* gene on chromosome 15. The fusion gene encodes an abnormal RAR that blocks myeloid cell differentiation. Pharmacologic doses of ATRA overcome the block, causing neutrophil differentiation. Although this "differentiation therapy" induces remission in most patients with acute promyelocytic leukemia, patients ultimately develop resistance to ATRA. The retinoic acid isomer 13-*cis* retinoic acid has been used with success in the treatment of neuroblastomas in children. Retinoic acid, it should be noted, has no effect on vision.

Vitamin A plays a role in host *resistance to infections*. Vitamin A supplementation can reduce morbidity and mortality from some forms of diarrhea, and supplementation in preschool children with measles can quickly improve the clinical outcome. The beneficial effect of vitamin A in diarrheal diseases may be related to the maintenance and restoration of the integrity of the epithelium of the gut. The effects of vitamin A on infections derive in part from its ability to stimulate the immune system, probably through an enhancement of humoral immunity, although the mechanisms are unclear. Another aspect of the relationship between vitamin A and infection is that infections may reduce the bioavailability of vitamin A. One possible mechanism for this effect is the inhibition of RBP synthesis in the liver by the acute-phase response associated with many infections. The drop in hepatic RBP causes a decrease in circulating retinol, which reduces the tissue availability of vitamin A.

Deficiency States. Vitamin A deficiency occurs worldwide either as a consequence of general poor nutrition or as a secondary deficiency in individuals with conditions that cause malabsorption of fats. In children, stores of vitamin A are depleted by infections, and the absorption of the vitamin is poor in newborn infants. In adults, patients with malaborption syndromes, such as celiac disease, Crohn disease, and colitis, may develop vitamin A deficiency, in conjunction with depletion of other fat-soluble vitamins. Bariatric surgery and, in elderly persons, continuous use of mineral oil as laxative may lead to deficiency.

As was already discussed, vitamin A is a component of rhodopsin and other visual pigments. Not surprisingly, one of the earliest manifestations of vitamin A deficiency is impaired vision, particularly in reduced light (*night blindness*). Other effects of vitamin A deficiency are related to the role of vitamin A in maintaining the differentiation of epithelial cells (Fig. 8–18). Persistent deficiency gives rise to a series of changes involving epithelial metaplasia and keratization. The most devastating changes occur in the eyes and are referred to as *xerophthalmia* (dry eye). First, there is dryness of the conjunctiva (xerosis conjunctivae) as the normal lachrymal and mucus-secreting epithelium is replaced by keratinized epithelium. This is followed by buildup of keratin debris in small opaque plaques (*Bitot spots*) and, eventually, erosion of the roughened corneal surface with softening and destruction of the cornea (*keratomalacia*) and total blindness.

In addition to the ocular epithelium, the epithelium lining the upper respiratory passage and urinary tract is replaced by keratinizing squamous cells (*squamous metaplasia*). Loss of the mucociliary epithelium of the

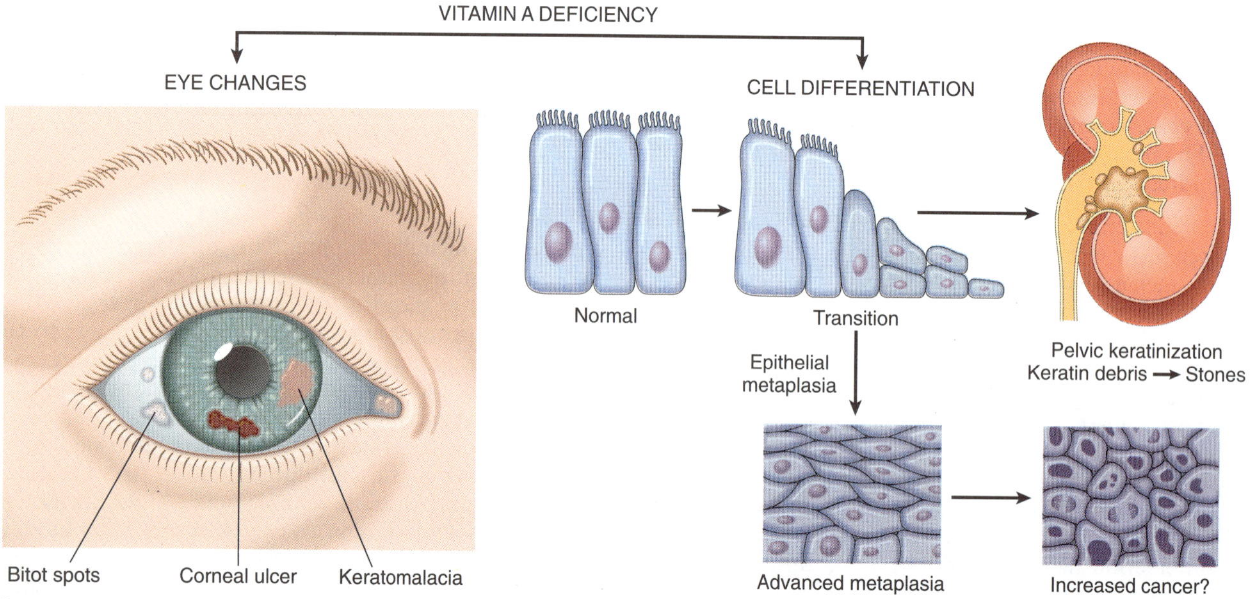

Figure 8–18

Vitamin A deficiency: its major consequences in the eye and in the production of keratinizing metaplasia of specialized epithelial surfaces, and its possible role in epithelial metaplasia. Not depicted are night blindness and immune deficiency.

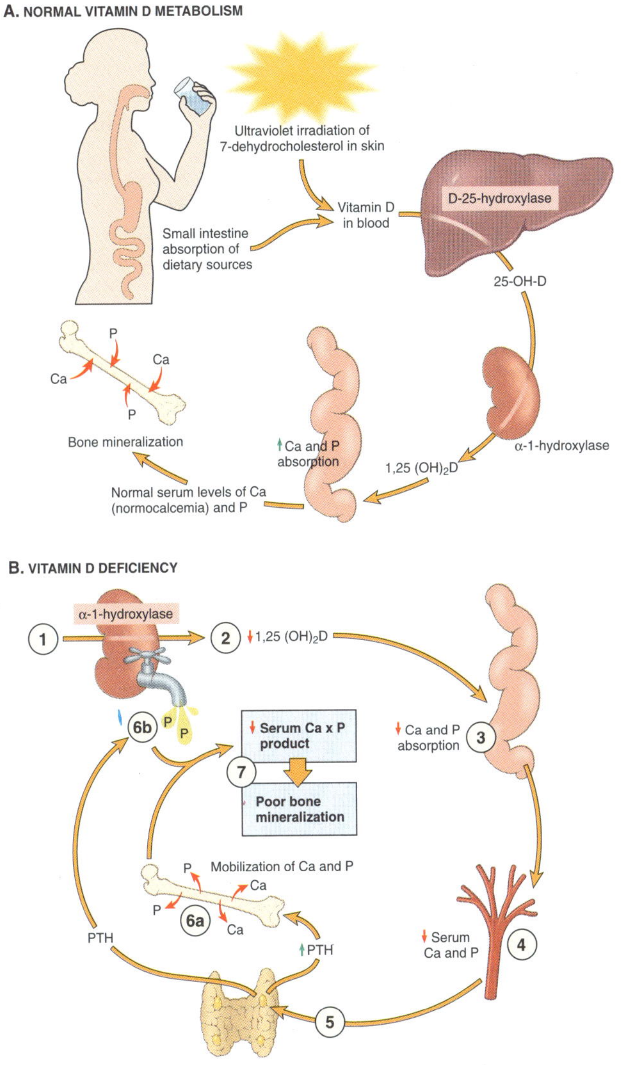

Figure 8–19

A, Normal vitamin D metabolism. **B,** Vitamin D deficiency. There is inadequate substrate for the renal hydroxylase (*1*), yielding a deficiency of 1,25(OH)$_2$-D (*2*), and deficient absorption of calcium and phosphorus from the gut (*3*), with consequent depressed serum levels of both (*4*). The hypocalcemia activates the parathyroid glands (*5*), causing mobilization of calcium and phosphorus from bone (*6a*). Simultaneously, the parathyroid hormone (PTH) induces wasting of phosphate in the urine (*6b*) and calcium retention. Consequently, the serum levels of calcium are normal or nearly normal, but the phosphate is low; hence, mineralization is impaired (*7*).

airways predisposes to secondary pulmonary infections, and desquamation of keratin debris in the urinary tract predisposes to renal and urinary bladder stones. Hyperplasia and *hyperkeratinization of the epidermis* with plugging of the ducts of the adnexal glands may produce follicular or papular dermatosis. Another very serious consequence of lack of vitamin A is immune deficiency. This impairment of immunity leads to higher mortality rates from common infections such as measles, pneumonia, and infectious diarrhea. In parts of the world where a deficiency of vitamin A is prevalent, dietary supplements reduce mortality by 20% to 30%.

In passing, we should note that despite past enthusiasms for the intake of megadoses of vitamin A to prevent cancer development, current evidence indicates that vitamin A and carotenes offer no protection from lung cancer.

Vitamin A Toxicity. Both short- and long-term excesses of vitamin A may produce toxic manifestations, a point of concern because of the megadoses being touted by certain sellers of supplements. The consequences of acute hypervitaminosis A were first described in 1597 by Gerrit de Veer, a ship's carpenter stranded in the Arctic, who recounted in his diary the serious symptoms that he and other members of the crew developed after eating polar bear liver. Keeping this in mind, eat with moderation when served this delicacy, but beware that acute vitamin A toxicity has also been described in individuals who ingested livers of whales, sharks, and even the lowly tuna! The symptoms of acute vitamin A toxicity include headache, dizziness, vomiting, stupor, and blurred vision, symptoms that may be confused with those of a brain tumor. Chronic toxicity is associated with weight loss, anorexia, nausea, vomiting, and bone and joint pain. Retinoic acid stimulates osteoclast production and activity, which lead to increased bone resorption and high risk of fractures. Although synthetic retinoids used for the treatment of acne are not associated with these complications, their use in pregnancy should be avoided because of the well-established effect of retinoids in increasing the risk of fetal malformations.

Vitamin D

The major function of the fat-soluble vitamin D is the maintenance of normal plasma levels of calcium and phosphorus. In this capacity, it is required for the prevention of bone diseases known as *rickets* (in children whose epiphyses have not already closed), *osteomalacia* (in adults), and hypocalcemic tetany. With respect to tetany, vitamin D maintains the correct concentration of ionized calcium in the extracellular fluid compartment required for normal neural excitation and relaxation of muscle. Insufficient ionized calcium in the extracellular fluid results in continuous excitation of muscle, leading to the convulsive state, hypocalcemic tetany. Our attention here will be focused on the function of vitamin D in the regulation of serum calcium levels.

Metabolism of Vitamin D. The major source of vitamin D for humans is its endogenous synthesis in the skin by photochemical conversion of a precursor, 7-dehydrocholesterol, via the energy of solar or artificial UV light. Irradiation of this compound forms *cholecalciferol* (known as vitamin D_3; for the sake of simplicity we will use the term vitamin D to refer to this compound). Under usual conditions of sun exposure about 90% of the vitamin D needed is endogenously derived from 7-dehydrocholesterol present in the skin. However, blacks may have a lower level of vitamin D production in the skin because of melanin pigmentation. The small remainder comes from dietary sources, such as deep-sea fish, plants, and grains; this requires normal fat absorption. In plant sources, vitamin D is present in its precursor form (ergosterol), which is converted to vitamin D in the body.

The metabolism of vitamin D can be outlined as follows (Fig. 8–19):

1. Absorption of vitamin D along with other fats in the gut or synthesis from precursors in the skin
2. Binding to plasma α_1-globulin (D-binding protein) and transport to liver
3. Conversion to 25-hydroxyvitamin D (25-OH-D) by 25-hydroxylase in the liver
4. Conversion of 25-OH-D to 1,25-dihydroxyvitamin D [1,25$(OH)_2$-D] by α_1-hydroxylase in the kidney (biologically the most active form of vitamin D).

The production of 1,25$(OH)_2$-D by the kidney is regulated by three mechanisms:

- *Hypocalcemia stimulates secretion of parathyroid hormone (PTH),* which in turn augments the conversion of 25-OH-D to 1,25$(OH)_2$-D by activating α_1-hydroxylase.
- *Hypophosphatemia directly activates α_1-hydroxylase* and thus increases formation of 1,25$(OH)_2$-D.
- In a feedback loop, increased levels of 1,25$(OH)_2$-D down-regulate synthesis of this metabolite by inhibiting the action of α_1-hydroxylase (a decrease in the levels of 1,25$(OH)_2$-D has the opposite effect).

Functions of Vitamin D. 1,25$(OH)_2$-D, the biologically active form of vitamin D, is best regarded as a steroid hormone. Like other steroid hormones, it acts by binding to a high-affinity nuclear receptor that in turn binds to regulatory DNA sequences, which induce transcription of genes coding for specific target proteins. The receptors for 1,25-$(OH)_2$-D are present in most nucleated cells of the body, and they transduce signals that result in various biologic activities, beyond those involved in calcium and phosphorus homeostasis. Nevertheless, the best understood functions of vitamin D relate to the maintenance of normal plasma levels of calcium and phosphorus, through action on the intestines, bones, and kidneys (see Fig. 8–19).

The active form of vitamin D

- Stimulates intestinal absorption of calcium and phosphorus
- Collaborates with PTH in the mobilization of calcium from bone
- Stimulates the PTH-dependent reabsorption of calcium in renal distal tubules.

We now consider these three functions of vitamin D.

How 1,25$(OH)_2$-D stimulates *intestinal absorption of calcium and phosphorus* is still somewhat unclear. The weight of evidence favors the view that it binds to the nuclear vitamin D receptor, activating the synthesis of proteins that participate in the transport of calcium from the intestinal lumen into the bloodstream. The increased absorption of phosphorus is independent of calcium transport.

The effects of vitamin D on bone depend on the plasma levels of calcium. On the one hand, with hypocalcemia, 1,25$(OH)_2$-D collaborates with PTH in the resorption of calcium and phosphorus from bone to support blood levels. On the other hand, vitamin D is required for normal mineralization of epiphyseal cartilage and osteoid matrix. It is still not clear how the resorptive function is mediated, but direct activation of osteoclasts is ruled out. More likely, vitamin D favors the formation of osteoclasts from their precursors (monocytes), possibly by influencing the production of RANK (receptor activator of NF-κB) ligand (Chapter 21). The precise details of mineralization of bone when vitamin D levels are adequate are also uncertain. The main function of vitamin D may be to maintain calcium and phosphorus at supersaturated levels in the plasma. However, vitamin D clearly activates osteoblasts to synthesize the calcium-binding protein osteocalcin, involved in the deposition of calcium into osteoid matrix, and may thus contribute to bone mineralization.

Equally unclear is the role of vitamin D in renal *reabsorption of calcium.* PTH is clearly necessary, but so is vitamin D. There is no substantial evidence that vitamin D participates in renal reabsorption of phosphorus.

Deficiency States. Rickets in growing children and osteomalacia in adults are skeletal diseases with worldwide distribution. They may result from diets deficient in calcium and vitamin D, but probably more important is limited exposure to sunlight (for instance, in heavily veiled women, children born to mothers who have frequent pregnancies followed by lactation that causes vitamin D deficiency, and inhabitants of northern climates with scant sunlight). Other less common causes of rickets and osteomalacia include renal disorders causing decreased synthesis of 1,25 $(OH)_2$-D or phosphate depletion and malabsorption disorders. Although rickets and osteomalacia rarely occur outside high-risk groups, milder forms of vitamin D deficiency (also called vitamin D insufficiency) leading to bone loss and hip fractures are quite common in the elderly. Whatever the basis, a deficiency of vitamin D tends to cause hypocalcemia. When hypocalcemia occurs, PTH production is increased, which (1) activates renal α_1-hydroxylase, thus increasing the amount of active vitamin D and calcium absorption, (2) mobilizes calcium from bone, (3) decreases renal calcium excretion, and (4) increases renal excretion of phosphate. Thus, the serum level of calcium is restored to near normal, but hypophosphatemia persists, and so mineralization of bone is impaired or there is high bone turnover.

An understanding of the morphologic changes in rickets and *osteomalacia* is facilitated by a brief summary of normal bone development and maintenance. The development of flat bones in the skeleton involves intramembranous ossification, while the formation of long tubular bones reflects endochondral ossification. With intramembranous bone formation, mesenchymal cells differentiate directly into osteoblasts, which synthesize the collagenous osteoid matrix on which calcium is deposited. In contrast, with endochondral ossification, growing cartilage at the epiphyseal plates is provisionally mineralized and then progressively resorbed and replaced by osteoid matrix, which undergoes mineralization to create bone (Fig. 8–20).

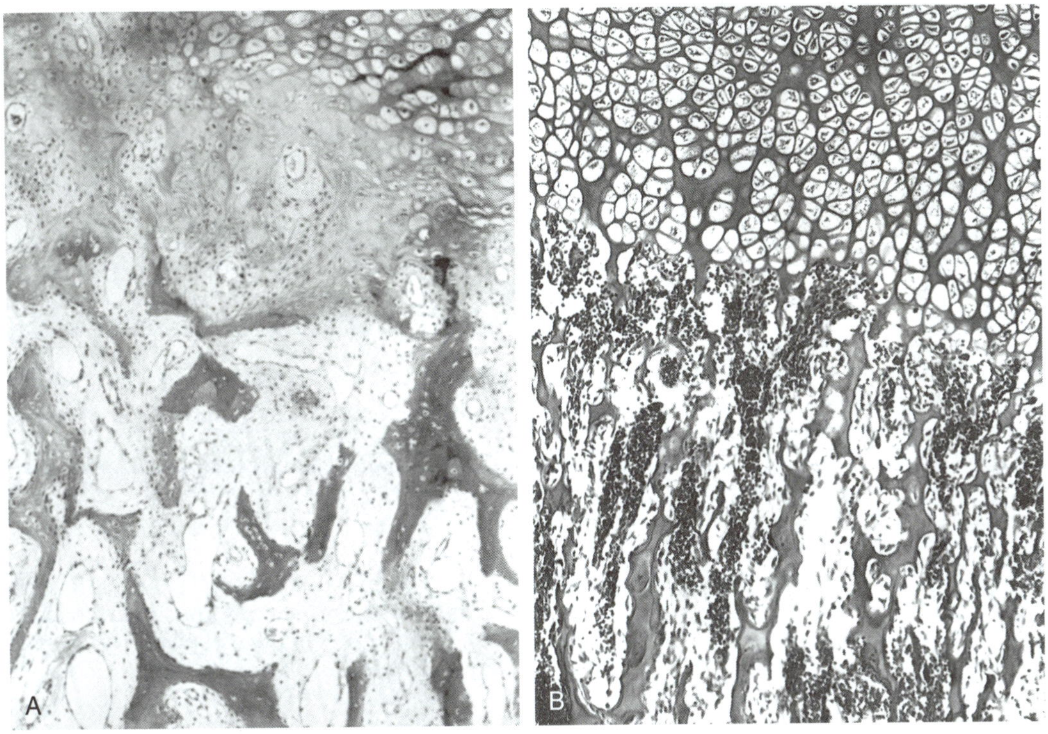

Figure 8–20

Rickets. **A,** Detail of costochondral junction in which the palisade of cartilage is lost. Darker trabeculae are well-formed bone; paler trabeculae consist of uncalcified osteoid. **B,** Compare with normal costochondral junction of a young child. Note cartilage palisade formation and orderly transition from cartilage to new bone.

Morphology

The basic derangement in both rickets and osteomalacia is an excess of unmineralized matrix. The changes that occur in the growing bones of children with rickets, however, are complicated by inadequate provisional calcification of epiphyseal cartilage, deranging endochondral bone growth. The following sequence ensues in rickets:

- Overgrowth of epiphyseal cartilage due to inadequate provisional calcification and failure of the cartilage cells to mature and disintegrate
- Persistence of distorted, irregular masses of cartilage, many of which project into the marrow cavity
- Deposition of osteoid matrix on inadequately mineralized cartilaginous remnants
- Disruption of the orderly replacement of cartilage by osteoid matrix, with enlargement and lateral expansion of the osteochondral junction (Fig. 8–20)
- Abnormal overgrowth of capillaries and fibroblasts in the disorganized zone resulting from microfractures and stresses on the inadequately mineralized, weak, poorly formed bone
- Deformation of the skeleton due to the loss of structural rigidity of the developing bones

The gross skeletal changes depend on the severity of the rachitic process; its duration; and, in particular, the stresses to which individual bones are subjected. During the nonambulatory stage of infancy, the head and chest sustain the greatest stresses. The softened occipital bones may become flattened, and the parietal bones can be buckled inward by pressure; with the release of the pressure, elastic recoil snaps the bones back into their original positions **(craniotabes)**. An excess of osteoid produces **frontal bossing** and a squared appearance to the head. Deformation of the chest results from overgrowth of cartilage or osteoid tissue at the costochondral junction, producing the "**rachitic rosary.**" The weakened metaphyseal areas of the ribs are subject to the pull of the respiratory muscles and thus bend inward, creating anterior protrusion of the sternum **(pigeon breast deformity)**. The inward pull at the margin of the diaphragm creates the **Harrison groove,** girdling the thoracic cavity at the lower margin of the rib cage. The pelvis may become deformed. When an ambulating child develops rickets, deformities are likely to affect the spine, pelvis, and long bones (e.g., tibia), causing, most notably, **lumbar lordosis** and **bowing of the legs** (Fig. 8–21).

In adults the lack of vitamin D deranges the normal bone remodeling that occurs throughout life. The newly formed osteoid matrix laid down by osteoblasts is inadequately mineralized, thus producing the excess of per-

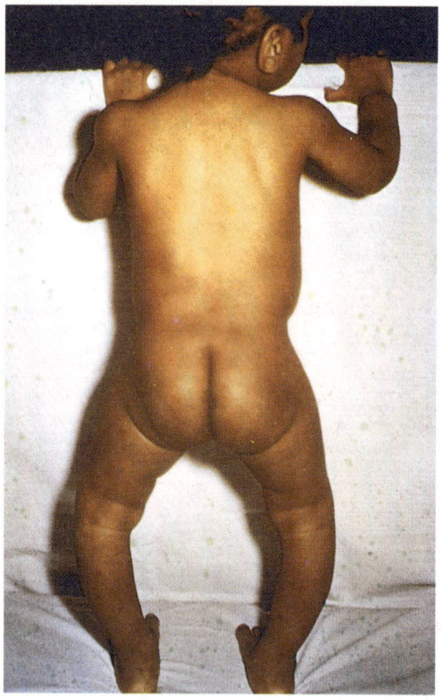

Figure 8–21

Rickets. Note bowing of legs due to the formation of poorly mineralized bones.

sistent osteoid that is characteristic of osteomalacia. Although the contours of the bone are not affected, the bone is weak and vulnerable to gross fractures or microfractures, which are most likely to affect vertebral bodies and femoral necks.

Histologically, the unmineralized osteoid can be visualized as a thickened layer of matrix (which stains pink in hematoxylin and eosin preparations) arranged about the more basophilic, normally mineralized trabeculae.

Studies also suggest that vitamin D may be important for preventing demineralization of bones. It appears that certain genetically determined variants of the vitamin D receptor are associated with an accelerated loss of bone minerals with aging. In certain familial forms of osteoporosis (Chapter 21), the defect has been localized to the vitamin D receptor.

Vitamin D Toxicity. Prolonged exposure to normal sunlight does not produce an excess of vitamin D, but megadoses of orally administered vitamin can lead to hypervitaminosis (the potentially harmful effects of exposure to high-intensity UV light in tanning salons remains a topic of continuous debate). In children, hypervitaminosis D may take the form of metastatic calcifications of soft tissues such as the kidney; in adults it causes bone pain and hypercalcemia. In passing, we might point out that the toxic potential of this vitamin is so great that in sufficiently large doses it is a potent rodenticide!

Vitamin C (Ascorbic Acid)

A deficiency of water-soluble vitamin C leads to the development of *scurvy,* characterized principally by bone disease in growing children and by hemorrhages and healing defects in both children and adults. Sailors of the British Royal Navy were nicknamed "limeys" because at the end of the 18th century the Navy began to provide lime and lemon juice to sailors to prevent scurvy during their long sojourn at sea. It was not until 1932 that ascorbic acid was identified and synthesized. Ascorbic acid is not synthesized endogenously in humans, and therefore we are entirely dependent on the diet for this nutrient. Ascorbic acid is present in milk and some animal products (liver, fish) and is abundant in a variety of fruits and vegetables. All but the most restricted diets provide adequate amounts of vitamin C.

Function. Ascorbic acid functions in a variety of biosynthetic pathways by accelerating hydroxylation and amidation reactions. The most clearly established function of vitamin C is the activation of prolyl and lysyl hydroxylases from inactive precursors, providing for hydroxylation of procollagen. Inadequately hydroxylated pro-collagen cannot acquire a stable helical configuration and cannot be adequately cross-linked, so it is poorly secreted from the fibroblasts. Those molecules that are secreted lack tensile strength, are more soluble, and are more vulnerable to enzymatic degradation. Collagen, which normally has the highest content of hydroxyproline, is most affected, particularly in blood vessels, accounting for the predisposition to hemorrhages in scurvy. In addition, it appears that a deficiency of vitamin C leads to suppression of the rate of synthesis of collagen peptides, independent of an effect on proline hydroxylation.

While the role of vitamin C in collagen synthesis has been known for many decades, it is only in recent years that its antioxidant properties have been recognized. Vitamin C can scavenge free radicals directly and can act indirectly by regenerating the antioxidant form of vitamin E.

Deficiency States. Consequences of vitamin C deficiency are illustrated in Figure 8–22. Fortunately, because of the abundance of ascorbic acid in so many foods, scurvy has ceased to be a global problem. It is sometimes encountered even in affluent populations as a secondary deficiency, particularly among elderly individuals, persons who live alone, and chronic alcoholics—groups that often have erratic and inadequate eating patterns. Occasionally, scurvy appears in patients undergoing peritoneal dialysis and hemodialysis and among food faddists.

Vitamin C Toxicity. The popular notion that megadoses of vitamin C protect against the common cold or at least allay the symptoms has not been borne out by controlled clinical studies. Such slight relief as may be experienced is probably a result of the mild antihistamine action of ascorbic acid. The large excess of vitamin C is promptly excreted in the urine, but may cause uricosuria and increased absorption of iron, with the potential of iron overload.

Other vitamins and some essential minerals are listed and briefly characterized in Tables 8–9 and 8–10. Folic acid and vitamin B_{12} are discussed in Chapter 12.

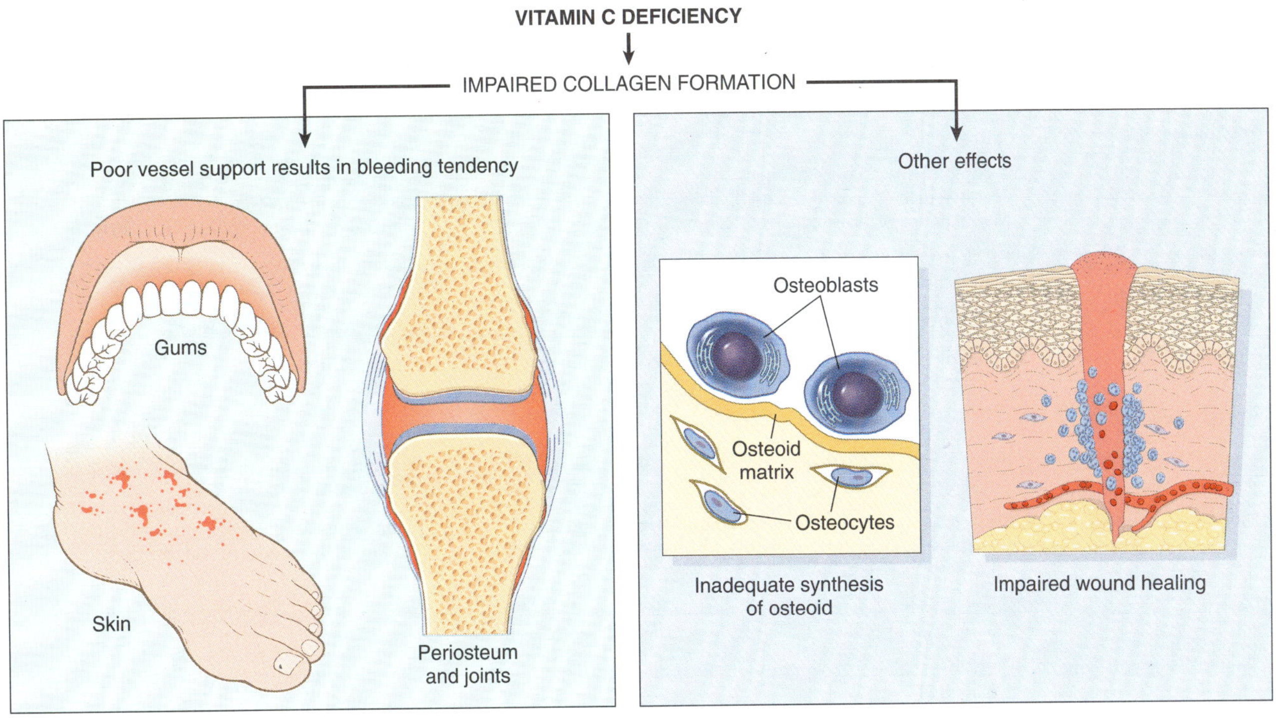

Figure 8–22

Major consequences of vitamin C deficiency caused by impaired formation of collagen. They include bleeding tendency because of poor vascular support, inadequate formation of osteoid matrix, and impaired wound healing.

SUMMARY

Nutritional Diseases

- Primary protein-energy malnutrition (PEM) is a common cause of children's mortality in poor countries. The two main primary PEM syndromes are marasmus and kwashiorkor. Secondary PEM occurs in chronically ill and advanced cancer patients (cachexia).
- Kwashiorkor is characterized by hypoalbuminemia, generalized edema, fatty liver, skin changes, and defects in immunity. It is caused by diets low in proteins but normal in calories.
- Marasmus is characterized by emaciation resulting from loss of muscle mass and fat with relative preservation of serum albumin. It is caused by diets severely lacking in calories—both protein and non-protein.
- Anorexia nervosa is self-induced starvation; it is characterized by amenorrhea and multiple consequences of low thyroid hormone levels. Bulimia is a condition in which food binges alternate with induced vomiting.
- Vitamins A and D are fat-soluble vitamins with a wide-range of activities. Vitamin C and members of the Vitamin B family are water-soluble (consult Table 8–9 for a listing of vitamin functions and deficiency syndromes).

Obesity

More than half of Americans between 20 and 75 years of age are overweight. Because obesity is highly correlated with an increased incidence of several diseases (e.g., diabetes, hypertension), it is important to define and recognize it, to understand its causes, and to be able to initiate appropriate measures to prevent it or to treat it.

Obesity is defined as a state of increased body weight, due to adipose tissue accumulation, that is of sufficient magnitude to produce adverse health effects. How does one measure fat accumulation? There are several highly technical ways to approximate the measurement, but for practical purposes the following are commonly used:

- Some expression of weight in relation to height, such as the measurement referred to as the body mass index (BMI) = (weight in kilograms)/(height in meters)^2
- Skinfold measurements
- Various body circumferences, particularly the ratio of the waist-to-hip circumference

The BMI, expressed in kilograms per square meter, is closely correlated with body fat. A BMI of approximately 25 kg/m^2 is considered normal. It is generally agreed that a 20% excess in body weight (BMI >27 kg/m^2) imparts a health risk.

The untoward effects of obesity are related not only to the total body weight but also to the distribution of the stored fat. *Central, or visceral, obesity,* in which fat accumulates in the trunk and in the abdominal cavity (in

Table 8–9 Vitamins: Major Functions and Deficiency Syndromes

Vitamin	Functions	Deficiency Syndromes
Fat-Soluble		
Vitamin A	A component of visual pigment Maintenance of specialized epithelia Maintenance of resistance to infection	Night blindness, xerophthalmia, blindness Squamous metaplasia Vulnerability to infection, particularly measles
Vitamin D	Facilitates intestinal absorption of calcium and phosphorus and mineralization of bone	Rickets in children Osteomalacia in adults
Vitamin E	Major antioxidant; scavenges free radicals	Spinocerebellar degeneration
Vitamin K	Cofactor in hepatic carboxylation of procoagulants – factors II (prothrombin), VII, IX, and X; and protein C and protein S	Bleeding diathesis
Water-Soluble		
Vitamin B_1 (thiamine)	As pyrophosphate, is coenzyme in decarboxylation reactions	Dry and wet beriberi, Wernicke syndrome, ? Korsakoff syndrome
Vitamin B_2 (riboflavin)	Converted to coenzymes flavin mononucleotide and flavin adenine dinucleotide, cofactors for many enzymes in intermediary metabolism	Ariboflavinosis, cheilosis, stomatitis, glossitis, dermatitis, corneal vascularization
Niacin	Incorporated into nicotinamide adenine dinucleotide (NAD) and NAD phosphate, involved in a variety of redox reactions	Pellagra – "three Ds": dementia, dermatitis, diarrhea
Vitamin B_6 (pyridoxine)	Derivatives serve as coenzymes in many intermediary reactions	Cheilosis, glossitis, dermatitis, peripheral neuropathy
Vitamin B_{12}	Required for normal folate metabolism and DNA synthesis Maintenance of myelinization of spinal cord tracts	Combined system disease (megaloblastic pernicious anemia and degeneration of posterolateral spinal cord tracts)
Vitamin C	Serves in many oxidation-reduction (redox) reactions and hydroxylation of collagen	Scurvy
Folate	Essential for transfer and use of 1-carbon units in DNA synthesis	Megaloblastic anemia, neural tube defects
Pantothenic acid	Incorporated in coenzyme A	No nonexperimental syndrome recognized
Biotin	Cofactor in carboxylation reactions	No clearly defined clinical syndrome

the mesentery and around viscera), is associated with a much higher risk for several diseases than is excess accumulation of fat diffusely in subcutaneous tissue.

The etiology of obesity is complex and incompletely understood. Involved are genetic, environmental, and psychological factors. However, simply put, obesity is a disorder of energy balance. The two sides of the energy equation, intake and expenditure, are finely regulated by neural and hormonal mechanisms, and body weight is thus maintained within a narrow range for many years. Apparently, this fine balance is maintained by an internal set point, or "lipostat," that can sense the quantity of energy stores (adipose tissue) and appropriately regulate food intake as well as energy expenditure. In recent years, several "obesity genes" have been identified. As might be expected, they encode the molecular components of the physiologic system that regulates energy balance. A key player in energy homeostasis is the *LEP* gene and its product, *leptin.* This unique member of the cytokine family, secreted by adipocytes, regulates both sides of the energy equation—intake of food and expenditure of energy. As discussed below, *the net effect of leptin is to reduce food intake and enhance the expenditure of energy.*

The neurohumoral mechanisms that regulate energy balance and body weight are very complex (Fig. 8–23). In a simplified way these mechanisms may be divided into three components:

- The afferent system, which generates signals from various sites. Its main components are *leptin* (adipose tissue), *insulin* (pancreas), *ghrelin* (stomach), and *peptide YY* (ileum and colon). Leptin reduces food intake and is discussed in detail below. Ghrelin secretion stimulates appetite, and it may function as a "meal-initiating signal." Peptide YY, which is released postprandially by endocrine cells in the ileum and colon, is a satiety signal.
- The hypothalamus processing system known as the *central melanocortin system,* which integrates the different types of afferent signals and generates efferent signals.
- The efferent system that carries the signals generated in the hypothalamus, which control food intake and energy expenditure.

Leptin. By mechanisms not clearly understood, the *output of leptin is regulated by the adequacy of fat stores.* With abundant adipose tissue, leptin secretion is stimu-

Table 8–10 Selected Trace Elements and Deficiency Syndromes

Element	Function	Basis of Deficiency	Clinical Features
Zinc	Component of enzymes, principally oxidases	Inadequate supplementation in artificial diets Interference with absorption by other dietary constituents Inborn error of metabolism	Rash around eyes, mouth, nose, and anus called acrodermatitis enteropathica Anorexia and diarrhea Growth retardation in children Depressed mental function Depressed wound healing and immune response Impaired night vision Infertility
Iron	Essential component of hemoglobin as well as several iron-containing metalloenzymes	Inadequate diet Chronic blood loss	Hypochromic microcytic anemia
Iodine	Component of thyroid hormone	Inadequate supply in food and water	Goiter and hypothyroidism
Copper	Component of cytochrome *c* oxidase, dopamine β-hydroxylase, tyrosinase, lysyl oxidase, and unknown enzyme involved in cross-linking collagen	Inadequate supplementation in artificial diet Interference with absorption	Muscle weakness Neurologic defects Abnormal collagen cross-linking
Fluoride	Mechanism unknown	Inadequate supply in soil and water Inadequate supplementation	Dental caries
Selenium	Component of glutathione peroxidase Antioxidant with vitamin E	Inadequate amounts in soil and water	Myopathy Cardiomyopathy (Keshan disease)

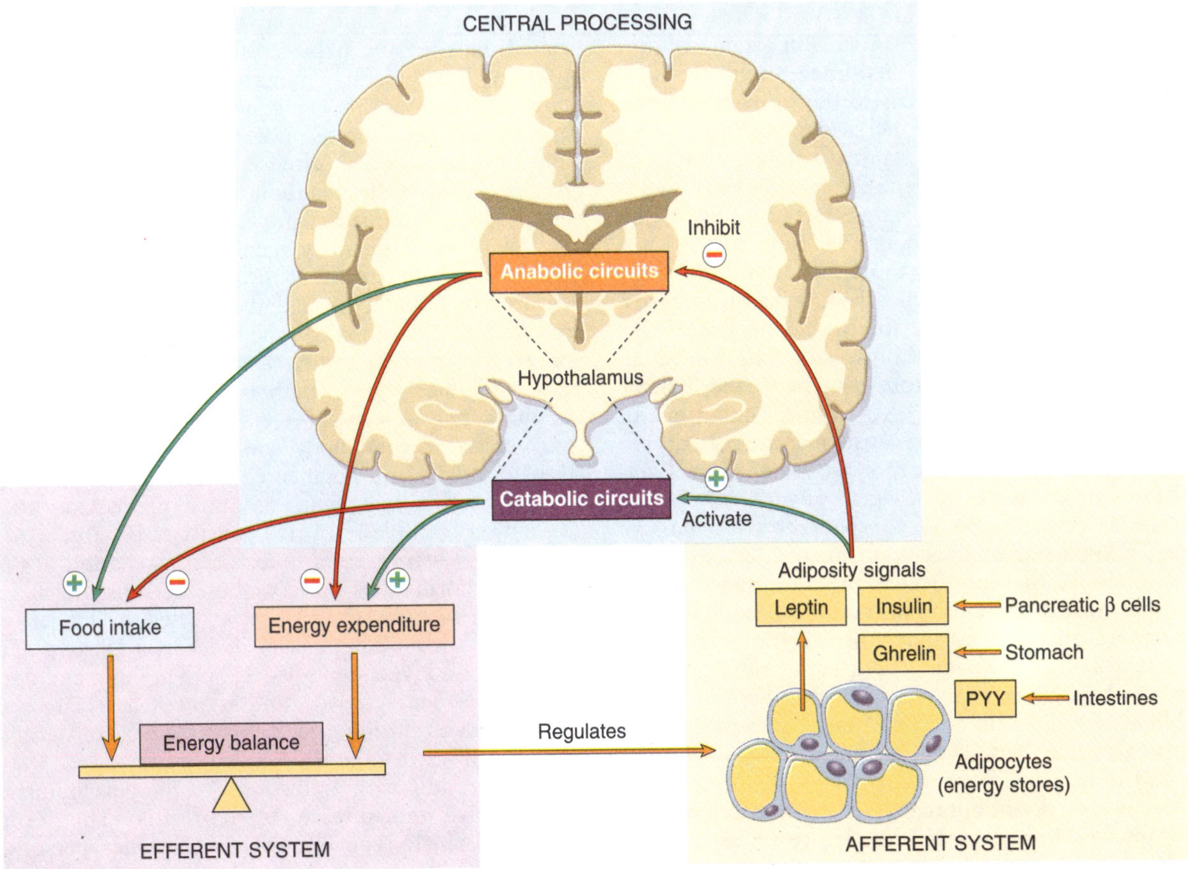

Figure 8–23

The circuitry that regulates energy balance. When sufficient energy is stored in adipose tissue and the individual is well fed, afferent adiposity signals (insulin, leptin, ghrelin, peptide YY) are delivered to the central neuronal processing units, in the hypothalamus. Here the adiposity signals inhibit anabolic circuits and activate catabolic circuits. The effector arms of these central circuits then influence energy balance by inhibiting food intake and promoting energy expenditure. This in turn reduces the energy stores, and the adiposity signals are blunted. Conversely, when energy stores are low, the available anabolic circuits take over at the expense of catabolic circuits to generate energy stores in the form of adipose tissue, thus generating an equilibrium.

lated, and the hormone travels to the hypothalamus, where it binds to leptin receptors on two classes of neurons. One class of leptin-sensitive neurons produces the feeding-inducing (*orexigenic*) neuropeptides, neuropeptide Y (NPY) and agouti-related protein (AgRP). The other class of leptin receptor–bearing neurons produces *anorexigenic* peptides, α-melanocyte-stimulating hormone (α-MSH) and cocaine- and amphetamine-related transcript (CART). The actions of the orexigenic and anorexigenic neuropeptides are exerted by binding to another set of receptors, the two most important being the NPY receptor and the melanocortin 4 receptor (MC4R), to which AgRP and α-MSH bind, respectively. *Leptin binding reduces food intake by stimulating the production of α-MSH and CART (anorexigenic peptides) and inhibiting the synthesis of NPY and AgRP (orexigenic peptides).* The opposite sequence of events occurs when there are inadequate stores of body fat: leptin secretion is diminished and food intake is increased. In individuals with stable weight, the activities of these pathways are balanced.

As indicated earlier, leptin regulates not only energy intake (appetite) but also energy expenditure, through a distinct set of pathways. Thus, abundance of leptin increases physical activity, production of heat, and energy expenditure. The neurohumoral mediators of leptin-induced energy expenditure are less well defined. *Thermogenesis* is probably the most important of the catabolic effects mediated by leptin through the hypothalamus. Thermogenesis seems to be controlled in part by hypothalamic signals that increase the release of norepinephrine from sympathetic nerve endings in adipose tissue. Fat cells express β_3-adrenergic receptors that, when stimulated by norepinephrine, cause fatty acid hydrolysis and also uncouple energy production from storage.

In rodents and humans, mutations that affect the central melanocortin circuit give rise to massive obesity. Mice with mutations that disable the leptin gene or its receptor continue to eat and gain weight. These mice fail to sense the adequacy of fat stores, and hence they behave as if they are undernourished. As in mice, mutations of the leptin gene or receptor cause massive obesity in humans. However, such patients are rare. More commonly, mutations of the MC4R gene give rise to obesity, as is the case in 4% to 5% of patients with massive obesity. While these monogenic forms of human obesity are uncommon, they underscore the importance of the leptin-melanocortin circuit in the control of body weight. Furthermore, they suggest that other acquired defects in these pathways may be pathogenetic in the more common forms of obesity. For example, in many obese individuals, blood leptin levels are high, suggesting that leptin resistance rather than leptin deficiency may be more prevalent in humans.

There is little doubt but that genetic influences play an important role in weight control. However, as with all complex traits, obesity is not merely a genetic disease. There are definite environmental influences; the prevalence of obesity in Asians who immigrate to the United States is much higher than in those who remain in their native land. These changes in all likelihood result from changes in the type and amount of dietary intake. After all, regardless of genetic makeup, obesity would not occur without intake of food!

Consequences of Obesity. Obesity, *particularly central obesity, increases the risk for a number of conditions,* including diabetes, hypertension, hypertriglyceridemia, and is associated with low HDL cholesterol (Chapter 10), which are major risk factors for coronary artery disease. The mechanisms underlying these associations are complex and probably interrelated. Obesity, for instance, is associated with *insulin resistance* and hyperinsulinemia, important features of type 2 diabetes (formerly known as non-insulin-dependent diabetes), and weight loss is associated with improvement (Chapter 20). It has been speculated that excess insulin, in turn, may play a role in the retention of sodium, expansion of blood volume, production of excess norepinephrine, and smooth muscle proliferation that are the hallmarks of hypertension. Whatever the mechanism, *the risk of developing hypertension among previously normotensive persons increases proportionately with weight.*

Obese persons are likely to have hypertriglyceridemia and a low HDL cholesterol value, and these factors may increase the risk of *coronary artery disease* in the very obese. It should be emphasized that the association between obesity and heart disease is not straightforward, and such linkage as there may be relates more to the associated diabetes and hypertension than to weight per se. Obesity, dyslipidemia, hypertension, and insulin resistance are components of a condition known as *metabolic syndrome,* which predisposes to cardiovascular disease and type 2 diabetes. Adipose tissue plays a role in the pathogenesis of the metabolic syndrome as a source of leptin, pro-inflammatory molecules such as TNF and IL-6, and anti-inflammatory agents such as adiponectin.

Nonalcoholic steatohepatitis is commonly associated with obesity and type 2 diabetes. This condition, also referred to as nonalcoholic fatty liver disease, can progress to fibrosis and cirrhosis.

Cholelithiasis (gallstones) is six times more common in obese than in lean subjects. The mechanism is mainly an increase in total body cholesterol, increased cholesterol turnover, and augmented biliary excretion of cholesterol in the bile, which in turn predisposes to the formation of cholesterol-rich gallstones (Chapter 16).

Hypoventilation syndrome is a constellation of respiratory abnormalities in very obese persons. It has been called the *pickwickian syndrome,* after the fat lad who was constantly falling asleep in Charles Dickens' *Pickwick Papers*. Hypersomnolence, both at night and during the day, is characteristic and is often associated with apneic pauses during sleep, polycythemia, and eventual right-sided heart failure.

Marked adiposity predisposes to the development of degenerative joint disease (*osteoarthritis*). This form of arthritis, which typically appears in older persons, is attributed in large part to the cumulative effects of wear and tear on joints. The greater the body burden of fat, the greater the trauma to joints with passage of time.

Obesity increases the risk of *ischemic stroke,* but the relationship between *obesity and stroke* is unclear, and opposing views can be found in the literature. According to some, the true relationship is between stroke and hypertension, not between stroke and obesity per se (i.e., obese patients who are not hypertensive are not at higher risk for stroke).

Equally controversial is the relationship between *obesity and cancer,* particularly cancers arising in the endometrium and breast. Here, the problem is complicated by the role of particular foods, such as animal fats, which may be independently associated with cancer and obesity. Nevertheless, it has been estimated that overweight and obesity may be associated with approximately 20% of cancer deaths in women and 14% of deaths in men. Obese women are at a higher risk of developing endometrial cancer than are lean women in the same age group. This relationship may be indirect; high estrogen levels are associated with increased risk of endometrial cancer (Chapter 19), and obesity is known to raise estrogen levels. With breast cancer the data are controversial. It seems that in postmenopausal women who live in countries with a moderate or low risk of breast cancer (e.g., Japan), central obesity is associated with an increased risk of breast cancer. Again, the role of sex hormones is a confounding variable.

SUMMARY

Obesity

- Obesity is a disorder of energy regulation. It increases the risk for a number of important conditions such as insulin resistance, type 2 diabetes, hypertension, and hypertriglyceridemia, which are associated with the development of coronary artery disease.
- The regulation of energy balance is very complex. It has three main components: (1) afferent signals provided mostly by insulin, leptin, ghrelin and PYY; (2) the central hypothalamic melanocortin system, which integrates afferent signals and triggers the efferent signals; and (3) efferent signals that control energy balance.
- Leptin plays a key role in energy balance. Its output from adipose tissues is regulated by the abundance of fat stores. Leptin binding to its receptors in the hypothalamus reduces food intake by stimulating anorexigenic peptides and inhibiting the synthesis of orexigenic peptides.
- Obesity contributes to the development of nonalcoholic fatty liver disease, which may progress to fibrosis and cirrhosis, and increases the formation of cholesterol gallstones.
- Obesity is associated with increased risk of endometrial and breast cancers, perhaps as a result of hormonal changes.

Diet and Systemic Diseases

The problems of under- and overnutrition, as well as specific nutrient deficiencies, have been discussed; however, the composition of the diet, even in the absence of any of these problems, may make a significant contribution to the causation and progression of a number of diseases. A few examples suffice here.

Currently, one of the most important and controversial issues is the contribution of diet to atherogenesis. The central question is "Can dietary modification—specifically, reduction in the consumption of cholesterol and saturated animal fats (e.g., eggs, butter, beef)—reduce serum cholesterol levels and prevent or retard the development of atherosclerosis (most importantly, coronary heart disease)?" The average adult in the United States consumes a large amount of fat and cholesterol daily, with a ratio of saturated fatty acids to polyunsaturated fatty acids of about 3:1. Lowering the level of saturates to the level of the polyunsaturates causes a 10% to 15% reduction in serum cholesterol level within a few weeks. Vegetable oils (e.g., corn and safflower oils) and fish oil contain polyunsaturated fatty acids and are good sources of such cholesterol-lowering lipids. Fish oil fatty acids belonging to the omega-3, or n-3, family have more double bonds than do the omega-6, or n-6, fatty acids found in vegetable oils. A study of Dutch men whose usual daily diet contained 30 gm of fish revealed a substantially lower frequency of death from coronary heart disease than that among comparable controls. Although dietary modification can affect heart disease, currently there are insufficient data to suggest that long-term supplementation of food with omega-3 fatty acids is of benefit in reducing coronary artery disease.

There are other examples of the effect of diet on disease.

- Hypertension is beneficially affected by restricting sodium intake.
- Dietary fiber, or roughage, resulting in increased fecal bulk, is thought by some to have a preventive effect against diverticulosis of the colon.
- Caloric restriction has been convincingly demonstrated to increase life span in experimental animals. The basis of this striking observation is not clear (Chapter 1).
- Even lowly garlic has been touted to protect against heart disease (and also, alas, against kisses—and the deveil), although research has yet to prove this effect unequivocally.

Diet and Cancer

With respect to carcinogenesis, three aspects of the diet are of concern: (1) the content of exogenous carcinogens, (2) the endogenous synthesis of carcinogens from dietary components, and (3) the lack of protective factors.

- Regarding *exogenous* substances, *aflatoxin* is clearly carcinogenic, and constitutes an important factor in the development of hepatocellular carcinomas in parts of Asia and Africa. Exposure to aflatoxin causes a specific mutation (codon 249) in the *p53* gene in tumor cells. The presence of the mutation can be used as a molecular signature for aflatoxin exposure in epidemiologic studies. Debate continues about the carcinogenicity of food additives, artificial sweeteners, and contaminating pesticides. Some artificial sweeteners (cyclamates and saccharin) have been implicated in bladder cancers, but convincing evidence is lacking.

- The concern about *endogenous* synthesis of carcinogens or promoters from components of the diet relates principally to gastric carcinomas. *Nitrosamines and nitrosamides* are implicated in the generation of these tumors in humans, because they have been clearly shown to induce gastric cancer in animals. These compounds can be formed in the body from nitrites and amines or amides derived from digested proteins. Sources of nitrites include sodium nitrite added to foods as a preservative, and nitrates, present in common vegetables, which are reduced in the gut by bacterial flora. There is, then, the potential for endogenous production of carcinogenic agents from dietary components, which might well have an effect on the stomach.
- High animal fat intake combined with low fiber intake has been implicated in the causation of colon cancer. The most convincing explanation of this association is as follows: High fat intake increases the level of bile acids in the gut, which in turn modifies intestinal flora, favoring the growth of microaerophilic bacteria. The bile acids or bile acid metabolites produced by these bacteria might serve as carcinogens or promoters. The protective effect of a high-fiber diet might relate to (1) increased stool bulk and decreased transit time, which decreases the exposure of mucosa to putative offenders, and (2) the capacity of certain fibers to bind carcinogens and thereby protect the mucosa. Attempts to document these theories in clinical and experimental studies have, on the whole, led to contradictory results.
- Vitamins C and E, β-carotenes, and selenium have been assumed to have anticarcinogenic effects because of their antioxidant properties. However, to date there is no convincing evidence that these antioxidants act as chemopreventive agents. As already mentioned, retinoic acid promotes epithelial differentiation and is believed to reverse squamous metaplasia. Better defined is its use for differentiation therapy in promyelocytic leukemia, as discussed earlier in this chapter.

Thus, we must conclude that despite many tantalizing trends and proclamations by "diet gurus," to date there is no definite proof that diet in general can cause or protect against cancer. Nonetheless, concern persists that carcinogens lurk in things as pleasurable as a juicy steak and rich ice cream.

BIBLIOGRAPHY

Anderson GL et al: Effects of estrogen plus progestins on gynecologic cancers and associated diagnostic procedures: the Women's Health Initiative randomized trial. JAMA 290:1739, 2003. *[A landmark report on the risk of ovarian cancer from HRT.]*

Badman MK, Flier JS: The gut and energy balance: visceral allies in the obesity wars. Science 307:1909, 2005. *[A review of the role of the gut in energy homeostasis.]*

Bellinger DC: Lead. Pediatrics 113:1016, 2004. *[An excellent overview of the subject.]*

Brass LM: Hormone replacement therapy and stroke: clinical trials review. Stroke 35 (Suppl 1):2644, 2004. *[Important data showing lack of protective of HRT on stroke.]*

Centers for Disease Control and Prevention: Third National Report on Human Exposure to Environmental Chemicals, 2005. *[A very important survey of environmental chemicals, with comments on exposure and health risk trends.]*

Clarkson TW et al: The toxicology of mercury, current exposures and clinical manifestations. N Engl J Med 349:1731, 2003. *[An excellent overview of the subject.]*

Cone RD: Anatomy and regulation of the central melanocortin system. Nat Neurosci 8:571, 2005. *[A review on the regulation of energy homeostasis by this system.]*

Creasman WT: WHI: Now that the dust has settled: a commentary. Am J Obstet Gynecol 189:621, 2003. *[A critical view on the Women's Health Initiative report on HRT effects.]*

Gomes MP, Deitcher SR: Risk of venous thromboembolic disease associated with hormonal contraceptives and hormone replacement therapy: a clinical review. Arch Intern Med 164:1965, 2004. *[A review of a very important clinical problem.]*

Hecht SS: Tobacco carcinogens, their biomarkers and tobacco-induced cancer. Nat Rev Cancer 3:733, 2003. *[An excellent review of the carcinogenic effects of tobacco smoke and unburned tobacco.]*

Hodgson E: A Textbook of Modern Toxicology, 3rd edition. Hoboken, N J, John Wiley & Sons, 2004. *[Concise textbook of toxicology with an excellent introductory chapter on the history and scope of toxicology.]*

Jarup L: Hazards of heavy metal contamination. Br Med Bull 68:167, 2003. *[A review of the health effects of exposure to lead, cadmium, mercury, and arsenic.]*

Kambhampati S et al: Signaling pathways activated by all-*trans*-retinoic acid in acute promyelocytic leukemia cells. Leuk Lymphoma 45:2175, 2004. *[An analysis of the mechanisms of action of retinoic acid therapy in acute promyelocytic leukemia.]*

Klaassen CD: Casarett and Doull's Toxicology, 6th edition. New York, McGraw-Hill, 2001. *[A comprehensive treatise on toxicology with excellent chapters on biotransformation of xenobiotics, toxic effects of metals, radiation toxicity, and air pollution.]*

La Vecchia C: Oral contraceptives and ovarian cancer: An update, 1998–2004. Eur J Cancer Prev 15:117, 2006. *[The most recent statistical analysis of the protective effect of oral contraceptive.]*

Lafontan M: Fat cells: afferent and efferent messages define new approaches to treat obesity. Annu Rev Pharmacol Toxicol 45:119, 2005. *[A review of the production of pro-inflammatory and other peptides by adipocytes, and the communication between these cells and other tissues.]*

Lips P: Vitamin D deficiency and secondary hyperparathyroidism in the elderly: consequences for bone loss and fractures and therapetic implications. Endocrine Rev 22:477, 2001. *[A comprehensive review of vitamin D deficiency, particularly in the elderly population.]*

Longnecker MP et al: The human health effects of DDT (dichlorodiphenyltrichloroethane), and PCBs (polychlorinated biphenyls) and an overview of organochlorines in public health. Annu Rev Public Health 18:211, 1997. *[A comprehensive review of the effects of organochlorines important for public health.]*

Manson JE et al: Estrogen plus progestin and the risk of coronary heart disease. N Engl J Med 349:523, 2003. *[A landmark study from the Women's Health Initiative.]*

Moelle DW: Environmental Health, 3rd edition. Cambridge, Harvard University Press, 2005 *[A concise textbook of environmental health with interesting introductory chapters and an excellent chapter on the effects of electromagnetic radiation.]*

Nagpal S: Retinoids: inducers of tumor/growth suppressors. J Invest Dermatol 123:1162, 2004.

Samet JM, et al: Fine particulate air pollution and mortality in 20 US cities 1987–1994. N Engl J Med 343:1742, 2000. *[A substantial study of the problem.]*

Sporer KA: Acute heroin overdose. Ann Intern Med 130:584, 1999. *[A good survey of a major problem.]*

Stewart BW, Kleihues P (eds): World Cancer Report, Lyon, IARC Press, 2003. *[A very useful report from the International Agency for Research on Cancer, with articles on the causes, mechanisms, and prevention of cancer, with excellent data on tobacco, alcohol consumption, and environmental/occupational carcinogenesis.]*

Wolf G: The visual cycle of the cone photoreceptors of the retina. Nutr Rev 62:283, 2004. *[An analysis of the role of retinol and derivatives in the visual cycle.]*

Chapter 9

General Pathology of Infectious Diseases*

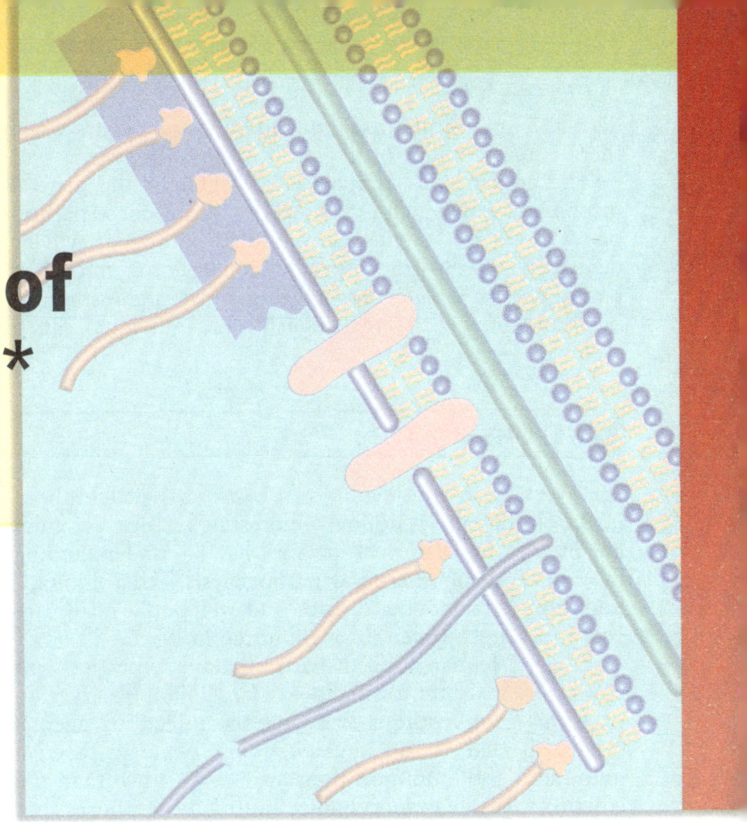

In many ways infectious diseases are as important to human history as wars and natural disasters; consider the Black Death of the Middle Ages, the wholesale death of Native Americans from measles and smallpox (many more than from bullets and starvation), or acquired immunodeficiency syndrome (AIDS). Infectious disease is also an important driving force in vertebrate evolution, underlying the development and progressive complexity of the human immune system. Despite medical advances, we have actually defeated only a handful of these diseases; notably, almost all the victories are due to immunization programs (e.g., smallpox, whooping cough, polio, and measles) that succeed by augmenting our own immunity. Although antibiotic usage has indeed contributed to the taming of some infectious diseases, indiscriminate use also has resulted, ironically, in the development of increasingly virulent, multiple drug-resistant pathogens. As a result, microbes once easily controlled have come roaring back: resistant strains of tuberculosis, malaria, salmonella, gonorrhea, and even the lowly streptococci.

Thus, infectious diseases remain important causes of death around the globe. In developing countries, unsanitary living conditions and malnutrition contribute to a massive burden of infectious disease responsible for more than 10 million deaths annually; most occur in children, especially from respiratory and diarrheal infections. Even in the United States, two of the top 10 leading causes of death are attributable to infection (pneumonia and sepsis). Infectious diseases are particularly important causes of death among the elderly and individuals with AIDS, as well as among those with chronic diseases. Medical advances like chemotherapy for tumors and immunosuppression for organ transplantation have also created a whole new class of patients vulnerable to usually innocuous but nevertheless *opportunistic* organisms.

In the face of what seems to be an overwhelming onslaught of microbes, it is well to remember that *cooperation* between microorganisms and humans is the rule; disease is the exception. Indeed, without our normal gut flora, we would be at risk for vitamin K deficiency and the normal vaginal flora prevent recurrent *Candida* ("yeast") infections. The majority of these relationships are *symbiotic* (of benefit to both partners) or, at worst, *commensal* (the fellow passenger shares the host's food without causing harm). When microbes cause disease, the nature and extent of the pathology depend on (1) the *virulence* (or pathogenicity) of the microorganism and (2) the *response of the host*. Consequently, infection in the microbiologic sense is not synonymous with infectious

*The contributions of Dr. John Samuelson to previous editions are gratefully acknowledged.

disease in a clinical sense; *infectious disease* occurs when there is tissue injury or altered host physiology.

The goal of this chapter is to highlight the general mechanisms by which infectious organisms cause pathology. Only a few of the many human pathogens will be described to illustrate specific concepts of microbial pathogenesis. Greater coverage of most organisms can be found in the chapters focusing on individual organ systems.

HISTORY

An overview of the evolution of our knowledge about infectious diseases is not only interesting but also provides an important historical perspective to understanding the concepts of microbial pathogenesis. Microbiology, immunology, infectious disease, and even public health are very much interwoven throughout the story.

Edward Jenner noticed that milkmaids working with cows were resistant to smallpox. His seminal observation in 1796 (even without knowing the infectious agent!) eventually led to an understanding of cross-reactive immunity and immunization; we know now that the cowpox virus (*Vaccinia*) induces antibody responses that neutralize subsequent infection with the considerably more virulent smallpox virus (*Variola*). Seventy years later (in 1865), Louis Pasteur was the first to demonstrate that microorganisms can in fact cause disease (germ theory of disease); he also created the first attenuated vaccines, including one for rabies in 1885. In 1882 Robert Koch championed the criteria for connecting a specific microorganism to a disease. Koch's postulates (interestingly enough, first applied in linking the anthrax bacillus to its specific disease constellation) require that (1) a causal organism be found in disease lesions, (2) the organism be isolable in culture, (3) secondary inoculation of the purified organism causes lesions (usually in experimental animals), and (4) the organism be recoverable from the experimental animal.

Modern microbiology, based on molecular genetics, arrived in 1944, when Oswald Avery demonstrated that transfer of deoxyribonucleic acid (DNA) from virulent to avirulent *Streptococcus pneumoniae* transformed the latter into a virulent phenotype. This conclusively proved that DNA is the material responsible for transmission of genetic traits, and it was the starting point for the explosion of research in molecular genetics that continues to this day.

Improved techniques in cell and tissue culture led to additional advances in infectious disease; previously, viral propagation relied on passage through animal hosts, making manipulation and observation problematic. The successful culture of polioviruses in human fetal tissues and foreskin fibroblasts in roller bottles by Enders and Weller in 1949 led to the development of formalin-killed and, eventually, attenuated live vaccines. Much later, identification of the human immunodeficiency virus (HIV) by Montagnier and Gallo in 1984 led to the subsequent development of diagnostic tests for screening blood, and to antiviral therapies based on understanding the structure of particular HIV enzymes; the race is on worldwide to develop an effective vaccine. Today, the entire genomic sequences of many species, including microbes and humans, are known, and this holds great promise for future research into the pathogenesis, diagnosis, and treatment of infectious diseases.

NEW AND EMERGING INFECTIOUS DISEASES

Some infectious diseases have coexisted with humans throughout our history; thus, leprosy has been known since at least biblical times, parasitic schistosomes have been found in Egyptian mummies, and many bacteria, fungi, and viruses probably plagued even prehistoric humans. Nevertheless, the arrival of new diseases has punctuated human history, and a surprising number of new infectious agents are described each year (Table 9–1). For example, venereal syphilis was unknown before the siege of Naples in 1494, Legionnaires' disease first appeared in 1976 in Philadelphia, Lyme disease first surfaced in the mid-1970s, AIDS was not recognized until the early 1980s, and "flesh-eating streptococci" are a recent popular staple of the tabloid press.

The infectious causes of some "new" diseases (e.g., *Helicobacter* gastritis, hepatitis B and C, rotavirus diarrhea, and Legionnaires' pneumonia) were previously unrecognized, largely because the infectious agents were difficult to culture. Other infections may genuinely be new to humans (e.g., HIV causing AIDS, *Borrelia*

Table 9–1 Some Recently Recognized Infectious Agents and the Diseases They Cause

Year	Agent	Disease
1977	Ebola Virus	Epidemic hemorrhagic fever
	Hanta virus	Hemorrhagic fever with renal disease
	Legionella pneumophila	Legionnaires' disease
	Campylobacter jejuni	Enteritis
1981	*Staphylococcus aureus*	Toxic shock syndrome
1982	*Escherichia coli* O157:H7	Hemolytic-uremic syndrome
	Borrelia burgdorferi	Lyme disease
1983	HIV	AIDS
	Helicobacter pylori	Gastric ulcers
1988	Hepatitis E	Enterically transmitted hepatitis
1989	Hepatitis C	Chronic hepatitis
1992	*Vibrio cholerae* O139	New epidemic cholera strain
	Bartonella henselae	Cat-scratch disease
1995	KSHV (HHV-8)	Kaposi sarcoma in AIDS
2002	West Nile virus	Acute flaccid paralysis
2003	SARS coronavirus	Severe acute respiratory syndrome

Adapted from Lederberg J: Infectious disease as an evolutionary paradigm. Emerg Infect Dis 3:417, 1997.

burgdorferi causing Lyme disease, and new exotic strains of *influenza*). Such apparently new entities probably arise from microbial mutations and/or recombinations among different organisms that alter their virulence factors or change their host specificity. Certain "new" disease entities are also being recognized only because of an expanding cohort of immunocompromised hosts (e.g., cytomegalovirus [CMV], Kaposi sarcoma herpesvirus [KSHV, or HHV-8], *Mycobacterium avium-intracellulare, Pneumocystis jiroveci [carinii]*, and *Cryptosporidium parvum*). Changes in the environment may increase the rates of other infectious diseases: reforestation of the eastern part of the United States led to massive increases in deer and mice carrying the ticks that transmit Lyme disease, babesiosis, and ehrlichiosis. Finally, as mentioned above, the emergence of multiple drug–resistant strains of *M. tuberculosis, Neisseria gonorrhoeae, Staphylococcus aureus*, and *Enterococcus faecium* also represents a challenge to medicine.

AGENTS OF BIOTERRORISM

The "weaponization" of biologic agents as a terrorist strategy has long been a theoretical threat; it unfortunately became reality with the US anthrax attacks in 2001. The Centers for Disease Control and Prevention have evaluated the microorganisms that pose the greatest danger as weapons (based on efficiency of disease transmission, difficulty of microbial propagation and distribution, difficulty of defending against, and potential for inciting fear in the public), ranking them in three categories (Table 9–2).

Category A agents are the highest risk agents, with easy dissemination and high potential for mortality, thus posing the greatest public panic and social disruption. Smallpox falls in this category because of its high transmissibility (respiratory aerosol or direct contact with skin lesions), low required infective dose, mortality rate of 30%, and lack of effective antiviral therapy. Since the United States stopped vaccinating for smallpox in 1972, with a subsequent drop in general immunity, the total population is highly susceptible. Category B agents are relatively easy to disseminate and produce moderate morbidity but low mortality (except in immune-compromised populations); many of these agents are food- or waterborne. Category C agents include emerging pathogens that have the potential for mass dissemination and high morbidity and mortality.

CATEGORIES OF INFECTIOUS AGENTS

Agents that cause infectious diseases range in size from the 27-kD prion protein to the 20-nm poliovirus to the 10-m tapeworm (Table 9–3). The following brief descriptions of the categories of infectious agents are not intended to be all-inclusive but rather to only convey important concepts.

Prions. Prions are abnormal forms of a normal host *prion protein* (PrP) found in high levels in neurons; the function of PrP is unknown. Prions (the name derives from proteinaceous infectious particles) cause transmissible spongiform encephalopathies, including kuru (associated with human cannibalism), Creutzfeldt-Jakob disease (CJD; associated with corneal transplants, among other procedures), bovine spongiform encephalopathy (BSE; popularly known as "mad cow disease"), and variant Creutzfeldt-Jakob disease (transmitted by consuming meat from BSE-infected cattle). The spongiform encephalopathies occur when a PrP undergoes a conformational (folding) change that confers protease resistance. The protease-resistant PrP then promotes conversion of the normal protease-sensitive PrP to the abnormal form, explaining the "infectious" nature of these diseases. Accumulation of abnormal PrP leads to neuronal damage and distinctive foamy "spongiform" changes in the brain. Spontaneous or inherited PrP mutations that make PrP intrinsically protease resistant have been observed in the sporadic and familial forms of CJD, respectively. These diseases are discussed in detail in Chapter 23.

Table 9–2 Potential Agents of Bioterrorism

Category A Diseases/Agents	Category B Diseases/Agents	Category C Diseases/Agents
• Anthrax (*Bacillus anthracis*) • Botulism (*Clostridium botulinum* toxin) • Plague (*Yersinia pestis*) • Smallpox (*Variola major* virus) • Tularemia (*Francisella tularensis*) • Viral hemorrhagic fevers: filoviruses (e.g., Ebola, Marburg), arenaviruses (Lassa fever virus and New World arenaviruses), bunyaviruses (e.g., Crimean-Congo hemorrhagic fever and Rift Valley Fever viruses)	• Brucellosis (*Brucella* species) • Epsilon toxin of *Clostridium perfringens* • Food safety threats (e.g., *Salmonella* species, *Escherichia coli* O157:H7, *Shigella*) • Glanders (*Burkholderia mallei*) • Melioidosis (*Burkholderia pseudomallei*) • Psittacosis (*Chlamydia psittaci*) • Q fever (*Coxiella burnetti*) • Ricin toxin from *Ricinus communis* (castor beans) • Staphylococcal enterotoxin B • Typhus fever (*Rickettsia prowazekii*) • Viral encephalitis: alphaviruses (e.g., Venezuelan equine encephalitis, eastern equine encephalitis, western equine encephalitis). • Water safety threats (e.g., *Vibrio cholerae, Cryptosporidium parvum*)	• Emerging infectious disease threats such as Nipah virus and Hantavirus

Adapted from Centers for Disease Control and Prevention information.

Table 9–3 Classes of Human Pathogens and Their Habitats

Taxonomic	Size	Site of Propagation	Sample Species	Disease
Prions	Proteins	Intracellular	PrP	Creutzfeld-Jakob disease
Viruses	20–300 nm	Obligate intracellular	Poliovirus	Poliomyelitis
Chlamydiae	200–1000 nm	Obligate intracellular	*Chlamydia trachomatis*	Trachoma, urethritis
Rickettsiae	300–1200 nm	Obligate intracellular	*Rickettsia prowazekii*	Typhus fever
Mycoplasmas	125–350 nm	Extracellular	*Mycoplasma pneumoniae*	Atypical pneumonia
Bacteria	0.8–15 µm	Cutaneous Mucosal Extracellular Facultative intracellular	*Staphylococcus aureus* *Vibrio cholerae* *Streptococcus pneumoniae* *Mycobacterium tuberculosis*	Wound Cholera Pneumonia Tuberculosis
Fungi	2–200 µm	Cutaneous Mucosal Extracellular Facultative intracellular	*Trichophyton* sp. *Candida albicans* *Sporothrix schenckii* *Histoplasma capsulatum*	Tinea pedis (athlete's foot) Thrush Sporotrichosis Histoplasmosis
Protozoa	1–50 µm	Mucosal Extracellular Facultative intracellular Obligate intracellular	*Giardia lamblia* *Trypanosoma gambiense* *Trypanosoma cruzi* *Leishmania donovani*	Giardiasis Sleeping sickness Chagas disease Kala-azar
Helminths	3 mm–10 m	Mucosal Extracellular Intracellular	*Enterobius vermicularis* *Wuchereria bancrofti* *Trichinella spiralis*	Enterobiasis Filariasis Trichinosis

Viruses. Viruses are obligate intracellular organisms that commandeer the host cell's biosythetic and replicative apparatus for their own proliferation. They consist of a nucleic acid genome surrounded by a protein coat (called a capsid) and, occasionally, a host-derived lipid membrane. Viruses may be classified by some combination of their nucleic acid genome (DNA or ribonucleic acid [RNA], but not both), the shape of the capsid (icosahedral or helical), the presence or absence of a lipid envelope, the mode of replication, the preferred host cell type (called *tropism*), or the type of pathology they cause (Table 9–4).

Because viruses are individually smaller than the limits of light microscopic resolution (20–300 nm in size), they are best visualized by electron microscopy. However, certain viruses have the propensity to aggregate within the cells they infect and form characteristic *inclusion bodies;* these may be visualized by light microscopy and may be diagnostically helpful. Thus, CMV-infected cells are markedly enlarged (hence the prefix *cytomegalo-*) and have characteristic inclusion bodies—both eosinophilic nuclear inclusions and smaller basophilic cytoplasmic inclusions (Fig. 9–1A). In comparison, herpesviruses can form a large nuclear inclusion surrounded by a clear halo (Fig. 9–1B), and in chronic hepatitis B virus (HBV) infections, accumulated hepatitis B surface antigen (HBsAg) forms so-called ground-glass hepatocytes (Fig. 9–1C). It should, however, be emphasized that most viruses do not give rise to readily demonstrable inclusions.

Viruses account for a large share of human infections. Different species of viruses can produce the same clinical picture (e.g., upper respiratory infection); conversely, a single virus can cause different clinical manifestations depending on host age or immune status (e.g., CMV). While many viruses cause transient illnesses (e.g., the

Table 9–4 Selected Human Viral Diseases

Viral Pathogen	Disease Expression
Respiratory	
Adenovirus	Upper and lower respiratory tract infections, conjunctivitis, diarrhea
Rhinovirus	Upper respiratory tract infection
Influenza viruses A, B	Influenza
Respiratory syncytial virus	Bronchiolitis, pneumonia
Digestive	
Mumps virus	Mumps, pancreatitis, orchitis
Rotavirus	Childhood diarrhea
Hepatitis A–E virus	Acute and chronic hepatitis
Systemic with Skin Eruptions	
Measles virus	Measles (rubeola)
Varicella-zoster virus	Chickenpox, shingles
Herpes simplex virus 1	"Cold sore"
Herpes simplex virus 2	Genital herpes
Systemic with Hematopoietic Disorders	
Cytomegalovirus	Cytomegalic inclusion disease
Epstein-Barr virus	Infectious mononucleosis
HIV-1 and HIV-2	AIDS
Arboviral and Hemorrhagic Fevers	
Dengue virus 1–4	Dengue, hemorrhagic fever
Yellow fever virus	Yellow fever
Warty Growths	
Papillomavirus	Condyloma; cervical carcinoma
Central Nervous System	
Poliovirus	Poliomyelitis
JC virus	Progressive multifocal leukoencephalopathy (opportunistic)

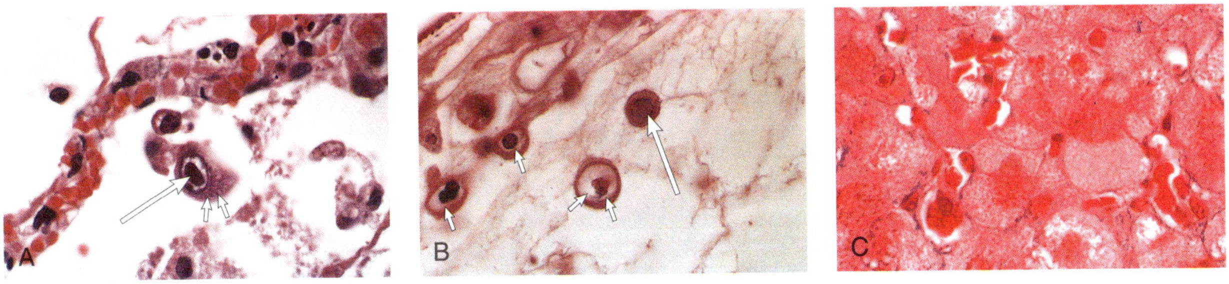

Figure 9–1

Examples of viral inclusions. **A,** Cytomegalovirus infection in the lung; infected cells show distinct nuclear (*long arrow*) and ill-defined (*short arrows*) cytoplasmic inclusions. **B,** Mucosal herpesvirus infection; infected cells show glassy nuclear inclusions (*long arrow*), frequently with a surrounding halo (*short arrows*). **C,** Hepatitis B viral infection in liver; in chronic infections, infected hepatocytes show diffuse granular (*ground-glass*) cytoplasm, reflecting accumulated hepatitis B surface antigen (HBsAg).

common cold and influenza), others can persist within cells of the host for years, either continuing to multiply (e.g., chronic HBV) or surviving in some nonreplicating form with potential for reactivation (*latent infection*). Thus, the herpes varicella-zoster (chickenpox) virus, establishes latency in the dorsal root ganglia; later reactivation results in *shingles*, an extremely painful cutaneous lesion. Some viruses also have the nasty capacity to transform host cells into neoplastic cells (see below).

Bacteriophages, Plasmids, and Transposons. These are mobile genetic elements that infect bacteria and can indirectly promulgate human disease by encoding bacterial virulence factors (e.g., adhesins, toxins, or enzymes). Exchange of these elements between bacteria often endows the recipient with a survival advantage (e.g., antibiotic resistance), and/or converts otherwise nonpathogenic bacteria into virulent ones.

Bacteria. Bacterial infections are common causes of disease (Table 9–5). Bacterial cells are prokaryotes: they have a cell membrane but lack membrane-bound nuclei and other membrane-enclosed organelles. They are also bound by a cell wall usually consisting of *peptidoglycan*, a polymer made up of a mixture of sugars and amino acids; many antibiotics function by inhibiting cell wall synthesis (e.g., penicillin). Bacterial cell walls generally occur in one of two varieties: a thick wall surrounding the cell membrane that retains crystal violet stain (*Gram-positive*) or a thin cell wall sandwiched between two phospholipid bilayer membranes (these do not retain crystal violet stain and are thus *Gram-negative*) (Fig. 9–2). Bacteria are classified by Gram staining (positive or negative), shape (e.g., spherical ones are *cocci*; rod-shaped ones are *bacilli*), and form of respiration (aerobic or anaerobic) (Fig. 9–3). Many bacteria have flagella that permit movement; others possess *pili* (see Fig. 9–2) that allow attachment to host cells. Most bacteria synthesize their own DNA, RNA, and proteins, but look to the host for their nutrition. Most bacteria remain *extracellular*, while some can grow only within host cells (*obligate intracellular* bacteria); still others can survive and replicate either outside or inside of host cells (*facultative intracellular* bacteria).

Normal healthy people are colonized by as many as 10^{10} bacteria in the mouth, 10^{12} bacteria on the skin, and 10^{14} bacteria in the gastrointestinal (GI) tract. Aerobic and anaerobic bacteria in the mouth, particularly *Streptococcus mutans*, contribute to dental plaque, a major cause of tooth decay. Bacteria colonizing the skin include *Staphylococcus epidermidis* and *Propionibacterium acnes*, the cause of acne. In the colon, 99.9% of bacteria are anaerobic.

Chlamydiae, Rickettsias, and Mycoplasmas. Like bacteria, these organisms divide by binary fission and are sensitive to antibiotics. However, they are considered separately here because they lack certain structures (e.g., *Mycoplasma* lack a cell wall) or metabolic capabilities (e.g., *Chlamydia* cannot synthesize adenosine triphosphate [ATP]) that distinguish them from bacteria. *Chlamydia* and *Rickettsia* species are obligate intracellular organisms that replicate in membrane-bound vacuoles in epithelial cells and the cytoplasm of endothelial cells, respectively. Rickettsiae are notable for their transmission by arthropod vectors, including lice, ticks, and mites.

Chlamydia trachomatis is the most frequent infectious cause of female sterility (by scarring fallopian tubes) and blindness (causing conjunctival inflammation that eventually scars and opacifies the cornea). By injuring endothelial cells, rickettsiae cause hemorrhagic vasculitis (often presenting as a rash), but they can also cause pneumonia or hepatitis (Q fever) or injure the central nervous system and cause death (Rocky Mountain spotted fever). *Mycoplasma* and the closely related genus *Ureaplasma* are the tiniest free-living organisms known; *M. pneumoniae* spreads from person to person by aerosols, binds to the surface of epithelial cells in the airways, and causes an atypical pneumonia characterized by peribronchiolar infiltrates of lymphocytes and plasma cells (Chapter 13). *Ureaplasma* infections are transmitted venereally and may cause nongonococcal urethritis (Chapter 18).

Fungi. Fungi are eukaryotes possessing thick chitin-containing cell walls and ergosterol-containing cell membranes; these unique wall and membrane constituents are the targets of most antifungal agents. Fungi can grow either as budding yeast forms or as slender filamentous hyphae. Hyphae may be septate (cell walls separate individual cells) or aseptate, a distinction important in clinical diagnosis. Many pathogenic fungi show *thermal dimorphism;* that is, they grow as hyphae at room tem-

Table 9–5 Examples of Bacterial, Spirochetal, and Mycobacterial Diseases

Clinical or Microbiologic Category	Species	Frequent Disease Presentations
Infections by pyogenic cocci	*Staphylococcus aureus, S. epidermidis*	Abscess, cellulitis, pneumonia, septicemia
	Streptococcus pyogenes, β-hemolytic	Upper respiratory tract infection, erysipelas, scarlet fever, septicemia
	Streptococcus pneumoniae (pneumoccoccus)	Lobar pneumonia, meningitis
	Neisseria meningitidis (meningococcus)	Cerebrospinal meningitis
	Neisseria gonorrhoeae (gonococcus)	Gonorrhea
Gram-negative infections, common	*Escherichia coli, Klebsiella pneumoniae Enterobacter* (*Aerobacter*) *aerogenes Proteus* spp. (*P. mirabilis, P. morgagni*) *Serratia marcescens, Pseudomonas* spp. (*P. aeruginosa*)	Urinary tract infection, wound infection, abscess, pneumonia, septicemia, endotoxemia, endocarditis
	Legionella spp. (*L. pneumophila*)	Legionnaires disease
Contagious and childhood bacterial diseases	*Haemophilus influenzae*	Meningitis, upper and lower respiratory tract infections
	Bordetella pertussis	Whooping cough
	Corynebacterium diphtheriae	Diphtheria
Enteropathic infections	Enteropathogenic *E. coli, Shigella* spp. *Vibrio cholerae, Campylobacter fetus, C. jejuni, Yersinia enterocolitica*	Invasive or noninvasive gastroenterocolitis, some with septicemia
	Salmonella typhi	Typhoid fever
Clostridial infections	*Clostridium tetani*	Tetanus (lockjaw)
	Clostridium botulinum	Botulism (paralytic food poisoning)
	Clostridium perfringens, C. septicum	Gas gangrene, necrotizing cellulitis
	Clostridium difficile	Pseudomembranous colitis
Zoonotic bacterial infections	*Bacillus anthracis*	Anthrax (malignant pustule)
	Yersinia pestis	Bubonic plague
	Francisella tularensis	Tularemia
	Brucella melitensis, B. suis, B. abortus	Brucellosis (undulant fever)
	Borrelia recurrentis	Relapsing fever
	Borrelia burgdorferi	Lyme borreliosis
Human treponemal infections	*Treponema pallidum*	Syphilis, bejel
Mycobacterial infections	*Mycobacterium tuberculosis, M. bovis*	Tuberculosis
	M. leprae	Leprosy
Actinomycetaceae	*Nocardia asteroides*	Nocardiosis
	Actinomyces israelii	Actinomycosis

perature but as yeast at body temperature. Fungi may produce spores sexually or, more commonly, asexual spores (*conidia*); the latter are produced on specialized structures or fruiting bodies arising along hyphal filaments.

Fungi may cause superficial or deep infections. Superficial infections typically involve the skin, hair, or nails. Dermatophytes ("skin lovers") are fungal species confined to superficial skin layers; these infections are commonly referred to by the term "tinea" (Latin for "grub" or "worm") followed by the area of the body affected (tinea pedis is "athlete's foot," while tinea capitis is "scalp ringworm"). Certain fungal species invade the subcutaneous tissue, causing abscesses or granulomas (e.g., sporotrichosis and tropical mycoses). Deep fungal infections usually heal or remain latent in normal hosts; in immunocompromised hosts, however, they can spread systemically and invade tissues, destroying vital organs. Some species responsible for deep fungal infections are limited to particular geographic regions (e.g., *Coccidioides* in the American Southwest and *Histoplasma* in the Ohio River Valley). By contrast, many fungi that cause deep infections in immunocompromised hosts (opportunistic fungi such as *Candida, Aspergillus, Mucor,* and *Cryptococcus*) are ubiquitous and colonize normal human epithelia without causing illness. In immunocompromised individuals these opportunistic fungi result in life-threatening infections characterized by tissue necrosis, hemorrhage, and vascular occlusion. AIDS patients in particular are frequent victims of the opportunistic fungus *Pneumocystis jiroveci* (formerly called *P. carinii*).

Protozoa. Protozoa, single-celled eukaryotes, are among the major causes of morbidity and mortality in developing countries. Parasitic protozoa can replicate intracellularly in many cell types (e.g., malaria in erythrocytes, *Leishmania* in macrophages) or extracellularly in the urogenital system, intestine, or blood. *Trichomonas vaginalis* is a sexually transmitted protozoan that can colonize the vagina and male urethra. The most prevalent intestinal protozoans, *Entamoeba histolytica* and *Giardia lamblia,* have two forms: (1) nonmotile cysts that are resistant to stomach acids and are infectious when ingested, and (2) motile trophozoites that multiply in the intestinal

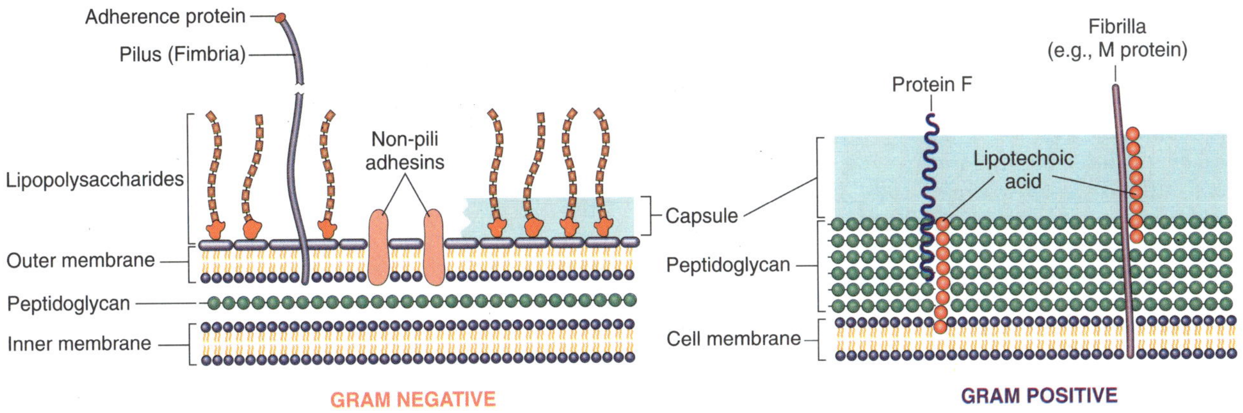

Figure 9–2

Wall structure of gram-negative and gram-positive bacteria, including several of the surface molecules involved in bacterial pathogenesis (see text).

lumen. Blood-borne protozoa (e.g., *Plasmodium, Trypanosoma,* and *Leishmania*) replicate within insect vectors before transmission to new human hosts. *Toxoplasma gondii* is acquired either by contact with oocyst-shedding kittens or by consumption of cyst-ridden undercooked meat.

Helminths. Parasitic worms are highly differentiated multicellular organisms with complex life cycles; most alternate between sexual reproduction in the definitive host and asexual multiplication in an intermediary host or vector. Thus, depending on the species, humans may harbor adult worms (e.g., *Ascaris lumbricoides*), imma-

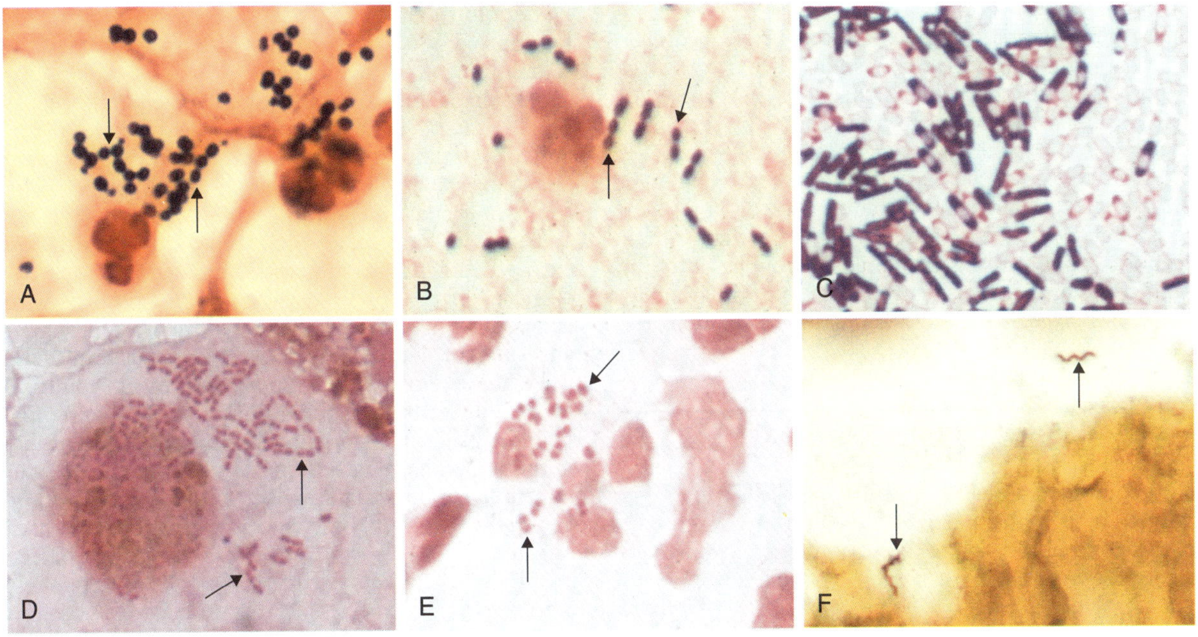

Figure 9–3

Bacterial morphology. **A,** Gram stain of sputum from a patient with *Staphylococcus aureus* pneumonia showing gram-positive cocci in clusters (*arrows*) among degenerating neutrophils. **B,** Gram stain of sputum from a patient with *Streptococcus pneumoniae* pneumonia showing gram-positive, elongated cocci in pairs and short chains (*arrows*). **C,** Gram stain of cultured *Clostridium sordellii* showing a mixture of gram-positive and gram-negative bacilli, many with subterminal spores (clear areas). **D,** Gram stain of a bronchoalveolar lavage specimen showing gram-negative intracellular bacilli (*arrows*) typical of *Klebsiella pneumoniae* or *Escherichia coli.* **E,** Gram stain of urethral discharge from a patient with *Neisseria gonorrhoeae* showing many gram-negative diplococci (*arrow*). **F,** Silver stain of brain tissue from a patient with Lyme disease meningoencephalitis; two helical spirochetes (*Borrelia burgdorferi*) are indicated by *arrows.* (**D,** Courtesy of Dr. Karen Krisher, Clinical Microbiology Institute, Wilsonville, Oregon. All other panels courtesy of Dr. Kenneth Van Horn, Westchester Medical Center, Valhalla, New York.)

ture forms (e.g., *Toxocara canis*), or asexual larval forms (e.g., *Echinococcus* species). Once adult worms take up residence in humans, they generate eggs or larvae destined for the next phase of the cycle. This is significant in that helminthic disease is usually proportionate to the number of infecting organisms (e.g., 10 hookworms cause little disease, whereas 1000 hookworms cause severe anemia by consuming 100 mL of blood per day). Moreover, pathology related to helminth infections is usually due to inflammatory responses to the eggs or larvae rather than to the adult forms (e.g., the robust granulomatous inflammation in schistosomiasis). *Strongyloides stercoralis* is an exception in that larvae can become infectious in the gut and cause overwhelming autoinfection in immunocompromised hosts.

Helminths comprise three classes:

- *Roundworms* (*nematodes*) have a collagenous tegument and a nonsegmented structure. These include *Ascaris* species, hookworms, and *Strongyloides* species among the intestinal worms and the filariae and *Trichinella* species among the tissue invaders.
- *Flatworms* (*cestodes*) are gutless worms whose head (scolex) sprouts a ribbon of flat segments (proglottids) covered by an absorptive tegument. They include the pork, beef, and fish tapeworms and the cystic tapeworm larvae (*cysticerci* and *hydatid* cysts).
- *Flukes* (*trematodes*) are primitive, leaflike worms with a syncytial integument; these include the Asian liver and lung flukes and the blood-dwelling schistosomes.

Ectoparasites. Ectoparasites are insects (lice, bedbugs, fleas) or arachnids (mites, ticks, spiders) that attach to and live on or in the skin. Arthropods may produce disease by direct tissue damage or indirectly by serving as the vectors for transmission of infectious agents (e.g., deer ticks transmit the Lyme disease spirochete *B. burgdorferi*). Some arthropods induce itching and excoriations (e.g., pediculosis caused by lice attached to hair shafts, or scabies caused by mites burrowing into the stratum corneum); at the site of the bite, mouthparts may be found associated with a mixed inflammatory infiltrate.

TRANSMISSION OF MICROBES

The outcome of infection depends on the ability of a microbe to breach host barriers and colonize and damage host tissues opposed to the ability of host defenses to eradicate the invader. *Host barriers to infection prevent microbes from entering the body and consist of innate and adaptive immune defenses* (see Chapter 5). Innate immunity is typically the first line of defense against microbes and does not adapt to repeated attacks; it includes physical barriers to infection, phagocytic and natural killer (NK) cells, complement, and inflammatory mediators (e.g., cytokines, collectins, acute-phase reactants). Adaptive immune responses—mediated by T and B lymphocytes and their products—are stimulated by microbial exposure and typically improve with successive contacts (Chapter 5).

Routes of Infection

Microbes can enter the host by inhalation, ingestion, sexual transmission, insect or animal bites, or injection. The first barriers to infection are intact host skin and mucosal surfaces and their secretory products (e.g., lysozyme in tears degrades the peptidoglycan wall of bacteria). These are formidable defenses against most infections; for example, only four of every 10 exposures to gonococci result in gonorrhea, and 10^{11} are required to produce vibrios cholera in human volunteers with normal gastric pH. Still, some infectious agents (having greater *virulence*) are able to overcome these barriers; thus, 100 *Shigella* organisms, *Giardia* cysts, or *M. tuberculosis* organisms can be sufficient to cause disease. In general, in healthy individuals, respiratory, GI, or genitourinary tract infections are caused by relatively virulent microorganisms that are capable of damaging or penetrating intact epithelial barriers. In contrast, most skin infections in healthy persons are caused by less virulent organisms entering the skin through damaged sites (cuts and burns). In the following sections we describe the common routes of entry of microbes, host barriers to infections, and some of the strategies used by microorganisms to overcome these barriers.

Skin. The dense, keratinized outer layer of skin is a natural barrier to infection; its low pH (about 5.5) and content of fatty acids inhibit microbial growth other than the normal bacterial and fungal flora adapted to that environment (including potential opportunists such as *S. epidermidis* and *Candida albicans*). Moreover, the keratinized outer layer is constantly shed and renewed so that colonization is difficult.

Although skin is usually an effective barrier, dermatophytes can infect the stratum corneum, hair, and nails, and a few microorganisms are able to traverse the unbroken skin. For example, *Schistosoma* larvae released from freshwater snails penetrate swimmers' skin by releasing collagenase, elastase, and other enzymes that dissolve the extracellular matrix. Superficial infections of the stratum corneum of the epidermis by *S. aureus* (impetigo) or by cutaneous fungi are all aggravated by heat and humidity, and human papillomavirus (HPV; cause of venereal warts), and *Treponema pallidum* (agent of syphilis) both penetrate warm, moist skin during sexual intercourse.

Most other microorganisms penetrate through breaks in the skin, including superficial cuts or abrasions (fungal infections), wounds (staphylococci), burns (*Pseudomonas aeruginosa*), and diabetic and pressure-related foot sores (multibacterial infections). Intravenous catheters in hospitalized patients frequently cause bacteremia with *Staphylococcus* species or gram-negative organisms. Needle sticks, whether deliberate (by needle-sharing drug abusers) or unintentional (accidental sticks by health care workers), expose the recipient to potentially infected blood and may transmit hepatitis B or C, or HIV. Bites by fleas, ticks, mosquitoes, mites, and lice break the skin and transmit diverse infectious organisms, including arboviruses (causes of yellow fever and encephalitis), rickettsiae, bacteria (Lyme disease), protozoans (malaria), and helminths (filariasis). Animal bites can lead to infections with bacteria or with rabies virus.

Respiratory Tract. Some 10,000 microorganisms, including viruses, bacteria, and fungi, are inhaled daily by every city inhabitant. The distance these microorganisms travel into the respiratory system is inversely proportional to their size. Large microbes are trapped in the nose and the upper respiratory tract in a mucus layer secreted by goblet cells; from there they are transported by the ciliary action of the respiratory epithelium to the back of the throat, where they are swallowed and cleared. Organisms smaller than 5 µm are inhaled directly into the alveoli, where they are phagocytosed by alveolar macrophages or by neutrophils recruited to the lung by cytokines.

The mucociliary clearance mechanism can be damaged by smoking (causing metaplasia of the normal bronchial epithelium with loss of cilia) or can be severely impeded by the hyperviscous mucus in cystic fibrosis. Intubation or gastric acid aspiration will also acutely interfere with normal mucociliary clearance. However, in normal hosts, virulent respiratory pathogens successfully evade the epithelial defenses by specifically adhering to respiratory epithelium. For example, influenza viruses express hemagglutinin proteins that bind to sialic acid residues on cell surface glycoproteins; once internalized, co-expressed viral neuraminidase releases the virus from the hemagglutinin. Viral neuraminidase also lowers the viscosity of mucus and facilitates viral transit in the respiratory tract. Taking a different tack, certain organisms (e.g., *Haemophilus influenzae* or *Bordetella pertussis*) elaborate toxins that directly paralyze mucosal cilia. Viral damage to epithelial cells also allows *secondary infection* by organisms that normally lack the necessary adherence capability (e.g., *S. pneumoniae* or *Staphylococcus* species).

M. tuberculosis causes respiratory infections because it is able to escape phagocytotic killing by alveolar macrophages. Finally, opportunistic fungi infect the lungs when cellular immunity is depressed or when leukocytes are deficient in number (e.g., *P. jiroveci* in AIDS patients and *Aspergillus* species in patients receiving chemotherapy).

Intestinal Tract. Most GI pathogens are transmitted by food or drink contaminated with fecal material. Where hygiene fails, diarrheal disease becomes rampant.

Normal defenses against ingested pathogens include (1) acidic gastric pH, (2) viscous mucus secretions, (3) lytic pancreatic enzymes and bile detergents, (4) antimicrobial peptides called defensins, (5) immunoglobulin A (IgA) antibodies, secreted by B cells located in mucosa-associated lymphoid tissues, and (6) the normal gut flora. Pathogenic organisms must compete for nutrients with abundant commensal bacteria resident in the lower gut, and all gut microbes are also intermittently expelled by defecation.

Infections of the GI tract occur when local defenses are undermined or organisms develop strategies to overcome the barriers. Host defenses are weakened by loss of gastric acidity, by antibiotics that unbalance the normal bacterial flora (e.g., in pseudomembranous colitis), or when there is stalled peristalsis or mechanical obstruction (e.g., in blind-loop syndrome).

Most enveloped viruses are killed by the bile and digestive enzymes, but nonenveloped viruses may be resistant (e.g., the hepatitis A virus, rotaviruses, reoviruses, and Norwalk agents).

Pathogenic bacteria in the GI tract cause disease by a variety of mechanisms:

- Staphylococcal strains growing in contaminated food release powerful enterotoxins that cause food poisoning symptoms without any bacterial multiplication in the gut.
- *Vibrio cholerae* and toxigenic *E. coli* multiply within the mucous layer, releasing exotoxins that cause the gut epithelium to secrete large volumes of watery diarrhea.
- *Shigella, Salmonella,* and *Campylobacter* invade and damage the intestinal mucosa and lamina propria, causing ulceration, inflammation, and hemorrhage, clinically manifesting as dysentery.
- *Salmonella typhi* passes from the damaged mucosa through Peyer's patches and mesenteric lymph nodes and into the bloodstream, resulting in a systemic infection.

Fungal infection of the GI tract occurs mainly in immunologically compromised hosts. *Candida* organisms have a predilection for stratified squamous epithelium, causing oral thrush or membranous esophagitis, but they may also disseminate to the stomach, lower GI tract, and systemic organs.

Intestinal protozoan infections particularly rely on cysts for transmission because they can resist stomach acid. Cysts eventually convert to motile trophozoites that attach to sugars on the intestinal epithelia via surface lectins. Other protozoa vary widely in how they traverse tissue barriers: *G. lamblia* attaches to the epithelial brush border, while *Cryptosporidium* organisms enter epithelial cells to form gametes and spores. *E. histolytica* causes contact-mediated cytolysis through a channel-forming pore protein and thereby invades and ulcerates the colonic mucosa.

Intestinal helminthes such as *Ascaris* typically cause disease only when present in large numbers or in ectopic sites (e.g., by obstructing the gut or invading and damaging the bile ducts). Hookworms may cause iron deficiency anemia by chronic loss of blood, which is sucked from intestinal villi. The fish tapeworm *Diphyllobothrium* can deplete its host of vitamin B_{12}, giving rise to an illness resembling pernicious anemia. Finally, the larvae of several helminth parasites pass through the gut briefly on their way to other organs; for example, *Trichinella* larvae preferentially encyst in muscle, while *Echinococcus* larvae travel to the liver or lungs.

Urogenital Tract. Even though urine can support the growth of many bacteria, the urinary tract is normally sterile because it is flushed many times per day; successful pathogens (e.g., *E. coli,* gonococci) are those that can adhere to the epithelium. Women have more than 10 times more urinary tract infections (UTIs) than men because the distance between the urinary bladder and the bacteria-laden skin (i.e., the length of the urethra) is 5 cm in women, compared with 20 cm in men. Obstruction of urinary flow and/or reflux of urine into the ureters also increases the risk of UTI. When a UTI spreads retrograde from the bladder into the kidney, it can cause acute and chronic pyelonephritis (Chapter 14).

From puberty until menopause, the vagina is protected from pathogens (mostly yeasts) by a low pH resulting from catabolism of glycogen in the normal epithelium by commensal lactobacilli. Antibiotics can kill the lactobacilli and make the vagina susceptible to infection. To be successful as pathogens, microorganisms have developed specific mechanisms for attaching to vaginal or cervical mucosa or for entering via local breaks in the mucosa during sexual intercourse (genital warts, syphilis).

Dissemination of Microbes Within the Body

Some microorganisms proliferate only locally at the site of infection, staying confined to the lumen of hollow viscera (e.g., cholera) or proliferate exclusively in or on epithelial cells (e.g., papillomaviruses, dermatophytes); others breach the epithelial barrier and spread to other sites via the lymphatics, blood, or nerves (Fig. 9–4).

A variety of pathogenic bacteria, fungi, and helminths are invasive by virtue of their motility or ability to secrete lytic enzymes (e.g., staphylococci secrete hyaluronidase that degrades the extracellular matrix). Microbial spread in these cases initially follows tissue planes of least resistance, but they can eventually involve lymphatics and the systemic vasculature. Thus, an initially localized staphylococcal infection *(abscess)* can progress to regional lymphadenitis to bacteremia and eventually to colonization of distant organs.

Within the blood, microorganisms may be transported free or intracellularly: some viruses (e.g., poliovirus and HBV), most bacteria and fungi, some protozoa (e.g., African trypanosomes), and all helminths are transported cell-free. Leukocytes can carry herpesviruses, HIV, mycobacteria, and *Leishmania* and *Toxoplasma* organisms, and transport some viruses (e.g., Colorado tick fever virus) and parasites (*Plasmodium* and *Babesia*). Viruses can also propagate by cell-cell fusion or by transport within neurons (e.g., rabies virus). Blood-disseminated foci of infection can be single and large (e.g., a solitary abscess or tuberculoma) or multiple and tiny (e.g., *Candida* microabscesses or miliary tuberculosis, miliary referring to the resemblance of foci infection to millet seeds). Sporadic bloodstream invasion by low-virulence or nonvirulent microbes occurs commonly (e.g., with vigorous tooth brushing!) but is quickly suppressed by the normal host defenses. By contrast, sustained bloodstream invasion with pathogens (viremia, bacteremia, fungemia, or parasitemia) is serious, manifested by fever, hypotension, and other systemic signs of sepsis. Massive bloodstream invasion by bacteria or their endotoxins can rapidly become fatal, even for previously healthy individuals.

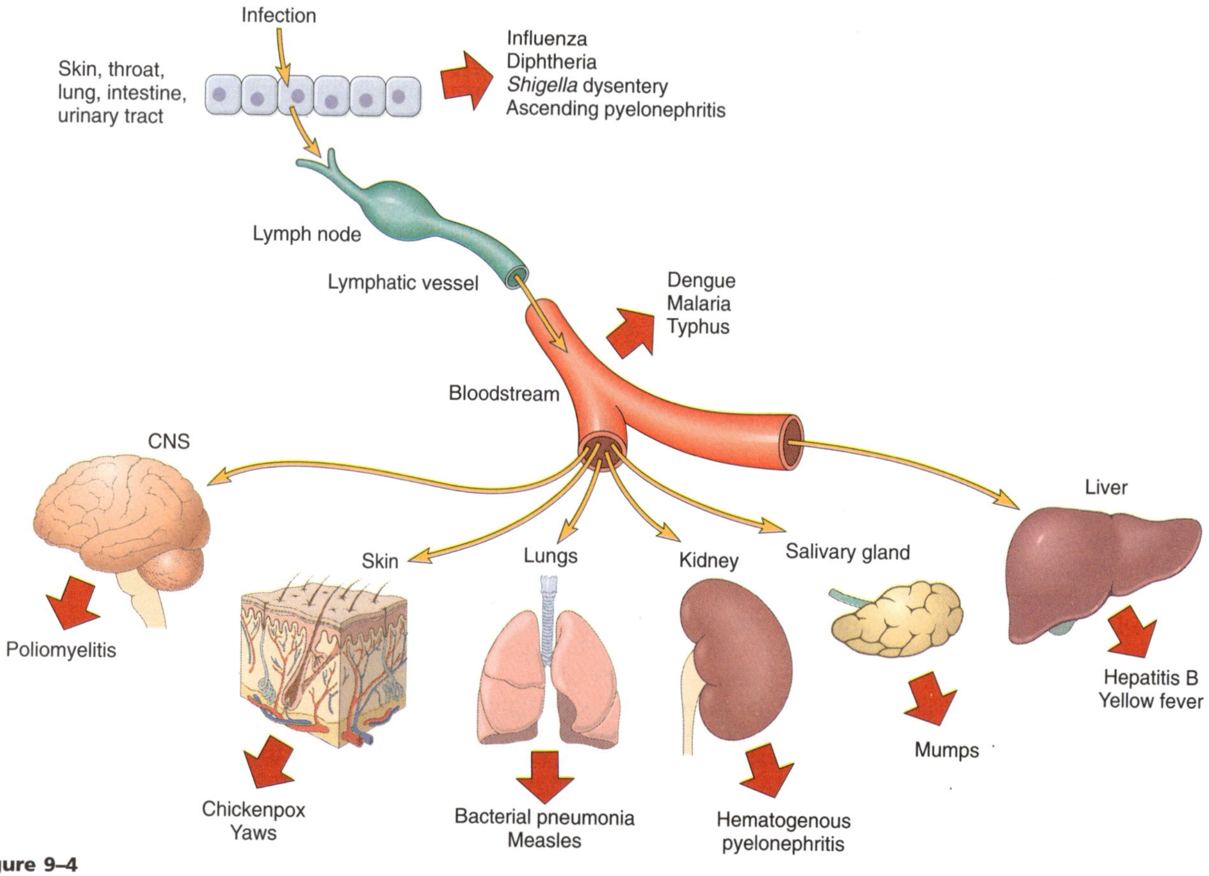

Figure 9–4

Entry and dissemination of microbes. (Adapted from Mims CA: The Pathogenesis of Infectious Disease. Orlando, Academic Press, 1987.)

The major manifestations of infectious disease can arise at sites distant from those of initial microbial entry. For example, chickenpox and measles viruses enter through the airways but chickenpox causes cutaneous rashes, and measles causes skin lesions, in addition to pneumonia; poliovirus enters through the intestine but kills motor neurons. *Schistosoma mansoni* parasites penetrate the skin but eventually localize in portal and mesenteric blood vessels, damaging the liver and intestine. The rabies virus travels from the skin to the brain in a retrograde fashion within nerves, while the varicella-zoster virus hibernates in dorsal root ganglia and, on reactivation, travels along nerves to cause skin shingles.

The placentofetal route is also an important mode of transmission (so-called *vertical transmission,* Chapter 7; *horizontal transmission* is the more common person-to-person mode of infectious disease transmission). Infectious organisms can reach the pregnant uterus through the cervical orifice or the bloodstream; if they traverse the placenta, severe fetal damage can result. Bacterial or mycoplasmal infections can cause premature delivery or stillbirth. Viral infections can cause fetal maldevelopment depending on the timing. Thus, rubella infection during the first trimester can cause congenital heart disease, mental retardation, cataracts, or deafness, while little damage occurs with third-trimester rubella infections. Infection also can occur during passage through the birth canal (e.g., gonoccocal or chlamydial conjunctivitis) or through breastfeeding (e.g., CMV, HBV in milk). Maternal transmission of HIV results in opportunistic infections in 50% of untreated children during the first year of life. Maternal transmission of HBV can result in chronic hepatitis or liver cancer.

Microbial Egress From the Body

For transmission of disease to occur, exit of microorganisms from the host is as important as the original entry. Release may occur through skin shedding, coughing, sneezing, urination, or defecation, or via insect vectors (as well as vertical transmission, described above). Some pathogens may be actively spread even though the host is asymptomatic (i.e., during an incubation period before symptoms start or in the instance of an immunologically unresponsive host).

Subsequent transmission to the next host depends very much on the hardiness of the particular microbe. Thus, some microbes can survive for extended periods in dust, food, or water; bacterial spores, protozoan cysts, and thick-shelled helminth eggs may be especially resilient outside of their original host. Following defecation many expelled pathogens will persist in fecally contaminated food or water, with subsequent transmission by ingestion (*fecal-oral route*); hepatitis A and E viruses, poliovirus, and rotavirus are examples. Eggs shed by some helminths (e.g., hookworms, schistosomes) into stool gain access to new hosts by larval penetration of the skin rather than by oral intake. Less hardy microorganisms must be quickly passed from person to person, often by direct contact (e.g., respiratory or sexual routes) or by blood-borne transmission. Bacteria and fungi can be spread by the respiratory route (e.g., *M. tuberculosis*) only if host lesions gain access to the airways. Viruses infecting the salivary glands (e.g., Epstein-Barr virus [EBV], CMV, mumps viruses) are transmitted principally by kissing or talking. Transmission of HBV, hepatitis C virus, and HIV infections through blood and blood products can occur through needle-sharing, cuts, or needle sticks and other accidents.

Microorganisms can be transmitted from animals to humans by invertebrate vectors such as insects (i.e., mosquitoes), ticks, or mites that either passively spread infection or occasionally serve as necessary hosts for microbial replication and development. Transmission can also occur directly from animals to humans (called *zoonotic infections*), either by direct contact (e.g., *leptospirosis, listeriosis*) or by eating the infected animal (e.g., *Trichinella spiralis*).

Prolonged intimate or mucosal contact during sexual activity allows the transmission of a variety of agents, including viruses (e.g., HPV, herpesviruses, HIV), bacteria (e.g., *T. pallidum, N. gonorrhoeae, Chlamydia trachomatis*), fungi (*Candida* species), protozoa (*Trichomonas* species), and arthropods (*Phthirus pubis,* or crab lice). The organisms that cause sexually transmitted infections (STIs) tend to be short-lived outside of the host and so depend on direct person-to-person spread. Many of these microbes are infectious in the absence of symptoms, so that transmission often occurs from individuals who are unaware of their illness. The initial site of infection may be the urethra, vagina, cervix, rectum, or oropharynx (Chapter 18).

SUMMARY

Transmission of Microbes

- The ability of a microbe to infect an individual depends on organism-specific virulence factors that allow it to breach host barriers and colonize the host.
- Host barriers include:
  - Skin: constantly sloughing keratin layer and normal skin flora
  - Respiratory system: alveolar macrophages and mucociliary clearance by bronchial epithelium
  - GI system: acidic gastric pH, viscous mucus secretions, pancreatic enzymes and bile, defensins, IgA, and normal gut flora
  - Urogenital tract: repeated flushing and commensal flora
- Microorganisms may proliferate locally or spread to other sites depending on microbial tissue tropisms.
- The route of secondary transmission of any given infection is related to the target tissue and the hardiness of the particular microbe. Transmission can involve direct contact, respiratory droplets, fecal-oral routes, blood-borne contact, sexual transmission, vertical transmission, or insect/arthropod vectors.

IMMUNE EVASION BY MICROBES

Once microorganisms have scaled host tissue barriers, the chief remaining obstacle between them and a permanent domicile is the immune system. Throughout evolution, microbes have been engaged in a struggle for survival against the arrayed forces of innate and adaptive immunity. Not surprisingly, microorganisms have developed many strategies to resist and evade these defenses, and such mechanisms are important determinants of microbial virulence and pathogenicity. These include:

- *Remaining inaccessible to the host immune system.* Microbes that propagate in the lumen of the intestine (e.g., toxin-producing *Clostridium difficile*) or gallbladder (e.g., *Salmonella typhi*) are concealed from many host immune defenses. Viruses that shed from epithelial luminal surfaces (e.g., CMV in urine or milk and poliovirus in stool) or those that infect keratinized epithelium (poxviruses) are inaccessible to antibodies and complement. Some organisms rapidly invade host cells before the humoral response becomes effective (e.g., malaria sporozoites enter hepatocytes; *Trichinella* enters skeletal muscles). Some larger parasites (e.g., tapeworm larvae) form cysts enshrouded in a dense fibrous capsule that renders the microbe largely inaccessible to host immune cells and antibodies. Viral latency within infected cells is the ultimate strategy; during the latent state (e.g., varicella-zoster virus in dorsal root ganglia), many viral genes are not expressed. Finally, some organisms can circumvent immune defenses by covering themselves with host proteins ("the wolf in sheep's clothing approach").
- *Varying or shedding antigens.* Neutralizing antibodies block the ability of microbes to infect cells; this is the basis for vaccination. However, neutralizing antibodies cannot effectively protect against microbes with the capacity to express multiple variants of their surface antigens. The low fidelity of viral RNA polymerases (e.g., in HIV and many respiratory viruses) and the ability to re-assort viral genomes (e.g., influenza viruses) leads to viral antigenic variation. Besides viruses, other classes of microbes also show antigenic variability, all using different strategies (Table 9–6). Thus, there are at least 80 different *S. pneumoniae* serotypes, distinguished by unique capsular polysaccharides; the problem is that an antibody produced in response to one serotype does not usually cross-react with another. Another approach is used by *Borrelia* spirochetes (including those that cause Lyme disease), which repeatedly switch their surface antigens. Yet another strategy is used by *S. mansoni,* which shed their antigens within minutes of penetrating the skin, preventing recognition by antibodies.
- *Resisting innate immune defenses.* Cationic antimicrobial peptides (CAMPs), including *defensins, cathelicidins,* and *thrombocidins,* provide important innate defenses against microbes; CAMP resistance is key to the virulence of many bacterial pathogens, allowing them to avoid neutrophil and macrophage killing. The carbohydrate capsules on many bacteria that cause pneumonia or meningitis shield bacterial antigens from circulating antibodies and complement proteins and also prevent neutrophil phagocytosis. Other bacteria make proteins that frustrate phagocytosis, kill phagocytes, prevent their migration, or diminish their oxidative burst. Thus, *S. aureus* expresses protein A molecules that bind the Fc portion of antibodies and so inhibit phagocytosis. *Neisseria, Haemophilus,* and *Streptococcus* all secrete proteases that can degrade antibodies. Several viruses, rickettsiae, some intracellular bacteria (including mycobacteria, *Listeria,* and *Legionella*), fungi (e.g., *Cryptococcus neoformans*), and protozoa (e.g., leishmania, trypanosomes, toxoplasmas) have developed strategies to resist intracellular killing and can, therefore, multiply within macrophages even after phagocytosis. Some viruses (e.g., herpesviruses and poxviruses) produce proteins that block complement activation. Other viruses have developed strategies to combat interferons (IFNs), an early host defense against viruses; inactive homologues of IFN-α/β or proteins that inhibit intracellular signaling downstream of IFN receptors can all block the antiviral effects of IFNs. Viruses also can produce inactive homologues of chemokines or chemokine receptors; these act as "decoys" and inhibit recruitment of inflammatory cells. Viruses also can produce soluble cytokine mimics; EBV produces a homologue of the immunosuppressive cytokine IL-10.
- *Inhibiting adaptive immunity.* Some microbes use a strategy of reducing the ability of CD4+ helper T cells and CD8+ cytotoxic T cells to recognize infected cells. For example, several DNA viruses (e.g., CMV and EBV) inhibit production of major histocompatibility complex (MHC) class I proteins or alter their intracellular trafficking, impairing peptide presentation to CD8+ T cells and preventing killing of infected cells. Although reduced MHC class I expression might be expected to trigger NK cell killing, herpesviruses are one step ahead in that they also express MHC class I homologues that inhibit NK activity (Chapter 5). Similarly, herpesviruses can target MHC class II molecules for early degradation, impairing antigen presentation to CD4+ T helper cells. Finally, viruses can directly infect lymphocytes and thereby compromise their function; HIV infection (with subsequent cell death) of CD4+ T cells, macrophages, and dendritic cells is but one example.

Table 9–6 Pathogens with Significant Antigenic Variation

Pathogen	Disease
Rhinoviruses	Colds
Influenza virus	Influenza
Neisseria gonorrhoeae	Gonorrhea
Borrelia hermsii	Relapsing fever
Borrelia burgdorferi	Lyme disease
Trypanosoma brucei	African sleeping sickness
HIV	AIDS

SUMMARY

Immune Evasion by Microbes

After bypassing host tissue barriers, infectious microorganisms must also evade host innate and adaptive immunity to successfully proliferate and be transmitted to the next host. Strategies include:

- Remaining inaccessible to host defenses, either in areas not reachable by antibodies or mononuclear cells (e.g., GI tract lumen or epidermis), inside cells, or enshrouded within host proteins
- Constantly changing antigenic repertoires
- Inactivating antibodies or complement, resisting phagocytosis, or growing within phagocytes after ingestion
- Suppressing the host adaptive immune response, e.g. by inhibiting MHC expression and antigen presentation.

HOW MICROORGANISMS CAUSE DISEASE

Infectious agents can be divided into those that are generally capable of causing disease (*pathogens*) and those that do not. All pathogens do not have the same probability of causing disease. This is partially a result of host variation in the general population (age, nutritional status, co-morbid disease, immune status). However, it is mostly because different organisms have different levels of *virulence,* that is, the ability to cause disease. High virulence connotes the capacity to cause disease in an otherwise healthy population; low virulence implies that the agent causes disease only in particularly susceptible populations (for example, certain bacterial strains can only infect previously damaged heart valves). *Opportunistic infections* are those in which normally nonpathogenic organisms produce disease in an immunocompromised host. As in real estate ("location is everything"), location in the body is also important in whether a pathogen causes disease. Thus, *E. coli* organisms in the colon are completely normal, whereas *E. coli* infecting the lungs is a cause of pneumonia, and *E. coli* infecting the urinary bladder causes cystitis.

Having reviewed the manner by which infectious agents breach host barriers, we next examine how they injure cells and cause tissue damage. There are three general mechanisms:

- Infectious agents can bind to or enter host cells and directly cause cell death or dysfunction.
- Pathogens can release endotoxins or exotoxins that kill cells (or affect their function) at a distance, release enzymes that degrade tissue components, or damage blood vessels and cause ischemic injury.
- Pathogens can induce host immune and inflammatory responses that may cause additional tissue damage.

Mechanisms of Viral Injury

Viruses can directly damage host cells by entering them and replicating at the host's expense. The predilection to infect certain cells and not others is called tissue tropism and is determined by several factors:

- *Host-cell receptors for a particular virus.* Viruses possess specific cell surface proteins that bind to selected host cell surface proteins. Many viruses use normal cellular receptors of the host to enter cells. Thus, HIV gp120 binds to CD4 (mostly on T cells) and to the chemokine receptors CXCR4 (T cells) or CCR5 (macrophages). Rhinoviruses bind to intercellular adhesion molecule-1, the same adhesion molecule used by lymphocytes to facilitate migration and activation at sites of inflammation (Chapter 2). In some cases, host proteases are needed to permit viral binding to host cells (e.g., a host protease cleaves and activates the influenza virus hemagglutinin).
- *Cell type–specific transcription factors that recognize viral enhancer and promoter sequences.* For example, the JC virus, which causes progressive multifocal leukoencephalopathy (Chapter 23), is restricted to oligodendroglia in the central nervous system, because the promoter and enhancer DNA sequences upstream from the viral genes are active in glial cells but not in neurons or endothelial cells.
- *Physical barriers.* For example, enteroviruses replicate in the intestine in part because they can resist inactivation by acids, bile, and digestive enzymes. Rhinoviruses replicate only within the upper respiratory tract, because they survive optimally at the lower temperature of the upper respiratory tract.

Once viruses are inside host cells, they can injure or kill in several ways (Fig. 9–5):

- *Lysis of host cells.* Viral replication interferes with normal cellular functions and may lead to cell death. For example, viral replication and release is the mechanism by which influenza virus kills respiratory epithelial cells, yellow fever virus kills hepatocytes, and poliovirus and rabies destroy neurons.
- *Immune cell–mediated killing.* Viral proteins expressed on host cell surfaces are recognized as foreign by the immune system and induce attack by cytotoxic T lymphocytes. Although this is a normal response to eliminate virally infected cells, it can clearly lead to significant host injury. Thus, liver cell injury during HBV infection is largely driven by cytotoxic T lymphocyte–mediated destruction of infected hepatocytes.
- *Alteration of apoptosis pathways.* Some virus-encoded proteins (including TAT and gp120 of HIV and adenovirus E1A) induce apoptosis. Indeed, this may be a protective host response to eliminate virus-infected cells. In contrast, some viruses encode genes that inhibit apoptosis (e.g., homologues of the cellular *BCL-2* gene). Such strategies may enhance viral replication and promote persistent viral infections, but they may also promote virus-induced cancers.
- *Induction of cell proliferation and transformation, resulting in cancer.* Examples include EBV, HBV, HCV, HPV, and human T-cell leukemia/lymphotropic virus-1.

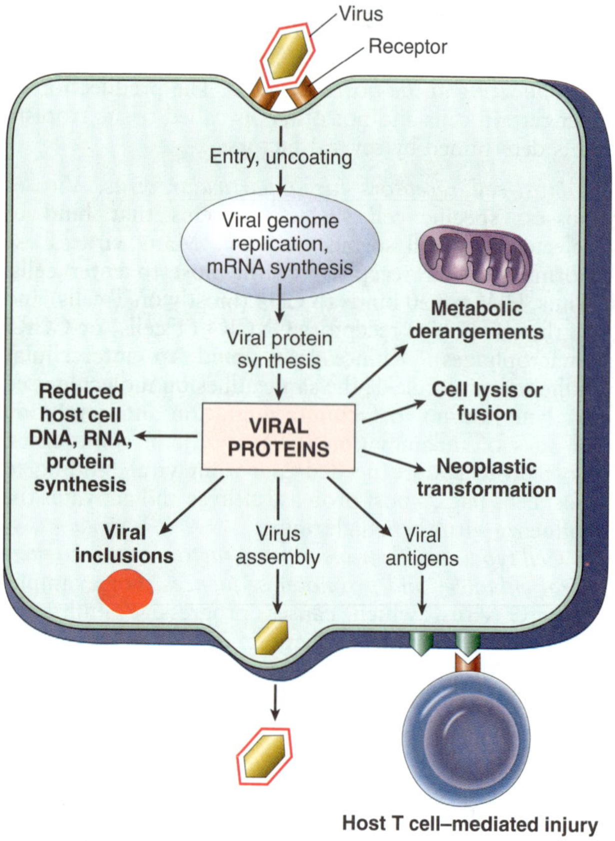

Figure 9–5

Mechanisms by which viruses cause injury to cells.

The mechanisms of viral transformation are discussed in Chapter 6.

- *Inhibition of host cell DNA, RNA, or protein synthesis.* These effects may eventually cause cell death, or they may lead to more subtle cellular dysfunction. For example, poliovirus inactivates a cap-binding protein essential for translation of host cell messenger RNA (mRNA); however, translation of poliovirus mRNA remains unaffected.
- *Damage to plasma membranes.* Viral proteins can insert into host plasma membranes and thereby alter their integrity or promote cell fusion (e.g., HIV, measles virus, and herpesviruses).
- *Damage to cells involved in antimicrobial defense, leading to secondary infections.* For example, viral damage to respiratory epithelium predisposes to subsequent bacterial pneumonia, and HIV depletion of CD4+ helper T lymphocytes leads to opportunistic infections.

Mechanisms of Bacterial Injury

The ability of bacteria to cause disease (virulence) depends on their ability to *(1) adhere to host cells, (2) invade cells and tissues, and/or (3) deliver toxins that damage cells and tissues.* Pathogenic bacteria have virulence genes that encode proteins that confer these properties. Differences in a small number of virulence genes determine whether an isolate of *Salmonella,* for example, will cause life-threatening infection or will be relatively benign. The coordination of bacterial adherence and toxin delivery is so important to bacterial virulence that the genes encoding the relevant proteins are frequently co-regulated by specific environmental signals. Thus, many bacteria induce expression of virulence factors as their concentration in the tissues increases, thereby overcoming host defenses.

Bacterial Adherence to Host Cells. *Adhesins* are bacterial surface molecules that bind to host cells; they typically have rather limited structural diversity but have broad host cell specificity.

Fibrillae cover the surface of gram-positive bacteria; fibrillae on *Streptococcus pyogenes* are composed of lipoteichoic acids and M protein (see Fig. 9–2). *Lipoteichoic acids* are hydrophobic and bind to fibronectin and buccal epithelial cells, while M proteins prevent macrophage phagocytosis. *Protein F* binds to fibronectin (see Fig. 9–2), and it may also help facilitate *S. pyogenes* entry into epithelial cells.

Fimbriae (or *pili*) are filamentous proteins on Gram-negative bacteria (see Fig. 9–2). Although some pili allow exchange of genes between bacteria, most are involved in adherence. Their stalks are composed of conserved repeating protein subunits, while the amino acids on the tips are variable and determine binding specificity. For example, *E. coli* strains that cause UTIs uniquely express a type P pilus that binds to a gal(α1–4)gal carbohydrate motif expressed on urothelium. Pili on *N. gonorrhoeae* mediate adherence of bacteria to host cells and can also act as targets for host antibody formation; subsequent variation in pili is an important mechanism by which *N. gonorrhoeae* can escape the immune response.

Virulence of Intracellular Bacteria. Facultative intracellular bacteria infect epithelial cells (*Shigella* and enteroinvasive *E. coli*), macrophages (*M. tuberculosis, Mycobacterium leprae*), or both (*S. typhi*). Intracellular growth is a strategy that not only allows escape from certain immune effector mechanisms (e.g., antibodies) but can also facilitate bacterial spread within the body; thus, macrophage migration carries *M. tuberculosis* from the lung to other sites. The virulence factors of intracellular bacteria concern their ability to (1) bind and enter cells, and (2) survive within them.

- *Entry into cells.* The host immune response is occasionally subverted to allow bacterial entry into macrophages; antibody- and/or complement C3b–coated (opsonized) bacteria are avidly phagocytized by macrophages. For example, *M. tuberculosis* can recruit a complement C2a fragment or activate the alternative complement pathway, with either pathway ultimately resulting in C3b opsonization; once coated with C3b, *M. tuberculosis* binds to the CR3 complement receptor on macrophages and is endocytosed.
- *Intracellular survival.* Once in the cytoplasm, bacteria have different strategies for interacting with the host cell. Inside their epithelial targets, *Shigella* and *E. coli* inhibit host protein synthesis, replicate rapidly, and lyse the host cell within a few hours. Macrophages

present a different obstacle; once phagocytosed by macrophages, most bacteria are killed by phagosome fusion with lysosomes. Thus, if bacteria are to thrive inside macrophages, they must escape this destruction. *Mycobacterium tuberculosis* accomplishes this by blocking phagosome-lysosome fusion, permitting unfettered intracellular proliferation. Other bacteria avoid macrophage annihilation by slipping out of the phagosome to proliferate in the cytoplasm; *Listeria monocytogenes* produces a pore-forming protein called listeriolysin O and two phospholipases that degrade the phagosome membrane and allow bacterial escape.

Bacterial Endotoxin. *Bacterial endotoxin* is a lipopolysaccharide (LPS) that is a major component of the outer cell wall of gram-negative bacteria (see Fig. 9–2). LPS is composed of a long-chain fatty acid anchor (lipid A) connected to a core sugar chain, both of which are similar in all gram-negative bacteria. Attached to the core sugar is a variable carbohydrate chain (O antigen), which can be used to distinguish different bacterial strains. Free LPS attaches to a circulating LPS-binding protein, and the complex then binds to a specific receptor (CD14) on monocytes, macrophages, and neutrophils. Engagement of CD14 results in intracellular signaling via an associated Toll-like receptor (TLR-4), causing cell activation and production of effector cytokines (Chapter 2). TLR-4 engagement on endothelial cells also causes endothelial activation and a net prothrombotic state (Chapter 4).

The host response to LPS can be both beneficial and harmful. At low levels, LPS induces many important cytokines and chemokines, as well as increased expression of costimulatory molecules, resulting in leukocyte recruitment and enhancement of T-lymphocyte activation. However, at high levels, LPS can precipitate septic shock, disseminated intravascular coagulation, and acute respiratory distress syndrome, mainly through overexuberant induction of cytokines such as tumor necrosis factor (TNF), IL-1, and IL-12 (Chapter 4).

Bacterial Exotoxins. Exotoxins are secreted proteins that directly cause cellular injury and frequently underlie disease manifestations.

- Some exotoxins are bacterial enzymes (proteases, hyaluronidases, coagulases, fibrinolysins) that act on target substrates and contribute to normal bacterial housekeeping and survival. Nevertheless, they can contribute significantly to pathologic manifestations of an infection. Thus, *Staphylococcus aureus* proteases cleave epidermal intercellular adhesion proteins and presumably lead to easier cutaneous invasion; at the same time they cause desquamation. *Clostridium perfringens*—the agent of gas gangrene—produces an α toxin (lecithinase) that disrupts plasma membranes, including those of circulating cells; this exotoxin literally digests host tissues, including the relatively resistant collagens.
- Other exotoxins are not as clearly related to bacterial adhesion or survival but nevertheless cause a distinct disease entity. Thus, the punctate, erythematous "scarlatiniform" rash of *scarlet fever* is due to a phage-encoded pyrogenic exotoxin made by only certain *Streptococcus pyogenes* strains.
- Many exotoxins alter intracellular signaling or regulatory pathways. Most of these have an enzymatically active (A) subunit linked by disulfide bridges to a B subunit that binds receptors on the cell surface and delivers the A subunit into the cell cytoplasm by endocytosis (Fig. 9–6). Within the cytoplasm, the disulfide bond of the toxin is reduced and broken, releasing the enzymatically active amino fragment A. In the case of diptheria toxin the A subunit catalyzes transfer of adenosine diphosphate (ADP)-ribose from nicotinamide adenine dinucleotide (NAD) to the EF-2 (an elongation factor that is critical for polypeptide synthesis), protein thus inactivating it (Fig. 9–6). One toxin molecule can thereby kill a cell by ADP-ribosylating more than 10^6 EF-2 molecules! *Corynebacterium diphtheriae* elaborates such a toxin to create a layer of dead cells in the throat, on which the bacteria outgrows its

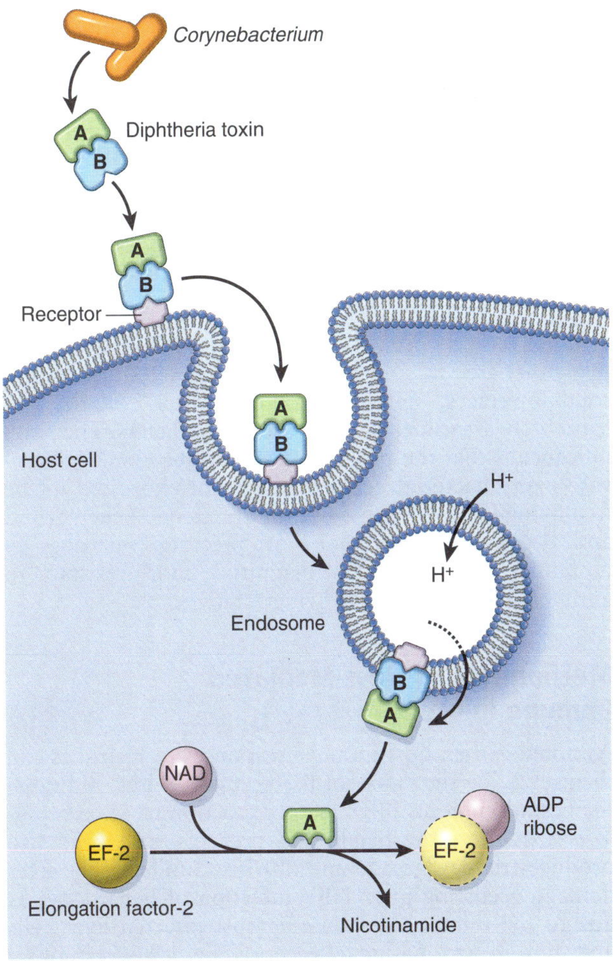

Figure 9–6

Inhibition of cellular protein synthesis by diphtheria toxin. See text for abbreviations. (Adapted from Collier RJ: Corynebacteria. In Davis BD, et al. [eds]: Microbiology. New York, Harper & Row, 1990.)

competition. Unfortunately, wider dissemination of diphtheria toxin causes serious disease manifestations through neural and myocardial dysfunction. The heat-labile enterotoxins of *V. cholerae* and *E. coli* also have an A-B structure and are ADP-ribosyl transferases; these enzymes, however, catalyze transfer from NAD to the guanyl nucleotide–dependent regulatory component of adenylate cyclase. This generates excess cyclic adenosine monophosphate (cAMP), causing intestinal epithelial cells to secrete isosmotic fluid and resulting in voluminous diarrhea and loss of water and electrolytes (Chapter 15).

- Neurotoxins, such as those produced by *Clostridium botulinum* and *Clostridium tetani,* inhibit release of neurotransmitters, resulting in paralysis. These toxins do not kill neurons; rather, their A domains interact specifically with proteins involved in synaptic neurotransmitter release. Both tetanus and botulism can result in death from respiratory failure due to paralysis of the chest and diaphragm muscles.
- *Superantigens* are bacterial toxins with the capacity to stimulate large populations of T lymphocytes, functionally resulting in a "cytokine storm." Superantigens bind to MHC class II molecules on antigen-presenting cells, without the usual internal processing, and then bind to conserved regions of T-cell receptors (TCRs). Such MHC II–TCR bridging through the superantigens leads to widespread T-cell activation and subsequent massive cytokine release, in particular TNF; the high cytokine levels in turn cause capillary leak and shock. Superantigens made by *Staphylococcus aureus* and *Streptococcus pyogenes* (i.e., the toxic shock syndrome toxin) cause toxic shock syndrome with fever, shock, and multisystem organ failure.

It has recently been appreciated that many bacteria can live either free in solution or in colonies coating liquid-solid interfaces, so-called *biofilms*. These colonies can form on heart values or intravascular catheters. Their significance is that the processes that produce biofilms activate many bacterial genes that are not expressed in the free-living forms. Because of the expression of such genes, and because of the colony architecture, microbes in biofilms may be orders of magnitude more resistant to antibiotics than their free-living relatives.

Mechanisms of Host-Mediated Immune Injury

As noted earlier, host immune responses to microbes can themselves be the cause of tissue injury. Thus, although the granulomatous inflammatory reaction to *M. tuberculosis* sequesters the bacilli and prevents spread, it also produces tissue damage and fibrosis. Similarly, the liver damage occurring after HBV infection of hepatocytes is due to the immune response against infected liver cells and not to cytopathic effects of the virus. Humoral immune responses can also have pathologic sequelae. For example, antibodies against bacterial M proteins that form in the setting of certain streptococcal infections can bind to cross-reactive cardiac proteins and lead to rheumatic fever (Chapter 11). β-hemolytic streptococcal infections can also induce the formation of streptococcal antigen-antibody complexes; these can deposit in renal glomeruli and lead to poststreptococcal glomerulonephritis (Chapter 14).

Patterns of Inflammatory Responses to Infection

Although infectious microorganisms themselves are wildly diverse, the infected host actually has relatively few ways that it can respond. Thus, at the microscopic level many pathogens evoke similar reaction patterns, rarely with any feature that is pathognomonic for a specific agent. Nevertheless, the different patterns of response do suggest particular classes of causative organisms and an astute observer can make an educated guess about the responsible microbe.

Broadly speaking, there are five histologic patterns of tissue reaction, described next.

Suppurative Inflammation. This pattern is the reaction to acute tissue damage (Chapter 2), characterized by increased vascular permeability and leukocytic exudates, predominantly neutrophils (Fig. 9–7). In many cases, this is a response to *extracellular bacteria*. The neutrophils are typically recruited to the site of infection by chemoattractants released from "pyogenic"organisms and from host cells.

Morphology

Collections of neutrophils may give rise to localized liquefactive necrosis, forming **abscesses.** The necrotic tissue and inflammatory cells constitute **pus,** and bacteria that evoke pus formation are called "pyogenic." Typically, these are extracellular Gram-positive cocci and Gram-negative rods. The sizes of such lesions can vary from tiny microabscesses formed by bacteria seeding from an infected heart valve, to distended, pus-filled fallopian tubes caused by *N. gonorrhoeae,* to diffuse involvement of the meninges during *H. influenzae* infection, to entire lobes of the lung during pneumonia. The extent to which the lesions are destructive depends on their location and the organism involved. Thus, *S. pneumoniae* usually spares alveolar walls in the lung, and even lobar streptococcal pneumonias typically resolve completely without permanent damage (Fig. 9–7). On the other hand, staphylococcal and *Klebsiella* species destroy alveolar walls and form abscesses that heal with scar formation. Bacterial pharyngitis resolves without sequelae, whereas untreated acute bacterial infection of a joint can destroy it in a few days.

Mononuclear and Granulomatous Inflammation. Diffuse mononuclear interstitial infiltrates are a common feature of all chronic inflammatory processes, but when they develop acutely, they often are a response to viruses, intracellular bacteria, or intracellular parasites. In addition, spirochetes and helminths provoke chronic inflammatory responses.

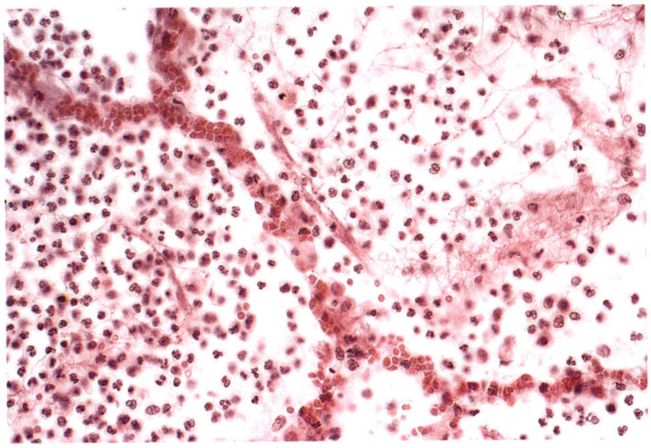

Figure 9–7

Suppurative (polymorphonuclear) inflammation occurring in a pneumococcal pneumonia. Note the intra-alveolar polymorphonuclear exudate and intact alveolar septa.

Morphology

Which mononuclear cell predominates within the inflammatory lesion depends on the host immune response to the organism. Thus, lymphocytes predominate in HBV infection (Fig. 9–8A), whereas plasma cells are common in the primary and secondary lesions of syphilis (Fig. 9–8B). The presence of these lymphocytes reflects cell-mediated immune responses against the pathogen or pathogen-infected cells. **Granulomatous inflammation** is a distinctive form of mononuclear inflammation usually evoked by infectious agents that resist eradication (e.g., *M. tuberculosis, Histoplasma capsulatum,* schistosome eggs) but are nevertheless capable of stimulating strong T cell–mediated immunity. Granulomatous inflammation (Chapter 2) is characterized by accumulation of activated macrophages called "epithelioid" cells, which may fuse to form giant cells. In some cases, there is a central area of caseous necrosis (Fig. 9–8C).

The final common pathway of many infections is chronic inflammation, which can lead to extensive scarring. For example, chronic HBV infection may cause cirrhosis of the liver, in which dense fibrous septae surround nodules of regenerating hepatocytes. Sometimes the exuberant scarring response is the major cause of dysfunction (e.g., the fibrosis of the urinary bladder wall caused by schistosomal eggs, Fig. 9–9) or the constrictive fibrous pericarditis caused by tuberculosis).

Cytopathic-Cytoproliferative Response. These reactions are usually produced by viruses and are characterized by sparse inflammation and either cell death (cytopathic response) or proliferation (cytoproliferative response).

Morphology

Some viruses replicate within cells and make viral aggregates that are visible as inclusion bodies (e.g., CMV, HSV, HBV; see Fig. 9–1) or induce cells to fuse and form polykaryons (e.g., measles, herpesviruses). Focal cell damage may cause epithelial cells to become discohesive and form blisters (e.g., varicella-zoster virus; Fig. 9–10). Viruses can also cause epithelial cells to proliferate and take unusual forms (e.g., venereal warts caused by HPV or the umbilicated papules of molluscum contagiosum caused by poxviruses; Chapter 22). Finally, viruses can cause dysplastic changes and cancers in epithelial cells and lymphocytes (Chapter 6).

Necrotizing Response. Some organisms produce potent toxins that cause such rapid and severe necrosis that tissue damage is the dominant feature (e.g., C. perfringens). Similarly, *E. histolytica* can cause colonic ulcers and liver abscesses with extensive tissue destruction and liquefactive necrosis without a prominent inflammatory infiltrate.

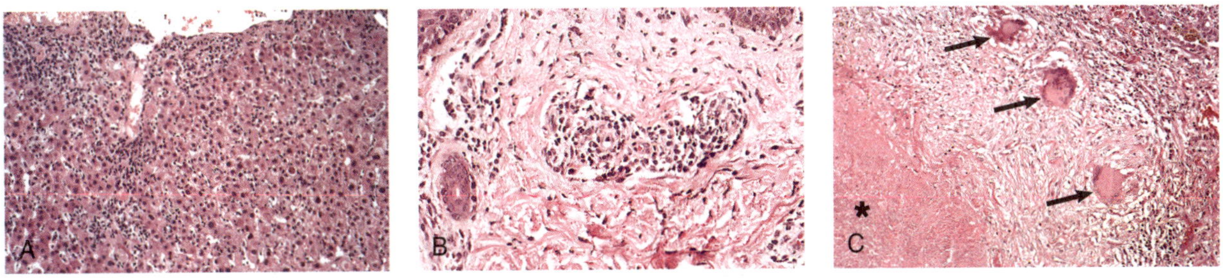

Figure 9–8

Mononuclear and granulomatous inflammation. **A,** Acute viral hepatitis characterized by a predominantly lymphocytic infiltrate. **B,** Secondary syphilis in the dermis with perivascular lymphoplasmacytic infiltrate and endothelial proliferation. **C,** Granulomatous inflammation in response to tuberculosis. Note the zone of caseation *(asterisk),* which normally forms the center of the granuloma, with a surrounding rim of activated epithelioid macrophages, some of which have fused to form giant cells *(arrows);* this, in turn, is surrounded by a zone of activated T lymphocytes. This is a high-magnification view to highlight the histologic features; the granulomatous response typically forms a three-dimensional sphere with the offending organism in the central area.

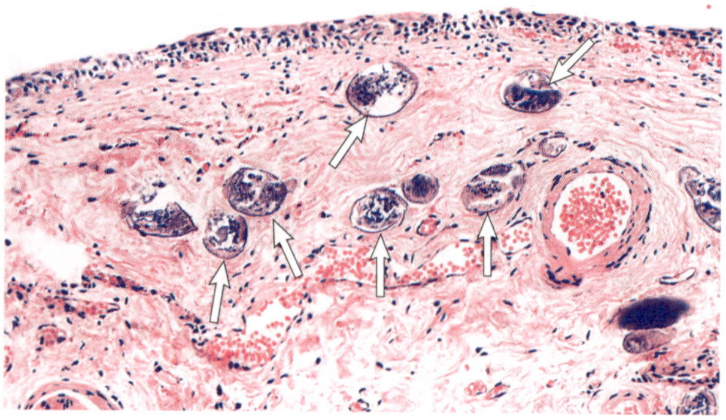

Figure 9–9

Schistosoma haematobium infection of the bladder with numerous calcified eggs *(arrows)* and extensive scarring.

Morphology

Because so few inflammatory cells are involved, these lesions resemble infarcts, with disruption or loss of basophilic nuclear staining and preservation of cellular outlines. Occasionally, by virtue of massive host inflammatory responses, viruses can cause widespread and severe necrosis of host cells, exemplified by total destruction of the temporal lobes of the brain by herpesvirus or the liver by HBV.

Infections in the Immunocompromised Host

Different types of immunodeficiency or immunosuppression affect different cells of the immune system (Chapter 5). The opportunistic infections that an immunocompromised individual contracts depend on the types of immune effector mechanisms that are not functioning. Patients with deficiencies in antibody production and in neutrophils are susceptible to infections with extracellular bacteria and some fungi. In contrast, deficiencies in T-cell–mediated immunity result in increased susceptibility mainly to viruses and intracellular bacteria.

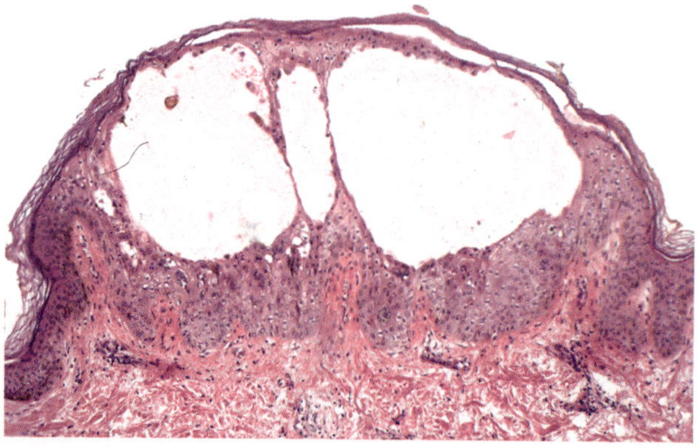

Figure 9–10

Skin lesion of chickenpox (varicella-zoster virus) with intraepithelial vesicle.

Diseases of organ systems other than the immune system can also make patients susceptible to specific microbes. Thus, patients with cystic fibrosis commonly develop respiratory infections with *Burkholderia capacia* (Chapter 13). Burns destroy skin, removing this barrier to microbes and allowing infection with pathogens such as *P. aeruginosa*. Loss of splenic function in individuals with sickle cell disease makes them susceptible to infection with encapsulated bacteria (e.g., *S. pneumoniae*) that are normally opsonized and phagocytosed by splenic macrophages. Finally, malnutrition may impair the immune response.

Morphology

In immunocompromised individuals, the absence of a host inflammatory response frequently eliminates some of the histologic clues about the potential nature of infecting microorganism(s). For example, patients with antibody, complement, or neutrophil defects may have severe local bacterial infections without eliciting any significant neutrophilic infiltrate. In these cases, the causal organism may only be inferred by culture or special stains. Although many viral cytopathic effects (e.g., cell fusion or inclusions, see Fig. 9–1) may still be present, viral infections in immunocompromised hosts may not engender the anticipated mononuclear inflammatory response. Indeed, hepatocytes in HBV "carriers" can have a substantial intracellular viral burden without inflammation—and without hepatocyte death (Chapter 16). Finally, in AIDS patients who have no helper T cells and cannot mount normal cellular responses, organisms that would otherwise cause granulomatous inflammation (e.g., ***M. avium-intracellulare***) present only as sheets of macrophages filled with acid-fast bacilli (Fig. 9–11A). A similar phenomenon occurs in some patients with leprosy; although most individuals have a strong cell-mediated immune response (so that their lesions contain many lymphocytes with few organisms, i.e., **tuberculoid leprosy**), others have a genetic predilection for mounting a weak immune response to these organisms. As a result, patients in the latter group have lesions that contain few lymphocytes with macrophages stuffed with copious organisms (**lepromatous leprosy;** Fig. 9–11B).

SUMMARY

How Microorganisms Cause Disease

- Diseases caused by microbes involve an interplay of microbial virulence and host responses.
  - Infectious agents can directly cause cell death or dysfunction by binding to or by entering host cells.
  - Injury may be due to local or systemic release of bacterial products, including endotoxins (LPS), exotoxins, or superantigens.
  - Pathogens can induce immune responses that cause tissue damage. Absence of an immune response may reduce the damage induced by

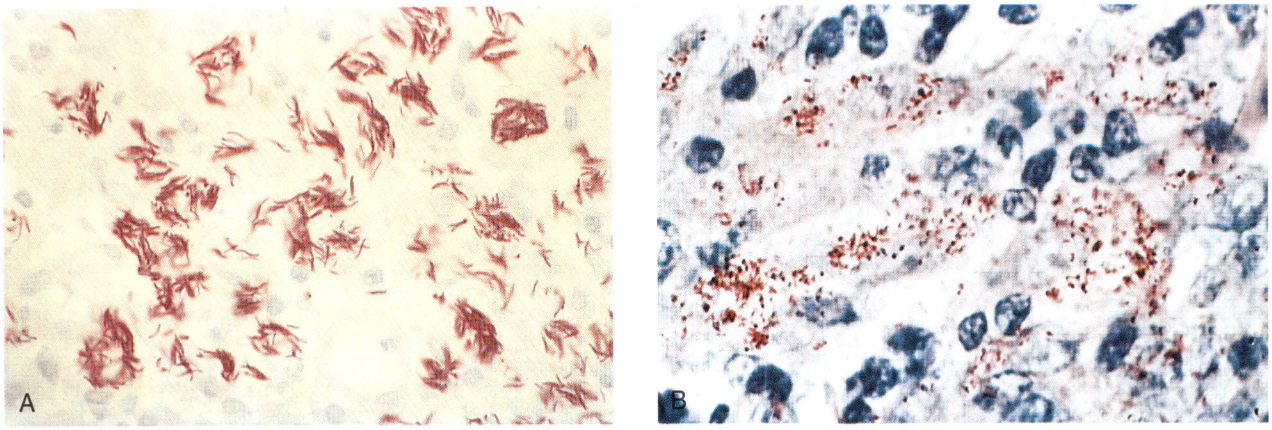

Figure 9–11

Host responses in the absence of appropriate T cell–mediated immunity. In both cases, there is no granulomatous response; the intracellular bacteria persist and even proliferate within macrophages, because either there are inadequate T cells (AIDS) or the T-cell responses do not appropriately activate macrophages to kill the intracellular pathogens (lepromatous leprosy). **A,** *Mycobacterium avium* infection in a patient with AIDS, showing massive intracellular macrophage infection with acid-fast organisms (filamentous and pink in this acid-fast stain). **B,** *M. leprae* infection in a patient with lepromatous leprosy; there are abundant acid-fast bacilli proliferating within macrophages.

some infections; conversely, immunocompromise can allow uncontrolled expansion of opportunistic agents or of microorganisms that can directly cause injury.

- In normal individuals, the patterns of host responses are fairly stereotyped for different classes of microbes; these patterns of responses can be used to infer causal organisms.
  - Neutrophil-rich acute suppurative inflammation is typical of many bacteria ("pyogenic" bacteria) and some fungi.
  - Mononuclear cell infiltrates are common in many chronic infections and some acute viral infections.
  - Granulomatous inflammation is the hallmark of *Mycobacterium tuberculosis* and certain fungi.
  - Cytopathic and proliferative lesions are caused by some viruses.

TECHNIQUES FOR DIAGNOSING INFECTIOUS AGENTS

As discussed above, the histopathology of various infections provides an important clue as to etiology. Moreover, some infectious agents can be directly identified in H+E-stained sections (e.g., CMV or herpesvirus inclusion bodies; bacterial clumps, which usually stain blue; *Candida* and *Mucor* among the fungi; most protozoans; and all helminths). However, many infectious agents are best visualized by special stains that identify organisms on the basis of their cell wall or cell coat characteristics (see Fig. 9–3), including Gram, acid-fast, silver, mucicarmine, and Giemsa stains; microorganisms can also be identified after labeling with specific antibody probes (Table 9–7). Regardless of the staining technique, organisms are usually best visualized at the advancing edge of a lesion rather than at its center, particularly if there is necrosis.

Nucleic acid amplification tests such as polymerase chain reaction (PCR) are now used for diagnosis of gonorrhea, chlamydial infection, tuberculosis, and herpes encephalitis; in many cases, molecular assays are much more sensitive than conventional testing. For example, PCR testing of cerebrospinal fluid for HSV encephalitis has a sensitivity of about 80%, while viral culture has a sensitivity of less than 10%. Similarly, PCR-based methods for detecting genital chlamydia identify 10% to 30% more infections than do conventional cultures. Not only are molecular techniques expanding our diagnostic capabilities, genomic sequencing of many pathogens is permitting ever better understanding of the pathogenesis and therapy of infectious diseases.

Nucleic acid–based tests are also useful for quantifying several pathogens. For example, the management of

Table 9–7 Special Techniques for Diagnosing Infectious Agents

Gram stain	Most bacteria
Acid-fast stain	Mycobacteria, nocardiae (modified)
Silver stains	Fungi, legionellae, pneumocystis
Periodic acid–Schiff	Fungi, amebae
Mucicarmine	Cryptococci
Giemsa	Campylobacteria, leishmaniae, malaria parasites
Antibody probes	Viruses, rickettsiae
Culture	All classes
DNA probes	Viruses, bacteria, protozoa

hepatitis B and C infections is guided by nucleic acid–based viral quantification or typing to predict resistance to antiviral drugs. In patients with HIV, viral RNA load is used routinely to guide antiretroviral therapy.

BIBLIOGRAPHY

Baker MD, Acharya KR: Superantigens: structure-function relationships. Int J Med Microbiol 293:529, 2004. *[Nice, succinct overview.]*

Falkow S: Molecular Koch's postulates applied to bacterial pathogenicity—a personal recollection 15 years later. Nat Rev Microbiol 2:67, 2004. *[A good summary from one of the earliest proponents of applying Koch's postulates to microbial pathogenesis.]*

Gatfield J, Pieters J: Molecular mechanisms of host-pathogen interaction: entry and survival of mycobacteria in macrophages. Adv Immunol 81:45, 2003. *[Review of the molecular and cellular biology of intracellular mycobacterial infections.]*

Glatzel M, et al.: Human prion diseases: molecular and clinical aspects. Arch Neurol 62:545, 2005. *[A thorough review of the nature and pathogenesis of prion-based disease, including current controversies in the field.]*

Hornef MW, et al.: Bacterial strategies for overcoming host innate and adaptive immune responses. Nat Immunol 3:1033, 2002. *[Well-written overview of examples of microbial resistance to host immune responses.]*

Kaufmann SHE, et al.: Immunology of Infectious Diseases. Washington, DC, ASM Press, 2002. *[A thorough and complete text examining the interplay of host immunity and microbial infection.]*

Koplan J: CDC's strategic plan for bioterrorism preparedness and response. Public Health Rep 116 Suppl 2:9, 2001. *[Overview of the CDC approach to bioterrorism.]*

Mims CA: The Pathogenesis of Infectious Disease, 5th ed. San Diego, CA, Academic Press, 2001. *[An extensive text discussing the mechanisms of microbial pathogenesis.]*

Morens DM, et al.: The challenge of emerging and re-emerging infectious diseases. Nature 430:242, 2004. *[Review of emerging infections and the evolutionary properties of pathogenic microorganisms.]*

O'Connor DH, et al.: Pathology of Infectious Diseases. Stamford, CT, Appleton & Lang, 1997. *[A classic; extensive descriptions and illustrations of the histopathology of infectious diseases.]*

Okeke IN, et al.: Antimicrobial resistance in developing countries. Part I: recent trends and current status. Lancet Infect Dis 5:481, 2005. *[An excellent two-part overview of the global problem of microbial resistance and the strategies that must be implemented to combat it.]*

Okeke IN, et al.: Antimicrobial resistance in developing countries. Part II: strategies for containment. Lancet Infect Dis 5:568, 2005.

Peschel A: How do bacteria resist human antimicrobial peptides? Trends Microbiol 10:179, 2002. *[Summary of many innate defenses and strategies used by microbes to overcome them.]*

Rappuoli R: From Pasteur to genomics: progress and challenges in infectious diseases. Nat Med 10:1177, 2004. *[Well-written, largely historical paper looking at our expanding abilities to detect, prevent, and treat infectious disease at the same time that newer, more virulent diseases are emerging.]*

Rotz LD, Hughes JM: Advances in detecting and responding to threats from bioterrorism and emerging infectious disease. Nat Med 10:S130–S136, 2004 *[An overview of the infrastructure underlying global preparedness for emerging infectious diseases.]*

Schoolnik GK: Microarray analysis of bacterial pathogenicity. Adv Microb Physiol 46:1, 2002. *[Exciting review about the potential use of gene array technology in understanding microbial pathogenesis.]*

Stein CE, et al.: The global mortality of infectious and parasitic diseases in children. Semin Pediatr Infect Dis 15: 125, 2004. *[A startling commentary on the effect of potentially treatable infectious diseases in third-world pediatric populations.]*

West SA, et al: Social evolution theory for microorganisms. Nat Rev Microbiol 4:597, 2006. *[A complete and nicely conceptualized review of the mechanisms and consequences of biofilm formation.]*

Yewdell JW, Hill AB: Viral interference with antigen presentation. Nat Immunol 3:1019, 2002. *[Excellent discussion of the mechanisms by which viruses can evade adaptive immunity.]*

Chapter 10

The Blood Vessels*

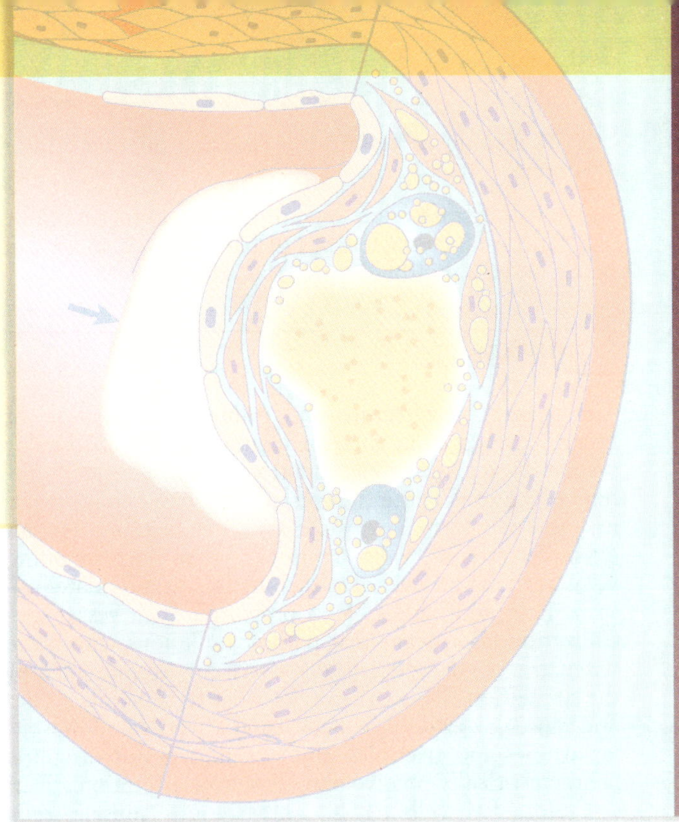

Vascular disease is responsible for more morbidity and mortality than any other category of human disease. Although the most clinically significant lesions involve arteries, venous pathology can also cause clinical disorders. Vascular pathology results in disease via two principal mechanisms:

- *Narrowing* or *complete obstruction* of vessel lumina, either progressively (e.g., by atherosclerosis) or precipitously (e.g., by thrombosis or embolism)

*The contributions of Dr. Frederick Schoen to the previous editions of this chapter are gratefully acknowledged.

- *Weakening* of vessel walls, causing dilation and/or rupture.

We will first describe some of the important anatomic and functional characteristics of blood vessels so we can better understand the diseases that affect them.

NORMAL VESSELS

The general architecture and cellular composition of blood vessels are the same throughout the cardiovascular system. However, distinct functional requirements in different locations within the vasculature (see below) result in multiple forms of vascular specialization. As an example, arterial walls are thicker than corresponding veins at the same level of branching to accommodate pulsatile flow and higher blood pressures. Such vessel specialization also means that pathologic lesions within the vascular tree characteristically affect only certain parts of the circulation. Thus, atherosclerosis affects mainly elastic and muscular arteries, hypertension affects small muscular arteries and arterioles, and specific types of vasculitis characteristically involve only vessels of a certain caliber.

Endothelial cells (ECs) and smooth muscle cells (SMCs) constitute the bulk of vessel wall cellularity; the remainder of the wall is composed of extracellular matrix (ECM) including elastin, collagen, and glycosaminoglycans. Vessel walls are organized into three concentric layers: *intima, media,* and *adventitia* (Fig. 10–1); these are present to some extent in all vessels but are most apparent in larger arteries and veins. In normal arteries, the intima consists of an EC monolayer overlying a thin ECM sheet; the intima is demarcated from the media by a dense elastic membrane called the *internal elastic lamina*. The media is composed predominantly of SMCs and ECM, surrounded by the relatively loose connective tissue, nerve fibers, and smaller vessels of the adventitia; an *external elastic lamina* is present in some arteries and defines the transition between media and adventitia. By virtue of *fenestrations* (holes) in the internal elastic membrane, the innermost medial SMCs receive oxygen and nutrients by direct diffusion from the vessel lumen. However, diffusion from the lumen is inadequate to sustain the SMCs in the outer media in large and medium-sized vessels; in that case, small arterioles within the adventitia (termed *vasa vasorum,* literally "vessels of the vessels") supply the outer 50% to 65% of the media.

Based on size and structural features, *arteries* are divided into three basic types:

- Large, or *elastic arteries,* including the aorta and its large branches (particularly the innominate, subclavian, common carotid, and iliac), and pulmonary arteries. In these arteries, elastic fibers alternate in layers with SMCs. Because of the high content of elastic fibers, the media expands during systole (storing some of the energy of each heartbeat), and elastic recoil of the vascular wall during diastole propels blood through the more distal vessels.
- Medium-sized, or *muscular, arteries,* including smaller branches off the aorta (e.g., coronary and renal arteries). Here, the media is composed primarily of SMCs, with elastin limited to the internal and external elastic lamina. Although arterial wall thickness diminishes with decreasing vessel size, the ratio of wall thickness to lumen diameter actually increases for these vessels.
- Small arteries (≤2 mm in diameter) and *arterioles* (20–100 µm in diameter), which lie within the interstitial connective tissue of organs. The media here is essentially all SMCs. *Arterioles are the principal control points for regulation of physiologic resistance to blood flow; in arterioles, the pressure and velocity of blood flow are both sharply reduced, and flow becomes steady rather than pulsatile.* The modulation of regional blood flow and blood pressure are accomplished by changes in lumen size through SMC contraction (*vasoconstriction*) or relaxation (*vasodilation*). Because the resistance to fluid flow in a tube is inversely proportional to the fourth power of the diameter (i.e., halving the diameter increases resistance 16-fold), small changes in arteriolar lumen size have profound flow-limiting effects.

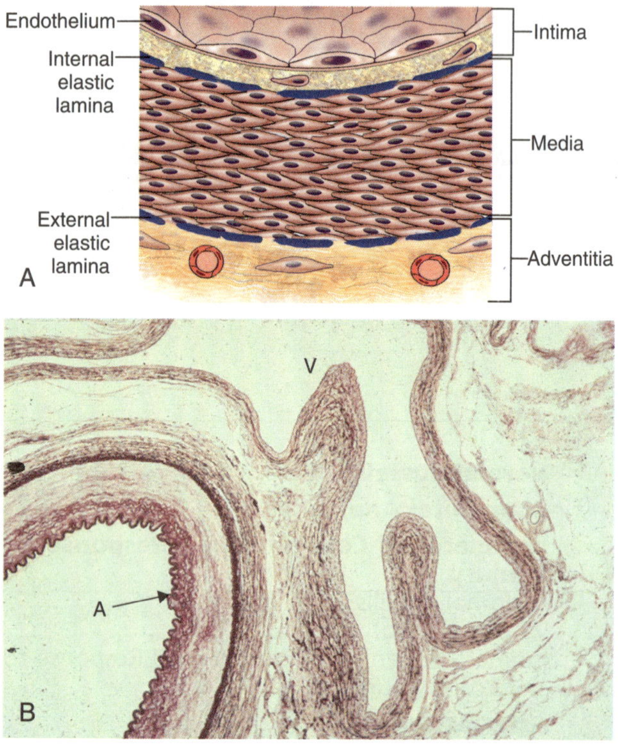

Figure 10–1

The vascular wall. **A,** Cross-section from a muscular artery (e.g., coronary artery). **B,** Histology showing an artery (A) and adjacent vein (V), with the elastic lamellae stained black (the *arrow* points to the arterial internal elastic lamina). Because it must sustain higher pressures, the artery has a thicker wall with more-organized elastin architecture than in the corresponding vein. Conversely, the vein has a larger lumen with diffusely distributed elastin, permitting greater capacitance. (**B,** Courtesy of Dr. Mark Flomenbaum, Office of the Chief Medical Examiner, Boston, Massachusetts.)

Capillaries represent the next level of vascular branching after arterioles. These are approximately the diameter of a red blood cell (7–8 μm) and have an endothelial cell lining but no media. Collectively, capillaries have a very large total cross-sectional area, and with thin walls (only one cell thick) and slow flow, they are ideally suited for the rapid exchange of diffusible substances between blood and tissue. Normal tissue function depends on adequate supplies of oxygen and nutrients, and since diffusion of these components is not efficient beyond 100 μm, the capillary network of most tissues is very rich; metabolically active tissues (e.g., heart) have the highest capillary density.

Blood flows from capillary beds into postcapillary venules and then sequentially through collecting venules to progressively larger veins. In the setting of inflammation, vascular leakage and leukocyte emigration occur preferentially in postcapillary venules (Chapter 2). Relative to corresponding arteries, veins have larger diameters, larger lumina, and thinner, less well-organized walls (Fig. 10–1B). Thus, veins are more prone to dilation, compression, and easy penetration by tumors and inflammatory processes. Venous pressure and flow velocities are very low; thus, where venous blood has to flow against gravity (e.g., leg veins), reversed flow is prevented by valves. Collectively, the venous system has a huge capacitance, containing approximately two-thirds of all systemic blood.

Lymphatics are thin-walled, endothelium-lined channels that drain excess interstitial tissue fluid (Chapter 2), eventually returning it to blood via the thoracic duct. Lymphatic flow also contains mononuclear inflammatory cells and a host of proteins; by passing through lymph nodes, lymphatics constitute an important pathway for continuous sampling of peripheral tissues for infection. *These channels can also disseminate disease by transporting microbes or tumor cells from distant sites to lymph nodes and eventually to the systemic circulation.*

CONGENITAL ANOMALIES

Although rarely symptomatic, variants of the usual anatomic pattern of vascular supply can become important during surgery when a vessel in an unexpected location is injured. Among the congenital vascular anomalies, three are particularly significant, though not necessarily common:

- *Developmental,* or *berry, aneurysms* occur in cerebral vessels. These are small, spherical dilatations typically in the circle of Willis; when ruptured, they can causes fatal intracerebral hemorrhage. They are discussed in greater detail in Chapter 23.

- *Arteriovenous fistulas* are abnormal, typically small, direct connections between arteries and veins that bypass the intervening capillaries. They occur most commonly as developmental defects but can also result from rupture of an arterial aneurysm into the adjacent vein, from penetrating injuries that pierce arteries and veins, or from inflammatory necrosis of adjacent vessels; intentionally created arteriovenous fistulas are used to provide vascular access for chronic hemodialysis. When arteriovenous fistulas are large or extensive, they can become clinically significant by shunting blood from the arterial to the venous circulations. This forces the heart to pump additional volume, and high-output cardiac failure can ensue.

- *Fibromuscular dysplasia* is a focal irregular thickening of the walls of medium and large muscular arteries, including renal, carotid, splanchnic, and vertebral vessels. The cause is unknown but is probably developmental. Segments of the vessel wall are focally thickened by some combination of irregular medial and intimal hyperplasia and fibrosis; this results in luminal stenosis and, in the renal arteries, may be a cause of renovascular hypertension (Chapter 14).

VASCULAR WALL CELLS AND THEIR RESPONSE TO INJURY

As the main cellular components of the blood vessel walls, ECs and SMCs play central roles in vascular biology and pathology. The integrated function of these cells is critical for vasculature to adapt to hemodynamic and biochemical stimuli.

Endothelial Cells

ECs form a single-cell-thick continuous sheet (the *endothelium*) that lines the entire vascular system and is critical for maintaining vessel wall homeostasis and circulatory function. ECs contain *Weibel-Palade bodies,* intracellular membrane-bound storage organelles for von Willebrand factor. Antibodies to von Willebrand factor and/or platelet–endothelial cell adhesion molecule 1 (PECAM-1 or CD31, a protein localized to interendothelial junctions) can be used to identify ECs immunohistochemically.

Vascular endothelium is a multifunctional tissue with a wealth of synthetic and metabolic properties; at baseline it has a number of constitutive activities critical for normal vessel homeostasis (Table 10–1). Thus, ECs maintain a nonthrombogenic blood-tissue interface (until clotting is necessitated by local injury, Chapter 4), modulate vascular resistance, metabolize hormones, regulate inflammation, and affect the growth of other cell types, particularly SMCs. As a selectively permeable monolayer, endothelium controls the transfer of small and large molecules into the vascular wall and beyond. In most regions, the interendothelial junctions are essentially impermeable. However, tight EC junctions can loosen under the influence of hemodynamic factors (e.g., high blood pressure) and/or vasoactive agents (e.g., histamine in inflammation), resulting in the flooding of adjacent tissues by electrolytes and protein; in inflammatory states, even leukocytes can slip between adjacent ECs (Chapter 2).

Although ECs share many general attributes, there is also substantial phenotypic variability depending on anatomic site and dynamic adaptation to local environmental cues. For example, endothelia lining hepatocyte cords or in renal glomeruli are fenestrated (i.e., they have holes), while endothelium (and associated perivascular cells) in the central nervous system create a very impermeable blood-brain barrier.

Table 10–1 Endothelial Cell Properties and Functions

Maintenance of Permeability Barrier
Elaboration of Anticoagulant, Antithrombotic, Fibrinolytic Regulators
Prostacyclin Thrombomodulin Heparin-like molecules Plasminogen activator
Elaboration of Prothrombotic Molecules
Von Willebrand factor Tissue factor Plasminogen activator inhibitor
Extracellular Matrix Production (Collagen, Proteoglycans)
Modulation of Blood Flow and Vascular Reactivity
Vasconstrictors: endothelin, ACE Vasodilators: NO, prostacyclin
Regulation of Inflammation and Immunity
IL-1, IL-6, chemokines Adhesion molecules: VCAM-1, ICAM, E-selectin P-selectin Histocompatibility antigens
Regulation of Cell Growth
Growth stimulators: PDGF, CSF, FGF Growth inhibitors: heparin, TGF-β
Oxidation of LDL

ACE, angiotensin-converting enzyme; CSF, colony-stimulating factor; FGF, fibroblast growth factor; ICAM, intercelluar adhesion molecule; IL, interleukin; LDL, low-density lipoprotein; NO, nitric oxide; PDGF, platelet-derived growth factor; TGF-β, transforming growth factor-β; VCAM, vascular cell adhesion molecule.

Endothelial injury contributes to a host of pathologies including thrombosis, atherosclerosis, and hypertensive vascular lesions. For example, EC denudation stimulates clotting (Chapter 4) and eventually SMC proliferation (see later). However, structurally intact ECs can also respond to various stimuli by modulating their constitutive activities and expressing new (induced) properties (e.g., increased adhesion and prothrombotic molecules, growth factors, and other products). *Endothelial dysfunction* is the term used to describe such reversible changes in the repertoire of ECs. It can be induced by hemodynamic stresses and lipid metabolites (contributing to the pathogenesis of atherosclerosis, see below) as well as by cytokines and bacterial products (contributing to the pathogenesis of septic shock; Chapter 4). Some changes are rapid (within minutes), reversible, and independent of new protein synthesis (e.g., EC contraction induced by histamine, causing venular gaps; Chapter 2). Other changes require new gene expression and protein synthesis and may take hours to days to manifest themselves. The consequences of endothelial dysfunction include impaired endothelium-dependent vasodilation, hypercoagulable states (Chapter 4), and leukocyte adhesion.

Vascular Smooth Muscle Cells

SMCs participate in both normal vascular repair and pathologic processes such as atherosclerosis. As stable cells, SMCs have the capacity to proliferate when appropriately stimulated; they can also synthesize ECM collagen, elastin, and proteoglycans and elaborate growth factors and cytokines. As the predominant cellular element of the vascular media, SMCs are also responsible for the vasoconstriction or dilation that occurs in response to physiologic or pharmacologic stimuli.

Intimal Thickening: A Stereotyped Response to Vascular Injury

Vascular injury—with EC loss or even merely dysfunction—stimulates SMC growth and associated matrix synthesis. Healing in injured vessels is very much analogous to the physiologic healing process that occurs in any damaged tissue composed of stable cell elements (Chapter 3). Following endothelial injury SMCs or SMC precursor cells migrate into the intima, proliferate, and synthesize ECM in much the same way that fibroblasts fill in a wound forming a neointima (Fig. 10–2). This neointimal response occurs with any form of vascular damage or dysfunction, including infection, inflammation, immune injury, physical trauma (e.g., balloon catheter or hypertension), or toxic exposure (e.g. oxidized lipids or cigarette smoke). Thus, intimal thickening is essentially the stereotyped response of the vessel wall to *any* insult.

It should be emphasized that the phenotype of neointimal SMCs is distinct from medial SMCs; neointimal SMCs cannot contract as can medial SMCs, but they do have the capacity to divide. Concurrently, there are decreased contractile filaments, while organelles involved in protein synthesis, such as rough endoplasmic reticulum and Golgi apparatus, increase.

With time and restoration and/or normalization of the endothelial layer, the intimal SMCs can return to a nonproliferative state. However, by that point, the stereotyped healing response has already resulted in intimal thickening that may be permanent. With persistent or recurrent insults, excessive thickening can cause stenosis of small and medium-sized blood vessels (e.g., atherosclerosis, see below) that impedes downstream tissue perfusion.

SUMMARY

Response of Vascular Wall Cells to Injury

- Injury (of almost any type) to the vessel wall results in a stereotypic healing response, involving intimal expansion by proliferating SMCs and newly synthesized ECM.
- The recruitment and activation of the SMCs in this process involves signals from cells (e.g., ECs, platelets, and macrophages), as well as mediators derived from coagulation and complement cascades.
- Excessive thickening of the intima can result in luminal stenosis that blocks vascular flow.

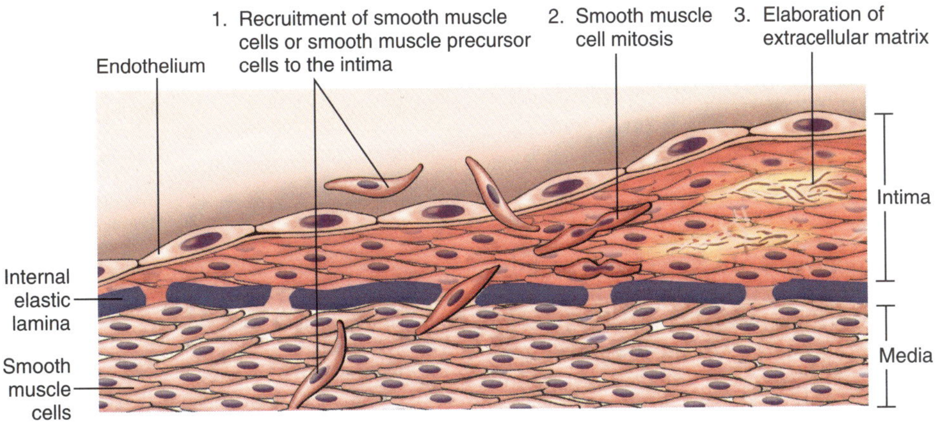

Figure 10–2

Stereotypic response to vascular injury: Intimal thickening, with smooth muscle cell (SMC) migration and proliferation within the intima, and associated ECM synthesis. Intimal SMCs may derive from the underlying media or may be recruited from circulating precursors; their color is different from the medial cells to emphasize that they have a proliferative, synthetic, and noncontractile phenotype distinct from medial SMCs. (Modified and redrawn from Schoen FJ: Interventional and Surgical Cardiovascular Pathology: Clinical Correlations and Basic Principles. Philadelphia, WB Saunders, 1989, p 254.)

ARTERIOSCLEROSIS

Arteriosclerosis literally means "hardening of the arteries"; it is a generic term reflecting arterial wall thickening and loss of elasticity. Three patterns are recognized, with different clinical and pathologic consequences:

- *Arteriolosclerosis* affects small arteries and arterioles. The two anatomic variants, hyaline and hyperplastic, are both associated with vessel wall thickening and luminal narrowing that may cause downstream ischemic injury. Arteriolosclerosis is most often associated with hypertension and/or diabetes mellitus and will be discussed in detail later in the section on hypertension.
- *Mönckeberg medial calcific sclerosis* is characterized by calcific deposits in muscular arteries, typically in persons older than age 50. The radiographically visible, often palpable calcifications, do not encroach on the vessel lumen and are usually not clinically significant.
- *Atherosclerosis*, from Greek root words for "gruel" and "hardening," is the most frequent and clinically important pattern (see below).

ATHEROSCLEROSIS

Atherosclerosis is characterized by intimal lesions called *atheromas* (also called *atheromatous* or *atherosclerotic plaques*), that protrude into vascular lumina. An atheromatous plaque consists of a raised lesion with a soft, yellow, grumous core of lipid (mainly cholesterol and cholesterol esters) covered by a firm, white fibrous cap (Fig. 10–3). Besides obstructing blood flow, atherosclerotic plaques weaken the underlying media and can themselves rupture, causing acute catastrophic vessel thrombosis. Atherosclerosis overwhelmingly causes more morbidity and mortality (roughly half of all deaths) in the Western world than any other disorder. Because coronary artery disease is an important manifestation of the disease, epidemiologic data related to atherosclerosis

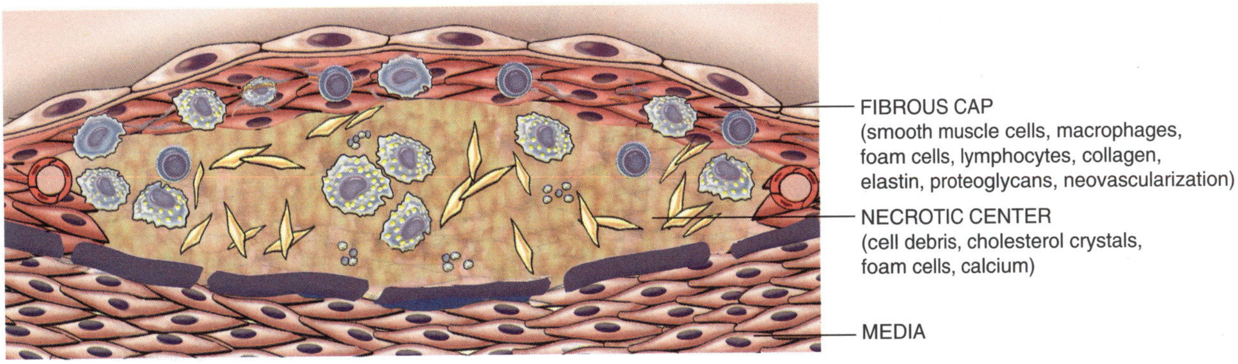

Figure 10–3

The major components of a well-developed intimal atheromatous plaque overlying an intact media.

mortality typically reflect deaths caused by ischemic heart disease (IHD) (Chapter 11); indeed, myocardial infarction is responsible for almost a quarter of all deaths in the United States. Not to be minimized, carotid atherosclerotic disease and stroke are also associated with significant morbidity and mortality (Chapter 23).

Epidemiology

Virtually ubiquitous among most developed nations, atherosclerosis is much less prevalent in Central and South America, Africa, and Asia. The mortality rate for IHD in the United States is among the highest in the world and is approximately five times higher than that in Japan. Nevertheless, IHD has been increasing in Japan and is now the second leading cause of death there. Moreover, Japanese who immigrate to the United States and adopt American lifestyles and dietary customs acquire the same predisposition to atherosclerosis as the homegrown population.

The prevalence and severity of atherosclerosis and IHD among individuals and groups are related to several risk factors, some constitutional (and therefore less controllable) but others acquired or related to behaviors and potentially amenable to manipulation (Table 10–2). Risk factors have been identified through a number of prospective studies in well-defined populations, most notably the Framingham (Massachusetts) Heart Study and Atherosclerosis Risk in Communities (Fig. 10–4). *Multiple risk factors have a multiplicative effect;* two risk factors increase the risk approximately fourfold. When three risk factors are present (e.g., hyperlipidemia, hypertension, and smoking), the rate of myocardial infarction is increased seven times.

Table 10–2 Risk Factors for Atherosclerosis

Major Risks	Lesser, Uncertain, or Nonquantitated Risks
Nonmodifiable	Obsesity
Increasing age	Physical inactivity
Male gender	Stress ("type A personality)
Family history	Postmenopausal estrogen deficiency
Genetic abnormalities	High carbohydrate intake
	Lipoprotein(a)
Potentially Controllable	Hardened (trans)unsaturated fat intake
Hyperlipidemia	*Chlamydia pneumoniae infection*
Hypertension	
Cigarette smoking	
Diabetes	
C-reactive protein	

Major Constitutional Risk Factors for IHD

Age. Age is a dominant influence. Although the accumulation of atherosclerotic plaque is typically a progressive process, it does not usually become clinically manifest until lesions reach a critical threshold and begin to precipitate organ injury in middle age or later. Thus, between ages 40 and 60, the incidence of myocardial infarction in men increases fivefold, even though the underlying arterial lesions were probably evolving before that. Death rates from IHD rise with each decade even into advanced age.

Gender. Other factors being equal, premenopausal women are relatively protected against atherosclerosis and its consequences compared with age-matched men. Thus, myocardial infarction and other complications of atherosclerosis are uncommon in premenopausal women unless they are otherwise predisposed by diabetes, hyperlipidemia, or severe hypertension. After menopause, however, the incidence of atherosclerosis-related diseases increases and with greater age eventually exceeds that of men. Although a favorable influence of estrogen has long been proposed to explain this effect, several clinical trials have failed to demonstrate any utility of hormonal therapy for vascular disease prevention in either sex; indeed, postmenopausal estrogen replacement probably

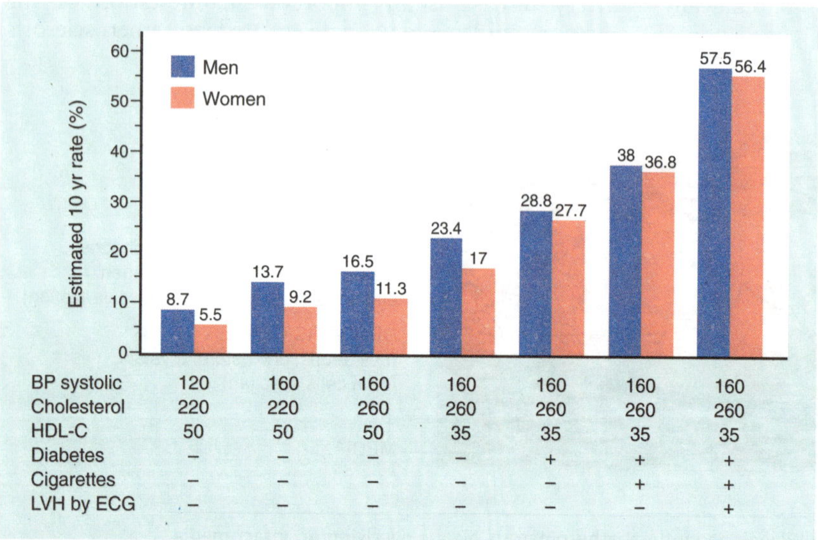

Figure 10–4

Estimated 10-year risk of coronary artery disease in hypothetical 55-year-old men and women as a function of traditional risk factors (hyperlipidemia, hypertension, smoking, and diabetes). BP, blood pressure; ECG, electrocardiogram; HDL-C, high-density lipoprotein cholesterol; LVH, left ventricular hypertrophy. (Adapted from O'Donnell CJ, Kannel WB: Cardiovascular risks of hypertension: lessons from observational studies. J Hypertension 16 (Suppl 6):3, 1998, with permission from Lippincott Williams & Wilkins.)

is associated with *increased* cardiovascular risk and is no longer recommended for preventing heart disease in women. Aside from atherosclerosis, gender also affects a number of parameters that can affect outcomes of IHD; thus, women show differences in hemostasis, infarct healing, and myocardium remodeling.

Genetics. The well-established familial predisposition to atherosclerosis and IHD is multifactorial. In some instances it relates to familial clustering of other risk factors, such as hypertension or diabetes, whereas in others it involves well-defined genetic derangements in lipoprotein metabolism, such as familial hypercholesterolemia (Chapter 7), that result in excessively high blood lipid levels.

Major Modifiable Risk Factors for IHD

Hyperlipidemia. *Hyperlipidemia*—more specifically, *hypercholesterolemia*—is a major risk factor for atherosclerosis; even in the absence of other risk factors, hyercholesterolemia is sufficient to stimulate lesion development. The major component of serum cholesterol associated with increased risk is low-density lipoprotein (LDL) cholesterol ("bad cholesterol"); LDL cholesterol has an essential physiologic role delivering cholesterol to peripheral tissues. In contrast, high-density lipoprotein (HDL, "good cholesterol") mobilizes cholesterol from developing and existing atheromas and transports it to the liver for excretion in the bile. Consequently, higher levels of HDL correlate with reduced risk.

Understandably, dietary and pharmacologic approaches that lower LDL or total serum cholesterol, and/or raise serum HDL are all of considerable interest. High dietary intake of cholesterol and saturated fats (present in egg yolks, animal fats, and butter, for example) raises plasma cholesterol levels. Conversely, diets low in cholesterol and/or with higher ratios of polyunsaturated fats lower plasma cholesterol levels. Omega-3 fatty acids (abundant in fish oils) are beneficial, whereas (*trans*)unsaturated fats produced by artificial hydrogenation of polyunsaturated oils (used in baked goods and margarine) adversely affect cholesterol profiles. Exercise and moderate consumption of ethanol both raise HDL levels, whereas obesity and smoking lower it. *Statins* are a class of drugs that lower circulating cholesterol levels by inhibiting hydroxymethylglutaryl coenzyme A reductase, the rate-limiting enzyme in hepatic cholesterol biosynthesis.

Hypertension. *Hypertension* (see below) is another major risk factor for atherosclerosis; both systolic and diastolic levels are important. On its own, hypertension can increase the risk of IHD by approximately 60% in comparison with normotensive populations (Fig. 10–4). Left untreated, roughly half of hypertensive patients will die of IHD or congestive heart failure, and another third will die of stroke. Left ventricular hypertrophy in many cases probably represents a marker of long-standing functional hypertension (see Fig. 10–4).

Cigarette Smoking. *Cigarette smoking* is a well-established risk factor in men, and an increase in the number of women who smoke probably accounts for the increasing incidence and severity of atherosclerosis in women. Prolonged (years) smoking of one pack of cigarettes or more daily increases the death rate from IHD by 200%. Smoking cessation reduces that risk substantially.

Diabetes Mellitus. *Diabetes mellitus* induces hypercholesterolemia (see Chapter 20) as well as a markedly increased predisposition to atherosclerosis. Other factors being equal, the incidence of myocardial infarction is twice as high in diabetic as in nondiabetic individuals. There is also an increased risk of strokes and a 100-fold increased risk of atherosclerosis-induced gangrene of the lower extremities.

Additional Risk Factors for IHD

Despite the identification of hypertension, diabetes, smoking, and hyperlipidemia as major risk factors, as many as 20% of all cardiovascular events occur in the absence of any of these. Indeed, even though hyperlipidemia is clearly contributory, more than 75% of cardiovascular events in previously healthy women occurred with LDL cholesterol levels below 160 mg/dL (a cutoff generally considered to connote low risk). Clearly, other "nontraditional" factors contribute to risk; the assessment of some of these has already entered clinical practice.

Inflammation as marked by C-reactive protein. Inflammation is present during all stages of atherogenesis and is intimately linked with atherosclerotic plaque formation and rupture (see below). With the increasing recognition that inflammation does play a significant causal role in IHD, assessing systemic inflammatory status has become important in overall risk stratification. While a number of systemic markers of inflammation correlate with IHD risk (e.g., interleukin-6 [IL-6], soluble intercellular adhesion molecule-1, CD40 ligand, etc.), C-reactive protein (CRP) has emerged as one of the cheapest and most sensitive.

CRP is an acute-phase reactant synthesized primarily by the liver. It is downstream of a number of inflammatory triggers and plays a major role in the innate immune response by opsonizing bacteria and activating complement (Chapter 5); when locally synthesized within atherosclerotic intima, it can also regulate local endothelial adhesion and thrombotic states. Most importantly, it strongly *and independently* predicts the risk of myocardial infarction, stroke, peripheral arterial disease, and sudden cardiac death, even among apparently healthy individuals (Fig. 10–5). Interestingly, although there is no direct evidence that lowering CRP reduces cardiovascular risk, smoking cessation, weight loss, and exercise all reduce CRP; moreover, statins reduce CRP levels largely independent of their effects on LDL cholesterol.

Hyperhomocystinemia. Clinical and epidemiologic studies show a strong relationship between total serum homocysteine levels and coronary artery disease, peripheral vascular disease, stroke, and venous thrombosis. Elevated homocysteine levels can be caused by low folate and vitamin B intake, although the jury is still out on whether supplemental folate and vitamin B_6 ingestion can reduce the incidence of cardiovascular disease. *Homocystinuria*, due to rare inborn errors of metabolism,

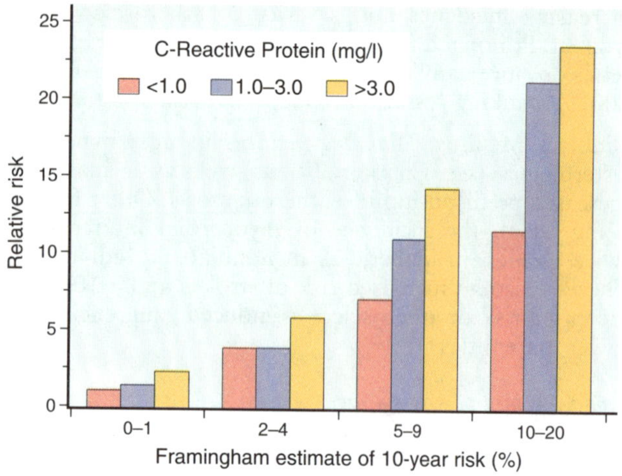

Figure 10–5

CRP adds prognostic information at all levels of traditional risk identified from the Framingham Heart Study. Relative risk (y-axis) refers to the risk of a cardiovascular event (e.g. myocardial infarction). The x-axis is the 10 year risk of a cardiovascular event derived from the traditional risk factor identified in the Framingham study. In each group of Framingham risk, CRP values further stratify the patients. For example, if a patient in the high-risk strata has low CRP (<1.0), his likelihood of developing a cardiovascular event is actually *less* than a patient in the lower risk group with high CRP (>3.0). (Adapted from Ridker PM, et al.: Comparison of C-reactive protein and low-density lipoprotein cholesterol levels in the prediction of first cardiovascular events. N Engl J Med 347:1557–1565, 2002. Copyright © 2002 Massachusetts Medical Society. All rights reserved.)

results in elevated levels of circulating homocysteine (>100 μmol/L) and premature vascular disease.

Lipoprotein a. *Lipoprotein a,* or *Lp(a),* is an altered form of LDL that contains the apolipoprotein B-100 portion of LDL linked to apolipoprotein A; increased Lp(a) levels are associated with a higher risk of coronary and cerebrovascular disease, independent of total cholesterol or LDL levels.

Factors Affecting Hemostasis. Several markers of hemostatic and/or fibrinolytic function (e.g., elevated plasminogen activator inhibitor 1) are strong predictors of risk for major atherosclerotic events, including myocardial infarction and stroke. The increased risk of ischemic heart disease resulting from use of selective cyclooxygenase 2 (COX-2) inhibitors is believed to be due to suppression of endothlium-derived prostacyclin without an inhibition of platelet-derived thromboxane A2, thus creating a prothrombotic state.

Other Factors. Factors associated with a less pronounced and/or difficult-to-quantitate risk include lack of exercise; competitive, stressful lifestyle ("type A" personality); and obesity (the latter due to hypertension, diabetes, hypertriglyceridemia, and decreased HDL).

Pathogenesis

The overwhelming clinical importance of atherosclerosis has stimulated enormous efforts to understand its cause. The contemporary view of atherogenesis is expressed by the *response-to-injury hypothesis.* This model views *atherosclerosis as a chronic inflammatory response of the arterial wall to endothelial injury. Lesion progression occurs through interactions of modified lipoproteins, monocyte-derived macrophages, T lymphocytes, and the normal cellular constituents of the arterial wall* (Fig. 10–6). The following are central tenets of the hypothesis:

- *Chronic endothelial injury,* with resultant endothelial dysfunction, causing (among other things) increased permeability, leukocyte adhesion, and thrombosis
- *Accumulation of lipoproteins* (mainly LDL and its oxidized forms) in the vessel wall
- *Monocyte adhesion to the endothelium,* followed by migration into the intima and transformation into *macrophages* and *foam cells*
- *Platelet adhesion*
- *Factor release* from activated platelets, macrophages, and vascular wall cells, inducing *SMC recruitment,* either from the media or from circulating precursors
- *SMC proliferation and ECM production*
- *Lipid accumulation* both extracellularly and within cells (macrophages and SMCs)

The accumulation of lipid-containing macrophages in the initima gives rise to "fatty streaks" (Fig. 10–6, step 4). With further evolution, a fibrofatty atheroma (Fig. 10–6, step 5) consisting of proliferated SMC, foam cells, extracellular lipid, and ECM is formed. Several aspects of atherogenesis will now be considered in detail.

Endothelial Injury

Chronic or repetitive endothelial injury is the cornerstone of the response-to-injury hypothesis. Endothelial loss due to *any* kind of injury—whether induced experimentally by mechanical denudation, hemodynamic forces, immune complex deposition, irradiation, or chemicals—results in intimal thickening; in the presence of high-lipid diets, typical atheromas ensue. However, *early human lesions begin at sites of morphologically intact endothelium.* Thus, non-denuding *endothelial dysfunction* underlies human atherosclerosis; in the setting of intact but dysfunctional ECs there is increased endothelial permeability, enhanced leukocyte adhesion, and altered gene expression.

The specific causes of endothelial dysfunction in early atherosclerosis are not completely understood. Etiologic culprits include toxins from cigarette smoke, homocysteine, and even infectious agents. Inflammatory cytokines (e.g., tumor necrosis factor, or TNF) can also stimulate the expression of pro-atherogenic genes in EC. Nevertheless, the two most important causes of endothelial dysfunction are hemodynamic disturbances and hypercholesterolemia. Inflammation is also an important contributor.

Hemodynamic Disturbance. The importance of hemodynamic turbulence in atherogenesis is illustrated by the observation that plaques tend to occur at ostia of exiting vessels, branch points, and along the posterior wall of the abdominal aorta, where there are disturbed flow patterns. In vitro studies further demonstrate that nonturbulent laminar flow in other parts of the normal vasculature

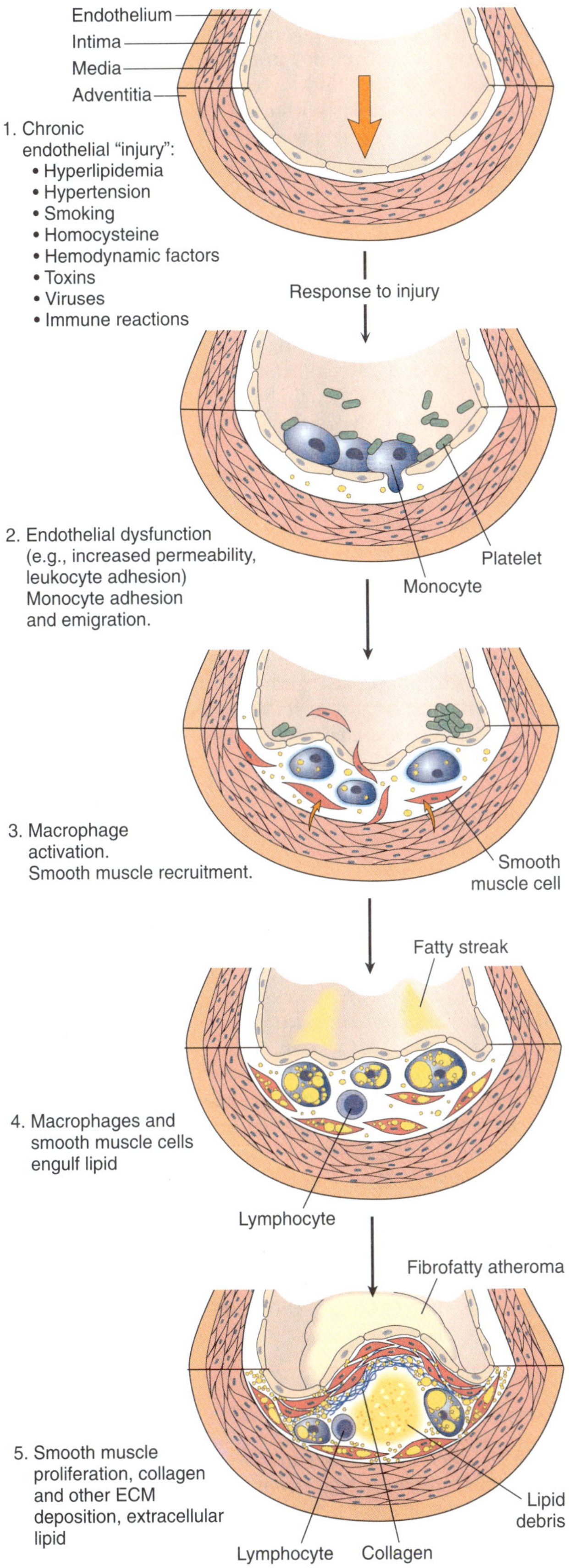

Figure 10–6

Evolution of arterial wall changes in the response to injury hypothesis. ***1,*** Normal. ***2,*** Endothelial injury with adhesion of monocytes and platelets (the latter to sites where endothelium has been lost). ***3,*** Migration of monocytes and SMCs into the intima. ***4,*** SMC proliferation in the intima with ECM elaboration. ***5,*** Well-developed plaque.

leads to the induction of endothelial genes whose products (e.g., the antioxidant superoxide dismutase) actually *protect* against atherosclerosis. Such "atheroprotective" genes could explain the nonrandom localization of early atherosclerotic lesions.

Lipids. Lipids are typically transported in the bloodstream bound to specific apoproteins (forming lipoprotein complexes). *Dyslipoproteinemias* can result from mutations that encode defective apoproteins or alter the lipoprotein receptors on cells, or from some other underlying disorder that affects the circulating levels of lipids (e.g., nephrotic syndrome, alcoholism, hypothyroidism, or diabetes mellitus). Common lipoprotein abnormalities in the general population (indeed, present in many survivors of myocardial infarction) include (1) increased LDL cholesterol levels, (2) decreased HDL cholesterol levels, and (3) increased levels of the abnormal Lp(a) (see earlier).

The evidence implicating hypercholesterolemia in atherogenesis includes the following observations:

- The dominant lipids in atheromatous plaques are cholesterol and cholesterol esters.
- Genetic defects in lipoprotein uptake and metabolism that cause hyperlipoproteinemia are associated with accelerated atherosclerosis. Thus, homozygous familial hypercholesterolemia, caused by defective LDL receptors and inadequate hepatic LDL uptake (Chapter 7), can lead to myocardial infarction before the age of 20 years. Similarly, accelerated atherosclerosis occurs in animal models with engineered deficiencies in apolipoproteins or LDL receptors.
- Other genetic or acquired disorders (e.g., diabetes mellitus, hypothyroidism) that cause hypercholesterolemia lead to premature atherosclerosis.
- Epidemiologic studies demonstrate a significant correlation between the severity of atherosclerosis and the levels of total plasma cholesterol or LDL.
- Lowering serum cholesterol by diet or drugs slows the rate of progression of atherosclerosis, causes regression of some plaques, and reduces the risk of cardiovascular events.

The mechanisms by which hyperlipidemia contributes to atherogenesis include the following:

- Chronic hyperlipidemia, particularly hypercholesterolemia, can directly impair EC function by increasing local production of reactive oxygen species. Among other effects, oxygen free radicals accelerate nitric oxide decay, damping its vasodilator activity and thereby increasing local shear stress.

- With chronic hyperlipidemia, lipoproteins accumulate within the intima. These lipids are *oxidized* through the action of oxygen free radicals locally generated by macrophages or ECs. Oxidized LDL is ingested by macrophages through a *scavenger receptor,* distinct from the LDL receptor (Chapter 7), resulting in foam-cell formation. In addition, oxidized LDL stimulates the release of growth factors, cytokines, and chemokines by ECs and macrophages that increase monocyte recruitment into lesions. Finally, oxidized LDL is cytotoxic to ECs and SMCs and can induce EC dysfunction.
- The importance of oxidized LDL in atherogenesis is suggested by its accumulation within macrophages at all stages of plaque formation. Moreover, antioxidant therapy (β-carotene and vitamin E) protects against atherosclerosis in animal models, but it does not appear to be effective for preventing IHD.

Inflammation. Inflammatory cells and mediators are involved in the initiation, progression, and the complications of atherosclerotic lesions. Although normal vessels do not bind inflammatory cells, early in atherogenesis dysfunctional arterial ECs express adhesion molecules that encourage leukocyte adhesion; vascular cell adhesion molecule 1 (VCAM-1) in particular binds monocytes and T cells. After these cells adhere to the endothelium, they migrate into the intima under the influence of locally produced chemokines.

- Monocytes transform into macrophages and avidly engulf lipoproteins, including oxidized LDL. Monocyte recruitment and differentiation into macrophages (and ultimately into foam cells) is theoretically protective, since these cells remove potentially harmful lipid particles. Over time, however, progressive accumulation of oxidized LDL drives lesion progression. Thus, macrophage activation (via oxidized LDL or T cells, see below) results in cytokine production (e.g., TNF) that further increases leukocyte adhesion and chemokine production that in turn propel mononuclear inflammatory cell recruitment. Activated macrophages also produce reactive oxygen species, aggravating LDL oxidation.
- T lymphocytes recruited to the intima interact with macrophages and can generate a chronic immune inflammatory state. It is not clear whether the T cells are responding to specific antigens (e.g., bacterial or viral antigens, heat-shock proteins [see below], or modified arterial wall constituents and lipoproteins) or are nonspecifically activated by the local inflammatory milieu. Nevertheless, activated T cells in the growing intimal lesions elaborate inflammatory cytokines, (e.g., interferon-γ), which in turn can stimulate macrophages as well as ECs and SMCs.
- As a consequence of the chronic inflammatory state, activated leukocytes and vascular wall cells release growth factors that promote SMC proliferation and ECM synthesis.

Infection. Although there is tantalizing evidence that infections may drive the local inflammatory process that results in atherosclerotic plaque, this hypothesis has yet to be definitively proven. Herpesvirus, cytomegalovirus, and *Chlamydia pneumoniae* have all been detected in atherosclerotic plaque but not in normal arteries, and seroepidemiologic studies find increased antibody titers to *C. pneumoniae* in patients with more severe atherosclerosis. However, a causal link between any of these infections and the development or progression of atherosclerosis remains to be established.

Smooth Muscle Proliferation

Intimal SMC proliferation and ECM deposition convert a fatty streak into a mature atheroma (see Fig. 10–6, steps 4 and 5) and contribute to the progressive growth of atherosclerotic lesions. Recall that the intimal SMCs have a proliferative and synthetic phenotype distinct from the underlying medial SMCs and, in fact, may substantially derive from the recruitment of circulating precursors. Several growth factors are implicated in SMC proliferation and ECM synthesis, including platelet-derived growth factor (PDGF, released by locally adherent platelets as well as by macrophages, ECs, and SMCs), fibroblast growth factor, and transforming growth factor α. The recruited SMCs synthesize ECM (notably collagen), which stabilizes atherosclerotic plaques. However, activated inflammatory cells in atheromas can cause intimal SMC apoptosis, and they also increase ECM catabolism, resulting in unstable plaques.

Figure 10–7 summarizes the major proposed cellular mechanisms of atherogenesis, emphasizing the multifactorial pathogenesis of this disease. This scheme highlights the canon that atherosclerosis is a chronic inflammatory response of the vascular wall to a variety of insults, including endothelial injury, lipid accumulation and oxidation, and thrombosis. Atheromas are dynamic lesions consisting of dysfunctional ECs, recruited and proliferating SMCs, and admixed chronic inflammation (macrophages and lymphocytes). All four cell types contribute mediators that influence atherogenesis. At early stages, intimal plaques are little more than aggregates of macrophage and SMC foam cells, some of which die, releasing lipid and necrotic debris. With progression, the atheroma is modified by collagen and proteoglycans synthesized by SMCs; connective tissue is particularly prominent on the intimal aspect, producing a fibrous cap, but lesions typically retain a central core of lipid-laden cells and fatty debris that may also become calcified over time. Disruption of the fibrous cap with superimposed thrombus is often associated with catastrophic clinical events.

With this overview of pathogenesis we can now discuss the morphologic evolution and correlates of atherosclerosis.

Morphology

Fatty Streaks. Fatty streaks are composed of lipid-filled foam cells but are not significantly raised and thus do not cause any disturbance in blood flow. They begin as multiple minute yellow, flat spots that can coalesce into elongated streaks, 1 cm long or longer (Fig. 10-8). Fatty streaks can appear in the aortas of infants younger than

1 year and are present in virtually all children older than 10 years, regardless of geography, race, sex, or environment. Coronary fatty streaks begin to form in adolescence, at the same anatomic sites that later tend to develop plaques. The relationship of fatty streaks to atherosclerotic plaques is uncertain; although they may evolve into precursors of plaques, not all fatty streaks are destined to become advanced atherosclerotic lesions.

Atherosclerotic Plaque. The key processes in atherosclerosis are intimal thickening and lipid accumulation (see Figs. 10–3 and 10–7). Atheromatous plaques (also called fibrous or fibrofatty plaques) impinge on the lumen of the artery and grossly appear white to yellow; thrombosis superimposed over the surface of ulcerated plaques is red-brown in color. Plaques vary from 0.3 to 1.5 cm in diameter but can coalesce to form larger masses (Fig. 10–9).

Atherosclerotic lesions are patchy, usually involving only a portion of any given arterial wall. On cross-section, the lesions therefore appear "eccentric" (Fig 10–10A). The focality of atherosclerotic lesions—despite the uniform exposure of vessel walls to such factors as cigarette smoke toxins, elevated LDL, and hyperglycemia—is almost certainly due to the vagaries of vascular hemodynamics. Local flow disturbances, such as turbulence at branch points, leads to certain portions of a vessel wall being more susceptible to plaque formation. Although focal and sparsely distributed at first, atherosclerotic lesions become more numerous and more diffuse with time.

In humans, the abdominal aorta is typically much more frequently involved than the thoracic aorta. In descending order, the **most extensively involved vessels are the lower abdominal aorta, the coronary arteries, the popliteal arteries, the internal carotid**

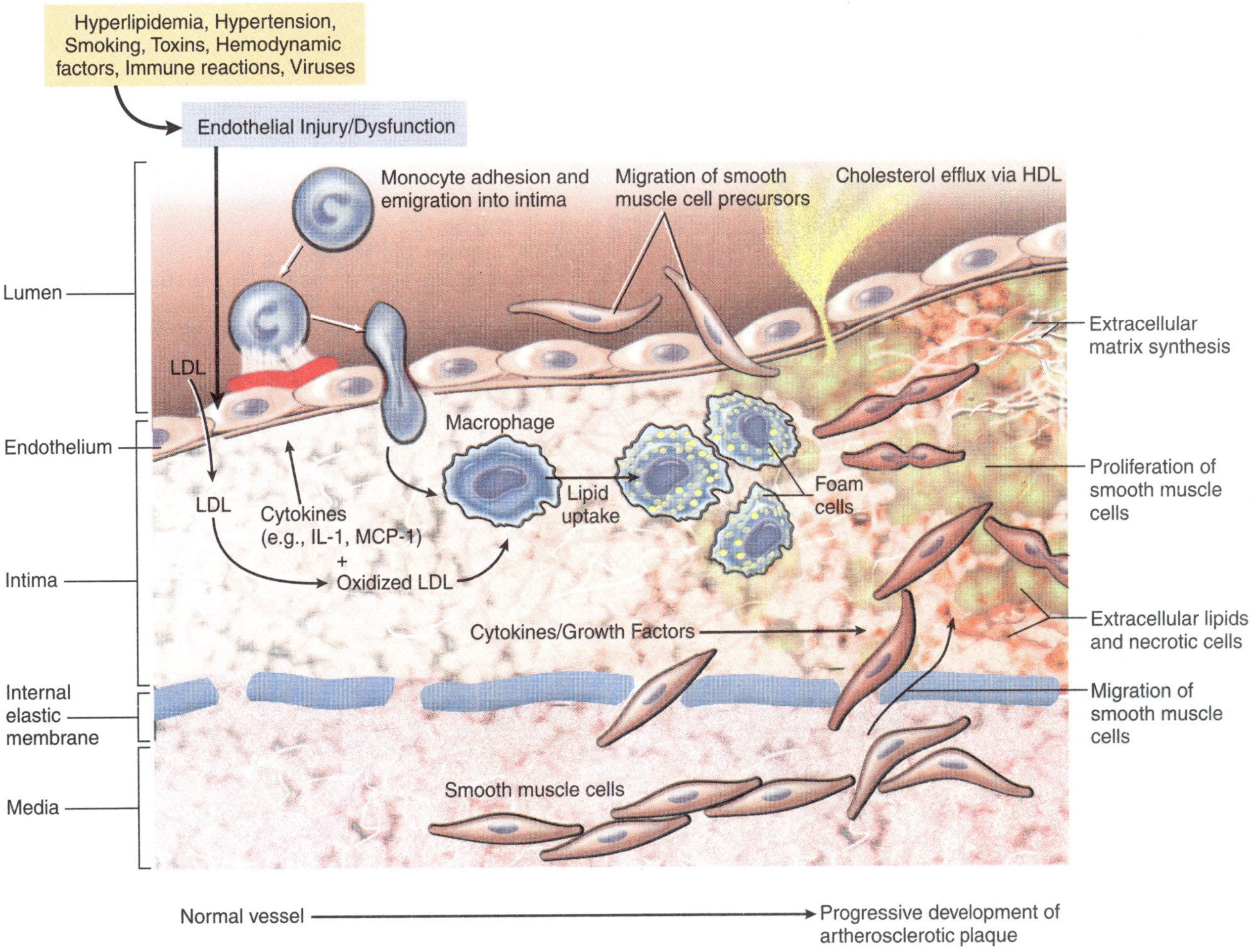

Figure 10–7

Hypothetical sequence of cellular interactions in atherosclerosis. Hyperlipidemia and other risk factors are thought to cause endothelial injury, resulting in adhesion of platelets and monocytes and release of growth factors, including platelet-derived growth factor (PDGF), which lead to SMC migration and proliferation. Foam cells of atheromatous plaques are derived from both macrophages and SMCs—from macrophages via the very-low-density lipoprotein (VLDL) receptor and low-density lipoprotein (LDL) modifications recognized by scavenger receptors (e.g., oxidized LDL), and from SMCs by less certain mechanisms. Extracellular lipid is derived from insudation from the vessel lumen, particularly in the presence of hypercholesterolemia, and also from degenerating foam cells. Cholesterol accumulation in the plaque reflects an imbalance between influx and efflux, and high-density lipoprotein (HDL) probably helps clear cholesterol from these accumulations. SMCs migrate to the intima, proliferate, and produce ECM, including collagen and proteoglycans.

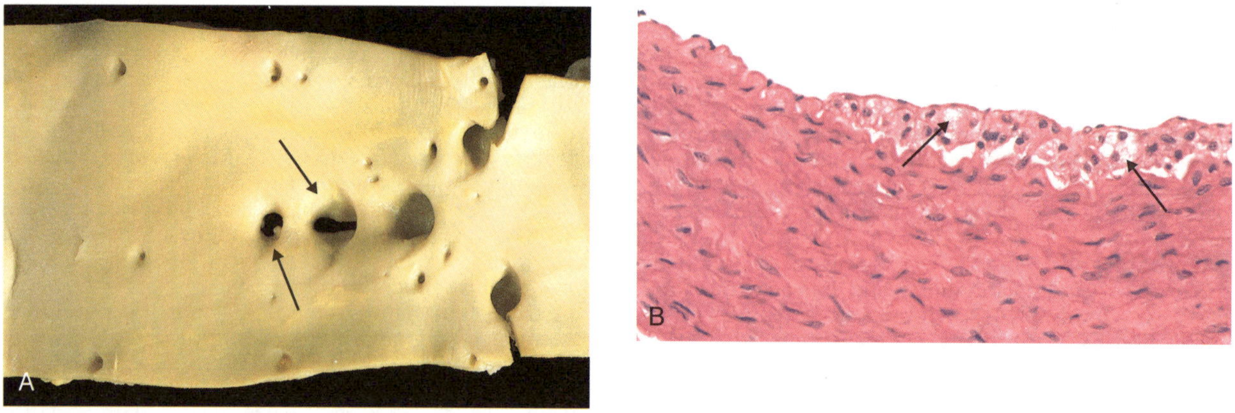

Figure 10–8

Fatty streak—a collection of foam cells in the intima. **A,** Aorta with fatty streaks (*arrows*), associated largely with the ostia of branch vessels. **B,** Photomicrograph of fatty streak in an experimental hypercholesterolemic rabbit, demonstrating intimal, macrophage-derived foam cells (*arrow*). (**B,** Courtesy of Dr. Myron I. Cybulsky, University of Toronto, Ontario, Canada.)

arteries, and the vessels of the circle of Willis. Vessels of the upper extremities are usually spared, as are the mesenteric and renal arteries, except at their ostia. Nevertheless, in an individual case, the severity of atherosclerosis in one artery does not predict its severity in another. Moreover, in any given vessel, lesions at various stages often coexist.

Atherosclerotic plaques have three principal components: (1) cells, including SMCs, macrophages, and T cells; (2) ECM, including collagen, elastic fibers, and proteoglycans; and (3) intracellular and extracellular lipid (Fig. 10–10). These components occur in varying proportions and configurations in different lesions. Typically, the superficial **fibrous cap** is composed of SMCs and relatively dense collagen. Beneath and to the side of the cap (the "**shoulder**") is a more cellular area containing macrophages, T cells, and SMCs. Deep to the fibrous cap is a **necrotic core,** containing lipid (primarily cholesterol and cholesterol esters), debris from dead cells, foam cells (lipid-laden macrophages and SMCs), fibrin, variably organized thrombus, and other plasma proteins; the cholesterol content is frequently present as crystalline aggregates that are washed out during routine tissue processing and leave behind only empty "clefts." At the periphery of the lesions, there is usually **neovascularization** (proliferating small blood vessels). Typical atheromas contain relatively abundant lipid, but some plaques ("fibrous plaques") are composed almost exclusively of SMCs and fibrous tissue.

Plaques generally continue to change and progressively enlarge through cell death and degeneration, synthesis and degradation (remodeling) of ECM, and organization of thrombi. Moreover, atheromas often undergo **calcification** (Fig. 10–10C). Patients with advanced coronary calcification appear to be at increased risk for coronary events.

Atherosclerotic plaques are susceptible to the following pathologic changes with clinical significance:

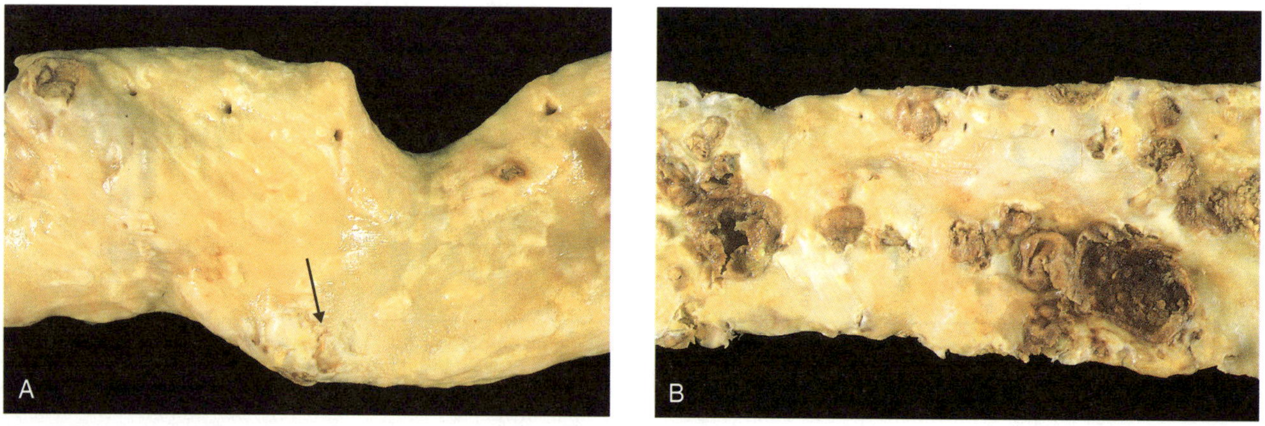

Figure 10–9

Gross views of atherosclerosis in the aorta. **A,** Mild atherosclerosis composed of fibrous plaques (*arrow*). **B,** Severe disease with diffuse and complicated lesions, some of which have coalesced.

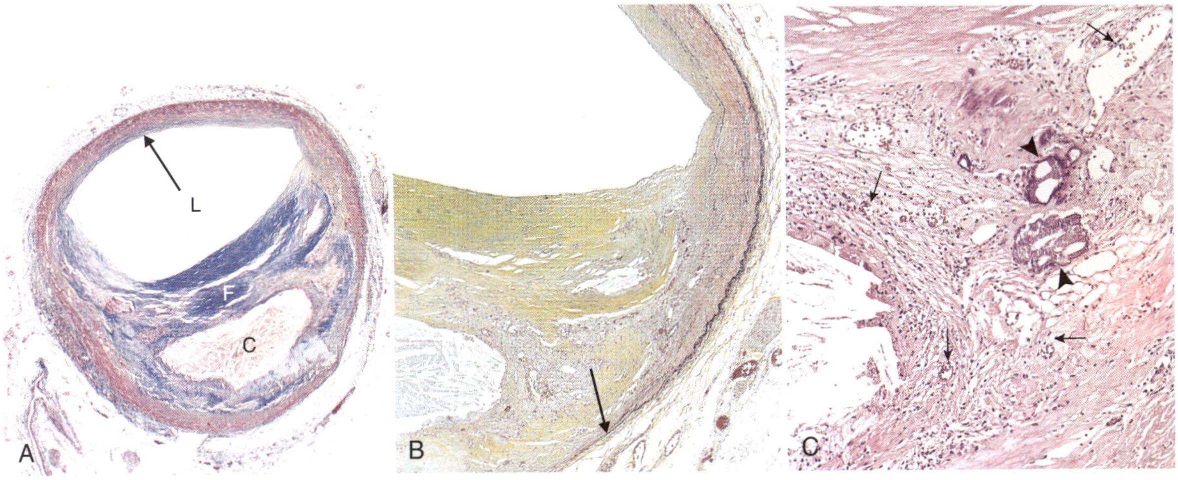

Figure 10–10

Histologic features of atheromatous plaque in the coronary artery. **A**, Overall architecture demonstrating fibrous cap (*F*) and a central necrotic (largely lipid) core (*C*). The lumen (*L*) has been moderately narrowed. Note that a segment of the wall is plaque free (*arrow*), so that there is an eccentric lesion. In this section, collagen has been stained blue (Masson's trichrome stain). **B**, Higher power photograph of a section of the plaque shown in **A**, stained for elastin (*black*), demonstrating that the internal and external elastic membranes are destroyed and the media of the artery is thinned under the most advanced plaque (*arrow*). **C**, Higher magnification photomicrograph at the junction of the fibrous cap and core, showing scattered inflammatory cells, calcification (*arrowhead*), and neovascularization (*small arrows*).

- **Rupture, ulceration, or erosion** of the luminal surface of atheromatous plaques exposes the bloodstream to highly thrombogenic substances and induces thrombus formation. Such thrombi can partially or completely occlude the lumen and lead to downstream ischemia (e.g., in the heart; Chapter 11) (Fig. 10–11). If the patient survives the initial vascular occlusion, thrombi may become organized and incorporated into the growing plaque.
- **Hemorrhage** into a plaque. Rupture of the overlying fibrous cap or of the thin-walled vessels in the areas of neovascularization can cause intra-plaque hemorrhage; a contained hematoma may expand the plaque or induce plaque rupture.
- **Atheroembolism.** Plaque rupture can discharge debris into the bloodstream, producing microemboli composed of plaque contents.
- **Aneurysm formation.** Atherosclerosis-induced pressure or ischemic atrophy of the underlying media, with loss of elastic tissue, causes weakness of the vessel wall and development of aneurysms that may rupture.

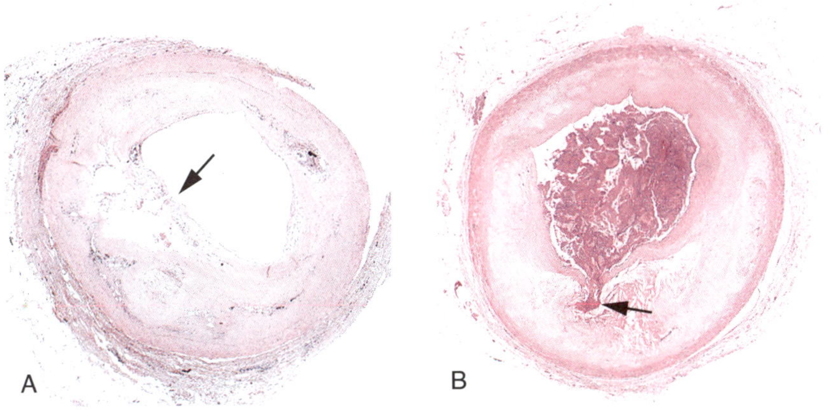

Figure 10–11

Atherosclerotic plaque rupture. **A**, Plaque rupture (*arrow*) without superimposed thrombus, in a patient who died suddenly. **B**, Acute coronary thrombosis superimposed on an atherosclerotic plaque with focal disruption of the fibrous cap (*arrow*), triggering fatal myocardial infarction. (**B**, From Schoen FJ: Interventional and Surgical Cardiovascular Patherosclerosisology: Clinical Correlations and Basic Principles. Philadelphia, WB Saunders, 1989, p 61.)

Natural History of Atherosclerosis

The natural history, morphologic features, and main pathogenic events of atherosclerosis are encapsulated in Figure 10–12. Atherosclerosis primarily affects elastic arteries (e.g., aorta, carotid, and iliac arteries) and large and medium-sized muscular arteries (e.g., coronary and popliteal arteries). In small arteries, atheromas can gradually occlude lumina, compromising blood flow to distal organs and cause ischemic injury. Moreover, atherosclerotic plaques can undergo acute disruption and precipitate thrombi that further obstruct blood flow. In large arteries, plaques are destructive, encroaching on the subjacent media and weakening the affected vessel wall, causing aneurysms that can rupture. Moreover, atheromas can be friable, fragmenting atheroemboli into downstream circulations. *It is important to emphasize that atherosclerosis is a slowly evolving lesion usually requiring many decades to become significant. However, acute plaque changes (e.g., rupture, thrombosis, or hematoma formation) can rapidly precipitate clinical sequelae (the so-called "clinical horizon";* see Fig. 10–12).

Symptomatic atherosclerotic disease most often involves the arteries supplying the heart, brain, kidneys, and lower extremities. *Myocardial infarction (heart attack), cerebral infarction (stroke), aortic aneurysms, and peripheral vascular disease (gangrene of the legs) are the major consequences of atherosclerosis.* Atherosclerosis also takes a toll through other consequences of acutely or chronically diminished arterial perfusion, *such as mesenteric occlusion, sudden cardiac death, chronic IHD, and ischemic encephalopathy.* The effects of vascular occlusion ultimately depend on arterial supply and tissue metabolic demand; details will be discussed in greater detail in subsequent organ-specific chapters.

Prevention of Atherosclerotic Vascular Disease

Efforts to reduce the consequences and impact of atherosclerosis include

- *Primary prevention* programs aimed at either delaying atheroma formation or encouraging regression of established lesions in persons who have not yet suffered a serious complication of atherosclerosis
- *Secondary prevention* programs intended to prevent recurrence of events such as myocardial infarction or stroke in symptomatic patients

Primary prevention of atherosclerosis-related complications typically involves risk factor identification and modification of those that are amenable to intervention: cessation of cigarette smoking, control of hypertension, weight loss, exercise, and lowering total and LDL blood cholesterol levels while increasing HDL (e.g., by diet or through statins). Interestingly, statin use may also modulate the inflammatory state of the vascular wall. Several lines of evidence suggest that risk factor stratification and reduction should even begin in childhood.

Secondary prevention involves the judicious use of aspirin (anti-platelet agent), statins, and beta blockers (to limit cardiac demand), as well as surgical interventions (e.g., coronary artery bypass surgery, carotid endarterec-

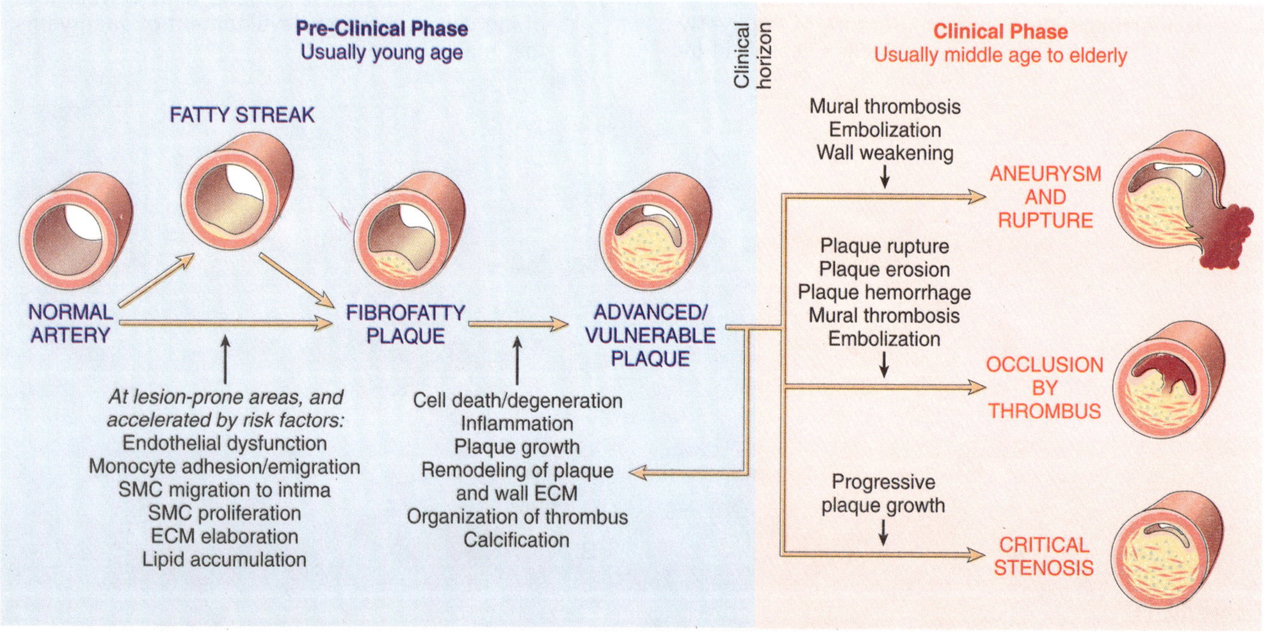

Figure 10–12

The natural history, morphologic features, main pathogenic events, and clinical complications of atherosclerosis.

tomy). These can successfully reduce recurrent myocardial or cerebral events.

Considerable progress on the health impact of atherosclerosis-related disease has been made over the past decades in the United States and elsewhere. Between 1963 (the peak year) and 2000 there has been an approximately 50% decrease in the death rate from IHD and a 70% decrease in deaths from strokes, a reduction in mortality that alone has largely increased the average life expectancy in the United States by 5 years. Three main contributors to this impressive improvement have been (1) prevention of atherosclerosis through recognition of risk factors and changes in life style (e.g., reduced cigarette smoking, reduced consumption of cholesterol, and control of hypertension); (2) improved methods of treatment of myocardial infarction and other complications of IHD; and (3) prevention of recurrences in patients who have previously suffered serious atherosclerosis-related clinical events.

SUMMARY

Atherosclerosis

- Atherosclerosis is an intima-based lesion organized into a fibrous cap and an atheromatous (gruel-like) core and composed of SMCs, ECM, inflammatory cells, lipids, and necrotic debris.
- Atherogenesis is driven by an interplay of inflammation and injury to vessel wall cells. Many known risk factors influence EC dysfunction, as well as SMC recruitment and stimulation.
- Atherosclerotic plaques accrue slowly over decades but may acutely cause symptoms due to rupture, thrombosis, hemorrhage, or embolization.
- Risk factor recognition and reduction can reduce the incidence and severity of atherosclerosis-related disease.

HYPERTENSIVE VASCULAR DISEASE

Systemic and local blood pressure must be tightly regulated. Low pressures result in inadequate organ perfusion, leading to dysfunction and/or tissue death. Conversely, high pressures that drive blood flow in excess of metabolic demands provide no additional benefit but result in blood vessel and end-organ damage. Elevated blood pressure is called *hypertension;* as we saw previously, it is one of the major risk factors for atherosclerosis. Here we will first discuss the mechanisms of normal blood pressure control, followed by pathways that may underlie hypertension, and finally the pathologic changes in vessels associated with hypertension.

Although hypertension is a common health problem with occasionally devastating outcomes, it typically remains asymptomatic until late in its course. Besides contributing to the pathogenesis of coronary heart disease and cerebrovascular accidents, hypertension can also cause cardiac hypertrophy and heart failure (*hypertensive heart disease*), aortic dissection, and renal failure. Although we have an improving understanding of the molecular pathways that regulate normal blood pressure, the mechanisms of hypertension in the vast majority of people remain unknown; consequently, we refer to most of these as "essential hypertension" (to mask our ignorance?).

Like height and weight, blood pressure is a continuously distributed variable, with essential hypertension at one end of the distribution rather than a distinct entity. The detrimental effects of blood pressure increase continuously as the pressure rises; no rigidly defined threshold level of blood pressure distinguishes risk from safety. Nevertheless, a sustained diastolic pressure greater than 90 mm Hg, or a sustained systolic pressure in excess of 140 mm Hg, constitutes hypertension; systolic blood pressure is more important than diastolic blood pressure in determining cardiovascular risk. By either criteria, some 25% of individuals in the general population are hypertensive. The prevalence and vulnerability to complications increase with age; they are also higher in African Americans. Reduction of blood pressure dramatically reduces the incidence and death rates from IHD, heart failure, and stroke.

Regulation of Blood Pressure

Blood pressure is a complex trait involving the interaction of multiple genetic and environmental factors that influence two hemodynamic variables: cardiac output and peripheral vascular resistance (Fig. 10–13). Cardiac output is affected by blood volume, itself strongly dependent on sodium concentrations. Peripheral resistance is regulated predominantly at the level of the arterioles and is influenced by neural and hormonal inputs. Normal vascular tone reflects an interplay between circulating factors that induce vasoconstriction (e.g., angiotensin II and catecholamines) and vasodilation (e.g., kinins, prostaglandins, and nitric oxide). Resistance vessels also exhibit autoregulation, whereby increased blood flow induces vasoconstriction to protect tissues against hyperperfusion. Other local factors such as pH and hypoxia, as well as neural interactions (α- and β-adrenergic systems), are also involved. The integrated function of these systems ensures adequate systemic perfusion, despite regional demand differences.

The kidneys (primarily) and adrenals (secondarily) are central players in blood pressure regulation; they interact with each other to modify vessel tone and blood volume, as follows (Fig. 10–14):

- The *kidney* influences peripheral resistance and sodium homeostasis primarily through the renin-angiotensin system. *Renin* is a proteolytic enzyme produced in the kidney by the juxtaglomerular cells—modified myoepithelial cells that surround the glomerular afferent arterioles.

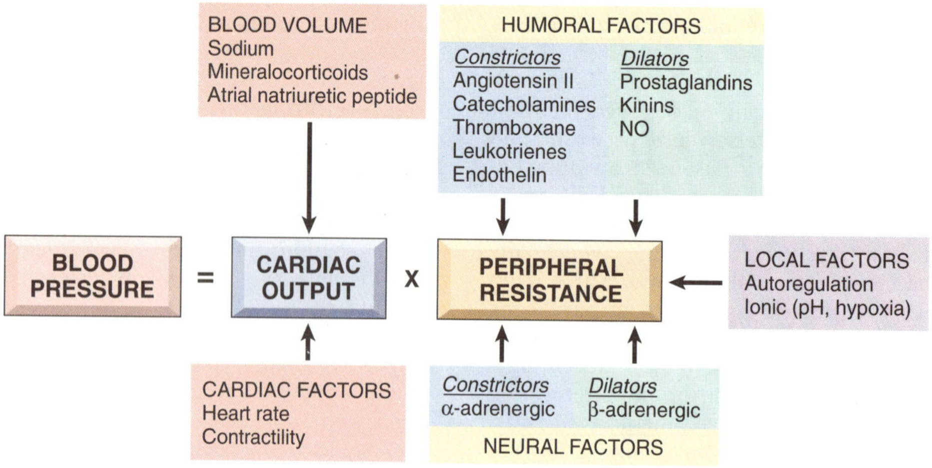

Figure 10–13

Blood pressure modulation by effects on cardiac output and peripheral resistance.

• When blood volume or pressure is reduced, the kidney senses this as a decreased pressure in the afferent arterioles. Moreover, lower volumes or pressures result in a reduced *glomerular filtration rate* in the kidney with *increased resorption* of sodium by proximal tubules; these latter two effects putatively conserve sodium and expand the blood volume.

• The juxtaglomerular cells respond to reduced intraluminal pressures in the afferent arterioles by releasing renin; they also produce renin when the cells of the macula densa sense decreased sodium concentration in the distal convoluted tubule.

• Renin catabolizes *plasma angiotensinogen* to *angiotensin I*, which in turn is converted to *angiotensin*

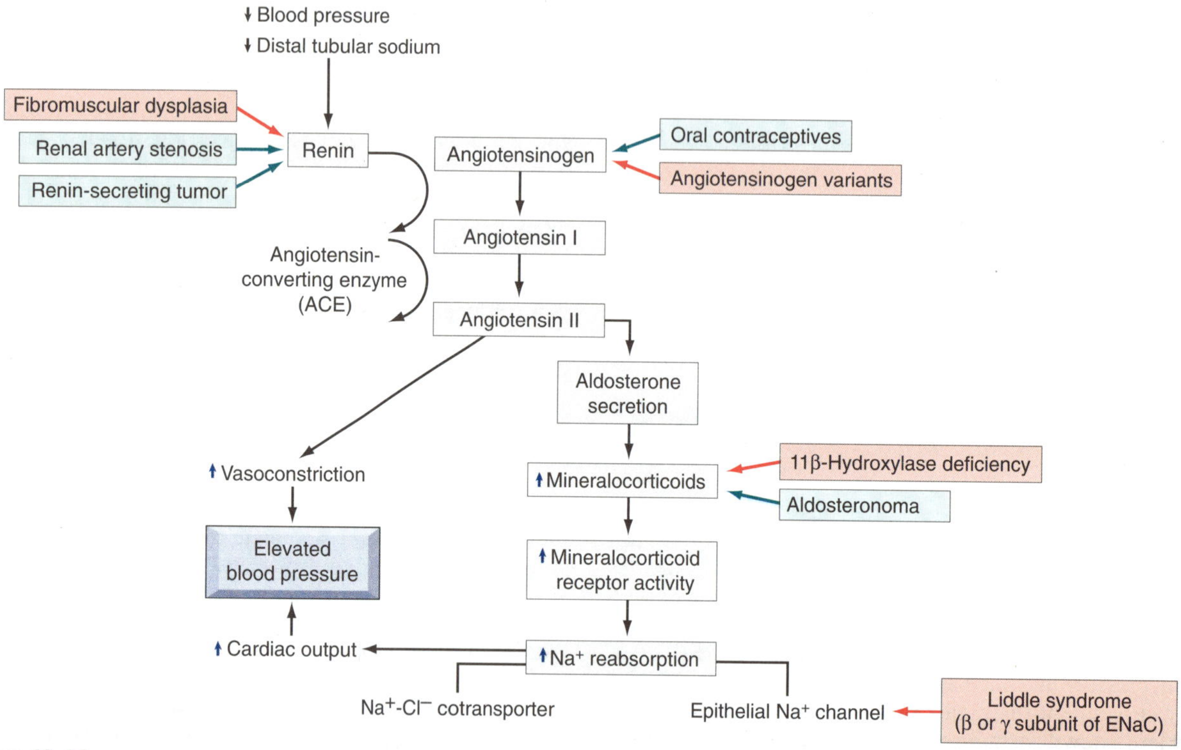

Figure 10–14

Blood pressure variation and the renin-angiotensin system. Components of the systemic renin-angiotensin system are shown in *black.* Some genetic disorders that affect blood pressure by altering activity of this pathway are indicated in *red; arrows* indicate sites in the pathway altered by mutation. Acquired disorders that alter blood pressure through effects on this pathway are indicated in *green.* ENaC, epithelial sodium channel. (Modified with permission from Lifton RP: Molecular genetics of human blood pressure variation. Science 272:676–680, 1996. Copyright 1996 AAAS.)

II by angiotensin-converting enzyme in the periphery. Angiotensin II raises blood pressure by: increasing peripheral resistance by inducing vascular SMC contraction; increasing blood volume by stimulating aldosterone secretion in the adrenals; increasing distal tubular reabsorption of sodium.

- The kidneys filter 170 liters of plasma containing 23 moles of salt daily! Moreover, 99.5% of the filtered salt must be reabsorbed to maintain homeostasis (assuming daily ingestion of only 100 mEq). *As it turns out, the absorption of the last 2% of sodium is the key to normal sodium homeostasis; this is regulated by the renin-angiotensin system acting on the epithelial Na^+ channel (ENaC)* (see Fig. 10–14).
- The kidney also produces a variety of vasorelaxant or antihypertensive substances (including prostaglandins and nitric oxide) that presumably counterbalance the vasopressor effects of angiotensin.
- When renal excretory function is impaired, increased arterial pressure is a compensatory mechanism that can help restore fluid and electrolyte balance.
- Other tissues can also influence influence blood pressure and volume. Thus, *atrial natriuretic peptide, secreted by heart atria in response to volume expansion* (e.g., in heart failure) inhibits sodium reabsorption in distal tubules and causes global vasodilation.

Pathogenesis of Hypertension

Table 10–3 lists the major causes of hypertension. *Ninety percent to 95% of hypertension is idiopathic (essential hypertension), which is compatible with long life, unless a myocardial infarction, cerebrovascular accident, or other complication supervenes.* Most of the remainder of "benign hypertension" is secondary to renal disease or, less often, to narrowing of the renal artery, usually by an atheromatous plaque (renovascular hypertension). Infrequently, hypertension is secondary to diseases of the adrenal glands, such as primary aldosteronism. Cushing syndrome, pheochromocytoma, or other disorders.

About 5% of hypertensive persons show a rapidly rising blood pressure that if untreated leads to death within 1 or 2 years. Termed *accelerated* or *malignant hypertension,* the clinical syndrome is characterized by severe hypertension (diastolic pressure over 120 mm Hg), renal failure, and retinal hemorrhages and exudates, with or without papilledema. It may develop in previously normotensive persons but more often is superimposed on preexisting benign hypertension, either essential or secondary.

Essential Hypertension. Even without knowing the specific lesion(s), it is reasonable to conclude that alterations in renal sodium homeostasis and/or vessel wall tone or structure underlie essential hypertension (Fig. 10–15). In established hypertension, both increased blood volume and increased peripheral resistance contribute to the increased pressure.

- *Reduced renal sodium excretion* in the presence of normal arterial pressure is probably a key initiating event; indeed, it is a final common pathway for the pathogenesis of most forms of hypertension (see bottom of Fig. 10–14). Decreased sodium excretion will cause an obligatory increase in fluid volume and increased cardiac output, thereby elevating blood pressure (see Fig. 10–15). At the higher setting of blood pressure, enough additional sodium will be excreted by the kidneys to equal intake and prevent fluid retention. Thus, a new steady state of sodium excretion would be achieved, but at the expense of an elevated blood pressure.
- *Vascular changes* may involve *functional vasoconstriction* or *changes in vascular wall structure that result in increased resistance.* Chronic functional vasoconstriction could also conceivably result in permanent structural thickening of the resistant vessels.

Although we frequently cannot point to a discrete cause, the accepted wisdom is that essential hypertension results from an interplay of multiple genetic and environmental factors affecting cardiac output and/or peripheral resistance.

- *Genetic factors.* Studies comparing blood pressure in monozygotic and dizygotic twins, and studies of famil-

Table 10–3 Types and Causes of Hypertension (Systolic and Diastolic)

Essential Hypertension (90% to 95% of Cases)
Secondary Hypertension
RENAL
Acute glomerulonephritis
Chronic renal disease
Polycystic disease
Renal artery stenosis
Renal vasculitis
Renin-producing tumors
ENDOCRINE
Adrenocortical hyperfunction (Cushing syndrome, primary aldosteronism, congenital adrenal hyperplasia, licorice ingestion)
Exogenous hormones (glucocorticoids, estrogen [including pregnancy-induced and oral contraceptives], sympathomimetics and tyramine-containing foods, monoamine oxidase inhibitors)
Pheochromocytoma
Acromegaly
Hypothyroidism (myxedema)
Hyperthyroidism (thyrotoxicosis)
Pregnancy-induced
CARDIOVASCULAR
Coarctation of aorta
Polyarteritis nodosa
Increased intravascular volume
Increased cardiac output
Rigidity of the aorta
NEUROLOGIC
Psychogenic
Increased intracranial pressure
Sleep apnea
Acute stress, including surgery

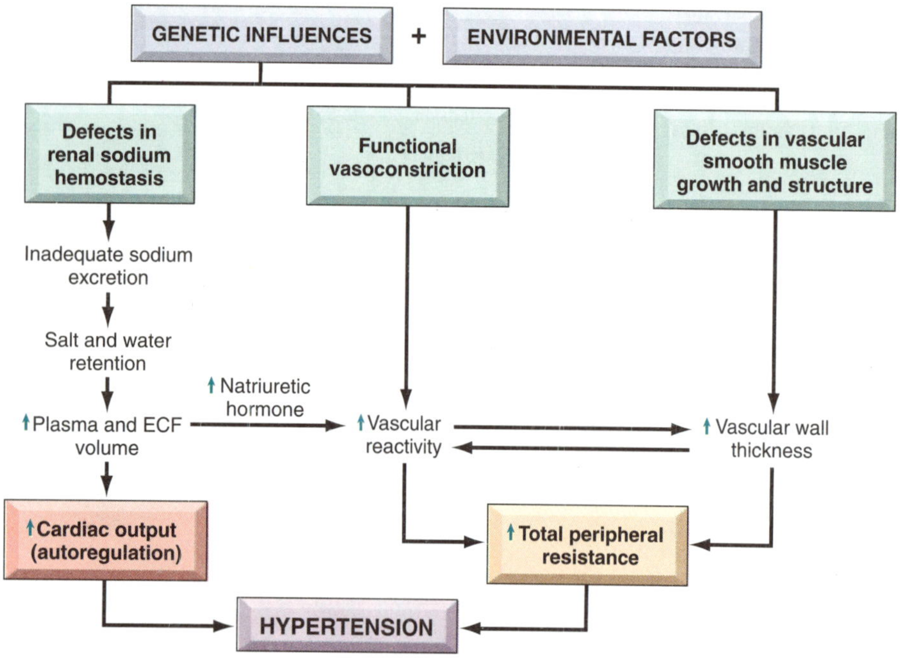

Figure 10–15

Hypothetical scheme for the pathogenesis of essential hypertension, implicating genetic defects in renal excretion of sodium, functional regulation of vascular tone, and structural regulation of vascular caliber. Environmental factors, especially increased salt intake, potentiate the effects of genetic factors. The resultant increase in cardiac output and peripheral resistance contributes to hypertension. ECF, extracellular fluid.

ial clustering of hypertension, clearly establish a strong genetic component. Moreover, several single-gene disorders cause relatively rare forms of hypertension (and hypotension) by altering net renal sodium resorption. Some of these are illustrated in Figure 10–14.

Allelic variations in the genes encoding components of the renin-angiotensin system. Hypertension is associated with polymorphisms in both the angiotensinogen locus and the angiotensin II type I receptor locus. Genetic variants in the renin-angiotensin system may contribute to the known racial differences in blood pressure regulation. Susceptibility genes for essential hypertension in the larger population are currently unknown, but may well include genes that govern responses to an increased renal sodium load, levels of pressor substances, reactivity of vascular SMCs to pressor agents, or SMC growth.

- *Environmental factors* modify the expression of any underlying genetic determinants of hypertension; stress, obesity, smoking, physical inactivity, and heavy consumption of salt are all implicated. Indeed, evidence linking dietary sodium intake with the prevalence of hypertension in different population groups is particularly impressive.

Vascular Pathology in Hypertension

In addition to accelerating atherogenesis, hypertension-associated degenerative changes in the walls of large and medium arteries can potentiate both aortic dissection and cerebrovascular hemorrhage. Hypertension is also associated with two forms of small blood vessel disease: hyaline arteriolosclerosis and hyperplastic arteriolosclerosis (Fig. 10–16).

Morphology

Hyaline Arteriolosclerosis. This vascular lesion consists of a homogeneous pink hyaline thickening of the walls of arterioles with loss of underlying structural detail and with narrowing of the lumen (Fig. 10–16A). Encountered frequently in elderly patients, whether normotensive or hypertensive, hyaline arteriolosclerosis is more generalized and more severe in patients with hypertension. It is also common as part of the characteristic microangiography in diabetes (Chapter 20).

The lesions reflect leakage of plasma components across vascular endothelium and excessive ECM production by SMCs secondary to the chronic hemodynamic stress of hypertension. Hyaline arteriolosclerosis is a major morphologic characteristic of benign nephrosclerosis, in which the arteriolar narrowing causes diffuse impairment of renal blood supply, with loss of nephrons (Chapter 14).

Hyperplastic Arteriolosclerosis. Related to more acute or severe elevations of blood pressure, hyperplastic arteriolosclerosis is characteristic of (but not limited to) malignant hypertension (typically, diastolic pressures over 120 mm Hg associated with acute cerebral and/or renal injury). Hyperplastic arteriolosclerosis is associated with "onion-skin," concentric, laminated thickening of the walls of arterioles with luminal narrowing (Fig. 10–16B). The laminations consist of SMCs and thickened, duplicated basement membrane. In malignant hypertension, these hyperplastic changes are accompanied by fibrinoid deposits and vessel wall necrosis (necrotizing arteriolitis), particularly prominent in the kidney (Chapter 14).

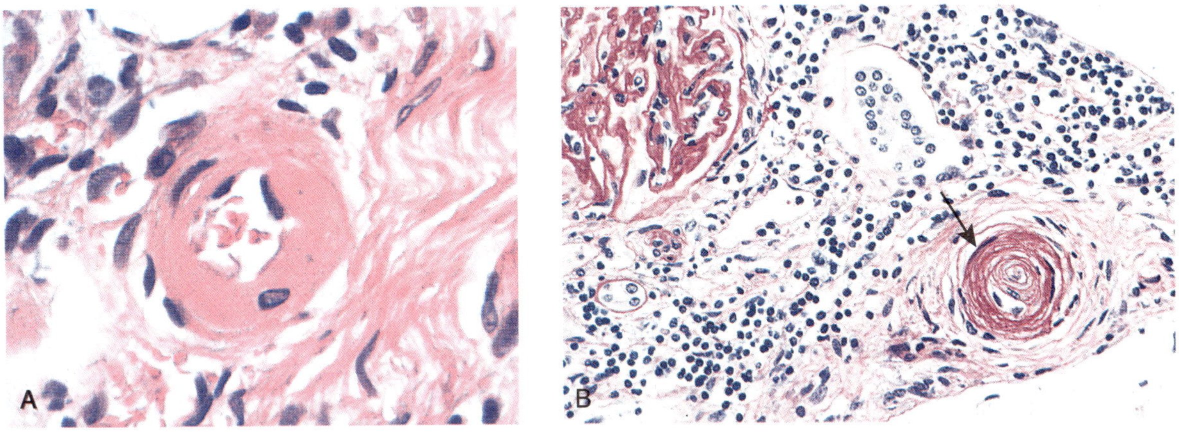

Figure 10–16

Vascular pathology in hypertension. **A,** Hyaline arteriolosclerosis. The arteriolar wall is hyalinized and the lumen is markedly narrowed. **B,** Hyperplastic arteriolosclerosis (onion-skinning) causing luminal obliteration (*arrow*), with secondary ischemic changes, manifest by wrinkling of the glomerular capillary vessels at the upper left (periodic acid–Schiff stain). (Courtesy of Dr. Helmut Rennke, Brigham and Women's Hospital, Boston, Massachusetts.)

SUMMARY

Hypertension

- Blood pressure is regulated by the combined influences of cardiac output (largely related to blood volume) and vascular resistance. Blood volume is dependent on renal sodium homeostasis, and arteriolar vascular resistance is regulated by neural and hormonal inputs.
- Renin is a major regulator of normal blood pressure; it is secreted by kidneys in response to reduced afferent aretriole pressure or glomerular filtration of sodium. Renin converts angiotensinogen to angiotensin II; angiotensin II regulates blood pressure by increasing vascular SMC contraction and by increasing aldosterone secretion to increase renal sodium resorption.
- Essential hypertension represents 90% to 95% of cases of hypertension and is a complex, multifactorial disorder resulting most likely from the combined effect of mutations or polymorphisms at several gene loci (e.g., sodium resorption, renin-angiotensin system, aldosterone) in association with a variety of environmental influences.
- Secondary hypertension is caused by diseases of the kidneys or endocrine glands.

ANEURYSMS AND DISSECTIONS

An *aneurysm* is a *localized abnormal dilation of a blood vessel or the heart* (Fig. 10–17). When an aneurysm involves all three layers of the arterial wall (intima, media, and adventitia) or the attenuated wall of the heart, it is called a "true" aneurysm. Atherosclerotic, syphilitic, and congenital aneurysms, and ventricular aneurysms that follow transmural myocardial infarctions, are of this type. In contrast, a *false aneurysm* (also called *pseudoaneurysm*) is a breach in the vascular wall leading to an extravascular hematoma that freely communicates with the intravascular space ("pulsating hematoma"). Examples include ventricular ruptures after myocardial infarctions that are contained by a pericardial adhesion, or a leak at the junction of a vascular graft with a natural artery. An arterial *dissection* arises when blood enters the wall of the artery, as a hematoma dissecting between its layers. Dissections are often but not always aneurysmal (see also below). Both true and false aneurysms as well as dissections can rupture, often with catastrophic consequences.

Descriptively, aneurysms are classified by macroscopic shape and size (see Fig. 10–17). *Saccular* aneurysms are essentially spherical outpouchings (involving only a portion of the vessel wall); they vary from 5 to 20 cm in diameter and often contain thrombi. *Fusiform* aneurysms involve diffuse, circumferential dilation of a long vascular segment; they vary in diameter (≤20 cm) and in length and can involve extensive portions of the aortic arch, abdominal aorta, or even the iliacs. Particular aspects of shape and size are not specific for any disease or clinical manifestations.

The two most important causes of aortic aneurysms are atherosclerosis and cystic medial degeneration of the arterial media. Other causes that weaken vessel walls and lead to aneurysms include trauma, congenital defects (e.g., *berry* aneurysms), infections (*mycotic* aneurysms), or syphilis. Arterial aneurysms can also be caused by systemic diseases, such as vasculitis (see later).

Infection of a major artery that weakens its wall is called a *mycotic aneurysm;* thrombosis and rupture are possible complications. Mycotic aneurysms can originate (1) from embolization of a septic thrombus, usually as a complication of infective endocarditis; (2) as an extension of an adjacent suppurative process; or (3) by circulating organisms directly infecting the arterial wall.

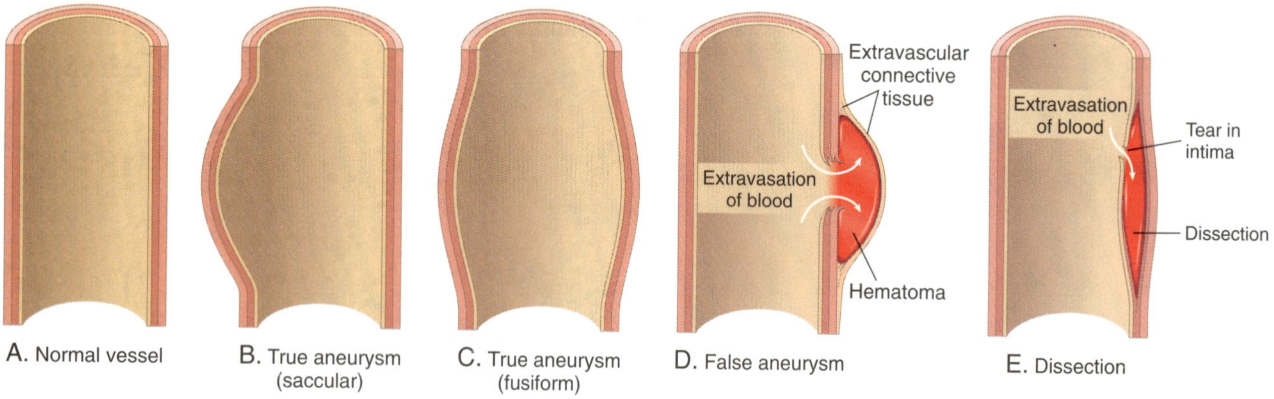

Figure 10–17

Aneurysms. **A.** Normal vessel. **B,** True aneurysm, saccular type. The wall focally bulges outward and may be attenuated but is otherwise intact. **C,** True aneurysm, fusiform type. There is circumferential dilation of the vessel, without rupture. **D,** False aneurysm. The wall is ruptured, and there is a collection of blood (hematoma) that is bounded externally by adherent extravascular tissues. **E,** Dissection. Blood has entered (*dissected*) the wall of the vessel and separated the layers. Although this is shown as occurring through a tear in the lumen, dissections can also occur by rupture of the vessels of the vaso vasorum within the media.

Abdominal Aortic Aneurysm

Atherosclerosis, the most common cause of aneurysms, causes thinning and weakening of the media secondary to intimal plaques. Such plaques compress the underlying media and also compromise nutrient and waste diffusion from the vascular lumen into the arterial wall. The media consequently undergoes degeneration and necrosis, thus allowing the dilation of the vessel. *Atherosclerotic aneurysms occur most frequently in the abdominal aorta* (*abdominal aortic aneurysm,* often abbreviated AAA), but the common iliac arteries, the arch, and descending parts of the thoracic aorta can also be involved.

Pathogenesis. AAA occurs more frequently in men and rarely develops before age 50. Atherosclerosis is a major cause of AAA, but there are clearly other contributors, since the incidence is less than 5% in men older than 60 years, despite almost universal abdominal aortic atherosclerosis in that population. There can be a familial predisposition independent of any genetic predilection to atherosclerosis or hypertension. In some cases, hereditary defects in structural components of the aorta can produce aneurysms (e.g., defective fibrillin production in Marfan disease affects elastic tissue synthesis; see below).

In the majority of cases, however, AAA results from an altered balance of collagen degradation and synthesis mediated by local inflammatory infiltrates and the destructive proteolytic enzymes they produce and regulate. Thus, abnormal collagen or elastic tissue—or inadequate remodeling of these ECM components—provide a background on which atherosclerosis or hypertension weaken the aortic wall. In this regard, matrix metalloproteinases (MMPs) have been increasingly implicated in AAA development. MMPs are expressed in aortic aneurysms at elevated levels compared with the normal vessel wall; macrophage MMP production is especially augmented. These enzymes have the capacity to degrade virtually all components of the ECM in the arterial wall (collagens, elastin, proteoglycans, laminin, fibronectin). Concurrently, decreased level of tissue inhibitor of metalloproteinases (TIMP) can also contribute to overall ECM degradation.

In this model of AAA pathogenesis, genetic predisposition may be related to the quality of the aortic connective tissue, to MMP and/or TIMP polymorphisms, or to the nature of local inflammatory responses. Indeed, evidence suggests that AAA is associated with local cytokine environments shifted toward the production of T_H2 cytokines (e.g., IL-4 and IL-10; Chapter 5). Both in vitro and in vivo, T_H2 cytokines drive macrophages to produce increased amounts of elastolytic MMPs.

Morphology

Usually positioned below the renal arteries and above the bifurcation of the aorta, AAA can be saccular or fusiform, as large as 15 cm in diameter, and as long as 25 cm (Fig. 10–18). There is severe complicated atherosclerosis with destruction and thinning of the underlying aortic media; the aneurysm frequently contains a bland, laminated, poorly organized mural thrombus that may fill some or all of the dilated segment. Occasionally, the aneurysm can affect the renal and superior or inferior mesenteric arteries, either by producing direct pressure or by narrowing or occluding vessel ostia with mural thrombi. Not infrequently, AAA is accompanied by smaller aneurysms of the iliac arteries.

Two AAA variants merit special mention:

- **Inflammatory AAAs** are characterized by dense periaortic fibrosis containing abundant lymphoplasmacytic infiltrate with many macrophages and often giant cells. Their cause is uncertain.
- **Mycotic AAAs** are atherosclerotic lesions infected by lodging of circulating microorganisms in the wall, particularly in the setting of bacteremia from a primary *Salmonella* gastroenteritis. In such cases, suppuration further destroys the media, potentiating rapid dilation and rupture.

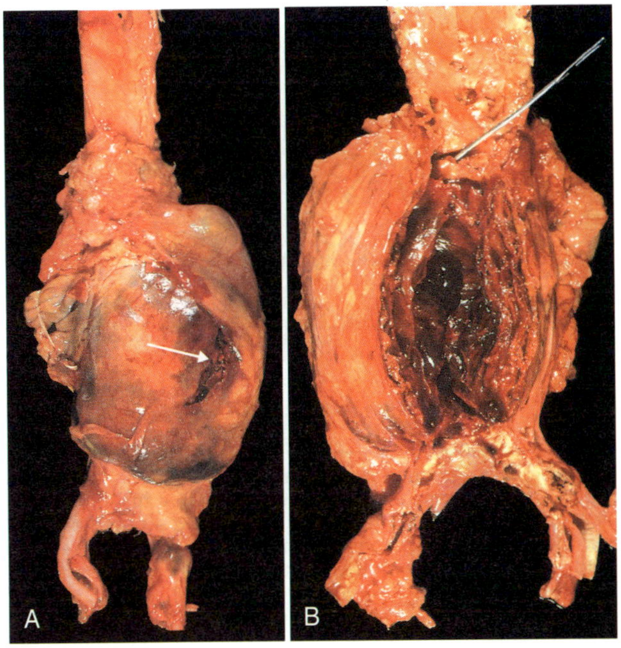

Figure 10–18

Abdominal aortic aneurysm. **A,** External view, gross photograph of a large aortic aneurysm that ruptured (*arrow*). **B,** Opened view, with the location of the rupture tract indicated by a probe. The wall of the aneurysm is exceedingly thin, and the lumen is filled by a large quantity of layered but largely unorganized thrombus.

Clinical Course. The clinical consequences of AAA include:

- Rupture into the peritoneal cavity or retroperitoneal tissues with massive, potentially fatal hemorrhage
- Obstruction of a branch vessel resulting in downstream tissue ischemic injury—for example, iliac (leg), renal (kidney), mesenteric (gastrointestinal [GI] tract), or vertebral (spinal cord) arteries
- Embolism from atheroma or mural thrombus
- Impingement on an adjacent structure (e.g., compression of a ureter or erosion of vertebrae)
- Presentation as an abdominal mass (often palpably pulsating) that simulates a tumor

The risk of rupture is directly related to the size of the aneurysm, varying from nil for AAAs of 4 cm or less in diameter, to 1% per year for AAAs between 4 and 5 cm, to 11% per year for AAAs between 5 and 6 cm, and 25% per year for aneurysms larger than 6 cm in diameter. Consequently, aneurysms of 5 cm or more in diameter are managed aggressively, usually by surgical bypass involving prosthetic grafts. Timely surgery is critical; operative mortality for unruptured aneurysms is approximately 5%, whereas emergency surgery after rupture carries a mortality rate of more than 50%. It is worth reiterating that because atherosclerosis is a systemic disease, a patient with an AAA is also very likely to have atherosclerosis in other vascular beds and is at a significantly increased risk of IHD and stroke.

Syphilitic Aneurysm

The *obliterative endarteritis* (see below) characteristic of the tertiary stage of syphilis (lues) can involve small vessels in any part of the body. Involvement of the vasa vasorum of the aorta is particularly devastating; this results in ischemic medial injury, leading to aneurysmal dilation of the aorta and aortic annulus, and eventually valvular insufficiency. Fortunately, better recognition and treatment of syphilis in its early stages have made this a vanishingly rare complication in the U.S. and Western Europe.

Morphology

T. pallidum has a prediliction to involve small blood vessels, the vasa vasorum, in the aortic adventitia. These vessels develop so-called **obliterative endarteritis.** The affected vessels show luminal narrowing and obliteration, scarring of the vessel wall, and a dense surrounding rim of lymphocytes and plasma cells that may extend into the media **(syphilitic aortitis).** The spirochetes are difficult to demonstrate in tissues.

The narrowing of the lumina of the vasa vasorum causes ischemic injury of the aortic media, with patchy loss of the medial elastic fibers and muscle cells, followed by inflammation and scarring. With destruction of the media, the aorta loses its elastic recoil and may become dilated, producing an aneurysm. Contraction of fibrous scars may lead to wrinkling of intervening segments of aortic intima, grossly reminiscent of "tree bark." Syphilitic involvement of the aorta favors the development of superimposed atherosclerosis of the aortic root, which can envelop and occlude the coronary ostia.

With weakening of the aortic root, the valvular annulus becomes dilated, resulting in valvular insufficiency and massive volume overload hypertrophy of the left ventricle. The greatly enlarged hearts are sometimes called "cor bovinum" (cow's heart).

Thoracic aortic aneurysms (regardless of etiology) cause signs and symptoms referable to (1) encroachment on mediastinal structures, (2) respiratory difficulties caused by encroachment on the lungs and airways, (3) difficulty in swallowing caused by compression of the esophagus, (4) persistent cough from irritation of the recurrent laryngeal nerves, (5) pain caused by erosion of bone (i.e., ribs and vertebral bodies), (6) cardiac disease due to valvular insufficiency or narrowing of the coronary ostia, and (7) aortic rupture. Most patients with syphilitic aneurysms die of heart failure induced by aortic valvular incompetence.

Aortic Dissection

Aortic dissection is a catastrophic event whereby blood splays apart the laminar planes of the media to form a blood-filled channel within the aortic wall (see Figs. 10–17 and 10–19); this channel often ruptures through the adventitia and into various spaces, where it causes either massive hemorrhage or cardiac tamponade (hemorrhage into the pericardial sac). In contrast to atherosclerotic and

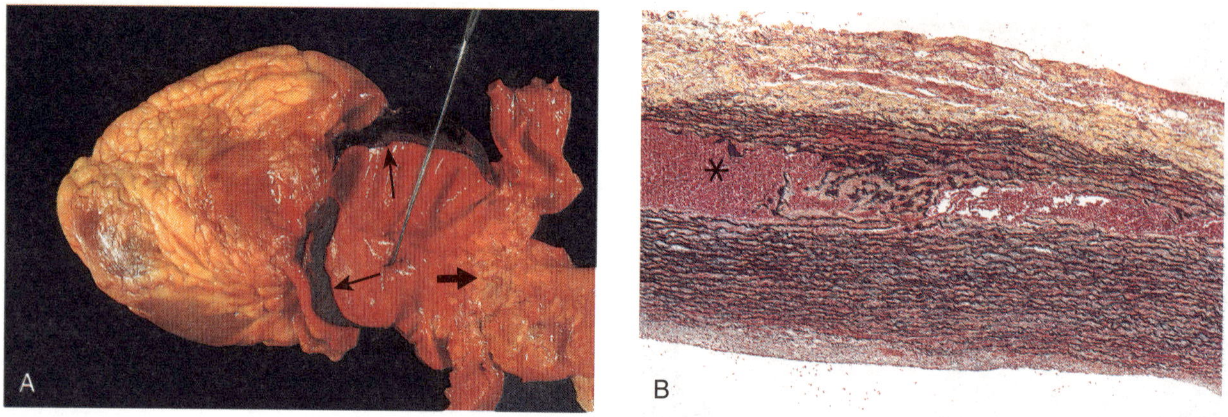

Figure 10–19

Aortic dissection. **A,** Gross photograph of an opened aorta with proximal dissection originating from a small, oblique intimal tear (identified by the probe), allowing blood to enter the media and create an intramural hematoma (*narrow arrows*). Note that the intimal tear has occurred in a region largely free of atherosclerotic plaque and that propagation of the intramural hematoma is arrested at a site more distally where atherosclerosis begins (*broad arrow*). **B,** Histologic view of the dissection demonstrating an aortic intramural hematoma (*asterisk*). Aortic elastic layers are *black* and blood is *red* in this section, stained with the Movat stain.

syphilitic aneurysms, aortic dissection may or may not be associated with aortic dilation. Consequently, the older term "dissecting aneurysm" is discouraged.

Aortic dissection occurs principally in two epidemiologic groups: (1) men aged 40 to 60 years, with antecedent hypertension (more than 90% of cases of dissection), and (2) younger patients with systemic or localized abnormalities of connective tissue affecting the aorta (e.g., Marfan syndrome; Chapter 7). Dissections can also be iatrogenic (e.g., complicating arterial cannulations during diagnostic catheterization or cardiopulmonary bypass). Rarely, for unknown reasons, dissection of the aorta or other branches, including the coronary arteries, occurs during or after pregnancy. Dissection is unusual in the presence of substantial atherosclerosis or other causes of medial scarring, such as syphilis, presumably because the medial fibrosis inhibits propagation of the dissecting hematoma.

Pathogenesis. Hypertension is *the* major risk factor for aortic dissection. Aortas in hypertensive patients show medial hypertrophy of the vasa vasorum associated with ECM degenerative changes and variable loss of medial SMCs, suggesting that pressure-related mechanical injury and/or ischemic injury (due to diminished flow through the vasa vasorum) is somehow contributory. Nevertheless, the pathways by which hypertension causes aortic medial damage remain ill-defined. Moreover, recognizable medial damage appears to be neither a prerequisite for dissection nor a guarantee that dissection is imminent. Occasionally, dissections occur in the setting of rather trivial medial degeneration, and conversely marked degenerative changes are frequently seen at autopsies of patients who are completely free from dissection.

A considerably smaller number of dissections is related to inherited or acquired connective tissue disorders causing abnormal vascular ECM (e.g., Marfan syndrome, Ehlers-Danlos syndrome, vitamin C deficiency, copper metabolic defects). Among these, Marfan syndrome is probably the most common; it is an autosomal dominant disease of fibrillin, an ECM scaffolding protein required for normal elastic tissue synthesis. Patients have skeletal abnormalities (elongated axial bones) and ocular findings (lens subluxation) in addition to the cardiovascular manifestations (Chapter 7).

Regardless of the underlying etiology that causes medial weakness, the trigger for the intimal tear and initial intramural aortic hemorrhage is not known in most cases. Nevertheless, once the tear has occurred, blood flow under systemic pressure dissects through the media, fostering progression of the medial hematoma. Accordingly, aggressive pressure-reducing therapy may be effective in limiting an evolving dissection. In some cases, disruption of penetrating vessels of the vasa vasorum can give rise to an intramural hematoma *without* an intimal tear.

Morphology

In the vast majority of spontaneous dissections, the intimal tear marking the point of origin of the dissection is found in the ascending aorta, usually within 10 cm of the aortic valve (see Fig. 10–19A). Such tears are usually transverse or oblique and 1 to 5 cm in length, with sharp, jagged edges. The dissection can extend along the aorta retrograde toward the heart as well as distally, sometimes all the way into the iliac and femoral arteries. The dissecting hematoma spreads characteristically along the laminar planes of the aorta, usually approximately between the middle and outer thirds (see Fig. 10–19B). It often ruptures out through the adventitia, causing massive hemorrhage. In some (lucky) instances, the dissecting hematoma reenters the lumen of the aorta, producing a second distal intimal tear and a new vascular channel within the media of the aortic wall (and resulting in a "double-barreled aorta" with a false channel). This averts a fatal extra-aortic hemorrhage. In the course of time, false channels may become endothelialized and can be recognized as chronic dissections.

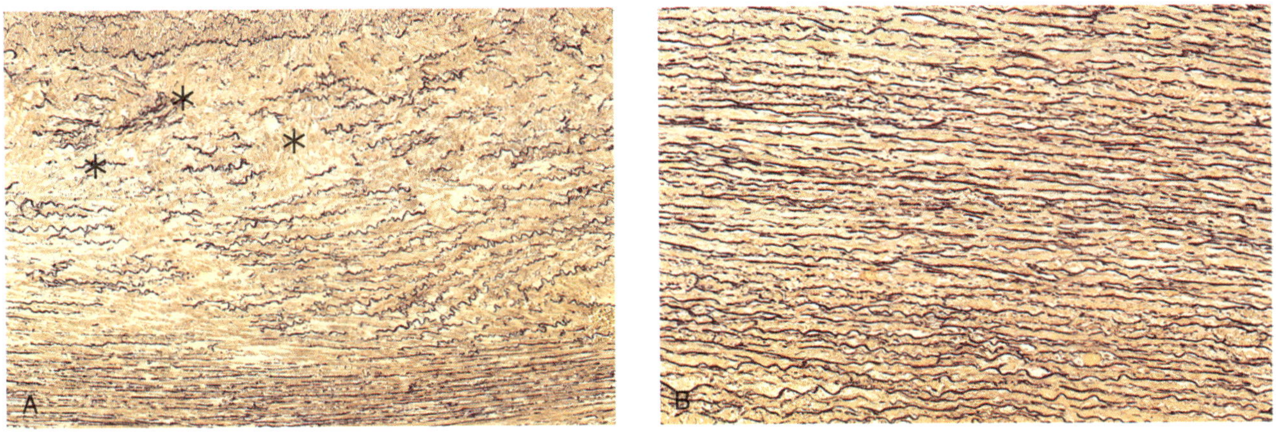

Figure 10–20

Cystic medial degeneration. Elastin is stained *black*. **A,** Cross-section of aortic media from a patient with Marfan syndrome, showing marked elastin fragmentation and formation of areas devoid of elastin that resemble cystic spaces (*asterisks*). **B,** Normal media for comparison, showing the regular layered pattern of elastic tissue.

In most cases, no specific underlying causal pathology can be identified in the aortic wall. The most frequent pre-existing histologically detectable lesion is cystic medial degeneration (CMD). CMD is characterized by elastic tissue fragmentation and separation of the elastic and SMC elements of the media by cystic spaces filled with the amorphous proteoglycan-rich ECM. Ultimately, there may be large-scale loss of elastic laminae (Fig. 10–20). Inflammation is characteristically absent. CMD of the aorta frequently accompanies Marfan syndrome, but patients with dissection caused by hypertension have variable nonspecific changes in aortic wall histology ranging from mild fragmentation of elastic tissue (most commonly) to overt CMD.

Clinical Course. The risk and nature of serious complications of dissection depend strongly on the level of the aorta affected; the most serious complications occur with dissections that involve the aorta from the aortic valve to the arch. Thus, aortic dissections are generally classified into two types (Fig. 10–21):

- The more common (and dangerous) *proximal* lesions (called *type A dissections*), involving either the ascending aorta only or both the ascending and descending aorta (types I and II of the DeBakey classification)
- *Distal lesions not involving the ascending part* and usually beginning distal to the subclavian artery (called *type B dissections* or DeBakey type III).

The classic clinical symptoms of aortic dissection are the *sudden onset of excruciating pain*, usually beginning in the anterior chest, radiating to the back between the scapulae, and moving downward as the dissection progresses; the pain can be confused with that of myocardial infarction.

The most common cause of death is rupture of the dissection outward into any of the three body cavities (i.e., pericardial, pleural, or peritoneal). Retrograde dissection into the aortic root can cause disruption of the aortic valvular apparatus. Thus, common clinical manifestations include *cardiac tamponade, aortic insufficiency,* and *myocardial infarction* or *extension of the dissection into the great arteries* of the neck or into the coronary, renal, mesenteric, or iliac arteries, causing critical vascular obstruction; compression of spinal arteries may cause transverse myelitis.

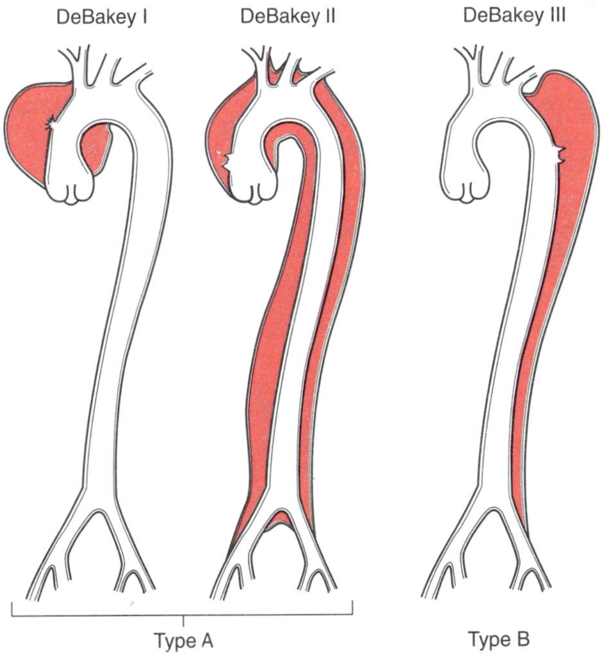

Figure 10–21

Classification of dissections. Type A (proximal) involves the ascending aorta, either in isolation (DeBakey I) or as part of a more extensive dissection (DeBakey II). Type B (distal, or DeBakey III) dissections arise after the take off of the great vessels. The serious complications predominantly occur in Type A dissections, which therefore mandate surgical intervention.

Previously, aortic dissection was typically fatal, but the prognosis has markedly improved. Rapid diagnosis and institution of intensive antihypertensive therapy, coupled with surgical procedures involving plication of the aorta permits survival of 65% to 75% of patients.

VASCULITIS

Vasculitis, or inflammation of vessel walls, occurs in diverse clinical settings. Depending on the vascular bed affected (e.g., central nervous system vs. heart vs. small bowel), the manifestations can be protean. Besides the findings referable to the specific tissue(s) involved, clinical manifestations common to these entities typically include constitutional signs and symptoms such as fever, myalgia, arthralgias, and malaise.

Vessels of any type in virtually any organ can be affected, and most vasculitides can affect all small vessels from arterioles to capillary to venules. Nevertheless, several of the vasculitides tend to affect only vessels of particular caliber or tissue beds; thus, there are vasculitic entities that primarily affect the aorta and medium-sized arteries, while others principally affect only smaller arterioles. Some 20 primary forms of vasculitis are recognized, and classifications schemes attempt (with variable success) to group them according to vessel size, role of immune complexes, presence of specific autoantibodies, granuloma formation, organ tropism, and even population demographics (Table 10–4). As we will see, there is considerable clinical and pathologic overlap among many of these disorders.

The two most common pathogenic mechanisms of vasculitis are immune-mediated inflammation and direct invasion of vascular walls by infectious pathogens. Predictably, *infections can also indirectly induce a noninfectious vasculitis,* for example, by generating immune complexes or triggering cross-reactivity. In any given patient, it is critical to distinguish between infectious and immunologic mechanisms, because immunosuppressive therapy is appropriate for immune-mediated vasculitis but could very well be counterproductive for infectious vasculitides. Physical and chemical injury, such as from irradiation, mechanical trauma, and toxins, can also cause vasculitis.

Noninfectious Vasculitis

The main immunologic mechanisms that initiate noninfectious vasculitis are (1) immune complex deposition, (2) antineutrophil cytoplasmic antibodies (ANCAs), and (3) anti-endothelial cell antibodies.

Immune Complex–Associated Vaculitis. The lesions resemble those found in experimental immune complex-mediated conditions (e.g., serum sickness; Chapter 5). Antibody and complement are typically detected in vasculitic lesions, although the nature of the antigens responsible for such deposition cannot usually be determined.

Table 10–4 Classification and Characteristics of Selected Immune-Mediated Vasculitides

Vasculitis type*	Examples	Description
Large-Vessel Vasculitis (Aorta and Large Branches to Extremities, Head, and Neck)	Giant-cell (temporal) arteritis	Granulomatous inflammation; also frequently involves the temporal artery. Usually occurs in patients older than age 50 and is associated with polymyalgia rheumatica.
	Takayasu arteritis	Granulomatous inflammation usually occurring in patients younger than age 50
Medium-Vessel Vasculitis (Main Visceral Arteries and Their Branches)	Polyarteritis nodosa	Necrotizing inflammation typically involving renal arteries but sparing pulmonary vessels
	Kawasaki disease	Arteritis with mucocutaneous lymph node syndrome; usually occurs in children. Coronary arteries can be involved with aneurysm formation and/or thrombosis.
Small-Vessel Vasculitis (Arterioles, Venules, Capillaries, and Occasionally Small Arteries)	Wegener granulomatosis	Granulomatous inflammation involving the respiratory tract and necrotizing vasculitis affecting small vessels, including glomerulonephritis. Associated with c-ANCAs.
	Churg-Strauss syndrome	Eosinophil-rich and granulomatous inflammation involving the respiratory tract and necrotizing vasculitis affecting small vessels. Associated with asthma and blood eosinophilia. Associated with p-ANCAs.
	Microscopic polyangiitis	Necrotizing small-vessel vasculitis with few or no immune deposits; necrotizing arteritis of small and medium-sized arteries can occur. Necrotizing glomerulonephritis and pulmonary capillaritis are common. Associated with p-ANCAs.

*Note that some small- and large-vessel vasculitides may involve medium-sized arteries, but large- and medium-sized vessel vasculitides do not involve vessels smaller than arteries.

Modified from Jennette JC, et al. Nomenclature of systemic vasculitides: The proposal of an international consensus conference. Arthritis Rheum 37:187, 1994.

c-ANCAs, antineutrophil cytoplasmic antibodies, cytoplasmic localization; p-ANCAs, antineutrophil cytoplasmic antibodies, perinuclear localization.

Circulating immune (antigen-antibody) complexes may also be seen—for example, DNA–anti-DNA complexes in systemic lupus erythematosus (SLE)–associated vasculitis (Chapter 5). Several examples follow:

- Immune complex deposition underlies the vasculitis associated with drug hypersensitivity. In some cases (e.g., penicillin), the drugs bind to serum proteins; other agents, like streptokinase, are themselves foreign proteins. In either event, antibodies directed against the drug-modified self proteins or foreign molecules lead to the formation of immune complexes. Manifestations range across the spectrum of vasculitides, frequently involving the skin (see below), and can be mild and self-limiting or severe and even fatal. It is important to identify such disorders as drug hypersensitivities, since discontinuation of the offending agent is often curative.
- In vasculitis associated *secondarily* with viral infections, antibody to viral proteins may form immune complexes detectable in the serum and in the vascular lesions; for example, as many as 30% of patients with polyarteritis nodosa (see below) have an underlying hepatitis B infection with vasculitis attributable to complexes of hepatitis B surface antigen (HBsAg) and antibodies to HBsAg.

In most cases, it is not clear whether the antigen-antibody complexes form elsewhere and then deposit in a particular vascular bed, or if they form in situ from the seeding of antigen in a vessel wall, with subsequent antibody binding (Chapter 5). Moreover, in many cases of presumed immune complex vasculitis, there is a distressing scarcity of antigen-antibody deposits. Either the immune complexes have been largely degraded at the time that the tissue diagnosis is made, or other mechanisms must be considered for such "pauci-immune" vasculitides.

Antineutrophil Cytoplasmic Antibodies. Many patients with vasculitis have circulating antibodies that react with neutrophil cytoplasmic antigens, so-called ANCAs. ANCAs are a heterogeneous group of autoantibodies directed against constituents (mainly enzymes) of neutrophil primary granules, monocyte lysosomes, and endothelial cells. Two general types of ANCAs are recognized based on immunofluorescence staining patterns:

- Cytoplasmic localization (c-ANCA), wherein the most common target antigen is proteinase-3 (PR3), a neutrophil granule constituent
- Perinuclear localization (p-ANCA), wherein most of the autoantibodies are specific for myeloperoxidase (MPO).

Either ANCA specificity can occur in ANCA-associated vasculitides, but *c-ANCA is typical of Wegener granulomatosis and p-ANCA is found in most cases of microscopic polyangiitis and Churg-Strauss syndrome* (see below).

ANCAs serve as useful quantitative diagnostic markers for the ANCA-associated vasculitides, and their levels can reflect the degree of inflammatory activity. Perhaps more significantly, the close association between ANCA titers and disease activity suggests an important pathogenic role. Although the precise mechanisms are unknown, ANCAs can directly activate neutrophils and thus may mimic an inflammatory state that continually recruits and stimulates neutrophils to release reactive oxygen species and proteolytic enzymes. Moreover, although the antigenic targets of ANCAs are primarily intracellular and therefore might not be expected to be accessible to circulating antibodies, newer evidence suggests that ANCA antigens (in particular PR3) may be either constitutively expressed at low levels on the plasma membrane or translocated to the cell surface in activated neutrophils.

A plausible mechanism for ANCA vasculitis is:

- Neutrophil release of PR3 and MPO (e.g., in the setting of infections) incites ANCA formation in a susceptible host.
- Some underlying disorder (e.g., infection, endotoxin exposure, etc.) elicits inflammatory cytokines, such as TNF, that result in surface expression of PR3 and MPO on neutrophils and other cell types.
- ANCAs react with these cytokine-primed cells and either cause direct injury (e.g., to endothelium) or induce activation (e.g., in neutrophils).
- ANCA-activated neutrophils degranulate and also cause injury by the release of reactive oxygen species, engendering EC toxicity and other direct tissue injury.

Interestingly, ANCAs directed against constituents other than PR3 and MPO are also found in some patients with inflammatory disorders that do not involve vasculitis (e.g., inflammatory bowel disease, primary sclerosing cholangitis, and rheumatoid arthritis).

Anti-Endothelial Cell Antibodies. Antibodies to ECs may predispose to certain vasculitides, for example Kawasaki disease (see below).

We will now briefly present several of the best-characterized and generally recognized vasculitides, emphasizing that there is substantial overlap among the different entities. Moreover, it should be kept in mind that any given patient may not have a classic constellation of findings that allows the clinician to settle on a specific diagnosis.

Giant-Cell (Temporal) Arteritis

Giant-cell (temporal) arteritis is the most common of the vasculitides. It is a chronic, typically granulomatous inflammation of large to small-sized arteries; it principally affects the arteries in the head—especially the temporal arteries—but also the vertebral and ophthalmic arteries, as well as the aorta (*giant-cell aortitis*). Ophthalmic artery involvement can lead to sudden and permanent blindness.

Pathogenesis. The cause of giant-cell arteritis remains elusive, although the bulk of the evidence supports a T cell–mediated immune response to an unknown, possibly vessel wall, antigen. An immune origin is supported by the characteristic granulomatous response with associated helper T cells, a correlation with certain major histocompatibility complex (MHC) class II haplotypes, and a therapeutic response to steroids. The extraordinary predilection for a single vascular site (temporal artery) remains unexplained.

Temporal Arteritis is T-cell mediated.

Morphology

Involved arterial segments in giant-cell arteritis develop **nodular intimal thickening** with reduction of the lumen and occasional thrombosis. Classical lesions show **granulomatous inflammation** within the inner media centered on the internal elastic membrane; there is a lymphocyte (CD4+ more than CD8+) and macrophage infiltrate, with multinucleated giant cells, and **fragmentation of the internal elastic lamina** (Fig. 10–22). Occasionally, granulomas and giant cells are rare or absent, and lesions show only a nonspecific panarteritis with a mixed infiltrate composed predominantly of lymphocytes and macrophages with scattered neutrophils and eosinophils. Inflammatory lesions are not continuous along the vessel, and long segments of relatively normal artery may separate areas of inflammation. The healed stage of either pattern is marked by collagenous thickening of the vessel wall; organization of a luminal thrombus can transform the artery into a fibrous cord. End-stage scarring may be difficult to distinguish from age-associated changes.

Clinical Features. Temporal arteritis occurs only rarely in persons younger than 50 years of age. Symptoms may be only vague and constitutional—fever, fatigue, weight loss—or may involve facial pain or headache, most intense along the course of the superficial temporal artery, which is painful to palpation. Ocular symptoms (associated with involvement of the ophthalmic artery) abruptly appear in about 50% of patients; these range from diplopia to complete vision loss. Diagnosis depends on biopsy and histologic confirmation. However, because temporal arteritis is extremely segmental, adequate biopsy requires at least a 2- to 3-cm length of artery; even then, a negative biopsy result does not exclude the diagnosis. Treatment with corticosteroids is generally effective.

Takayasu Arteritis

This is a granulomatous vasculitis of medium and larger arteries characterized principally by ocular disturbances and marked weakening of the pulses in the upper extremities (hence its other name, "pulseless disease"). Takayasu arteritis manifests with transmural fibrous thickening of the aorta—particularly the aortic arch and great vessels—with severe luminal narrowing of the major branch vessels (Fig. 10–23). It occurs most frequently in women younger than 40 years of age; although traditionally associated with the Japanese population, it has a global distribution. The cause and pathogenesis are unknown, although immune mechanisms are suspected.

Morphology

Takayasu arteritis classically involves the **aortic arch** but in a third of cases also affects the remainder of the aorta and its branches; pulmonary arteries are involved in 50% of patients. Gross changes include intimal hyperplasia and irregular thickening of the vessel wall; when the aortic arch is involved, the origin for the great

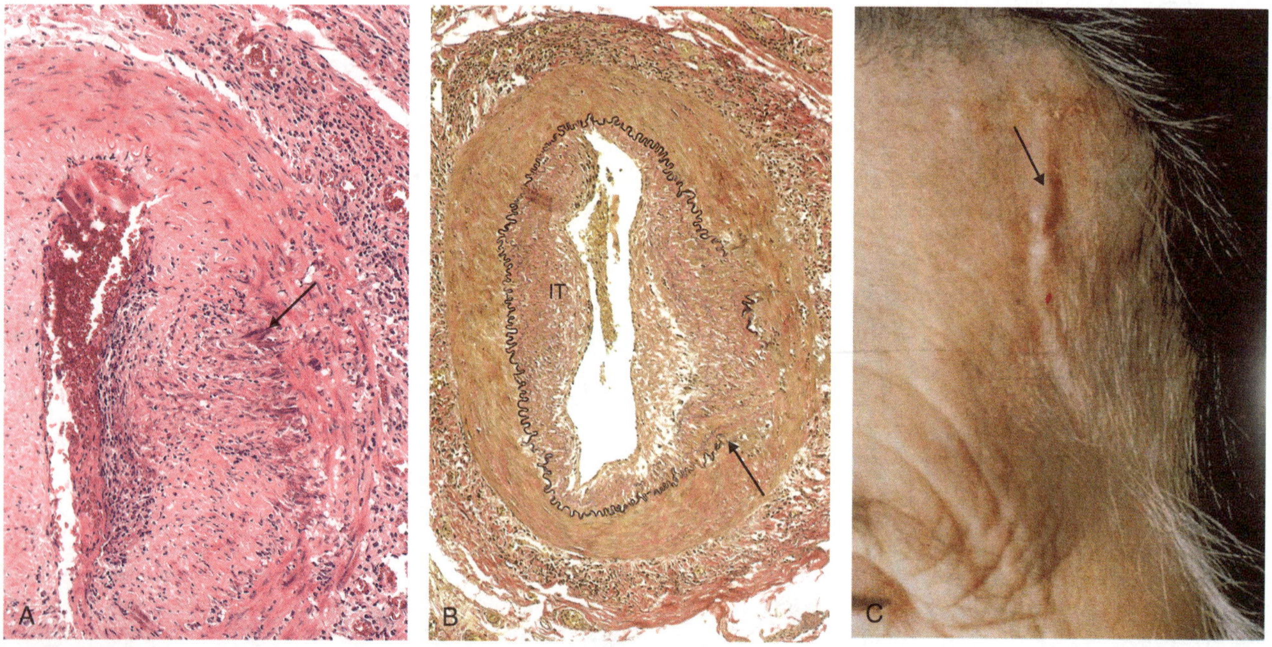

Figure 10–22

Temporal (giant-cell) arteritis. **A,** H+E-stained section of temporal artery showing giant cells at the degenerating internal elastic membrane (*arrow*). **B,** Elastic tissue stain demonstrating focal destruction of internal elastic membrane (*arrow*) and intimal thickening (*IT*) characteristic of long-standing or healed arteritis. **C,** Temporal artery of a patient with temporal arteritis showing a thickened, nodular, and tender segment of a vessel on the surface of head (*arrow*). (**C,** From Salvarani C, et al.: Polymyalgia rheumatica and giant-cell arteritis. N Engl J Med 347:261–271, 2002. Copyright © 2002 Massachusetts Medical Society. All rights reserved.)

vessels can be markedly narrowed or even obliterated (Fig. 10–23A and B). Such narrowing explains the weakness of the peripheral pulses; coronary and renal arteries may be similarly affected. Histologically, the changes range from adventitial mononuclear infiltrates with perivascular cuffing of the vasa vasorum, to intense mononuclear inflammation in the media, to granulomatous inflammation, replete with giant cells and patchy medial necrosis. The histology (Fig. 10–23C) may be indistinguishable from temporal arteritis. **Thus, distinctions between active giant-cell lesions of the aorta are based largely on the age of the patient; most aortic giant-cell lesions in young patients (age 40 years and younger) are designated as Takayasu aortitis.** As the disease progresses, collagenous scarring, with admixed chronic inflammatory infiltrates, occurs in all three layers of the vessel wall. Prominent intimal involvement causes the luminal narrowing and obliteration. Occasionally, aortic root involvement causes dilation and aortic valve insufficiency.

Clinical Features. Initial symptoms are usually nonspecific, including fatigue, weight loss, and fever. With progression, vascular symptoms appear and dominate the clinical picture. These include *reduced blood pressure and weaker pulses in the upper extremities relative to the lower extremities,* with coldness or numbness of the fingers; ocular disturbances, including visual defects, retinal hemorrhages, and total blindness; and neurologic deficits. Involvement of the more distal aorta may lead to claudication of the legs; pulmonary artery involvement may cause pulmonary hypertension. Narrowing of the coronary ostia may lead to myocardial infarction, and involvement of the renal arteries leads to systemic hypertension in roughly half of patients. The course of the disease is variable. In some persons there is rapid progression, but in others a quiescent stage is reached in 1 to 2 years, permitting long-term survival, albeit sometimes with visual or neurologic deficits.

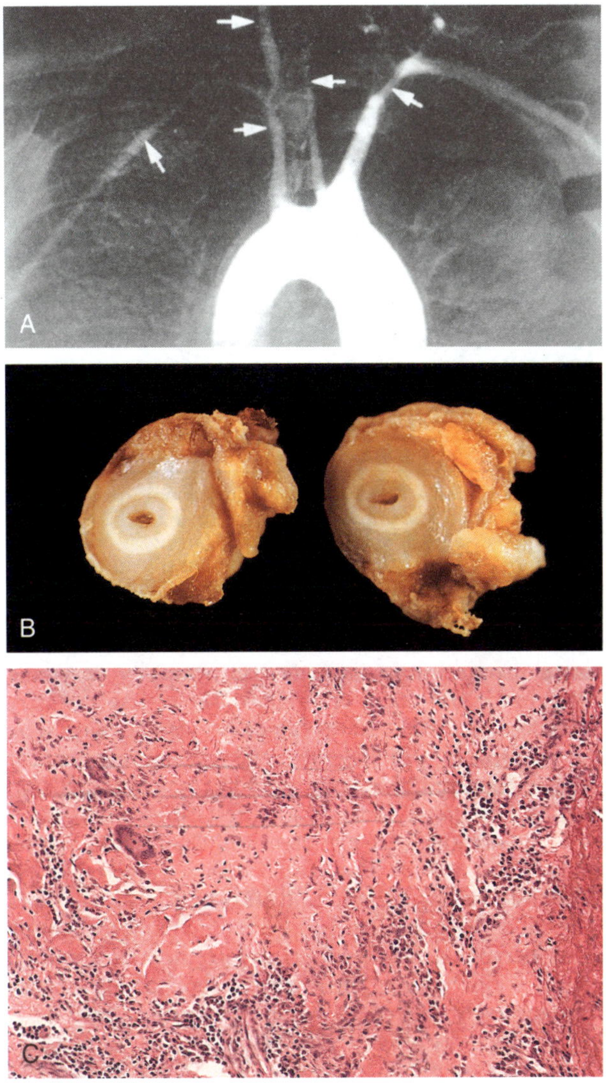

Figure 10–23

Takayasu arteritis. **A,** Aortic arch angiogram showing narrowing of the brachiocephalic, carotid, and subclavian arteries (*arrows*). **B,** Gross photograph of two cross-sections of the right carotid artery from the patient shown in **A**, demonstrating marked intimal thickening with minimal residual lumen. **C,** Histologic view of active Takayasu aortitis, illustrating destruction and fibrosis of the arterial media and an infiltrate of mononuclear inflammation, including giant cells.

Polyarteritis Nodosa

Polyarteritis nodosa (PAN) is a systemic vasculitis of small or medium-sized muscular arteries (but not arterioles, capillaries, or venules), typically involving renal and visceral vessels but sparing the pulmonary circulation.

Morphology

Classic PAN is characterized by segmental transmural necrotizing inflammation of **small to medium-sized arteries.** Vessels of the kidneys, heart, liver, and GI tract are involved in descending order of frequency. Lesions usually involve only **part of the vessel circumference,** with a predilection for branch points. The inflammatory process weakens the arterial wall and can lead to aneurysms or even rupture. Impaired perfusion with ulcerations, infarcts, ischemic atrophy, or hemorrhages in the distribution of affected vessels may be the first sign of disease.

During the acute phase there is **transmural inflammation** of the arterial wall with a mixed infiltrate of neutrophils, eosinophils, and mononuclear cells, frequently accompanied by **fibrinoid necrosis** (Fig. 10–24). Luminal thrombosis can occur. Later, the acute inflammatory infiltrate is replaced by fibrous (occasionally nodular) thickening of the vessel wall that can extend into the adventitia. Characteristically, all stages of activity (from early to late) may coexist in different vessels or even within the same vessel, suggesting ongoing and recurrent pathogenic insults.

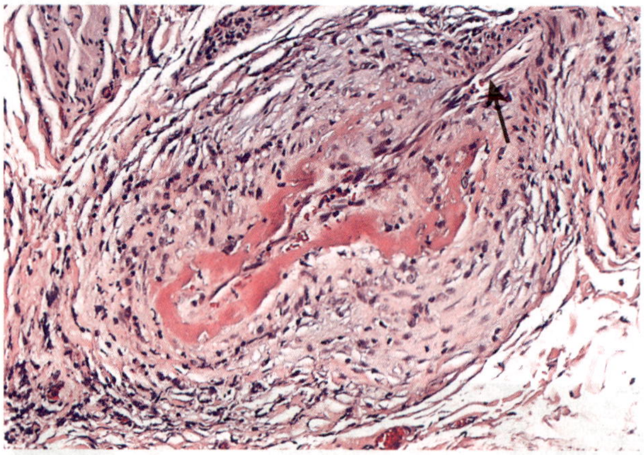

Figure 10–24

Polyarteritis nodosa. There is segmental fibrinoid necrosis and thrombotic occlusion of the lumen of this small artery. Note that part of the vessel wall at the upper right (*arrow*) is uninvolved. (Courtesy of Dr. Sidney Murphree, Department of Pathology, University of Texas, Southwestern Medical School, Dallas, Texas.)

Clinical Course. PAN is a disease primarily of young adults, but it can occur at all ages. The course can vary from acute to chronic but is typically episodic, with long symptom-free intervals. Because the vascular involvement is widely scattered, the clinical findings may be varied and puzzling. The most common manifestations are malaise, fever, and weight loss; hypertension, usually developing rapidly; abdominal pain and melena (bloody stool) caused by vascular GI lesions; diffuse muscular aches and pains; and peripheral neuritis, predominantly affecting motor nerves. Renal (arterial) involvement is common and a major cause of death, although glomerular arteriolar involvement (and thus, glomerulonephritis) is absent. Biopsy is often necessary to confirm the diagnosis. There is no association with ANCA, but some 30% of patients with PAN have hepatitis B antigenemia, and HBsAg-HBsAb immune complexes can be demonstrated in their lesions. If untreated, the disease is fatal in most cases; therapy with corticosteroids and cyclophosphamide results in remissions or cures in 90%.

Kawasaki Disease

Kawasaki disease is an acute febrile, usually self-limited illness of infancy and childhood (80% of patients are younger than 4 years) associated with an arteritis affecting large to medium-sized, and even small vessels. Its clinical significance stems from the involvement of coronary arteries; coronary arteritis can result in aneurysms that rupture or thrombose, causing acute myocardial infarctions. Kawasaki disease is the leading cause of acquired heart disease in children. Originally described in Japan, the disease is now increasingly reported in the United States and other countries.

Pathogenesis. The etiology is uncertain, but the vasculitis is thought to result from a delayed-type hypersensitivity response of T cells to an as yet uncharacterized vascular antigen. This leads to cytokine production, with B-cell activation and the formation of autoantibodies to ECs and SMCs. The autoantibodies precipitate the acute vasculitis. It is speculated that in genetically susceptible persons, a variety of infectious agents (most likely viral) can trigger the disease.

Morphology

The vasculitis of Kawasaki disease is PAN-like, with pronounced inflammation affecting the entire thickness of the vessel wall; nevertheless, the fibrinoid necrosis is usually less prominent in Kawasaki disease than in PAN. Although the acute vasculitis subsides spontaneously or in response to treatment, aneurysm formation, or thrombosis and myocardial infarction, can supervene. As with other causes of arteritis, healed lesions may have obstructive intimal thickening. Pathologic changes outside the cardiovascular system are rarely significant.

Clinical Course. Kawasaki disease is also called *mucocutaneous lymph node syndrome,* so named because it presents with conjunctival and oral erythema and erosion, edema of the hands and feet, erythema of the palms and soles, a desquamative rash, and cervical lymph node enlargement. Approximately 20% of untreated patients develop cardiovascular sequelae, ranging from asymptomatic coronary arteritis, to coronary artery ectasia and aneurysm formation, to giant coronary artery aneurysms (7–8 mm) with rupture or thrombosis, myocardial infarction, and sudden death. With intravenous immunoglobulin therapy, the rate of coronary artery disease is reduced to about 4%.

Microscopic Polyangiitis

This is a necrotizing vasculitis that generally affects capillaries as well as arterioles and venules of a size smaller than those involved in PAN; rarely, larger arteries may be involved. It is also called hypersensitivity vasculitis or leukocytoclastic vasculitis. *Unlike PAN, all lesions of microscopic polyangiitis tend to be of the same age in any given patient*. The skin, mucous membranes, lungs, brain, heart, GI tract, kidneys, and muscle can all be involved; *in contrast to PAN, necrotizing glomerulonephritis (90% of patients) and pulmonary capillaritis are particularly common*. Disseminated vascular lesions of hypersensitivity angiitis can also occur as a presentation of other disorders (e.g., Henoch-Schönlein purpura, essential mixed cryoglobulinemia, and vasculitis associated with connective tissue disorders).

Pathogenesis. In many cases, an antibody response to antigens such as drugs (e.g., penicillin), microorganisms (e.g., streptococci), heterologous proteins, or tumor proteins is the presumed cause. This can result in immune complex deposition, or it may trigger secondary immune responses that are ultimately causal; in this regard it is noteworthy that p-ANCAs are present in more than 70% of patients. Recruitment and activation of neutrophils within a particular vascular bed are probably responsible for the manifestations of the disease.

Morphology

Microscopic polyangiitis is characterized by segmental fibrinoid necrosis of the media with focal transmural necrotizing lesions; granulomatous inflammation is absent. These lesions morphologically resemble PAN but typically spare medium-sized and larger arteries; consequently, PAN-like macroscopic infarcts are uncommon. In some areas (typically post-capillary venules), only infiltrating and fragmenting neutrophils are seen, giving rise to the term **leukocytoclastic vasculitis** (Fig. 10–25A). Although immunoglobulins and complement components can be demonstrated in early skin lesions, **little or no immunoglobulin can be seen in most lesions (so-called "pauci-immune" injury).**

Clinical Course. Depending on the vascular bed involved, major clinical features include hemoptysis, hematuria, and proteinuria; bowel pain or bleeding; muscle pain or weakness; and palpable cutaneous purpura. With the exception of those who develop widespread renal or brain involvement, most patients respond to simple removal of the offending agent.

Wegener Granulomatosis

Wegener granulomatosis is a necrotizing vasculitis characterized by a triad of

- *Acute necrotizing granulomas* of the upper respiratory tract (ear, nose, sinuses, throat) or the lower respiratory tract (lung) or both
- *Necrotizing or granulomatous vasculitis* affecting small to medium-sized vessels (e.g., capillaries, venules, arterioles, and arteries), most prominent in the lungs and upper airways but affecting other sites as well
- Renal disease in the form of *focal necrotizing, often crescentic, glomerulonephritis*.

"Limited" forms of Wegener granulomatosis may be restricted to the respiratory tract. Conversely, a widespread form of the disease can affect eyes, skin, and other organs, notably the heart; clinically, this resembles PAN except that there is also respiratory involvement.

Pathogenesis. Wegener granulomatosis probably represents some form of cell-mediated hypersensitivity response, possibly to an inhaled infectious or other environmental agent; such a pathogenesis is supported by the presence of granulomas and a dramatic response to immunosuppressive therapy. c-ANCAs are present in up to 95% of cases; they are a useful marker of disease activity, and may participate in disease pathogenesis. Following immunosuppressive treatment, a rising c-ANCA titer suggests a relapse; most patients in remission have a negative test, or the titer falls significantly.

Morphology

The **upper respiratory** tract lesions of Wegener granulomatosis range from **inflammatory sinusitis with mucosal granulomas to ulcerative lesions of the nose, palate, or pharynx, rimmed by granulomas with geographic patterns of central necrosis** and accompanying vasculitis (Fig. 10–25B). The necrotizing granulomas are surrounded by a zone of fibroblastic proliferation with giant cells and leukocyte infiltrate, suggesting the possibility of mycobacterial or fungal infections. Multiple granulomata can coalesce to produce radiographically visible nodules that can also cavitate; late-stage disease

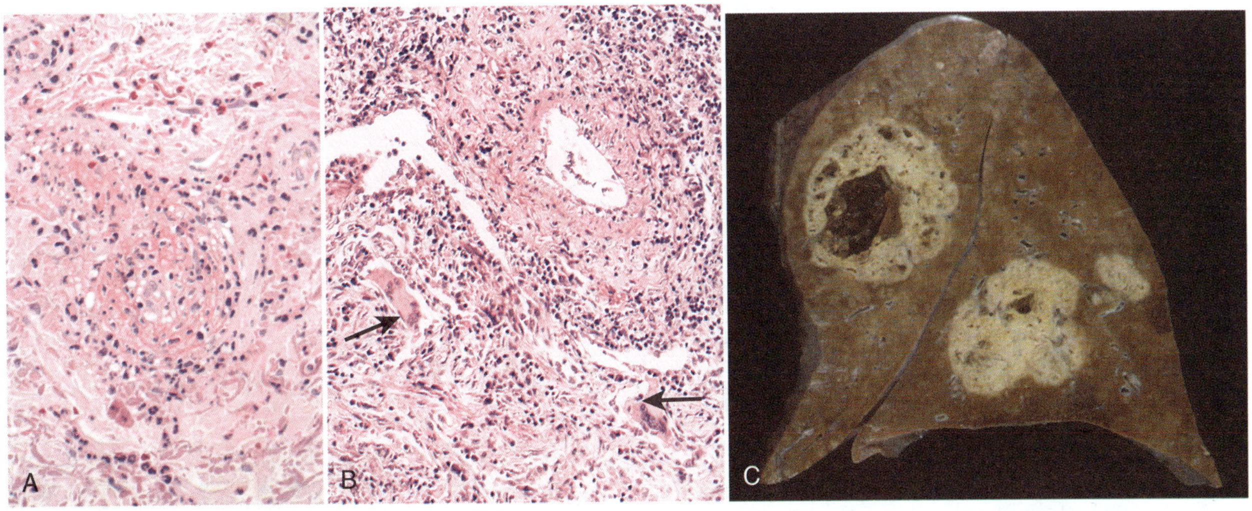

Figure 10–25

Representative forms of ANCA-associated small-vessel vasculitis. **A,** Microscopic polyangiitis (leukocytoclastic vasculitis) with fragmentation of neutrophils in and around blood vessel walls. **B** and **C,** Wegener granulomatosis. **B,** Vasculitis of a small artery with adjacent granulomatous inflammation including epithelioid cells and giant cells (*arrows*). **C,** Gross photo from the lung of a patient with fatal Wegener granulomatosis, demonstrating large nodular centrally cavitating lesions. (**A,** Courtesy of Dr. Scott Granter, Brigham and Women's Hospital, Boston, Massachusetts. **C,** Courtesy of Dr. Sidney Murphree, Department of Pathology, University of Texas Southwestern Medical School, Dallas, Texas.)

may be marked by extensive necrotizing granulomatous involvement of the parenchyma (Fig. 10–25C), and alveolar hemorrhage. Lesions may ultimately undergo progressive fibrosis and organization.

The **renal lesions** (Chapter 14) range over a spectrum. At one end, there is mild or early disease, where glomeruli show acute focal necrosis with thrombosis of isolated glomerular capillary loops (focal and segmental necrotizing glomerulonephritis). More advanced glomerular lesions are characterized by diffuse necrosis and parietal cell proliferation to form crescents (**crescentic glomerulonephritis**). Patients with focal lesions may have only hematuria and proteinuria responsive to therapy, whereas those with diffuse disease can develop rapidly progressive renal failure.

Clinical Features. Males are affected more often than are females, at an average age of about 40 years. Classical features include persistent pneumonitis with bilateral nodular and cavitary infiltrates (95%), chronic sinusitis (90%), mucosal ulcerations of the nasopharynx (75%), and evidence of renal disease (80%). Other features include rashes, muscle pains, articular involvement, mononeuritis or polyneuritis, and fever. If untreated, the course of the disease is malignant; 80% of patients die within 1 year.

Allergic granulomatosis and angiitis (Churg-Strauss syndrome) is a related entity distinguished by a strong association with *allergic rhinitis, bronchial asthma,* and *peripheral eosinophilia;* p-ANCAs are present in roughly half the patients. In Churg-Strauss syndrome, vascular lesions can resemble PAN and microscopic polyangiitis, but in the lung, heart, spleen, peripheral nerves, and skin there are also intravascular and extravascular granulomas, with striking infiltration of vessels and perivascular tissues by eosinophils. Unlike Wegener granulomatosis, severe renal disease is infrequent in Churg-Strauss syndrome; instead, coronary arteritis and myocarditis are the principal causes of morbidity and mortality.

Thromboangiitis Obliterans (Buerger Disease)

Thromboangiitis obliterans (Buerger disease) is a distinctive disease that often leads to vascular insufficiency; it is characterized by segmental, thrombosing acute and chronic inflammation of medium-sized and small arteries, principally the tibial and radial arteries, with occasional secondary extension into extremity veins and nerves. Buerger disease is a condition that occurs almost exclusively in heavy smokers of cigarettes, usually beginning before age 35.

Pathogenesis. The strong relationship to cigarette smoking is thought to involve direct toxicity to endothelium by some tobacco products, or an idiosyncratic immune response to the same agents. Most Buerger patients have hypersensitivity to intradermally injected tobacco extracts, and their vessels show impaired endothelium-dependent vasodilation when challenged with acetylcholine. Genetic influences are suggested by an increased prevalence in certain ethnic groups (Israeli, Indian subcontinent, Japanese) and an association with certain MHC haplotypes.

Morphology

Thromboangiitis obliterans is characterized by a **sharply segmental acute and chronic vasculitis of medium-sized and small arteries, predominantly of the extremities.** Microscopically, there is acute and chronic inflammation, accompanied by luminal thrombosis. Typically, the thrombus contains small **microabscesses** composed of neutrophils surrounded by granulomatous inflammation (Fig. 10–26); the thrombus may eventually organize and recanalize. The inflammatory process extends into contiguous veins and nerves (rare with other forms of vasculitis), and in time all three structures become encased in fibrous tissue.

Clinical Features. The early manifestations are a superficial nodular phlebitis, cold sensitivity of the Raynaud type (see below) in the hands, and pain in the instep of the foot induced by exercise (so-called *instep claudication*). In contrast to the vascular insufficiency caused by atherosclerosis, in Buerger disease the insufficiency tends to be accompanied by severe pain, even at rest, related undoubtedly to the neural involvement. Chronic ulcerations of the toes, feet, or fingers may appear, perhaps followed in time by frank gangrene. Abstinence from cigarette smoking in the early stages of the disease often brings dramatic relief from further attacks.

Vasculitis Associated with Other Disorders

Vasculitis resembling hypersensitivity angiitis or classic PAN may sometimes be associated with some other disorder, such as rheumatoid arthritis, SLE, malignancy,

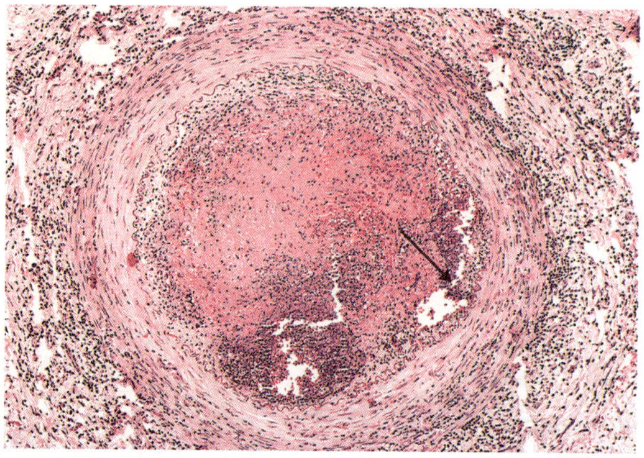

Figure 10–26

Thromboangiitis obliterans (Buerger disease). The lumen is occluded by a thrombus containing abscesses (*arrow*), and the vessel wall is infiltrated with leukocytes.

or systemic illnesses such as mixed cryoglobulinemia, antiphospholipid antibody syndrome (Chapter 4), and Henoch-Schönlein purpura. *Rheumatoid vasculitis* occurs predominantly after long-standing, severe rheumatoid arthritis and usually affects small and medium-sized arteries, leading to visceral infarction; it may also cause a clinically significant aortitis. Identifying the underlying pathology may be therapeutically important. For example, distinguishing between *lupus vasculitis* (Chapter 5) and the morphologically similar antiphospholipid antibody syndrome is clinically important, as aggressive anti-inflammatory therapy is required in the former, and aggressive anticoagulant therapy is indicated in the latter.

Infectious Vasculitis

Localized arteritis may be caused by the direct invasion of infectious agents, usually bacteria or fungi, and in particular *Aspergillus* and *Mucor* species. Vascular invasion can be part of a more general tissue infection (e.g., bacterial pneumonia or adjacent to abscesses), or—less commonly—it may arise from hematogenous spread of bacteria during septicemia or embolization from infective endocarditis.

Vascular infections can weaken arterial walls and give rise to *mycotic aneurysms* (see earlier), or they can induce thrombosis and infarction. Thus, involvement of meningeal vessels in bacterial meningitis can cause thrombosis and infarction, ultimately extending a subarachnoid infection into the brain parenchyma.

SUMMARY

Vasculitis

- Vasculitis is inflammation of the vessel wall; although there are frequently systemic manifestations (including fever, malaise, myalgias, and arthralgias), specific symptoms depend on the vascular bed that is involved.
- Vasculitis can result from infections, but it more commonly has an immunologic basis such as immune complex deposition, ANCAs, or anti-EC antibodies.
- Different forms of vasculitis tend to specifically affect vessels of a particular caliber and location (summarized in Table 10–4).

RAYNAUD PHENOMENON

Raynaud phenomenon results from an exaggerated vasoconstriction of digital arteries and arterioles. These vascular changes induce paroxysmal pallor or cyanosis of the digits of the hands or feet; infrequently, the nose, earlobes, or lips can also be involved. Characteristically, the involved digits show red, white, and blue color changes from most proximal to most distal, correlating with proximal vasodilation, central vasoconstriction, and more distal cyanosis (Fig. 10–27). Raynaud phenomenon may be a primary disease entity or be secondary to a variety of conditions.

Primary Raynaud phenomenon (previously called Raynaud disease) reflects an exaggeration of central and local vasomotor responses to cold or emotion, with a prevalence in the general population of 3% to 5% and a predilection for young women. Structural changes in the arterial walls are absent except late in the course, when intimal thickening can appear. The course of primary Raynaud phenomenon is usually benign, but long-standing, chronic cases can result in atrophy of the skin, subcutaneous tissues, and muscles. Ulceration and ischemic gangrene are rare.

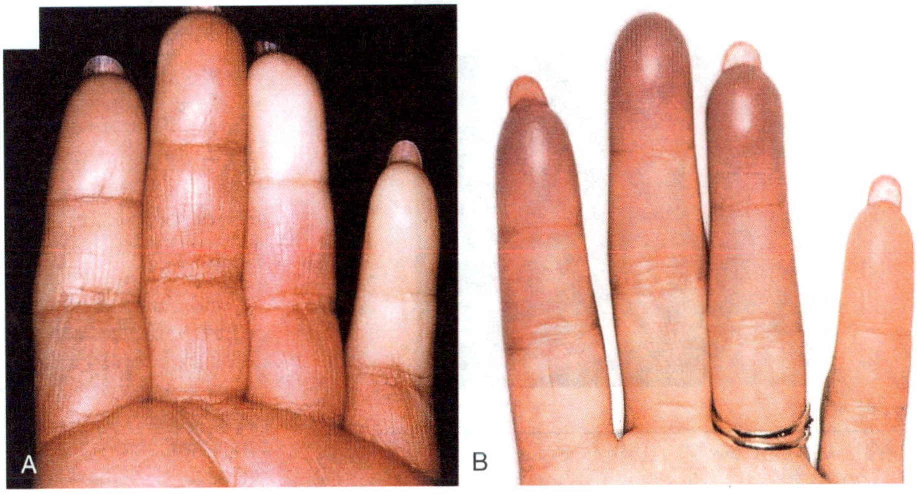

Figure 10–27

Raynaud phenomenon. **A,** Sharply demarcated pallor of the distal fingers resulting from the closure of digital arteries. **B,** Cyanosis of the fingertips. (From Salvarani C, et al.: Polymyalgia rheumatica and giant-cell arteritis. N Engl J Med 347:261, 2002.)

In contrast, *secondary Raynaud phenomenon* refers to vascular insufficiency of the extremities in the context of arterial disease caused by other entities including SLE, scleroderma, Buerger disease, or even atherosclerosis. Indeed, since Raynaud phenomenon may be the first manifestation of such conditions, any patient with symptoms should be evaluated; 10% will eventually manifest their underlying disease.

VEINS AND LYMPHATICS

Varicose veins and phlebothrombosis/thrombophlebitis together account for at least 90% of clinical disease associated with veins.

Varicose Veins

Varicose veins are abnormally dilated, tortuous veins produced by prolonged increase in intraluminal pressure and loss of vessel wall support. The *superficial veins* of the upper and lower leg are typically involved (Fig. 10–28). When legs are dependent for long periods, venous pressures in these sites can be markedly elevated (up to 10 times normal) and can lead to venous stasis and pedal edema, even in essentially normal veins (*simple orthostatic edema*). Some 10% to 20% of adult males and 25% to 33% of adult females develop lower extremity varicose veins; obesity increases the risk, and the higher incidence in women is a reflection of the elevated venous pressure in lower legs caused by pregnancy. A *familial tendency* toward premature varicosities results from imperfect venous wall development.

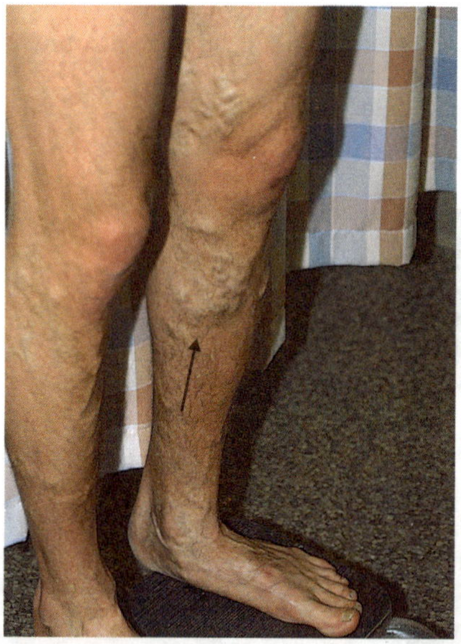

Figure 10–28

Varicose veins of the leg (*arrow*). (Courtesy of Dr. Magruder C. Donaldson, Brigham and Women's Hospital, Boston, Massachusetts.)

Morphology

Varicose veins show wall thinning at the points of maximal dilation with smooth muscle hypertrophy and intimal fibrosis in adjacent segments; elastic tissue degeneration and spotty medial calcifications (phlebosclerosis) also occur. Focal intraluminal thrombosis (due to stasis) and venous valve deformities (rolling and shortening) are common.

Clinical Course. Varicose dilation renders the venous valves incompetent and leads to stasis, congestion, edema, pain, and thrombosis. The most disabling sequelae include persistent edema in the extremity and secondary ischemic skin changes including stasis dermatitis and ulcerations; poor wound healing and superimposed infections can become chronic *varicose ulcers. Notably, embolism from these superficial veins is very rare. This is in sharp contrast to the relatively frequent thromboembolism that arises from thrombosed deep veins* (see below and Chapter 4).

Varicosities also occur in two other sites that deserve mention:

- *Esophageal varices.* Liver cirrhosis (less frequently, portal vein obstruction or hepatic vein thrombosis) causes portal vein hypertension (Chapter 16). Portal hypertension leads to the opening of porto-systemic shunts, increasing blood flow into veins at the gastroesophageal junction (forming *esophageal varices*), the rectum (forming *hemorrhoids*), and periumbilical veins of the abdominal wall (forming a *caput medusa*). Esophageal varices are the most important, since their rupture can lead to massive (even fatal) upper GI hemorrhage.
- *Hemorrhoids* can also result from primary varicose dilation of the venous plexus at the anorectal junction (e.g., through prolonged pelvic vascular congestion due to pregnancy or straining to defecate). Hemorrhoids are uncomfortable and may be a source of bleeding; they can also thrombose and are prone to painful ulceration.

Thrombophlebitis and Phlebothrombosis

The deep leg veins account for more than 90% of cases of thrombophlebitis and *phlebothrombosis;* the two terms are largely interchangeable designations for venous thrombosis and inflammation. The periprostatic venous plexus in males and the pelvic venous plexus in females are additional sites, as are the large veins in the skull and the dural sinuses (especially in the setting of infection or inflammation). Peritoneal infections (e.g., peritonitis, appendicitis, salpingitis, and pelvic abscesses) can lead to portal vein thrombosis. For deep venous thrombosis (DVT) of legs, *congestive heart failure, neoplasia* (see below), *pregnancy, obesity, the postoperative state, and prolonged bed rest or immobilization are the most important clinical predispositions.* Genetic hypercoagulability syndromes (Chapter 4) can also be associated with venous thrombosis.

In patients with cancer, particularly adenocarcinomas, hypercoagulability occurs as a paraneoplastic syndrome related to tumor elaboration of procoagulant factors (Chapter 6). In this setting, venous thromboses classically appear in one site, disappear, and then reoccur in other veins, so-called *migratory thrombophlebitis (Trousseau sign).*

Thrombi in the legs tend to produce few, if any, reliable signs or symptoms. Indeed, local manifestations, including distal edema, cyanosis, superficial vein dilation, heat, tenderness, redness, swelling, and pain may be entirely absent, especially in bedridden patients. In some cases, pain can be elicited by pressure over affected veins, squeezing the calf muscles, or forced dorsiflexion of the foot *(Homan sign); absence of these findings does not exclude a diagnosis of DVT.*

Pulmonary embolism is a common and serious clinical complication of DVT (Chapter 4), resulting from fragmentation or detachment of the venous thrombus. In many cases, the first manifestation of thrombophlebitis is a pulmonary embolus. Depending on the size and number of emboli, the outcome can range from no symptoms at all to death.

Superior and Inferior Vena Caval Syndromes

The *superior vena caval syndrome* is usually caused by neoplasms that compress or invade the superior vena cava (e.g., bronchogenic carcinoma or mediastinal lymphoma). The resulting obstruction produces a characteristic clinical complex including marked dilation of the veins of the head, neck, and arms with cyanosis. Pulmonary vessels can also become compressed, inducing respiratory distress.

The *inferior vena caval syndrome* can be caused by neoplasms that compress or invade the inferior vena cava (IVC) or by a thrombus from the hepatic, renal, or lower extremity veins that propagates upward. Certain neoplasms—particularly hepatocellular carcinoma and renal cell carcinoma—show a striking tendency to grow within veins, and these may ultimately occlude the IVC. IVC obstruction induces marked lower extremity edema, distention of the superficial collateral veins of the lower abdomen, and—with renal vein involvement—massive proteinuria.

Lymphangitis and Lymphedema

Primary disorders of lymphatic vessels are extremely uncommon; secondary processes are much more common and develop in association with inflammation or malignancies.

Lymphangitis is the acute inflammation elicited when bacterial infections spread into and through the lymphatics; the most common agents are group A β-hemolytic streptococci, although any microbe can cause acute lymphangitis. The affected lymphatics are dilated and filled with an exudate of neutrophils and monocytes; these infiltrates can extend through the vessel wall into the perilymphatic tissues and, in severe cases, produce cellulitis or focal abscesses. Clinically, lymphangitis is recognized by red, painful subcutaneous streaks (the inflamed lymphatics), with painful enlargement of the draining lymph nodes *(acute lymphadenitis).* If bacteria are not contained within the lymph nodes, subsequent passage into the venous circulation can result in bacteremia or sepsis.

Primary lymphedema can occur as an isolated congenital defect (simple congenital lymphedema) or as the familial *Milroy disease (heredofamilial congenital lymphedema),* resulting from lymphatic agenesis or hypoplasia. *Secondary* or *obstructive lymphedema* represents the accumulation of interstitial fluid behind a blockage of a previously normal lymphatic; such obstruction can result from

- Malignant tumors obstructing either the lymphatic channels or the regional lymph nodes
- Surgical procedures that remove regional groups of lymph nodes (e.g., axillary lymph nodes in radical mastectomy)
- Postirradiation fibrosis
- Filariasis
- Postinflammatory thrombosis and scarring

Regardless of the cause, lymphedema increases the hydrostatic pressure in the lymphatics behind the obstruction and causes increased interstitial fluid. Persistence of this edema leads to increased deposition of interstitial connective tissue, with tissue expansion, *brawny induration* or *peau d'orange* appearance of the overlying skin, and eventually ulcers due to inadequate tissue perfusion. Milky accumulations of lymph in various spaces are designated *chylous ascites* (abdomen), *chylothorax,* and *chylopericardium;* these are caused by rupture of dilated lymphatics, typically obstructed secondary to an infiltrating tumor mass.

TUMORS

Tumors of blood vessels and lymphatics range from benign hemangiomas, to intermediate lesions that are locally aggressive but infrequently metastatic, to relatively rare, highly malignant angiosarcomas (Table 10–5). Primary tumors of large vessels (aorta, pulmonary artery, and vena cava) are extremely rare and are mostly connective tissue sarcomas. Congenital or developmental malformations and non-neoplastic reactive vascular proliferations (e.g., *bacillary angiomatosis*) can also present as tumor-like lesions.

Vascular neoplasms can be derived from ECs (e.g., hemangioma, lymphangioma, angiosarcoma) or can arise from cells that support and/or surround blood vessels (e.g., glomus tumor, hemangiopericytoma). Although a benign, well-differentiated hemangioma can usually be readily discriminated from an anaplastic, high-grade angiosarcoma, the distinction between benign and malignant can occasionally be difficult. General rules of thumb:

- Benign tumors usually produce obvious vascular channels filled with blood cells (lymphatics are filled with lymph), lined by a monolayer of normal ECs, without atypia.

Table 10–5 Classification of Vascular Tumors and Tumor-like Conditions

Benign Neoplasms, Developmental and Acquired Conditions
Hemangioma
Capillary hemangioma
Cavernous hemangioma
Pyogenic granuloma
Lymphangioma
Simple (capillary) lymphangioma
Cavernous lymphangioma (cystic hygroma)
Glomus tumor
Vascular ectasias
Nevus flammeus
Spider telangiectasia (arterial spider)
Hereditary hemorrhagic telangiectasis (Osler-Weber-Rendu disease)
Reactive vascular proliferations
Bacillary angiomatosis
Intermediate-Grade Neoplasms
Kaposi sarcoma
Hemangioendothelioma
Malignant Neoplasms
Angiosarcoma
Hemangiopericytoma

- Malignant tumors are more solidly cellular with cytologic anaplasia, including mitotic figures; they usually do not form well-organized vessels. The endothelial origin of neoplastic proliferations that do not form distinct vascular lumina can usually be confirmed by immunohistochemical demonstration of EC-specific markers such as CD31 or von Willebrand factor.

Because vascular tumors result from dysregulated vascular proliferation, the possibility of controlling such growth by inhibitors of blood vessel formation (antiangiogenic factors) is particularly exciting.

Benign Tumors and Tumor-like Conditions

Hemangioma

Hemangiomas are very common tumors characterized by increased numbers of normal or abnormal vessels filled with blood (Fig. 10–29); they may be difficult to distinguish from vascular malformations. These lesions constitute 7% of all benign tumors of infancy and childhood (Chapter 7). Most are present from birth and expand along with the growth of the child, but many of the capillary lesions eventually regress spontaneously. Although some hemangiomas can involve large portions of the body (called *angiomatosis*), most are localized; the majority are superficial lesions, often of the head or neck, but they can occur internally, with nearly one-third being found in the liver. Malignant transformation occurs rarely, if at all. There are several histologic and clinical variants:

Capillary Hemangioma. The most common variant, *capillary hemangiomas* occur in the skin, subcutaneous tissues, and mucous membranes of the oral cavities and lips, as well as in the liver, spleen, and kidneys. The "strawberry type," or *juvenile, hemangioma* of the skin of newborns is extremely common (1 in 200 births) and may be multiple. It grows rapidly in the first few months but then fades at 1 to 3 years of age and completely regresses by age 7 in 75% to 90% of cases.

Morphology

Capillary hemangiomas are bright red to blue and vary from a few millimeters to several centimeters in diameter; hemangiomas can be level with the surface of the skin or slightly elevated and have an intact overlying epithelium (Fig. 10–29A). Histologically, these are unencapsulated aggregates of closely packed, thin-walled capillaries, usually blood filled and lined by flattened endothelium; vessels are separated by scant connective tissue stroma (Fig. 10–29B). The lumina may be partially or completely thrombosed and organized. Vessel rupture accounts for hemosiderin pigment in these lesions as well as focal scarring.

Cavernous Hemangioma. These are characterized by large, dilated vascular channels; compared with capillary hemangiomas, *cavernous hemangiomas* are less well circumscribed and more frequently involve deep structures. Because they may be locally destructive and show no spontaneous tendency to regress, some may require surgery.

Morphology

Grossly, cavernous hemangiomas appear as red-blue, soft, spongy masses 1 to 2 cm in diameter; rare giant forms can affect large subcutaneous areas of the face, extremities, or other body regions. Histologically, the mass is sharply defined but not encapsulated, and it is composed of large, cavernous blood-filled vascular spaces separated by a mild-to-moderate amount of connective tissue stroma (Fig. 10–29C). Intravascular thrombosis with associated dystrophic calcification is common.

In most cases, the tumors are of little clinical significance; however, they can be a cosmetic disturbance and are vulnerable to traumatic ulceration and bleeding. Moreover, visceral hemagiomas detected by imaging studies may need to be distinguished from more ominous (e.g., malignant) lesions. Brain hemangiomas are most problematic, because they can cause pressure symptoms or rupture. Cavernous hemangiomas are a component of **von Hippel–Lindau disease** (Chapter 23), occurring within the cerebellum or brain stem and eye grounds, along with similar angiomatous lesions or cystic neoplasms in the pancreas and liver; von Hippel–Lindau disease is also associated with renal neoplasms (Chapter 14).

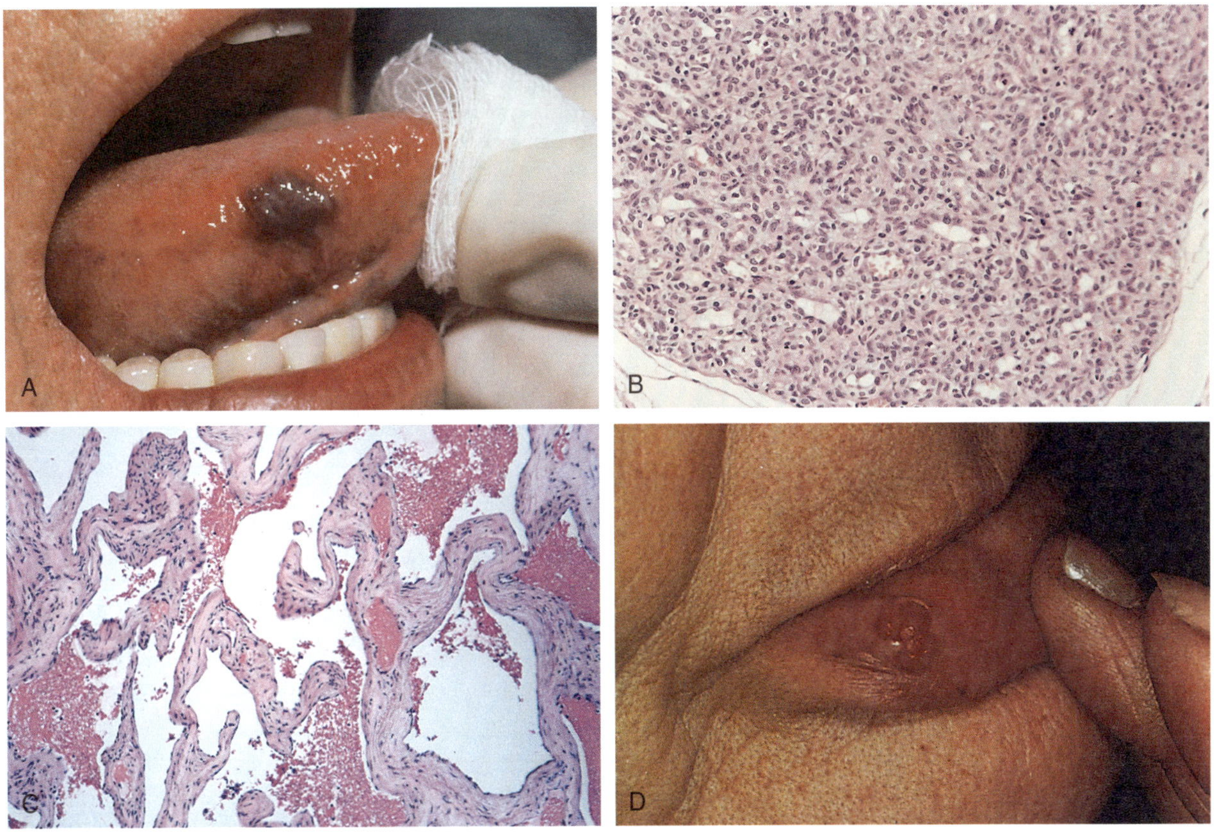

Figure 10–29

Hemangiomas. **A,** Hemangioma of the tongue. **B,** Histology of juvenile capillary hemangioma. **C,** Histology of cavernous hemangioma. **D,** Pyogenic granuloma of the lip. (**A** and **D,** Courtesy of Dr. John Sexton, Beth Israel Hospital, Boston, Massachusetts. **B,** Courtesy of Dr. Christopher D.M. Fletcher, Brigham and Women's Hospital, Boston, Massachusetts. **C,** Courtesy of Dr. Thomas Rogers, University of Texas Southwestern Medical School, Dallas, Texas.)

Pyogenic Granuloma. This form of capillary hemangioma is a rapidly growing peduncular red nodule on the skin, gingival, or oral mucosa; it bleeds easily and is often ulcerated (Fig. 10–29D). Roughly a third of lesions develop after trauma, reaching a size of 1 to 2 cm within a few weeks. The proliferating capillaries are often accompanied by extensive edema and an acute and chronic inflammatory infiltrate, an appearance with striking similarity to exuberant granulation tissue. *Pregnancy tumor* (granuloma gravidarum) is a pyogenic granuloma that occurs in the gingiva of 1% of pregnant women. These lesions can spontaneously regress (especially after pregnancy) or undergo fibrosis; in some cases surgical excision is required. Recurrence is rare.

Lymphangioma

Lymphangiomas are the benign lymphatic analogue of hemangiomas.

Simple (Capillary) Lymphangioma. These are composed of small lymphatic channels predominantly occurring in the head, neck, and axillary subcutaneous tissues. They are slightly elevated or sometimes pedunculated lesions that may reach 1 to 2 cm in diameter. Histologically, lymphangiomas show networks of endothelium-lined spaces that can be *distinguished from capillary channels only by the absence of blood cells.*

Cavernous Lymphangioma (Cystic Hygroma). These lesions are typically found in the neck or axilla of children and, rarely, in the retroperitoneum; cavernous lymphangiomas of the neck are common in Turner syndrome (Chapter 7). These lesions can occasionally be enormous (≤15 cm in diameter) and may fill the axilla or produce gross deformities about the neck. Tumors are composed of massively dilated lymphatic spaces lined by ECs and separated by intervening connective tissue stroma containing lymphoid aggregates. The tumor margins are not discrete and the lesions are not encapsulated, making resection difficult.

Glomus Tumor (Glomangioma)

Glomus tumors are biologically benign but often exquisitely painful tumors *arising from modified SMCs of the glomus body,* a specialized arteriovenous structure involved in thermoregulation. Although they can resemble cavernous hemangiomas, glomus tumors constitute a distinct entity by virtue of their constituent cells. They are most commonly found in the distal portion of the digits, especially under the fingernails. Excision is curative.

Morphology

Glomus tumors are round, slightly elevated, red-blue, firm nodules (generally much less than 1 cm in diameter) that can initially resemble a minute focus of hemorrhage under the nail. Histologically, these are aggregates, nests, and masses of specialized glomus cells intimately associated with branching vascular channels, all within a connective tissue stroma. Individual tumor cells are small, uniform, and round or cuboidal, with scant cytoplasm and ultrastructural features similar to SMCs.

Vascular Ectasias

Vascular ectasias are common lesions characterized by local dilation of preexisting vessels; *they are not true neoplasms. Telangiectasia* is a term used for a congenital anomaly or acquired exaggeration of preformed vessels—usually in the skin or mucous membranes—composed of capillaries, venules, and arterioles that creates a discrete red lesion.

Nevus Flammeus. This lesion is the ordinary "birthmark" and is the most common form of ectasia; it is characteristically a flat lesion on the head or neck, ranging in color from light pink to deep purple. Histologically, there is only vascular dilation; most ultimately regress.

The so-called *port wine stain* is a special form of nevus flammeus; these lesions tend to grow with a child, thicken the skin surface, and demonstrate no tendency to fade. In most cases, the reason(s) for this distinct behavior of port wine nevi is not known; however, such lesions in a trigeminal nerve distribution are occasionally associated with the *Sturge-Weber syndrome* (also called *encephalotrigeminal angiomatosis*). Sturge-Weber syndrome is an uncommon congenital disorder with aberrant mesoderm and ectoderm development associated with venous angiomatous masses in the cortical leptomeninges and ipsilateral facial port wine nevi; mental retardation, seizures, hemiplegia, and skull radio-opacities. Thus, *a large facial vascular malformation in a child with mental deficiency may indicate more extensive vascular malformations.*

Spider Telangiectasia. This non-neoplastic vascular lesion grossly resembles a spider; there is a radial, often pulsatile array of dilated subcutaneous arteries or arterioles (resembling legs) about a central core (resembling a body) that blanches when pressure is applied to its center. It is commonly seen on the face, neck, or upper chest and is most frequently associated with hyperestrogenic states such as pregnancy or cirrhosis; how elevated estrogen levels contribute to "spider" formation is not known.

Hereditary Hemorrhagic Telangiectasia (Osler-Weber-Rendu Disease). In this autosomal dominant disorder, the telangiectasias are malformations composed of dilated capillaries and veins. Present from birth, they are widely distributed over the skin and oral mucous membranes, as well as in the respiratory, GI, and urinary tracts. Occasionally, these lesions rupture, causing serious epistaxis (nosebleeds), GI bleeding, or hematuria.

Bacillary Angiomatosis

Bacillary angiomatosis is an opportunistic infection in immunocompromised persons that manifests as vascular proliferations involving skin, bone, brain, and other organs; there is a closely related vascular lesion of liver and spleen called *bacillary peliosis.* First described in patients with acquired immunodeficiency syndrome, bacillary angiomatosis is caused by infection with gram-negative bacilli of the *Bartonella* genus. Two species are implicated: *Bartonella henselae,* the organism responsible for cat-scratch disease (the domestic cat is the principal reservoir), and *B. quintana,* the cause of "trench fever" in World War I (the organism is transmitted by human body lice).

Morphology

Grossly, the skin lesions in bacillary angiomatosis are characterized by red papules and nodules, or rounded subcutaneous masses; histologically, there is capillary proliferation with prominent epithelioid ECs showing nuclear atypia and mitoses (Fig. 10–30). Lesions contain stromal neutrophils, nuclear dust, and purplish granular material representing the causal bacteria.

Although difficult to cultivate in the laboratory, the causal organisms can be unequivocally demonstrated using molecular methods such as polymerase chain reaction and species-specific primers. Very recent evidence suggests that the vascular proliferation occurs by bacterial induction of host tissue production of hypoxia-inducible factor 1, which in turn drives vascular endothelial growth factor (VEGF) production. The infections are cleared by macrolide antibiotics (including erythromycin).

Intermediate-Grade (Borderline Low-Grade Malignant) Tumors

Kaposi Sarcoma

Though rare in other populations, Kaposi sarcoma (KS) used to be fairly common in patients with acquired immunodeficiency syndrome (AIDS) prior to the advent of effective antiretroviral therapy; indeed, its presence is used as a criterion for diagnosing AIDS (Chapter 5). While four forms of the disease are recognized (based on population demographics and risks), all of these share the same underlying viral pathogenesis (see below):

- *Chronic KS* (also called *classic* or *European KS*) was first described by Kaposi in 1872; it characteristically occurs in older men of Eastern European (especially Ashkenazi Jews) or Mediterranean descent and is uncommon in the United States. While chronic KS can be associated with an underlying second malignancy or altered immunity, it is not associated with human immunodeficiency virus (HIV). Chronic KS presents with multiple red to purple skin plaques or nodules, usually in the distal lower extremities; these slowly

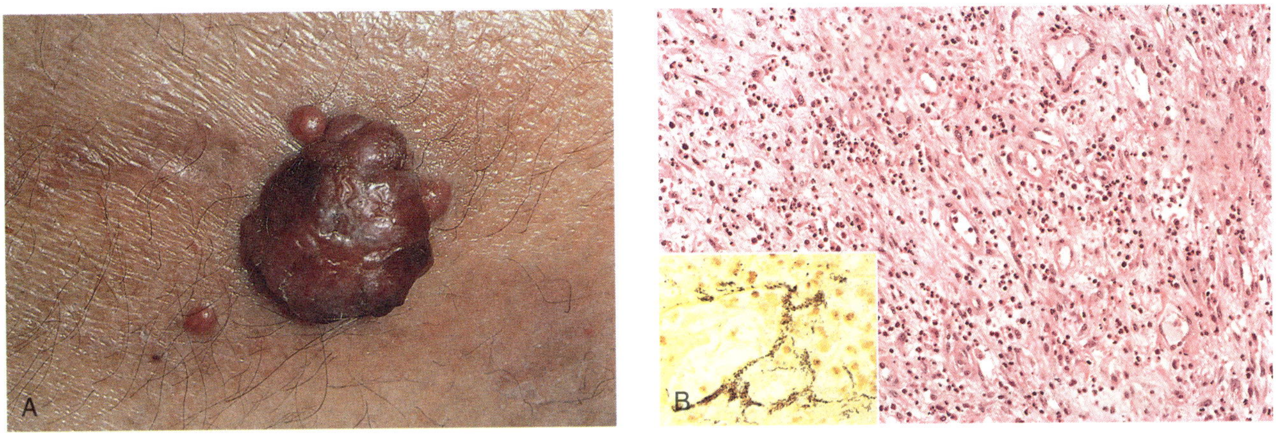

Figure 10–30

Bacillary angiomatosis. **A,** Photograph of a moist, erosive cutaneous lesion. **B,** Histologic appearance with acute neutrophilic inflammation and vascular (capillary) proliferation. Inset, Demonstration by modified silver (Warthin-Starry) stain of clusters of tangled bacilli (*black*). (**A,** Courtesy of Dr. Richard Johnson, Beth Israel Deaconess Medical Center, Boston, Massachusetts. **B** and **inset,** Courtesy of Dr. Scott Granter, Brigham and Women's Hospital, Boston, Massachusetts.)

increase in size and number and spread more proximally. Though locally persistent, the tumors are typically asymptomatic and remain localized to the skin and subcutaneous tissue.

- *Lymphadenopathic KS* (also called *African* or *endemic KS*) has the same general geographic distribution as Burkitt lymphoma and is particularly prevalent among South African Bantu children; it is also not associated with HIV. Skin lesions are sparse, and patients present instead with lymphadenopathy due to KS involvement; the tumor occasionally involves the viscera and is extremely aggressive. In combination with AIDS-associated KS (see below), KS is now the most common tumor in central Africa (50% of all tumors in men in some countries).
- *Transplant-associated KS* occurs in the setting of solid-organ transplantation with its attendant long-term immunosuppression. It tends to be aggressive (even fatal) with nodal, mucosal, and visceral involvement; cutaneous lesions may be absent. Lesions occasionally regress when immunosuppressive therapy is attenuated, but at the risk of organ rejection.
- *AIDS-associated (epidemic) KS* was originally found in a third of AIDS patients, particularly male homosexuals. However, with current regimens of intensive antiretroviral therapy, KS incidence is now less than 1% (although it is still the most prevalent malignancy in AIDS patients in the United States). AIDS-associated KS can involve lymph nodes and viscera, with wide dissemination early in the course of disease. Most patients eventually die of opportunistic infectious rather than from KS.

Pathogenesis. In 1994 a previously unrecognized herpesvirus (*human herpesvirus 8 [HHV-8]* or KS-associated herpesvirus [KSHV]) was identified in a cutaneous KS lesion in an AIDS patient. Indeed, regardless of the clinical subtype (described above), 95% of KS lesions have subsequently been shown to be KSHV infected. Like Epstein-Barr virus, KSHV is a member of the γ-herpesvirus subfamily; it is transmitted sexually and by poorly understood nonsexual routes. The role of KSHV in the pathogenesis of KS was discussed in Chapter 5 along with other manifestations of HIV infection.

Morphology

In the indolent, classic KS of older men (and sometimes in other variants), three stages are recognized: patch, plaque, and nodule.

Patches are solitary or multiple pink, red, or purple macules typically confined to the distal lower extremities (Fig. 10–31A). Microscopic examination discloses only dilated, irregular, and angulated blood vessels lined by ECs with an interspersed infiltrate of lymphocytes, plasma cells, and macrophages (sometimes containing hemosiderin). These lesions are difficult to distinguish from granulation tissue.

With time, lesions spread proximally and convert into larger, violaceous, raised **plaques** (Fig. 10–31A) composed of dermal accumulations of dilated, jagged vascular channels lined by plump spindle cells and perivascular aggregates of similar spindled cells. Scattered between the vascular channels are red blood cells (escaping from leaky vessels), hemosiderin-laden macrophages, lymphocytes, and plasma cells. Pink hyaline globules of uncertain nature may be found in the spindled cells and macrophages.

At a still later stage, lesions become **nodular** and more distinctly neoplastic. These lesions are composed of sheets of plump, proliferating spindle cells, mostly in the dermis or subcutaneous tissues (Fig. 10–31B), encompassing small vessels and slitlike spaces containing rows of red cells. More marked hemorrhage, hemosiderin pigment, lymphocytes, and occasional macrophages are seen; mitotic figures are common, as are the round, pink, cytoplasmic globules. The nodular stage is often accompanied by nodal and visceral involvement, particularly in the African and AIDS-associated variants.

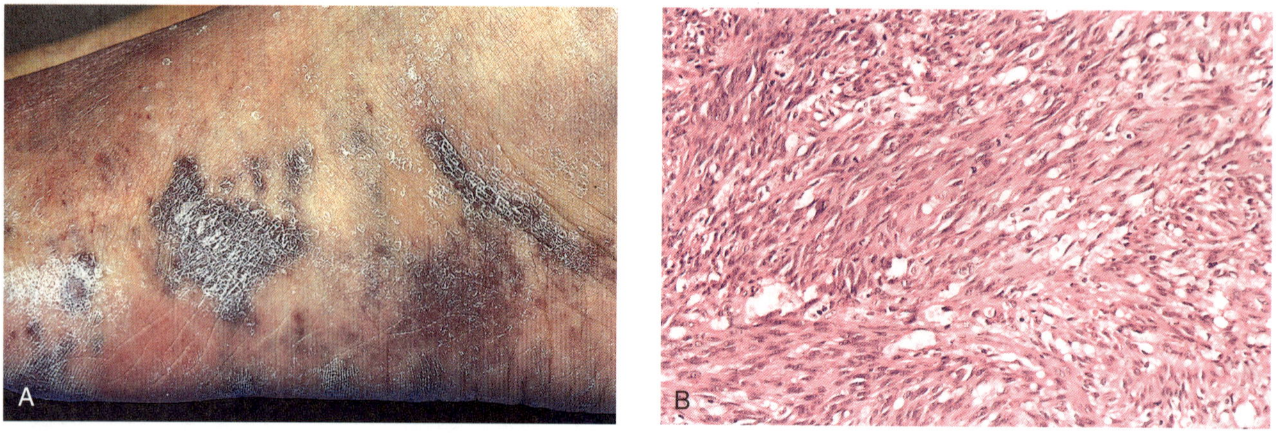

Figure 10–31

Kaposi sarcoma. **A,** Gross photograph, illustrating coalescent red-purple macules and plaques of the skin. **B,** Histologic view of the nodular form demonstrating sheets of plump, proliferating spindle cells and vascular spaces. (Courtesy of Dr. Christopher D.M. Fletcher, Brigham and Women's Hospital, Boston, Massachusetts.)

Clinical Course. The course of KS varies widely and is significantly affected by the clinical setting. Most primary KSHV infections are asymptomatic. Classic KS is—at least initially—largely restricted to the surface of the body, and surgical resection is usually adequate with an excellent prognosis. Radiation can be used for multiple lesions in a restricted area, and chemotherapy yields satisfactory results for more disseminated disease. Lymphadenopathic KS can also be treated with chemotherapy or radiotherapy with good results. In immunosuppression-associated KS, withdrawal of immunosuppression (perhaps with adjunct chemotherapy or radiotherapy) is often effective. For AIDS-associated KS, antiretroviral therapy for HIV is usually helpful, with or without therapy targeted to the KS lesions. Interferon-α and angiogenesis inhibitors have also proved somewhat effective.

Hemangioendothelioma

Hemangioendothelioma denotes a wide spectrum of vascular neoplasms with histology and clinical behaviors intermediate between benign, well-differentiated hemangiomas and frankly anaplastic angiosarcomas (see below).

Epithelioid hemangioendothelioma is an example of this group; it is a vascular tumor of adults occurring around medium-sized and large veins. The tumor cells are plump and often cuboidal (resembling epithelial cells); well-defined vascular channels are inconspicuous. The differential diagnosis includes other epithelioid tumors including metastatic carcinoma, melanoma, and sarcomas. Clinical behavior is variable; most are cured by excision, but up to 40% recur, 20% to 30% eventually metastasize, and perhaps 15% of patients die of the tumors.

Malignant Tumors

Angiosarcoma

Angiosarcomas are malignant endothelial neoplasms (Fig. 10–32) with histology varying from highly differentiated tumors that resemble hemangiomas (*hemangiosarcoma*) to anaplastic lesions difficult to distinguish from carcinomas or melanomas. Older adults are more commonly affected, with equal gender predilections; they occur at any site but most often involve skin, soft tissue, breast, and liver.

Hepatic angiosarcomas are associated with carcinogenic exposures, including arsenic (arsenical pesticides), Thorotrast (a radioactive contrast agent formerly used for radiologic imaging), and polyvinyl chloride (PVC; a widely used plastic). All of these agents have long latencies between initial exposure and eventual tumor development. The increased frequency of angiosarcomas among PVC workers is one of the truly well-documented instances of human chemical carcinogenesis.

Angiosarcomas can also arise in the setting of lymphedema, classically in the ipsilateral upper extremity several years after radical mastectomy (i.e., with lymph node resection) for breast cancer; the tumor presumably arises from lymphatic vessels (*lymphangiosarcoma*). Angiosarcomas can also be induced by radiation and are associated with foreign material introduced into the body either iatrogenically or accidentally.

Morphology

Cutaneous angiosarcomas can begin as deceptively small, sharply demarcated, asymptomatic, often multiple red nodules; most eventually become large, fleshy masses of red-tan to gray-white tissue (see Fig. 10–32A). The margins blend imperceptibly with surrounding structures. Central areas of necrosis and hemorrhage are frequent.

Microscopically, all degrees of differentiation can be seen, from plump, anaplastic but recognizable ECs producing vascular channels (see Fig. 10–32B) to wildly undifferentiated tumors having a solid spindle cell appearance and producing no definite blood vessels. The EC origin of these tumors can be demonstrated by staining with CD31 or von Willebrand factor (see Fig. 10–32C).

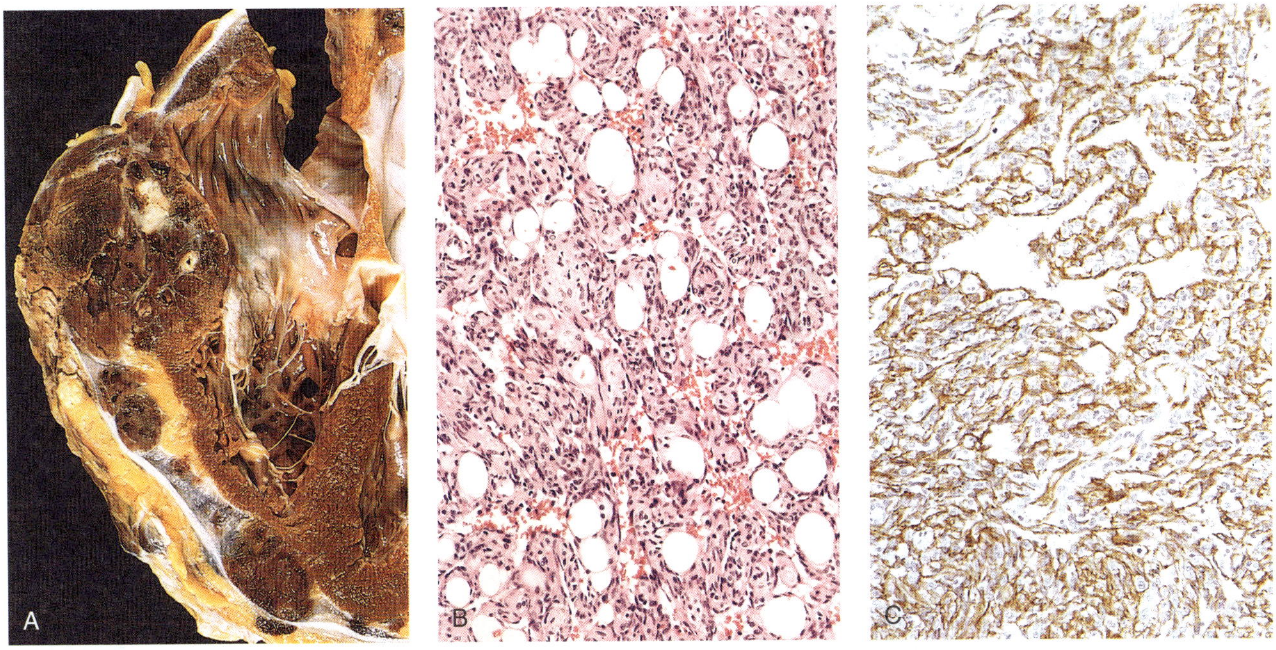

Figure 10–32

Angiosarcoma. **A,** Gross photograph of angiosarcoma of the heart (right ventricle). **B,** Photomicrograph of moderately well-differentiated angiosarcoma with dense clumps of irregular, moderate anaplastic cells and distinct vascular lumens. **C,** Positive immunohistochemical staining of angiosarcoma for the EC marker CD31, proving the endothelial nature of the tumor cells.

Clinically, angiosarcomas are locally invasive and can metastasize readily. Although patients with angiosarcomas have historically done quite poorly, current 5-year survival rates approach 30%.

Hemangiopericytoma

Hemangiopericytomas are rare tumors derived from pericytes—myofibroblast-like cells that are normally arranged around capillaries and venules. Hemangiopericytomas can occur as slowly enlarging, painless masses at any anatomic site, but they are most common on the lower extremities (especially the thigh) and in the retroperitoneum. They consist of numerous branching capillary channels and gaping sinusoidal spaces enclosed within nests of spindle-shaped to round cells. Special stains confirm that these cells are outside the EC basement membrane and are therefore pericytes. The tumors may recur after excision, and roughly half metastasize, usually hematogenously to lungs, bone, or liver.

SUMMARY

Vascular Tumors

- Neoplasms of vessels can derive from either blood vessels or lymphatics, and can be composed of EC (hemangioma, lymphangioma, angiosarcoma) or vascular support cells (glomus tumor or hemangiopericytoma).
- Vascular tumors are predominantly benign (e.g., hemangiomas) but can also be intermediate, locally aggressive lesions (e.g. Kaposi sarcoma), or rarely, highly malignant neoplasms (e.g. angiosarcoma).
- Benign tumors usually form obvious vascular channels lined by normal-appearing EC. Malignant tumors are more typically solid and cellular, without well-organized vessels, and with cytologic atypia.

PATHOLOGY OF VASCULAR INTERVENTION

The morphologic changes that occur in vessels following therapeutic intervention (i.e., balloon angioplasty, stenting, or bypass surgery) typically recapitulate many of the changes that occur in the setting of any vascular insult. Local EC trauma (e.g., due to a stent), vascular thrombosis (after angioplasty), and abnormal mechanical forces (e.g., a saphenous vein inserted into the arterial circulation as a coronary artery bypass graft) all elicit similar responses characteristic of vessel wall healing. As with atherosclerosis, the traumas of vascular intervention tend to induce a concentric intimal thickening composed of recruited SMCs and their associated matrix deposition (Fig. 10–33).

Endovascular Stenting

Coronary stents are expandable tubes of metallic mesh that are inserted to preserve luminal patency during angioplasty dilation of arterial stenoses; stents are used

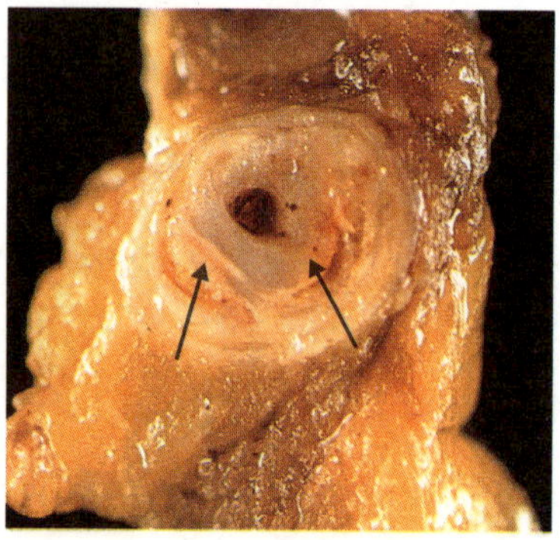

Figure 10–33

Gross photograph of restenosis subsequent to balloon angioplasty, demonstrating residual atherosclerotic plaque (*left arrow*) and a new, glistening proliferative lesion (*right arrow*).

fairly routinely in all angioplasty procedures. Stents provide a larger and more regular lumen, "tack down" the intimal flaps and vascular dissections that occur during angioplasty, and mechanically limit vascular spasm. Nevertheless, both early thrombosis and late intimal thickening can occur within stents and can lead to proliferative restenosis much like that seen with angioplasty alone (Fig. 10–33). Potent antithrombotic agents (platelet antagonists) are taken to minimize thrombosis, and the newest generation of stents release antiproliferative drugs (e.g., paclitaxel or sirolimus); these combined interventions result in markedly diminished intimal hyperplasia.

Vascular Replacement

Synthetic or autologous vascular grafts are increasingly used to replace damaged vessels or bypass diseased arteries. Of the synthetic grafts, large-bore (12- to 18-mm) conduits function well in high-flow locations such as the aorta, while small-diameter artificial grafts (≤8 mm in diameter) generally fail because of acute thrombosis.

Consequently, for coronary artery bypass surgery (>400,000 per year in the United States), grafts are composed of either reversed autologous saphenous vein (taken from the patient's own leg) or left internal mammary artery (because of its proximity to the heart). The long-term patency of saphenous vein grafts is only 50% at 10 years; grafts occlude as a result of thrombosis (typically early), intimal thickening (months to years postoperatively), and graft atherosclerosis—sometimes with superimposed plaque rupture, thrombi, or aneurysms (usually more than 2 to 3 years). In contrast, more than 90% of internal mammary artery grafts are patent at 10 years.

BIBLIOGRAPHY

Aikawa M, Libby P: The vulnerable atherosclerotic plaque: pathogenesis and therapeutic approach. Cardiovasc Pathol 13:125, 2004. *[Current and extensive overview of the concept, diagnosis, and treatment of vulnerable atherosclerotic plaque.]*

Chambless LE, et al.: Coronary heart disease risk prediction in the Atherosclerosis Risk in Communities (ARIC) study. J Clin Epidemiol 56:880, 2003.

Ganem D: KSHV infection and pathogenesis of Kaposi's sarcoma. Ann Rev Pathol: Mech Dis 1:273, 2006. *[A good review of the role of KSHV in the pathogenesis of Kaposi Sarcoma.]*

Gimbrone MA Jr, et al.: Endothelial dysfunction, hemodynamic forces, and atherogenesis. Ann NY Acad Sci 902:230, 2000. *[An excellent discussion of endothelial dysfunction and vascular disease.]*

Hansson GK, et al: Inflammation and atherosclerosis. Ann Review Pathol: Mech Dis 1:297, 2006. *[A terrific review of the role of inflammation in atherosclerosis.]*

Harper L, Savage COS: Leukocyte-endothelial interactions in antineutrophil cytoplasmic antibody–associated systemic vasculitis. Rheum Dis Clin North Am 27:887, 2001. *[A model for ANCA-mediated vasculitis.]*

Kaplan NM: Systemic hypertension: mechanisms and diagnosis. In Zipes DP, et al. (eds): Heart Disease, 7th ed. Philadelphia, Elsevier Saunders, 2005, p 959. *[A recent chapter in hypertension, covering all aspects.]*

Kempf VA, et al.: Activation of hypoxia-inducible factor-1 in bacillary angiomatosis: evidence for a role of hypoxia-inducible factor-1 in bacterial infections. Circulation 111:1054, 2005. *[New evidence for the mechanism underlying bacillary angiomatosis.]*

Libby P, Theroux P: Pathophysiology of coronary artery disease. Circulation 111:3481, 2005. *[An excellent review of cardiac vascular disease.]*

Lifton RP, et al.: Molecular mechanisms of human hypertension. Cell 104:545, 2001. *[A scholarly overview of the genetics and molecular pathways that underlie hypertension.]*

Rarok AA, et al.: Neutrophil-activating potential of antineutrophil cytoplasm autoantibodies. J Leukoc Biol 74:3, 2003. *[A review of the evidence for ANCA-driven neutrophil activation.]*

Ridker PM, et al.: Comparison of C-reactive protein and low-density lipoprotein cholesterol levels in the prediction of first cardiovascular events. N Engl J Med 347:1557, 2002.

Ridker PM, Libby P: Risk factors for atherothrombotic disease. In Zipes DP, et al. (eds): Braunwald's Heart Disease, 7th ed. Philadelphia, Elsevier Saunders, 2005, p 939. *[A detailed discussion of risk factors for atherosclerosis.]*

Ross R: Atherosclerosis—an inflammatory disease. N Engl J Med 340:115, 1999. *[The original, elegant, and compelling description of the response-to-injury hypothesis regarding atherogenesis; still worth a read.]*

Sakalihasan N, et al.: Abdominal aortic aneurysm. Lancet 365:1577, 2005. *[A good current review of diagnosis, treatment, and pathogenesis.]*

Saleh A, Stone JH: Classification and diagnostic criteria in systemic vasculitis. Best Pract Res Clin Rheumatol 19:209, 2005. *[Good overview of the complexity and the controversies in the classification of vasculitides.]*

Savige J, et al.: Antineutrophil cytoplasmic antibodies and associated diseases: a review of the clinical and laboratory features. Kidney Int 57:846, 2000. *[An excellent review of this complicated subject.]*

Shimizu K, et al.: Local cytokine environments drive aneurysm formation in allografted aortas. Trends Cardiovasc Med 15:142, 2005. *[A nice summary of the data on AAA pathogenesis.]*

Sweitzer NK, Douglas PS: Cardiovascular disease in women. In Zipes DP, et al. (eds): Braunwald's Heart Disease, 7th ed. Philadelphia, Elsevier Saunders, 2005, p 1951. *[An excellent discussion of the multiple issues relating to gender in atherosclerosis and other cardiovascular diseases.]*

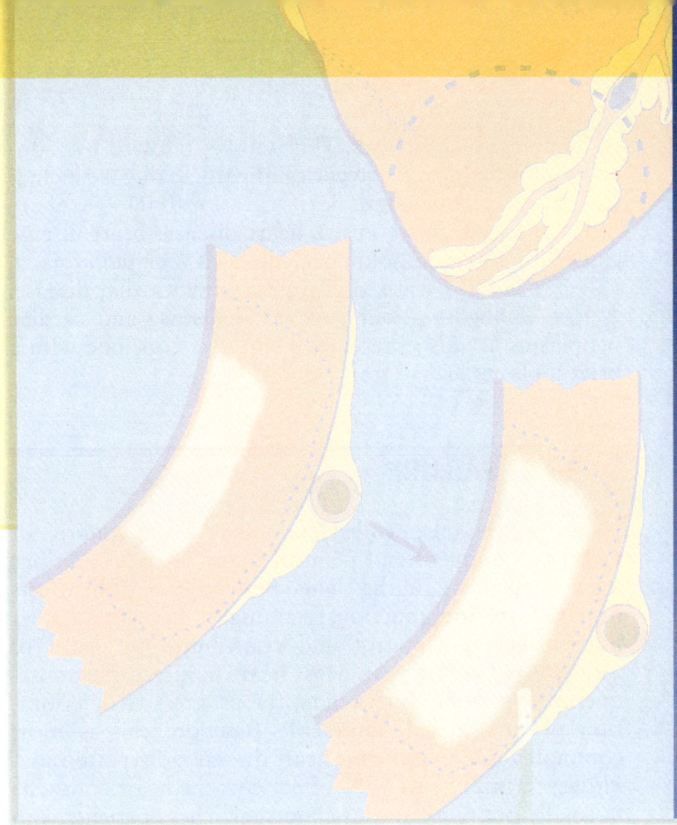

Chapter 11

The Heart*

In addition to its historical association with human emotions (as well as compassion, strength, and resolve—indeed, Aristotle felt it was the seat of the soul!), the heart is a vitally life-sustaining organ; it is responsible for pumping more than 6000 liters of blood daily through the body. In its normal, healthy state, the heart perfuses tissues with a steady supply of vital nutrients and facilitates the removal of waste products. When pathology supervenes, cardiac dysfunction is associated with devastating physiologic consequences. Heart disease remains the leading cause of morbidity and mortality in industrialized nations; it accounts for nearly 40% of all postnatal deaths in the United States, totaling about 750,000 individuals annually (nearly twice the number of deaths caused by all forms of cancer combined). The yearly economic burden of ischemic heart disease (IHD) alone is in excess of $100 billion.

In this chapter we will first review the salient features of congestive heart failure (CHF), the common end point

*The authors acknowledge and thank Dr. Dennis Burns for his previous contributions to many aspects of this chapter.

of many cardiac diseases. This will be followed by a discussion of the major categories of cardiac disease including selected congenital heart dieases, IHD (coronary artery disease), hypertensive heart disease, heart disease caused by intrinsic pulmonary diseases *(cor pulmonale)*, valvular heart disease, and primary myocardial disease. A few highlights about pericardial disease and cardiac neoplasms are also presented before we conclude with a brief look at cardiac transplantation.

HEART FAILURE

Heart failure (also called *congestive heart failure*, or *CHF*) is a frequent end point of many of the conditions mentioned above. In the United States alone, CHF affects nearly 5 million individuals annually, necessitating >1 million hospitalizations, and contributes to death of 300,000 patients a year. Most heart failure is the consequence of *systolic dysfunction*, the progressive deterioration of myocardial contractile function; this is most commonly due to ischemic heart disease or hypertension. However, in 20% to 50% of patients the heart contracts normally but relaxation is abnormal. These patients with "diastolic" failure are generally older and more likely to be female with hypertension or diabetes mellitus. Heart failure may be caused by valve failure (e.g., endocarditis) or can also occur in normal hearts suddenly burdened with an abnormal load (e.g., fluid or pressure overload).

In heart failure, the heart is unable to pump blood at a rate that meets the requirements of the metabolizing tissues, or can only do so only with filling pressures that are higher than normal. Onset may be insidious or acute. In most cases of CHF the heart cannot keep pace with basic peripheral demands; in a minority of cases, heart failure results from greatly increased tissue demands for blood *(high-output failure)*. Excluded from the definition are conditions in which inadequate cardiac output occurs because of blood loss or some other process that impairs blood return to the heart.

In a mechanical sense, the failing heart in CHF can no longer pump the blood delivered to it by the venous circulation. Inadequate cardiac output—called *forward failure*—is almost always accompanied by increased congestion of the venous circulation *(backward failure)*, because the failing ventricle is unable to eject the venous blood delivered to it. This results in an increased end-diastolic ventricular volume, leading to increased end-diastolic pressures and, finally, elevated venous pressures. Although the root problem in CHF is typically abnormal cardiac function, virtually every other organ is eventually affected by some combination of forward and backward failure.

The cardiovascular system can adapt to reduced myocardial contractility or increased hemodynamic burden by a few different pathways. The most important are

- *Activation of neurohumoral systems*, especially (1) release of the neurotransmitter norepinephrine by the sympathetic nervous system (increases heart rate and augments myocardial contractility and vascular resistance), (2) activation of the renin-angiotensin-aldosterone system, and (3) release of atrial natriuretic peptide (ANP). This is a polypeptide hormone secreted by the atria in the setting of atrial distension. It causes vasodilation, naturiuresis, and diuresis that help alleviate volume or pressure overload states.
- *The Frank-Starling mechanism.* As cardiac failure progresses, end-diastolic pressures increase, causing individual cardiac muscle fibers to stretch; this ultimately increases the volume of the cardiac chamber. In accordance with the Frank-Starling relationship, these lengthened fibers initially contract more forcibly, thereby increasing cardiac output. If the dilated ventricle is able to maintain cardiac output at a level that meets the needs of the body, the patient is said to be in *compensated heart failure*. However, increasing dilation increases ventricular wall tension, which increases the oxygen requirements of an already compromised myocardium. With time, the failing myocardium is no longer able to propel sufficient blood to meet the needs of the body, even at rest. At this point, patients enter a phase termed *decompensated heart failure*.
- *Myocardial structural changes, including augmented muscle mass (hypertrophy)*, to increase the mass of contractile tissue. Because adult cardiac myocytes cannot proliferate, adaptation to a chronically increased workload involves hypertrophy of individual muscle cells. In pressure overload states (e.g., hypertension, valvular stenosis), the hypertrophy is characterized by increased diameter of individual muscle fibers. This yields *concentric hypertrophy*, in which the thickness of the ventricular wall increases without an increase in the size of the chamber. In volume overload states (e.g., valvular regurgitation or abnormal shunts), it is the length of individual muscle fibers that increases. This results in *eccentric hypertrophy*, characterized by an increase in heart size as well as an increase in wall thickness.

Initially, these adaptive mechanisms may be adequate to maintain cardiac output in the face of declining cardiac performance. However, with sustained or worsening heart function, pathologic changes may eventually supervene, resulting in structural and functional disturbances; such degenerative changes include myocyte apoptosis, cytoskeletal alterations, and altered extracellular matrix synthesis and remodeling. Even hypertrophy comes at a significant cost to the cell. Oxygen requirements of the hypertrophic myocardium are increased as a result of increased myocardial cell mass and increased tension of the ventricular wall. Because the myocardial capillary bed does not always increase in step with the increased oxygen demands of the hypertrophic muscle fibers, the myocardium becomes vulnerable to *ischemic* injury.

Heart failure can affect predominantly the left side or the right side, or both sides of the heart. The most common causes of left-sided cardiac failure are (1) IHD, (2) systemic hypertension, (3) mitral or aortic valve disease, and (4) primary diseases of the myocardium. The most common cause of right-sided heart failure is left ventricular failure, with its associated pulmonary congestion and elevation in pulmonary arterial pressure.

Right-sided failure can also occur in the absence of left-sided heart failure in patients with intrinsic diseases of the lung parenchyma and/or pulmonary vasculature (cor pulmonale) and in patients with primary pulmonic or tricuspid valve disease. It sometimes follows congenital heart diseases, i.e., in the setting of left-to-right shunts with chronic volume and pressure overloads.

Left-Sided Heart Failure

The morphologic and clinical effects of left-sided CHF primarily result from progressive damming of blood within the pulmonary circulation and the consequences of diminished peripheral blood pressure and flow.

Morphology

Findings in the heart depend on the underlying disease process; for example, myocardial infarction or valvular deformities may be present. Except in cases of mitral valve stenosis (or other processes that restrict left ventricular size), the left ventricle is usually **hypertrophied** and often **dilated,** sometimes quite massively. There are usually nonspecific changes of hypertrophy and fibrosis in the myocardium. Secondary enlargement of the left atrium with resultant atrial fibrillation (i.e., uncoordinated, chaotic contraction of the atrium) can reduce stroke volume or lead to blood stasis and **thrombus formation** (particularly in the atrial appendage); a fibrillating left atrium carries a substantially increased risk of embolic stroke. The extracardiac effects of left-sided heart failure are manifested most prominently in the lungs.

Rising pressure in the pulmonary veins is ultimately transmitted retrogradely to the capillaries, resulting in **pulmonary congestion and edema.** The lungs are heavy and boggy, and histologically there are perivascular and interstitial transudate, alveolar septal edema, and intra-alveolar edema (see also Chapters 4 and 13). Moreover, capillary leakiness leads to the accumulation of erythrocytes (containing hemoglobin) that are phagocytosed by macrophages. Within macrophages, hemoglobin is converted to hemosiderin and hence hemosiderin-containing macrophages in the alveoli (called **heart failure cells**) are evidence of prior of pulmonary edema.

Clinical Features. *Dyspnea* (breathlessness) is usually the earliest and most significant complaint of patients in left-sided heart failure; cough is also a common accompaniment of left heart failure due to fluid transudation into airspaces. With further cardiac impairment, patients develop dyspnea when recumbent (so-called *orthopnea*); this occurs because of increased venous return from the lower extremities and by elevation of the diaphragm when in the supine position. Orthopnea is typically relieved by sitting or standing, so that such patients usually sleep while sitting upright. *Paroxysmal nocturnal dyspnea* is a particularly dramatic form of breathlessness awakening patients from sleep with attacks of extreme dyspnea bordering on suffocation.

Other manifestations of left ventricular failure include an enlarged heart (cardiomegaly), tachycardia, a third heart sound (S_3), and fine rales at the lung bases, produced by respirations through edematous pulmonary alveoli. With progressive ventricular dilation, the papillary muscles are displaced laterally, causing mitral regurgitation and a systolic murmur. Subsequent chronic dilation of the left atrium is often associated with *atrial fibrillation,* manifested by an "irregularly irregular" heartbeat.

Right-Sided Heart Failure

Right-sided heart failure is usually the consequence of left-sided heart failure; any pressure increase in the pulmonary circulation inevitably produces an increased burden on the right side of the heart. Isolated right-sided heart failure is less common and it occurs in patients with intrinsic disease of lung parenchyma and/or pulmonary vasculature that result in chronic pulmonary hypertension (cor pulmonale). It can also occur in patients with pulmonic or tricuspid valve disease. Congenital heart diseases with right-to-left shunt can cause isolated right-sided heart failure, as well. Hypertrophy and dilation are generally confined to the right ventricle and atrium, although bulging of the ventricular septum to the left can cause dysfunction of the left ventricle.

The major morphologic and clinical effects of pure right-sided heart failure differ from those of left-sided heart failure in that pulmonary congestion is minimal, whereas engorgement of the systemic and portal venous systems is typically pronounced.

Morphology

Liver and Portal System. The liver is usually increased in size and weight (congestive hepatomegaly), and a cut section displays prominent passive congestion, a pattern referred to as **nutmeg liver** (see Chapter 4); congested red centers of the liver lobules are surrounded by paler, sometimes fatty, peripheral regions. In some instances, especially when left-sided heart failure is also present, severe central hypoxia produces **centrilobular necrosis** along with the sinusoidal congestion. With long-standing severe right-sided heart failure, the central areas can become fibrotic, creating so-called **cardiac cirrhosis** (Chapter 16).

Right-sided heart failure also leads to elevated pressure in the portal vein and its tributaries. Congestion produces a tense, enlarged spleen (**congestive splenomegaly**). With long-standing congestion, the enlarged spleen can achieve weights of 300 to 500 gm (normal <150 gm). Microscopically, there can be marked sinusoidal dilation. Chronic edema of the bowel wall may interfere with absorption of nutrients. Accumulations of transudate in the peritoneal cavity can cause ascites.

Pleural and Pericardial Spaces. Fluid may accumulate in the pleural space (particularly right) and pericardial space (effusions). Thus, while pulmonary edema indicates left-sided heart failure, pleural effusions accompany both right-sided and left-sided heart failure. Pleural effusions (typically serous) can range from 100 mL to well over 1 L and can cause partial atelectasis of the affected lung. Unlike inflammatory edema, the edema fluid in CHF has a low protein content.

Subcutaneous Tissues. Peripheral edema of dependent portions of the body, especially ankle (pedal) and pretibial edema, is a hallmark of right-sided heart failure. In chronically bedridden patients, the edema may be primarily presacral. Generalized massive edema is called **anasarca**.

Clinical Features. While the symptoms of left-sided heart failure are largely due to pulmonary congestion and edema, pure right-sided heart failure typically causes very few respiratory symptoms. Instead, there is systemic and portal venous congestion, with hepatic and splenic enlargement, peripheral edema, pleural effusion, and ascites. It is worth emphasizing, however, that in most cases of chronic cardiac decompensation, patients present with *biventricular CHF, encompassing the clinical syndromes of both right-sided and left-sided heart failure.* As CHF progresses, patients can become frankly cyanotic and acidotic, as a result of decreased tissue perfusion.

SUMMARY

Heart Failure

- CHF occurs when the heart is unable to pump blood at a rate that meets the metabolic requirements of the peripheral tissue; inadequate cardiac output is usually accompanied by increased congestion of the relevant venous circulation.
- Left-sided heart failure is most commonly due to IHD, systemic hypertension, mitral or aortic valve disease, and primary diseases of the myocardium; symptoms are primarily related to pulmonary congestion and edema.
- Right-sided heart failure is most commonly due to left-sided heart failure or to primary pulmonary diseases; it is associated with peripheral edema and visceral congestion.

CONGENITAL HEART DISEASE

Congenital heart diseases are abnormalities of the heart or great vessels that are present at birth. Most such disorders arise from faulty embryogenesis during gestational weeks 3 through 8, when major cardiovascular structures develop. Congenital malformations of the heart encompass a broad spectrum of defects, ranging from severe anomalies that cause death in the perinatal period, to mild lesions that produce only minimal symptoms, even in adult life. Although figures vary, a generally accepted incidence is approximately 1% of live births; the incidence is higher in premature infants and in stillborns. As might be expected, congenital heart disease is the most common type of heart disease among children.

Because of clinical advances, the number of patients surviving with congenital heart disease is increasing rapidly; by 2020 there will be an estimated 750,000 adults with congenital heart disease. Although surgery can correct the hemodynamic abnormalities, the repaired heart may still not be completely normal. Myocardial hypertrophy and a cardiac remodeling brought about by the congenital defect may be irreversible. Although adaptive initially, such changes can elicit late-onset arrhythmias, ischemia, or myocardial dysfunction, sometimes many years after surgery.

Pathogenesis. General concepts regarding the etiology of congenital malformations were discussed in Chapter 7. We will therefore focus here on factors relevant to congenital cardiac disease, keeping in mind that the cause is unknown in almost 90% of cases. *Environmental factors,* such as congenital rubella infection, are causal in many instances. *Genetic factors* are also clearly involved, as evidenced by familial forms of congenital heart disease and by well-defined associations with certain chromosomal abnormalities (e.g., trisomies 13, 15, 18, and 21 and Turner syndrome).

Cardiac morphogenesis involves multiple genes and is tightly regulated to ensure an effective embryonic circulation. Key steps involve specifying cardiac cell fate, morphogenesis and looping of the heart tube, segmentation and growth of the cardiac chambers, cardiac valve formation, and connection of the great vessels to the heart. The molecular pathways controlling such cardiac development provide a foundation for understanding the basis of some congenital heart defects. Several congenital heart diseases are associated with mutations in transcription factors. Mutations of the TBX5 transcription factor cause the atrial and ventricular septal defects seen in Holt-Oram syndrome. Mutations in the transcription factor NKX2.5 are associated with isolated atrial septal defects (ASDs).

Since different cardiac structures can share the same developmental pathways, dissimilar lesions may nevertheless be related to a common genetic defect. The unifying feature of many outflow tract defects is the abnormal development of neural crest–derived cells, whose migration into the embryonic heart is required for outflow tract formation. In particular, genes located on chromosome 22 have a major role in forming the conotruncus, the branchial arches, and the human face; we now know that deletions of chromosome 22q11.2 underlie 15% to 50% of outflow tract abnormalities. Moreover, these deletions can also cause developmental anomalies of the fourth branchial arch and derivatives of the third and fourth pharyngeal pouches leading to thymic and parathyroid hypoplasia with resultant immune deficiency (Di George syndrome, Chapter 5) and hypocalcemia.

Twelve disorders account for 85% of congenital heart disease; their frequencies are shown in Table 11–1. For purposes of discussion, congenital heart diseases can be subdivided into three major groups:

Table 11–1 Frequencies of Congenital Cardiac Malformations*

Malformation	Incidence per Million Live Births	%
Ventricular septal defect	4482	42
Atrial septal defect	1043	10
Pulmonary stenosis	836	8
Patent ductus arteriosus	781	7
Tetralogy of Fallot	577	5
Coarctation of aorta	492	5
Atrioventricular septal defect	396	4
Aortic stenosis	388	4
Transposition of great arteries	388	4
Truncus arteriosus	136	1
Total anomalous pulmonary venous connection	120	1
Tricuspid atresia	118	1
TOTAL	9757	

*Presented as upper quartile of 44 published studies. Percentages do not add to 100% owing to rounding.

Source: Hoffman JIE, Kaplan S: The incidence of congenital heart disease. J Am Coll Cardiol 39:1890, 2002.

- Malformations causing a *left-to-right shunt*
- Malformations causing a *right-to-left shunt* (cyanotic congenital heart diseases)
- Malformations causing *obstruction*

A *shunt* is an abnormal communication between chambers or blood vessels. Depending on pressure relationships, shunts permit the flow of blood from the left heart to the right heart (or vice versa). When there is a *right-to-left shunt,* a dusky blueness of the skin *(cyanosis)* results because the pulmonary circulation is bypassed and poorly oxygenated blood enters the systemic circulation. In contrast, *left-to-right shunts* increase pulmonary blood flow and are not associated (at least initially) with cyanosis. However, they expose the low-pressure, low-resistance pulmonary circulation to increased pressure and volume, resulting in right ventricular hypertrophy and—eventually—right-sided failure. Some developmental anomalies obstruct vascular flow by narrowing the chambers, valves, or major blood vessels; these are called *obstructive congenital heart disease.* A complete obstruction is called an *atresia.* In some disorders (e.g., tetralogy of Fallot), an obstruction (pulmonary stenosis) is associated with a shunt (right-to-left through a ventricular septal defect [VSD]).

Left-to-Right Shunts

Left-to-right shunts represent the most common type of congenital cardiac malformation (Fig. 11–1). They include atrial and ventricular septal defects, and *patent ductus arteriosus.* Atrial septal defects are typically associated with increased pulmonary blood volumes, while ventricular septal defects and patent ductus arteriosus result in both increased pulmonary blood flow and pressure. These malformations can be asymptomatic or can cause fulminant CHF at birth.

Cyanosis is not an early feature of these defects, but it can occur late, after prolonged left-to-right shunting has produced pulmonary hypertension sufficient to yield right-sided pressures that exceed those on the left and thus result in a reversal of blood flow through the shunt. Such reversal of flow and shunting of unoxygenated blood to the systemic circulation is called *Eisenmenger syndrome.* Once significant pulmonary hypertension develops, the structural defects of congenital heart disease are considered irreversible. This is the rationale for early intervention, either surgical or nonsurgical.

Atrial Septal Defects

ASDs are perhaps best understood from the perspective of normal atrial septation (Fig. 11–2). The atrial septum begins as an ingrowth of the *septum primum* from the dorsal wall of the common atrial chamber toward the developing *endocardial cushion;* a gap, termed the *ostium primum,* initially separates the two. Continued growth

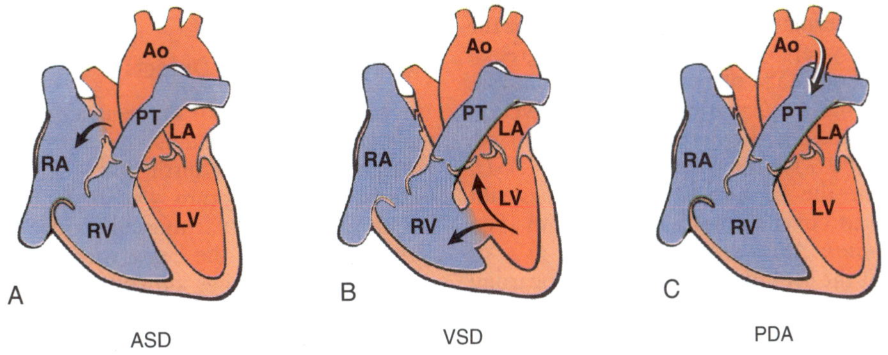

Figure 11–1

Congenital left-to-right shunts (see *arrows*). **A,** Atrial septal defect (ASD). **B,** Ventricular septal defect (VSD). With VSD the shunt is left to right, and the pressures are the same in both ventricles. Pressure hypertrophy of the right ventricle and volume hypertrophy of the left ventricle are generally present. **C,** Patent ductus arteriosus (PDA).

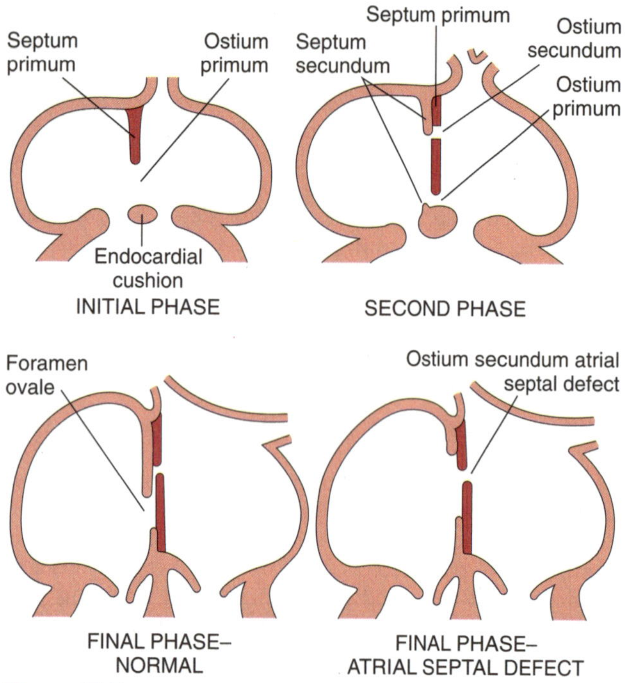

Figure 11–2

Embryogenesis of an atrial septal defect, ostium secundum type. The right atrium is to the left of the septum primum.

and fusion of the septum with the endocardial cushion ultimately obliterates the ostium primum; however, a second opening, *ostium secundum,* now appears in the central area of the primary septum (allowing continued flow of oxygenated blood from the right to left atria, essential for fetal life). As the ostium secundum enlarges, the *septum secundum* makes its appearance adjacent to the septum primum. This septum secundum proliferates to form a crescent-shaped structure overlapping a space termed the *foramen ovale.* The foramen ovale is closed on its left side by a flap of tissue derived from the primary septum; this flap acts as a one-way valve that allows right-to-left blood flow during intrauterine life. At the time of birth, falling pulmonary vascular resistance and rising systemic arterial pressure causes left atrial pressures to exceed those in the right atrium; the result is a functional closure of the foramen ovale. In most individuals the foramen ovale is permanently sealed by fusion of the primary and secondary septa, although a minor degree of patency persists in about 25% of the general population.

Abnormalities in this sequence result in the development of the various ASDs; three types are recognized. The most common (90%) is the *ostium secundum ASD,* which occurs when the septum secundum does not enlarge sufficiently to cover the ostium secundum (Fig. 11–2). *Ostium primum ASDs* are less common (5% of cases); these occur if the septum primum and endocardial cushion fail to fuse and are often associated with abnormalities in other structures derived from the endocardial cushion (e.g., mitral and tricuspid valves). The *sinus venosus ASDs* (5% of cases) are located near the entrance of the superior vena cava and have been associated with frameshift mutations in the NKX2.5 transcription factor.

Morphology

Ostium secundum ASDs are typically smooth-walled defects near the foramen ovale, usually without other associated cardiac abnormalities. Because of the left-to-right shunt, hemodynamically significant lesions are accompanied by right atrial and ventricular dilation, right ventricular hypertrophy, and dilation of the pulmonary artery, reflecting the effects of a chronically increased volume load on the right side of the heart. **Ostium primum** ASDs occur at the lowest part of the atrial septum and can extend to the mitral and tricuspid valves, reflecting the close relationship between development of the septum primum and endocardial cushion. Abnormalities of the atrioventricular valves are usually present, typically in the form of a cleft in the anterior leaflet of the mitral valve or septal leaflet of the tricuspid valve. In more severe cases, the ostium primum defect is accompanied by a VSD and severe mitral and tricuspid valve deformities, with a resultant common atrioventricular canal. Sinus venosus ASDs are located high in the atrial septum and are often accompanied by anomalous drainage of the pulmonary veins into the right atrium or superior vena cava.

Clinical Features. Although VSDs are the most common congenital malformations at birth (Table 11–1), many of these close spontaneously. Consequently, ASDs (which are less likely to spontaneously close) are the most common defects to be first diagnosed in adults. ASDs initially cause left-to-right shunts, as a result of the lower pressures in the pulmonary circulation and right side of the heart. In general these defects are well tolerated, especially if they are less than 1 cm in diameter; even larger lesions do not usually produce any symptoms in childhood. With time, however, pulmonary vascular resistance can increase, resulting in pulmonary hypertension. This occurs in less than 10% of patients with uncorrected ASD. The objectives of surgical closure of ASDs are the reversal of the hemodynamic abnormalities and the prevention of complications, including heart failure, paradoxical embolization, and irreversible pulmonary vascular disease. Mortality is low, and postoperative survival is comparable to that of a normal population. Ostium primum defects are more likely to be associated with evidence of CHF, in part because of the high frequency of associated mitral insufficiency.

Ventricular Septal Defects

Incomplete closure of the ventricular septum allows left-to-right shunting and is the most common congenital cardiac anomaly at birth (Table 11–1 and Fig. 11–1B). The ventricular septum is normally formed by the fusion of an intraventricular muscular ridge that grows upward from the apex of the heart with a thinner membranous partition that grows downward from the endocardial cushion. The basal (membranous) region is the last part of the septum to develop and is the site of approximately 90% of VSDs. Although more common at birth than ASDs, most VSDs close spontaneously in childhood, so that the overall incidence in adults is lower than that of ASDs. Roughly 30% of VSDs occur in isolation; more commonly, they are associated with other cardiac malformations.

Morphology

The size and location of VSDs are variable, ranging from minute defects in the muscular or membranous portions of the septum (Fig. 11–3) to large defects involving virtually the entire septum. In defects associated with a significant left-to-right shunt, the right ventricle is hypertrophied and often dilated. The diameter of the pulmonary artery is increased because of the increased volume ejected by the right ventricle. Vascular changes typical of pulmonary hypertension are common (Chapter 13).

Clinical Features. Small VSDs may be asymptomatic, and those in the muscular portion of the septum may close spontaneously during infancy or childhood. Larger defects, however, cause a severe left-to-right shunt, often complicated by pulmonary hypertension and CHF. Progressive pulmonary hypertension, with resultant reversal of the shunt and cyanosis, occurs earlier and more frequently in patients with VSDs than in those with ASDs; hence, early surgical correction is indicated for such lesions. Small- or medium-sized defects that produce jet lesions in the right ventricle are also prone to superimposed infective endocarditis.

Patent Ductus Arteriosus

During intrauterine life, the ductus arteriosus permits blood flow from the pulmonary artery to the aorta, thereby bypassing the unoxygenated lungs. Shortly after birth, however, the ductus constricts; this occurs in response to increased arterial oxygenation, decreased pulmonary vascular resistance, and declining local levels of prostaglandin E_2. In healthy term infants, the ductus is functionally nonpatent within 1 to 2 days after birth; complete, structural obliteration occurs within the first few months of extrauterine life to form the *ligamentum arteriosum.* Ductal closure is often delayed (or even absent) in infants with hypoxia (resulting from respiratory distress or heart disease). PDAs account for about 7% of cases of congenital heart lesions (Table 11–1 and Fig. 11–1C); 90% of these are isolated defects. The remaining occur with other congenital defects, most commonly VSDs.

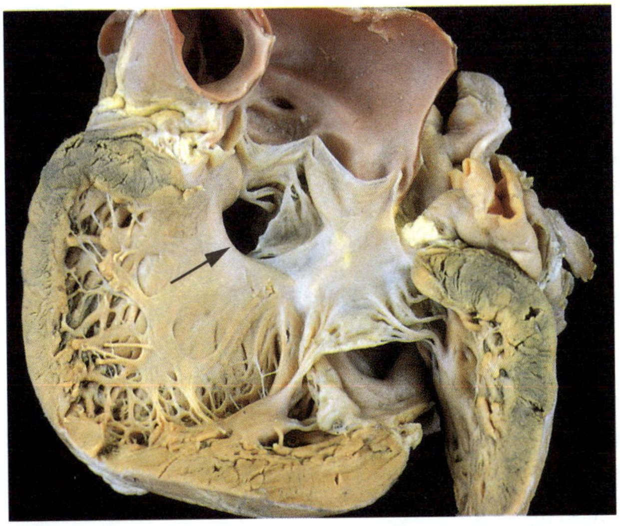

Figure 11–3

Gross photograph of a ventricular septal defect (membranous type, *arrow*). (Courtesy of Dr. William D. Edwards, Mayo Clinic, Rochester, Minnesota.)

Morphology

The ductus arteriosus arises from the left pulmonary artery and joins the aorta just distal to the origin of the left subclavian artery. In PDAs some of the oxygenated blood flowing out from the left ventricle is shunted back to the lungs (Fig. 11–1C). Because of the resultant volume overload, the proximal pulmonary arteries, left atrium, and ventricle can become dilated. With the development of pulmonary hypertension, atherosclerosis of the main pulmonary arteries and proliferative changes in more distal pulmonary vessels are seen, followed by right heart hypertrophy and dilation.

Clinical Features. PDAs are high-pressure left-to-right shunts, audible as harsh "machinery-like" murmurs. A small PDA generally causes no symptoms, although larger bore defects can eventually lead to the Eisenmenger syndrome with cyanosis and CHF. The high-pressure shunt also predisposes affected individuals to infective endocarditis. While there is general agreement that isolated PDAs should be closed as early in life as is feasible, preservation of ductal patency (by administering prostaglandin E) may be critically important for infants with various forms of congenital heart disease wherein the PDA is the only means to provide systemic or pulmonary blood flow (e.g., aortic or pulmonic atresia). Ironically, then, the ductus can be either life threatening or lifesaving.

Right-to-Left Shunts

Cardiac malformations associated with right-to-left shunts are distinguished by *cyanosis at or near the time of birth.* This occurs because poorly oxygenated blood from the right side of the heart is introduced directly into the arterial circulation. Two of the most important conditions associated with cyanotic congenital heart disease are *tetralogy of Fallot* and *transposition of the great vessels* (Fig. 11–4). Clinical findings associated with severe, long-standing cyanosis include clubbing of the fingertips *(hypertrophic osteoarthropathy)* and *polycythemia.* In addition, right-to-left shunts permit venous emboli to bypass the lungs and directly enter the systemic circulation *(paradoxical embolism).*

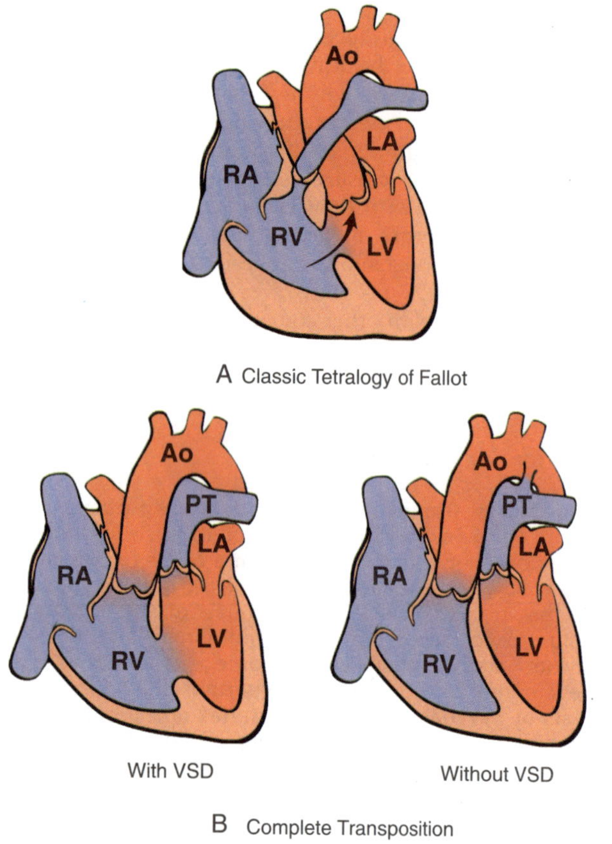

Figure 11–4

Schematic diagram of the most important right-to-left shunts (*cyanotic congenital heart disease*). **A,** Tetralogy of Fallot. Arrow indicates the direction of the blood flow. **B,** Transposition of the great vessels with and without VSD. (Ao, aorta; LA, left atrium; LV, left ventricle; PT, pulmonary trunk; RA, right atrium; RV, right ventricle.) (Courtesy of Dr. William D. Edwards, Mayo Clinic, Rochester, Minnesota.)

Tetralogy of Fallot

Accounting for about 5% of all congenital cardiac malformations, *tetralogy of Fallot is the most common cause of cyanotic congenital heart disease* (Table 11–1). The four features of the tetralogy are (1) VSD, (2) obstruction to the right ventricular outflow tract (subpulmonic stenosis), (3) an aorta that overrides the VSD, and (4) right ventricular hypertrophy (Fig. 11–4). All of the features result from anterosuperior displacement of the infundibular septum, so that there is abnormal division into the pulmonary trunk and aortic root. Even untreated, some tetralogy patients can survive into adult life; the clinical severity largely depends on the degree of the pulmonary outflow obstruction.

Morphology

The heart is large and "boot shaped" in tetralogy of Fallot as a result of right ventricular hypertrophy; the proximal aorta is typically larger than normal, with a diminished pulmonary trunk. The left-sided cardiac chambers are normal sized, while the right ventricular wall is markedly thickened and may even exceed that of the left. The VSD lies in the vicinity of the membranous portion of the interventricular septum, and the aortic valve lies immediately over the VSD. The pulmonary outflow tract is narrowed, and, in a few cases, the pulmonic valve may be stenotic. Additional abnormalities are present in many cases, including PDA or ASD; these are actually beneficial in many respects, because they permit pulmonary blood flow.

Clinical Features. The hemodynamic consequences of tetralogy of Fallot are right-to-left shunting, decreased pulmonary blood flow, and increased aortic volumes. *The extent of shunting* (and the clinical severity) *is determined by the amount of right ventricular outflow obstruction.* If the pulmonic obstruction is mild, the condition resembles an isolated VSD, because the high left-sided pressures on the left side cause a left-to-right shunt with no cyanosis. More commonly, marked stenosis causes significant right-to-left shunting and consequent cyanosis early in life. As patients with tetralogy grow, the pulmonic orifice does not enlarge, despite an overall increase in the size of the heart. Hence, the degree of stenosis typically worsens with time resulting in increasing cyanosis. The lungs are protected from hemodynamic overload by the pulmonic stenosis, so that pulmonary hypertension does not develop. As with any cyanotic heart disease, patients develop erythrocytosis with attendant hyperviscosity, and hypertrophic osteoarthropathy; the right-to-left shunting also increases the risk for infective endocarditis, systemic emboli, and brain abscesses. Surgical correction of this defect is now possible in most instances.

Transposition of the Great Arteries

Transposition of the great arteries (TGA) is a discordant connection of the ventricles to their vascular outflow. The embryologic defect is an abnormal formation of the truncal and aortopulmonary septa, so that the aorta arises from the right ventricle and the pulmonary artery emanates from the left ventricle (Fig. 11–4B). The atrium-to-ventricle connections, however, are normal (concordant), with right atrium joining right ventricle and left atrium emptying into left ventricle.

The functional outcome is separation of the systemic and pulmonary circulations, a condition incompatible with postnatal life unless a shunt exists for adequate mixing of blood and delivery of oxygenated blood to the aorta. Patients with TGA and a VSD (~35%) tend to have a relatively stable shunt. However, those individuals with only a patent foramen ovale or PDA (~65%) tend to have unstable shunts that can close and often require surgical intervention within the first few days of life.

Morphology

TGA has many variants, but a detailed review of them should really be left to the cognoscenti. The fundamental lesion is the abnormal origin of the pulmonary trunk and aortic root. Varying combinations of ASD, VSD, and PDA are seen in patients surviving beyond the neonatal period. Right ventricular hypertrophy becomes prominent because this chamber functions as the systemic ventricle. Concurrently the left ventricle becomes somewhat atrophic, since it only has to support the low-resistance pulmonary circulation.

Clinical Features. The predominant manifestation of TGA is early cyanosis. The outlook for neonates with TGA depends on the degree of the shunting, the magnitude of the tissue hypoxia, and the ability of the right ventricle to maintain systemic pressures. Infusions of prostaglandin E_2 can be used to maintain patency of the ductus arteriosus, and maneuvers such as atrial septostomy are performed to create ASDs that enhance arterial oxygen saturation. Even with stable shunting, most uncorrected TGA patients still die within the first months of life. Consequently, affected individuals usually undergo corrective surgery (switching the great arteries) within weeks of birth.

Obstructive Lesions

Congenital obstruction to blood flow can occur at the level of the heart valves or within a great vessel. Obstruction can also occur within a chamber, as with subpulmonic stenosis in tetralogy of Fallot. Relatively common examples of congenital obstruction include pulmonic valve stenosis, aortic valve stenosis or atresia, and coarctation of the aorta.

Aortic Coarctation

Coarctation (narrowing, or constriction) of the aorta is a relatively common structural anomaly (Table 11–1) and is the most important form of obstructive congenital heart disease. Males are affected twice as often as females, although females with Turner syndrome frequently have aortic coarctation. Two classic forms have been described (Fig. 11–5): an "infantile" form with hypoplasia of the aortic arch proximal to a PDA, and an "adult" form in which there is a discrete ridgelike infolding of the aorta, just opposite the ligamentum arteriosum distal to the arch vessels. Coarctation of the aorta may occur as a solitary defect, but in more than 50% of cases, it is accompanied by a bicuspid aortic valve. Congenital aortic stenosis, ASD, VSD, or mitral regurgitation may also occur. In some cases berry aneurysms in the circle of Willis coexist.

Morphology

Preductal ("infantile") coarctation is characterized by tubular narrowing of the aortic segment between the left subclavian artery and the ductus arteriosus. The ductus arteriosus is usually patent and is the main source of blood delivered to the distal aorta. Because the right side of the heart must perfuse the body distal to the narrowing, the right ventricle is typically hypertrophied and dilated; the pulmonary trunk is also dilated to accommodate the increased blood flow.

In the more common postductal ("adult") coarctation, the aorta is sharply constricted by a ridge of tissue at or just distal to the ligamentum arteriosum (Fig. 11–6). The constricted segment is made up of smooth muscle and elastic fibers that are continuous with the aortic media and are lined by a thickened layer of intima. The ductus arteriosus is closed. Proximal to the coarct, the aortic arch and its branch vessels are dilated and, in older patients, often atherosclerotic. The left ventricle is hypertrophic.

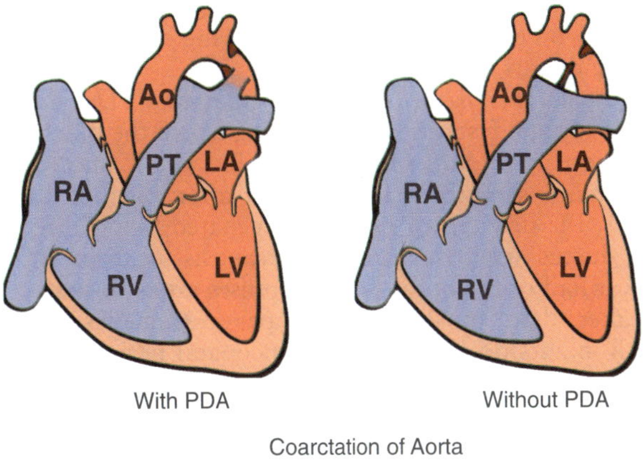

Figure 11–5

Coarctation of the aorta with and without a patent ductus arteriosus (PDA). Ao, aorta; LA, left atrium; LV, left ventricle; PT, pulmonary trunk; RA, right atrium; RV, right ventricle. (Courtesy of Dr. William D. Edwards, Mayo Clinic, Rochester, Minnesota.)

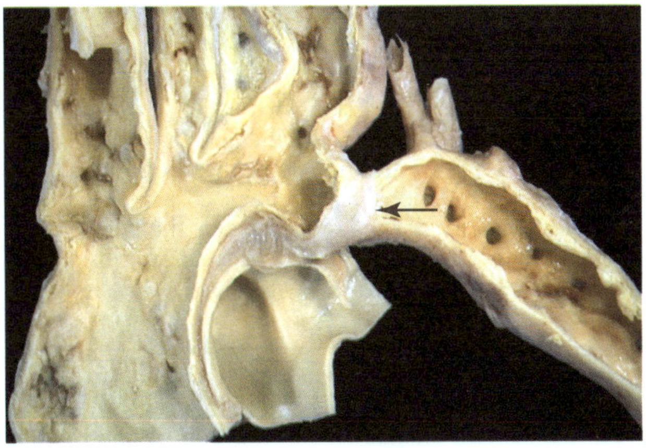

Figure 11–6

Coarctation of the aorta, postductal type. The area of coarctation is visible here as a segmental narrowing of the aorta *(arrow)*. Such lesions typically present later in life than do preductal coarctations. Note the dilated ascending aorta and major branch vessels to the left of the coarctation. A large amount of blood reaches the lower extremities via dilated, tortuous collateral channels. (Courtesy of Dr. Sid Murphree, Department of Pathology, University of Texas Southwestern Medical School, Dallas, Texas.)

Clinical Features. Clinical manifestations depend almost entirely on the severity of the narrowing and the patency of the ductus arteriosus.

Preductal coarctation of the aorta with a PDA usually leads to manifestations early in life, hence the older designation of *infantile* coarctation; indeed, it may cause signs and symptoms immediately after birth. In such cases, the delivery of poorly oxygenated blood through the ductus arteriosus produces cyanosis localized to the lower half of the body. Femoral pulses are almost always weaker than those of the upper extremeties. Many such infants do not survive the neonatal period without intervention.

Postductal coarctation of the aorta without a PDA is usually asymptomatic, and the disease may go unrecognized until well into adult life. Typically, there is upper extremity hypertension, due to poor perfusion of the kidneys, but weak pulses and a lower blood pressure in the lower extremities. Claudication and coldness of the lower extremeties result from arterial insufficiency. Adults tend to show exuberant collateral circulation "around" the coarctation involving markedly enlarged intercostal and internal mammary arteries; expansion of the flow through these vessels leads to radiographically visible "notching" of the ribs.

SUMMARY

Congenital Heart Disease

- Congenital heart diseases consist of defects of cardiac chambers or the great vessels; these either result in shunting of blood between the right and left circulation or cause outflow obstructions.
- Left-to-right shunts are most common and typically involve ASDs, VSDs, or a PDA. These lesions result in chronic right-sided pressure and volume overload that eventually causes pulmonary hypertension with reversal of flow and right-to-left shunts with cyanosis (Eisenmenger syndrome).
- Right-to-left shunts are typically caused by tetralogy of Fallot or transposition of great vessels. These are cyanotic lesions from the outset and are associated with polycythemia, hypertrophic osteoarthropathy, and paradoxical emboli.
- Obstructive lesions include aortic coarctation; the clinical severity of the lesion depends the degree of stenosis and the patency of the ductus arteriosus.

ISCHEMIC HEART DISEASE (IHD)

IHD is a generic designation for a group of related syndromes resulting from myocardial *ischemia*—an imbalance between cardiac blood supply (perfusion) and myocardial oxygen demand. Although ischemia can result from increased demand (e.g., increased heart rate or hypertension), or diminished oxygen-carrying capacity (e.g., anemia, carbon monoxide poisoning), in the vast majority of cases, IHD is due to a reduction in coronary blood flow caused by obstructive atherosclerotic disease (Chapter 10). Thus, IHD is also frequently called coronary artery disease (CAD). Despite dramatic improvement over the past 3 to 4 decades, IHD in its various forms still represents the leading cause of death in the United States and other industrialized nations.

The clinical manifestations of IHD are a direct consequence of insufficient blood supply to the heart. There are four basic clinical syndromes of IHD:

- *Angina pectoris* (literally *chest pain*), wherein the ischemia causes pain but is insufficient to lead to death of myocardium; as we will discuss, angina may be *stable* (occurring reliably after certain levels of exertion), may be due to vessel spasm *(variant angina or Prinzmetal angina),* or may be *unstable* (occurring with progressively less exertion or even at rest).
- *Acute myocardial infarction (MI),* wherein the severity or duration of ischemia is enough to cause cardiac muscle death
- *Chronic IHD* refers to progressive cardiac decompensation (heart failure) following MI.
- *Sudden cardiac death (SCD),* can result from a lethal arrhythmia following myocardial ischemia. As discussed later, there are other causes of SCD as well.

These syndromes are all relatively late manifestations of coronary atherosclerosis that begins early in life but manifests only after the vascular occlusions reach a critical stage. The term *acute coronary syndrome* is applied to three catastrophic manifestations of IHD: unstable angina, acute MI, and SCD.

Epidemiology. Nearly 500,000 Americans die of IHD annually; nevertheless, this represents a spectacular improvement over previous eras. After peaking in 1963, the overall death rate from IHD has fallen in the United States by approximately 50%. The decline can be attributed largely to the recognition of cardiac risk factors (that is, risk factors leading to atherosclerotic disease; Chapter 10) and interventions such as stopping smoking, treating hypertension and diabetes, and lowering cholesterol. To a lesser extent, *diagnostic and therapeutic advances* are also contributory; these include coronary angiography, aspirin prophylaxis, newer medications like statins, better arrhythmia control, coronary care units, angioplasty and endovascular stents, thrombolysis for MI, and coronary artery bypass surgery. Nevertheless, continuing this progress in the 21st century will be particularly challenging in view of the predicted increased longevity of "baby boomers."

Pathogenesis. In most cases IHD occurs because of inadequate coronary perfusion relative to myocardial demand. This may result from a combination of preexisting ("fixed") atherosclerotic occlusion of coronary arteries and new superimposed thrombosis and/or vasospasm (Fig. 11–7).

A lesion obstructing 70% to 75% or more of a vessel lumen—so-called critical stenosis—generally causes symptomatic ischemia (angina) only in the setting of increased demand (Fig. 11–7); a fixed 90% stenosis can lead to inadequate coronary blood flow even at rest. Importantly, if a coronary artery develops atherosclerotic occlusion at a sufficiently slow rate, it may be able to

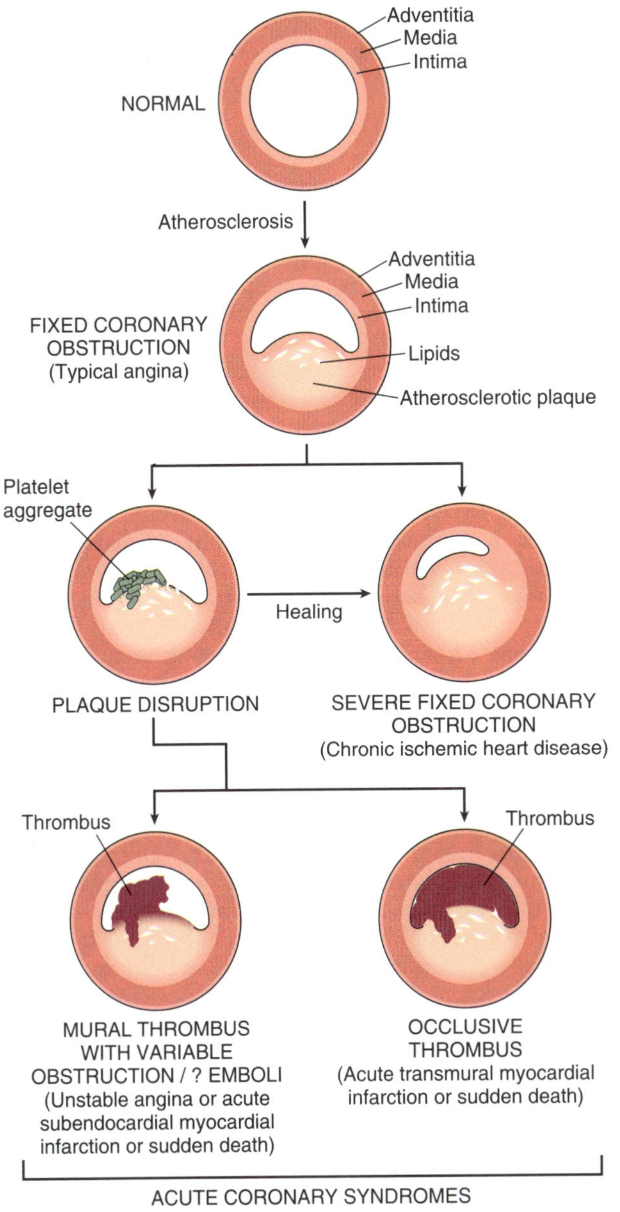

Figure 11–7

Sequential progression of coronary artery lesion morphology, beginning with stable chronic plaque, responsible for typical angina, and leading to the various acute coronary syndromes. (Modified and redrawn from Schoen FJ: Interventional and Surgical Cardiovascular Pathology: Clinical Correlations and Basic Principles. Philadelphia, WB Saunders, 1989, p 63.)

stimulate collateral blood flow from other major epicardial vessels; such *collateral perfusion* can then protect against MI even in the setting of a complete vascular occlusion. Unfortunately, acute coronary occlusions cannot spontaneously recruit collateral flow and will result in infarction (see below).

Although only a single major coronary epicardial artery may be affected by atherosclerotic narrowing, two or all three arteries—left anterior descending (LAD), left circumflex (LCX), and right coronary artery (RCA)—can be concurrently involved. Clinically significant plaques can be located anywhere but tend to predominate within the first several centimeters of the LAD and LCX, and along the entire length of the RCA. Sometimes, secondary branches are also involved (i.e., diagonal branches of the LAD, obtuse marginal branches of the LCX, or posterior descending branch of the RCA). It should be emphasized that symptom onset depends not only on the extent and severity of fixed atherosclerotic disease but also critically on dynamic changes in coronary plaque morphology (see below).

Role of Acute Plaque Change. In most patients, unstable angina, infarction, and many cases of SCD all occur because of abrupt plaque change followed by thrombosis (Fig. 11–7), hence the term acute coronary syndrome. The initiating event is typically disruption of a plaque due to:

- *Rupture, fissuring, or ulceration* of plaques exposing highly thrombogenic plaque constituents or underlying subendothelial basement membrane.
- *Hemorrhage into the core of plaques* with expansion of plaque volume and worsening of the luminal occlusion.

The events that trigger the abrupt plaque changes are complex. They may be intrinsic to the structure of the plaque or extrinsic to it. Basically, rupture reflects the inability of a plaque to withstand mechanical stresses.

Plaques that contain a large atheromatous core or those in which the overlying fibrous caps are thin are more likely to rupture and are therefore denoted as "vulnerable." Fissures frequently occur at the junction of the fibrous cap and the adjacent normal plaque-free arterial segment, a location at which the mechanical stresses are highest and the fibrous cap is thinnest. Fibrous caps are also continuously remodeling; the balance of collagen synthesis and degradation determines its mechanical strength and thus plaque stability. Collagen is produced by smooth muscle cells and degraded by the action of metalloproteinases elaborated by macrophages in the plaque. Consequently, a paucity of smooth muscle cells or an increase in inflammatory cell activity in atherosclerotic lesions is associated with plaque vulnerability. Interestingly, statins (inhibitors of HMG Co-A reductase, a key enzyme in the synthesis of cholesterol) may reduce clinical events associated with IHD by their lipid-lowering effect, as well as by reducing plaque inflammation.

Influences extrinsic to the plaque are also important. Adrenergic stimulation can elevate physical stresses on the plaque through systemic hypertension or local vasospasm. Indeed, the adrenergic stimulation associated with awakening and rising may underlie the known peak incidence (between 6 AM and 12 noon) of acute MIs. Intense emotional stress can also contribute to plaque disruption.

Such acute changes often develop in plaques not initially critically stenotic or even symptomatic before rupture. Recall that anginal symptoms typically occur with fixed lesions that cause greater than 70% to 75% occlusion. Pathologic and clinical studies show that two-thirds of ruptured plaques are ≤50% stenotic before plaque rupture, and 85% have initial stenosis ≤70%. Thus, the worrisome conclusion is that a rather large number of now asymptomatic adults in the industrial world have a significant but unpredictable risk of a catastrophic coronary event. Regrettably, it is presently impossible to reliably predict plaque rupture in any given patient.

Accumulating evidence also indicates that plaque disruption with ensuing platelet aggregation and thrombosis are common, repetitive, and often clinically silent complications of atherosclerosis. Moreover, healing of subclinical plaque disruptions and overlying thrombosis is an important mechanism by which atherosclerotic lesions progressively enlarge.

Role of Inflammation. Inflammation plays an essential role at all stages of atherosclerosis, from inception to plaque rupture. As described in Chapter 10, atherosclerosis begins with the interaction of endothelial cells and circulating leukocytes, resulting in T-cell and macrophage recruitment and activation. These cells subsequently drive smooth muscle cell proliferation, with variable amounts of extracellular matrix (ECM) accumulating over an atheromatous core of lipid, cholesterol, calcification, and necrotic debris. At later stages, destabilization of atherosclerotic plaque occurs through metalloproteinase secretion.

Role of Thrombus. Thrombosis associated with a disrupted plaque is critical to the pathogenesis of acute coronary syndromes. Partial vascular occlusion by a newly formed thrombus on a disrupted atherosclerotic plaque can wax and wane with time and lead to unstable angina or sudden death; alternatively, even partial luminal occlusion by thrombus can compromise blood flow sufficiently to cause a small infarction of the innermost zone of the myocardium (subendocardial infarct). Mural thrombus in a coronary artery can also embolize; indeed, small fragments of thrombotic material, along with associated microinfarcts, can be found in the distal intramyocardial circulation at autopsy of patients who experienced unstable angina or sudden death. In the most serious extreme, completely obstructive thrombus over a disrupted plaque can cause a massive MI. Since blood flow is abruptly blocked by thrombosis, collateral circulation cannot develop. Finally, organizing thrombi produce potent activators of smooth muscle proliferation, which can contribute to the growth of atherosclerotic lesions (Chapter 10).

Role of Vasoconstriction. Vasoconstriction directly compromises lumen diameter; and by increasing local mechanical shear forces, it can potentiate plaque disruption. Vasoconstriction in atherosclerotic plaques can be stimulated by (1) circulating adrenergic agonists, (2) locally released platelet contents, (3) an imbalance between endothelial cell relaxing factors (e.g., nitric oxide) versus contracting factors (e.g., endothelin) (see Chapter 10), and (4) mediators released from perivascular inflammatory cells.

Other Pathologic Processes. Rarely, processes other than atherosclerosis and superimposed thrombi can compromise coronary perfusion. These include emboli originating from valve vegetations, coronary vasculitis, and systemic hypotension. Myocardial hypertrophy (e.g., hypertrophic cardiomyopathy, see below) can also increase myocardial demand beyond what even relatively normal coronaries can provide.

Angina Pectoris

Angina pectoris is intermittent chest pain caused by transient, reversible myocardial ischemia. There are three variants:

- *Typical* or *stable angina* is episodic chest pain associated with exertion or some other form of increased myocardial oxygen demand (e.g., tachycardia or hypertension due to fever, anxiety, fear). The pain is classically described as a crushing or squeezing substernal sensation, which can radiate down the left arm or to the left jaw *(referred pain)*. Stable angina pectoris is usually associated with a fixed atherosclerotic narrowing (≥75%) of one or more coronary arteries. With this degree of critical stenosis, the myocardial oxygen supply may be sufficient under basal conditions but cannot be adequately augmented to meet any increased requirements. The pain is usually relieved by rest (reducing demand) or by administering agents such as nitroglycerin; such drugs cause peripheral vasodilation and thus reduce venous blood delivered to the heart (hence reducing cardiac work); in larger doses, nitroglycerin also increases blood supply to the myocardium by direct coronary vasodilation.
- *Prinzmetal, or variant angina* is angina occurring at rest due to coronary artery spasm. Although such spasms typically occur on or near an existing atherosclerotic plaque, completely normal vessels can be affected. The etiology is not clear, but Prinzmetal angina typically responds promptly to the administration of vasodilators such as nitroglycerin or calcium channel blockers.
- *Unstable angina* (also called *crescendo angina*) is characterized by increasing frequency of pain, precipitated by progressively less exertion; the episodes also tend to be more intense and longer lasting than stable angina. As discussed above, unstable angina is associated with plaque disruption and superimposed partial thrombosis, distal embolization of the thrombus, and/or vasospasm. Unstable angina is the harbinger of more serious, potentially irreversible ischemia (due to complete luminal occlusion by thrombus) and is therefore sometimes called *pre-infarction angina.*

Myocardial Infarction

MI, popularly called *heart attack, is necrosis of heart muscle resulting from ischemia.* Roughly 1.5 million people in the United States suffer an MI every year; of these, one-third die—half before they can reach the hospital. The major underlying cause of IHD is atherosclerosis and therefore *the frequency* of MIs *rises progressively with increasing age* and presence of other risk factors such as hypertension, smoking, and diabetes discussed in Chapter 10. Approximately 10% of MIs occur in people younger than 40 years, and 45% occur in people younger than age 65. Blacks and whites are equally affected. Men are at significantly greater risk than women, although the gap progressively narrows with age. In general, women are remarkably protected against MI during their reproductive years. Nevertheless, menopause—and presumably declining estrogen production—is associated with exacerbation of coronary atherosclerosis.

Pathogenesis. Although any form of coronary artery occlusion can cause acute MI, angiographic studies demonstrate that *most MIs are caused by acute coronary artery thrombosis.* In most cases, disruption of an atherosclerotic plaque results in the formation of thrombus. Vasospasm and/or platelet aggregation can contribute but are infrequently the sole cause of an occlusion. Sometimes, particularly with infarcts limited to the innermost (subendocardial) myocardium, thrombi may be absent. In these cases, severe diffuse coronary atherosclerosis significantly limits coronary vessel perfusion, and a prolonged period of increased demand (e.g., due to tachycardia or hypertension) may be sufficient to cause necrosis of myocytes most distal to the epicardial vessels.

Coronary Artery Occlusion. In a *typical MI,* the following sequence of events transpires:

- There is a sudden disruption of an atheromatous plaque—for example, intraplaque hemorrhage, erosion or ulceration, or rupture or fissuring—exposing subendothelial collagen and necrotic plaque contents.
- Platelets adhere, aggregate, become activated, and release potent secondary aggregators including thromboxane A_2, adenosine diphosphate, and serotonin.
- Vasospasm is stimulated by platelet aggregation and mediator release.
- Other mediators activate the extrinsic pathway of coagulation, adding to the bulk of the thrombus.
- Within minutes the thrombus can evolve to completely occlude the coronary lumen of the coronary vessel.

The evidence for this series of events derives from (1) autopsy studies of patients dying with acute MI, (2) angiographic studies demonstrating a high frequency of thrombotic occlusion early after MI, (3) the high success rate of therapeutic thrombolysis and primary angioplasty, and (4) the demonstration of residual disrupted atherosclerotic lesions by angiography after thrombolysis. Interestingly, coronary angiography performed within 4 hours of the onset of MI shows a thrombosed coronary artery in almost 90% of cases. However, when angiography is delayed until 12 to 24 hours after onset of symptoms, occlusions are observed in only 60% of patients, *even without intervention.* Thus, at least some occlusions seem to clear spontaneously as a result of lysis of the thrombus and/or relaxation of spasm; as noted previously, any residual thrombus is likely to be incorporated into the growing atherosclerotic plaque.

Myocardial Response to Ischemia. Coronary artery obstruction blocks the myocardial blood supply, leading to profound functional, biochemical, and morphologic consequences. Within seconds of vascular obstruction, cardiac myocyte aerobic glycolysis ceases, leading to inadequate production of adenosine triphosphate (ATP) and accumulation of potentially noxious breakdown products (e.g., lactic acid). The *functional* consequence is a striking loss of contractility, occurring within a minute or so of the onset of ischemia. Ultrastructural changes including myofibrillar relaxation, glycogen depletion, and cell and mitochondrial swelling also become rapidly apparent. However, these early changes are potentially *reversible,* and myocardial cell death is not immediate (Chapter 1). Only severe ischemia lasting at least 20 to 40 minutes causes *irreversible* injury and myocyte death; the predominant pattern is coagulation necrosis (Chapter 1). With longer periods of ischemia, microvasculature injury ensues.

If myocardial blood flow is restored anywhere along this timeline (*reperfusion*), cell viability may be preserved. This provides the rationale for early clinical detection of acute MI, and prompt intervention by angioplasty or thrombolysis, to restore blood flow to the at-risk areas. Ischemic but still viable myocardium can be salvaged by early reperfusion. However, as discussed later, reperfusion can also have some untoward effects.

Myocardial ischemia also contributes to arrhythmias, probably by causing *electrical instability (irritability)* of ischemic regions of the heart. Although massive myocardial damage can clearly cause a fatal mechanical failure, SCD in the setting of myocardial ischemia is most often (80% to 90% of cases) due to ventricular fibrillation caused by myocardial irritability.

Irreversible injury of ischemic myocytes first occurs in the subendocardial zone (Fig. 11–8). Not only is this region the last area to receive blood delivered by the epicardial vessels, the relatively higher intramural pressures there further compromise blood inflow. With more prolonged ischemia, a wavefront of cell death moves through the myocardium to involve progressively more of the transmural thickness of the ischemic zone, so that an infarct usually reaches its full size within 3 to 6 hours. Any intervention in this time frame can potentially limit the final extent of necrosis.

The final location, size, and specific morphologic features of an acute MI depend on:

- Location, severity, and rate of development of the coronary occlusion
- Size of the vascular bed perfused by the obstructed vessels
- Duration of the occlusion
- Metabolic demands of the myocardium (affected, e.g., by blood pressure and heart rate)
- Extent of collateral supply.

Morphology

Nearly all transmural infarcts (defined as involving ≥50% of the myocardial wall thickness) affect at least a portion of the left ventricle and/or ventricular septum. Roughly 15% to 30% of MIs affecting the posterior or posteroseptal wall also extend into the adjacent right ventricular wall. Isolated right ventricle infarcts, however, occur in only 1% to 3% of cases. Even in transmural infarcts, a narrow rim (~0.1 mm) of viable subendocardial myocardium is preserved by diffusion of oxygen and nutrients from the ventricular lumen.

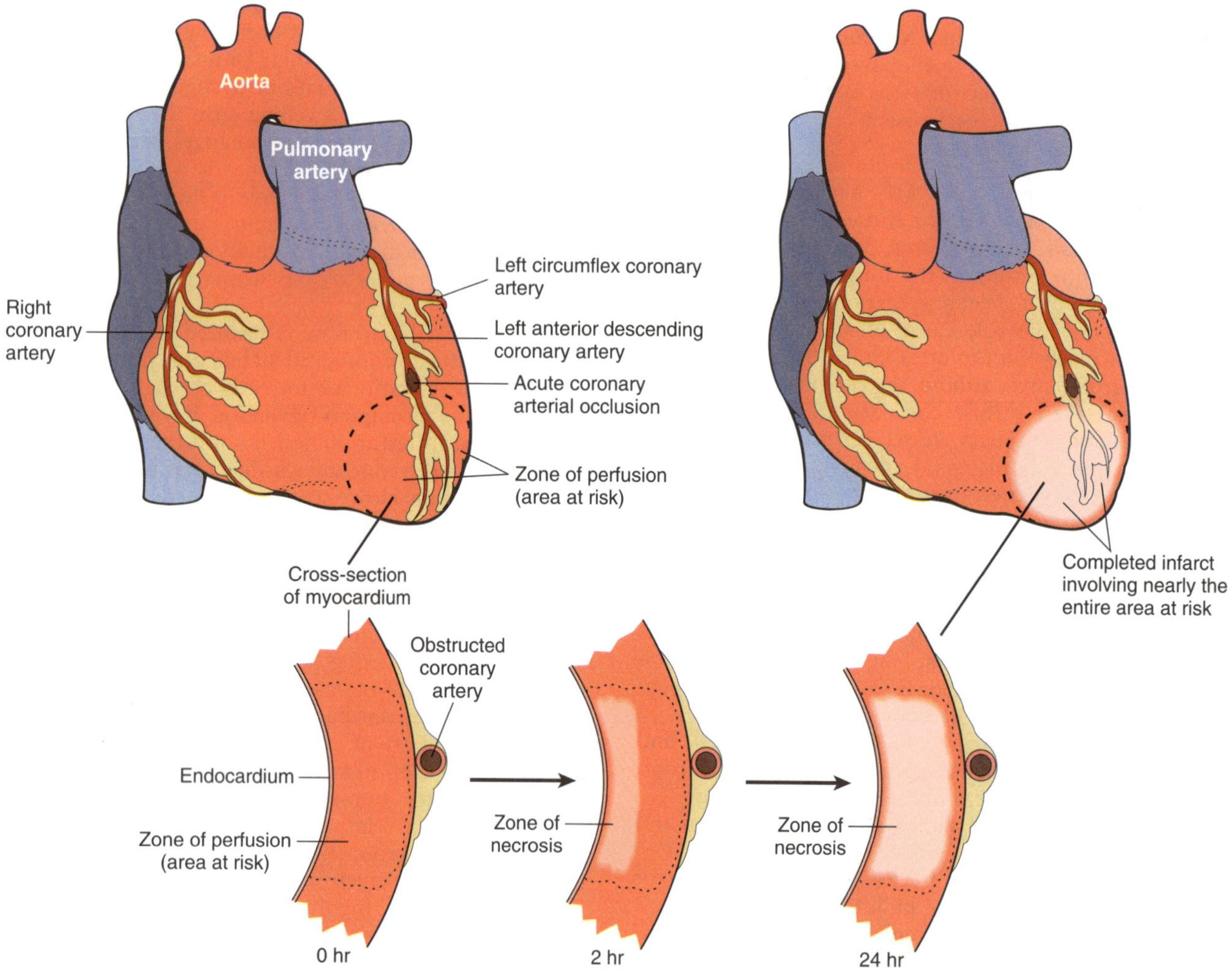

Figure 11–8

Progression of myocardial necrosis after coronary artery occlusion. Necrosis begins in a small zone of the myocardium beneath the endocardial surface in the center of the ischemic zone. This entire region of myocardium depends on the occluded vessel for perfusion and is the area at risk. Note that a very narrow zone of myocardium immediately beneath the endocardium is spared from necrosis because it can be oxygenated by diffusion from the ventricle. The end result of obstruction to blood flow is necrosis of the muscle that was dependent on perfusion from the coronary artery obstructed. Nearly the entire area at risk loses viability.

In 90% of the population the posterior descending artery is supplied by the right coronary artery. In such individuals (said to have right dominant coronary artery), the following distribution of infarcts is seen:

Left anterior descending artery (40% to 50%): infarct involves anterior left ventricle, anterior septum, and apex circumferentially.

Right coronary artery (30% to 40%): infarct involves posterior left ventricle, posterior septum, and right ventricular free wall in some cases.

Left circumflex artery (15% to 20%): infarct involves lateral left ventricle except the apex.

Other coronary occlusions are occasionally encountered. These include the left main coronary artery or secondary branches, such as the diagonal branches of the LAD artery or marginal branches of the LCX artery. In contrast, significant atherosclerosis or thrombosis of penetrating intramyocardial branches of coronary arteries rarely occur. Severe coronary occlusion without associated myocardial damage suggests the prior formation of protective collateral connections.

The gross and microscopic appearance of an MI depends on the interval of time since the original injury (Table 11–2). Areas of damage undergo a progressive and highly characteristic sequence of morphologic changes. Despite recent excitement about potential myocardial repopulation by resident or circulating stem cells, myocardial necrosis proceeds invariably to scar formation without any significant regeneration.

Early recognition of acute MIs can be challenging, particularly when death occurs within a few hours after symptom onset. **MIs less than 12 hours old are usually not grossly apparent.** However, infarcts more than 3 hours old can be visualized by exposing heart slices to vital stains (e.g., triphenyl tetrazolium chloride, a substrate for lactate dehyrogenase in viable heart). Because dehydrogenases are depleted in the area of

Table 11–2 Evolution of Morphologic Changes in Myocardial Infarction

Time	Gross Features	Light Microscopic Findings	Electron Microscopic Findings
Reversible Injury			
0–½ hr	None	None	Relaxation of myofibrils; glycogen loss; mitochondrial swelling
Irreversible Injury			
½–4 hr	None	Usually none; variable waviness of fibers at border	Sarcolemmal disruption; mitochondrial amorphous densities
4–12 hr	Occasionally dark mottling	Beginning coagulation necrosis; edema; hemorrhage	
12–24 hr	Dark mottling	Ongoing coagulation necrosis; pyknosis of nuclei; myocyte hypereosinophilia; marginal contraction band necrosis; beginning neutrophilic infiltrate	
1–3 days	Mottling with yellow-tan infarct center	Coagulation necrosis, with loss of nuclei and striations; interstitial infiltrate of neutrophils	
3–7 days	Hyperemic border; central yellow-tan softening	Beginning disintegration of dead myofibers, with dying neutrophils; early phagocytosis of dead cells by macrophages at infarct border	
7–10 days	Maximally yellow-tan and soft, with depressed red-tan margins	Well-developed phagocytosis of dead cells; early formation of fibrovascular granulation tissue at margins	
10–14 days	Red-gray depressed infarct borders	Well-established granulation tissue with new blood vessels and collagen deposition	
2–8 wk	Gray-white scar, progressive from border toward core of infarct	Increased collagen deposition, with decreased cellularity	
>2 mo	Scarring complete	Dense collagenous scar	

ischemic necrosis (they leak through damaged cell membranes and can actually form the basis for detecting MI in peripheral blood samples; Chapter 1), an infarcted area is revealed as an unstained pale zone (old scars appear white and glistening; Fig. 11–9). By **12 to 24 hours after MI, an infarct can usually be grossly identified by a reddish blue discoloration** caused by stagnant, trapped blood. Progressively thereafter, an infarct becomes more sharply delineated as a yellow-tan, softened area; by 10 to 14 days infarcts become rimmed by hyperemic (highly vascularized) granulation tissue. Over the succeeding weeks the MI evolves to a fibrous scar.

The microscopic appearance also undergoes a characteristic sequence of changes (Table 11–2 and Fig. 11–10). Typical features of **coagulative necrosis** (Chapter 1) become detectable within 4 to 12 hours of infarction. "**Wavy fibers**" can also be present at the edges of an infarct; these reflect the stretching and buckling of noncontractile dead fibers but are considered "soft" findings of acute infarction. Sublethal ischemia can also induce myocyte vacuolization. These are large cleared intracellular spaces, probably containing water; such myocytes are still alive but are poorly contractile.

Necrotic myocardium elicits **acute inflammation** (typically most prominent 1–3 days after MI), followed

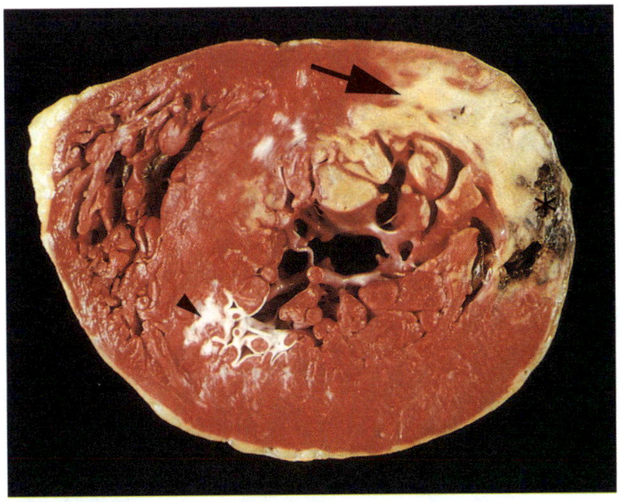

Figure 11–9

Acute myocardial infarct of the posterolateral left ventricle demonstrated by a lack of triphenyl tetrazolium chloride staining in areas of necrosis *(arrow);* the staining defect is due to leakage of lactate dehydrogenase after cell death. Note the anterior scar *(arrowhead),* indicative of old infarct. The myocardial hemorrhage at the right edge of the infarct *(asterisk)* is due to ventricular rupture and was the acute cause of death in this patient (specimen is oriented with the posterior wall at the top).

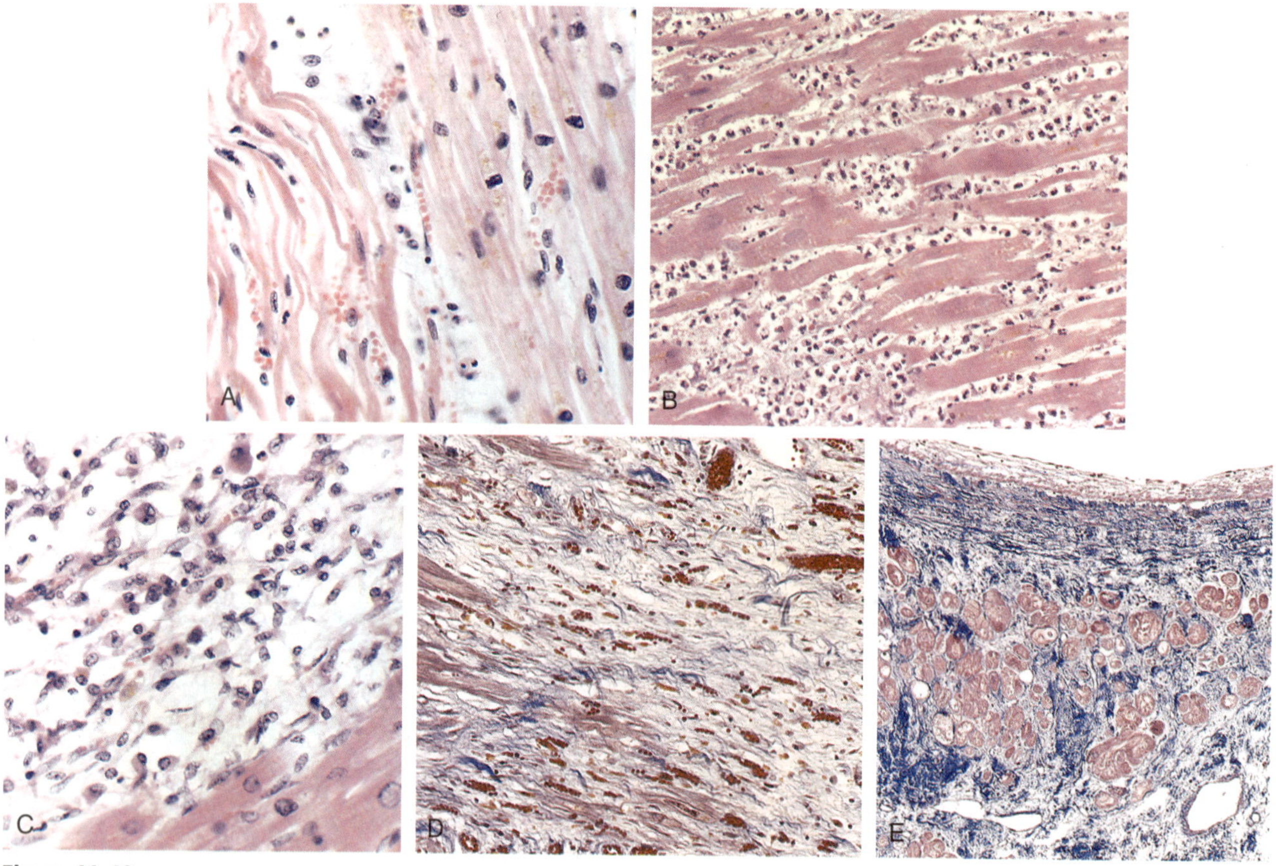

Figure 11–10

Microscopic features of MI and its repair. **A,** One-day-old infarct showing coagulative necrosis along with wavy fibers, compared with adjacent normal fibers (at right). Widened spaces contain edema fluid and scattered neutrophils. **B,** Dense polymorphonuclear leukocytic infiltrate in area of 2- to 3-day-old MI. **C,** Nearly complete removal of necrotic myocytes by macrophage phagocytosis (7–10 days). **D,** Granulation tissue characterized by loose collagen and abundant capillaries. **E,** Well-healed myocardial infarct with replacement of the necrotic fibers by dense collagenous scar. A few residual cardiac muscle cells are present. **D** and **E,** Masson's trichrome stain to accentuate the collagen (staining peacock blue).

by a wave of macrophages to remove necrotic myocytes and neutrophil fragments (most pronounced 5–10 days after MI). The infarcted zone is progressively replaced by **granulation tissue** (most prominent 2–3 weeks after MI), which in turn forms the provisional scaffolding upon which dense **collagenous scar** is formed. In most instances scarring is well advanced by the end of the sixth week, but the efficiency of repair depends on the size of the original lesion. Healing requires the migration of inflammatory cells and ingrowth of new vessels that can access infarcts only from the intact vasculature at the infarct margins. Thus, an **MI heals from its borders toward the center,** and a large infarct may not heal as readily or as completely as a small one. Once an MI is completely healed, it is impossible to distinguish its age (i.e., the dense fibrous scars of 8-week-old and 10-year-old lesions look similar).

Changes in an Infarct due to Reperfusion. The current therapeutic goal in acute MIs is to salvage the maximal amount of ischemic myocardium by restoration of tissue perfusion as quickly as possible. Such *reperfusion* is achieved by thrombolysis (dissolution of thrombus by streptokinase or tissue plasminogen activator), balloon angioplasty (with or without stenting), or coronary arterial bypass graft. Unfortunately, while preservation of viable (but at-risk) heart can improve both short- and long-term outcomes, reperfusion is not a completely innocuous process. Indeed, there is a distinct entity of *reperfusion injury* that can incite *greater* local damage than might have otherwise occurred without rapid restoration of blood flow. As discussed in Chapter 1, reperfusion injury is mediated in part by oxygen free radicals generated by the increased number of infiltrating leukocytes facilitated by reperfusion. Reperfusion-induced microvascular injury causes not only hemorrhage but also endothelial swelling that occludes capillaries and may prevent local blood flow (called *no-reflow*).

The typical appearance of ischemic and reperfused myocardium is shown in Figure 11–11A and B. A reperfused infarct usually has hemorrhage because the vasculature injured during the period of ischemia is leaky after flow is restored. Irreversibly damaged myocytes subjected to reperfusion also show *contraction band necrosis*. Contraction bands are intensely eosinophilic transverse bands

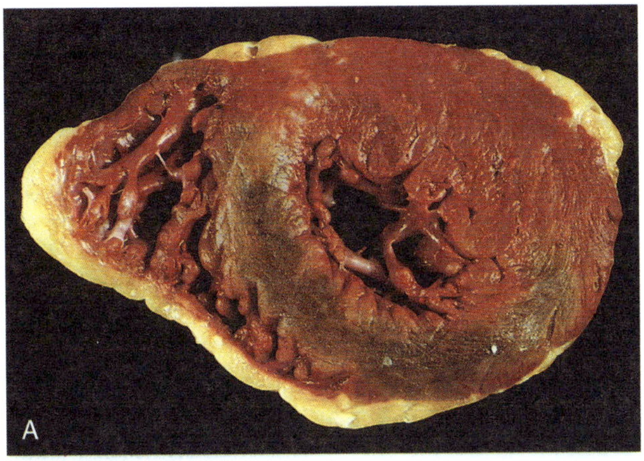

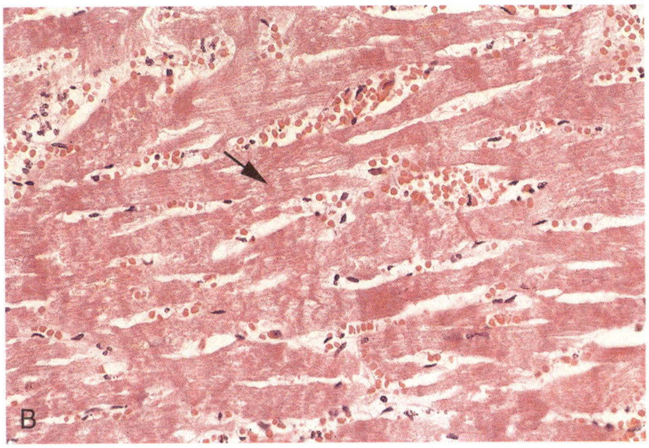

Figure 11–11

Consequences of myocardial ischemia followed by reperfusion. **A** and **B,** Gross and microscopic appearance of myocardium modified by reperfusion. **A,** Large, hemorrhagic, anterior-wall MI from patient treated with streptokinase (triphenyl tetrazolium chloride–stained transverse section; posterior wall at top.) **B,** Myocardial necrosis with hemorrhage and contraction bands, visible as hypereosinophilic bands spanning myofibers *(arrow).*

composed of hypercontracted sarcomeres. These are due to exaggerated contraction of myofibrils occurring when high extracellular calcium concentrations in the restored blood flow are able to cross damaged plasma membranes and drive actin-myosin interactions. In the absence of ATP to allow relaxation, the sarcomeres are stuck in this final agonal tetanic state. Thus, *reperfusion not only salvages reversibly injured cells but also alters the morphology of cells already lethally injured at the time of reflow.*

It should be noted that despite timely reperfusion and salvage, ischemic (but viable) myocardium can show profound dysfunction. Although most of this viable myocardium can ultimately recover normal function, abnormalities in cellular biochemistry may persist for several days after ischemia and lead to a noncontractile state *(stunned myocardium).* Such stunning can produce a state of transient reversible cardiac failure that may require pump assistance to support the patient until cardiac function returns.

Clinical Features. An MI is usually heralded by severe, crushing substernal chest pain or discomfort that can radiate to the neck, jaw, epigastrium, or left arm. In contrast to the pain of angina pectoris, the pain of an MI typically lasts from 20 minutes to several hours and is not significantly relieved by nitroglycerin or rest. In a substantial minority of patients (10% to 15%) MIs can be entirely asymptomatic. Such "silent" infarcts are particularly common in patients with underlying diabetes mellitus (with peripheral neuropathies) and in the elderly.

With MIs the pulse is generally rapid and weak, and patients can be diaphoretic and nauseated particularly with posterior-wall MIs. Dyspnea is common and is caused by impaired myocardial contractility and dysfunction of the mitral valve apparatus, with resultant pulmonary congestion and edema. With massive MIs (>40% of the left ventricle) cardiogenic shock develops.

Electrocardiographic abnormalities are important markers of MIs; these include changes such as Q waves (indicating transmural infarcts), and ST-segment abnormalities and T-wave inversion (representing abnormalities in myocardial repolarization). Arrhythmias caused by electrical abnormalities of the ischemic myocardium and conduction system are common, and indeed, SCD due to a lethal arrhythmia accounts for the vast majority of deaths occurring before hospitalization.

Laboratory evaluation of MI is based on measuring the blood levels of intracellular macromolecules that leak out of injured myocardial cells through damaged cell membranes; these molecules include myoglobin, cardiac troponins T and I (TnT, TnI), creatine kinase (CK, and more specifically the myocardial-specific isoform, CK-MB), lactate dehydrogenase, and many others. Troponins and CK-MB have high specificity and sensitivity for myocardial damage.

TnI and TnT are not normally detectable in the circulation, but after acute MI both troponins become detectable after 2 to 4 hours and peak at 48 hours; their levels remain elevated for 7 to 10 days. CK-MB is the second best marker after the cardiac-specific troponins. Since various forms of CK are found in brain, myocardium, and skeletal muscle, total CK activity is not a reliable marker of cardiac injury (i.e., it could come from skeletal muscle injury). Thus, the CK-MB isoform—principally derived from myocardium but also present at low levels in skeletal muscle—is the more specific indicator of heart damage. CK-MB activity begins to rise within 2 to 4 hours of MI, peaks at 24 to 48 hours, and returns to normal within approximately 72 hours. Although cardiac troponin and CK-MB are equally sensitive at early stages of an MI, persistence of elevated troponin levels for approximately 10 days allows the diagnosis of an acute MI long after CK-MB levels have returned to normal. With reperfusion, both troponin and CK-MB peaks occur earlier as a result of washout of the enzyme from the necrotic tissue.

Consequences and Complications of MI. Extraordinary progress has been made in patient outcomes subsequent to acute MI; since the 1960s the *in-hospital death rate* has declined from approximately 30% to an overall rate of between 10% and 13% today (and to ~7% for patients receiving aggressive reperfusion therapy). Unfortunately, half of the deaths associated with acute MI occur in individuals who never reach the hospital; such patients generally die within 1 hour of symptom onset—usually as a result of arrhythmias. The variables associated with a poor prognosis include advanced age, female gender, diabetes mellitus, and previous MI.

Nearly three-fourths of patients have one or more complications after acute MI (some are illustrated in Fig. 11–12):

- *Contractile dysfunction.* An MI affects left ventricular pump function approximately proportional to its size. Typically, there is some degree of left ventricular failure, with hypotension, pulmonary vascular congestion, and fluid transudation into the pulmonary interstitial and alveolar spaces. Severe "pump failure" *(cardiogenic shock)* occurs in 10% to 15% of patients after acute MI, generally with a large infarct (often >40% of the left ventricle). Cardiogenic shock has a nearly 70% mortality rate and accounts for two-thirds of in-hospital deaths.
- *Arrhythmias.* Following an MI, many patients develop arrhythmias, which undoubtedly are responsible for many of the sudden deaths. MI-associated arrhythmias include sinus bradycardia, heart block, tachycardia, ventricular premature contractions or ventricular tachycardia, and ventricular fibrillation.
- *Myocardial rupture.* Rupture complicates somewhere between 1% and 5% of MIs but is a frequent cause (7% to 25%) of MI-associated demise. Complications include (1) rupture of the ventricular free wall, with hemopericardium and cardiac tamponade, usually fatal (Fig. 11–12A); (2) rupture of the ventricular septum, leading to a new VSD and left-to-right shunt (Fig. 11–12B); and (3) papillary muscle rupture, resulting in severe mitral regurgitation (Fig. 11–12C). Rupture can occur at almost any time after MI but is most common 3 to 7 days after infarction; it is at this point in the healing process that lysis of the myocardial connective tissue is maximal and the

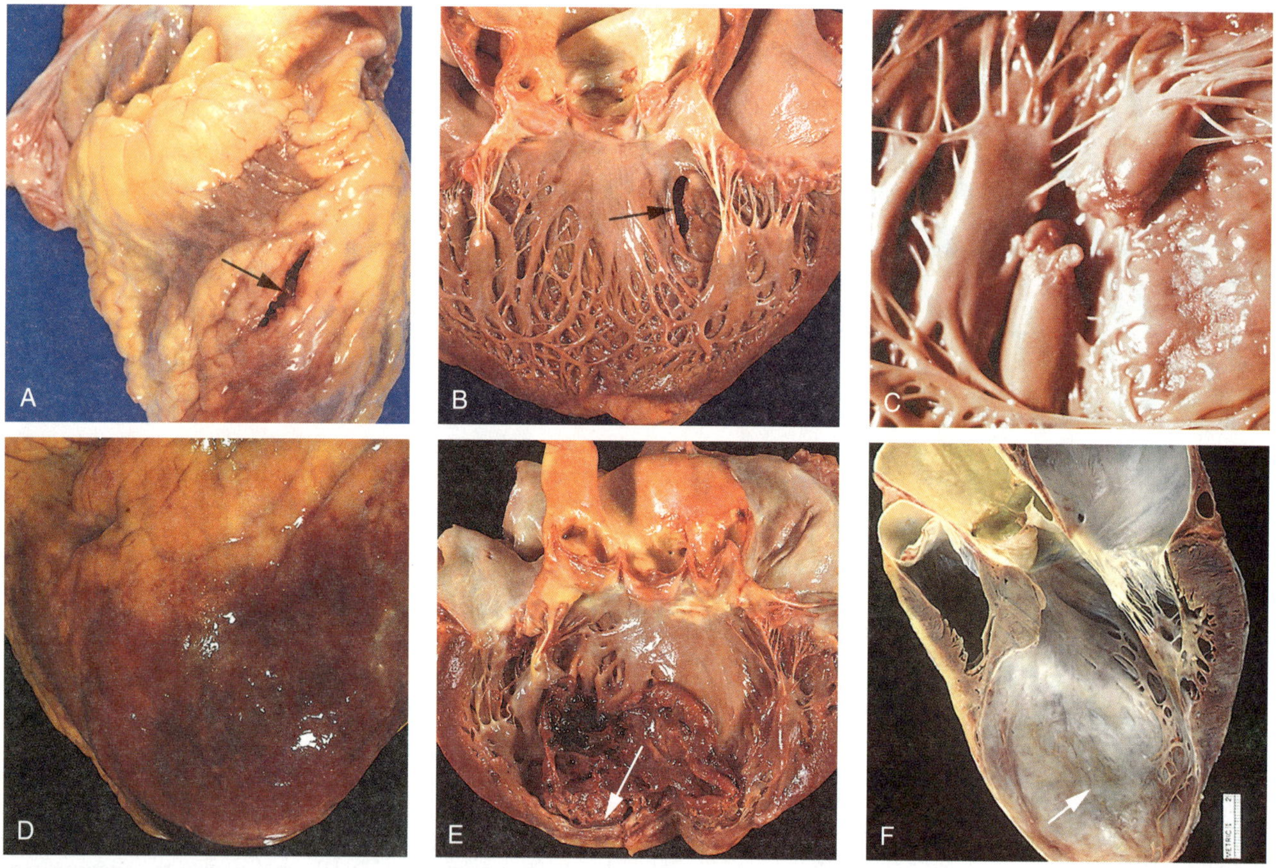

Figure 11–12

Complications of MI. **A–C,** Cardiac rupture. **A,** Anterior myocardial rupture in an acute infarct *(arrow).* **B,** Rupture of the ventricular septum *(arrow).* **C,** Complete rupture of a necrotic papillary muscle. **D,** Fibrinous pericarditis, showing a dark, roughened epicardial surface overlying an acute infarct. **E,** Early expansion of anteroapical infarct with wall thinning *(arrow)* and mural thrombus. **F,** Large apical left ventricular aneurysm *(arrow).* (**A–E,** From Schoen FJ: Interventional and Surgical Cardiovascular Pathology: Clinical Correlations and Basic Principles. Philadelphia, WB Saunders, 1989. **F,** Courtesy of Dr. William D. Edwards, Mayo Clinic, Rochester, Minnesota.)

granulation tissue has not deposited sufficient collagenous matrix to buttress the wall. Risk factors for free-wall rupture include age older than 60 years, female gender, pre-existing hypertension, lack of left ventricular hypertrophy, and no previous MI (pre-existing scarring tends to prevent myocardial tearing).

• *Pericarditis.* A fibrinous or hemorrhagic pericarditis usually develops within 2 to 3 days of a transmural MI and typically spontaneously resolves with time (Fig. 11–12D); it is the epicardial manifestation of the underlying myocardial inflammation.

• *Infarct expansion.* Because of the weakening of necrotic muscle, there may be disproportionate stretching, thinning, and dilation of the infarct region (especially with anteroseptal infarcts); this is often associated with mural thrombus (Fig. 11–12E).

• *Mural thrombus.* With any infarct, the combination of a local loss of contractility (causing stasis) with endocardial damage (causing a thrombogenic surface) can foster *mural thrombosis* (Chapter 4) and, potentially, *thromboembolism* (Fig. 11–12E).

• *Ventricular aneurysm.* A late complication, aneurysms of the ventricular wall most commonly result from a large transmural anteroseptal infarct that heals with the formation of thin scar tissue (Fig. 11–12F). Complications of ventricular aneurysms include mural thrombus, arrhythmias, and heart failure, but rupture of the fibrotic wall does not occur.

• *Papillary muscle dysfunction.* As mentioned above, dysfunction of a papillary muscle after MI occurs rarely as a result of rupture. More frequently, postinfarct mitral regurgitation results from ischemic dysfunction of a papillary muscle and underlying myocardium, and later from papillary muscle fibrosis and shortening, or ventricular dilation.

• *Progressive late heart failure* is discussed as chronic IHD below.

The risk of developing complications and the prognosis after MI depend on infarct size, site, and fractional thickness of the myocardial wall that is damaged (subendocardial or transmural infarct). Large transmural infarcts have a higher probability of cardiogenic shock, arrhythmias, and late CHF. Patients with anterior transmural infarcts are at greatest risk for free-wall rupture, expansion, mural thrombi, and aneurysm. In contrast, posterior transmural infarcts are more likely to be complicated by serious conduction blocks, right ventricular involvement, or both; when acute ventricular septal defects occur in this area they are more difficult to manage. Overall, however, patients with anterior infarcts have a substantially worse clinical course than those with posterior infarcts. With subendocardial infarcts thrombi may form on the endocardial surface, but pericarditis, rupture, and aneurysms rarely occur.

Long-term prognosis after MI depends on many variables, the most important of which are the quality of left ventricular function and the extent of vascular obstructions in vessels that perfuse the remaining viable myocardium. The overall total mortality within the first year is about 30%, including those who die before reaching the hospital. Thereafter, there is a 3% to 4% per year mortality.

Chronic Ischemic Heart Disease

Chronic IHD, also called *ischemic cardiomyopathy,* is essentially progressive heart failure as a consequence of ischemic myocardial damage. In most instances there is a history of MI. Chronic IHD usually results from postinfarction cardiac decompensation that follows exhaustion of the hypertrophy of the viable myocardium. In other cases severe obstructive CAD may be present without prior infarction, but with diffuse myocardial dysfunction.

Morphology

Hearts from patients with chronic IHD are usually **enlarged** and heavy from **left ventricular dilation and hypertrophy.** Invariably there is moderate to severe atherosclerosis of the coronary arteries, sometimes with total occlusion. Discrete, gray-white scars of healed infarcts are usually present. The endocardium generally shows patchy, fibrous thickening, and mural thrombi may be present. The major microscopic findings include myocardial hypertrophy, diffuse subendocardial myocyte vacuolization, and fibrosis from previous infarcts.

Clinical Features. Chronic IHD is characterized by the development of severe, progressive heart failure, sometimes punctuated by episodes of angina or MI. Arrhythmias are common and, along with CHF and intercurrent MI, account for many deaths.

Sudden Cardiac Death (SCD)

Affecting some 300,000 to 400,000 individuals annually in the United States, SCD is most commonly defined as unexpected death from cardiac causes either without symptoms or within 1 to 24 hours of symptom onset (different authors use different time points). Coronary artery disease is the most common underlying cause, and in many adults SCD is the first clinical manifestation of IHD. With younger victims other nonatherosclerotic causes are more common:

- Congenital coronary arterial abnormalities
- Aortic valve stenosis
- Mitral valve prolapse
- Myocarditis or sarcoidosis
- Dilated or hypertrophic cardiomyopathy
- Pulmonary hypertension
- Hereditary or acquired abnormalities of the cardiac conduction system. Of these, the most important cause is the autosomal dominant long-QT syndrome, due to mutations in various cardiac ion channels.
- Isolated myocardial hypertrophy, hypertensive or of unknown cause. Increased cardiac mass is an independent risk factor for SCD; thus, some young individuals

who die suddenly (including athletes) have unsuspected hypertrophic cardiomyopathy, myocarditis, or congenital abnormalities of coronary arteries.

The ultimate mechanism of SCD is most often a lethal arrhythmia, such as *ventricular fibrillation.* Although ischemic injury, as well as other pathologies, can directly affect the conduction system, most cases of fatal arrhythmia are triggered by electrical irritability of myocardium distant from the conduction system. The prognosis of patients vulnerable to SCD, especially those with chronic IHD, is markedly improved by automatic cardioverter defibrillators, which sense and electrically terminate episodes of ventricular fibrillation.

Morphology

Severe coronary atherosclerosis with critical (≥75%) stenosis involving one or more of the three major vessels is present in 80% to 90% of SCD victims; acute plaque disruption is found in only 10% to 20% of these. A healed MI is present in about 40%, but in those who were successfully resuscitated from sudden cardiac arrest, new MI is found in only 25% or less. Subendocardial myocyte vacuolization indicative of severe chronic ischemia is common. Only a minority (10% to 20%) of cases of SCD are of nonatherosclerotic origin.

SUMMARY

Ischemic Heart Disease

- The vast majority of ischemic heart disease is due to coronary artery atherosclerosis, with less frequent contributions of vasospasm, vasculitis, or embolism.
- Cardiac ischemia represents a mismatch in coronary supply and myocardial demand, and presents as different, albeit overlapping, syndromes:
    - *Angina pectoris* is chest pain due to inadequate perfusion and is typically due to atherosclerotic disease with ≥75% fixed stenosis (so-called critical stenosis).
    - *Unstable angina* results from a small fissure or rupture of atherosclerotic plaque triggering platelet aggregation, vasoconstriction, and formation of a mural thrombus that may not be occlusive.
    - *Acute myocardial infarction* typically results from acute thromboses that follow plaque disruption.
    - *Sudden cardiac death* results from a fatal arrhythmia, most commonly in patients with severe coronary artery disease.
    - *Chronic ischemic heart disease* is progressive heart failure due to ischemic injury, either from prior infarction(s) or chronic low-grade ischemia.
- Ischemia to myocardium rapidly (minutes) leads to loss of function and causes necrosis after 20 to 40 minutes. The diagnosis of MI is based on symptoms, electrocardiographic changes, and measurement of serum CK-MB and troponins. Gross and histologic changes of infarction require hours to days to develop.
- Complications of infarction include rupture of ventricle, free wall, septum, or papillary muscle; aneurysm formation; mural thrombus; arrhythmia; pericarditis; and CHF.

HYPERTENSIVE HEART DISEASE

As discussed in Chapter 10, chronic hypertension is a common disorder associated with considerable morbidity affecting many organs, including heart, brain, and kidneys. We will begin this section by first discussing the pathophysiology of myocardial hypertrophy, even though such hypertrophy can be caused by many stressors in addition to hypertension. The comments will then focus specifically on the cardiac complications of hypertension and will consider the effects of high blood pressure systemically, as well as of isolated pulmonary hypertension *(cor pulmonale).*

The Pathophysiology of Cardiac Hypertrophy

Cardiac myocytes are terminally differentiated cells without the capacity to divide; consequently, increase in myocyte number *(hyperplasia)* cannot occur in response to exogenous stresses. Instead, increased work—resulting from pressure or volume overload or from trophic signals (e.g., hyperthyroidism)—induces an increased myocyte mass and heart size *(hypertrophy).*

The extent of hypertrophy varies with the underlying cause. Thus, heart weights usually range from 350 to 600 gm (as much as twice normal) in pulmonary hypertension and IHD, from 400 to 800 gm (two to three times normal) in systemic hypertension, aortic stenosis, mitral regurgitation, or dilated cardiomyopathy, and from 600 to 1000 gm (three to four times normal) in aortic regurgitation or hypertrophic cardiomyopathy.

The pattern of hypertrophy reflects the nature of the initiating stimulus (Fig. 11–13). *Pressure-overloaded ventricles* (e.g., in hypertension or aortic valve stenosis) develop *concentric hypertrophy,* with an increased wall thickness; in the left ventricle the augmented muscle can even reduce the cavity diameter. In contrast, *volume overload* (e.g., aortic valve insufficiency) is characterized by hypertrophy associated with ventricular dilation. In volume overload, muscle mass increases roughly in proportion to chamber diameter; thus, in these severely dilated hearts there can actually be a substantial hyper-

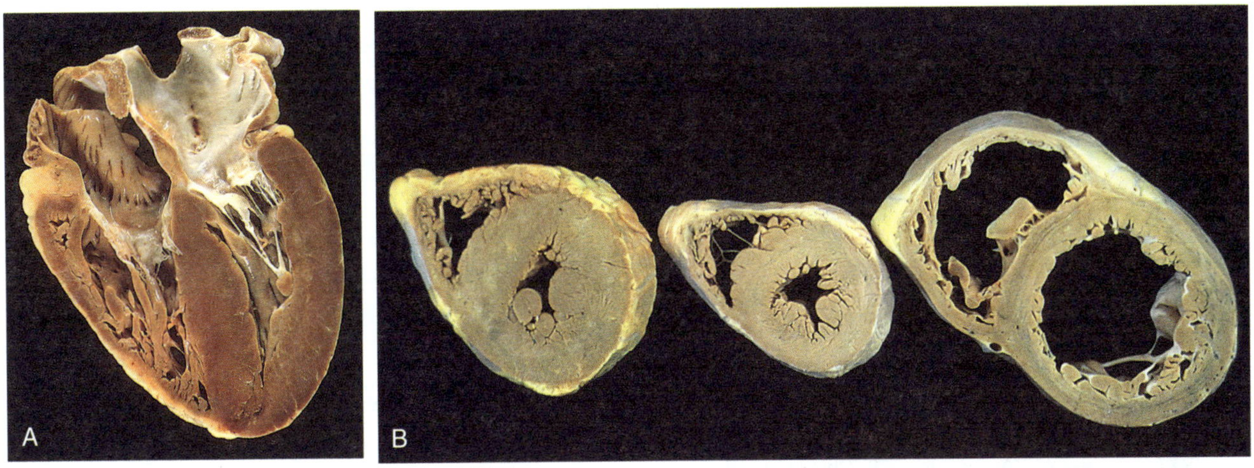

Figure 11–13

Left ventricular hypertrophy (LVH). **A,** Pressure hypertrophy due to left ventricular outflow obstruction. The left ventricle is on the lower right in this apical four-chamber view of the heart. **B,** Altered cardiac configuration in LVH without and with dilation, viewed in transverse heart sections. Compared with a normal heart *(center),* the pressure-hypertrophied hearts (*left* and in **A**) have increased mass and a thick left ventricular wall, but the hypertrophied and dilated heart *(right)* has increased mass but a normal wall thickness. (From Edwards WD: Cardiac anatomy and examination of cardiac specimens. In Emmanouilides GC, Riemenschneider TA, Allen HD, Gutgesell HP (eds): Moss and Adams Heart Disease in Infants, Children, and Adolescents: Including the Fetus and Young Adults, 5th ed. Philadelphia, Williams & Wilkins, 1995, p 86.)

trophy without increased wall thickness. Thus wall thickness is by itself not an adequate measure of hypertrophy due to volume overload.

While initially compensatory, prolonged or excessive hypertrophy can eventually result in myocyte contractile failure. However, the structural, biochemical, and molecular bases for this failure remain obscure. What is known is that cardiac hypertrophy is accompanied by numerous changes in gene expression, typically with patterns of protein synthesis recapitulating fetal cardiac development. The fetal isoforms of proteins may either be less functional than the adult isoforms, or may be expressed in different amounts. Alternatively, different intracellular handling of calcium ions could conceivably contribute to impaired contraction and relaxation. Myocyte hypertrophy is usually not accompanied by a commensurate increase in the vascular supply. Thus, there is a relative decrease in capillary density. The resultant chronic ischemia causes deposition of fibrous tissue, which limits diastolic relaxation. At the same time, the enlarged muscle mass has increased metabolic requirements that increase oxygen consumption. This sequence of events leads, eventually, to cardiac decompensation.

Systemic Hypertensive Heart Disease

Systemic hypertensive heart disease is diagnosed when there is (1) left ventricular hypertrophy (usually concentric) in the absence of other causal cardiovascular pathology (e.g., valvular stenosis), and (2) a history or pathologic evidence of hypertension. The Framingham Heart Study established unequivocally that even mild hypertension (levels only slightly above 140/90 mm Hg), if sufficiently prolonged, induces left ventricular hypertrophy. Roughly 25% of the US population suffers from at least this degree of hypertension.

Morphology

The essential feature of hypertensive heart disease is left ventricular hypertrophy, typically without ventricular dilation (Fig. 11–14). The left ventricular wall thickness may exceed 2.0 cm and the heart weight may exceed 500 gm. In time, the increased thickness of the left ventricular wall imparts a stiffness that impairs diastolic filling. This often induces left atrial enlargement.

Microscopically, myocyte diameter increases, typically associated with prominent, somewhat irregular nuclear enlargement and hyperchromasia ("box-car nuclei"); there is also increased interstitial fibrosis.

Clinical Features. Compensated hypertensive heart disease may be asymptomatic and suspected only by electrocardiographic or echocardiographic indications of left ventricular hypertrophy. In a subset of patients, the disease comes to attention only after the onset of atrial fibrillation (resulting from left atrial enlargement) and/or CHF. Depending on the severity, duration, and underlying cause of hypertension, and on the adequacy of therapeutic control, the patient may (1) enjoy normal longevity and die of unrelated causes, (2) develop progressive IHD by potentiating coronary atherosclerosis, (3) suffer progressive renal damage or cerebrovascular stroke, or (4) experience progressive heart failure. As mentioned earlier, increased cardiac mass is an independent risk factor for sudden cardiac death. Effective control of hypertension can prevent or lead to regression of cardiac hypertrophy and its associated risks.

Pulmonary Hypertensive Heart Disease (Cor Pulmonale)

Cor pulmonale consists of right ventricular hypertrophy and dilation due to *pulmonary hypertension caused by*

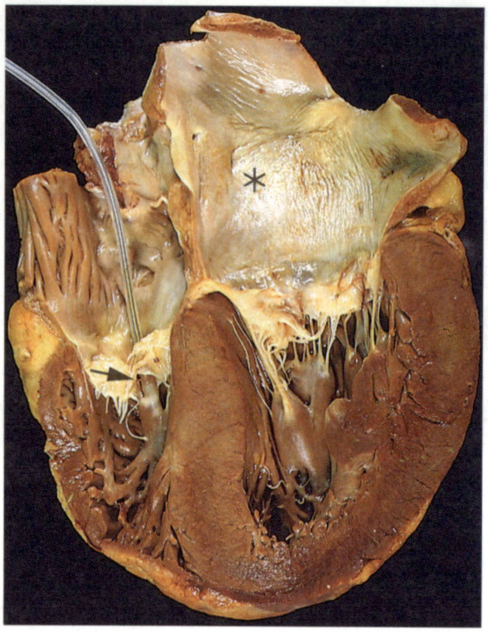

Figure 11–14

Hypertensive heart disease with marked concentric thickening of the left ventricular wall causing reduction in lumen size. The left ventricle is on the right in this apical four-chamber view of the heart. A pacemaker is incidentally present in the right ventricle *(arrow)*. Note also the left atrial dilation *(asterisk)* due to relative stiffening of the left ventricle causing impaired diastolic relaxation and subsequent atrial volume overload.

Table 11–3 Disorders Predisposing to Cor Pulmonale

Diseases of the Pulmonary Parenchyma
Chronic obstructive pulmonary disease
Diffuse pulmonary interstitial fibrosis
Pneumoconioses
Cystic fibrosis
Bronchiectasis
Diseases of the Pulmonary Vessels
Recurrent pulmonary thromboembolism
Primary pulmonary hypertension
Extensive pulmonary arteritis (e.g., Wegener granulomatosis)
Drug-, toxin-, or radiation-induced vascular obstruction
Extensive pulmonary tumor microembolism
Disorders Affecting Chest Movement
Kyphoscoliosis
Marked obesity (pickwickian syndrome)
Neuromuscular diseases
Disorders Inducing Pulmonary Arterial Constriction
Metabolic acidosis
Hypoxemia
Chronic altitude sickness
Obstruction to major airways
Idiopathic alveolar hypoventilation

primary *disorders of the lung parenchyma or pulmonary vasculature* (Table 11–3). Generally, right ventricular dilation and hypertrophy caused by congenital heart disease or by left ventricular failure are excluded by this definition.

Cor pulmonale may be acute or chronic, depending on the tempo by which the pulmonary hypertension develops. *Acute cor pulmonale* most commonly follows massive pulmonary embolism with obstruction of >50% of the pulmonary vascular bed. *Chronic cor pulmonale* occurs secondary to prolonged pressure overload caused by obstruction of the pulmonary vasculature, or compression or obliteration of septal capillaries (resulting from emphysema, interstitial pulmonary fibrosis, or primary pulmonary hypertension).

Morphology

In acute cor pulmonale the right ventricle is usually dilated but does not show hypertrophy; if an embolism causes sudden death the heart may even be of normal size. Chronic cor pulmonale is characterized by right ventricular (and often right atrial) hypertrophy. In extreme cases the thickness of the right ventricular wall may be comparable to or even exceed that of the left ventricle (Fig. 11–15). When ventricular failure develops the right ventricle and atrium may also be dilated. Such dilation may mask right ventricular hypertrophy. Because chronic cor pulmonale occurs in the setting of chronically elevated pulmonary arterial pressure, the pulmonary arteries often contain atheromatous plaques and other lesions reflecting long-standing pulmonary hypertension (Chapter 13).

SUMMARY

Hypertensive Heart Disease

- Hypertensive heart disease can affect either the left or the right ventricle; the latter is called cor pulmonale. The response of the heart to increased pressures is myocyte hypertrophy.
- In chronic pressure overload, as with hypertension or aortic stenosis, there is concentric hypertrophy of the affected ventricle. With volume overload (e.g., valvular incompetence), ventricular hypertrophy is accompanied by dilation.
- The mechanisms that result in heart failure due to hypertension are poorly understood; they probably involve the synthesis of relatively less efficient myocyte proteins, as well as a diminished vascular supply relative to the increased myocyte mass.
- Cor pulmonale results from pulmonary hypertension caused by primary disorders of lung parenchyma (e.g., emphysema) or pulmonary vasculature.

VALVULAR HEART DISEASE

Valvular disease results in stenosis or insufficiency (regurgitation or incompetence), or both.

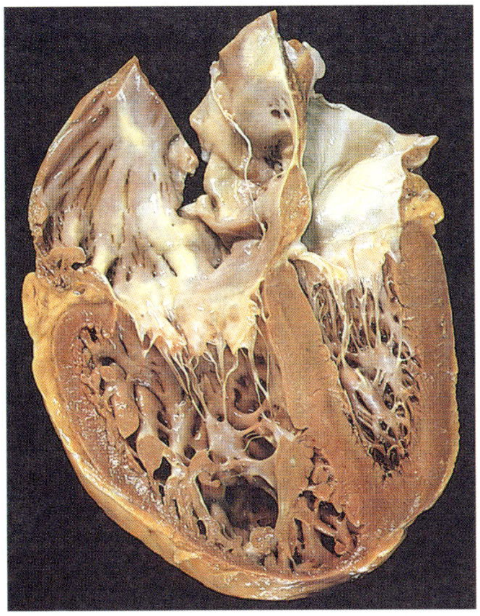

Figure 11–15

Chronic cor pulmonale, characterized by a markedly dilated and hypertrophied right ventricle, with thickened free wall and hypertrophied trabeculae (apical four-chamber view of heart, right ventricle on *left*). The shape of the left ventricle (to the *right*) has been distorted by the right ventricular enlargement. Compare with Figure 11–16.

- *Stenosis is the failure of a valve to open completely, obstructing forward flow.* Valvular stenosis is almost always a chronic process caused by a primary cuspal abnormality (e.g., calcification or valve scarring).
- *Insufficiency results from failure of a valve to close completely, thereby allowing reversed flow.* Valvular insufficiency may result from either intrinsic disease of the valve cusps (e.g., valve destruction) or distortion of the supporting structures (e.g., the aorta, mitral annulus, tendinous cords, papillary muscles, ventricular free wall) without primary changes in the cusps. It can appear acutely, as with chordal rupture, or chronically due to leaflet scarring and retraction.

Stenosis or regurgitation can occur in pure forms, or may coexist in the same valve. Valvular disease may affect only a single valve (the mitral valve is most commonly affected), or more than one valve. The outcome of valvular disease depends on the valve involved, the degree of impairment, the tempo of its development, and the rate and quality of compensatory mechanisms. For example, sudden destruction of an aortic valve cusp by infection may cause massive regurgitation and rapid cardiac failure. In contrast, rheumatic mitral stenosis usually develops over years, and its clinical effects are remarkably well tolerated. Abnormal flow through diseased valves typically produces abnormal heart sounds called *murmurs*.

Valve abnormalities can be caused by congenital disorders or by a variety of acquired diseases. The most important causes of acquired valve diseases are summarized in Table 11–4; *acquired stenoses of the aortic and mitral valves account for approximately two-thirds of all valve disease.*

Calcific Aortic Stenosis

Degenerative changes in the cardiac valves are an almost inevitable part of the aging process, given the repetitive mechanical stresses to which they are subjected during life (>40 million cardiac cycles per year with substantial deformations during each cycle). Cuspal fibrosis and calcification can be thought of as valvular counterparts of age-related arteriosclerosis.

The most common degenerative valvular disease is calcific aortic stenosis. *It is the most common cause of aortic stenosis in the United States* and is usually the consequence of calcification from progressive age-associated "wear and tear" of either anatomically normal aortic valves or congenitally bicuspid valves (Fig. 11–16). *Congenitally bicuspid valves* (i.e., valves with only two functional cusps) occur with an estimated frequency of approximately 1.4% of live births. The two cusps are usually of unequal size, with the larger cusp having a midline *raphe,* resulting from incomplete cuspal separation during development. Bicuspid aortic valves are generally neither stenotic nor symptomatic throughout early life. However, they are more prone to progressive degenerative calcification (Fig. 11–16B). *Mitral valve calcification* primarily involves the valve annulus and is usually asymptomatic unless the calcifications encroach on the adjacent conduction system (Fig. 11–6C, D).

Table 11–4 Major Etiologies of Acquired Heart Valve Disease

Mitral Valve Disease	Aortic Valve Disease
Mitral Stenosis	**Aortic Stenosis**
Postinflammatory scarring (rheumatic heart disease)	Postinflammatory scarring (rheumatic heart disease) Senile calcific aortic stenosis Calcification of congenitally deformed valve
Mitral Regurgitation	**Aortic Regurgitation**
ABNORMALITIES OF LEAFLETS AND COMMISSURES	INTRINSIC VALVULAR DISEASE
Postinflammatory scarring Infective endocarditis Mitral valve prolapse Fen-phen-induced valvular fibrosis	Postinflammatory scarring (rheumatic heart disease) Infective endocarditis
ABNORMALITIES OF TENSOR APPARATUS	AORTIC DISEASE
Rupture of papillary muscle Papillary muscle dysfunction (fibrosis) Rupture of chordae tendineae	Degenerative aortic dilation Syphilitic aortitis Ankylosing spondylitis Rheumatoid arthritis Marfan syndrome
ABNORMALITIES OF LEFT VENTRICULAR CAVITY AND/OR ANNULUS	
LV enlargement (myocarditis, dilated cardiomyopathy) Calcification of mitral ring	

LV, left ventricular.

Modified from Schoen FJ: Surgical pathology of removed natural and prosthetic valves. Hum Pathol 18:558, 1987.

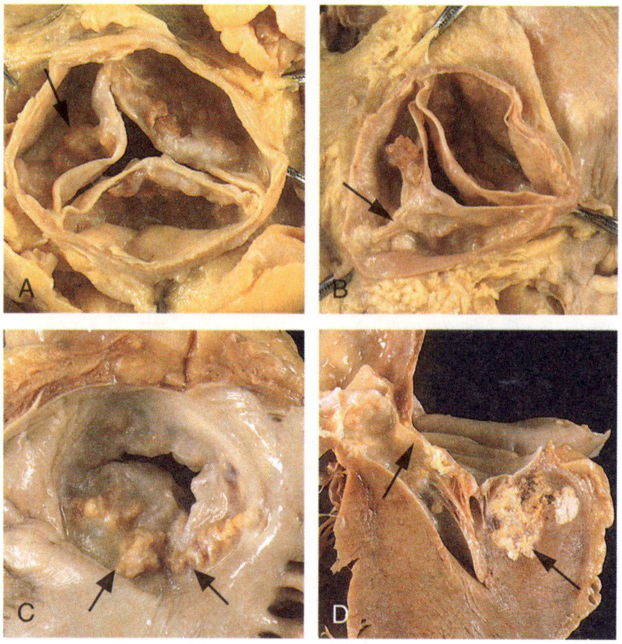

Figure 11–16

Calcific valvular degeneration. **A,** Calcific aortic stenosis of a previously normal valve having three cusps (viewed from aortic aspect). Nodular masses of calcium are heaped up within the sinuses of Valsalva *(arrow).* Note that the commissures are not fused, as in rheumatic aortic valve stenosis (see Fig. 11–20E). **B,** Calcific aortic stenosis occurring on a congenitally bicuspid valve. One cusp has a partial fusion at its center, called a raphe *(arrow).* **C–D,** Mitral annular calcification, with calcific nodules at the base (attachment margin) of the anterior mitral leaflet *(arrows).* **C,** Left atrial view. **D,** Cut section of myocardium. Arrows indicate leaflet and annular calcification.

The incidence of calcific aortic stenosis is increasing with the rising average age of the US population. In anatomically normal valves, it typically begins to manifest when patients reach their 70s and 80s; onset with bicuspid aortic valves is at a much earlier age (40–50 years).

Morphology

The hallmark of calcific aortic stenosis (with either normal or bicuspid valves) is **heaped-up calcified masses** on the outflow side of the cusps; these protrude into the sinuses of Valsalva and mechanically impede valve opening (see Fig. 11–16A); commissural fusion is not a usual feature of degenerative aortic stenosis, although the cusps may become secondarily fibrosed and thickened. An earlier, hemodynamically inconsequential stage of the calcification process is called aortic valve sclerosis. In calcific aortic stenosis, significant outflow obstruction leads to left ventricular pressure overload with concentric hypertrophy.

Clinical Features. In severe calcific aortic stenosis, valve orifices can be compromised by as much as 70% to 80%. The resulting left ventricular outflow obstruction leads to left ventricular pressures as high as 200 mm Hg or more; cardiac output is maintained only by virtue of concentric left ventricular hypertrophy. The hypertrophied myocardium tends to be relatively ischemic (see discussion above regarding hypertensive heart disease), and angina can develop. Syncope may develop due to poor perfusion of the brain. Systolic and diastolic dysfunction collude to cause CHF, and cardiac decompensation eventually ensues. The onset of symptoms (angina, CHF, or syncope) in aortic stenosis heralds the exhaustion of compensatory cardiac hyperfunction and carries a poor prognosis if not treated by surgery (50% mortality within 2 years of CHF inception).

Myxomatous Mitral Valve

In *myxomatous degeneration of the mitral valve,* one or both mitral leaflets are "floppy" and *prolapse,* meaning that they balloon back into the left atrium during systole. *Mitral valve prolapse* is a primary form of myxomatous mitral degeneration affecting 3% to 5% of adults in the United States, women seven times more frequently than men; as such, it is one of the most common forms of valvular heart disease in the industrialized world. Secondary myxomatous mitral degeneration can occur in any of a number of settings in which mitral regurgitation is caused by some other entity (e.g., IHD).

Morphology

Myxomatous degeneration of the mitral valve is characterized by ballooning (hooding) of the mitral leaflets (Fig. 11–17). The affected leaflets are enlarged, redundant, thick, and rubbery; the tendinous cords also tend to be elongated, thinned, and occasionally ruptured. In mitral valve prolapse, concomitant tricuspid valve involvement is common (20% to 40% of cases), and aortic and pulmonic valves can also be affected. Histologically, the essential change is thinning of the fibrosa layer of the valve, on which the structural integrity of the leaflet depends, accompanied by expansion of the middle spongiosa layer with increased deposition of myxomatous (mucoid) material. The same changes occur whether the myxomatous degeneration is due to an intrinsic defect (primary) or is caused by regurgitation due to another etiology (e.g., ischemic dysfunction).

Pathogenesis. The basis for primary myxomatous degeneration of the mitral valve is unknown. Nevertheless, there is almost certainly some underlying (possibly systemic) intrinsic defect of connective tissue—either in its synthesis or remodeling. Thus, myxomatous degeneration of the mitral valve is a common feature of Marfan syndrome (due to fibrillin-1 mutations; Chapter 7) and occasionally occurs in other connective tissue disorders. In some patients, there are additional hints of systemic connective tissue structural abnormalities, such as scoliosis and high-arched palates. Subtle defects in structural proteins or the cells that make them may predispose hemodynamically stressed connective tissues (e.g., cardiac valves) to defective synthesis or catabolism of

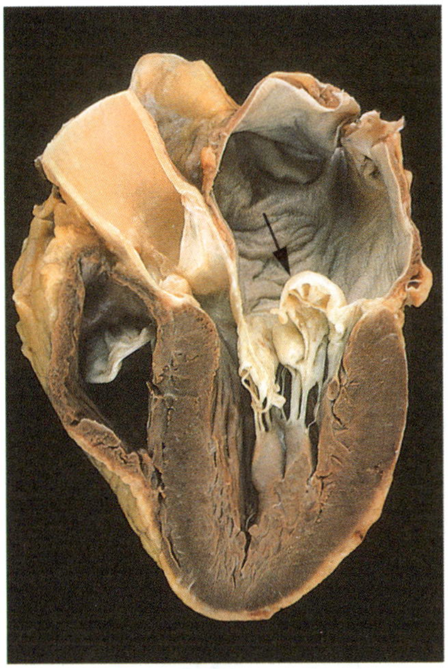

Figure 11–17

Myxomatous degeneration of the mitral valve. Long axis of left ventricle demonstrating hooding with prolapse of the posterior mitral leaflet into the left atrium *(arrow)*. The left ventricle is on the right in this apical four-chamber view. (Courtesy of Dr. William D. Edwards, Mayo Clinic, Rochester, Minnesota.)

extracellular matrix. Secondary myxomatous change presumably results from "degenerative" changes in the valve myofibroblasts, responding to chronically aberrant hemodynamic forces.

Clinical Features. Most patients with mitral valve prolapse are asymptomatic, and the valvular abnormality is usually discovered only incidentally on physical examination. A minority of patients may complain of palpitations, dyspnea, or atypical chest pain. Auscultation discloses midsystolic click(s) caused by abrupt tension on the redundant valve leaflets and chordae tendineae as the valve attempts to close; there may or may not be an associated regurgitant murmur. Although the majority of patients with mitral valve prolapse have a relatively benign course, approximately 3% experience one of several complications. These include hemodynamically significant mitral regurgitation and CHF, particularly if the chordae or valve leaflets rupture. Patients with mitral valve prolapse and valvular insufficiency are also at increased risk for the development of infective endocarditis (see below) and sudden death caused by ventricular arrhythmias. Stroke or other systemic infarction may occur from embolism of thrombi formed in the left atrium.

Rheumatic Valvular Disease

Rheumatic fever (RF) is an acute, immunologically mediated, multisystem inflammatory disease that occurs a few weeks after an episode of group A β-hemolytic streptococcal pharyngitis; it can also rarely occur with streptococcal infections at other sites (e.g., skin). Acute rheumatic heart disease (RHD) is the cardiac manifestation of RF and is associated with inflammation of the valves, myocardium, or pericardium.

Chronic valvular deformities are the most important consequences of RHD; these are characterized by diffuse and dense scarring of valves resulting in permanent dysfunction (mitral stenosis being most common). The incidence of RF, and thus RHD, has declined in many parts of the industrialized world over the past 30 years; this is due to a combination of improved socioeconomic conditions, rapid diagnosis and treatment of streptococcal pharyngitis, and a fortuitous (and unexplained) decline in the virulence of group A streptococci. Nevertheless, in economically depressed urban areas or developing countries, RF and RHD remain important public health problems.

Morphology

The cardiac manifestations of acute RF and chronic RHD are shown in Fig. 11–18. During **acute RF,** discrete inflammatory lesions are found in various tissues throughout the body. Within the heart these are called **Aschoff bodies** and are pathognomonic for RF (Fig. 11–18A). Aschoff bodies consist of a central zone of degenerating, hypereosinophilic extracellular matrix infiltrated by lymphocytes (primarily T cells), occasional plasma cells, and plump activated macrophages called **Anitschkow cells.** The Anitschkow cells have abundant cytoplasm and central nuclei with chromatin arrayed in a slender, wavy ribbon (so-called caterpillar cells); these activated macrophages can also fuse to form giant cells. Aschoff bodies can be found in any of the three layers of the heart—pericardium, myocardium, or endocardium (including valves)—so-called **pancarditis.** The pericardium shows a fibrinous or serofibrinous exudate, which generally resolves without sequelae. The myocardial involvement (myocarditis) takes the form of scattered Aschoff bodies within the interstitial connective tissue. Valve involvement results in fibrinoid necrosis along the lines of closure (Fig. 11–18B) forming 1- to 2-mm vegetations (verrucae) that have little effect on cardiac function. These irregular, warty projections probably arise from the precipitation of fibrin at sites of erosion caused by underlying inflammation and collagen degeneration.

Chronic RHD is characterized by organization of the acute inflammation and subsequent scarring. The cardinal anatomic changes of the mitral (or tricuspid) valve include leaflet thickening, commissural fusion and shortening, and thickening and fusion of the chordae tendineae (Fig. 11–18C–D). Fibrous bridging across the valvular commissures and calcification create "fish mouth" or "buttonhole" stenoses (Fig. 11–18C). Microscopically there is neovascularization (grossly evident in Fig. 11–18D), with diffuse fibrosis that obliterates the normal leaflet architecture. Aschoff bodies are replaced by fibrous scar, so diagnostic forms of these lesions are rarely seen in chronic RHD.

The functional consequence of RHD is **valvular stenosis and regurgitation** (stenosis tends to predominate); indeed, RHD is overwhelmingly the most frequent cause of mitral stenosis accounting for 99% of cases. The **mitral valve alone is involved in 70% of cases** of RHD, with combined mitral and aortic disease

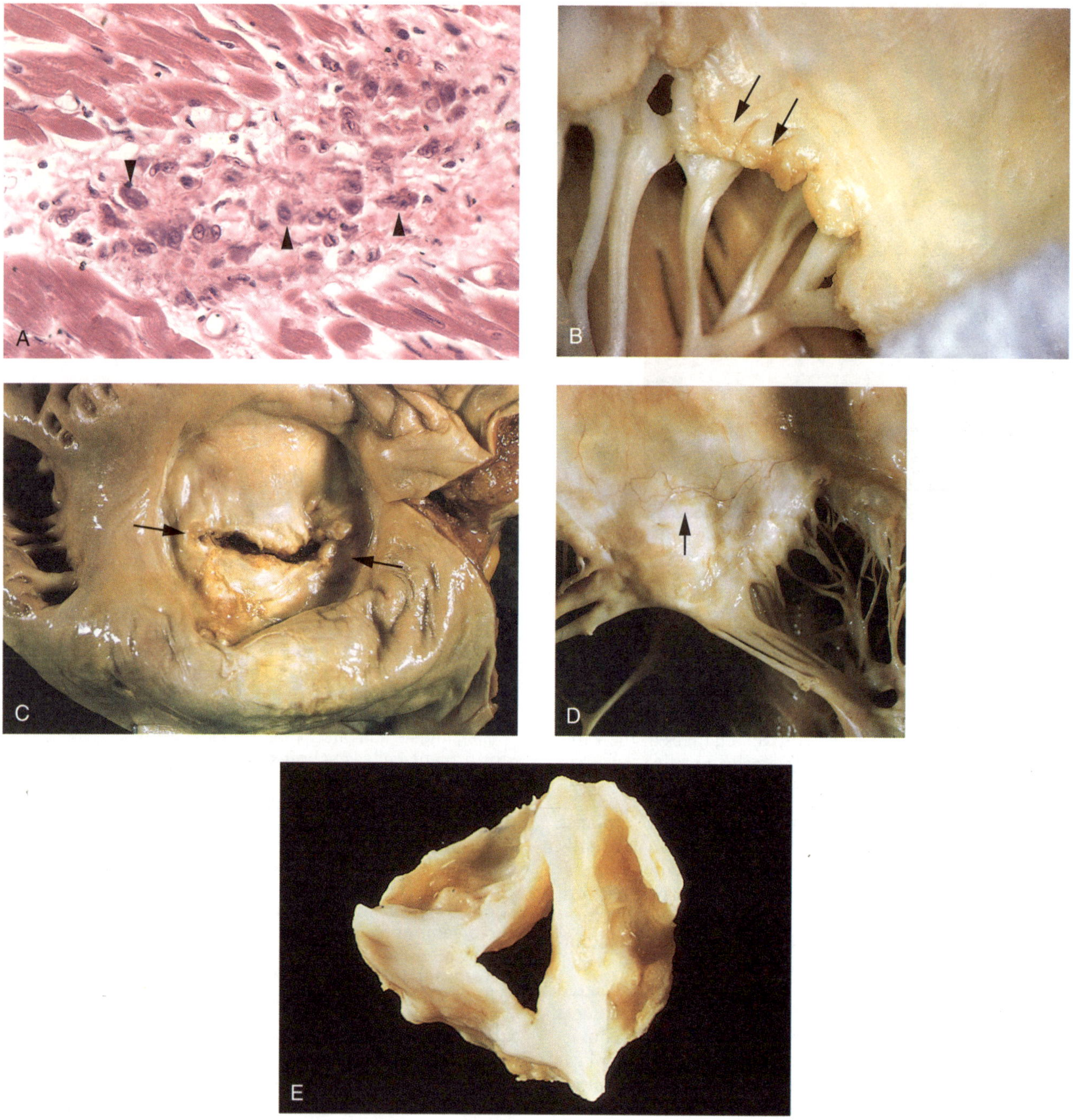

Figure 11–18

Acute and chronic rheumatic heart disease. **A,** Microscopic appearance of an Aschoff body in a patient with acute rheumatic carditis; there is central necrosis with a circumscribed collection of mononuclear inflammatory cells, with some activated macrophages (Anitschkow cells) with prominent nucleoli *(arrowheads)*. **B,** Acute rheumatic mitral valvulitis superimposed on chronic rheumatic heart disease. Small vegetations (verrucae) are visible along the line of closure of the mitral valve leaflet *(arrows)*. Previous episodes of rheumatic valvulitis have caused fibrous thickening and fusion of the chordae tendineae. **C–D,** Mitral stenosis with diffuse fibrous thickening and distortion of the valve leaflets, commissural fusion *(arrows)*, and thickening and shortening of the chordae tendineae. **D,** Opened valve. Note neovascularization of anterior mitral leaflet *(arrow)*. **E,** Surgically removed specimen of rheumatic aortic stenosis, demonstrating thickening and distortion of the cusps with commissural fusion (**E,** From Schoen FJ, St. John-Sutton M: Contemporary issues in the pathology of valvular heart disease. Human Pathol 18:568, 1967.)

in another 25%; the tricuspid valve is usually less frequently and less severely involved, and the pulmonic valve almost always escapes injury. With tight mitral stenosis, the left atrium progressively dilates and may harbor **mural thrombi.** Long-standing congestive changes in the lungs may induce pulmonary vascular and parenchymal changes and in time lead to right ventricular hypertrophy. With pure mitral stenosis, the left ventricle is generally normal.

Pathogenesis. *Acute RF is a hypersensitivity reaction induced by host antibodies elicited by group A streptococci.* However, many details of the pathogenesis remain uncertain despite years of investigation. It appears that the M proteins of certain streptococcal strains induce host antibodies that cross-react with glycoprotein antigens in the heart, joints, and other tissues. This explains the typical 2- to 3-week delay in symptom onset after the original infection, and the absence of streptococci in the lesions. Since only a small minority of infected patients ever experience RF (estimated at 3%), a genetic susceptibility is likely to influence the development of the pathogenic antibodies. The proposed sequence of events in acute RHD is summarized in Fig. 11–19. The chronic sequelae result from progressive fibrosis due to healing of the acute inflammatory lesions.

Clinical Features. Acute RF appears most often in children aged 5 to 15 years, but about 20% of first attacks

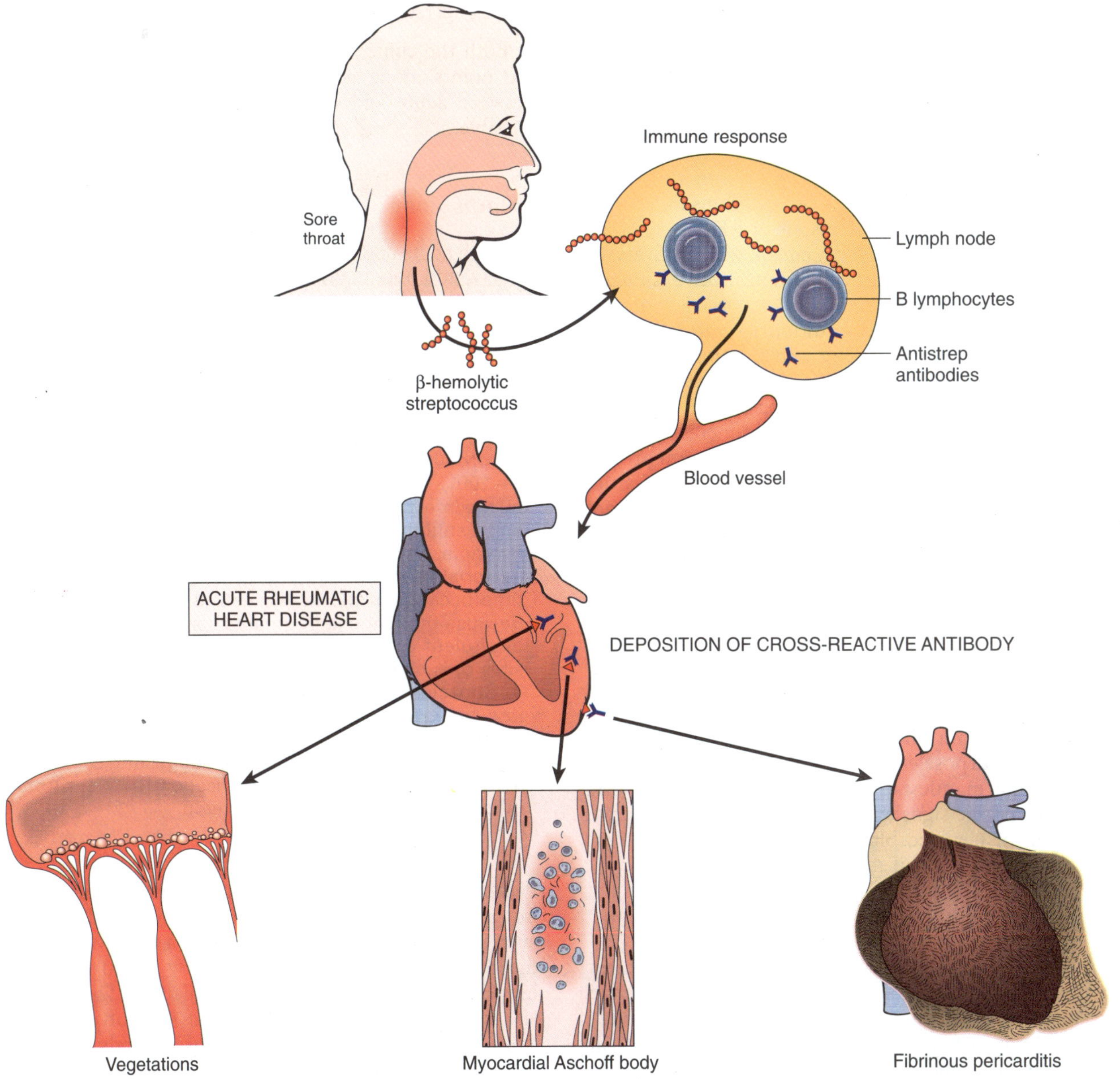

Figure 11–19

Pathogenesis and key morphologic changes of acute rheumatic heart disease. Acute rheumatic fever causes changes in the endocardium, myocardium, and epicardium. Chronic rheumatic heart disease is almost always caused by deformity of the heart valves, particularly the mitral and aortic valves.

occur in adults. Typically, the symptoms occur two to three weeks after an episode of streptococcal pharyngitis. Although cultures for streptococci are negative by the time clinical illness begins, antibodies to one or more streptococcal antigens (streptolysin O or DNAase) can be detected in most patients. The predominant clinical manifestations are arthritis and carditis; arthritis is far more common in adults. It typically begins with migratory polyarthritis accompanied by fever in which one large joint after another becomes painful and swollen for a period of days and then subsides spontaneously, leaving no residual disability. Clinical features of the carditis include pericardial friction rubs and arrhythmias. Myocarditis can be so severe that resulting cardiac dilation causes functional mitral insufficiency and even CHF. Nevertheless, fewer than 1% of patients die of acute RF.

After an initial attack there is increased vulnerability to disease reactivation with subsequent pharyngeal infections. Carditis is likely to worsen with each recurrence, and damage is cumulative. Other hazards include embolization from mural thrombi, primarily within the atria or their appendages, and infective endocarditis superimposed on deformed valves. *Chronic rheumatic carditis* usually does not cause clinical manifestations for years or even decades after the initial episode of RF. The signs and symptoms of valvular disease depend on which valve(s) are involved. As mentioned earlier, the mitral valve is the one most commonly involved and its stenosis is the most common manifestation. In addition to various cardiac murmurs, cardiac hypertrophy and dilation, and CHF, patients with chronic RHD often have arrhythmias (particularly atrial fibrillation in the setting of mitral stenosis), thromboembolic complications, and an increased risk of subsequent infective endocarditis. The long-term prognosis is highly variable. In some cases, there is a relentless cycle of valvular deformity yielding hemodynamic abnormality, which begets further deforming fibrosis. Surgical repair or replacement of diseased valves has greatly improved the outlook for patients with RHD.

Diagnosis of acute RHD is made by serologic evidence of a previous streptococcal infection, in conjunction with two or more of the following *Jones criteria:* (1) carditis, (2) migratory polyarthritis of the large joints, (3) subcutaneous nodules, (4) erythema marginatum of the skin, and (5) Sydenham chorea, a neurologic disorder with involuntary purposeless, rapid movements. One of the Jones criteria manifestations and two minor manifestations (nonspecific signs and symptoms that include fever, arthralgia, or elevated blood levels of acute-phase reactants) are also sufficient to make the diagnosis.

Infective Endocarditis

Infective endocarditis (IE) is a serious infection requiring prompt diagnosis and intervention. It is characterized by microbial invasion of heart valves or mural endocardium—often with destruction of the underlying cardiac tissues—and results in bulky, friable *vegetations* composed of necrotic debris, thrombus, and organisms. Although fungi, rickettsiae (Q fever), and chlamydiae can cause endocarditis, the vast majority of cases are caused by extracellular bacteria.

IE is traditionally classified into *acute and subacute forms,* mostly on the basis of clinical tempo and severity; the distinctions are attributable to the intrinsic microbial virulence and whether underlying cardiac disease is present.

- *Acute endocarditis* usually suggests a tumultuous, destructive infection, frequently involving a highly virulent organism attacking a previously normal valve, and causing death within days to weeks in more than 50% of patients despite antibiotics and surgery.
- *Subacute endocarditis* refers to infections by organisms of low virulence colonizing a previously abnormal heart, especially when there are deformed valves. The disease typically appears insidiously and follows a protracted course of weeks to months with most patients recovering after appropriate antibiotic therapy.

Both the clinical and morphologic patterns, however, are points along a spectrum, and a clear delineation between acute and subacute endocarditis is not always possible.

Morphology

In both acute and subacute forms of the disease, **friable, bulky,** and potentially **destructive vegetations** containing fibrin, inflammatory cells, and microorganisms are present on the heart valves (Fig. 11–20). The aortic and mitral valves are the most common sites of infection, although the tricuspid valve is a frequent target in the setting of intravenous drug abuse. Vegetations may be single or multiple and may involve more than one valve; they can erode into the underlying myocardium to produce an abscess cavity (ring abscess) (Fig. 11–20B). The appearance of vegetations is influenced by the infecting organism, the degree of host response, and antibiotic therapy. Fungal endocarditis, for example, tends to cause larger vegetations than does bacterial infection. **Systemic emboli** may occur at any time because of the friable nature of the vegetations. Because the embolic fragments contain large numbers of virulent organisms, abscesses often develop at the sites of such infarcts (**septic infarcts**).

Subacute endocarditis is typically associated with less valvular destruction than is acute endocarditis. Microscopically, in subacute IE vegetations often have granulation tissue at their bases, suggesting chronicity. As time passes, fibrosis, calcification, and a chronic inflammatory infiltrate may develop.

Pathogenesis. IE can develop on previously normal valves, but the presence of cardiac abnormalities predisposes to such infections. RHD was previously a major antecedent disorder, but it has been displaced by mitral valve prolapse, bicuspid aortic valves, and calcific valvular stenosis. Sterile platelet-fibrin deposits at sites of jet streams caused by pre-existing cardiac disease or indwelling vascular catheters may also be important sites for seeding of bacteria and development of endocarditis. With increasing use of prosthetic heart valves (discussed later), they now account for 10% to 20% of all cases of IE. Host factors such as neutropenia, immunodeficiency, malig-

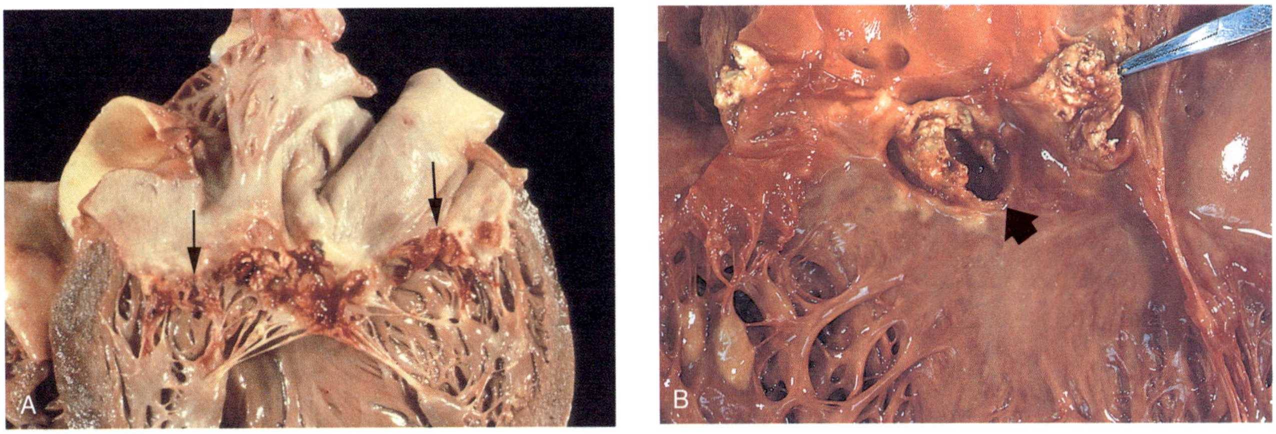

Figure 11–20

Infective (bacterial) endocarditis. **A,** Endocarditis of mitral valve (subacute, caused by *Streptococcus viridans*). The large, friable vegetations are denoted by arrows. **B,** Acute endocarditis of congenitally bicuspid aortic valve (caused by *Staphylococcus aureus*) with extensive cuspal destruction and ring abscess *(arrow).*

nancy, therapeutic immunosuppression, diabetes mellitus, and alcohol or intravenous drug abuse also increase the risk of IE.

The causative organisms differ depending on the underlying risk factors. Thus, endocarditis of previously damaged or otherwise abnormal valves is caused most commonly (50% to 60% of cases) by *viridans Streptococci,* a relatively banal group of normal oral flora. In contrast, the more virulent *S. aureus* (common to skin) can attack *deformed and healthy* valves and is responsible for 10% to 20% of cases overall; it is also the major offender in intravenous drug abusers. Additional bacterial agents include enterococci and the so-called HACEK group (*Haemophilus, Actinobacillus, Cardiobacterium, Eikenella,* and *Kingella*), all commensals in the oral cavity. More rarely, gram-negative bacilli and fungi are involved. In about 10% of cases, no organism can be isolated from the blood ("culture-negative" endocarditis). This is attributed to previous antibiotic therapy or difficulties in isolating the offending agent, or because deeply embedded organisms within the enlarging vegetation are not released into the blood.

Foremost among the conditions predisposing to endocarditis is seeding of the blood with microbes. The portal of entry of the agent into the bloodstream may be an obvious infection elsewhere, a dental or surgical procedure that causes a transient bacteremia, injection of contaminated material directly into the bloodstream by intravenous drug users, or an occult source from the gut, oral cavity, or trivial injuries. Recognition of predisposing cardiac abnormalities and clinical conditions causing bacteremia allows appropriate antibiotic prophylaxis.

Clinical Features. Fever is the most consistent sign of IE. However, in subacute disease (particularly in the elderly) fever may be absent, and the only manifestations may be nonspecific fatigue, weight loss, and a flulike syndrome. Splenomegaly is common in subacute IE. In contrast, acute endocarditis has a stormy onset with rapidly developing fever, chills, weakness, and lassitude. Murmurs are present in 90% of patients with left-sided lesions, but these may merely relate to the pre-existing cardiac abnormality predisposing to IE. Diagnosis is largely made on the basis of positive blood cultures, echocardiographic findings, and other clinical and laboratory findings.

Complications generally begin within the first weeks of the onset of IE. These include glomerulonephritis due to glomerular trapping of antigen-antibody complexes, thus giving rise to hematuria, albuminuria, or renal failure (*glomerulonephritis;* see Chapter 14). Septicemia, arrhythmias (suggesting invasion into underlying myocardium), and systemic embolization all bode ill. With prompt antibiotic therapy, previously common clinical findings due to microemboli are no longer seen frequently. These include petechiae, hemorrhages under the nail bed, and subcutaneous nodules in the pulp of digits.

Noninfected Vegetations

Nonbacterial Thrombotic Endocarditis

Nonbacterial thrombotic endocarditis (NBTE) is characterized by the deposition of variably sized masses of fibrin, platelets, and other blood components on cardiac valves. In contrast to IE, the valvular lesions of NBTE are sterile and do not contain microorganisms. Valvular damage is not a prerequisite for NBTE; indeed, the condition is usually found on previously normal valves. Although NBTE may occur in otherwise healthy individuals, a wide variety of diseases associated with general debility or wasting are associated with an increased risk of NBTE, hence the alternative term *marantic endocarditis.*

Morphology

NBTE vegetations are **sterile, nondestructive, and small** (1 mm); they occur singly or multiply along the line of closure of the leaflets or cusps (Fig. 11–21). Histologically they are composed of bland thrombus without accompanying inflammation or valve damage. With time, they can organize into delicate strands of fibrous tissue (so-called Lambl excrescences).

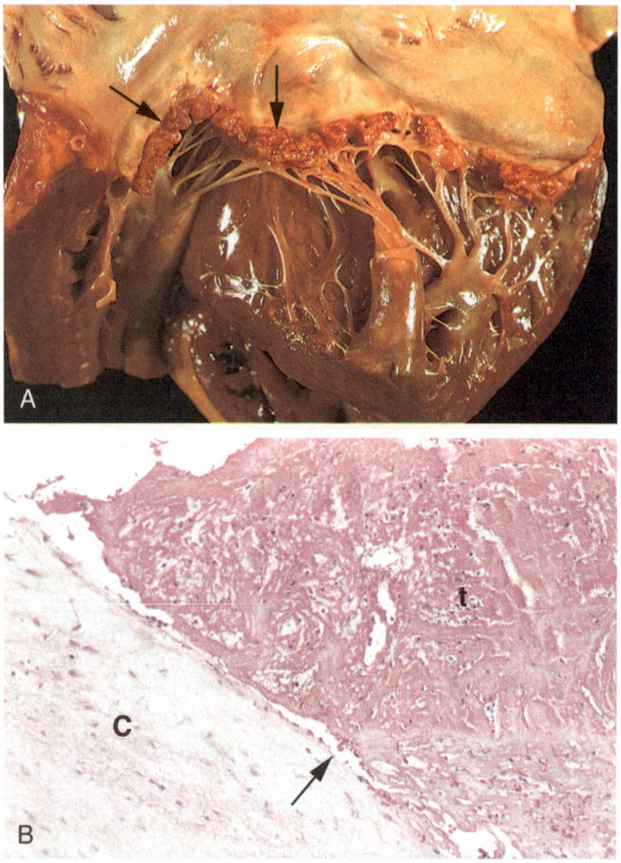

Figure 11–21

Nonbacterial thrombotic endocarditis. **A,** Nearly complete row of thrombotic vegetations along the line of closure of the mitral valve leaflets *(arrows).* **B,** Photomicrograph of nonbacterial thrombotic endocarditis, showing bland thrombus, with virtually no inflammation in the valve cusp (c) or the thrombotic deposit (t). The thrombus is only loosely attached to the cusp *(arrow).*

Pathogenesis. NBTE typically occurs in the setting of hypercoagulable states, for example, sepsis with disseminated intravascular coagulation (Chapter 4), hyperestrogenic states, or underlying malignancy, particularly mucinous adenocarcinomas. The latter association probably relates to the procoagulant effect of circulating mucin and/or tissue factor elaborated by these tumors; indeed, NBTE can be part of Trousseau syndrome (Chapter 6). Endocardial trauma (e.g., from an indwelling catheter) is also a well-recognized predisposing condition.

Clinical Features. Although the local effect on the valve is usually trivial, NBTE lesions can become clinically significant by embolizing to the brain, heart, or other organs. NBTE can also serve as a potential nidus for bacterial colonization and thus the development of IE.

Libman-Sacks Endocarditis

Libman-Sacks endocarditis refers to sterile vegetations that can develop on the valves of patients with systemic lupus erythematosus. These lesions presumably occur because of immune complex deposition and thus have associated inflammation. With increasing use of steroids for treatment of lupus, Libman-Sacks endocarditis has become fairly uncommon.

Morphology

The lesions in Libman-Sacks endocarditis are small sterile, granular pink vegetations 1–4 mm in diameter; they have no special predilection for the lines of valve closure and can be located on the undersurfaces of the atrioventricular valves, on the cords, or even on the atrial or ventricular endocardium. Histologically the lesions are finely granular, fibrinous eosinophilic vegetations containing nuclear debris. An intense valvulitis is often present, with fibrinoid necrosis of the valve substance adjacent to the vegetation. Subsequent fibrosis and serious deformity can result that resemble chronic RHD.

Figure 11–22 compares the appearance of the various vegetations, including acute RHD, IE, NBTE, and Libman-Sacks endocarditis.

Carcinoid Heart Disease

Carcinoid heart disease refers to the cardiac manifestation of a systemic syndrome that includes flushing, diarrhea, dermatitis, and bronchoconstriction, and is caused by bioactive compounds released by *carcinoid tumors.* Cardiac lesions do not typically occur until there is a massive hepatic metastatic burden and presumably the causal mediators are no longer catabolized by the liver. Classically, the endocardium and valves of the right heart are primarily affected, because they are the first cardiac tissues bathed by the bioactive substances released into the venous circulation. Carcinoid lesions on the left side of the heart can occur in the setting of a patent foramen ovale and right-to-left flow, or with pulmonary carcinoids.

Morphology

The cardiovascular lesions associated with the carcinoid syndrome are distinctive, glistening white intimal plaquelike thickenings on the endocardial surfaces of the cardiac chambers and valve leaflets. The lesions are composed of smooth muscle cells and sparse collagen fibers embedded in an acid mucopolysaccharide-rich matrix. Underlying structures are intact. With right-sided involvement there is typically tricuspid insufficiency and pulmonic stenosis.

Pathogenesis. The mediators elaborated in carcinoid tumors include serotonin (5-hydroxytryptamine), kallikrein, bradykinin, histamine, prostaglandins, and tachykinins. Although it is not clear which of these causes the lesions, plasma levels of serotonin and urinary excretion of the serotonin metabolite 5-hydroxyindoleacetic acid correlate with the severity of cardiac lesions. The valvular plaqûes in carcinoid syndrome are also histologically similar to the lesions that occasionally compli-

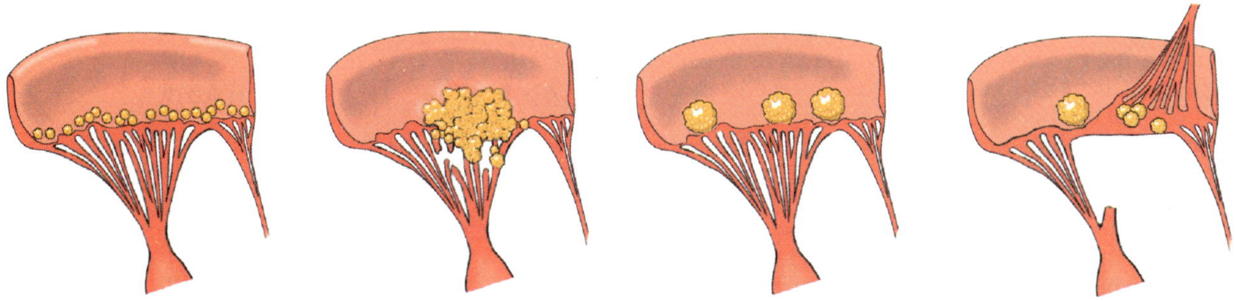

Figure 11–22

Comparison of the lesions in the four major forms of vegetative endocarditis. The acute rheumatic heart disease (RHD) is marked by a row of small, warty verrucae along the lines of closure of the valve leaflets. Infective endocarditis (IE) typically shows large, irregular, and destructive masses that can extend onto the chordae. Nonbacterial thrombotic endocarditis (NBTE) typically shows small, bland vegetations, usually attached at the line of closure. One or many may be present. Libman-Sacks endocarditis (LSE) has small or medium-sized vegetations on either or both sides of the valve leaflets, or elsewhere on the endocardial surface.

cate the use of the appetite suppressants fenfluramine and phentermine (fen-phen); interestingly, these agents affect systemic serotonin metabolism. Similar left-sided plaques can also occur following methysergide or ergotamine therapy for migraines; these drugs are metabolized to serotonin as they pass through the pulmonary vasculature. How serotonin may damage the valves is unknown.

Prosthetic Cardiac Valves

Although prosthetic heart valves are less than perfect substitutes for the native tissues, their introduction has radically altered the prognosis of patients with valve disease. Two types of prosthetic valves are currently used, each with its own advantages and disadvantages:

- *Mechanical valves:* most commonly double tilting disk devices made of pyrolytic carbon. They have excellent durability but require chronic anticoagulation, with the attendant risks of hemorrhage (or valve thrombosis if anticoagulation is inadequate). Mechanical aortic valves can also cause significant red cell hemolysis due to shear stresses.
- *Bioprosthetic valves:* glutaraldehyde-fixed porcine or bovine tissues, or cryopreserved human valves. These do not require anticoagulation but are less durable and can fail because of matrix deterioration. Virtually all biologic valve leaflets undergo some degree of stiffening after implantation; the loss of mobility may be sufficient to cause significant stenosis. Calcification of bioprosthetic leaflets is also common and can contribute to the stenosis. Bioprosthetic valves can perforate or tear, resulting in valvular insufficiency.

Prosthetic valves are also subject to infection. In mechanical valves, IE typically involves the suture line and adjacent perivalvular tissue and may cause the valve to detach *(paravalvular leak)*. In bioprosthetic valves, the valve leaflets as well as the perivalvular tissues can become infected.

SUMMARY

Valvular Heart Disease

- Valve pathology can lead to occlusion *(stenosis)* and/or to regurgitation *(insufficiency);* acquired aortic and mitral valve stenoses account for approximately two-thirds of all valve disease.
- Calcification of valve substance typically results in stenosis; abnormal extracellular matrix synthesis and turnover can result in myxomatous degeneration and insufficiency.
- Rheumatic heart disease results from formation of anti-streptococcal antibodies that cross-react with cardiac tissue. Pericardium, myocardium, and the valves are involved by acute inflammation; healing is associated with mitral and, less commonly, aortic valve disease.
- Infective endocarditis can be aggressive and rapidly destroy normal valves (acute IE) or can be indolent and minimally destructive of previously abnormal valves (subacute IE). Systemic embolization may produce septic infarcts.
- Nonbacterial thrombotic endocarditis (NBTE) gives rise to sterile vegetations on previously normal valves in states of general debility. Embolic complications can occur.

CARDIOMYOPATHIES

Most cardiac disease is secondary to some other condition (e.g., coronary atherosclerosis, hypertension, or valvular heart disease). However, there are some that are attributable to intrinsic myocardial dysfunction. Such myocardial diseases are termed *cardiomyopathies* (literally, *heart muscle diseases*). They are a diverse group that includes inflammatory disorders (*myocarditis;* see below), immunologic diseases (e.g., sarcoidosis), systemic metabolic disorders (e.g., hemochromatosis), muscular dystrophies, and genetic disorders of cardiac muscle cells. In many cases, cardiomyopathies are of unknown etiology (termed *idiopathic*); however, several previously "idiopathic" cardiomyopathies have been shown to be caused by specific genetic abnormalities in cardiac energy metabolism or structural and contractile proteins.

Cardiomyopathies can be subdivided by a variety of criteria. The 2006 American Heart Association classification divides them into two major groups: (1) *Primary* includes those entities in which the disease is solely or predominantly confined to the heart muscle and (2) *Secondary* in which heart is involved as a part of a generalized multiorgan disorder. Within each of these two groups, some diseases are genetic, others are acquired, and many are idiopathic. A more clinical and functional classification divides cardiomyopathies into three groups (Fig. 11–23 and Table 11–5) as follows:

- Dilated cardiomyopathy
- Hypertrophic cardiomyopathy
- Restrictive cardiomyopathy

Among these, dilated cardiomyopathy is most common (90% of cases), and restrictive cardiomyopathy is the least frequent. Within each pattern there is a spectrum of clinical severity, and each of these three patterns can be caused by a specific identifiable cause or can be idiopathic (Table 11–5). While the recent American Heart Association classification is intellectually more satisfying, we follow here the time-honored clinicopathologic classification since, at present, it is more useful for patient management.

Before we go into further details, some comments are in order about myocarditis. They are included here under the umbrella of cardiomyopathies since there is clinical overlap between some cases of myocarditis and dilated cardiomyopathy and in a proportion of cases, dilated cardiomyopathy can be shown to evolve from acute myocarditis. Indeed, since experts at the American Heart Association also include myocarditis among cardiomyopathies, we seem to be in good company!

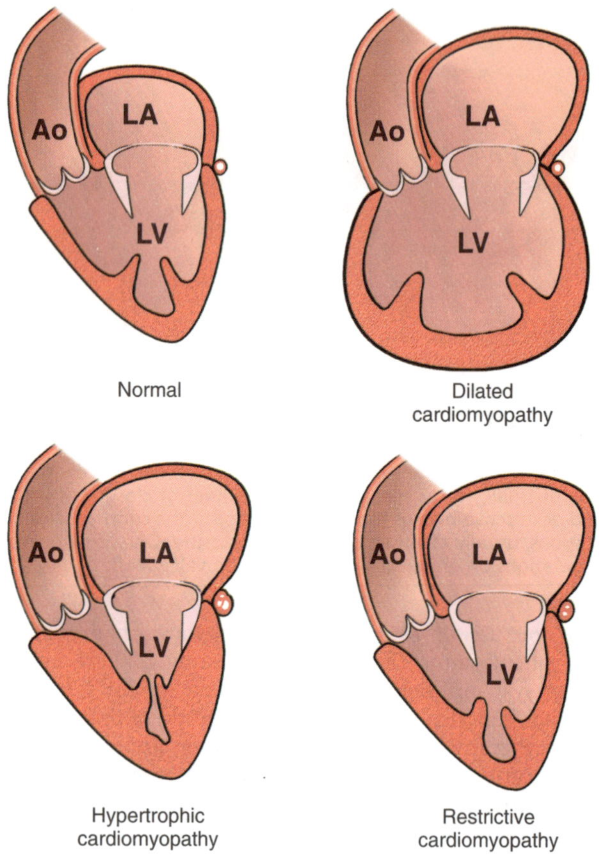

Figure 11–23

The three distinctive and predominant clinical-pathologic-functional forms of myocardial disease.

Dilated Cardiomyopathy

Dilated cardiomyopathy (DCM) is characterized by progressive cardiac dilation and *contractile (systolic) dysfunction,* usually with concurrent hypertrophy. It is sometimes called congestive cardiomyopathy. Approximately 25% to 35% of DCM cases have a familial (genetic) basis. Others result from a variety of acquired myocardial insults including toxic exposures (e.g., chronic alcoholism), myocarditis, and pregnancy-associated changes (see later). In some patients, the cause of DCM is unknown. Such cases are appropriately called *idio-*

Table 11–5 Cardiomyopathy and Indirect Myocardial Dysfunction: Functional Patterns and Causes

Functional Pattern	Left Ventricular Ejection Fraction*	Mechanisms of Heart Failure	Causes	Indirect Myocardial Dysfunction (Not Cardiomyopathy)
Dilated	<40%	Impairment of contractility (systolic dysfunction)	Idiopathic; alcohol; peripartum; genetic; myocarditis; chronic anemia; doxorubicin (Adriamycin)	Ischemic heart disease; valvular heart disease; hypertensive heart disease; congenital heart disease
Hypertrophic	50% to 80%	Impairment of compliance (diastolic dysfunction)	Genetic; Friedreich ataxia; storage diseases; infants of diabetic mothers	Hypertensive heart disease; aortic stenosis
Restrictive	45% to 90%	Impairment of compliance (diastolic dysfunction)	Idiopathic; amyloidosis; hemochromatosis; sarcoidosis; radiation-induced fibrosis	Pericardial constriction

*Normal, ≥65%.

pathic dilated cardiomyopathy. Many in this category are likely to be of genetic origin. Regardless of the cause, all share a similar clinicopathologic picture.

Morphology

The heart in DCM is characteristically **enlarged** (two to three times its normal weight) and **flabby, with dilation of all chambers** (Fig. 11–24). Because of the wall thinning that accompanies dilation, the ventricular thickness may be less than, equal to, or greater than normal. **Mural thrombi** are common and may be a source of thromboemboli. By definition there is no primary valve pathology; consequently, any valvular insufficiency is a secondary consequence of ventricular chamber dilation. The coronary arteries are usually free of significant atherosclerotic stenosis.

The histologic abnormalities in DCM are nonspecific. Microscopically most myocytes are **hypertrophied** with **enlarged nuclei,** but many are attenuated, stretched, and irregular. There is variable interstitial and endocardial fibrosis; scattered scars are also often present, probably marking previous myocyte ischemic necrosis caused by reduced perfusion (due to poor contractile function) and increased demand (due to myocyte hypertrophy). The extent of the changes frequently does not reflect the degree of dysfunction or the patient's prognosis.

Pathogenesis. When discovered clinically, DCM is frequently at its end stage, and many hearts show only the nonspecific findings described above. As a result the etiology can often only be inferred by the patient's medical history, or it is based on epidemiologic evidence. The causes of DCM can be grouped into four broad categories:

- *Viral.* The nucleic acid "footprints" from coxsackievirus B and other enteroviruses can occasionally be detected in the myocardium. Moreover, sequential endomyocardial biopsies have documented cases where there is progression from myocarditis to DCM. Consequently, some cases of DCM are attributed to myocarditis (discussed in greater detail below); even without direct evidence of inflammation, simply finding viral transcripts may be sufficient to invoke a myocarditis that was "missed" in its early stages.
- *Alcohol or other toxic exposure.* Alcohol abuse is strongly associated with development of DCM. Alcohol and its metabolites, especially acetaldehyde, have a direct toxic effect on myocardium (Chapter 8). Moreover, chronic alcoholism can be associated with thiamine deficiency, introducing an element of beriberi heart disease (Chapter 8). Nevertheless, the cause-and-effect relationship with alcohol alone is debated, and no morphologic features serve to distinguish *alcoholic cardiomyopathy* from DCM of any other cause. Nonalcoholic toxic insults include certain chemotherapeutic agents, particularly doxorubicin (Adriamycin), and cobalt.
- *Genetic influences.* Familial forms of DCM account for 25% to 35% of cases; autosomal dominant inheritance is the predominant pattern; X-linked, autosomal recessive, and mitochondrial inheritances are less common. Most of the genetic abnormalities seem to involve the myocyte cytoskeleton. Although not the most common form, X-linked DCM caused by mutation in the *dystrophin* gene is the best understood. Dystrophin is an intracellular structural protein that plays a critical role in linking the cytoskeleton of striated muscle with the extracellular matrix; indeed, dystrophin is mutated in the most common muscular dys-

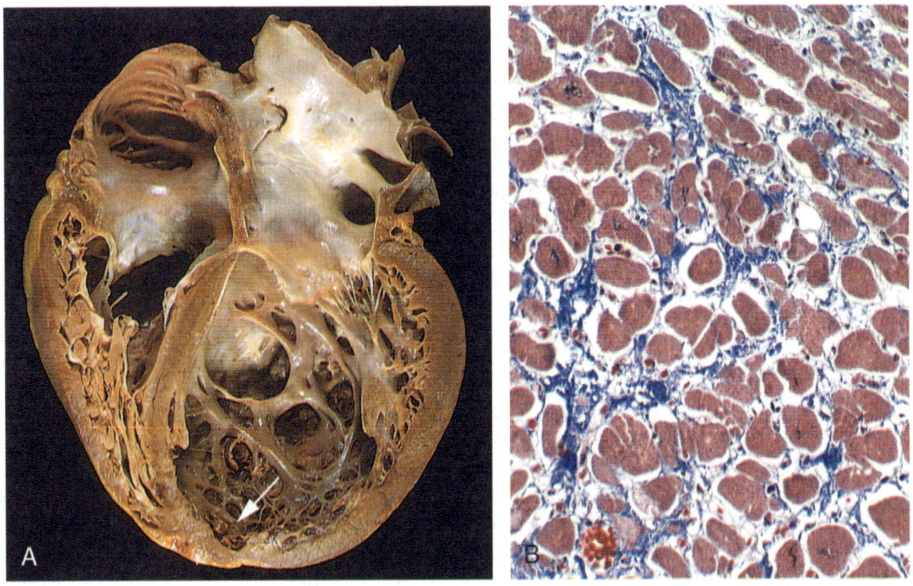

Figure 11–24

Dilated cardiomyopathy (DCM). **A,** Four-chamber dilatation and hypertrophy are evident. There is a small mural thrombus (*arrow*) at the apex of the left ventricle (on the right in this apical four-chamber view). There was no coronary artery disease. **B,** Histology of typical DCM demonstrating variable myocyte hypertrophy and interstitial fibrosis (collagen is highlighted as blue in this Masson trichrome stain).

trophies (see Chapter 21). Interestingly, some patients with dystrophin gene mutations have DCM as the primary clinical feature. Other cytoskeletal proteins involved in DCM include α-cardiac actin (links the sarcomere with dystrophin), desmin (the principal intermediate-filament protein in cardiac myocytes), and the nuclear lamins A and C. Mitochondrial gene deletions and mutations in genes encoding enzymes involved in fatty acid beta-oxidation can presumably cause DCM by altering myocardial ATP generation.

• *Peripartum cardiomyopathy* occurs late in gestation or several weeks to months postpartum. The etiology is multifactorial, including pregnancy-associated hypertension, volume overload, nutritional deficiency, other metabolic derangement, and/or an immunologic response (e.g., abnormal cytokine production). Fortunately, approximately half of these patients spontaneously recover normal function.

Clinical Features. DCM can occur at any age, including in childhood, but it most commonly occurs between ages 20 and 50 years. It typically presents with slowly progressing CHF (e.g., shortness of breath and poor exertional capacity), but patients can slip precipitously from a compensated to a decompensated state. The fundamental defect in DCM is ineffective contraction. Hence in end-stage DCM, the cardiac ejection fraction is typically less than 25%. Secondary mitral regurgitation and abnormal cardiac rhythms are common, and embolism from intracardiac thrombi can occur. Fifty percent of patients die within 2 years, and only 25% survive longer than 5 years; death is usually due to progressive cardiac failure or arrhythmia. In most cases cardiac transplantation is the only definitive treatment.

Arrhythmogenic Right Ventricular Cardiomyopathy

Arrhythmogenic right ventricular cardiomyopathy is a unique (albeit uncommon) entity with a clinical presentation involving right-sided heart failure and various rhythm disturbances (including SCD). Morphologically the right ventricular wall is severely thinned as a result of myocyte replacement by massive fatty infiltration and lesser amounts of fibrosis. Most cases are sporadic, but familial forms do occur with gene defects localized to chromosome 14 (autosomal dominant inheritance with variable penetrance). Most of the mutations seem to involve desmosomal junctional proteins.

Hypertrophic Cardiomyopathy

Hypertrophic cardiomyopathy (HCM) (also known as idiopathic hypertrophic subaortic stenosis) is characterized by *myocardial hypertrophy, abnormal diastolic filling,* and—in a third of cases—*ventricular outflow obstruction.* As discussed below, the obstruction, in some cases, is dynamic, caused by the anterior leaflet of the mitral valve. The heart is thick-walled, heavy, and hypercontracting, in striking contrast to the flabby, poorly contractile heart in DCM. Systolic function is usually preserved in HCM, but the myocardium does not relax and therefore shows primary diastolic dysfunction.

Morphology

The essential gross feature of HCM is massive myocardial hypertrophy without ventricular dilation (Fig. 11–25A). The classic pattern of HCM involves disproportionate thickening of the ventricular septum relative to the left ventricle free wall (so-called **asymmetrical septal hypertrophy**); nevertheless, in about 10% of cases there is concentric hypertrophy. On longitudinal sectioning, the ventricular cavity loses its usual round-to-ovoid shape and is compressed into a "banana-like" configuration (Fig. 11–25A). Often present is an endocardial plaque in the left ventricular outflow tract, as well as a thickening of the anterior mitral leaflet. Both findings reflect contact of the anterior mitral leaflet with the septum during ventricular systole and correlate with functional left ventricular outflow tract obstruction.

The characteristic histologic features in HCM are **severe myocyte hypertrophy, myocyte (and myofiber) disarray,** and interstitial and replacement fibrosis (Fig. 11–25B).

Pathogenesis. Almost all cases of HCM are caused by missense point mutations in one of several genes encoding the sarcomeric proteins that form the contractile apparatus of striated muscle (Fig. 11–25C). In most cases, the pattern of transmission is autosomal dominant with variable expression. Greater than 100 causal mutations have been identified in at least 12 sarcomeric genes (Fig. 11–25C), with the β-myosin heavy chain being most frequently affected, followed by myosin-binding protein C and troponin T. These three genes account for 70% to 80% of all cases of HCM.

Although it is clear that these genetic defects underlie HCM, the sequence of events leading from mutations to disease is still poorly understood. A current proposal suggests that HCM represents a compensatory change in response to impaired contractility. In this model, ineffective myocyte contraction triggers exuberant growth factor release with subsequent intense compensatory hypertrophy (causing myofiber disarray) and fibroblast proliferation (causing interstitial fibrosis).

Clinical Features. *HCM is characterized by a massively hypertrophied left ventricle that paradoxically provides a markedly reduced stroke volume.* This pathophysiologic effect is a direct consequence of *impaired diastolic filling* and overall smaller chamber size. In addition, roughly 25% of patients have dynamic obstruction to the left ventricular outflow by the anterior leaflet of the mitral valve. Reduced cardiac output and a secondary increase in pulmonary venous pressure cause exertional dyspnea, and there is a *harsh systolic ejection murmur.* A combination of massive hypertrophy, high left ventricular pressures, and compromised intramural coronary arteries frequently leads to myocardial ischemia (with angina), even in the absence of concomitant coronary artery disease. Major clinical problems include atrial fibrillation with mural thrombus formation, IE of the mitral valve, CHF, arrhythmias, and sudden death. Most patients are improved by therapy that promotes ventricular

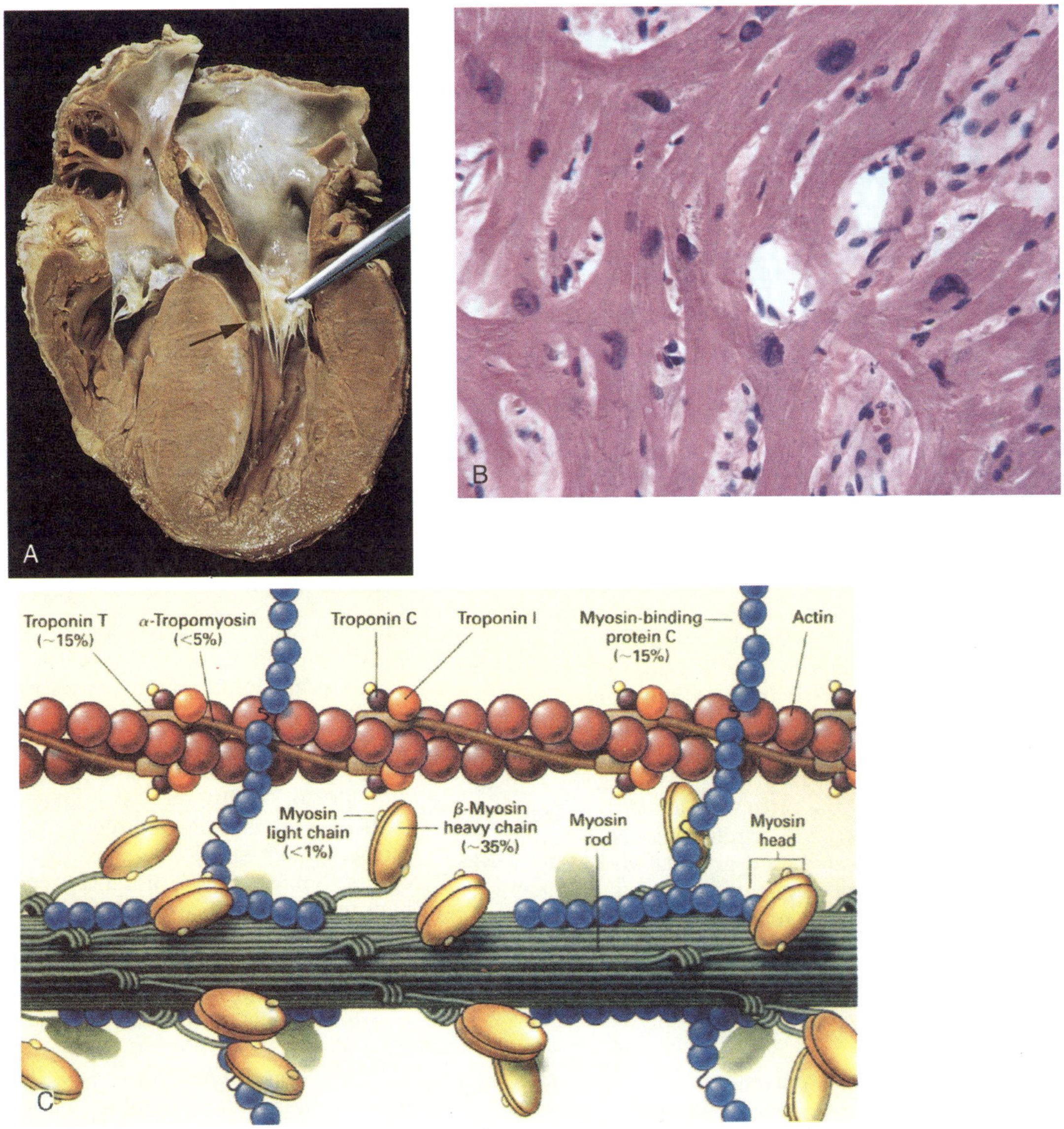

Figure 11–25

Hypertrophic cardiomyopathy (HCM) with asymmetric septal hypertrophy. **A,** The septal muscle bulges into the left ventricular outflow tract, and the left atrium is enlarged. The anterior mitral leaflet has been moved away from the septum to reveal a fibrous endocardial plaque *(arrow)*. See text. **B,** Histologic appearance demonstrating disarray, extreme hypertrophy, and characteristic branching of myocytes. **C,** Sarcomere of cardiac muscle, showing proteins in which mutations cause defective contraction, hypertrophy, and myocyte disarray in HCM. The frequency of a particular gene mutation is indicated as a percentage of all cases of HCM; most common are mutations in β-myosin heavy chain. Normal contraction of the sarcomere involves myosin-actin interaction initiated by calcium binding to troponin C, I, and T, and α-tropomyosin. Actin stimulates adenosine triphosphatase activity in the myosin head and produces force along the actin filaments. Myocyte-binding protein C modulates contraction. (**A,** From Schoen FJ: Interventional and Surgical Cardiovascular Pathology: Clinical Correlations and Basic Principles. Philadelphia, WB Saunders, 1989. **C,** From Spirito P, et al.: The management of hypertrophic cardiomyopathy. N Engl J Med 336:775, 1997.)

relaxation; occasionally, partial surgical excision of septal muscle is necessary to relieve the outflow tract obstruction.

Restrictive Cardiomyopathy

Restrictive cardiomyopathy is characterized by a *primary decrease in ventricular compliance, resulting in impaired ventricular filling during diastole* (simply put, the wall is *stiffer*). The contractile (systolic) function of the left ventricle is usually unaffected. Thus, the functional state can be confused with that of constrictive pericarditis or hypertrophic cardiomyopathy. Restrictive cardiomyopathy can be idiopathic or associated with systemic diseases that also happen to affect the myocardium—for example, radiation fibrosis, amyloidosis, hemochromatosis, sarcoidosis, or products of inborn errors of metabolism. For each of these causes, the curious reader is referred to the more complete discussion in the relevant chapters. Genetic factors are less clearly defined in restrictive cardiomyopathy.

Morphology

In idiopathic restrictive cardiomyopathy the ventricles are of approximately normal size or slightly enlarged, the cavities are not dilated, and the myocardium is firm. Biatrial dilation is commonly observed. Microscopically there is interstitial fibrosis, varying from minimal and patchy to extensive and diffuse. Restrictive cardiomyopathy of disparate causes may have similar gross morphology. However, endomyocardial biopsy can reveal disease-specific features (e.g., amyloid, iron overload, sarcoid granulomas).

Two other forms of restrictive cardiomyopathy merit brief mention:

- *Endomyocardial fibrosis* is principally a disease of children and young adults in Africa and other tropical areas; it is characterized by dense fibrosis of the ventricular endocardium and subendocardium extending from the apex up to the tricuspid and mitral valves. The fibrous tissue markedly diminishes the volume and compliance of affected chambers and so causes a restrictive physiology. Worldwide, this is the most common form of restrictive cardiomyopahy.
- *Loeffler endomyocarditis* also causes endocardial fibrosis, typically with large mural thrombi; however, Loeffler endomyocarditis is not geographically restricted. There is often an associated peripheral hypereosinophilia; the circulating eosinophils are abnormal, and many are degranulated. Release of the eosinophil granule contents, especially major basic protein, is speculated to initiate endocardial damage, with subsequent endomyocardial necrosis followed by scarring of the necrotic area.

Myocarditis

In myocarditis there is inflammation of the myocardium with resulting injury. It is important, however, to emphasize that the presence of inflammation alone is *not* diagnostic of myocarditis; for example, inflammatory infiltrates can also occur as a secondary response to ischemic injury. *In myocarditis, the inflammatory process is the cause of—rather than a response to—myocardial injury.*

Morphology

During active myocarditis the heart may appear normal or dilated. The ventricular myocardium is typically flabby and often mottled by patchy or diffuse foci of pallor and/or hemorrhage. Mural thrombi can be present.

Microscopically, active myocarditis shows an interstitial inflammatory infiltrate, with focal necrosis of myocytes adjacent to the inflammatory cells (Fig. 11–26).

Lymphocytic myocarditis is most common (Fig. 11–26A). If the patient survives the acute phase of myocarditis, the inflammatory lesions either resolve, leaving no residual changes, or heal by progressive fibrosis.

Hypersensitivity myocarditis has interstitial and perivascular infiltrates composed of lymphocytes, macrophages, and a high proportion of eosinophils (Fig. 11–26B).

Giant-cell myocarditis is a morphologically distinctive entity characterized by widespread inflammatory cellular infiltrates containing multinucleate giant cells (formed by macrophage fusion) interspersed with lymphocytes, eosinophils, and plasma cells. Giant-cell myocarditis probably represents the aggressive end of the spectrum of lymphocytic myocarditis, and there is at least focal—and frequently extensive—necrosis (Fig. 11–26C). This variant carries a poor prognosis.

Chagas myocarditis is distinctive by virtue of the parasitization of scattered myofibers by trypanosomes accompanied by an inflammatory infiltrate of neutrophils, lymphocytes, macrophages, and occasional eosinophils (Fig. 11–26D).

Pathogenesis. In the United States, viral infections are the most common cause of myocarditis. Coxsackieviruses A and B and other enteroviruses probably account for most of the cases. Less common agents include cytomegalovirus, human immunodeficiency virus, and a long list of other agents (Table 11–6). Although it is often difficult to isolate the offending virus from infected tissues, serologic and molecular techniques (e.g., polymerase chain reaction) can occasionally point to the culprit. Some viruses cause direct cytolytic injury; others may induce cross-reactive antibodies or T lymphocytes. In most cases, however, the injury is caused by an immune response directed against virally infected cells (Chapter 5); this is analogous to the damage inflicted by virus-specific T cells on hepatitis virus–infected liver cells (Chapter 16).

The *nonviral infectious causes of myocarditis* run the entire gamut of the microbial world (Table 11–6). The protozoan *Trypanosoma cruzi* is the agent of Chagas disease. Although uncommon in the northern hemisphere, Chagas disease affects as much as half the population in endemic areas of South America, and myocardial involvement can be found in 80% of infected individuals. About 10% of patients die during an acute attack; others enter a chronic immune-mediated phase and develop progressive signs of congestive heart failure and arrhythmias 10 to 20 years later. *Toxoplasma gondii* (household cats are the most common vector) can also cause myocarditis, particularly in immunocompromised hosts. *Trichinosis* is the most common helminthic disease with associated cardiac involvement.

Myocarditis occurs in approximately 5% of patients with Lyme disease, a systemic illness caused by the bacterial spirochete *Borrelia burgdorferi*. Lyme myocarditis manifests primarily as a self-limited conduction system disease. A temporary pacemaker may be required for AV block in approximately 30% of patients.

Noninfectious causes of myocarditis include systemic diseases of immune origin, such as lupus erythematosus and polymyositis. Drug hypersensitivity reactions *(hyper-*

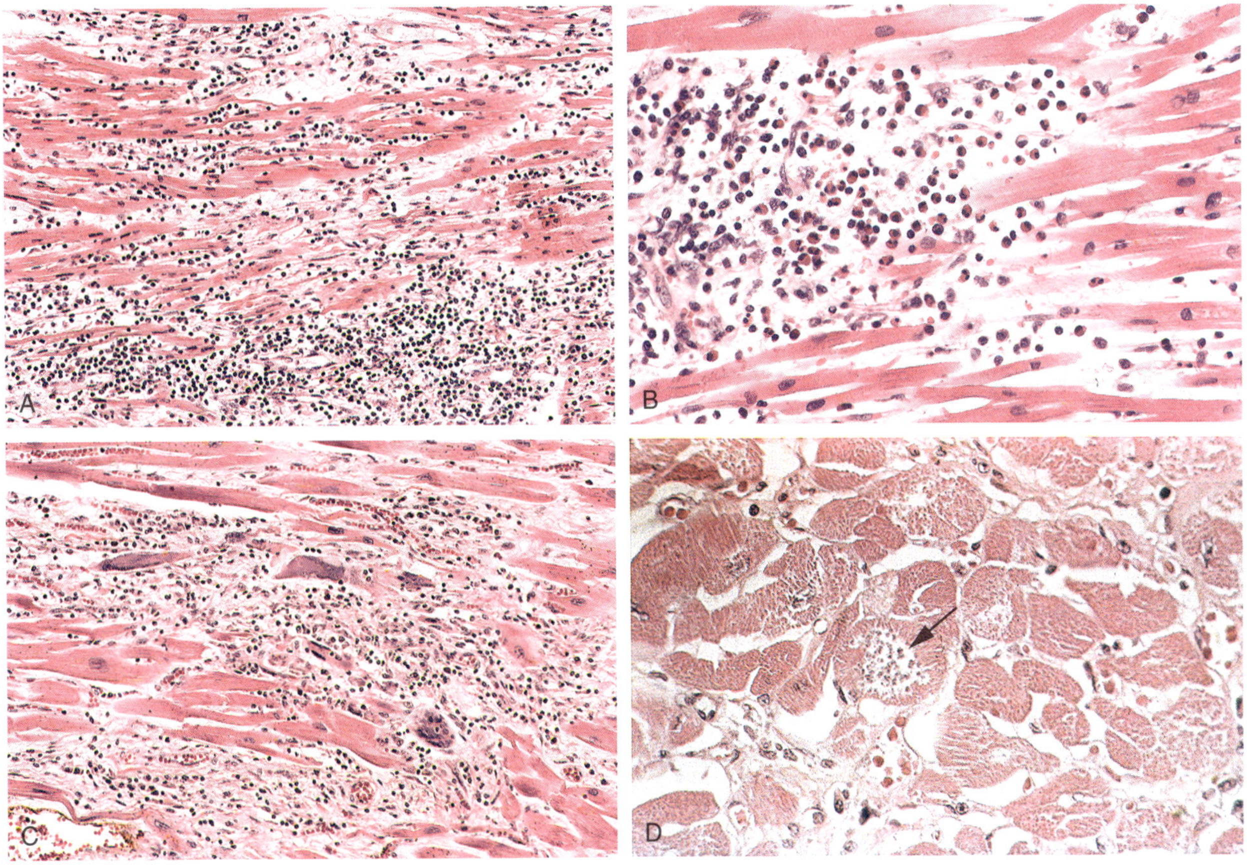

Figure 11–26

Myocarditis. **A,** Lymphocytic myocarditis, with mononuclear inflammatory cell infiltrate and associated myocyte injury. **B,** Hypersensitivity myocarditis, characterized by interstitial inflammatory infiltrate composed largely of eosinophils and mononuclear inflammatory cells, predominantly localized to perivascular and large interstitial spaces. This form of myocarditis is associated with drug hypersensitivity. **C,** Giant-cell myocarditis, with mononuclear inflammatory infiltrate containing lymphocytes and macrophages, extensive loss of muscle, and multinucleated giant cells. **D,** The myocarditis of Chagas disease. A myofiber is distended with trypanosomes *(arrow).* There is a surrounding inflammatory reaction and individual myofiber necrosis.

Table 11–6 Major Causes of Myocarditis

Infections
Viruses e.g., coxsackievirus, ECHO, influenza, HIV, cytomegalovirus
Chlamydiae e.g., *C. psittaci*
Rickettsiae e.g., *R. typhi*, typhus fever
Bacteria e.g., *Corynebacterium diphtheriae*, *Neisseria meningococcus*, *Borrelia* (Lyme disease)
Fungi e.g., *Candida*
Protozoa e.g., *Trypanosoma* (Chagas disease), toxoplasmosis
Helminths e.g., trichinosis
Immune-Mediated Reactions
Postviral
Poststreptococcal (rheumatic fever)
Systemic lupus erythematosus
Drug hypersensitivity (e.g., methyldopa, sulfonamides)
Transplant rejection
Unknown
Sarcoidosis
Giant-cell myocarditis

HIV, human immunodeficiency virus.

sensitivity myocarditis) can also occur in response to any of a wide range of agents; these are typically benign and only in rare circumstances lead to CHF or sudden death.

Clinical Features. The clinical spectrum of myocarditis is broad. At one end, the disease is asymptomatic and patients recover without sequelae, and at the other end is the precipitous onset of heart failure or arrhythmias, occasionally with sudden death. Between these extremes are the many forms of presentation, associated with a variety of symptoms (e.g., fatigue, dyspnea, palpitations, pain, and fever). The clinical features of myocarditis can even mimic those of acute MI. Occasionally, over many years, patients can progress from myocarditis to DCM.

SUMMARY

Cardiomyopathy

- Cardiomyopathy is a term applied to intrinsic disease of the cardiac muscle; there may be specific causes, or it may be idiopathic.

- There are three general pathophysiologic categories of cardiomyopathy: dilated (90%), hypertrophic, and restrictive (least common).
- Dilated cardiomyopathy results in systolic (contractile) dysfunction. It may be acquired, for example, following myocarditis, toxic exposures (e.g., alcohol), or pregnancy (peripartum). In 25% to 35% of cases genetic defects in cytoskeletal proteins are causal.
- Hypertrophic cardiomyopathy results in diastolic (relaxation) dysfunction. The vast majority of cases are due to autosomal dominant mutations in the genes encoding the contractile apparatus, in particular β-myosin heavy chain.
- Restrictive cardiomyopathy results in a stiff, noncompliant myocardium and can be due to depositions (e.g., amyloidosis and hemochromatosis), increased interstitial fibrosis (e.g., caused by irradiation), or to endomyocardial scarring.
- Myocarditis results from muscle injury caused by an inflammatory process that may be secondary to infections or immune reactions. Coxsackieviruses A and B are the most common causes in the U.S. Clinically, myocarditis may be asymptomatic, give rise to acute heart failure, or evolve into dilated cardiomyopathy.

PERICARDIAL DISEASE

Diseases of the pericardium include inflammatory conditions and effusions. Isolated pericardial disease is unusual, and pericardial lesions are almost always associated with disease in other portions of the heart or surrounding structures, or are secondary to a systemic disorder.

Pericarditis

Primary pericarditis is uncommon; in most cases it is caused by infection. *Viruses are usually responsible,* although other organisms (e.g., bacteria and fungi) can be involved. Myocarditis can also be present, especially with viral disease.

In most cases pericarditis is secondary to acute MI, cardiac surgery, irradiation to the mediastinum, or processes involving other thoracic structures (e.g., pneumonia or pleuritis). *Uremia* is the most common systemic disorder associated with pericarditis. Less common secondary causes include rheumatic fever, systemic lupus erythematosus, and metastatic malignancies. Pericarditis can (1) cause immediate hemodynamic complications if a significant effusion is present (see below), (2) resolve without significant sequelae, or (3) progress to a chronic fibrosing process.

Morphology

The appearance of **acute pericarditis** varies slightly depending on its cause. In patients with viral pericarditis or uremia, the exudate is typically **fibrinous,** imparting an irregular (even shaggy) appearance to the pericardial surface (so-called bread-and-butter pericarditis). In acute bacterial pericarditis the exudate is **fibrinopurulent** (suppurative), often with areas of frank pus (Fig. 11–27); tuberculous pericarditis can show areas of caseation. Pericarditis due to malignancy is often associated with an exuberantly shaggy fibrinous exudate and a bloody effusion; metastases can be grossly evident as irregular excrescences or may be relatively inapparent, especially in the case of leukemia. In most cases, acute fibrinous or fibrinopurulent pericarditis resolves without any sequelae. However, when there is extensive suppuration or caseation, healing can result in fibrosis **(chronic pericarditis).**

The appearance of chronic pericarditis ranges from delicate adhesions to dense, fibrotic scars that obliterate the pericardial space. In extreme cases the heart is so completely encased by dense fibrosis that it cannot expand normally during diastole, so-called **constrictive pericarditis.**

Clinical Features. Pericarditis classically presents with atypical chest pain, not related to exertion and often worse on reclining, and a prominent friction rub. When associated with significant fluid accumulation, acute pericarditis can cause cardiac tamponade, with declining cardiac output and shock. Chronic constrictive pericarditis produces a combination of right-sided venous distention and low cardiac output, similar to restrictive cardiomyopathy.

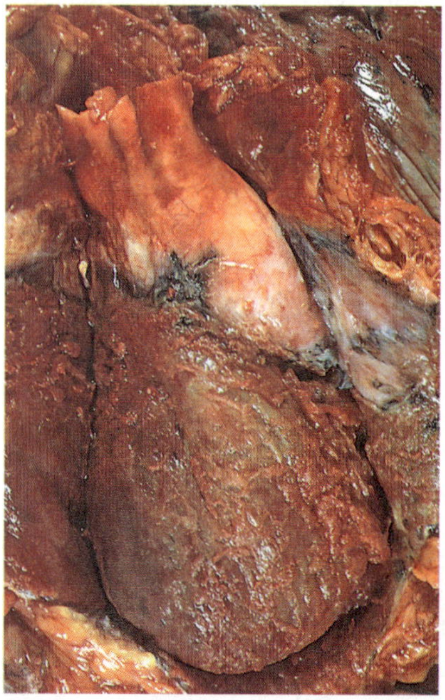

Figure 11–27

Acute suppurative pericarditis as an extension from a pneumonia. Extensive purulent exudate is evident in this in situ photograph.

Pericardial Effusions

Normally, there is about 30 to 50 mL of thin, clear, straw-colored (serous) fluid in the pericardial sac. Pericardial effusions in excess of this amount occur in a number of settings, in addition to the inflammatory states described above. The major types and some of their more common causes include:

- *Serous:* CHF, hypoalbuminemia of any cause
- *Serosanguinous:* blunt chest trauma, malignancy, ruptured MI, or aortic dissection
- *Chylous:* mediastinal lymphatic obstruction

The consequences of pericardial effusions depend on the ability of the parietal pericardium to stretch. This, in turn, depends on the amount of fluid and the tempo of its accumulation. Thus, slowly accumulating effusions—even as large as 1000 mL—can be tolerated without clinical manifestation. In contrast, rapidly developing collections of as little as 250 mL (e.g., ruptured MI or ruptured aortic dissection) can restrict diastolic cardiac filling to produce fatal *cardiac tamponade.*

CARDIAC TUMORS

Metastatic Neoplasms

The most common tumor of the heart is a metastatic tumor; tumor metastases to the heart occur in about 5% of patients dying of cancer. Although any malignancy can secondarily involve the heart, certain tumors have a higher predilection to spread to the heart. In descending order these tumors are carcinoma of the lung, lymphoma, breast cancer, leukemia, melanoma, carcinomas of the liver, and colon.

Primary Neoplasms

Primary cardiac tumors are uncommon; in addition, most primary cardiac tumors are also (thankfully) benign. The five most common have no malignant potential and account for 80% to 90% of all primary heart tumors. In descending order of frequency (adults) the primary cardiac tumors are: myxomas, fibromas, lipomas, papillary fibroelastomas, rhabdomyomas, and angiosarcomas (this last one is malignant). Only the myxomas and rhabdomyomas will receive any significant attention here.

Myxomas. Myxomas are the most common primary tumor of the adult heart (Fig. 11–28). Roughly 90% are located in the atria, with the left atrium accounting for 80% of those.

Morphology

Myxomas are almost always single and are most commonly located at the fossa ovalis (atrial septum). They range from small (<1 cm) to impressive (≤10 cm), sessile or pedunculated masses (Fig. 11–28A) and can vary from globular hard masses to soft, translucent, villous lesions with a gelatinous appearance. Pedunculated forms are often sufficiently mobile to swing into the mitral or tricuspid valves during systole, causing intermittent obstruction. Sometimes such mobility exerts a "wrecking-ball" effect, causing damage to the valve leaflets.

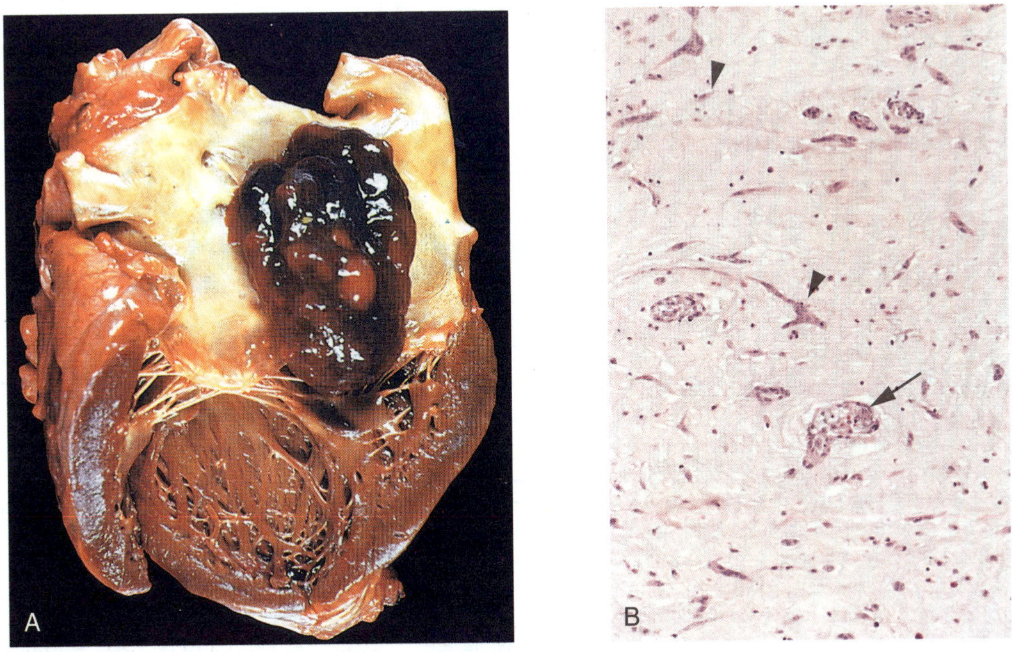

Figure 11–28

Left atrial myxoma. **A,** Gross photograph showing large pedunculated lesion arising from the region of the fossa ovalis and extending into the mitral valve orifice. **B,** Microscopic appearance, with abundant amorphous extracellular matrix in which are scattered collections of multinucleated myxoma cells *(arrowheads)* in various groupings, including abnormal vascular formations *(arrow).*

Histologically myxomas are composed of stellate, multinucleated myxoma cells with hyperchromatic nuclei, admixed with cells showing endothelial, smooth muscle, and/or fibroblastic differentiation, all embedded in an abundant acid mucopolysaccharide ground substance (Fig. 11–28B). Hemorrhage, poorly organizing thrombus, and mononuclear inflammation are also usually present.

Clinical Features. The major clinical manifestations are due to valvular "ball-valve" obstruction, embolization, or a syndrome of constitutional symptoms, such as fever and malaise. Constitutional symptoms are probably due to the elaboration of interleukin-6, a major mediator of the acute-phase response. Echocardiography is the diagnostic modality of choice, and surgical resection is almost uniformly curative.

Rhabdomyomas. Rhabdomyomas are the most frequent primary tumor of the heart in infants and children; they are frequently discovered because of an obstruction of a valvular orifice or cardiac chamber. Cardiac rhabdomyomas occur with high frequency in patients with tuberous sclerosis (Chapter 7). Rhabdomyomas are probably better classified as hamartomas or malformations rather than true neoplasms; recent work suggests that these lesions may be caused by defective apoptosis during developmental remodeling.

Morphology

Rhabdomyomas are generally small, gray-white myocardial masses up to several centimeters in diameter that protrude into the ventricular chambers. Histologically they have a mixed population of cells; the most characteristic of which are large, rounded, or polygonal cells containing numerous glycogen-laden vacuoles separated by strands of cytoplasm running from the plasma membrane to the more or less centrally located nucleus. These are the so-called **spider cells.**

Other Primary Cardiac Tumors

- *Lipomas* are localized, poorly encapsulated masses of adipose tissue, which can be asymptomatic, can create ball-valve obstructions (as with myxomas), or can produce arrhythmias. Lipomas are typically located in the left ventricle, right atrium, or atrial septum.
- *Papillary fibroelastomas* are curious, usually incidental, lesions that can sometimes embolize. They are generally located on valves, forming hairlike projections that grossly resemble sea anemones. Histologically there is myxoid connective tissue containing abundant mucopolysaccharide matrix and laminated elastic fibers, all surrounded by endothelium. While these masses are called neoplasms, it is possible that at least some fibroelastomas represent organized thrombi.
- *Cardiac angiosarcomas* and other sarcomas are not clinically or morphologically distinctive from their counterparts in other locations and therefore need no further comments.

CARDIAC TRANSPLANTATION

An estimated five million people in the United States have heart failure, and 300,000 die each year as a direct consequence. Cardiac transplantation is increasingly an option for these patients (mostly for IHD and dilated cardiomyopathy), with roughly 2000 performed annually in the U.S. (3000 a year worldwide). A brief look at the numbers suggests that *many* more patients die while on a waiting list (estimated at 50,000 per year) than are successfully transplanted. Indeed, even though the demand for hearts has doubled in the last decade, largely as a result of better ways to support patients in severe failure, the actual supply has dropped.

Beyond the issues of supply and demand, the major complications of cardiac transplantation are acute cardiac rejection and graft coronary arteriosclerosis (Fig. 11–29).

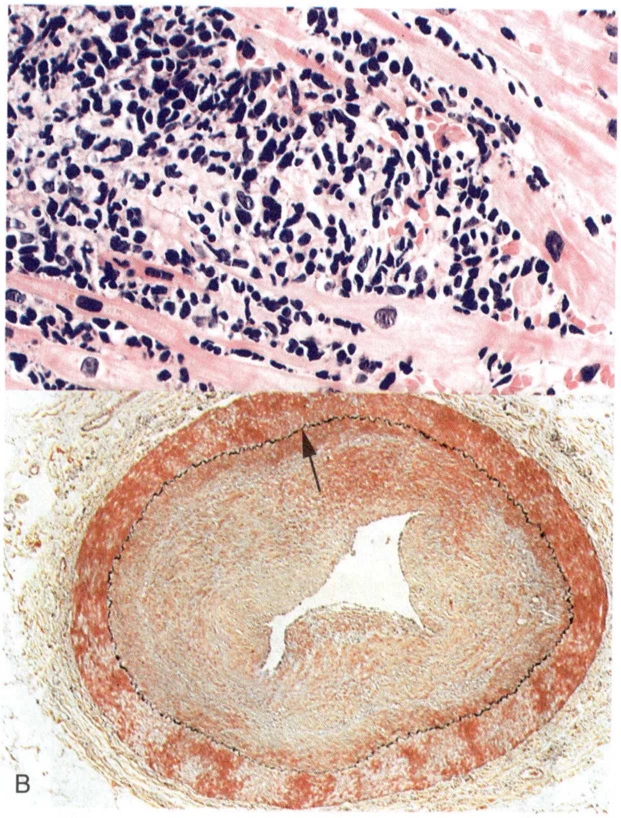

Figure 11–29

Complications of heart transplantation. **A,** Cardiac allograft rejection typified by lymphocytic infiltrate, with associated damage to cardiac myocytes. Note the similarity between rejection and typical viral myocarditis (see Fig. 11–26A). **B,** Graft coronary arteriosclerosis, demonstrating severe diffuse concentric intimal thickening producing critical stenosis. The internal elastic lamina *(arrow)* and media are intact (Movat pentachrome stain, elastin black). (**B,** From Salomon RN, et al.: Human coronary transplantation-associated arteriosclerosis. Evidence for chronic immune reaction to activated graft endothelial cells. Reprinted from Am J Pathol 138:791, 1991 with permission from the American Society for Investigative Pathology.)

• *Rejection* is typically diagnosed by endomyocardial biopsy of the transplanted heart; it is characterized by an interstitial lymphocytic inflammation with associated myocyte damage (Fig. 11–29A). The histology is similar to that seen in viral myocarditis (Fig. 11–26A). In both instances, T-cell–mediated killing and local cytokine production can materially compromise cardiac function. When myocardial injury is not extensive, the "rejection episode" can be reversed by immunosuppressive therapy. Advanced rejection can be irreversible and fatal.

• *Graft coronary arteriosclerosis* (GCA) is the single most important long-term limitation for cardiac transplantation. It is a late, progressive, diffusely stenosing intimal proliferation in the coronary arteries (Fig. 11–29B), leading to ischemic injury. Within 5 years of transplantation, 50% of patients have significant GCA, and virtually all patients have lesions within 10 years. The pathogenesis of GCA involves immunologic responses that induce local production of growth factors that promote intimal smooth muscle cell recruitment and proliferation with extracellular matrix synthesis. GCA is a particularly vexing problem, because it can lead to silent MI (transplant patients have denervated hearts and do not experience angina), progressive CHF, or SCD.

Despite these problems, the outlook for transplanted patients is generally good, with a 1-year survival of 80% and 5-year survivals of more than 60% (compared with 50% and <10%, respectively, in medically managed end-stage heart failure).

BIBLIOGRAPHY

Ahmad F, et al: The genetic basis for cardiac remodeling. Annu Rev Genomics Hum Genet 6:185, 2005. *[A review from one of the preeminent cardiac genetics groups regarding mutations that lead to hypertrophic and dilated phenotypes, as well as rhythm disturbances.]*

Aurigemma GP: Diastolic heart failure—a common lethal condition by any name. New Engl J Med 355:308, 2006. *[A review that emphasizes the importance of diastolic heart failure.]*

Brickner ME, et al: Congenital heart disease in adults. N Engl J Med 342:256 and 334, 2000. *[A nice two-part review of congenital cardiac malformations; despite the date, this is still a useful and highly accessible summary of the various conditions.]*

Calkins H: Arrhythmogenic right-ventricular dysplasia/cardiomyopathy. Curr Opin Cardiol 21:55, 2006. *[Excellent review of the theories of pathogenesis, as well as the diagnosis and treatment of this newly recognized entity.]*

Cannon RO III: Mechanisms, management and future directions for reperfusion injury after acute myocardial infarction. Nat Clin Pract Cardiovasc Med 2:88, 2005. *[Great review of the mechanisms and therapeutic approaches to limiting reperfusion injury after MI.]*

Corti R, et al: Pathogenetic concepts of acute coronary syndromes. J Am Coll Cardiol 41:7S, 2003. *[An excellent review of the acute coronary syndromes.]*

Feldman AM, McNamara D: Myocarditis. N Engl J Med 343:1388, 2000. *[A nice review of etiology, pathogenesis, and clinical features. Even given the date this was published, it is still quite relevant and authoritative.]*

Guilherme L, Kalil J: Rheumatic fever: from sore throat to autoimmune heart lesions. Int Arch Allergy Immunol 134:56, 2004. *[A well-written and scholarly discussion of the pathogenic mechanisms emerging about rheumatic heart disease.]*

Hill EE, et al: Evolving trends in infective endocarditis. Clin Microbiol Infect 12:5, 2006. *[Good, clinically oriented overview of the developments in microorganisms, diagnosis, and therapies for infective endocarditis.]*

Hughes BR, et al: Aortic stenosis: is it simply a degenerative process or an active atherosclerotic process? Clin Cardiol 28:111, 2005. *[A provocative look at the etiology for calcific degeneration in the aortic valve.]*

Kass M, Haddad H: Cardiac allograft vasculopathy: pathology, prevention and treatment. Curr Opin Cardiol 21:132, 2006. *[Timely review of this entity.]*

Kostin S, et al: The cytoskeleton and related proteins in the human failing heart. Heart Fail Rev 5:271, 2000. *[A good overview of the cytoskeletal remodeling that underlies dilated cardiomyopathies, in an issue of the journal with several other good articles about heart failure pathogenesis.]*

Loe MJ, Edwards WD: A light-hearted look at a lion-hearted organ (or a perspective from three standard deviations beyond the norm). Cardiovasc Pathol 13:282 and 334, 2004. *[An entertaining compendium of all matters involving the heart, including medical, historical, poetic, and popular references.]*

Maron BJ, et al.: AHA Scientific statement. Contemporary definitions and clarification of cardiomyopathies. Circulation 113:1087, 2006. *[A consensus statement by the American Heart Association, it includes details of the genes involved.]*

Rabkin E, et al: Activated interstitial myofibroblasts express catabolic enzymes and mediate matrix remodeling in myxomatous heart valves. Circulation 104:2525, 2001. *[Interesting paper suggesting a mechanism by which myxomatous valvular degeneration can occur.]*

Ro A, Frishman WH: Peripartum cardiomyopathy. Cardiol Rev 14:35, 2006. *[A succinct and up-to-date account of this enigmatic entity.]*

Roberts R, Sigwart U: Current concepts of the pathogenesis and treatment of hypertrophic cardiomyopathy. Circulation 112:293, 2005. *[A focused and scholarly review of hypertrophic cardiomyopathy.]*

Schoen FJ: Pathology of heart valve substitution with mechanical and tissue prostheses. In Silver MD, et al. (eds): Cardiovascular Pathology, 3rd ed. Philadelphia, Churchill Livingstone, 2001, pp 629–677. *[Extensive scholarly overview of prosthetic valve pathology.]*

Troughton RW, et al: Pericarditis. Lancet 363:717, 2004. *[Solid review of the causes, diagnosis, and therapy for pericarditis.]*

Wu JC, Child JS: Common congenital heart disorders in adults. Curr Probl Cardiol 29:641, 2004. *[Exhaustively thorough overview of the congenital heart disorders seen in the adult population, often as a consequence of improved pediatric therapies.]*

Zipe DP, et al. (eds): Braunwald's Heart Disease: A Textbook of Cardiovascular Medicine, 7th ed. Philadelphia, Saunders, 2005. *[An outstanding and authoritative text, with excellent sections on heart failure and atherosclerotic cardiovascular disease.]*

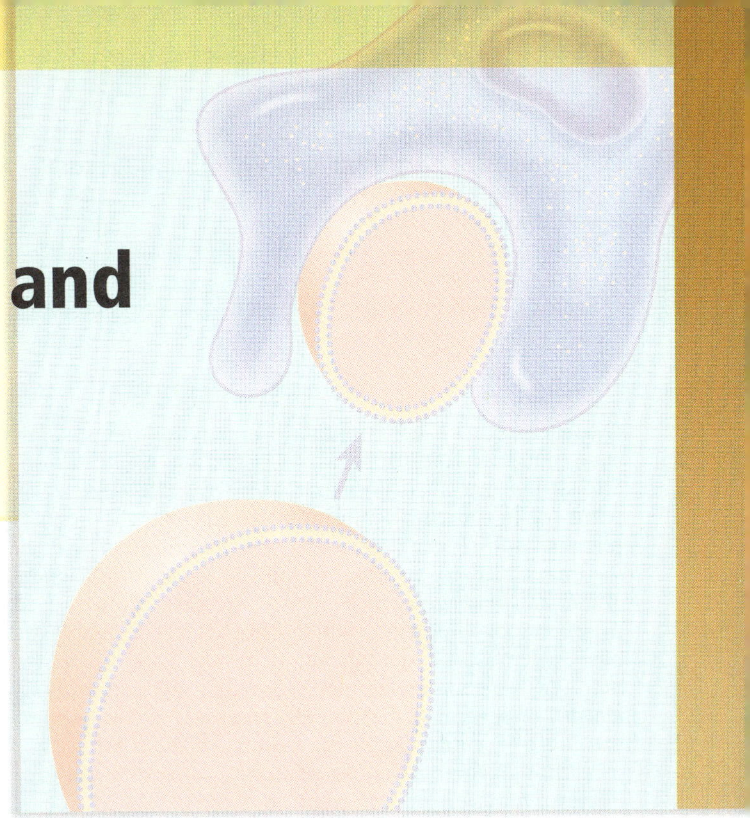

Chapter 12

The Hematopoietic and Lymphoid Systems

JON C. ASTER, MD, PhD

Disorders of the hematopoietic and lymphoid systems encompass a wide range of diseases that are traditionally sorted into disorders that primarily affect red cells, white cells, or the hemostatic system, which includes platelets and clotting factors. The most common *red cell disorders* lead to *anemia,* a state of red cell deficiency. *White cell disorders,* in contrast, are most often caused by excess proliferation, which usually has a neoplastic basis. Hemostatic derangements result in *hemorrhagic diatheses* (bleeding disorders). Finally, splenomegaly, a feature of several hematopoietic diseases, is discussed at the end of the chapter, as are tumors of the thymus.

Although these divisions are useful, in reality the production, function, and destruction of red cells, white cells, and components of the hemostatic system are closely linked, and pathogenic derangements primarily affecting one cell type or component of the system often lead to alterations in others. For example, in certain conditions B lymphocytes make autoantibodies against components of the red cell membrane. The opsonized red cells are recognized and destroyed by phagocytes in the spleen, which becomes enlarged. The increased red cell destruction causes anemia, which in turn drives a compensatory hyperplasia of red cell progenitors in the bone marrow.

Other levels of interplay and complexity stem from the dispersed nature of the lymphohematopoietic system, which is not confined to a single anatomic site. When considering hematopoietic disorders, it is important to remember that both normal and malignant lymphoid and hematopoietic cells "traffic" between various compartments. Hence, a patient who is diagnosed by lymph node biopsy to have a malignant lymphoma may also be found to have neoplastic lymphocytes in the bone marrow and blood. The malignant lymphoid cells in the marrow may suppress hematopoiesis, giving rise to cytopenias, and the further seeding of tumor cells to the liver and spleen may cause organomegaly. Thus, in both benign and malignant hematolymphoid disorders, a single underlying abnormality can result in diverse, systemic manifestations.

RED CELL DISORDERS

Disorders of red cells can result in anemia or, less commonly, polycythemia (i.e., an increase in the number of red cells). *Anemia* is a reduction in the oxygen-transporting capacity of blood, which usually stems from a reduction of the total circulating red cell mass to below-normal amounts.

Anemia can result from excessive bleeding, increased red cell destruction, or decreased red cell production. These mechanisms serve as a basis for classifying anemias (Table 12–1). With the exception of the anemia of chronic renal failure, in which erythropoietin-producing cells in the kidney are lost, the decrease in tissue oxygen tension that attends anemia usually triggers increased erythropoietin production. This drives a compensatory hyperplasia of erythroid precursors in the bone marrow and, in severe anemias, the appearance of extramedullary hematopoiesis within the secondary hematopoietic organs (the spleen, liver, and lymph nodes). In well-nourished individuals who become anemic because of acute bleeding or increased red cell destruction (hemolysis), the compensatory response can increase the regeneration of red cells fivefold to eightfold. The hallmark of increased marrow output is reticulocytosis, the appearance of increased numbers of newly formed red cells (reticulocytes) in the peripheral blood. In contrast, disorders of decreased red cell production (aregenerative anemias) are characterized by reticulocytopenia.

Another classification of anemias is based on the morphology of red cells, which often correlates with the cause of their deficiency. Specific red cell features that provide etiologic clues include the cell size (normocytic, microcytic, or macrocytic), the degree of hemoglobinization—which is reflected in the color of the cells (normochromic or hypochromic)—and the shape of the cells. These features are judged subjectively by visual inspection of peripheral smears and are also expressed quantitatively through the following indices:

- *Mean cell volume* (MCV): the average volume per red cell, expressed in femtoliters (cubic microns)
- *Mean cell hemoglobin* (MCH): the average content (mass) of hemoglobin per red cell, expressed in picograms
- *Mean cell hemoglobin concentration* (MCHC): the average concentration of hemoglobin in a given volume of packed red cells, expressed in grams per deciliter

Table 12–1 Classification of Anemia According to Underlying Mechanism

Blood Loss

- Acute: trauma
- Chronic: lesions of gastrointestinal tract, gynecologic disturbances

Increased Destruction (Hemolytic Anemias)

- Intrinsic (intracorpuscular) abnormalities
  - Hereditary
    - Membrane abnormlities
      - Membrane skeleton proteins: spherocytosis, elliptocytosis
      - Membrane lipids: abetalipoproteinemia
    - Enzyme deficiencies
      - Glycolytic enzymes: pyruvate kinase, hexokinase
      - Enzymes of hexose monophosphate shunt: glucose-6-phosphate dehydrogenase, glutathione synthetase
    - Disorders of hemoglobin synthesis
      - Deficient globin synthesis: thalassemia syndromes
      - Structurally abnormal globin synthesis (hemoglobinopathies): sickle cell anemia, unstable hemoglobins
  - Acquired
    - Membrane defect: paroxysmal nocturnal hemoglobinuria
- Extrinsic (extracorpuscular) abnormalities
  - Antibody mediated
    - Isohemagglutinins: transfusion reactions, erythroblastosis fetalis (Rh disease of the newborn)
    - Autoantibodies: idiopathic (primary), drug-associated, systemic lupus erythematosus
  - Mechanical trauma to red cells
    - Microangiopathic hemolytic anemias: thrombotic thrombocytopenic purpura, disseminated intravascular coagulation
    - Infections: malaria

Impaired Red Cell Production

- Disturbance of proliferation and differentiation of stem cells: aplastic anemia, pure red cell aplasia, anemia of renal failure, anemia of endocrine disorders
- Disturbance of proliferation and maturation of erythroblasts
  - Defective DNA synthesis: deficiency or impaired utilization of vitamin B_{12} and folic acid (megaloblastic anemias)
  - Defective hemoglobin synthesis
    - Deficient heme synthesis: iron deficiency
    - Deficient globin synthesis: thalassemias
    - Anemia of renal failure
  - Unknown or multiple mechanisms: myelodysplastic syndrome, anemia of chronic inflammation, myelophthisic anemias due to marrow infiltrations

- *Red cell distribution width* (RDW): the coefficient of variation of red cell volume.

In modern clinical laboratories, specialized instruments directly measure or automatically calculate the red cell indices. Adult reference ranges are shown in Table 12–2.

As we will discuss, the clinical consequences of anemia are determined by its severity, speed of onset, and underlying pathogenic mechanism. If the onset is slow, adaptations take place that partially compensate for the deficit in O_2 carrying capacity, such as increases in plasma volume, cardiac output, respiratory rate, and red cell 2,3-diphosphoglycerate levels. These changes can largely mitigate the effects of mild to moderate anemia in otherwise healthy individuals, but are less effective in those with compromised pulmonary or cardiac function. *Pallor, fatigue,* and *lassitude* are common to all anemias, and are the primary presenting symptoms of the most common types, such as that caused by iron deficiency. Anemias caused by the premature destruction of red cells in the peripheral blood (*hemolytic anemias*) are associated with *hyperbilirubinemia, jaundice,* and *pigment gallstones.* Anemias that stem from *ineffective hematopoiesis* (the premature death of erythroid progenitors in the marrow) are associated with inappropriately high levels of iron absorption from the gut, which can lead to iron overload (*secondary hemochromatosis*) and eventual damage to endocrine organs and the heart. If left untreated, *severe congenital anemias,* such as β-thalassemia major, inevitably result in *growth retardation, skeletal abnormalities,* and *cachexia.*

SUMMARY

Pathology of Anemias

CAUSES

- Blood loss (hemorrhage)
- Increased red cell destruction (hemolysis)
- Decreased red cell production

MORPHOLOGY

- Microcytic (iron deficiency, thalassemia)
- Macrocytic (folate or B_{12} deficiency)
- Normocytic but with abnormal shapes (hereditary spherocytosis, sickle cell disease)

CLINICAL MANIFESTATIONS

- Acute: shortness of breath, organ failure, shock
- Chronic:
  - With hemolysis: skeletal abnormalities because of expansion of marrow; growth retardation; jaundice and gallstones
  - With defective erythropoiesis: iron overload, heart and endocrine failure

ANEMIA OF BLOOD LOSS: HEMORRHAGE

With acute blood loss, the immediate threat to the patient is hypovolemia (shock) rather than anemia. If the patient survives, hemodilution begins at once and achieves its full effect within 2 to 3 days, unmasking the extent of the red cell loss. *The anemia is normocytic and normochromic.* Recovery from blood loss anemia is enhanced by a rise in the erythropoietin level, which stimulates increased red cell production within several days. The onset of the marrow response is marked by reticulocytosis.

With chronic blood loss, iron stores are gradually depleted. Iron is essential for hemoglobin synthesis and effective erythropoiesis, and its deficiency thus leads to a chronic anemia of underproduction. Iron deficiency

Table 12–2 Adult Reference Ranges for Red Blood Cells*

	Units	Men	Women
Hemoglobin (Hb)	g/dL	13.6–17.2	12.0–15.0
Hematocrit (HCT)	%	39–49	33–43
Red cell count	$\times 10^6/mm^3$	4.3–5.9	3.5–5.0
Reticulocyte count	%	0.5–1.5	0.5–1.5
Mean cell volume (MCV)	fL	76–100	76–100
Mean cell Hb (MCH)	pg	27–33	27–33
Mean cell Hb concentration (MCHC)	g/dL	33–37	33–37
Red cell distribution width (RDW)		11.5–14.5	

*Reference ranges vary among laboratories. The reference ranges for the laboratory providing the result should always be used when interpreting a laboratory test.

anemia can occur in other clinical settings as well, and it is described later in this chapter along with other anemias of diminished erythropoiesis.

THE HEMOLYTIC ANEMIAS

Normal red cells have a life span of about 120 days. Anemias that are associated with accelerated destruction of red cells are termed *hemolytic anemias.* Destruction can be caused by either inherent (intracorpuscular) red cell defects, which are usually inherited, or external (extracorpuscular) factors, which are usually acquired. Several examples are listed in Table 12–1.

Before discussing the various disorders individually, we will describe certain general features of hemolytic anemias. All are characterized by (1) an increased rate of red cell destruction, (2) a compensatory increase in erythropoiesis that results in reticulocytosis, and (3) the retention by the body of the products of red cell destruction (including iron). Because the iron is conserved and recycled readily, red cell regeneration can keep pace with the hemolysis. Consequently, these anemias are almost invariably associated with a marked *erythroid hyperplasia within the marrow* and an *increased reticulocyte count in peripheral blood.* In severe hemolytic anemias, extramedullary hematopoiesis often develops in the spleen, liver, and lymph nodes.

Destruction of red cells can occur within the vascular compartment (intravascular hemolysis) or within the cells of the mononuclear phagocyte (reticuloendothelial) system (extravascular hemolysis). *Intravascular hemolysis* can result from mechanical trauma (e.g., a defective heart valve) or biochemical or physical agents that damage the red cell membrane (e.g., fixation of complement, exposure to clostridial toxins, or heat). Regardless of cause, hemolysis leads to hemoglobinemia, hemoglobinuria, and hemosiderinuria. The conversion of the heme pigment to bilirubin can result in unconjugated hyperbilirubinemia and jaundice. Massive intravascular hemolysis sometimes leads to acute tubular necrosis (Chapter 14). *Haptoglobin,* a circulating protein that binds and clears free hemoglobin, is often absent from the plasma.

Extravascular hemolysis, the more common mode of red cell destruction, takes place largely within the phagocytic cells of the spleen and liver. The mononuclear phagocyte system removes damaged or immunologically targeted red cells from the circulation. Because extreme alterations of shape are necessary for red cells to successfully navigate the splenic sinusoids, any reduction in red cell deformability makes this passage difficult and leads to splenic sequestration, followed by phagocytosis. As will be described, diminished deformability is an important cause of red cell destruction in a variety of hemolytic anemias. Extravascular hemolysis is not associated with hemoglobinemia and hemoglobinuria, but it often produces jaundice and, if long-standing, can lead to the formation of bilirubin-rich gallstones (so-called pigment stones). *Haptoglobin* amounts are always decreased, because some hemoglobin invariably escapes into the plasma. In most forms of hemolytic anemia there is a reactive hyperplasia of the mononuclear phagocyte system, which results in splenomegaly.

In chronic hemolytic anemias, changes in iron metabolism lead to increases in iron absorption from the gut. Because the pathways for the excretion of excess iron are limited, this often causes iron to accumulate, giving rise to systemic hemosiderosis (Chapter 1) or, in very severe cases, secondary hemochromatosis (Chapter 16).

We will now discuss some of the common hemolytic anemias.

Hereditary Spherocytosis

This disorder is characterized by an inherited (intrinsic) defect in the red cell membrane that renders the cells spheroidal, less deformable, and vulnerable to splenic sequestration and destruction. Hereditary spherocytosis (HS) is transmitted most commonly as an autosomal dominant trait; approximately 25% of patients have a more severe autosomal recessive form of the disease.

Pathogenesis. In HS the primary abnormality resides in one of a group of proteins that form a meshlike supportive skeleton on the intracellular face of the red cell membrane (Fig. 12–1). The major protein in this skeleton is spectrin, a long, flexible heterodimer that is linked to the membrane at two points: through ankyrin and band 4.2 to the intrinsic membrane protein band 3; and through band 4.1 to the intrinsic membrane protein glycophorin. The horizontal spectrin–spectrin and vertical spectrin–intrinsic membrane protein interactions serve to stabilize the membrane and are responsible for the normal shape, strength, and flexibility of the red cell.

The common pathogenic feature of all HS mutations is that they weaken the vertical interactions between the membrane skeleton and the intrinsic membrane proteins. The mutations most frequently involve ankyrin, band 3, and spectrin, but mutations in other components of the skeleton have also been described. In all types of HS the red cells have reduced membrane stability and conse-

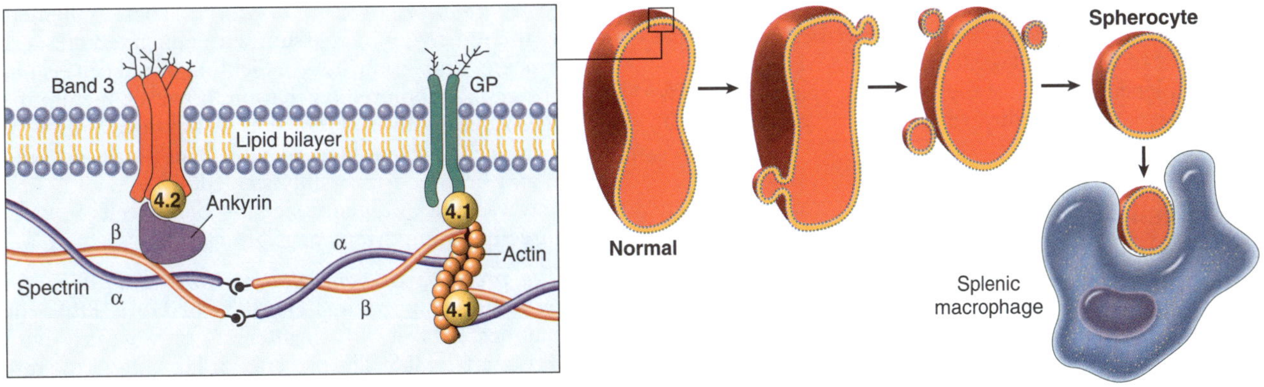

Figure 12–1

The red cell membrane cytoskeleton and the effect of alterations in the cytoskeleton proteins on red cell shape. With mutations that affect the integrity of the membrane cytoskeleton, the normal biconcave erythrocyte loses membrane fragments. To accommodate the loss of surface area, the cell adopts a spherical shape. Such spherocytic cells are less deformable than normal and are therefore trapped in the splenic cords, where they are phagocytosed by macrophages. GP, glycophorin.

quently lose membrane fragments after their release into the periphery, while retaining most of their volume. As a result, the ratio of surface area to volume of HS cells decreases until the cells become spherical, at which point no further membrane loss is possible (see Fig. 12–1).

The spleen plays a major role in the destruction of spherocytes. Red cells must undergo extreme degrees of deformation to leave the cords of Billroth and enter the splenic sinusoids. The discoid shape of normal red cells allows considerable latitude for changes in cell shape. In contrast, because of their spheroidal shape and limited deformability, spherocytes are sequestered in the splenic cords and eventually destroyed by macrophages, which are plentiful. *The critical role of the spleen is illustrated by the invariably beneficial effect of splenectomy; although the red cell defect and spherocytes persist, the anemia is corrected.*

Morphology

On smears, the red cells lack the central zone of pallor because of their spheroidal shape (Fig. 12–2). Spherocytosis, though distinctive, is not diagnostic; it is seen in other conditions, such as immune hemolytic anemias (discussed later), in which there is a loss of cell membrane relative to cell volume. The excessive red cell destruction and resultant anemia lead to a compensatory hyperplasia of marrow red cell progenitors and an increase in red cell production, which is marked by peripheral blood reticulocytosis. Splenomegaly is greater and more common in HS than in any other form of hemolytic anemia. The splenic weight is usually between 500 and 1000 gm and can be even greater. The enlargement results from marked congestion of the cords of Billroth and increased numbers of mononuclear phagocytes. Phagocytosed red cells are frequently seen within macrophages lining the sinusoids and, in particular, within the cords. In long-standing cases there is prominent systemic hemosiderosis. The other general features of hemolytic anemias described earlier are also present, including cholelithiasis, which occurs in 40% to 50% of HS patients.

Clinical Course. The characteristic clinical features are *anemia, splenomegaly,* and *jaundice.* The severity of the anemia is highly variable, ranging from subclinical to profound; most commonly it is moderate in severity. Because of their spheroidal shape, HS red cells show *increased osmotic fragility* when placed in hypotonic salt solutions, a characteristic that is helpful for diagnosis.

The clinical course is often stable but may be punctuated by aplastic crises. Such episodes are often triggered by the infection of bone marrow erythroblasts by parvovirus B19, which causes a transient cessation of red cell production. Because HS red cells have a shortened life span, the failure of erythropoiesis for even a few days results in a rapid worsening of the anemia. Such episodes are self-limited, but some patients need blood transfusions until the infection clears.

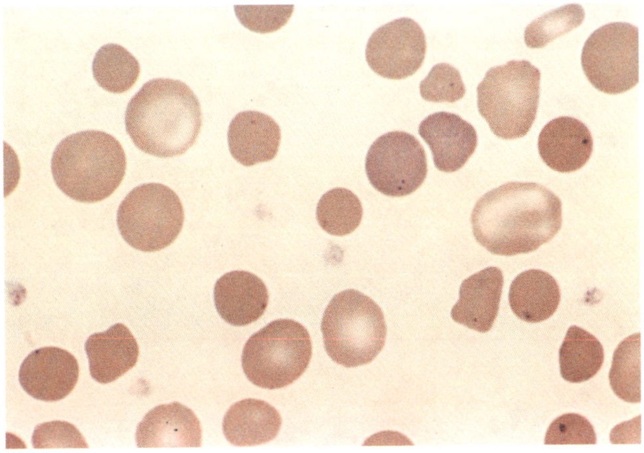

Figure 12–2

Hereditary spherocytosis (peripheral smear). Note the anisocytosis and several dark-appearing spherocytes with no central pallor. Howell-Jolly bodies (small dark nuclear remnants) are also present in the red cells. (Courtesy of Dr. Robert W. McKenna, Department of Pathology, University of Texas Southwestern Medical School, Dallas, Texas.)

There is no specific treatment for HS. Splenectomy is beneficial for those who are symptomatic, because the major site of red cell destruction is removed. The benefits of splenectomy must be weighed against the risk of increased susceptibility to infections, particularly in children.

Sickle Cell Anemia

The hemoglobinopathies are a group of hereditary disorders that are defined by the presence of structurally abnormal hemoglobins. Of the more than 300 variant hemoglobins that have been discovered, one-third are associated with significant clinical manifestations. The prototypical (and most prevalent) hemoglobinopathy is caused by a mutation in the β-globin chain gene that creates sickle hemoglobin (HbS). The disease associated with HbS, sickle cell anemia, is discussed here; other hemoglobinopathies are infrequent and beyond our scope.

HbS, like 90% of other abnormal hemoglobins, results from a single amino acid substitution in the globin chain. Normal hemoglobins, as may be recalled, are tetramers composed of two pairs of similar chains. On average, the normal adult red cell contains 96% HbA ($\alpha2\beta2$), 3% HbA_2 ($\alpha2\delta2$), and 1% fetal Hb (HbF, $\alpha2\gamma2$). Substitution of valine for glutamic acid at the sixth position of the β-chain produces HbS. In homozygotes all HbA is replaced by HbS, whereas in heterozygotes only about half is replaced.

Incidence. Approximately 8% of American blacks are heterozygous for HbS. In parts of Africa where malaria is endemic the gene frequency approaches 30%, as a result of a small but significant protective effect of HbS against *Plasmodium falciparum* malaria. In the United States sickle cell anemia affects approximately one of every 600 blacks, and worldwide, sickle cell anemia is the most common form of familial hemolytic anemia.

Etiology and Pathogenesis. Upon deoxygenation, HbS molecules undergo polymerization, a process also referred to as *gelation* or *crystallization*. These polymers distort the red cell, which assumes an elongated crescentic, or sickle, shape (Fig. 12–3). Sickling of red cells is initially reversible upon reoxygenation; however, membrane damage occurs with each episode of sickling, and eventually the cells accumulate calcium, lose potassium and water, and become irreversibly sickled.

Many variables influence sickling of red cells in vivo. The three most important ones are as follows:

- *The presence of hemoglobins other than HbS.* In heterozygotes approximately 40% of Hb is HbS; the remainder is HbA, which interacts only weakly with deoxygenated HbS. The presence of HbA slows the rate of polymerization greatly, and as a result the red cells of heterozygotes have little tendency to sickle in vivo. Such individuals are said to have the *sickle cell trait.* HbC, another mutant β-globin, is fairly common. The carrier rate for HbC in American blacks is about 2.3%; as a result about one in 1250 newborns are double heterozygotes because they have inherited HbS from one parent and HbC from the other. HbC has a greater tendency to aggregate with HbS than does HbA, and those with HbS and HbC (called *HbSC disease*) are symptomatic. Conversely, HbF interacts more weakly with HbS, and therefore newborns with sickle cell anemia do not manifest the disease until they are 5 to 6 months old, when the HbF falls to adult levels.
- *The concentration of HbS in the cell.* The tendency for deoxygenated HbS to form the insoluble polymers that create sickle cells is strongly dependent on the concentration of HbS. Thus, red cell dehydration, which increases the Hb concentration, greatly facilitates sickling and can trigger occlusion of small blood vessels. Conversely, the coexistence of α-thalassemia (described later) reduces the Hb concentration and therefore the severity of sickling. The relatively low concentration of HbS also contributes to the lack of sickling in heterozygotes with sickle cell trait.
- *The length of time that red cells are exposed to low oxygen tension.* Normal transit times for red cells

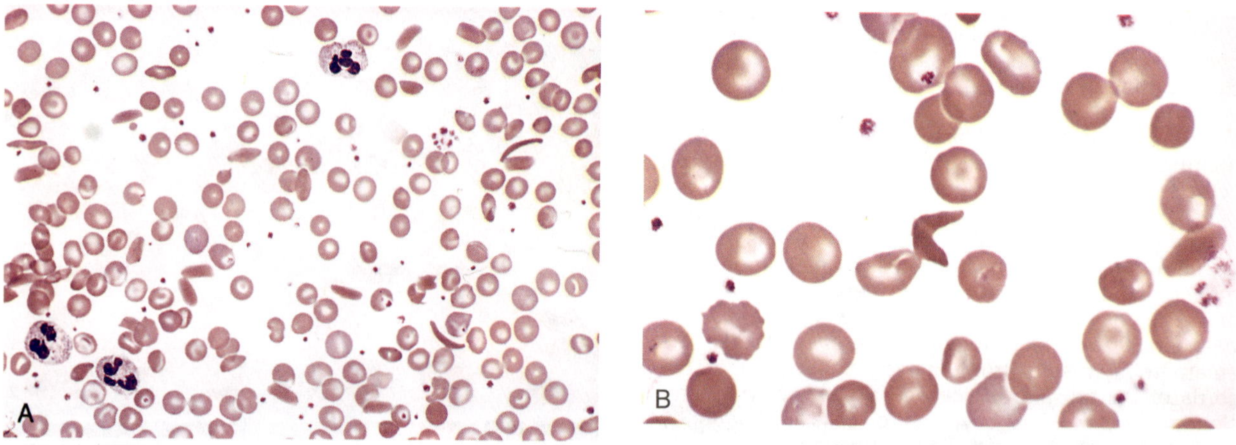

Figure 12–3

Peripheral blood smear from a patient with sickle cell anemia. **A,** Low magnification shows sickle cells, anisocytosis, poikilocytosis, and target cells. **B,** Higher magnification shows an irreversibly sickled cell in the center. (Courtesy of Dr. Robert W. McKenna, Department of Pathology, University of Texas Southwestern Medical School, Dallas, Texas.)

passing through capillaries are not sufficient for significant aggregation of deoxygenated HbS to occur. Hence, sickling is confined to microvascular beds where blood flow is sluggish. This is normally the case in the spleen and the bone marrow, which are prominently affected by sickle cell disease. In other vascular beds, it has been suggested that particularly important pathogenic roles are played by two factors: inflammation and increased red cell adhesion. As you will recall, blood flow in inflamed tissues is slowed, as a result of the adhesion of leukocytes and red cells to activated endothelium and the exudation of fluid through leaky vessels. This prolongs the red cell transit times, making clinically significant sickling more likely. Sickle red cells also have a greater tendency than normal red cells to adhere to endothelial cells, apparently because membrane damage makes them sticky. In fact, the adhesion of sickle red cells to cultured endothelial cells correlates with clinical severity, presumably because this "stickiness" reflects a greater risk for delays in transit across microvascular beds in vivo.

Two major consequences stem from the sickling of red cells (Fig. 12–4). First, repeated episodes of deoxygenation cause membrane damage and dehydration of red cells, which become rigid and irreversibly sickled. These dysfunctional red cells are recognized and removed by mononuclear phagocyte cells, producing a chronic extravascular hemolytic anemia. Overall, the mean life span of red cells in sickle cell anemia patients averages only 20 days (one-sixth of normal). Second, the sickling of red cells produces widespread *microvascular obstructions,* which result in ischemic tissue damage and pain crises. Vaso-occlusion does not correlate with the number of irreversibly sickled cells and therefore appears to result from factors, such as infection, inflammation, dehydration, and acidosis, that trigger the sickling of reversibly sickled cells.

Morphology

The anatomic alterations in sickle cell anemia stem from the following three aspects of the disease: (1) the severe chronic hemolytic anemia; (2) the increased breakdown of heme pigments, which are processed into bilirubin; and (3) the microvascular obstruction, which provokes tissue ischemia and infarction. In peripheral smears, bizarre elongated, spindled, or boat-shaped irreversibly sickled red cells are evident (see Fig. 12–3). Both the anemia and the vascular stasis lead to fatty changes in the heart, liver, and renal tubules. There is a compensatory hyperplasia of erythroid progenitors in the marrow. The burgeoning marrow often causes bone resorption and secondary new bone formation, resulting in prominent cheekbones and changes in the skull resembling a "crew-cut" in roentgenograms. Extramedullary hematopoiesis can also appear in the spleen and liver.

In children there is moderate **splenomegaly** (splenic weight as great as 500 gm) caused by congestion of the red pulp, which is stuffed with sickled red cells. However, the chronic splenic erythrostasis results in

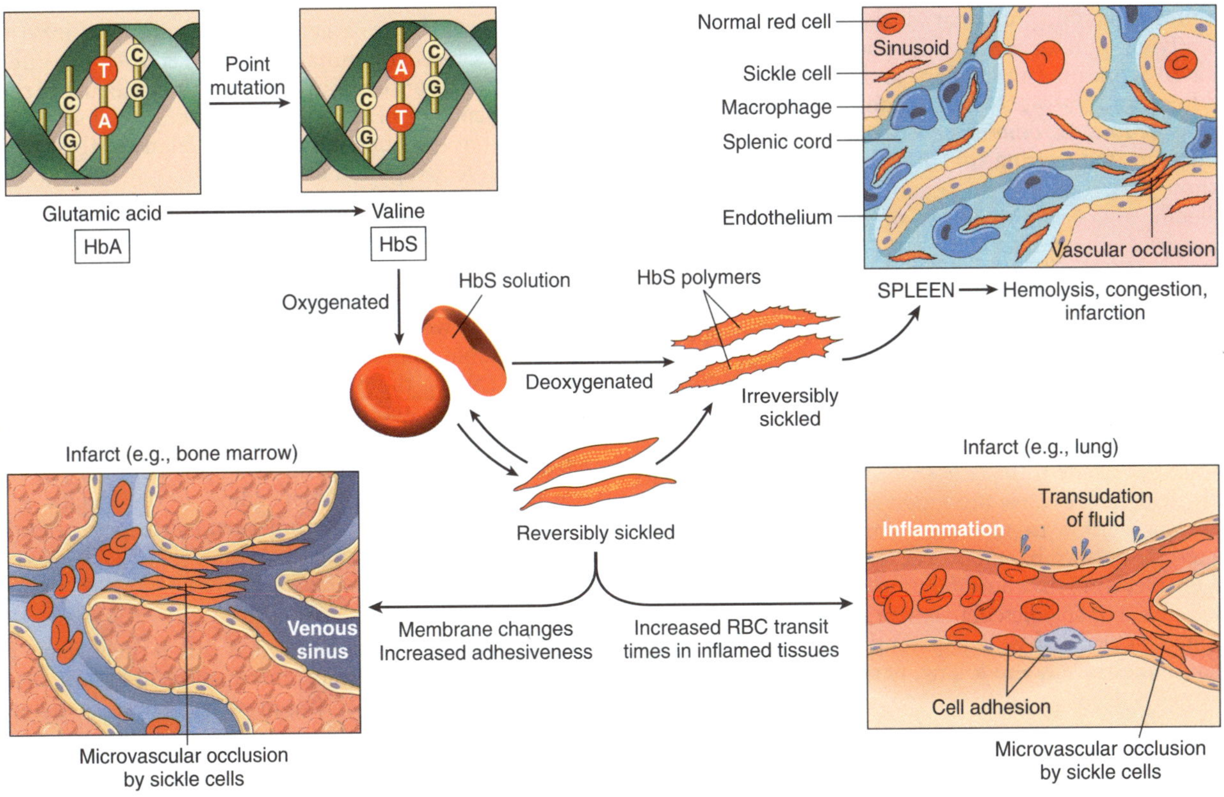

Figure 12–4

Pathophysiology and morphologic consequences of sickle cell anemia.

progressive hypoxic tissue damage, which eventually reduces the spleen to a functionally useless nubbin of fibrous tissue. This process, referred to as **autosplenectomy,** is complete by adulthood.

Vascular congestion, thrombosis, and **infarction** can affect any organ, including bones, liver, kidney, retina, brain, lung, and skin. The bone marrow is particularly prone to ischemia, because of its relatively sluggish blood flow and high rate of metabolism. Priapism, another common problem, can lead to penile fibrosis and eventual erectile dysfunction. As with the other hemolytic anemias, **hemosiderosis** and **gallstones** are common.

Clinical Course. Homozygous sickle cell disease usually becomes apparent after the sixth month of life, since HbF is gradually replaced by HbS. The anemia is severe; most patients have hematocrit values of 18% to 30% (normal range, 35%–45%). The chronic hemolysis is associated with marked reticulocytosis and hyperbilirubinemia. From the time of onset, the process runs an unremitting course, punctuated by sudden crises. The most serious of these are the *vaso-occlusive,* or *pain, crises.* Pain crises can involve many sites but are most common in the bone marrow, where they often progress to infarction and necrosis.

A feared complication is the *acute chest syndrome,* which can be triggered by pulmonary infections or fat emboli from necrotic marrow that secondarily involve the lung. The blood flow in the inflamed, ischemic lung becomes sluggish and "spleenlike," leading to sickling within hypoxemic pulmonary beds. This exacerbates the underlying pulmonary dysfunction, creating a vicious cycle of worsening pulmonary and systemic hypoxemia, sickling, and vaso-occlusion. Another major complication is *central nervous system stroke,* which sometimes occurs in the setting of the acute chest syndrome. Although virtually any organ can be damaged by ischemic injury in the course of the disease, *the acute chest syndrome and stroke are the two leading causes of ischemia-related death.*

A second acute event, the *aplastic crisis,* represents a sudden but usually temporary cessation of erythropoiesis. As in hereditary spherocytosis, these are usually triggered by parvovirus infection of erythroblasts, and, while severe, are self-limited.

In addition to these crises, patients with sickle cell disease are prone to *infections.* Both children and adults with sickle cell disease are functionally asplenic, making them susceptible to infections caused by encapsulated bacteria, such as pneumococci. In adults the basis for "hyposplenism" is autoinfarction. In the earlier childhood phase of splenic enlargement, congestion caused by trapped sickled red cells apparently interferes with bacterial sequestration and killing; hence, even children with enlarged spleens are at risk for fatal septicemia. Defects in the alternative complement pathway that impair the opsonization of encapsulated bacteria are also observed. For reasons that are not entirely clear, patients with sickle cell disease are particularly predisposed to *Salmonella* osteomyelitis.

In full-blown sickle cell disease, at least some irreversibly sickled red cells can be seen on an ordinary peripheral blood smear. In sickle cell trait, sickling can be induced in vitro by exposing cells to marked hypoxia. Ultimately, the diagnosis depends on the electrophoretic demonstration of HbS. Prenatal diagnosis of sickle cell anemia can be performed by analyzing the DNA in fetal cells obtained by amniocentesis or biopsy of chorionic villi (Chapter 7).

The clinical course of patients with sickle cell anemia is highly variable. As a result of improvements in supportive care, an increasing number of patients are surviving into adulthood and producing offspring. Of particular importance is prophylactic treatment with penicillin to prevent pneumococcal infections. Approximately 50% of patients survive beyond the fifth decade. In contrast, sickle cell trait causes symptoms rarely and only under extreme conditions, such as following vigorous exertion at high altitudes.

Hydroxyurea, a "gentle" inhibitor of DNA synthesis, has been shown to reduce pain crises and lessen the anemia. Hydroxyurea increases the red cell levels of HbF, acts as an anti-inflammatory agent by inhibiting the production of white cells, increases the MCV, and is oxidized by heme groups to produce NO, a potent vasodilator and inhibitor of platelet aggregation. These complementary intracorpuscular and extracorpuscular effects are believed to work together to lessen microvascular sickling and its attendant signs and symptoms.

Thalassemia

The thalassemias are a heterogeneous group of inherited disorders caused by mutations that decrease the rate of synthesis of α- or β-globin chains. As a consequence there is a deficiency of hemoglobin, with additional secondary red cell abnormalities caused by the relative excess of the other unaffected globin chain.

Molecular Pathogenesis. A diverse collection of molecular defects underlies the thalassemias, which are inherited as autosomal codominant conditions. Recall that adult hemoglobin, or HbA, is a tetramer composed of two α chains and two β chains. The α chains are encoded by two α-globin genes, which lie in tandem on chromosome 11, while the β chains are encoded by a single β-globin gene located on chromosome 16. The mutations that cause thalassemia are particularly common among Mediterranean, African, and Asian populations. The clinical features vary widely depending on the specific combination of alleles that are inherited by the patient (Table 12–3), as will be described below.

β-Thalassemia

The β-globin mutations associated with β-thalassemia fall into two categories: (1) β^0, in which no β-globin chains are produced; and (2) β^+, in which there is reduced (but detectable) β-globin synthesis. Sequencing of β-thalassemia genes has revealed more than 100 different responsible mutations, the majority of which consist of single-base changes. Individuals inheriting one abnormal allele have *thalassemia minor* or *thalassemia trait,* which

Table 12–3 Clinical and Genetic Classification of Thalassemias

Clinical Nomenclature	Genotype	Disease	Molecular Genetics
β-Thalassemias			
Thalassemia major	Homozygous or compound heterozygous (β^0/β^0, β^0/β^+, or β^+/β^+)	Severe, requires blood transfusions regularly	Defects in transcription, processing, or translation of mRNA, resulting in absent (β^0) or decreased (β^+) synthesis of β-globin
β-thalassemia trait	β/β^+ or β/β^0	Asymptomatic, with mild microcytic anemia, or microcytosis without anemia	
α-Thalassemias			
Hydrops fetalis	–/–	Fatal in utero	Gene deletions spanning one or both α-globin loci
HbH disease	–/–α	Moderately severe anemia	
α-thalassemia trait	–/αα (Asian) or –α/–α (black African)	Similar to β-thalassemia trait	
Silent carrier	–α/αα	Asymptomatic, normal red cells	

is asymptomatic or mildly symptomatic. Most individuals inheriting any two β^0 and β^+ alleles have β-thalassemia major; occasionally, individuals inheriting two β^+ alleles have a milder disease termed β-thalassemia intermedia. In contrast to α-thalassemias, described later, *gene deletions rarely underlie β-thalassemias* (Table 12–3).

Most of the mutations in β-thalassemia fall into one of three molecular subtypes (Fig. 12–5):

- The promoter region controls the initiation and rate of transcription. Some mutations lie within promoter regions and typically lead to reduced globin gene transcription. Because some β-globin is synthesized, such alleles are designated β^+.
- Mutations in the coding sequences are usually associated with more serious consequences. For example, in some cases a single-nucleotide change in one of the exons leads to the formation of a termination, or "stop" codon, which interrupts translation of β-globin messenger RNA (mRNA) and completely prevents the synthesis of β-globin. Such alleles are designated β^0.
- *Mutations that lead to aberrant mRNA processing are the most common cause of β-thalassemia.* Most of these affect introns, but some have been located within exons. If the mutation alters the normal splice junctions, splicing does not occur, and all of the mRNA formed is abnormal. Unspliced mRNA is degraded within the nucleus, and no β-globin is made. However, some mutations affect the introns at locations away from the normal intron-exon splice junction. These mutations create new sites that are substrates for the action of splicing enzymes at abnormal locations-within an intron, for example. Because normal splice sites remain intact, both normal and abnormal splicing occur, and normal β-globin mRNA is decreased but not absent. Thus, depending on their position, splice junction mutations can create either β^0 or β^+ alleles.

Two conditions contribute to the pathogenesis of the anemia in β-thalassemia. The reduced synthesis of β-globin leads to inadequate HbA formation, so that the MCHC is low, and the cells appear *hypochromic* and

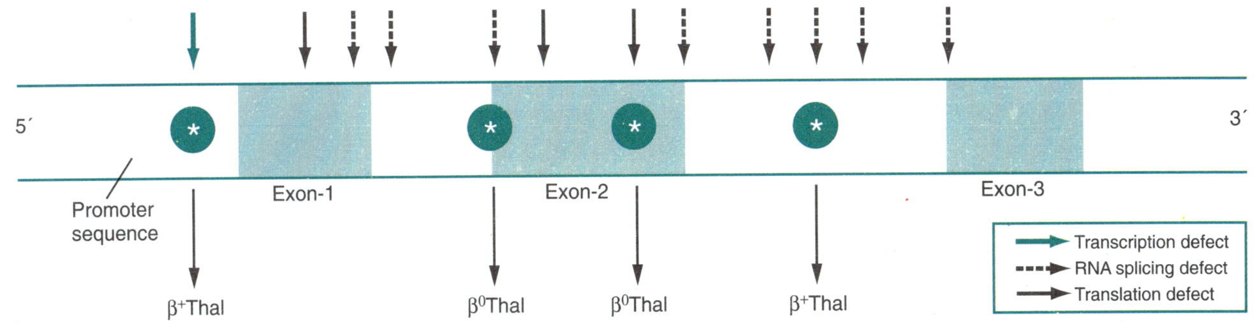

Figure 12–5

The β-globin gene and some sites at which point mutations giving rise to β-thalassemia have been localized. Asterisks within circles indicate the most common sites of mutations that cause different types of β-thalassemia. (Modified from Wyngaarden JB, Smith LH, Bennett JC [eds]: Cecil Textbook of Medicine, 19th ed. Philadelphia, WB Saunders, 1992.)

microcytic. Even more important is *red cell hemolysis,* which results from the unbalanced rates of β-globin and α-globin chain synthesis. Unpaired α chains form insoluble aggregates that precipitate within the red cells and cause membrane damage that is severe enough to provoke extravascular hemolysis (Fig. 12–6). Erythroblasts in the bone marrow are also susceptible to damage through the same mechanism, which in severe β-thalassemia results in the destruction of the majority of erythroid progenitors before their maturation into red cells. This intramedullary destruction of erythroid precursors (*ineffective erythropoiesis*) has another untoward effect: it is associated with an inappropriate increase in the absorption of dietary iron, which often leads to iron overload.

α-Thalassemia

The molecular basis of α-thalassemia is quite different from that of β-thalassemia. Most of the α-thalassemias are caused by deletions that remove one or more of the α-globin gene loci. The severity of the disease that results from these lesions is directly proportional to the number of α-globin genes that are missing (see Table 12–3). For example, the loss of a single α-globin gene is associated with a silent-carrier state, whereas the deletion of all four α-globin genes is associated with fetal death in

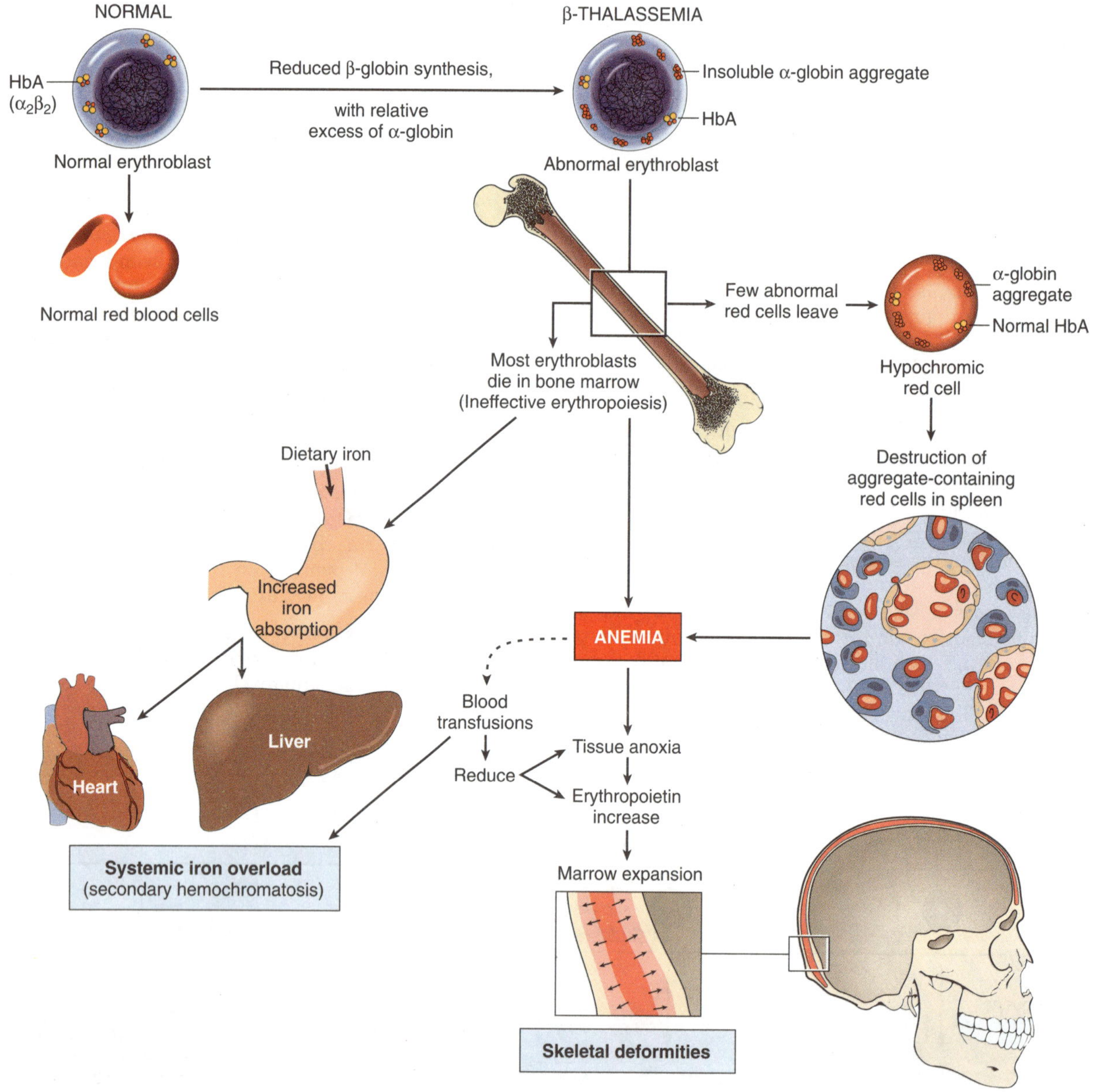

Figure 12–6

Pathogenesis of β-thalassemia major. Note that aggregates of excess α-globin are not visible on routine blood smears. Blood transfusions, on the one hand, correct the anemia and reduce stimulus for erythropoietin secretion and deformities induced by marrow expansion; on the other hand, they add to systemic iron overload.

utero, because the blood has virtually no oxygen-delivering capacity. With loss of three α-globin genes there is a relative excess of β-globin or chains other than α-globin. Excess β-globin (or γ-globin chains early in life) forms relatively stable β4 and γ4 tetramers known as HbH and Hb Bart, respectively, that cause less membrane damage than do free α-globin chains. Therefore, the hemolytic anemia and ineffective erythropoiesis tend be less severe in α-thalassemia than in β-thalassemia. Unfortunately, both HbH and Hb Bart have an abnormally high affinity for oxygen, which renders them ineffective at delivering oxygen to the tissues.

Morphology

Only the morphologic changes in β-thalassemia, which is more common in the United States, will be described. In β-thalassemia minor the abnormalities are confined to the peripheral blood. In smears the red cells appear small (microcytic), pale (hypochromic), and regular in shape. Target cells are often seen, a feature that results from the relatively large surface area-to-volume ratio, which leads Hb to collect in a central, dark-red "puddle." In smears from patients with β-thalassemia major the **microcytosis** and **hypochromia** are much more pronounced, and there is marked poikilocytosis, anisocytosis, and reticulocytosis. Nucleated red cells (normoblasts) are also seen, which reflect the underlying erythropoietic drive.

The anatomic changes in β-thalassemia major are similar to those seen in other hemolytic anemias but extreme in degree. The combination of ineffective erythropoiesis and hemolysis results in a striking hyperplasia of erythroid progenitors, with a shift toward early forms. The expanded erythropoietic marrow may completely fill the intramedullary space of the skeleton, invade the bony cortex, impair bone growth, and produce **skeletal deformities**. The extramedullary hematopoiesis and the hyperplasia of the mononuclear phagocytes result in prominent splenomegaly, **hepatomegaly**, and **lymphadenopathy**. The ineffective erythropoietic precursors consume nutrients and produce growth retardation and a degree of **cachexia** reminiscent of that seen in cancer patients. Unless steps are taken to prevent iron overload, over the span of years **severe hemosiderosis** develops (see Fig. 12–6).

Clinical Course. β-thalassemia major manifests itself postnatally as HbF synthesis diminishes. Affected children fail to develop normally, and their growth is retarded from shortly after birth. They are sustained only by repeated blood transfusions, which improve the anemia and reduce the skeletal deformities associated with excessive erythropoiesis. With transfusions alone survival into the second or third decade is possible, but gradually systemic iron overload develops. The combination of iron present in transfused red cells and the increased uptake of dietary iron from the gut lead inevitably to iron overload. The latter stems from inappropriately low levels of plasma hepcidin, a negative regulator of iron uptake that is "underexpressed" in conditions (such as β-thalassemia major) that are associated with ineffective erythropoiesis. Unless patients are treated aggressively with iron chelators, cardiac failure from secondary hemochromatosis commonly occurs and often causes death in the second or third decade of life. When feasible, bone marrow transplantation at an early age is the treatment of choice.

In β-thalassemia minor there is usually only a mild microcytic hypochromic anemia; generally, these patients have a normal life expectancy. Iron deficiency anemia is associated with a similar red cell appearance and must be excluded by appropriate laboratory tests, described later in this chapter. The diagnosis of β-thalassemia minor is made by Hb electrophoresis. In addition to reduced amounts of HbA (α2β2), the level of HbA_2 (α2δ2) is increased. The diagnosis of β-thalassemia major can generally be made on clinical grounds. The peripheral blood shows a severe microcytic hypochromic anemia, with marked variation in cell shapes (poikilocytosis). The reticulocyte count is increased. Hb electrophoresis shows profound reduction or absence of HbA and increased levels of HbF. The HbA_2 level may be normal or increased. Prenatal diagnosis of both forms of thalassemia can be made by DNA analysis.

HbH disease (caused by deletion of three α-globin genes) is not as severe as β-thalassemia major, since α- and β-globin chain synthesis is not as imbalanced and hematopoiesis is effective. Anemia is moderately severe, but patients usually do not require transfusions. Thus, the iron overload that is so common in β-thalassemia major is rarely seen. α-Thalassemia trait (caused by deletion of two α-globin genes) is often an asymptomatic condition associated with microcytic red cells and mild anemia.

Glucose-6-Phosphate Dehydrogenase Deficiency

The red cell is vulnerable to injury by endogenous and exogenous oxidants, which are normally inactivated by reduced glutathione (GSH). Abnormalities affecting the enzymes that are required for GSH production reduce the ability of red cells to protect themselves from oxidative injury and lead to hemolytic anemias. The prototype (and most prevalent) of these anemias is that associated with a deficiency of glucose-6-phosphate dehydrogenase (G6PD). The G6PD gene is on the X chromosome. More than 400 G6PD variants have been identified, but only a few are associated with disease. One of the most important is the G6PD A^- variant, which is carried by approximately 10% of black males in the United States. G6PD A^- has normal enzymatic activity but a decreased half-life. Because red cells lack the capacity for protein synthesis, older G6PD A^- red cells become progressively deficient in enzyme activity and more vulnerable to oxidant stress.

G6PD deficiency produces no symptoms until the patient is exposed to an environmental factor (most commonly infectious agents or drugs) that results in increased oxidant stress. The drugs incriminated include antimalarials (e.g., primaquine), sulfonamides, nitrofurantoin, phenacetin, aspirin (in large doses), and vitamin K derivatives. More commonly, episodes of hemolysis are triggered by infections, which induced phagocytes to produce free radicals as part of the normal host response. These offending agents produce oxidants such as hydrogen peroxide that are sopped up by GSH, which is converted to oxidized glutathione in the process. Because regeneration of GSH is impaired in G6PD-deficient cells, hydrogen peroxide is free to "attack" other red cell components, including globin chains, which have sulfhydryl groups that are susceptible to oxidation. Oxidized Hb denatures and precipitates, forming intracellular inclusions called Heinz bodies, which can damage the cell membrane sufficiently to cause intravascular hemolysis. Other cells that are less severely damaged neverthelss suffer from a loss of deformability, and their cell membranes are further damaged when splenic phagocytes attempt to "pluck out" the Heinz bodies, creating so-called bite cells (Fig. 12–7). All of these changes predispose the red cells to becoming trapped in the splenic sinusoids and destroyed by the phagocytes (extravascular hemolysis).

Drug-induced hemolysis is acute and of variable clinical severity. Typically, patients develop evidence of hemolysis after a lag period of 2 or 3 days. Because the G6PD gene is on the X chromosome, all the red cells of affected males are affected. However, because of random inactivation of one X chromosome in women (Chapter 7), heterozygous females have two distinct populations of red cells, one normal and the other deficient in G6PD activity. Thus, affected males are more vulnerable to oxidant injury, whereas most carrier females are asymptomatic, except those with a very large proportion of deficient red cells (a chance situation known as *unfavorable lyonization*). In G6PD A^-, the enzyme deficiency is most marked in older red cells, which are thus more susceptible to lysis. Since the marrow compensates by producing new (young) resistant red cells, hemolysis tends to abate

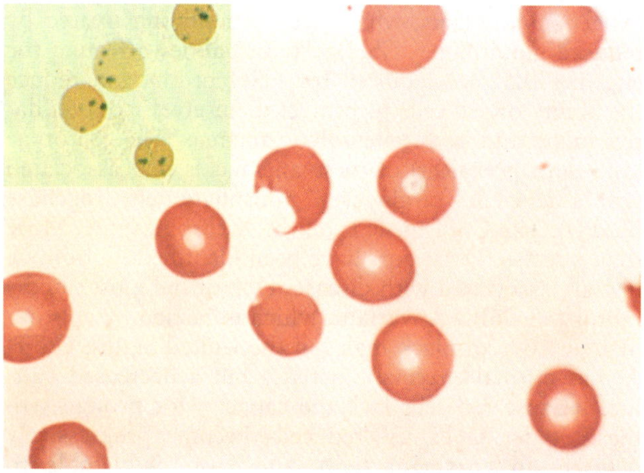

Figure 12–7

Peripheral blood smear from a patient with glucose-6-phosphate dehydrogenase deficiency after exposure to an oxidant drug. *Inset,* red cells with precipitates of denatured globin (Heinz bodies) revealed by supravital staining. As the splenic macrophages pluck out these inclusions, "bite cells" like the one in this smear are produced. (Courtesy of Dr. Robert W. McKenna, Department of Pathology, University of Texas Southwestern Medical School, Dallas, Texas.)

even if drug exposure continues. In other variants, such as G6PD Mediterranean, found mainly in the Middle East, the enzyme deficiency and the hemolysis that occur upon exposure to oxidants are more severe.

Paroxysmal Nocturnal Hemoglobinuria

A rare disorder of unknown etiology, paroxysmal nocturnal hemoglobinuria (PNH) is mentioned here because it is the only form of hemolytic anemia that results from an *acquired membrane defect secondary to a mutation that affects myeloid stem cells.* The mutant gene, called *PIGA,* is required for the synthesis of a specific type of intramembranous glycolipid anchor, phosphatidylinositol glycan (PIG), which is a component of diverse membrane-associated proteins. Without the membrane anchor, these "PIG-tailed" proteins cannot be expressed on the surface of cells. The affected proteins include several that limit the spontaneous activation of complement on the surface of cells. As a result, PIG-deficient precursors give rise to red cells that are inordinately sensitive to the lytic activity of complement. It is believed that the hemolysis is nocturnal because the blood becomes acidic during sleep (because of CO_2 retention) and an acid pH may promote hemolysis. It is not known why red cell destruction is paroxysmal. Several other PIG-tailed proteins are deficient from the membranes of granulocytes and platelets, possibly explaining the striking susceptibility of these patients to *infections* and intravascular *thromboses.*

PIGA is X-linked, and thus normal cells have only a single active *PIGA* gene, mutation of which is sufficient to give rise to PIG deficiency. Because all myeloid lineages are affected in PNH, the responsible mutations must occur in a multipotent stem cell. Remarkably, most, if not all, normal individuals harbor small numbers of PIG-deficient bone marrow cells that have mutations identical to those that cause PNH. It is believed that clinically evident PNH occurs only in rare instances in which the PIG-deficient clone has a survival advantage. One is the setting of primary bone marrow failure (aplastic anemia), which appears most often to be caused by immune-mediated destruction or suppression of marrow stem cells. It is hypothesized that in PNH patients, autoreactive T cells specifically recognize PIG-tailed surface antigens on normal bone marrow progenitors. Because PIG-deficient stem cells do not express these targets, they escape immune attack and eventually replace the normal marrow elements. Therapy with an antibody that inhibits the C5–9 complement membrane complex (and thereby red cell hemolysis) is currently under evaluation.

Immunohemolytic Anemias

Antibodies that recognize determinants on red cell membranes cause these uncommon forms of hemolytic anemia. The antibodies may arise spontaneously or be induced by exogenous agents such as drugs or chemicals. Immunohemolytic anemias are classified based on (1) the nature of the antibody and (2) the presence of certain predisposing conditions (summarized in Table 12–4).

Whatever the cause of antibody formation, the diagnosis of immunohemolytic anemias depends on the detec-

Table 12–4 Classification of Immunohemolytic Anemias

Warm Antibody Type
Primary (idiopathic)
Secondary: B-cell lymphoid neoplasms (e.g., chronic lymphocytic leukemia), autoimmune disorders (e.g., systemic lupus erythematosus), drugs (e.g., α-methyldopa, penicillin, quinidine)
Cold Antibody Type
Acute: *Mycoplasma* infection, infectious mononucleosis
Chronic: idiopathic, B-cell lymphoid neoplasms (e.g., lymphoplasmacytic lymphoma)

tion of antibodies and/or complement on patient red cells. This is done using the *direct Coombs antiglobulin test,* which measures the capacity of antibodies raised in animals against human immunoglobulins or complement to agglutinate red cells from the patient. The indirect Coombs test, in which patient serum is tested for the ability to agglutinate defined red cells, can then be used to characterize the target of the autoantibody.

Warm Antibody Immunohemolytic Anemias. These are caused by immunoglobulin G (IgG) or, rarely, immunoglobulin A (IgA) antibodies that are active at 37°C. More than 60% of cases are idiopathic (primary), while another 25% are associated with an underlying disease affecting the immune system (e.g., systemic lupus erythematosus [SLE]) or are induced by drugs. *The hemolysis usually results from the opsonization of red cells by the autoantibodies,* which leads to erythrophagocytosis in the spleen and elsewhere. Spheroidal cells resembling those seen in hereditary spherocytosis are often found in the peripheral blood smear. Presumably, cell membrane is removed during attempted phagocytosis of antibody-coated cells. This reduces the surface area-to-volume ratio and leads to the formation of *spherocytes,* which are rapidly destroyed in the spleen, as described earlier. The clinical severity of immunohemolytic anemias is quite variable. Most patients have chronic mild anemia with moderate splenomegaly and often require no treatment.

The mechanisms of hemolysis induced by drugs are varied and in some cases poorly understood. Drugs such as α-methyldopa induce autoantibodies that are directed against intrinsic red cell antigens, in particular Rh blood group antigens, producing an anemia that is indistinguishable from primary idiopathic immunohemolytic anemia. Presumably, the drug alters native epitopes and thus allows a bypass of T-cell tolerance to the membrane proteins (see Chapter 5). In other cases, drugs such as penicillin act as haptens and induce an antibody response by binding to a red cell membrane protein. Sometimes antibodies bind to a drug in the circulation and form immune complexes, which are then deposited on red cell membranes. Here they may fix complement or act as opsonins, either of which can damage red cells and lead to hemolysis.

Cold Antibody Immunohemolytic Anemias. These anemias are caused by low-affinity immunoglobulin M (IgM) antibodies, which bind to red cell membranes only at temperatures below 30°C, which are commonly experienced in distal parts of the body (e.g., ears, hands, and toes). Although IgM fixes complement well, the later steps of complement fixation occur inefficiently at temperatures below 37°C. As a result, most cells with bound IgM pick up some C3b but are not lysed in the periphery. When these cells travel to warmer areas, the weakly bound IgM antibody is released, but the coating of C3b remains. Because C3b is an opsonin (Chapter 2), the cells are phagocytosed by the mononuclear phagocyte system, especially Kupffer cells; hence, the *hemolysis is extravascular.* Cold agglutinins sometimes develop transiently during recovery from pneumonia caused by *Mycoplasma* sp. and infectious mononucleosis, producing a mild anemia of little clinical importance. A chronic cold agglutinin hemolytic anemia occurs in association with lymphoid neoplasms or as an idiopathic condition. In addition to anemia, Raynaud phenomenon often occurs in these patients as a result of the agglutination of red cells in the capillaries of exposed parts of the body.

Hemolytic Anemias Resulting from Mechanical Trauma to Red Cells

Red cells are disrupted by physical trauma in a variety of circumstances. Clinically important hemolytic anemias are sometimes caused by cardiac valve prostheses or by the narrowing and partial obstruction of the vasculature. *Traumatic hemolytic anemia* can be seen incidentally following any activity that produces repeated physical blows (e.g., marathon racing and bongo drumming) but is of clinical importance mainly in patients with mechanical heart valves, which can cause sufficiently tubulent blood flow to shear red cells. *Microangiopathic hemolytic anemia* is observed in a variety of pathologic states in which small vessels become partially obstructed. The most frequent of these conditions is disseminated intravascular coagulation (DIC; see later), in which the narrowing is caused by the intravascular deposition of fibrin. Other causes of microangiopathic hemolytic anemia include malignant hypertension, SLE, thrombotic thrombocytopenic purpura, hemolytic-uremic syndrome, and disseminated cancer, all of which produce vascular lesions that predispose the circulating red cells to mechanical injury. The morphologic alterations in the injured red cells (schistocytes) are striking and quite characteristic; "burr cells," "helmet cells," and "triangle cells" may be seen (Fig. 12–8). While the recognition of microangiopathic hemolysis often provides an important diagnostic clue, in and of itself it is not usually a major clinical problem.

Malaria

It has been estimated that 200 million persons suffer from this infectious disease, which is one of the most widespread afflictions of humans. Malaria is endemic in Asia and Africa, but with widespread jet travel, cases now occur all over the world. Malaria is caused by one of four types of protozoa. Of these, the most important is *Plasmodium falciparum,* which causes tertian malaria (falci-

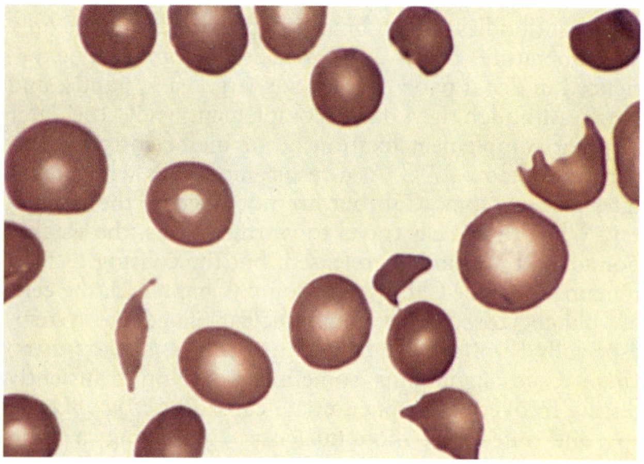

Figure 12–8

Microangiopathic hemolytic anemia. The peripheral blood smear from a patient with hemolytic-uremic syndrome shows several fragmented red cells. (Courtesy of Dr. Robert W. McKenna, Department of Pathology, University of Texas Southwestern Medical School, Dallas, Texas.)

parum malaria), a serious disorder with a high fatality rate. The other three species of *Plasmodium* that infect humans (*P. malariae, P. vivax,* and *P. ovale*) cause relatively benign disease. All forms are transmitted only by the bite of female *Anopheles* mosquitoes, and humans are the only natural reservoir.

Etiology and Pathogenesis. The life cycle of plasmodia is complex. As mosquitoes feed on human blood, sporozoites are introduced from the saliva and within a few minutes infect liver cells. Here, the parasites multiply rapidly to form a schizont containing thousands of merozoites. After a period of days to several weeks that varies with the *Plasmodium* species, the infected hepatocytes release the merozoites, which quickly infect red cells. Intraerythrocytic parasites either continue asexual reproduction to produce more merozoites or give rise to gametocytes that are capable of infecting the next hungry mosquito. During their asexual reproduction in red cells, the parasites first develop into trophozoites that are somewhat distinctive for each of the four forms of malaria. Thus, *the species of malaria that is responsible for an infection can be identified in appropriately stained thick smears of peripheral blood.* The asexual phase is completed when the trophozoites give rise to new merozoites, which escape by lysing the red cells.

Clinical Features. The distinctive clinical and anatomic features of malaria are related to the following:

- Showers of new merozoites are released from the red cells at intervals of approximately 48 hours for *P. vivax, P. ovale,* and *P. falciparum,* and 72 hours for *P. malariae.* The clinical spikes of shaking, chills, and fever coincide with this release.
- The parasites destroy large numbers of red cells and thus cause hemolytic anemia.
- A characteristic brown malarial pigment, probably a derivative of Hb that is identical to hematin, is released from the ruptured red cells along with the merozoites, discoloring principally the spleen, but also the liver, lymph nodes, and bone marrow.
- Activation of the phagocytic defense mechanisms of the host leads to marked hyperplasia of the mononuclear phagocyte system throughout the body, reflected in massive splenomegaly. Less frequently, the liver may also be enlarged.

Fatal falciparum malaria often involves the brain, a complication known as cerebral malaria. Normally, red cells bear negatively charged surfaces that interact poorly with endothelial cells. Infection of red cells with *P. falciparum* induces the appearance of positively charged surface knobs containing parasite-encoded proteins, which bind to adhesion molecules expressed on activated endothelium. Several endothelial cell adhesion molecules have been proposed to mediate this interaction, including intercellular adhesion molecule 1, which leads to the sequestration of red cells in postcapillary venules. In the brain this process gives rise to engorged cerebral vessels that are full of parasitized red cells and often occluded by microthrombi. Cerebral malaria is rapidly progressive; convulsions, coma, and death usually occur within days to weeks. Fortunately, falciparum malaria more commonly pursues a more chronic course that may be punctuated at any time by a dramatic complication known as *blackwater fever.* The trigger for this uncommon complication is obscure, but it is associated with massive hemolysis, leading to jaundice, hemoglobinemia, and hemoglobinuria.

With appropriate chemotherapy, the prognosis for patients with most forms of malaria is good; however, treatment of falciparum malaria is becoming more difficult, as a result of the emergence of drug-resistant strains. Because of the potentially serious consequences of this disease, early diagnosis and treatment are particularly important but are sometimes delayed in nonendemic settings. The ultimate solution is an effective vaccine, which is long sought but still elusive.

SUMMARY

Hemolytic Anemias

- *Hereditary Spherocytosis*:
  - Autosomal dominant disorder caused by inherited mutations that affect the red cell membrane skeleton, leading to loss of membrane and eventual conversion of red cells to spherocytes, which are phagocytosed and removed in the spleen.
  - Manifested by anemia, splenomegaly.
- *Sickle Cell Anemia*:
  - Autosomal recessive disorder that results from a mutation in β-globin that causes deoxygenated hemoglobin to self-associate into long polymers that distort (sickle) the red cell.
  - Blockage of vessels by aggregates of sickled cells causes acute pain crises and tissue infarction.

- Red cell membrane damage that attends repeated bouts of sickling results in a moderate to severe hemolytic anemia.
- *Thalassemias*:
  - Group of autosomal co-dominant disorders in which mutations in the α- or β-globin genes result in reduced hemoglobin synthesis, causing a microcytic, hypochromic anemia. In β-thalassemia unpaired α-globin chains form aggregates that damage red cell precursors and further impair erythropoiesis.
- *Glucose-6-Phosphate Dehydrogenase (G6PD) Deficiency*:
  - X-linked disorder in which red cells are unusually susceptible to damage caused by oxidants.
- *Immunohemolytic Anemias*:
  - Caused by antibody binding to red cell surface antigens, which may be normal red cell constituents or antigens that are modified by haptens (such as drugs).
  - Antibody binding can result in red cell opsonization and phagocytosis in the spleen or complement fixation and intravascular hemolysis.

ANEMIAS OF DIMINISHED ERYTHROPOIESIS

This category includes anemias that are caused by an inadequate dietary supply of substances that are needed for hematopoiesis, particularly iron, folic acid, and vitamin B_{12}. Other disorders that suppress erythropoiesis include those associated with bone marrow failure (aplastic anemia) or the replacement of the bone marrow by tumor or inflammatory cells (myelophthisic anemia). In the following sections some common examples of anemias resulting from nutritional deficiencies and marrow suppression are discussed individually.

Iron Deficiency Anemia

It is estimated that anemia affects about 10% of the population in developed countries and 25% to 50% in developing countries. In both settings the most common cause of anemia is iron deficiency, which is without question *the most common form of nutritional deficiency.* The factors responsible for iron deficiency differ in various populations and can be best considered in the context of normal iron metabolism.

Total body iron content is about 2 gm for women and 6 gm for men. Approximately 80% of functional body iron is found in hemoglobin, with the remainder being found in myoglobin and iron-containing enzymes (e.g., catalase and cytochromes). The iron storage pool, represented by hemosiderin and ferritin-bound iron, contains on average 15% to 20% of total body iron. Stored iron is found mainly in the liver, spleen, bone marrow, and skeletal muscle. Because *serum ferritin* is largely derived from the storage pool of iron, its concentration is a good indicator of the adequacy of body iron stores. *Assessment of bone marrow iron stores* is another reliable, but more invasive, method for estimating body iron content. Iron is transported in the plasma by an iron-binding protein called *transferrin.* In normal persons, transferrin is about 33% saturated with iron, yielding serum iron levels that average 120 μg/dL in men and 100 μg/dL in women. Thus, the total iron-binding capacity of serum is in the range of 300 μg/dL to 350 μg/dL.

As might be expected given the very high prevalence of iron deficiency in human populations, evolutionary pressures have yielded metabolic pathways that are strongly biased toward the retention of iron. There is no regulated pathway for iron excretion, which is limited to the 1 to 2 mg/day that is lost by the shedding of mucosal and skin epithelial cells. *Iron balance therefore is maintained largely by regulating the absorption of dietary iron.* The normal daily western diet contains 10 mg to 20 mg of iron. Most of this is in the form of heme contained in animal products, with the remainder being inorganic iron in vegetables. About 20% of heme iron (in contrast to 1% to 2% of nonheme iron) is absorbable, so the average western diet contains sufficient iron to balance fixed daily losses.

Iron is absorbed in the duodenum, where it must pass through the apical and basolateral membranes of enterocytes (Fig. 12–9). Nonheme iron is carried across each of these two membranes by distinct transporters. After reduction by ferric reductase, the reduced iron is transported by the divalent metal transporter (DMT1) across the apical membrane into the cytoplasm. At least two additional proteins are then required for the basolateral transfer of iron to transferrin in the plasma: ferroportin, which acts as a transporter; and hephaestin, which oxidizes the iron. Both DMT1 and ferroportin are widely distributed in the body and are involved in iron transport in other tissues as well. As depicted in Figure 12–9, only a fraction of the iron that enters the cell is delivered to plasma transferrin by the action of ferroportin. The remainder is bound to ferritin and lost through the exfoliation of mucosal cells.

When the body is replete with iron, most of the iron that enters duodenal cells is bound to ferritin and never transferred to transferrin; in iron deficiency, or when there is ineffective erythropoiesis, transfer to plasma transferrin is enhanced. This balance is regulated by hepcidin, a small hepatic peptide that is synthesized and secreted in an iron-dependent fashion. Plasma hepcidin binds to ferroportin and induces its internalization and degradation; thus, when hepcidin concentrations are high, ferroportin levels fall, and less iron is transferred out of the enterocytes to transferrin. Conversely, when hepcidin levels are low, as occurs in hemochromatosis (Chapter 16), transport of iron from the enterocytes to plasma is increased, resulting eventually in systemic iron overload.

Negative iron balance and consequent anemia can result from a variety of causes:

- Low dietary intake alone is rarely the cause of iron deficiency in the United States, because the average daily dietary intake of 10 mg to 20 mg is more than

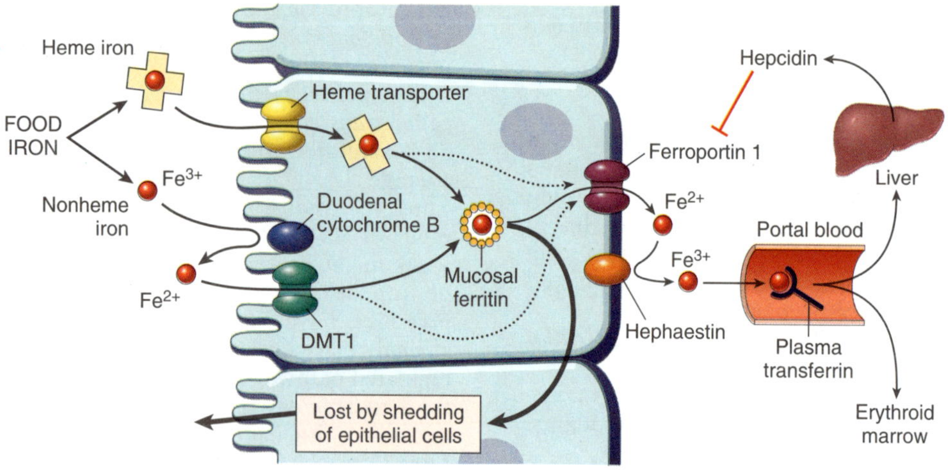

Figure 12–9

Iron absorption. Mucosal uptake of heme and nonheme iron is depicted. When the storage sites of the body are replete with iron and erythropoietic activity is normal, most of the absorbed iron is lost into the gut by shedding of the epithelial cells. Conversely, when body iron requirements increase or when erythropoiesis is stimulated, a greater fraction of the absorbed iron is transferred into plasma transferrin, with a concomitant decrease in iron loss through mucosal ferritin. DMT1, divalent metal transporter 1.

enough for males and adequate for females. In other parts of the world, however, low intake and poor bioavailability from predominantly vegetarian diets are an important cause of iron deficiency.

- Malabsorption can occur with sprue and celiac disease or after gastrectomy (Chapter 15).
- Increased demands not met by normal dietary intake occur around the world during pregnancy and infancy.
- Chronic blood loss is the most important cause of iron deficiency anemia in the western world; this loss may occur from the gastrointestinal tract (e.g., peptic ulcers, colonic cancer, hemorrhoids, hookworm disease) or the female genital tract (e.g., menorrhagia, metrorrhagia, cancers).

Regardless of the cause, iron deficiency develops insidiously. At first iron stores are depleted, leading to a decline in serum ferritin and the absence of stainable iron in the bone marrow. This is followed by a decrease in serum iron and a rise in the serum iron-binding capacity. Ultimately the capacity to synthesize hemoglobin, myoglobin, and other iron-containing proteins is diminished, leading to anemia, impaired work and cognitive performance, and even reduced immunocompetence.

Morphology

Except in unusual circumstances, iron deficiency anemia is relatively mild. The red cells are **microcytic and hypochromic,** reflecting the reductions in MCV and MCHC (Fig. 12–10). For unclear reasons, iron deficiency is often accompanied by an increase in the platelet count. Although erythropoietin levels are increased, the marrow response is blunted by the iron deficiency, and thus the marrow cellularity is usually only slightly increased. Extramedullary hematopoiesis is uncommon.

Clinical Course. In most instances, iron deficiency anemia is asymptomatic. Nonspecific manifestations, such as weakness, listlessness, and pallor, may be present in severe cases. With long-standing severe anemia, thinning, flattening, and eventually "spooning" of the fingernails sometimes appears. A curious but characteristic neurobehavioral complication is *pica,* the compunction to consume non-foodstuffs such as dirt or clay.

Diagnostic criteria include anemia, hypochromic and microcytic red cell indices, low serum ferritin and serum iron levels, low transferrin saturation, increased total iron-binding capacity, and, ultimately, response to iron therapy. Persons frequently die *with* this form of anemia but rarely *of* it. It is important to remember that in reasonably well-nourished persons, microcytic hypochromic

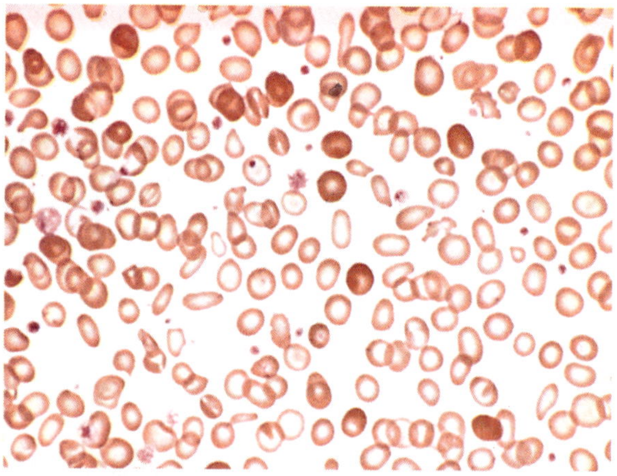

Figure 12–10

Hypochromic microcytic anemia of iron deficiency. Note the small red cells containing a narrow rim of hemoglobin at the periphery. Compare to the scattered, fully hemoglobinized cells derived from a recent blood transfusion given to the patient. (Courtesy of Dr. Robert W. McKenna, Department of Pathology, University of Texas Southwestern Medical School, Dallas, Texas.)

anemia is not a disease but rather a symptom of some underlying disorder.

Anemia of Chronic Disease

This is the most common form of anemia in hospitalized patients. It superficially resembles the anemia of iron deficiency, but it stems from inflammation-induced sequestration of iron within the cells of the mononuclear phagocyte (reticuloendothelial) system. It occurs in a variety of chronic inflammatory disorders, including the following:

- Chronic microbial infections, such as osteomyelitis, bacterial endocarditis, and lung abscess
- Chronic immune disorders, such as rheumatoid arthritis and regional enteritis
- Neoplasms, such as Hodgkin lymphoma and carcinomas of the lung and breast

The serum iron levels are usually low, and the red cells can be normocytic and normochromic, or, as in anemia of iron deficiency, hypochromic and microcytic. However, the anemia of chronic disease is associated with *increased storage iron in the bone marrow, a high serum ferritin concentration, and a reduced total iron-binding capacity,* all of which readily rule out iron deficiency. This combination of findings is attributable to high concentrations of circulating hepcidin, which inhibits ferroportin and thereby block the transfer of iron from the mononuclear phagocyte storage pool to the erythroid precursors. The elevated hepcidin concentrations are caused by proinflammatory cytokines, which enhance the synthesis of hepcidin by the liver. In addition, chronic inflammation also blunts the compensatory increase in erythropoietin levels, which is not adequate for the degree of anemia. The teleologic explanation for iron sequestration in the presence of a wide variety of chronic inflammatory disorders is unclear; it may serve to inhibit the growth of iron-dependent microorganisms or to augment certain aspects of host immunity. Administration of erythropoietin and iron can improve the anemia, but only effective treatment of the underlying condition is curative.

Megaloblastic Anemias

There are two principal causes of megaloblastic anemia: folate deficiency and vitamin B_{12} deficiency. Both vitamins are required for DNA synthesis, and, hence, the effects of their deficiency on hematopoiesis are quite similar. However, as will be described, the causes and consequences of folate and vitamin B_{12} deficiency differ in important ways.

Pathogenesis. The morphologic hallmark of megaloblastic anemias is an enlargement of erythroid precursors (*megaloblasts*), which gives rise to abnormally large red cells (macrocytes). The other myeloid lineages are also affected. Most notably, granulocyte precursors are enlarged (*giant metamyelocytes*) and yield highly characteristic *hypersegmented neutrophils.* Underlying the cellular gigantism is an impairment of DNA synthesis, which results in a delay in nuclear maturation and cell division. Because the synthesis of RNA and cytoplasmic elements proceeds at a normal rate and thus outpaces that of the nucleus, the hematopoietic precursors show *nuclear-cytoplasmic asynchrony.* This maturational derangement contributes to anemia in several ways. Some megaloblasts are so defective in DNA synthesis that they undergo apoptosis in the marrow (ineffective hematopoiesis). Others succeed in maturing into red cells but do so after fewer cell divisions; as a result, the total output from these precursors is diminished. Granulocyte and platelet precursors are similarly affected. As a result, most patients with megaloblastic anemia develop pancytopenia (anemia, thrombocytopenia, and granulocytopenia).

Morphology

Certain morphologic features are common to all forms of megaloblastic anemias. The **bone marrow** is markedly hypercellular, as a result of increased numbers of **megaloblasts.** These cells are larger than normoblasts and have a delicate, finely reticulated nuclear chromatin (suggestive of nuclear immaturity) and an abundant, strikingly basophilic cytoplasm (Fig. 12–11). As the megaloblasts differentiate and begin to acquire hemoglobin, the nucleus retains its finely distributed chromatin and fails to undergo the chromatin clumping typical of an orthochromatic normoblast. Similarly, the granulocytic precursors also demonstrate nuclear-cytoplasmic asynchrony, yielding giant metamyelocytes. Megakaryocytes, too, may be abnormally large and have bizarre multilobed nuclei.

In the **peripheral blood** the earliest change is usually the appearance of **hypersegmented neutrophils,** which appear even before the onset of anemia. Normally, neutrophils have three or four nuclear lobes, but in megaloblastic anemias neutrophils often have five or more. **The red cells typically include large, egg-shaped macro-ovalocytes; the MCV is often greater than 110 fL** (normal, 82–92 fL). Although macrocytes appear hyperchromic, in reality the MCHC is normal. Large, misshapen platelets may also be seen. Morphologic changes in other systems, especially the gastrointestinal tract, also occur, giving rise to some of the clinical features.

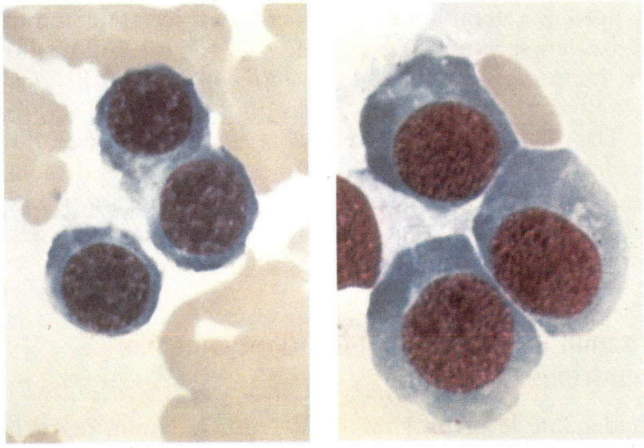

Figure 12–11

Comparison of normoblasts (*left*) and megaloblasts (*right*). The megaloblasts are larger, have relatively immature nuclei with finely reticulated chromatin, and have an abundant basophilic cytoplasm. (Courtesy of Dr. José Hernandez, Department of Pathology, University of Texas Southwestern Medical School, Dallas, Texas.)

Folate (Folic Acid) Deficiency Anemia

Megaloblastic anemia secondary to folate deficiency is not common, but marginal folate stores occur with surprising frequency even in apparently healthy individuals. The risk of clinically significant folate deficiency is high in those with a poor diet (the economically deprived, the indigent, and the elderly) or increased metabolic needs (pregnant women and patients with chronic hemolytic anemias).

Ironically, folate is widely prevalent in nearly all foods but is readily destroyed by 10 to 15 minutes of cooking. Thus, the best sources of folate are fresh uncooked vegetables and fruits. Food folates are predominantly in polyglutamate form and must be split into monoglutamates for absorption, a conversion that is hampered by acidic foods and substances found in beans and other legumes. Phenytoin (Dilantin) and a few other drugs also inhibit folate absorption, while others, such as methotrexate, inhibit folate metabolism. The principal site of intestinal absorption is the upper third of the small intestine; thus, malabsorptive disorders that affect this level of the gut, such as celiac disease and tropical sprue, can impair folate uptake.

The metabolism and physiologic functions of folate are complex. Here, it is sufficient to note that, after absorption, folate is transported in the blood mainly as a monoglutamate. Within cells it is further metabolized to several derivatives, but its conversion from dihydrofolate to tetrahydrofolate by the enzyme dihydrofolate reductase is particularly important. Tetrahydrofolate acts as an acceptor and donor of one-carbon units in a variety of steps involved in the synthesis of purines and thymidylate, the building blocks of DNA, and its deficiency accounts for the inadequate DNA synthesis that is characteristic of megaloblastic anemia.

The onset of the anemia is insidious and is associated with nonspecific symptoms such as weakness and easy fatigability. The clinical picture may be complicated by the coexistent deficiency of other vitamins, especially in alcoholics. Because the gastrointestinal tract, like the hematopoietic system, is a site of rapid cell turnover, symptoms referable to the alimentary tract are common and often severe. These include sore tongue and cheilosis. *It should be stressed that, unlike in vitamin B_{12} deficiency, neurologic abnormalities do not occur.*

The diagnosis of a megaloblastic anemia is readily made from examination of a smear of peripheral blood and bone marrow. The anemia of folate deficiency is best distinguished from that of vitamin B_{12} deficiency by measuring serum and red cell folate and vitamin B_{12} levels.

Vitamin B_{12} (Cobalamin) Deficiency Anemia: Pernicious Anemia

Inadequate levels of vitamin B_{12}, or cobalamin, result in a megaloblastic macrocytic anemia similar to that caused by folate deficiency. However, vitamin B_{12} deficiency can also cause a demyelinating disorder involving the peripheral nerves and, ultimately and most importantly, the spinal cord. There are many causes of vitamin B_{12} deficiency. The term *pernicious anemia,* a relic of the days when the cause and therapy of this condition were unknown, is used to describe vitamin B_{12} deficiency resulting from inadequate gastric production or defective function of intrinsic factor. Intrinsic factor plays a critical role in the absorption of vitamin B_{12}, a complex multistep process that proceeds as follows:

1. Peptic digestion releases dietary vitamin B_{12}, which then binds to salivary B_{12}-binding proteins called *cobalophilins,* or *R binders.*
2. R-B_{12} complexes are transported to the duodenum and processed by pancreatic proteases; this releases B_{12}, which attaches to intrinsic factor secreted from the parietal cells of the gastric fundic mucosa.
3. The intrinsic factor–B_{12} complex passes to the distal ileum and attaches to the epithelial intrinsic factor receptors, which leads to absorption of vitamin B_{12}.
4. The absorbed B_{12} is bound to transport proteins called *transcobalamins,* which then deliver it to the liver and other cells of the body.

Etiology. *Among the many potential causes of cobalamin deficiency, long-standing malabsorption is the most common and important.* Vitamin B_{12} is abundant in all animal foods, including eggs and dairy products, and is resistant to cooking and boiling. Even bacterial contamination of water and nonanimal foods can provide adequate amounts. As a result, deficiencies due to diet are rare and are virtually confined to strict vegans. Once vitamin B_{12} is absorbed, the body handles it very efficiently. It is stored in the liver, which normally contains reserves that are sufficient to support bodily needs for 5 to 20 years.

Until proved otherwise, *a deficiency of vitamin B_{12} (in the western world) is caused by pernicious anemia.* This disease seems to stem from an autoimmune reaction against parietal cells and intrinsic factor itself, which produces gastric mucosal atrophy (Chapter 15). Several associations favor an autoimmune basis:

- Autoantibodies are present in the serum and gastric juice of most patients with pernicious anemia. Three types of antibodies have been found: *parietal canalicular antibodies,* which bind to the mucosal parietal cells; *blocking antibodies,* which block the binding of vitamin B_{12} to intrinsic factor; and *binding antibodies* that react with intrinsic factor–B_{12} complex and prevent it from binding to the ileal receptor.
- An occurrence of pernicious anemia with other autoimmune diseases such as Hashimoto thyroiditis, Addison disease, and type I diabetes mellitus is well documented.
- The frequency of serum antibodies to intrinsic factor is increased in patients with other autoimmune diseases.

Chronic vitamin B_{12} malabsorption is also seen following gastrectomy (which leads to loss of cells producing intrinsic factor) or resection of ileum (which prevents absorption of intrinsic factor–B_{12} complex), and in disorders that involve the distal ileum (such as Crohn disease, tropical sprue, and Whipple disease). In individuals older than 70 years of age, gastric atrophy and achlorhydria can interfere with the production of acid and pepsin, which are needed to release the vitamin from its bound form in the diet.

The metabolic defects that are responsible for the anemia are intertwined with folate metabolism. Vitamin B_{12} is required for recycling of tetrahydrofolate, and hence its deficiency reduces the availability of the form of folate that is required for DNA synthesis. As expected, given this relationship, the anemia of vitamin B_{12} deficiency improves with administration of folates. In contrast, the biochemical basis of the neuropathy in vitamin B_{12} deficiency is unclear, and administration of folate may actually exacerbate the neurologic disease. The principal neurologic lesions associated with vitamin B_{12} deficiency are *demyelination of the posterior and lateral columns of the spinal cord,* sometimes beginning in the peripheral nerves. In time, axonal degeneration may supervene. The severity of neurologic manifestations is not related to the degree of anemia. Indeed, uncommonly, the neurologic disease occurs in the absence of overt megaloblastic anemia.

Clinical Features. Manifestations of vitamin B_{12} deficiency are nonspecific. As with any other anemia, there is pallor, easy fatigability, and, in severe cases, dyspnea and even congestive heart failure. The increased destruction of erythroid progenitors may give rise to mild jaundice. Gastrointestinal symptoms similar to those seen in folate deficiency are seen. The spinal cord disease begins with symmetric numbness, tingling, and burning in feet or hands, followed by unsteadiness of gait and loss of position sense, particularly in the toes. Although the anemia responds dramatically to parenteral vitamin B_{12}, the neurologic manifestations often fail to resolve. As discussed in Chapter 15, patients with pernicious anemia have an increased risk of gastric carcinoma.

The diagnostic features of pernicious anemia include (1) low serum vitamin B_{12} levels, (2) normal or elevated serum folate levels, (3) serum antibodies to intrinsic factor, (4) moderate to severe megaloblastic anemia, (5) leukopenia with hypersegmented granulocytes, and (6) a dramatic reticulocytic response (within 2–3 days) to parenteral administration of vitamin B_{12}.

Aplastic Anemia

Aplastic anemia is a disorder in which *multipotent myeloid stem cells are suppressed, leading to marrow failure and pancytopenia.* Notwithstanding its name, aplastic anemia should not be confused with selective suppression of erythroid stem cells (pure red cell aplasia), in which anemia is the only manifestation.

Etiology and Pathogenesis. In more than half of cases, aplastic anemia is idiopathic. In the remainder, an exposure to known myelotoxic agents, such as drugs or chemicals, can be identified. With some agents, the marrow damage is predictable, dose related, and usually reversible. Included in this category are antineoplastic drugs (e.g., alkylating agents, antimetabolites), benzene, and chloramphenicol. In other instances marrow toxicity occurs as an apparent "idiosyncratic" or hypersensitivity reaction to small doses of known myelotoxic drugs (e.g., chloramphenicol) or to drugs such as sulfonamides, which are not myelotoxic in other persons.

Aplastic anemia sometimes arises after certain viral infections, most often community-acquired viral hepatitis. The specific virus responsible is not known; hepatitis viruses A, B, and C are apparently not the culprits. Marrow aplasia develops insidiously several months after recovery from the hepatitis and follows a relentless course.

The pathogenetic events leading to marrow failure remain vague, but it seems that autoreactive T cells may play an important role. This is supported by a variety of experimental data and clinical experience, which has shown that in 70% to 80% of cases aplastic anemia responds to immunosuppressive therapy aimed at T cells. Much less clear are the events that trigger the T-cell attack on marrow stem cells; perhaps viral antigens, drug-derived haptens, and/or genetic damage create neoantigens within stem cells that serve as targets for the immune system.

Rare but interesting genetic conditions are also associated with marrow failure. Of note, a small fraction of patients with "acquired" aplastic anemia have inherited defects in telomerase, which you will recall is needed for the maintenance and stability of chromosomes. In these settings intrinsic defects lead directly to damage and senescence of hematopoietic stem cells.

Morphology

The bone marrow in aplastic anemia typically is markedly hypocellular, with greater than 90% of the intertrabecular space being occupied by fat. The limited cellularity often consists of only lymphocytes and plasma cells. These changes are better appreciated in bone marrow biopsy specimens than in marrow aspirates, which often yield a "dry tap." A number of secondary changes often accompany marrow failure. Anemia may cause fatty change in the liver, and thrombocytopenia and granulocytopenia may result in hemorrhages and bacterial infections, respectively. The requirement for transfusions may eventually cause hemosiderosis.

Clinical Course. Aplastic anemia affects persons of all ages and both sexes. The slowly progressive *anemia* causes the insidious development of weakness, pallor, and dyspnea. *Thrombocytopenia* often presents with petechiae and ecchymoses. *Granulocytopenia* may be manifested only by frequent and persistent minor infections or by the sudden onset of chills, fever, and prostration. It is important to distinguish aplastic anemia from anemias caused by marrow infiltration (myelophthisic anemia), "aleukemic leukemia," and granulomatous diseases. Because pancytopenia is common to these conditions, their clinical manifestations may be indistinguishable, but they are easily distinguished by examination of the bone marrow. *Splenomegaly* is characteristically absent in aplastic anemia; if it is present, the diagnosis of aplastic anemia should be seriously questioned. Typically, the red cells are normocytic and normochromic, although slight macrocytosis is occasionally present; *reticulocytes are reduced in number.*

The prognosis of marrow aplasia is quite unpredictable. As mentioned earlier, withdrawal of toxic drugs may lead to recovery in some cases. The idiopathic form has a poor prognosis if left untreated. Bone marrow transplantation is an extremely effective form of therapy, especially if performed in nontransfused patients younger than 40 years of age. It is proposed that transfusions sensitize patients to alloantigens, producing a high engraftment failure rate following bone marrow transplantation. As mentioned earlier, patients who are poor transplant candidates may benefit from immunosuppressive therapy.

Myelophthisic Anemia

This form of anemia is caused by the extensive replacement of the marrow by tumors or other lesions. It is most commonly associated with metastatic breast, lung, or prostate cancer, but other cancers, advanced tuberculosis, lipid storage disorders, and osteosclerosis can produce a similar clinical picture. The principal manifestations of marrow infiltration include anemia and thrombocytopenia; in general, the white cell series is less affected. Characteristically, misshapen red cells, some resembling teardrops, are seen in the peripheral blood. Immature granulocytic and erythrocytic precursors may also be seen (leukoerythroblastosis), along with a slightly elevated white cell count. Treatment is focused on the management of the underlying condition.

SUMMARY

Anemias of Diminished Erythropoiesis

- *Iron Deficiency Anemia*:
  - Inadequate intake of iron results in insufficient hemoglobin synthesis and hypochromic and microcytic red cells.
- *Anemia of Chronic Disease*:
  - Caused by production of inflammatory cytokines, which cause iron to be sequestered in macrophages, resulting in an anemia that is usually normochromic and normocytic.
- *Megaloblastic Anemia*:
  - Caused by deficiencies of folate or vitamin B_{12}, which lead to inadequate synthesis of thymidine and defective DNA replication.
  - Results in enlarged abnormal hematopoietic precursors (megaloblasts) in the bone marrow, ineffective hematopoiesis, and (in most cases) pancytopenia.
- *Aplastic Anemia*:
  - Caused by bone marrow failure (hypocellularity) due to diverse causes, including exposures to toxins and radiation, idiosyncratic reactions to drugs and viruses, and inherited defects in DNA repair and the enzyme telomerase.
- *Myelophthisic Anemia*:
  - Caused by replacement of the bone marrow by infiltrative processes such as metastatic carcinoma and granulomatous disease.
  - Leads to the release of early erythroid and granulocytic precursors (leukoerythroblastosis) and the appearance of tear-drop red cells in the peripheral blood.

Laboratory Diagnosis of Anemias

The diagnosis of anemia is established by a decrease in the hemoglobin and the hematocrit to levels that are below normal. Based on the red cell hemoglobin content and size, anemias can be placed into three major subgroups: normocytic normochromic, microcytic hypochromic, and macrocytic. The presence of red cells with a particular morphology, such as spherocytes, sickled cells, and fragmented cells, provide additional etiologic clues. The specialized tests cited below are particularly important in establishing the diagnosis of certain classes of anemia:

- Gel electrophoresis: used to detect abnormal hemoglobins, such as HbS
- Coombs test: used to diagnose immunohemolytic anemias
- Reticulocyte counts: used to distinguish between anemias caused by red cell destruction (hemolysis) and depressed production (marrow failure)
- Iron indices (serum iron, serum iron-binding capacity, transferrin saturation, and serum ferritin concentrations): used to distinguish between hypochromic microcytic anemias caused by iron deficiency, anemia of chronic disease, and thalassemia minor
- Serum and red cell folate and vitamin B_{12} concentrations: used to identify the cause of megaloblastic anemia
- Plasma unconjugated bilirubin and haptogloblin concentrations: used to support the diagnosis of hemolytic anemia

In isolated anemia, tests performed on the peripheral blood usually suffice to establish a cause. In contrast, when anemia occurs in combination with thrombocytopenia and/or granulocytopenia, it is much more likely to be associated with marrow aplasia or infiltration; in these instances, a marrow examination is often critical for diagnosis.

POLYCYTHEMIA

Polycythemia, or *erythrocytosis,* as it is sometimes referred to, denotes an increase in the blood concentration of red cells, which usually correlates with an increase in the hemoglobin concentration. Polycythemia may be *relative,* when there is hemoconcentration caused by a decrease in plasma volume, or *absolute,* when there is an increase in the total red cell mass. Relative polycythemia results from any cause of dehydration, such as water deprivation, prolonged vomiting, diarrhea, or the excessive use of diuretics. Absolute polycythemia is said to be *primary* when the increase in red cell mass results from an autonomous proliferation of the myeloid stem cells, and *secondary* when the red cell progenitors are proliferating in response to an increase in erythropoietin. Primary polycythemia (polycythemia vera [PCV]) is a clonal, neoplastic proliferation of myeloid progenitors, which is considered later in this chapter with the other myeloproliferative disorders. The increases in erythropoietin that are seen in secondary polycythemias have a variety of causes (Table 12–5).

Table 12–5 Pathophysiologic Classification of Polycythemia

Relative
Reduced plasma volume (hemoconcentration)
Absolute
Primary: Abnormal proliferation of myeloid stem cells, normal or low erythropoietin levels (polycythemia vera); inherited activating mutations in the erythropoietin receptor (rare)
Secondary: Increased erythropoietin levels Appropriate: lung disease, high-altitude living, cyanotic heart disease Inappropriate: erythropoietin-secreting tumors (e.g., renal cell carcinoma, hepatoma, cerebellar hemangioblastoma); surreptitious erythropoietin use (e.g., in endurance athletes)

WHITE CELL DISORDERS

Disorders of white cells include deficiencies (leukopenias) and proliferations, which may be reactive or neoplastic. Reactive proliferation in response to an underlying primary, often microbial, disease is fairly common. Neoplastic disorders, though less common, are more ominous; they cause approximately 9% of all cancer deaths in adults and a staggering 40% in children younger than 15 years. In the following discussion we first describe some non-neoplastic conditions and then consider in some detail the malignant proliferations of white cells.

NON-NEOPLASTIC DISORDERS OF WHITE CELLS

Leukopenia

Leukopenia results most commonly from a decrease in granulocytes, which are the most prevalent circulating white cells. Lymphopenias are much less common; they are associated with congenital immunodeficiency diseases or are acquired in association with specific clinical states, such as advanced human immunodeficiency virus (HIV) infection or treatment with corticosteroids. Only the more common leukopenias that affect granulocytes are discussed here.

Neutropenia/Agranulocytosis

A reduction in the number of granulocytes in blood is known as *neutropenia* or sometimes, when severe, as *agranulocytosis*. Characteristically, the total white cell count is reduced to 1000 cells/μL and in some instances to as few as 200 to 300 cells/μL. Affected persons are extremely susceptible to bacterial and fungal infections, which can be severe enough to cause death.

Etiology and Pathogenesis. The mechanisms that cause neutropenia can be broadly divided into two categories:

- *Inadequate or ineffective granulopoiesis.* Reduced granulopoiesis is a manifestation of generalized marrow failure, which occurs in aplastic anemia and a variety of leukemias. Cancer chemotherapy agents also produce neutropenia by inducing transient marrow aplasia. Alternatively, some neutropenias are isolated, with only the differentiation of committed granulocytic precursors being affected. These forms of neutropenia are most often caused by certain drugs or, more uncommonly, by neoplastic proliferations of cytotoxic T cells and natural killer (NK) cells.
- *Accelerated removal or destruction of neutrophils.* This can be encountered with immune-mediated injury to neutrophils (triggered in some cases by drugs), or it may be idiopathic. Increased peripheral utilization can occur in overwhelming bacterial, fungal, or rickettsial infections. An enlarged spleen can also lead to sequestration and accelerated removal of neutrophils.

Morphology

The anatomic alterations in the bone marrow depend on the underlying basis of the neutropenia. **Marrow hypercellularity** is seen when the neutropenia results from excessive destruction of the mature neutrophils or from ineffective granulopoiesis, such as occurs in megaloblastic anemia. In contrast, agents such as drugs that suppress granulocytopoiesis are associated with **a marked decrease in maturing granulocytic precursors in the marrow.** Erythropoiesis and megakaryopoiesis can be normal if the responsible agent specifically affects the granulocytes, but with most myelotoxic drugs all marrow elements are affected.

Clinical Course. The initial symptoms are often malaise, chills, and fever, with subsequent marked weakness and fatigability. Infections constitute the major problem. They commonly take the form of ulcerating, necrotizing lesions of the gingiva, floor of the mouth, buccal mucosa, pharynx, or other sites within the oral cavity (agranulocytic angina). These lesions often show a massive growth of microorganisms, due to the inability to mount a leukocyte response. In addition to removal of the offending drug and control of infections, treatment efforts may also include the administration of granulocyte colony-stimulating factor, which stimulates neutrophil production by the bone marrow.

Reactive Leukocytosis

An increase in the number of white cells is common in a variety of reactive inflammatory states caused by microbial and nonmicrobial stimuli. Leukocytoses are relatively nonspecific and can be classified on the basis of the particular white cell series affected (Table 12–6). As will be discussed later, in some cases reactive leukocytosis may mimic leukemia. Such *leukemoid reactions* must be distinguished from true malignancies of the white cells. Infectious mononucleosis, a form of lymphocytosis caused by Epstein-Barr virus (EBV) infection, merits separate consideration because it gives rise to a distinctive syndrome.

Table 12–6 Causes of Leukocytosis

Neutrophilic Leukocytosis
Acute bacterial infections, especially those caused by pyogenic organisms; sterile inflammation caused by, for example, tissue necrosis (myocardial infarction, burns)
Eosinophilic Leukocytosis (Eosinophilia)
Allergic disorders such as asthma, hay fever, allergic skin diseases (e.g., pemphigus, dermatitis herpetiformis); parasitic infestations; drug reactions; certain malignancies (e.g., Hodgkin disease and some non-Hodgkin lymphomas); collagen vascular disorders and some vasculitides; atheroembolic disease (transient)
Basophilic Leukocytosis (Basophilia)
Rare, often indicative of a myeloproliferative disease (e.g., chronic myelogenous leukemia)
Monocytosis
Chronic infections (e.g., tuberculosis), bacterial endocarditis, rickettsiosis, and malaria; collagen vascular diseases (e.g., systemic lupus erythematosus); and inflammatory bowel diseases (e.g., ulcerative colitis)
Lymphocytosis
Accompanies monocytosis in many disorders associated with chronic immunologic stimulation (e.g., tuberculosis, brucellosis); viral infections (e.g., hepatitis A, cytomegalovirus, Epstein-Barr virus); *Bordetella pertussis* infection

Infectious Mononucleosis

In the Western world, infectious mononucleosis is an acute, self-limited disease of adolescents and young adults that is caused by B lymphocytotropic EBV, a member of the herpesvirus family. The infection is characterized by (1) fever, sore throat, and generalized lymphadenitis; (2) an increase of lymphocytes in blood, many of which have an atypical morphology; and (3) an antibody and T cell response to EBV. It should be noted that cytomegalovirus infection induces a similar syndrome, which can be differentiated only by serologic methods.

Epidemiology and Immunology. EBV is ubiquitous in all human populations. Where economic deprivation results in inadequate living standards, EBV infection early in life is nearly universal. At this age, symptomatic disease is uncommon, and, even though infected hosts develop an immune response (described later), more than half continue to shed virus. In contrast, in developed countries that enjoy better standards of hygiene, infection is usually delayed until adolescence or young adulthood. For reasons that are not clear, only about 20% of healthy seropositive persons in developed countries shed the virus, and only about 50% of those who are exposed to the virus acquire the infection. Transmission to a seronegative "kissing cousin" usually involves direct oral contact. It is hypothesized (but not proven) that the virus initially infects oropharyngeal epithelial cells and then spreads to underlying lymphoid tissue (tonsils and adenoids), where B lymphocytes, which have receptors for EBV, are infected. The infection of B cells takes one of two forms. In a minority of cells, the infection leads to viral replication and eventual cell lysis accompanied by the release of virions. In most cells, however, the infection is nonproductive, and the virus persists in latent form as an extrachromosomal episome. *B cells that are latently infected with EBV undergo polyclonal activation and proliferation,* as a result of the action of several EBV proteins (Chapter 6). These cells disseminate in the circulation and secrete antibodies with several specificities, including the well-known heterophil anti-sheep red cell antibodies that are recognized in diagnostic tests for mononucleosis. During this early acute infection, EBV is shed in the saliva; it is not known if the source of these virions is oropharyngeal epithelial cells or B cells.

A normal immune response is extremely important in controlling the proliferation of EBV-infected B cells and spread of virus. Early in the course of the infection, IgM, and, later, IgG, antibodies are formed against viral capsid antigens. The latter persist for life. More important in the control of polyclonal B-cell proliferation are cytotoxic CD8+ T cells and NK cells. *Virus-specific cytotoxic T cells appear as atypical lymphocytes in the circulation, a finding that is characteristic of acute mononucleosis.* In otherwise healthy persons, the fully developed humoral and cellular responses to EBV act as brakes on viral shedding, limiting the number of infected B cells rather than eliminating them. Latent EBV remains in a few B cells and possibly oropharyngeal epithelial cells as well. As will be seen, impaired immunity in the host can have disastrous consequences.

Morphology

The major alterations involve the blood, lymph nodes, spleen, liver, central nervous system, and, occasionally, other organs. There is peripheral blood **leukocytosis,** with a white cell count that is usually between 12,000 and 18,000 cells/μL. Typically more than half of these cells are large, **atypical lymphocytes,** 12 to 16 μm in diameter, with an abundant cytoplasm that often contains azurophilic granules and an oval, indented, or folded nucleus (Fig. 12–12). These atypical lymphocytes, which are sufficiently distinctive to suggest the diagnosis, are mainly cytotoxic CD8+ T cells.

The **lymph nodes** are enlarged throughout the body, including the posterior cervical, axillary, and groin regions. Histologically, the enlarged nodes are flooded by atypical lymphocytes, which occupy the paracortical (T-cell) areas. Occasionally, cells resembling Reed-Sternberg cells, the hallmark of Hodgkin lymphoma, are present. Because of these atypical features, special tests are sometimes needed to distinguish the reactive changes of mononucleosis from malignant lymphoma.

The **spleen** is enlarged in most cases, weighing between 300 and 500 gm. The histologic changes are analogous to those of the lymph nodes, showing a heavy infiltration of atypical lymphocytes. As a result of the increase in splenic size and the infiltration of the trabeculae and capsule by the lymphocytes, such spleens are fragile and prone to rupture after even minor trauma.

Liver function is almost always transiently impaired to some degree. Histologically, atypical lymphocytes are seen in the portal areas and sinusoids, and scattered, isolated cells or foci of parenchymal necrosis filled with lymphocytes may be present. This histologic picture can be difficult to distinguish from other forms of viral hepatitis.

Clinical Course. Although mononucleosis classically presents as fever, sore throat, lymphadenitis, and the other features mentioned earlier, atypical presentations are not unusual. It can appear with little or no fever and only malaise, fatigue, and lymphadenopathy, raising the specter of lymphoma; as a fever of unknown origin, unassociated with significant lymphadenopathy or other localized findings; as hepatitis that is difficult to differentiate from one of the hepatotropic viral syndromes (Chapter 16); or as a febrile rash resembling rubella. Ultimately, the diagnosis depends on the following findings, in increasing order of specificity: (1) lymphocytosis with the characteristic atypical lymphocytes in the peripheral blood, (2) a positive heterophil reaction (monospot test), and (3) a rising titer of antibodies specific for EBV antigens (viral capsid antigens, early antigens, or Epstein-Barr nuclear antigen). In most patients, mononucleosis resolves within 4 to 6 weeks, but sometimes the fatigue lasts longer. Occasionally, one or more complications supervene. Perhaps the most common of these is hepatic dysfunction, associated with jaundice, elevated hepatic enzyme levels, disturbed appetite, and, rarely, even liver failure. Other complications involve the nervous system, kidneys, bone marrow, lungs, eyes, heart, and spleen (including fatal splenic rupture).

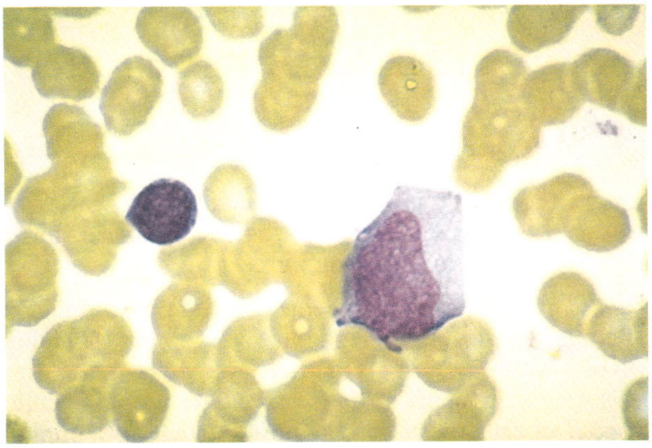

Figure 12–12

Atypical lymphocytes in infectious mononucleosis. The cell on the left is a normal small lymphocyte with a compact nucleus filling the entire cytoplasm. In contrast, an atypical lymphocyte on the right has abundant cytoplasm and a large nucleus with fine chromatin.

EBV is a potent transforming virus that plays a role in a number of human malignancies, including several types of B-cell lymphoma (Chapter 6). A serious complication in those lacking T-cell immunity (particularly organ and bone marrow transplant recipients) is that the EBV-driven B-cell proliferation can run amok, leading to death. This process can be initiated by an acute infection or the reactivation of a latent B-cell infection and generally begins as a polyclonal proliferation that progresses to overt monoclonal B-cell lymphoma over time. Reconstitution of immunity (e.g., by cessation of immunosuppressive therapy) is sometimes sufficient to cause complete regression of the B-cell proliferation, which is uniformly fatal if left untreated.

The importance of T cells and NK cells in the control of EBV infection is driven home by X-linked lymphoproliferative syndrome, a rare inherited immunodeficiency characterized by inability to mount an immune response against EBV. Most affected boys have a mutation in the *SH2D1A* gene, which encodes a signaling protein that is important in the activation of T cells and NK cells. On exposure to EBV, more than 50% of these boys develop an overwhelming infection that is usually fatal. Of the remainder, some develop lymphoma or hypogammaglobulinemia, the basis of which is not understood.

Reactive Lymphadenitis

Infections and nonmicrobial inflammatory stimuli not only cause leukocytosis but also involve the lymph nodes, which act as defensive barriers. Any immune response against foreign antigens is often associated with lymph node enlargement (lymphadenopathy). The infections that cause lymphadenitis are numerous and varied and may be acute or chronic. In most instances, the histologic appearance of the nodes is entirely nonspecific. A somewhat distinctive form of lymphadenitis that occurs with cat scratch disease will be described separately.

Acute Nonspecific Lymphadenitis

This form of lymphadenitis may be confined to a local group of nodes draining a focal infection, or be generalized in systemic bacterial or viral infections.

Morphology

Macroscopically, inflamed nodes in acute nonspecific lymphadenitis are swollen, gray-red, and engorged. Histologically, there are **large germinal centers** containing numerous mitotic figures. When the cause is a pyogenic organism, a neutrophilic infiltrate is seen about the follicles and within the lymphoid sinuses. With severe infections, the centers of follicles can undergo necrosis, resulting in the formation of an abscess.

Affected nodes are tender and, when abscess formation is extensive, become fluctuant. The overlying skin is frequently red, and penetration of the infection to the skin can produce draining sinuses. With control of the infection, the lymph nodes can revert to their normal appearance or, if damaged by the immune response, undergo scarring.

Chronic Nonspecific Lymphadenitis

This condition can assume one of three patterns, depending on the causative agent: follicular hyperplasia, paracortical hyperplasia, or sinus histiocytosis.

Morphology

Follicular Hyperplasia. This pattern is associated with infections or inflammatory processes that activate B cells, which enter into B-cell follicles and create the **follicular (or germinal center) reaction.** The cells in the reactive follicles include the activated B cells, scattered phagocytic macrophages containing nuclear debris (tingible body macrophages), and an inconspicuous meshwork of follicular dendritic cells that function in antigen display to the B cells. Causes of follicular hyperplasia include **rheumatoid arthritis, toxoplasmosis,** and **the early stages of HIV infection.** This form of lymphadenitis can be confused morphologically with follicular lymphomas (discussed later). Findings that favor a diagnosis of follicular hyperplasia are (1) the preservation of the lymph node architecture, with normal lymphoid tissue between germinal centers; (2) variation in the shape and size of the lymphoid nodules; (3) a mixed population of lymphocytes at various stages of differentiation; and (4) prominent phagocytic and mitotic activity in germinal centers.

Paracortical Hyperplasia. This pattern is characterized by reactive changes within the **T-cell regions** of the lymph node. On immune activation parafollicular T cells transform into large proliferating immunoblasts that can efface the B-cell follicles. Paracortical hyperplasia is encountered in **viral infections** (such as EBV), following certain **vaccinations** (e.g., smallpox), and in immune reactions induced by certain **drugs** (especially phenytoin).

Sinus Histiocytosis. This reactive pattern is characterized by distention and prominence of the lymphatic sinusoids, owing to a marked **hypertrophy of lining endothelial cells** and an infiltrate of **macrophages** (histiocytes). Sinus histiocytosis is often encountered in lymph nodes draining cancers and may represent an immune response to the tumor or its products.

Cat Scratch Disease

Cat scratch disease is a self-limited lymphadenitis caused by the bacterium *Bartonella henselae*. It is primarily a disease of childhood; 90% of the patients are younger than 18 years of age. It presents as regional lymphadenopathy, most frequently in the axilla and neck. The nodal enlargement appears approximately 2 weeks after a feline scratch or, uncommonly, after a splinter or thorn injury. A raised, inflammatory nodule, vesicle, or eschar is sometimes visible at the site of skin injury. In most patients the lymph node enlargement regresses over the next 2 to 4 months. Rarely, patients develop encephalitis, osteomyelitis, or thrombocytopenia.

Morphology

The anatomic changes in the lymph node in cat scratch disease are quite characteristic. Initially, **sarcoid-like granulomas** are formed, but these then undergo central necrosis associated with the accumulation of neutrophils. These **irregular stellate necrotizing granulomas** are similar in appearance to those seen in certain other infections, such as lymphogranuloma venereum. The microbe is extracellular and can be visualized only with silver stains or electron microscopy. The diagnosis is based on a history of exposure to cats, the clinical findings, a positive skin test to the microbial antigen, and the distinctive morphologic changes in the lymph nodes.

NEOPLASTIC PROLIFERATIONS OF WHITE CELLS

Tumors represent the most important of the white cell disorders. They can be divided into three broad categories based on the origin of the tumor cells:

- *Lymphoid neoplasms,* which include non-Hodgkin lymphomas (NHLs), Hodgkin lymphomas, lymphocytic leukemias, and plasma cell dyscrasias and related disorders. In many instances these tumors are composed of cells that resemble normal stages of lymphocyte differentiation, a feature that serves as one of the bases for their classification.
- *Myeloid neoplasms* arise from stem cells that normally give rise to the formed elements of the blood: granulocytes, red cells, and platelets. The myeloid neoplasms fall into three fairly distinct subcategories: *acute myelogenous leukemias,* in which immature progeni-

tor cells accumulate in the bone marrow; *chronic myeloproliferative disorders,* in which inappropriately increased production of formed blood elements leads to elevated blood cell counts; and *myelodysplastic syndromes,* which are characteristically associated with ineffective hematopoiesis and cytopenias.

- *Histiocytic neoplasms* represent proliferative lesions of histiocytes. Of special interest is a spectrum of proliferations comprising Langerhans cells (the *Langerhans cell histiocytoses*).

Lymphoid Neoplasms

The lymphoid neoplasms encompass a group of entities that vary widely in their clinical presentation and behavior, thus presenting challenges to students and clinicians alike. Some of these neoplasms characteristically appear as *leukemias,* tumors that primarily involve the bone marrow with spillage of neoplastic cells into the peripheral blood. Others tend to present as *lymphomas,* tumors that produce masses in involved lymph nodes or other tissues. Plasma cell tumors, the *plasma cell dyscrasias,* usually present within the bones as discrete masses and cause systemic symptoms related to the production of a complete or partial monoclonal immunoglobulin. Despite these tendencies, all lymphoid neoplasms have the potential to spread to lymph nodes and various tissues throughout the body, especially the liver, spleen, and bone marrow. In some cases lymphomas or plasma cell tumors spill over into the peripheral blood, creating a leukemia-like picture. Conversely, leukemias of lymphoid cells, originating in the bone marrow, can infiltrate lymph nodes and other tissues, creating the histologic picture of lymphoma. *Because of the overlap in clinical presentations, the various lymphoid neoplasms can only be distinguished based on the appearance and molecular characteristics of the tumor cells.* Stated another way, for purposes of diagnosis and prognostication, it is most helpful to focus on what the tumor cell is, not where it resides in the patient.

Two groups of lymphomas are recognized: Hodgkin lymphoma and non-Hodgkin lymphomas. Although both arise most commonly in lymphoid tissues, Hodgkin lymphoma is set apart by the presence of distinctive neoplastic Reed-Sternberg giant cells (see below), which in involved nodes are usually greatly outnumbered by non-neoplastic inflammatory cells. The biologic behavior and clinical treatment of Hodgkin lymphoma are also different from those of most NHLs, making the distinction of practical importance.

Historically, few areas of pathology have evoked as much controversy and confusion as the classification of lymphoid neoplasms, which is perhaps inevitable given the intrinsic complexity of the immune system from which they arise. Great progress has been made over the last decade in this area, however, and an international working group of pathologists, molecular biologists, and clinicians working on behalf of the World Health Organization (WHO) has formulated a widely accepted classification scheme that relies on a combination of morphologic, phenotypic, genotypic, and clinical features. Before we delve into the classification of lymphoid neoplasms, certain important relevant principles should be emphasized:

- B- and T-cell tumors are often composed of cells that are arrested or derived from specific stages of their normal differentiation pathways (Fig. 12–13). The diagnosis and classification of these tumors relies heavily on tests (either immunohistochemistry or flow cytometry) that detect lineage-specific antigens (e.g., B-cell, T-cell, and NK-cell markers) and markers of maturity. As will become evident, many such markers are identified according to their cluster of differentiation (CD) number.
- The most common lymphomas of adults are derived from follicular center or post-follicular center B cells. This conclusion is drawn from molecular analyses, which have shown that most B-cell lymphomas have undergone somatic hypermutation, an activity that is confined to follicular center B cells. Follicular center B cells also undergo immunoglobulin class switching, and together with somatic hypermutation, these forms of regulated genomic instability seem to place B cells at a relatively high risk for mutations that can lead to transformation. In fact, many recurrent chromosomal translocations that are commonly seen in mature B-cell malignancies involve the immunoglobulin (Ig) loci and seem to stem from mistakes that are made during attempted recombination events involving Ig genes. In this regard, it is interesting that mature T cells (which are genomically stable) give rise to lymphomas much less frequently and very rarely have chromosomal translocations involving the T-cell receptor loci.
- All lymphoid neoplasms are derived from a single transformed cell and are therefore monoclonal. As will be recalled from Chapter 5, during the differentiation of precursor B and T cells there is a somatic rearrangement of their antigen receptor genes. This process ensures that each lymphocyte makes a single, unique antigen receptor. Because antigen receptor gene rearrangement precedes transformation, the daughter cells derived from a given malignant progenitor share the same antigen receptor gene configuration and synthesize identical antigen receptor proteins (either immunoglobulins or T-cell receptors). For this reason, *analysis of antigen receptor genes and their protein products is frequently used to differentiate monoclonal neoplasms from polyclonal, reactive processes.*
- As tumors of the immune system, lymphoid neoplasms often disrupt normal immune regulatory mechanisms. Both immunodeficiency (as evidenced by susceptibility to infection) and autoimmunity can be seen, sometimes in the same patient. Ironically, patients with inherited or acquired immunodeficiency are themselves at high risk of developing certain lymphoid neoplasms, particularly those associated with EBV infection.
- Although NHLs often present at a particular tissue site, sensitive molecular assays usually show that the tumor is widely disseminated at the time of diagnosis. As a result, with few exceptions, only systemic therapies are curative. In contrast, Hodgkin lymphoma often presents at a single site and spreads in a pre-

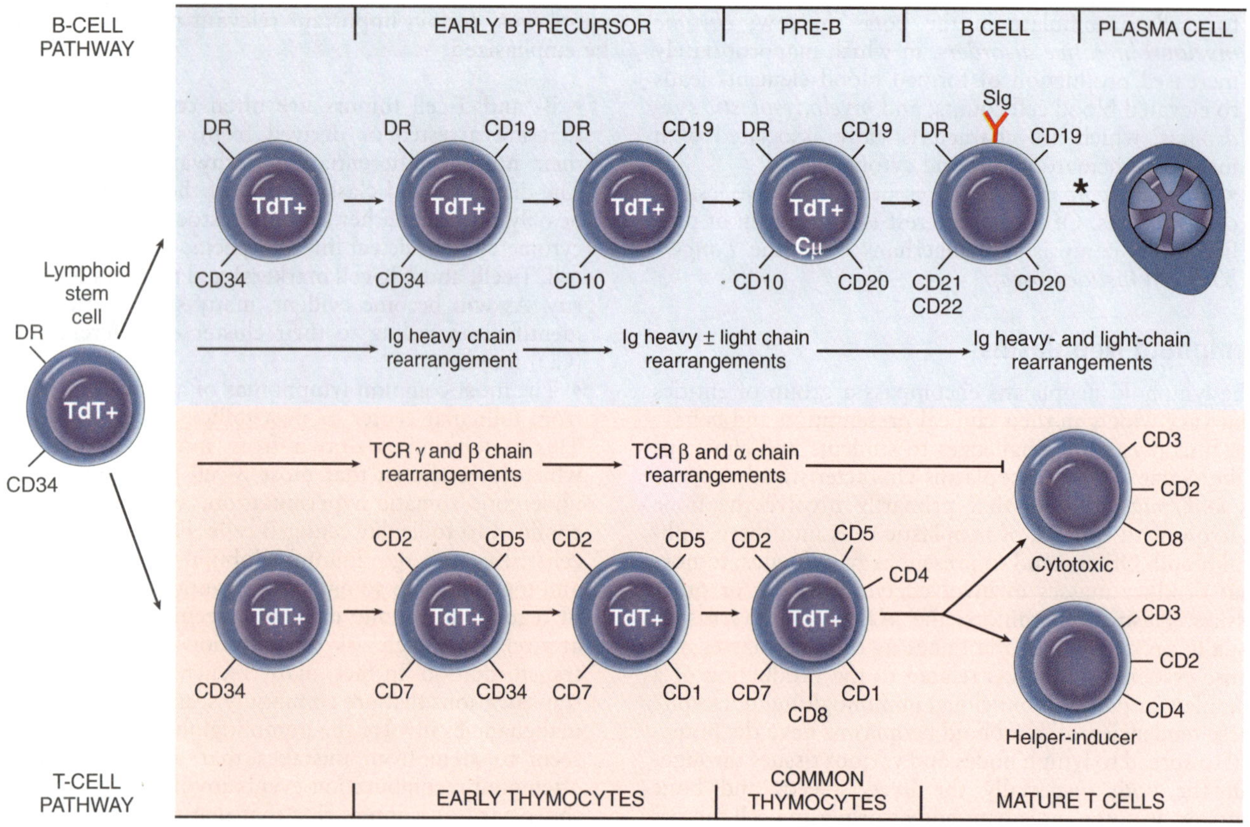

Figure 12–13

Origin of lymphoid neoplasms. Stages of B- and T-cell differentiation from which specific lymphoid and tumors emerge are shown. CD, cluster of differentiation; DR, human lymphocyte antigen–class II antigens; Ig, immunoglobulin; TCR, T-cell receptor; TdT, terminal deoxyribonucleotidyl transferase.

dictable fashion to contiguous lymph node groups. For this reason, early in its course, local therapy may be indicated.

The WHO classification of lymphoid neoplasms considers the morphology, cell of origin (determined in practice by immunophenotyping), clinical features, and genotype (e.g., karyotype, presence of viral genomes) of each entity. It includes all lymphoid neoplasms, including leukemias and multiple myeloma, and segregates them on the basis of origin into three major categories: (1) tumors of B cells, (2) tumors of T cells and NK cells, and (3) Hodgkin lymphoma.

An updated version of the WHO classification of lymphoid neoplasms is presented in Table 12–7. As can be seen, the diagnostic entities are numerous. Our focus will be on the subset of neoplasms listed below, which together constitute more than 90% of the lymphoid neoplasms seen in the United States:

- Precursor B- and T-cell lymphoblastic leukemia/lymphoma (commonly called acute lymphoblastic leukemia, or ALL)
- Small lymphocytic lymphoma/chronic lymphocytic leukemia
- Follicular lymphoma
- Mantle cell lymphoma
- Diffuse large B-cell lymphomas
- Burkitt lymphoma
- Multiple myeloma and related plasma cell dyscrasias
- Hodgkin lymphoma

The salient features of the more common lymphoid neoplasms are summarized in Table 12–8. We will also touch on a few of the uncommon entities that have distinctive clinicopathologic features.

Precursor B- and T-Cell Lymphoblastic Leukemia/Lymphoma

These are aggressive tumors, composed of immature lymphocytes (lymphoblasts), which occur predominantly in children and young adults. The various lymphoblastic tumors are morphologically indistinguishable and often cause similar signs and symptoms. Because precursor B- and T-cell neoplasms have overlapping features, we will consider them together.

Just as B-cell precursors normally develop within the bone marrow, pre–B-lymphoblastic tumors characteristically appear in bone marrow and peripheral blood as leukemias. Similarly, pre–T-lymphoblastic tumors commonly present as masses involving the thymus, which is the

Table 12–7 The WHO Classification of Lymphoid Neoplasms*

Precursor B-Cell Neoplasms
Precursor B-cell leukemia/lymphoma (B-cell ALL)
Peripheral B-Cell Neoplasms
B-cell chronic lymphocytic leukemia/small lymphocytic lymphoma (CLL)
B-cell prolymphocytic leukemia
Lymphoplasmacytic lymphoma
Mantle cell lymphoma
Follicular lymphoma
Extranodal marginal zone lymphoma (MALT lymphoma)
Splenic marginal zone lymphoma
Nodal marginal zone lymphoma
Hairy cell leukemia
Plasmacytoma/plasma cell myeloma
Diffuse large B-cell lymphoma
Burkitt lymphoma
Precursor T-Cell Neoplasms
Precursor T-cell leukemia/lymphoma (T-cell ALL)
Peripheral T-/NK-Cell Neoplasms
T-cell prolymphocytic leukemia
T-cell granular lymphocytic leukemia
Mycosis fungoides/Sézary syndrome
Peripheral T-cell lymphoma, not otherwise specified (NOS)
Angioimmunoblastic T-cell lymphoma
Anaplastic large-cell lymphoma, primary systemic type
Enteropathy-type T-cell lymphoma
Panniculitis-like T-cell lymphoma
Hepatosplenic $\gamma\delta$ T-cell lymphoma
Adult T-cell lymphoma/leukemia (HTLV1)
NK/T-cell lymphoma, nasal type
NK-cell leukemia
Hodgkin Lymphoma
Lymphocyte predominance, nodular
Nodular sclerosis
Mixed cellularity
Lymphocyte-rich
Lymphocyte depletion

*Entries in italics are among the most common lymphoid tumors.

site of early stages of normal T-cell differentiation. However, pre–T-cell "lymphomas" often progress rapidly to a leukemic phase, and other pre–T-cell tumors seem to involve only the marrow at presentation. Hence, *both pre–B- and pre–T-lymphoblastic tumors usually take on the clinical appearance of an acute lymphoblastic leukemia (ALL) at some time during their course.* As a group, ALLs constitute 80% of childhood leukemia, peaking in incidence at age 4, with most of the cases being of pre–B-cell origin. The pre–T-cell tumors are most common in adolescent males of between 15 and 20 years of age.

The pathophysiology, laboratory findings, and clinical features of ALL closely resemble those of acute myelogenous leukemia (AML), the other major type of acute leukemia. Because of these similarities, we will first step back to review the features common to the acute leukemias before discussing those that are specific to ALL.

Pathophysiology of Acute Leukemias. Although acute leukemias are rapidly growing tumors, normal bone marrow progenitors grow at an even more rapid rate. *The principal pathogenetic problem in acute leukemia is a block in differentiation.* This leads to the accumulation of immature leukemic blasts in the bone marrow, which suppress the function of normal hematopoietic stem cells by physical displacement and other poorly understood mechanisms. Eventually bone marrow failure results, which accounts for the major clinical manifestations of acute leukemia. Thus, the therapeutic goal is to reduce the leukemic clone sufficiently to allow normal hematopoiesis to resume.

Clinical Features of Acute Leukemias. The acute leukemias have the following characteristics:

- *Abrupt stormy onset.* Most patients present within 3 months of the onset of symptoms.
- *Symptoms related to depression of normal marrow function.* These include fatigue (due mainly to anemia), fever (reflecting infections resulting from the absence of mature leukocytes), and bleeding (petechiae, ecchymoses, epistaxis, gum bleeding) secondary to thrombocytopenia.
- *Bone pain and tenderness.* These result from marrow expansion and infiltration of the subperiosteum.
- *Generalized lymphadenopathy, splenomegaly, and hepatomegaly.* These reflect dissemination of the leukemic cells, and are more pronounced in ALL than in AML.
- *Central nervous system manifestations.* These include headache, vomiting, and nerve palsies resulting from meningeal spread; these features are more common in children than in adults and are more common in ALL than AML.

Laboratory Findings of Acute Leukemias. The diagnosis of acute leukemia rests on the identification of blast forms in the peripheral blood and the bone marrow. The white cell count is variable; it is somtimes elevated to more than 100,000 cells/μL, but in about 50% of patients it is less than 10,000 cells/μL. Anemia is almost always present, and the platelet count is usually below 100,000 platelets/μL. Neutropenia is also a common finding in the peripheral blood. Uncommonly the peripheral blood examination shows pancytopenia but no blasts (aleukemic leukemia); here, the diagnosis can only be established by examining the bone marrow.

Morphology

Because of different responses to therapy, it is of great practical importance to distinguish ALL from AML. By definition, in ALL, blasts compose more than 25% of the marrow cellularity. The nuclei of lymphoblasts in Wright-Giemsa–stained preparations have somewhat coarse and clumped chromatin and one or two nucleoli (Fig. 12–14A); myeloblasts tend to have finer chromatin and more cytoplasm, which may contain granules (Fig. 12–14B). The cytoplasm of lymphoblasts often contains large aggregates of periodic acid–Schiff–positive material, whereas myeloblasts are often peroxidase positive.

Table 12–8 Summary of the More Common Lymphoid Neoplasms

Entity	Frequency	Salient Morphology
Precursor B-cell lymphoblastic leukemia/lymphoma	85% of childhood acute leukemia	Lymphoblasts with irregular nuclear contours, condensed chromatin, small nucleoli, and scant agranular cytoplasm
Precursor T-cell leukemia/lymphoma	15% of childhood acute leukemia; 40% of childhood lymphomas	Identical to precursor B-cell lymphoblastic leukemia/lymphoma
Small lymphocytic lymphoma/chronic lymphocytic leukemia	3% to 4% of adult lymphomas; 30% of all leukemias	Small resting lymphocytes mixed with variable numbers of large activated cells; lymph nodes diffusely effaced
Follicular lymphoma	40% of adult lymphomas	Frequent small "cleaved" cells mixed with large cells; growth pattern is usually nodular (follicular)
Mantle cell lymphoma	3% to 4% of adult lymphomas	Small to intermediate-sized irregular lymphocytes growing in a diffuse pattern
Extranodal marginal zone lymphoma	~5% of adult lymphomas	Variable cell size and differentiation; 40% show plasmacytic differentiation; B cells home to epithelium, creating "lymphoepithelial lesions"
Diffuse large B-cell lymphoma	40% to 50% of adult lymphomas	Variable; most resemble large germinal center B cells; diffuse growth pattern
Burkitt lymphoma	<1% of lymphomas in the United States	Intermediate-sized round lymphoid cells with several nucleoli; diffuse tissue involvement associated with apoptosis produces a "starry-sky" appearance
Plasmacytoma/plasma cell myeloma	Most common lymphoid neoplasm in older adults	Plasma cells in sheets, sometimes with prominent nucleoli or inclusions containing Ig
Mycosis fungoides	Most common cutaneous lymphoid malignancy	In most cases, small lymphoid cells with markedly convoluted nuclei; cells often infiltrate the epidermis (Pautrier microabscesses)
Peripheral T-cell lymphoma, not otherwise specified (NOS)	Most common adult T-cell lymphoma	Variable; usually a spectrum of small to large lymphoid cells with irregular nuclear contours
Hodgkin lymphoma, nodular sclerosis type	Most common type of Hodgkin lymphoma	Lacunar Reed-Sternberg cell variants in a mixed inflammatory background; broad sclerotic bands of collagen usually also present
Hodgkin lymphoma, mixed cellularity type	Second most common form of Hodgkin lymphoma	Frequent classic Reed-Sternberg cells in a mixed inflammatory background

GI, gastrointestinal; Ig, immunoglobulin.

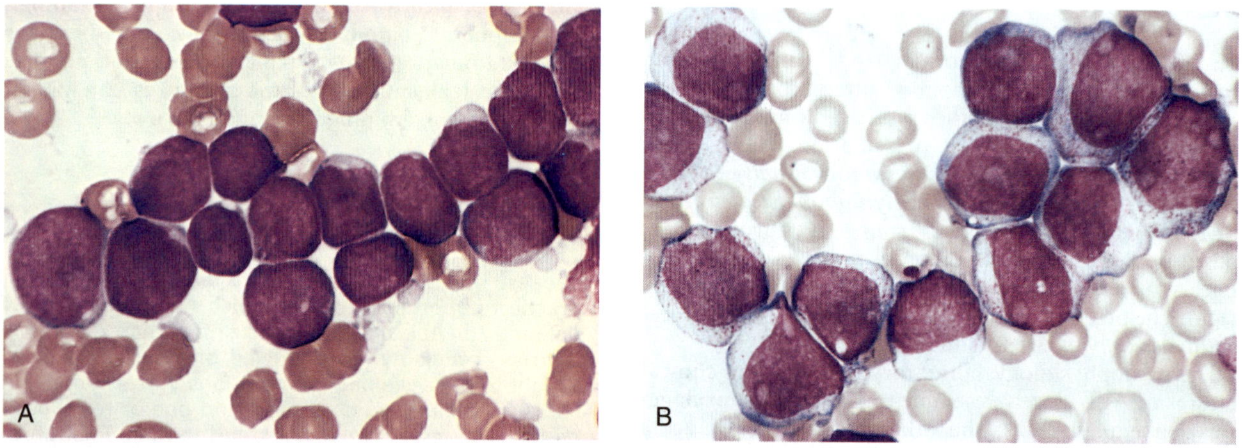

Figure 12–14

Morphologic comparison of lymphoblasts and myeloblasts. **A,** Lymphoblastic leukemia/lymphoma. Lymphoblasts have fewer nucleoli than do myeloblasts, and the nuclear chromatin is more condensed. Cytoplasmic granules are absent. **B,** Acute myeloblastic leukemia (M1 subtype). Myeloblasts have delicate nuclear chromatin, prominent nucleoli, and fine azurophilic granules in the cytoplasm. (Courtesy of Dr. Robert W. McKenna, Department of Pathology, University of Texas Southwestern Medical School, Dallas, Texas.)

Immunophenotype	Comments
TdT+ immature B cells (CD19+, variable expression of other B-cell markers)	Usually presents as acute leukemia; less common in adults; prognosis is predicted by karyotype
TdT+ immature T cells (CD2+, CD7+, variable expression of other T-cell markers)	Most common in adolescent males; often presents as a mediastinal mass due to thymic involvement; highly associated with mutations in *NOTCH1*
CD5+ B-cell expressing surface Ig	Occurs in older adults; usually involves nodes, marrow, and spleen; most patients have peripheral blood involvement; indolent
CD10+ BCL2+ mature B cells that express surface Ig	Occurs in older adults; usually involves nodes, marrow, and spleen; associated with t(14;18); indolent
CD5+ mature B cells that express cyclin D1 and have surface Ig	Occurs mainly in older males; usually involves nodes, marrow, and spleen; GI tract also commonly affected; t(11;14) is characteristic; moderately aggressive
CD5- CD10- mature B cells with surface Ig	Frequently occurs at extranodal sites involved by chronic inflammation; very indolent; may be cured by local excision
Mature B cells with variable expression of CD10 and surface Ig	Occurs in all ages, but most common in older adults; often arise at extranodal sites; aggressive
Mature CD10+ B cells expressing surface Ig	Endemic in Africa, sporadic elsewhere; increased frequency in immunosuppressed patients; predominantly affects children; often presents with visceral involvement; highly aggressive
Terminally differentiated plasma cells containing cytoplasmic Ig	Myeloma presents as disseminated bone disease, often with destructive lytic lesions Hypercalcemia, renal insufficiency, and bacterial infections are common
CD4+ mature T cells	Presents with localized or more generalized skin involvement; generally indolent. Sézary syndrome, a more aggressive variant, is characterized by diffuse skin erythema and peripheral blood involvement
Mature T-cell phenotype (CD3+)	Probably spans a diverse collection of rare tumors. Often disseminated, generally aggressive
CD15+, CD30+ Reed-Sternberg cells	Most common in young adults, often arises in the mediastinum or cervical lymph nodes
CD15+, CD30+ Reed-Sternberg cells	Most common in men, more likely to present at advanced stages than the nodular sclerosis type EBV+ in 70% of cases

Having completed our "short course" in acute leukemia, we will return to lymphoblastic leukemia/lymphoma; the AMLs are discussed later.

Immunophenotyping. Immunophenotyping is very useful in subtyping lymphoblastic tumors and distinguishing them from AML. Terminal deoxytransferase, an enzyme that is specifically expressed in pre-B and pre-T cells, is present in more than 95% of cases. Further subtyping of ALL into pre-B- and pre-T-cell types relies on stains for lineage-specific markers, such as CD19 (B cell) and CD3 (T cell). Although immunophenotyping has historically proven somewhat useful in predicting clinical outcome, the tumor karyotype provides more robust and specific prognostic information.

Karyotypic Changes. Approximately 90% of patients with lymphoblastic leukemia/lymphoma have nonrandom karyotypic abnormalities. Most common in pre–B-cell tumors is hyperdiploidy (>50 chromosomes/cell), which is associated with the presence of a cryptic (12;21) chromosomal translocation involving the *TEL1* and *AML1* genes. The presence of these aberrations correlates with a good outcome. Poor outcomes are observed with pre–B-cell tumors that have translocations involving the *MLL* gene on chromosome 11q23 or the Philadelphia (Ph) chromosome. Pre–T-cell tumors are associated with a group of chromosomal rearrangements that are completely different than those found in pre–B-cell tumors, but none is predictive of outcome.

Activating Mutations in *NOTCH1*. NOTCH1 is a transmembrane receptor whose activity is essential for normal T-cell development. NOTCH1 signals promote the proliferation and survival of pre-T cells and are capable of causing stem cells to differentiate into pre-T cells outside of the thymus. Interestingly, 55% to 60% of pre–T-cell tumors have activating point mutations in *NOTCH1*, indicating that the NOTCH1 signaling pathway plays a central role in the development of many pre-T ALLs. The ability of NOTCH1 to promote T-cell development outside the thymus may explain why some patients with pre–T-cell tumors have bone marrow disease and no thymic involvement.

Prognosis. Treatment of lymphoblastic tumors of childhood represents one of the great success stories in oncology. Children 2 to 10 years of age have the best prognosis; most can be cured. Other groups of patients do less well. Variables correlated with worse outcomes include male gender, age younger than 2 or older than 10 years, and a high leukocyte count at diagnosis. Age-dependent differences in the frequencies of various karyotypic abnormalities are likely to explain the relationship of age to outcome. Tumors with rearrangements of *MLL* or the Ph chromosome (both associated with a poor outcome) are most common in children younger than age 2 and adults, respectively, whereas tumors with "good prognosis" chromosomal aberrations (such as the t[12;21] and hyperdiploidy) are common in the 2- to 10-year age group.

Small Lymphocytic Lymphoma/Chronic Lymphocytic Leukemia

These two disorders are morphologically, phenotypically, and genotypically identical, differing only in the extent of peripheral blood involvement. Arbitrarily, if the peripheral blood lymphocytosis exceeds 4000 cells/mm^3, the patient is diagnosed with chronic lymphocytic leukemia (CLL); if not, a diagnosis of small lymphocytic lymphoma (SLL) is made. Most patients fit the criteria for CLL, which is the most common leukemia of adults in the western world. In contrast, SLL constitutes only 4% of NHLs. For unclear reasons, both CLL and SLL are much less common in Asia.

Pathophysiology. The neoplastic B cells, through mechanisms that are not understood, suppress normal B-cell function, often resulting in hypogammaglobulinemia. Paradoxically, approximately 15% of patients have autoantibodies against autologous red cells; other autoantibodies can also be detected. When present, these autoantibodies are made by nontumor B cells, indicating that there is a general breakdown in immune regulation. As time passes the tumor cells tend to displace the normal marrow elements, leading to anemia, neutropenia, and eventual thromobocytopenia.

Morphology

In SLL/CLL, sheets of small round lymphocytes and scattered ill-defined foci of larger, actively dividing cells diffusely efface involved lymph nodes (Fig. 12–15A). The predominant cells are compact, small, resting lymphocytes with dark-staining round nuclei, scanty cytoplasm, and little variation in size (Fig. 12–15B). The foci of mitotically active cells are called **proliferation centers;** their presence is pathognomonic for CLL/SLL. Mitotic figures are rare except in the proliferation centers, and there is little or no cytologic atypia. In addition to the lymph nodes, the bone marrow, spleen, and liver are involved in almost all cases. In most patients there is an **absolute lymphocytosis** of small, mature-looking lymphocytes. The neoplastic lymphocytes are fragile and are frequently disrupted during the preparation of smears, which produces characteristic **smudge cells.** Variable numbers of larger activated lymphocytes are also usually present in the blood smear.

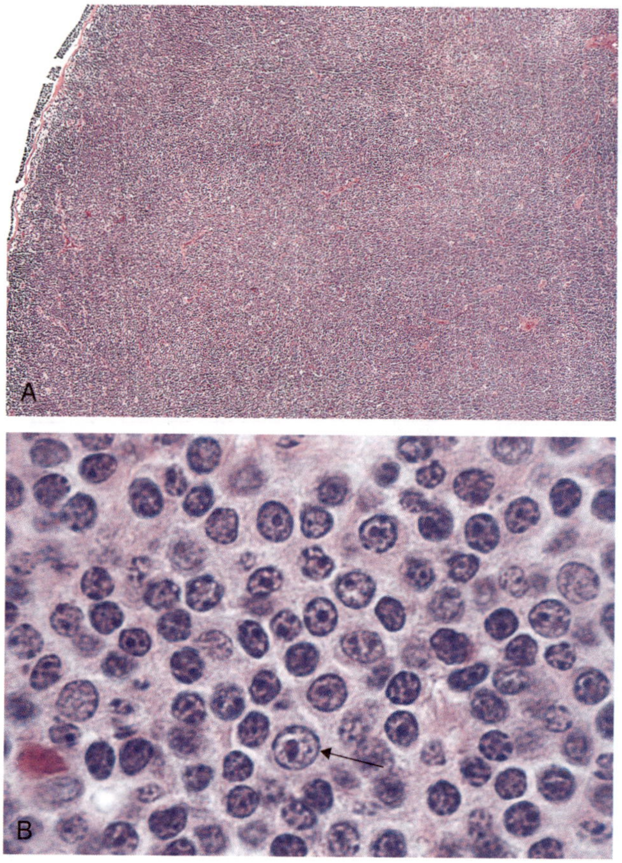

Figure 12–15

Nodal involvement by small lymphocytic lymphoma/chronic lymphocytic leukemia. **A,** Low-power view shows diffuse effacement of nodal architecture. **B,** At high power, the majority of the tumor cells have the appearance of small, round lymphocytes. A single "prolymphocyte," a larger cell with a centrally placed nucleolus, is also present in this field. (**A,** Courtesy of Dr. José Hernandez, Department of Pathology, University of Texas Southwestern Medical School, Dallas, Texas.)

Immunophenotype, Karyotype, and Molecular Features. CLL/SLL is a neoplasm of mature B cells expressing the pan–B-cell markers CD19, CD20, and CD23 and surface immunoglobulin heavy and light chains. The tumor cells also express CD5, a tendency that is shared (among the B-cell neoplasms) only by mantle cell lymphoma. Approximately 50% of patients have karyotypic abnormalities, the most common of which are trisomy 12 and deletions of chromosomes 11 and 12. Unlike other lymphoid neoplasms, chromosomal translocations are rare. Of interest, most CLL/SLLs have undergone somatic hypermutation of their immunoglobulin segments, a finding that is consistent with an origin from a post–follicular center B cell (possibly a memory cell). Less commonly these tumors are derived from naive B cells that have not undergone a follicular center reaction; such tumors appear to have a substantially worse prognosis.

Clinical Features. CLL/SLL is often asymptomatic at presentation. The most common symptoms are nonspecific and include easy fatigability, weight loss, and anorexia. Generalized *lymphadenopathy* and *hepato-*

splenomegaly are present in 50% to 60% of cases. The total leukocyte count may be increased only slightly (in SLL) or may exceed 200,000 cells/μL. *Hypogammaglobulinemia* develops in more than 50% of the patients, usually late in the course of the disease, and is responsible for increased susceptibility to bacterial infections. Less commonly, *autoimmune hemolytic anemia* and *thrombocytopenia* are seen. The course and prognosis are extremely variable. Many patients live more than 10 years after diagnosis and die of unrelated causes; the median survival is 4 to 6 years. However, as time passes CLL/SLL tends to transform to more aggressive tumors that resemble either pro-lymphocytic leukemia or diffuse large B-cell lymphoma. Once transformation occurs, the median survival is less than 1 year.

Follicular Lymphoma

These are relatively common tumors that constitute 40% of the adult NHLs in the United States. Like CLL/SLL, they occur much less frequently in Asian populations.

Morphology

Lymph nodes are effaced by proliferations that usually have a distinctly **nodular appearance** (Fig 12–16A). The tumor cells resemble normal follicular center B cells. Most commonly, the predominant neoplastic cells are "centrocyte-like" cells slightly larger than resting lymphocytes that have angular "cleaved" nuclear contours with prominent indentations and linear infoldings (see Fig. 12–16B). The nuclear chromatin is coarse and condensed, and nucleoli are indistinct. These small, cleaved cells are mixed with variable numbers of larger "centroblast-like" cells that have vesicular chromatin, several nucleoli, and modest amounts of cytoplasm. In most tumors, centroblast-like cells are a minor component of the overall cellularity, mitoses are infrequent, and single necrotic cells (cells undergoing apoptosis) are not seen. These findings help to distinguish neoplastic follicles from reactive follicles, in which mitoses and apoptosis are prominent. Uncommonly, centroblast-like cells predominate, a histology that correlates with a more aggressive clinical behavior.

Immunophenotype and Molecular Features. These tumors express the pan–B-cell markers CD19 and CD20, CD10, and BCL6, a transcription factor that is required for follicular center formation. In addition, the neoplastic cells characteristically express BCL2, a protein that is absent from normal follicular B cells. As would be expected of a B cell–derived tumor, the immunoglobulin genes show evidence of somatic hypermutation.

Karyotype. The majority of tumors have a characteristic t(14;18) translocation. This translocation fuses the *BCL2* gene on chromosome 18q21 to the IgH locus on chromosome 14 and leads to the inappropriate expression of BCL2 protein, which functions to prevent apoptosis (Chapter 6).

Clinical Features. Follicular lymphoma occurs predominantly in older persons (rarely before age 20 years) and affects males and females equally. It usually presents as *painless lymphadenopathy,* which is frequently generalized. Involvement of visceral sites is uncommon, but the *bone marrow almost always contains lymphoma* at the time of diagnosis. The natural history is prolonged (median survival, 7–9 years), but *follicular lymphoma is not easily curable,* a feature that is common to most of the indolent lymphoid malignancies. Their incurability may be related in part to the elevated levels of BCL2, which may protect tumor cells from the effects of chemotherapeutic agents. In about 40% of patients, follicular lymphoma progresses to a diffuse large B-cell lymphoma, with or without treatment. This is an ominous transition, because tumors arising from such conversions are much less curable than de novo diffuse large B-cell lymphomas, described later.

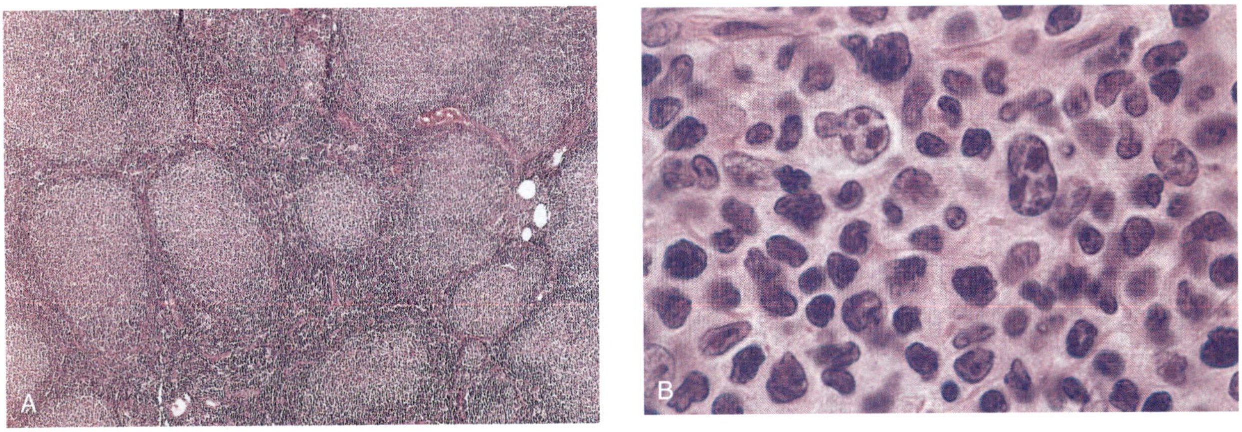

Figure 12–16

Follicular lymphoma, involving a lymph node. **A,** Nodular aggregates of lymphoma cells are present throughout. **B,** At high magnification, small lymphoid cells with condensed chromatin and irregular or cleaved nuclear outlines (centrocytes) are mixed with a population of larger cells with nucleoli (centroblasts). (**A,** Courtesy of Dr. Robert W. McKenna, Department of Pathology, University of Texas Southwestern Medical School, Dallas, Texas.)

Mantle Cell Lymphoma

Mantle cell lymphomas are composed of B cells that resemble cells in the mantle zone of normal lymphoid follicles. They constitute approximately 4% of all NHLs and occur mainly in older males.

Morphology

Mantle cell lymphomas involve lymph nodes in a diffuse or vaguely nodular pattern. The tumor cells are usually slightly larger than normal lymphocytes and have an irregular nucleus and inconspicuous nucleoli. Less commonly, the cells are larger and morphologically resemble lymphoblasts. The bone marrow is involved in the majority of cases, and about 20% of patients have peripheral blood involvement. One unexplained but characteristic tendency is the frequent involvement of the gastrointestinal tract, sometimes in the form of multifocal submucosal nodules that grossly resemble polyps (lymphomatoid polyposis).

Immunophenotype. The tumor cells usually coexpress surface IgM and IgD, the pan–B-cell antigens CD19 and CD20, and (like CLL/SLL) CD5. Mantle cell lymphoma is distinguished from CLL/SLL by the absence of proliferation centers and the *presence of cyclin D1 protein.*

Karyotype and Molecular Features. Most (and possibly all) tumors have a t(11;14) translocation that fuses the cyclin D1 gene on chromosome 11 to the IgH locus on chromosome 14. This translocation dysregulates the expression of cyclin D1, a cell cycle regulator (Chapter 6), and explains the characteristically increased cyclin D1 protein levels. The immunoglobulin loci have not undergone somatic hypermutation, consistent with an origin from a naive B cell.

Clinical Features. Most patients present with fatigue and lymphadenopathy and are found to have generalized disease involving the bone marrow, spleen, liver, and (often) the gastrointestinal tract. These tumors are aggressive and incurable, and are associated with a median survival of 3 to 5 years.

Diffuse Large B-Cell Lymphoma

This diagnostic category includes several forms of NHL that share certain features, including a B-cell phenotype, a diffuse growth pattern, and an aggressive clinical history. As a group, *this is the most important type of lymphoma in adults, as it accounts for approximately 50% of adult NHL.*

Morphology

The nuclei of the neoplastic B cells are large (at least three to four times the size of resting lymphocytes) and can take a variety of forms. In many tumors, cells with round, irregular, or cleaved nuclear contours, dispersed chromatin, several distinct nucleoli, and modest amounts of pale cytoplasm predominate (Fig. 12–17). Such cells resemble "centroblasts," the large cells that are seen in reactive lymphoid follicles. In other tumors, the cells have a large round or multilobulated vesicular nucleus, one or two centrally placed prominent nucleoli, and abundant cytoplasm that can be either pale or intensely staining. These cells resemble an "immunoblast," a type of antigen-activated lymphocyte that is normally found in the paracortex of lymph nodes.

Immunophenotype and Molecular Features. These are mature B-cell tumors that express pan–B-cell antigens, such as CD19 and CD20. Many also express surface IgM and/or IgG. Other antigens (e.g., CD10) are variably expressed. These tumors uniformly demonstrate somatic hypermutation of immunoglobulin genes, consistent with an origin from a follicular or post-follicular center B cell.

Karyotype. Approximately 30% of tumors have a t(14;18) translocation involving the *BCL2* gene. Such tumors may represent "transformed" follicular lymphomas. About one-third have rearrangements of the *BCL6* gene, located on 3q27, and mutations in *BCL6* are seen in an even higher fraction of tumors. Both the translocations and the mutations seem to cause inappropriate increases in BCL6 protein levels.

Distinct Subtypes. Several distinctive clinicopathologic subtypes are included in the general category of diffuse large B-cell lymphoma. *EBV* is implicated in the pathogenesis of diffuse large B-cell lymphomas that arise in the setting of the acquired immunodeficiency syndrome (AIDS) and iatrogenic immunosuppression (e.g., in transplant patients). In the post-transplant setting, these tumors often begin as EBV-driven polyclonal B-cell proliferations that may regress if immune function is restored. Otherwise, with time, progression to mono-

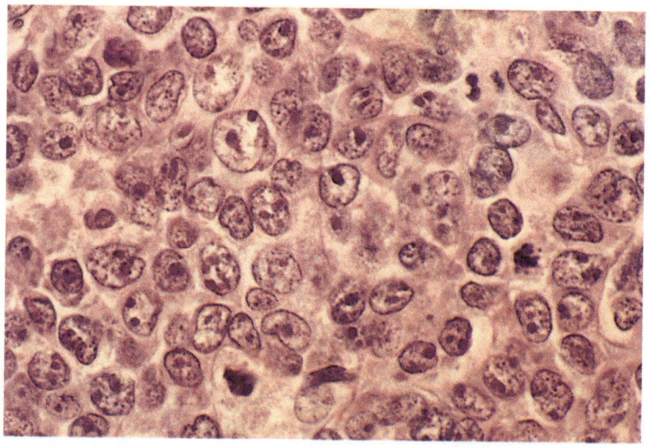

Figure 12–17

Diffuse large B-cell lymphoma. The tumor cells have large nuclei with open chromatin and prominent nucleoli. (Courtesy of Dr. Robert W. McKenna, Department of Pathology, University of Texas Southwestern Medical School, Dallas, Texas.)

clonal large B-cell lymphoma is observed. *Kaposi sarcoma herpesivirus (KSHV),* also called *human herpesvirus type 8 (HHV-8)* is associated with a rare group of tumors that present as *primary effusion lymphomas* within the pleura, pericardium, or peritoneum. The tumor cells are latently infected with KSHV, which encodes proteins homologous to several known oncoproteins, including cyclin D1. Patients with these primary effusion lymphomas are usually immunosuppressed. Note that this virus is also associated with Kaposi sarcoma in AIDS patients (Chapter 5). *Mediastinal large B-cell lymphoma* usually presents in young females and shows a predilection for spread to abdominal viscera and the central nervous system.

Clinical Features. Although the median age at presentation is about 60 years, diffuse large B-cell lymphomas can arise at any age; they constitute about 15% of childhood lymphomas. Patients typically present with a rapidly enlarging, often symptomatic mass at one or several sites. Extranodal presentations are common. Although the gastrointestinal tract and the brain are among the more frequent extranodal sites, these tumors can arise in virtually any organ or tissue. Unlike the more indolent lymphomas (e.g., follicular lymphoma), involvement of the liver, spleen, and bone marrow is not common at the time of diagnosis.

Diffuse large cell B-cell lymphomas are *aggressive tumors that are rapidly fatal if untreated.* With intensive combination chemotherapy, however, complete remission can be achieved in 60% to 80% of the patients; of these, approximately 50% remain free of disease for several years and are often cured. For those not cured with conventional therapy, other more aggressive treatments (e.g., high-dose therapy and bone marrow transplantation) offer some hope. Microarray-based molecular profiling of these tumors may improve the ability to predict the response to current therapies and perhaps even identify targets for new therapeutic approaches (Chapter 6).

Burkitt Lymphoma

Burkitt lymphoma is endemic in some parts of Africa and sporadic in other areas, including the United States. Histologically, the African and nonendemic diseases are identical, although there are clinical and virologic differences. The relationship of these disorders to EBV is discussed in Chapter 6.

Morphology

The tumor cells are uniform and intermediate in size and have round or oval nuclei containing two to five **prominent nucleoli** (Fig. 12–18). The nuclear size approximates that of benign macrophages within the tumor. There is a moderate amount of basophilic or amphophilic cytoplasm, which on smears is often seen to contain small, lipid-filled vacuoles. A **high mitotic rate** is very characteristic of this tumor, as is cell death, accounting for the presence of numerous tissue macrophages containing ingested nuclear debris. Because these benign macrophages are often surrounded by a clear space, they create a **"starry sky" pattern.**

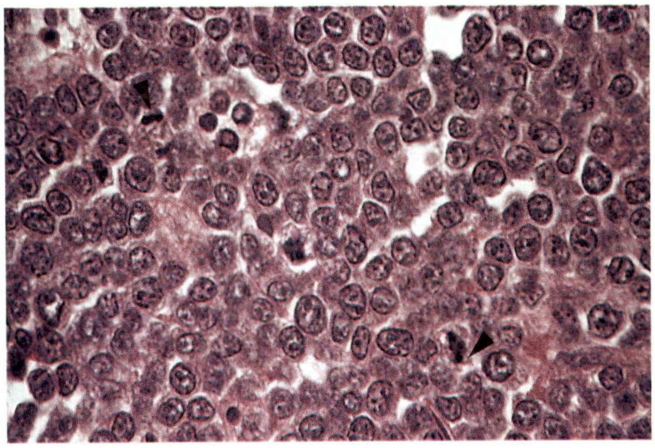

Figure 12–18

Burkitt lymphoma. The tumor cells and their nuclei are fairly uniform, giving a monotonous appearance. Note the high mitotic activity (*arrowheads*) and prominent nucleoli. The "starry sky" pattern produced by interspersed, lightly staining, normal macrophages is better appreciated at a lower magnification. (Courtesy of Dr. Robert W. McKenna, Department of Pathology, University of Texas Southwestern Medical School, Dallas, Texas.)

Immunophenotype and Molecular Features. These B-cell tumors express surface IgM, κ or λ light chain, the pan–B-cell markers CD19 and CD20, and CD10. The immunoglobulin genes are somatically hypermutated, consistent with an origin from a follicular center B cell.

Karyotype. Burkitt lymphoma is always associated with translocations involving the *MYC* gene on chromosome 8. Most translocations fuse *MYC* with the *IgH* gene on chromosome 14, but variant translocations involving the κ or λ light chain loci on chromosomes 2 and 22, respectively, are also observed. The net result of each is the dysregulation and overexpression of the MYC protein. The role of Myc in transformation was discussed in Chapter 6.

Clinical Features. Both the endemic and nonendemic forms affect mainly children and young adults. Burkitt lymphoma accounts for approximately 30% of childhood NHLs in the United States. In both forms, the disease usually arises at extranodal sites. In African patients, involvement of the maxilla or mandible is the common mode of presentation, whereas abdominal tumors involving the bowel, retroperitoneum, and ovaries are more common in North America. Leukemic presentations are uncommon, especially in the endemic form, but do occur and must be distinguished from acute lymphoblastic leukemias, which respond to different drug regimens. Burkitt lymphoma is a high-grade tumor that is among the fastest growing human neoplasms; however, with very aggressive chemotherapy regimens, the majority of patients can be cured.

Multiple Myeloma and Related Plasma Cell Disorders

The common feature that is shared among multiple myeloma and the plasma cell dyscrasias is that all originate from a clone of B cells that differentiates into plasma cells and secretes a single complete or partial immunoglobulin. Because the serum usually contains excessive amounts of immunoglobulins, these disorders have also been called monoclonal gammopathies, and the associated immunoglobulin is often referred to as an M component. Although the presence of an M component may be indicative of an overt B-cell malignancy, M components are fairly common in otherwise normal elderly persons, a condition called monoclonal gammopathy of undetermined significance. Collectively these disorders account for about 15% of deaths from tumors of white blood cells; they are most common in middle-aged and elderly persons.

The plasma cell dyscrasias can be divided into six major variants: (1) multiple myeloma, (2) localized plasmacytoma (solitary myeloma), (3) lymphoplasmacytic lymphoma, (4) heavy-chain disease, (5) primary or immunocyte-associated amyloidosis, and (6) monoclonal gammopathy of undetermined significance. In all forms, the immunoglobulin genes are somatically hypermutated, consistent with an origin from a post-follicular center B cell. Each of these disorders will be briefly described, and then the morphologic features of the more common forms will be presented.

Multiple Myeloma. Multiple myeloma, by far the most common of the malignant plasma cell dyscrasias, is a clonal proliferation of neoplastic plasma cells in the bone marrow that is usually associated with *multifocal lytic lesions throughout the skeletal system.* The proliferation of neoplastic plasma cells, also called myeloma cells, is supported by the cytokine interleukin 6 (IL-6), which is produced by fibroblasts and macrophages in the bone marrow stroma. As is true of other B-cell malignancies, it has been appreciated recently that many myelomas have chromosomal translocations involving the IgH locus on chromosome 14. The identified fusion partners include the cyclin D1, fibroblast growth factor receptor 3, and cyclin D3 genes; late in the course, translocations involving MYC are sometimes observed. As might be surmised by the list of genes involved by chromosomal translocations, dysregulation of D cyclins seems to be of general importance in multiple myeloma.

The most common M component is IgG (60%), followed by IgA (20% to 25%); only rarely is it IgM, IgD, or IgE. In the remaining 15% to 20% of cases, the plasma cells produce *only* κ or λ light chains. Because of their low molecular weight, the free light chains are rapidly excreted in the urine, where they are termed *Bence-Jones proteins.* Even more commonly, malignant plasma cells secrete complete immunoglobulin molecules and free light chains and thus produce both serum M components and Bence-Jones proteins. As will be seen, the excess light chains have untoward effects on renal function and are an important aspect of the pathophysiology of multiple myeloma.

Localized Plasmacytoma. These are solitary lesions involving the skeleton or the soft tissues. Skeletal plasmacytomas tend to occur in the same locations as multiple myeloma, whereas extraosseous lesions occur mainly in the upper respiratory tract (sinuses, nasopharynx, larynx). Modestly elevated M proteins are demonstrable in some of these patients. Those with solitary skeletal plasmacytomas usually have occult disease elsewhere, and most develop full-blown multiple myeloma over a period of 5 to 10 years. Extraosseous (soft tissue) plasmacytomas spread less commonly and are often cured by local resection.

Lymphoplasmacytic Lymphoma. This tumor is composed of a mixed proliferation of B cells that range from small round lymphocytes to plasmacytic lymphocytes to plasma cells. It behaves like an *indolent B-cell lymphoma* and commonly involves multiple lymph nodes, the bone marrow, and the spleen at the time of presentation. It is included in the plasma cell dyscrasias because the tumor produces an M component, but, unlike multiple myeloma, it consists in most cases of IgM. Often, the large amount of IgM causes the blood to become viscous, producing a syndrome called *Waldenström macroglobulinemia,* described below. Other symptoms are related to the infiltation of various tissues, particularly the bone marrow, by tumor cells. The synthesis of immunoglobulin heavy and light chains is balanced, so free light chains and Bence-Jones proteinuria are not seen. Unlike myeloma, this disease *does not produce lytic bone lesions.*

Heavy-Chain Disease. This is not a specific entity but a group of proliferations in which only heavy chains are produced, most commonly IgA. IgA heavy-chain disease shows a predilection for the lymphoid tissues where IgA is normally produced, such as the small intestine and respiratory tract, and may represent a variant of MALT lymphoma (discussed later). The less common IgG heavy-chain disease often presents as diffuse lymphadenopathy and hepatosplenomegaly and histologically resembles lymphoplasmacytic lymphoma.

Primary or Immunocyte-Associated Amyloidosis. It may be recalled that a monoclonal proliferation of plasma cells that secrete free light chains underlies this form of amyloidosis (Chapter 5). The amyloid deposits (of AL type) consist of partially degraded light chains.

Monoclonal Gammopathy of Undetermined Significance. Monoclonal gammopathy of undetermined significance (MGUS) is the term applied to monoclonal gammopathies that are detected in asymptomatic individuals. M proteins are found in the serum of 1% to 3% of asymptomatic healthy persons older than age 50 years, making this the most common plasma cell dyscrasia. Despite the name, it is increasingly apparent that *MGUS is a precursor lesion that should be considered a form of neoplasia.* Patients with MGUS develop a well-defined plasma cell dyscrasia (myeloma, lymphoplasmacytic lymphoma, or amyloidosis) at a rate of 1% per year. Moreover, MGUS cells often contain the same chromosomal translocations that are found in full-blown multiple myeloma. Thus, the diagnosis of MGUS should be made with caution and only after careful exclusion of all other forms of monoclonal gammopathies, particularly multiple myeloma. In general, patients with MGUS have less than 3 gm/dL of monoclonal protein in the serum and no Bence-Jones proteinuria.

Morphology

Multiple myeloma presents most often as multifocal destructive bone lesions throughout the skeletal system. Although any bone can be affected, the following distribution was found in a large series of cases: vertebral column, 66%; ribs, 44%; skull, 41%; pelvis, 28%; femur, 24%; clavicle, 10%; and scapula, 10%. These focal lesions generally begin in the medullary cavity, erode the cancellous bone, and progressively destroy the cortical bone. The bone resorption results from the secretion of certain cytokines (e.g., IL-1β, tumor necrosis factor, IL-6) by myeloma cells. These cytokines stimulate production of another cytokine called RANK-ligand, which promotes the differentiation and activation of osteoclasts (Chapter 21). Plasma cell lesions often lead to **pathologic fractures,** which occur most frequently in the vertebral column. The bone lesions usually appear radiographically as **punched-out defects** of 1 to 4 cm in diameter (Fig. 12–19A), but in some cases diffuse skeletal demineralization is evident. Microscopic examination of the marrow reveals an increased number of plasma cells, which constitute 10% to 90% of the cellularity. The neoplastic cells can resemble normal mature plasma cells, but they more often show abnormal features, such as prominent nucleoli or abnormal cytoplasmic inclusions containing immunoglobulin (Fig. 12–19B). With progressive disease, plasma cell infiltrations of soft tissues can be encountered in the spleen, liver, kidneys, lungs, and lymph nodes, or they may be more widely distributed. Terminally, a leukemic picture may emerge.

Renal involvement, generally called **myeloma nephrosis,** is a distinctive feature of multiple myeloma. Proteinaceous casts are prominent in the distal convoluted tubules and collecting ducts. Most of these casts are made up of Bence-Jones proteins, but they may also contain complete immunoglobulins, Tamm-Horsfall protein, and albumin. Some casts have tinctorial properties of amyloid. This is not surprising, in that AL amyloid is derived from Bence-Jones proteins (Chapter 5). Multinucleate giant cells created by the fusion of infiltrating macrophages usually surround the casts. **Very often the epithelial cells lining the cast-filled tubules become necrotic or atrophic because of the toxic actions of the Bence-Jones proteins.** Metastatic calcification stemming from bone resorption and hypercalcemia may be encountered. When complicated by systemic amyloidosis, nodular glomerular lesions are present. **Pyelonephritis** can also occur as a result of the increased susceptibility to bacterial infections. Less commonly, interstitial infiltrates of abnormal plasma cells are seen.

In contrast to multiple myeloma, lymphoplasmacytic lymphoma is not associated with lytic skeletal lesions. Instead, the neoplastic cells diffusely infiltrate the bone marrow, lymph nodes, spleen, and sometimes the liver. Infiltrations of other organs also occur, particularly with disease progression. The cellular infiltrate consists of lymphocytes, plasma cells, and plasmacytoid lymphocytes of intermediate differentiation. The remaining forms of plasma cell dyscrasias have either already been described (e.g., primary amyloidosis; Chapter 5) or are too rare for further description.

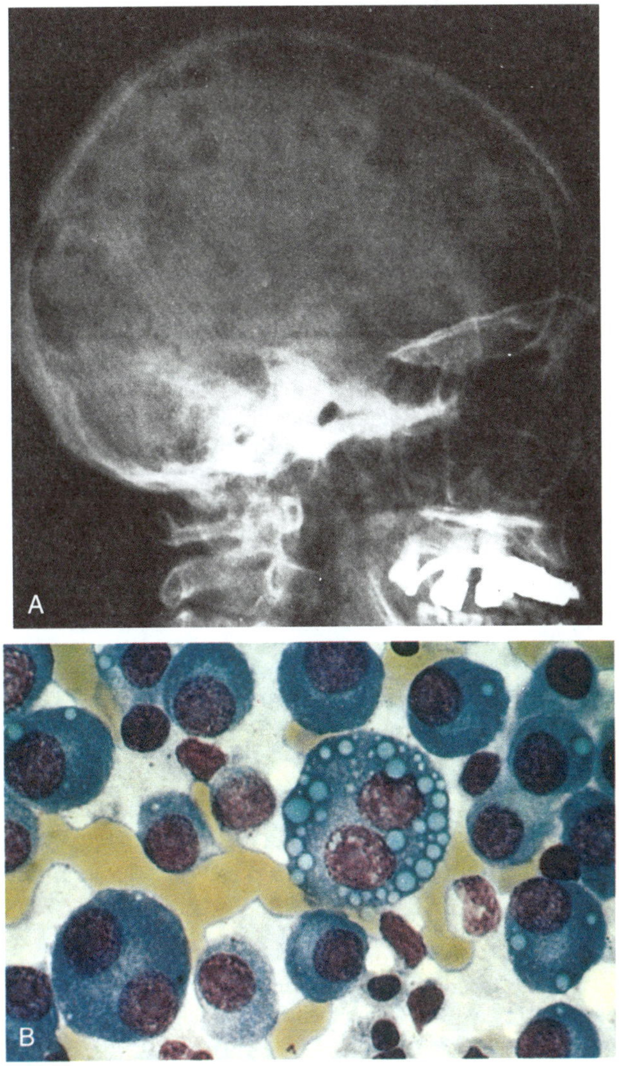

Figure 12–19

Multiple myeloma. **A,** Radiograph of the skull (lateral view). The sharply punched-out bone defects are most obvious in the calvarium. **B,** Bone marrow aspirate. Normal marrow cells are largely replaced by plasma cells, including atypical forms with multiple nuclei, prominent nucleoli, and cytoplasmic droplets containing immunoglobulin.

Clinical Course. The clinical manifestations of the plasma cell dyscrasias are varied. They result from the destructive or otherwise damaging effect of the infiltrating neoplastic cells in various tissues and the abnormal immunoglobulins secreted by the tumors. In multiple myeloma the pathologic effects of plasma cell tumors predominate, whereas in lymphoplasmacytic lymphoma most of the signs and symptoms result from the IgM macroglobulins in the serum.

The peak age of incidence of multiple myeloma is between 50 and 60 years. The major clinicopathologic features of this disease can be summarized as follows:

- *Bone pain,* resulting from infiltration by neoplastic plasma cells, is extremely common. Pathologic fractures and hypercalcemia occur, with focal bone destruction and diffuse resorption. Hypercalcemia can cause neurologic manifestations such as confusion and lethargy; it also contributes to renal disease. Anemia results from marrow replacement as well as from inhibition of hematopoiesis by tumor cells.

- *Recurrent infections* with bacteria such as *Staphylococcus aureus, Streptococcus pneumoniae,* and *Escherichia coli* are serious clinical problems. They result from severe suppression of normal immunoglobulin secretion.
- *Hyperviscosity syndrome* may occur due to excessive production and aggregation of myeloma proteins, but this is much more characteristic of lymphoplasmacytic lymphoma.
- *Renal insufficiency* occurs in as many as 50% of patients. It results from multiple conditions, such as recurrent bacterial infections and hypercalcemia, but most importantly from the toxic effects of Bence-Jones proteins on cells lining the tubules.
- Amyloidosis develops in 5% to 10% of patients.

The diagnosis of multiple myeloma can be strongly suspected when the characteristic focal, punched-out radiologic defects in the bone are present—especially when located in the vertebrae or calvarium. Electrophoresis of the serum and urine is an important diagnostic tool. In 99% of cases a monoclonal spike of complete immunoglobulin or immunoglobulin light chain can be detected in the serum, in the urine, or in both. In the remaining 1% of cases, monoclonal immunoglobulins can be found within the plasma cells but not in the serum or urine. Such cases are sometimes called *nonsecretory myelomas.* Examination of the bone marrow is used to confirm the presence of a plasma cell proliferation.

Lymphoplasmacytic lymphoma affects older persons, with the peak incidence being between the sixth and seventh decades. Most clinical symptoms of this disease can be traced to the presence of large amounts of IgM (macroglobulin). Because of their size, the macroglobulins greatly increase blood viscosity. This gives rise to the *hyperviscosity syndrome* known as *Waldenström macroglobulinemia,* which is characterized by the following features:

- *Visual impairment,* related to the striking tortuosity and distention of retinal veins; retinal hemorrhages and exudates can also contribute to the visual problems
- *Neurologic problems* such as headaches, dizziness, tinnitus, deafness, and stupor, stemming from sluggish blood flow and sludging
- *Bleeding,* related to the formation of complexes between macroglobulins and clotting factors as well as interference with platelet functions
- *Cryoglobulinemia,* related to precipitation of macroglobulins at low temperatures and producing symptoms such as Raynaud phenomenon and cold urticaria.

Multiple myeloma is a progressive disease, with median survival ranging from 4 to 5 years. The median survival in lymphoplasmacytic lymphoma is somewhat longer, in the range of 4 to 5 years. Although aggressive therapies are being tried in both, neither disease is presently curable.

Hodgkin Lymphoma

Hodgkin lymphoma encompasses a distinctive group of neoplasms that arise almost invariably in a single lymph node or chain of lymph nodes and spread characteristically in a stepwise fashion to the anatomically contiguous nodes. It is separated from the non-Hodgkin lymphomas for several reasons. First, it is *characterized morphologically by the presence of distinctive neoplastic giant cells called Reed-Sternberg (RS) cells,* which are admixed with reactive, nonmalignant inflammatory cells. Second, it is often associated with somewhat distinctive clinical features, including systemic manifestations such as fever. Third, its stereotypical pattern of spread allows it to be treated differently than most other lymphoid neoplasms. Despite these distinguishing features, molecular studies have shown that it is a tumor of B-cell origin.

Classification. Five subtypes of Hodgkin lymphoma are recognized: (1) nodular sclerosis, (2) mixed cellularity, (3) lymphocyte predominance, (4) lymphocyte rich, and (5) lymphocyte depletion. The latter two subtypes are uncommon and will not be mentioned further. Before delineating the remaining three, however, we should describe the common denominator among all—RS cells and variants thereof—and the staging system used to characterize the extent of the disease in an individual.

Morphology

The sine qua non for Hodgkin lymphoma is the **Reed-Sternberg (RS) cell** (Fig. 12–20). This is a large cell (15–45 μm in diameter) with an enlarged multilobated nucleus, exceptionally prominent nucleoli, and abundant, usually slightly eosinophilic, cytoplasm. **Particularly characteristic are cells with two mirror-image nuclei or nuclear lobes, each containing a large (inclusion-like) acidophilic nucleolus surrounded by a distinctive clear zone; together they impart an owl-eye appearance. The nuclear membrane is distinct.** As we will see, such "classic" RS cells are common in the mixed-cellularity subtype, uncommon in the nodular sclerosis subtype, and rare in the lymphocyte-predominance subtype; in these latter two subtypes, other characteristic RS cell variants predominate.

The staging of Hodgkin lymphoma (Table 12–9) is of clinical importance, because the course, choice of therapy, and prognosis are all intimately related to the distribution of the disease.

With this background we can turn to the morphologic classification of Hodgkin lymphoma into its subgroups and point out some of the salient clinical features of each. Later the manifestations common to all will be presented. The essential features that serve to differentiate the major subgroups (lymphocyte predominance, nodular sclerosis, and mixed cellularity) are the morphology, immunophenotype, and frequency of the neoplastic elements (RS cells) and the nature of the tissue response.

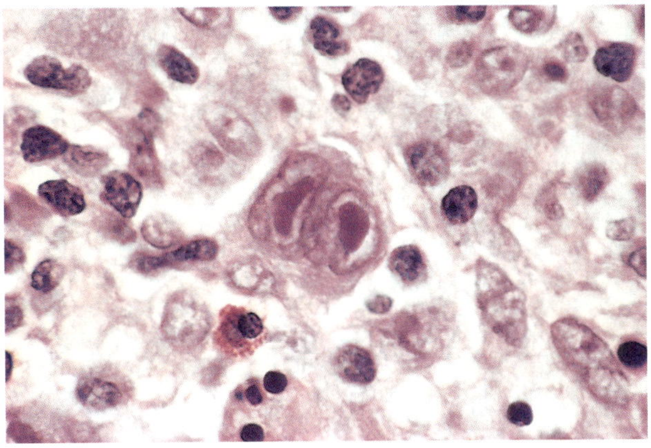

Figure 12–20

Hodgkin lymphoma. A binucleate Reed-Sternberg cell with large, inclusion-like nucleoli and abundant cytoplasm is surrounded by lymphocytes, and an eosinophil can be seen below. (Courtesy of Dr. Robert W. McKenna, Department of Pathology, University of Texas Southwestern Medical School, Dallas, Texas.)

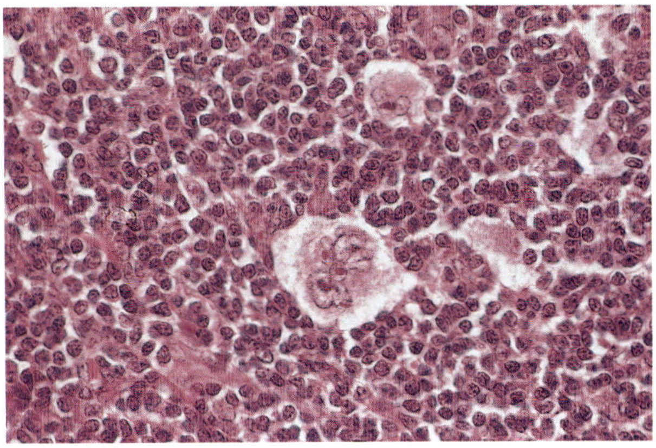

Figure 12–21

Hodgkin lymphoma, nodular sclerosis type. A distinctive "lacunar cell" with multilobed nucleus containing many small nucleoli is seen lying within a clear space created by retraction of its cytoplasm. It is surrounded by lymphocytes. (Courtesy of Dr. Robert W. McKenna, Department of Pathology, University of Texas Southwestern Medical School, Dallas, Texas.)

Nodular Sclerosis Hodgkin Lymphoma. This is the most common form. It is equally frequent in men and women and has a striking propensity to involve the lower cervical, supraclavicular, and mediastinal lymph nodes. Most of the patients are adolescents or young adults, and the overall prognosis is excellent. It is characterized morphologically by:

- The presence of a particular variant of the RS cell, the **lacunar cell** (Fig. 12–21). This cell is large and has a single multilobate nucleus with multiple small nucleoli and an abundant, pale-staining cytoplasm. In formalin-fixed tissue, the cytoplasm often retracts, giving rise to the appearance of cells lying in empty spaces, or lacunae.
- The presence of collagen bands that divide the lymphoid tissue into circumscribed nodules (Fig. 12–22). The fibrosis may be scant or abundant, and the cellular infiltrate may show varying proportions of lymphocytes, eosinophils, histiocytes, and lacunar cells. Classic RS cells are infrequent.

The immunophenotype of the lacunar variants is identical to that of classic RS cells. These cells express CD15 and CD30 and usually do not express B- and T-cell–specific antigens.

Mixed-Cellularity Hodgkin Lymphoma. This is the most common form of Hodgkin lymphoma in patients older than the age of 50 and overall comprises about 25% of

Table 12–9 Clinical Staging of Hodgkin and Non-Hodgkin Lymphomas (Ann Arbor Classification)*

Stage	Distribution of Disease
I	Involvement of a single lymph node region (I) or involvement of a single extralymphatic organ or tissue (I_E)
II	Involvement of two or more lymph node regions on the same side of the diaphragm alone (II) or with involvement of limited contiguous extralymphatic organs or tissue (II_E)
III	Involvement of lymph node regions on both sides of the diaphragm (III), which may include the spleen (III_S), limited contiguous extralymphatic organ or site (III_E), or both (III_{ES})
IV	Multiple or disseminated foci of involvement of one or more extralymphatic organs or tissues with or without lymphatic involvement

*All stages are further divided on the basis of the absence (A) or presence (B) of the following systemic symptoms: significant fever, night sweats, unexplained loss of more than 10% of normal body weight.

From Carbone PT, et al.: Symposium (Ann Arbor): staging in Hodgkin disease. Cancer Res 31:1707, 1971.

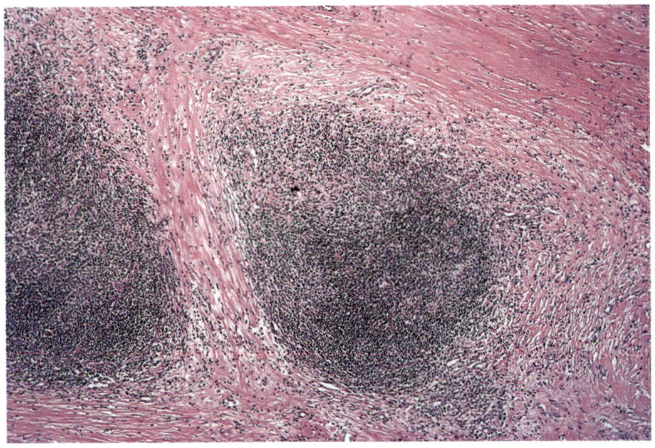

Figure 12–22

Hodgkin lymphoma, nodular sclerosis type. A low-power view shows well-defined bands of pink, acellular collagen that have subdivided the tumor cells into nodules. (Courtesy of Dr. Robert W. McKenna, Department of Pathology, University of Texas Southwestern Medical School, Dallas, Texas.)

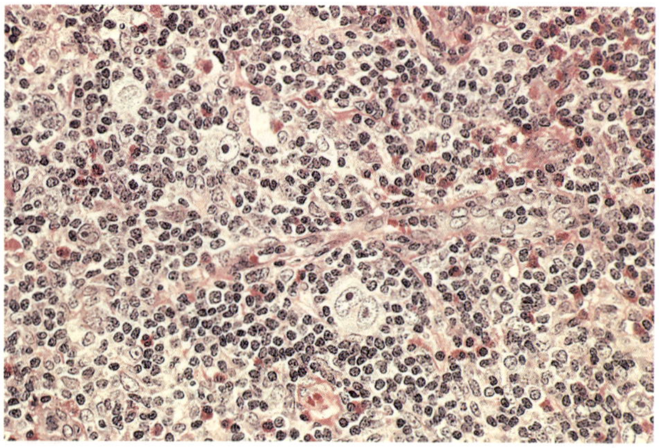

Figure 12–23

Hodgkin disease, mixed-cellularity type. A diagnostic, binucleate Reed-Sternberg cell is surrounded by multiple cell types, including eosinophils (bright-red cytoplasm), lymphocytes, and histiocytes. (Courtesy of Dr. Robert W. McKenna, Department of Pathology, University of Texas Southwestern Medical School, Dallas, Texas.)

cases. There is a male predominance. Classic RS cells are plentiful within a distinctive heterogeneous cellular infiltrate, which includes small lymphocytes, eosinophils, plasma cells, and benign histiocytes (Fig. 12–23). Compared with the other common subtypes, more patients with mixed cellularity have disseminated disease and systemic manifestations.

Lymphocyte-Predominance Hodgkin Lymphoma. This subgroup, comprising about 5% of Hodgkin lymphoma, is characterized by a large number of small resting lymphocytes admixed with a variable number of benign histiocytes (Fig. 12–24), often within large, poorly defined nodules. Other types of reactive cells, such as eosinophils, neutrophils, and plasma cells, are scanty or absent, and classic RS cells are extremely difficult to find. Scattered among the reactive cells are lymphohistiocytic (L&H) variant RS cells that have a delicate multilobed, puffy nucleus that has been likened in appearance to popcorn (**"popcorn cell"**). The typical nodular growth pattern of lymphocyte-predominance Hodgkin lymphoma has long suggested that this might be a neoplasm of follicular B cells; indeed, phenotypic studies have revealed that the L&H variants express B-cell markers (e.g., CD20). Furthermore, L&H variants have rearranged and somatically hypermutated IgH genes, which strongly supports a follicular B-cell origin. Most individuals with this form of the disease present with isolated cervical or axillary lymphadenopathy and have an excellent prognosis.

It is apparent that Hodgkin lymphoma spans a wide range of histologic patterns and that certain forms, with their characteristic fibrosis, eosinophils, neutrophils, and plasma cells, come deceptively close to simulating an inflammatory reactive process. **The histologic diagnosis of Hodgkin lymphoma rests on the definitive identification of RS cells or their variants in the appropriate background of reactive cells.** Immunophenotyping plays an important adjunct role in helping to distinguish Hodgkin lymphoma from reactive conditions and other forms of lymphoma.

In all forms, involvement of the spleen, liver, bone marrow, and other organs may appear in due course and take the form of irregular nodules that are composed of a mixture of RS cells and reactive cells similar to that observed in lymph nodes. In advanced disease, the spleen and the liver can be enlarged by tumor.

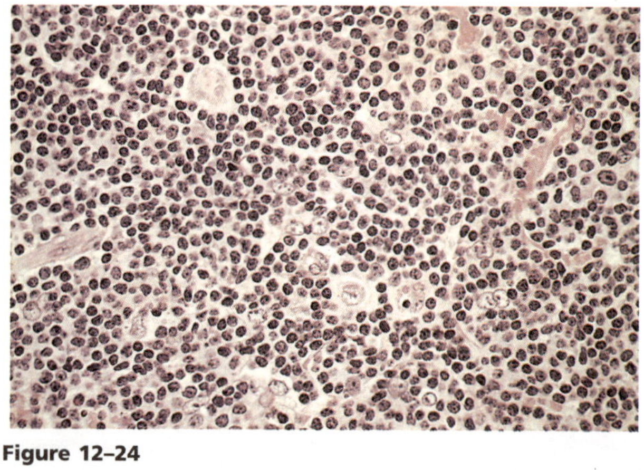

Figure 12–24

Hodgkin disease, lymphocyte-predominance type. Numerous mature-looking lymphocytes surround scattered, large, pale-staining lymphocytic and histiocytic variants ("popcorn" cells). (Courtesy of Dr. Robert W. McKenna, Department of Pathology, University of Texas Southwestern Medical School, Dallas, Texas.)

Etiology and Pathogenesis. Determining the origin of the neoplastic RS cells of Hodgkin lymphoma has proved daunting, in part because these cells are rare compared with the surrounding reactive inflammatory infiltrate. It has been recognized for some time that the L&H variants of RS cells found in nodular lymphocyte-predominance Hodgkin lymphoma express B-cell markers, supporting a B-cell origin. By contrast, the RS cells in other forms of Hodgkin lymphoma have been enigmatic, in that they generally do not express lineage-specific lymphoid markers. This uncertainty was finally resolved by elegant studies performed on single microdissected RS cells obtained from cases of mixed-cellularity and nodular-sclerosis Hodgkin lymphoma. Sequence analysis of DNA amplified from such cells has shown that each RS cell from any given case possesses the same immunoglobulin gene rearrangements as its neighbor and that the rearranged immunoglobulin genes have undergone somatic hypermutation. As a result, it is now agreed that *Hodgkin lymphoma is a neoplasm arising from germinal center B cells.*

This said, many puzzles remain to be answered. RS cells are aneuploid but lack the chromosomal translocations that are common in other germinal center B-cell lymphomas and have patterns of gene expression that bear little resemblance to normal B cells. The events that transform these cells and alter their appearance and gene expression programs are still unknown. One clue stems from the involvement of EBV. The EBV genome is present in the RS cells in as many as 70% of cases of the mixed-cellularity type and a smaller fraction of the nodular sclerosis type. More importantly, the integration of the EBV genome is identical in all RS cells in a given tumor, indicating that infection precedes (and therefore may be related to) transformation. Thus, as in Burkitt lymphoma and B-cell lymphomas in immunodeficient patients, EBV infection is likely to be one of several steps contributing to the development of Hodgkin lymphoma, particularly the mixed-cellularity type.

If EBV is playing a causative role, are there common oncogenic signals in EBV-positive and EBV-negative tumors? A possible lead stems from the observation that the RS cells in classical forms of Hodgkin lymphoma, regardless of their EBV status, contain high levels of activated NF-κB, a transcription factor that normally stimulates B-cell proliferation and protects B cells from pro-apoptotic signals. Several EBV proteins that are known to activate NF-κB are expressed in EBV-positive RS cells. Somatic mutations that abolish the function of IκB, an important inhibitor of NF-κB, have been found in EBV-negative RS cells. Thus, hyperactivation of NF-κB may be a central event in the genesis, growth, and survival of RS cells.

The characteristic non-neoplastic, inflammatory-cell infiltrate seems to result from a number of cytokines secreted by RS cells, including IL-5 (which attracts and activates eosinophils), transforming growth factor β (a fibrogenic factor), and IL-13 (which may stimulate RS cells through an autocrine mechanism). Conversely, the responding inflammatory cells, rather than being innocent bystanders, produce factors (such as CD30 ligand) that can aid the growth and survival of RS cells, and contribute further to the tissue reaction.

Clinical Course. Hodgkin lymphomas, like NHLs, usually present as a painless enlargement of the lymph nodes. Although a definitive distinction from NHL can be made only by examination of a lymph node biopsy specimen, several clinical features favor the diagnosis of Hodgkin lymphoma (Table 12–10). Younger patients with the more favorable histologic types tend to present in clinical stages I or II and are usually free of systemic manifestations. Patients with disseminated disease (stages III and IV) are more likely to have systemic complaints such as fever, unexplained weight loss, pruritus, and anemia. As mentioned earlier, these patients generally have the histologically less favorable variants. The outlook after aggressive radiotherapy and chemotherapy for patients with this disease, including those with disseminated disease, is generally very good. *With current modalities of therapy, the clinical stage is the most important prognostic indicator.* The 5-year survival rate of patients with stage I-A or II-A disease is close to 100%. Even with advanced disease (stage IV-A or IV-B), the overall 5-year disease-free survival rate is around 50%. However, therapeutic successes have also brought problems. Long-term survivors of radiotherapy protocols are at much higher risk of developing certain malignancies, including lung cancer, melanoma, and breast cancer. As a result, current efforts are aimed at developing less genotoxic therapeutic regimens that decrease therapy-related complications while preserving a high cure rate.

Table 12–10 Clinical Differences Between Hodgkin and Non-Hodgkin Lymphomas

Hodgkin Lymphoma	Non-Hodgkin Lymphoma
More often localized to a single axial group of nodes (cervical, mediastinal, para-aortic)	More frequent involvement of multiple peripheral nodes
Orderly spread by contiguity	Noncontiguous spread
Mesenteric nodes and Waldeyer ring rarely involved	Mesenteric nodes and Waldeyer ring commonly involved
Extranodal involvement uncommon	Extranodal involvement common

Miscellaneous Lymphoid Neoplasms

Of the many remaining forms of lymphoid neoplasia within the WHO classification, several with distinctive or clinically important features merit brief discussion.

Extranodal Marginal Zone Lymphoma. This is a special category of low-grade mature B-cell tumors that arise most commonly in mucosal-associated lymphoid tissue (MALT), such as salivary glands, small and large bowel, and lungs, and some nonmucosal sites such as the orbit and breast. Extranodal marginal zone lymphomas tend to develop in the setting of autoimmune disorders (such as Sjögren syndrome and Hashimoto thyroiditis) or chronic infections with such organisms as *Helicobacter pylori* and *Campylobacter jejuni*), suggesting that sustained antigenic stimulation contributes to lymphomagenesis. In the case of *H. pylori*–associated gastric MALT lymphoma, eradication of the organism with antibiotic therapy often leads to regression of the tumor cells, which seem to depend on cytokines secreted by *H. pylori*–specific T cells for their growth and survival (Chapter 6). When arising at other sites, MALT tumors can often be cured by local excision or radiotherapy. Two recurrent cytogenetic abnormalities are recognized: t(1;14), involving the *BCL10* and *IgH* genes; and t(11;18), involving the *MALT1* and *IAP2* genes.

Hairy Cell Leukemia. This uncommon, indolent B-cell neoplasm is distinguished by the presence of leukemic cells that have fine, hairlike cytoplasmic projections. The tumor cells express pan–B-cell markers, including CD19 and CD20, surface immunoglobulin, and, characteristically, CD11c and CD103; these two antigens are not present on most other B-cell tumors, making them diagnostically useful.

This tumor occurs mainly in older males, and its *manifestations result largely from infiltration of bone marrow and spleen.* Splenomegaly, which is often massive, is the most common and sometimes the only abnormal physical finding. *Pancytopenia,* resulting from marrow infiltration and splenic sequestration, is seen in more than half the cases. Hepatomegaly is less common and not as marked, and lymphadenopathy is distinctly rare. *Leukocytosis is not a common feature,* being present in only 15% to 20% of patients, but hairy cells can be identified in the peripheral blood smear in most cases. The disease is indolent but progressive if untreated; pancytopenia and infections are major problems. Unlike most other low-grade lymphoid neoplasms, this tumor is extremely sensitive to chemotherapeutic agents, particularly purine nucleosides. Complete durable responses are the rule, and the overall prognosis is excellent.

Mycosis Fungoides and Sézary Syndrome. These are composed of neoplastic CD4+ T cells that home to the skin; as a result, they are often referred to as *cutaneous T-cell lymphomas.*

Mycosis fungoides usually presents as a nonspecific erythrodermic rash, which over time tends to progress through a plaque phase to a tumor phase. Histologically, there is infiltration of the epidermis and upper dermis by neoplastic T cells, which often have a cerebriform nucleus characterized by marked infolding of the nuclear membrane. With progressive disease, both nodal and visceral dissemination appear. Sézary syndrome is a clinical variant characterized by the presence of (1) a generalized exfoliative erythroderma and (2) tumor cells (Sézary cells) in the peripheral blood. Circulating tumor cells are also present in as many as 25% of cases of plaque- or tumor-phase mycosis fungoides. Patients with erythrodermic-phase mycosis fungoides often survive for many years, whereas survival is generally 1 to 3 years for patients with tumor-phase disease, visceral disease, or Sézary syndrome.

Adult T-Cell Leukemia/Lymphoma. This T-cell neoplasm is caused by a retrovirus, human T-cell leukemia virus type 1 (HTLV-1). It is endemic in southern Japan, the Caribbean basin, and West Africa and occurs sporadically elsewhere, including in the southeastern United States. The pathogenesis of this tumor is discussed in Chapter 6. In addition to causing lymphoid malignancies, HTLV-1 infection can also give rise to transverse myelitis, a progressive demyelinating disease that affects the central nervous system and the spinal cord.

Adult T-cell leukemia/lymphoma is characterized by skin lesions, generalized lymphadenopathy, hepatosplenomegaly, hypercalcemia, and variable numbers of malignant CD4+ lymphocytes in the peripheral blood. The leukemic cells express high levels of CD25, the IL-2 receptor α chain. In most cases this is an extremely aggressive disease, with a median survival time of about 8 months. In 15% to 20% of patients the course of the disease is chronic; their disease is clinically indistinguishable from cutaneous T-cell lymphoma.

Peripheral T-Cell Lymphomas. This is a heterogeneous group of tumors that together make up about 15% of adult NHLs. Although several rare distinctive subtypes fall under this heading, most tumors in this group are unclassifiable. In general, they present as disseminated disease, are aggressive, and respond poorly to therapy.

SUMMARY

Lymphoid Neoplasms

- *Classified based on cell of origin and stage of differentiation*
- *Most common types in children are acute lymphoblastic leukemias and lymphomas, which are derived from B- and T-cell precursors.*
  - Highly aggressive tumors that present with symptoms of bone marrow failure, or as rapidly growing masses
  - Tumor cells contain genetic lesions that block differentiation, leading to the accumulation of immature blasts that cannot function as immune cells.
- *Most common types in adults are non-Hodgkin lymphomas derived from germinal center B cells.*
  - May be indolent (e.g., follicular lymphoma) or aggressive (e.g., diffuse large B-cell lymphoma)
  - Sometimes interfere with the immune system by dysregulating the function of normal B and T cells (e.g., chronic lymphocytic leukemia, multiple myeloma)
  - Often contain chromosomal translocations or mutations involving genes (such as *BCL2* and *BCL6*) that regulate normal mature B-cell development and survival
- *Precursor B- and T-Cell Lymphoblastic Leukemia/Lymphoma*:
  - Aggressive tumors of pre-B or pre-T cells that are most common in childhood and young adults, but which occur throughout life.
  - Most patients present with bone marrow failure caused by extensive marrow replacement by leukemic cells, resulting in pancytopenia.
- *Small Lymphocytic Lymphoma/Chronic Lymphocytic Leukemia*:
  - Tumor of mature B cells that usually presents with involvement of the bone marrow and the lymph nodes.
  - Follows an indolent course, commonly associated with immune abnormalities, including an increased susceptibility to infection and autoimmune disorders.
- *Follicular Lymphoma*:
  - Tumor cells recapitulate the growth pattern of normal germinal center B cells; more than 80% of cases are associated with a t(14;18) translocation that results in the over-expression of the anti-apoptotic protein BCL2.
- *Mantle Cell Lymphoma*:
  - Tumor of mature B cells that usually presents with advanced disease involving lymph nodes,

bone marrow, and extranodal sites such as the gut.
  - Highly associated with a t(11;14) translocation that results in over-expression of cyclin D1, a regulator of cell cycle progression.
- *Diffuse Large B-Cell Lymphoma*:
  - Heterogeneous group of mature B cell tumors that share a similar large-cell morphology and aggressive clinical behavior; the most common type of lymphoma.
  - Highly associated with rearrangements or mutations of *BCL6* gene; one-third arise from follicular lymphomas and carry a t(14;18) translocation.
- *Burkitt Lymphoma*:
  - Very aggressive tumor of mature B cells that usually arises at extranodal sites, is uniformly associated with translocations involving the *c-MYC* proto-oncogene, and is often associated with latent infection by Epstein-Barr virus (EBV).
- *Multiple Myeloma*:
  - Plasma cell tumor that usually presents as multiple lytic bone lesions with pathologic fractures and hypercalcemia.
  - Neoplastic plasma cells may suppress normal humoral immunity and secrete partial immunoglobulins that are often nephrotoxic.
- *Hodgkin Lymphoma*:
  - Unusual tumor mostly comprised of reactive lymphocytes, macrophages, and stromal cells; the malignant cell, the Reed-Sternberg cell (which is derived from B cells), typically makes up a minor fraction of the tumor mass.

See also Table 2–8 for features of different tumors.

Myeloid Neoplasms

Myeloid neoplasms arise from hematopoietic stem cells and typically give rise to monoclonal proliferations that replace normal bone marrow cells. There are three general categories of myeloid neoplasia. In the *AMLs,* the neoplastic cells are blocked at some early stage of myeloid cell development. Immature myeloid cells (blasts), which can exhibit evidence of granulocytic, erthroid, monocytic, or megakaryoctyic differentiation, accumulate in the marrow, replacing normal elements, and frequently circulate in the peripheral blood. In the *chronic myeloproliferative disorders,* the neoplastic clone retains the capacity to undergo terminal differentiation but exhibits increased or dysregulated growth. Commonly there is an increase in one or more of the formed elements (red cells, platelets, and/or granulocytes) in the peripheral blood. In the *myelodysplastic syndromes,* terminal differentiation occurs but in a disordered and ineffective fashion, leading to the appearance of dysplastic marrow precursors and peripheral blood cytopenias.

Although these three categories provide a useful starting point when considering the myeloid neoplasms, the divisions between them sometimes blur. Both myelodysplastic syndromes and myeloproliferative disorders often transform to a picture identical to acute myelogenous leukemia, and some patients present with disorders that have features of both myelodysplastic and myeloproliferative disorders. Given that all arise from hematopoietic stem cells, the close relationship among these disorders is not surprising.

Acute Myelogenous Leukemia

AML primarily affects older adults, with the median age being 50 years. It is an extremely heterogeneous disorder, as will be discussed below. The clinical signs and symptoms, which closely resemble those produced by ALL, are usually related to marrow failure caused by the replacement of normal marrow elements by leukemic blasts. Fatigue and pallor, abnormal bleeding, and infections are common in newly diagnosed patients, who typically present within a few weeks of the onset of symptoms. Splenomegaly and lymphadenopathy are in general less prominent than in ALL, but, rarely, AML presents as a discrete tissue mass (a so-called granulocytic sarcoma). Ideally the diagnosis and classification of AML are based on the results of morphologic, histochemical, immunophenotypic, and karyotypic studies. Of these tests, karyotyping is most predictive of outcome.

Pathophysiology. Most AMLs are associated with acquired mutations in transcription factors that inhibit normal myeloid differentiation, leading to the accumulation of cells at earlier stages of development. Of particular interest is the t(15;17) translocation in acute promyelocytic leukemia. This translocation results in the fusion of the retinoic acid receptor α (*RARA*) gene on chromosome 17 with the *PML* gene on chromosome 15. The chimeric gene(s) produce abnormal PML/RARA fusion proteins that block myeloid differentiation at the promyelocytic stage, probably by inhibiting the function of normal RARA receptors. Remarkably, pharmacologic doses of retinoic acid (Chapter 8), a vitamin A analogue, overcome this block and cause the neoplastic promyelocytes to terminally differentiate into neutrophils and die. Because neutrophils live, on average, for 6 hours, the result is the rapid clearance of tumor cells and remission in a high fraction of patients. The effect is very specific; AMLs without translocations involving *RARA* do not respond to retinoic acid. Sufferers relapse if treated with retinoic acid alone, possibly because the neoplastic progenitor that gives rise to the promyelocytes is resistant to the pro-differentiative effects of retinoic acid. However, when combined with chemotherapy, the prognosis is excellent. Nonetheless, this is an important example of an effective therapy that is targeted at a tumor-specific molecular defect.

Other work using transgenic or gene knock-in mice has generally suggested that the mutated transcription factors found in AML are not sufficient, in and of themselves, to cause the disease. Complementary mutations have been described in a number of genes that have no effect on maturation but instead promote enhanced proliferation and survivial. One example is gain-of-function mutations in FLT3 (a surface receptor with tyrosine kinase activity), which are seen in a number of AML subtypes, including acute promyelocytic leukemia.

Morphology

By definition, in AML myeloid blasts or promyelocytes make up more than 20% of the bone marrow cellularity. **Myeloblasts** (precursors of granulocytes) have delicate nuclear chromatin; three to five nucleoli; and fine, azurophilic granules in the cytoplasm (see Fig. 12–14B). Distinctive red-staining rodlike structures **(Auer rods)** may be present in myeloblasts or more differentiated cells; they are particularly prevalent in the progranulocytes found in acute promyelocytic leukemia (Fig. 12–25). Auer rods are found only in neoplastic myeloblasts and are thus a helpful diagnostic clue when present. In other subtypes of AML, monoblasts, erythroblasts, or megakaryoblasts predominate.

Classification. *AMLs are diverse in terms of genetics, the predominant line of differentiation, and the maturity of cells.* The latter two features serve as the basis for the Revised French-American-British (FAB) classification (Table 12–11A), which is still used widely. However, experience has shown that the FAB classification has limited prognostic value, whereas *certain recurrent chromosomal abnormalities, prior drug exposure, and a history of a myelodyplastic syndrome are predictive of outcome.* As a result, a new WHO classification has been proposed that takes these variables into account (Table 12–11B). The FAB categories are used within the WHO classification for tumors that lack these strong prognostic factors.

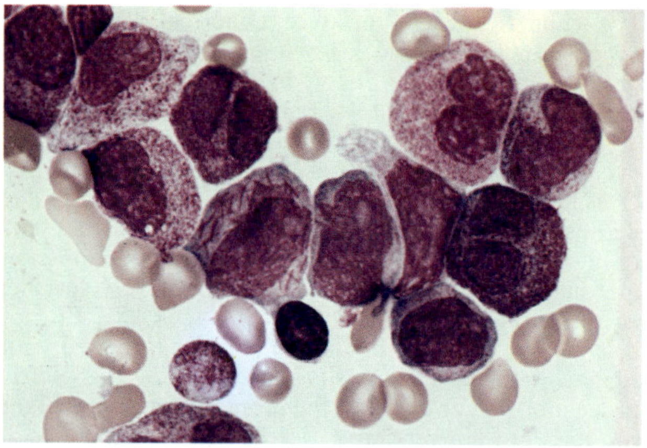

Figure 12–25

Acute promyelocytic leukemia (M3 subtype). Bone marrow aspirate shows neoplastic promyelocytes with abnormally coarse and numerous azurophilic granules. Other characteristic findings include the presence of several cells with bilobed nuclei and a cell in the center of the field that contains multiple needle-like Auer rods. (Courtesy of Dr. Robert W. McKenna, Department of Pathology, University of Texas Southwestern Medical School, Dallas, Texas.)

Histochemistry. Cases with granulocytic differentiation are typically positive for the enzyme myeloperoxidase, which is detected by incubation of cells with peroxidase substrates. Auer rods are intensely peroxidase positive, which can help bring out their presence when they are rare. Monocytic differentiation is demonstrated by staining for lysosomal nonspecific esterases.

Immunophenotype. The expression of immunologic markers is heterogeneous in AML. Most express some combination of myeloid-associated antigens, such as CD13, CD14, CD15, CD64, or CD117 (cKIT). CD33 is expressed on pluripotent stem cells but is retained on myeloid progenitor cells. Such markers are helpful in distinguishing AML from ALL (as shown in Fig. 12–14) and identifying primitive AMLs (e.g., the M0 subtype). In addition, monoclonal antibodies reactive with platelet-associated antigens are very helpful in the diagnosis of the M7 subtype, acute megakaryocytic leukemia.

Prognosis. AML is a devastating disease. Tumors with "good-risk" karyotypic aberrations (t[8;21], inv[16]) are associated with a 50% chance of long-term disease-free survival, but the overall long-term disease-free survival is only 15% to 30% with conventional chemotherapy. An increasing number of patients with AML are being treated with more aggressive approaches, such as allogeneic bone marrow transplantation.

Myelodysplastic Syndromes

In patients with these disorders, the bone marrow is partly or wholly replaced by the clonal progeny of a transformed multipotent stem cell that retains the capacity to differentiate into red cells, granulocytes, and platelets, but in a manner that is both ineffective and disordered. As a result the bone marrow is usually hypercellular or normocellular, but the peripheral blood shows one or more cytopenias. The abnormal stem cell clone in the bone marrow is genetically unstable, which leads to acquisiton of additional mutations and the eventual transformation to AML. Most cases are idiopathic, but some develop after chemotherapy with alkylating agents or exposure to ionizing radiation therapy.

Cytogenetic studies reveal that a chromosomally abnormal clone of cells is present in the marrow of as many as 70% of individuals with this disease. Some common karyotypic abnormalities include loss of chromosomes 5 or 7, or deletions of 5q or 7q. Morphologically, the marrow is populated by abnormal-appearing hematopoietic precursors. Some of the more common abnormalities include megaloblastoid erythroid precursors resembling those seen in the megaloblastic anemias, erythroid forms with iron deposits within their mitochondria (ringed sideroblasts), granulocyte precursors with abnormal granules or nuclear maturation, and small megakaryocytes with single small nuclei.

Table 12–11A Revised FAB Classification of Acute Myelogenous Leukemias (AML)

Class	Definition	Incidence (% of AML)	Morphology/Comments
M0	Minimally differentiated AML	2–3	Blasts lack Auer rods and myeloperoxidase but express myeloid lineage surface markers.
M1	AML without maturation	20	Some blasts (≥3%) are myeloperoxidase positive; few granules or Auer rods and very little maturation beyond the myeloblast stage of differentiation.
M2	AML with maturation	30–40	>20% of marrow cells are myeloblasts, but many cells are seen at later stages of granulocyte differentiation; Auer rods are usually present; often associated with t(8;21).
M3	Acute promyelocytic leukemia	5–10	Most cells are abnormal promyelocytes, often containing many Auer rods per cell; patients are younger on average (median age 35–40 yr); high incidence of DIC; strongly associated with t(15;17).
M4	Acute myelomonocytic leukemia	15–20	Myelocytic and monocytic differentiation evident by cytochemical stains; monoblasts are positive for nonspecific esterase; myeloid cells show a range of maturation; variable numbers of Auer rods; subset associated with inv(16).
M5	Acute monocytic leukemia	10	Monoblasts and immature monocytic cells (myeloperoxidase negative, nonspecific esterase positive) predominate; Auer rods are usually absent; older patients; more likely to be associated with organomegaly, lymphadenopathy, and tissue infiltration; the M5b subtype is defined by the predominance of mature-appearing monocytes in the peripheral blood, whereas only immature cells are seen in the M5a subtype.
M6	Acute erythroleukemia	5	Most commonly associated with abundant dysplastic erythroid progenitors; >20% of cells of the marrow nonerythroid cells are myeloblasts, which may contain Auer rods; usually occurs in advanced age or following exposure to mutagens (e.g., chemotherapy).
M7	Acute megakaryocytic leukemia	1	Blasts of megakaryocytic lineage predominate, as judged by expression of platelet-specific antigens; myelofibrosis or increased marrow reticulin often present; Auer rods are absent.

DIC, disseminated intravascular coagulation.

Table 12–11B Proposed WHO Classification of Acute Myelogenous Leukemia (AML)

Class	Prognosis
I. AML with Recurrent Chromosomal Translocations	
AML with t(8;21)(q22;q22); *CBFa/ETO* fusion gene	Favorable
AML with inv(16)(p13;q22); *CBFb/MYH11* fusion gene	Favorable
AML with t(15;17)(q22;q21.1); PML/RARa	Favorable
AML with t(11q23;variant)	Poor
II. AML with Multilineage Dysplasia	
With prior myelodysplastic syndrome	Very poor
Without prior myelodysplastic syndrome	Poor
III. AML, Therapy-Related	
Alkylating agent related	Very poor
Epipodophyllotoxin related	Very poor
IV. AML, Not Otherwise Classified	
Subclasses defined by extent and type of differentiation (M0–M7)	Intermediate

Most individuals with this disease are between 50 and 70 years of age. AML develops in 10% to 40%. The others suffer from infections, anemia, and hemorrhages, as a result of the defective bone marrow function. The response to chemotherapy is usually poor, lending support to the idea that myelodysplasia arises in a background of stem cell failure. It is of interest in this regard that some patients with aplastic anemia eventually develop a myelodysplastic syndrome, and a significant minority of patients with myelodysplasia respond to T-cell immunosuppressants. In this subset of patients, it is possible that the malignant clone "grows out" because normal stem cells are under attack by T cells. As discussed earlier, a similar mechanism seems to underlie paroxysmal nocturnal hemoglobinuria. The prognosis is variable; the median survival time varies from 9 to 29 months and is worse in those with increased marrow blasts or cytogenetic abnormalities at the time of diagnosis.

Chronic Myeloproliferative Disorders

These disorders are marked by the hyperproliferation of neoplastic myeloid progenitors that retain the capacity for terminal differentiation; as a result, there is an increase in one or more formed elements of the peripheral blood. The neoplastic progenitors tend to seed secondary hematopoietic organs (the spleen, liver, and lymph nodes), resulting in hepatosplenomegaly (caused by neoplastic extramedullary hematopoiesis) and mild lymphadenopathy. A common theme is the association of these disorders with mutated tyrosine kinases, which generate high-intensity constitutive signals that mimic those that regulate the growth and survival of normal myeloid cells. This insight provides a satisfying explanation for the observed overproduction of myeloid cells and is important therapeutically because of the availability of tyrosine kinase inhibitors.

Most patients with this disease subgroup fall into one of four diagnostic entities: chronic myelogenous leukemia (CML), polycythemia vera (PCV), primary myelofibrosis, and essential thrombocythemia. CML is clearly separated from the other disorders by being associated with a characteristic abnormality, the presence of a *BCR-ABL* fusion gene. In contrast, the other myeloproliferative disorders show considerable overlap clinically and genetically. Mutations of the JAK2 kinase are the single most common genetic abnormality in this group. It is seen in >90% of cases of polycythemia vera, 50% of primary myelofibrosis, and 30% of essential thrombocythemias. Additional rarer types of myeloproliferative disorders are associated with activating mutations in still other tyrosine kinases, such as platelet derived growth factor receptor alpha and beta. Thus, an evolving theme is that *most, if not all, myeloproliferative disorders are associated with an abnormal increase in the activity of one or another tyrosine kinase, which appears to stimulate the same signaling pathways that are normally activated by hematopoietic growth factors.* Only CML, PCV, and primary myelofibrosis are presented here. Essential thrombocythemia and other myeloproliferative disorders occur too infrequently to merit discussion.

Chronic Myelogenous Leukemia

CML principally affects adults between 25 and 60 years of age and accounts for 15% to 20% of all cases of leukemia. The peak incidence is in the fourth and fifth decades of life.

Pathophysiology. *CML is uniformly associated with the presence of an acquired genetic abnormality, a BCR-ABL fusion gene.* In about 95% of cases the *BCR-ABL* fusion gene is the product of a (9;22) translocation that moves the *ABL* gene from chromosome 9 to a position on chromosome 22 adjacent to the *BCR* gene. The derivative chromosome 22 is often referred to as the Philadelphia (Ph) chromosome, because it was discovered in Philadelphia. In the remaining 5% of patients, the *BCR-ABL* fusion gene is created by rearrangements that are cytogenetically cryptic or obscured by the involvement of more than two chromosomes. In individuals with CML the *BCR-ABL* fusion gene is present in granulocytic, erythroid, megakaryocytic, and B-cell precursors, and in some cases T-cell precursors as well. This finding is *firm evidence for the origin of CML from a pluripotent stem cell.* As you recall from Chapter 6, the *BCR-ABL* gene encodes a fusion protein consisting of portions of BCR and the tyrosine kinase domain of ABL that is critical for neoplastic transformation. Although the Ph chromosome is highly characteristic of CML, it should be remembered that it is also present in 25% of adults with ALL and rare cases of adults with AML.

Normal myeloid progenitors depend on signals generated by growth factors and their receptors for growth and survival, but CML progenitors have much decreased requirements. This altered growth-factor dependence is due to the presence of the BCR-ABL tyrosine kinase, which generates constitutive signals that mimic the effects of growth-factor receptor activation. Although the *BCR-ABL* fusion gene is present in multiple lineages, for unclear reasons the granulocyte precursors are most affected. As is evident from the markedly elevated number of granulocytes in the bone marrow and peripheral blood, *the proliferating CML progenitors retain the capacity for terminal differentiation.*

Morphology

The peripheral blood findings are highly characteristic. The leukocyte count is elevated, often exceeding 100,000 cells/μL. The circulating cells are **predominantly neutrophils, metamyelocytes, and myelocytes** (Fig. 12–26), but basophils and eosinophils are also prominent. A small proportion of **myeloblasts, usually less than 5%,** can be seen in the peripheral blood. An increased number of platelets (thrombocytosis) is also typical. The bone marrow is hypercellular as a result of a hyperplasia of granulocytic and megakaryocytic precursors. Myeloblasts are usually only slightly increased, and there is frequently an increase in the number of phagocytes. The red pulp of the enlarged spleen has an appearance that resembles bone marrow because of the extensive extramedullary hematopoiesis. This burgeoning mass of hematopoietic cells often compromises the local blood supply, leading to splenic infarcts.

Clinical Features. The onset of CML is usually slow, and the initial symptoms are often nonspecific (e.g., easy fatigability, weakness, and weight loss). Sometimes the first

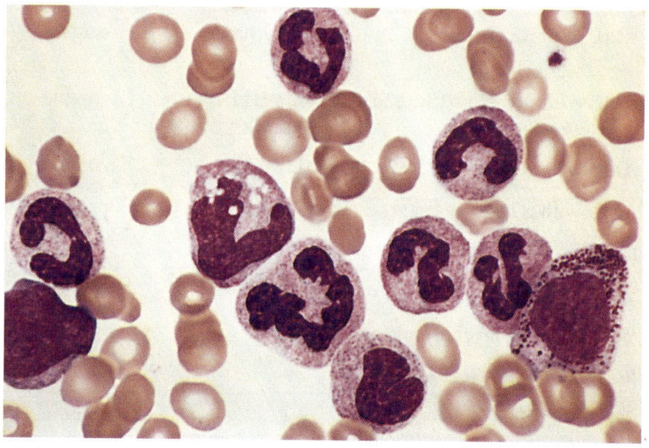

Figure 12–26

Chronic myelogenous leukemia. Peripheral blood smear shows many mature neutrophils, some metamyelocytes, and a myelocyte. (Courtesy of Dr. Robert W. McKenna, Department of Pathology, University of Texas Southwestern Medical School, Dallas, Texas.)

symptom is a dragging sensation in the abdomen, caused by the *extreme splenomegaly* that is characteristic of this condition. On occasion it may be necessary to distinguish CML from a "leukemoid reaction," a dramatic elevation of the granulocyte count in response to infection, stress, chronic inflammation, and certain neoplasms. *The presence of the Ph chromosome* is the most definitive way of distinguishing CML from leukemoid reactions (and the other chronic myeloproliferative diseases). Measurement of leukocyte alkaline phosphatase can also be helpful, because the granulocytes in CML are almost completely devoid of this enzyme, whereas it is increased in leukemoid reactions and other myeloproliferative disorders (such as PCV).

The course of CML is one of slow progression. Even without treatment, the median survival is 3 years. After a variable (and unpredictable) period, approximately 50% of individuals with CML enter an accelerated phase, during which there is a gradual failure in the response to treatment; increasing anemia and new thrombocytopenia; the appearance of additional cytogenetic abnormalities; and, finally, *transformation into a picture resembling acute leukemia* (i.e., blast crisis). In the remaining 50% blast crisis occurs abruptly, without an intermediate accelerated phase. Notably, in 30% of patients, the blast crisis is of a pre–B-cell type, further attesting to the origin of CML from a pluripotent stem cell. In the remaining 70% of patients, the blast crisis resembles AML. Less commonly, CML progresses to a phase of extensive bone marrow fibrosis resembling that seen in other myeloproliferative disorders, most notably myeloid metaplasia with myelofibrosis.

Treatment of CML is evolving rapidly. Most patients were formerly treated with palliative "gentle" chemotherapy, which unfortunately did not prevent the development of blast crisis. Bone marrow transplantation was (and remains) a definitive form of therapy, being curative in 70% of patients, but it carries a high risk of death in patients without a matched donor and in the aged. An inhibitor of the BCR-ABL tyrosine kinase, Gleevec (imantinib mesylate), induces complete remission in a high fraction of individuals with stable-phase CML with little of the toxicity associated with nonspecific chemotherapeutic agents. When CML sufferers on imantinib mesylate relapse, they often have new mutations in the active site of BCR-ABL that prevent the binding of imantinib mesylate; this proves that the drug is working by "hitting the target." Further work is needed to determine whether imantinib mesylate is curative, but it is an excellent therapy for persons who cannot undergo bone marrow transplantation and has stimulated great interest in the development of other targeted cancer therapies.

Polycythemia Vera

The hallmark of PCV is the excessive neoplastic proliferation and maturation of erythroid, granulocytic, and megakaryocytic elements, producing a *panmyelosis*. Although platelet and granulocyte numbers are increased, the most obvious clinical signs and symptoms are related to the *absolute increase in red cell mass*. This must be distinguished from *relative polycythemia*, which results from hemoconcentration. Unlike reactive forms of absolute polycythemia, PCV is associated with *low levels of erythropoietin in the serum*, which is a reflection of the hypersensitivity of the neoplastic clone to erythropoietin and other growth factors. Recently it was observed that in nearly all cases, PCV cells carry a particular mutation in JAK2, a tyrosine kinase that acts in the signaling pathways downstream of the erythropoietin receptor and other growth factor receptors. This mutation, which results in a valine-to-phenylalanine substitution at residue 617, is sufficient to render cells expressing the erythropoietic receptor hypersensitive to erythropoietin, suggesting that it is probably an important part of the pathogenesis of PCV.

Morphology

The major anatomic changes in PCV stem from the increase in blood volume and viscosity brought about by the polycythemia. Plethoric congestion of all tissues and organs is characteristic. The liver is enlarged and frequently contains foci of extramedullary hematopoiesis. The spleen is slightly enlarged (250–300 gm) in about 75% of patients, because of the vascular congestion. **As a result of the increased viscosity and vascular stasis, thromboses and infarctions are common, particularly in the heart, spleen, and kidneys.** Hemorrhages occur in about a third of these individuals, probably as a result of excessive distention of blood vessels and abnormal platelet function. They usually affect the gastrointestinal tract, oropharynx, or brain. Although these hemorrhages may occasionally be spontaneous, they more often follow some minor trauma or surgical procedure. Platelets produced from the neoplastic clone are often dysfunctional. Depending on their nature, the platelet defects can either exacerbate the tendency for thrombosis or lead to abnormal bleeding. As in CML, the peripheral blood often shows increased basophils.

The bone marrow is hypercellular due to the hyperplasia of erythroid, myeloid, and megakaryocytic forms. In addition, some degree of marrow fibrosis is present in 10% of patients at the time of diagnosis. In a subset of patients, the disease progresses to myelofibrosis, where the marrow space is largely replaced by fibroblasts and collagen.

Clinical Course. PCV appears insidiously, usually in late middle age. Patients are plethoric and often somewhat cyanotic. Histamine release from the neoplastic basophils may contribute to *pruritus*, which can be intense. Excessive histamine release may also account for the *peptic ulceration* seen in these individuals. Other complaints are referable to the thrombotic and hemorrhagic tendencies and to hypertension. *Headache, dizziness, gastrointestinal symptoms, hematemesis, and melena are common.* Because of the high rate of cell turnover, symptomatic gout is seen in 5% to 10% of cases, and many more patients have asymptomatic hyperuricemia.

The diagnosis is usually made in the laboratory. Red cell counts range from 6 to 10 million per microliter, and the hematocrit often approaches 60%. The other myeloid lineages are also hyperproliferative: the granulocyte count can be as high as 50,000 cells/mm^3, and the platelet count is often greater than 400,000 cells/mm^3. The basophil count is also frequently elevated. The platelets are functionally abnormal in most cases, and giant forms and megakaryocyte fragments are seen in the blood. About 30% of patients develop *thrombotic complications,* usually affecting the brain or heart. Hepatic vein thrombosis, giving rise to the Budd-Chiari syndrome (Chapter 16), is an uncommon but grave complication. Minor *hemorrhages* (e.g., epistaxis and bleeding from gums) are common, and life-threatening hemorrhages occur in 5% to 10% of patients. In those receiving no treatment, death occurs from vascular complications within months after diagnosis; however, if the red cell mass is maintained at near normal levels by phlebotomies, the median survival is around 10 years.

Prolonged survival with treatment has revealed that PCV tends to evolve to a "spent phase," during which the clinical and anatomic features of primary myelofibrosis develop. After an average interval of 10 years, 15% to 20% of tumors undergo such a transformation. This transition is marked by creeping fibrosis in the bone marrow and a shift of hematopoiesis to the spleen, which enlarges markedly. Transformation to a "blast crisis" identical to AML also occurs but much less frequently than in CML. Targeted molecular therapy with JAK2 inhibitors is presently under consideration.

Myeloid Metaplasia with Primary Myelofibrosis

In this chronic myeloproliferative disorder, a "spent phase" of marrow fibrosis supervenes early in the disease course, often following a brief period in which the peripheral blood white cell and platelet counts are elevated. As hematopoiesis shifts from the fibrotic marrow to the spleen, liver, and lymph nodes, extreme splenomegaly and hepatomegaly develop. Hematopoiesis in these extramedullary sites tends to be disordered and inefficient and, together with the marrow fibrosis, leads to moderate-to-severe anemia and thrombocytopenia in most patients.

Although marrow fibrosis is characteristic, the fibroblasts that lay down the collagen are not clonal descendants of the transformed stem cells. Instead, marrow fibrosis is secondary to derangements confined to the hematopoietic cells, particularly the megakaryocytes. It is believed that *marrow fibroblasts are stimulated to proliferate by platelet-derived growth factor and transforming growth factor β* released from neoplastic megakaryocytes. These two growth factors are known to be mitogenic for fibroblasts. By the time patients come to clinical attention, marrow fibrosis and marked extramedullary hematopoiesis are usually evident. More uncommonly, marrow fibrosis is less advanced at diagnosis, and the clinical picture resembles that seen in other "hyperproliferative" myeloproliferative disorders.

It is of pathogenic and possibly therapeutic importance that the same JAK2 mutation that is found in PCV (a valine-to-phenylalanine mutation at amino residue 617) is present in around half of the cases of primary myelofibrosis (as well as a similar proportion of individuals with essential thrombocytosis), findings that emphasize the extent of the overlap between these entities. It is not yet known why tumors with the same mutation have such varied clinical pictures. Perhaps the JAK2 mutation occurs in a different stem cell population in primary myelofibrosis, or the unknown mutations that promote progression to the spent phase occur much earlier in some individuals by chance.

Morphology

The principal site of the extramedullary hematopoiesis in myeloid metaplasia with primary myelofibrosis is the **spleen,** which is usually markedly enlarged, sometimes weighing as much as 4000 gm. As is always true when splenomegaly is massive, multiple **subcapsular infarcts** are often present. Histologically the spleen contains normoblasts, granulocyte precursors, and megakaryocytes, which are often prominent in terms of their numbers and bizarre morphology. Sometimes disproportional activity of any one of the three major cell lines is seen.

The **liver** is often moderately enlarged, with foci of extramedullary hematopoiesis. Microscopically, the **lymph nodes** also contain foci of extramedullary hematopoiesis, but these are insufficient to cause appreciable enlargement.

The **bone marrow** in a typical case is **hypocellular and diffusely fibrotic.** However, early in the course the marrow can be hypercellular, with equal representation of the three major cell lines. Both early and late in the disease, megakaryocytes are often prominent and are usually dysplastic.

Clinical Course. Primary myelofibrosis can begin with a blood picture suggestive of PCV or CML, but it more commonly has progressed to marrow fibrosis by the time it comes to clinical attention. Most patients have moderate-to-severe anemia. The white cell count can be normal, reduced, or markedly elevated. Early in the disease course, the platelet count is normal or elevated, but eventually patients develop thrombocytopenia. The *peripheral blood smear appears markedly abnormal* (Fig. 12–27). Red cell abnormalities include bizarre shapes (poikilocytes, teardrop cells). Nucleated erythroid precursors are often found in the peripheral blood as well. Immature white cells (myelocytes and metamyelocytes) are also seen, and basophils are sometimes increased as well. The presence of nucleated red cell precursors and immature white cells is referred to as *leukoerythrocytosis.* Platelets are often abnormal in size and shape and defective in function. In some cases the clinical and blood picture resembles CML, but the *Ph chromosome is absent.* Because of a high rate of cell turnover, *hyperuricemia and gout* may also complicate the picture.

The outcome of this disease is variable, but the median survival time is 4 to 5 years. There is a constant threat of infections, as well as thrombotic and hemorrhagic episodes stemming from platelet abnormalities. Splenic infarctions are common. In 5% to 15% of individuals, there is eventually a blast crisis resembling AML.

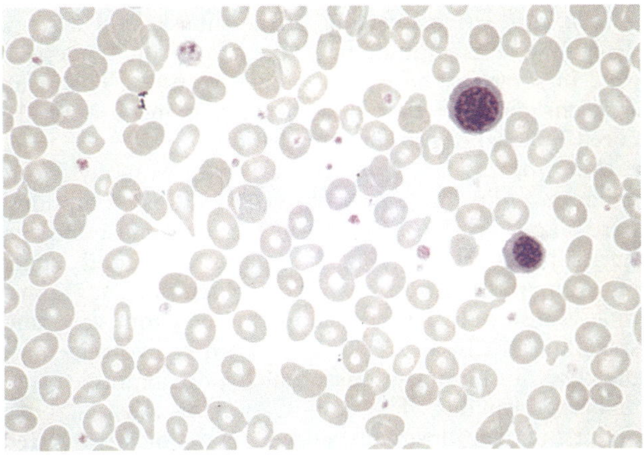

Figure 12–27

Myelofibrosis with myeloid metaplasia (peripheral blood smear). Two nucleated erythroid precursors and several teardrop-shaped red cells (dacryocytes) are evident. Immature myeloid cells were present in other fields. An identical picture can be seen in other diseases producing marrow distortion and fibrosis.

SUMMARY

Myeloid Neoplasms

Myeloid tumors are mainly tumors of adults that fall into three groups.

- *Acute Myelogenous Leukemias* (AML):
  - Collection of aggressive tumors that are comprised of immature myeloid lineage cells (myeloblasts), which replace the marrow and suppress normal hematopoiesis.
  - AML cells contain diverse genetic lesions that often lead to the expression of abnormal transcription factors that block myeloid cell differentiation.
- *Chronic Myeloproliferative Disorders*:
  - Indolent tumors in which production of cells is initially increased, leading to high blood counts and extramedullary hematopoiesis
  - Commonly associated with acquired genetic lesions that lead to constitutive activation of tyrosine kinases, which mimic signals from normal growth factors; treated with kinase inhibitors.
  - Two main types are:
    - *Chronic Myelogenous Leukemia* (CML): myeloid tumor arising from a pluripotent stem cell; associated with chromosome rearrangements that cause the formation of a *BCR-ABL* fusion gene, which encodes a constitutively active tyrosine kinase; causes increased hematopoiesis, particularly in the granulocytic and thrombocytic lineages; if untreated, inevitably progresses to a blast crisis phase that can resemble either AML or lymphoblastic leukemia.
    - *Polycythemia Vera*: myeloid tumor associated with point mutations that activate JAK2, a tyrosine kinase; causes increased hematopoiesis with high white cell, platelet, and red cell counts; the latter is responsible for most of the clinical symptoms.
- *Myelodysplastic Syndromes*: group of myeloid tumors characterized by disordered and ineffective hematopoiesis. Most patients present with pancytopenia, and many progress to a disease state that is identical to AML.
  - *Myeloid Metaplasia with Myelofibrosis* is the most common myelodysplastic syndrome. It is a myeloid tumor in which abnormal megakaryocytes release growth factors that stimulate reactive marrow fibroblasts to deposit collagen, and the resulting fibrosis slowly replaces the marrow space, leading to pancytopenia and extramedullary hematopoiesis, which can produce massive splenomegaly.

Histiocytic Neoplasms

Langerhans Cell Histiocytoses

The term *histiocytosis* is an "umbrella" designation for a variety of proliferative disorders of histiocytes, or macrophages. Some, such as very rare histiocytic lymphomas, are clearly malignant neoplasms. Others, such as most histiocytic proliferations in lymph nodes, are completely benign and reactive. Between these two extremes lies a group of relatively rare tumors, *the Langerhans cell histiocytoses,* which are derived from Langerhans cells. You will recall that the Langerhans cell is an immature dendritic cell that is found normally in many organs, most prominently the skin (Chapter 5).

These proliferations take on different clinical forms, but all are believed to be variations of the same basic disorder. The proliferating Langerhans cells are human leukocyte antigen DR (HLA-DR) positive and express the CD1 antigen. *Characteristically, these cells have HX bodies (Birbeck granules) in their cytoplasm. Under the electron microscope these are seen to have a pentalaminar, rodlike, tubular structure, with characteristic periodicity and sometimes a dilated terminal end ("tennis racket" appearance).* Under the light microscope the proliferating Langerhans cells in these disorders do not resemble their normal dendritic counterparts. Instead, they have abundant, often vacuolated, cytoplasm with vesicular nuclei. This appearance is more akin to that of tissue histiocytes (macrophages), hence the term *Langerhans cell histiocytosis.*

Acute disseminated Langerhans cell histiocytosis (Letterer-Siwe disease) usually occurs in children younger than 2 years of age but may occasionally been seen in adults. The dominant clinical feature is the development of multifocal cutaneous lesions composed of Langerhans cells that grossly resemble seborrheic skin eruptions. Most of those affected have concurrent hepatosplenomegaly, lymphadenopathy, pulmonary lesions, and, eventually, destructive osteolytic bone lesions. Extensive infiltration of the marrow often leads to anemia, thrombocytopenia, and predisposition to recurrent infections such as otitis media and mastoiditis. Thus, the clinical picture may resemble that of an acute leukemia. The course of untreated disease is rapidly fatal. With intensive chemotherapy, 50% of patients survive 5 years.

Both unifocal and multifocal Langerhans cell histiocytosis (unifocal and multifocal eosinophilic granuloma) are characterized by expanding, erosive accumulations of Langerhans cells, usually within the medullary cavities of bones. Histiocytes are variably admixed with eosinophils, lymphocytes, plasma cells, and neutrophils. The eosinophilic component ranges from scattered mature cells to sheetlike masses of cells. Virtually any bone in the skeletal system may be involved; the calvarium, ribs, and femur are most commonly affected. Similar lesions may be found in the skin, lungs, or stomach, either as unifocal lesions or as components of the multifocal disease.

Unifocal lesions usually affect the skeletal system. They may be asymptomatic or cause pain and tenderness and, in some instances, pathologic fractures. This is an indolent disorder that may heal spontaneously or be cured by local excision or irradiation.

Multifocal Langerhans cell histiocytosis usually affects children, who present with fever; diffuse eruptions, particularly on the scalp and in the ear canals; and frequent bouts of otitis media, mastoiditis, and upper respiratory tract infections. The proliferation may sometimes cause mild lymphadenopathy, hepatomegaly, and splenomegaly. In about 50% of patients, involvement of the posterior pituitary stalk of the hypothalamus leads to diabetes insipidus. The combination of calvarial bone defects, diabetes insipidus, and exophthalmos is referred to as the *Hand-Schüller-Christian triad.* Many patients experience spontaneous regressions; others are treated effectively with chemotherapy.

BLEEDING DISORDERS

These disorders are characterized clinically by abnormal bleeding, which can either be spontaneous or become evident after some inciting event (e.g., trauma or surgery). It should be recalled from the discussion in Chapter 4 that the normal hemostatic response involves the blood vessel wall, the platelets, and the clotting cascade, and abnormalities in any of these three components can be associated with clinically significant bleeding. Before embarking on a discussion of disorders of coagulation, we should first review normal hemostasis and the common laboratory tests used in the evaluation of a bleeding diathesis. The various tests used in the initial evaluation of patients with bleeding disorders are as follows:

- *Bleeding time.* This represents the time taken for a standardized skin puncture to stop bleeding. Measured in minutes, this procedure provides an in vivo assessment of platelet response to limited vascular injury. The reference range depends on the actual method used and varies from 2 to 9 minutes. It is abnormal when there is a defect in platelet numbers or function. Bleeding time is fraught with variability and poor reproducibility. Hence, new instrument-based assays that provide quantitative measures of platelet function are being introduced.
- *Platelet counts.* These are obtained on anticoagulated blood by using an electronic particle counter. The reference range is 150×10^3 to 450×10^3 cells/mm^3. Counts outside this range must be confirmed by a visual inspection of a peripheral blood smear.
- *Prothrombin time (PT).* This procedure tests the adequacy of the extrinsic and common coagulation pathways. It represents the time needed for plasma to clot in the presence of an exogenously added source of tissue thromboplastin (e.g., brain extract) and Ca^{2+} ions. A prolonged PT can result from a deficiency of factors V, VII, or X, prothrombin, or fibrinogen.
- *Partial thromboplastin time (PTT).* This test is designed to assess the integrity of the intrinsic and common clotting pathways. In this test the time needed for the plasma to clot in the presence of kaolin, cephalin, and calcium is measured. Kaolin serves to activate the contact-dependent factor XII, and cephalin substitutes for platelet phospholipids. Prolongation of PTT can be caused by a deficiency of factors V, VIII, IX, X, XI, or XII or prothrombin or fibrinogen or an acquired inhibitor (typically an antibody) that interferes with the intrinsic pathway.

Additional, more specialized tests are available that measure the levels of specific clotting factors, fibrinogen, and fibrin split products; assess the presence of circulating anticoagulants; and evaluate platelet function. With this overview we can return to the three important categories of bleeding disorders.

Abnormalities of vessels can contribute to bleeding in several ways. *Increased fragility* of the vessels is associated with severe vitamin C deficiency (scurvy) (Chapter 8), systemic amyloidosis (Chapter 5), chronic glucocorticoid use, rare inherited conditions affecting the connective tissues, and a large number of infectious and hypersensitivity vasculitides. The latter include meningococcemia, infective endocarditis, the rickettsial diseases, typhoid, and Henoch-Schönlein purpura. Some of these conditions are discussed in other chapters; others are beyond the scope of this book. A hemorrhagic diathesis that is purely the result of vascular fragility is characterized by the apparently spontaneous appearance of petechiae and ecchymoses in the skin and mucous membranes (probably resulting from minor trauma). In most instances, the laboratory tests of coagulation are normal. *Bleeding can also be triggered by systemic conditions that activate or damage endothelial cells.* If severe enough, such insults convert the vascular lining to a prothrombotic surface that activates coagulation throughout the circulatory system. Paradoxically, in such *consumptive coagulopathies* platelets and coagulation factors are used up faster than they can be replaced, and the resulting deficiencies (which are readily identified in laboratory tests of coagulation) often lead to severe bleeding.

Deficiencies of platelets (thrombocytopenia) are important causes of hemorrhage. They can occur in a variety of clinical settings that are discussed later. Other disorders are characterized by *qualitative defects in platelet function*. These include defects that are *acquired*, as in uremia, after aspirin ingestion, and in certain myeloproliferative disorders, or *inherited*, as in von Willebrand disease and other rare congenital disorders. The clinical signs of inadequate platelet function include easy bruising, nosebleeds, excessive bleeding from minor trauma, and menorrhagia. The PT and PTT are normal, but *the bleeding time is prolonged.*

Bleeding diatheses based purely on a *derangement of blood clotting* differ in several respects from those resulting from defects in the vessel walls or in platelets. The PT, PTT, or both, are prolonged, whereas the bleeding time is normal. Petechiae and other evidence of bleeding from very minor surface trauma are usually absent. However, massive hemorrhage can occur subsequent to operative or dental procedures or severe trauma. Moreover, hemorrhages into areas of the body subject to trauma, such as the joints of the lower extremities, are characteristic. This category includes the hemophilias, an important group of inherited coagulation disorders.

Disseminated intravascular coagulation, one of the most common consumptive coagulopathies, presents with laboratory and clinical features related to both thrombocytopenia and coagulation factor deficiencies. Von Willebrand disease is a fairly common inherited disorder in which both platelet and (to a lesser degree) coagulation factor function are abnormal. With this as an overview, we will now turn to specific bleeding disorders.

DISSEMINATED INTRAVASCULAR COAGULATION

An acute, subacute, or chronic thrombohemorrhagic disorder, disseminated intravascular coagulation (DIC) occurs as a secondary complication in a variety of diseases. *It is caused by the systemic activation of the coagulation pathways, leading to the formation of thrombi throughout the microcirculation. As a consequence of the widespread thromboses, there is consumption of platelets and coagulation factors and, secondarily, activation of fibrinolysis.* Thus, DIC can give rise to either tissue hypoxia and microinfarcts caused by myriad microthrombi or to a bleeding disorder related to pathologic activation of fibrinolysis and the depletion of the elements required for hemostasis (hence the term *consumptive coagulopathy*). This entity is probably a more common cause of bleeding than all of the congenital coagulation disorders combined.

Etiology and Pathogenesis. Before presenting the specific disorders associated with DIC, we will discuss in a general way the pathogenetic mechanisms by which intravascular clotting can occur. Reference to earlier comments on normal blood coagulation (Chapter 4) may be helpful at this point. It suffices here to recall that clotting can be initiated by either of two pathways: the extrinsic pathway, which is triggered by the release of tissue factor (tissue thromboplastin), or the intrinsic pathway, which involves the activation of factor XII by surface contact, collagen, or other negatively charged substances. Both pathways lead to the generation of thrombin. Clot-inhibiting influences include the rapid clearance of activated clotting factors by the mononuclear phagocytic system or by the liver, activation of endogenous anticoagulants (e.g., protein C), and activation of fibrinolysis.

Two major mechanisms can trigger DIC: (1) the release of tissue factor or thromboplastic substances into the circulation, and (2) widespread endothelial cell damage (Fig. 12–28). Thromboplastic substances can be released into the circulation from a variety of sources—for example, the placenta in obstetric complications, the cytoplasmic granules of acute promyelocytic leukemia cells, or mucin-secreting adenocarcinoma cells. Carcinomas can also release other procoagulant substances, such as proteolytic enzymes, and other still-undefined tumor products. Some tumors express tissue factor on the cell membrane. In gram-negative and gram-positive sepsis (important causes of DIC), endotoxins or exotoxins cause increased synthesis, surface expression, and release of tissue factor from monocytes. Furthermore, activated monocytes release IL-1 and tumor necrosis factor, both of which increase the expression of tissue factor on endothelial cells and simultaneously decrease the expression of thrombomodulin. The latter, you may recall, activates protein C, an anticoagulant (Chapter 4). The net result is the enhanced activation of the extrinsic clotting system and the blunting of inhibitory pathways that tend to prevent coagulation.

Severe endothelial cell injury can initiate DIC by causing the release of tissue factor and by exposing subendothelial collagen and von Willebrand factor (vWF), which act together to promote platelet aggregation and the activation of the intrinsic coagulation cascade. Even subtle endothelial damage can unleash procoagulant activity by stimulating the increased expression of tissue factor on endothelial cell surfaces. Widespread endothelial injury can be produced by the deposition of antigen-antibody complexes (e.g., in SLE), by temperature extremes (e.g., following heat stroke or burns), or by infections (e.g., meningococci and rickettsiae). As discussed in Chapter 4, endothelial injury is an important consequence of endotoxemia, and, not surprisingly, DIC is a frequent complication of gram-negative sepsis.

Several additional disorders associated with DIC are listed in Table 12–12. Of these, *DIC is most likely to occur after sepsis, obstetric complications, malignancy, and major trauma (especially trauma to the brain).* The initiating events in these conditions are multiple and often

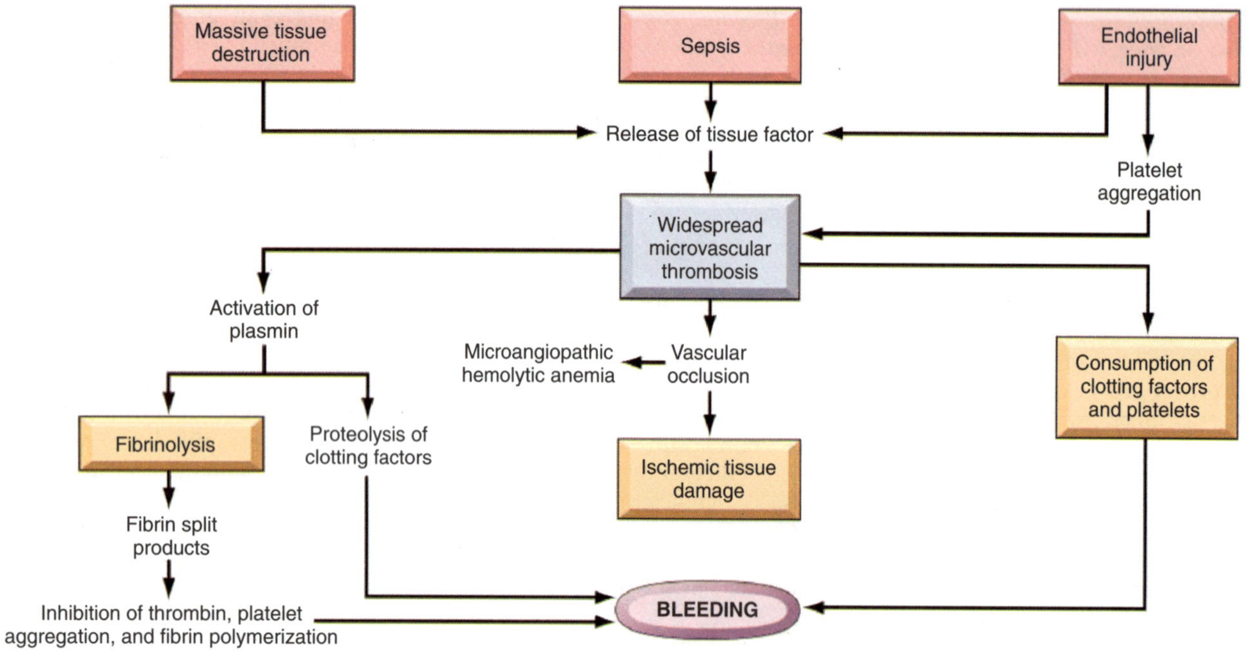

Figure 12–28

Pathophysiology of disseminated intravascular coagulation.

interrelated. For example, in obstetric conditions, tissue factor derived from the placenta, retained dead fetus, or amniotic fluid enters the circulation; however, shock, hypoxia, and acidosis often coexist and can lead to widespread endothelial injury. Trauma to the brain releases fat and phospholipids, which can act as contact factors and thereby activate the intrinsic arm of the coagulation cascade.

Table 12–12 Major Disorders Associated with Disseminated Intravascular Coagulation

Obstetric Complications	
	Abruptio placentae
	Retained dead fetus
	Septic abortion
	Amniotic fluid embolism
	Toxemia
Infections	
	Sepsis (gram-negative and gram-positive)
	Meningococcemia
	Rocky Mountain spotted fever
	Histoplasmosis
	Aspergillosis
	Malaria
Neoplasms	
	Carcinomas of pancreas, prostate, lung, and stomach
	Acute promyelocytic leukemia
Massive Tissue Injury	
	Trauma
	Burns
	Extensive surgery
Miscellaneous	
	Acute intravascular hemolysis, snakebite, giant hemangioma, shock, heat stroke, vasculitis, aortic aneurysm, liver disease

Whatever the pathogenetic mechanism, DIC has two consequences. First, *there is widespread fibrin deposition within the microcirculation.* This leads to ischemia in the more severely affected or vulnerable organs and to hemolysis as red cells are traumatized while passing through vessels narrowed by fibrin thrombi (*microangiopathic hemolytic anemia*). Second, a *bleeding diathesis* results from the depletion of platelets and clotting factors and the secondary release of plasminogen activators. Plasmin cleaves not only fibrin (fibrinolysis) but also factors V and VIII, thereby reducing their concentration further. In addition, fibrinolysis creates fibrin degradation products, which inhibit platelet aggregation, have antithrombin activity, and impair fibrin polymerization, all of which contribute to the hemostatic failure (see Fig. 12–28).

Morphology

In DIC **microthrombi** are found principally in the arterioles and capillaries of the kidneys, adrenals, brain, and heart, but no organ is spared, and the lungs, liver, and gastrointestinal mucosa can be prominently involved. The glomeruli contain small fibrin thrombi. These may be associated with only a subtle, reactive swelling of the endothelial cells, or varying degrees of focal glomerulitis. The microvascular occlusions lead to small infarcts in the renal cortex. In severe cases, the ischemia can destroy the entire cortex and cause bilateral renal cortical necrosis. Involvement of the adrenal glands can produce the **Waterhouse-Friderichsen**

syndrome (Chapter 20). Microinfarcts are also commonly encountered in the brain, surrounded by microscopic or gross foci of hemorrhage. These can give rise to bizarre neurologic signs. Similar changes are seen in the heart and often in the anterior pituitary. It has been suggested that DIC contributes to **Sheehan postpartum pituitary necrosis** (Chapter 20).

When the underlying disorder is toxemia of pregnancy, the placenta is the site of capillary thromboses and, occasionally, florid degeneration of the vessel walls. Such changes are in all likelihood responsible for the premature loss of cytotrophoblasts and syncytiotrophoblasts that characterizes this condition.

The bleeding tendency associated with DIC is manifested not only by larger than expected hemorrhages near foci of infarction but also by diffuse petechiae and ecchymoses, which can be found on the skin, serosal linings of the body cavities, epicardium, endocardium, lungs, and mucosal lining of the urinary tract.

Clinical Course. As might be imagined, depending on the balance between clotting and bleeding tendencies, the range of possible clinical manifestations is enormous. In general, *acute DIC (e.g., that associated with obstetric complications) is dominated by a bleeding diathesis, whereas chronic DIC (e.g., as occurs in an individual with cancer) tends to present with symptoms related to thrombosis.* Typically, the abnormal clotting occurs only in the microcirculation, although large vessels are involved occasionally. The manifestations may be minimal, or there may be shock, with acute renal failure, dyspnea, cyanosis, convulsions, and coma. Most often, attention is called to the presence of DIC by prolonged and copious postpartum bleeding or by the presence of petechiae and ecchymoses on the skin. These may be the only manifestations, or there may be severe hemorrhage into the gut or urinary tract. Laboratory evaluation reveals *thrombocytopenia and prolongation of PT and PTT* (resulting from depletion of platelets, clotting factors, and fibrinogen). Fibrin split products are increased in the plasma.

The prognosis for patients with DIC is highly variable, and depends on the nature of the underlying disorder and the severity of the intravascular clotting and fibrinolysis. In some acute cases it can be life-threatening and must be treated aggressively with anticoagulants such as heparin or the coagulants contained in fresh-frozen plasma. Conversely, in more chronic forms DIC is sometimes identified as a laboratory abnormality. In either circumstance, definitive treatment must be directed at the cause of the DIC, not at its hemostatic consequences.

THROMBOCYTOPENIA

Thrombocytopenia is characterized by spontaneous bleeding, a prolonged bleeding time, and a normal PT and PTT. A platelet count of 100,000 cells/μL or less is generally considered to constitute thrombocytopenia. Platelet counts in the range of 20,000 to 50,000 cells/μL are associated with an increased risk of post-traumatic bleeding, and spontaneous bleeding becomes evident when counts fall below 20,000 cells/μL. Most bleeding tends to occur from small, superficial blood vessels and produces petechiae or large ecchymoses in the skin, the mucous membranes of the gastrointestinal and urinary tracts, and other sites. Larger hemorrhages into the central nervous system are a major hazard in patients with markedly depressed platelet counts.

The major causes of thrombocytopenia are listed in Table 12–13. Clinically important thrombocytopenias are confined to those disorders in which there is reduced production or increased destruction of platelets. In most cases in which the cause is accelerated destruction, the bone marrow reveals a compensatory increase in the number of megakaryocytes. Hence, bone marrow examination can help to distinguish the two major categories of thrombocytopenia. It is also worth emphasizing that *thrombocytopenia is one of the most common hematologic manifestations of AIDS.* It can occur early in the course of HIV infection and has multifactorial bases, including immune complex–mediated platelet destruction, antiplatelet autoantibodies, and HIV-mediated suppression of megakaryocyte development and survival.

Immune Thrombocytopenic Purpura

Immune thrombocytopenic purpura (ITP), also called idiopathic thrombocytopenic purpura, can occur in the setting of a variety of conditions and exposures (secondary ITP) or in the absence of any known risk factors (primary or idiopathic ITP). There are two clinical sub-

Table 12–13 Causes of Thrombocytopenia

Decreased Production of Platelets
Generalized disease of bone marrow
Aplastic anemia: congenital and acquired
Marrow infiltration: leukemia, disseminated cancer
Selective impairment of platelet production
Drug-induced: alcohol, thiazides, cytotoxic drugs
Infections: measles, HIV infection
Ineffective megakaryopoiesis
Megaloblastic anemia
Paroxysmal nocturnal hemoglobinuria
Decreased Platelet Survival
Immunologic destruction
Autoimmune: immune thrombocytopenic purpura, systemic lupus erythematosus
Isoimmune: post-transfusion and neonatal
Drug-associated: quinidine, heparin, sulfa compounds
Infections: infectious mononucleosis, HIV infection, cytomegalovirus infection
Nonimmunologic destruction
Disseminated intravascular coagulation
Thrombotic thrombocytopenic purpura
Giant hemangiomas
Microangiopathic hemolytic anemias
Sequestration
Hypersplenism
Dilutional

HIV, human immunodeficiency virus.

types of primary ITP: chronic primary ITP, a relatively common disorder that tends to affect adult females between the ages of 20 and 40 years; and acute ITP, a self-limited form that is most commonly seen in children subsequent to viral infections.

Antiplatelet immunoglobulins directed against platelet membrane glycoproteins IIb/IIIa or Ib/IX complexes can be identified in 80% of patients with chronic ITP. The spleen is an important site of antiplatelet antibody production and the major site of destruction of the IgG-coated platelets. It is usually normal in size and shows only subtle evidence of increased platelet destruction; thus, splenic enlargement or lymphadenopathy should lead one to consider other possible diagnoses. Nonetheless, the importance of the spleen in this disorder is confirmed by the clinical benefits produced by splenectomy, which normalizes the platelet count and induces a complete remission in more than two-thirds of patients. The bone marrow usually contains increased numbers of megakaryocytes, a finding that is common to all forms of thrombocytopenia that are caused by accelerated platelet destruction. A marrow examination can be helpful in excluding marrow failure as a cause of the thrombocytopenia.

The onset of chronic ITP is insidious. Common findings include petechiae, easy bruisability, epistaxis, gum bleeding, and hemorrhages after minor trauma. Fortunately, more serious intracerebral or subarachnoid hemorrhages occur much less commonly. The diagnosis rests on the clinical features, the presence of thrombocytopenia, examination of the marrow, and the exclusion of secondary ITP. Reliable clinical tests for antiplatelet antibodies are not widely available.

Heparin-Induced Thrombocytopenia

This special type of drug-induced thrombocytopenia merits brief mention because of its clinical importance. Moderate to severe thrombocytopenia develops in 3% to 5% of individuals treated with unfractionated heparin after 1 to 2 weeks of therapy. The disorder is caused by IgG antibodies that bind to platelet factor IV on platelet surfaces in a heparin-dependent fashion. This activates platelets and induces their aggregation, thus exacerbating the condition that heparin is used to treat—thrombosis. Both venous and arterial thromboses occur, even in the setting of marked thrombocytopenia, and can cause severe morbidity (e.g., loss of limbs because of vascular insufficiency) and death. Cessation of heparin therapy breaks the cycle of platelet activation and consumption.

Thrombotic Microangiopathies: Thrombotic Thrombocytopenic Purpura and Hemolytic-Uremic Syndrome

The term *thrombotic microangiopathies* encompasses a spectrum of clinical syndromes that include thrombotic thrombocytopenic purpura (TTP) and hemolytic-uremic syndrome (HUS). As originally defined, TTP is associated with the pentad of fever, thrombocytopenia, microangiopathic hemolytic anemia, transient neurologic deficits, and renal failure. HUS is also associated with microangiopathic hemolytic anemia and thrombocytopenia but is distinguished from TTP by the absence of neurologic symptoms, the dominance of acute renal failure, and an onset in childhood (Chapter 14). Clinical experience has blurred these distinctions, because many adults with TTP lack one or more of the five criteria, and some patients with HUS have fever and neurologic dysfunction. *Fundamental to both of these conditions is the widespread formation of hyaline thrombi in the microcirculation that are composed primarily of dense aggregates of platelets surrounded by fibrin.* The consumption of platelets leads to thrombocytopenia, and the narrowing of blood vessels by the platelet-rich thrombi results in a microangiopathic hemolytic anemia.

For many years the pathogenesis of TTP was enigmatic, although treatment with plasma exchange (initiated in the early 1970s) converted it from a disease that was almost uniformly fatal to one that is successfully treated in more than 80% of individuals. Recently, the underlying cause of most cases of TTP has been elucidated. In brief, *symptomatic patients are deficient in a metalloprotease called ADAMTS13.* This enzyme degrades very-high-molecular-weight multimer of vWF, and hence the absence of ADAMTS13 activity allows multimers of vWF to accumulate in plasma. Under some circumstances, these colossal vWF multimers promote platelet microaggregate formation throughout the circulation. The superimposition of an endothelial cell injury (caused by some other condition) can further promote microaggregate formation, thus initiating or exacerbating clinically evident TTP.

The deficiency of ADAMTS13 activity can be an inherited condition, but it is more commonly caused by an acquired autoantibody that binds and inhibits the metalloprotease. TTP must be considered in any individual who presents with unexplained thrombocytopenia and microangiopathic hemolytic anemia, because the failure to make an early diagnosis can be fatal.

Although clinically similar to TTP, HUS has a different basis, because ADAMTS13 levels are normal in this disorder. HUS in children and the elderly usually occurs subsequent to infectious gastroenteritis caused by *E. coli* strain O157:H7. This organism elaborates a Shiga-like toxin that damages endothelial cells, which initiates platelet activation and aggregation. Affected individuals often present with bloody diarrhea, which is followed a few days later by HUS. With supportive care and plasma exchange, recovery is possible, but irreversible renal damage and death can occur in more severe cases. About 10% of cases in children are not preceded by infection with Shiga toxin-producing bacteria. Some of these patients have mutations in the gene encoding complement regulatory proteins, notably factor H. Deficiency of this protein leads to uncontrolled complement activation after minor endothelial injury, resulting in thrombosis. HUS can also be seen after exposures to other factors (e.g., certain drugs, radiation therapy) that damage endothelial cells. Here the prognosis is more guarded, in part because the underlying conditions are often chronic or life-threatening.

Although DIC and the thrombotic microangiopathies share features such as microvascular occlusion and microangiopathic hemolytic anemia, they are pathogenetically distinct. In TTP and HUS, unlike in DIC, activation of the coagulation cascade is not of primary importance, and thus the laboratory tests of coagulation (such as the PT and the PTT) are usually normal.

COAGULATION DISORDERS

These disorders result from either congenital or acquired deficiencies of clotting factors. Most common are the *acquired coagulation factor deficiencies,* which typically affect many factors simultaneously. As was discussed in Chapter 8, *vitamin K* is essential for the synthesis of prothrombin and clotting factors VII, IX, and X, and its deficiency causes a severe coagulation defect. The liver is the site of both the synthesis of several coagulation factors and the removal of many activated coagulation factors; thus, *parenchymal diseases of the liver* are common causes of complex hemorrhagic diatheses.

Hereditary deficiencies have been identified for each of the coagulation factors. These deficiencies characteristically occur singly. Hemophilia A, resulting from deficiency of factor VIII, and hemophilia B (Christmas disease), resulting from deficiency of factor IX, are transmitted as X-linked recessive disorders, whereas most others are autosomal disorders. These inherited deficiencies are rare; only von Willebrand disease, hemophilia A, and hemophilia B are sufficiently common to warrant further consideration here.

Deficiencies of Factor VIII–vWF Complex

Hemophilia A and von Willebrand disease, two of the most common inherited disorders of bleeding, are caused by qualitative or quantitative defects involving the factor VIII–vWF complex. Before we can discuss these disorders, it is useful to review the structure and function of these proteins.

Plasma factor VIII–vWF complex is made up of two proteins (Fig. 12–29). One, which is required for the activation of factor X in the intrinsic coagulation pathway, is called *factor VIII procoagulant protein,* or *factor VIII.* Deficiency of factor VIII gives rise to hemophilia A. Factor VIII is associated noncovalently with a much larger protein, vWF, that forms high-molecular-weight multimers of sizes that range as high as 20 megadaltons. vWF is found normally in the plasma (in association with factor VIII), in platelet granules, in endothelial cells in unusual cytoplasmic vesicles called Weibel-Palade bodies, and in the subendothelium, where it binds to collagen.

When endothelial cells are stripped away by trauma or injury, subendothelial vWF becomes exposed and binds to platelets through the receptors glycoproteins Ib and IIb/IIIa (see Fig. 12–29). *The most important function of vWF is to facilitate the adhesion of platelets to damaged blood vessel walls,* which is a crucial early event in the formation of a hemostatic plug. It is this activity that is believed to be deficient in von Willebrand disease. In addition to its function in platelet adhesion, vWF also serves as a carrier for factor VIII.

The various forms of von Willebrand disease can be characterized by immunologic techniques and the so-called ristocetin agglutination test. Ristocetin (developed as an antibiotic) binds platelets and promotes the interaction between vWF and platelet membrane glycoprotein Ib. The binding of vWF creates interplatelet "bridges" that lead to the formation of platelet clumps (agglutination), an event that can be measured easily. Thus, ristocetin-dependent platelet agglutination serves as a useful bioassay for vWF.

The two components of the factor VIII–vWF complex are encoded by separate genes and are synthesized by different cells. vWF is produced by both megakaryocytes and endothelial cells. The latter are the major source of

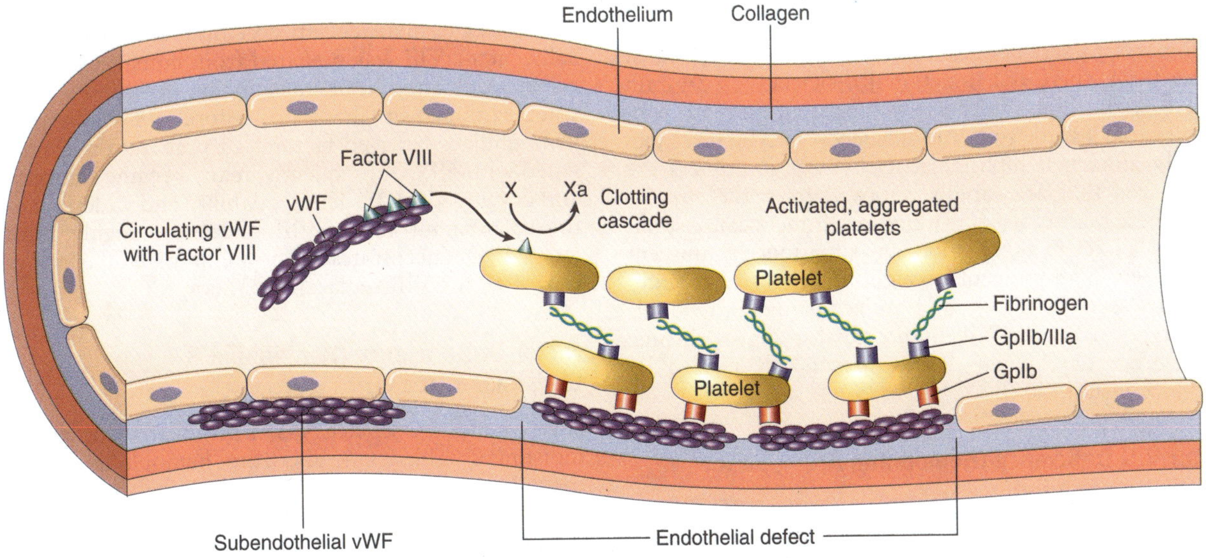

Figure 12–29

Structure and function of factor VIII–von Willebrand factor (vWF) complex. Factor VIII and vWF are synthesized in the liver and in endothelial cells, respectively. The two circulate as a complex in the circulation. vWF is also present in the subendothelial matrix of normal blood vessels. Factor VIII takes part in the coagulation cascade by activating factor X. vWF causes adhesion of platelets to subendothelial collagen, primarily through the glycoprotein Ib (GpIb) platelet receptor. Ristocetin activates GpIb receptors in vitro and causes platelet aggregation if vWF is present.

plasma vWF, whereas most factor VIII is synthesized in the liver. *To summarize, the two components of factor VIII–vWF complex, synthesized separately, come together and circulate in the plasma as a unit that serves to promote clotting as well as the platelet-vessel wall interactions necessary to ensure hemostasis.*

With this background we can turn to the discussion of diseases resulting from deficiencies of factor VIII–vWF complex.

von Willebrand Disease

von Willebrand disease is marked by spontaneous bleeding from mucous membranes, excessive bleeding from wounds, menorrhagia, and a prolonged bleeding time in the presence of a normal platelet count. In most cases it is transmitted as an autosomal dominant disorder. Its precise incidence is difficult to estimate, because in many instances the clinical manifestations are mild and the diagnosis requires sophisticated tests; it may well be the most common inherited bleeding disorder.

Individuals with von Willebrand disease have a compound defect involving platelet function and the coagulation pathway. The amounts of factor VIII are only moderately depressed, and it is the defect in platelet function that dominates the clinical picture. Except for rare homozygous patients with type III von Willebrand disease, the effects of factor VIII deficiency that characterize hemophilia are not seen.

The classic and most common variant of *von Willebrand disease (type I) is an autosomal dominant disorder characterized by a reduced quantity of circulating vWF.* Because vWF stabilizes factor VIII by binding to it, its deficiency causes a secondary decrease in factor VIII levels, but not to levels that are clinically significant. The other, less common, varieties of von Willebrand disease tend to show both qualitative and quantitative defects in vWF. *Type II* is divided into several subtypes that are all *characterized by a selective loss of high-molecular-weight multimers of vWF.* Because these multimers are the most active form, there is a functional deficiency of vWF. In type IIA, the high-molecular-weight multimers are not synthesized, leading to a true deficiency. In type IIB, functionally abnormal high-molecular-weight multimers are synthesized that are rapidly removed from the circulation. These high-molecular-weight multimers cause spontaneous platelet aggregation (a situation reminiscent of the very-high-molecular-weight multimer aggregates that are seen in TTP), and indeed some individuals with type IIB von Willebrand disease have chronic mild thrombocytopenia that is presumably caused by platelet consumption.

Factor VIII Deficiency (Hemophilia A, Classic Hemophilia)

Hemophilia A is the most common hereditary disease associated with serious bleeding. It is an X-linked recessive disorder that is caused by reduction in factor VIII activity. It primarily affects males, but much less commonly excessive bleeding also occurs in heterozygous females, presumably as a result of extremely unfavorable lyonization (inactivation of the normal X chromosome in most of the cells). *Approximately 30% of cases are caused by new mutations;* in the remainder, there is a positive family history. Severe hemophilia A is observed in individuals with a marked degree of factor VIII deficiency (activity levels of <1% of normal). Milder deficiencies may only become apparent when a major hemodynamic stress supervenes, such as trauma. The varying degrees of factor VIII deficiency are for the most part explained by the existence of many different causative mutations. As in the thalassemias, several types of genetic lesions (e.g., deletions, splice junction mutations, nonsense mutations) have been identified. In about 10% of patients, the factor VIII concentration is normal by immunoassay, but the coagulant activity detected by bioassay is low because of a mutation that causes the synthesis of functionally abnormal protein.

In all symptomatic cases there is a tendency toward easy bruising and massive hemorrhage after trauma or operative procedures. In addition, "spontaneous" hemorrhages are frequently encountered in regions of the body that are normally subject to trauma, particularly the joints, where recurrent bleeds into the joints (*hemarthroses*) lead to progressive deformities that can be crippling. *Petechiae are characteristically absent.* Typically, patients with hemophilia A have a prolonged PTT that is corrected by mixing the patient's plasma with normal plasma. In approximately 15% of the most severely affected patients, replacement therapy is complicated by the development of neutralizing antibodies against factor VIII, perhaps because factor VIII is seen as foreign in severely deficient individuals. In these persons the PTT fails to correct in mixing studies. Specific factor VIII assays are required to confirm the diagnosis on hemophilia A.

Treatment involves infusion of factor VIII. Historically, factor VIII was prepared from human plasma, carrying with it the risk of transmission of viral diseases. As was mentioned in Chapter 5, before 1985 thousands of hemophiliacs received factor VIII preparations contaminated with HIV. Subsequently, many became seropositive and developed AIDS. The availability and widespread use of recombinant factor VIII and more highly purified factor VIII concentrates has now eliminated the infectious risk of factor VIII replacement therapy.

Factor IX Deficiency (Hemophilia B, Christmas Disease)

Severe factor IX deficiency is an X-linked disorder that is indistinguishable clinically from hemophilia A but is much less common. The PTT is prolonged, and the bleeding time is normal. The diagnosis of Christmas disease (named after the first patient with this condition) is made with specific assays of factor IX. It is treated by infusion of recombinant factor IX.

SUMMARY

Bleeding Disorders

- *Disseminated Intravascular Coagulation*:
  - Syndrome in which systemic activation of the coagulation cascade by various stimuli, including sepsis, massive tissue injury, and release of procoagulant factors from tumor cells, leads to consumption of coagulation factors and platelets.
  - The clinical picture can be dominated by bleeding, vascular occlusion and tissue hypoxemia, or both. Common stimuli include sepsis, major trauma, certain cancers, and obstetric complications.
- *Immune Thrombocytopenia Purpura* (ITP): is caused by autoantibodies against platelet antigens; may be triggered by drugs, infections, or lymphomas, or be idiopathic.
- *Thrombotic Thromobocytopenia Purpura* (TTP):
  - Caused most commonly by acquired or inherited deficiencies of ADAMTS13, a plasma metalloprotease that normally prevents the accumulation of very high molecular weight multimers of von Willebrand factor (vWF). Deficiency of ADAMTS13 results in abnormally large vWF multimers, which lead to the formation of platelet-rich thrombi, particularly in the kidney and the central nervous system.
  - Manifested as thrombocytopenia and microangiopathic hemolytic anemia.
  - Hemolytic Uremic Syndrome resembles TTP clinically, but is caused by deficiencies of complement regulatory protein factor H, or agents that damage endothelial cells, such as a Shiga-like toxin elaborated by *E. coli* strain O157: H7. The endothelial injury initiates platelet activation, platelet aggregation, and microvasculature thrombosis.
- *von Willebrand Disease*:
  - Autosomal dominant disorder caused by mutations in vWF, which normally functions as a bridging molecule between platelets and subendothelial collagen.
  - Typically causes a mild to moderate bleeding disorder that mimics that caused by thrombocytopenia.
- *Hemophilia A* is an X-linked disorder caused by mutations in coagulation factor VIII. Affected males typically present with severe bleeding into soft tissues and joints, and have a prolonged partial thromboplastin time (PTT).
- *Hemophilia B* is an X-linked disorder caused by mutations in coagulation factor IX; clinically, it is identical to hemophilia A.

DISORDERS THAT AFFECT THE SPLEEN AND THYMUS

SPLENOMEGALY

The spleen is frequently secondarily involved in a wide variety of systemic diseases. In virtually all instances, the response of the spleen causes its enlargement (splenomegaly), which produces a set of stereotypical signs and symptoms. Evaluation of splenomegaly is a common clinical problem that is aided considerably by knowledge of the usual limits of the splenic enlargement that is seen in the context of specific disorders. It would be erroneous to attribute enlargement of the spleen into the pelvis to vitamin B_{12} deficiency, or to entertain a diagnosis of CML in the absence of significant splenomegaly. As an aid to diagnosis, then, we present the following list of disorders, classified according to the degree of splenomegaly that is characteristically produced:

A. Massive splenomegaly (weight more than 1000 gm)
   1. Chronic myeloproliferative disorders (chronic myeloid leukemia, myeloid metaplasia with myelofibrosis)
   2. Chronic lymphocytic leukemia
   3. Hairy cell leukemia
   4. Lymphomas
   5. Malaria
   6. Gaucher disease
   7. Primary tumors of the spleen (rare)

B. Moderate splenomegaly (weight 500–1000 gm)
   1. Chronic congestive splenomegaly (portal hypertension or splenic vein obstruction)
   2. Acute leukemias (inconstant)
   3. Hereditary spherocytosis
   4. Thalassemia major
   5. Autoimmune hemolytic anemia
   6. Amyloidosis
   7. Niemann-Pick disease
   8. Langerhans histiocytosis
   9. Chronic splenitis (especially with infective endocarditis)
   10. Tuberculosis, sarcoidosis, typhoid
   11. Metastatic carcinoma or sarcoma

C. Mild splenomegaly (weight <500 gm)
   1. Acute splenitis
   2. Acute splenic congestion
   3. Infectious mononucleosis

4. Miscellaneous acute febrile disorders, including septicemia, SLE, and intra-abdominal infections

The microscopic changes associated with these diseases need not be described here, because they have been discussed in the relevant sections of this and other chapters.

An enlarged spleen often removes excessive numbers of one or more of the formed elements of blood, resulting in anemia, leukopenia, or thrombocytopenia. This is referred to as *hypersplenism,* a state that can be associated with many of the diseases affecting the spleen listed previously. In addition, platelets are particularly susceptible to sequestration in the interstices of the red pulp; as a result, thrombocytopenia is more prevalent and severe in individuals with splenomegaly than are anemia or neutropenia.

DISORDERS OF THE THYMUS

As is well known, the thymus is a central lymphoid organ that has a crucial role in T-cell differentiation. It is not surprising, therefore, that the thymus can be involved by lymphomas, particularly those of T-cell lineage, which were discussed earlier in this chapter. Here we will focus on the two most frequent (albeit uncommon) disorders of the thymus: thymic hyperplasia and thymoma.

Thymic Hyperplasia

Hyperplasia of the thymus is often associated with the appearance of lymphoid follicles, or germinal centers, within the medulla. These germinal centers contain reactive B cells, which are normally present in only low numbers in the thymus. Thymic follicular hyperplasia is present in most patients with myasthenia gravis and is sometimes also found in other autoimmune diseases, such as SLE and rheumatoid arthritis. The relationship between the thymus and myasthenia gravis is discussed in Chapter 21. Significantly, removal of the hyperplastic thymus is often beneficial early in the disease.

Thymoma

The term *thymoma* is restricted to tumors in which epithelial cells constitute the neoplastic element. Scant or abundant precursor T cells (thymocytes) are present in these tumors, but these are non-neoplastic. Several classification systems for thymoma have been proposed on the basis of cytologic and biologic criteria. One simple and clinically useful classification is as follows:

- Benign or encapsulated thymoma: cytologically and biologically benign
- Malignant thymoma
  - Type I: cytologically benign but biologically aggressive and capable of local invasion and, rarely, distant spread
  - Type II, also called *thymic carcinoma:* cytologically malignant with all of the features of cancer and comparable behavior

Morphology

Macroscopically, thymomas are lobulated, firm, gray-white masses up to 15 to 20cm in longest dimension. Most appear encapsulated, but in 20% to 25% there is apparent penetration of the capsule and infiltration of perithymic tissues and structures.

Microscopically, virtually all thymomas are made up of a mixture of epithelial cells and a variable infiltrate of non-neoplastic thymocytes. The relative proportions of the epithelial and lymphocytic components are of little significance. In **benign thymomas** the epithelial cells are spindled or elongated and resemble those that normally populate the medulla. As a result, these are sometimes referred to as **medullary thymomas.** In other tumors there is an admixture of the plumper, rounder, cortical-type epithelial cells; this pattern is sometimes referred to as a **mixed thymoma.** The medullary and mixed patterns account for 60% to 70% of all thymomas.

Malignant thymoma type I is a tumor that is cytologically bland but locally invasive. These tumors occasionally (and unpredictably) metastasize and account for 20% to 25% of all thymomas. They are composed of varying proportions of epithelial cells and reactive thymocytes; the epithelial cells usually resemble those that are normally found in the cortex, in that they have abundant cytoplasm and rounded vesicular nuclei. The neoplastic epithelial cells often form palisades around blood vessels. Sometimes spindled epithelial cells are present as well. **The critical distinguishing feature is the penetration of the capsule and the invasion of surrounding structures.**

Malignant thymoma type II is perhaps better thought of as a form of **thymic carcinoma.** These represent about 5% of thymomas and, in contrast to the type I malignant thymomas, are malignant cytologically. Macroscopically, they are usually fleshy, obviously invasive masses sometimes accompanied by metastases to such sites as the lungs. Most resemble either poorly or well-differentiated **squamous cell carcinomas.** The next most common malignant pattern is **lymphoepithelioma-like carcinoma,** which is composed of anaplastic cortical-type epithelial cells mixed with large numbers of benign thymocytes. Tumors of this type are more common in Asian populations and sometimes contain the EBV genome.

Clinical Features. All thymomas are rarities, the malignant more so than the benign. They may arise at any age but typically occur in middle adult life. In a large series, about 30% were asymptomatic; 30% to 40% produced local manifestations such as a mass demonstrable on computed tomography in the anterosuperior mediastinum associated with cough, dyspnea, and superior vena caval syndrome; and the remainder were associated with some systemic disease, principally myasthenia gravis. Fifteen to 20% of patients with this disorder have a thymoma. Removal of the tumor often leads to improvement in the neuromuscular disorder. Additional associations with thymomas include hypogammaglobulinemia, SLE, pure red cell aplasia, and nonthymic cancers.

BIBLIOGRAPHY

Red Cell Disorders

Beutler E, Luzzatto L: Hemolytic anemia. Semin Hematol 36:38, 1999. *[An excellent overview of the hemolytic anemias.]*

Brodsky RA, Jones RJ: Aplastic anemia. Lancet 365:1647, 2005. *[An updated perspective on the causes of aplastic anemia.]*

Hunt NH, Grau GE: Cytokines: accelerators and brakes in the pathogenesis of cerebral malaria. Trends Immunol 24:491, 2003. *[A review of the importance of the immune response in induction of endothelial cell–red cell interactions in cerebral malaria.]*

Stuart MJ, Nagel RL: Sickle-cell disease. Lancet 363:1343, 2004. *[A review focused on recent pathogenic insights and their translation into new therapies.]*

Weiss G, Goodnough LT: Anemia of chronic disease. N Engl J Med 352:1011, 2005. *[An excellent update on the anemia of chronic disease, with a particular focus on the role of perturbed iron metabolism.]*

Young NS, Maciejewski JP: Genetic and environmental effects in paroxysmal nocturnal hemoglobinuria: this little PIG-A goes "Why? Why? Why?." J Clin Invest 106:637, 2000. *[Discussion of the dual role of somatic mutation and autoimmunity in PNH.]*

White Cell Disorders

Harris NL, et al.: World Health Organization classification of neoplastic diseases of the hematopoietic and lymphoid tissues: report of the Clinical Advisory Committee meeting, Airlie House, Virginia, November 1997. J Clin Oncol 17:3835, 1999. *[A progress report confirming the utility of the WHO classification for lymphoid neoplasms.]*

Harris NL, Brunning RD: The World Health Organization (WHO) classification of the myeloid neoplasms. Blood 100:2292, 2002. *[A proposed updated classification system for acute myelogenous leukemias, myeloproliferative disorders, and myelodysplastic syndromes.]*

Kantargian H, et al.: Hematologic and cytogenetic responses to imatinib mesylate in chronic myelogenous leukemia. N Engl J Med 346:645, 2002. *[An elegant example of how understanding the molecular biology of CML has led to improved treatment.]*

Krause DS, Van Etten RA: Tyrosine kinases as targets for cancer therapy. N Engl J Med 353:172, 2005. *[A timely and thorough review of the increasing number of mutations that activate tyrosine kinases in cancer, many of which occur in acute leukemia and myeloproliferative disorders.]*

Kuppers R: Mechanisms of B-cell lymphoma pathogenesis. Nat Rev Cancer 5:251, 2005. *[A lucid discussion of the origin of diverse B-cell malignancies.]*

Mitsiades CS, Mitsiades N, Munshi NC, Anderson KC. Focus on multiple myeloma. Cancer Cell 6:439, 2004. *[A review of recent advances in understanding the molecular pathogenesis of multiple myeloma.]*

Pui CH, Relling MV, Downing JR: Acute lymphoblastic leukemia. N Engl J Med 350:1535, 2004. *[A recent review of the molecular pathogenesis, diagnosis, and treatment of ALL.]*

Re D, Thomas, RK, Behringer K, Diehl V: From Hodgkin disease to Hodgkin lymphoma: biologic insights and therapeutic potential. Blood 105:4553, 2005. *[A current concise review of Hodgkin lymphoma pathogenesis and therapy.]*

Reilly JT: Pathogenesis of acute myeloid leukaemia and inv(16)(p13;q22): a paradigm for understanding leukaemogenesis? Br J Haematol 128:18, 2005. *[A review discussing the evidence supporting the idea that mutations of two types, one anti-differentiative and the second pro-proliferative, collaborate to induce and maintain AML.]*

Coagulation Disorders

Levi GG, Motto DG, Ginsberg D: ADAMTS13 turns 3. Blood 106:11, 2005. *[An excellent review of ADAM-TS13 and its deficiency in TTP.]*

Levi M, Cate HT: Disseminated intravascular coagulation. N Engl J Med 341:586, 1999. *[A clinically oriented review of the causes, pathogenesis, and treatment of this disorder.]*

Jang IK, Hursting MJ: When heparins promote thrombosis: review of the pathogenesis of heparin-induced thrombocytopenia. Circulation 111:2671, 2005. *[A discussion of the role of autoantibodies against platelet factor 4 and heparin in heparin-induced thrombocytopenia.]*

Schneppenheim R, Budde U: Phenotypic and genotypic diagnosis of von Willebrand disease: a 2004 update. Semin Hematol 42:12, 2005. *[An update on this disorder.]*

Siegler R, Oakes R: Hemolytic uremic syndrome; pathogenesis, treatment, and outcome. Curr Opin Pediatr 17:200, 2005. *[An article on the etiology and pathogenesis of the hemolytic-uremic syndrome.]*

Disorders That Affect the Spleen and Thymus

Choi SS, Kim KD, Chung KY: Prognostic and clinical relevance of the World Health Organization schema for the classification of thymic epithelial tumors: a clinicopathologic study of 108 patients and literature review. Chest 127:755, 2005. *[A large clinicopathologic series that shows that stage is the best predictor of outcome in thymoma.]*

Chapter 13

The Lung

ANIRBAN MAITRA, MBBS
VINAY KUMAR, MD*

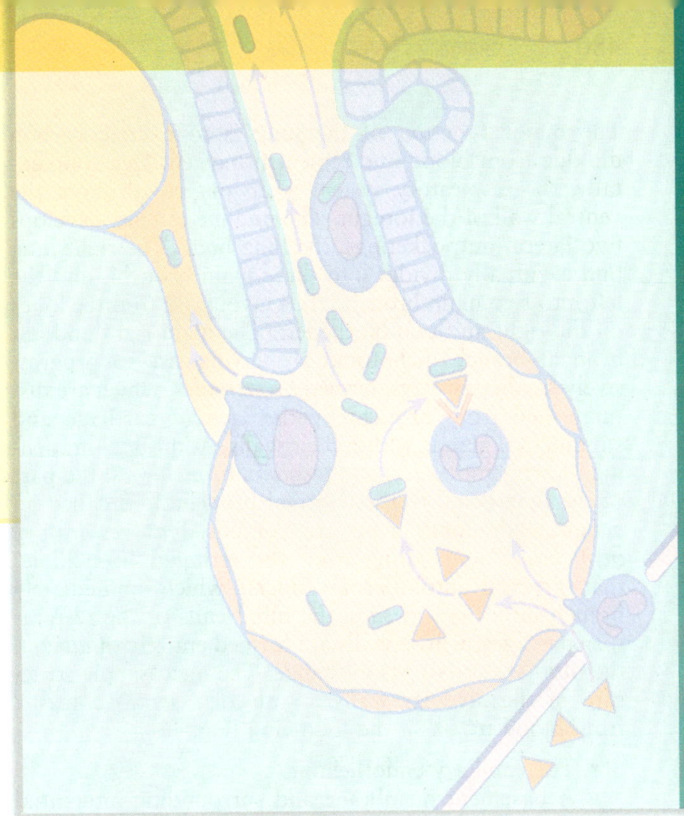

*The contributions of Aliya Hussain, MD, and Tamara Lotan, MD, to this chapter are gratefully acknowledged.

The major function of the lung is to excrete carbon dioxide from blood and replenish oxygen. Developmentally, the respiratory system is an outgrowth from the ventral wall of the foregut. The midline trachea develops two lateral outpocketings, the lung buds. The right lung bud eventually divides into three main bronchi, and the left into two main bronchi, thus giving rise to three lobes on the right and two on the left. The main right and left bronchi branch dichotomously, giving rise to progressively smaller airways, termed *bronchioles,* which are distinguished from bronchi by the lack of cartilage and submucosal glands within their walls. Additional branching of bronchioles leads to *terminal bronchioles;* the part of the lung distal to the terminal bronchiole is called an *acinus.* Pulmonary acini are composed of *respiratory bronchioles* (emanating from the terminal bronchiole) that proceed into *alveolar ducts,* which immediately branch into *alveolar sacs,* the blind ends of the respiratory passages, whose walls are formed entirely of *alveoli,* the ultimate site of gas exchange. The microscopic structure of the alveolar walls (or alveolar septa) consists, from blood to air, of the following (Fig. 13–1):

- The capillary endothelium
- A basement membrane and surrounding interstitial tissue separating the endothelium from the alveolar lining epithelium. The pulmonary interstitium, composed of fine elastic fibers, small bundles of collagen, a few fibroblast-like cells, smooth muscle cells, mast cells, and rare mononuclear cells, is most prominent in thicker portions of the alveolar septum.
- Alveolar epithelium, which contains a continuous layer of two principal cell types: flattened, platelike type I pneumocytes covering 95% of the alveolar surface and rounded type II pneumocytes. The latter cells are the source of pulmonary surfactant and are the main cell type involved in repair of alveolar epithelium in the wake of damage to type I pneumocytes. The alveolar walls are not solid but are perforated by numerous pores of Kohn, which permit passage of bacteria and exudates between adjacent alveoli.
- Alveolar macrophages, mononuclear cells of phagocytic lineage, usually lie free within the alveolar space. Often these macrophages contain phagocytosed carbon particles.

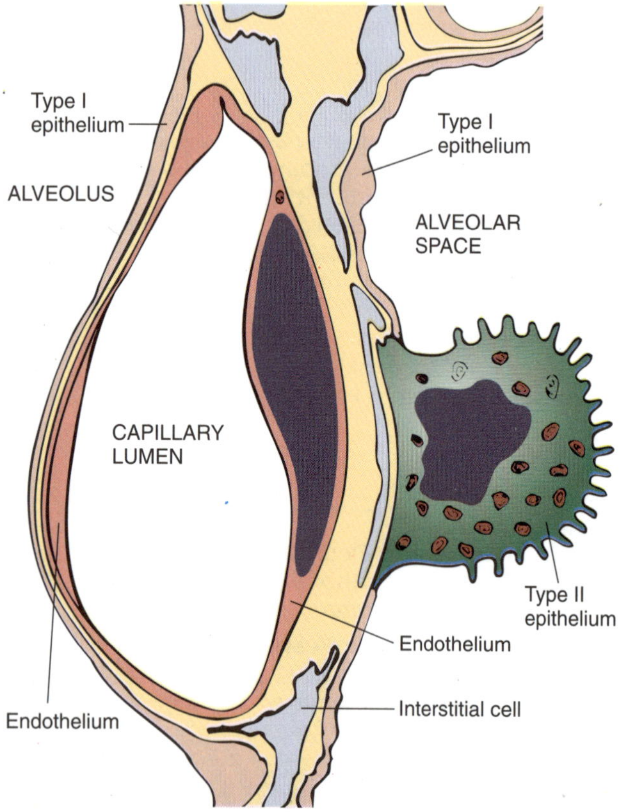

Figure 13–1

Microscopic structure of the alveolar wall. Note that the basement membrane *(yellow)* is thin on one side and widened where it is continuous with the interstitial space. Portions of interstitial cells are shown.

Obviously, opportunities for disease in this important organ system are legion. A common approach in the study of lung pathology, and one that provides the framework for this chapter, is to organize lung diseases into those affecting (1) the airways, (2) the interstitium, and (3) the pulmonary vascular system. This division into discrete compartments is, of course, deceptively neat. In reality, disease in one compartment is generally accompanied by alterations of morphology and function in another. We begin our discussion with atelectasis, because it can complicate many primary lung disorders.

ATELECTASIS (COLLAPSE)

Atelectasis, also known as collapse, is loss of lung volume caused by *inadequate expansion of airspaces.* It results in shunting of inadequately oxygenated blood from pulmonary arteries into veins, thus giving rise to a ventilation-perfusion imbalance and hypoxia. On the basis of the underlying mechanism or the distribution of alveolar collapse, atelectasis is classified into three forms (Fig.13–2).

Resorption Atelectasis. Resorption atelectasis occurs when an obstruction prevents air from reaching distal airways. The air already present gradually becomes absorbed, and alveolar collapse follows. Depending on the level of airway obstruction, an entire lung, a complete lobe, or one or more segments may be involved. The most common cause of resorption collapse is obstruction of a bronchus by a mucous or mucopurulent plug. This frequently occurs postoperatively but may also complicate bronchial asthma, bronchiectasis, chronic bronchitis, or the aspiration of foreign bodies, particularly in children.

Compression Atelectasis. Compression atelectasis (sometimes called *passive* or *relaxation atelectasis*) is usually associated with accumulations of fluid, blood, or air within the pleural cavity, which mechanically collapse the adjacent lung. This is a frequent occurrence with pleural effusions, caused most commonly by congestive heart failure (CHF). Leakage of air into the pleural cavity (pneumothorax) also leads to compression atelectasis.

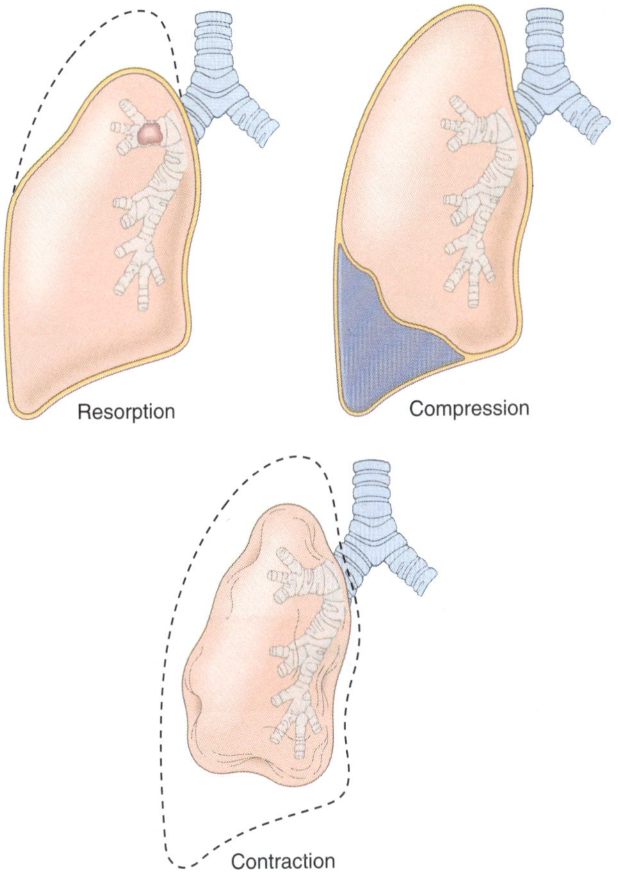

Figure 13–2

Various forms of atelectasis in adults.

Basal atelectasis resulting from the elevated position of the diaphragm commonly occurs in bedridden patients, in patients with ascites, and in patients during and after surgery.

Contraction Atelectasis. Contraction (or *cicatrization*) atelectasis occurs when either local or generalized fibrotic changes in the lung or pleura hamper expansion and increase elastic recoil during expiration.

Atelectasis (except that caused by contraction) is potentially reversible and should be treated promptly to prevent hypoxemia and superimposed infection of the collapsed lung.

ACUTE LUNG INJURY

The term *acute lung injury* encompasses a spectrum of pulmonary lesions (endothelial and epithelial), which can be initiated by numerous conditions. Clinically, acute lung injury manifests as (1) the acute onset of dyspnea, (2) decreased arterial oxygen pressure (hypoxemia), (3) development of bilateral pulmonary infiltrates on radiographs, and (4) absence of clinical evidence of primary left-sided heart failure. Since the pulmonary infiltrates in acute lung injury are usually caused by damage to the alveolar capillary membrane rather than left-sided heart failure (Chapter 11), they represent an example of *noncardiogenic pulmonary edema.* Acute lung injury can progress to the more severe *acute respiratory distress syndrome,* described below.

Acute Respiratory Distress Syndrome (ARDS)

ARDS is a clinical syndrome caused by diffuse alveolar capillary and epithelial damage. There is usually rapid onset of life-threatening respiratory insufficiency, cyanosis, and severe arterial hypoxemia that is refractory to oxygen therapy and that may progress to multisystem organ failure. The histologic manifestation of ARDS in the lungs is known as *diffuse alveolar damage.* ARDS can occur in a multitude of clinical settings and is associated with either direct injury to the lung or indirect injury in the setting of a systemic process (Table 13–1).

Pathogenesis. The alveolar capillary membrane is formed by two separate barriers: the microvascular endothelium and the alveolar epithelium. *In ARDS the integrity of this barrier is compromised by either endothelial or epithelial injury, or, more commonly, both.* The acute consequences of damage to the alveolar capillary membrane include increased vascular permeability and alveolar flooding, loss of diffusion capacity, and widespread surfactant abnormalities caused by damage to type II pneumocytes (Fig. 13–3). Although the cellular and molecular basis of acute lung injury and ARDS remains an area of active investigation, recent work suggests that in ARDS, *lung injury is caused by an imbalance of pro-inflammatory and anti-inflammatory mediators.* The most proximate signals leading to uncontrolled activation of the acute inflammatory response are not yet understood. However, *nuclear factor κB* (NF-κB), a transcription factor whose activation itself is tightly regulated under normal conditions, has emerged as a likely candidate shifting the balance in favor of pro-inflammatory state. As early as

Table 13–1 Clinical Disorders Associated with the Development of Acute Respiratory Distress Syndrome

Direct Lung Injury	Indirect Lung Injury
Common Causes	
Pneumonia	Sepsis
Aspiration of gastric contents	Severe trauma with shock
Uncommon Causes	
Pulmonary contusion	Cardiopulmonary bypass
Fat embolism	Acute pancreatitis
Near-drowning	Drug overdose
Inhalational injury	Transfusion of blood products
Reperfusion injury after lung transplantation	Uremia

Modified from Ware LB, Matthay MA: The acute respiratory distress syndrome. N Engl J Med 342:1334, 2000.

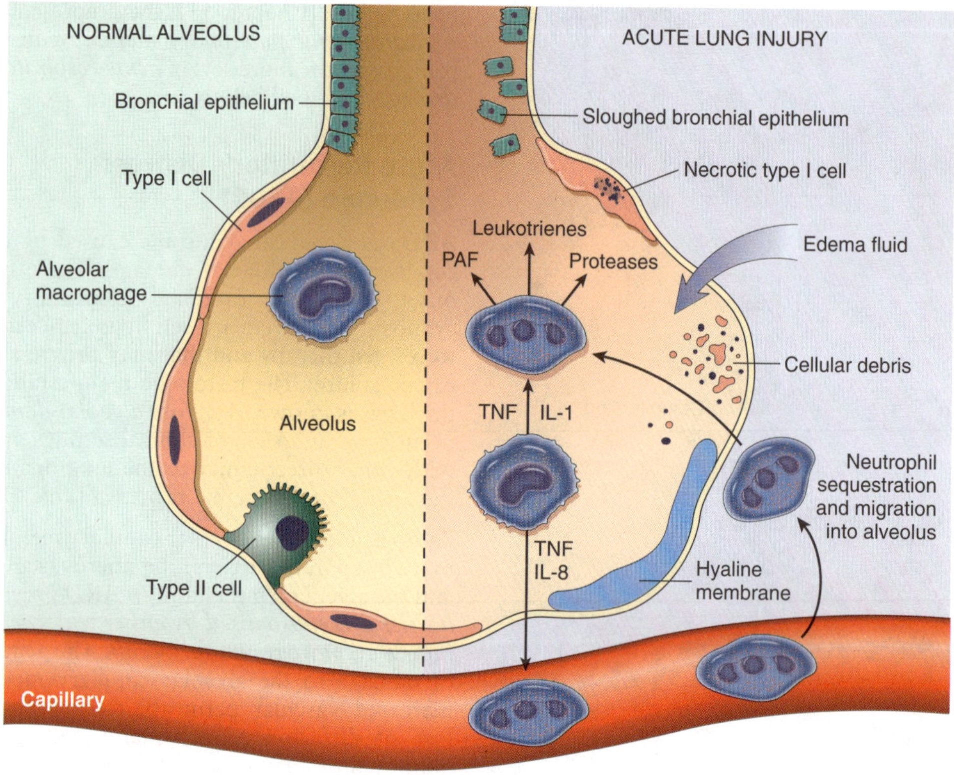

Figure 13–3

The normal alveolus *(left)* compared with the injured alveolus in the early phase of acute lung injury and the acute respiratory distress syndrome. Under the influence of proinflammatory cytokines such as IL-8, IL-1, and TNF (released by macrophages), neutrophils initially undergo sequestration in the pulmonary microvasculature, followed by margination and egress into the alveolar space, where they undergo activation. Activated neutrophils release a variety of factors such as leukotrienes, oxidants, proteases, and platelet-activating factor (PAF), which contribute to local tissue damage, accumulation of edema fluid in the airspaces, surfactant inactivation, and hyaline membrane formation. Subsequently, the release of macrophage-derived fibrogenic cytokines such as transforming growth factor β (TGF-β) and platelet-derived growth factor (PGDF) stimulate fibroblast growth and collagen deposition associated with the healing phase of injury. (Modified from Ware LB, Matthay MA: The acute respiratory distress syndrome. N Engl J Med 342:1334, 2000.)

30 minutes after an acute insult, there is increased synthesis of interleukin 8 (IL-8), a potent neutrophil chemotactic and activating agent, by pulmonary macrophages. Release of this and similar compounds, such as IL-1 and tumor necrosis factor (TNF), leads to endothelial activation, and pulmonary microvascular sequestration and activation of neutrophils. *Neutrophils are thought to have an important role in the pathogenesis of ARDS.* Histologic examination of lungs early in the disease process shows increased numbers of neutrophils within the vascular space, the interstitium, and the alveoli. Activated neutrophils release a variety of products (e.g., oxidants, proteases, platelet-activating factor, and leukotrienes) that cause damage to the alveolar epithelium and maintain the inflammatory cascade. Combined assault on the endothelium and epithelium perpetuate vascular leakiness and loss of surfactant that render the alveolar unit unable to expand. It should be noted that the destructive forces unleashed by neutrophils can be counteracted by an array of endogenous antiproteases, antioxidants, and anti-inflammatory cytokines (e.g. IL-10) that are upregulated by pro-inflammatory cytokines. In the end, it is the balance between the destructive and protective factors that determines the degree of tissue injury and clinical severily of ARDS.

Morphology

In the **acute phase of ARDS** the lungs are dark red, firm, airless, and heavy. Microscopically, there is capillary congestion, necrosis of alveolar epithelial cells, interstitial and intra-alveolar edema and hemorrhage, and (particularly with sepsis) collections of neutrophils in capillaries. The most characteristic finding is the presence of **hyaline membranes,** particularly lining the distended alveolar ducts (Fig. 13–4). Such membranes consist of fibrin-rich edema fluid admixed with remnants of necrotic epithelial cells. Overall, the picture is remarkably similar to that seen in respiratory distress syndrome in the newborn (Chapter 7). In the **organizing stage** there is marked proliferation of type II pneumocytes in an attempt to regenerate the alveolar lining. Resolution is unusual; more commonly there is organization of the fibrin exudates, with resultant intra-alveolar fibrosis. Marked thickening of the alveolar septa ensues, caused by proliferation of interstitial cells and deposition of collagen.

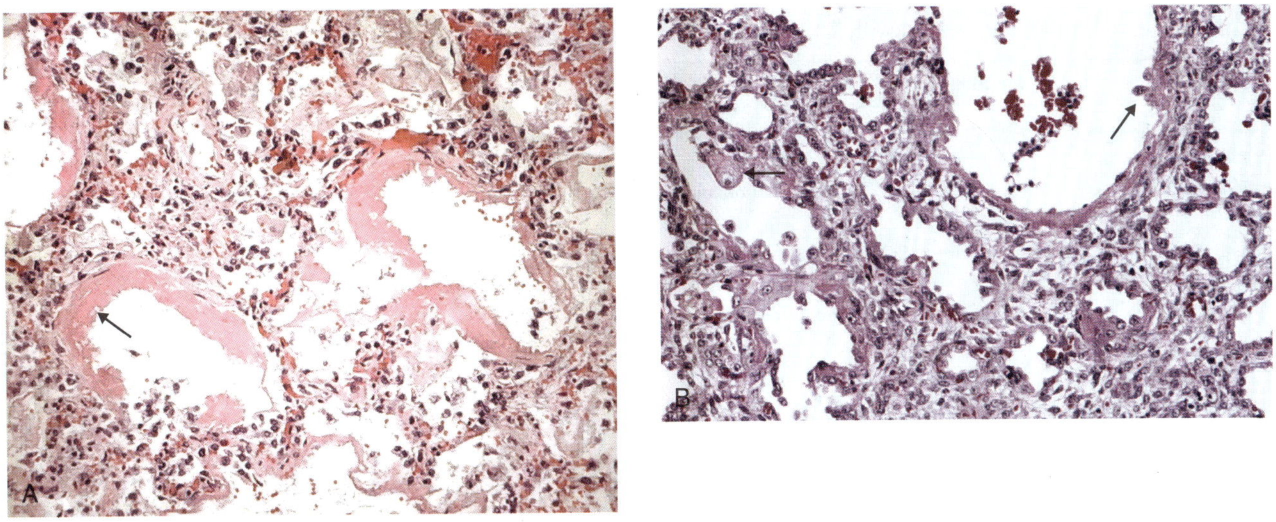

Figure 13–4

A, Diffuse alveolar damage in acute lung injury and ARDS. Some alveoli are collapsed; others are distended. Many are lined by bright pink hyaline membranes *(arrow).* **B,** In the healing stage there is resorption of hyaline membranes with thickened alveolar septa containing inflammatory cells, fibroblasts, and collagen. Numerous atypical type II pneumocytes are seen at this stage *(arrows),* associated with regeneration and repair.

Clinical Course. Approximately 85% of patients develop the clinical syndrome of acute lung injury or ARDS within 72 hours of the initiating insult. The prognosis of ARDS is grim, and mortality rates have historically approached 100%. Despite improvements in supportive therapy the mortality rate among the 150,000 ARDS cases seen yearly is still about 60%. Predictors of poor prognosis in ARDS include advanced age, underlying bacteremia (sepsis), and the development of multisystem (especially cardiac, renal, or hepatic) failure. Should the patient survive the acute stage, diffuse interstitial fibrosis may occur and continue to compromise respiratory function. However, in most patients who survive the acute insult and are spared the chronic sequela, normal respiratory function returns within 6 to 12 months.

SUMMARY

ARDS

- ARDS is a clinical syndrome of progressive respiratory insufficiency caused by diffuse alveolar damage in the setting of sepsis, severe trauma, and diffuse pulmonary infections.
- There is an imbalance of pro- and anti-inflammatory mediators causing acute inflammatory injury to the alveolar epithelium and capillary endothelium.
- Neutrophils and their products have a crucial role in the pathogenesis of ARDS.
- The characteristic histologic picture is that of alveolar edema, epithelial necrosis, accumulation of neutrophils, and presence of hyaline membranes lining the alveolar ducts.

OBSTRUCTIVE VERSUS RESTRICTIVE PULMONARY DISEASES

Diffuse pulmonary diseases can be classified in two categories: (1) obstructive disease (airway disease), characterized by limitation of airflow usually resulting from an increase in resistance caused by partial or complete obstruction at any level, and (2) restrictive disease, characterized by reduced expansion of lung parenchyma accompanied by decreased total lung capacity.

The major diffuse obstructive disorders are *emphysema, chronic bronchitis, bronchiectasis, and asthma.* In patients with these diseases, total lung capacity and forced vital capacity (FVC) are either normal or increased, and the hallmark is a decreased expiratory flow rate, usually measured by forced expiratory volume at 1 second (FEV_1). Thus, *the ratio of* FEV_1 *to FVC is characteristically decreased.* Expiratory obstruction may result either from anatomic airway narrowing, classically observed in asthma, or from loss of elastic recoil, characteristic of emphysema.

In contrast, in *diffuse restrictive diseases,* FVC is reduced and the expiratory flow rate is normal or reduced proportionately. Hence, *the ratio of* FEV_1 *to FVC is near normal.* The restrictive defect occurs in two general conditions: (1) *chest wall disorders in the presence of normal lungs* (e.g., severe obesity, diseases of the pleura, and neuromuscular disorders, such as the Guillain-Barré syndrome [Chapter 23], that affect the respiratory muscles) and (2) *acute or chronic interstitial lung diseases.* The classic acute restrictive disease is ARDS, discussed above. *Chronic restrictive diseases* include the pneumoconioses (see below), interstitial fibrosis of unknown etiology, and most of the infiltrative conditions (e.g., sarcoidosis).

Table 13–2 Disorders Associated with Airflow Obstruction: The Spectrum of Chronic Obstructive Pulmonary Disease

Clinical Term	Anatomic Site	Major Pathologic Changes	Etiology	Signs/Symptoms
Chronic bronchitis	Bronchus	Mucus gland hyperplasia, hypersecretion	Tobacco smoke, air pollutants	Cough, sputum production
Bronchiectasis	Bronchus	Airway dilation and scarring	Persistent or severe infections	Cough, purulent sputum, fever
Asthma	Bronchus	Smooth muscle hyperplasia, excessive mucus, inflammation	Immunologic or undefined causes	Episodic wheezing, cough, dyspnea
Emphysema	Acinus	Airspace enlargement, wall destruction	Tobacco smoke	Dyspnea
Small-airway disease, bronchiolitis*	Bronchiole	Inflammatory scarring, obliteration of bronchioles	Tobacco smoke, air pollutants	Cough, dyspnea

*A feature of chronic bronchitis (see text).

OBSTRUCTIVE PULMONARY DISEASE

In their prototypal forms, these individual disorders—emphysema, chronic bronchitis, asthma, and chronic bronchiectasis—have distinct anatomic and clinical characteristics (Table 13–2). The relationship between chronic bronchitis and emphysema is complicated, but the use of precise definitions has helped bring some order to what was once chaos. At the outset, it should be *emphasized that the definition of emphysema is morphologic, whereas chronic bronchitis is defined on the basis of clinical features* such as the presence of chronic and recurrent cough with excessive mucus secretion. Second, the anatomic distribution is also different; chronic bronchitis affects both the large and small airways (the latter component has been called *chronic bronchiolitis* to indicate the level of involvement); by contrast, emphysema is restricted to the *acinus* (Fig. 13–5). Although chronic bronchitis may exist without demonstrable emphysema, and almost pure emphysema may occur (particularly in patients with inherited α_1-antitrypsin deficiency, see below), the two diseases usually coexist. This is almost certainly because one extrinsic trigger—cigarette smoking, especially long-term, heavy tobacco exposure—is a common underlying theme in both disorders. Given their propensity to coexist, emphysema and chronic bronchitis are often clinically grouped together under the rubric of *chronic obstructive pulmonary disease (COPD)*. COPD affects more than 10% of the US adult population and is the fourth leading cause of death in this country. The primarily *irreversible* airflow obstruction of

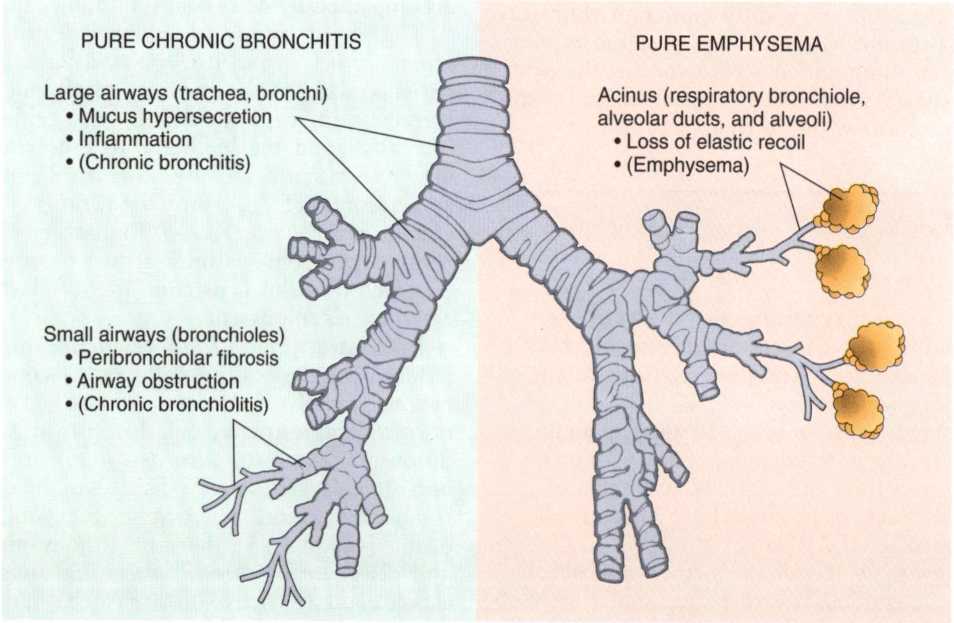

Figure 13–5

Anatomic distribution of pure chronic bronchitis and pure emphysema. In chronic bronchitis the small-airway disease (chronic bronchiolitis) results in airflow obstruction, while the large-airway disease is primarily responsible for the mucus hypersecretion.

COPD distinguishes it from asthma, which, as discussed later, is characterized largely by *reversible* airflow obstruction.

Emphysema

Emphysema is characterized by *abnormal permanent enlargement of the airspaces* distal to the terminal bronchioles, accompanied by *destruction of their walls* without obvious fibrosis. There are several conditions in which enlargement of airspaces is not accompanied by destruction; this is more correctly called *overinflation.* For example, the distention of airspaces in the opposite lung after unilateral pneumonectomy is compensatory overinflation rather than emphysema.

Types of Emphysema. Emphysema is classified according to its *anatomic distribution* within the *lobule;* recall that the acinus is the structure distal to terminal bronchioles, and a cluster of three to five acini is called a *lobule.* There are four major types of emphysema: (1) centriacinar, (2) panacinar, (3) distal acinar, and (4) irregular. Only the first two cause clinically significant airway obstruction, with centriacinar emphysema being about 20-fold more common than panacinar disease.

Centriacinar (Centrilobular) Emphysema. The distinctive feature of this type of emphysema is the pattern of involvement of the lobules: the central or proximal parts of the acini, formed by respiratory bronchioles, are affected, while distal alveoli are spared. Thus, both emphysematous and normal airspaces exist within the same acinus and lobule (Fig. 13–6B). The lesions are more common and severe in the upper lobes, particularly in the apical segments. In severe centriacinar emphysema the distal acinus also becomes involved, and so, as noted, the differentiation from panacinar emphysema becomes difficult. This type of emphysema is most commonly seen as a consequence of cigarette smoking in people who do not have congenital deficiency of α_1-antitrypsin.

Panacinar (Panlobular) Emphysema. In this type of emphysema, the acini are uniformly enlarged from the level of the respiratory bronchiole to the terminal blind alveoli (Fig. 13–6C). In contrast to centriacinar emphysema, panacinar emphysema tends to occur more commonly in the lower lung zones and is the type of emphysema that occurs in α_1-antitrypsin deficiency.

Distal Acinar (Paraseptal) Emphysema. In this form, the proximal portion of the acinus is normal but the distal part is primarily involved. The emphysema is more striking adjacent to the pleura, along the lobular connective tissue septa, and at the margins of the lobules. It occurs adjacent to areas of fibrosis, scarring, or atelectasis and is usually more severe in the upper half of the lungs. The

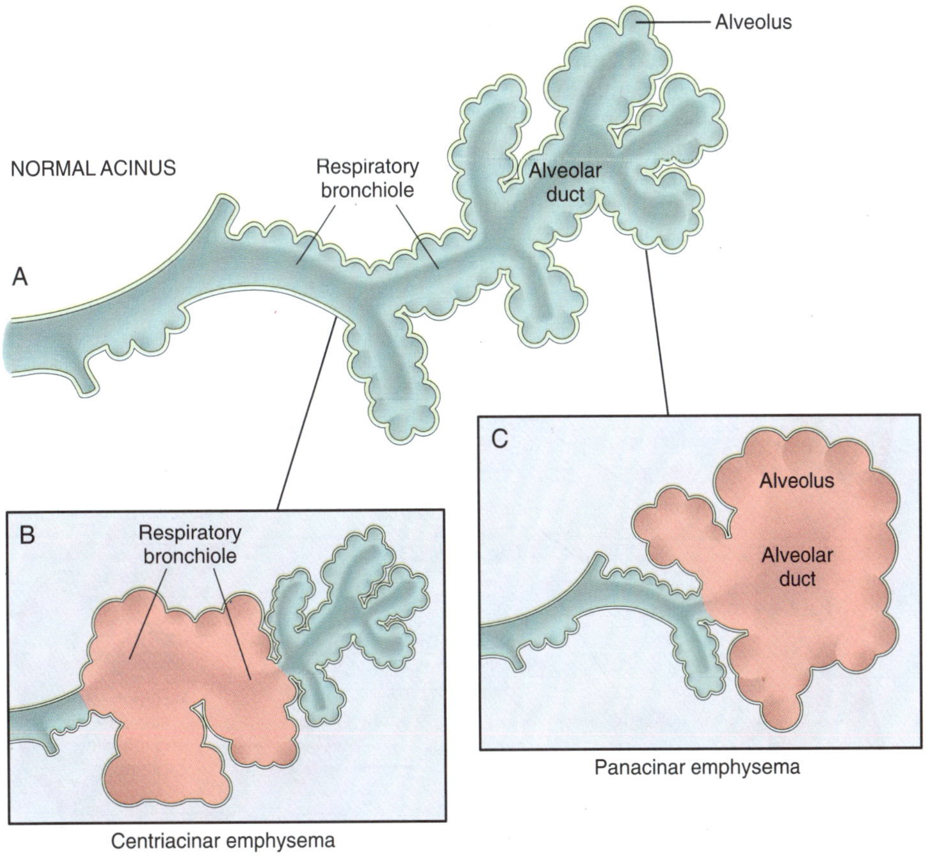

Figure 13–6

A, Diagram of normal structures within the acinus, the fundamental unit of the lung. A terminal bronchiole (not shown) is immediately proximal to the respiratory bronchiole. **B,** Centrilobular emphysema with dilation that initially affects the respiratory bronchioles. **C,** Panacinar emphysema with initial distention of the peripheral structures (i.e., the alveolus and alveolar duct); the disease later extends to affect the respiratory bronchioles.

characteristic findings are the presence of multiple, contiguous, enlarged airspaces that range in diameter from less than 0.5 mm to more than 2.0 cm, sometimes forming cystlike structures that with progressive enlargement are referred to as *bullae*. This type of emphysema probably underlies many of the cases of spontaneous pneumothorax in young adults.

Irregular Emphysema. *Irregular emphysema, so named because the acinus is irregularly involved, is almost invariably associated with scarring,* such as resulting from healed inflammatory diseases. Although clinically asymptomatic, this may be the most common form of emphysema.

Pathogenesis. The genesis of the two common forms of emphysema, centriacinar and panacinar, is not completely understood. Current opinion favors emphysema arising as a consequence of *two critical imbalances:* the protease-antiprotease imbalance and oxidant-antioxidant imbalance (Fig. 13–7). Such imbalances almost always coexist, and in fact, their effects are additive in producing the end result of tissue damage.

The *protease-antiprotease imbalance* hypothesis is based on the observation that patients with a genetic deficiency of the antiprotease α_1-antitrypsin have a markedly enhanced tendency to develop pulmonary emphysema, which is compounded by smoking. About 1% of all patients with emphysema have this defect. α_1-Antitrypsin, normally present in serum, tissue fluids, and macrophages, is a major inhibitor of proteases (particularly elastase) secreted by neutrophils during inflammation. α_1-Antitrypsin is encoded by codominantly expressed genes on the proteinase inhibitor *(Pi)* locus on chromosome 14. The *Pi* locus is extremely polymorphic, with many different alleles. Most common is the normal *(M)* allele and the corresponding phenotype. Approximately 0.012% of the US population is homozygous for the *Z* allele, associated with markedly decreased serum levels of α_1-antitrypsin. More than 80% of these individuals develop symptomatic emphysema, which occurs at an earlier age and with greater severity if the individual smokes.

The following sequence is postulated:

1. Neutrophils (the principal source of cellular proteases) are normally sequestered in peripheral capillaries, including those in the lung, and a few gain access to the alveolar spaces.
2. Any stimulus that increases either the number of leukocytes (neutrophils and macrophages) in the lung or the release of their protease-containing granules increases proteolytic activity.
3. With low levels of serum α_1-antitrypsin, elastic tissue destruction is unchecked and emphysema results.

Thus, emphysema is seen to result from the destructive effect of high protease activity in subjects with low antiprotease activity. The protease-antiprotease imbalance hypothesis also helps explain the effect of cigarette smoking in the development of emphysema, particularly the centriacinar form in subjects with normal amounts of α_1-antitrypsin:

- *In smokers, neutrophils and macrophages accumulate in alveoli.* The mechanism of inflammation is not entirely clear, but possibly involves the direct chemoattractant effects of nicotine as well as the effects of reactive oxygen species contained in smoke. These activate the transcription factor NF-κB, which switches on genes that encode TNF and chemokines, including IL-8. These, in turn, attract and activate neutrophils.
- Accumulated neutrophils are activated and release their granules, rich in a variety of cellular proteases (neutrophil elastase, proteinase 3, and cathepsin G), resulting in tissue damage.
- Smoking also enhances elastase activity in macrophages; macrophage elastase is not inhibited by α_1-

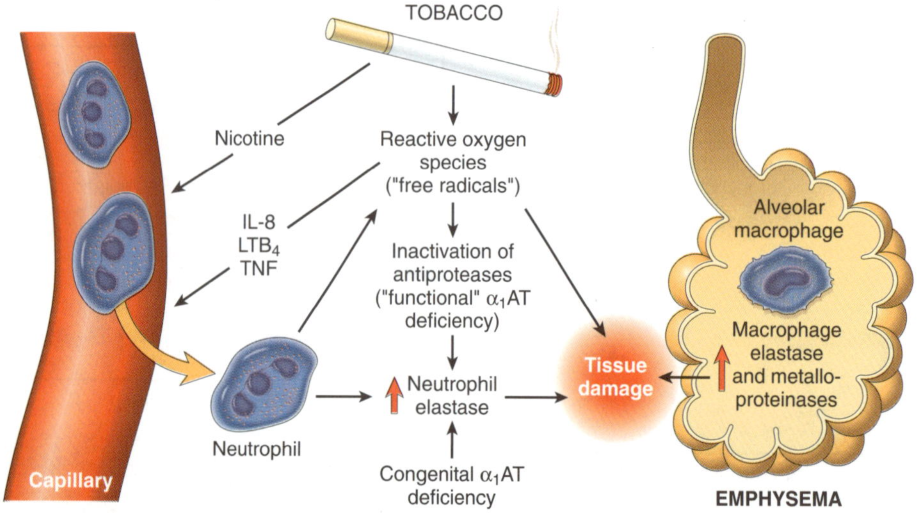

Figure 13–7

Pathogenesis of emphysema. The protease-antiprotease imbalance and oxidant-antioxidant imbalance are additive in their effects and contribute to tissue damage. α_1-Antitrypsin (α_1AT) deficiency can be either congenital or "functional" as a result of oxidative inactivation. See text for details. IL-8, interleukin 8; LTB_4, leukotriene B_4; TNF, tumor necrosis factor.

antitrypsin and, indeed, can proteolytically digest this antiprotease. There is increasing evidence that in addition to elastase, matrix metalloproteinases derived from macrophages and neutrophils have a role in tissue destruction.

Smoking also has a seminal role in perpetuating the *oxidant-antioxidant imbalance* in the pathogenesis of emphysema. Normally, the lung contains a healthy complement of antioxidants (superoxide dismutase, glutathione) that keep oxidative damage to a minimum. Tobacco smoke contains abundant reactive oxygen species (free radicals), which deplete these antioxidant mechanisms, thereby inciting tissue damage (Chapter 1). Activated neutrophils also add to the pool of reactive oxygen species in the alveoli. A secondary consequence of oxidative injury is inactivation of native antiproteases, resulting in "functional" α_1-antitrypsin deficiency even in patients without enzyme deficiency.

Morphology

The diagnosis and classification of emphysema depend largely on the macroscopic appearance of the lung. **Panacinar emphysema,** when well developed, produces pale, voluminous lungs that often obscure the heart when the anterior chest wall is removed at autopsy. The macroscopic features of **centriacinar emphysema** are less impressive. The lungs are a deeper pink than in panacinar emphysema and less voluminous, unless the disease is well advanced. Generally, in centriacinar emphysema the upper two-thirds of the lungs is more severely affected than the lower lungs. Histologically there is **thinning and destruction of alveolar walls.** With advanced disease, adjacent alveoli become confluent, creating large airspaces (Fig. 13–8). Terminal and respiratory bronchioles may be deformed because of the loss of septa that help tether these structures in the parenchyma. With the **loss of elastic tissue** in the surrounding alveolar septa, there is reduced radial traction on the small airways. As a result, they tend to collapse during expiration—an important cause of chronic airflow obstruction in severe emphysema. In addition to alveolar loss, the number of alveolar capillaries is diminished.

Clinical Course. *Dyspnea* is usually the first symptom; it begins insidiously but is steadily progressive. In patients with underlying chronic bronchitis or chronic asthmatic bronchitis, cough and wheezing may be initial complaints. Weight loss is common and may be so severe as to suggest a hidden malignant tumor. Pulmonary function tests reveal reduced FEV_1 with normal or near-normal FVC. *Hence, the ratio of FEV_1 to FVC is reduced.*

The classic presentation in individuals who have no "bronchitic" component is one in which the patient is barrel-chested and dyspneic, with obviously prolonged expiration, sitting forward in a hunched-over position, attempting to squeeze the air out of the lungs with each expiratory effort. In these patients, airspace enlargement is severe and diffusing capacity is low. Dyspnea and hyperventilation are prominent, so that until very late in the disease, gas exchange is adequate and blood gas values are relatively normal. Because of prominent dyspnea and adequate oxygenation of hemoglobin, these patients are sometimes called *"pink puffers."*

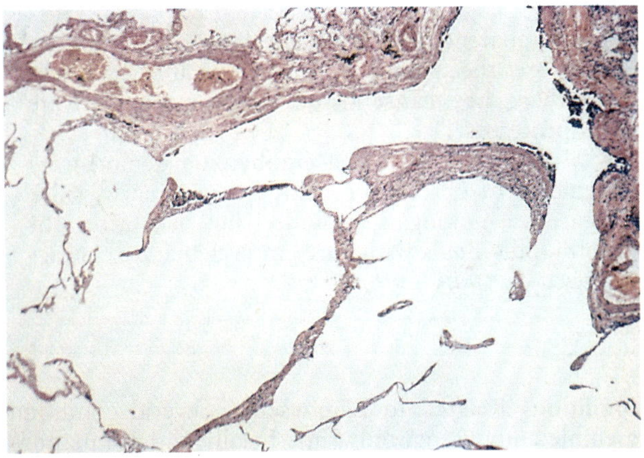

Figure 13–8

Pulmonary emphysema. There is marked enlargement of airspaces, with thinning and destruction of alveolar septa. (From the teaching collection of the Department of Pathology, University of Texas Southwestern Medical School, Dallas, Texas.)

On the other extreme are patients with emphysema who also have pronounced chronic bronchitis and a history of recurrent infections with purulent sputum. They usually have less prominent dyspnea and respiratory drive, so they retain carbon dioxide, become hypoxic, and are often cyanotic. For reasons not entirely clear, they tend to be obese. Often they seek medical help after the onset of CHF (cor pulmonale; Chapter 11) and associated edema. Patients with this clinical picture are sometimes called *"blue bloaters."*

Most individuals with emphysema and COPD fall somewhere between these two classic extremes. In all, *secondary pulmonary hypertension develops gradually,* arising from both hypoxia-induced pulmonary vascular spasm and loss of pulmonary capillary surface area from alveolar destruction. Death from emphysema is related to either pulmonary failure with respiratory acidosis, hypoxia, and coma, or right-sided heart failure (cor pulmonale).

SUMMARY

Emphysema

- Emphysema is a chronic obstructive airway disease characterized by permanent enlargement of airspaces distal to terminal bronchioles.
- Subtypes include centriacinar (most common; smoking related), panacinar (seen in α_1-antitrypsin deficiency), distal acinar, and irregular.
- The two key pathogenic mechanisms are an excess of cellular proteases with low antiprotease levels (protease-antiprotease imbalance), and an excess of reactive oxygen species (oxidant-antioxi-

dant imbalance). The accumulated inflammatory cells are the source of proteases and oxidants; together, they cause tissue injury and inactivate antiproteases.

• Most individuals with emphysema demonstrate elements of chronic bronchitis concurrently, since cigarette smoking is an underlying risk factor for both; individuals with pure emphysema are characterized as "*pink puffers.*"

Conditions Related to Emphysema. Several conditions resemble emphysema only superficially and are inappropriately referred to as such.

Compensatory emphysema is a term used to designate the compensatory dilation of alveoli in response to loss of lung substance elsewhere, such as occurs in residual lung parenchyma after surgical removal of a diseased lung or lobe.

Obstructive overinflation refers to the condition in which the lung expands because air is trapped within it. A common cause is subtotal obstruction by a tumor or foreign object. Obstructive overinflation can be a life-threatening emergency if the affected portion extends sufficiently to compress the remaining normal lung.

Bullous emphysema refers merely to any form of emphysema that produces large subpleural blebs or bullae (spaces >1 cm in diameter in the distended state) (Fig. 13–9). They represent localized accentuations of one of the four forms of emphysema, are most often subpleural, and on occasion, rupture leading to pneumothorax.

Mediastinal (interstitial) emphysema designates the entrance of air into the connective tissue stroma of the lung, mediastinum, and subcutaneous tissue. This may occur spontaneously with a sudden increase in intra-alveolar pressure (as with vomiting or violent coughing) that causes a tear, with dissection of air into the interstitium. Sometimes it occurs in children with whooping cough. It is particularly likely to occur in patients on respirators who have partial bronchiolar obstruction or in persons who suffer a perforating injury (e.g., a fractured rib). When the interstitial air enters the subcutaneous tissue, the patient may literally blow up like a balloon, with marked swelling of the head and neck and crackling crepitation all over the chest. In most instances, the air is resorbed spontaneously when the site of entry is sealed.

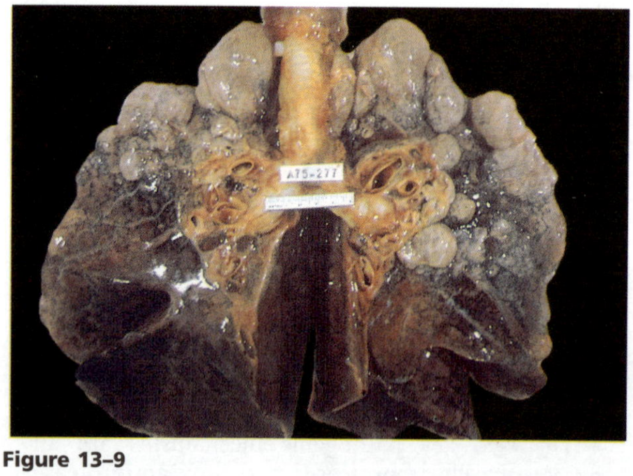

Figure 13–9

Bullous emphysema with large apical and subpleural bullae. (From the teaching collection of the Department of Pathology, University of Texas Southwestern Medical School, Dallas, Texas.)

Chronic Bronchitis

Chronic bronchitis is common among cigarette smokers and urban dwellers in smog-ridden cities; some studies of men in the 40- to 65-year age group indicate that 20% to 25% have the disease. The diagnosis of chronic bronchitis is made on clinical grounds: it is defined as *a persistent productive cough for at least 3 consecutive months in at least 2 consecutive years.* It can occur in several forms:

• Most patients have *simple chronic bronchitis:* the productive cough raises mucoid sputum, but airflow is not obstructed.

• Some patients with chronic bronchitis may demonstrate hyper-responsive airways with intermittent bronchospasm and wheezing, a condition referred to as *chronic asthmatic bronchitis.*

• A subpopulation of bronchitic patients, especially heavy smokers, develops chronic outflow obstruction, usually with evidence of associated emphysema, and these individuals are said to have *chronic obstructive* bronchitis.

Pathogenesis. The distinctive feature of chronic bronchitis is *hypersecretion of mucus,* beginning in the large airways. Although the single most important cause is cigarette smoking, other air pollutants, such as sulfur dioxide and nitrogen dioxide, may contribute. These environmental irritants induce hypertrophy of mucous glands in the trachea and main-stem bronchi and lead to a marked increase in mucin-secreting goblet cells in the surface epithelium of smaller bronchi and bronchioles. In addition, these irritants cause inflammation with infiltration of CD8+ T cells, macrophages, and neutrophils. In contrast to asthma, eosinophils are lacking in chronic bronchitis unless the patient has asthmatic bronchitis. Whereas the defining feature of chronic bronchitis (mucus hypersecretion) is primarily a reflection of large bronchial involvement, *the morphologic basis of airflow obstruction in chronic bronchitis is more peripheral and results from (1) so-called "small airway disease,"* induced by goblet cell metaplasia with mucus plugging of the bronchiolar lumen, inflammation, and bronchiolar wall fibrosis, and (2) *coexistent emphysema.* It is generally believed that while small airway disease (also known as chronic bronchiolitis) is an important component of early and relatively mild airflow obstruction, chronic bronchitis with significant airflow obstruction is almost always complicated by emphysema. It is postulated that many of the respiratory epithelial effects of environmental irritants (e.g., mucus hypersecretion) are mediated by local release of T cell cytokines such as IL-13. The transcription of the mucin gene, and neutrophil elastase *MUC5AC,* which is increased as a consequence of exposure to tobacco smoke in both in vitro and in vivo experimental models, is in part mediated by signaling via the epidermal growth factor receptor pathways. *Microbial infection* is often present but has a secondary role, chiefly by maintaining the inflammation and exacerbating symptoms.

Morphology

Grossly, the mucosal lining of the larger airways is usually **hyperemic and swollen** by edema fluid. It is often covered by a layer of mucinous or mucopurulent **secretions.** The smaller bronchi and bronchioles may also be filled with similar secretions. Histologically, the diagnostic feature of chronic bronchitis in the trachea and larger bronchi is **enlargement of the mucus-secreting glands** (Fig. 13–10). The magnitude of the increase in size is assessed by the ratio of the thickness of the submucosal gland layer to that of the bronchial wall (Reid index; normally 0.4). A variable density of inflammatory cells, largely mononuclear but sometimes admixed with neutrophils, is frequently present in the bronchial mucosa. The tissue neutrophilia increases markedly during bronchitic exacerbations, and some studies have shown a relationship between the intensity of neutrophilic infiltrate and severity of disease. **Chronic bronchiolitis** (small airway disease), characterized by goblet cell metaplasia, mucus plugging, inflammation, and fibrosis, is also present. In the most severe cases, there may be complete obliteration of the lumen due to fibrosis (bronchiolitis obliterans). As was previously stated, it is the peribronchiolar fibrosis and luminal narrowing that results in airway obstruction.

Clinical Course. In individuals with chronic bronchitis, a prominent cough and the production of sputum may persist indefinitely without ventilatory dysfunction. However, as alluded to earlier, some sufferers develop significant COPD with outflow obstruction. This is accompanied by hypercapnia, hypoxemia, and (in severe cases) cyanosis (*"blue bloaters"*). Differentiation of this form of COPD from that caused by emphysema can be made in the classic case (*"pink puffers,"* see above), but, as mentioned, many individuals have both conditions. With progression, chronic bronchitis is complicated by pulmonary hypertension and cardiac failure (Chapter 11). Recurrent infections and respiratory failure are constant threats.

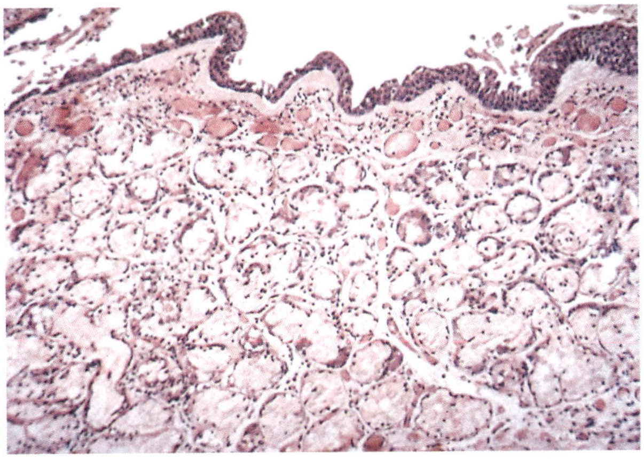

Figure 13–10

Chronic bronchitis. The lumen of the bronchus is above. Note the marked thickening of the mucous gland layer (approximately twice normal) and squamous metaplasia of lung epithelium. (From the teaching collection of the Department of Pathology, University of Texas, Southwestern Medical School, Dallas, Texas.)

SUMMARY

Chronic Bronchitis

- Chronic bronchitis is defined as persistent productive cough for at least 3 consecutive months in at least 2 consecutive years.
- Cigarette smoking is the most important underlying risk factor; air pollutants also contribute.
- Chronic obstructive component largely results from small airway disease (chronic bronchiolitis) and coexistent emphysema.
- Histology demonstrates enlargement of mucus-secreting glands, goblet cell metaplasia, and bronchiolar wall fibrosis.

Asthma

Asthma is a chronic inflammatory disorder of the airways that causes recurrent episodes of wheezing, breathlessness, chest tightness, and cough, particularly at night and/or early in the morning. This clinical picture is caused by repeated immediate hypersensitivity and late-phase reactions in the lung that give rise to the *triad of intermittent and reversible airway obstruction, chronic bronchial inflammation with eosinophils, and bronchial smooth muscle cell hypertrophy and hyperreactivity.* It is thought that inflammation causes an increase in airway responsiveness (bronchospasm) to a variety of stimuli, which would cause no ill effects in the normal airways of nonasthmatic individuals. The underlying genetic basis for hyper-responsive airways is not entirely clear, although significant advances have been made in understanding the pathogenesis and environmental triggers of asthma "attack." In some cases, the attacks are triggered by exposure to an allergen to which the person has been previously sensitized, but often no trigger can be identified. Of note, there has been a significant increase in the incidence of asthma in the Western world over the past 3 decades.

Because asthma is a heterogeneous disease triggered by a variety of inciting agents, there is no universally accepted classification scheme. About 70% of cases are said to be "extrinsic" or "atopic" and are due to IgE and T_H2-mediated immune responses to environmental antigens. In the remaining 30% of patients, asthma is said to be "intrinsic" or "non-atopic" and is triggered by nonimmune stimuli such as aspirin; pulmonary infections, especially those caused by viruses; cold; psychological stress; exercise; and inhaled irritants. While this distinction is useful from the point of pathophysiology, in clinical practice it is not always possible to classify asthma.

Pathogenesis. The major etiologic factors of asthma are genetic predisposition to type I hypersensitivity ("atopy"), acute and chronic airway inflammation, and bronchial hyper-responsiveness to a variety of stimuli. *The inflammation involves many cell types and numerous inflammatory mediators, but the role of type 2 helper T (T_H2) cells may be critical to the pathogenesis of asthma.* The classic "atopic" form of asthma is associated with an excessive T_H2 reaction against environmental antigens. Cytokines produced by T_H2 cells account for most of the features of asthma—IL-4 stimulates IgE production, IL-5 activates eosinophils, and IL-13 stimulates mucus production. All three of these cytokines are produced by T_H2 cells. In addition, epithelial cells are activated to produce chemokines that promote recruitment of more T_H2 cells and eosinophils, as well as other leukocytes, thus amplifying the inflammatory reaction. In addition to the inflammatory responses mediated by T_H2 type cells, asthma is characterized by structural changes in the bronchial wall, referred to as *"airway remodeling."* These changes include hypertrophy of bronchial smooth muscle and deposition of subepithelial collagen. Until recently, airway remodeling was considered a late, secondary change of asthma; the current view suggests that it may occur over several years before initiation of symptoms. The etiologic basis for remodeling is not clear, although there may be an *inherited predisposition* associated with polymorphisms in genes that result in accelerated proliferation of bronchial smooth muscle cells and fibroblasts. One candidate gene that has emerged in recent years is *ADAM33*, which is expressed by the cell types implicated in airway remodeling (smooth muscle cells and fibroblasts), although there are undoubtedly other genetic factors involved in this process. *Mast cells*, part of the inflammatory infiltrate in asthma, are also thought to contribute to airway remodeling by secreting growth factors that stimulate smooth muscle proliferation.

Atopic asthma. This most common type of asthma usually begins in childhood. A positive family history of atopy is common, and asthmatic attacks are often preceded by allergic rhinitis, urticaria, or eczema. The disease is triggered by environmental antigens, such as dusts, pollen, animal dander, and foods, but potentially any antigen is implicated. A skin test with the offending antigen results in an immediate wheal-and-flare reaction, a classic example of the *type I IgE–mediated hypersensitivity reaction* (Chapter 5). In the airways there is an initial *sensitization* to the inhaled inciting antigens, which stimulates induction of T_H2-type cells and release of interleukins IL-4 and IL-5 (Fig. 13–11A). This leads to synthesis of IgE that binds to mucosal mast cells. Subsequent IgE-mediated reaction to inhaled allergens elicits an *immediate response* and a *late-phase reaction* (Fig. 13–11B). Exposure of *IgE-coated mast cells* to the same antigen causes cross-linking of IgE and the release of chemical mediators. Mast cells on the respiratory mucosal surface are initially activated; the resultant mediator release opens mucosal intercellular junctions, allowing penetration of the antigen to more numerous mucosal mast cells. In addition, direct stimulation of *subepithelial vagal (parasympathetic) receptors* provokes reflex bronchoconstriction through both central and local reflexes. This occurs within minutes after stimulation and is therefore called the *acute*, or *immediate, response*, which consists of bronchoconstriction, edema (due to increased vascular permeability), and mucus secretion. A variety of inflammatory mediators have been implicated in the acute-phase response, although their relative importance in an actual asthma attack varies widely. Nevertheless, a partial list includes:

- *Leukotrienes C_4, D_4, and E_4*: extremely potent mediators that cause prolonged bronchoconstriction, increase vascular permeability, and increase mucin secretion.
- *Acetylcholine:* released from intrapulmonary motor nerves, resulting in airway smooth muscle constriction by direct stimulation of muscarinic receptors.
- *Histamine:* causes bronchospasm and increases vascular permeability, but is not considered an important mediator since antihistamine drugs do not provide benefit.
- *Prostaglandin D_2*: elicits bronchoconstriction and vasodilatation.
- *Platelet-activating factor:* causes aggregation of platelets and release of histamine from their granules.

Mast cells also release additional cytokines that cause the influx of other leukocytes, including neutrophils and mononuclear cells, and particularly *eosinophils*. These inflammatory cells set the stage for the *late-phase reaction*, which starts 4 to 8 hours later and may persist for 12 to 24 hours, or more (Fig. 13–11C). *Eosinophils* are particularly important in the late phase. As mentioned, their accumulation at sites of allergic inflammation is favored by several mast cell–derived chemotactic factors, as well as chemokines (e.g., *eotaxin*) produced by activated bronchial epithelial cells themselves. The accumulated eosinophils exert a variety of effects. Their armamentarium of mediators is as extensive as that of mast cells and includes *major basic protein* and *eosinophil cationic protein*, which are directly toxic to airway epithelial cells. *Eosinophil peroxidase* causes tissue damage through oxidative stress. Activated eosinophils are also a rich source of leukotrienes, especially leukotriene C_4, which contribute to bronchoconstriction. Thus, *eosinophils can amplify and sustain the inflammatory response* without additional exposure to the triggering antigen. The appreciation of the importance of inflammatory cells and mediators in asthma has led to greater emphasis on anti-inflammatory therapeutics in clinical practice.

Non-Atopic Asthma. The mechanism of bronchial inflammation and hyper-responsiveness is much less clear in individuals with non-atopic asthma. Incriminated in such cases are *viral infections of the respiratory tract* (most common) and *inhaled air pollutants* such as sulfur dioxide, ozone, and nitrogen dioxide. These agents increase airway hyper-reactivity in both normal and asthmatic subjects. In the latter, however, the bronchial response, manifested as spasm, is much more severe and sustained. A positive family history is uncommon, serum IgE levels are normal, and there are no associated allergies. *It is thought that virus-induced inflammation of the respiratory mucosa lowers the threshold of the subepithelial vagal receptors to irritants.* Although the connections are not well understood, the ultimate humoral and cellular mediators of

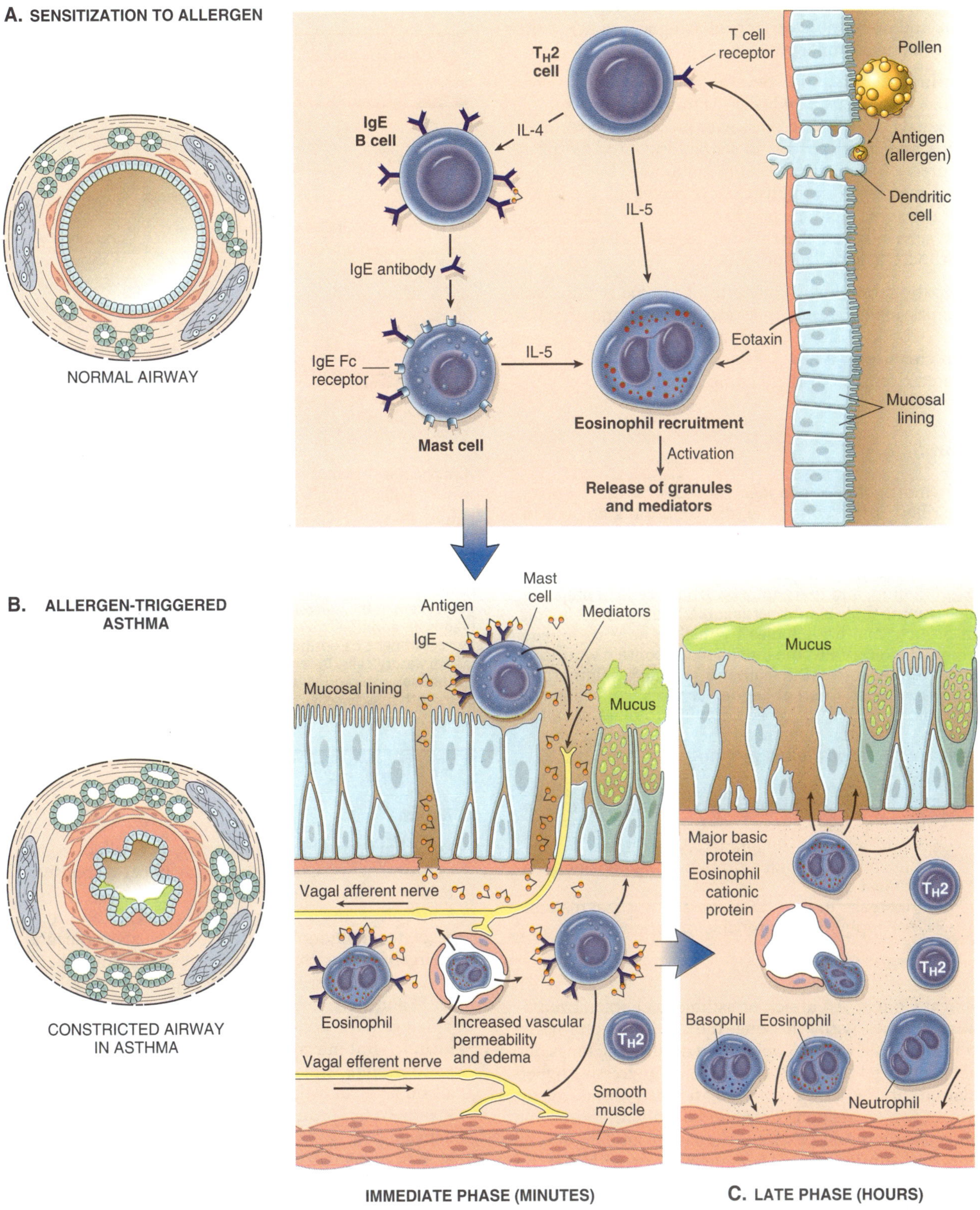

Figure 13–11

A model for allergic asthma. **A,** Sensitization to allergen. Inhaled allergens (antigens) elicit a T_H2-dominated response favoring IgE production and eosinophil recruitment (priming or sensitization). **B,** Allergen-triggered asthma. On re-exposure to antigen (Ag) the immediate reaction is triggered by Ag-induced cross-linking of IgE bound to IgE receptors on mast cells in the airways. These cells release preformed mediators that open tight junctions between epithelial cells. Antigen can then enter the mucosa to activate mucosal mast cells and eosinophils, which in turn release additional mediators. Collectively, either directly or through neuronal reflexes, the mediators induce bronchospasm, increased vascular permeability, and mucus production, besides recruiting additional mediator-releasing cells from the blood. **C,** Late phase (hours). The arrival of recruited leukocytes (neutrophils, eosinophils, basophils, and T_H2 cells) signals the initiation of the late phase of asthma and a fresh round of mediator release from leukocytes, endothelium, and epithelial cells. Factors, particularly from eosinophils (e.g., major basic protein, eosinophil cationic protein), also cause damage to the epithelium.

airway obstruction (e.g., eosinophils) are common to both atopic and non-atopic variants of asthma, and hence they are treated in a similar way.

Drug-Induced Asthma. Several pharmacologic agents provoke asthma, *aspirin* being the most striking example. Individuals with aspirin sensitivity present with recurrent rhinitis and nasal polyps, urticaria, and bronchospasm. The precise mechanism remains unknown, but it is presumed that aspirin inhibits the cyclooxygenase pathway of arachidonic acid metabolism without affecting the lipoxygenase route, thereby shifting the balance toward bronchoconstrictor leukotrienes.

Occupational Asthma. This form of asthma is stimulated by fumes (epoxy resins, plastics), organic and chemical dusts (wood, cotton, platinum), gases (toluene), and other chemicals. Asthma attacks usually develop after repeated exposure to the inciting antigen(s).

Morphology

The morphologic changes in asthma have been described in persons who die of prolonged severe attacks (status asthmaticus) and in mucosal biopsy specimens of persons challenged with allergens. In fatal cases, grossly, the lungs are overdistended because of overinflation, and there may be small areas of atelectasis. The most striking macroscopic finding is occlusion of bronchi and bronchioles by thick, tenacious **mucus plugs.** Histologically, the mucus plugs contain whorls of shed epithelium **(Curschmann spirals).** Numerous eosinophils and **Charcot-Leyden crystals** (collections of crystalloids made up of eosinophil proteins) are also present. The other characteristic findings of asthma, collectively called "airway remodeling" include (Fig. 13–12):

- Thickening of the basement membrane of the bronchial epithelium.
- Edema and an inflammatory infiltrate in the bronchial walls, with a prominence of eosinophils and mast cells.
- An increase in the size of the submucosal glands.
- Hypertrophy of the bronchial muscle walls.

Clinical Course. An attack of asthma is characterized by severe dyspnea with wheezing; the chief difficulty lies in expiration. The victim labors to get air into the lungs and then cannot get it out, so that there is progressive hyperinflation of the lungs with air trapped distal to the bronchi, which are constricted and filled with mucus and debris. In the usual case, attacks last from 1 to several hours and subside either spontaneously or with therapy, usually bronchodilators and corticosteroids. Intervals between attacks are characteristically free from respiratory difficulty, but persistent, subtle respiratory deficits can be detected by spirometric methods. Occasionally a severe paroxysm occurs that does not respond to therapy and persists for days and even weeks *(status asthmaticus)*. The associated hypercapnia, acidosis, and severe hypoxia may be fatal, although in most cases the disease is more disabling than lethal.

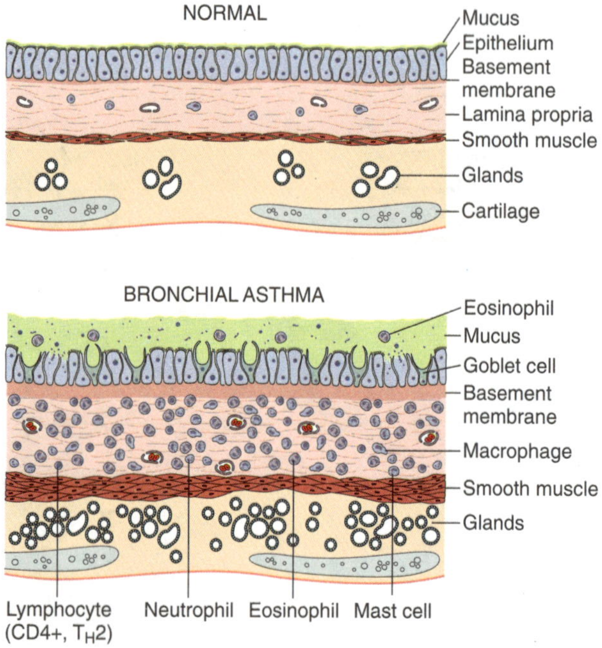

Figure 13–12

Comparison of a normal bronchiole with that in a person with asthma. Note the accumulation of mucus in the bronchial lumen resulting from an increase in the number of mucus-secreting goblet cells in the mucosa and hypertrophy of submucosal mucous glands. In addition, there is intense chronic inflammation caused by recruitment of eosinophils, macrophages, T_H2 cells and other inflammatory cells. Basement membrane underlying the mucosal epithelium is thickened, and there is hypertrophy and hyperplasia of smooth muscle cells.

SUMMARY

Asthma

- Asthma is characterized by reversible bronchoconstriction caused by airway hyper-responsiveness to a variety of stimuli.
- Atopic asthma is caused by a T_H2 and IgE-mediated immunologic reaction to environmental allergens and is characterized by acute (immediate) and late-phase reactions. The T_H2 cytokines IL-4, IL-5, and IL-13 are important mediators.
- Triggers for non-atopic asthma are less clear but include viral infections and inhaled air pollutants.
- *Eosinophils* are key inflammatory cells found in all subtypes of asthma; eosinophil products such as major basic protein are responsible for airway damage.
- Airway remodeling (basement membrane thickening and hypertrophy of bronchial smooth muscle) adds to the element of obstructive disease.

Bronchiectasis

Bronchiectasis is the permanent dilation of bronchi and bronchioles caused by destruction of the muscle and elastic supporting tissue, resulting from or associated with chronic necrotizing infections. It is not a primary disease but rather is secondary to persisting infection or obstruction caused by a variety of conditions. Once developed, it gives rise to a characteristic symptom complex dominated by cough and expectoration of copious amounts of purulent sputum. Diagnosis depends on an appropriate history along with radiographic demonstration of bronchial dilation. The conditions that most commonly predispose to bronchiectasis include the following:

- *Bronchial obstruction.* Common causes are tumors, foreign bodies, and occasionally impaction of mucus. Under these conditions, the bronchiectasis is localized to the obstructed lung segment. Bronchiectasis can also complicate atopic asthma and chronic bronchitis.
- *Congenital or hereditary conditions.* Only a few are cited:
  - In cystic fibrosis, widespread severe bronchiectasis results from obstruction and infection caused by the secretion of abnormally viscid mucus. This is an important and serious complication (Chapter 7).
  - In immunodeficiency states, particularly immunoglobulin deficiencies, bronchiectasis is likely to develop because of an increased susceptibility to repeated bacterial infections; localized or diffuse bronchiectasis can occur.
  - Kartagener syndrome, an autosomal recessive disorder, is frequently associated with bronchiectasis and with sterility in males. Structural abnormalities of the cilia impair mucociliary clearance in the airways, leading to persistent infections, and reduce the mobility of spermatozoa.
- *Necrotizing,* or *suppurative, pneumonia,* particularly with virulent organisms such as *Staphylococcus aureus* or *Klebsiella* spp., may predispose to bronchiectasis. In the past, postinfective bronchiectasis was sometimes a sequel to the childhood pneumonias that complicated measles, whooping cough, and influenza, but this has substantially decreased with the advent of successful immunization. Post-tubercular bronchiectasis continues to be a significant cause of morbidity in endemic areas.

Pathogenesis. Two processes are crucial and intertwined in the pathogenesis of bronchiectasis: *obstruction and chronic persistent infection.* Either of these two processes may come first. Normal clearance mechanisms are hampered by obstruction, so secondary infection soon follows; conversely, chronic infection in time causes damage to bronchial walls, leading to weakening and dilation. For example, obstruction caused by a bronchogenic carcinoma or a foreign body impairs clearance of secretions, providing a fertile soil for superimposed infection. The resultant inflammatory damage to the bronchial wall and the accumulating exudate further distend the airways, leading to irreversible dilation. Conversely, a persistent necrotizing inflammation in the bronchi or bronchioles may cause obstructive secretions, inflammation throughout the wall (with peribronchial fibrosis and traction on the walls), and eventually the train of events already described.

Morphology

Bronchiectatic involvement of the lungs usually affects the **lower lobes** bilaterally, particularly those air passages that are most vertical. When tumors or aspiration of foreign bodies lead to bronchiectasis, involvement may be sharply localized to a single segment of the lungs. Usually, the most severe involvement is found in the more distal bronchi and bronchioles. The airways may be **dilated** to as much as four times their usual diameter and on gross examination of the lung can be followed almost to the pleural surfaces (Fig. 13–13). (By contrast, in normal lungs, the bronchioles cannot be followed by ordinary gross examination beyond a point 2–3 cm from the pleural surfaces.) The histologic findings vary with the activity and chronicity of the disease. In the full-blown active case, an **intense acute and chronic inflammatory exudate within the walls of the bronchi and bronchioles** and the desquamation of lining epithelium cause extensive areas of ulceration. In the usual case, a **mixed** flora can be cultured from the involved bronchi, including staphylococci, streptococci, pneumococci, enteric organisms, anaerobic and microaerophilic bacteria, and (particularly in children) *Haemophilus influenzae* and *Pseudomonas aeruginosa.* When healing occurs, the lining epithelium may regenerate completely; however, usually so much injury has occurred that abnormal dilation and scarring persist. Fibrosis of the bronchial and bronchiolar walls and **peribronchiolar fibrosis** develop in more chronic cases. In some instances, the necrosis destroys the bronchial or bronchiolar walls and forms a lung abscess.

Clinical Course. The clinical manifestations consist of severe, persistent cough with expectoration of mucopurulent, sometimes fetid, sputum. The sputum may contain flecks of blood; frank hemoptysis can occur. Symptoms are often episodic and are precipitated by upper respiratory tract infections or the introduction of new pathogenic agents. Clubbing of the fingers may develop. In cases of severe, widespread bronchiectasis, significant

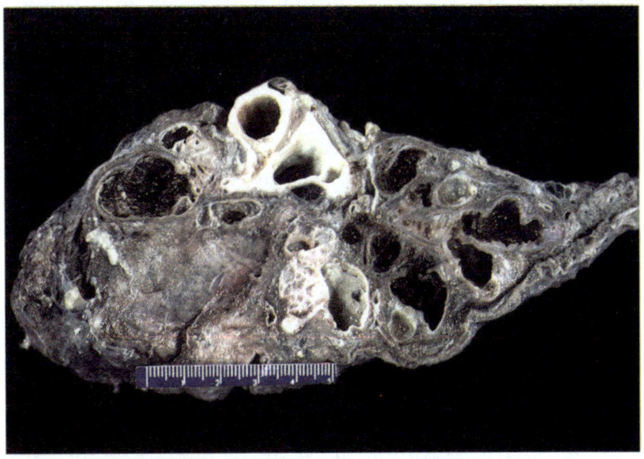

Figure 13–13

Bronchiectasis. Cross-section of lung demonstrating dilated bronchi extending almost to the pleura. (Courtesy of Dr. Linda Margraf, Department of Pathology, University of Texas Southwestern Medical School, Dallas, Texas.)

obstructive ventilatory defects develop, with hypoxemia, hypercapnia, pulmonary hypertension, and (rarely) cor pulmonale. Metastatic brain abscesses and reactive amyloidosis (Chapter 5) are other, less frequent complications of bronchiectasis.

DIFFUSE INTERSTITIAL (RESTRICTIVE, INFILTRATIVE) LUNG DISEASES

Diffuse interstitial (restrictive) lung diseases are a heterogeneous group of disorders *characterized predominantly by diffuse and usually chronic involvement of the pulmonary connective tissue, principally the most peripheral and delicate interstitium in the alveolar walls.* As noted in Fig. 13–1, the pulmonary interstitium is composed of the basement membrane of the endothelial and epithelial cells (fused in the thinnest portions), collagen fibers, elastic tissue, fibroblasts, a few mast cells, and occasional mononuclear cells. Many of the entities in this group are of unknown cause and pathogenesis; some have an intra-alveolar as well as an interstitial component, and there is frequent overlap in histologic features among the different conditions. Nevertheless, the presence of similar clinical signs, symptoms, radiographic alterations, and pathophysiologic changes justifies their consideration as a group. Although chest wall abnormalities, some of which were mentioned earlier, can also cause restrictive disease, this discussion will concentrate on parenchymal causes. The important signs and symptoms of restrictive lung disease can be inferred from the morphologic changes. *The hallmark of these disorders is reduced compliance* (i.e., more pressure is required to expand the lungs because they are stiff), which in turn necessitates increased effort of breathing (dyspnea). Furthermore, damage to the alveolar epithelium and interstitial vasculature produces abnormalities in the ventilation-perfusion ratio, leading to *hypoxia.* Chest radiographs show diffuse infiltration by small nodules, irregular lines, or "ground-glass shadows." With progression, individuals can develop respiratory failure, often in association with pulmonary hypertension and cor pulmonale (Chapter 11).

Diffuse infiltrative diseases are categorized either as clinicopathologic syndromes or as having characteristic histology (Table 13–3). While the end stage of most chronic restrictive lung diseases, irrespective of etiology, is diffuse interstitial pulmonary fibrosis with or without *honeycombing,* there are often sufficient histologic pointers in biopsy material (e.g., the existence of granulomas or telltale foreign material) to narrow, if not pinpoint, the diagnosis. An accurate social and occupational history is indispensable for the surgical pathologist examining the histologic tissue.

Pathogenesis. It is now thought that regardless of the type of interstitial disease or specific cause, the earliest common manifestation of most of the interstitial diseases is *alveolitis,* that is, accumulation of inflammatory and immune effector cells within the alveolar walls and spaces. If the injury is mild and self-limited, resolution with restoration of normal architecture follows. However, with persistence of the injurious agent, *cellular interactions involving lymphocytes, macrophages, and neutrophils lead to parenchymal injury, proliferation of fibroblasts, and progressive interstitial fibrosis* (Fig. 13–14). *Activation of pulmonary macrophages is a key event in the pathogenesis of interstitial fibrosis.* Activated macrophages secrete chemoattractants (e.g., IL-8 and leukotriene B_4) that recruit and activate neutrophils. The soluble mediators (oxidants, proteases) released from macrophages and recruited neutrophils injure alveolar

Table 13–3 Major Categories of Chronic Interstitial Lung Disease

Fibrosing
Usual interstitial pneumonia (idiopathic pulmonary fibrosis)
Nonspecific interstitial pneumonia
Cryptogenic organizing pneumonia
Associated with collagen vascular disease
Pneumoconiosis
Associated with therapies (drugs, radiation)
Granulomatous
Sarcoidosis
Hypersensitivity pneumonia
Eosinophilic
Smoking Related
Desquamative interstitial pneumonia
Respiratory bronchiolitis

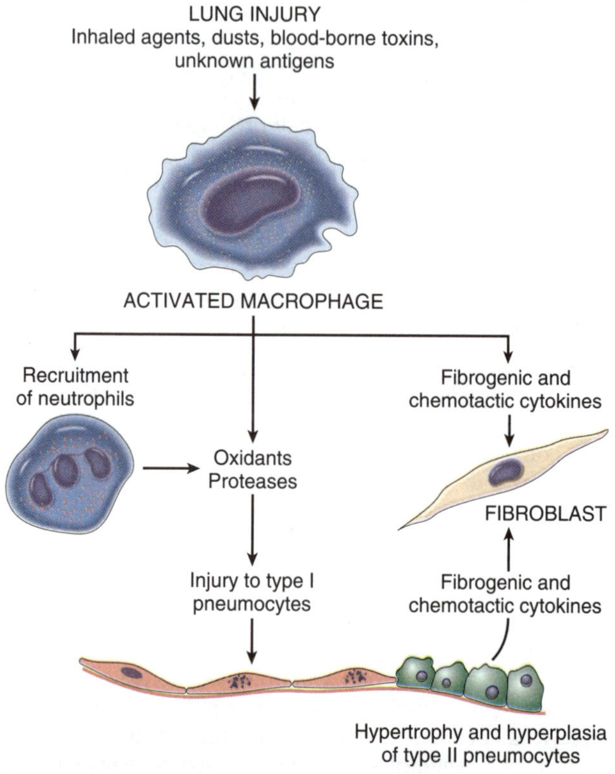

Figure 13–14

General scheme for the pathogenesis of chronic restrictive lung disease. See text for details.

epithelial cells and degrade connective tissue. Alveolar macrophages also secrete a host of "fibrogenic" factors, including fibroblast growth factor, transforming growth factor β (TGF-β), and platelet-derived growth factor, which can attract *fibroblasts* as well as stimulate their proliferation, thus setting in motion a repair response. It is now believed that alveolar epithelial cells are not merely passive targets in this process. Destruction of type I pneumocytes is often accompanied by proliferation of type II pneumocytes. These cells secrete chemotactic factors (e.g., macrophage chemotactic protein 1) that attract additional macrophages to the alveolar milieu. In addition, they can contribute to fibrosis by secreting platelet-derived growth factor and other fibrogenic cytokines, such as TGF-β. Drugs to inhibit TGF-β induced fibrosis are being developed.

Fibrosing Diseases

Idiopathic Pulmonary Fibrosis

Idiopathic pulmonary fibrosis (IPF), also known as *cryptogenic fibrosing alveolitis,* refers to a pulmonary disorder of unknown etiology characterized histologically by diffuse interstitial fibrosis, which in advanced cases results in severe hypoxemia and cyanosis. The inciting agent for recurrent alveolitis in IPF is unknown. Males are affected more often than are females, and approximately two-thirds of patients are older than 60 years of age at presentation. The histologic pattern of fibrosis is referred to as *usual interstitial pneumonia* (UIP), which is required for the diagnosis of IPF. It should be stressed, however, that similar pathologic findings in the lung may be noted with well-defined entities such as asbestosis, the collagen-vascular diseases, and a number of other conditions. Therefore, known causes must be ruled out before the appellation of "idiopathic" is used.

Morphology

Grossly, the pleural surfaces of the lung have the appearance of cobblestones because of the retraction of scars along the interlobular septa. The cut surface shows fibrosis (firm, rubbery white areas), with lower lobe predominance and a distinctive distribution in the subpleural regions and along the interlobular septa. The pattern of fibrosis in IPF is referred to as **usual interstitial pneumonia** (UIP). The histologic hallmark of UIP is **patchy interstitial fibrosis,** which varies in intensity (Fig. 13–15) and with time. The earliest lesions contain exuberant fibroblastic proliferation and appear as **fibroblastic foci** (Fig. 13–16). With time these areas become more collagenous and less cellular. Quite typical is the existence of both early and late lesions **(temporal heterogeneity).** The dense fibrosis causes collapse of alveolar walls and formation of cystic spaces lined by hyperplastic type II pneumocytes or bronchiolar epithelium **(honeycomb fibrosis).** The interstitial inflammation is usually patchy and consists of an alveolar septal infiltrate of mostly lymphocytes and occasional plasma cells, mast cells, and eosinophils. Secondary pulmonary hypertensive changes (intimal fibrosis and medial thickening of pulmonary arteries) are often present.

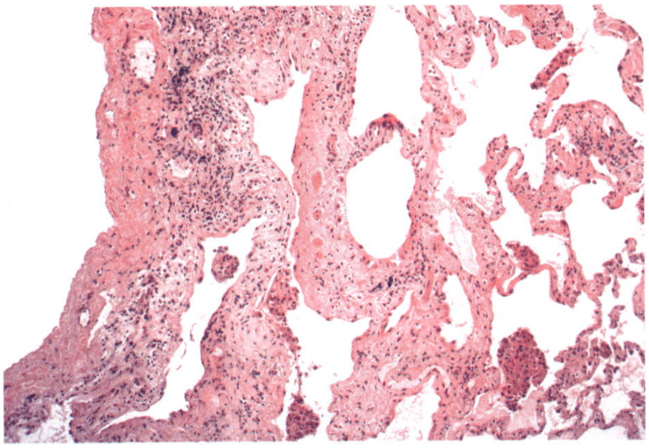

Figure 13–15

Usual interstitial pneumonia. The fibrosis, which varies in intensity, is more pronounced in the subpleural region.

Clinical Course. IPF usually presents insidiously, with the gradual onset of a nonproductive cough and progressive dyspnea. On physical examination, most individuals with IPF have characteristic "dry" or "Velcro"-like crackles during inspiration. Cyanosis, cor pulmonale, and peripheral edema may develop in the later stages of the disease. Surgical lung biopsy remains the gold standard for diagnosing IPF and for excluding other causes of pulmonary fibrosis. Unfortunately, the progress of IPF is relentless despite therapy, and the mean survival is 3 years or less. Lung transplantation is the only definitive therapy available.

Nonspecific Interstitial Pneumonia

Patients with nonspecific interstitial pneumonia have a diffuse interstitial lung disease of unknown etiology wherein the lung biopsies fail to show diagnostic features of any of the other well-characterized interstitial diseases. Though a "wastebasket" type of diagnosis, it is important to differentiate non-specific interstitial fibrosis from UIP, since the former has a better prognosis. On the basis of histology, non-specific interstitial pneumonia is divided into cellular and fibrosing patterns. The *cellular pattern*

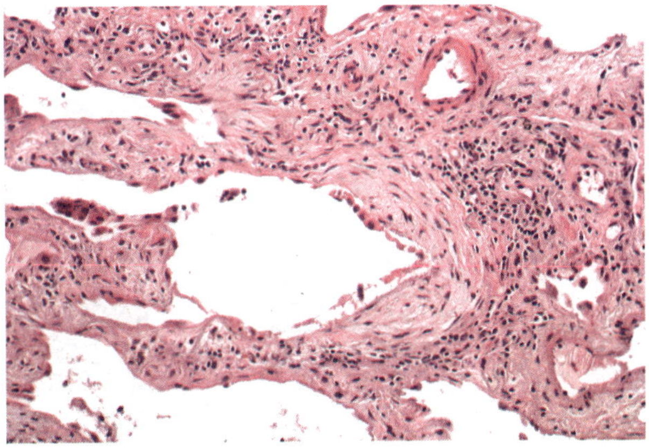

Figure 13–16

Usual interstitial pneumonia. Fibroblastic focus with fibers running parallel to surface and bluish myxoid extracellular matrix.

of non-specific interstitial fibrosis is composed of mild-to-moderate chronic interstitial inflammation (lymphocytes and a few plasma cells) in a uniform or patchy distribution. The *fibrosing pattern* consists of diffuse or patchy interstitial fibrosis, *without the temporal heterogeneity characteristic of UIP.* Fibroblastic foci are typically absent. Patients present with dyspnea and cough of several months' duration. Patients with the cellular pattern have a better outcome than those with the fibrosing pattern and UIP.

Cryptogenic Organizing Pneumonia

Cryptogenic organizing pneumonia is synonymous with "bronchiolitis obliterans organizing pneumonia"; however, the former term is now preferred, since it emphasizes the unknown etiology of this clinicopathologic entity. Patients present with cough and dyspnea and radiographically have subpleural or peribronchial patchy areas of airspace consolidation. Histologically, cryptogenic organizing pneumonia is characterized by the presence of polypoid plugs of loose organizing connective tissue within alveolar ducts, alveoli, and often bronchioles (Fig. 13–17). The connective tissue is all of the same age, and the underlying lung architecture is normal. Some individuals recover spontaneously, but most require treatment with oral steroids for 6 months or longer. Of note, organizing pneumonia with intra-alveolar fibrosis can also be seen as a response to infections (e.g., pneumonia) or inflammatory injury (e.g., collagen vascular disease, transplantation injury) to the lung; in these cases the etiology is obviously not "cryptogenic."

Pulmonary Involvement in Collagen Vascular Diseases

Many collagen vascular diseases (e.g., systemic lupus erythematosus, rheumatoid arthritis, systemic sclerosis, and dermatomyositis-polymyositis) are associated with pulmonary manifestations. Several histologic variants can be seen depending on the underlying disorder, with NSIP, UIP-pattern (similar to what is seen in IPF), vascular sclerosis, organizing pneumonia, and bronchiolitis (small airway disease, with or without fibrosis) being the most common. Pleural involvement (pleuritis, pleural nodules, and pleural effusion) may also be present. Pulmonary involvement in these diseases is usually associated with a poor prognosis, although it is still better than that of idiopathic IPF.

SUMMARY

Diffuse Interstitial Fibrosis

- Diffuse interstitial fibrosis of the lung gives rise to restrictive lung diseases characterized by reduced lung compliance and reduced forced vital capacity (FVC). Ratio of FEV to FVC is normal.
- The diseases that cause diffuse interstitial fibrosis are heterogeneous. The unifying pathogenetic factor is injury to the alveoli with activation of macrophages and release of fibrogenic cytokines such as TFG-β.
- Idiopathic pulmonary fibrosis, is prototypic of restrictive lung diseases. It is characterized by patchy lung fibrosis and formation of cystic spaces (honeycomb lung). This histologic pattern is known as *usual interstitial pneumonia.*

Pneumoconioses

Pneumoconiosis is a term originally coined to describe the non-neoplastic lung reaction to inhalation of mineral dusts. The term has been broadened to include diseases induced by organic as well as inorganic particulates, and some experts also regard chemical fume- and vapor-induced non-neoplastic lung diseases as pneumoconioses. The mineral dust pneumoconioses—the three most common of which result from exposure to coal dust, silica, and asbestos—nearly always result from exposure in the workplace. However, the increased risk of cancer as a result of asbestos exposure extends to family members of asbestos workers and to other individuals

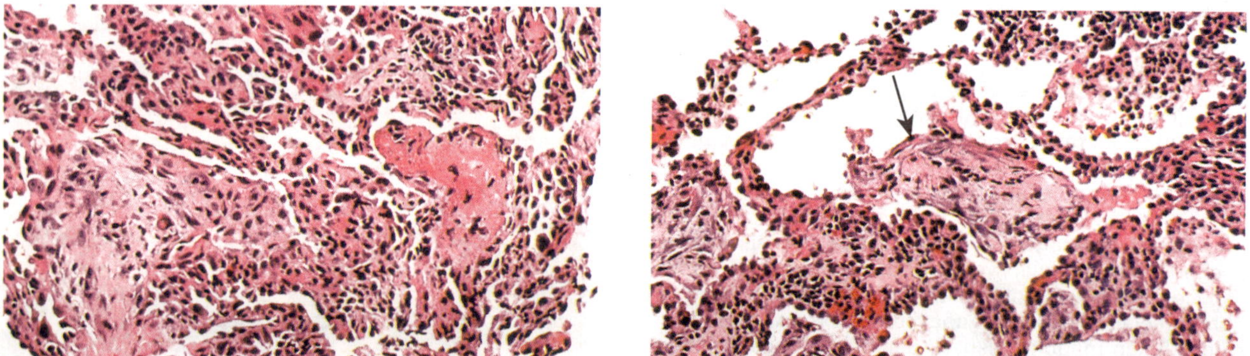

Figure 13–17

Cryptogenic organizing pneumonia. Alveolar spaces are filled with balls of fibroblasts (*arrow*).

Table 13–4 Mineral Dust-Induced Lung Disease

Agent	Disease	Exposure
Coal dust	Simple coal workers' pneumoconiosis: macules and nodules Complicated coal workers' pneumoconiosis: PMF	Coal mining
Silica	Silicosis	Sandblasting, quarrying, mining, stone cutting, foundry work, ceramics
Asbestos	Asbestosis pleural effusions, pleural plaques, or diffuse fibrosis; mesothelioma; carcinoma of the lung and larynx	Mining, milling, and fabrication of ores and materials; installation and removal of insulation

PMF, progressive massive fibrosis.

exposed to asbestos outside the workplace. Table 13–4 indicates the pathologic conditions associated with each mineral dust and the major industries in which the dust exposure is sufficient to produce disease.

Pathogenesis. The reaction of the lung to mineral dusts depends on many variables, including size, shape, solubility, and reactivity of the particles. For example, particles greater than 5 to 10 µm are unlikely to reach distal airways, whereas particles smaller than 0.5 µm tend to act like gases and move into and out of alveoli, often without substantial deposition and injury. *Particles that are 1 to 5 µm are the most dangerous, because they get lodged at the bifurcation of the distal airways.* Coal dust is relatively inert, and large amounts must be deposited in the lungs before lung disease is clinically detectable. Silica, asbestos, and beryllium are more reactive than coal dust, resulting in fibrotic reactions at lower concentrations. Most inhaled dust is entrapped in the mucus blanket and rapidly removed from the lung by ciliary movement. However, some of the particles become impacted at alveolar duct bifurcations, where macrophages accumulate and endocytose the trapped particulates. *The pulmonary alveolar macrophage is a key cellular element in the initiation and perpetuation of lung injury and fibrosis.* The more reactive particles trigger the macrophages to release a number of products that mediate an inflammatory response and initiate fibroblast proliferation and collagen deposition. Some of the inhaled particles may reach the lymphatics either by direct drainage or within migrating macrophages and thereby initiate an immune response to components of the particulates and/or to self-proteins that are modified by the particles. This then leads to an amplification and extension of the local reaction. *Tobacco smoking worsens the effects of all inhaled mineral dusts,* more so with asbestos than with any other particle.

Coal Workers' Pneumoconiosis

A number of British novels, including D. H. Lawrence's *Sons and Lovers,* poignantly describe the tragedy of the coal miners at the turn of the twentieth century who toiled underground all their lives, only to die of "black lung" complicated by tuberculosis. Dust reduction in the coal mines has drastically reduced the incidence of coal dust–induced disease. The spectrum of lung findings in coal workers is wide, ranging from *asymptomatic anthracosis,* in which pigment accumulates without a perceptible cellular reaction, to *simple coal workers' pneumoconiosis* (CWP), in which accumulations of macrophages occur with little to no pulmonary dysfunction, to *complicated CWP* or *progressive massive fibrosis* (PMF), in which fibrosis is extensive and lung function is compromised (see Table 13–4). Although statistics vary, it seems that fewer than 10% of cases of simple CWP progress to PMF. It should be noted that PMF is a generic term that applies to a confluent fibrosing reaction in the lung; this can be a complication of any one of the three pneumoconioses discussed here.

Although coal is mainly carbon, coal mine dust contains a variety of trace metals, inorganic minerals, and crystalline silica. The ratio of carbon to contaminating chemicals and minerals ("coal rank") increases from bituminous to anthracite coal; in general, anthracite mining has been associated with a higher risk of CWP.

Morphology

Pulmonary anthracosis is the most innocuous coal-induced pulmonary lesion in coal miners and is also commonly seen in all urban dwellers and tobacco smokers. Inhaled carbon pigment is engulfed by alveolar or interstitial macrophages, which then accumulate in the connective tissue along the lymphatics, including the pleural lymphatics, or in lymph nodes.

Simple CWP is characterized by **coal macules** and the somewhat larger **coal nodule.** The coal macule consists of dust-laden macrophages; in addition the nodule contains small amounts of a delicate network of collagen fibers. Although these lesions are scattered throughout the lung, the upper lobes and upper zones of the lower lobes are more heavily involved. In due course, **centrilobular emphysema** can occur. Functionally significant emphysema is more common in the United Kingdom and Europe, probably because the coal rank is higher than in the United States.

Complicated CWP (PMF) occurs on a background of simple CWP by coalescence of coal nodules and generally requires many years to develop. It is characterized by intensely blackened scars larger than 2 cm, sometimes up to 10 cm in greatest diameter. They are usually multiple (Fig. 13–18). Microscopically the lesions consist of dense collagen and pigment.

Clinical Course. CWP is usually a benign disease that produces little decrement in lung function. In those in whom PMF develops, there is increasing pulmonary dysfunction, pulmonary hypertension, and cor pulmonale. Progression

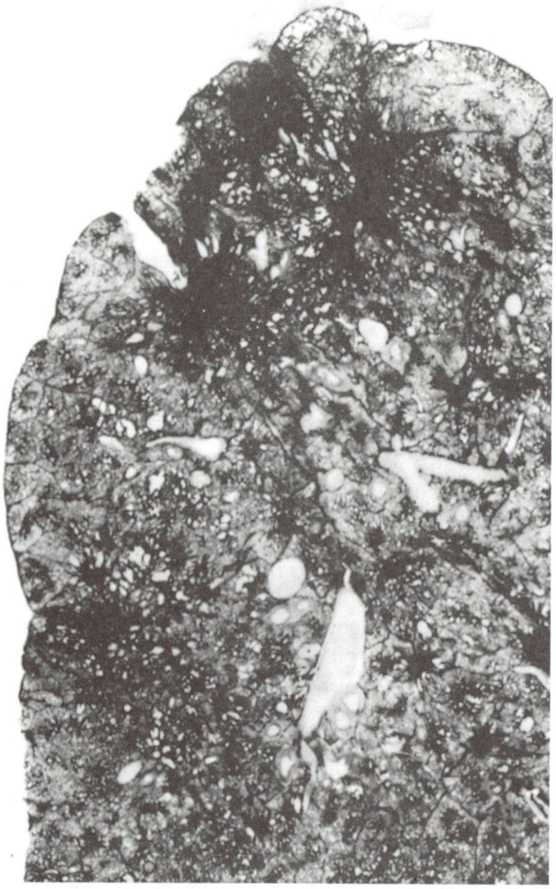

Figure 13–18

Progressive massive fibrosis superimposed on coal workers' pneumoconiosis. The large blackened scars are principally in the upper lobe. Note the extensions of scars into surrounding parenchyma and retraction of adjacent pleura. (Courtesy of Dr. Werner Laquer, Dr. Jerome Kleinerman, and the National Institute of Occupational Safety and Health.)

from CWP to PMF has been linked to a variety of conditions including coal dust exposure level and total dust burden. Unfortunately, PMF has a tendency to progress even in the absence of further exposure. Once smoking-related risk has been taken into account, there is no increased frequency of bronchogenic carcinoma in coal miners, a feature that distinguishes CWP from both silica and asbestos exposures (see below).

Silicosis

Silicosis *is currently the most prevalent chronic occupational disease in the world.* It is caused by inhalation of crystalline silica, mostly in occupational settings. Silica occurs in both crystalline and amorphous forms, but crystalline forms (including quartz, cristobalite, and tridymite) are by far the most toxic and fibrogenic. Of these, quartz is most commonly implicated in silicosis. After inhalation the particles interact with epithelial cells and macrophages. *Ingested silica particles cause activation and release of mediators by pulmonary macrophages,* including IL-1, TNF, fibronectin, lipid mediators, oxygen-derived free radicals, and fibrogenic cytokines. Especially compelling is the evidence incriminating TNF, since anti-TNF monoclonal antibodies can block lung collagen accumulation in mice that are given silica intratracheally. *It has been noted that when mixed with other minerals, quartz has a reduced fibrogenic effect.* This phenomenon is of practical importance because quartz in the workplace is rarely pure. Thus, miners of the iron-containing ore hematite may have more quartz in their lungs than some quartz-exposed workers and yet have relatively mild lung disease because the hematite provides a protective effect.

Morphology

Silicotic nodules are characterized grossly in their early stages by tiny, barely palpable, discrete, pale-to-blackened (if coal dust is also present) nodules in the upper zones of the lungs (Fig. 13–19). Microscopically, the silicotic nodule demonstrates **concentrically arranged hyalinized collagen fibers** surrounding an amorphous center. The "whorled" appearance of the collagen fibers is quite distinctive for silicosis (Fig. 13–20). Examination of the nodules by **polarized microscopy reveals weakly birefringent silica** particles, primarily in the center of the nodules. As the disease progresses, the individual nodules may coalesce into hard, collagenous scars, with eventual progression to PMF. The intervening lung parenchyma may be compressed or overexpanded, and a honeycomb pattern may develop. Fibrotic lesions may also occur in the hilar lymph nodes and pleura. Sometimes, thin sheets of calcification occur in the lymph nodes and are appreciated radiographically as "eggshell" calcification (e.g., calcium surrounding a zone lacking calcification).

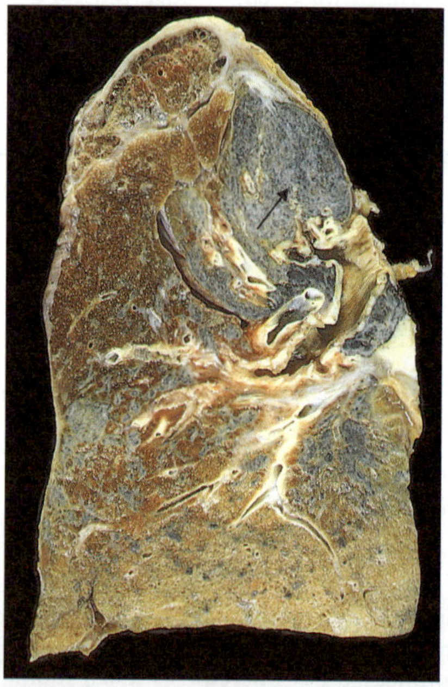

Figure 13–19

Advanced silicosis seen on transection of lung. Scarring has contracted the upper lobe into a small dark mass *(arrow).* Note the dense pleural thickening. (Courtesy of Dr. John Godleski, Brigham and Women's Hospital, Boston, Massachusetts.)

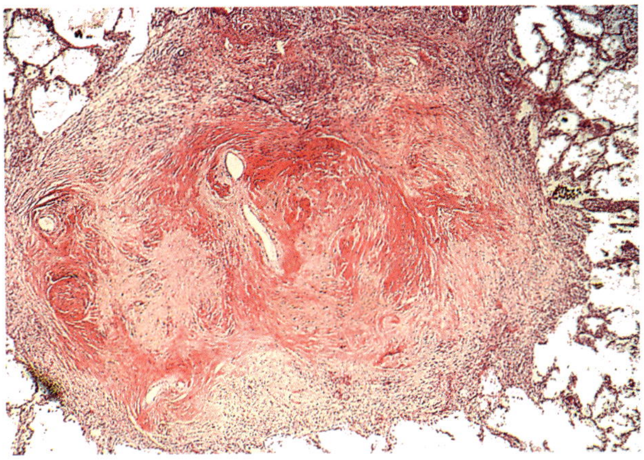

Figure 13–20

Several coalescent collagenous silicotic nodules. (Courtesy of Dr. John Godleski, Brigham and Women's Hospital, Boston, Massachusetts.)

Clinical Course. Silicosis is usually detected in routine chest radiographs performed on asymptomatic workers. The radiographs typically show a fine nodularity in the upper zones of the lung, but pulmonary function is either normal or only moderately affected. Most individuals do not develop shortness of breath until late in the course, after PMF is present. At this time, the disease may be progressive, even if the person is no longer exposed. Many individuals with PMF develop pulmonary hypertension and cor pulmonale, as a result of chronic hypoxia-induced vasoconstriction and parenchymal destruction. The disease is slow to kill, but impaired pulmonary function may severely limit activity. *Silicosis is associated with an increased susceptibility to tuberculosis.* It is postulated that silicosis results in a depression of cell-mediated immunity, and crystalline silica may inhibit the ability of pulmonary macrophages to kill phagocytosed mycobacteria. Nodules of silicotuberculosis often display a central zone of caseation. The relationship between silica and *lung cancer* has been a contentious issue, but in 1997, based on evidence from several epidemiologic studies, the International Agency for Research on Cancer concluded that *crystalline silica* from occupational sources is carcinogenic in humans. However, this subject continues to be controversial.

Asbestosis and Asbestos-Related Diseases

Asbestos is a family of crystalline hydrated silicates with a fibrous geometry. On the basis of epidemiologic studies, occupational exposure to asbestos is linked to (1) parenchymal interstitial fibrosis *(asbestosis);* (2) localized fibrous plaques or, rarely, diffuse fibrosis in the pleura; (3) pleural effusions; (4) bronchogenic carcinoma; (5) malignant pleural and peritoneal mesotheliomas; and (6) laryngeal carcinoma. An increased incidence of asbestos-related cancers in family members of asbestos workers has alerted the general public to the potential hazards of asbestos in the environment.

Pathogenesis. Concentration, size, shape, and solubility of the different forms of asbestos dictate whether disease will occur. There are two distinct forms of asbestos: *serpentine* (in which the fiber is curly and flexible) and *amphibole* (in which the fiber is straight, stiff, and brittle). There are several subtypes of curly and straight asbestos fibers. The serpentine *chrysotile* accounts for most of the asbestos used in industry. Amphiboles, even though less prevalent, are more pathogenic than the serpentine chrysotile, but both types can produce asbestosis, lung cancer, and mesothelioma. The greater pathogenicity of straight and stiff amphiboles is apparently related to their structure. The serpentine chrysotiles, with their more flexible, curled structure, are likely to become impacted in the upper respiratory passages and removed by the mucociliary elevator. Those that are trapped in the lungs are gradually leached from the tissues, because they are more soluble than amphiboles. The straight, stiff amphiboles, in contrast, align themselves in the airstream and are hence delivered deeper into the lungs, where they may penetrate epithelial cells and reach the interstitium. Despite these differences, both asbestos forms are fibrogenic, and increasing exposure to either is associated with a higher incidence of all asbestos-related diseases. Asbestosis, like other pneumoconioses, causes fibrosis by interacting with lung macrophages.

In addition to cellular and fibrotic lung reactions, asbestos probably also functions as both a tumor initiator and a promoter. Some of the oncogenic effects of asbestos on the mesothelium are mediated by reactive free radicals generated by asbestos fibers, which preferentially localize in the distal lung close to the mesothelial layer. However, potentially toxic chemicals adsorbed onto the asbestos fibers undoubtedly contribute to the pathogenicity of the fibers. For example, *the adsorption of carcinogens in tobacco smoke onto asbestos fibers may well be important to the remarkable synergy between tobacco smoking and the development of bronchogenic carcinoma in asbestos workers.*

Morphology

Asbestosis is marked by diffuse pulmonary interstitial fibrosis. These changes are indistinguishable from those resulting from other causes of diffuse interstitial fibrosis, except for the presence of **asbestos bodies,** which are seen as golden brown, fusiform or beaded rods with a translucent center. They consist of asbestos fibers coated with an iron-containing proteinaceous material (Fig. 13–21). Asbestos bodies apparently arise when macrophages attempt to phagocytose asbestos fibers; the iron is derived from phagocyte ferritin. Asbestos bodies can sometimes be found in the lungs of normal persons, but usually in much lower concentrations and without an accompanying interstitial fibrosis.

In contrast to CWP and silicosis, asbestosis begins in the lower lobes and subpleurally, but the middle and upper lobes of the lungs become affected as fibrosis progresses. Contraction of the fibrous tissue distorts the native architecture, creating enlarged airspaces enclosed within thick fibrous walls. In this way the affected regions become honeycombed. Simultaneously, the visceral pleura undergoes fibrous thickening and sometimes binds the lungs to the chest wall. The scarring may trap and narrow pulmonary arteries and arterioles, causing pulmonary hypertension and cor pulmonale.

Pleural plaques are the most common manifestation of asbestos exposure and are well-circumscribed plaques of dense collagen (Fig. 13–22), often containing calcium. They develop most frequently on the anterior and posterolateral aspects of the **parietal pleura** and over the domes of the diaphragm. They do not contain asbestos bodies, and only rarely do they occur in persons who have no history or evidence of asbestos exposure. Uncommonly, asbestos exposure induces pleural effusions, which are usually serous but may be bloody. Rarely, diffuse visceral pleural fibrosis may occur and, in advanced cases, bind the lung to the thoracic cavity wall.

Clinical Course. The clinical findings in asbestosis are indistinguishable from those of any other diffuse interstitial lung disease. Typically, progressively worsening dyspnea appears 10 to 20 years after exposure. The dyspnea is usually accompanied by a cough associated with production of sputum. The disease may remain static or progress to CHF, cor pulmonale, and death. Pleural plaques are usually asymptomatic and are detected on radiographs as circumscribed densities. *Both bronchogenic carcinomas and malignant mesotheliomas develop in workers exposed to asbestos.* The risk of bronchogenic carcinoma is increased about fivefold for asbestos workers; the relative risk for mesotheliomas, normally a very rare tumor (2–17 cases per 1 million persons), is more than 1000-fold greater. Both pleural and peritoneal mesotheliomas have an association with asbestos exposure. Concomitant cigarette smoking greatly increases the risk of bronchogenic carcinoma but not that of mesothelioma. Lung or pleural cancer associated with asbestos exposure has a particularly grim prognosis.

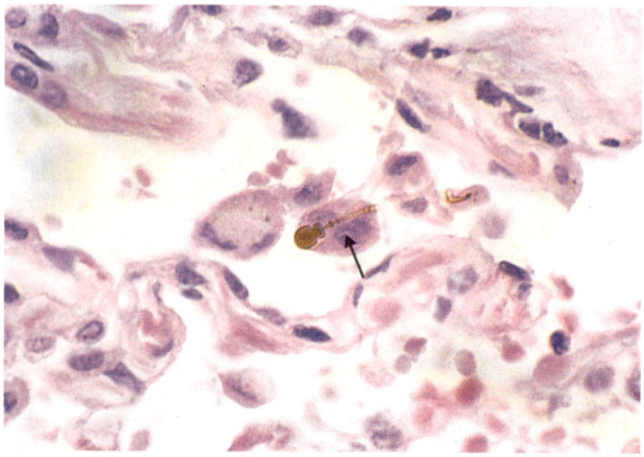

Figure 13–21

High-power detail of an asbestos body, revealing the typical beading and knobbed ends *(arrow)*.

SUMMARY

Pneumoconioses

- Pneumoconioses encompass a group of chronic fibrosing diseases of the lung resulting from exposure to organic and inorganic particulates, most commonly mineral dust.
- Pulmonary alveolar macrophages play a central role in the pathogenesis of lung injury by promoting inflammation and producing reactive oxygen species and fibrogenic cytokines.
- Coal dust-induced disease varies from *asymptomatic anthracosis*, to *simple coal workers pneumoconiosis* (coal macules or nodules, and centrilobular emphysema), to progressive massive fibrosis (PMF), manifested by increasing pulmonary dysfunction, pulmonary hypertension, and cor pulmonale.
- Silicosis is the most common pneumoconiosis in the world, and crystalline silica (e.g., quartz) is the usual suspect.
- The manifestations of silicosis can range from asymptomatic silicotic nodules to PMF; individuals with silicosis also have an increased susceptibility to tuberculosis. The relationship between silica exposure and subsequent lung cancer is controversial.
- Asbestos fibers come in two forms: the stiff *amphiboles* have a greater fibrogenic and carcinogenic potential than the serpentile *chrysotiles*.
- Asbestos exposure is linked with six disease processes: (1) parenchymal interstitial fibrosis *(asbestosis)*; (2) localized fibrous plaques or, rarely, diffuse pleural fibrosis; (3) pleural effusions; (4) lung cancer; (5) malignant pleural and peritoneal mesotheliomas; and (6) laryngeal cancer.
- Cigarette smoking increases the risk of lung cancer in the setting of asbestos exposure; moreover, even family members of workers exposed to asbestos are at increased risk for cancer.

Drug- and Radiation-Induced Pulmonary Diseases

Drugs can cause a variety of both acute and chronic alterations in respiratory structure and function. For example, *bleomycin*, an anticancer agent, causes pneumonitis and interstitial fibrosis, as a result of direct toxicity of the drug and by stimulating the influx of inflammatory cells into the alveoli. Similarly, *amiodarone*, an anti-arrhythmic agent, is also associated with pneumonitis and fibrosis. *Radiation pneumonitis* is a well-known complication of therapeutic radiation of pulmonary and other thoracic tumors. *Acute radiation pneumonitis*, which typically occurs 1 to 6 months after therapy in as many as 20% of individuals, is manifested by fever, dyspnea out of proportion to the volume of irradiated lung, pleural effusion, and pulmonary infiltrates corresponding to the area of radiation. These symptoms may resolve with corticosteroid therapy or progress to *chronic radiation pneumonitis*, associated with pulmonary fibrosis.

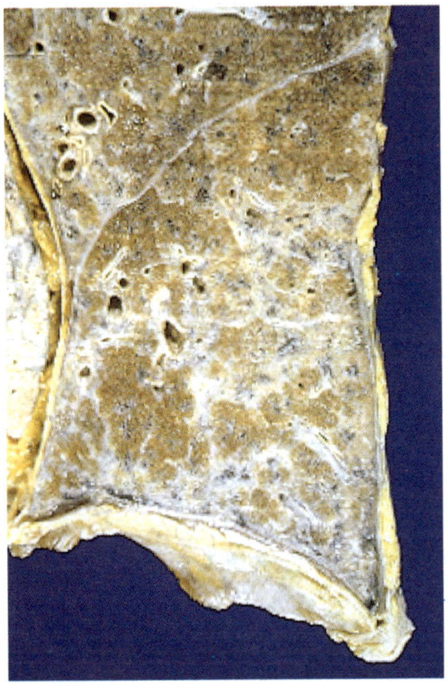

Figure 13–22

Asbestosis. Markedly thickened visceral pleura covers the lateral and diaphragmatic surface of lung. Note also severe interstitial fibrosis diffusely affecting the lower lobe of the lung.

Granulomatous Diseases

Sarcoidosis

Although sarcoidosis is considered here as an example of a restrictive lung disease, it is important to remember that sarcoidosis is a *multisystem disease of unknown etiology characterized by noncaseating granulomas in many tissues and organs.* Other diseases, including mycobacterial or fungal infections and berylliosis, sometimes also produce noncaseating granulomas; therefore, the histologic *diagnosis of sarcoidosis is one of exclusion.* Although the multisystemic involvement of sarcoidosis can present in many clinical guises, bilateral hilar lymphadenopathy or lung involvement (or both), visible on chest radiographs, is the major presenting manifestation in most cases. Eye and skin involvement each occurs in about 25% of cases and may occasionally be the presenting feature of the disease.

Epidemiology. Sarcoidosis occurs throughout the world, affecting both sexes and all races and ages. There are, however, certain interesting epidemiologic trends, including the following:

- There is a consistent predilection for adults younger than 40 years of age.
- A high incidence has been noted in the Danish and Swedish populations and among US African Americans (in whom the frequency of involvement is 10 times greater than in US Caucasians).
- Sarcoidosis is one of the few pulmonary diseases with a higher prevalence among *nonsmokers.*

Etiology and Pathogenesis. Although the etiology of sarcoidosis remains unknown, several lines of evidence suggest that it is a disease of disordered immune regulation in genetically predisposed individuals exposed to certain environmental agents. The role of each of these three contributory influences is summarized below.

There are several *immunologic abnormalities* in sarcoidosis that suggest the development of a cell-mediated response to an unidentified antigen. The process is driven by CD4+ helper T cells. These include:

- Intra-alveolar and interstitial accumulation of CD4+ T_H1 cells.
- Oligoclonal expansion of T-cell subsets as determined by analysis of T-cell receptor rearrangement.
- Increases in T cell-derived T_H1 cytokines such as IL-2 and IFN-γ, resulting in T-cell expansion and macrophage activation, respectively.
- Increases in several cytokines in the local environment (IL-8, TNF, macrophage inflammatory protein 1α) that favor recruitment of additional T cells and monocytes and contribute to the formation of granulomas.
- Anergy to common skin test antigens such as *Candida* or purified protein derivative (PPD), that may result from pulmonary recruitment of CD4+ T cells and consequent peripheral depletion.
- Polyclonal hypergammaglobulinemia, another manifestation of T_H-cell dysregulation.
- Genetic influences in individuals with sarcoidosis are suggested by familial and racial clustering of cases and association with certain human leukocyte antigen (HLA) genotypes (e.g., class I HLA-A1 and HLA-B8).

Finally, several putative "antigens" have been proposed as the inciting agent for sarcoidosis (e.g., viruses, mycobacteria, *Borrelia,* pollen), but thus far *there is no unequivocal evidence to suggest that sarcoidosis is caused by an infectious agent.*

Morphology

The histopathologic sine qua non of sarcoidosis is the **noncaseating epithelioid granuloma,** irrespective of the organ involved (Fig. 13–23). This is a discrete, compact collection of epithelioid cells rimmed by an outer zone of largely CD4+ T cells. The epithelioid cells are derived from macrophages and are characterized by abundant eosinophilic cytoplasm and vesicular nuclei. It is not uncommon to see intermixed multinucleated giant cells formed by fusion of macrophages. A thin layer of laminated fibroblasts is present peripheral to the granuloma; over time, these proliferate and lay down collagen that replaces the entire granuloma with a hyalinized scar. Two other microscopic features are sometimes seen in the granulomas: (1) **Schaumann bodies,** laminated concretions composed of calcium and proteins; and (2) **asteroid bodies,** stellate inclusions enclosed within giant cells. Their presence is not required for diagnosis of sarcoidosis; they may also occur in granulomas of other origins. Rarely, foci of central necrosis may be present in sarcoid granulomas, suggesting an infectious process. Caseation necrosis typical of tuberculosis is absent.

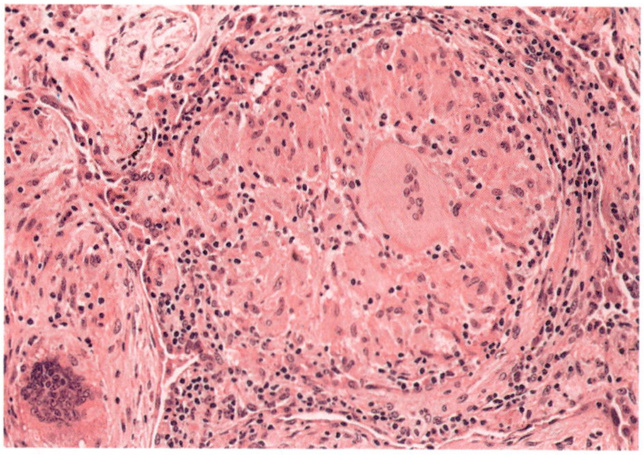

Figure 13–23

Characteristic sarcoid noncaseating granulomas in lung with many giant cells. (Courtesy of Dr. Ramon Blanco, Department of Pathology, Brigham and Women's Hospital, Boston, Massachusetts.)

The **lungs** are involved at some stage of the disease in 90% of patients. The granulomas predominantly involve the interstitium rather than airspaces, with some tendency to localize in the connective tissue around bronchioles and pulmonary venules and in the pleura ("lymphangitic" distribution). The bronchoalveolar lavage (BAL) contains abundant CD4+T cells. In 5% to 15% of patients, the granulomas are eventually replaced by **diffuse interstitial fibrosis** resulting in a honeycomb lung.

Intrathoracic **hilar and paratracheal lymph nodes** are enlarged in 75% to 90% of patients, while a third present with peripheral lymphadenopathy. The nodes are characteristically painless and have a firm, rubbery texture. Unlike in tuberculosis, lymph nodes in sarcoidosis are "nonmatted" (nonadherent) and do not ulcerate.

Skin lesions are encountered in approximately 25% of patients. **Erythema nodosum,** the hallmark of acute sarcoidosis, consists of raised, red, tender nodules on the anterior aspects of the legs. Sarcoidal granulomas are uncommon in these lesions. In contrast, discrete painless subcutaneous nodules can also occur in sarcoidosis, and these usually reveal abundant noncaseating granulomas. Another characteristic skin lesion of sarcoidosis consists of indurated plaques associated with a violaceous discoloration in the region of the nose, cheeks, and lips **(lupus pernio).**

Involvement of the eye and lacrimal glands occurs in about one-fifth to one-half of patients. The ocular involvement takes the form of iritis or iridocyclitis and may be unilateral or bilateral. As a consequence, corneal opacities, glaucoma, and (less commonly) total loss of vision may develop. The posterior uveal tract is also affected, with resultant **choroiditis, retinitis,** and **optic nerve involvement.** These ocular lesions are frequently accompanied by inflammation in the lacrimal glands, with suppression of lacrimation **(sicca syndrome). Unilateral or bilateral parotitis with painful enlargement of the parotid glands** occurs in less than 10% of the individuals with sarcoidosis; some go on to develop xerostomia (dry mouth). Combined uveoparotid involvement is designated **Mikulicz syndrome.**

The spleen may appear unaffected grossly, but in about three-fourths of cases it contains granulomas. In approximately 10% it becomes clinically enlarged. **The liver** demonstrates microscopic granulomatous lesions, usually in the portal triads, about as often as the spleen, but only about one-third of the patients demonstrate hepatomegaly or abnormal liver function. Sarcoid involvement of **bone marrow** is reported in as many as 40% of patients, although it rarely causes severe manifestations. Sometimes there is hypercalcemia and hypercalciuria. This is not related to bone destruction but rather is caused by increased calcium absorption secondary to production of active vitamin D by the mononuclear phagocytes in the granulomas.

Clinical Course. In many individuals the disease is entirely asymptomatic, discovered on routine chest films as bilateral hilar adenopathy or as an incidental finding at autopsy. In others, peripheral lymphadenopathy, cutaneous lesions, eye involvement, splenomegaly, or hepatomegaly may be presenting manifestations. In about two-thirds of symptomatic cases there is a gradual appearance of respiratory symptoms (shortness of breath, dry cough, or vague substernal discomfort) or constitutional signs and symptoms (fever, fatigue, weight loss, anorexia, night sweats). Because of the variable and nondiagnostic clinical features, resort is frequently made to lung or lymph node biopsy. *The presence of noncaseating granulomas is suggestive of sarcoidosis, but other identifiable causes of granulomatous inflammation must be excluded.*

Sarcoidosis follows an unpredictable course characterized by either progressive chronicity or periods of activity interspersed with remissions. The remissions may be spontaneous or initiated by steroid therapy and are often permanent. Overall, 65% to 70% of affected individuals recover with minimal or no residual manifestations. Twenty percent develop permanent lung dysfunction or visual impairment. Of the remaining 10% to 15%, most succumb to progressive pulmonary fibrosis and cor pulmonale.

SUMMARY

Sarcoidosis

- Multisystemic disease of unknown etiology; histopathologic sine qua non is noncaseating granulomas in various tissues.
- Immunologic abnormalities include high levels of CD4+ T cells in the lung that secrete T_H1-dependent cytokines such as IFN-γ and IL-2 locally.
- Clinical manifestations include lymph node enlargement, eye involvement (sicca syndrome [dry eyes], iritis, or iridocyclitis), skin lesions (erythema nodosum, lupus pernio), and visceral (liver, skin, marrow) involvement. Lung involvement occurs in 90% of cases with formation of granulomas and interstitial fibrosis.

Hypersensitivity Pneumonitis

Hypersensitivity pneumonitis is an immunologically mediated inflammatory lung disease that primarily affects the alveoli and is therefore often called *allergic alveolitis.* Most often it is an occupational disease that results from heightened sensitivity to inhaled antigens such as moldy hay (Table 13–5). Unlike bronchial asthma, in which *bronchi are the focus of immunologically mediated injury, the damage in hypersensitivity pneumonitis occurs at the level of alveoli.* Hence, it presents as a predominantly restrictive lung disease with decreased diffusion capacity, lung compliance, and total lung volume. The occupational exposures are diverse, but the syndromes share common clinical and pathologic findings and probably have very similar pathophysiology.

Several lines of evidence suggest that hypersensitivity pneumonitis is an immunologically mediated disease:

- Bronchioalveolar lavage specimens consistently demonstrate increased numbers of T lymphocytes of both CD4+ and CD8+ phenotype.
- Most individuals with hypersensitivity pneumonitis have specific precipitating antibodies in their serum, and complement and immunoglobulins have been demonstrated within vessel walls by immunofluorescence, indicating a type III hypersensitivity. The presence of noncaseating granulomas in two-thirds of individuals with this disorder suggests development of a type IV hypersensitivity against the implicated antigen(s).

In summary, hypersensitivity pneumonitis is an immunologically mediated response to an extrinsic antigen that involves both immune-complex and delayed-type hypersensitivity reactions.

Morphology

The histopathology of both acute and chronic forms of hypersensitivity pneumonitis demonstrates patchy mononuclear cell infiltrates in the pulmonary interstitium, with a characteristic peribronchiolar accentuation. Lymphocytes predominate, but plasma cells and epithelioid cells are also present. In acute forms of the disease, variable numbers of neutrophils also may be seen. **Interstitial noncaseating granulomas** are present in more than two-thirds of cases, usually in a peribronchiolar location. In advanced chronic cases, diffuse interstitial fibrosis occurs.

Clinical Course. Hypersensitivity pneumonitis may present either as an *acute reaction* with fever, cough, dyspnea, and constitutional complaints 4 to 8 hours after exposure or as a *chronic disease* with insidious onset of cough, dyspnea, malaise, and weight loss. The diagnosis of the acute form of this disease is usually obvious because of the temporal relationship of symptoms to exposure to the incriminating antigen. *If antigenic exposure is terminated after acute attacks of the disease,* there is complete resolution of pulmonary symptoms within days. Failure to remove the inciting agent from the environment eventually results in a chronic interstitial pulmonary disease without the acute exacerbations seen on antigen re-exposure.

Pulmonary Eosinophilia

A number of clinical and pathologic pulmonary entities are characterized by an infiltration and activation of eosinophils, the latter by elevated levels of alveolar IL-5. These diverse diseases are generally of immunologic origin, but are incompletely understood. Pulmonary eosinophilia is divided into the following categories:

- *Acute eosinophilic pneumonia with respiratory failure,* characterized by rapid onset of fever, dyspnea, hypoxia, and diffuse pulmonary infiltrates on chest radiograms. The bronchioalveolar lavage fluid typically contains more than 25% eosinophils. There is prompt response to corticosteroids.

Table 13–5 Selected Causes of Hypersensitivity Pneumonitis

Syndrome	Exposure	Antigens
Fungal and Bacterial Antigens		
Farmer's lung	Moldy hay	*Micropolyspora faeni*
Bagassosis	Moldy pressed sugar cane (bagasse)	Thermophilic actinomycetes
Maple bark disease	Moldy maple bark	*Cryptostroma corticale*
Humidifier lung	Cool-mist humidifier	Thermophilic actinomycetes, *Aureobasidium pullulans*
Malt worker's lung	Moldy barley	*Aspergillus clavatus*
Cheese washer's lung	Moldy cheese	*Penicillium casei*
Insect Products		
Miller's lung	Dust-contaminated grain	*Sitophilus granarius* (wheat weevil)
Animal Products		
Pigeon breeder's lung	Pigeons	Pigeon serum proteins in droppings
Chemicals		
Chemical worker's lung	Chemical industry	Trimellitic anhydride, isocyanates

- *Simple pulmonary eosinophilia* (Löffler syndrome), characterized by transient pulmonary lesions, eosinophilia in the blood, and a benign clinical course. The alveolar septa are thickened by an infiltrate containing eosinophils and occasional giant cells.
- *Tropical eosinophilia,* caused by infection with microfilariae, a parasite.
- *Secondary eosinophilia,* seen, for example, in association with asthma, drug allergies, and certain forms of vasculitis.
- *Idiopathic chronic eosinophilic pneumonia,* characterized by aggregates of lymphocytes and eosinophils within the septal walls and the alveolar spaces, typically in the periphery of the lung fields, and accompanied by high fever, night sweats, and dyspnea. This is a disease of exclusion, once other causes of pulmonary eosinophilia have been ruled out.

Smoking-Related Interstitial Diseases

The role of cigarette smoking in causing obstructive pulmonary disease (emphysema and chronic bronchitis) has been discussed. Smoking is also associated with restrictive or interstitial lung diseases. *Desquamative interstitial pneumonia* (DIP) and *respiratory bronchiolitis* are the two related examples of smoking-associated interstitial lung disease. The most striking histologic feature of DIP is the accumulation of large numbers of macrophages with abundant cytoplasm containing dusty brown pigment *(smoker's macrophages)* in the airspaces (Fig. 13–24). The alveolar septa are thickened by a sparse inflammatory infiltrate (usually lymphocytes), and interstitial fibrosis, when present, is mild. Pulmonary functions usually show a mild restrictive abnormality, and patients with DIP typically have a good prognosis with excellent response to steroid therapy and smoking cessation. Respiratory bronchiolitis is a common histologic lesion found in smokers, characterized by the presence of pigmented intraluminal macrophages akin to DIP, but in a "bronchiolocentric" distribution (first- and second-order respiratory bronchioles). Mild peribronchiolar fibrosis is also seen. As with DIP, individuals present with gradual onset of dyspnea and dry cough, and the symptoms recede with cessation of smoking.

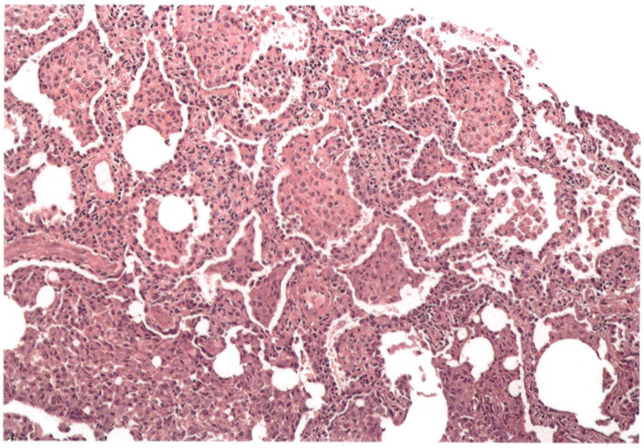

Figure 13–24

Desquamative interstitial pneumonia. Medium-power detail of lung to demonstrate the accumulation of large numbers of mononuclear cells within the alveolar spaces with only mild fibrous thickening of the alveolar walls.

DISEASES OF VASCULAR ORIGIN

Pulmonary Embolism, Hemorrhage, and Infarction

Blood clots that occlude the large pulmonary arteries are almost always embolic in origin. More than 95% of all pulmonary emboli arise from thrombi within the large deep veins of the lower legs, typically originating in the popliteal vein and larger veins above it. Thromboembolism causes approximately 50,000 deaths per year in the United States. Even when not directly fatal, it can complicate the course of other diseases. The true incidence of nonfatal pulmonary embolism is not known. Some emboli undoubtedly occur outside the hospital in ambulatory patients and are small and clinically silent. Even among hospitalized individuals, no more than one-third are diagnosed before death. Autopsy data on the incidence of pulmonary emboli vary widely, ranging from 1% in the general hospitalized population, to 30% in individuals dying after severe burns, trauma, or fractures. The influences that predispose to venous thrombosis in the legs were discussed in Chapter 4, but the following risk factors should be emphasized: (1) prolonged bedrest (particularly with immobilization of the legs), (2) surgery, especially orthopedic surgery, of knee and hip, (3) severe trauma (including burns or multiple fractures), (4) congestive heart failure, (5) women in the period around parturition or who take birth control pills with high estrogen content, (6) disseminated cancer, and (7) primary disorders of hypercoagulability (e.g., factor V Leiden; see Chapter 4).

The pathophysiologic consequences of thromboembolism in the lung depend largely on the size of the embolus, which in turn dictates the size of the occluded pulmonary artery, and on the cardiopulmonary status of the patient. There are two important consequences of embolic pulmonary arterial occlusion: (1) an increase in pulmonary artery pressure from blockage of flow and, possibly, vasospasm caused by neurogenic mechanisms and/or release of mediators (e.g., thromboxane A_2 and serotonin); and (2) ischemia of the down-stream pulmonary parenchyma. Thus, occlusion of a *major vessel* results in a sudden increase in pulmonary artery pressure, diminished cardiac output, right-sided heart failure *(acute cor pulmonale),* or even death. Usually hypoxemia develops, as a result of multiple mechanisms:

- *Perfusion of lung zones that have become atelectatic.* The alveolar collapse occurs in the ischemic areas because of a reduction in surfactant production and because pain associated with embolism leads to reduced movement of the chest wall; in addition, some of the pulmonary blood flow is redirected through areas of the lung that are normally hypoventilated.

- The decrease in cardiac output causes a *widening of the difference in arterial-venous oxygen saturation.*
- *Right-to-left shunting* of blood may occur in some persons through a patent foramen ovale, present in 30% of normal individuals.
- If *smaller vessels* are occluded, the result is less catastrophic, and the event may even be clinically silent.

Recall that lung is oxygenated not only by the pulmonary arteries but also by bronchial arteries and directly from air in the alveoli. If the bronchial circulation is normal and adequate ventilation is maintained, the resultant decrease in blood flow does not cause tissue necrosis. Indeed, ischemic necrosis (infarction) resulting from pulmonary thromboembolism is the exception rather than the rule, occurring in as few as 10% of cases. It occurs only if there is compromise in cardiac function or bronchial circulation, or if the region of the lung at risk is underventilated as a result of underlying pulmonary disease.

Morphology

The morphologic consequences of pulmonary embolism, as noted, depend on the size of the embolic mass and the general state of the circulation. Large emboli impact in the main pulmonary artery or its major branches or lodge astride the bifurcation as a **saddle embolus** (Fig. 13–25). Death usually follows so suddenly from hypoxia or acute failure of the right side of the heart (acute cor pulmonale) that there is no time for morphologic alterations in the lung. Smaller emboli become impacted in medium-sized and small pulmonary arteries. With adequate circulation and bronchial arterial flow, the vitality of the lung parenchyma is maintained, but the alveolar spaces may fill with blood to produce pulmonary hemorrhage as a result of ischemic damage to the endothelial cells.

With compromised cardiovascular status, as may occur with congestive heart failure, **infarction** results. The more peripheral the embolic occlusion, the more likely is infarction. About three-fourths of all infarcts affect the lower lobes, and more than half are multiple. Characteristically, they are wedge shaped, with their base at the pleural surface and the apex pointing toward the hilus of the lung. Pulmonary infarcts are typically hemorrhagic and appear as raised, red-blue areas in the early stages (Fig. 13–26). The adjacent pleural surface is often covered by a fibrinous exudate. If the occluded vessel can be identified, it is usually found near the apex of the infarcted area. The red cells begin to lyse within 48 hours, and the infarct pales, eventually becoming red-brown as hemosiderin is produced. In time, fibrous replacement begins at the margins as a gray-white peripheral zone and eventually converts the infarct into a scar that is contracted below the level of the lung substance. Histologically, the hallmark of fresh infarcts is coagulative necrosis of the lung parenchyma in the area of hemorrhage.

Clinical Course. The clinical consequences of pulmonary thromboembolism are summarized here:

- Most pulmonary emboli (60% to 80%) are clinically silent because they are small; the embolic mass is rapidly removed by fibrinolytic activity, and the bronchial circulation sustains the viability of the affected lung parenchyma until this is accomplished.
- In 5% of cases, sudden death, acute right-sided heart failure (acute cor pulmonale), or cardiovascular collapse (shock) may occur when more than 60% of the total pulmonary vasculature is obstructed by a large embolus or multiple simultaneous small emboli. Massive pulmonary embolism is one of the few causes of literally instantaneous death, even before the person experiences chest pain or dyspnea.
- Obstruction of relatively small to medium pulmonary branches (10% to 15% of cases) that behave

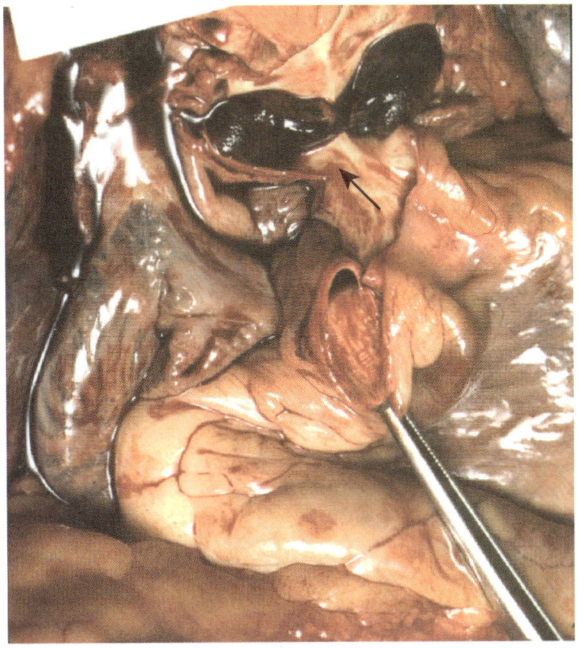

Figure 13–25

Large saddle embolus from the femoral vein lying astride the main left and right pulmonary arteries. (Courtesy of Dr. Linda Margraf, Department of Pathology, University of Texas Southwestern Medical School, Dallas, Texas.)

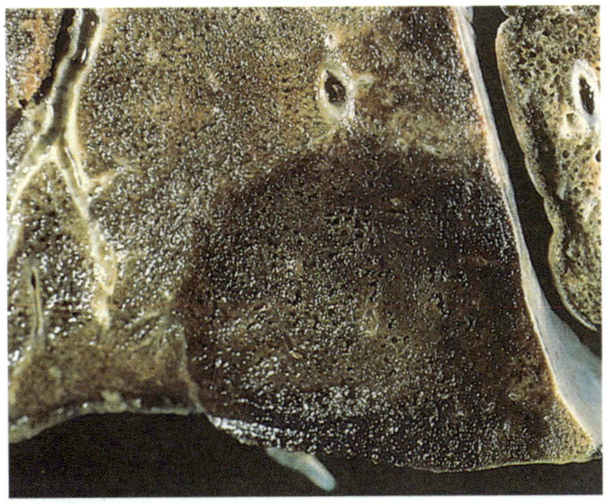

Figure 13–26

A recent small, roughly wedge-shaped hemorrhagic pulmonary infarct.

as end arteries causes pulmonary infarction when some element of circulatory insufficiency is present. Typically, persons who sustain an infarct manifest dyspnea, the basis of which is not fully understood.

- In a small but significant subset of persons (<3%), recurrent multiple emboli lead to pulmonary hypertension, chronic right-sided heart strain (chronic cor pulmonale), and, in time, pulmonary vascular sclerosis with progressively worsening dyspnea.

Emboli usually resolve after the initial acute insult. They contract, and endogenous fibrinolytic activity may cause total lysis of the thrombus. However, in the presence of an underlying predisposing factor, a small innocuous embolus may presage a larger one, and *patients who have experienced one pulmonary embolism have a 30% chance of developing a second.* Thus, recognition and appropriate preventive treatment are essential. Prophylactic therapy includes early ambulation for postoperative and postpartum patients, elastic stockings, intermittent pneumatic compression and isometric leg exercises for bedridden patients. Anticoagulation is warranted for persons at high risk. Patients with pulmonary embolism are given anticoagulation therapy. Patients with massive pulmonary embolism are candidates for thrombolytic therapy.

In passing, mention should be made of nonthrombotic forms of pulmonary embolism, which include several uncommon but potentially lethal forms, such as air embolism, fat embolism, and amniotic fluid embolism, which were discussed in Chapter 4. Intravenous drug abuse is often associated with foreign body embolism in the pulmonary microvasculature; the presence of magnesium trisilicate (talc) in the intravenous mixture elicits a granulomatous response within the interstitium or pulmonary arteries. Involvement of the interstitium may lead to fibrosis, while the latter leads to pulmonary hypertension. Residual talc crystals can be demonstrated within the granulomas using polarized light. Bone marrow embolism (presence of hematopoietic and fat elements within pulmonary circulation) can occur after massive trauma and in patients with bone infarction secondary to sickle cell anemia.

SUMMARY

Pulmonary Embolism

- Almost all large pulmonary artery thrombi are embolic in origin, usually arising from the deep veins of the lower leg.
- Risk factors include prolonged bedrest, leg surgery, severe trauma, CHF, oral contraceptives (especially those containing high estrogen), disseminated cancer, and genetic diseases of hypercoagulability.
- The vast majority (60% to 80%) of emboli are clinically silent, a minority (5%) cause acute cor pulmonale, shock, or death (typically large "saddle emboli"), and the remaining cause pulmonary infarction.
- Individuals who have experienced one episode of pulmonary embolism are at high risk for recurrences.

Pulmonary Hypertension

The pulmonary circulation is normally one of low resistance, with pulmonary blood pressures being only about one-eighth of systemic pressure. Pulmonary hypertension (when mean pulmonary pressures reach one-fourth or more of systemic levels) is most often *secondary* to a decrease in the cross-sectional area of the pulmonary vascular bed, or to increased pulmonary vascular blood flow. The causes of secondary pulmonary hypertension include:

- *Chronic obstructive or interstitial lung disease,* which is accompanied by destruction of lung parenchyma and consequent reduction in alveolar capillaries. This causes increased pulmonary arterial resistance and secondarily, elevated arterial pressure.
- *Recurrent pulmonary emboli,* which lead to a reduction in the functional cross-sectional area of the pulmonary vascular bed, in turn, leading to increased vascular resistance
- *Antecedent heart disease,* for example, *mitral stenosis,* which increases left atrial pressure, leading to higher pulmonary venous pressures, and ultimately pulmonary arterial hypertension. *Congenital left-to-right shunts* are another cause of secondary pulmonary hypertension.

Uncommonly, pulmonary hypertension exists even though all known causes of increased pulmonary pressure can be excluded; this is referred to as *primary,* or *idiopathic, pulmonary hypertension.* Of these, the vast majority of cases are sporadic and only 6% have the familial form with an autosomal dominant mode of inheritance.

Pathogenesis. According to current thinking, *pulmonary endothelial cell and/or vascular smooth muscle dysfunction* is the probable underlying basis for most forms of pulmonary hypertension.

- In states of *secondary pulmonary hypertension,* endothelial cell dysfunction arises as a consequence of the underlying disorder (e.g., shear and mechanical injury due to increased blood flow in left-to-right shunts, or biochemical injury produced by fibrin in recurrent thromboembolism). Endothelial cell dysfunction reduces production of vasodilatory agents (e.g., nitric oxide, prostacyclin) while increasing synthesis of vasoconstrictive mediators like endothelin. In addition, there is production of growth factors and cytokines that induce the migration and replication of vascular smooth muscle and elaboration of extracellular matrix.
- In *primary pulmonary hypertension,* especially in the uncommon *familial form,* the TGF-β signaling pathway has emerged as a key mediator of endothelial and smooth muscle dysfunction. Specifically, germ-line mutations of *bone morphogenetic protein receptor, type 2 (BMPR2),* a cell surface molecule that binds to a variety of TGF-β pathway ligands, have been demonstrated in 50% of familial cases. The *BMPR2* gene product is inhibitory in its effects on proliferation; hence, loss-of-function mutations of this gene result in abnormal vascular endothelial and pulmonary smooth muscle proliferation. The endothelial proliferations in these instances are usually *monoclonal,* reiterating the

genetic basis of their origin. Not all individuals with germ-line mutations of *BMPR2* develop primary pulmonary hypertension, however, suggesting the existence of *"modifier genes"* that probably affect penetrance of this particular phenotype.

- Studies on sporadic forms of primary pulmonary hypertension have also elucidated the possible role of the *serotonin transporter gene (5-HTT)*. Specifically, pulmonary smooth muscle cells from some individuals with primary pulmonary hypertension demonstrate increased proliferation on exposure to serotonin or serum. Genetic polymorphisms of *5-HTT* that lead to enhanced expression of the transporter protein on vascular smooth muscle are postulated to cause their proliferation. Aberrant 5-HTT function may also be the basis for pulmonary hypertension arising in persons taking the anti-obesity drug fenfluramine and its derivatives.

Morphology

Vascular alterations in all forms of pulmonary hypertension (primary and secondary) involve the entire arterial tree (Fig. 13–27) and include: (1) in the **main elastic arteries,** atheromas similar to those in systemic atherosclerosis; (2) **in medium-sized muscular arteries,** proliferation of myointimal cells and smooth muscle cells, causing thickening of the intima and media with narrowing of the lumina; and (3) in **smaller arteries and arterioles,** thickening, medial hypertrophy, and reduplication of the internal and external elastic membranes. In these vessels, the wall thickness may exceed the diameter of the lumen, which is sometimes narrowed to the point of near-obliteration. Individuals with severe, long-standing primary pulmonary hypertension may develop **plexogenic pulmonary arteriopathy,** so called because a tuft of capillary formations is present, producing a network, or web, that spans the lumens of dilated thin-walled, small arteries.

Clinical Course. Secondary pulmonary hypertension may develop at any age. The clinical features reflect the underlying disease, usually pulmonary or cardiac, with accentuation of respiratory insufficiency and right-sided heart strain. Primary pulmonary hypertension, on the other hand, is almost always encountered in young persons, more commonly women, and is marked by fatigue, syncope (particularly on exercise), dyspnea on exertion, and sometimes chest pain. These persons eventually develop severe respiratory insufficiency and cyanosis, and death usually results from right-sided heart failure (decompensated cor pulmonale) within 2 to 5 years of the diagnosis. Some amelioration of the respiratory distress can be achieved by vasodilators and antithrombotic agents, but without lung transplantation the prognosis is grim.

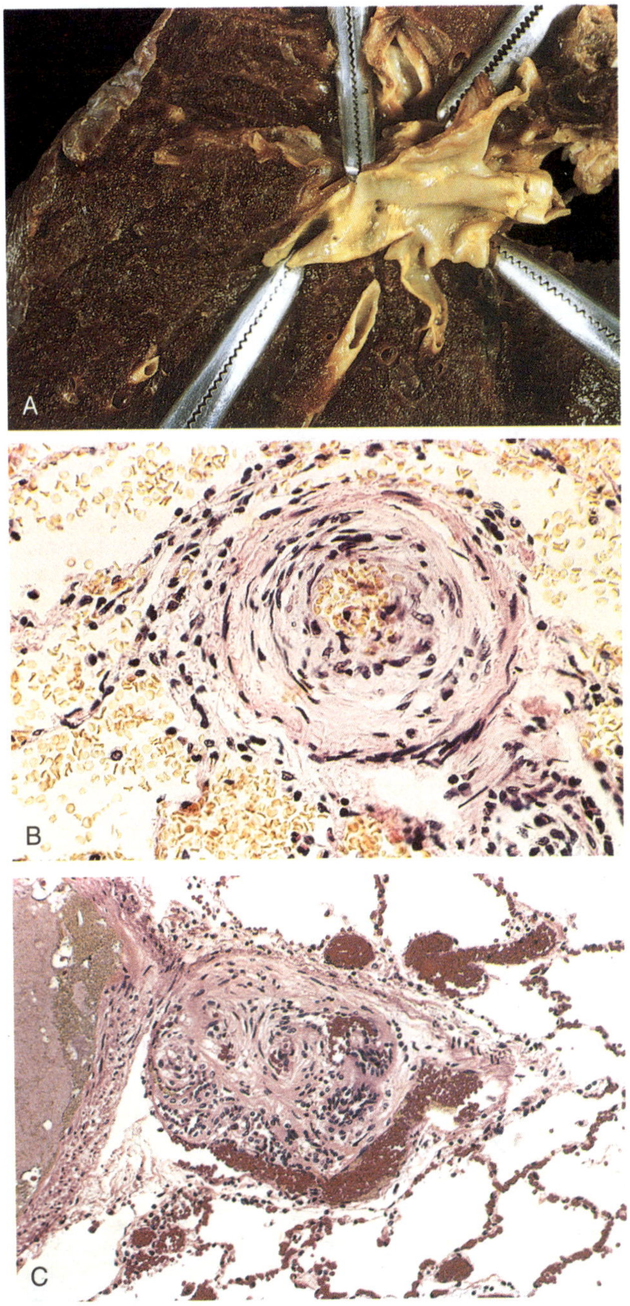

Figure 13–27

Vascular changes in pulmonary hypertension. **A,** Gross photograph of atheroma formation, a finding usually limited to large vessels. **B,** Marked medial hypertrophy. **C,** Plexogenic lesion characteristic of advanced pulmonary hypertension seen in small arteries.

Diffuse Alveolar Hemorrhage Syndromes

While there may be several "secondary" causes of pulmonary hemorrhage (necrotizing bacterial pneumonia, passive venous congestion, bleeding diathesis), the diffuse alveolar hemorrhage syndromes are a group of "primary" immune-mediated diseases that present as the *triad of hemoptysis, anemia, and diffuse pulmonary infiltrates.*

Goodpasture Syndrome

Goodpasture syndrome, the prototype disorder of this group, is an uncommon but intriguing condition characterized by a *proliferative, usually rapidly progressive, glomerulonephritis* (Chapter 14) and *hemorrhagic interstitial pneumonitis*. Both the renal and the pulmonary lesions are caused by antibodies targeted against the noncollagenous domain of the α3 chain of collagen IV. These antibodies can be detected in the serum of more than 90% of persons with Goodpasture syndrome.

Morphology

In the classic case of **diffuse alveolar hemorrhage,** the lungs are heavy, with areas of red-brown consolidation. Microscopic examination of the lungs demonstrates focal necrosis of alveolar walls associated with intra-alveolar hemorrhages, fibrous thickening of the septa, and hypertrophy of septal lining cells. The presence of **hemosiderin,** either within macrophages or extracellularly, is characteristically seen for a few days after an acute presentation (Fig. 13–28). The immunopathogenesis of Goodpasture syndrome and the changes in the glomeruli are discussed in Chapter 14. Suffice it to say here that the characteristic **linear pattern of immunoglobulin deposition** (usually IgG, sometimes IgA or IgM) that is the sine qua non of diagnosis in renal biopsy specimens is also seen along the alveolar septa.

Plasmapheresis and immunosuppressive therapy have markedly improved the once dismal prognosis for this disease. Plasma exchange removes offending antibodies, and immunosuppressive drugs inhibit antibody production. With severe renal disease, renal transplantation is eventually required.

Idiopathic Pulmonary Hemosiderosis

Idiopathic pulmonary hemosiderosis is a disease of uncertain etiology that has pulmonary manifestations and histology similar to those of Goodpasture syndrome, but there is no associated renal disease or circulating anti–basement membrane antibody. Clinically, the course is usually mild to moderate, with periods of activity followed by prolonged, often spontaneous, remissions. Most cases occur in children, although the disease is reported in adults as well.

Pulmonary Angiitis and Granulomatosis (Wegener Granulomatosis)

Wegener granulomatosis (WG) is the prototype of the group of vasculitides known as pulmonary angiitis and granulomatosis and has been discussed in Chapter 10. In this section we will focus on the manifestations of WG in the respiratory system. More than 80% of patients with WG develop upper respiratory or pulmonary manifestations at some time in the course of their disease. The lung lesions in WG are characterized by a combination of necrotizing vasculitis ("angiitis") and parenchymal necrotizing granulomatous inflammation. The pulmonary vessels may also show necrotizing granulomas, although most often acute and chronic inflammation are intermingled with fibrinoid necrosis. The manifestations of WG can include both upper respiratory symptoms (chronic sinusitis, epistaxis, nasal perforation) and pulmonary symptoms (cough, hemoptysis, chest pain). Radiologically, multiple nodular densities, representing confluence of the necrotizing granulomas, are seen, some of which may undergo cavitation. Although WG is classically a multisystemic disease, it may be restricted to the lung without upper respiratory tract or renal involvement ("limited" WG).

PULMONARY INFECTIONS

Pulmonary infections in the form of pneumonia are responsible for one-sixth of all deaths in the United States. This is not surprising because (1) the epithelial sur-

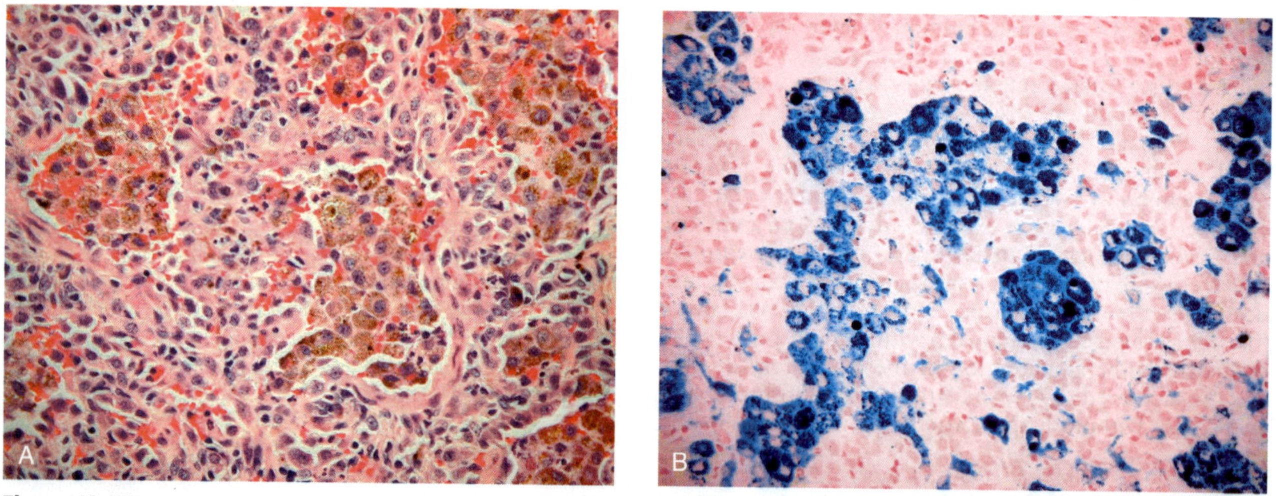

Figure 13–28

A, Lung biopsy specimen from a person with a diffuse alveolar hemorrhage syndrome demonstrates large numbers of intra-alveolar hemosiderin-laden macrophages on a background of thickened fibrous septa. **B,** The tissue has been stained with Prussian blue, an iron stain that highlights the abundant intracellular hemosiderin. (From the teaching collection of the Department of Pathology, Children's Medical Center, Dallas, Texas.)

faces of the lung are constantly exposed to liters of variously contaminated air; (2) nasopharyngeal flora are regularly aspirated during sleep, even by healthy persons; and (3) other common lung diseases render the lung parenchyma vulnerable to virulent organisms. It is therefore a small miracle that the normal lung parenchyma remains sterile. This attests to the efficiency of a series of pulmonary defense mechanisms. A plethora of immune and nonimmune defense mechanisms exists in the respiratory system, extending from the nasopharynx all the way into the alveolar airspaces (Table 13–6, Fig. 13–29). They pose an impressive barrier to an infectious onslaught.

Despite the multitude of defense mechanisms, "chinks in the armor" do exist, and they predispose the individual to infections. Defects in innate immunity (including neutrophil and complement defects) and humoral immunodeficiency typically lead to an increased incidence of infections with pyogenic bacteria. On the other hand, cell-mediated immune defects lead to increased infections with intracellular microbes such as mycobacteria and herpesviruses as well as with microorganisms of very low virulence such as *Pneumocystis jiroveci*. Several exogenous aspects of lifestyle interfere with host immune defense mechanisms and facilitate infections. For example, cigarette smoke compromises mucociliary clearance and pulmonary macrophage activity, while alcohol not only impairs cough and epiglottic reflexes, thereby increasing the risk of aspiration, but also interferes with neutrophil mobilization and chemotaxis.

Table 13–6 Pulmonary Host Defenses

Location	Host Defense Mechanism
Upper Airways	
Nasopharynx	Nasal hair Turbinates Mucociliary apparatus Immunoglobulin A (IgA) secretion
Oropharynx	Saliva Sloughing of epithelial cells Local complement production Interference from resident flora
Conducting Airways	
Trachea, bronchi	Cough, epiglottic reflexes Sharp-angled branching of airways Mucociliary apparatus Immunoglobulin production (IgG, IgM, IgA)
Lower Respiratory Tract	
Terminal airways, alveoli	Alveolar lining fluid (surfactant, Ig, complement, fibronectin) Cytokines (interleukin 1, tumor necrosis factor) Alveolar macrophages Polymorphonuclear leukocytes Cell-mediated immunity

Reproduced from Mandell GL, et al. (eds): Mandell, Douglas and Bennett's Principles and Practice of Infectious Diseases, 5th ed. Philadelphia, Churchill Livingstone, p 718.

Pneumonia can be very broadly defined as any infection in the lung. It may present as acute, fulminant clinical disease or as chronic disease with a more protracted course. The histologic spectrum of pneumonia may vary from a fibrinopurulent alveolar exudate seen in acute bacterial pneumonias, to mononuclear interstitial infiltrates in viral and other atypical pneumonias, to granulomas and cavitation seen in many of the chronic pneumonias. Acute bacterial pneumonias can present as one of two anatomic and radiographic patterns, referred to as *bronchopneumonia* and *lobar pneumonia.* Bronchopneumonia implies a patchy distribution of inflammation that generally involves more than one lobe (Fig. 13–30). This pattern results from an initial infection of the bronchi and bronchioles with extension into the adjacent alveoli. By contrast, in lobar pneumonia the contiguous airspaces of part or all of a lobe are homogeneously filled with an exudate that can be visualized on radiographs as a lobar or segmental consolidation (see Fig. 13–30). *Streptococcus pneumoniae* is responsible for more than 90% of lobar pneumonias. The anatomic distinction between lobar pneumonia and bronchopneumonia can often become blurry, because (1) many organisms present with either of the two patterns of distribution and (2) confluent bronchopneumonia can be hard to distinguish radiologically from lobar pneumonia. *Therefore, it is best to classify pneumonias either by the specific etiologic agent or, if no pathogen can be isolated, by the clinical setting in which infection occurs.* Classifying pneumonias by the setting in which they arise considerably narrows the list of suspected pathogens for administering empirical antimicrobial therapy. As illustrated in Table 13–7, pneumonia can arise in seven distinct clinical settings ("pneumonia syndromes"), and the implicated pathogens are reasonably specific to each category.

Community-Acquired Acute Pneumonias

Most community-acquired acute pneumonias are bacterial in origin. Not uncommonly, the infection follows a viral upper respiratory tract infection. The onset is usually abrupt, with high fever, shaking chills, pleuritic chest pain, and a productive mucopurulent cough; occasional patients may have hemoptysis. *S. pneumoniae* (or *pneumococcus*) is the most common cause of community-acquired acute pneumonia; hence, pneumococcal pneumonia will be discussed as the prototype for this subgroup.

Streptococcus pneumoniae

Pneumococcal infections occur with increased frequency in three groups of individuals: (1) those with underlying chronic diseases such as CHF, COPD, or diabetes; (2) those with either congenital or acquired immunoglobulin defects (e.g., the acquired immune deficiency syndrome); and (3) those with decreased or absent splenic function (e.g., sickle cell disease or after splenectomy). The last occurs because the spleen contains the largest collection of phagocytes and is, therefore, the major organ responsible for removing pneumococci from the blood.

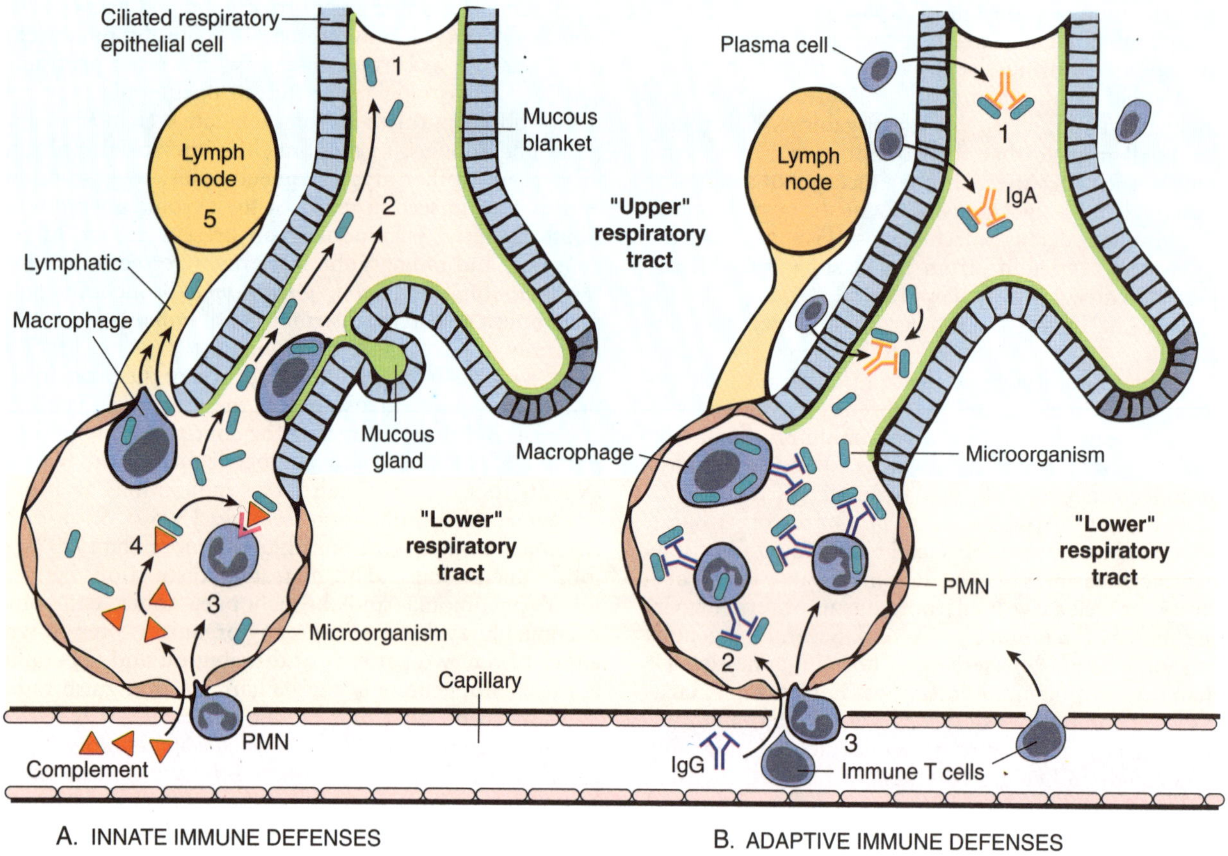

Figure 13–29

Lung defense mechanisms. **A,** (1) In the nonimmune lung, removal of microbial organisms depends on entrapment in the mucous blanket and removal via the mucociliary elevator, (2) phagocytosis by alveolar macrophages that can kill and degrade organisms and remove them from the airspaces by migrating onto the mucociliary elevator, or (3) phagocytosis and killing by neutrophils recruited by macrophage factors. (4) Serum complement may enter the alveoli and be activated by the alternative pathway to provide the opsonin C3b that enhances phagocytosis. (5) Organisms, including those ingested by phagocytes, may reach the draining lymph nodes to initiate immune responses. **B,** Additional mechanisms operate after development of adaptive immunity. (1) Secreted IgA can block attachment of the microorganism to epithelium in the upper respiratory tract. (2) In the lower respiratory tract, serum antibodies (IgM, IgG) are present in the alveolar lining fluid. They activate complement more efficiently by the classic pathway, yielding C3b (not shown). In addition, IgG is opsonic. (3) The accumulation of immune T cells is important for controlling infections by viruses and other intracellular microorganisms. PMN, polymorphonuclear cells.

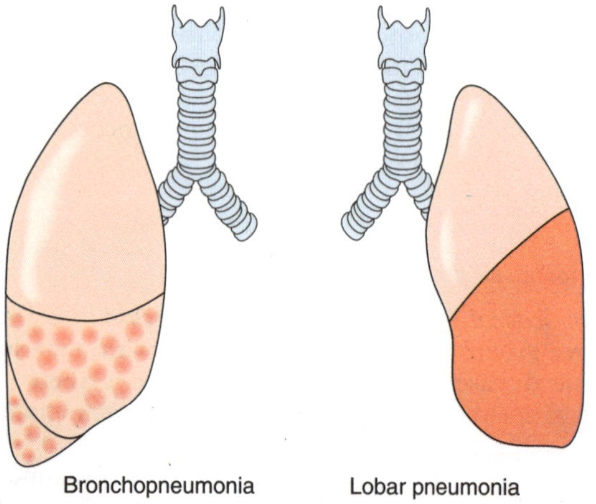

Figure 13–30

The anatomic distribution of bronchopneumonia and lobar pneumonia.

Morphology

With pneumococcal lung infection, either pattern of pneumonia, lobar or bronchopneumonia, may occur; the latter is much more prevalent at the extremes of age. Regardless of the distribution of the pneumonia, because pneumococcal lung infections usually originate by aspiration of pharyngeal flora (20% of adults harbor *S. pneumoniae* in their throats), the lower lobes or the right middle lobe are most frequently involved.

In the era before antibiotics, pneumococcal pneumonia involved entire or almost entire lobes and evolved through four stages: **congestion, red hepatization, gray hepatization,** and **resolution.** Early antibiotic therapy alters or halts this typical progression, so if the person dies, the anatomic changes seen at autopsy may not conform to the classic stages.

During the first stage, that of **congestion,** the affected lobe(s) is (are) heavy, red, and boggy; histologically, vascular congestion can be seen, with pro-

Table 13–7 The Pneumonia Syndromes

Community-Acquired Acute Pneumonia
Streptococcus pneumoniae *Haemophilus influenzae* *Moraxella catarrhalis* *Staphylococcus aureus* *Legionella pneumophila* Enterobacteriaceae (*Klebsiella pneumoniae*) and *Pseudomonas* spp.
Community-Acquired Atypical Pneumonia
Mycoplasma pneumoniae *Chlamydia* spp. (*C. pneumoniae, C. psittaci, C. trachomatis*) *Coxiella burnetti* (Q fever) Viruses: respiratory syncytial virus, parainfluenza virus (children); influenza A and B (adults); adenovirus (military recruits)
Nosocomial Pneumonia
Gram-negative rods belonging to Enterobacteriaceae (*Klebsiella* spp., *Serratia marcescens, Escherichia coli*) and *Pseudomonas* spp. *S. aureus* (usually methicillin-resistant)
Aspiration Pneumonia
Anaerobic oral flora (*Bacteroides, Prevotella, Fusobacterium, Peptostreptococcus*), admixed with aerobic bacteria (*S. pneumoniae, S. aureus, H. influenzae,* and *Pseudomonas aeruginosa*)
Chronic Pneumonia
Nocardia *Actinomyces* Granulomatous: *Mycobacterium tuberculosis* and atypical mycobacteria, *Histoplasma capsulatum, Coccidioides immitis, Blastomyces dermatitidis*
Necrotizing Pneumonia and Lung Abscess
Anaerobic bacteria (extremely common), with or without mixed aerobic infection *S. aureus, K. pneumoniae, Streptococcus pyogenes,* and type 3 pneumococcus (uncommon)
Pneumonia in the Immunocompromised Host
Cytomegalovirus *Pneumocystis jiroveci* *Mycobacterium avium-intracellulare* Invasive aspergillosis Invasive candidiasis "Usual" bacterial, viral, and fungal organisms (listed above)

teinaceous fluid, scattered neutrophils, and many bacteria in the alveoli. Within a few days, the stage of **red hepatization** ensues, in which the lung lobe has a liver-like consistency; the alveolar spaces are packed with neutrophils, red cells, and fibrin (Fig. 13–31A). In the next stage, **gray hepatization,** the lung is dry, gray, and firm, because the red cells are lysed, while the fibrinosuppurative exudate persists within the alveoli (Figs. 13–31B and 13–32). **Resolution** follows in uncomplicated cases, as exudates within the alveoli are enzymatically digested to produce granular, semifluid debris that is resorbed, ingested by macrophages, coughed up, or organized by fibroblasts growing into it (Fig. 13–31C). The pleural reaction (fibrinous or fibrinopurulent **pleuritis**) may similarly resolve or undergo organization, leaving fibrous thickening or permanent adhesions.

In the **bronchopneumonic** pattern, foci of inflammatory consolidation are distributed in patches throughout one or several lobes, most frequently bilateral and basal. Well-developed lesions up to 3 or 4 cm in diameter are slightly elevated and are gray-red to yellow; confluence of these foci may occur in severe cases, producing the appearance of a lobar consolidation. The lung substance immediately surrounding areas of consolidation is usually hyperemic and edematous, but the

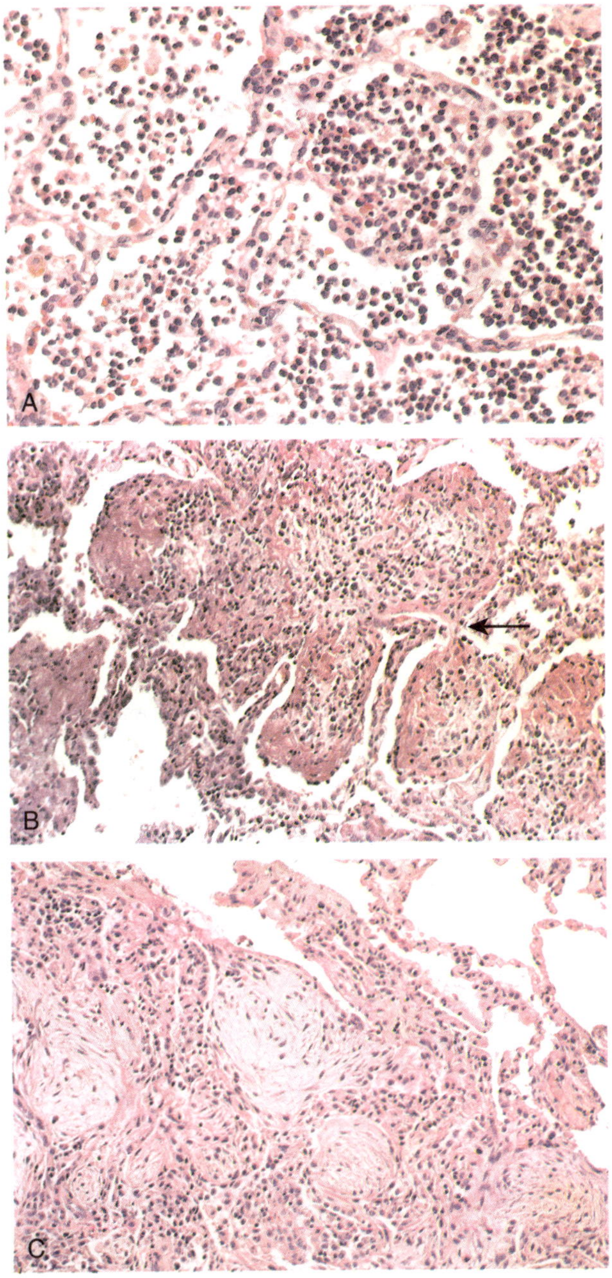

Figure 13–31

A, Acute pneumonia. The congested septal capillaries and extensive neutrophil exudation into alveoli corresponds to early red hepatization. Fibrin nets have not yet formed. **B,** Early organization of intra-alveolar exudates, seen in areas to be streaming through the pores of Kohn *(arrow).* **C,** Advanced organizing pneumonia, featuring transformation of exudates to fibromyxoid masses richly infiltrated by macrophages and fibroblasts.

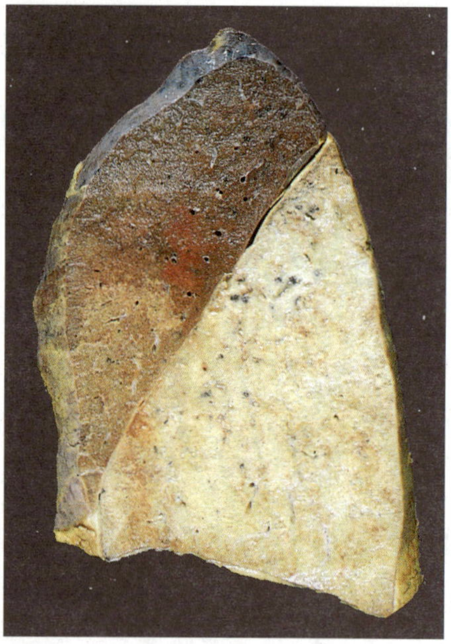

Figure 13–32

Gross view of lobar pneumonia with gray hepatization. The lower lobe is uniformly consolidated.

large intervening areas are generally normal. Pleural involvement is less common than in lobar pneumonia. Histologically, the reaction consists of focal suppurative exudate that fills the bronchi, bronchioles, and adjacent alveolar spaces.

With appropriate therapy, complete restitution of the lung is the rule for both forms of pneumococcal pneumonia, but in occasional cases complications may occur: (1) tissue destruction and necrosis may lead to **abscess** formation; (2) suppurative material may accumulate in the pleural cavity, producing an **empyema;** (3) organization of the intra-alveolar exudate may convert areas of the lung into solid fibrous tissue; and (4) bacteremic dissemination may lead to **meningitis, arthritis,** or **infective endocarditis.** Complications are much more likely with serotype 3 pneumococci.

Examination of Gram-stained sputum is an important step in the diagnosis of acute pneumonia. The presence of numerous neutrophils containing the typical gram-positive, lancet-shaped diplococci is good evidence of pneumococcal pneumonia, but it must be remembered that *S. pneumoniae* is a part of the endogenous flora and therefore false-positive results may be obtained by this method. Isolation of pneumococci from blood cultures is more specific. During early phases of illness, blood cultures may be positive in 20% to 30% of persons with pneumonia. Whenever possible antibiotic sensitivity should be determined. Commercial pneumococcal vaccines containing capsular polysaccharides from the common serotypes of the bacteria are available, and their proven efficacy mandates their use in those at risk for pneumococcal infections (see above).

Other organisms commonly implicated in community-acquired acute pneumonias include the following.

Haemophilus influenzae

- Both *encapsulated* and *unencapsulated* forms are important causes of community-acquired pneumonias. The former can cause a particularly life-threatening form of pneumonia in children, often following a respiratory viral infection.
- Adults at risk for developing infections include those with chronic pulmonary diseases such as chronic bronchitis, cystic fibrosis, and bronchiectasis. *H. influenzae is the most common bacterial cause of acute exacerbation of COPD.*
- Encapsulated *H. influenzae* type b was formerly an important cause of epiglottitis and suppurative meningitis in children, although vaccination against this organism in infancy has significantly reduced the risk.

Moraxella catarrhalis

- *M. catarrhalis* is being increasingly recognized as a cause of bacterial pneumonia, especially in the elderly.
- It is the second most common bacterial cause of acute exacerbation of COPD in adults.
- Along with *S. pneumoniae* and *H. influenzae, M. catarrhalis* constitutes one of the three most common causes of otitis media (infection of the middle ear) in children.

Staphylococcus aureus

- *S. aureus* is an important cause of secondary bacterial pneumonia in children and healthy adults after viral respiratory illnesses (e.g., measles in children and influenza in both children and adults).
- Staphylococcal pneumonia is associated with a high incidence of complications, such as lung abscess and empyema.
- Staphylococcal pneumonia occurring in association with right-sided staphylococcal endocarditis is a serious complication of *intravenous drug abuse.*
- It is also an important cause of nosocomial pneumonia (see below).

Klebsiella pneumoniae

- *K. pneumoniae* is the most frequent cause of gram-negative bacterial pneumonia.
- It frequently afflicts debilitated and malnourished persons, particularly *chronic alcoholics.*
- Thick and gelatinous sputum is characteristic, because the organism produces an abundant viscid capsular polysaccharide, which the individual may have difficulty coughing up.

Pseudomonas aeruginosa

- Although discussed here with community-acquired pathogens because of its association with infections in cystic fibrosis, *P. aeruginosa* is most commonly seen in nosocomial settings (see below).

- *Pseudomonas* pneumonia is also common in persons who are neutropenic, usually secondary to chemotherapy; in victims of extensive burns; and in those requiring mechanical ventilation.
- *P. aeruginosa* has a propensity to invade blood vessels at the site of infection with consequent extrapulmonary spread; *Pseudomonas* bacteremia is a fulminant disease, with death often occurring within a matter of days.
- Histologic examination reveals coagulation necrosis of the pulmonary parenchyma with organisms invading the walls of necrotic blood vessels (*Pseudomonas* vasculitis).

Legionella pneumophila

- *L. pneumophila* is the agent of legionnaire disease, an eponym for the epidemic and sporadic forms of pneumonia caused by this organism. Pontiac fever is a related self-limited upper respiratory tract infection caused by *L. pneumophila,* without pneumonic symptoms.
- *L. pneumophila* flourishes in artificial aquatic environments, such as water-cooling towers and within the tubing system of domestic (potable) water supplies. The mode of transmission is thought to be either inhalation of aerosolized organisms or aspiration of contaminated drinking water.
- *Legionella* pneumonia is common in persons with some predisposing condition such as cardiac, renal, immunologic, or hematologic disease. *Organ transplant recipients are particularly susceptible.*
- *Legionella* pneumonia can be quite severe, frequently requiring hospitalization, and immunosuppressed individuals may have a fatality rate of 30% to 50%.
- Rapid diagnosis is facilitated by demonstration of *Legionella* antigens in the urine or by a positive fluorescent antibody test on sputum samples; culture remains the gold standard of diagnosis.

Community-Acquired Atypical Pneumonias

The term "primary atypical pneumonia" was initially applied to an acute febrile respiratory disease characterized by patchy inflammatory changes in the lungs, largely confined to the alveolar septa and pulmonary interstitium. The term "atypical" denotes the moderate amounts of sputum, absence of physical findings of consolidation, only moderate elevation of white cell count, and lack of alveolar exudates. Atypical pneumonia is caused by a variety of organisms, *Mycoplasma pneumoniae* being the most common. *Mycoplasma* infections are particularly common among children and young adults. They occur sporadically or as local epidemics in closed communities (schools, military camps, prisons). Other etiologic agents are *viruses,* including influenza types A and B, the respiratory syncytial viruses, adenovirus, rhinoviruses, rubeola, and varicella viruses; *Chlamydia pneumoniae* and *Coxiella burnetti* (Q fever) (see Table 13–7). Nearly all of these agents can also cause a primarily upper respiratory tract infection ("common cold").

The common pathogenetic mechanism is attachment of the organisms to the respiratory epithelium followed by necrosis of the cells and an inflammatory response. When the process extends to alveoli there is usually *interstitial* inflammation, but there may also be some outpouring of fluid into alveolar spaces so that on chest films the changes may mimic bacterial pneumonia. Damage to and denudation of the respiratory epithelium inhibits mucociliary clearance and predisposes to secondary bacterial infections. Viral infections of the respiratory tract are well known for this complication. More serious lower respiratory tract infection is more likely to occur in infants, the elderly, the malnourished, alcoholics, and the immunosuppressed. Not surprisingly, viruses and mycoplasmas are frequently involved in outbreaks of infection in hospitals.

Morphology

Regardless of cause, the morphologic patterns in atypical pneumonias are similar. The process may be patchy, or it may involve whole lobes bilaterally or unilaterally. Macroscopically, the affected areas are red-blue, congested, and subcrepitant. Histologically the **inflammatory reaction is largely confined within the walls of the alveoli** (Fig. 13–33). The septa are widened and edematous; they usually contain a mononuclear inflammatory infiltrate of lymphocytes, histiocytes, and, occasionally, plasma cells. In contrast to bacterial pneumonias, alveolar spaces in atypical pneumonias are remarkably free of cellular exudate. In severe cases, however, full-blown diffuse alveolar damage with hyaline membranes may develop. In less severe, uncomplicated cases, subsidence of the disease is followed by reconstitution of the native architecture. Superimposed bacterial infection, as expected, results in a mixed histologic picture.

Clinical Course. The clinical course of primary atypical pneumonia is extremely varied. It may masquerade as a severe upper respiratory tract infection or "chest cold" that goes undiagnosed, or it may present as a fulminant,

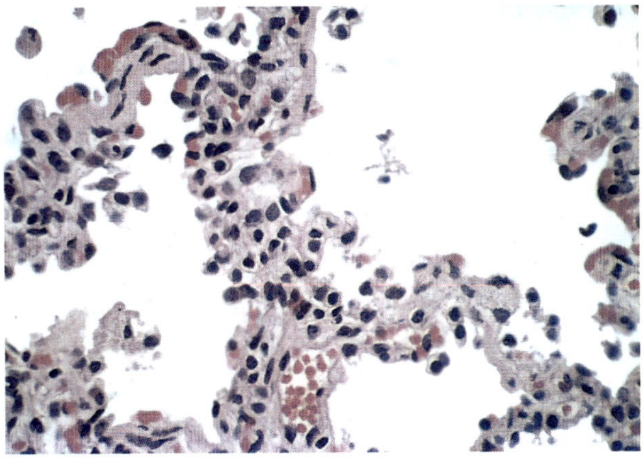

Figure 13–33

Atypical pneumonia. The thickened alveolar walls are heavily infiltrated with mononuclear leukocytes.

life-threatening infection in immunocompromised patients. The onset is usually that of an acute, nonspecific febrile illness characterized by fever, headache, and malaise and, later, cough with minimal sputum. Because the edema and exudation are both in a strategic position to cause an alveolocapillary block, there may be *respiratory distress seemingly out of proportion to the physical and radiographic findings*. Identifying the causative agent can be difficult. Tests for *Mycoplasma* antigens and polymerase chain reaction (PCR) testing for *Mycoplasma* DNA are available. As a practical matter, patients with community-acquired pneumonia for which a bacterial agent seems unlikely are treated with a macrolide antibiotic effective against *Mycoplasma* and *Chlamydia pneumoniae,* because these are the most common treatable pathogens.

Influenza Infections

Perhaps no other communicable disorder causes as much public distress in the developed world as the threat of an influenza epidemic. The influenza virus is a single-stranded RNA virus, bound by a nucleoprotein that determines the virus type (A, B, or C). The spherical surface of the virus is a lipid bilayer containing the viral hemagglutinin and neuraminidase, which determine the subtype (e.g., H1N1, H3N2, etc.). Host antibodies to the hemagglutinin and neuraminidase prevent and ameliorate, respectively, future infection with the influenza virus. The type A viruses infect humans, pigs, horses, and birds and are the major cause of *pandemic* and *epidemic* influenza infections. Epidemics of influenza occur through mutations of the hemagglutinin and neuraminidase antigens that allow the virus to escape most host antibodies *(antigenic drift)*. Pandemics, which last longer and are more widespread than epidemics, may occur when both the hemagglutinin and neuraminidase are replaced through recombination of RNA segments with those of animal viruses, making all animals susceptible to the new influenza virus *(antigenic shift)*. Commercially available influenza vaccines provide reasonable protection against the disease, especially in vulnerable infants and elderly individuals. A particular subtype of avian influenza ("bird flu," H5N1) has caused massive outbreaks in domesticated poultry in parts of Southeast Asia in the last few years; this strain is particularly dangerous, since it has the potential to "jump" to humans and thereby cause an unprecedented, worldwide influenza pandemic.

Severe Acute Respiratory Syndrome (SARS)

The severe acute respiratory syndrome (SARS) first appeared in November 2002 in the Guangdong Province of China, and subsequently spread to Hong Kong, Taiwan, Singapore, Vietnam, and Toronto, where large outbreaks also occurred. Between the fall of 2002 and July 2003, when the outbreak culminated, over 8,000 cases and 774 deaths had been ascribed to SARS. The cause of SARS is a previously undiscovered coronavirus (SARS-CoV). Nearly a third of upper respiratory tract infections are caused by coronaviruses, but the SARS-CoV differs in its ability to infect the lower respiratory tract and induce viremia. The SARS-CoV appears to have been first transmitted to humans through contact with wild masked palm civets that are eaten in China. Subsequent cases were spread person-to-person, mainly through infected secretions, although some cases may have been contracted through fecal-oral transmission. Patients typically become ill 2 to 10 days after exposure to the virus, and symptoms include fever, myalgias, headache, chills, and occasionally diarrhea. Respiratory symptoms typically follow systemic manifestations, and include dry cough and dyspnea, but unlike other atypical pneumonias, upper respiratory tract symptoms are rare. The lungs of patients dying of SARS usually demonstrate diffuse alveolar damage and multinucleated giant cells. The unraveling the cause of SARS, including complete sequencing of the SARS-CoV genome, within a few weeks of issuance of a WHO "global alert" represents a triumph of molecular medicine and the collaborative scientific spirit.

SUMMARY

Acute Pneumonias

- *S. pneumoniae* (pneumococcus) is the most common cause of community-acquired acute pneumonia, and the distribution of inflammation is usually lobar.
- Morphologically, lobar pneumonias evolve through four stages: congestion, red hepatization, gray hepatization, and resolution.
- Other common causes of acute pneumonias in the community include *H. influenzae* and *M. catarrhalis* (both associated with acute exacerbations of COPD), *S. aureus* (usually secondary to viral respiratory infections), *K. pneumoniae* (observed in chronic alcoholics), *P. aeruginosa* (seen in individuals with cystic fibrosis, in burn patients and in neutropenics), and *L. pneumophila,* seen particularly in individuals who have undergone organ transplants.
- In contrast to acute pneumonias, *atypical pneumonias* are characterized by respiratory distress out of proportion to the clinical and radiologic signs, and inflammation that is predominantly confined to alveolar septa, with generally clear alveoli.
- The most common causes of atypical pneumonias include those caused by *M. pneumoniae,* viruses, including influenza types A and B, *C. pneumoniae,* and *C. burnetti* (Q fever).

Nosocomial Pneumonia

Nosocomial, or hospital-acquired, pneumonias are defined as pulmonary infections acquired in the course of a hospital stay. The specter of nosocomial pneumonia places an immense burden on the burgeoning costs of health care, besides the expected adverse impact on illness outcome. Nosocomial infections are common in hospitalized persons with severe underlying disease, immune suppression, or prolonged antibiotic therapy. Those on mechanical ventilation represent a particularly high-risk group, and infections acquired in this setting are given the distinctive designation *ventilator-associated pneumonia.* Gram-negative rods (Enterobacteriaceae and *Pseudomonas* spp.) and *S. aureus* are the most common isolates; unlike community-acquired pneumonias, *S. pneumoniae* is not a major pathogen in nosocomial infections.

Aspiration Pneumonia

Aspiration pneumonia occurs in markedly debilitated patients or those who aspirate gastric contents either while unconscious (e.g., after a stroke) or during repeated vomiting. These individuals have abnormal gag and swallowing reflexes that facilitate aspiration. The resultant pneumonia is partly chemical, resulting from the extremely irritating effects of the gastric acid, and partly bacterial. Although it is commonly assumed that anaerobic bacteria predominate, recent studies implicate aerobes more commonly than anaerobes (see Table 13–7). This type of pneumonia is often necrotizing, pursues a fulminant clinical course, and is a frequent cause of death in persons predisposed to aspiration. In those who survive, abscess formation is a common complication.

Lung Abscess

Lung abscess refers to a localized area of suppurative necrosis within the pulmonary parenchyma, resulting in the formation of one or more large cavities. The term *necrotizing pneumonia* has been used for a similar process resulting in multiple small cavitations; necrotizing pneumonia often coexists or evolves into lung abscess, making this distinction somewhat arbitrary. The causative organism may be introduced into the lung by any of the following mechanisms:

- *Aspiration of infective material* from carious teeth or infected sinuses or tonsils, particularly likely during oral surgery, anesthesia, coma, or alcoholic intoxication and in debilitated patients with depressed cough reflexes.
- *Aspiration of gastric contents,* usually accompanied by infectious organisms from the oropharynx.
- *As a complication of necrotizing bacterial pneumonias,* particularly those caused by *S. aureus, Streptococcus pyogenes, K. pneumoniae, Pseudomonas* spp., and, rarely, type 3 pneumococci. Mycotic infections and bronchiectasis may also lead to lung abscesses.
- *Bronchial obstruction,* particularly with bronchogenic carcinoma obstructing a bronchus or bronchiole. Impaired drainage, distal atelectasis, and aspiration of blood and tumor fragments all contribute to the development of abscesses. An abscess may also form within an excavated necrotic portion of a tumor.
- *Septic embolism,* from septic thrombophlebitis or from infective endocarditis of the right side of the heart.
- In addition, lung abscesses may result from *hematogenous spread of bacteria* in disseminated pyogenic infection. This occurs most characteristically in staphylococcal bacteremia and often results in multiple lung abscesses.
- *Anaerobic bacteria are present in almost all lung* abscesses, sometimes in vast numbers, and they are the exclusive isolates in one-third to two-thirds of cases. The most frequently encountered anaerobes are commensals normally found in the oral cavity, principally species of *Prevotella, Fusobacterium, Bacteroides, Peptostreptococcus,* and microaerophilic streptococci.

Morphology

Abscesses vary in diameter from a few millimeters to large cavities of 5 to 6 cm. The localization and number of abscesses depend on their mode of development. Pulmonary abscesses resulting from aspiration of infective material are much **more common on the right side** (more vertical airways) than on the left, and most are single. On the right side, they tend to occur in the posterior segment of the upper lobe and in the apical segments of the lower lobe, because these locations reflect the probable course of aspirated material when the patient is recumbent. Abscesses that develop in the course of pneumonia or bronchiectasis are commonly multiple, basal, and diffusely scattered. Septic emboli and abscesses arising from hematogenous seeding are commonly multiple and may affect any region of the lungs.

As the focus of suppuration enlarges, it almost inevitably ruptures into airways. Thus, the contained exudate may be partially drained, producing an air-fluid level on radiographic examination. Occasionally, abscesses rupture into the pleural cavity and produce bronchopleural fistulas, the consequence of which is **pneumothorax** or **empyema.** Other complications arise from embolization of septic material to the brain, giving rise to meningitis or brain abscess. Histologically, as expected with any abscess, there is suppuration surrounded by variable amounts of fibrous scarring and mononuclear infiltration (lymphocytes, plasma cells, macrophages), depending on the chronicity of the lesion.

Clinical Course. The manifestations of a lung abscess are much like those of bronchiectasis and include a prominent cough that usually yields copious amounts of foul-smelling, purulent, or sanguineous sputum; occasionally, hemoptysis occurs. Spiking fever and malaise are common. Clubbing of the fingers, weight loss, and anemia may all occur. Infective abscesses occur in 10% to 15% of persons with bronchogenic carcinoma; thus, when a lung abscess is suspected in an older person, underlying carcinoma must be considered. Secondary amyloidosis (Chapter 5) may develop in chronic cases. Treatment includes antibiotic therapy and, if needed, surgical drainage. Overall, the mortality rate is in the range of 10%.

Chronic Pneumonia

Chronic pneumonia is most often a localized lesion in an immunocompetent person, with or without regional lymph node involvement. There is typically granulomatous inflammation, which may be due to bacteria (e.g., *M. tuberculosis*) or fungi. In the immunocompromised, such as those with debilitating illness, on immunosuppressive agents, or with human immune deficiency virus (HIV) infection (see below), there is usually systemic dissemination of the causative organism, accompanied by widespread disease. Tuberculosis is by far the most important entity within the spectrum of chronic pneumonias, with the World Health Organization (WHO) estimating that tuberculosis causes 6% of all deaths worldwide, *making it the most common cause of death resulting from a single infectious agent.*

Tuberculosis

Tuberculosis is a communicable chronic granulomatous disease caused by *Mycobacterium tuberculosis*. It usually involves the lungs but may affect any organ or tissue in the body. Typically, the centers of tubercular granulomas undergo *caseous necrosis*.

Epidemiology. Among medically and economically deprived persons throughout the world, tuberculosis remains a leading cause of death. It is estimated that 1.7 billion individuals are infected worldwide, with 8 to 10 million new cases and 3 million deaths per year. In the Western world, deaths from tuberculosis peaked in 1800 and steadily declined throughout the 1800s and 1900s. However, in 1984 the decline in new cases stopped abruptly, a change that resulted from the increased incidence of tuberculosis in HIV-infected persons. Following intensive surveillance and tuberculosis prophylaxis among immunosuppressed individuals, the incidence of tuberculosis in US-born individuals has declined since 1992. Currently, it is estimated that about 25,000 new cases with active tuberculosis arise in the United States annually, and nearly 40% of these are in immigrants from countries where tuberculosis is highly prevalent.

Tuberculosis flourishes wherever there is poverty, crowding, and chronic debilitating illness. Similarly, elderly persons, with their weakened defenses, are vulnerable. In the United States, tuberculosis is a disease of the elderly, the urban poor, patients with AIDS, and those belonging to minority communities. African Americans, Native Americans, the Inuit (from Alaska), Hispanics, and immigrants from Southeast Asia have higher attack rates than other segments of the population. *Certain disease states also increase the risk:* diabetes mellitus, Hodgkin disease, chronic lung disease (particularly silicosis), chronic renal failure, malnutrition, alcoholism, and immunosuppression. In areas of the world where HIV infection is prevalent, *it has become the single most important risk factor for the development of tuberculosis.* Most, perhaps all, of these predisposing conditions are related to a decrease in the capacity to develop and maintain T cell–mediated immunity against the infectious agent.

It is important that *infection* be differentiated from *disease.* Infection implies seeding of a focus with organisms, which may or may not cause clinically significant tissue damage (i.e., disease). Although other routes may be involved, most infections are acquired by direct person-to-person transmission of airborne droplets of organisms from an active case to a susceptible host. In most persons, an asymptomatic focus of pulmonary infection appears that is self-limited, although, uncommonly, primary tuberculosis may result in the development of fever and pleural effusion. Generally, the only evidence of infection, if any remains, is a tiny, telltale fibrocalcific nodule at the site of the infection. Viable organisms may remain dormant in such loci for decades, and possibly for the life of the host. Such persons are infected but do not have active disease and so cannot transmit organisms to others. Yet when their defenses are lowered, the infection may reactivate to produce communicable and potentially life-threatening disease.

Infection with *M. tuberculosis* typically leads to the development of delayed hypersensitivity, which can be detected by the tuberculin (Mantoux) test. About 2 to 4 weeks after the infection has begun, intracutaneous injection of 0.1 mL of PPD induces a visible and palpable induration (at least 5 mm in diameter) that peaks in 48 to 72 hours. Sometimes, more PPD is required to elicit the reaction, and unfortunately, in some responders, the standard dose may produce a large, necrotizing lesion. *A positive tuberculin test result* signifies cell-mediated hypersensitivity to tubercular antigens. It does not differentiate between infection and disease. It is well recognized that *false-negative reactions (or skin test anergy) may be produced by certain viral infections, sarcoidosis, malnutrition, Hodgkin's lymphoma, immunosuppression, and (notably) overwhelming active tuberculous disease.* False-positive reactions may also result from infection by atypical mycobacteria.

About 80% of the population in certain Asian and African countries is tuberculin positive. By contrast, in 1980, 5% to 10% of the US population reacted positively to tuberculin, indicating the marked difference in rates of exposure to the tubercle bacillus. In general, 3% to 4% of previously unexposed individuals acquire active tuberculosis during the first year after "tuberculin conversion," and no more than 15% do so thereafter. Thus, *only a small fraction of those who contract an infection develop active disease.*

Etiology. Mycobacteria are slender rods that are acid fast (i.e., they have a high content of complex lipids that readily bind the Ziehl-Neelsen [carbol fuchsin] stain and subsequently stubbornly resist decolorization). *M. tuberculosis hominis* is responsible for most cases of tuberculosis; the reservoir of infection is usually found in humans with active pulmonary disease. Transmission is usually direct, by inhalation of airborne organisms in aerosols generated by expectoration or by exposure to contaminated secretions of infected persons. Oropharyngeal and intestinal tuberculosis contracted by drinking milk contaminated with *Mycobacterium bovis* is now rare in developed nations, but it is still seen in countries that have tuberculous dairy cows and unpasteurized milk. Both *M.*

tuberculosis hominis and *M. bovis* species are obligate aerobes whose slow growth is retarded by a pH lower than 6.5 and by long-chain fatty acids, hence the difficulty of finding tubercle bacilli in the centers of large caseating lesions where anaerobiosis, low pH, and increased levels of fatty acids are present. Other mycobacteria, particularly *M. avium-intracellulare,* are much less virulent than *M. tuberculosis* and rarely cause disease in immunocompetent individuals. However, in patients with AIDS, these strains are frequently found, affecting 10% to 30% of sufferers.

Pathogenesis. The pathogenesis of tuberculosis in the previously *unexposed immunocompetent* individual is centered on the development of a targeted cell-mediated immunity that confers *resistance* to the organism and results in development of *tissue hypersensitivity* to tubercular antigens. The pathologic features of tuberculosis, such as caseating granulomas and cavitation, are the result of the destructive tissue hypersensitivity that is part and parcel of the host immune response. Because the effector cells for both processes are the same, the appearance of tissue hypersensitivity also signals the acquisition of immunity to the organism. The sequence of events from inhalation of the infectious inoculum to containment of the primary focus is illustrated in Fig. 13–34A and B and outlined in the text below.

- Once virulent strains of mycobacteria gain entry into the macrophage endosomes (a process mediated by several macrophage receptors, including the macrophage mannose receptor and complement receptors that recognize several components of the mycobacterial cell walls), the organisms are able to inhibit normal microbicidal responses by manipulation of endosomal pH and arrest of endosomal maturation. The end result of this "endosomal manipulation" is impairment of effective phagolysosome formation and unhindered mycobacterial proliferation. Thus, the earliest phase of primary tuberculosis (<3 weeks) in the nonsensitized individual is characterized by bacillary proliferation within the pulmonary alveolar macrophages and airspaces, with resulting bacteremia and seeding of multiple sites. *Despite the bacteremia, most persons at*

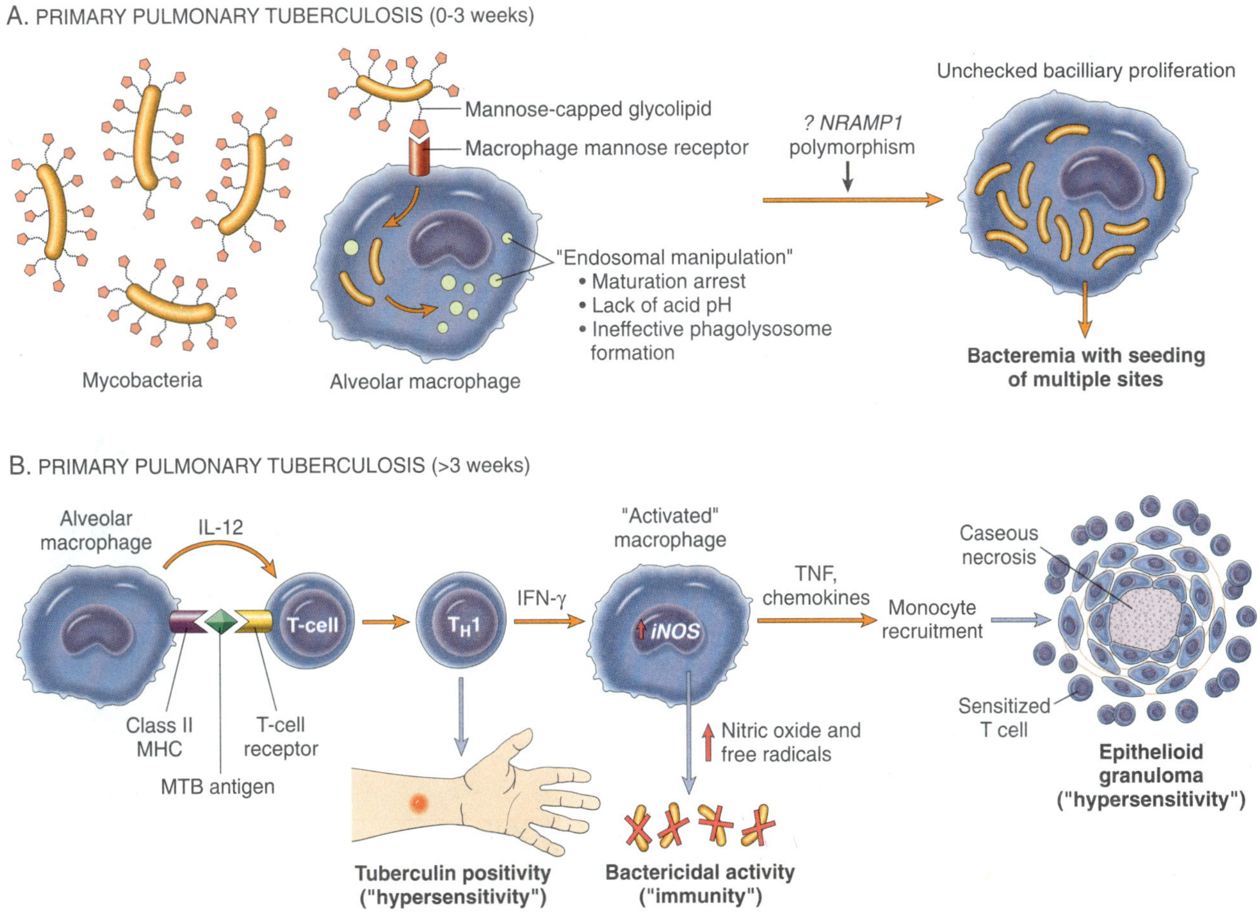

Figure 13–34

The sequence of events in primary pulmonary tuberculosis, commencing with inhalation of virulent strains of *Mycobacterium* and culminating with the development of immunity and delayed hypersensitivity to the organism. **A,** Events occurring in the first 3 weeks after exposure. **B,** Events thereafter. The development of resistance to the organism is accompanied by the appearance of a positive tuberculin test. Cells and bacteria not drawn to scale. iNOS, inducible nitric oxide synthase; IFN-γ, interferon γ; MHC, major histocompatibility complex; MTB, *Mycobacterium tuberculosis; NRAMP1,* natural resistance–associated macrophage protein; TNF, tumor necrosis factor.

this stage are asymptomatic or have a mild flulike illness.

- The genetic makeup of the individual may influence the course of the disease. In some people with polymorphisms of the *NRAMP1* (natural resistance–associated macrophage protein 1) gene, the disease may progress from this point without development of an effective immune response. NRAMP1 is a transmembrane ion transport protein found in endosomes and lysosomes that is believed to contribute to microbial killing.
- The development of *cell-mediated immunity* occurs approximately 3 weeks after exposure. Processed mycobacterial antigens reach the draining lymph nodes and are presented in a major histocompatibility class II context by dendritic cell macrophages to CD4+ T cells. Under the influence of macrophage-secreted IL-12, CD4+ T cells of the T_H1 subset are generated, capable of secreting IFN-γ.
- *IFN-γ released by the CD4+ T cells of the T_H1 subset is crucial in activating macrophages.* Activated macrophages, in turn, release a variety of mediators with important down-stream effects, including (a) secretion of TNF, which is responsible for recruitment of monocytes, which in turn undergo activation and differentiation into the "epithelioid histiocytes" that characterize the granulomatous response; (b) expression of the *inducible nitric oxide synthase (iNOS)* gene, which results in elevated *nitric oxide* levels at the site of infection. Nitric oxide is a powerful oxidizing agent and results in generation of reactive nitrogen intermediates and other free radicals capable of oxidative destruction of several mycobacterial constituents, from cell wall to DNA; (c) generation of reactive oxygen species that can have antibacterial activity.
- Defects in any of the steps of a T_H1 response (including IL-12, IFN-γ, TNF, or nitric oxide production) result in poorly formed granulomas, absence of resistance, and disease progression.

In summary, immunity to a tubercular infection is primarily mediated by T_H1 cells, which stimulate macrophages to kill bacteria. This immune response, while largely effective, comes at the cost of hypersensitivity and the accompanying tissue destruction. Reactivation of the infection or re-exposure to the bacilli in a previously sensitized host results in rapid mobilization of a defensive reaction but also increased tissue necrosis. Just as hypersensitivity and resistance appear in parallel, so, too, the loss of hypersensitivity (indicated by tuberculin negativity in a tuberculin-positive individual) may be an ominous sign that resistance to the organism has faded.

Primary Tuberculosis

Primary tuberculosis is the form of disease that develops in a previously unexposed, and therefore unsensitized, person. Elderly persons and profoundly immunosuppressed persons may lose their sensitivity to the tubercle bacillus and so may develop primary tuberculosis more than once. With primary tuberculosis, the source of the organism is exogenous. About 5% of those newly infected develop significant disease.

Morphology

In countries where bovine tuberculosis and infected milk have largely disappeared, primary tuberculosis almost always begins in the lungs. Typically, the inhaled bacilli implant in the distal airspaces of the lower part of the upper lobe or the upper part of the lower lobe, usually close to the pleura. As sensitization develops, a 1- to 1.5-cm area of gray-white inflammatory consolidation emerges, the **Ghon focus.** In most cases the center of this focus undergoes caseous necrosis. Tubercle bacilli, either free or within phagocytes, drain to the regional nodes, which also often caseate. **This combination of parenchymal lesion and nodal involvement** is referred to as the Ghon complex (Fig. 13–35). During the first few weeks, there is also lymphatic and hematogenous dissemination to other parts of the body. In approximately 95% of cases, development of cell-mediated immunity controls the infection. Hence, the Ghon complex undergoes progressive fibrosis, often followed by radiologically detectable calcification **(Ranke complex),** and, despite seeding of other organs, no lesions develop.

Histologically, sites of active involvement are marked by a characteristic granulomatous inflammatory reaction that forms both caseating and noncaseat-

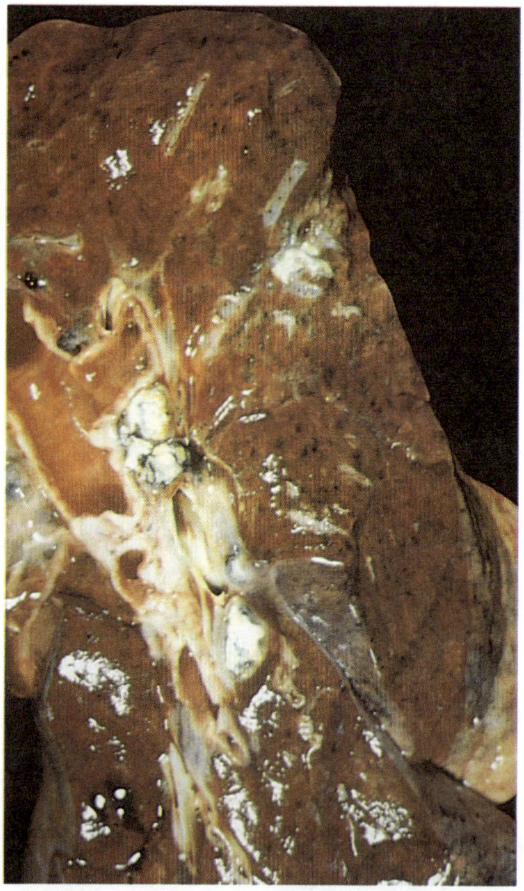

Figure 13–35

Primary pulmonary tuberculosis, Ghon complex. The gray-white parenchymal focus is under the pleura in the lower part of the upper lobe. Hilar lymph nodes with caseation are seen on the left.

ing tubercles (Fig. 13–36A–C). Individual tubercles are microscopic; it is only when multiple granulomas coalesce that they become macroscopically visible. The granulomas are usually enclosed within a fibroblastic rim punctuated by lymphocytes. Multinucleate giant cells are present in the granulomas.

The chief implications of primary tuberculosis are that (1) it induces hypersensitivity and increased resistance; (2) the foci of scarring may harbor viable bacilli for years, perhaps for life, and thus be the nidus for *reactivation* at a later time when host defenses are compromised; and (3) uncommonly, the disease may develop without interruption into so-called *progressive primary tuberculosis.* This occurs in individuals who are immunocompromised because of a defined illness such as AIDS or because of nonspecific impairment of host defenses, as may occur in malnourished children or in the elderly. Certain racial groups, such as Inuit, are also more prone to develop progressive primary tuberculosis. The incidence of progressive primary tuberculosis is particularly high in HIV-positive patients with an advanced degree of immunosuppression (i.e., CD4+ counts <200 cells/mm^3). Immunosuppression results in an inability to mount a CD4+ T cell–mediated immunologic reaction that would contain the primary focus; because hypersensitivity and resistance are most often concomitant, the lack of a tissue hypersensitivity reaction results in the absence of the characteristic caseating granulomas *(nonreactive tuberculosis)* (Fig. 13–36D).

The diagnosis of progressive primary tuberculosis in adults can be difficult. Contrary to the usual picture of

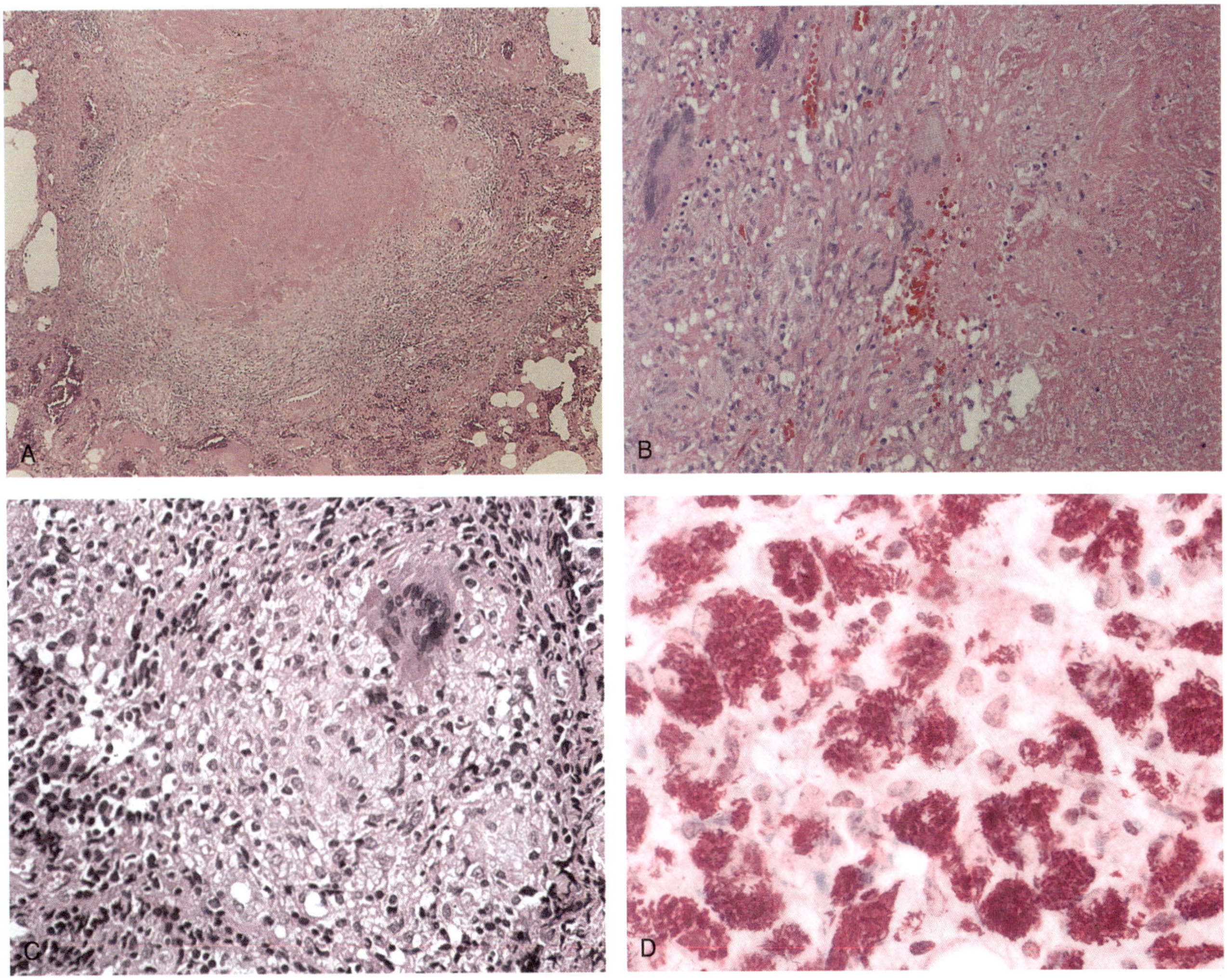

Figure 13–36

The morphologic spectrum of tuberculosis. A characteristic tubercle at low magnification **(A)** and in detail **(B)** illustrates central granular caseation *(right)* that is surrounded by epithelioid and multinucleated giant cells *(left)*. This is the usual response seen in individuals who have developed cell-mediated immunity to the organism. **C,** Occasionally, even in immunocompetent individuals, tubercular granulomas may not show central caseation; hence, irrespective of the presence or absence of caseous necrosis, special stains for acid-fast organisms must be performed when granulomas are present in histologic sections. **D,** In immunosuppressed individuals, tuberculosis may not elicit a granulomatous response ("nonreactive tuberculosis"); instead, sheets of foamy histiocytes are seen, packed with mycobacteria that are demonstrable with acid-fast stains. (**D,** Courtesy of Dr. Dominick Cavuoti, Department of Pathology, University of Texas Southwestern Medical School, Dallas, Texas.)

"adult-type" (or reactivation) tuberculosis (apical disease with cavitation, see below), progressive primary tuberculosis more often resembles an acute bacterial pneumonia, with lower and middle lobe consolidation, hilar adenopathy, and pleural effusion; cavitation is rare, especially in persons with severe immunosuppression. Lymphohematogenous dissemination is a dreaded complication and may result in the development of *tuberculous meningitis* and *miliary* tuberculosis. Because similar lesions also occur after progression of secondary tuberculosis, these will be discussed later.

Secondary Tuberculosis (Reactivation Tuberculosis)

Secondary (or postprimary) tuberculosis is the pattern of disease that arises in a previously sensitized host. It may follow shortly after primary tuberculosis, but more commonly it arises from reactivation of dormant primary lesions many decades after initial infection, particularly when host resistance is weakened. It may also result from exogenous reinfection because of waning of the protection afforded by the primary disease or because of a large inoculum of virulent bacilli. Reactivation of endogenous tuberculosis is more common in low-prevalence areas, whereas reinfection plays an important role in regions of high contagion. Whatever the source of the organism, only a few individuals (less than 5%) with primary disease subsequently develop secondary tuberculosis.

Secondary pulmonary tuberculosis is classically localized to the apex of one or both upper lobes. The reason is obscure but may relate to high oxygen tension in the apices. Because of the preexistence of hypersensitivity, the bacilli excite a prompt and marked tissue response that tends to wall off the focus. As a result of this localization, the regional lymph nodes are less prominently involved early in the developing disease than they are in primary tuberculosis. On the other hand, *cavitation occurs readily in the secondary form,* resulting in dissemination along the airways. Indeed, cavitation is almost inevitable in neglected secondary tuberculosis, and erosion into an airway becomes an important source of infectivity, because the person now raises sputum containing bacilli.

Secondary tuberculosis should always be an important consideration in HIV-positive patients who present with pulmonary disease. It is noteworthy that *while an increased risk of tuberculosis exists at all stages of HIV disease, the manifestations differ depending on the degree of immunosuppression.* For example, persons with less severe immunosuppression (CD4+ counts >300 cells/mm^3) present with "usual" secondary tuberculosis (apical disease with cavitation). On the contrary, persons with more advanced immunosuppression (CD4+ counts <200 cells/mm^3) present with a clinical picture that resembles progressive primary tuberculosis (lower and middle lobe consolidation, hilar lymphadenopathy, and noncavitary disease). The extent of immunosuppression also determines the frequency of extrapulmonary involvement, rising from 10% to 15% in mildly immunosuppressed patients to greater than 50% in those with severe immune deficiency. *Other atypical features* in HIV-positive patients that make the diagnosis of tuberculosis particularly challenging include an increased frequency of sputum-smear negativity for acid-fast bacilli compared with HIV-negative controls. This is because the incidence of cavitation and endobronchial damage is more in immunocompetent individuals and therefore induced sputum elicits more AFB. In contrast, despite the higher tissue bacillary load, the absence of tissue (bronchial wall) destruction due to suppressed type IV hypersensitivity results in fewer bacilli in the sputum. In addition, false-negative PPD because of tuberculin anergy, and the lack of characteristic granulomas in tissues, particularly in the late stages of HIV infection, also render diagnosis more difficult.

Morphology

The initial lesion is usually a small focus of consolidation, less than 2 cm in diameter, within 1 to 2 cm of the **apical pleura.** Such foci are sharply circumscribed, firm, gray-white to yellow areas that have a variable amount of central caseation and peripheral fibrosis. In favorable cases, the initial parenchymal focus undergoes progressive fibrous encapsulation, leaving only fibrocalcific scars. Histologically, the active lesions show characteristic coalescent tubercles with central caseation. Although tubercle bacilli can be demonstrated by appropriate methods in early exudative and caseous phases of granuloma formation, it is usually impossible to find them in the late, fibrocalcific stages. Localized, apical, secondary pulmonary tuberculosis may heal with fibrosis either spontaneously or after therapy, or the disease may progress and extend along several different pathways:

Progressive pulmonary tuberculosis may ensue. The apical lesion enlarges with expansion of the area of caseation. Erosion into a bronchus evacuates the caseous center, creating a ragged, **irregular cavity lined by caseous material** that is poorly walled off by fibrous tissue (Fig. 13–37). Erosion of blood vessels results in hemoptysis. With adequate treatment, the process may be arrested, although healing by fibrosis often distorts the pulmonary architecture. Irregular cavities, now free of caseation necrosis, may remain or collapse in the surrounding fibrosis. If the treatment is inadequate, or if host defenses are impaired, the infection may spread by direct expansion, via dissemination through airways, lymphatic channels, or the vascular system. **Miliary pulmonary disease** occurs when organisms drain through lymphatics into the lymphatic ducts, which empty into the venous return to the right side of the heart and thence into the pulmonary arteries. Individual lesions are either microscopic or small, visible (2-mm) foci of yellow-white consolidation scattered through the lung parenchyma (the word *miliary* is derived from the resemblance of these foci to millet seeds). Miliary lesions may expand and coalesce to yield almost total consolidation of large regions or even whole lobes of the lung. With progressive pulmonary tuberculosis, the pleural cavity is invariably involved and serous **pleural effusions, tuberculous empyema,** or **obliterative fibrous pleuritis** may develop.

Endobronchial, endotracheal, and **laryngeal tuberculosis** may develop when infective material is spread either through lymphatic channels or from expectorated infectious material. The mucosal lining may be

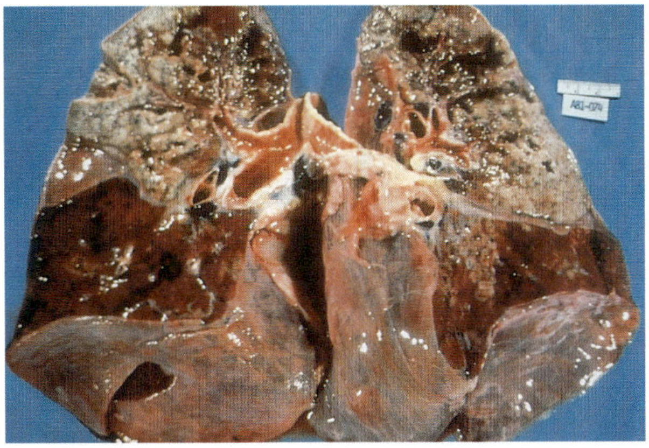

Figure 13–37

Secondary pulmonary tuberculosis. The upper parts of both lungs are riddled with gray-white areas of caseation and multiple areas of softening and cavitation.

studded with minute granulomatous lesions, sometimes apparent only on microscopic examination.

Systemic miliary tuberculosis ensues when infective foci in the lungs seed the pulmonary venous return to the heart; the organisms subsequently disseminate through the systemic arterial system. Almost every organ in the body may be seeded. Lesions resemble those in the lung. Miliary tuberculosis is most prominent in the liver, bone marrow, spleen, adrenals, meninges, kidneys, fallopian tubes, and epididymis (Fig. 13–38).

Isolated-organ tuberculosis may appear in any one of the organs or tissues seeded hematogenously and may be the presenting manifestation of tuberculosis. Organs typically involved include the meninges (tuberculous meningitis), kidneys (renal tuberculosis), adrenals (formerly an important cause of Addison disease), bones (osteomyelitis), and fallopian tubes (salpingitis). When the vertebrae are affected, the disease is referred to as Pott disease. Paraspinal "cold" abscesses in persons with this disorder may track along the tissue planes to present as an abdominal or pelvic mass.

Lymphadenitis is the most frequent form of extrapulmonary tuberculosis, usually occurring in the cervical region ("scrofula"). In HIV-negative individuals, lymphadenopathy tends to be unifocal, and most individuals do not have evidence of ongoing extranodal disease. HIV-positive persons, on the other hand, almost always demonstrate multifocal disease, systemic symptoms, and either pulmonary or other organ involvement by active tuberculosis.

In years past, **intestinal tuberculosis** contracted by the drinking of contaminated milk was fairly common as a primary focus of tuberculosis. In developed countries today, intestinal tuberculosis is more often a complication of protracted advanced secondary tuberculosis, secondary to the swallowing of coughed-up infective material. Typically, the organisms are trapped in mucosal lymphoid aggregates of the small and large bowel, which then undergo inflammatory enlargement with ulceration of the overlying mucosa, particularly in the ileum.

The many patterns of tuberculosis are depicted in Figure 13–39.

Clinical Course. Localized secondary tuberculosis may be asymptomatic. When manifestations appear, they are usually *insidious* in onset; there is gradual development of both systemic and localizing symptoms. Systemic symptoms, probably related to cytokines released by activated macrophages (e.g., TNF and IL-1), often appear early in the course and include malaise, anorexia, weight loss, and fever. Commonly, the *fever is low grade* and remittent (appearing late each afternoon and then subsiding), and *night sweats* occur. With progressive pulmonary involvement, increasing amounts of sputum, at first mucoid and later purulent, appear. When cavitation is present, the sputum contains tubercle bacilli. Some degree of *hemoptysis* is present in about half of all cases of pulmonary tuberculosis. *Pleuritic pain* may result from extension of the infection to the pleural surfaces. Extrapulmonary manifestations of tuberculosis are legion and depend on the organ system involved (for example, tuberculous salpingitis may present as infertility, tuberculous meningitis with headache and neurologic deficits, Pott disease with paraplegia). The diagnosis of pulmonary disease is based in part on the history and on physical and radiographic findings of *consolidation or cavitation in the apices of the lungs.* Ultimately, however, *tubercle bacilli must be identified.*

The most common methodology for diagnosis of tuberculosis remains demonstration of acid-fast organisms in sputum by acid-fast stains or by use of fluorescent auramine rhodamine; most protocols require at least two sputum examinations prior to conferring a diagnosis of sputum negativity. Conventional cultures for mycobacteria require up to 10 weeks, but recent liquid media–based radiometric assays that detect mycobacterial metabolism are able to provide an answer within 2 weeks. PCR amplification of *M. tuberculosis* DNA allows for even greater rapidity of diagnosis, and two such assays are currently approved for use in the United States. PCR assays can detect as few as 10 organisms in clinical specimens, compared with greater than 10,000 organisms required for smear positivity. However, culture remains the gold standard because it also allows testing of drug susceptibility. Multidrug resistance (MDR), defined as resistance of mycobacteria to two or more of the primary drugs used for treatment of tuberculosis, is now seen more

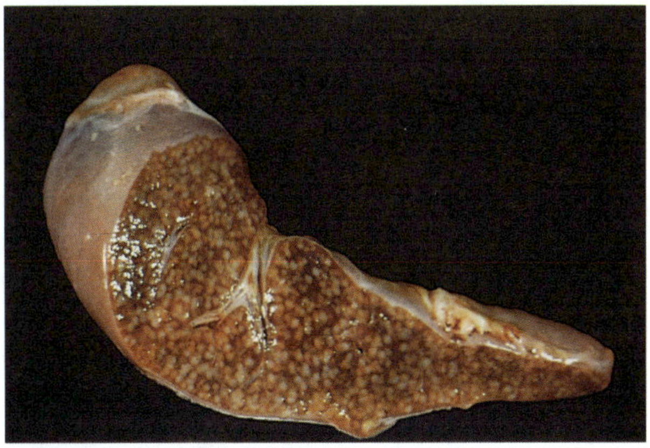

Figure 13–38

Miliary tuberculosis of the spleen. The cut surface shows numerous gray-white granulomas.

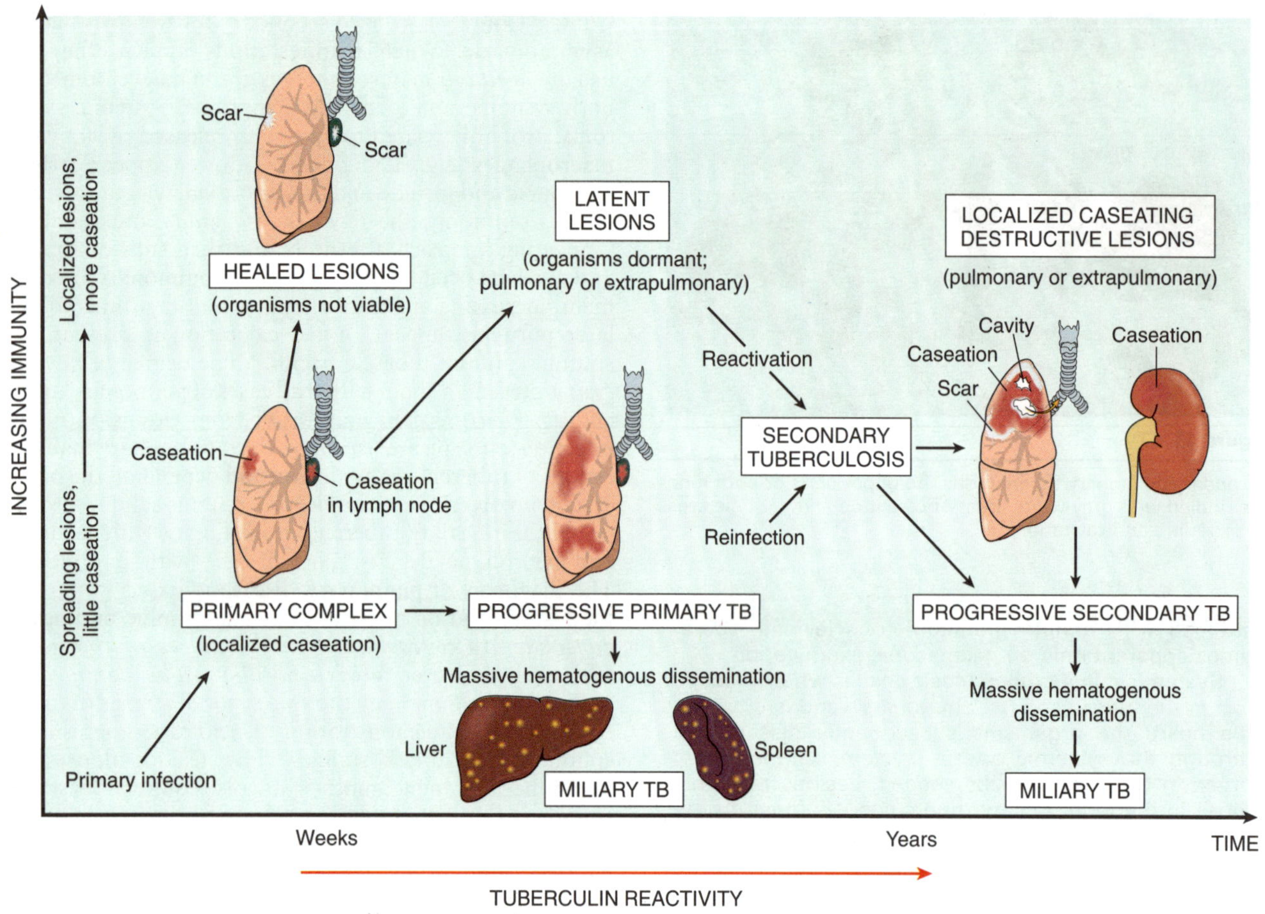

Figure 13–39

The natural history and spectrum of tuberculosis. (Adapted from a sketch provided by Dr. R. K. Kumar, The University of New South Wales, School of Pathology, Sydney, Australia.)

commonly, and the WHO estimates that 50 million people worldwide may be infected with MDR-TB. This form of tuberculosis is of particular concern in patients with HIV infection.

The prognosis of tuberculosis is generally favorable if infections are localized to the lungs, but it worsens significantly when the disease occurs in the setting of aged, debilitated, or immunosuppressed persons, who are at high risk for developing miliary tuberculosis, and in those with MDR-TB. Amyloidosis may appear in persistent cases.

SUMMARY

Tuberculosis

- It is a chronic granulomatous disease caused by *M. tuberculosis,* usually affecting the lungs, but virtually any extra-pulmonary organ can be involved by isolated tuberculosis.
- Initial exposure to mycobacteria results in development of an immune response that confers resistance but also leads to hypersensitivity (as determined by a positive *tuberculin test*).
- CD4+ T cells of the T_H1 subset have a crucial role in the cell-mediated immunity against mycobacteria; mediators of inflammation and bacterial containment include IFN-γ, IL-12, TNF, and nitric oxide synthase.
- The histopathologic sine qua non of host reaction to tuberculosis in immunocompetent individuals is the presence of *granulomas,* usually with central caseating necrosis.
- Secondary (reactivation) tuberculosis arises in previously exposed individuals when host immune defenses are compromised, and usually manifests as cavitary lesions in the lung apices.
- Both progressive primary tuberculosis and secondary tuberculosis can result in systemic seeding, causing life-threatening forms such as miliary tuberculosis and tuberculous meningitis.
- HIV is a well known risk factor for development or recrudescence of active tuberculosis.

Nontuberculous Mycobacterial Disease

Nontuberculous mycobacteria most commonly cause chronic but clinically localized pulmonary disease in immunocompetent individuals. In the United States, strains implicated most frequently include *M. avium-intracellulare* (also called *M. avium* complex), *M. kansasii*, and *M. abscessus*. It is not uncommon for nontuberculous mycobacteria to present as upper lobe cavitary disease, mimicking tuberculosis, especially in individuals with a long-standing history of smoking or alcoholism. The presence of concomitant chronic pulmonary disease (COPD, cystic fibrosis, pneumoconiosis) is an important risk factor associated with nontuberculous mycobacterial infection.

In *immunosuppressed individuals* (primarily, HIV-positive patients), *M. avium* complex presents as disseminated disease, associated with systemic symptoms (fever, night sweats, weight loss). Hepatosplenomegaly and lymphadenopathy, signifying involvement of the mononuclear phagocyte system by the opportunistic pathogen, is common, as are gastrointestinal symptoms such as diarrhea and malabsorption. Pulmonary involvement is often indistinguishable from tuberculosis in AIDS patients. Disseminated *M. avium* complex infection in AIDS patients tends to occur late in the course of the disease, when CD4 counts have fallen below 100 cells/mm^3; hence, tissue examination usually does not reveal granulomas and, instead, foamy histiocytes "plugged" with atypical mycobacteria are typically seen.

Histoplasmosis, Coccidioidomycosis, and Blastomycosis

The dimorphic fungi, which include *Histoplasma capsulatum, Coccidioides immitis,* and *Blastomyces dermatitidis,* present either with isolated pulmonary involvement as commonly seen in infected immunocompetent individuals, or with disseminated disease in immunocompromised persons. T cell–mediated immune responses are critical for containing the infection, and therefore, persons with compromised cell-mediated immunity, such as those with HIV, are more prone to systemic disease. In part because of the overlap in clinical presentations, all three dimorphic fungi will be considered together in this section.

Epidemiology. Each of the dimorphic fungi has a typical geographic distribution.

H. capsulatum: endemic in the Ohio and central Mississippi River valleys and along the Appalachian mountains in the southeastern United States. Warm, moist soil, enriched by droppings from bats and birds, provides the ideal medium for the growth of the mycelial form, which produces infectious spores.

C. immitis: endemic in the Southwest and Far West of the United States, particularly in California's San Joaquin Valley, where it is known as "valley fever."

B. dermatitidis: endemic area is confined in the United States to areas overlapping with those where histoplasmosis is found.

Morphology

The yeast forms are fairly distinctive, which helps in the identification of individual fungi in tissue sections.

- *H. capsulatum:* round to oval and small yeast forms measuring 2 to 5 μm in diameter (Fig. 13–40A).
- *C. immitis:* thick-walled, nonbudding spherules, 20 to 60 μm in diameter, often filled with small endospores (Fig. 13–40B).
- *B. dermatitidis:* round to oval and larger than *Histoplasma* (5–25 μm in diameter); reproduce by characteristic "broad-based" budding (Fig. 13–40C, D).

Clinical Features. Clinical manifestations may take the form of (1) *acute (primary) pulmonary infection,* (2) *chronic (cavitary) pulmonary disease,* or (3) *disseminated miliary disease.* The primary pulmonary nodules, composed of aggregates of macrophages stuffed with organisms, are associated with similar lesions in the regional lymph nodes. These lesions develop into small granulomas complete with giant cells, and may develop central necrosis and later fibrosis and calcification. *The similarity to primary tuberculosis is striking,* and differentiation requires identification of the yeast forms (best seen with periodic acid–Schiff or silver stains). The clinical symptoms resemble a "flulike" syndrome, most often self limited. In the vulnerable host, chronic cavitary pulmonary disease develops, with a predilection for the upper lobe, resembling the secondary form of tuberculosis. It is not uncommon for these fungi to give rise to perihilar mass lesions that resemble bronchogenic carcinoma radiologically. At this stage, cough, hemoptysis, and even dyspnea and chest pain may appear.

In infants or immunocompromised adults, particularly those with HIV infection, disseminated disease (analogous to miliary tuberculosis) may develop. Under these circumstances there are no well-formed granulomas. Instead, focal collections of phagocytes stuffed with yeast forms are seen within cells of the mononuclear phagocyte system, including in the liver, spleen, lymph nodes, lymphoid tissue of the gastrointestinal tract, and bone marrow. The adrenals and meninges may also be involved, and in a minority of cases ulcers form in the nose and mouth, on the tongue, or in the larynx. Disseminated disease is a hectic, febrile illness with hepatosplenomegaly, anemia, leukopenia, and thrombocytopenia. Cutaneous infections with disseminated *Blastomyces* organisms frequently induce striking epithelial hyperplasia, which may be mistaken for squamous cell carcinoma.

Pneumonia in the Immunocompromised Host

The appearance of a pulmonary infiltrate and signs of infection (e.g., fever) are some of the most common and serious complications in persons whose immune and

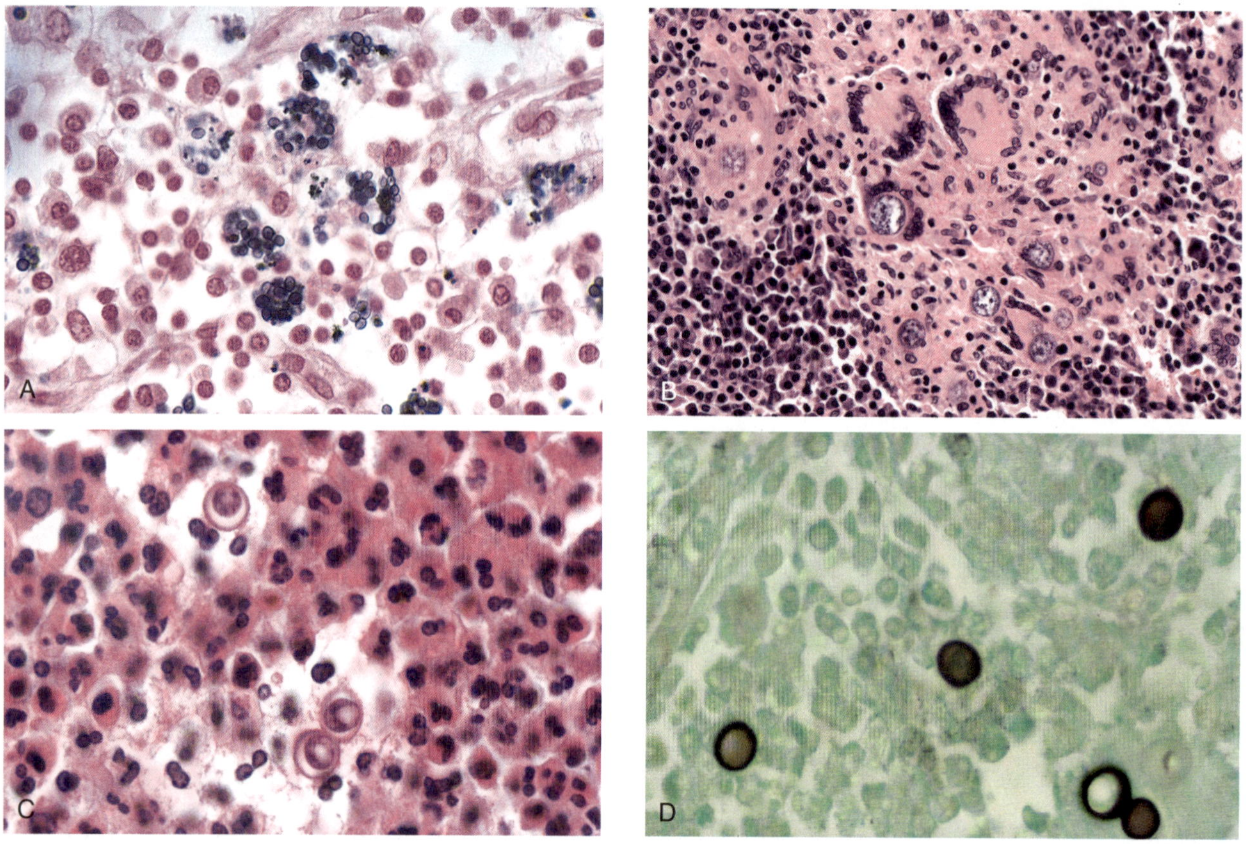

Figure 13–40

A, *Histoplasma capsulatum* yeast forms fill phagocytes in a lymph node of a person with disseminated histoplasmosis. **B,** Coccidioidomycosis with intact spherules within multinucleated giant cells. **C,** Blastomycosis, with rounded budding yeasts, larger than neutrophils. Note the characteristic thick wall and nuclei (not seen in other fungi). **D,** Silver stain highlighting broad-based budding.

defense systems are suppressed by disease, immunosuppression for organ transplants and tumors, or irradiation. A wide variety of so-called opportunistic agents, many of which rarely cause infection in normal hosts, can cause these pneumonias, and often more than one agent is involved. Examples of pulmonary opportunistic pathogens include (1) bacteria (*P. aeruginosa, Mycobacterium* spp., *L. pneumophila,* and *Listeria monocytogenes*); (2) viruses (cytomegalovirus and herpesvirus); and (3) fungi (*P. jiroveci, Candida* spp., *Aspergillus* spp., and *Cryptococcus neoformans*). Of these, we will discuss here cytomegalovirus, *P. jiroveci,* and the opportunistic fungal infections.

Cytomegalovirus Infections

Cytomegalovirus (CMV), a member of the herpesvirus family, may produce a variety of disease manifestations, depending partly on the age of the infected host but even more on the host's immune status. Cells infected by the virus exhibit gigantism of both the entire cell and its nucleus. Within the nucleus is an enlarged inclusion surrounded by a clear halo ("owl's eye"), which gives the name to the classic form of symptomatic disease that occurs in neonates, cytomegalic inclusion disease. Although classic cytomegalic inclusion disease involves many organs, CMV infections are discussed here because in immunosuppressed adults, particularly AIDS patients and recipients of allogeneic bone marrow transplants, CMV pneumonitis is a serious problem.

Transmission of CMV can occur by several mechanisms, depending on the age group affected:

- A fetus can be infected transplacentally from a newly acquired or primary infection in the mother ("congenital CMV").
- The virus can be transmitted to the fetus through cervical or vaginal secretions at birth, or, later, through breast milk from a mother who has active infection ("perinatal CMV").
- Preschool children, especially in day care centers, can acquire it through saliva. Toddlers so infected readily transmit the virus to their parents.
- In individuals over 15 years of age, the venereal route is the dominant mode of transmission, but spread may also occur via respiratory secretions and the fecal-oral route.
- Iatrogenic transmission can occur at any age through organ transplants or by blood transfusions.

Morphology

Histologically, the characteristic enlargement of cells can be appreciated. In the glandular organs, the parenchymal epithelial cells are affected; in the brain, the neurons; in the lungs, the alveolar macrophages and epithelial and endothelial cells; and in the kidneys, the tubular epithelial and glomerular endothelial cells. **Affected cells are strikingly enlarged, often to a diameter of 40μm, and they show cellular and nuclear polymorphism.** Prominent intranuclear basophilic inclusions spanning half the nuclear diameter are usually set off from the nuclear membrane by a clear halo (Fig. 13–41). Within the cytoplasm of these cells, smaller basophilic inclusions may also be seen.

Cytomegalovirus Mononucleosis. In healthy young children and adults, the disease is nearly always asymptomatic. In surveys around the world, 50% to 100% of adults demonstrate anti-CMV antibodies in the serum, indicating previous exposure. The most common *clinical manifestation of CMV* infection in immunocompetent hosts beyond the neonatal period is an infectious mononucleosis-like illness, with fever, atypical lymphocytosis, lymphadenopathy, and hepatomegaly accompanied by abnormal liver function test results, suggesting mild hepatitis. Most individuals recover from CMV mononucleosis without any sequelae, although excretion of the virus may occur in body fluids for months to years. Irrespective of the presence or absence of symptoms after infection, a person once infected becomes seropositive for life. The virus remains latent within leukocytes, which are the major reservoirs.

CMV in Immunosuppressed Individuals. This occurs most commonly in three groups:

- *Recipients of organ transplants* (heart, liver, kidney) from seropositive donors. These individuals typically receive immunosuppressive therapy, and the CMV is usually derived from the donor organ, but reactivation of latent CMV infection in the host may also occur.
- *Recipients of allogeneic bone marrow transplants.* These people are immunosuppressed not only because of drug therapy but also because of graft-versus-host disease. In this setting there is usually reactivation of latent CMV in the recipient.
- *Persons with AIDS.* These immunosuppressed individuals have reactivation of latent infection and are also infected by their sexual partners. *CMV is the most common opportunistic viral pathogen in AIDS.*

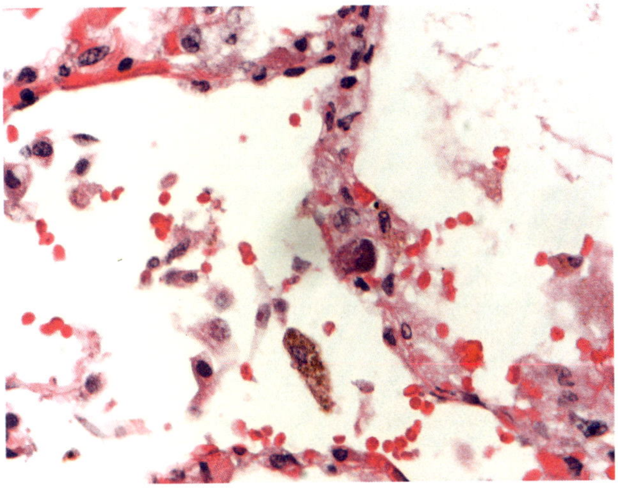

Figure 13–41

Cytomegalovirus infection of the lung. A typical distinct nuclear and ill-defined cytoplasmic inclusion is seen. (Courtesy of Dr. Arlene Sharpe, Brigham and Women's Hospital, Boston, Massachusetts.)

In all these settings, serious, life-threatening disseminated CMV infections primarily affect the lungs (pneumonitis), gastrointestinal tract (colitis), and retina (retinitis); the central nervous system is usually spared. In the pulmonary infection, an interstitial mononuclear infiltrate with foci of necrosis develops, accompanied by the typical enlarged cells with inclusions. The pneumonitis can progress to full-blown acute respiratory distress syndrome. Intestinal necrosis and ulceration can develop and be extensive, leading to the formation of "pseudomembranes" (Chapter 15) and debilitating diarrhea. CMV retinitis, by far the most common form of opportunistic CMV disease, can occur either alone or in combination with involvement of the lungs and intestinal tract. Diagnosis of CMV infections is made by demonstration of characteristic morphologic alterations in tissue sections, successful viral culture, rising antiviral antibody titer, and qualitative or quantitative PCR-based detection of CMV DNA. The last approach has revolutionized the approach to monitoring patients after transplantation.

Pneumocystis Pneumonia

P. jiroveci (formerly known as *P. carinii*), an opportunistic infectious agent long considered to be a protozoan, is now believed to be more closely related to fungi. Serologic evidence indicates that virtually all persons are exposed to *Pneumocystis* during the first few years of life, but in most the infection remains latent. Reactivation and clinical disease occurs almost exclusively in those who are immunocompromised. Indeed, *P. jiroveci* is an extremely common cause of infection in persons with AIDS, and it may also infect severely malnourished infants and immunosuppressed individuals (especially after organ transplantation or in individuals receiving cytotoxic chemotherapy or corticosteroids). In AIDS patients, the risk of acquiring *P. jiroveci* infections increases in direct proportion to the reduction in the CD4 count, with counts of less than 200 cells/mm^3 having a strong predictive value. *Pneumocystis* infections are largely confined to the lung, where they produce an interstitial pneumonitis.

Morphology

Microscopically, involved areas of the lung demonstrate a characteristic **intra-alveolar foamy, pink-staining exudate** with H&E stains ("cotton candy" exudate) (Fig. 13–42A), and the septa are thickened by edema and a minimal mononuclear infiltrate. Special stains are required to visualize the organism in either the trophozoite or encysted form. Silver stains of tissue sections reveal **cup-shaped cyst walls** (5–8 μm in diameter) in the alveolar exudates (Fig. 13–42B). If sputum production can be successfully induced, Giemsa or methylene blue stains can demonstrate the trophozoite forms of the organism (~4 μm in diameter with long filopodia) in about 50% of patients.

The diagnosis of *Pneumocystis* pneumonia should be considered in any immunocompromised individual with respiratory symptoms and an abnormal chest radiograph. Fever, dry cough, and dyspnea occur in 90% to 95% of patients, who typically demonstrate bilateral perihilar and basilar infiltrates. Hypoxia is frequent; pulmonary function studies show a restrictive lung defect. The most sensitive and effective method of diagnosis is to identify the organism in bronchoalveolar lavage fluids or in a transbronchial biopsy specimen. Besides the histologic stains mentioned already, immunofluorescence antibody kits and PCR-based assays have also become available for use on clinical specimens. If treatment is initiated before widespread involvement, the outlook for recovery is good; however, because residual organisms are likely to remain, particularly in AIDS patients, relapses are common unless the underlying immunodeficiency is corrected or suppressive therapy is given.

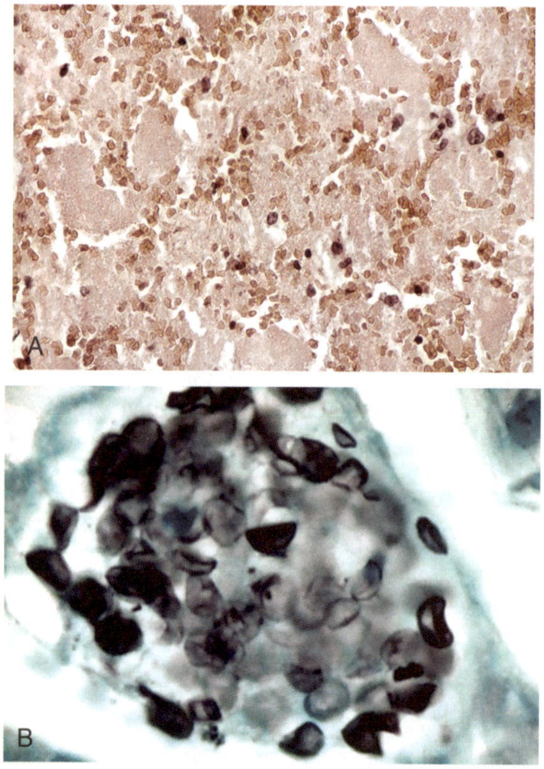

Figure 13–42

Pneumocystis pneumonia. **A,** The alveoli are filled with a characteristic foamy "cotton candy" exudate. **B,** Silver stain demonstrates cup-shaped cyst walls within the exudate.

Opportunistic Fungal Infection

Candidiasis

Candida albicans is the most frequent disease-causing fungus. It is a normal inhabitant of the oral cavity, gastrointestinal tract, and vagina in many individuals. Even though systemic candidiasis (with associated pneumonia) is a disease that is restricted to immunocompromised patients, we will consider the protean manifestations of *Candida* species in this section.

Morphology

In tissue sections, *C. albicans* demonstrates yeastlike forms (blastoconidia), pseudohyphae, and true hyphae (Fig. 13–43*A*). Pseudohyphae are an important diagnostic clue for *C. albicans* and represent budding yeast cells joined end to end at constrictions, thus simulating true fungal hyphae. The organisms may be visible with routine hematoxylin and eosin stains, but a variety of special "fungal" stains (Gomori methenamine-silver, periodic acid–Schiff) are commonly used to better highlight the pathogens.

Clinical Syndromes. Candidiasis can involve the mucous membranes, skin, and deep organs (invasive candidiasis).

- *The most common pattern of candidiasis takes the form of a superficial infection on mucosal surfaces of the oral cavity (thrush).* Florid proliferation of the fungi creates gray-white, dirty-looking pseudomembranes composed of matted organisms and inflammatory debris. Deep to the surface, there is mucosal hyperemia and inflammation. This form of candidiasis is seen in newborns, debilitated patients, children receiving oral corticosteroids for asthma, and after a course of broad-spectrum antibiotics that destroy competing normal bacterial flora. *The other major risk group includes HIV-positive patients;* patients with oral thrush for no obvious reason should be evaluated for HIV infection.
- *Candida vaginitis* is an extremely common form of vaginal infection in women, especially those who are diabetic or pregnant or on oral contraceptive pills. It is usually associated with intense itching and a thick, curdlike discharge.
- *Candida esophagitis* is common in AIDS patients and in those with hematolymphoid malignancies. These patients present with dysphagia (painful swallowing) and retrosternal pain; endoscopy demonstrates white plaques and pseudomembranes resembling oral thrush on the esophageal mucosa.
- *Cutaneous candidiasis* can present in many different forms, including infection of the nail proper ("onychomycosis"), nail folds ("paronychia"), hair follicles ("folliculitis"), moist, intertriginous skin such as armpits or webs of the fingers and toes ("intertrigo"), and penile skin ("balanitis"). "Diaper rash" is often a cutaneous candidal infection seen in the perineum of infants, in the region of contact of wet diapers.

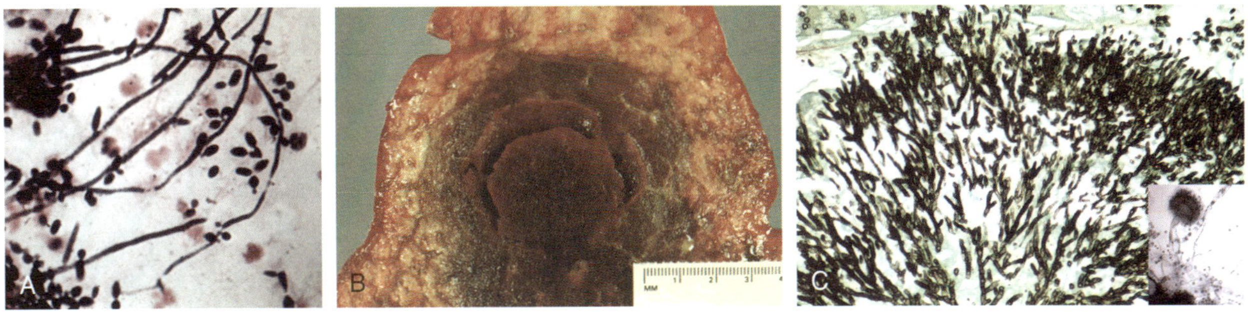

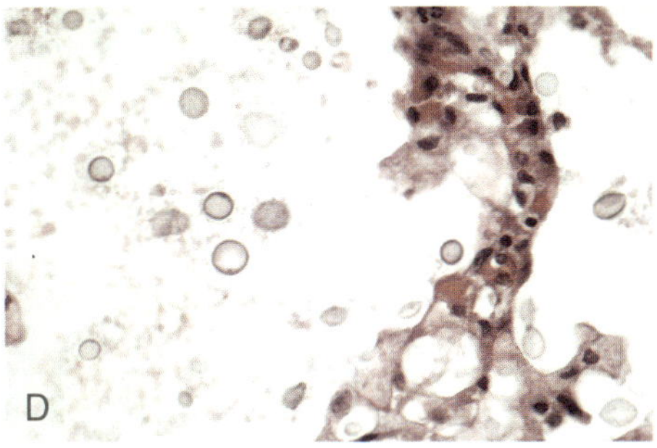

Figure 13–43

The morphology of fungal infections. **A,** The diagnosis of candidiasis is made by observing the characteristic pseudohyphae and blastoconidia (budding yeasts) in tissue sections or exudates. **B,** Invasive aspergillosis of the lung in a bone marrow transplant patient. **C,** Histologic sections from this case, stained with Gomori methenamine-silver (GMS) stain, show septate hyphae with acute-angle branching, features consistent with *Aspergillus.* Occasionally, *Aspergillus* may demonstrate so-called fruiting bodies (*inset*) when it grows in areas that are well-aerated (such as the upper respiratory tract). **D,** Cryptococcosis of the lung in a patient with AIDS. The yeast forms are somewhat variable in size; unlike in *Candida,* pseudohyphae are not seen. (All Figures courtesy of Dr. Dominick Cavuoti, Department of Pathology, University of Texas Southestern Medical School, Dallas, Texas.)

- *Chronic mucocutaneous candidiasis* is a chronic refractory disease afflicting the mucous membranes, skin, hair, and nails; it is associated with underlying T-cell defects. Associated conditions include endocrinopathies (most commonly hypoparathyroidism and Addison disease) and the presence of autoantibodies. Disseminated candidiasis is rare in this disease.
- *Invasive candidiasis* implies bloodborne dissemination of organisms to various tissues or organs. Common patterns include (1) renal abscesses, (2) myocardial abscesses and endocarditis, (3) brain involvement (most commonly meningitis, but parenchymal microabscesses occur), (4) endophthalmitis (virtually any eye structure can be involved), (5) hepatic abscesses, and (6) *Candida* pneumonia, usually presenting as bilateral nodular infiltrates, resembling *Pneumocystis* pneumonia (see above). Patients with acute leukemias who are profoundly neutropenic post chemotherapy are particularly prone to developing systemic disease. *Candida* endocarditis is the most common fungal endocarditis, usually occurring in patients with prosthetic heart valves or in intravenous drug abusers.

Cryptococcosis

Cryptococcosis, caused by *C. neoformans,* rarely occurs in healthy persons. It almost exclusively presents as an opportunistic infection in immunocompromised hosts, particularly those with AIDS or hematolymphoid malignancies.

Morphology

The fungus, a 5- to 10-μm yeast, has a thick, gelatinous capsule and reproduces by budding (Fig. 13–43*D*). Unlike in *Candida,* however, pseudohyphal or true hyphal forms are not seen. **The capsule is invaluable to diagnosis:** (1) In routine H & E stains, the capsule is not directly visible but often a clear "halo" can be seen surrounding the individual fungi representing the area occupied by the capsule. It is stained by India ink or periodic acid–Schiff stains and effectively highlights the fungus; and (2) the capsular polysaccharide antigen is the substrate for the cryptococcal latex agglutination assay, which is positive in greater than 95% of patients infected with the organism.

Clinical Syndromes. Human cryptococcosis usually manifests as *pulmonary, central nervous system, or disseminated disease. Cryptococcus* is most likely acquired by inhalation from the soil or from bird droppings. *The fungus initially localizes in the lungs and then disseminates to other sites, particularly the meninges.* Sites of involvement are marked by a variable tissue response, which ranges from florid proliferation of gelatinous organisms with a minimal or absent inflammatory cell infiltrate (in immunodeficient hosts) to a granulomatous reaction (in the more reactive host). In immunosuppressed patients, fungi grow in gelatinous masses within the meninges or expand the perivascular Virchow-Robin spaces, producing the so-called soap-bubble lesions.

The Opportunistic Molds

Mucormycosis and *invasive aspergillosis* are uncommon infections almost always limited to immunocompromised hosts, particularly those with hematolymphoid malignancies, profound neutropenia, corticosteroid therapy, or post allogeneic bone marrow transplantation.

Morphology

Mucormycosis is caused by the class of fungi known as Zygomycetes. Their hyphae are **nonseptate** and branch at right angles; in contrast, the hyphae of *Aspergillus* species are **septate** and branch at more acute angles (Fig. 13–43*C*).

Rhizopus and *Mucor* are the two fungi of medical importance within the Zygomycetes class. Both Zygomycetes and *Aspergillus* cause a nondistinctive, suppurative, sometimes granulomatous reaction with a **predilection for invading blood vessel walls, causing vascular necrosis and infarction.**

Clinical Syndromes

Rhinocerebral and *pulmonary mucormycosis:* Zygomycetes have a propensity to colonize the nasal cavity or sinuses and then spread by direct extension into the brain, orbit, and other head and neck structures. Patients with diabetic ketoacidosis are most likely to develop a fulminant invasive form of rhinocerebral mucormycosis. Pulmonary disease can be localized (e.g., cavitary lesions) or may present radiologically with diffuse "miliary" involvement.

Invasive aspergillosis occurs almost exclusively in patients who are immunosuppressed. The fungus preferentially localizes to the lungs, and it most often presents as a necrotizing pneumonia (see Fig. 13–43*B*). As mentioned previously, *Aspergillus* species have a propensity to invade blood vessels, and thus systemic dissemination, especially to the brain, is often a fatal complication.

Allergic bronchopulmonary aspergillosis occurs in patients with asthma who develop an exacerbation of symptoms caused by a type I hypersensitivity against the fungus growing in the bronchi. These patients often have circulating IgE antibodies against *Aspergillus* and peripheral eosinophilia.

Aspergilloma ("fungus ball") occurs by colonization of preexisting pulmonary cavities (e.g., ectatic bronchi or lung cysts, post-tuberculous cavitary lesions) by the fungus; these may act as ball valves, occluding the cavity and thus predisposing to infection and hemoptysis.

Pulmonary Disease in HIV Infection

Pulmonary disease continues to be the leading cause of morbidity and mortality in HIV-infected persons. Although the use of potent antiretroviral agents and effective chemoprophylaxis has markedly altered the incidence and outcome of pulmonary disease in HIV-infected persons, the plethora of entities involved makes diagnosis and treatment a distinct challenge. Some of the individual microbial agents afflicting HIV-infected persons have already been discussed; this section will focus only on the general principles of HIV-associated pulmonary disease.

- Despite the emphasis on "opportunistic" infections, it must be remembered that bacterial lower respiratory tract infection caused by the "usual" pathogens is one of the most serious pulmonary disorders in HIV infection. The implicated organisms include *S. pneumoniae, S. aureus, H. influenzae,* and gram-negative rods. Bacterial pneumonias in HIV-infected persons are more common, more severe, and more often associated with bacteremia than in those without HIV infection.
- Not all pulmonary infiltrates in HIV-infected individuals are infectious in etiology. A host of noninfectious diseases, including Kaposi sarcoma (Chapters 5 and 10), pulmonary non-Hodgkin lymphoma (Chapter 12), and primary lung cancer, occur with increased frequency and must be excluded.
- *The CD4+ T cell count is often useful in narrowing the differential diagnosis.* As a rule of thumb, bacterial and tubercular infections are more likely at higher CD4 counts (>200 cells/mm^3); *Pneumocystis* pneumonia usually strikes at CD4 counts below 200 cells/mm^3, while CMV and *M. avium* complex infections are uncommon until the very late stages of immunosuppression (CD4 counts <50 cells/mm^3).

Finally, it is useful to remember that pulmonary disease in HIV-infected individuals may result from more than one cause, and even common pathogens may present with atypical manifestations. Therefore, the diagnostic work-up of these persons may be more extensive than would be mandated in an immunocompetent individual.

LUNG TUMORS

Although lungs are frequently the site of metastases from cancers in extrathoracic organs, primary lung cancer is also a common disease. Bronchial epithelium is the site of origin of 95% of primary lung tumors (carcinomas); the remaining 5% are a miscellaneous group that includes bronchial carcinoids, mesenchymal malignancies (e.g., fibrosarcomas, leiomyomas), lymphomas, and a few benign lesions. The most common benign lesions are spherical, small (3–4 cm), discrete hamartomas that often show up as "coin" lesions on chest radiographs. They consist mainly of mature cartilage but are often admixed with fat, fibrous tissue, and blood vessels in varying proportions.

Carcinomas

Carcinoma of the lung (also known as "lung cancer") is without doubt the number one cause of cancer-related deaths in industrialized countries. It has long held this position among males in the United States, accounting for about one-third of cancer deaths in men, and has become the leading cause of cancer deaths in women as well. The American Cancer Society estimates that in 2006 approximately 172,570 individuals were diagnosed with lung cancer and 163,510 will die from it. The rate of increase among males is slowing down, but it continues to accelerate among females, with more women dying each year from lung cancer than breast cancers, since 1987. These statistics are undoubtedly related to the causal relationship of cigarette smoking and lung cancer. The peak incidence of lung cancer occurs in persons in their 50s and 60s. At diagnosis, more than 50% of individuals already have distant metastatic disease, while a fourth have disease in the regional lymph nodes. The prognosis of lung cancer is dismal: the 5-year survival rate for all stages of lung cancer combined is about 15%; even those with disease localized to the lung have a 5-year survival of approximately 45%.

The four major histologic types of carcinomas of the lung are squamous cell carcinoma, adenocarcinoma, small-cell carcinoma, and large-cell carcinoma (Table 13–8). In some cases there is a combination of histologic patterns (e.g., combined small-cell carcinoma, adenosquamous carcinoma). For reasons not entirely understood, but probably due to changes in smoking patterns, adenocarcinoma has replaced squamous cell carcinoma as the most common primary lung tumor in recent years. Adenocarcinomas are also by far the most common primary tumors arising in women, in lifetime nonsmokers, and in persons younger than 45 years. Before the individual histologic types are discussed, some general principles underlying classification of lung tumors are presented.

- For therapeutic purposes, carcinomas of the lung are classified into two broad groups: small-cell lung cancer (SCLC) and non-small-cell lung cancer (NSCLC). The latter category includes squamous cell, adenocarcinomas, and large-cell carcinomas.
- *The key reason for this distinction is that virtually all SCLCs have metastasized by the time of diagnosis and hence are not curable by surgery. Therefore, they are best treated by chemotherapy, with or without radiation.* In contrast, NSCLCs usually respond poorly to chemotherapy and are better treated by surgery.
- In addition to the differences in morphology, immunophenotypic characteristics, and response to treatment (Table 13–9), there are also pertinent genetic differences between SCLCs and NSCLCs. For example, although the G_1-S cell cycle checkpoint is abrogated in most lung carcinomas, it occurs via different genetic mechanisms; SCLCs are characterized by a high frequency of *RB* gene mutations, while the *p16/CDKN2A* gene is commonly inactivated in NSCLCs. Similarly, activating *KRAS* and *EGFR* oncogene mutations are virtually restricted to adenocarcinomas within the NSCLC group and are rare in SCLCs.

Table 13–8 Histologic Classification of Malignant Epithelial Lung Tumors

Squamous cell carcinoma
Adenocarcinoma Acinar, papillary, solid, bronchioloalveolar, mixed subtypes
Large-cell carcinoma Large-cell neuroendocrine carcinoma
Small-cell carcinoma Combined small-cell carcinoma
Adenosquamous carcinoma
Carcinomas with pleomorphic, sarcomatoid, or sarcomatous elements Spindle cell carcinoma Giant-cell carcinoma
Carcinoid tumor Typical, atypical
Carcinomas of salivary gland type
Unclassified carcinoma

Squamous cell, adenocarcinoma, large cell carcinoma are collectively referred to as non-small-cell lung carcinoma (NSLC).

Etiology and Pathogenesis. Carcinomas of the lung, similar to cancers at many other anatomic sites, arise by a stepwise accumulation of genetic abnormalities that result in transformation of benign bronchial epithelium into neoplastic tissue. The sequence of molecular changes is not random but follows a predictable sequence that parallels the histologic progression toward cancer. Thus, inactivation of the putative tumor suppressor genes located on chromosome 3p is a very early event, whereas *p53* mutations or activation of the *KRAS* oncogene occurs relatively late. More importantly, it seems that certain genetic changes such as loss of chromosome 3p material, can be found even in benign bronchial epithelium of individuals with lung cancer, as well as in the respiratory epithelium of smokers *without* lung cancers, suggesting that large areas of the respiratory mucosa are mutagenized after exposure to carcinogens ("field effect"). On this fertile soil, those cells that accumulate additional mutations ultimately develop into cancer. A subset of adenocarcinomas, particularly those arising in non-smoking women of Far Eastern origin, harbor activating mutations of the *epidermal growth factor receptor (EGFR)*. Notably, these tumors are profoundly susceptible to a class of agents that inhibit EGFR signaling, probably because the *EGFR*-mutant cancer cells become "addicted" to the presence of a constitutively activated oncogene. The identification of a defined genetic alteration in lung cancer that can guide therapy represents one of the successes in the rapidly expanding field of molecular medicine.

With regard to carcinogenic influences, there is strong evidence that *cigarette smoking* and, to a much lesser extent, other environmental insults are the main culprits responsible for the genetic changes that give rise to lung cancers. First, the evidence relating to cigarette smoking will be given, followed by a few brief comments on the less important influences.

An impressive body of statistical, clinical, and experimental evidence incriminates cigarette smoking in the causation of lung cancer. Statistically, about 90% of lung cancers occur in active smokers or those who stopped recently. There is a nearly linear correlation between the frequency of lung cancer and pack-years of cigarette smoking. The increased risk becomes 60 times greater among habitual heavy smokers (two packs a day for 20 years) compared with nonsmokers. For reasons not entirely clear, women have a higher susceptibility to carcinogens in tobacco than men. Although cessation of smoking decreases the risk of developing lung cancer over time, it may never return to baseline levels. In fact, genetic changes that predate lung cancer can persist for many years in the bronchial epithelium of former smokers. Passive smoking (proximity to cigarette smokers) increases the risk of developing lung cancer to approximately twice that of nonsmokers. The smoking of pipes and cigars also increases the risk, but only modestly.

The *clinical evidence* is largely composed of the documentation of progressive morphologic alterations in the

Table 13–9 Comparison of Small-Cell Lung Carcinoma (SCLC) and Non–Small Cell Lung Carcinoma (NSCLC)

	SCLC	NSCLC
Histology		
	Scant cytoplasm; small, hyperchromatic nuclei with fine chromatin pattern; nucleoli indistinct; diffuse sheets of cells	Abundant cytoplasm; pleomorphic nuclei with coarse chromatin pattern; nucleoli often prominent; glandular or squamous architecture
Neuroendocrine Markers		
For example, dense core granules on electron microscopy; expression of chromogranin, neuron-specific enolase and synaptophysin	Usually present	Usually absent
Epithelial Markers		
Epithelial membrane antigen, carcinoembryonic antigen, and cytokeratin intermediate filaments	Present	Present
Mucin		
	Absent	Present in adenocarcinomas
Peptide Hormone Production		
	Adrenocorticotropic hormone, antidiuretic hormone, gastrin-releasing peptide, calcitonin	Parathyroid hormone–related peptide (PTH-rp) in squamous cell carcinoma
Tumor Suppressor Gene Abnormalities		
3p deletions	>90%	>80%
RB mutations	~90%	~20%
p16/CDKN2A mutations	~10%	>50%
p53 mutations	>90%	>50%
Dominant Oncogene Abnormalities		
KRAS mutations	Rare	~30% (adenocarcinomas)
EGFR mutations	Absent	~20% (adenocarcinomas, nonsmokers, women)
Response to Chemotherapy and Radiotherapy		
	Often complete response but recur invariably	Uncommonly complete response

Adapted and modified with permission from Minna JD: Neoplasms of the lung. In Fauci A, et al. (eds): In Harrison's Principles of Internal Medicine, 14th ed. New York, McGraw-Hill, 1998.

lining epithelium of the respiratory tract in habitual cigarette smokers. These sequential changes have been best documented for squamous cell carcinomas, but they may also be present in other histologic subtypes. In essence, there is a linear correlation between the intensity of exposure to cigarette smoke and the appearance of ever more worrisome epithelial changes that begin with rather innocuous basal cell hyperplasia and squamous metaplasia and progress to squamous dysplasia and carcinoma in situ, before culminating in invasive cancer. *Among the major histologic subtypes of lung cancer, squamous and small-cell carcinomas show the strongest association with tobacco exposure.*

The *experimental evidence,* although it mounts with each passing year, lacks one important link: it has not so far been possible to produce lung cancer in an experimental animal by exposing it to cigarette smoke. Nonetheless, cigarette smoke condensate is a witches' brew of tumorigenic delicacies such as polycyclic hydrocarbons and other potent mutagens and carcinogens. Despite the lack of an experimental model, the chain of evidence linking cigarette smoking to lung cancer grows ever stronger.

Other influences may act in concert with smoking or may by themselves be responsible for some lung cancers; witness the increased incidence of this form of neoplasia in miners of radioactive ores; asbestos workers; and workers exposed to dusts containing arsenic, chromium, uranium, nickel, vinyl chloride, and mustard gas. Exposure to asbestos increases the risk of lung cancer fivefold in nonsmokers. By contrast, *heavy smokers exposed to asbestos have an approximately 55 times greater risk of lung cancer than do nonsmokers not exposed to asbestos.*

Even though smoking and other environmental influences are paramount in the causation of lung cancer, it is well known that all persons exposed to tobacco smoke do not develop cancer. It is very likely that the mutagenic effect of carcinogens is conditioned by hereditary (genetic) factors. Recall that many chemicals (procarcinogens) require metabolic activation via the P-450 monooxygenase enzyme system for conversion into ultimate carcinogens (Chapter 6). There is evidence that persons with specific genetic polymorphisms involving the P-450 genes have an increased capacity to metabolize procarcinogens derived from cigarette smoke and, conceivably, incur the greatest risk of developing lung cancer.

Similarly, individuals whose peripheral blood lymphocytes undergo chromosomal breakages after exposure to tobacco-related carcinogens (mutagen sensitivity genotype) have a greater than 10-fold risk of developing lung cancer as compared with controls.

Morphology

Carcinomas of the lung begin as small mucosal lesions that are usually firm and gray-white. They may form intraluminal masses, invade the bronchial mucosa, or form large bulky masses pushing into adjacent lung parenchyma. Some large masses undergo cavitation caused by central necrosis or develop focal areas of hemorrhage. Finally, these tumors may extend to the pleura, invade the pleural cavity and chest wall, and spread to adjacent intrathoracic structures. More distant spread can occur via the lymphatics or the hematogenous route.

Squamous cell carcinomas are more common in men than in women and are closely correlated with a smoking history; they tend to **arise centrally in major bronchi** and eventually spread to local hilar nodes, but they disseminate outside the thorax later than other histologic types. Large lesions may undergo central necrosis, giving rise to **cavitation.** The preneoplastic lesions that antedate, and usually accompany, invasive squamous cell carcinoma are well characterized. Squamous cell carcinomas are often preceded for years by **squamous metaplasia or dysplasia** in the bronchial epithelium, which then transforms to **carcinoma in situ,** a phase that may last for several years (Fig. 13–44). By this time, atypical cells may be identified in cytologic smears of sputum or in bronchial lavage fluids or brushings, although the lesion is asymptomatic and undetectable on radiographs. Eventually, the small neoplasm reaches a symptomatic stage, when a well-defined tumor mass begins to obstruct the lumen of a major bronchus, often producing distal atelectasis and infection. Simultaneously, the lesion invades surrounding pulmonary substance (Fig. 13–45). Histologically, these tumors range from well-differentiated squamous cell neoplasms showing keratin pearls and intercellular bridges to poorly differentiated neoplasms having only minimal residual squamous cell features.

Adenocarcinomas may occur as central lesions like the squamous cell variant but are usually more **peripherally located,** many arising in relation to peripheral lung scars ("scar carcinomas"). The etiologic basis for this association is not clear, although the current thinking is that the scarring probably occurred secondary to the tumor, rather than being contributory. Adenocarcinomas are the most common type of lung cancer in women and nonsmokers. In general, adenocarcinomas grow slowly and form smaller masses than do the other subtypes, but they tend to metastasize widely at an early stage. Histologically, they assume a variety of forms, including **acinar (gland forming)** (Fig. 13–46C), **papillary,** and **solid types.** The solid variant often requires demonstration of intracellular mucin production by special stains to establish its adenocarcinomatous lineage. Although foci of squamous metaplasia and dysplasia may be present in the epithelium proximal to resected adenocarcinomas, these are not the precursor lesions for this tumor. The putative precursor of peripheral adenocarcinomas has been described as **atypical adenomatous hyperplasia** (AAH) (Fig. 13–46A). Microscopically, AAH is recognized as a well-demarcated focus of epithelial proliferation composed of cuboidal to low-columnar cells resembling Clara cells or type 2 alveolar pneumocytes, which demonstrate various degrees of cytologic atypia (nuclear hyperchromasia, pleomorphism, prominent nucleoli), but not to the extent seen in frank adenocarcinomas. Genetic analyses have shown that lesions of AAH are monoclonal, and they share many of the molecular aberrations associated with adenocarcinomas (e.g., *KRAS* mutations).

Bronchioloalveolar carcinomas (BACs) are included as a subtype of adenocarcinomas in the current WHO classification of lung tumors. They involve peripheral parts of the lung, either as a single nodule or, more often, as multiple diffuse nodules that may coalesce to produce pneumonia-like consolidation. **The key feature of BACs is their growth along preexisting structures and preservation of alveolar architecture** (see Fig. 13–46B). The tumor cells grow in a monolayer on top of the alveolar septa, which serves as a scaffold (this has been termed a "lepidic" growth pattern, an allusion to the neoplastic cells resembling butterflies sitting on a fence). By definition, BACs do not demonstrate destruction of alveolar architecture or stromal invasion with desmoplasia, features that would merit their classification as frank adenocarcinomas. The two subtypes of BACs are mucinous and nonmucinous, with the former comprising tall, columnar cells with prominent cytoplasmic and intra-alveolar mucin. Analogous to the adenoma-carcinoma sequence in the colon, it is proposed that some invasive adenocarcinomas of the lung may arise through an **atypical adenomatous hyperplasia–bronchioloalveolar carcinoma–invasive adenocarcinoma sequence.** It is important to stress, however, that not all adenocarcinomas arise in this manner, nor do all BACs become invasive if left untreated. While the cell types giving rise to the centrally located squamous cell carcinoma (metaplastic squamous cells in the main stem bronchi) and small cell lung carcinoma (native neuroendocrine cells, *see below*) were recognized for a while, the "cell of origin" for peripheral adenocarcinomas remained unclear until recently. Studies of lung injury models in mice have now identified a population of multipotent cells at the bronchioalveolar duct junction, termed **bronchioalveolar stem cells** (BASCs). Following peripheral lung injury, the multipotent BASCs undergo expansion, replenishing the normal cell types (bronchiolar Clara cells and alveolar cells) found in this location, thereby facilitating epithelial regeneration. It is postulated that BASCs incur the initiating oncogenic event (for example, a somatic *K-RAS* mutation) that enable these cells to escape normal "checkpoint" mechanisms and result in pulmonary adenocarcinomas.

Large-cell carcinomas are undifferentiated malignant epithelial tumors that lack the cytologic features of small-cell carcinoma and glandular or squamous differentiation. The cells typically have large nuclei, prominent nucleoli, and a moderate amount of cytoplasm. Large-cell carcinomas probably represent squamous cell or adenocarcinomas that are so undifferentiated that they can no longer be recognized by light microscopy. Ultrastructurally, however, minimal glandular or squamous differentiation is common.

Small-cell lung carcinomas generally appear as pale gray, **centrally located masses** with extension into the lung parenchyma and early involvement of the hilar and mediastinal nodes. These cancers are composed of tumor cells with a round to fusiform shape, scant cytoplasm, and finely granular chromatin. Mitotic figures are frequently seen (Fig. 13–47A). Despite the appellation of "small," the neoplastic cells are usually twice the size of resting lymphocytes. Necrosis is invariably present and may be extensive. The tumor cells are markedly fragile and often show fragmentation and "crush artifact" in small biopsy specimens. Another feature of small-cell carcinomas, best appreciated in cytologic specimens, is nuclear molding resulting from close apposition of tumor cells that have scant cytoplasm (Fig. 13–47B). These tumors are derived from neuroendocrine cells of the lung, and hence they express a variety of neuroendocrine markers (see Table 13–9) in addition to a host of polypeptide hormones that may result in paraneoplastic syndromes (see below).

Combined patterns require no further comment, but it should be noted that a significant minority of bronchogenic carcinomas reveal more than one line of differentiation, sometimes several (see Table 13–8), suggesting that all are derived from a multipotential progenitor cell.

For all of these neoplasms, one can trace involvement of successive chains of nodes about the carina, in the mediastinum, and in the neck (scalene nodes) and clavicular regions and, sooner or later, distant metastases. Involvement of the left supraclavicular node (Virchow node) is particularly characteristic and sometimes calls attention to an occult primary tumor. These cancers, when advanced, often extend into the pericardial or pleural spaces, leading to inflammation and effusions. They may compress or infiltrate the superior vena cava to cause either venous congestion or the full-blown vena caval syndrome (Chapter 10). Apical neoplasms may invade the brachial or cervical sympathetic plexus to cause severe pain in the distribution of the ulnar nerve or to produce Horner syndrome (ipsilateral enophthalmos, ptosis, miosis, and anhidrosis). Such apical neoplasms are sometimes called **Pancoast tumors,** and the combination of clinical findings is known as Pancoast syndrome. Pancoast tumor is often accompanied by destruction of the first and second ribs and sometimes thoracic vertebrae. As with other cancers, tumor-node-metastasis (TNM) categories have been established to indicate the size and spread of the primary neoplasm.

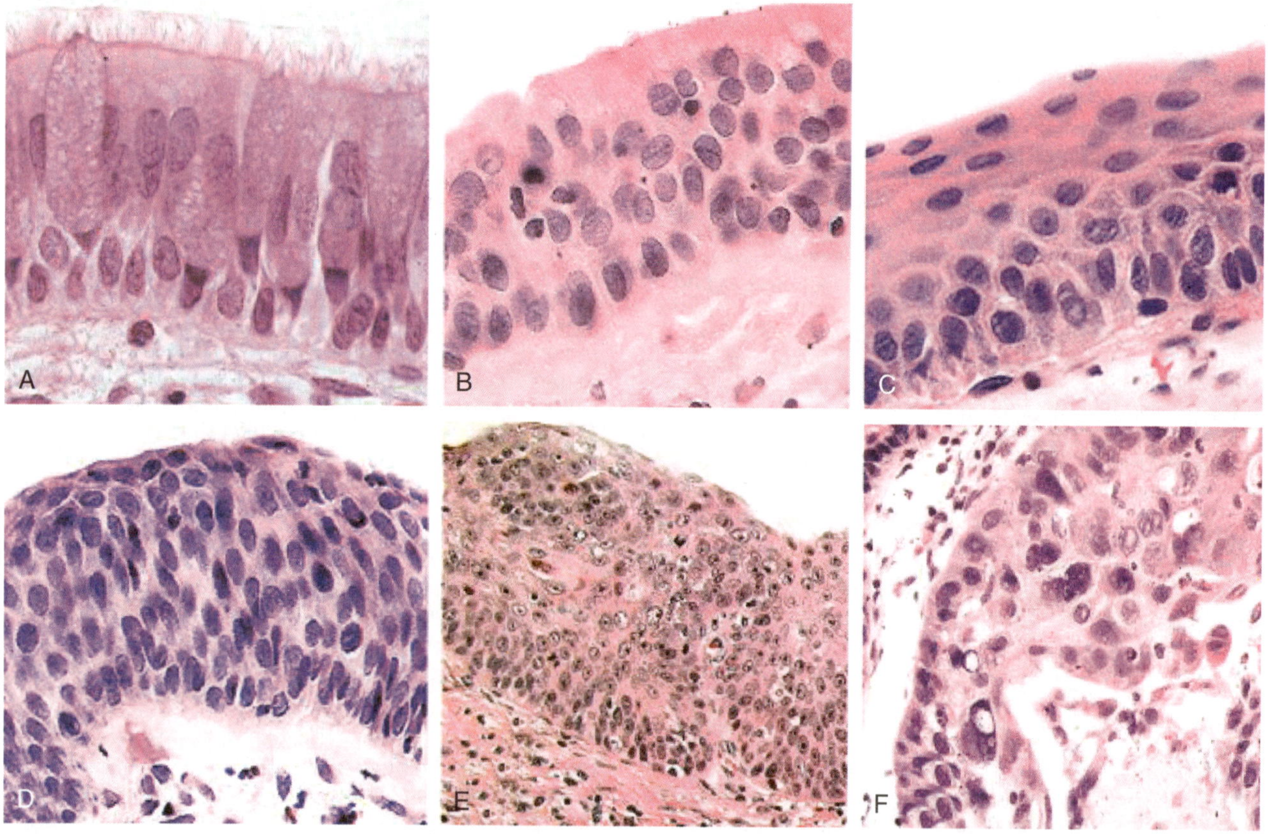

Figure 13–44

The precursor lesions of squamous cell carcinomas may antedate the appearance of invasive tumor by years. Some of the earliest (and "mild") changes in smoking-damaged respiratory epithelium include goblet cell hyperplasia **(A),** basal cell (or reserve cell) hyperplasia **(B),** and squamous metaplasia **(C).** More ominous changes include the appearance of squamous dysplasia **(D),** characterized by the presence of disordered squamous epithelium, with loss of nuclear polarity, nuclear hyperchromasia, pleomorphism, and mitotic figures. Squamous dysplasia may, in turn, progress through the stages of mild, moderate, and severe dysplasia. Carcinoma-in-situ (CIS) **(E)** is the stage that immediately precedes invasive squamous carcinoma **(F),** and apart from the lack of basement membrane disruption in CIS, the cytologic features are similar to those in frank carcinoma. Unless treated, CIS will eventually progress to invasive cancer. (**A–E,** Courtesy of Dr. Adi Gazdar, Department of Pathology, University of Texas, Southwestern Medical School, Dallas. **F,** reproduced with permission from Travis WD, et al [eds]: World Health Organization Histological Typing of Lung and Pleural Tumors. Heidelberg, Springer, 1999.)

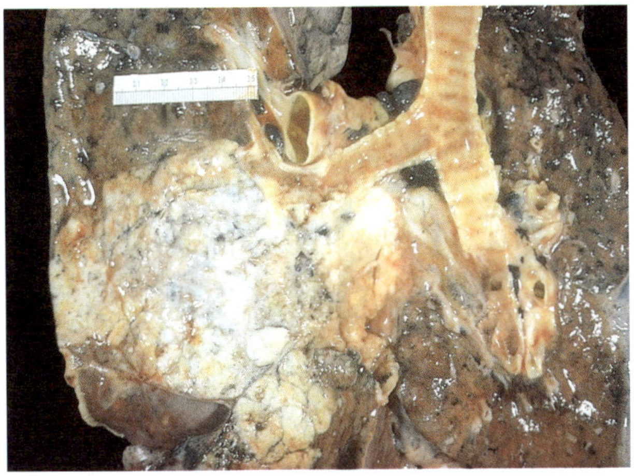

Figure 13–45

Squamous cell carcinomas usually begin as central (hilar) masses and grow contiguously into the peripheral parenchyma. It is not uncommon for squamous cell carcinomas to undergo cavitary necrosis during intrapulmonary spread.

Clinical Course. Carcinomas of the lung are silent, insidious lesions that more often than not have spread so as to be unresectable before they produce symptoms. In some instances, chronic cough and expectoration call attention to still localized, resectable disease. By the time hoarseness, chest pain, superior vena caval syndrome, pericardial or pleural effusion, or persistent segmental atelectasis or pneumonitis makes its appearance, the prognosis is grim. Too often, the tumor presents with symptoms emanating from metastatic spread to the brain (mental or neurologic changes), liver (hepatomegaly), or bones (pain). Although the adrenals may be nearly obliterated by metastatic disease, adrenal insufficiency (Addison disease) is uncommon because islands of cortical cells sufficient to maintain adrenal function usually persist.

Overall, NSCLCs have a better prognosis than SCLCs. When NSCLCs (squamous cell carcinomas or adenocarci-

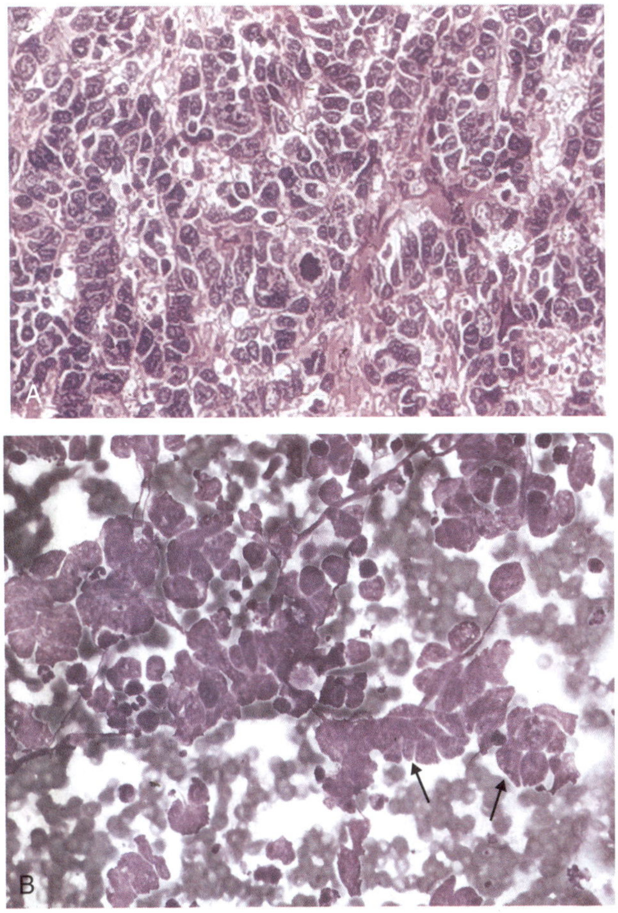

Figure 13–47

Small-cell lung carcinoma. **A,** Nests and cords of round to polygonal cells with scant cytoplasm, granular chromatin, and inconspicuous nucleoli. Note mitotic figure in center. **B,** Cytologic preparation from a case of small-cell carcinoma demonstrating "nuclear molding" of adjacent cells *(arrows)*. This is a useful feature in bronchioloalveolar lavage samples or fine-needle aspiration specimens for diagnosing small-cell carcinoma.

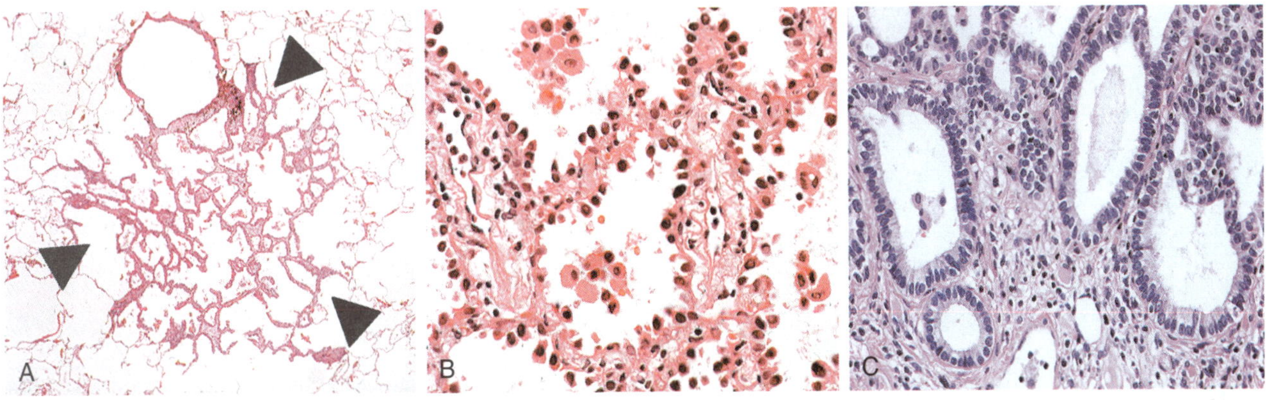

Figure 13–46

Glandular lesions of the lung. **A,** The putative precursor lesion of invasive adenocarcinomas is known as atypical adenomatous hyperplasia, *(arrowheads)*, which presents typically as multifocal nodules. **B,** Bronchioloalveolar carcinomas are a variant of adenocarcinoma that grow along existing structures and do not demonstrate evidence of stromal, vascular, or pleural invasion. **C,** Invasive adenocarcinoma, with stromal invasion and desmoplasia. (**A** and **B**, From Travis WD, et al [eds]: World Health Organization Histological Typing of Lung and Pleural Tumors. Heidelberg, Springer, 1999. **C,** Courtesy of Dr. Adi Gazdar, Department of Pathology, University of Texas Southwestern Medical School, Dallas, Texas.)

nomas) are detected before metastasis or local spread, cure is possible by lobectomy or pneumonectomy. SCLCs, on the other hand, have invariably spread by the time they are first detected, even if the primary tumor appears small and localized. Thus, surgical resection is not a viable treatment. They are very sensitive to chemotherapy but invariably recur. Median survival even with treatment is 1 year.

It is variously estimated that 3% to 10% of all patients with lung cancer develop clinically overt *paraneoplastic syndromes.* These include (1) hypercalcemia caused by secretion of a parathyroid hormone–related peptide (osteolytic lesions may also cause hypercalcemia, but this would not be a paraneoplastic syndrome [Chapter 6]); (2) Cushing syndrome (from increased production of adrenocorticotropic hormone); (3) syndrome of inappropriate secretion of antidiuretic hormone; (4) neuromuscular syndromes, including a myasthenic syndrome, peripheral neuropathy, and polymyositis; (5) clubbing of the fingers and hypertrophic pulmonary osteoarthropathy; and (6) hematologic manifestations, including migratory thrombophlebitis, nonbacterial endocarditis, and disseminated intravascular coagulation. Secretion of calcitonin and other ectopic hormones has also been documented by assays, but these products usually do not provoke distinctive syndromes. Hypercalcemia is most often encountered with squamous cell neoplasms, the hematologic syndromes with adenocarcinomas. The remaining syndromes are much more common with small-cell neoplasms, but exceptions abound.

SUMMARY

Carcinomas of the Lung

- The four major histologic subtypes are adenocarcinomas (most common), squamous cell carcinoma, large-cell carcinoma, and small-cell carcinoma (SCLC). Together the first three are designated as non-small-cell lung cancer (NSCLC).
- SCLC and NSCLC are clinically and genetically distinct. SCLC are best treated by chemotherapy because all are metastatic at presentation. NSCLCs, by contrast, are curable by surgery (if limited to the lung).
- Smoking is most important risk factor for lung cancer; adenocarcinomas are most common cancers to arise in women and nonsmokers.
- Precursor lesions include squamous dysplasia (for squamous cancer) and atypical adenomatous hyperplasia (for some adenocarcinomas).
- Bronchioloalveolar carcinomas are a subtype of adenocarcinomas characterized by absence of stromal invasion and growth along preexisting structures.
- Lung cancers, particularly SCLCs, can cause *paraneoplastic syndromes.*

Bronchial Carcinoids

Bronchial carcinoids are thought to arise from the Kulchitsky cells (neuroendocrine cells) that line the bronchial mucosa and resemble intestinal carcinoids (Chapter 15). The neoplastic cells contain dense-core neurosecretory granules in their cytoplasm and, rarely, may secrete hormonally active polypeptides. They occasionally occur as part of the multiple endocrine neoplasia syndrome (Chapter 20). Bronchial carcinoids appear at an early age (mean 40 years) and represent about 5% of all pulmonary neoplasms. In happy contrast to their more ominous neuroendocrine counterpart, small-cell carcinomas, carcinoids are often resectable and curable.

Morphology

Most bronchial carcinoids originate in main-stem bronchi and grow in one of two patterns: (1) an obstructing polypoid, spherical, intraluminal mass (Fig. 13–48A); or (2) a mucosal plaque penetrating the bronchial wall to fan out in the peribronchial tissue—the so-called collar-button lesion. Even these penetrating lesions push into the lung substance along a broad front and are therefore reasonably well demarcated. Although 5% to 15% of these tumors have metastasized to the hilar nodes at presentation, distant metastasis is rare. Histologically, these neoplasms, like their counterparts in the intestinal tract, are composed of nests of uniform cells that have regular round nuclei with "salt-and-pepper" chromatin, absent or rare mitoses, and little pleomorphism (Fig. 13–48B). Occasional tumors display a higher mitotic rate, increased cytologic variability, and focal necrosis—features that qualify for a designation of **atypical carcinoid.** The latter tumors have a higher incidence of lymph node and distant metastasis than "typical" carcinoids, and understandably persons with atypical carcinoids fare worse in the long run. Unlike typical carcinoids, the atypical subset demonstrates *p53* mutations in 20% to 40% of cases. **Typical carcinoid, atypical carcinoid, and small-cell carcinoma can be considered to represent a continuum of increasing histologic aggressiveness and malignant potential within the spectrum of pulmonary neuroendocrine neoplasms.**

Most bronchial carcinoids present with findings related to their intraluminal growth (i.e., they cause cough, hemoptysis, and recurrent bronchial and pulmonary infections). Some are asymptomatic and discovered by chance on chest radiographs. Only rarely do they induce the *carcinoid syndrome,* characterized by intermittent attacks of diarrhea, flushing, and cyanosis. The reported 10-year survival rates for typical carcinoids is above 85%, while it drops to 56% and 35%, respectively for atypical carcinoids. Only 5% of patients with the most aggressive neuroendocrine lung tumor—SCLC—are alive at 10 years.

PLEURAL LESIONS

Pathologic involvement of the pleura is, with rare exceptions, a secondary complication of some underlying pulmonary disease. Secondary infections and pleural adhesions are particularly common findings at autopsy.

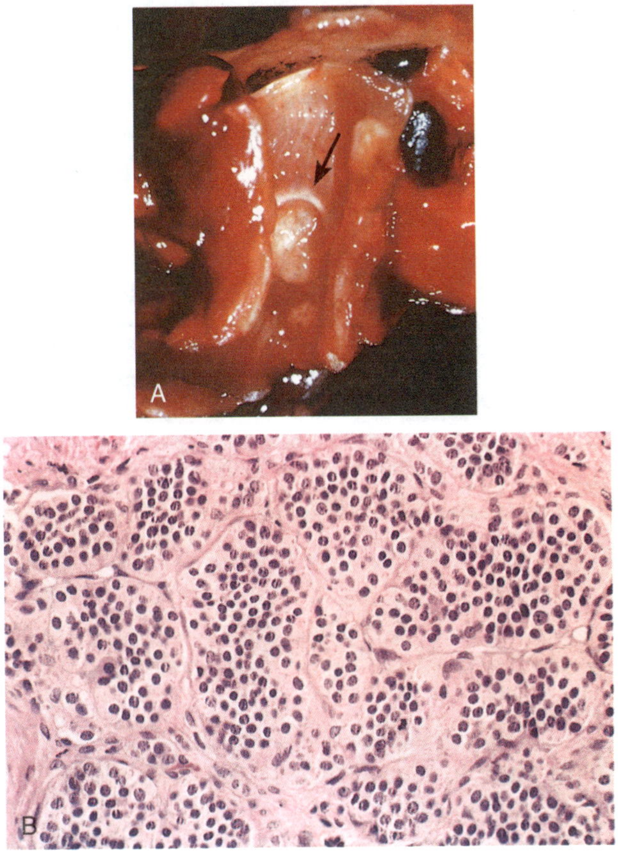

Figure 13–48

A, Bronchial carcinoid growing as a spherical, pale mass *(arrow)* protruding into the lumen of the bronchus. **B,** Histologic appearance of bronchial carcinoid demonstrating small, rounded, uniform cells.

Important primary disorders include (1) primary intrapleural bacterial infections and (2) a primary neoplasm of the pleura known as *malignant mesothelioma.*

Pleural Effusion and Pleuritis

Pleural effusion, the presence of fluid in the pleural space, can be either a transudate or an exudate. A pleural effusion that is a transudate is termed *hydrothorax.* Hydrothorax from CHF is probably the most common cause of fluid in the pleural cavity. An exudate, characterized by protein content >2.9 gm/dL and, often, inflammatory cells, suggests pleuritis. The four principal causes of *pleural exudate* are (1) microbial invasion through either direct extension of a pulmonary infection or blood-borne seeding (*suppurative pleuritis* or *empyema*); (2) cancer (bronchogenic carcinoma, metastatic neoplasms to the lung or pleural surface, mesothelioma); (3) pulmonary infarction; and (4) viral pleuritis. Other, less common causes of exudative pleural effusions are systemic lupus erythematosus, rheumatoid arthritis, or uremia and previous thoracic surgery. Cancer should be suspected as the underlying cause of an exudative effusion in any patient older than the age of 40, particularly when there is no febrile illness, no pain, and a negative tuberculin test result. These effusions characteristically are large and frequently are bloody *(hemorrhagic pleuritis).* Cytologic examination may reveal malignant and inflammatory cells.

Whatever the cause, transudates and serous exudates are usually resorbed without residual effects if the inciting cause is controlled or remits. In contrast, fibrinous, hemorrhagic, and suppurative exudates may lead to fibrous organization, yielding adhesions or fibrous pleural thickening, and sometimes minimal to massive calcifications.

Pneumothorax, Hemothorax, and Chylothorax

Pneumothorax refers to air or other gas in the pleural sac. It may occur in young, apparently healthy adults, usually men without any known pulmonary disease (simple or spontaneous pneumothorax), or as a result of some thoracic or lung disorder (secondary pneumothorax), such as emphysema or a fractured rib. Secondary pneumothorax occurs with rupture of any pulmonary lesion situated close to the pleural surface that allows inspired air to gain access to the pleural cavity. Such pulmonary lesions include emphysema, lung abscess, tuberculosis, carcinoma, and many other, less common, processes. Mechanical ventilatory support with high pressure may also trigger secondary pneumothorax.

There are several possible complications of pneumothorax. A ball-valve leak may create a tension pneumothorax that shifts the mediastinum. Compromise of the pulmonary circulation may follow and may even be fatal. If the leak seals and the lung is not re-expanded within a few weeks (either spontaneously or through medical or surgical intervention), so much scarring may occur that it can never be fully re-expanded. In these cases, serous fluid collects in the pleural cavity and creates hydropneumothorax. With prolonged collapse, the lung becomes vulnerable to infection, as does the pleural cavity when communication between it and the lung persists. Empyema is thus an important complication of pneumothorax (pyopneumothorax). Secondary pneumothorax tends to be recurrent if the predisposing condition remains. What is less well recognized is that simple pneumothorax is also recurrent.

Hemothorax, the collection of whole blood (in contrast to bloody effusion) in the pleural cavity, is a complication of a ruptured intrathoracic aortic aneurysm that is almost always fatal. With hemothorax, in contrast to bloody pleural effusions, the blood clots within the pleural cavity.

Chylothorax is a pleural collection of a milky lymphatic fluid containing microglobules of lipid. The total volume of fluid may not be large, but chylothorax is always significant because it implies obstruction of the major lymph ducts, usually by an intrathoracic cancer (e.g., a primary or secondary mediastinal neoplasm, such as a lymphoma).

Malignant Mesothelioma

Malignant mesothelioma is a rare cancer of mesothelial cells, usually arising in the parietal or visceral pleura, although it also occurs, much less commonly, in the peritoneum and pericardium. It has assumed great importance because it is related to occupational exposure to asbestos in the air. Approximately 50% of individuals with this cancer have a history of exposure to asbestos. Those who work directly with asbestos (shipyard workers, miners, insulators) are at greatest risk, but malignant mesotheliomas have appeared in persons whose only exposure was living in proximity to an asbestos factory or being a relative of an asbestos worker. The latent period for developing malignant mesotheliomas is long, often 25 to 40 years after initial asbestos exposure, suggesting that multiple somatic genetic events are required for tumorigenic conversion of a mesothelial cell. As stated earlier, *the combination of cigarette smoking and asbestos exposure greatly increases the risk of bronchogenic carcinoma, but it does not increase the risk of developing malignant mesotheliomas.*

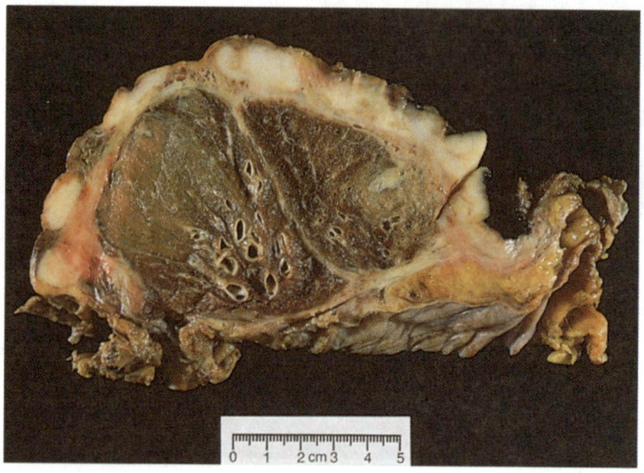

Figure 13–49

Malignant mesothelioma. Note the thick, firm, white, pleural tumor that ensheaths this bisected lung.

Morphology

Malignant mesotheliomas are often preceded by extensive **pleural fibrosis and plaque formation,** readily seen in computed tomographic scans. These tumors begin in a localized area and in the course of time spread widely, either by contiguous growth or by diffusely seeding the pleural surfaces. At autopsy, the affected lung **is typically ensheathed by a yellow-white, firm, sometimes gelatinous layer of tumor** that obliterates the pleural space (Fig. 13–49). Distant metastases are rare. The neoplasm may directly invade the thoracic wall or the subpleural lung tissue. Normal mesothelial cells are biphasic, giving rise to pleural lining cells as well as the underlying fibrous tissue. Therefore, histologically, mesotheliomas conform to one of three patterns: (1) **epithelial,** in which cuboidal cells line tubular and microcystic spaces, into which small papillary buds project; this is the most common pattern and also the one most likely to be confused with a pulmonary adenocarcinoma; (2) **sarcomatoid,** in which spindled and sometimes fibroblastic-appearing cells grow in nondistinctive sheets; and (3) **biphasic,** having both sarcomatoid and epithelioid areas.

The basis for the carcinogenicity of asbestos is still a mystery. Asbestos is not removed or metabolized from the lung, and hence the fibers remain in the body for life. Thus, there is a lifetime risk after exposure that does not diminish with time (unlike smoking, in which the risk decreases after cessation). It has been hypothesized that asbestos fibers preferentially gather near the mesothelial cell layer, where they generate reactive oxygen species that cause DNA damage and potentially oncogenic mutations. Somatic mutations of two tumor suppressor genes (*p16/CDKN2A* on chromosome 9p21 and *NF2* on chromosome 22q12) have been observed in malignant mesotheliomas. Recent work has demonstrated the presence of simian virus 40 viral DNA sequences in 60% to 80% of pleural malignant mesotheliomas and in a smaller fraction of peritoneal cases. The simian virus 40 T-antigen is a potent carcinogen that binds to and inactivates several essential regulators of growth, such as p53 and RB. Not everyone is convinced that this association is causal and currently, the interaction of asbestos and simian virus 40 in mesothelioma pathogenesis is an area of active investigation.

LESIONS OF THE UPPER RESPIRATORY TRACT

Acute Infections

Acute infections of the upper respiratory tract are among the most common afflictions of humans, most frequently presenting as the "common cold." The clinical features are well known to all: nasal congestion accompanied by watery discharge; sneezing; scratchy, dry sore throat; and a slight increase in temperature that is more pronounced in young children. The most common pathogens are rhinoviruses, but coronaviruses, respiratory syncytial viruses, parainfluenza and influenza viruses, adenoviruses, enteroviruses, and sometimes even group A β-hemolytic streptococci have been implicated. In a significant number of cases (around 40%) the cause cannot be determined; perhaps new viruses will be discovered. Most of these infections occur in the fall and winter and are self-limiting (usually lasting for a week or less). In a minority of cases, colds may be complicated by the development of bacterial otitis media or sinusitis.

In addition to the common cold, infections of the upper respiratory tract may present as signs and symptoms localized to the pharynx, epiglottis, or larynx. *Acute pharyngitis,* manifesting as a sore throat, may be caused by a host of agents. Mild pharyngitis with minimal physical findings frequently accompanies a cold and is the most common form of pharyngitis. More severe forms with tonsillitis, associated with marked hyperemia and exudates, occur with β-hemolytic streptococci and adenovirus infections. Streptococcal tonsillitis is important to recognize and treat early, because of its potential to develop peritonsillar abscesses ("quinsy") or result in post-streptococcal glomerulonephritis and acute rheumatic fever. Coxsackievirus A may produce pharyngeal vesicles and ulcers (herpangina). Infectious mononucleosis, caused by Epstein-Barr virus (EBV), is an important cause of pharyngitis and bears the moniker of "kissing disease," a reflection on the common mode of transmission in previously nonexposed individuals.

Acute *bacterial epiglottitis* is a syndrome predominantly of young children who have an infection of the epiglottis by *H. influenzae,* in which pain and airway obstruction are the major findings. The onset is abrupt. Failure to appreciate the need to maintain an open airway for a child with this condition can be fatal. The advent of vaccination against *H. influenzae* has greatly decreased the incidence of this disease.

Acute laryngitis can result from inhalation of irritants or may be caused by allergic reactions. It may also be caused by the agents that produce the common cold and usually involve the pharynx and nasal passages as well as the larynx. Brief mention should be made of two uncommon but important forms of laryngitis: *tuberculous* and *diphtheritic.* The former is almost always a consequence of protracted active tuberculosis, during which infected sputum is coughed up. Diphtheritic laryngitis has fortunately become uncommon because of the widespread immunization of young children against diphtheria toxin. After it is inhaled, *Corynebacterium diphtheriae* implants on the mucosa of the upper airways and elaborates a powerful exotoxin that causes necrosis of the mucosal epithelium accompanied by a dense fibrinopurulent exudate that creates the classic superficial, dirty-gray pseudomembrane of diphtheria. The major hazards of this infection are sloughing and aspiration of the pseudomembrane (causing obstruction of major airways) and absorption of bacterial exotoxins (producing myocarditis, peripheral neuropathy, or other tissue injury).

In children, parainfluenza virus is the most common cause of laryngotracheobronchitis, more commonly known as *croup,* but other agents such as respiratory syncytial virus may also precipitate this condition. Although self-limited, croup may cause frightening inspiratory stridor and harsh, persistent cough. In occasional cases the laryngeal inflammatory reaction may narrow the airway sufficiently to cause respiratory failure. Viral infections in the upper respiratory tract predispose the patient to secondary bacterial infection, particularly by staphylococci, streptococci, and *H. influenzae.*

Nasopharyngeal Carcinoma

This rare neoplasm merits comment because of (1) the strong epidemiologic links to EBV and (2) the high frequency of this form of cancer in the Chinese, which raises the possibility of viral oncogenesis on a background of genetic susceptibility. EBV infects the host by first replicating in the nasopharyngeal epithelium and then infecting nearby tonsillar B lymphocytes. In some persons this leads to transformation of the epithelial cells. Unlike the case with Burkitt lymphoma (Chapter 12), another EBV-associated tumor, the EBV genome is found in virtually all nasopharyngeal carcinomas, including those that occur outside the endemic areas in Asia.

The three histologic variants are keratinizing squamous cell carcinoma, nonkeratinizing squamous cell carcinoma, and undifferentiated carcinoma; the last-mentioned is the most common and the one most closely linked with EBV. The undifferentiated neoplasm is characterized by large epithelial cells having indistinct cell borders ("syncytial" growth) and prominent eosinophilic nucleoli. It should be recalled that in infectious mononucleosis, EBV directly infects B lymphocytes, after which a marked proliferation of reactive T lymphocytes causes atypical lymphocytosis, seen in the peripheral blood, and enlarged lymph nodes (Chapter 12). Similarly, in nasopharyngeal carcinomas a striking influx of mature lymphocytes can often be seen. These neoplasms are therefore referred to as "lymphoepitheliomas," a misnomer because the lymphocytes are not part of the neoplastic process, nor are the tumors benign. The presence of large neoplastic cells in a background of reactive lymphocytes may give rise to an appearance similar to non-Hodgkin lymphomas, and immunohistochemical stains may be required to prove the epithelial nature of the malignant cells. Nasopharyngeal carcinomas invade locally, spread to cervical lymph nodes, and then metastasize to distant sites. They tend to be radiosensitive, and 5-year survival rates of 50% are reported for even advanced cancers.

Laryngeal Tumors

A variety of non-neoplastic, benign, and malignant neoplasms of squamous epithelial and mesenchymal origin may arise in the larynx, but only vocal cord nodules, papillomas, and squamous cell carcinomas are sufficiently common to merit comment. In all these conditions, the most common presenting feature is hoarseness.

Nonmalignant Lesions

Vocal cord nodules ("polyps") are smooth, hemispherical protrusions (usually less than 0.5 cm in diameter) located, most often, on the true vocal cords. The nodules are composed of fibrous tissue and covered by stratified squamous mucosa that is usually intact but can be ulcerated by contact trauma with the other vocal cord. These lesions occur chiefly in heavy smokers or singers (singer's nodes), suggesting that they are the result of chronic irritation or abuse.

Laryngeal papilloma or *squamous papilloma* of the larynx is a benign neoplasm, usually on the true vocal cords, that forms a soft, raspberry-like excrescence rarely more than 1 cm in diameter. Histologically, it consists of multiple, slender, finger-like projections supported by central fibrovascular cores and covered by an orderly, typical, stratified squamous epithelium. When the papilloma is on the free edge of the vocal cord, trauma may lead to ulceration that can be accompanied by hemoptysis.

Papillomas are usually single in adults but are often multiple in children, in whom they are referred to as *recurrent respiratory papillomatosis* (RRP), since they typically tend to recur after excision. These lesions are caused by human papillomavirus (HPV) types 6 and 11, do not become malignant, and often spontaneously regress at puberty. Cancerous transformation is rare. The most likely cause for their occurrence in children is believed to be vertical transmission from an infected mother during delivery. Therefore, the recent availability of an HPV vaccine that can protect women in the reproductive age group against types 6 and 11 provides a unique opportunity for prevention of RRP in children.

Carcinoma of the Larynx

Carcinoma of the larynx represents only 2% of all cancers. It most commonly occurs after age 40 years and is more common in men (7:1) than in women. Environmental influences are very important in its causation; nearly all cases occur in smokers, and alcohol and asbestos exposure may also play roles.

About 95% of laryngeal carcinomas are typical squamous cell lesions. Rarely, adenocarcinomas are seen, presumably arising from mucous glands. The tumor develops directly on the vocal cords (glottic tumors) in 60% to 75% of cases, but it may arise above the cords (supraglottic; 25% to 40%) or below the cords (subglottic; less then 5%). The major etiologic factors associated with laryngeal squmaous carcinomas include most importantly smoking, but also alcohol and previous radiation exposure. Human papillomavirus sequences have been detected in a minority of cases. Squmaous cell carcinomas of the larynx follow the growth pattern of all squamous cell carcinomas. They begin as in situ lesions that later appear as pearly gray, wrinkled plaques on the mucosal surface, ultimately ulcerating and fungating (Fig. 13–50). The glottic tumors are usually keratinizing, well- to moderately differentiated squamous cell carcinomas, although neonkeratinizing, poorly differentiated carcinomas may also be seen. As expected with lesions arising from recurrent exposure to environmental carcinogens, adjacent mucosa may demonstrate squamous cell hyperplasia with foci of dysplasia, or even carcinoma in situ.

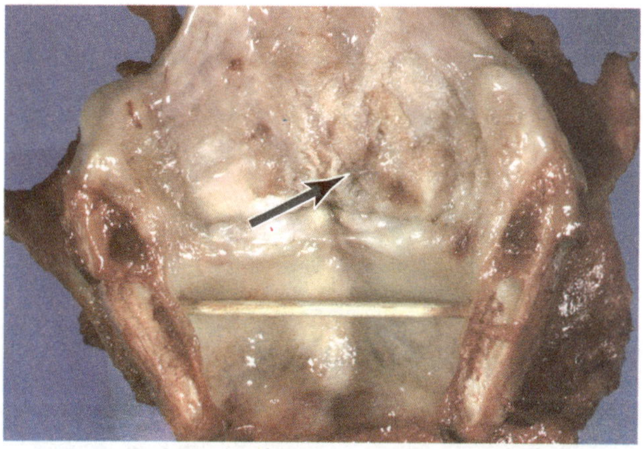

Figure 13–50

Laryngeal squamous cell carcinoma (*arrow*) arising in a supraglottic location (above the true vocal cord).

Carcinoma of the larynx manifests itself clinically by persistent hoarseness. The location of the tumor within the larynx has a significant bearing on prognosis. For example, about 90% of glottic tumors are confined to the larynx at diagnosis. First, as a result of interference with vocal cord mobility, they develop symptoms early in the course of disease; second, the glottic region has a sparse lymphatic supply, and spread beyond the larynx is uncommon. By contrast, the supraglottic larynx is rich in lymphatic spaces, and nearly a third of these tumors metastasize to regional (cervical) lymph nodes. The subglottic tumors tend to remain clinically quiescent, usually presenting as advanced disease. With surgery, radiation, or combined therapeutic treatments, many patients can be cured, but about one third die of the disease. The usual cause of death is infection of the distal respiratory passages or widespread metastases and cachexia.

BIBLIOGRAPHY

American Thoracic Society/European Respiratory Society: International Multidisciplinary Consensus Classification of the Idiopathic Interstitial Pneumonias. Am J Respir Crit Care Med 165:277, 2002. *[The authoritative classification of interstitial pneumonias from the two major trans-Atlantic pulmonary societies.]*

Barker A: Bronchiectasis. N Engl J Med 18:1383, 2002. *[A clinicopathologic review of bronchiectasis.]*

Baughman RP, et al: Sarcoidosis. Lancet 361:1111, 2003. *[A recent review of this subject, including emerging evidence on the role of genetic polymorphisms that determine susceptibility to sarcoidosis, and newer treatment options.]*

Collard HR, King TE Jr: Demystifying idiopathic interstitial pneumonia. Arch Intern Med 163:17, 2003. *[A review on the histopathologic and clinical features distinguishing interstitial pneumonias, with particular emphasis on idiopathic pulmonary fibrosis and the importance of recognizing this pattern from other causes of pulmonary fibrosis.]*

Davies D, et al: Airway remodeling in asthma: new insights. J Allergy Clin Immunol 111:215, 2003. *[A review on the structural changes involved in asthma pathogenesis, and the role of candidate gene polymorphisms that may confer potential susceptibility to airway remodeling and asthma.]*

Fan J, et al: Transcriptional mechanisms of acute lung injury. Am J Physiol Lung Cell Mol Physiol 281:L1037, 2001. *[A review outlining transcriptional pathways activated in acute lung injury, with emphasis on the seminal role of NFκB-mediated signaling in this process.]*

Fraig M, et al: Respiratory bronchiolitis: a clinicopathologic study in current smokers, ex-smokers, and never-smokers. Am J Surg Pathol 26:647, 2002. *[A study that demonstrates respiratory bronchiolitis is a reliable marker of smoking and may persist for many years after smoking cessation.]*

Frieden TR, et al: Tuberculosis. Lancet 362:887, 2003. *[A clinical review on global trends in tuberculosis, emergence of multi-drug resistance, and measures for primary prevention of this disease from a public health perspective.]*

Hogg JC: Pathophysiology of airflow limitation in chronic obstructive pulmonary disease. Lancet 364:709, 2004 *[A comprehensive review on the pathogenesis of COPD, stressing the roles of inflammation and oxidative stress in inducing pulmonary injury and airflow limitation.]*

Jeffery PK: Comparison of the structural and inflammatory features of COPD and asthma. Chest 117:S251, 2000. *[A comparison of the histopathologic features in the two obstructive airway diseases, with a concurrent discussion of the underlying pathogenetic mechanisms.]*

Marik PE: Aspiration pneumonitis and aspiration pneumonia. N Engl J Med 344:665, 2001. *[A clinically oriented review of the subject.]*

Mutsaers SE, et al: Pathogenesis of pleural fibrosis. Respirology 9:428, 2004. *[A review on the etiologic bases of pleural fibrosis, and cell types implicated in this process.]*

Peiris JS, et al: The severe acute respiratory syndrome. N Engl J Med 349:2431, 2003. *[An overview of the current definition, epidemiology, pathology, and clinical features of ARDS.]*

Rabinovitch M: Pathobiology of Pulmonary Hypertension. Annual Review of Pathology: Mechanisms of Disease, Vol. 2:369, 2007. *[Current concepts in the causation of pulmonary hypertension.]*

Rimal B, et al: Basic pathogenetic mechanisms in silicosis: current understanding. Curr Opin Pulm Med 11:169; 2005 *[A review on how silica exposure leads to pulmonary disease, including discussions on the controversy surrounding the potential carcinogenic role of this mineral dust.]*

Runo J, Loyd J: Primary pulmonary hypertension. Lancet 361:1533, 2003. *[A comprehensive review on the genetics, pathophysiology, clinical manifestations and treatment options for this entity.]*

Sekido, Y, et al: Molecular genetics of lung cancer. Annu Rev Med 54:73, 2003. *[An outstanding review on the molecular abnormalities underlying lung cancers, particularly those differentiating small cell cancers from NSCLCs.]*

Shaw RJ, et al: The role of small airways in lung disease. Respir Med 96:67, 2002. *[A review on the emerging importance of small airway inflammation not only in asthma, but also COPD and other pulmonary disorders.]*

Walter MJ, Holtzmann MJ: A centennial history of research on asthma pathogenesis. Am J Respir Cell Mol Biol 32:483, 2005. *[An excellent summary paper describing important milestones in 100 years of research on the pathogenesis of asthma.]*

Ware LB: Pathophysiology of acute lung injury and the acute respiratory distress syndrome. Semin Respir Crit Care Med 27:337, 2006. *[An excellent discussion of the pathogenesis of ARDS.]*

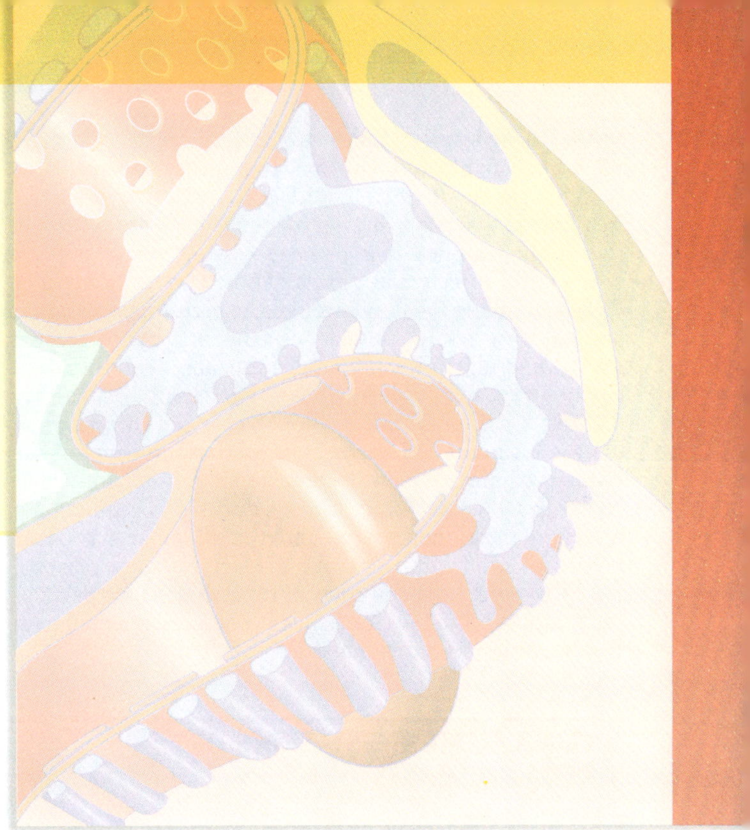

Chapter 14

The Kidney and Its Collecting System

CHARLES E. ALPERS, MD
AGNES B. FOGO, MD

The kidney is a structurally complex organ that has evolved to carry out a number of important functions: excretion of the waste products of metabolism, regulation of body water and salt, maintenance of appropriate acid balance, and secretion of a variety of hormones and autacoids. Diseases of the kidney are as complex as its structure, but their study is facilitated by dividing them into those that affect the four basic morphologic components: glomeruli, tubules, interstitium, and blood vessels. This traditional approach is useful because the early manifestations of diseases that affect each of these components tend to be distinctive. Furthermore, some components seem to be more vulnerable to specific forms of renal injury; for example, glomerular diseases are often immunologically mediated, whereas tubular and interstitial disorders are more likely to be caused by toxic or infectious agents. Nevertheless, some disorders affect more than one structure. In addition, the anatomic interdependence of structures in the kidney implies that damage to one almost always secondarily affects the others. Thus, severe glomerular damage impairs the flow through the peritubular vascular system; conversely, tubular destruction, by increasing intraglomerular pressure and inducing cytokines and chemokines, may induce glomerular sclerosis. Whatever the origin, there is a tendency for all forms of chronic renal disease ultimately to damage all four components of the kidney, culminating in chronic renal failure and what has been called *end-stage kidney disease.* The functional reserve of the kidney is large, and much damage may occur before functional impairment is evident. For these reasons, the early signs and symptoms of renal disease are particularly important to the clinician, and these are referred to in the discussion of individual diseases.

CLINICAL MANIFESTATIONS OF RENAL DISEASES

The clinical manifestations of renal disease can be grouped into reasonably well-defined syndromes. Some are peculiar to glomerular diseases; others are present in diseases that affect any one of the components. Before we list the syndromes, a few terms must be clarified.

Azotemia refers to an elevation of blood urea nitrogen and creatinine levels and is largely related to a decreased glomerular filtration rate (GFR). Azotemia is produced by many renal disorders, but it also arises from extrarenal disorders. *Prerenal azotemia* is encountered when there is hypoperfusion of the kidneys, which decreases GFR *in the absence of parenchymal damage. Postrenal azotemia* can result when urine flow is obstructed below the level of the kidney. Relief of the obstruction is followed by correction of the azotemia.

When azotemia progresses to clinical manifestations and systemic biochemical abnormalities, it is termed *uremia.* Uremia is characterized not only by failure of renal excretory function but also by a host of metabolic and endocrine alterations incident to renal damage. There is, in addition, secondary gastrointestinal (e.g., uremic gastroenteritis), neuromuscular (e.g., peripheral neuropathy), and cardiovascular (e.g., uremic fibrinous pericarditis) involvement.

We can now turn to a brief description of the major renal syndromes:

1. *Acute nephritic syndrome* is a glomerular syndrome dominated by the acute onset of usually grossly visible hematuria (red blood cells in urine), mild to moderate proteinuria, azotemia, edema, and hypertension; it is the classic presentation of acute post-streptococcal glomerulonephritis.
2. The *nephrotic syndrome* is a glomerular syndrome characterized by heavy proteinuria (excretion of >3.5 gm of protein/day in adults), hypoalbuminemia, severe edema, hyperlipidemia, and lipiduria (lipid in the urine).
3. *Asymptomatic hematuria* or *proteinuria,* or a combination of these two, is usually a manifestation of subtle or mild glomerular abnormalities.
4. *Rapidly progressive glomerulonephritis* results in loss of renal function in a few days or weeks and is manifested by microscopic hematuria, dysmorphic red blood cells and red blood cell casts in the urine sediment, and mild-to-moderate proteinuria.
5. *Acute renal failure* is dominated by oliguria or anuria (no urine flow), with recent onset of azotemia. It can result from glomerular injury (such as crescentic glomerulonephritis), interstitial injury, vascular injury (such as thrombotic microangiopathy), or acute tubular necrosis.
6. *Chronic renal failure,* characterized by prolonged symptoms and signs of uremia, is the end result of all chronic renal diseases.
7. *Urinary tract infection* is characterized by bacteriuria and pyuria (bacteria and leukocytes in the urine). The infection may be symptomatic or asymptomatic, and it may affect the kidney *(pyelonephritis)* or the bladder *(cystitis)* only.
8. *Nephrolithiasis* (renal stones) is manifested by renal colic, hematuria, and recurrent stone formation.

In addition to these renal syndromes, *urinary tract obstruction* and *renal tumors,* discussed later, represent specific anatomic lesions that often have varied manifestations.

GLOMERULAR DISEASES

Glomerular diseases constitute some of the major problems encountered in nephrology; indeed, chronic glomerulonephritis is one of the most common causes of chronic kidney disease in humans. Recall that the glomerulus consists of an anastomosing network of capillaries invested by two layers of epithelium. The visceral epithelium (podocytes) is an intrinsic part of the capillary wall, whereas the parietal epithelium lines Bowman space (urinary space), the cavity in which plasma ultrafiltrate first collects. The glomerular capillary wall is the filtration unit and consists of the following structures (Figs. 14–1 and 14–2):

1. A thin layer of fenestrated *endothelial cells,* each fenestra 70 to 100 nm in diameter.
2. A *glomerular basement membrane* (GBM) with a thick, electron-dense central layer, the *lamina densa,* and thinner, electron-lucent peripheral layers, the *lamina rara interna* and *lamina rara externa.* The GBM consists of collagen (mostly type IV), laminin, polyanionic proteoglycans, fibronectin, and several other glycoproteins.
3. The *visceral epithelial cells* (podocytes), structurally complex cells that possess interdigitating processes embedded in and adherent to the lamina rara externa of the basement membrane. Adjacent *foot processes* are separated by 20- to 30-nm-wide *filtration slits,* which are bridged by a thin slit diaphragm composed in large part of nephrin (see below).

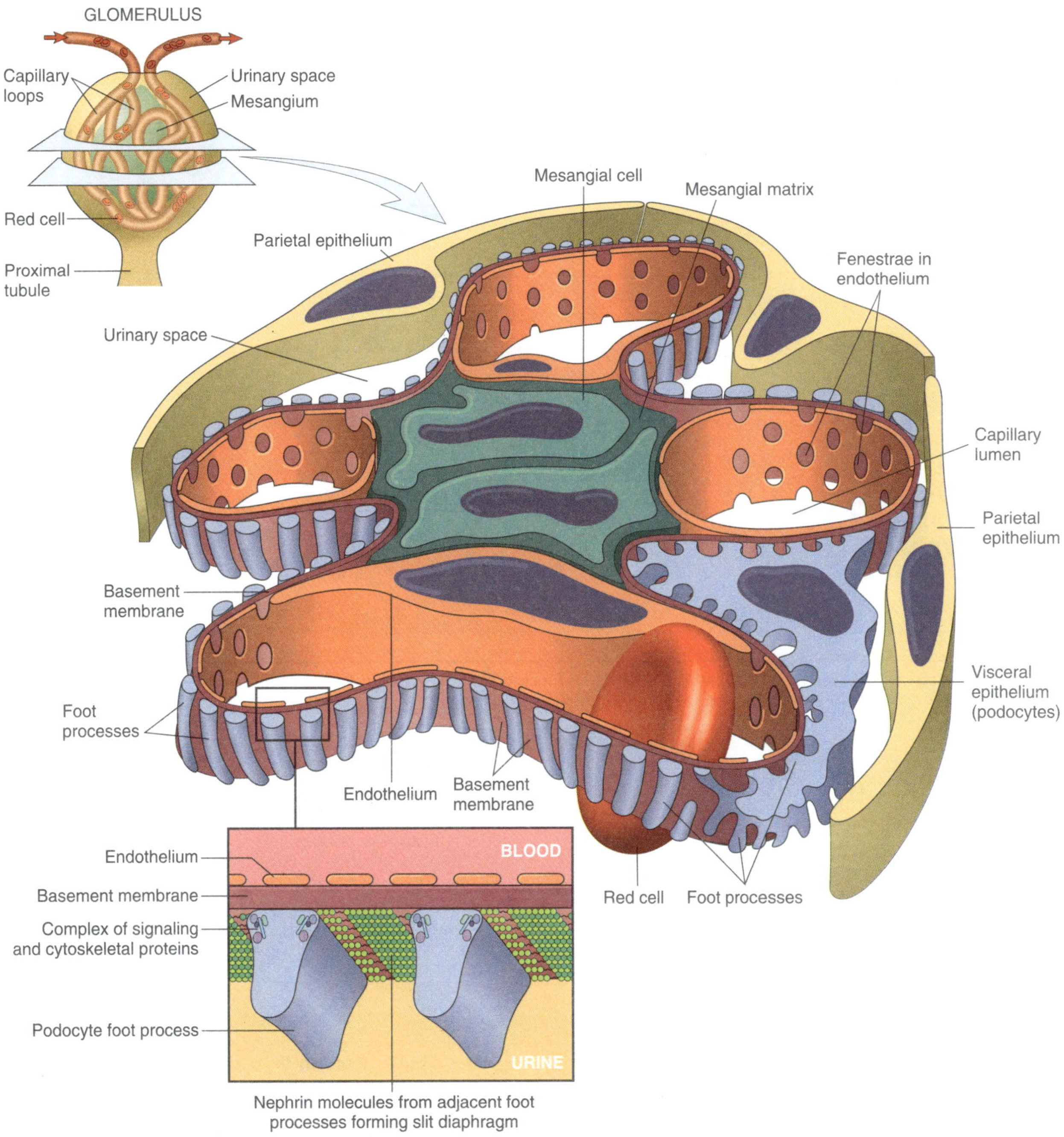

Figure 14–1

Schematic diagram of a lobe of a normal glomerulus.

4. The entire glomerular tuft is supported by *mesangial cells* lying between the capillaries. Basement membrane–like mesangial matrix forms a meshwork through which the mesangial cells are scattered. These cells, of mesenchymal origin, are contractile and are capable of proliferation, of laying down both matrix and collagen, and of secreting a number of biologically active mediators, as we shall see.

The major characteristics of glomerular filtration are an extraordinarily high permeability to water and small solutes and an almost complete impermeability to molecules of the size and molecular charge of albumin (size: 3.6 nm radius; 70,000 kD). The selective permeability, called glomerular barrier function, discriminates among protein molecules depending on their size (the larger, the less permeable), their charge (the more cationic, the more permeable), and their configuration. This size-dependent and charge-dependent barrier function is accounted for by the complex structure of the capillary wall, the integrity of the GBM, and the many anionic molecules present within the wall, including the

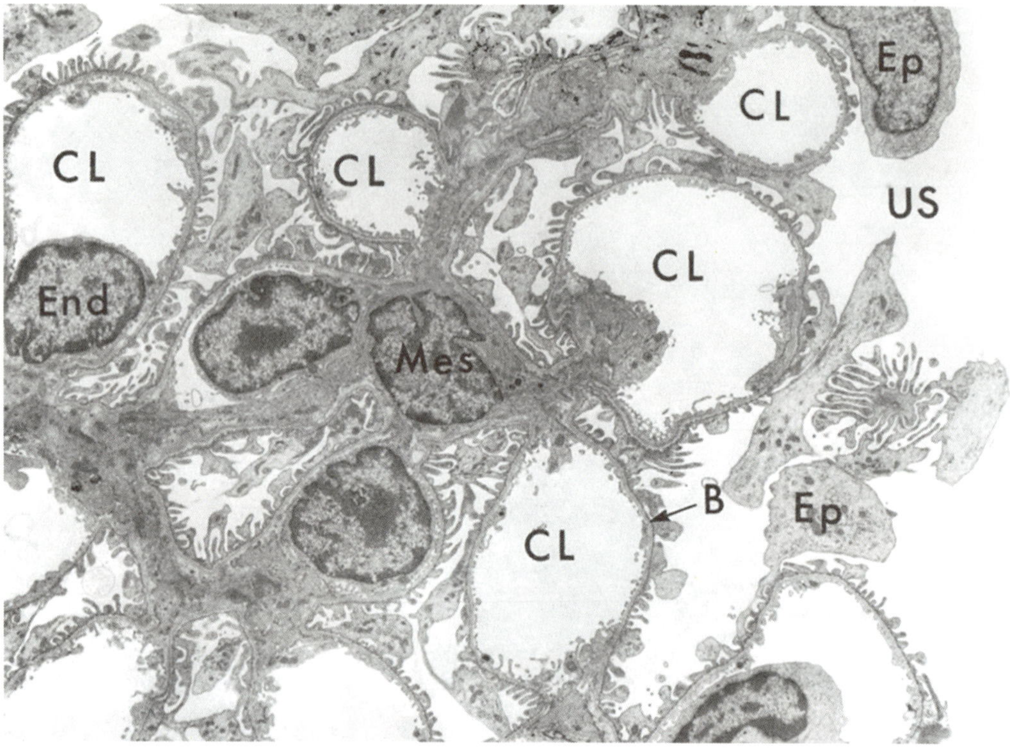

Figure 14–2

Low-power electron micrograph of rat glomerulus. B, basement membrane; CL, capillary lumen; End, endothelium; Ep, visceral epithelial cells (podocytes) with foot processes; Mes, mesangium; US, urinary space.

acidic proteoglycans of the GBM and the sialoglycoproteins of epithelial and endothelial cell coats. The *podocyte* is crucial to the maintenance of glomerular barrier function: its filtration slit diaphragm presents a distal resistance to the flow of water and a diffusion barrier to the filtration of proteins, and it is largely responsible for synthesis of GBM components.

In the past few years much has been learned about the molecular architecture of the glomerular filtration barrier. *Nephrin,* a transmembrane glycoprotein, is the major component of the slit diaphragms between adjacent foot processes. Nephrin molecules from adjacent foot processes bind to each other through disulfide bridges at the center of the slit diaphragm. The intracellular part of nephrin molecules binds to and interacts with several cytoskeletal and signaling proteins (see Fig. 14–1). Nephrin and its associated proteins, including *podocin,* have a crucial role in maintaining the selective permeability of the glomerular filtration barrier. This is dramatically illustrated by rare hereditary diseases in which mutations of nephrin or its partner proteins are associated with abnormal leakage of plasma proteins, giving rise to the nephrotic syndrome (discussed below). This suggests that acquired defects in the function or structure of slit diaphragms may constitute an important mechanism of proteinuria, which is the hallmark of the nephrotic syndrome.

Glomeruli may be injured by diverse mechanisms and in the course of a number of systemic diseases (Table 14–1). Immunologically mediated diseases such as sys-

Table 14–1 Glomerular Diseases

Primary Glomerular Diseases
Minimal-change disease
Focal and segmental glomerulosclerosis
Membranous nephropathy
Acute postinfectious GN
Membranoproliferative GN
IgA nephropathy
Chronic GN
Glomerulopathies Secondary to Systemic Diseases
Lupus nephritis (systemic lupus erythematosus)
Diabetic nephropathy
Amyloidosis
GN secondary to lymphoplasmacytic disorders
Goodpasture syndrome
Microscopic polyangiitis
Wegener's granulomatosis
Henoch-Schönlein purpura
Bacterial endocarditis—related GN
GN secondary to extrarenal infection
Thrombotic microangiopathy
Hereditary Disorders
Alport syndrome
Fabry disease
Podocyte/slit-diaphragm protein mutations

GN, glomerulonephritis.

temic lupus erythematosus (SLE), vascular disorders such as hypertension and hemolytic-uremic syndrome, metabolic diseases such as diabetes mellitus, and some purely hereditary conditions such as Alport syndrome often affect the glomerulus. These are termed *secondary glomerular diseases* to differentiate them from those in which the kidney is the only or predominant organ involved. The latter constitute the various types of *primary glomerular diseases*, which we shall discuss here. The glomerular alterations in systemic diseases are discussed in other parts of this book.

Pathogenesis of Glomerular Diseases

Although we know little about the etiologic agents or triggering events, it is clear that immune mechanisms underlie most types of primary glomerular diseases and many of the secondary glomerular diseases. Experimentally, GN can be readily induced by antibodies, and glomerular deposits of immunoglobulins, often with various components of complement, are found frequently in patients with glomerulonephritis. Cell-mediated immune mechanisms may also play a role in certain glomerular diseases.

Two forms of antibody-associated injury have been established: (1) injury resulting from deposition of soluble circulating antigen-antibody complexes in the glomerulus, and (2) injury by antibodies reacting in situ within the glomerulus, either with insoluble fixed (intrinsic) glomerular antigens or with molecules planted within the glomerulus (Fig. 14–3). In addition, antibodies directed against glomerular cell components may cause

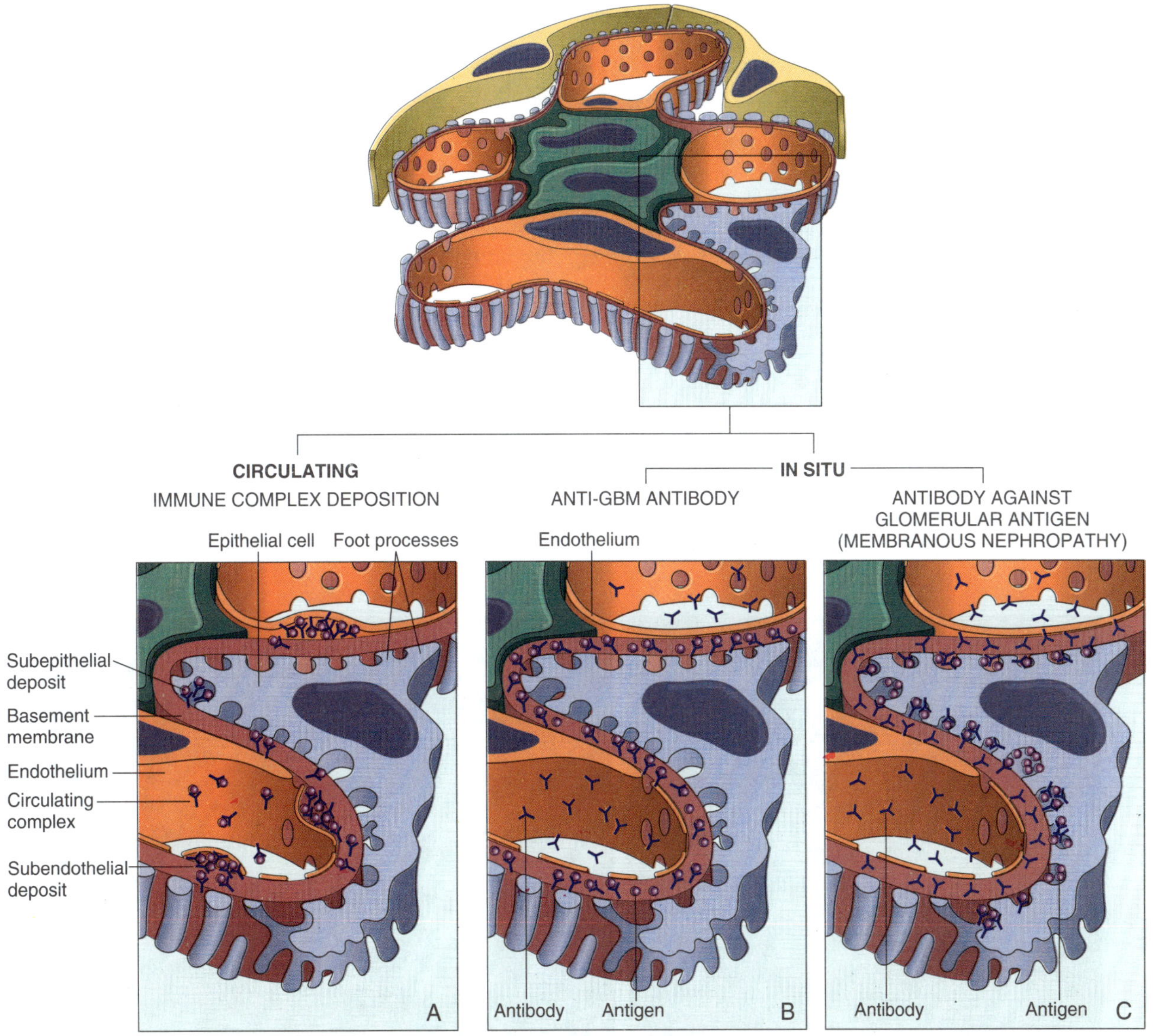

Figure 14–3

Antibody-mediated glomerular injury. Injury can result either from the deposition of circulating immune complexes or from formation in situ of complexes. **A**, Deposition of circulating immune complexes gives a granular immunofluorescence pattern. **B**, Anti-GBM antibody GN is characterized by a linear immunofluorescence pattern. **C**, Antibodies against some glomerular components deposit in a granular pattern.

glomerular injury. These pathways are not mutually exclusive, and in humans all may contribute to injury.

Nephritis Caused by Circulating Immune Complexes

The pathogenesis of immune complex diseases (type III hypersensitivity reactions) was discussed in detail in Chapter 5. Here we briefly review the salient features that relate to glomerular injury in glomerulonephritis (GN). With circulating immune complex–mediated disease, the glomerulus may be considered an "innocent bystander" because it does not incite the reaction. The antigen is not of glomerular origin. It may be endogenous, as in the GN associated with SLE, or it may be exogenous, as is probable in the GN that follows certain bacterial (streptococcal), viral (hepatitis B), parasitic (*Plasmodium falciparum* malaria), and spirochetal *(Treponema pallidum)* infections. Often the inciting antigen is unknown, as in most cases of membranous nephropathy.

Whatever the antigen may be, antigen-antibody complexes are formed in situ or in the circulation and are then trapped in the glomeruli, where they produce injury, in large part through the activation of complement and the recruitment of leukocytes. Injury may also occur through the engagement of Fc receptors on leukocytes independent of complement activation. Regardless of the mechanism, the glomerular lesions usually consist of leukocytic infiltration (exudation) into glomeruli and variable proliferation of endothelial, mesangial, and parietal epithelial cells. Electron microscopy reveals the immune complexes as electron-dense deposits or clumps that lie at one of three sites: in the mesangium, between the endothelial cells and the GBM (subendothelial deposits), or between the outer surface of the GBM and the podocytes (subepithelial deposits). Deposits may be located at more than one site in a given case. The presence of immunoglobulins and complement in these deposits can be demonstrated by immunofluorescence microscopy. *When fluoresceinated anti-immunoglobulin or anti-complement antibodies are used, the immune complexes are seen as granular deposits in the glomerulus* (Fig. 14–4A). The pattern of immune complex deposition is helpful in distinguishing various types of GN. Once deposited in the kidney, immune complexes may eventually be degraded or phagocytosed, mostly by infiltrating leukocytes and mesangial cells, and the inflammatory changes may then subside. Such a course occurs when the exposure to the inciting antigen is short-lived and limited, as in most cases of poststreptococcal or acute infection-related GN. However, if the shower of antigens is continuous, repeated cycles of immune complex formation, deposition, and injury may occur, leading to chronic GN. In some cases the source of chronic antigenic exposure is clear, such as in hepatitis B virus infection and self nuclear antigens in SLE. In other cases, however, the antigen is unknown.

Nephritis Caused by In Situ Immune Complexes

As noted, antibodies in this form of injury react directly with fixed or planted antigens in the glomerulus.

Anti–Glomerular Basement Membrane (GBM) Antibody Glomerulonephritis. The best-characterized disease in this group is classic anti-GBM antibody GN (see Fig. 14–3B). In this type of injury, antibodies are directed against fixed antigens in the GBM. It has its experimental counterpart in the nephritis of rodents called *nephrotoxic serum nephritis*. This is produced by injecting rats with anti-GBM antibodies produced by immunization of rabbits or other species with rat kidney. Although in the experimental model anti-GBM antibodies are produced by injecting "foreign" kidney antigens into an animal, *spontaneous anti-GBM antibody GN in humans results from the formation of autoantibodies directed against the GBM*. Deposition of these antibodies creates a *linear*

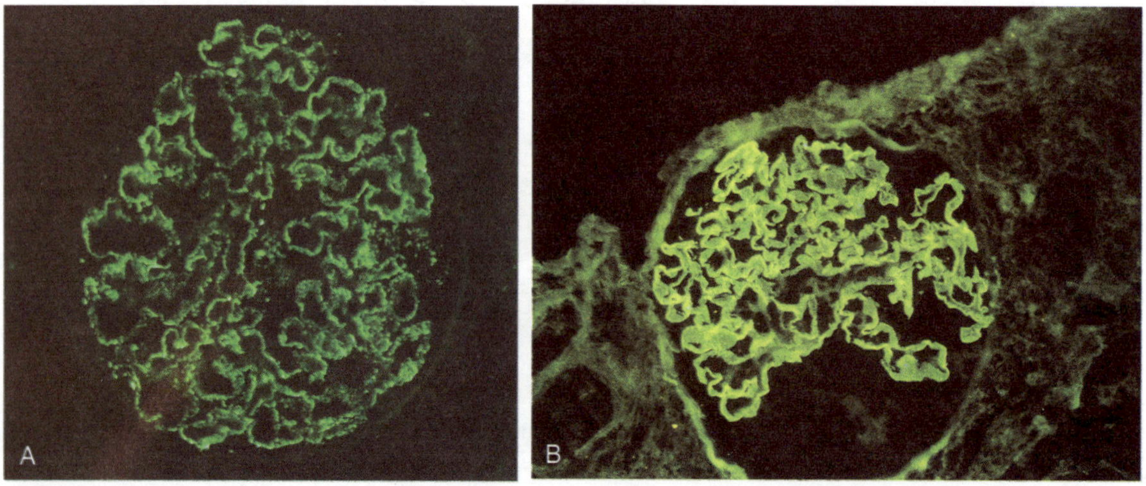

Figure 14–4

Two patterns of deposition of immune complexes as seen by immunofluorescence microscopy. **A,** Granular, characteristic of circulating and in situ immune complex deposition. **B,** Linear, characteristic of classic anti-GBM antibody GN. (**A,** Courtesy of Dr. J. Kowalewska, Department of Pathology, University of Washington, Seattle, Washington.)

pattern of staining when the bound antibodies are visualized with immunofluorescence microscopy, in contrast to the granular pattern described for other forms of immune complex–mediated nephritis (see Fig. 14–4B). This distinction is useful in the diagnosis of glomerular disease. The basement membrane antigen responsible for classic anti-GBM antibody GN is a component of the noncollagenous domain of the α3 chain of collagen type IV. Sometimes the anti-GBM antibodies cross-react with basement membranes of lung alveoli, resulting in simultaneous lung and kidney lesions *(Goodpasture syndrome)*. It is clear that this form of GN is an autoimmune disease, so any one of the several mechanisms discussed earlier in relation to autoimmunity (Chapter 5) may be involved in triggering the disease.

Although anti-GBM antibody GN accounts for less than 1% of human GN cases, the resulting disease can be very serious. It is established as the cause of renal injury in Goodpasture syndrome (Chapter 13). Many instances of anti-GBM antibody GN are characterized by very severe glomerular damage with crescents and the development of the clinical syndrome of rapidly progressive GN. This distinction is useful in the diagnosis of glomerular disease.

Antibodies may also react in situ with previously "planted" nonglomerular antigens, which may localize in the kidney by interacting with various intrinsic components of the glomerulus. Planted antigens include DNA, which has an affinity for GBM components; bacterial products, such as endostreptosin, a protein of group A streptococci; large aggregated proteins (e.g., aggregated IgG), which deposit in the mesangium because of their size; and immune complexes themselves, because they continue to have reactive sites for further interactions with free antibody, free antigen, or complement. Most of these planted antigens induce a granular pattern of immunoglobulin deposition as seen by immunofluorescence microscopy.

Several factors affect glomerular localization of antigen, antibody, or complexes. The molecular charge and size of these reactants are clearly important. The pattern of localization is also affected by changes in glomerular hemodynamics, mesangial function, and the integrity of the charge-selective barrier in the glomerulus. The localization of antigen, antibody, or immune complexes in turn determines the glomerular injury response. Studies in experimental models have shown that complexes deposited in the proximal zones of the GBM (endothelium or subendothelium) elicit an inflammatory reaction in the glomerulus with infiltration of leukocytes. In contrast, antibodies directed to distal zones of the GBM (epithelium and subepithelium) are largely noninflammatory and elicit lesions similar to those of Heymann nephritis or membranous nephropathy.

To conclude the discussion of antibody-mediated injury, it should be clear that *antibody deposition in the glomerulus is a major pathway of glomerular injury* and that immune reactions in situ, trapping of circulating complexes, interactions between these two events, and local hemodynamic and structural determinants in the glomerulus all contribute to the morphologic and functional alterations in GN.

Cell-Mediated Immune Glomerulonephritis

It has often been suggested that sensitized T cells, formed during the course of a cell-mediated immune reaction, can cause glomerular injury. In some forms of experimental GN in rodents, the disease can be induced by transfer of sensitized T cells. T cell-mediated injury may account for the instances of GN in which either there are no deposits of antibodies or immune complexes or the deposits do not correlate with the severity of damage. Even when antibodies are present, T-cell-mediated injury cannot be excluded. However, despite these intriguing hypotheses, it has been difficult to establish a causal role of T cells or cell-mediated immune responses in any form of GN in humans.

Mediators of Immune Injury

Glomerular damage, reflected by loss of glomerular barrier function, is manifested by proteinuria and, in some instances, by reductions in GFR. Once immune reactants are localized in the glomerulus, how does glomerular damage ensue? A major pathway of antibody-initiated injury is complement-leukocyte–mediated (Fig. 14–5A). Activation of complement leads to the generation of chemotactic agents (mainly C5a) and the recruitment of neutrophils and monocytes. Neutrophils release proteases, which cause GBM degradation; oxygen-derived free radicals, which cause cell damage; and arachidonic acid metabolites, which contribute to reduction in GFR. However, this mechanism applies only to some types of GN, because many types show few neutrophils in the damaged glomeruli. Some models suggest complement-dependent but not neutrophil-dependent injury, due to an effect of the C5-C9 lytic component (membrane attack complex) of complement, which causes epithelial cell detachment and stimulates mesangial and epithelial cells to secrete various mediators of cell injury. The membrane attack complex also up-regulates transforming growth factor-β (TGF-β) receptors on podocytes; TGF-β stimulates synthesis of extracellular matrix, thus giving rise to altered GBM composition and thickening.

Antibodies directed to glomerular cell antigens may also be directly cytotoxic to glomerular cells. Such cytotoxic antibodies may mediate damage in those disorders in which immune complexes are not found. Other mediators of glomerular damage include (1) *monocytes and macrophages,* which infiltrate the glomerulus in antibody- and cell-mediated reactions and, when activated, release a vast number of biologically active molecules; (2) *platelets,* which aggregate in the glomerulus during immune-mediated injury and release prostaglandins and growth factors; (3) *resident glomerular cells* (epithelial, mesangial, and endothelial), which can be stimulated to secrete mediators such as cytokines (interleukin 1), arachidonic acid metabolites, growth factors, nitric oxide, and endothelin; and (4) *fibrin-related products,* which cause leukocyte infiltration and glomerular cell proliferation as a consequence of intraglomerular thrombosis. In essence, virtually all the mediators described in our discussion of inflammation in Chapter 2 may contribute to glomerular injury.

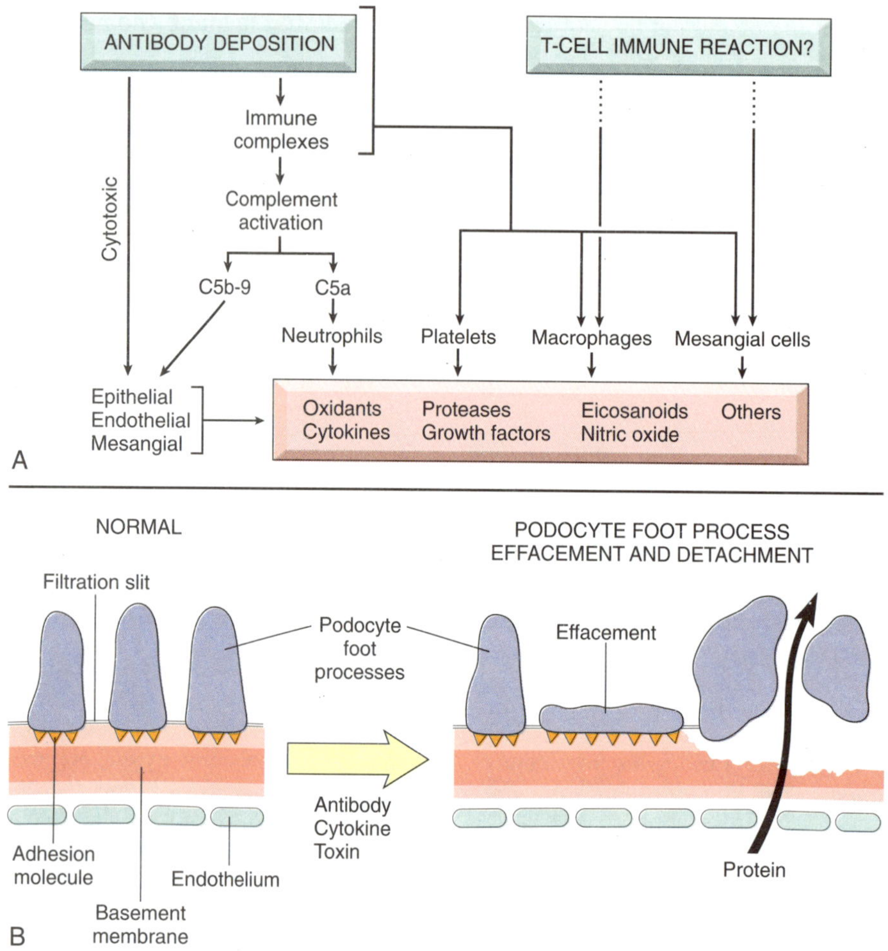

Figure 14–5

A, Mediators of immune glomerular injury (see text). Note that the role of T cells is not clearly established. **B,** Podocyte injury. The postulated sequence is a consequence of antibodies to podocyte antigens, or toxins, cytokines, or other factors causing injury with foot process effacement and sometimes detachment of epithelial cells, and protein leakage through defective GBM and filtration slits. (Adapted from Couser WG: Mediation of immune glomerular injury. J Am Soc Nephrol 1:13, 1990.)

Other Mechanisms of Glomerular Injury

Other mechanisms may contribute to glomerular damage in certain primary renal disorders. Two that deserve special mention are podocyte injury and injury secondary to nephron loss.

Podocyte Injury. This can be induced by antibodies to visceral epithelial cell antigens; by toxins, as in an experimental model of proteinuria induced by puromycin aminonucleoside; conceivably by certain cytokines; or by still poorly characterized factors, as in some cases of focal and segmental glomerulosclerosis (see below). Such injury is reflected by morphologic changes in the podocytes, which include effacement of foot processes, vacuolization, and retraction and detachment of cells from the GBM, and functionally by proteinuria. In most forms of glomerular injury, loss of normal slit diaphragms is key in the development of proteinuria (Fig. 14–5B). Functional abnormalities of the slit diaphragm may also result from mutations in its components, such as nephrin and the associated podocin, without actual inflammatory damage to the glomerulus. Such mutations are the cause of rare hereditary forms of the nephrotic syndrome.

Nephron Loss. Once any renal disease, glomerular or otherwise, destroys sufficient functioning nephrons to reduce the GFR to 30% to 50% of normal, progression to end-stage renal failure often proceeds inexorably, although the rate varies. Such individuals develop proteinuria, and their kidneys show widespread *glomerulosclerosis*. Such progressive sclerosis may be initiated, at least in part, by the adaptive changes that occur in the remaining glomeruli not destroyed by the initial disease. These remaining glomeruli undergo hypertrophy to maintain renal function. This is associated with hemodynamic changes, including increases in single-nephron GFR, blood flow, and transcapillary pressure (capillary hypertension). These adaptations in the intact glomeruli are ultimately maladaptive and lead to further endothelial and epithelial cell injury, increased glomerular permeability to proteins, and accumulation of proteins and lipids in the mesangial matrix. This is followed by capillary collapse and obliteration, hyaline entrapment, increased deposition of mesangial matrix, and ultimately by segmental or global sclerosis of glomeruli. The last results in further reductions in nephron mass and a vicious cycle of continuing glomerulosclerosis.

SUMMARY

Pathogenesis of Glomerular Injury

- Antibody-mediated immune injury is an important mechanism of glomerular damage, mainly via complement- and leukocyte-mediated pathways. Antibodies may also be directly cytotoxic to cells in the glomerulus.
- The most common forms of antibody-mediated GN are caused by the deposition of circulating immune complexes, which may involve exogenous (e.g. microbial) antigens or endogenous antigens (e.g. in SLE). Immune complexes show a granular pattern of deposition.
- Autoantibodies against components of the GBM are the cause of anti-GBM–mediated disease, often associated with severe injury. The pattern of antibody deposition is linear.
- Antibodies may also be formed against antigens that are planted in the GBM. The resultant in situ immune complexes may show a granular pattern of deposition.

We now turn to a consideration of specific types of GN and the glomerular syndromes they produce.

The Nephrotic Syndrome

The nephrotic syndrome refers to a clinical complex that includes the following: (1) massive proteinuria, with daily protein loss in the urine of 3.5 gm or more in adults; (2) hypoalbuminemia, with plasma albumin levels less than 3 gm/dL; (3) generalized edema, the most obvious clinical manifestation; and (4) hyperlipidemia and lipiduria. At the onset there is little or no azotemia, hematuria, or hypertension.

The components of the nephrotic syndrome bear a logical relationship to one another. The initial event is a derangement in the capillary walls of the glomeruli, resulting in increased permeability to plasma proteins. It will be remembered from the previous discussion of the normal kidney that the glomerular capillary wall, with its endothelium, GBM, and podocytes, acts as a barrier through which the glomerular filtrate must pass. Any increased permeability resulting from either structural or physicochemical alterations allows protein to escape from the plasma into the glomerular filtrate. With long-standing or extremely heavy proteinuria, serum albumin is decreased, resulting in hypoalbuminemia. The generalized edema of the nephrotic syndrome is, in turn, a consequence of the drop in plasma colloid osmotic pressure as a result of hypoalbuminemia, and primary retention of salt and water by the kidney. As fluid escapes from the vascular tree into the tissues, there is a concomitant drop in plasma volume, with diminished glomerular filtration. Compensatory secretion of aldosterone, along with the reduced GFR and reduction of secretion of natriuretic peptides, promotes retention of salt and water by the kidneys, thus further aggravating the edema. By repetition of this chain of events, generalized edema (termed *anasarca*) may develop. The genesis of the hyperlipidemia is more obscure. Presumably, hypoalbuminemia triggers increased synthesis of lipoproteins in the liver. There is also abnormal transport of circulating lipid particles and impairment of peripheral breakdown of lipoproteins. The lipiduria, in turn, reflects the increased permeability of the GBM to lipoproteins.

The relative frequencies of the several causes of the nephrotic syndrome vary according to age (Table 14–2). In children 1 to 7 years of age, for example, the nephrotic syndrome is almost always caused by a lesion primary to the kidney, whereas among adults it is often due to renal manifestations of a systemic disease. The most frequent systemic causes of the nephrotic syndrome in adults are diabetes, amyloidosis, and SLE. The renal lesions produced by these disorders are described in Chapter 5. The most important of the primary glomerular lesions that characteristically lead to the nephrotic syndrome are focal and segmental glomerulosclerosis (FSGS) and minimal-change disease (MCD). The latter is more important in children; the former in adults. Two other primary lesions, membranous nephropathy and membranoproliferative GN, also produce the nephrotic syndrome. These four lesions are discussed individually below.

Table 14–2 Causes of Nephrotic Syndrome

	Prevalence (%)*	
Cause	**Children**	**Adults**
Primary Glomerular Disease		
Membranous GN	5	30
Minimal-change disease	65	10
Focal segmental glomerulosclerosis	10	–35
Membranoproliferative GN	10	10
IgA nephropathy and others	10	15
Systemic Diseases with Renal Manifestations		
Diabetes mellitus‡		
Amyloidosis‡		
Systemic lupus erythematosus		
Ingestion of drugs (gold, penicillamine, "street heroin")		
Infections (malaria, syphilis, hepatitis B, HIV)		
Malignancy (carcinoma, melanoma)		
Miscellaneous (bee-sting allergy, hereditary nephritis)		

GN, glomerulonephritis; HIV, human immunodeficiency virus.
*Approximate prevalence of primary disease is 95% of the cases in children, 60% in adults. Approximate prevalence of systemic disease is 5% of the cases in children, 40% in adults.

Minimal-Change Disease (Lipoid Nephrosis)

This relatively benign disorder is the most frequent cause of the nephrotic syndrome in children. It is characterized by glomeruli that have a normal appearance by light microscopy but show diffuse effacement of podocyte foot processes when viewed with the electron microscope. Although it may develop at any age, this condition is most common between ages 1 and 7 years.

Pathogenesis. The pathogenesis of proteinuria in minimal change disease remains to be clearly elucidated. Based on some experimental studies, the proteinuria has been attributed to a T-cell derived factor that causes podocyte damage and effacement of foot processes. However, neither the nature of such a putative factor nor a causal role of T cells is established in the human disease, and there is no good experimental model of minimal change disease.

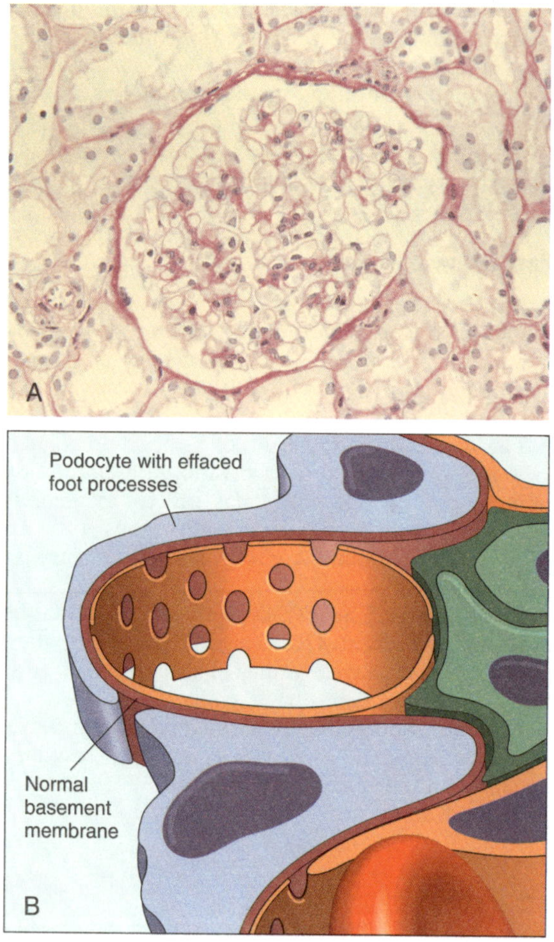

Figure 14–6

Minimal change disease. **A,** Under the light microscope the PAS-stained glomerulus appears normal, with a delicate basement membrane. **B,** Schematic diagram illustrating diffuse effacement of foot processes of podocytes with no immune deposits.

Morphology

With the light microscope, the glomeruli in minimal change disease appear normal (Fig. 14–6A). The cells of the proximal convoluted tubules are often heavily laden with protein droplets and lipids, but this is secondary to tubular reabsorption of the lipoproteins passing through the diseased glomeruli. This appearance of the proximal convoluted tubules is the basis for the older term for this disorder, **lipoid nephrosis.** Even with the electron microscope, the GBM appears normal. The only obvious glomerular abnormality is the **uniform and diffuse effacement of the foot processes of the podocytes** (Fig. 14–6B). The cytoplasm of the podocytes thus appears flattened over the external aspect of the GBM, obliterating the network of arcades between the podocytes and the GBM. There are also epithelial cell vacuolization, microvillus formation, and occasional focal detachments. When the changes in the podocytes reverse (e.g., in response to corticosteroids), the proteinuria remits.

Clinical Course. The disease manifests itself by the insidious development of the nephrotic syndrome in an otherwise healthy child. There is no hypertension, and renal function is preserved in most individuals. The protein loss is usually confined to the smaller serum proteins, chiefly albumin (selective proteinuria). The prognosis in children with this disorder is good. More than 90% of cases respond to a short course of corticosteroid therapy; however, proteinuria recurs in more than two-thirds of the initial responders, some of whom become steroid dependent. Less than 5% develop chronic renal failure after 25 years, and it is likely that most persons in this subgroup had nephrotic syndrome caused by focal and segmental glomerulosclerosis not detected by biopsy. Because of its responsiveness to therapy in children, minimal change disease must be differentiated from other causes of the nephrotic syndrome in nonresponders. Adults with minimal change disease also respond to steroid therapy, but the response is slower and relapses are more common.

Focal and Segmental Glomerulosclerosis

Focal segmental glomerulosclerosis (FSGS) is a lesion characterized histologically by sclerosis affecting some but not all glomeruli (focal involvement) and involving only segments of each affected glomerulus. This histologic picture is often associated with the nephrotic syndrome and can occur (1) in association with other known conditions, such as human immunodeficiency virus infection or heroin abuse (human immunodeficiency virus nephropathy, heroin nephropathy); (2) as a secondary event in other forms of GN (e.g., immunoglobulin A [IgA] nephropathy); (3) as a maladaptation after nephron loss (described above); (4) in inherited or congenital forms resulting from mutations affecting cytoskeletal or related proteins expressed in podocytes (e.g., nephrin); or (5) as a primary disease.

Primary (or idiopathic) FSGS accounts for approximately 20% to 30% of all cases of the nephrotic syndrome. It is becoming an increasingly common cause of nephrotic syndrome in adults and remains a frequent cause in children. *In children it is important to distinguish this cause of the nephrotic syndrome from MCD,* because the clinical courses are markedly different. Unlike MCD, there is a higher incidence of hematuria and hypertension in persons with this lesion; their proteinuria is nonselective, and in general their response to corticosteroid therapy is poor. At least 50% of individuals with FSGS develop end-stage renal failure within 10 years of diagnosis. Adults in general fare even less well than children.

Pathogenesis. The pathogenesis of primary FSGS is unknown. Some investigators have suggested that FSGS and MCD are part of a continuum and that MCD may transform into FSGS. Others believe them to be distinct clinicopathologic entities from the outset. In any case, *injury to the podocytes is thought to represent the initiating event of primary FSGS.* As with MCD, permeability-increasing factors produced by lymphocytes have been proposed. The deposition of hyaline masses in the glomeruli represents the entrapment of plasma proteins and lipids in foci of injury where sclerosis develops. IgM and complement proteins commonly seen in the lesion are also believed to result from nonspecific entrapment in damaged glomeruli. The recurrence of proteinuria in some persons with FSGS who receive renal allografts, sometimes within 24 hours of transplantation, supports the idea that a circulating mediator is the cause of the damage to podocytes.

Morphology

In FSGS, the disease first affects only some of the glomeruli (hence the term "**focal**") and initially only the juxtamedullary glomeruli. With progression, eventually all levels of the cortex are affected. Histologically, FSGS is characterized by lesions occurring in some tufts within a glomerulus and sparing of the others (hence the term "**segmental**"). Thus, the involvement is both focal and segmental (Fig. 14–7). The affected glomeruli exhibit **increased mesangial matrix, obliterated capillary lumens, and deposition of hyaline masses (hyalinosis) and lipid droplets.** Occasionally, glomeruli are completely sclerosed (global sclerosis). In affected glomeruli, immunofluorescence microscopy often reveals nonspecific trapping of immunoglobulins, usually IgM, and complement in the areas of hyalinosis. On electron microscopy, the podocytes exhibit **effacement of foot processes,** as in MCD.

In time, progression of the disease leads to global sclerosis of the glomeruli with pronounced tubular atrophy and interstitial fibrosis. This advanced picture is difficult to differentiate from other forms of chronic glomerular disease, described below.

A morphologic variant called **collapsing glomerulopathy** is being increasingly reported. It is characterized by collapse of the entire glomerular tuft and podocyte hyperplasia. This is a more severe manifestation of FSGS that may be idiopathic or associated with human immunodeficiency virus infection or drug-induced toxicities. It carries a particularly poor prognosis.

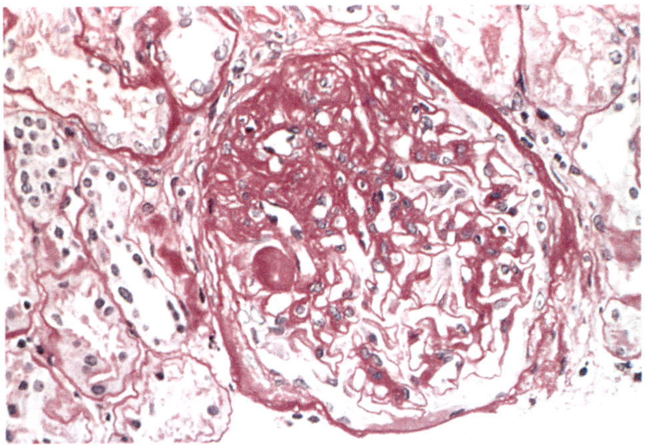

Figure 14–7

High-power view of focal and segmental glomerulosclerosis (PAS stain), seen as a mass of scarred, obliterated capillary lumens with accumulations of matrix material, that has replaced a portion of the glomerulus. (Courtesy of Dr. H. Rennke, Department of Pathology, Brigham and Women's Hospital, Boston, Massachusetts.)

Clinical Course. There is little tendency for spontaneous remission of idiopathic FSGS, and responses to corticosteroid therapy are usually poor. Progression to renal failure occurs at varying rates, and about 50% of individuals suffer renal failure after 10 years.

Membranous Nephropathy (Membranous Glomerulonephritis)

This slowly progressive disease, most common between 30 and 50 years of age, *is characterized morphologically by the presence of subepithelial immunoglobulin-containing deposits along the GBM.* Early in the disease, the glomeruli may appear normal by light microscopy, but well-developed cases show *diffuse thickening of the capillary wall.*

Membranous nephropathy is idiopathic in about 85% of cases. In the remainder (secondary membranous nephropathy), it may be secondary to other disorders, including: (1) infections (chronic hepatitis B, syphilis, schistosomiasis, malaria); (2) malignant tumors, particularly carcinoma of the lung and colon and melanoma; (3) SLE and other autoimmune conditions; (4) exposure to inorganic salts (gold, mercury); and (5) drugs (penicillamine, captopril, nonsteroidal anti-inflammatory agents).

Pathogenesis. Membranous GN is a form of chronic immune complex nephritis. Although circulating complexes of known exogenous (e.g., hepatitis B virus) or endogenous (DNA in SLE) antigen can cause membranous nephropathy, it is now thought that most idiopathic forms are induced by antibodies reacting in situ to endogenous or planted glomerular antigens.

The experimental model of membranous GN is Heymann nephritis, which is induced in animals by immunization with renal tubular brush border proteins. The antibodies that are produced react with an antigen located in the GBM, resulting in granular deposits ("in situ immune complex formation") and proteinuria without severe inflammation. Idiopathic membranous nephropathy in humans is considered an autoimmune disease caused by antibodies to a renal autoantigen that remains unidentified.

In the presence of immune deposits, how does the glomerular capillary wall become leaky? In the absence of neutrophils, monocytes, or platelets and in the virtually uniform presence of complement, current work points to a direct action of C5b-C9, the membrane attack complex of complement, on the podocyte. The membrane attack complex causes activation of glomerular mesangial cells and podocytes, inducing them to liberate proteases and oxidants that can damage capillary walls, with consequent perturbations in filtration.

Morphology

Seen by light microscopy with H&E stain, the basic change in membranous nephropathy appears to be **diffuse thickening of the GBM** (Fig. 14–8A). By electron microscopy, this apparent thickening is determined to be caused in part by **subepithelial deposits** that nestle against the GBM and are separated from each other by small, spikelike protrusions of GBM matrix that form in reaction to the deposits (**"spike and dome" pattern**) (Fig. 14–8B). As the disease progresses, these spikes close over the deposits, incorporating them into the GBM. In addition, the podocytes show **effacement of foot processes.** Later in the disease, the incorporated deposits may be catabolized and eventually disappear, leaving cavities within the GBM. Continued deposition of basement membrane matrix leads to progressively thicker basement membranes. With further progression, the glomeruli can become sclerosed. Immunofluorescence microscopy shows typical **granular deposits** of immunoglobulins and complement along the GBM (see Fig. 14–4A).

Clinical Course. The onset in idiopathic cases is characterized by the insidious development of the nephrotic syndrome, usually without antecedent illness; however, some individuals with membranous nephropathy may have lesser degrees of proteinuria rather than the full-blown nephrotic syndrome. In contrast to minimal change disease, the proteinuria is nonselective, with urinary loss of globulins as well as smaller albumin molecules, and does not usually respond to corticosteroid therapy. Secondary causes of membranous nephropathy should be ruled out. Membranous nephropathy follows a notoriously variable and often indolent course. Overall, although proteinuria persists in over 60% of individuals with membranous nephropathy, only about 40% suffer progressive disease terminating in renal failure after 2 to 20 years. An additional 10% to 30% have a more benign course with partial or complete remission of proteinuria.

Membranoproliferative Glomerulonephritis

Membranoproliferative GN (MPGN) is manifested histologically by alterations in the GBM and mesangium and by proliferation of glomerular cells. It accounts for 5% to 10% of cases of idiopathic nephrotic syndrome in children and adults. Some individuals present only with hematuria or proteinuria in the non-nephrotic range; others have a combined nephrotic-nephritic picture. Two major types of MPGN (I and II) are recognized on the basis of distinct ultrastructural, immunofluorescence microscopic, and pathogenic findings. Of the two types, type I is far more common (about 80% of cases).

Pathogenesis. Different pathogenic mechanisms are involved in the development of type I and type II disease. Most cases of type I MPGN seem to be caused by circulating immune complexes, akin to chronic serum sickness, but the inciting antigen is not known. Type I MPGN

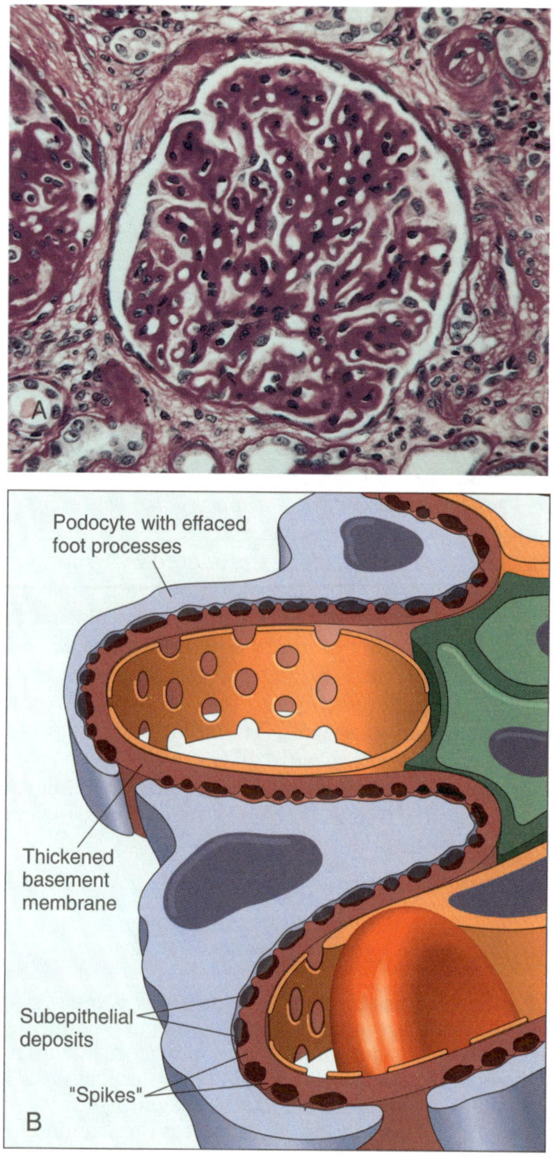

Figure 14–8

Membranous nephropathy. **A,** Diffuse thickening of the glomerular basement membrane. **B,** Schematic diagram illustrating subepithelial deposits, effacement of foot processes, and the presence of "spikes" of basement membrane material between the immune deposits.

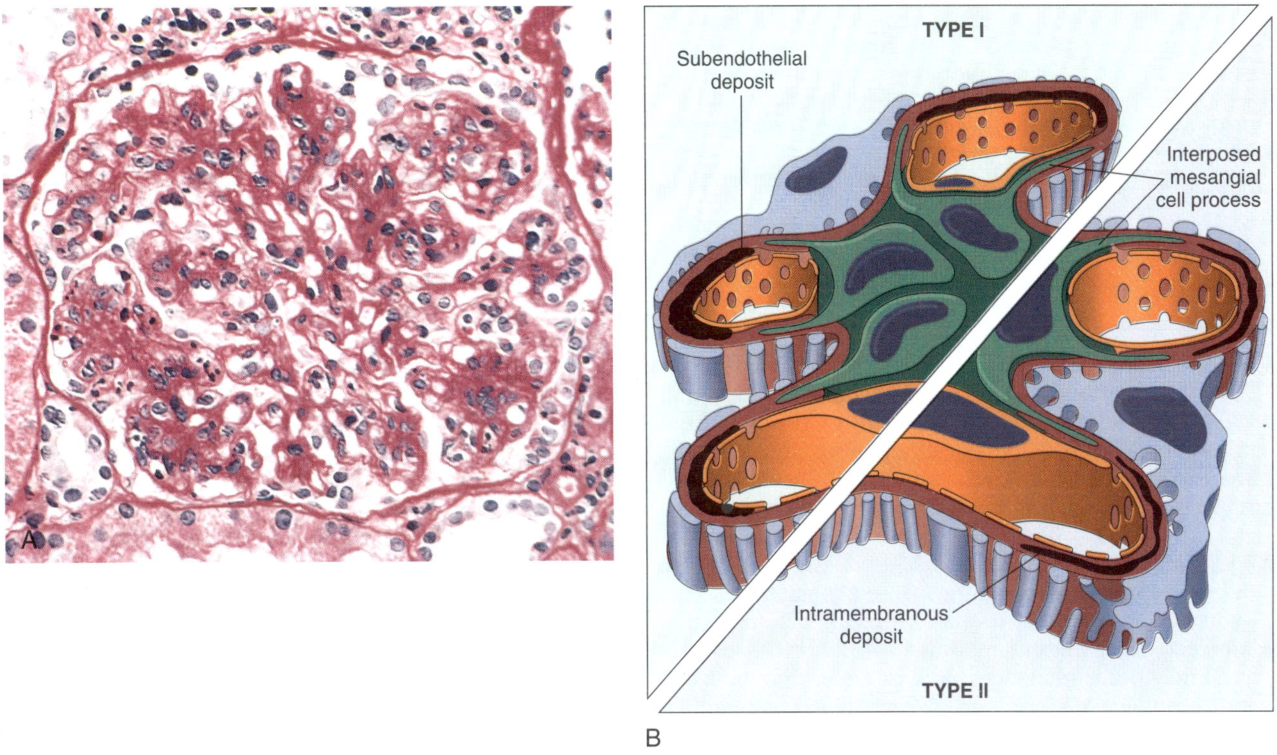

Figure 14–9

A, Membranoproliferative GN, showing mesangial cell proliferation, basement membrane thickening, leukocyte infiltration, and accentuation of lobular architecture. **B,** Schematic representation of patterns in the two types of membranoproliferative GN. In type I there are subendothelial deposits; type II is characterized by intramembranous dense deposits (dense-deposit disease). In both, mesangial interposition gives the appearance of split basement membranes when viewed by light microscopy.

also occurs in association with hepatitis B and C antigenemia, SLE, infected atrioventricular shunts, and extrarenal infections with persistent or episodic antigenemia. The pathogenesis of type II MPGN, also known as *dense-deposit disease,* is less clear. *The fundamental abnormality appears to be excessive complement activation*, which may be caused by several mechanisms not involving antibodies. Some patients have an autoantibody against C3 convertase, called *C3 nephritic factor*, which is believed to stabilize the enzyme and lead to uncontrolled cleavage of C3 and activation of the alternative complement pathway. Mutations in the gene encoding the complement regulatory protein *Factor H* have been described in some patients. These mutations may lead to a deficiency of plasma Factor H or defective function of the protein, again resulting in excessive complement activation. Functional impairment of Factor H may also be caused by autoantibodies, or abnormalities in the C3 protein that prevent its interaction with Factor H. Hypocomplementemia, more marked in type II, is produced in part by excessive consumption of C3 and in part by reduced synthesis of C3 by the liver. It is still not clear how the complement abnormality induces the glomerular changes. Because of these important differences in pathogenesis and major differences in ultrastructural appearance, there is a growing trend to separate this diagnostic category and consider dense-deposit disease as an entity distinct from MPGN type I.

Morphology

By light microscopy, both types of MPGN are similar. The glomeruli are large, with an accentuated **lobular appearance,** and show **proliferation of mesangial and endothelial cells** as well as infiltrating leukocytes (Fig. 14–9A). The **GBM is thickened,** and the glomerular capillary wall often shows a double contour, or "tram track," appearance, especially evident in silver or periodic acid–Schiff (PAS) stains. This is caused by **"splitting" of the GBM** due to the inclusion within it of processes of mesangial and inflammatory cells extending into the peripheral capillary loops (Fig. 14–9B).

Types I and II have different ultrastructural and immunofluorescence microscopic features (see Fig. 14–9B). **Type I MPGN** is characterized by discrete **subendothelial electron-dense deposits.** By immunofluorescence microscopy, C3 is deposited in an irregular granular pattern, and IgG and early complement components (C1q and C4) are often also present, indicative of an immune complex pathogenesis.

In **type II lesions** the lamina densa and the subendothelial space of the GBM are transformed into an irregular, ribbon-like, extremely electron-dense structure, resulting from the deposition of material of unknown composition, giving rise to the term **dense-deposit disease.** C3 is present in irregular chunky and segmental linear foci in the basement membranes and in the mesangium in characteristic circular aggregates (mesangial rings). IgG is usually absent, as are the early components of the classical complement pathway (C1q and C4).

Clinical Course. The principal mode of presentation (in ~50% of cases) is the nephrotic syndrome, although MPGN may begin as acute nephritis or mild proteinuria. The prognosis of MPGN is generally poor. In one study, none of 60 patients followed for 1 to 20 years showed complete remission. Forty percent progressed to end-stage renal failure, 30% had variable degrees of renal insufficiency, and the remaining 30% had persistent nephrotic syndrome without renal failure. Dense-deposit disease has a worse prognosis, and it tends to recur in renal transplant recipients. Like many other GNs, MPGN, usually type I, may occur in association with other known disorders *(secondary MPGN),* such as SLE, hepatitis B and C, chronic liver disease, and chronic bacterial infections. Indeed, many so-called idiopathic cases are believed to be associated with hepatitis C and related cryoglobulinemia.

SUMMARY

The Nephrotic Syndrome

- The nephrotic syndrome is characterized by proteinuria, which results in hypoalbuminemia and edema.
- Podocyte injury is an underlying mechanism of proteinuria, and may be the result of nonimmune causes (as in MCD and FSGS) or immune mechanisms (as in MN).
- *Minimal change disease (MCD)* is the most frequent cause of nephrotic syndrome in children; it is manifested by proteinuria and effacement of glomerular foot processes without antibody deposits; the pathogenesis is unknown; the disease responds well to steroid therapy.
- *Focal and segmental glomerulosclerosis (FSGS)* may be primary (podocyte injury by unknown mechanisms) or secondary (e.g. as a consequence of prior glomerulonephritis, hypertension or infection such as HIV); glomeruli show focal obliteration of capillary lumens, hyaline deposits and loss of foot processes; the disease is often resistant to therapy and may progress to end stage renal disease.
- *Membranous nephropathy (MN)* is caused by an autoimmune response against an unknown renal antigen; it is characterized by granular subepithelial deposits of antibodies with GBM thickening and loss of foot processes but little or no inflammation; the disease is often resistant to steroid therapy.

The Nephritic Syndrome

The nephritic syndrome is a clinical complex, usually of acute onset, characterized by (1) *hematuria* with dysmorphic red cells and red blood cell casts in the urine, (2) some degree of *oliguria* and azotemia, and (3) *hypertension.* Although there may also be some proteinuria and even edema, these are usually not as severe as in the nephrotic syndrome. The lesions that cause the nephritic syndrome have in common proliferation of the cells within the glomeruli, accompanied by a leukocytic infiltrate. This inflammatory reaction injures the capillary walls, permitting escape of red cells into the urine, and induces hemodynamic changes that lead to a reduction in the GFR. The reduced GFR is manifested clinically by oliguria, reciprocal fluid retention, and azotemia. Hypertension is probably a result of both the fluid retention and some augmented renin release from the ischemic kidneys.

The acute nephritic syndrome may be produced by systemic disorders such as SLE, or it may be the result of primary glomerular disease. The latter is exemplified by acute postinfectious GN.

Acute Postinfectious (Poststreptococcal) Glomerulonephritis

Acute postinfectious GN, one of the more frequently occurring glomerular disorders, is typically caused by glomerular deposition of immune complexes resulting in diffuse proliferation and swelling of resident glomerular cells and frequent infiltration of leukocytes, especially neutrophils. The inciting antigen may be exogenous or endogenous. The prototypic exogenous pattern is seen in poststreptococcal GN. A similar proliferative GN may occur with other exogenous or endogenous antigens. Infections by organisms other than the streptococci may also be associated with diffuse postinfectious GN. These include certain pneumococcal and staphylococcal infections as well as several common viral diseases such as mumps, measles, chickenpox, and hepatitis B and C. Endogenous antigens, as occur in SLE, may also cause a proliferative GN, but more commonly in a membranous nephropathy pattern (see above), without the typical neutrophil abundance characteristic of postinfectious GN.

The classic case of poststreptococcal GN develops in a child 1 to 4 weeks after the individual recovers from a group A streptococcal infection. Only certain "nephritogenic" strains of β-hemolytic streptococci are capable of evoking glomerular disease. In most cases the initial infection is localized to the pharynx or skin.

Pathogenesis. It is generally agreed that immune complex deposition is involved in the pathogenesis of acute poststreptococcal GN. Typical features of immune complex disease, such as hypocomplementemia and granular deposits of IgG and complement on the GBM, are seen. The relevant antigens are probably streptococcal proteins, but their identity is not established. It is also not clear if immune complexes are formed mainly in the circulation or in situ (the latter by binding of antibodies to bacterial antigens "planted" in the GBM). Studies indicate that C3 may be deposited on the GBM before IgG; hence, the primary injury might be by complement activation. Eventually, immune complexes are formed.

Morphology

By light microscopy, the most characteristic change in postinfectious GN is a fairly **uniformly increased cellularity** of the glomerular tufts that affects nearly all glomeruli, hence the term "diffuse" (Fig. 14–10A). The increased cellularity is caused both by proliferation and swelling of endothelial and mesangial cells and by a neutrophilic and monocytic infiltrate. Sometimes there is necrosis of the capillary walls. In a few cases there may also be "crescents" (described next) within the urinary space in response to the severe inflammatory injury. In general, these findings are ominous. Electron microscopy shows deposited immune complexes arrayed as subendothelial, intramembranous, or, most often, **subepithelial "humps"** nestled against the GBM (Fig. 14–10B). Mesangial deposits are also occasionally present. Immunofluorescence studies reveal scattered **granular deposits of IgG and complement** within the capillary walls and some mesangial areas, corresponding to the deposits visualized by electron microscopy. These deposits are usually cleared over a period of about 2 months.

Clinical Course. The onset of the kidney disease tends to be abrupt, heralded by malaise, a slight fever, nausea, and the nephritic syndrome. In the usual case, oliguria, azotemia, and hypertension are only mild to moderate. Characteristically, there is gross hematuria, the urine appearing smoky brown rather than bright red. Some proteinuria is a constant feature of the disease, and as mentioned earlier it may occasionally be severe enough to produce the nephrotic syndrome. Serum complement levels are low during the active phase of the disease, and serum anti–streptolysin O antibody titers are elevated in poststreptococcal cases.

Recovery occurs in most children in epidemic cases. Some children develop rapidly progressive GN due to severe injury with crescents or chronic renal disease due to secondary scarring. The prognosis in sporadic cases is less clear. In adults, 15% to 50% of individuals develop end-stage renal disease over the ensuing few years or 1 to 2 decades, depending on the clinical and histologic severity. In contrast, in children, the prevalence of chronicity after sporadic cases of acute postinfectious GN is much lower.

IgA Nephropathy (Berger Disease)

This condition usually affects children and young adults and begins as an episode of gross hematuria that occurs within 1 or 2 days of a nonspecific upper respiratory tract infection. Typically, the hematuria lasts several days and then subsides, only to recur every few months. It is often associated with loin pain. *IgA nephropathy is one of the most common causes of recurrent microscopic or gross hematuria and is the most common glomerular disease revealed by renal biopsies worldwide.*

The pathogenic hallmark is the deposition of IgA in the mesangium. Some have considered IgA nephropathy to be a localized variant of *Henoch-Schönlein purpura,* also characterized by IgA deposition in the mesangium. In contrast to IgA nephropathy, which is purely a renal disorder, Henoch-Schönlein purpura is a systemic syndrome involving the skin (purpuric rash), gastrointestinal tract (abdominal pain), joints (arthritis), and kidneys.

Pathogenesis. Accumulating evidence suggests that IgA nephropathy is associated with an abnormality in IgA

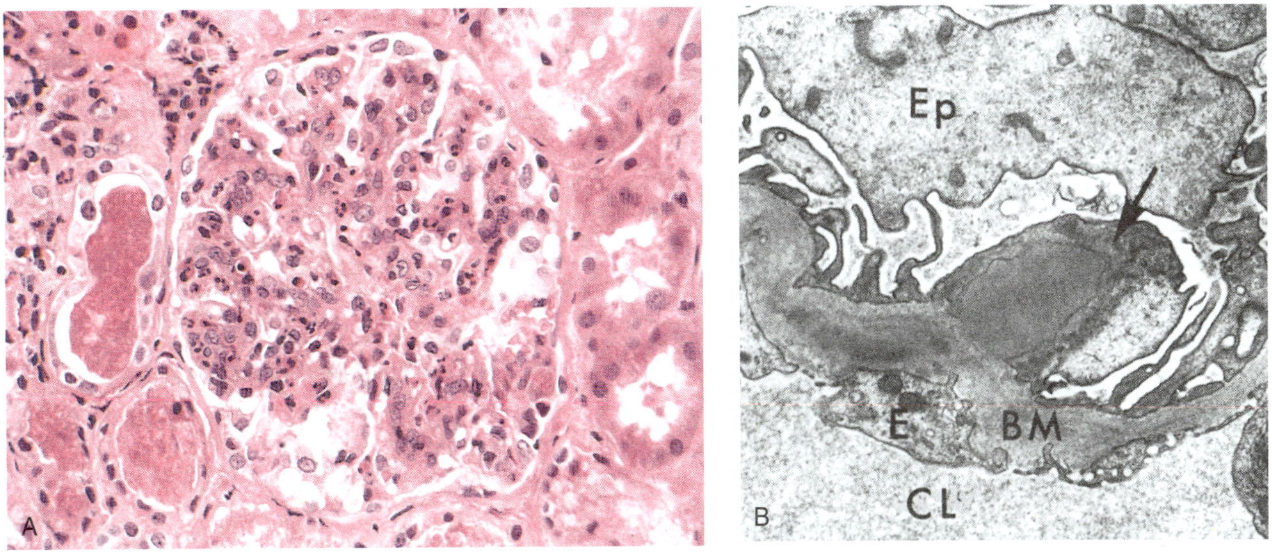

Figure 14–10

Poststreptococcal GN. **A,** Glomerular hypercellularity is caused by intracapillary leukocytes and proliferation of intrinsic glomerular cells. Note the red cell casts in the tubules. **B,** Typical electron-dense subepithelial "hump" *(arrow)* and intramembranous deposits. BM, basement membrane; CL, capillary lumen; E, endothelial cell; Ep, visceral epithelial cells (podocytes).

production and clearance. IgA, the main immunoglobulin in mucosal secretions, is at low levels in normal serum but increased in 50% of patients with IgA nephropathy due to increased production in the marrow. In addition, circulating IgA-containing immune complexes are present in some individuals. A genetic influence is suggested by the occurrence of this condition in families and in HLA–identical siblings, and by the increased frequency of certain HLA and complement phenotypes in some populations. Studies also suggest an abnormality in glycosylation of the IgA immunoglobulin, a process that would reduce plasma clearance of IgA, thus favoring deposition in the mesangium. The prominent mesangial deposition of IgA suggests entrapment of IgA immune complexes in the mesangium, and the absence of C1q and C4 in glomeruli points to activation of the alternative complement pathway. Taken together, these clues suggest that increased IgA synthesis in response to respiratory or gastrointestinal exposure to environmental agents (e.g., viruses, bacteria, food proteins) may lead to deposition of IgA and IgA-containing immune complexes in the mesangium, where they activate the alternative complement pathway and initiate glomerular injury. In support of this scenario, IgA nephropathy occurs with increased frequency in individuals with celiac disease, in whom intestinal mucosal defects are seen, and in liver disease where there is defective hepatobiliary clearance of IgA complexes *(secondary IgA nephropathy).*

Morphology

Histologically, the lesions in IgA nephropathy vary considerably. The glomeruli may be normal or may show mesangial widening and segmental inflammation confined to some glomeruli (focal proliferative GN); diffuse mesangial proliferation (mesangioproliferative); or (rarely) overt crescentic GN. The characteristic immunofluorescence picture is of **mesangial deposition of IgA,** often with C3 and properdin and smaller amounts of IgG or IgM (Fig. 14–11). Early components of the classical complement pathway are usually absent. Electron microscopy confirms the presence of electron-dense deposits in the mesangium. The deposits may extend to the subendothelial area of adjacent capillary walls in a minority of cases, usually those with focal proliferation.

Clinical Course. The disease most often affects children and young adults. More than half of those with IgA nephropathy present with gross hematuria after an infection of the respiratory or, less commonly, gastrointestinal or urinary tract; 30% to 40% have only microscopic hematuria, with or without proteinuria; and 5% to 10% develop a typical acute nephritic syndrome. The hematuria typically lasts for several days and then subsides, only to return every few months. The subsequent course is highly variable. Many individuals maintain normal renal function for decades. Slow progression to chronic renal failure occurs in 25% to 50% of cases during a period of 20 years.

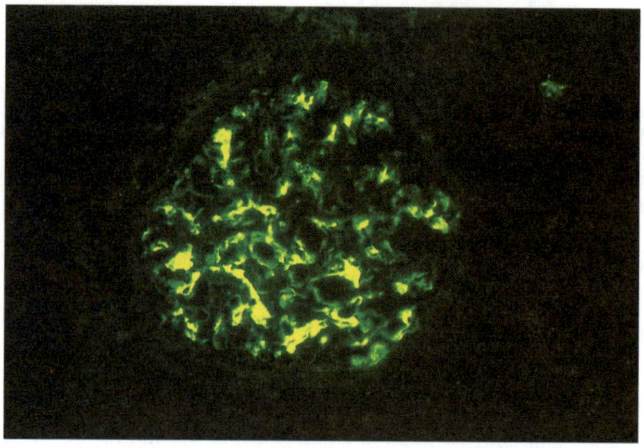

Figure 14–11

IgA nephropathy showing characteristic immunofluorescence deposition of IgA, principally in mesangial regions.

Hereditary Nephritis

Hereditary nephritis refers to a group of hereditary glomerular diseases caused by mutations in GBM proteins. The best-studied entity is *Alport syndrome,* in which nephritis is accompanied by nerve deafness and various eye disorders, including lens dislocation, posterior cataracts, and corneal dystrophy.

Pathogenesis. The GBM is largely composed of type IV collagen, which is made up of heterotrimers of α3, α4, and α5 type IV collagen. This form of type IV collagen is crucial for normal function of the lens, cochlea, and glomerulus. Mutation of any one of the α chains results in defective heterotrimer assembly, and thus the disease manifestations of Alport syndrome.

Morphology

Histologically, glomeruli in hereditary nephritis appear unremarkable until late in the course, when secondary sclerosis may occur. In some kidneys, interstitial cells take on a foamy appearance as a result of accumulation of neutral fats and mucopolysaccharides **(foam cells)** as a reaction to marked proteinuria. With progression, there is increasing glomerulosclerosis, vascular sclerosis, tubular atrophy, and interstitial fibrosis. With the electron microscope, the basement membrane of glomeruli appears thin and attenuated early in the course. Late in the course, the GBM develops irregular foci of thickening or attenuation with pronounced splitting and lamination of the lamina densa, yielding a "basket-weave" appearance.

Clinical Course. The inheritance is heterogeneous, being most commonly X-linked as a result of mutation of the gene encoding α5 type IV collagen. Males therefore tend to be affected more frequently and more severely than females and are more likely to develop renal failure. Rarely, inheritance is autosomal recessive or dominant, linked to defects in the genes that encode α3 or α4 type IV collagen. Individuals with hereditary nephritis present at age 5 to 20 years with gross or microscopic hematuria and proteinuria, and overt renal failure occurs between 20 and 50 years of age.

Female carriers of X-linked Alport syndrome or carriers of either gender of the autosomal forms usually present with persistent hematuria, which is most often asymptomatic and follows a benign course.

In a few instances, a heterozygous defect in the α3 or α4 chains is associated with persistent, often familial hematuria and a benign course (so-called benign familial hematuria, or thin basement membrane lesion).

SUMMARY

The Nephritic Syndrome

- The nephritic syndrome is characterized by hematuria, oliguria with azotemia, proteinuria, and hypertension.
- The most common causes are immunologically mediated glomerular injury; lesions are characterized by proliferative changes and leukocyte infiltration.
- *Acute post-infectious glomerulonephritis* typically occurs after streptococcal infection in children and young adults but may occur following infection with many other organisms; it is caused by deposition of immune complexes mainly in the subepithelial spaces, with abundant neutrophils and proliferation of glomerular cells. Most affected children recover; the prognosis is worse in adults.
- *IgA nephropathy,* characterized by mesangial deposits of IgA-containing immune complexes, is the most common cause of the nephritic syndrome worldwide; it is also a common cause of recurrent hematuria; it commonly affects children and young adults and has a variable course.
- *Hereditary nephritis* is caused by mutations in genes encoding GBM collagen; it manifests as hematuria and slowly progressing poteinuria and declining renal function; glomeruli appear normal until late in the disease course.

Rapidly Progressive (Crescentic) Glomerulonephritis

RPGN is a clinical syndrome and not a specific etiologic form of GN. Clinically, it is characterized by rapid and progressive loss of renal function with features of the nephritic syndrome, often with severe oliguria and (if untreated) death from renal failure within weeks to months. *Regardless of the cause, the histologic picture is characterized by the presence of crescents* (crescentic GN). These are produced in part by proliferation of the parietal epithelial cells of Bowman's capsule in response to injury and in part by infiltration of monocytes and macrophages.

Pathogenesis. Crescentic glomerulonephritis (CrGN) may be caused by a number of different diseases, some restricted to the kidney and others systemic. Although no single mechanism can explain all cases, there is little doubt that in most cases the glomerular injury is immunologically mediated. Thus, a practical classification divides CrGN into three groups on the basis of immunologic findings (Table 14–3). In each group, the disease may be associated with a known disorder or it may be idiopathic.

It will be obvious from the discussion below that although all three types of CrGN may be associated with a well-defined renal or extrarenal disease, in some cases CrGN is idiopathic. When the cause can be identified, about 12% of individuals have anti-GBM antibody-mediated GN (type I CrGN) with or without lung involvement; 44% have type II CrGN; and the remaining 44% have pauci-immune type III CrGN. All have severe glomerular injury.

Anti–Glomerular Basement Membrane Antibody (Type I) Crescentic Glomerulonephritis

Anti-GBM antibody crescentic glomerulonephritis, or type I CrGN, is characterized by linear deposits of IgG and, in many cases, C3 on the GBM, as described above. In some of these individuals the anti-GBM antibodies also bind to pulmonary alveolar capillary basement membranes to produce the clinical picture of pulmonary hemorrhages associated with renal failure. These persons are said to have *Goodpasture syndrome,* to distinguish their condition from so-called idiopathic cases in which renal involvement occurs in the absence of pulmonary disease. Anti-GBM antibodies are present in the serum and are helpful in diagnosis. It is important to recognize type I CrGN because these individuals benefit from plasmapheresis, which removes pathogenic antibodies from the circulation.

Table 14–3 Crescentic Glomerulonephritis

Type I (Anti-GBM Antibody)
Idiopathic
Goodpasture syndrome
Type II (Immune Complex)
Idiopathic
Postinfectious/infection related
Systemic lupus erythematosus
Henoch-Schönlein purpura/IgA nephropathy
Type III (Pauci-Immune) ANCA Associated
Idiopathic
Wegener granulomatosis
Microscopic angiitis

ANCA, antineutrophil cytoplasmic antibody; Anti-GBM, anti–glomerular basement membrane.

Morphology

The kidneys are enlarged and pale, often with **petechial hemorrhages** on the cortical surfaces. Glomeruli show segmental necrosis and GBM breaks, with resulting proliferation of the parietal epithelial cells in response to the exudation of plasma proteins including fibrin into Bowman's space. These distinctive lesions of proliferation are called **crescents** due to their shape as they fill Bowman's space. Crescents are formed both by proliferation of parietal cells and by migration of monocytes/macrophages into Bowman's space (Fig. 14–12). Smaller numbers of other types of leukocytes may also be present. The uninvolved portion of the glomerulus shows no proliferation. Immunofluorescence is characteristic with strong **linear staining** of deposited IgG and C3 along the GBM. However, deposits are not visualized by electron microscopy, because the endogenous collagen IV antigen to which the antibody is reacting is diffusely distributed, and so the large lattices of antigens and antibodies that occur in deposited immune complexes are not formed. Electron microscopy may show distinct ruptures in the GBM. The crescents eventually obliterate Bowman's space and compress the glomeruli. Fibrin strands are prominent between the cellular layers in the crescents. In time, crescents may undergo scarring.

Immune Complex–Mediated (Type II) Crescentic Glomerulonephritis

Type II CrGNs are immune complex–mediated disorders. This can be a complication of any of the immune complex nephritides, including poststreptococcal GN, SLE, IgA nephropathy, and Henoch-Schönlein purpura. In some cases, immune complexes can be demonstrated but the underlying cause is undetermined. In all of these cases, immunofluorescence studies reveal the characteristic granular ("lumpy bumpy") pattern of staining of the GBM and/or mesangium for immunoglobulin and/or complement. These individuals cannot usually be helped by plasmapheresis.

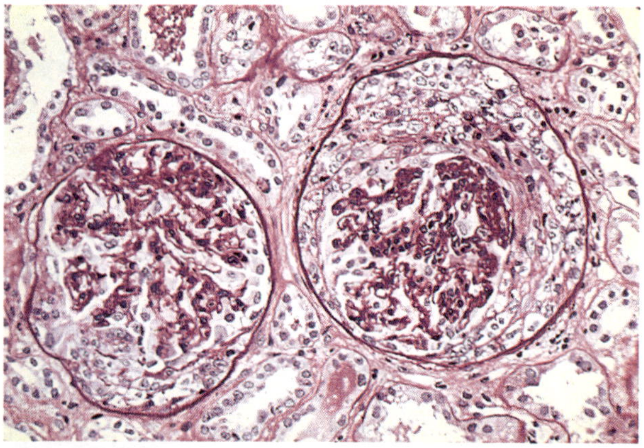

Figure 14–12

Crescentic GN (PAS stain). Note the collapsed glomerular tufts and the crescent-shaped mass of proliferating cells and leukocytes internal to Bowman's capsule. ANCA, antineutrophil cytoplasmic antibody. (Courtesy of Dr. M. A. Venkatachalam, Department of Pathology, University of Texas Health Sciences Center, San Antonio, Texas.)

Morphology

There is severe injury with **segmental necrosis** and GBM breaks with resultant crescent formation, as described above. However, in contrast to type I CrGN (anti-GBM antibody disease), segments of glomeruli without necrosis show evidence of the underlying immune complex GN (e.g., diffuse proliferation and leukocyte exudation in postinfectious GN or SLE, and mesangial proliferation in IgA nephropathy or Henoch-Schönlein purpura). Immunofluorescence shows the characteristic **granular pattern** of the underlying immune complex disease, and electron microscopy demonstrates discrete deposits.

Pauci-Immune (Type III) Crescentic Glomerulonephritis

Type III CrGN, also called *pauci-immune type CrGN,* is defined by the lack of anti-GBM antibodies or significant immune complex deposition detectable by immunofluorescence and electron microscopy. Most of these individuals have antineutrophil cytoplasmic antibodies in the serum, which, as we have seen (Chapter 10), have a role in some vasculitides. Therefore, in some cases type III CrGN is a component of a systemic vasculitis such as microscopic polyangiitis or Wegener granulomatosis. In many cases, however, pauci-immune CrGN is limited to the kidney and is thus called idiopathic.

Morphology

Glomeruli show **segmental necrosis** and GBM breaks with resulting crescent formation (see above). Uninvolved segments of glomeruli appear normal without proliferation or prominent inflammatory cell influx. However, in contrast to anti-GBM antibody disease, immunofluorescence studies for immunoglobulin and complement are negative or nearly so, and there are no deposits detectable by electron microscopy.

Clinical Course. The onset of RPGN is much like that of the nephritic syndrome except that the oliguria and azotemia are more pronounced. Proteinuria sometimes approaching nephrotic range may occur. Some of these persons become anuric and require long-term dialysis or transplantation. The prognosis can be roughly related to the number of crescents: those with crescents in less than 80% of the glomeruli have a better prognosis than those with higher percentages of crescents. Plasma exchange benefits some individuals, particularly those with anti-GBM antibody GN and Goodpasture syndrome.

SUMMARY

Rapidly Progressive Glomerulonephritis

- RPGN is a clinical entity with features of the nephritic syndrome and rapid loss of renal function.
- RPGN is commonly associated with severe glomerular injury with necrosis and GBM breaks and subsequent proliferation of parietal epithelium (crescents).
- RPGN may be immune mediated, as when autoantibodies develop to the GBM in anti-GBM antibody disease or when it develops consequent to immune complex deposition; it can also be pauci-immune, associated with antineutrophil cytoplasmic antibodies.

Chronic Glomerulonephritis

Having discussed various forms of glomerular disease, we should now turn to one of their unfortunate outcomes, chronic glomerular disease, which is also referred to as chronic GN by some, irrespective of whether there has been preceding glomerular inflammatory injury. It is an important cause of end-stage renal disease presenting as chronic renal failure. Among all individuals who require chronic hemodialysis or renal transplantation, 30% to 50% have the diagnosis of chronic GN.

By the time chronic GN is discovered, the glomerular changes are so far advanced that it is difficult to discern the nature of the original lesion. It probably represents the end stage of a variety of entities, prominent among which are the CrGNs, FSGS, MN, IgA nephropathy, and MPGN. It has been estimated that perhaps 20% of cases arise with no history of symptomatic renal disease. Although chronic GN may develop at any age, it is usually first noted in young and middle-aged adults.

Morphology

Classically, the kidneys are **symmetrically contracted** and their surfaces are red-brown and **diffusely granular.**

Microscopically, the feature common to all cases is advanced scarring of the glomeruli, sometimes to in the point of complete sclerosis (Fig. 14–13). This **obliteration of the glomeruli** is the end point of many diseases, and it is impossible to ascertain from such kidneys the nature of the earlier lesion.

There is also marked **interstitial fibrosis,** associated with atrophy and dropout of many of the tubules in the cortex, and diminution and loss of portions of the peritubular capillary network. The small and medium-sized arteries are frequently thick walled, with narrowed lumina, secondary to hypertension. Lymphocytic (and, rarely, plasma cell) infiltrates are present in the fibrotic interstitial tissue. As damage to all structures progresses, it may become difficult to ascertain whether the primary lesion was glomerular, vascular, tubular, or interstitial. Such markedly damaged kidneys are designated "end-stage kidneys."

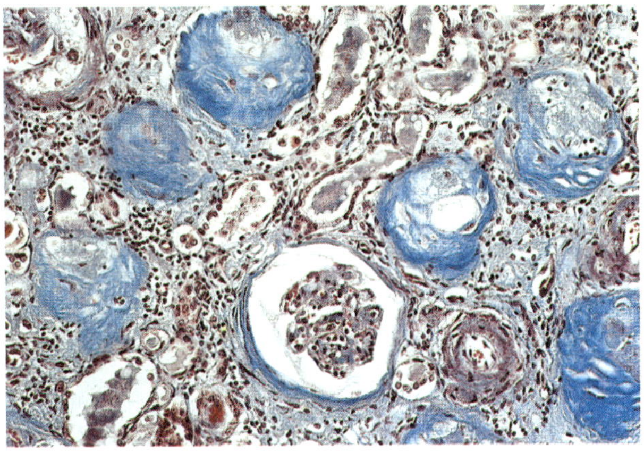

Figure 14–13

Chronic GN. A Masson trichrome preparation shows complete replacement of virtually all glomeruli by blue-staining collagen. (Courtesy of Dr. M. A. Venkatachalam, Department of Pathology, University of Texas Health Sciences Center, San Antonio, Texas.)

Clinical Course. Most often, chronic GN develops insidiously and is discovered only late in its course, after the onset of renal insufficiency. Very frequently, renal disease is first detected with the discovery of proteinuria, hypertension, or azotemia on routine medical examination. In some individuals the course is punctuated by transient episodes of either the nephritic or the nephrotic syndrome. Some of these persons may seek medical attention for the edema. As the glomeruli become obliterated, the avenue for protein loss is progressively closed and the nephrotic syndrome thus becomes less severe with more advanced disease. Some proteinuria, however, is constant in all cases. Hypertension is very common, and its effects may dominate the clinical picture. Although microscopic hematuria is usually present, grossly bloody urine is infrequent at this late stage.

Without treatment, the prognosis is poor; relentless progression to uremia and death is the rule. The rate of progression is extremely variable, however, and 10 years or more may elapse between onset of the first symptoms and terminal renal failure. Renal dialysis and kidney transplantation, of course, alter this course and allow long-term survival.

DISEASES AFFECTING TUBULES AND INTERSTITIUM

Most forms of tubular injury also involve the interstitium, so the two are discussed together. Under this heading we present diseases characterized by (1) inflammatory involvement of the tubules and interstitium (interstitial nephritis) and (2) ischemic or toxic tubular injury, leading to *acute tubular necrosis* and *acute renal failure.*

Tubulointerstitial Nephritis

Tubulointerstitial nephritis (TIN) refers to a group of inflammatory diseases of the kidneys that primarily involve the interstitium and tubules. The glomeruli may be spared altogether or affected only late in the course. In most cases of TIN caused by bacterial infection, the renal pelvis is prominently involved—hence the more descriptive term *pyelonephritis* (from *pyelo,* "pelvis"). The term *interstitial nephritis* is generally reserved for cases of TIN that are nonbacterial in origin. These include tubular injury resulting from drugs, metabolic disorders such as hypokalemia, physical injury such as irradiation, viral infections, and immune reactions. On the basis of clinical features and the character of the inflammatory exudate, TIN, regardless of the etiologic agent, can be divided into acute and chronic categories. In the following section we present pyelonephritis first, followed by other, nonbacterial forms of interstitial nephritis.

Acute Pyelonephritis

Acute pyelonephritis, a common suppurative inflammation of the kidney and the renal pelvis, is caused by bacterial infection. It is an important manifestation of urinary tract infection (UTI), which implies involvement of the lower (cystitis, prostatitis, urethritis) or upper (pyelonephritis) urinary tract, or both. As we will see, the great majority of cases of pyelonephritis are associated with infection of the lower urinary tract. The latter, however, may remain localized without extending to involve the kidney. UTIs are extremely common clinical problems.

Pathogenesis. The principal causative organisms are the enteric gram-negative rods. *Escherichia coli* is by far the most common one. Other important organisms are species of *Proteus, Klebsiella, Enterobacter,* and *Pseudomonas;* these are usually associated with recurrent infections, especially in persons who undergo urinary tract manipulations or have congenital or acquired anomalies of the lower urinary tract (see below). Staphylococci and *Streptococcus faecalis* may also cause pyelonephritis, but they are uncommon.

There are two routes by which bacteria can reach the kidneys: through the bloodstream (hematogenous) and from the lower urinary tract (ascending infection). Although *hematogenous spread* is the far less common of the two, acute pyelonephritis may result from seeding of the kidneys by bacteria in the course of septicemia or infective endocarditis (Fig. 14–14). *Ascending infection* from the lower urinary tract is the most important and common route by which the bacteria reach the kidney. The first step in the pathogenesis of ascending infection seems to be adhesion of bacteria to mucosal surfaces, followed by colonization of the distal urethra (and the introitus in females). Genetically determined properties of both the urothelium and of bacterial pathogens may facilitate adhesion to the urothelial lining by bacterial fimbriae (proteins that attach to receptors on the surface of urothelial cells), conferring susceptibility to infection. From here the organisms must gain access to the bladder, by expansive growth of the colonies and by moving against the flow of urine. This may occur during urethral instrumentation, including catheterization and cystoscopy, which are important predisposing factors in the

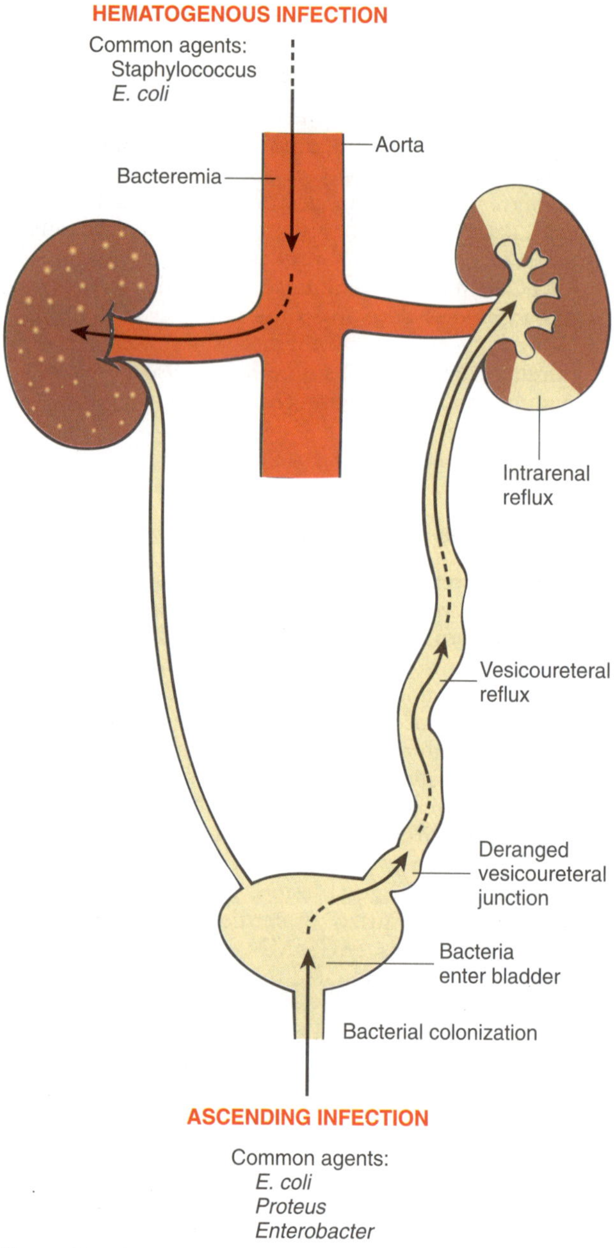

Figure 14–14

Pathways of renal infection. Hematogenous infection results from bacteremic spread. More common is ascending infection, which results from a combination of urinary bladder infection, vesicoureteral reflux, and intrarenal reflux.

pathogenesis of UTIs. In the absence of instrumentation, UTI most commonly affects females. Because of the close proximity of the urethra to the rectum, colonization by enteric bacteria is favored. Furthermore, the short urethra, and trauma to the urethra during sexual intercourse, facilitate the entry of bacteria into the urinary bladder. Ordinarily, bladder urine is sterile, and remains so, as a result of the antimicrobial properties of the bladder mucosa and the flushing action associated with periodic voiding of urine. With outflow obstruction or bladder dysfunction, however, the natural defense mechanisms of the bladder are overwhelmed, setting the stage for UTI. Obstruction at the level of the urinary bladder results in incomplete emptying and increased residual volume of urine. In the presence of stasis, bacteria introduced into the bladder can multiply undisturbed, without being flushed out or destroyed by the bladder wall. From the contaminated bladder urine, the bacteria ascend along the ureters to infect the renal pelvis and parenchyma. Accordingly, UTI is particularly frequent among individuals with urinary tract obstruction, as may occur with benign prostatic hyperplasia and uterine prolapse. UTI is also increased in diabetes because of the increased susceptibility to infection and neurogenic bladder dysfunction, which in turn predisposes to stasis.

Although obstruction is an important predisposing factor in the pathogenesis of ascending infection, it is the *incompetence of the vesicoureteral orifice* that allows bacteria to ascend the ureter into the pelvis. The normal ureteral insertion into the bladder is a competent one-way valve that prevents retrograde flow of urine, especially during micturition, when the intravesical pressure rises. An incompetent vesicoureteral orifice allows the reflux of bladder urine into the ureters, termed *vesicoureteral reflux (VUR)*. This condition is present in 20% to 40% of young children with UTI. It is usually a congenital defect that results in incompetence of the ureterovesical valve. VUR can also be acquired in individuals with a flaccid bladder resulting from spinal cord injury and with neurogenic bladder dysfunction secondary to diabetes. The effect of VUR is similar to that of an obstruction in that after voiding there is residual urine in the urinary tract, which favors bacterial growth. Furthermore, VUR affords a ready mechanism by which the infected bladder urine can be propelled up to the renal pelvis and farther into the renal parenchyma through open ducts at the tips of the papillae *(intrarenal reflux)*.

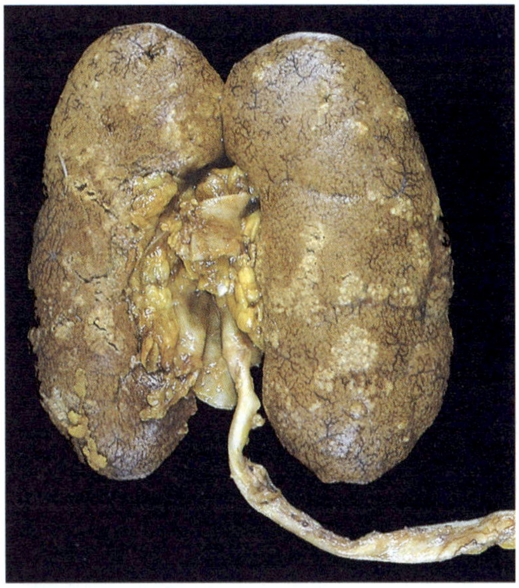

Figure 14–15

Acute pyelonephritis. The cortical surface is studded with focal pale abscesses, more numerous in the upper pole and middle region of the kidney; the lower pole is relatively unaffected. Between the abscesses there is dark congestion of the renal surface.

Morphology

One or both kidneys may be involved. The affected kidney may be normal in size or enlarged. **Characteristically, discrete, yellowish, raised abscesses are grossly apparent on the renal surface** (Fig. 14–15). They may be widely scattered or limited to one region of the kidney, or they may coalesce to form a single large area of suppuration.

The characteristic histologic feature of acute pyelonephritis is suppurative necrosis or abscess formation within the renal parenchyma. In the early stages the suppuration is limited to the interstitial tissue, but later abscesses rupture into tubules. **Large masses of intratubular neutrophils** frequently extend within involved nephrons into the collecting ducts, giving rise to the characteristic white cell casts found in the urine. Typically, the glomeruli are not affected.

When obstruction is prominent, the pus may be unable to drain and thus fills the renal pelvis, calyces, and ureter, producing pyonephrosis.

A second (and fortunately infrequent) form of pyelonephritis is necrosis of the renal papillae, known as **papillary necrosis.** This is particularly common among diabetics who develop acute pyelonephritis and may also complicate acute pyelonephritis when there is significant urinary tract obstruction. It is also seen with the chronic interstitial nephritis associated with analgesic abuse (described below). This lesion consists of a combination of ischemic and suppurative necrosis of the tips of the renal pyramids (renal papillae). The pathognomonic gross feature of papillary necrosis is sharply defined gray-white to yellow necrosis of the apical two-thirds of the pyramids. One papilla or several or all papillae may be affected. Microscopically, the papillary tips show characteristic coagulative necrosis, with surrounding neutrophilic infiltrate.

When the bladder is involved in a UTI, as is often the case, **acute** or **chronic cystitis** results. In long-standing cases associated with obstruction, the bladder may be grossly hypertrophic, with trabeculation of its walls, or it may be thinned and markedly distended from retention of urine.

Clinical Course. Acute pyelonephritis is often associated with predisposing conditions, which were covered in the discussion of pathogenetic mechanisms. These include the following:

- *Urinary obstruction,* either congenital or acquired
- *Instrumentation* of the urinary tract, most commonly catheterization
- *Vesicoureteral reflux.* Increased VUR contributes to the risk of developing pyelonephritis.
- *Pregnancy.* 4% to 6% of pregnant women develop bacteriuria sometime during pregnancy, and 20% to 40% of these eventually develop symptomatic urinary infection if not treated.

- *Patient's sex and age.* After the first year of life (when congenital anomalies in males commonly become evident) and as far as around age 40 years, infections are much more frequent in females. With increasing age, the incidence in males rises as a result of the development of prostatic hyperplasia and frequent instrumentation.
- *Preexisting renal lesions,* causing intrarenal scarring and obstruction
- *Diabetes mellitus,* in which acute pyelonephritis is caused by increased susceptibility to infection and neurogenic bladder dysfunction
- *Immunosuppression and immunodeficiency.*

The onset of uncomplicated acute pyelonephritis is usually sudden, with pain at the costovertebral angle and systemic evidence of infection, such as chills, fever, and malaise. *Urinary* findings include pyuria and bacteriuria. In addition, there are usually indications of bladder and urethral irritation (dysuria, frequency, urgency). Even without antibiotic treatment, the disease tends to be benign and self-limited. The symptomatic phase of the disease usually lasts no longer than a week, although bacteriuria may persist much longer. The disease is usually unilateral, and individuals thus do not develop renal failure because they still have one unaffected kidney. In cases with predisposing influences, the disease may become recurrent or chronic, particularly when it is bilateral. The development of papillary necrosis is associated with a much poorer prognosis. These persons have evidence of overwhelming sepsis and, often, renal failure. The diagnosis of acute pyelonephritis is established by finding leukocytes ("pus cells") by urinalysis and urine culture.

Chronic Pyelonephritis and Reflux Nephropathy

Chronic pyelonephritis is defined here as a morphologic entity in which predominantly interstitial inflammation and scarring of the renal parenchyma is associated with grossly visible scarring and deformity of the pelvicalyceal system. Chronic pyelonephritis is an important cause of chronic renal failure. It can be divided into two forms: chronic obstructive pyelonephritis and chronic reflux-associated pyelonephritis.

Chronic Obstructive Pyelonephritis. We have seen that obstruction predisposes the kidney to infection. Recurrent infections superimposed on diffuse or localized obstructive lesions lead to recurrent bouts of renal inflammation and scarring, which eventually cause chronic pyelonephritis. The disease can be bilateral, as with congenital anomalies of the urethra (posterior urethral valves), resulting in fatal renal insufficiency unless the anomaly is corrected; or unilateral, such as occurs with calculi and unilateral obstructive lesions of the ureter.

Chronic Reflux-Associated Pyelonephritis (Reflux Nephropathy). This is the more common form of chronic pyelonephritic scarring and results from superimposition of a UTI on congenital vesicoureteral reflux and intrarenal reflux. Reflux may be unilateral or bilateral; thus, the resultant renal damage either may cause scarring and atrophy of one kidney or may involve both and lead to chronic renal insufficiency. Whether VUR causes renal damage in the absence of infection (sterile reflux) is uncertain, because it is difficult clinically to rule out remote infections in a person first seen with pyelonephritic scarring.

Morphology

One or both kidneys may be involved, either diffusely or in patches. Even when involvement is bilateral, the kidneys are not equally damaged and therefore are not equally contracted. This **uneven scarring** is useful in differentiating chronic pyelonephritis from the more symmetrically contracted kidneys associated with vascular sclerosis (often referred to as "benign nephrosclerosis") and chronic GN. The hallmark of chronic pyelonephritis is **scarring involving the pelvis or calyces,** or both, leading to papillary blunting and marked **calyceal deformities** (Fig. 14–16).

The microscopic changes are largely nonspecific, and similar alterations may be seen with other tubulointerstitial disorders such as analgesic nephropathy. The parenchyma shows the following features:

- Uneven interstitial fibrosis and an inflammatory infiltrate of lymphocytes, plasma cells, and occasionally neutrophils.
- Dilation or contraction of tubules, with atrophy of the lining epithelium. Many of the dilated tubules contain pink to blue, glassy-appearing PAS-positive casts known as colloid casts that suggest the appearance of thyroid tissue, hence the descriptive term thyroidization. Often, neutrophils are seen within tubules.
- Chronic inflammatory infiltration and fibrosis involving the calyceal mucosa and wall.
- Vascular changes similar to those of benign arteriolosclerosis caused by the frequently associated hypertension.
- Although glomeruli may be normal, in most cases, glomerulosclerosis is seen in areas of better preserved renal parenchyma. Such changes represent secondary sclerosis caused by maladaptive changes secondary to nephron loss.

Clinical Course. Many persons with chronic pyelonephritis come to medical attention relatively late in the course of the disease, because of the gradual onset of renal insufficiency or because signs of kidney disease are noticed on routine laboratory tests. Often the renal disease is heralded by the development of hypertension. Ultrasonography can be used to determine the size and shape of the kidneys. Pyelograms are characteristic: they show the affected kidney to be asymmetrically contracted, with some degree of blunting and deformity of the calyceal system (caliectasis). Renal cortical scanning with radioactive technetium can also detect early scarring. The presence or absence of significant bacteriuria is not particularly helpful diagnostically; its absence certainly should not rule out chronic

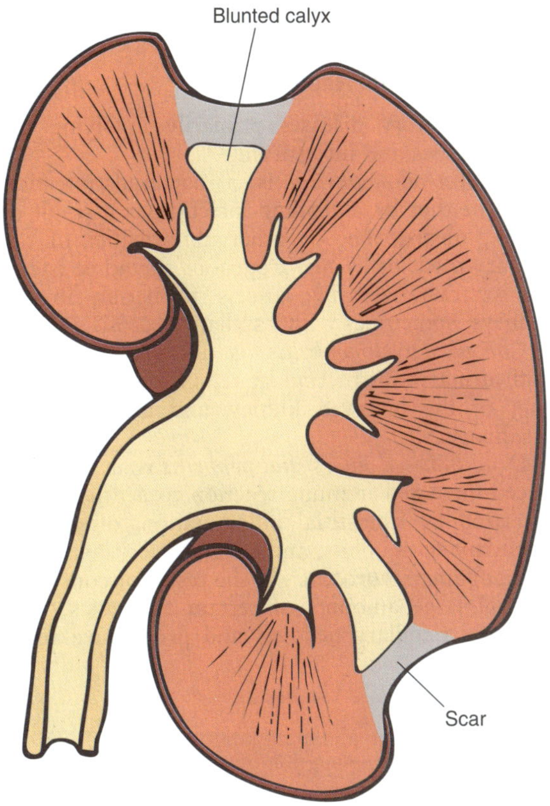

Figure 14–16

Typical coarse scars of chronic pyelonephritis associated with vesicoureteral reflux. The scars are usually located at the upper or lower poles of the kidney and are associated with underlying blunted calyces.

pyelonephritis. If the disease is bilateral and progressive, tubular dysfunction occurs with loss of concentrating ability, manifested by polyuria and nocturia.

As noted earlier, some persons with chronic pyelonephritis or reflux nephropathy ultimately develop glomerular lesions of global sclerosis and secondary FSGS. These are associated with proteinuria and eventually contribute to progressive chronic renal failure.

Drug-Induced Interstitial Nephritis

In this era of antibiotics and analgesics, drugs have emerged as important causes of renal injury. Two forms of TIN caused by drugs are discussed below.

Acute Drug-Induced Interstitial Nephritis

This is an adverse reaction to any of an increasing number of drugs. Acute TIN most frequently occurs with synthetic penicillins (methicillin, ampicillin), other synthetic antibiotics (rifampin), diuretics (thiazides), nonsteroidal anti-inflammatory agents, and numerous other drugs (phenindione, cimetidine).

Pathogenesis. Many features of the disease suggest an immune mechanism. Clinical evidence of hypersensitivity includes a latent period, the eosinophilia and rash, the information that the onset of nephropathy is not dose related, and the recurrence of hypersensitivity after re-exposure to the same or a cross-reactive drug. Serum IgE levels are increased in some persons, suggesting type I hypersensitivity. The mononuclear or granulomatous infiltrate, together with positive skin tests to drugs, suggests a T cell-mediated (type IV) hypersensitivity reaction.

The most likely sequence of pathogenetic events is that the drugs act as haptens that, during secretion by tubules, covalently bind to some cytoplasmic or extracellular component of tubular cells and become immunogenic. The resultant tubulointerstitial injury is then caused by IgE- and cell-mediated immune reactions to tubular cells or their basement membranes.

Morphology

The abnormalities in drug-induced nephritis are in the interstitium, which shows pronounced edema and infiltration by mononuclear cells, principally lymphocytes and macrophages (Fig. 14–17). Eosinophils and neutrophils may be present, often in large numbers. With some drugs (e.g., methicillin, thiazides, rifampin), interstitial non-necrotizing granulomas with giant cells may be seen. The glomeruli are normal except in some cases caused by nonsteroidal anti-inflammatory agents when the hypersensitivity reaction also leads to podocyte foot process effacement (MCD-like lesion), and the nephrotic syndrome develops concurrently.

Clinical Course. The disease begins about 15 days (range, 2–40 days) after exposure to the drug and is characterized by *fever, eosinophilia* (which may be transient), *a rash* in about 25% of persons, and *renal abnormalities.* Renal findings include hematuria, minimal or no proteinuria, and leukocyturia (sometimes including

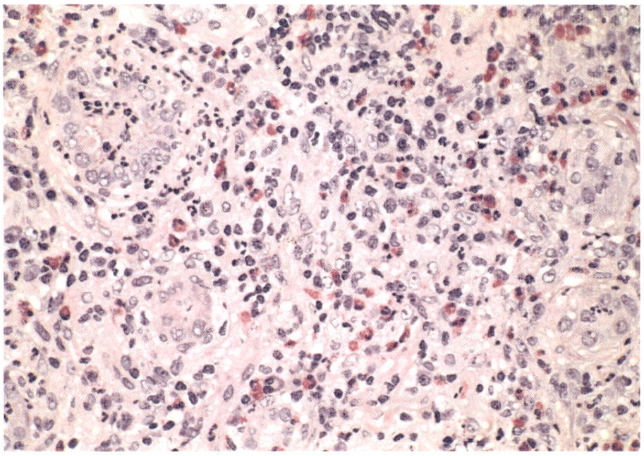

Figure 14–17

Drug-induced interstitial nephritis, with prominent eosinophilic and mononuclear infiltrate. (Courtesy of Dr. H. Rennke, Department of Pathology, Brigham and Women's Hospital, Boston, Massachussetts.)

eosinophils). A rising serum creatinine or acute renal failure with oliguria develops in about 50% of cases, particularly in older patients. It is important to recognize drug-induced renal failure, because withdrawal of the offending drug is followed by recovery, although it may take several months for renal function to return to normal.

Analgesic Nephropathy

Individuals who consume large quantities of analgesics may develop chronic interstitial nephritis, *often associated with renal papillary necrosis.* Although at times ingestion of single types of analgesics has been incriminated, most people who develop this nephropathy consume mixtures containing some combination of phenacetin, aspirin, acetaminophen, caffeine, and codeine for long periods. Aspirin and acetaminophen are the major culprits. While they can cause renal disease in apparently healthy individuals, preexisting renal disease seems to be a necessary precursor to analgesic-induced renal failure.

Pathogenesis. The pathogenesis of the renal lesions is not entirely clear. Papillary necrosis is the initial event, and the interstitial nephritis in the overlying renal parenchyma is a secondary phenomenon. Acetaminophen, a phenacetin metabolite, injures cells by both *covalent binding* and *oxidative damage.* The ability of aspirin to inhibit prostaglandin synthesis suggests that this drug may induce its potentiating effect by inhibiting the vasodilatory effects of prostaglandin and predisposing the papilla to ischemia. Thus, the papillary damage may be caused by a combination of direct toxic effects of phenacetin metabolites as well as ischemic injury to both tubular cells and vessels.

Morphology

The necrotic papillae appear yellowish brown, as a result of the accumulation of breakdown products of phenacetin and other lipofuscin-like pigments. Later on, the papillae may shrivel, be sloughed off, and drop into the pelvis. Microscopically, the papillae show coagulative necrosis associated with loss of cellular detail but preservation of tubular outlines. Foci of dystrophic calcification may occur in the necrotic areas. The cortex drained by the necrotic papillae shows tubular atrophy, interstitial scarring, and inflammation. The small vessels in the papillae and urinary tract submucosa exhibit characteristic PAS-positive basement membrane thickening.

Clinical Course. Common clinical features of analgesic nephropathy include chronic renal failure, hypertension, and anemia. The anemia results in part from damage to red cells by phenacetin metabolites. Cessation of analgesic intake may stabilize or even improve renal function. A complication of analgesic abuse is the increased incidence of *transitional-cell carcinoma* of the renal pelvis or bladder in persons who survive the renal failure.

SUMMARY

Tubulointerstitial Nephritis

- Inflammatory diseases primarily involving the renal tubules and interstitum.
- *Acute pyelonephritis* is a bacterial infection caused either by ascending infection as a result of reflux, obstruction, or other abnormality of the urinary tract, or by hematogenous spread of bacteria; characterized by abscess formation in the kidneys, sometimes with papillary necrosis.
- *Chronic pyelonephritis* is usually associated with urinary obstruction or reflux; results in scarring of the involved kidney, and gradual renal insufficiency.
- *Drug-induced interstitial nephritis* is an IgE- and T cell-mediated immune reaction to a drug; characterized by interstitial inflammation, often with abundant eosinophils, and edema.
- *Analgesic nephropathy* is the result of consumption of large amounts of certain analgesics; may result in papillary necrosis and progressive renal dysfunction.

Acute Tubular Necrosis (ATN)

ATN is a clinicopathologic entity characterized morphologically by damaged tubular epithelial cells and clinically by acute suppression of renal function. *It is the most common cause of acute renal failure.* In acute renal failure, urine flow falls within 24 hours to less than 400 mL per day (oliguria). Other causes of acute renal failure include (1) severe glomerular diseases manifesting as RPGN, (2) diffuse renal vascular diseases such as microscopic polyangiitis and thrombotic microangiopathies, (3) acute papillary necrosis associated with acute pyelonephritis, (4) acute drug-induced interstitial nephritis, and (5) diffuse cortical necrosis. Here we discuss ATN; the other causes of acute renal failure are discussed elsewhere in this chapter.

ATN is a reversible renal lesion that arises in a variety of clinical settings. Most of these, ranging from severe trauma to acute pancreatitis to septicemia, have in common a period of inadequate blood flow to the peripheral organs, often in the setting of marked hypotension and shock. The pattern of ATN associated with shock is called *ischemic ATN.* Mismatched blood transfusions and other hemolytic crises, as well as myoglobinuria, also produce a picture resembling ischemic ATN. A second pattern, called *nephrotoxic ATN,* is caused by a variety of poisons, including heavy metals (e.g., mercury); organic solvents (e.g., carbon tetrachloride); and a multitude of drugs such as gentamicin and other antibiotics, and radiographic contrast agents. Because of the many precipitating factors, ATN occurs quite frequently. Moreover, its reversibility adds to its clinical importance, because proper management can mean the difference between full recovery and death.

Pathogenesis. The decisive events in both ischemic and nephrotoxic ATN are believed to be (1) tubular injury and (2) persistent and severe disturbances in blood flow resulting in diminished oxygen and substrate delivery to tubular cells, as depicted in Figure 14–18.

Tubular epithelial cells are particularly sensitive to anoxia and are also vulnerable to toxins. Several factors predispose the tubules to toxic injury, including a vast electrically charged surface for fluid reabsorption, active transport systems for ions and organic acids, and the capability for effective concentration. Ischemia causes numerous structural alterations in epithelial cells. *Loss of cell polarity* seems to be a functionally important (but reversible) early event. This leads to redistribution of membrane proteins (e.g., Na^+, K^+-ATPase) from the basolateral to the luminal surface of tubular cells, resulting in decreased sodium reabsorption by proximal tubules and hence increased sodium delivery to distal tubules. The latter, through a tubuloglomerular feedback system, contributes to vasoconstriction. Redistribution or alteration of integrins that anchor tubular cells to their underlying basement membranes results in shedding of tubular cells into the urine. Further damage to the tubules and the resultant tubular debris can block urine outflow and eventually increase intratubular pressure, thereby decreasing GFR. Additionally, fluid from the damaged tubules could leak into the interstitium, resulting in increased interstitial pressure and collapse of the tubules. Ischemic tubular cells also express chemokines, cytokines, and adhesion molecules such as P-selectin that recruit and immobilize leukocytes that can participate in tissue injury.

Ischemic renal injury is also characterized by severe hemodynamic alterations that cause reduced GFR. The major one is intrarenal *vasoconstriction*, which results in both reduced glomerular plasma flow and reduced oxygen delivery to the functionally important tubules in the outer medulla (thick ascending limb and straight segment of the proximal tubule) (see Fig. 14–18). Although a number of vasoconstrictor pathways have been implicated in this phenomenon (e.g., renin-angiotensin, thromboxane A2, sympathetic nerve activity), some triggered by the increased distal sodium delivery, the current opinion is that vasoconstriction is mediated by *sublethal endothelial injury*, leading to increased release of the endothelial vasoconstrictor *endothelin* and decreased production of vasodilatory *nitric oxide and prostaglandins*. Finally, there is also some evidence of a direct effect of ischemia or toxins on the glomerulus, causing a reduced effective glomerular filtration surface.

Morphology

Ischemic ATN is characterized by **necrosis of short segments** of the tubules. Most of the lesions are seen in the straight portions of the proximal tubule and the ascending thick limbs, but no segment of the proximal

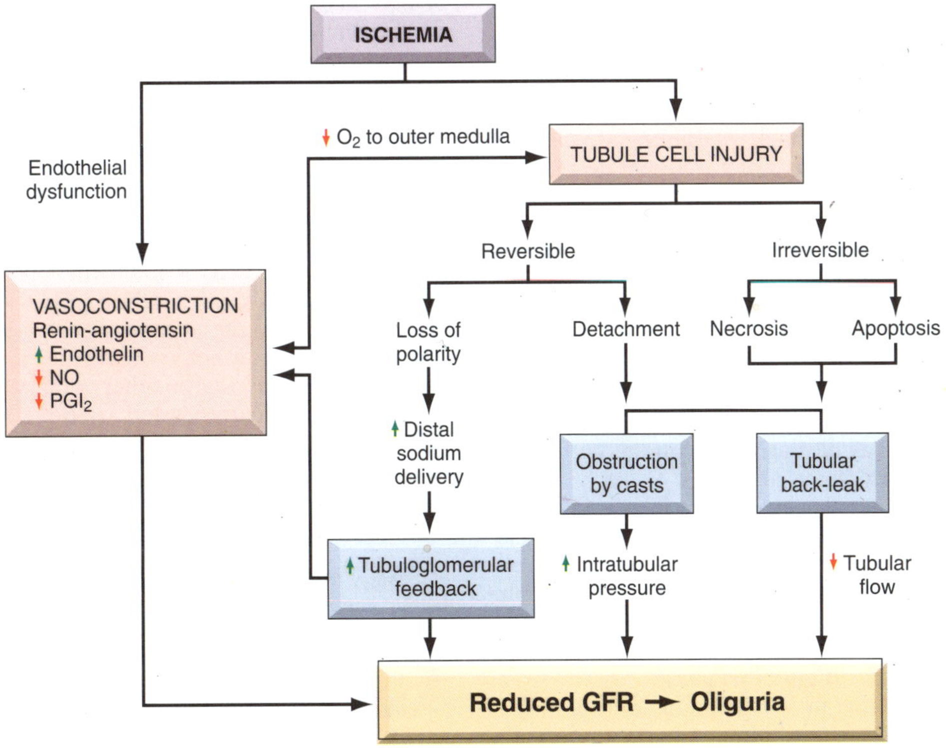

Figure 14–18

Postulated sequence in acute renal failure (see text). NO, nitric oxide; GFR, glomerular filtration rate; PGI_2, prostaglandin I_2 (prostacyclin). (Modified from Brady HR, et al.: Acute renal failure. In Brenner BM [ed]: Brenner and Rector's The Kidney, 5th ed, vol II. Philadelphia, WB Saunders, 1996, p 1210.)

or distal tubules is spared. Despite the long-standing nomenclature indicating cell death, widespread overt necrosis of tubular cells is uncommonly seen in renal biopsy samples from persons with clinically diagnosed ATN. Instead, there is often a variety of **tubular injuries,** including attenuation of proximal tubular brush borders, blebbing and sloughing of brush borders, vacuolization of cells, and detachment of tubular cells from their underlying basement membranes with sloughing of cells into the urine. A striking additional finding is the presence of proteinaceous casts in the distal tubules and collecting ducts. They consist of Tamm-Horsfall protein (secreted normally by tubular epithelium) along with hemoglobin and other plasma proteins. When crush injuries have produced ATN, the casts are composed of myoglobin. The interstitium usually shows generalized edema along with a mild inflammatory infiltrate consisting of polymorphonuclear leukocytes, lymphocytes, and plasma cells. The histologic picture in **toxic ATN** is basically similar, with some differences. Necrosis is most prominent in the proximal tubule, and the tubular basement membranes are generally spared.

If the patient survives for a week, epithelial regeneration becomes apparent in the form of a low cuboidal epithelial covering and mitotic activity in the persisting tubular epithelial cells. Except where the basement membrane is destroyed, regeneration is total and complete.

Clinical Course. The clinical course of ATN may be divided into initiation, maintenance, and recovery stages. The *initiation* phase, lasting about 36 hours, is usually dominated by the inciting medical, surgical, or obstetric event in the ischemic form of ATN. The only indication of renal involvement is a slight decline in urine output with a rise in serum creatinine. At this point, oliguria could be explained on the basis of a transient decrease in blood flow to the kidneys.

The *maintenance* phase begins anywhere from the second to the sixth day. Urine output falls markedly, usually to between 50 and 400 mL per day (oliguria). Sometimes it declines to only a few milliliters per day, but complete anuria is rare. Oliguria may last only a few days or may persist as long as 3 weeks. The clinical picture is dominated by the signs and symptoms of uremia and fluid overload. In the absence of careful supportive treatment or dialysis, patients may die during this phase. With good care, however, survival is the rule.

The *recovery* is ushered in by a steady increase in urine volume, reaching as much as about 3 L/day over the course of a few days. Because tubular function is still deranged, serious electrolyte imbalances may occur during this phase. There also seems to be increased vulnerability to infection. For these reasons, about 25% of deaths from ATN occur during this phase.

During the final phase there is a gradual return of the individual's well-being. Urine volume returns to normal; however, subtle functional impairment of the kidneys, particularly of the tubules, may persist for months. With modern methods of care, patients who do not die from the underlying precipitating problem have a 90% to 95% chance of recovering from ATN.

SUMMARY

Acute Tubular Necrosis

- ATN is the most common cause of acute renal failure; its clinical manifestations are oliguria, uremia, and signs of fluid overload.
- ATN results from ischemic or toxic injury to renal tubules, associated with intrarenal vasoconstriction resulting in reduced GFR and diminished delivery of oxygen and nutrients to tubular epithelial cells.
- ATN is characterized morphologically by necrosis of segments of the tubules (typically the proximal tubules), proteinaceous casts in distal tubules, and interstitial edema.

DISEASES INVOLVING BLOOD VESSELS

Nearly all diseases of the kidney involve the renal blood vessels secondarily. Systemic vascular diseases, such as various forms of arteritis, also involve renal blood vessels, and often the effects on the kidney are clinically important (see Chapter 10). The kidney is intimately involved in the pathogenesis of both essential and secondary hypertension. Here we will cover the renal lesions associated with benign and malignant hypertension.

Benign Nephrosclerosis

Benign nephrosclerosis, the term used for the renal changes in benign hypertension, is always associated with hyaline arteriolosclerosis. Some degree of benign nephrosclerosis, albeit mild, is present at autopsy in many persons older than 60 years of age. The frequency and severity of the lesions are increased at any age when hypertension or diabetes mellitus are present.

Pathogenesis. It should be remembered that many renal diseases cause hypertension, which in turn is associated with benign nephrosclerosis. Whether hypertension causes the nephrosclerosis, or a subtle primary microvascular renal injury causes the hypertension, which in turn accelerates the sclerosis, is not known. Thus, this renal lesion is often seen superimposed on other primary kidney diseases. Similar changes in arteries and arterioles are seen in individuals with chronic thrombotic microangiopathies.

Morphology

Grossly, the kidneys are **symmetrically atrophic,** each weighing 110 to 130 gm, with a surface of diffuse, fine granularity that resembles grain leather. Microscopically, the basic anatomic change is hyaline thickening of the walls of the small arteries and arterioles, known as **hyaline arteriolosclerosis.** This appears as a homogeneous, pink hyaline thickening, at the expense of the vessel lumina, with loss of underlying cellular detail (Fig. 14–19). The narrowing of the lumen results in markedly decreased blood flow through the affected vessels and thus produces ischemia in the organ served. All structures of the kidney show ischemic

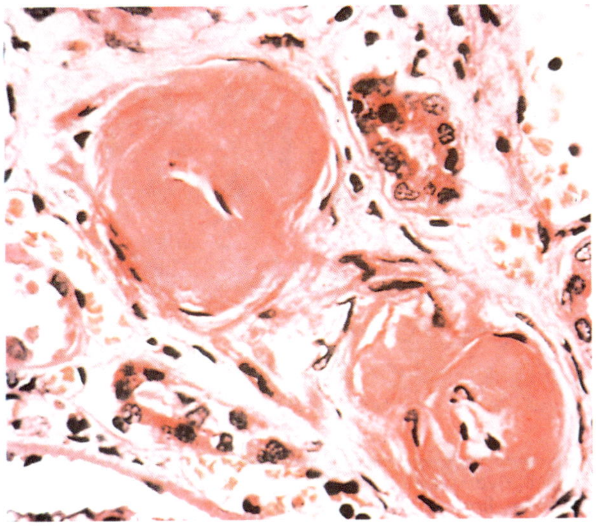

Figure 14–19

Benign nephrosclerosis. High-power view of two arterioles with hyaline deposition, marked thickening of the walls, and a narrowed lumen. (Courtesy of Dr. M. A. Venkatachalam, Department of Pathology, University of Texas Health Sciences Center, San Antonio, Texas.)

atrophy. In advanced cases of benign nephrosclerosis the glomerular tufts may become globally sclerosed. Diffuse tubular atrophy and interstitial fibrosis are present. Often there is a scant interstitial lymphocytic infiltrate. The larger blood vessels (interlobar and arcuate arteries) show reduplication of internal elastic lamina along with fibrous thickening of the media **(fibroelastic hyperplasia)** and the subintima.

Clinical Course. This renal lesion alone rarely causes severe damage to the kidney except in susceptible populations, such as African Americans, where it may lead to uremia and death. However, all persons with this lesion usually show some functional impairment, such as loss of concentrating ability or a variably diminished GFR. A mild degree of proteinuria is a frequent finding.

Malignant Hypertension and Malignant Nephrosclerosis

Malignant hypertension is far less common in the United States than benign hypertension and occurs in only about 5% of persons with elevated blood pressure. It may arise de novo (i.e., without preexisting hypertension), or it may appear suddenly in a person who had mild hypertension. In less developed countries, it occurs more commonly.

Pathogenesis. The basis for this turn for the worse in hypertensive subjects is unclear, but the following sequence of events is suggested. The initial event seems to be some form of vascular damage to the kidneys. This most commonly results from long-standing benign hypertension, with eventual injury to the arteriolar walls. The result is increased permeability of the small vessels to fibrinogen and other plasma proteins, endothelial injury, and platelet deposition. This leads to the appearance of *fibrinoid necrosis* of arterioles and small arteries and intravascular thrombosis. Mitogenic factors from platelets (e.g., platelet-derived growth factor) and plasma cause intimal smooth hyperplasia of vessels, resulting in the *hyperplastic arteriolosclerosis* typical of malignant hypertension and of morphologically similar thrombotic microangiopathies (see below) and further narrowing of the lumina. The kidneys become markedly ischemic. With severe involvement of the renal afferent arterioles, the renin-angiotensin system receives a powerful stimulus, and indeed *persons with malignant hypertension have markedly elevated levels of plasma renin.* This then sets up a self-perpetuating cycle in which angiotensin II causes intrarenal vasoconstriction, and the attendant renal ischemia perpetuates renin secretion. Aldosterone levels are also elevated, and salt retention undoubtedly contributes to the elevation of blood pressure. The consequences of the markedly elevated blood pressure on the blood vessels throughout the body are known as *malignant arteriolosclerosis,* and the renal disorder is referred to as *malignant nephrosclerosis.*

Morphology

The kidney may be essentially normal in size or slightly shrunken, depending on the duration and severity of the hypertensive disease. Small, **pinpoint petechial hemorrhages** may appear on the cortical surface from rupture of arterioles or glomerular capillaries, giving the kidney a peculiar, **flea-bitten appearance.**

The microscopic changes reflect the pathogenetic events described earlier. Damage to the small vessels is manifested as **fibrinoid necrosis** of the arterioles (Fig. 14–20A). The vessel walls show a homogeneous, granular eosinophilic appearance masking underlying detail. In the interlobular arteries and larger arterioles, proliferation of intimal cells produces an onion-skin appearance (Fig. 14–20B). This name is derived from the concentric arrangement of cells whose origin is believed to be intimal smooth muscle, although this issue is not finally settled. This lesion, called **hyperplastic arteriolosclerosis,** causes marked narrowing of arterioles and small arteries, to the point of total obliteration. Necrosis may also involve glomeruli, with microthrombi within the glomeruli as well as necrotic arterioles. Similar lesions are seen in persons with acute thrombotic microangiopathies.

Clinical Course. The full-blown syndrome of malignant hypertension is characterized by diastolic pressures greater than 120 mm Hg, papilledema, encephalopathy, cardiovascular abnormalities, and renal failure. Most often, the early symptoms are related to *increased intracranial pressure* and include headache, nausea, vomiting, and visual impairment, particularly the development of scotomas, or spots before the eyes. At the onset of rapidly mounting blood pressure there is marked proteinuria and microscopic, or sometimes macroscopic, hematuria but no significant alteration in renal function. Soon, however, *renal failure* makes its appearance. The syndrome is a true medical emergency that requires prompt and aggressive antihypertensive therapy before irreversible renal lesions develop. About 50% of patients survive at least 5 years, and further progress is still being made. Ninety percent of deaths are caused by uremia and the other 10% by cerebral hemorrhage or cardiac failure.

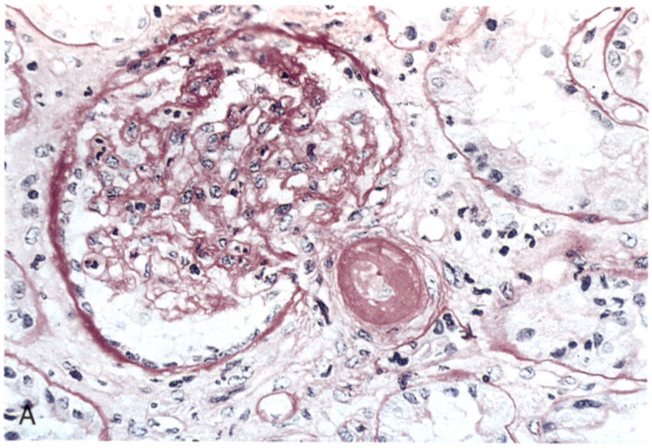

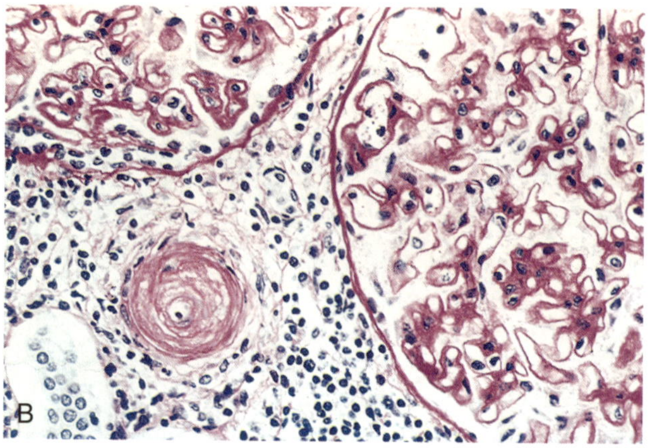

Figure 14–20

Malignant hypertension. **A,** Fibrinoid necrosis of afferent arteriole (PAS stain). **B,** Hyperplastic arteriolosclerosis (onion-skin lesion). (Courtesy of Dr. H. Rennke, Department of Pathology, Brigham and Women's Hospital, Boston, Massachusetts.)

Thrombotic Microangiopathies

As described in Chapter 12, this term describes lesions seen in various clinical syndromes, characterized morphologically by widespread thrombosis in the microcirculation and clinically by *microangiopathic hemolytic anemia, thrombocytopenia,* and, in certain instances, *renal failure.* Common diseases that cause lesions of thrombotic microangiopathy include (1) childhood hemolytic uremic syndrome (HUS), (2) various forms of adult HUS, and (3) thrombotic thrombocytopenic purpura (TTP).

Pathogenesis. Although clinically overlapping, HUS and TTP are pathogenetically distinct. Central to the pathogenesis of HUS is *endothelial injury and activation,* with resultant intravascular thrombosis. TTP is now known to be caused by an acquired defect in proteolytic cleavage of von Willebrand factor (vWF) multimers, or more rarely, an inherited defect as seen in familial TTP (Chapter 12). The defect involves a von Willebrand factor protease referred to as ADAMTS 13 (a disintegrin and metalloprotease with thrombospondin-like motifs).

Childhood HUS is the best characterized of the renal syndromes. As many as 75% of cases follow intestinal infection with Shiga toxin–producing *E. coli,* such as occurs in epidemics caused by ingestion of infected ground meat (e.g., hamburgers) and infections with *Shigella dysenteriae* type I. The pathogenesis of this syndrome is related to the effects of Shiga toxin, which is carried by neutrophils in the circulation. Renal glomerular endothelial cells are targets of this toxin because the cells express the membrane receptor for the toxin. The toxin has multiple effects on the endothelium, including increased adhesion of leukocytes, increased endothelin production, and loss of endothelial nitric oxide (both favoring vasoconstriction), and (in the presence of cytokines, such as tumor necrosis factor) endothelial damage. The toxin also gains entry to the cells and directly causes cell death. The resultant endothelial damage leads to thrombosis, which is most prominent in glomerular capillaries, afferent arterioles, and interlobular arteries, as well as vasoconstriction, resulting in the characteristic thrombotic microangiopathy.

Approximately 10% of the cases of HUS in children are not preceded by diarrhea caused by Shiga toxin–producing bacteria. In a subset of these patients there is mutational inactivation of complement regulatory proteins (e.g. factor H), which allows uncontrolled complement activation following minor vascular injuries. This then promotes the formation of thrombi.

Morphology

In childhood HUS, there are lesions of classic **thrombotic microangiopathy** with fibrin thrombi predominantly involving glomeruli, and extending into arterioles and larger arteries in severe cases. Cortical necrosis may be present. Morphologic changes in glomeruli resulting from endothelial injury include widening of the subendothelial space in glomerular capillaries, duplication or splitting of GBMs, and lysis of mesangial cells with mesangial disintegration. Chronically, scarring of glomeruli may develop.

Clinical Course. Typically, childhood HUS is characterized by the sudden onset, usually after a gastrointestinal or flulike prodromal episode, of bleeding manifestations (especially hematemesis and melena), severe oliguria, hematuria, microangiopathic hemolytic anemia, and (in some persons) prominent neurologic changes. *This disease is one of the main causes of acute renal failure in children.* If the renal failure is managed properly with dialysis, most patients recover in a matter of weeks. The long-term (15- to 25-year) prognosis, however, is not uniformly favorable, because about 25% of children eventually develop renal insufficiency due to the secondary scarring.

SUMMARY

Vascular Diseases of the Kidney

- *Benign nephrosclerosis:* Progressive, chronic renal damage associated with benign hypertension; characterized by hyaline arteriolosclerosis and narrowing of vascular lumens with resultant cortical atrophy.

- *Malignant nephrosclerosis:* Acute renal injury associated with malignant hypertension; arteries and arterioles show fibrinoid necrosis and hyperplasia of smooth muscle cells; petechial hemorrhages on the cortical surface; often culminates in acute renal failure.
- *Thrombotic microangiopathies:* Disorders characterized by fibrin thrombi in glomeruli and small vessels resulting in acute renal failure; childhood hemolytic uremic syndrome is caused by endothelial injury by an *E. coli* toxin; thrombotic thrombocytopenic purpura is caused by defects in von Willebrand factor leading to excessive thrombosis, with platelet consumption.

CYSTIC DISEASES OF THE KIDNEY

Cystic diseases of the kidney are a heterogeneous group comprising hereditary, developmental but nonhereditary, and acquired disorders. As a group, they are important for several reasons: (1) they are reasonably common and often present diagnostic problems for clinicians, radiologists, and pathologists; (2) some forms, such as adult polycystic disease, are major causes of chronic renal failure; and (3) they can occasionally be confused with malignant tumors. *An emerging theme in the pathophysiology of the hereditary cystic diseases is that the underlying defect is in the cilia-centrosome complex of tubular epithelial cells.* Such defects may interfere with fluid absorption or cellular maturation, resulting in cyst formation. Here we briefly mention simple cysts, the most common form, and discuss in some detail polycystic kidney disease.

Simple Cysts

These generally innocuous lesions occur as multiple or single cystic spaces that vary widely in diameter. Commonly, they are 1 to 5 cm in diameter; translucent; lined by a gray, glistening, smooth membrane; and filled with clear fluid. Microscopically, these membranes are composed of a single layer of cuboidal or flattened cuboidal epithelium, which in many instances may be completely atrophic. The cysts are usually confined to the cortex. Rarely, massive cysts as large as 10 cm in diameter are encountered.

Simple cysts are a common post-mortem finding that has no clinical significance. The main importance of cysts lies in their differentiation from kidney tumors, when they are discovered either incidentally or because of hemorrhage and pain. Radiographic studies show that, in contrast to renal tumors, renal cysts have smooth contours, are almost always avascular, and give fluid rather than solid tissue signals on ultrasonography.

Dialysis-associated acquired cysts occur in the kidneys of patients with end-stage renal disease who have undergone prolonged dialysis. They are present in both cortex and medulla and may bleed, causing hematuria. Occasionally, renal adenomas or even adenocarcinomas arise in the walls of these cysts.

Autosomal Dominant (Adult) Polycystic Kidney Disease

Adult polycystic kidney disease is characterized by multiple expanding cysts of both kidneys that ultimately destroy the intervening parenchyma. It is seen in approximately 1 in 500 to 1000 persons and accounts for 10% of cases of chronic renal failure. This disease is genetically heterogeneous. It can be caused by inheritance of one of at least two autosomal dominant genes of very high penetrance. In 85% to 90% of families, *PKD1,* the defective gene is on the short arm of chromosome 16. This gene encodes a large (460-kD) and complex cell membrane-associated protein, called polycystin-1, that is mainly extracellular.

Pathogenesis. The polycystin molecule has regions of homology with proteins involved in cell-cell or cell-matrix adhesion (e.g., domains that bind collagen, laminin, and fibronectin). It also has several other domains including those that can bind receptor tyrosine phosphatases. How mutations in this protein cause cyst formation is at present unclear, but it is thought that the resultant defects in cell-matrix interactions may lead to alterations in proliferation, adhesion, differentiation, and matrix production by tubular epithelial cells, and to cyst formation. The polycystins have also been localized in tubular cilia, like the nephrocystins linked to medullary cystic disease that are discussed below. It is interesting to note that whereas germ-line mutations of the *PKD1* gene are present in all renal tubular cells of affected persons, cysts develop in only some tubules. This is most likely due to loss of both alleles of *PKD1*. Thus, as with tumor suppressor genes, a second "somatic hit" is required for expression of the disease. The *PKD2* gene, implicated in 10% to 15% of cases, resides on chromosome 4 and encodes *polycystin 2,* a smaller, 110-kD protein. Polycystin 2 is thought to function as a calcium-permeable membrane channel. Although structurally distinct, polycystins 1 and 2 are believed to act together by forming heterodimers. Thus, mutation in either gene gives rise to essentially the same phenotype, although patients with *PKD2* mutations have a slower rate of disease progression as compared with patients with *PKD1* mutations.

Morphology

In autosomal dominant adult polycystic kidney disease, the kidney may reach enormous size, and weights of up to 4 kg for each kidney have been recorded. These **very large kidneys** are readily palpable abdominally as masses extending into the pelvis. On gross examination the kidney seems to be composed solely of a mass of cysts of varying sizes up to 3 or 4 cm in diameter with no intervening parenchyma. The cysts are filled with fluid, which may be clear, turbid, or hemorrhagic (Fig. 14–21).

Microscopic examination reveals some normal parenchyma dispersed among the cysts. Cysts may arise at any level of the nephron, from tubules to collecting ducts, and therefore they have a variable, often atrophic, lining. Occasionally, Bowman's capsules are involved in the cyst formation, and in these cases glomerular tufts may be seen within the cystic space.

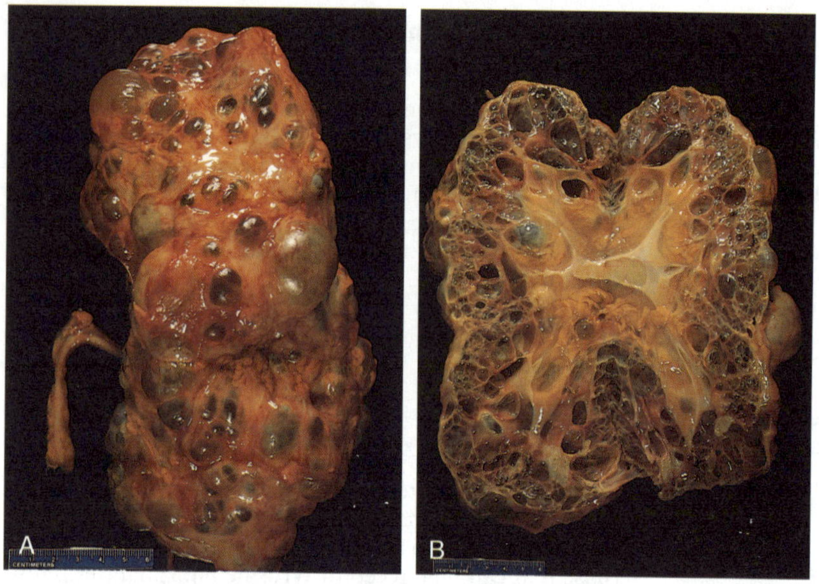

Figure 14–21

Autosomal dominant adult polycystic kidney, viewed from the external surface **(A)** and bisected **(B)**. The kidney is markedly enlarged (note the centimeter rule) with numerous dilated cysts.

The pressure of the expanding cysts leads to ischemic atrophy of the intervening renal substance. Evidence of superimposed hypertension or infection is common. Asymptomatic liver cysts occur in one-third of patients.

Clinical Course. Polycystic kidney disease in adults usually *does not produce symptoms until the fourth decade,* by which time the kidneys are quite large, although small cysts start to develop in adolescence. The most common presenting complaint is *flank pain* or a heavy, dragging sensation. Acute distention of a cyst, either by intracystic hemorrhage or by obstruction, may cause excruciating pain. Sometimes attention is first drawn to the lesion by palpation of an abdominal mass. *Intermittent gross hematuria* commonly occurs. The most important complications, because of their deleterious effect on already marginal renal function, are *hypertension and urinary infection.* Hypertension of varying severity develops in about 75% of persons with this disorder. Saccular aneurysms of the circle of Willis (Chapter 23) are present in 10% to 30% of patients, and these individuals have a high incidence of subarachnoid hemorrhage.

Although the disease is ultimately fatal, the outlook is generally better than with most chronic renal diseases. The condition tends to be relatively stable and progresses very slowly. End-stage renal failure occurs at about age 50, but there is wide variation in the course of this disorder, and nearly normal life spans are reported. Those who develop renal failure are treated by renal transplantation. Death usually results from uremia or hypertensive complications.

Autosomal Recessive (Childhood) Polycystic Kidney Disease

This rare developmental anomaly is genetically distinct from adult polycystic kidney disease, having autosomal recessive inheritance. It occurs in approximately 1 in 20,000 live births. Perinatal, neonatal, infantile, and juvenile subcategories have been defined, depending on time of presentation and the presence of associated hepatic lesions. All result from mutations in a gene *PKHD1,* coding for a putative membrane receptor protein called *fibrocystin,* localized to chromosome 6p. Fibrocystin may be involved in the function of cilia in tubular epithelial cells (see below).

Morphology

In autosomal recessive polycystic kidney disease, **numerous small cysts** in the cortex and medulla give the kidney a spongelike appearance. Dilated, elongated channels at right angles to the cortical surface completely replace the medulla and cortex. The cysts have a uniform lining of cuboidal cells, reflecting their origin from the collecting tubules. The disease is invariably bilateral. In almost all cases there are multiple epithelium-lined **cysts in the liver** as well as proliferation of portal bile ducts.

Clinical Course. Perinatal and neonatal forms are most common; serious manifestations are usually present at birth, and young infants may die quickly from hepatic or renal failure. Patients who survive infancy develop liver cirrhosis (congenital hepatic fibrosis).

Medullary Cystic Disease

There are two major types of medullary cystic disease: *medullary sponge kidney,* a relatively common and usually innocuous condition, which will not be discussed further, and *nephronophthisis-medullary cystic disease complex,* which is almost always associated with renal dysfunction.

Nephronophthisis-medullary cystic disease complex is an under-recognized cause of chronic kidney disease that usually begins in childhood. Four variants of this disease complex are recognized on the basis of the time of onset: infantile, juvenile, adolescent, and adult. The juvenile form is the most common. Approximately 15% to 20% of individuals with juvenile nephronophthisis have extrarenal manifestations, which most often appear as retinal abnormalities, including retinitis pigmentosa, but can extend to early blindness in their most severe form. Other abnormalities found in some persons include oculomotor apraxia, mental retardation, cerebellar malformations, and liver fibrosis. In aggregate, the various forms of nephronophthisis are now thought to be the most common genetic cause of end-stage renal disease in children and young adults.

Pathogenesis. At least seven gene loci have been identified for this complex, with both autosomal dominant and recessive modes of inheritance. Five genes, *NPHP1* through *NPHP5,* define the infantile, juvenile, and adolescent forms of nephronophthisis and cause autosomal recessive disease. The protein products of *NPHP1* and *NPHP3* through *NPHP5* (nephrocystins 1 and 3–5) have been identified as components of epithelial cell cilia, which in turn has led to a currently attractive hypothesis that ciliary dysfunction may underlie this and the other types of polycystic kidney disease. However, the normal functions of nephrocystins and their specific roles in disease pathogenesis are not clear. Two genes (*MCKD1* and *MCKD2*), with autosomal dominant transmission, cause medullary cystic disease in adult life.

Morphology

Pathologic features of medullary cystic disease include **small contracted kidneys.** Numerous small cysts lined by flattened or cuboidal epithelium are present, typically at the cortico-medullary junction. Other pathologic changes are nonspecific, but most notably they include a chronic tubulointerstital nephritis with tubular atrophy and thickened tubular basement membranes and progressive interstitial fibrosis.

Clinical Course. The initial manifestations are usually polyuria and polydipsia, a consequence of diminished tubular function. Progression to end-stage renal disease ensues over a 5- to 10-year period. The disease is difficult to diagnose, since there are no serologic markers and the cysts may be too small to be seen with radiologic imaging. Adding to this difficulty, cysts may not be apparent on renal biopsy if the cortico-medullary junction is not well sampled. A positive family history and unexplained chronic renal failure in young patients should lead to suspicion of medullary cystic disease.

SUMMARY

Cystic Diseases

- *Adult polycystic kidney disease* is an autosomal dominant disease caused by mutations in the genes encoding polycystin-1 or -2; it accounts for about 10% of cases of chronic renal failure; kidneys may be very large and contain many cysts.
- *Autosomal recessive (childhood) polycystic kidney disease* is caused by mutations in the gene encoding fibrocystin; it is less common than the adult form and strongly associated with liver abnormalities; kidneys contain numerous small cysts.
- *Medullary cystic disease* is being increasingly recognized as a cause of chronic renal failure in children and young adults; it has a complex inheritance, and is associated with mutations in several genes that encode epithelial cell proteins called nephrocystins that may be involved in ciliary function; kidneys are contracted and contain multiple small cysts.

URINARY OUTFLOW OBSTRUCTION

Renal Stones

Urolithiasis is calculus formation at any level in the urinary collecting system, but most often the calculi arise in the kidney. They occur frequently, as is evidenced by the finding of stones in about 1% of all autopsies. Symptomatic urolithiasis is more common in men than in women. A familial tendency toward stone formation has long been recognized.

Pathogenesis. About 80% of renal stones are composed of either calcium oxalate or calcium oxalate mixed with calcium phosphate. Another 10% are composed of magnesium ammonium phosphate, and 6% to 9% are either uric acid or cystine stones. In all cases, there is an organic matrix of mucoprotein that makes up about 2.5% of the stone by weight (Table 14–4).

The cause of stone formation is often obscure, particularly in the case of calcium-containing stones. Probably involved is a confluence of predisposing conditions. *The most important cause is increased urine concentration of the stone's constituents, so that it exceeds their solubility in urine (supersaturation).* As shown in Table 14–4, 50% of patients who develop *calcium stones* have hypercalciuria that is not associated with hypercalcemia. Most in this group absorb calcium from the gut in excessive amounts (absorptive hypercalciuria) and promptly

Table 14–4 Prevalence of Various Types of Renal Stones

Stone	Percentage of All Stones
Calcium Oxalate and/or Calcium Phosphate	**80**

Idiopathic hypercalciuria (50%)
Hypercalcemia and hypercalciuria (10%)
Hyperoxaluria (5%)
  Enteric (4.5%)
  Primary (0.5%)
Hyperuricosuria (20%)
No known metabolic abnormality (15% to 20%)	

Struvite (Mg, NH_3, Ca, PO_4)	**10**
Renal infection	
Uric Acid	**6–7**
Associated with hyperuricemia Associated with hyperuricosuria Idiopathic (50% of uric acid stones)	
Cystine	**1–2**
Others or Unknown	**±1–2**

excrete it in the urine, and some have a primary renal defect of calcium reabsorption (renal hypercalciuria). In 5% to 10% of persons with this diagnosis there is hypercalcemia (due to hyperparathyroidism, vitamin D intoxication, or sarcoidosis) and consequent hypercalciuria. In 20% of this subgroup, there is excessive excretion of uric acid in the urine, which favors calcium stone formation; presumably the urates provide a nidus for calcium deposition. In 5% there is hyperoxaluria or hypercitraturia, and in the remainder there is no known metabolic abnormality. A high urine pH favors crystallization of calcium phosphate and stone formation.

The causes of the other types of renal stones are better understood. *Magnesium ammonium phosphate (struvite) stones* almost always occur in persons with a persistently alkaline urine due to UTIs. In particular, the urea-splitting bacteria, such as *Proteus vulgaris* and the staphylococci, predispose the person to urolithiasis. Moreover, bacteria may serve as particulate nidi for the formation of any kind of stone. In avitaminosis A, desquamated cells from the metaplastic epithelium of the collecting system act as nidi.

Gout and diseases involving rapid cell turnover, such as the leukemias, lead to high uric acid levels in the urine and the possibility of *uric acid stones*. About half of the individuals with uric acid stones, however, have neither hyperuricemia nor increased urine urate but an unexplained tendency to excrete a persistently acid urine (under pH 5.5). This low pH favors uric acid stone formation—in contrast to the high pH that favors formation of stones containing calcium phosphate. *Cystine stones* are almost invariably associated with a genetically determined defect in the renal transport of certain amino acids, including cystine. In contrast to magnesium ammonium phosphate stones, both uric acid and cystine stones are more likely to form when the urine is relatively acidic.

Urolithiasis may also result from the lack of substances that normally inhibit mineral precipitation. Inhibitors of crystal formation in urine include Tamm-Horsfall protein, osteopontin, pyrophosphate, mucopolysaccharides, diphosphonates, and a glycoprotein called nephrocalcin, but no deficiency of any of these substances has been consistently demonstrated in individuals with urolithiasis.

Morphology

Stones are unilateral in about 80% of patients. Common sites of formation are renal pelves and calyces and the bladder. Often, many stones are found in one kidney. They tend to be small (average diameter 2–3 mm) and may be smooth or jagged. Occasionally, progressive accretion of salts leads to the development of branching structures known as **staghorn calculi,** which create a cast of the renal pelvis and calyceal system. These massive stones are usually composed of magnesium ammonium phosphate.

Clinical Course. Stones may be present without producing either symptoms or significant renal damage. This is particularly true with large stones lodged in the renal pelvis. Smaller stones may pass into the ureter, producing a typical intense pain known as *renal or ureteral colic,* characterized by paroxysms of flank pain radiating toward the groin. Often at this time there is *gross hematuria.* The clinical significance of stones lies in their capacity to obstruct urine flow or to produce sufficient trauma to cause ulceration and bleeding. In either case, they *predispose the sufferer to bacterial infection.* Fortunately, in most cases the diagnosis is readily made radiologically.

Hydronephrosis

Hydronephrosis refers to dilation of the renal pelvis and calyces, with accompanying atrophy of the parenchyma, caused by obstruction to the outflow of urine. The obstruction may be sudden or insidious, and it may occur at any level of the urinary tract, from the urethra to the renal pelvis. The most common causes are as follows:

- *Congenital:* Atresia of the urethra, valve formations in either ureter or urethra, aberrant renal artery compressing the ureter, renal ptosis with torsion, or kinking of the ureter
- *Acquired:*
  - Foreign bodies: Calculi, necrotic papillae
  - Tumors: Benign prostatic hyperplasia, carcinoma of the prostate, bladder tumors (papilloma and carcinoma), contiguous malignant disease (retroperitoneal lymphoma, carcinoma of the cervix or uterus)
  - Inflammation: Prostatitis, ureteritis, urethritis, retroperitoneal fibrosis
  - Neurogenic: Spinal cord damage with paralysis of the bladder
  - Normal pregnancy: Mild and reversible

Bilateral hydronephrosis occurs only when the obstruction is below the level of the ureters. If blockage is at the ureters or above, the lesion is unilateral. Sometimes obstruction is complete, allowing no urine to pass; usually it is only partial.

Pathogenesis. Even with complete obstruction, glomerular filtration persists for some time, and the filtrate subsequently diffuses back into the renal interstitium and perirenal spaces, whence it ultimately returns to the lymphatic and venous systems. Because of the continued filtration, the *affected calyces and pelvis become dilated,* often markedly so. The unusually high pressure thus generated in the renal pelvis, as well as that transmitted back through the collecting ducts, causes compression of the renal vasculature. Both arterial insufficiency and venous stasis result, although the latter is probably more important. The most severe effects are seen in the papillae, because they are subjected to the greatest increases in pressure. Accordingly, *the initial functional disturbances are largely tubular, manifested primarily by impaired concentrating ability.* Only later does glomerular filtration begin to diminish. Experimental studies indicate that serious irreversible damage occurs in about 3 weeks with complete obstruction, and in 3 months with incomplete obstruction. However, functional impairment can be demonstrated only a few hours after ureteral ligation. The obstruction also triggers an interstitial inflammatory reaction, leading eventually to interstitial fibrosis.

Morphology

Bilateral hydronephrosis (as well as unilateral hydronephrosis when the other kidney is already damaged or absent) leads to renal failure, and the onset of uremia tends to abort the natural course of the lesion. In contrast, **unilateral** involvements display the full range of morphologic changes, which vary with the degree and speed of obstruction. With subtotal or intermittent obstruction, the kidney may be massively enlarged (lengths in the range of 20 cm), and the organ may consist almost entirely of the greatly distended pelvicalyceal system. The renal parenchyma itself is compressed and atrophied, with obliteration of the papillae and flattening of the pyramids (Fig. 14–22). On the other hand, **when obstruction is sudden and complete, glomerular filtration is compromised relatively early, and as a consequence, renal function may cease while dilation is still comparatively slight**. Depending on the level of the obstruction, one or both ureters may also be dilated **(hydroureter).**

Microscopically the early lesions show tubular dilation, followed by atrophy and fibrous replacement of the tubular epithelium with relative sparing of the glomeruli. Eventually, in severe cases the glomeruli also become atrophic and disappear, converting the entire kidney into a thin shell of fibrous tissue. With sudden and complete obstruction, there may be coagulative necrosis of the renal papillae, similar to the changes of papillary necrosis. In uncomplicated cases the accompanying inflammatory reaction is minimal. Complicating pyelonephritis, however, is common.

Clinical Course. *Bilateral* complete obstruction produces anuria, which is soon brought to medical attention. When the obstruction is below the bladder, the dominant symptoms are those of bladder distention. Paradoxically, incomplete bilateral obstruction causes polyuria rather than oliguria, as a result of defects in tubular concentrating mechanisms, and this may obscure the true nature of the disturbance. Unfortunately, *unilateral* hydronephrosis may remain completely silent for long periods unless the other kidney is for some reason not functioning. Often the enlarged kidney is discovered on routine physical examination. Sometimes the basic cause of the hydronephrosis, such as renal calculi or an obstructing tumor, produces symptoms that indirectly draw attention to the hydronephrosis. Removal of obstruction within a few weeks usually permits full return of function; however, with time the changes become irreversible.

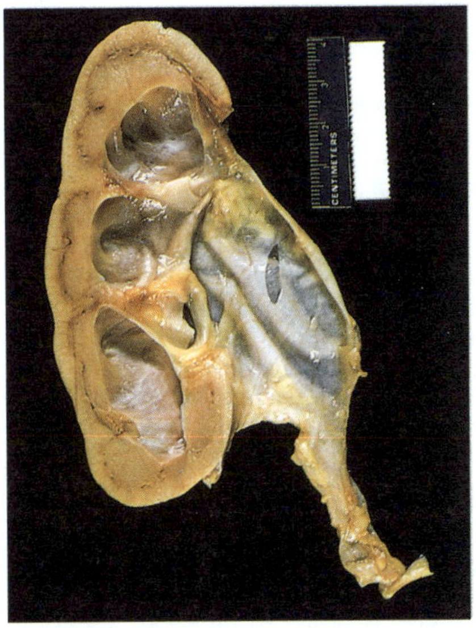

Figure 14–22

Hydronephrosis of the kidney, with marked dilation of the pelvis and calyces and thinning of renal parenchyma.

TUMORS

Many types of benign and malignant tumors occur in the urinary tract. In general, benign tumors such as small (<0.5 cm) cortical papillary adenomas or medullary fibromas (interstitial cell tumors) have no clinical significance. The most common malignant tumor of the kidney is renal cell carcinoma, followed in frequency by nephroblastoma (Wilms tumor) and by primary tumors of the calyces and pelvis. Other types of renal cancer are rare and need not be discussed here. *Tumors of the lower urinary tract are about twice as common as renal cell carcinomas.* They are described at the end of this section.

Renal Cell Carcinoma

These tumors are derived from the renal tubular epithelium, and hence they are located predominantly in the cortex. Renal carcinomas represent 80% to 85% of all primary malignant tumors of the kidney, and 2% to 3% of all cancers in adults. This translates into about 30,000 cases per year; 40% of patients die of the disease. Carcinomas of the kidney are most common from the sixth to seventh decades, and men are affected about twice as commonly as women. The risk of developing these tumors is higher in smokers, hypertensive or obese patients, and those who have had occupational exposure to cadmium. Smokers who are exposed to cadmium have a particularly high incidence of renal cell carcinomas. The risk of developing renal cell cancer is increased 30-fold in individuals who develop acquired polycystic disease as a complication of chronic dialysis. The role of genetic factors in the causation of these cancers is discussed below.

Renal cell cancers were formerly classified on the basis of morphology and growth patterns. However, recent advances in the understanding of the genetic basis of renal carcinomas have led to a new classification based on the molecular origins of these tumors. The three most common forms are as follows:

Clear Cell Carcinomas

These are the most common type, accounting for 70% to 80% of renal cell cancers. Histologically, they are made up of cells with clear or granular cytoplasm. Whereas the majority of them are sporadic, they also occur in familial forms or in association with von Hippel-Lindau (VHL) disease. It is the study of VHL disease that has provided molecular insights into the causation of clear cell carcinomas. VHL disease is autosomal dominant and is characterized by predisposition to a variety of neoplasms, but particularly to hemangioblastomas of the cerebellum and retina. Hundreds of bilateral renal cysts and bilateral, often multiple, clear cell carcinomas develop in 40% to 60% of individuals. Those with VHL syndrome inherit a germ-line mutation of the *VHL* gene on chromosome 3p25 and lose the second allele by somatic mutation. Thus, the loss of both copies of this tumor suppressor gene gives rise to clear cell carcinoma. The *VHL* gene is also involved in the majority of sporadic clear cell carcinomas. Cytogenetic abnormalities giving rise to loss of chromosomal segment 3p14 to 3p26 are often seen in sporadic renal cell cancers. This region harbors the *VHL* gene (3p25.3). The second, nondeleted allele is inactivated by a somatic mutation or hypermethylation in 60% of sporadic cases. Thus, homozygous loss of the *VHL* gene seems to be the common underlying molecular abnormality in both sporadic and familial forms of clear cell carcinomas. The VHL protein is involved in limiting the angiogenic response to hypoxia; thus, its absence may lead to increased angiogenesis and tumor growth (see Chapter 6). An uncommon familial form of clear cell carcinoma unrelated to VHL disease also involves cytogenetic abnormalities involving chromosome 3p.

Papillary Renal Cell Carcinomas

These comprise 10% to 15% of all renal cancers. As the name indicates, they show a papillary growth pattern. These tumors are frequently multifocal and bilateral and appear as early-stage tumors. Like clear cell carcinomas they occur in familial and sporadic forms, but unlike these tumors, papillary renal cancers have no abnormality of chromosome 3. The culprit in the case of papillary renal cell cancers is the *MET* proto-oncogene, located on chromosome 7q31. The *MET* gene is a tyrosine kinase receptor for the growth factor called hepatocyte growth factor. It is an increased gene dosage of the *MET* gene due to duplications of chromosome 7 that seems to spur abnormal growth in the proximal tubular epithelial cell precursors of papillary carcinomas. In keeping with this, trisomy of chromosome 7 is seen commonly in the familial cases. In these individuals, along with increased gene dosage there are activating mutations of the *MET* gene. By contrast, in sporadic cases there is duplication or trisomy of chromosome 7 but there is no mutation of the *MET* gene. Another chromosomal translocation, involving chromosome 8q24 close to the c-*MYC* gene, is also associated with some cases of papillary carcinoma.

Chromophobe Renal Carcinomas

These are the least common, representing 5% of all renal cell carcinomas. They arise from intercalated cells of collecting ducts. Their name denotes the observation that the tumor cells stain more darkly (i.e., they are less clear) than cells in clear cell carcinomas. These tumors are unique in having multiple losses of entire chromosomes, including chromosomes 1, 2, 6, 10, 13, 17, and 21. Thus, they show extreme hypodiploidy. Because of multiple losses, the "critical hit" has not been determined. In general, chromophobe renal cancers have a good prognosis.

Morphology

Clear cell cancers (the most common form) are usually solitary and large when symptomatic (spherical masses 3–15 cm in diameter), but increased use of high-resolution radiographic techniques for investigation of unrelated problems has led to the detection of even smaller lesions. They may arise anywhere in the cortex. The cut surface of clear cell renal cell carcinomas is **yellow to orange to gray-white, with prominent areas of cystic softening or of hemorrhage,** either fresh or old (Fig. 14–23). The margins of the tumor are well defined. However, at times small processes project into the surrounding parenchyma and small satellite nodules are found in the surrounding substance, providing clear evidence of the aggressiveness of these lesions. As the tumor enlarges, it may fungate through the walls of the collecting system, extending through the calyces and pelvis as far as the ureter. Even more frequently, the **tumor invades the renal vein** and grows as a solid column within this vessel, sometimes extending in serpentine fashion as far as the inferior vena cava and even into the right side of the heart. Occasionally, there is direct invasion into the perinephric fat and adrenal gland.

Depending on the amounts of lipid and glycogen present, **the tumor cells of clear cell renal cell carcinoma may appear almost vacuolated or may be solid.** The classic vacuolated (lipid-laden), or clear cells are demarcated only by their cell membranes. The nuclei are usually small and round (Fig. 14–24). At the other extreme are granular cells, resembling the tubular epithelium, which have small, round, regular nuclei enclosed within granular pink cytoplasm. Some tumors exhibit marked degrees of anaplasia, with numerous mitotic figures and markedly enlarged, hyperchromatic, pleomorphic nuclei. Between the extremes of clear cells and solid, granular cells, all intergradations may be found. The cellular arrangement, too, varies widely. The cells may form abortive tubules or may cluster in cords or disorganized masses. The stroma is usually scant but highly vascularized.

Papillary renal cell carcinomas exhibit varying degrees of papilla formation with fibrovascular cores. They tend to be bilateral and multiple. They may also show gross evidence of necrosis, hemorrhage, and cystic degeneration, but they are less vibrantly orange-yellow because of their lower lipid content. The cells can have clear or, more commonly, pink cytoplasm. **Chromophobe-type renal cell carcinoma** tends to be grossly tan-brown. The cells usually have clear, flocculent cytoplasm with very prominent, distinct cell membranes. The nuclei are surrounded by halos of cleared cytoplasm. Ultrastructurally, large numbers of characteristic macrovesicles are seen.

Clinical Course. Renal cell carcinomas have several peculiar clinical characteristics that create especially difficult and challenging diagnostic problems. The symptoms vary, but the *most frequent presenting manifestation is hematuria, occurring in more than 50% of cases.* Macro-

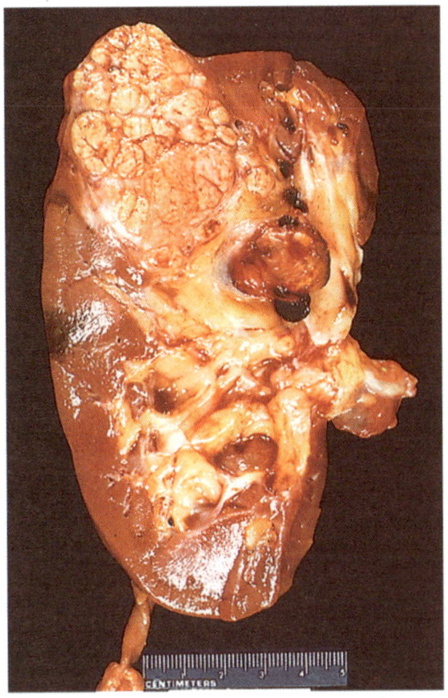

Figure 14–23

Renal cell carcinoma: typical cross-section of yellowish, spherical neoplasm in one pole of the kidney. Note the tumor in the dilated, thrombosed renal vein.

scopic hematuria tends to be intermittent and fleeting, superimposed on a steady microscopic hematuria. Less commonly (because of wide use of imaging studies for unrelated conditions), the tumor may declare itself simply by virtue of its size, when it has grown large enough to produce flank pain and a *palpable mass*. Extra-renal effects are *fever* and *polycythemia*, both of which may be associated with a renal cell carcinoma but which, because they are nonspecific, may be misinterpreted for some time before their true significance is appreciated. Polycythemia affects 5% to 10% of persons with this disease. It results from elaboration of erythropoietin by the renal tumor. Uncommonly, these tumors produce a variety of hormone-like substances, resulting in hypercalcemia, hypertension, Cushing syndrome, or feminization or masculinization. These, as will be recalled from Chapter 6, are *paraneoplastic syndromes*. In many individuals the primary tumor remains silent and is discovered only after its metastases have produced symptoms. The prevalent locations for metastases are the lungs and the bones. It must be apparent that renal cell carcinoma presents in many fashions, some quite devious, *but the triad of painless hematuria, a palpable abdominal mass, and dull flank pain is characteristic.*

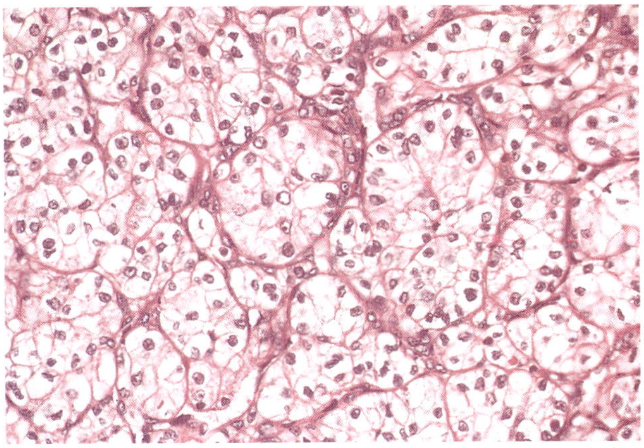

Figure 14–24

High-power detail of the clear cell pattern of renal cell carcinoma.

Wilms Tumor

Although Wilms tumor occurs infrequently in adults, it is the third most common organ cancer in children younger than the age of 10 years. It is therefore one of the major cancers of children. These tumors contain a variety of cell and tissue components, all derived from the mesoderm. Wilms tumor, like retinoblastoma, may arise sporadically or be familial, with the susceptibility to tumorigenesis inherited as an autosomal dominant trait. This tumor is discussed in greater detail in Chapter 7 along with other tumors of childhood.

SUMMARY

Renal Cell Carcinoma

- Renal cell carcinomas account for 2–3% of all cancers in adults; classified into three types.
  - *Clear cell carcinomas* are the most common; associated with homozygous loss of the VHL tumor suppressor protein; tumors frequently invade the renal vein.
  - *Papillary renal cell carcinomas* are frequently associated with increased expression and activating mutations of the *MET* oncogene; tend to be bilateral and multiple, and show varying papilla formation.
  - *Chromophobe renal cell carcinomas* are less common; tumor cells are not as clear as in the other renal cell carcinomas.

Tumors of the Urinary Bladder and Collecting System (Renal Calyces, Renal Pelvis, Ureter, and Urethra)

The entire urinary collecting system from renal pelvis to urethra is lined with transitional epithelium, so its epithelial tumors assume similar morphologic patterns. Tumors in the collecting system above the bladder are relatively uncommon; those in the bladder, however, are an even more frequent cause of death than are kidney tumors. Nevertheless, in the individual case a small lesion in the ureter, for example, may cause urinary outflow obstruction and have greater clinical significance than a much larger mass in the capacious bladder. We consider first the range of histologic patterns *as they occur in the urinary bladder* and then their clinical implications.

Morphology

Tumors arising in the urinary bladder range from small benign papillomas to large invasive cancers (Fig. 14–25). These tumors are classified into a rare benign papilloma, a group of papillary urothelial neoplasms of low malignant potential, and two grades of urothelial carcinoma (low and high grade).

The very rare benign **papillomas** are 0.2- to 1.0-cm frondlike structures having a delicate fibrovascular core covered by multilayered, well-differentiated transitional epithelium. In some of these lesions, the covering epithelium appears as normal as the mucosal surface from whence the tumors arose. Such lesions are usually solitary. They almost invariably noninvasive and benign, and they rarely recur once removed.

Urothelial (transitional) cell carcinomas range from papillary to flat, noninvasive to invasive, and low grade to high grade. Low-grade carcinomas (Fig. 14–26) are always papillary and are rarely invasive, but they may recur after removal. Whether the regrowth is a true recurrence or a second primary growth is uncertain. Increasing degrees of cellular atypia and anaplasia are encountered in papillary exophytic growths, accompanied by an increase in the size of the lesion and evidence of invasion of the submucosal or muscular layers. High-grade cancers can be papillary or occasionally flat; they may cover larger areas of the mucosal surface, invade deeper, and have a shaggier necrotic surface than do low-grade tumors. Occasionally, these cancers show foci of squamous cell differentiation, but only 5% of bladder cancers are true **squamous cell carcinomas.** Carcinomas of grades II and III infiltrate surrounding structures, spread to regional nodes, and, on occasion, metastasize widely.

In addition to overt carcinoma, an **in situ stage of bladder carcinoma** can be recognized, often in individuals with previous or simultaneous papillary or invasive tumors. Indeed, wide areas of atypical hyperplasia and dysplasia may be present. It is now thought that these epithelial changes and cancers in situ are caused by the generalized influence of a putative carcinogen on urothelium and that they may be the precursors of invasive carcinomas in some persons. However, despite the presence of wide areas of epithelial lesions, the bladder tumors, even when multiple, are monoclonal in origin. Apparently, clonal descendants of a single transformed cell can seed multiple areas of the mucosa.

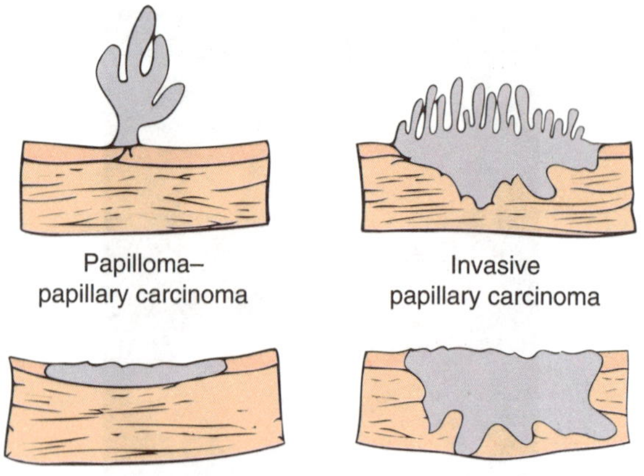

Figure 14–25

Four morphologic patterns of bladder tumor.

Clinical Course. *Painless hematuria is the dominant clinical presentation* of all these tumors. Because most arise in the bladder, we will consider these first. They affect men about three times as frequently as women and usually develop between the ages of 50 and 70 years. Although most occur in persons with no known history of exposure to industrial solvents, bladder tumors are 50 times more common in those exposed to β-naphthylamine. Cigarette smoking, chronic cystitis, schistosomiasis of the bladder, and certain drugs (cyclophosphamide) are also believed to induce higher rates of this cancer. A wide variety of genetic abnormalities are seen in bladder cancers; of these, mutations involving several genes on chromosome 9 (including p16), p53, and FGFR3 are the most common.

The clinical significance of bladder tumors depends on their histologic grade and differentiation and, most importantly, on the depth of invasion of the lesion. Except for the clearly benign papillomas, all tend stubbornly to recur after removal. Lesions that invade the ureteral or urethral orifices cause urinary tract obstruction. In general, with low-grade shallow lesions, the prognosis after removal is good, but when deep penetration of the bladder wall has occurred, the 5-year survival rate is less than 20%. Overall 5-year survival is 57%.

Although papillary and cancerous neoplasms of the lining epithelium of the collecting system occur much less frequently in the renal pelvis than in the bladder, they nonetheless make up 5% to 10% of primary renal tumors. Painless hematuria is the most characteristic feature of these lesions, but in their critical location they produce pain in the costovertebral angle as hydronephrosis develops. Infiltration of the walls of the pelvis, calyces, and renal vein worsens the prognosis. Despite removal of

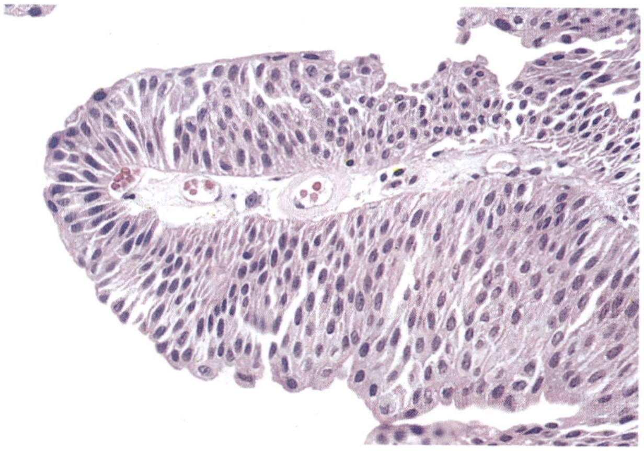

Figure 14–26

Low-grade papillary urothelial carcinoma of the bladder. The delicate papilla is covered by orderly transitional epithelium.

the tumor by nephrectomy, fewer than 50% of patients survive for 5 years. Cancer of the ureter is fortunately the rarest of the tumors of the collecting system. The 5-year survival rate is less than 10%.

BIBLIOGRAPHY

Appel GB, et al: Membranoproliferative glomerulonephritis type II (dense deposit disease): an update. J Am Soc Nephrol 16:1392, 2005. *[A comprehensive review of the pathophysiology, pathology, and clinical manifestations of this disease.]*

Barratt J, Feehally J: IgA nephropathy. J Am Soc Nephrol 16:2088, 2005. *[A comprehensive update on the pathogenesis, clinical manifestations and treatment of this disease.]*

Cattran DC: Idiopathic membranous glomerulonephritis. Kidney Int 59:1983, 2001. *[A clinically oriented review of diagnosis and management of this disease.]*

Coe FL, et al: Kidney stone disease. J Clin Invest 115:2598, 2005. *[A detailed discussion of cases of renal stones.]*

Cohen HT, Mc Govern FJ: Renal-cell carcinoma. N Engl J Med 353:2477, 2005. *[An excellent review of the genetic basis for renal cell carcinoma.]*

Fored CM, et al: Acetaminophen, aspirin, and chronic renal failure. N Engl J Med 345:1801, 2001. *[An important paper that analyzes the factors underlying analgesic nephropathy.]*

Grimbert P, et al: Recent approaches to the pathogenesis of minimal change nephrotic syndrome. Nephrol Dial Transplant 18:245, 2005. *[A paper that focuses on the evidence for an immune etiology of minimal-change disease.]*

Guay-Woodford LM: Renal cystic diseases: diverse phenotypes converge on the cilium/centrosome complex. Pediatr Nephrol 21:1369, 2006. *[An excellent review on the pathophysiology of renal cystic diseases, with emphasis on the role of ciliary dysfunction in tubular epithelial cells.]*

Hudson BG, et al: Alport's syndrome, Goodpasture's syndrome, and type IV collagen. N Engl J Med 348:2543, 2003. *[An insightful review by major investigators in the area, of renal basement membrane composition and its role in the pathogenesis of two different but linked renal diseases.]*

Jennette JC: Rapidly progressive crescentic glomerulonephritis. Kidney Int 63:1164, 2003. *[An excellent discussion of the differential diagnosis and pathogenesis of rapidly progressive glomerulonephritis.]*

Knowles MA: Molecular subtypes of bladder cancer: Jekyll and Hyde or chalk and cheese. Carcinogenesis 27:371, 2006. *[Comprehensive review of molecular changes in different types of bladder cancer.]*

Manthey DE, Teichman J: Nephrolithiasis. Emerg Med Clin North Am 19:633, 2001. *[A clinically oriented review of renal stones.]*

Miller O, Hemphill RR: Urinary tract infection and pyelonephritis. Emerg Med Clin North Am 19:655, 2001. *[An excellent review of acute urinary tract infections.]*

Pavenstadt H, et al: Cell biology of the glomerular podocyte. Physiol Rev 83:253, 2003. *[A comprehensive review of the structure and function of podocytes and the slit diaphragm and the basis for the nephrotic syndrome.]*

Piccoli G, et al: Acute pyelonephritis: a new approach to an old clinical entity. J Nephrol 18:474, 2005. *[A clinically oriented update on diagnosis and management of pyelonephritis.]*

Pollack MR: The genetic basis of FSGS and steroid-resistant nephrosis. Semin Nephrol 23:141, 2003. *[A discussion of the rapidly evolving field of genetic mutations that lead to FSGS and the nephrotic syndrome.]*

Reuter VE, Prestic JC: Contemporary approach to the classification of renal epithelial tumors. Semin Oncol 27:124, 2000. *[A nice discussion of morphology, clinical features, and genetic attributes of renal cell cancer.]*

Schrier RW, et al: Acute renal failure: definitions, diagnosis, pathogenesis, and therapy. J Clin Invest 114:5, 2004. *[An insightful review covering all aspects of acute renal failure.]*

Tryggvason K, Patrakka J, Wartiovaava J: Hereditary proteinuria syndromes and mechanisms of proteinuria. New Engl J Med 354:1387, 2006. *[An excellent review of the pathophysiology of defects in glomerular permeability.]*

Tsai HM: The molecular biology of thrombotic microangiopathy. Kidney Int 70:16, 2006. *[An excellent review of the pathogenesis of HUS and TTP.]*

Wilson PD: Polycystic kidney disease. N Engl J Med 350:151, 2004. *[A review emphasizing the molecular and structural biology underlying the development of polycystic kidney disease.]*

Wilson PD, Goilav B: Cystic disease of the kidney. Annual Review of Pathology: Mechanisms of Disease, Vol. 2:341, 2007. *[Pathobiology of a common condition affecting the kidney.]*

Chapter 15

The Oral Cavity and the Gastrointestinal Tract*

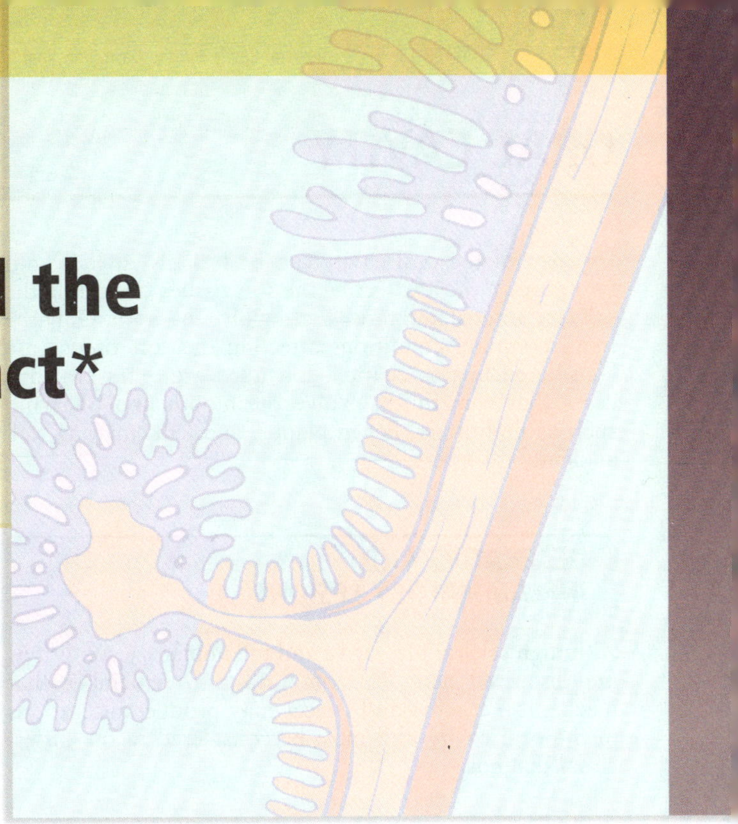

*The contributions of Dr. James M. Crawford to this chapter in previous editions are greatly appreciated.

ORAL CAVITY

Diseases of the oral cavity can be broadly divided into two groups: those affecting the soft tissues (including the salivary glands) and those that involve the teeth. Only the more common conditions affecting the soft tissues are considered in this chapter. Excluded are extra-oral diseases that sometimes involve the mouth and pharynx, such as diphtheria, lichen planus, and leukemia, as well as dental disorders.

ULCERATIVE AND INFLAMMATORY LESIONS

Although several ulcerative and inflammatory conditions are discussed here, it is important to remember that mechanical trauma and cancer may produce ulcerations in the oral cavity and must be considered in the differential diagnosis.

Aphthous Ulcers (Canker Sores)

These lesions are extremely common, small (usually <5 mm in diameter), painful, shallow ulcers. Characteristically, they take the form of rounded, superficial erosions, often covered with a gray-white exudate and having an erythematous rim. The lesions appear singly or in groups on the nonkeratinized oral mucosa, particularly the soft palate, buccolabial mucosa, floor of the mouth, and lateral borders of the tongue. They are more common in the first 2 decades of life and are often triggered by stress, fever, ingestion of certain foods, and activation of inflammatory bowel disease. In patients who are not immunosuppressed or do not have known viral infection such as with herpesvirus, an autoimmune basis is suspected. The canker sores are self-limited and usually resolve within a few weeks, but they may recur in the same or a different location in the oral cavity.

Herpesvirus Infection

Herpetic stomatitis is an extremely common infection caused by herpes simplex virus (HSV) type 1. The pathogen is transmitted from person to person, most often by kissing; by middle life over three-fourths of the population have been infected. In most adults the primary infection is asymptomatic, but the virus persists in a dormant state within ganglia about the mouth (e.g., trigeminal ganglia). With reactivation of the virus (which may be caused by fever, sun or cold exposure, respiratory tract infection, trauma), solitary or multiple small (<5 mm in diameter) vesicles containing clear fluid appear. They occur most often on the lips or about the nasal orifices and are well known as *cold sores* or *fever blisters*. They soon rupture, leaving shallow, painful ulcers that heal within a few weeks, but recurrences are common.

Morphology

The vesicles begin as an intraepithelial focus of intercellular and intracellular edema. The infected cells become ballooned and develop **intranuclear acidophilic viral inclusions.** Sometimes adjacent cells fuse to form giant cells known as **multinucleated polykaryons.** Necrosis of the infected cells and the focal collections of edema fluid account for the intraepithelial vesicles detected clinically (Fig. 15–1). Identification of the inclusion-bearing cells or polykaryons in smears of blister fluid constitutes the diagnostic *Tzanck test* for HSV infection.

Antiviral agents may accelerate healing of the lesions. In 10% to 20% of those with this condition—particularly in the immunocompromised—a more virulent disseminated eruption develops, producing multiple vesicles throughout the oral cavity, including the gingiva and pharynx (*herpetic gingivostomatitis*), and lymphadenopathy. In particularly severe cases, viremia may

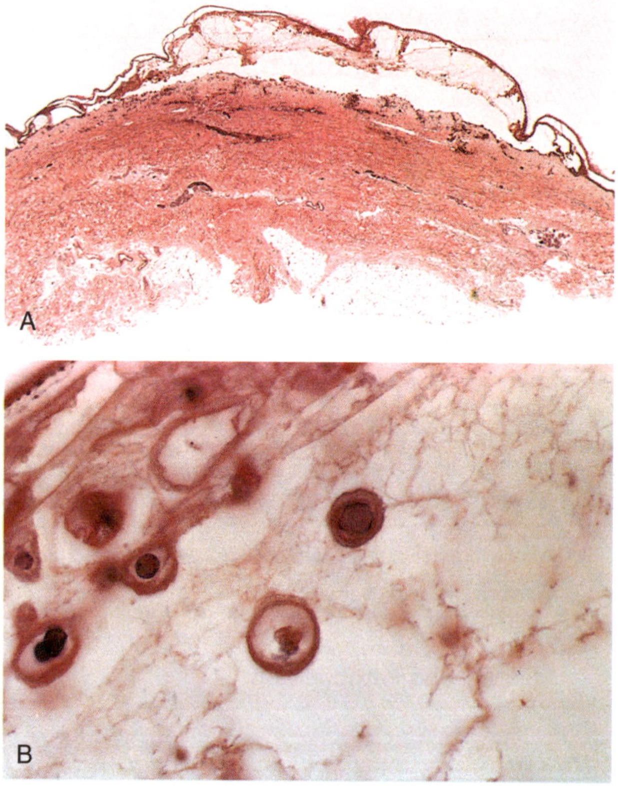

Figure 15–1

Herpesvirus pharyngitis. **A,** Herpesvirus blister in mucosa. **B,** High-power view of cells from blister in **A,** showing glassy intranuclear herpes simplex inclusion bodies.

seed the brain (causing encephalitis) or produce disseminated visceral lesions. HSV type 1 may localize in many other sites, including the conjunctivae (keratoconjunctivitis) and the esophagus when a nasogastric tube is introduced through an infected oral cavity. As a result of changes in sexual practices, genital herpes produced by HSV type 2 (the agent of *herpes genitalis*) is increasingly seen in the oral cavity. The infection produces vesicles in the mouth, which have the same histologic characteristics as those that develop on the genital mucous membranes and external genitalia.

Oral Candidiasis

Candida albicans is a normal inhabitant of the oral cavity found in 30% to 40% of the population; it causes disease only when there is some impairment of the usual protective mechanisms. *Pseudomembranous candidiasis (thrush, moniliasis)* is the most common fungal infection of the oral cavity and is particularly common among persons rendered vulnerable by diabetes mellitus, anemia, antibiotic or glucocorticoid therapy, immunodeficiency, or debilitating illnesses such as disseminated cancer. Persons with the acquired immunodeficiency syndrome (AIDS) are at particular risk.

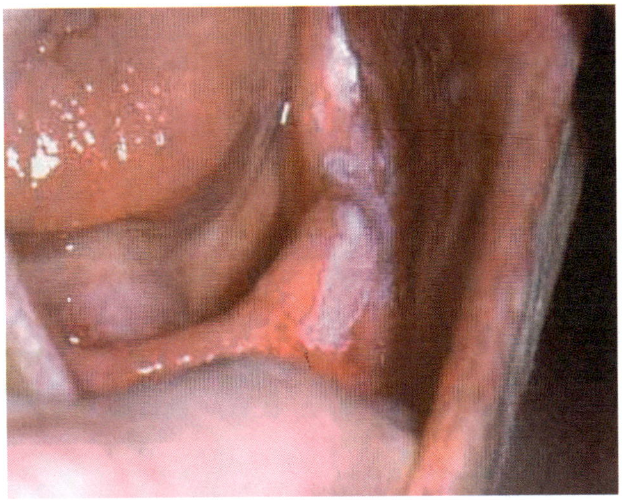

Figure 15–2

Oral candidiasis ("thrush"). A white plaquelike membrane coats the gingival mucosa of the left lower jaw. This pseudomembrane is composed of a layer of candidal pseudohyphae. (Courtesy of Dr. Harvey P. Kessler, Department of Oral Surgery, College of Dentistry, University of Florida, Gainesville, Florida.)

Morphology

Typically, **oral candidiasis takes the form of an adherent white, curdlike, circumscribed plaque anywhere within the oral cavity** (Fig. 15–2). The pseudomembrane can be scraped off to reveal an underlying granular erythematous inflammatory base. Histologically, the pseudomembrane is composed of a myriad of fungal organisms superficially attached to the underlying mucosa. In milder infections there is minimal ulceration, but in severe cases the entire mucosa may be denuded. The fungi can be identified within these pseudomembranes as boxcar-like chains of tubular cells producing pseudohyphae from which bud ovoid yeast forms, typically 2 to 4 μm in greatest diameter.

In the particularly vulnerable host, candidiasis may spread into the esophagus, especially when a nasogastric tube has been introduced, or it may produce widespread visceral lesions when the fungus gains entry into the bloodstream. Disseminated candidiasis is a life-threatening infection that must be treated aggressively. For poorly understood reasons, local candidal lesions may appear in the vagina, not only in predisposed females but also in apparently healthy young women, particularly during pregnancy, or in women who are using oral contraceptives or broad-spectrum antibiotics.

AIDS and Kaposi Sarcoma

AIDS and less advanced forms of human immune deficiency virus (HIV) infection are often associated with lesions in the oral cavity. They may take the form of candidiasis, herpetic vesicles, or some other microbial infection (producing gingivitis or glossitis). *Hairy leukoplakia* is an uncommon lesion seen virtually only in persons infected with HIV. It consists of white confluent patches, anywhere on the oral mucosa, that have a "hairy" or corrugated surface resulting from marked epithelial thickening. It is caused by Epstein-Barr virus infection of epithelial cells. Occasionally, the development of hairy leukoplakia calls attention to the existence of the underlying HIV infection.

More than 50% of individuals with *Kaposi sarcoma* (see Chapter 10) develop intraoral purpuric discolorations or violaceous, raised, nodular masses; sometimes this involvement constitutes the presenting manifestation.

LEUKOPLAKIA AND ERYTHROPLAKIA

As generally used, the term *leukoplakia refers to a whitish, well-defined mucosal patch or plaque caused by epidermal thickening or hyperkeratosis*. As defined by the World Health Organization, leukoplakia is a white patch or plaque that can not be scraped off and cannot be characterized as any other disease. Thus, the term is not applied to other white lesions, such as those caused by candidiasis, lichen planus, or many other disorders.

The plaques are more frequent among older men and are most often on the vermilion border of the lower lip, buccal mucosa, the hard and soft palates, and less frequently on the floor of the mouth and other intraoral sites. They appear as localized, sometimes multifocal or even diffuse, smooth or roughened, leathery, white, discrete areas of mucosal thickening. On microscopic evaluation they vary from banal hyperkeratosis without underlying epithelial dysplasia to mild to severe dysplasia bordering on carcinoma in situ (Fig. 15–3). Only histologic evaluation distinguishes these lesions. The lesions

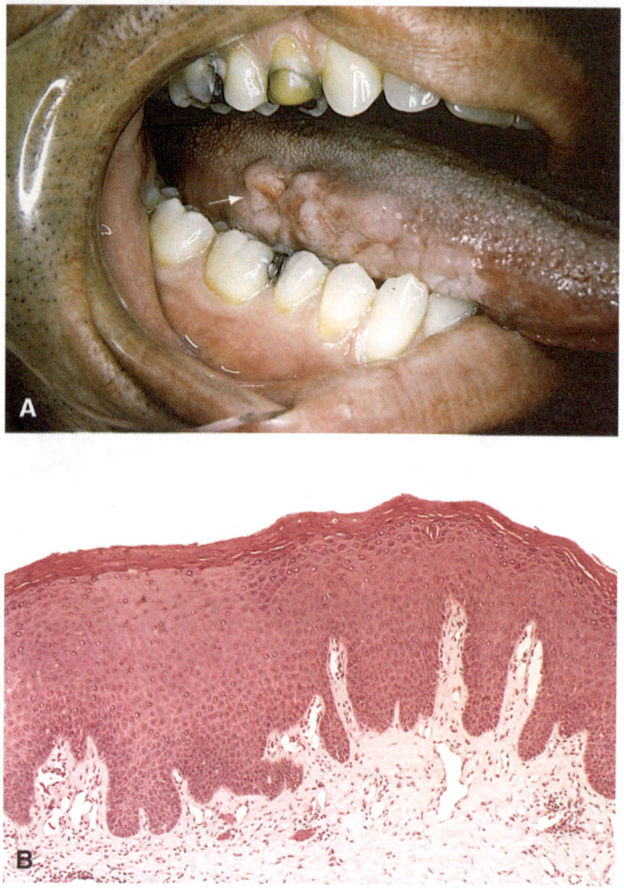

Figure 15–3

A, Leukoplakia of the tongue in a smoker. Microscopically, this lesion showed severe dysplasia with transformation to squamous cell carcinoma in the posterior elevated portion (*arrow*). **B,** Leukoplakia with marked epithelial thickening and hyperkeratosis.

are of unknown cause except that there is a *strong association with the use of tobacco*, particularly pipe smoking and smokeless tobacco (pouches, snuff, chewing). Less strongly implicated are *chronic friction*, as from ill-fitting dentures or jagged teeth; *alcohol abuse*; and irritant foods. More recently, human papillomavirus antigen has been identified in some tobacco-related lesions, raising the possibility that the virus and tobacco act in concert in the induction of these lesions.

Oral leukoplakia is an important finding because 3% to 25% (depending somewhat on location) undergo transformation to squamous cell carcinoma (see Fig. 15–3A). It is impossible to distinguish the innocent lesion from the ominous one on visual inspection. The transformation rate is greatest with lip and tongue lesions and lowest with those on the floor of the mouth. Those lesions that display significant dysplasia on microscopic examination have a greater probability of cancerous transformation.

Three somewhat related lesions must be differentiated from the usual oral leukoplakia. Hairy leukoplakia, described earlier and seen virtually only in persons with AIDS, has a corrugated or "hairy" surface rather than the white, opaque thickening of oral leukoplakia and has not been related to the development of oral cancer. *Verrucous leukoplakia* shows a corrugated surface caused by excessive hyperkeratosis. This seemingly innocuous form of leukoplakia recurs and insidiously spreads over time, resulting in a diffuse warty-type of oral lesion that may yet harbor squamous cell carcinoma. *Erythroplakia* refers to red, velvety, often granular, circumscribed areas that may or may not be elevated, having poorly defined, irregular boundaries. Histologically, erythroplakia almost invariably reveals marked epithelial dysplasia (the malignant transformation rate is >50%), so recognition of this lesion becomes even more important than identification of oral leukoplakia.

CANCERS OF THE ORAL CAVITY AND TONGUE

The overwhelming preponderance of oral cavity cancers are squamous cell carcinomas. Although they represent only about 3% of all cancers in the United States, they are disproportionately important clinically. Almost all are readily accessible to biopsy and early identification, but about half result in death within 5 years and indeed may have already metastasized by the time the primary lesion is discovered. These cancers tend to occur late in life and rarely before the age of 40 years. The various influences thought to be important in development of these cancers are summarized in Table 15–1.

Clinical Features. These lesions may cause local pain or difficulty in chewing, but many are relatively asymptomatic and so the lesion (very familiar to the exploring tongue) is ignored. As a result, a significant number are not discovered until beyond cure. The overall 5-year survival rates after surgery and adjuvant radiation and chemotherapy are about 40% for cancers of the base of the tongue, pharynx, and floor of the mouth without lymph node metastasis, compared with less than 20% for those with lymph node metastasis. When these cancers are discovered at an early stage, 5-year survival can exceed 90%.

Table 15–1 Risk Factors for Oral Cancer

Factor	Comments
Leukoplakia, erythroplakia	Risk of transformation in leukoplakia 3% to 25%
	More than 50% risk in erythroplakia
Tobacco use	Best-established influence, particularly pipe smoking and smokeless tobacco
Human papillomavirus types 16 and 18	Identified by molecular probes in 30% to 50% of cases; probably have a role in a subset of cases
Alcohol abuse	Weaker influence than tobacco use, but the two habits interact to greatly increase risk
Protracted irritation	Weakly associated

Morphology

The three predominant sites of origin of oral cavity carcinomas are (in order of frequency) the (1) vermilion border of the lateral margins of the lower lip, (2) floor of the mouth, and (3) lateral borders of the mobile tongue. Early lesions appear as pearly white to gray, circumscribed thickenings of the mucosa closely resembling leukoplakic patches. They then may grow in an exophytic fashion to produce readily visible and palpable nodular and eventually fungating lesions, or they may assume an endophytic, invasive pattern with central necrosis to create a cancerous ulcer. The squamous cell carcinomas are usually moderately to well-differentiated keratinizing tumors (Fig. 15–4). Before the lesions become advanced it may be possible to identify epithelial atypia, dysplasia, or carcinoma in situ in the margins, suggesting origin from leukoplakia or erythroplakia. Spread to regional nodes is present at the time of initial diagnosis only rarely with lip cancer, in about 50% of cases of tongue cancer, and in more than 60% of those with cancer of the floor of the mouth. More remote spread to tissues or organs in the thorax or abdomen is less common than extensive regional spread.

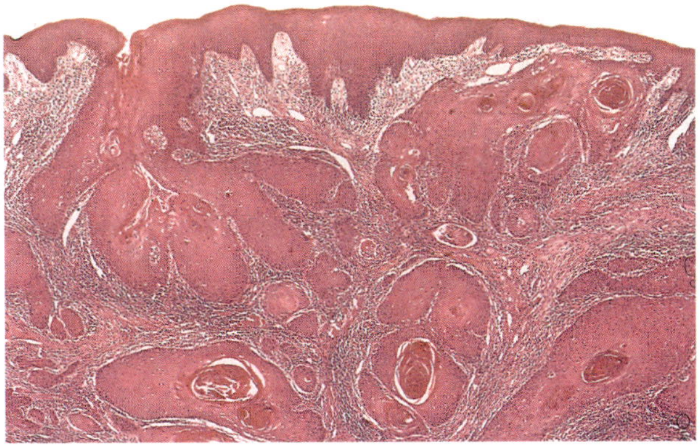

Figure 15–4

Oral squamous cell carcinoma. Invasive tumor islands show formation of keratin pearls.

SUMMARY

Diseases of the Oral Cavity

- *Aphthous ulcers* are painful superficial ulcers of unknown etiology that are often triggered by stress.
- *Herpes simplex virus infection* causes a usually self-limited infection with vesicles (cold sores, fever blisters) that typically rupture and heal but may leave latent virus in nerve ganglia.
- Oral *Candida infection* is seen in immunosuppressed individuals and manifests as a plaque; fungal dissemination is a potentially serious outcome.
- *Leukoplakia* is a mucosal plaque caused by epidermal thickening; depending on the location 3% to 25% may progress to squamous cell carcinoma.
- The majority of oral cancers are *squamous cell carcinomas.*

SALIVARY GLAND DISEASES

Although diseases primary to the major salivary glands are in general uncommon, the parotids bear the brunt of these involvements. Among the many possible disorders, attention is restricted here to sialadenitis and salivary gland tumors.

Sialadenitis

Inflammation of the major salivary glands may be of traumatic, viral, bacterial, or autoimmune origin. The most common lesion of the salivary glands is *mucocele*, resulting from blockage or rupture of a salivary gland duct, with consequent leakage of saliva into the surrounding tissues. Mucoceles are most often found in the lower lip, as a consequence of trauma. Dominant among other causations of sialadenitis is the infectious viral disease *mumps*, which may produce enlargement of all the major salivary glands but predominantly the parotids. Although several viruses may cause mumps, the most important cause is a paramyxovirus, an RNA virus related to the influenza and parainfluenza viruses. It usually produces a diffuse, interstitial inflammation marked by edema and a mononuclear cell infiltration and, sometimes, by focal necrosis. Although childhood mumps is self-limited and rarely creates residual problems, mumps in adults may be accompanied by pancreatitis or orchitis; the latter sometimes causes permanent sterility.

Bacterial sialadenitis most often occurs secondary to ductal obstruction resulting from stone formation (*sialolithiasis*), but it may also arise after retrograde entry of oral cavity bacteria under conditions of severe systemic dehydration such as the postoperative state. The most common bacteria causing the infection are *Staphylococcus aureus* and *Streptococcus viridans*. Persons with chronic, debilitating medical conditions, compromised immune function, or on medications contributing to oral or systemic dehydration are at increased risk for acute bacterial sialadenitis. The sialadenitis may be largely interstitial, or it may cause focal areas of suppurative necrosis or even abscess formation.

Chronic sialadenitis arises from decreased production of saliva with subsequent inflammation. The dominant cause is *autoimmune sialadenitis*, which is almost invariably bilateral. This is seen in Sjögren syndrome, discussed in Chapter 5. All of the salivary glands (major and minor), as well as the lacrimal glands, may be affected in this disorder, which presents with dry mouth (*xerostomia*) and dry eyes (*keratoconjunctivitis sicca*). The combination of salivary and lacrimal gland inflammatory enlargement, which is usually painless, and xerostomia, whatever the cause, is sometimes referred to as *Mikulicz syndrome*. The causes include sarcoidosis, leukemia, lymphoma, and idiopathic lymphoepithelial hyperplasia.

Salivary Gland Tumors

The salivary glands give rise to a diversity of tumors. About 80% of tumors occur within the parotid glands and most of the others in the submandibular glands. Males and females are affected about equally, usually in the sixth or seventh decade of life. In the parotids 70% to 80% of these tumors are benign, whereas in the submaxillary glands only half are benign. Thus, it is evident that *a neoplasm in the submaxillary glands is more ominous than one in the parotids*. The dominant tumor arising in the parotids is the benign *pleomorphic adenoma*, which is sometimes called a mixed tumor of salivary gland origin. Much less frequent is the *papillary cystadenoma lymphomatosum (Warthin tumor)*. Collectively, these two types account for three-fourths of parotid tumors. Whatever the type, they present clinically as a mass causing a swelling at the angle of the jaw. The most *malignant tumor of the salivary gland is mucoepidermoid carcinoma*, which occurs mainly in the parotids. When primary or recurrent benign tumors are present for many (10–20) years, malignant transformation may occur, referred to then as a *malignant mixed* salivary gland tumor. Malignancy is less common in the parotid gland (15%) than in the submandibular glands (40%). Only the benign pleomorphic adenoma and Warthin tumor are sufficiently common to merit description.

Pleomorphic Adenoma (Mixed Tumor of Salivary Glands). This tumor accounts for more than 90% of benign tumors of the salivary glands. It is a slow-growing, well-demarcated, apparently encapsulated lesion rarely exceeding 6 cm in greatest dimension. Most often arising in the superficial parotid, it usually causes painless swelling at the angle of the jaw and can be readily palpated as a discrete mass. It is nonetheless often present for years before being brought to medical attention. Despite the tumor's encapsulation, histologic examination often reveals multiple sites where the tumor penetrates the capsule. Adequate margins of resection are thus necessary to prevent recurrences. This may require sacrifice of the facial nerve, which courses through the parotid gland. On average, about 10% of excisions are followed by recurrence.

Morphology

The characteristic histologic feature of pleomorphic adenoma is **heterogeneity.** The tumor cells form ducts, acini, tubules, strands, or sheets of cells. The epithelial cells are small and dark and range from cuboidal to spindle forms. These epithelial elements are intermingled with a loose, often myxoid connective tissue stroma sometimes containing islands of apparent cartilage or, rarely, bone (Fig. 15–5). Immunohistochemical evidence suggests that all of the diverse cell types within pleomorphic adenoma, including those within the stroma, are of myoepithelial derivation.

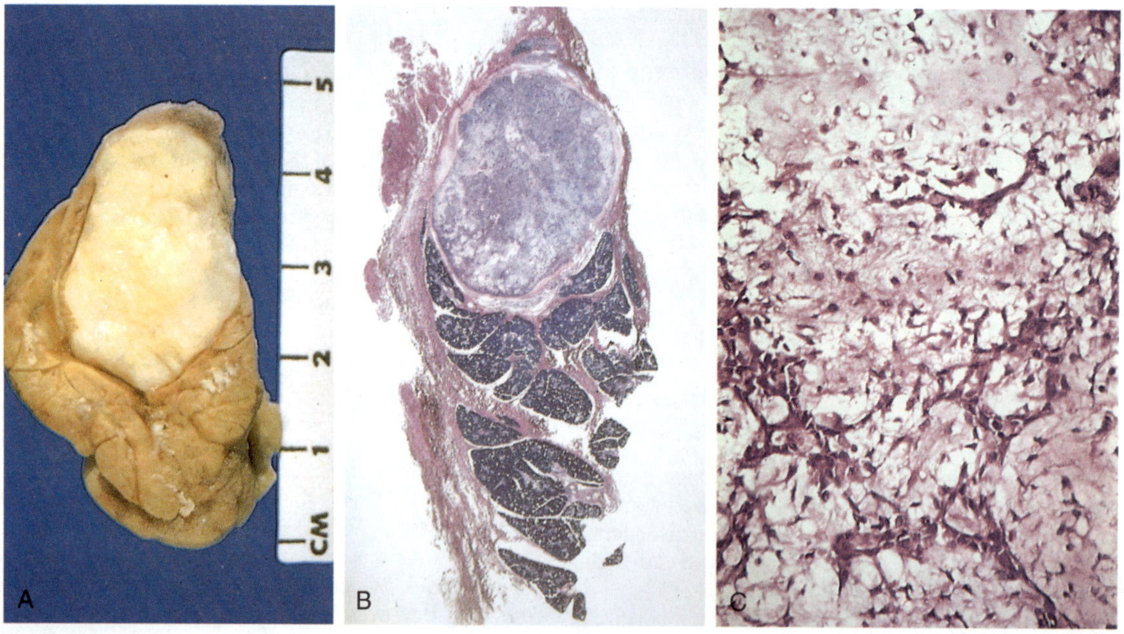

Figure 15–5

Pleomorphic adenoma. **A,** A well-demarcated tumor in the parotid gland. **B,** Low-power view showing a well-demarcated tumor with normal parotid acini below. **C,** High-power view showing amorphous myxoid stroma resembling cartilage, with interspersed islands and strands of myoepithelial cells. (Courtesy of Dr. E. Lee, Department of Pathology, University of Texas Southwestern Medical Center, Dallas, Texas.)

Warthin Tumor (Papillary Cystadenoma Lymphomatosum, Cystadenolymphoma). This infrequent benign tumor occurs virtually only in the region of the parotid gland and is thought to arise from heterotopic salivary tissue trapped within a regional lymph node during embryogenesis. This tumor is generally a small, well-encapsulated, round to ovoid mass that on transection often reveals mucin-containing cleftlike or cystic spaces within a soft gray background. Microscopically, it exhibits two characteristic features: (1) a two-tiered epithelial layer lining the branching, cystic, or cleftlike spaces; and (2) an immediately subjacent, well-developed lymphoid tissue sometimes forming germinal centers. A recurrence rate of about 10% is attributed to incomplete excision, multicentricity, or a second primary tumor. Malignant transformation is rare; about half of reported cases have had prior radiation exposure.

SUMMARY

Salivary Gland Diseases

- *Sialedinitis:* inflammation caused by infection (e.g. mumps, various bacteria) or autoimmune reaction (as in Sjögren syndrome).
- *Pleomorphic adenoma (mixed salivary gland tumor):* slow growing locally infiltrative tumor composed of heterogeneous epithelial elements and an often myxoid stroma.
- *Warthin tumor:* benign tumor composed of epithelial cells and dense lymphoid tissue.

ESOPHAGUS

Lesions of the esophagus run the gamut from bland esophagitis to lethal cancers, yet they evoke a similar and remarkably limited range of symptoms. All produce *dysphagia* (difficulty in swallowing), which is attributed either to deranged esophageal motor function or to narrowing or obstruction of the lumen. *Heartburn* (retrosternal burning pain) usually reflects regurgitation of gastric contents into the lower esophagus. Less commonly, *hematemesis* (vomiting of blood) and *melena* (blood in the stools) are evidence of severe inflammation, ulceration, or laceration of the esophageal mucosa. Massive hematemesis may reflect life-threatening rupture of esophageal varices.

ANATOMIC AND MOTOR DISORDERS

Both esophageal anatomy and motor function may be affected secondarily by many esophageal disorders. The more common anatomic disorders are described here. Infrequent conditions are listed in Table 15–2.

Achalasia

The term *achalasia* means "failure to relax," and in the present context, denotes incomplete relaxation of the lower esophageal sphincter in response to swallowing. This produces functional obstruction of the esophagus, with consequent dilation of the more proximal esophagus (Fig. 15–6). Manometric studies show three major abnormalities in achalasia: (1) aperistalsis, (2) partial or incomplete relaxation of the lower esophageal sphincter with swallowing, and (3) increased resting tone of the lower esophageal sphincter. It is now generally accepted that in primary achalasia there is loss of intrinsic inhibitory innervation of the lower esophageal sphincter and smooth muscle segment of the esophageal body. Secondary achalasia may arise from diverse pathologic processes that impair esophageal function. The classic example is Chagas disease, caused by *Trypanosoma cruzi*, which causes destruction of the myenteric plexus of the esophagus, duodenum, colon, and ureter. Disorders of the dorsal motor nuclei such as polio, and autonomic neuropathy in diabetes, can cause secondary achalasia. *In most instances, however, achalasia occurs as a primary disorder of uncertain etiology.* Autoimmunity and previous viral infection have been hypothesized but remain unproven.

In primary achalasia there is progressive dilation of the esophagus above the level of the lower esophageal sphincter. The wall of the esophagus may be of normal thick-

Table 15–2 Selected (Infrequent) Anatomic Disorders of the Esophagus

Disorder	Clinical Presentation and Anatomy
Stenosis	Adult with progressive dysphagia to solids and eventually to all foods; a lower esophageal narrowing, which is usually the result of chronic inflammatory disease, including gastroesophageal reflux
Atresia, fistula	Newborn with aspiration, paroxysmal suffocation, pneumonia; esophageal atresia (absence of a lumen) and tracheoesophageal fistula may occur together
Webs, rings	Episodic dysphagia to solid foods; an (presumably) acquired mucosal web or mucosal and submucosal concentric ring partially occluding the esophagus
Diverticula	Episodic food regurgitation, especially nocturnal; sometimes pain is present; an acquired outpouching of the esophageal wall

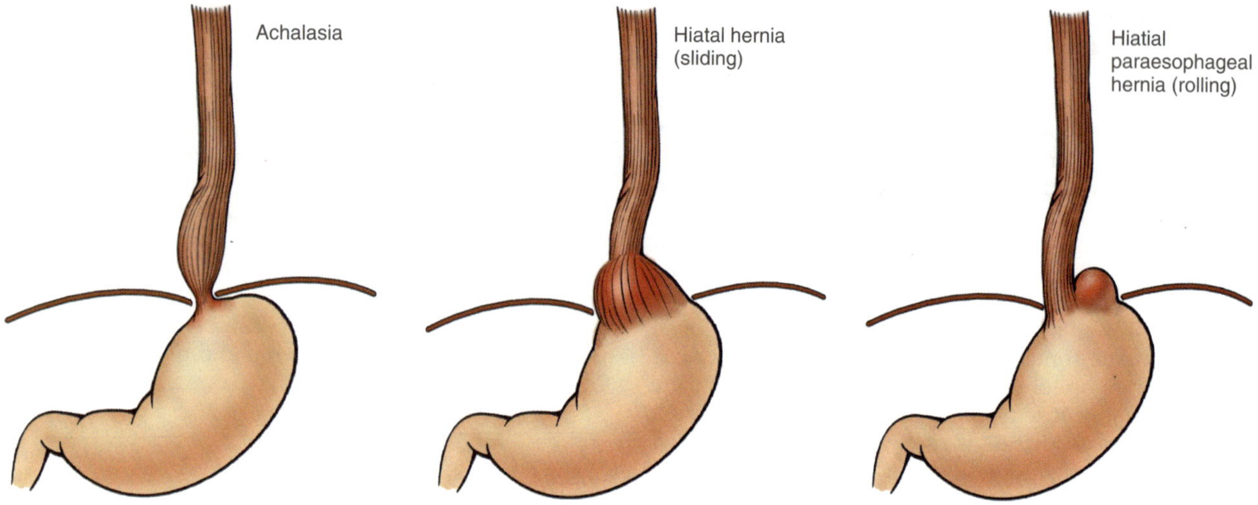

Figure 15–6

Achalasia and hiatal hernias. Comparison between sliding and paraesophageal (rolling) hiatal hernias.

ness, thicker than normal because of hypertrophy of the muscularis, or markedly thinned by dilation. The myenteric ganglia are usually absent from the body of the esophagus but may or may not be reduced in number in the region of the lower esophageal sphincter. Inflammation in the location of the esophageal myenteric plexus is pathognomonic of the disease. Although achalasia is not a mucosal disease, stasis of food may produce mucosal inflammation and ulceration proximal to the lower esophageal sphincter.

Achalasia is characterized clinically by progressive dysphagia and inability to completely convey food to the stomach. Nocturnal regurgitation and aspiration of undigested food may occur. It usually becomes manifest in young adulthood, but it may appear in infancy or childhood. The most serious aspect of this condition is the hazard of developing esophageal squamous cell carcinoma, reported to occur in about 5% of patients and typically at an earlier age than in those without achalasia.

Hiatal Hernia

In hiatal hernia, separation of the diaphragmatic crura and widening of the space between the muscular crura and the esophageal wall permits a dilated segment of the stomach to protrude above the diaphragm. Two anatomic patterns are recognized (Fig. 15–6): the axial, or sliding, hernia and the nonaxial, or paraesophageal, hernia. The *sliding hernia* constitutes 95% of cases; protrusion of the stomach above the diaphragm creates a bell-shaped dilation, bounded below by the diaphragmatic narrowing. In *paraesophageal hernias*, a separate portion of the stomach, usually along the greater curvature, enters the thorax through the widened foramen. The cause of this deranged anatomy, whether congenital or acquired, is unknown.

On the basis of radiographic studies, hiatal hernias are reported in 1% to 20% of adult subjects, increasing in incidence with age. Only about 9% of these adults, however, suffer from heartburn or regurgitation of gastric juices into the mouth. These symptoms more likely result from incompetence of the lower esophageal sphincter than from the hiatal hernia per se and are accentuated by positions favoring reflux (bending forward, lying supine) and obesity. Although most individuals with sliding hiatal hernias do not have reflux esophagitis (discussed later), those with severe reflux esophagitis are likely to have a sliding hiatal hernia. Other complications affecting both types of hiatal hernias include mucosal ulceration, bleeding, and even perforation. Paraesophageal hernias rarely induce reflux, but they can become strangulated or obstructed.

Lacerations (Mallory-Weiss Syndrome)

Longitudinal tears in the esophagus at the esophagogastric junction are termed *Mallory-Weiss tears* (Fig. 15–7). They are encountered in chronic alcoholics after a bout of severe retching or vomiting, but they may also occur during acute illnesses with severe vomiting. The presumed pathogenesis is inadequate relaxation of the musculature of the lower esophageal sphincter during vomiting, with stretching and tearing of the esophagogastric junction at the moment of propulsive expulsion of gastric contents. In support of this explanation, a hiatal hernia is found in more than 75% of patients with Mallory-Weiss tears. Notably, almost half of individuals presenting with upper gastrointestinal bleeding attributable to a Mallory-Weiss tear have no antecedent history of nausea, retching, abdominal pain, or vomiting. One must hypothesize that normal variability in intra-abdominal pressure can be transduced through a hiatal hernia, occasionally leading to a Mallory-Weiss tear. Tears may involve only the mucosa or may penetrate the wall. Infection of the defect may lead to an inflammatory ulcer or to mediastinitis.

Esophageal lacerations account for 5% to 10% of upper gastrointestinal bleeding episodes. Most often bleeding is not profuse and ceases without surgical intervention, but life-threatening hematemesis may occur.

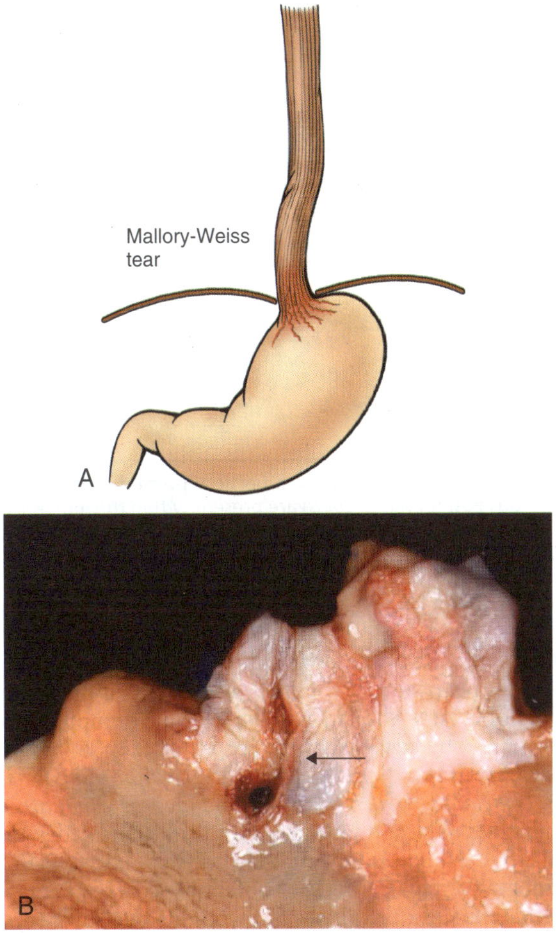

Figure 15–7

Esophageal lacerations (Mallory-Weiss syndrome). **A,** Longitudinal tears in the esophagogastric junction. **B,** Gross photograph demonstrating longitudinal lacerations oriented in the axis of the esophageal lumen (*arrow*), extending from the esophageal mucosa to the stomach mucosa. (Photograph courtesy of Dr. Richard Harruff, King County Medical Examiner's Office, Seattle, Washington.)

Even with severe blood loss, supportive therapy with vasoconstrictive medications, transfusions, and sometimes balloon tamponade, is usually all that is required. Healing is usually prompt, with minimal to no residual problems.

VARICES

One of the few potential sites for communication between the intra-abdominal splanchnic circulation and the systemic venous circulation is through the esophagus. When portal venous blood flow into the liver is impeded by cirrhosis or other causes, the resultant portal hypertension induces the formation of collateral bypass channels wherever the portal and systemic systems communicate. Portal blood flow is thereby diverted through the stomach veins into the plexus of esophageal subepithelial and submucosal veins, thence into the azygos veins and the superior vena cava. The increased pressure in the esophageal plexus produces dilated tortuous vessels called varices. *Persons with cirrhosis develop varices at a rate of 5% to 15% per year, so that varices are present in approximately two-thirds of all cirrhotic patients.* In the United States, esophageal varices are most often associated with alcoholic cirrhosis.

Morphology

Varices appear as tortuous dilated veins lying primarily within the submucosa of the distal esophagus and proximal stomach. The net effect is irregular protrusion of the overlying mucosa into the lumen, although varices are collapsed in surgical or postmortem specimens (Fig. 15–8). When the varix is unruptured, the mucosa may be normal, but often it is eroded and inflamed because of its exposed position, further weakening the tissue support of the dilated veins.

Variceal rupture produces massive hemorrhage into the lumen, *as well as suffusion of blood into the esophageal wall.* Varices produce no symptoms until they rupture. Among persons with advanced cirrhosis of the liver, half the deaths result from rupture of a varix, either as a direct consequence of the hemorrhage or from the hepatic coma triggered by the hemorrhage. However, even when varices are present, they account for less than half of all episodes of hematemesis. Bleeding from concomitant gastritis, peptic ulcer, or esophageal laceration accounts for most of the remainder.

The conditions leading to initial rupture of a varix are unclear: silent erosion of overlying thinned mucosa,

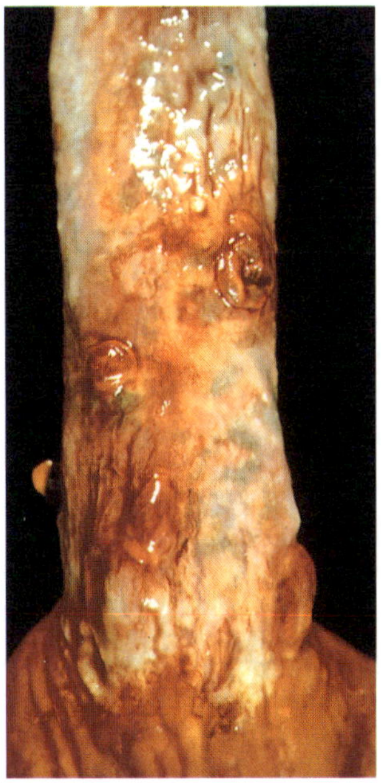

Figure 15–8

Esophageal varices: a view of the everted esophagus and gastroesophageal junction, showing dilated submucosal veins (varices). The blue-colored varices have collapsed in this postmortem specimen.

increased tension in progressively dilated veins, and vomiting with increased intra-abdominal pressure are likely to be involved. One-half of those affected are found to have coexistent hepatocellular carcinoma, suggesting that a progressive decrease in hepatic functional reserve from tumor growth enhances the likelihood of variceal rupture. Once begun, variceal hemorrhage subsides spontaneously in only 50% of cases; endoscopic injection of thrombotic agents (sclerotherapy) or balloon tamponade is often required. When varices bleed, 20% to 30% of patients die during the first episode. Among those who survive, rebleeding occurs in approximately 70% within 1 year, with a similar rate of mortality for each episode.

ESOPHAGITIS

Injury to the esophageal mucosa with subsequent inflammation is a common condition worldwide. The inflammation may have many origins: prolonged gastric intubation, uremia, ingestion of corrosive or irritant substances, and radiation or chemotherapy, among others. In northern Iran the prevalence of esophagitis is more than 80%; it is also extremely high in regions of China. The basis of this prevalence is unknown. *The overwhelming preponderance of cases in Western countries are attributable to reflux of gastric contents (reflux esophagitis).* Gastroesophageal reflux disease, as it is known clinically, affects about 0.5% of the US adult population and has recurrent heartburn as its dominant symptom. There are many presumed contributory factors:

- Decreased efficacy of esophageal antireflux mechanisms. Central nervous system depressants, alcohol or tobacco exposure may be some of the contributing causes, but most often no obvious etiology is identifiable.
- Inadequate or slowed esophageal clearance of refluxed material
- The presence of a sliding hiatal hernia
- Increased gastric volume, contributing to the volume of refluxed material
- Impaired reparative capacity of the esophageal mucosa by prolonged exposure to gastric juices

Any one of these influences may assume primacy in an individual case, but more than one is likely to be involved in most instances.

Morphology

The anatomic changes depend on the causative agent and on the duration and severity of the exposure. Mild esophagitis may appear macroscopically as simple hyperemia, with virtually no histologic abnormality. In contrast, the mucosa in severe esophagitis shows confluent epithelial erosions or total ulceration into the submucosa. Three histologic features are characteristic of uncomplicated **reflux esophagitis** (Fig. 15–9), although only one or two may be present: (1) eosinophils, with or without neutrophils, in the epithelial layer; (2) basal zone hyperplasia; and (3) elongation of lamina propria papillae. Intraepithelial neutrophils are markers of more severe injury.

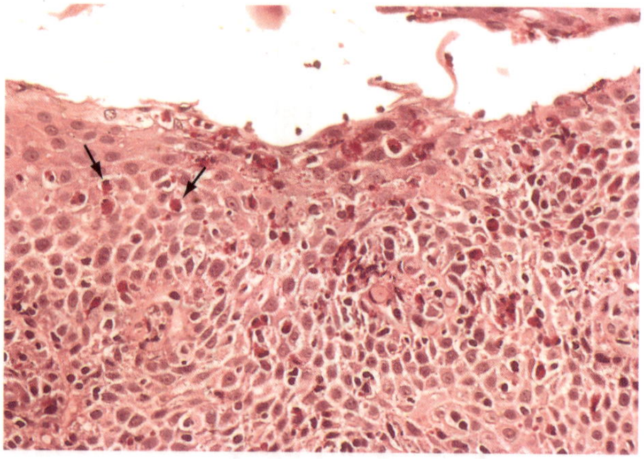

Figure 15–9

Reflux esophagitis showing the superficial portion of the mucosa. Numerous eosinophils (*arrows*) are present within the mucosa, and the stratified squamous epithelium has not undergone complete maturation because of ongoing inflammatory damage.

Clinical Features. The dominant manifestation of reflux disease is heartburn, sometimes accompanied by regurgitation of a sour brash. Rarely, chronic symptoms are punctuated by attacks of severe chest pain mimicking a heart attack. *The severity of symptoms is not closely related to the presence and degree of anatomic esophagitis.* Though largely limited to adults older than age 40, reflux esophagitis is occasionally seen in infants and children. The potential consequences of severe reflux esophagitis are bleeding, development of stricture, and Barrett esophagus, with its predisposition to malignancy.

BARRETT ESOPHAGUS

Barrett esophagus is defined as the replacement of the normal distal stratified squamous mucosa by metaplastic columnar epithelium containing goblet cells. It is a complication of long-standing gastroesophageal reflux, occurring in as many as 5% to 15% of persons with persistent symptomatic reflux disease. However, Barrett esophagus has been detected in about the same proportions in asymptomatic populations. It is unclear why individuals with few symptoms and little inflammation develop Barrett esophagus, and, conversely, why others have erosive esophagitis without Barrett esophagus. Barrett esophagus affects males more often than females (ratio of 4:1) and is much more common in whites than in other races. Prolonged and recurrent gastroesophageal reflux is thought to produce inflammation and eventually ulceration of the squamous epithelial lining. Healing occurs by ingrowth of progenitor cells and re-epithelialization. In the microenvironment of an abnormally low pH in the distal esophagus caused by acid reflux, the cells differentiate into columnar epithelium. Metaplastic columnar epithelium is thought to be more resistant to injury from refluxing gastric contents. However, the metaplastic epithelium is not a typical intestinal epithelium, as absorptive enterocytes are not observed.

Ulcer and stricture may develop as a complication of Barrett esophagus. However, *the chief clinical significance of Barrett esophagus is the risk for the development of adenocarcinoma*. Persons with Barrett esophagus have a 30- to 100-fold greater risk of developing esophageal adenocarcinoma than do normal populations, the greatest risk being associated with high-grade dysplasia. Hence, periodic screening for high-grade dysplasia with esophageal biopsy is recommended for Barrett esophagus sufferers. Persistence of high-grade dysplasia requires therapeutic interventions, such as surgery, photodynamic ablation, or very careful surveillance.

Morphology

Barrett esophagus is apparent as a salmon-pink, velvety mucosa between the smooth, pale-pink esophageal squamous mucosa and the more lush light brown gastric mucosa (Fig. 15–10). It may exist as "tongues" extending up from the gastroesophageal junction, as an irregular circumferential band displacing the squamocolumnar junction cephalad, or as isolated patches (islands) in the distal esophagus. The length of the changes is not as important as the presence in the anatomic esophagus of metaplastic mucosa containing goblet cells. **Microscopically, the esophageal squamous epithelium is replaced by metaplastic columnar epithelium,** as depicted in Figure 15–11. **Barrett mucosa may be quite focal and variable from one site to the next,** often necessitating repeated endoscopy and biopsy for definitive diagnosis. Critical to the pathologic evaluation of individuals with Barrett mucosa is the recognition of dysplastic changes in the mucosa that may be precursors of cancer.

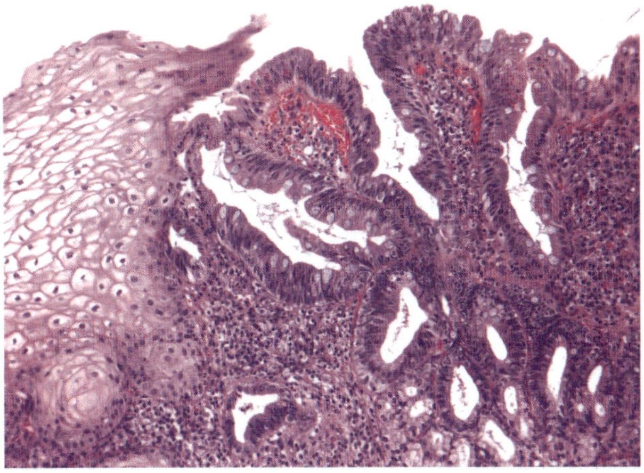

Figure 15–11

Barrett esophagus. Microscopic view showing squamous mucosa (*left*) and intestinal-type columnar epithelial cells in glandular mucosa (*right*).

ESOPHAGEAL CARCINOMA

Benign tumors may arise in the esophagus from both the squamous mucosa and underlying mesenchyme. However, these are overshadowed by cancer of the esophagus, of which there are two types: *squamous cell carcinomas and adenocarcinomas*. Worldwide, squamous cell carcinomas constitute 90% of esophageal cancers, but in the United States there has been a very large increase (three- to fivefold in the last 40 years) in the incidence of adenocarcinomas associated with Barrett esophagus. Indeed, this form of cancer has surpassed squamous cell carcinoma in incidence in the United States. Adenocarcinoma arising in Barrett esophagus is more common in

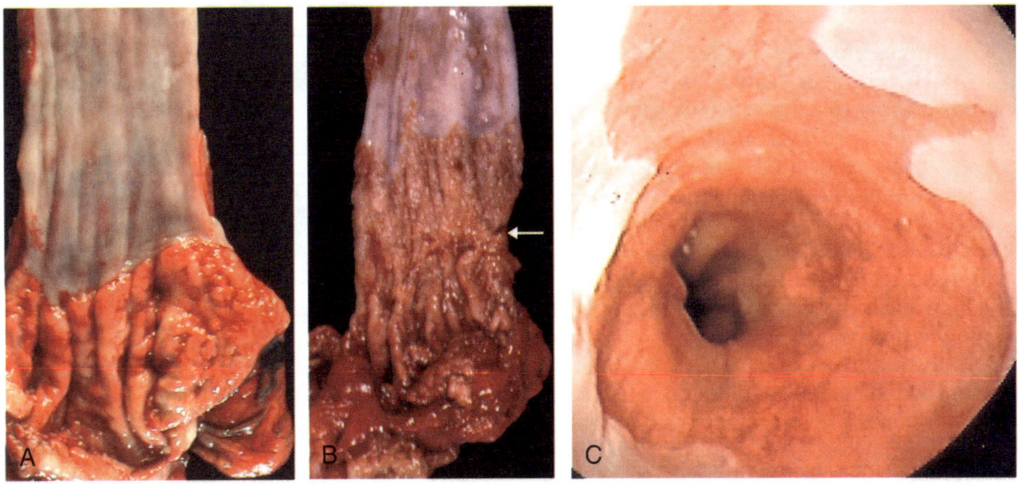

Figure 15–10

Barrett esophagus. **A–B,** Gross view of distal esophagus (*top*) and proximal stomach (*bottom*) showing (**A**) normal gastroesophageal junction and (**B**) the granular zone of Barrett esophagus (*arrow*). **C,** Endoscopic view showing red velvety gastrointestinal-type mucosa extending from the gastroesophageal orifice. Note paler squamous esophageal mucosa. (**C,** Courtesy of Dr. F. Farraye, Brigham and Women's Hospital, Boston, Massachusetts.)

Table 15–3 Risk Factors for Squamous Cell Carcinoma of the Esophagus

Esophageal Disorders	
Long-standing esophagitis	
Achalasia	
Plummer-Vinson syndrome (esophageal webs, microcytic hypochromic anemia, atrophic glossitis)	
Life-style	
Alcohol consumption	
Tobacco abuse	
Dietary	
Deficiency of vitamins (A, C, riboflavin, thiamine, pyridoxine)	
Deficiency of trace metals (zinc, molybdenum)	
Fungal contamination of foodstuffs	
High content of nitrites/nitrosamines	
Genetic Predisposition	
Tylosis (hyperkeratosis of palms and soles)	

whites than in blacks. By contrast, squamous cell carcinomas are more common in blacks worldwide. There are striking and puzzling differences in the geographic incidence of esophageal carcinoma. In the United States, there are about 6 new cases per 100,000 population per year, accounting for 1% to 2% of all cancer deaths. In regions of Asia extending from the northern provinces of China to the Caspian littoral in Iran, the prevalence is well over 100 per 100,000, and 20% of cancer deaths are caused by esophageal carcinoma (mainly squamous cell type).

Squamous Cell Carcinoma

An important contributing variable is retarded passage of food through the esophagus, prolonging mucosal exposure to potential carcinogens such as those contained in tobacco and alcoholic beverages (Table 15–3). There is a well-defined predisposing role for chronic esophagitis, which is often the consequence of alcohol and tobacco use. These two agents are associated with the majority of squamous cell carcinoma in Europe and the United States. However, other influences, perhaps in the diet, must underlie the very high incidence of this tumor among the orthodox Moslems of Iran, who neither drink nor smoke. The high levels of nitrosamines and fungi contained in some foods probably account for the very high incidence of this tumor in some regions of China. A strong association with human papillomavirus occurs only in high-incidence areas. Abnormalities affecting the *p16/INK4* tumor suppressor gene and the epidermal growth factor receptor are frequently present in squamous cell carcinoma of the esophagus. Mutations in *p53* are detected in as many as 50% of these tumors and are generally correlated with the use of tobacco and alcohol. Unlike in colon carcinomas, mutations in the *K-RAS* and *APC* genes are uncommon.

Morphology

Squamous cell carcinomas are usually preceded by a long prodrome of mucosal **epithelial dysplasia** followed by **carcinoma in situ** and, ultimately, by the emergence of **invasive cancer.** Early overt lesions appear as small, gray-white, plaquelike thickenings or elevations of the mucosa. In months to years, these lesions become tumorous, taking one of three forms: (1) **polypoid exophytic masses** that protrude into the lumen; (2) necrotizing cancerous **ulcerations** that extend deeply and sometimes erode into the respiratory tree, aorta, or elsewhere (Fig. 15–12); and (3) **diffuse infiltrative neoplasms** that cause thickening and rigidity of the wall and narrowing of the lumen. Whichever the pattern, about 20% arise in the cervical and upper thoracic esophagus, 50% in the middle third, and 30% in the lower third.

Adenocarcinoma

Barrett esophagus is the only recognized precursor of esophageal adenocarcinoma. The development of adenocarcinomas from Barrett esophagus is a multistep process

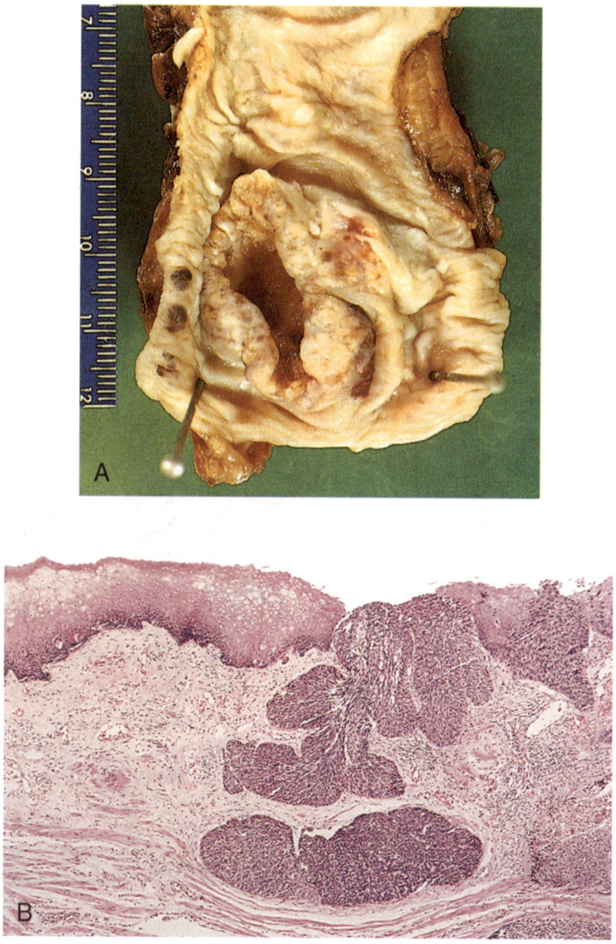

Figure 15–12

A, Large ulcerated squamous cell carcinoma of the esophagus. **B,** Low power view of cancer invasion of the submucosa.

that unfolds over many years. The degree of dysplasia is the strongest predictor of the progression to cancer. Individuals with low-grade dysplasia have very low rates of progression to adenocarcinomas but the progression to cancer may be 10% or more per year in individuals with high-grade dysplasia. Overall, the risk for developing adenocarcinoma varies from 30-fold to more than 100-fold above normal. In Barrett esophagus tissue there is increased cell proliferation, and chromosomal abnormalities become apparent in high-grade dysplasia. Mutations in *p53* progressively accumulate, and aneuploidy is commonly found. Additional genetic abnormalities, such as alterations in *HER-2/NEU* and *β-catenin*, are present in the carcinomas, but there are no specific markers that precisely identify the transition from high-grade dysplasia to cancer.

Morphology

Adenocarcinomas seem to arise from dysplastic mucosa in the setting of **Barrett esophagus.** Unlike squamous cell carcinomas, they are usually in the distal one-third of the esophagus and may invade the subjacent gastric cardia. Initially appearing as flat or raised patches on an otherwise intact mucosa, they may develop into **large nodular masses** or show deeply **ulcerative** or **diffusely infiltrative** features. Microscopically, most tumors are mucin-producing glandular tumors showing intestinal-type features, in keeping with the morphology of the preexisting metaplastic mucosa.

Clinical Features. Esophageal carcinoma is insidious in onset and produces dysphagia and obstruction gradually and late. Weight loss, anorexia, fatigue, and weakness appear, followed by pain, usually related to swallowing. Diagnosis is usually made by imaging techniques and endoscopic biopsy. Because these cancers extensively invade the rich esophageal lymphatic network and adjacent structures relatively early in their development, surgical excision is rarely curative. Thus, much emphasis is placed on surveillance procedures for individuals with persistent manifestations of chronic esophagitis or known Barrett esophagus. Esophageal cancer confined to the mucosa or submucosa is amenable to surgical treatment.

SUMMARY

Diseases of the Esophagus

- *Hiatal hernia:* protrusion of segment of the stomach above the diaphragm; occasionally results in reflux and esophagitis.
- *Lacerations (Mallory-Weiss syndrome):* longitudinal tears at the esophago-gastric junction caused by severe retching and vomiting; may cause upper GI bleeding.
- *Varices:* tortuous dilated veins at the distal esophagus and proximal stomach; caused by increased portal pressure (most often due to cirrhosis), leading to increased pressure in the esophageal venous plexus; may cause severe bleeding.
- *Esophagitis:* Inflammation of the esophageal mucosa most often caused by reflux of gastric contents; inflammatory infiltrate often contains abundant eosinophils.
- *Barrett esophagus:* replacement of stratified squamous epithelium of distal esophagus by metaplastic columnar epithelium containing goblet cells; associated with gastroesophageal reflux in ~15% of cases; main harmful consequence is the development of dysplasia and 30- to 100-fold increased risk for adenocarcinoma.
- *Esophageal carcinoma:*
  - Squamous cell carcinomas arise from dysplastic epithelium, associated with esophagitis, smoking; may be locally invasive.
  - Adenocarcinomas arise usually in Barrett esophagus, now more frequent in the US.

STOMACH

Gastric disorders frequently cause clinical disease, ranging from bland chronic gastritis to the anything but bland gastric carcinoma. Gastric infection with *Helicobacter pylori* represents the most common gastrointestinal infection. Occasionally, congenital anomalies are encountered; these are summarized in Table 15–4.

Gastric disorders give rise to symptoms similar to esophageal disorders, primarily *heartburn* and *vague epigastric pain.* With breach of the gastric mucosa and bleeding, *hematemesis* or *melena* may ensue. Unlike esophageal bleeding, however, blood quickly congeals and turns brown in the acid environment of the stomach lumen. Vomited blood hence has the appearance of coffee grounds.

GASTRITIS

This diagnosis is both overused and often missed—overused when it is applied loosely to any transient upper abdominal complaint in the absence of validating evidence, and missed because most persons with chronic gastritis are asymptomatic. *Gastritis is simply defined as inflammation of the gastric mucosa.* By far the majority

Table 15–4 Congenital Gastric Anomalies

Condition	Comment
Pyloric stenosis	1 in 300–900 live births Male-to-female ratio 3:1 Pathology: muscular hypertrophy of pyloric smooth muscle wall Symptoms: persistent, nonbilious projectile vomiting in young infant
Diaphragmatic hernia	Rare Pathology: herniation of stomach and other abdominal contents into thorax through a diaphragmatic defect Symptoms: acute respiratory distress in newborn
Gastric heterotopia	Uncommon Pathology: a nidus of gastric mucosa in the esophagus or small intestine ("ectopic rest") Symptoms: asymptomatic, or an anomalous peptic ulcer in adult

of cases are *chronic gastritis*, but occasionally, distinct forms of *acute gastritis* are encountered. These two conditions are discussed below.

Chronic Gastritis

Chronic gastritis is defined as the presence of chronic inflammatory changes in the mucosa leading eventually to mucosal atrophy and epithelial metaplasia. It is notable for distinct causal subgroups and for patterns of histologic alterations that vary in different parts of the world. In the Western world, the prevalence of histologic changes indicative of chronic gastritis is higher than 50% in the later decades of life.

Pathogenesis. By far the most important etiologic association is chronic infection by the bacillus *H. pylori*. This organism is a worldwide pathogen that has the highest infection rates in developing countries. American adults older than age 50 show prevalence rates approaching 50%. In areas where the infection is endemic, it seems to be acquired in childhood and persists for decades. *Most individuals with the infection also have the associated gastritis but are asymptomatic.* (Robin Warren, a pathologist, and Barry Marshall, a medical student at the time of the discovery, received the 2005 Nobel prize in Medicine for their identification in 1982 of *H. pylori*, originally called *Campylobacter.*)

H. pylori is a noninvasive, non–spore-forming, S-shaped gram-negative rod measuring approximately 3.5 µm × 0.5 µm. The mechanisms by which *H. pylori* causes tissue injury are discussed in detail in the section below on Peptic Ulcers. Suffice it to say that gastritis develops as a result of the combined influence of bacterial enzymes and toxins and release of noxious chemicals by the recruited neutrophils. After initial exposure to *H. pylori*, gastritis may develop in two patterns: (1) an antral-type with high acid production and higher risk for the development of duodenal ulcer, and (2) a pangastritis with multifocal mucosal atrophy, with low acid secretion and increased risk for adenocarcinoma. Persons with chronic gastritis and *H. pylori* usually improve symptomatically when treated with antibiotics and proton pump inhibitors. Improvement in the underlying chronic gastritis may take much longer. Relapses are associated with reappearance of this organism.

Other forms of chronic gastritis are much less common in the United States. *Autoimmune gastritis*, which represents no more than 10% of cases of chronic gastritis, results from the production of autoantibodies to the gastric gland parietal cells, in particular to the acid-producing enzyme H^+,K^+-ATPase. The autoimmune injury leads to gland destruction and mucosal atrophy, with concomitant loss of acid and intrinsic factor production. The resultant deficiency of intrinsic factor leads to *pernicious anemia*, discussed in Chapter 12. This form of gastritis is seen most often in Scandinavia, in association with other autoimmune disorders such as Hashimoto thyroiditis and Addison disease (see Chapter 20).

Morphology

Regardless of the cause or histologic distribution of chronic gastritis, the inflammatory changes consist of a lymphocytic and plasma cell infiltrate in the lamina propria (Fig. 15–13), occasionally accompanied by neutrophilic inflammation of the neck region of the mucosal pits. The inflammation may be accompanied by variable gland loss and mucosal atrophy. When present, *H. pylori* organisms are found nestled within the mucus layer overlying the superficial mucosal epithelium (Fig. 15–14). In the autoimmune variant, loss of parietal cells is particularly prominent. Two additional features are of note. **Intestinal metaplasia** refers to the replacement of gastric epithelium with columnar and goblet cells of intestinal variety. This is significant, because gastrointestinal-type carcinomas (see later) seem to arise from **dysplasia** of this metaplastic epithelium. Second, *H. pylori*–induced proliferation of **lymphoid tissue** within the gastric mucosa has been implicated as a precursor of gastric lymphoma.

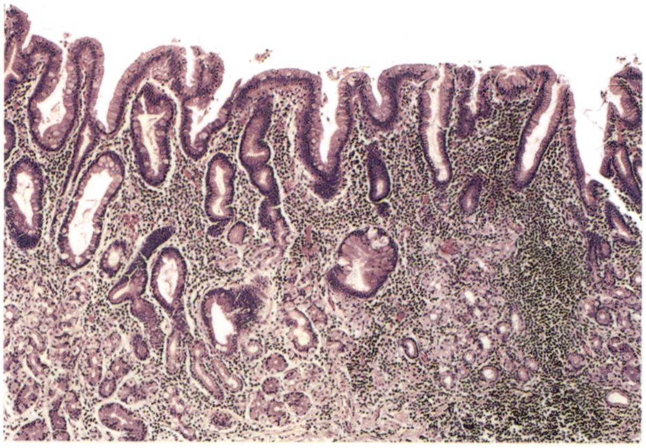

Figure 15–13

Chronic gastritis, showing partial replacement of the gastric mucosal epithelium by intestinal metaplasia (*upper left*), and inflammation of the lamina propria containing lymphocytes and plasma cells (*right*).

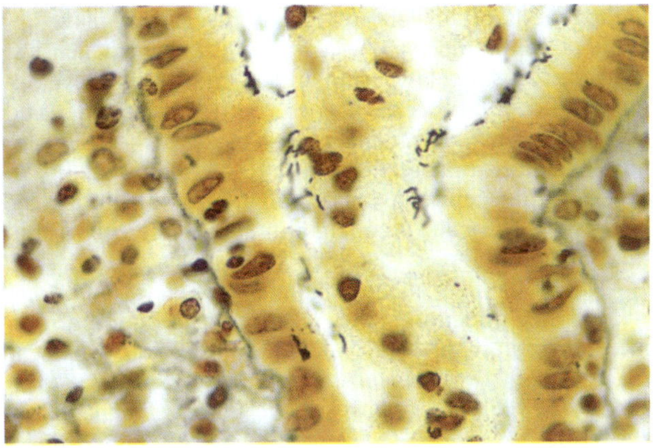

Figure 15–14

Helicobacter pylori gastritis. A Steiner silver stain demonstrates the numerous darkly stained *Helicobacter* organisms along the luminal surface of the gastric epithelial cells. There is no tissue invasion by bacteria. (Courtesy of Dr. Melissa Upton, Department of Pathology, University of Washington, Seattle, Washington.)

Clinical Features. Chronic gastritis usually causes few or no symptoms; upper abdominal discomfort and nausea and vomiting can occur. When severe parietal cell loss occurs in the setting of autoimmune gastritis, hypochlorhydria or achlorhydria (referring to concentrations of gastric luminal hydrochloric acid) and hypergastrinemia are characteristically present. Individuals with chronic gastritis from other causes may be hypochlorhydric, but because parietal cells are never completely destroyed, these persons do not develop achlorhydria or pernicious anemia. Serum gastrin levels are either normal or only modestly elevated. Most important is the relationship of chronic gastritis to the development of peptic ulcer and gastric carcinoma. Most individuals with a peptic ulcer, whether duodenal or gastric, have *H. pylori* infection. The long-term risk of gastric carcinoma for persons with *H. pylori*–associated chronic gastritis is increased about fivefold relative to the normal population. For autoimmune gastritis, the risk for cancer is in the range of 2% to 4% of affected individuals, which is well above that of the normal population.

Acute Gastritis

Acute gastritis is an acute mucosal inflammatory process, usually of a transient nature. The inflammation may be accompanied by hemorrhage into the mucosa and, in more severe circumstances, by sloughing of the superficial mucosal epithelium (*erosion*). This severe erosive form of the disease is an important cause of acute gastrointestinal bleeding.

Pathogenesis. The pathogenesis is poorly understood, in part because normal mechanisms for gastric mucosal protection are not totally clear. Acute gastritis is frequently associated with:

- Heavy use of nonsteroidal anti-inflammatory drugs (NSAIDs), particularly aspirin
- Excessive alcohol consumption
- Heavy smoking
- Treatment with cancer chemotherapeutic drugs
- Uremia
- Systemic infections (e.g., salmonellosis)
- Severe stress (e.g., trauma, burns, surgery)
- Ischemia and shock
- Suicide attempts with acids and alkali
- Mechanical trauma (e.g., nasogastric intubation)
- Reflux of bilious material after distal gastrectomy

One or more of the following influences are thought to be operative in these varied settings: disruption of the adherent mucous layer, stimulation of acid secretion with hydrogen ion back-diffusion into the superficial epithelium, decreased production of bicarbonate buffer by superficial epithelial cells, reduced mucosal blood flow, and direct damage to the epithelium. Not surprisingly, mucosal insults can act synergistically. Finally, acute infection with *H. pylori* induces neutrophilic inflammation of the gastric mucosa, but this event usually escapes the notice of the individual.

Morphology

Acute gastritis ranges from extremely localized (as occurs in NSAID-induced injury) to diffuse, and from superficial inflammation to involvement of the entire mucosal thickness with hemorrhage and focal erosions. Concurrent erosion and hemorrhage are readily visible by endoscopy and termed **acute erosive gastritis.** All variants are marked by mucosal edema and an inflammatory infiltrate of neutrophils and possibly by chronic inflammatory cells. Regenerative replication of epithelial cells in the gastric pits is usually prominent. Provided that the noxious event is short lived, acute gastritis may disappear within days with complete restitution of the normal mucosa.

Clinical Features. Depending on the severity of the anatomic changes, acute gastritis may be entirely asymptomatic, may cause variable epigastric pain with nausea and vomiting, or may present as overt hematemesis, melena, and potentially fatal blood loss. Overall, *it is one of the major causes of hematemesis, particularly in alcoholics.* Even in certain other settings, the condition is quite common; as many as 25% of persons who take daily aspirin for rheumatoid arthritis develop acute gastritis at some time in their course, many with occult or overt bleeding. The risk of gastric bleeding from NSAID-induced gastritis is dose related, thus increasing the likelihood of this complication in persons requiring long-term use of such drugs.

GASTRIC ULCERATION

Ulcers of the alimentary tract are defined histologically as a breach in the mucosa that extends through the muscularis mucosae into the submucosa or deeper. This is to be contrasted to *erosions*, in which there is a breach in the epithelium of the mucosa only. Erosions may heal within days, whereas healing of ulcers takes much longer. Although ulcers may occur anywhere in the alimentary tract, by far, the most common are the peptic ulcers that occur in the duodenum and stomach. Here we discuss peptic ulcers and acute gastric ulceration.

Peptic Ulcers

Peptic ulcers are chronic, most often solitary, lesions that occur in any portion of the gastrointestinal tract exposed to the aggressive action of acidic peptic juices. At least 98% of peptic ulcers are either in the first portion of the duodenum or in the stomach, in a ratio of about 4:1.

Epidemiology. Peptic ulcers are remitting, relapsing lesions that are most often diagnosed in middle-aged to older adults, but they may first become evident in young adult life. They often appear without obvious precipitating influences and may then heal after a period of weeks to months of active disease. *Even with healing, however, the propensity to develop peptic ulcers remains, in part because of recurrent infection with H. pylori.* Thus, it is difficult to obtain accurate data on the prevalence of active disease. Best estimates suggest that in the American population, 6% to 14% of males and 2% to 6% of females have peptic ulcers. The male/female ratio for duodenal ulcers is about 3:1. For both men and women in the United States, the lifetime risk of developing peptic ulcer disease is about 10%.

Genetic or racial influences seem to have little or no role in the causation of peptic ulcers. Duodenal ulcers are more frequent in persons with alcoholic cirrhosis, chronic obstructive pulmonary disease, chronic renal failure, and hyperparathyroidism. With respect to the last two conditions, hypercalcemia, whatever its cause, stimulates gastrin production and therefore acid secretion.

Pathogenesis. Two conditions are key for the development of peptic ulcers: (1) *H. pylori* infection, which has a strong causal relationship with peptic ulcer development, and (2) mucosal exposure to gastric acid and pepsin. Nevertheless, many aspects of the pathogenesis of mucosal ulceration remain murky. It is best perhaps to consider that peptic ulcers are created by an imbalance between the gastroduodenal mucosal defenses and the damaging forces that overcome such defenses (Fig. 15–15). Both sides of the imbalance are considered.

H. pylori infection is the most important condition in the pathogenesis of peptic ulcer. The infection is present in 70% to 90% of persons with duodenal ulcers and in about 70% of those with gastric ulcers. Furthermore, antibiotic treatment of *H. pylori* infection promotes healing of ulcers and tends to prevent their recurrence. Hence, much interest is focused on the possible mechanisms by which this tiny noninvasive spiral organism tips the balance of mucosal defenses. Here are the possible mechanisms:

- Although *H. pylori* does not invade the tissues, it induces an intense inflammatory and immune response. There is increased production of proinflammatory cytokines such as interleukin (IL)-1, IL-6, tumor necrosis factor, and, most notably, IL-8. IL-8 is produced by the mucosal epithelial cells, and it recruits and activates neutrophils.
- Several bacterial gene products are involved in causing epithelial cell injury and induction of in-

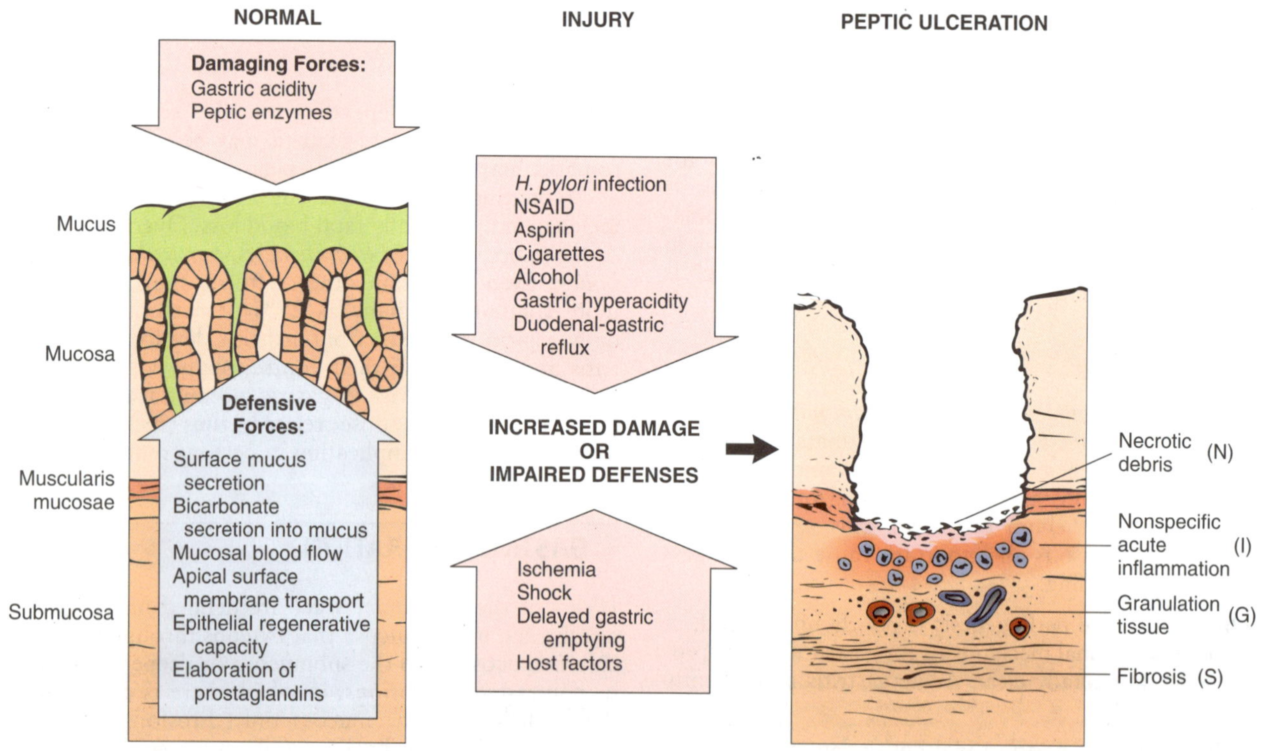

Figure 15–15

Aggravating causes of, and defense mechanisms against, peptic ulceration. The right panel shows the basis of a nonperforated ulcer, demonstrating necrosis (N), inflammation (I), granulation tissue (G), and fibrosis (S).

flammation. Epithelial injury is mostly caused by a vacuolating toxin called VacA, which is regulated by the cytotoxin-associated gene A (*CagA*). This gene is a component of the *Cag* pathogenicity island, a cluster of 29 genes, some of which encode pro-inflammatory proteins. In addition, *H. pylori* secretes a urease that breaks down urea to form toxic compounds such as ammonium chloride and monochloramine. The organisms also elaborate phospholipases that damage surface epithelial cells. Bacterial proteases and phospholipases break down the glycoprotein-lipid complexes in the gastric mucus, thus weakening the first line of mucosal defense.

- *H. pylori* enhances gastric acid secretion and impairs duodenal bicarbonate production, thus reducing luminal pH in the duodenum. This altered milieu seems to favor gastric metaplasia (the presence of gastric epithelium) in the first part of the duodenum. Such metaplastic foci provide areas for *H. pylori* colonization.
- Several *H. pylori* proteins are immunogenic, and they evoke a robust immune response in the mucosa. Both activated T cells and B cells can be seen in chronic gastritis caused by *H. pylori*. The B lymphocytes aggregate to form follicles. The role of T and B cells in causing epithelial injury is not established, but T-cell–driven activation of B cells may be involved in the pathogenesis of gastric lymphomas (MALT lymphomas, discussed later in this chapter).

Only 10% to 20% of individuals worldwide who are infected with *H. pylori* actually develop peptic ulcer. Hence, a key enigma is why most are spared and some are susceptible. Perhaps there are interactions between *H. pylori* and the mucosa that occur only in some individuals. Emerging evidence also strongly implicates bacterial factors. Thus, strains producing VacA and CagA cause more intense tissue inflammation, more severe epithelial damage, and higher cytokine production. Recent molecular analyses are beginning to uncover subtle genetic differences between different strains that may influence their pathogenicity. Suffice it to say that *while the link between H. pylori infection and gastric and duodenal ulcers is well established, variability in host-pathogen interactions leading to ulceration remains to be deciphered.*

NSAIDs are the major cause of peptic ulcer disease in persons who do not have H. pylori infection. The gastroduodenal effects of NSAIDs range from acute erosive gastritis and acute gastric ulceration to peptic ulceration in 1% to 3% of users. Because NSAIDs are among the most commonly used medications, the magnitude of gastroduodenal toxicity caused by these agents is quite large. Risk factors for NSAID-induced gastroduodenal toxicity are increasing age, higher dose, and prolonged usage. Thus, those who take these drugs for chronic rheumatic conditions are at particularly high risk. Suppression of mucosal prostaglandin synthesis, which increases secretion of hydrochloric acid and reduces bicarbonate and mucin production, is the key to NSAID-induced peptic ulceration. Loss of mucin degrades the mucosal barrier that normally prevents acid from reaching the epithelium. Synthesis of glutathione, a free-radical scavenger, is also reduced. Some NSAIDs can penetrate the gut mucosal cells as well. Whether coexisting *H. pylori* infection affects NSAID-induced ulceration is not entirely settled.

Other events may act alone or in concert with *H. pylori* and NSAIDs to promote peptic ulceration. Gastric *hyperacidity* may be strongly ulcerogenic. Excess production of gastric acid from a tumor in individuals with the *Zollinger-Ellison syndrome* (Chapter 20) causes multiple peptic ulcerations in the stomach, duodenum, and even the jejunum. *Cigarette smoking* impairs mucosal blood flow and healing. Alcohol has not been proved to directly cause peptic ulceration, but alcoholic cirrhosis is associated with an increased incidence of peptic ulcers. *Corticosteroids* in high dose and with repeated use promote ulcer formation. There are also compelling arguments that personality and psychological stress are important contributing variables. Although this is now accepted as "common wisdom," actual data on cause and effect are lacking.

Morphology

All peptic ulcers, whether gastric or duodenal, have an identical gross and microscopic appearance. **By definition, they are defects in the mucosa that penetrate at least into the submucosa, and often into the muscularis propria or deeper. Most are round, sharply punched-out craters 2 to 4 cm in diameter** (Fig. 15–16); those in the duodenum tend to be smaller, and occasional gastric lesions are significantly larger. Favored sites are the anterior and posterior walls of the first portion of the duodenum and the lesser curvature of the stomach. The location within the stomach is dictated by the extent of the associated gastritis: antral gastritis is most common, and the ulcer is often along the lesser curvature at the margin of the inflamed area and the upstream acid-secreting mucosa of the corpus. Occasional gastric ulcers occur on the greater curvature or anterior or posterior walls of the stomach, the very same locations of most ulcerative cancers.

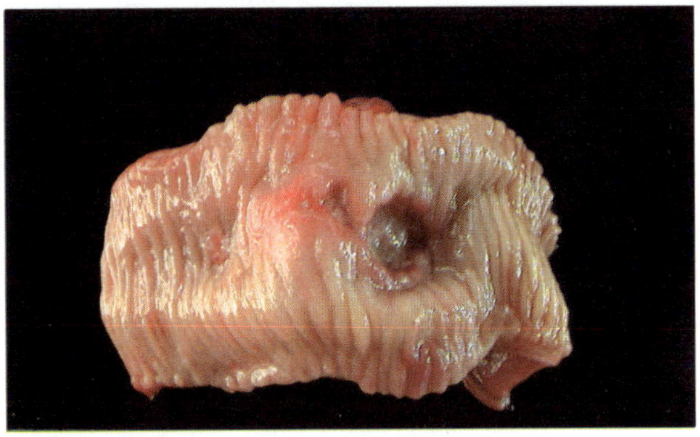

Figure 15–16

Peptic ulcer of the duodenum. Note that the ulcer is small (2 cm) with a sharply punched-out appearance. Unlike cancerous ulcers, the margins are not elevated. The ulcer base is clean (compare with the ulcerated carcinoma in Fig. 15–19). (Courtesy of Dr. Robin Foss, University of Florida, Gainesville, Florida).

Classically, **the margins of the crater are perpendicular and there is some mild edema of the immediately adjacent mucosa, but unlike ulcerated cancers there is no significant elevation or beading of the edges.** The surrounding mucosal folds may radiate like wheel spokes. The base of the crater appears remarkably clean, as a result of peptic digestion of the inflammatory exudate and necrotic tissue. Infrequently, an eroded artery is visible in the ulcer (usually associated with a history of significant bleeding). If the ulcer crater penetrates through the duodenal or gastric wall, a localized or generalized peritonitis may develop. Alternatively, the perforation is sealed by an adjacent structure such as adherent omentum, liver, or pancreas.

The histologic appearance varies with the activity, chronicity, and degree of healing. In a chronic, open ulcer, four zones can be distinguished (Fig. 15–17): (1) the base and margins have a thin layer of necrotic fibrinoid debris underlain by (2) a zone of active nonspecific inflammatory infiltration with neutrophils predominating, underlain by (3) granulation tissue, deep to which is (4) fibrous, collagenous scar that fans out widely from the margins of the ulcer. Vessels trapped within the scarred area are characteristically thickened and occasionally thrombosed, but in some instances they are widely patent. With healing, the crater fills with granulation tissue, followed by re-epithelialization from the margins and more or less restoration of the normal architecture (hence the prolonged healing times). Extensive fibrous scarring remains.

Chronic gastritis is extremely common among persons with peptic ulcer disease, and *H. pylori* infection is almost always demonstrable in those persons with gastritis. Similarly, individuals with NSAID-associated peptic ulcers do not have gastritis unless there is coexistent *H. pylori* infection. This feature is helpful in distinguishing peptic ulcers from acute gastric ulceration (discussed later), because gastritis in adjacent mucosa is generally absent in the latter condition.

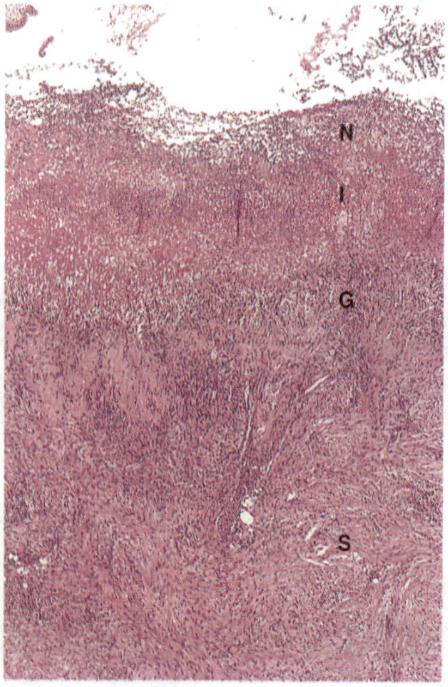

Figure 15–17

Medium-power detail of the base of a nonperforated peptic ulcer, demonstrating the layers of necrosis (N), inflammation (I), granulation tissue (G), and scar (S) moving from the luminal surface at the top to the muscle wall at the bottom.

Clinical Features. Most peptic ulcers cause epigastric pain, often described as gnawing, burning, or boring, but a significant minority first come to light with complications such as hemorrhage or perforation. The pain tends to be worse at night and occurs usually 1 to 3 hours after meals during the day. Classically, the pain is relieved by alkalis or food, but there are many exceptions. Nausea, vomiting, bloating, belching, and significant weight loss (raising the specter of some hidden malignancy) are additional manifestations.

Bleeding is the chief complication, occurring in as many as one-third of patients, and may be life-threatening. Perforation occurs in about 5% of patients but accounts for two-thirds of deaths from this disease in the United States. Obstruction of the pyloric channel is rare. Malignant transformation occurs in about 2% of patients, generally from ulcers in the pyloric channel, and is very rare with gastric ulcers. In the latter event, it is often difficult to exclude the possibility that carcinoma was present from the outset.

Peptic ulcers are notoriously chronic, recurrent lesions; they more often impair the quality of life than shorten it. Nevertheless, with present-day therapies (including antibiotics active against *H. pylori*, proton pump inhibitors, and hydrogen receptor antagonists), most ulcer victims can be helped if not cured, and they usually escape the surgeon's knife.

Acute Gastric Ulceration

Focal, acutely developing gastric mucosal defects that may appear after severe physiologic stress are called *stress ulcers*. Generally, there are many lesions located mainly in the stomach and occasionally in the duodenum. Stress ulcers are most commonly encountered in these conditions:

- Severe trauma, including major surgical procedures, sepsis, shock, or grave illness of any type
- Chronic exposure to gastric irritant drugs, particularly NSAIDs and corticosteroids
- Extensive burns (these ulcers are known as Curling ulcers)
- Traumatic or surgical injury to the central nervous system or an intracerebral hemorrhage (called Cushing ulcers; carry high risk of perforation).

The pathogenesis of these lesions is uncertain and may vary with the setting. NSAID-induced ulcers are linked to decreased prostaglandin production. The systemic acidosis that can accompany severe trauma and burns may contribute to mucosal injury presumably by lowering the intracellular pH of mucosal cells already rendered hypoxic by impaired mucosal blood flow. With cranial lesions, direct stimulation of vagal nuclei by increased intracranial pressure may cause gastric acid hypersecretion, which is common in these patients.

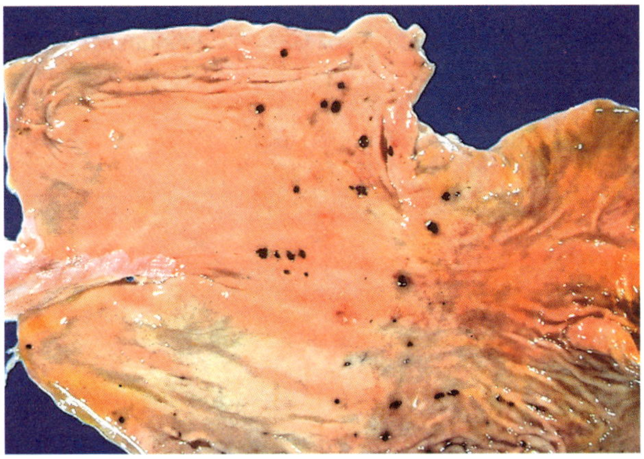

Figure 15–18

Multiple stress ulcers of the stomach, highlighted by the dark digested blood in their bases.

Morphology

Acute stress ulcers are usually circular and small (<1 cm in diameter). The ulcer base is frequently stained dark brown by the acid digestion of extruded blood. Unlike chronic peptic ulcers, acute stress ulcers are found anywhere in the stomach. They may occur singly, but more often there are several, located throughout the stomach and duodenum (Fig. 15–18). Microscopically, acute stress ulcers are abrupt lesions, with essentially unremarkable adjacent mucosa. They range in depth from very superficial lesions (erosion) to deeper lesions that involve the entire mucosal thickness (true ulceration). The shallow erosions are, in essence, an extension of acute erosive gastritis. The deeper lesions comprise well-defined ulcerations but are not precursors of chronic peptic ulcers. Even the deeper lesions do not penetrate the muscularis propria.

Clinical Features. A high percentage of persons admitted to hospital intensive care units with sepsis, severe burns, or trauma develop superficial gastric erosions or ulcers. These may be of limited clinical consequence or may be life-threatening. Although prophylactic antacid regimens and blood transfusions may blunt the impact of stress ulceration, the single most important determinant of clinical outcome is the ability to correct the underlying condition. The gastric mucosa can recover completely if the person does not die from the primary disease.

SUMMARY

Inflammatory Diseases of the Stomach

- *Chronic gastritis:* major cause is infection by *Helicobacter pylori,* less commonly autoimmune in origin; characterized by mononuclear cell infiltration in the lamina propria with intestinal metaplasia and frequently, proliferation of lymphoid tissue; may be the precursor of peptic ulcer and carcinoma.
- *Acute gastritis:* acute mucosal inflammation, usually transient, associated with use of NSAIDs, alcohol, heavy smoking, and various systemic abnormalities.
- *Peptic ulcer:* breach in the epithelium caused most commonly by *H. pylori* infection and mucosal exposure to gastric acid and enzymes (pepsin), or less frequently by use of NSAIDs; *H. pylori* elicits inflammatory reaction and damages epithelial cells; typically, sharply demarcated mucosal defects with underlying necrosis, acute inflammation, granulation tissue, and scarring; manifested by bleeding and, less commonly, rupture.
- *Stress ulcers (acute gastric ulcers):* associated with severe trauma, burns, CNS trauma or hemorrhage; usually small, multiple, hemorrhagic ulcers that are often shallow.

GASTRIC TUMORS

As with the remainder of the gastrointestinal tract, tumors arising from the mucosa predominate over mesenchymal tumors. Mucosal tumors are classified into polyps and carcinoma.

Gastric Polyps

The term polyp is applied to any nodule or mass that projects above the level of the surrounding mucosa. Occasionally, a lipoma or leiomyoma arising in the wall of the stomach may protrude from under the mucosa to produce an apparent polypoid lesion. However, *the use of the term polyp in the gastrointestinal tract is generally restricted to mass lesions arising in the mucosa.* Gastric polyps are uncommon and are found in about 0.4% of adult autopsies, as compared with colonic polyps, which are seen in 25% to 50% of older persons. In the stomach, these lesions are most frequently (1) hyperplastic polyps (80% to 85%), (2) fundic gland polyps (~10%), and (3) adenomatous polyps (~5%). All three types arise in the setting of chronic gastritis and so are seen in the same patient populations. Hyperplastic and fundic gland polyps are essentially innocuous. In contrast, there is a definite risk of an adenomatous polyp harboring adenocarcinoma, which increases with polyp size. Because the different types of gastric polyps cannot be reliably distinguished by endoscopy, histologic examination is mandatory.

Morphology

Hyperplastic polyps arise from an exuberant reparative response to chronic mucosal damage and hence are composed of a hyperplastic mucosal epithelium and an inflamed edematous stroma. They are not true neoplasms. Fundic gland polyps are small collections of dilated corpus-type glands thought to be small hamartomas. On the other hand, the less common adenomas contain dysplastic epithelium. As with colonic adenomas, to be described later, adenomas are true neoplasms.

Gastric Carcinoma

Among the malignant tumors that occur in the stomach, carcinoma is overwhelmingly the most important and the most common (90% to 95%). Next in order of frequency are lymphomas (4%), carcinoids (3%), and stromal tumors (2%). This discussion of gastric tumors focuses on gastric carcinomas, with only a brief mention of the other types. Gastrointestinal stromal tumors, carcinoids, and lymphomas are discussed later in this chapter, after the presentation of intestinal tumors.

Epidemiology and Classification. Gastric carcinoma is the second leading cause of cancer-related deaths in the world, with a widely varying geographic incidence. Japan and South Korea have the highest incidence (eight to nine times higher than in the United States and Western Europe), and the incidence in many other countries, such as China and Chile and Costa Rica, is also high. Nevertheless, in most countries there has been a steady decline in the overall incidence and the mortality of gastric cancer. Yet it remains the leading killer among cancers, as a result of its discouraging 5-year survival rate, which remains at less than 20%. It is responsible for approximately 2% of all cancer deaths in the United States.

Gastric cancers show two morphologic types, called *intestinal* and *diffuse*. The *intestinal type* is thought to arise from gastric mucous cells that have undergone intestinal metaplasia in the setting of chronic gastritis. This pattern of cancer tends to be better differentiated and is the more common type in high-risk populations. The *diffuse variant* is thought to arise de novo from native gastric mucous cells, is not associated with chronic gastritis, and tends to be poorly differentiated. Whereas the intestinal-type carcinoma occurs primarily after age 50 years with a 2:1 male predominance, the diffuse carcinoma occurs at an earlier age with female predominance. *The incidence of intestinal-type carcinoma has progressively diminished in the United States. By contrast, the incidence of diffuse gastric carcinoma has not significantly changed in the past 60 years* and now constitutes approximately half of gastric carcinomas in the United States. The intestinal and diffuse forms of gastric carcinomas can be considered as distinct entities, although their clinical outcome is similar.

Etiology and Pathogenesis

Intestinal-Type Adenocarcinoma. Several major variables are thought to affect the genesis of this form of cancer (Table 15–5). The predisposing influences are many, but their relative importance is changing. For example, dietary influences have changed drastically in recent years with the increased use of refrigeration worldwide, markedly decreasing the need for food preservation by nitrates, smoking, and salt. On the other hand, chronic gastritis associated with *H. pylori* infection constitutes a major risk factor for gastric carcinoma. The risk is particularly high in individuals with chronic gastritis limited to the gastric pylorus and antrum. Gastritis is generally accompanied by severe gastric atrophy and intestinal metaplasia, which are ultimately followed by dysplasia and cancer. The mechanisms of neoplastic transformation are not entirely clear. Chronic inflammation induced by *H. pylori* may release reactive oxygen species, which eventually cause DNA damage, leading to an imbalance between cell proliferation and apoptosis, particularly in areas of tissue repair. Notably, individuals with *H. pylori*–associated duodenal ulcers are largely protected from developing gastric cancer. Amplification of *HER-2/NEU* and increased expression of β-catenin are present in 20% to 30% of cases and are absent in diffuse carcinoma.

Table 15–5 Risk Factors for Gastric Carcinoma

Intestinal-Type Adenocarcinoma
Chronic gastritis with intestinal metaplasia
Infection with *Helicobacter pylori*
Nitrites derived from nitrates (found in food and drinking water, and used as preservatives in prepared meats, may undergo nitrosation to form nitrosamines and nitrosamides)
Diets containing foods that may generate nitrites (smoked foods, pickled vegetables and excessive salt intake)
Decreased intake of fresh vegetables and fruits (antioxidants present in these foods may inhibit nitrosation)
Partial gastrectomy
Pernicious anemia
Diffuse Carcinoma
Risk factors undefined, except for a rare inherited mutation of E-cadherin
Infection with *H. pylori* and chronic gastritis often absent

Diffuse Adenocarcinoma. The risk factors for this type of cancer remain undefined (Table 15–5), and precursor lesions have not been identified. Mutations in *E-cadherin*, which are not detectable in intestinal-type cancers, are present in 50% of diffuse cancers. A subset of patients may have a hereditary form of diffuse gastric cancer, caused by germ-line mutation in *E-cadherin*. Mutations in *FGFR2*, a member of the fibroblast growth factor receptor family, and increased expression of metalloproteinases are present in about one-third of cases, but are absent in intestinal-type carcinomas.

Morphology

The location of gastric carcinomas within the stomach is as follows: pylorus and antrum, 50% to 60%; cardia, 25%; and the remainder in the body and fundus. The lesser curvature is involved in about 40% and the greater curvature in 12%. **Thus, a favored location is the lesser curvature of the antropyloric region.** Though less frequent, an ulcerative lesion on the greater curvature is more likely to be malignant than benign.

Gastric carcinoma is classified on the basis of depth of invasion, macroscopic growth pattern, and histologic subtype. The morphologic feature having the greatest impact on clinical outcome is the **depth of invasion. Early gastric carcinoma is defined as a lesion confined to the mucosa and submucosa, regardless of the pres-**

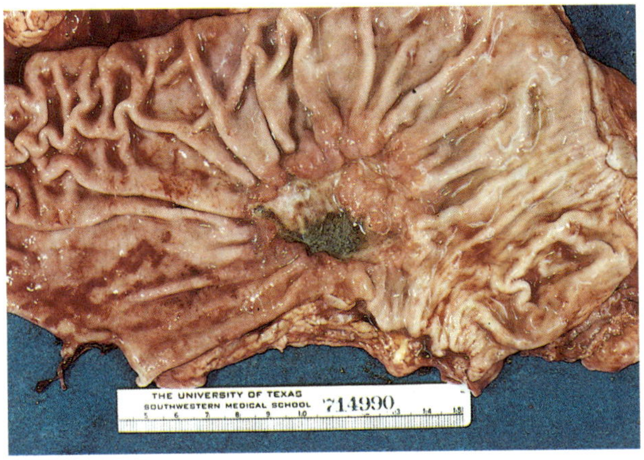

Figure 15–19

Ulcerative gastric carcinoma. The ulcer is large with irregular, heaped-up margins. There is extensive excavation of the gastric mucosa with a necrotic gray area in the deepest portion. Compare with the benign peptic ulcer in Figure 15–16.

ence or absence of perigastric lymph node metastases. Advanced gastric carcinoma is a neoplasm that has extended below the submucosa into the muscular wall and has perhaps spread more widely. Gastric mucosal **dysplasia** is the presumed precursor lesion of early gastric cancer, which then in turn progresses to "advanced" lesions.

The three macroscopic growth patterns of gastric carcinoma, which may be evident at both the early and advanced stages, are (1) **exophytic**, with protrusion of a tumor mass into the lumen; (2) **flat or depressed**, in which there is no obvious tumor mass within the mucosa; and (3) **excavated**, whereby a shallow or deeply erosive crater is present in the wall of the stomach. Exophytic tumors may contain portions of an adenoma. Flat or depressed malignancy presents only as regional effacement of the normal surface mucosal pattern. Excavated cancers may mimic, in size and appearance, chronic peptic ulcers, although more advanced cases show heaped-up margins (Fig. 15–19). Uncommonly, a broad region of the gastric wall, or the entire stomach, is extensively infiltrated by malignancy. The rigid and thickened stomach is termed a leather bottle stomach, or **linitis plastica**; metastatic carcinoma from the breast and lung may generate a similar picture.

As mentioned earlier, histologic appearances of gastric cancer are best classified into the intestinal type and diffuse type (Fig. 15–20). The **intestinal variant** is composed of malignant cells forming neoplastic intestinal glands resembling those of colonic adenocarcinoma. The **diffuse variant** is composed of gastric-type mucous cells that generally do not form glands but rather permeate the mucosa and wall as scattered individual **"signet-ring" cells** or small clusters in an "infiltrative" growth pattern.

Whatever the histologic variant, all gastric carcinomas eventually penetrate the wall to involve the serosa, spread to regional and more distant lymph nodes, and metastasize widely. For obscure reasons, the earliest lymph node metastasis may sometimes involve a supraclavicular lymph node (Virchow node). Another somewhat unusual mode of intraperitoneal spread in females is to both the ovaries, giving rise to the so-called **Krukenberg tumor** (Chapter 19).

Clinical Features. Both intestinal-type and diffuse gastric carcinoma are generally asymptomatic and can be discovered only by repeated endoscopic examinations in persons at high risk. Advanced carcinoma also may be asymptomatic, but it often first comes to light because of abdominal discomfort or weight loss. Uncommonly, these neoplasms cause dysphagia when they are located in the cardia or obstructive symptoms when they arise in the pyloric canal. The only hope for cure is early detection and surgical removal, because the most important prognostic indicator is stage of the tumor at the time of resection.

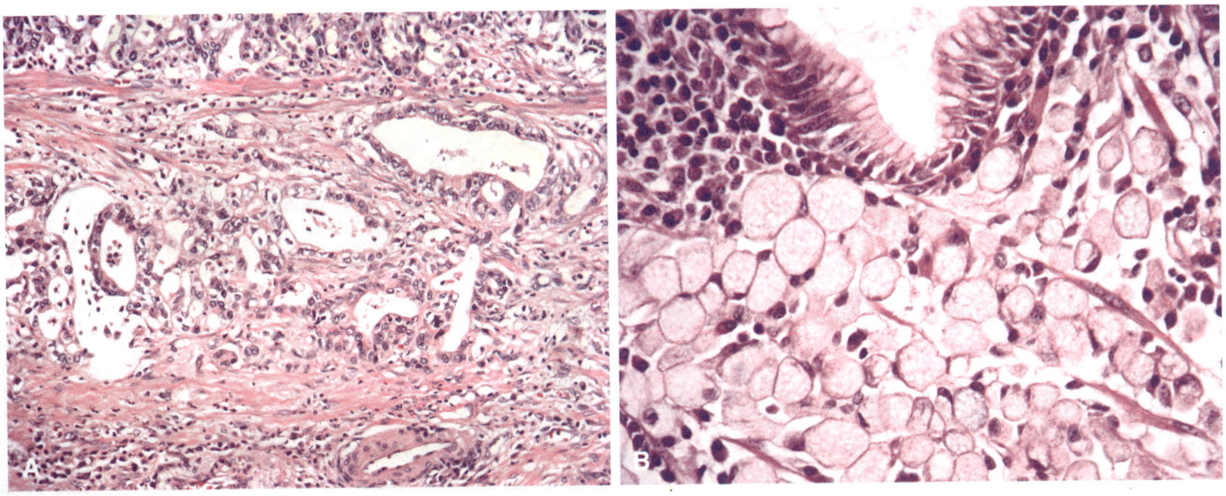

Figure 15–20

Gastric cancer. **A,** H&E stain demonstrating intestinal type of gastric carcinoma with gland formation by malignant cells that are invading the muscular wall of the stomach. **B,** Diffuse type of gastric carcinoma with signet-ring tumor cells.

SUMMARY

Gastric Tumors

- More than 90% of gastric tumors are carcinomas; lymphomas, carcinoids and stromal tumors are relatively infrequent.
- The two main types of gastric adenocarcinomas are the intestinal and diffuse types; macroscopic patterns of both types may be exophytic, flat or depressed, or excavating.
- *Intestinal type of adenocarcinoma* is associated with chronic gastritis caused by *H. pylori* infection, with gastric atrophy and intestinal metaplasia; composed of malignant cells forming intestinal glands.
- *Diffuse type of adenocarcinoma* is not associated with *H. pylori* infection; composed of gastric type of mucous cells (signet ring cells) that permeate the mucosa without forming glands.

SMALL AND LARGE INTESTINES

Many conditions, such as infections, inflammatory diseases, and tumors, affect both the small and large intestines. These two organs are therefore considered together. Collectively, disorders of the intestines account for a large portion of human disease.

DEVELOPMENTAL ANOMALIES

These defects are uncommon but sometimes result in serious clinical disease.

- *Atresia*, the complete failure of development of the intestinal lumen, and *stenosis*, narrowing of the intestinal lumen with incomplete obstruction, may affect any segment of the small intestine, but duodenal atresia is the most common.
- *Duplication* usually takes the form of well-formed saccular to tubular cystic structures, which may or may not communicate with the lumen of the small intestine.
- *Meckel diverticulum* is the most common and innocuous of the anomalies. It results from failure of involution of the omphalomesenteric duct, leaving a persistent blind-ended tubular protrusion as long as 5 to 6 cm (Fig. 15–21). The diameter is variable, sometimes approximating that of the small intestine itself. Such diverticula are usually in the ileum, about 80 cm proximal to the ileocecal valve, and are composed of all layers of the normal small intestine. They generally are asymptomatic, except when they permit bacterial overgrowth that depletes vitamin B_{12}, producing a syndrome similar to pernicious anemia. Rarely, pancreatic rests are found in a Meckel diverticulum, and in about half of the cases there are heterotopic islands of functioning gastric mucosa. Peptic ulceration in the adjacent intestinal mucosa sometimes is responsible for mysterious intestinal bleeding or symptoms resembling acute appendicitis.
- *Omphalocele* is a congenital defect of the periumbilical abdominal musculature that creates a membranous sac, into which the intestines herniate. In *gastroschisis*, extrusion of the intestines is caused by lack of formation of a portion of the abdominal wall.
- *Malrotation* of the developing bowel can prevent the intestines from assuming their normal intra-abdominal positions. The cecum, for example, may be found anywhere in the abdomen, including the left upper quadrant, rather than in its normal position in the right lower quadrant. The large intestine is predisposed to volvulus (discussed below). Confusing clinical syndromes may arise when appendicitis presents as left upper quadrant pain.
- *Hirschsprung disease*, leading to congenital megacolon. This condition is discussed separately.

Hirschsprung Disease: Congenital Megacolon

Distention of the colon to greater than 6 or 7 cm in diameter (megacolon) occurs as a congenital and as an acquired disorder. Hirschsprung disease (congenital megacolon) results when, during development, the migration of neural crest–derived cells along the alimentary tract arrests at some point before reaching the anus. Hence, an *aganglionic* segment is formed that lacks both the Meissner submucosal and Auerbach myenteric plexuses. This

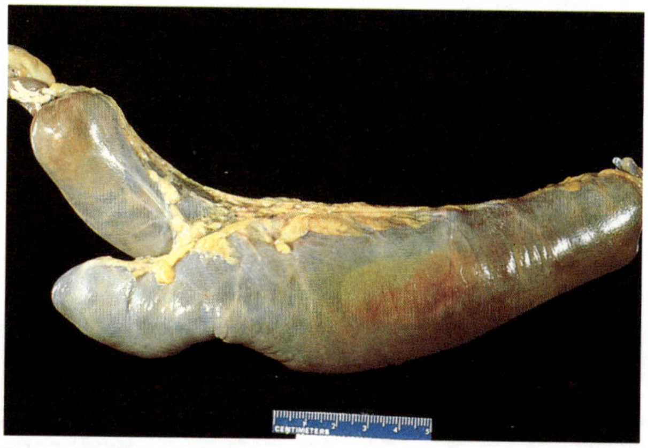

Figure 15–21

Meckel diverticulum. The blind pouch is located on the antimesenteric side of the small bowel.

causes functional obstruction and progressive distention of the colon proximal to the affected segment. Ganglia are absent from the muscle wall and submucosa of the constricted segment but may be present in the dilated portion.

Genetically, Hirschsprung disease is heterogeneous, and several different defects that lead to the same outcome have been identified. Approximately 50% of familial cases result from mutations in *RET* genes and RET ligands, because this signaling pathway is required for development of the myoenteric nerve plexus and provides direction to migrating neural crest cells. Many of the remaining cases arise from mutations in endothelin 3 and endothelin receptors. Hirschsprung disease occurs in approximately 1 in 5000 to 8000 live births; it predominates in males in a ratio of 4:1. It is much more frequent in those with other congenital anomalies such as hydrocephalus, ventricular septal defect, and Meckel diverticulum.

Morphology

The critical lesion in Hirschsprung disease is the lack of ganglion cells, and of ganglia, in the muscle wall and submucosa of the affected segment. The affected segment is not distended; it is the up-stream, properly innervated segment that undergoes dilation. Thus, when only the distal colon is affected, the remainder of the colon becomes massively distended, sometimes achieving a diameter of 15 to 20 cm. The wall may be thinned by distention or in some cases is thickened by compensatory muscle hypertrophy. The mucosal lining of the distended portion may be intact or have shallow, so-called **stercoral ulcers** produced by impacted, inspissated feces.

Clinical Features. In most cases a delay occurs in the initial passage of meconium, which is followed by vomiting in 48 to 72 hours. When a very short distal segment of the rectum alone is involved, the obstruction may not be complete and may not produce manifestations until later in infancy, in the form of alternating periods of obstruction and passage of diarrheal stools. The principal threat to life is superimposed enterocolitis with fluid and electrolyte disturbances. More rarely, the distended colon perforates, usually in the thin-walled cecum. The diagnosis is established by documenting the absence of ganglion cells in the *nondistended* bowel segment.

Acquired megacolon may result from (1) Chagas disease, in which the trypanosomes directly invade the bowel wall to destroy the plexuses, (2) organic obstruction of the bowel by a neoplasm or inflammatory stricture, (3) toxic megacolon complicating ulcerative colitis or Crohn disease (discussed later), or (4) a functional psychosomatic disorder. Except for the trypanosomal Chagas disease, in which the inflammatory involvement of the ganglia is evident, the remaining forms of megacolon are not associated with any deficiency of mural ganglia.

VASCULAR DISORDERS

Ischemic Bowel Disease

Ischemic lesions may be restricted to the small or large intestine or may affect both, depending on the particular vessel or vessels involved. Acute occlusion of one of the three major supply trunks of the intestines—celiac, superior, and inferior mesenteric arteries—may lead to infarction of extensive segments of intestine. However, insidious loss of one vessel may be without effect, thanks to the rich anastomoses between the vascular beds. Lesions within the end-arteries that penetrate the gut wall produce small, focal ischemic lesions. As illustrated in Figure 15–22, the severity of injury ranges from *transmural infarction* of the gut, involving all visceral layers, to *mural infarction* of the mucosa and submucosa, sparing the muscular wall, to *mucosal infarction*, if the lesion extends no deeper than the muscularis mucosae.

Almost always, transmural infarction is caused by acute occlusion of a major mesenteric artery. Mural or mucosal infarction more often results from either physiologic hypoperfusion or more localized anatomic defects, and may be acute or chronic. Mesenteric venous thrombosis is a less frequent cause of vascular compromise. The predisposing conditions for all three forms of ischemia are as follows:

- *Arterial thrombosis:* severe atherosclerosis (usually at the origin of the mesenteric vessel), systemic vasculitis, dissecting aneurysm, angiographic procedures, aortic reconstructive surgery, surgical accidents, hypercoagulable states, and oral contraceptives
- *Arterial embolism*: cardiac vegetations (as with endocarditis, or myocardial infarction with mural thrombosis), angiographic procedures, and aortic atheroembolism
- *Venous thrombosis*: hypercoagulable states induced, for example, by oral contraceptives or antithrombin III deficiency, intraperitoneal sepsis, the postoperative state, vascular-invasive neoplasms (particularly hepatocellular carcinoma), cirrhosis, and abdominal trauma

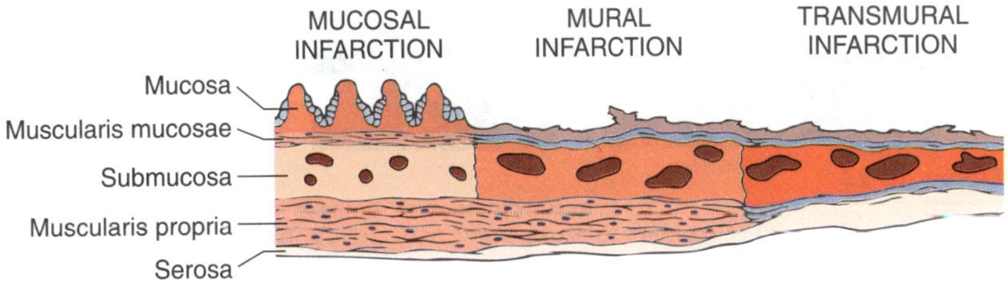

Figure 15–22

Acute ischemic bowel disease. Note the three levels of severity, represented for the small intestine.

- *Nonocclusive ischemia:* cardiac failure, shock, dehydration, vasoconstrictive drugs (e.g., digitalis, vasopressin, propranolol)
- *Miscellaneous:* radiation injury, volvulus, stricture, and internal or external herniation

Morphology

Transmural intestinal infarction may involve a short or long segment, depending on the particular vessel affected and the patency of the anastomotic supply. Whether the occlusion is arterial or venous, the infarction always has a dark red hemorrhagic appearance because of reflow of blood into the damaged area (Fig. 15–23). The ischemic injury usually begins in the mucosa and extends outward; within 18 to 24 hours there is a thin, fibrinous exudate over the serosa. With arterial occlusion the demarcation from adjacent normal bowel is fairly sharply defined, but with venous occlusion the margins are less distinct. Histologically, the changes are typical of ischemic damage with marked edema, interstitial hemorrhage, necrosis, and sloughing of the mucosa. Within 24 hours intestinal bacteria produce outright gangrene and sometimes perforation of the bowel.

Mural and mucosal infarctions are recognized by multi-focal lesions interspersed with spared areas. Their location depends in part on the extent of preexisting atherosclerotic narrowing of the arterial supply; lesions can be scattered over large regions of the small or large intestines. Affected foci may or may not be visible from the serosal surface, because by definition the ischemia does not affect the entire thickness of the bowel. When the bowel is opened, hemorrhagic edematous thickening of the mucosa, sometimes with superficial ulcerations, is seen. Histologic features are those of acute injury: edema, hemorrhage, and outright necrosis of the affected tissue layers (Fig. 15–24). Inflammation develops at the margins of the lesions, and an inflammatory fibrin-containing exudate (**pseudomembrane**), usually secondary to bacterial superinfection, may coat the affected mucosa. Alternatively, **chronic vascular insufficiency** may produce a chronic inflammatory and ulcerative condition, mimicking idiopathic inflammatory bowel disease (discussed below).

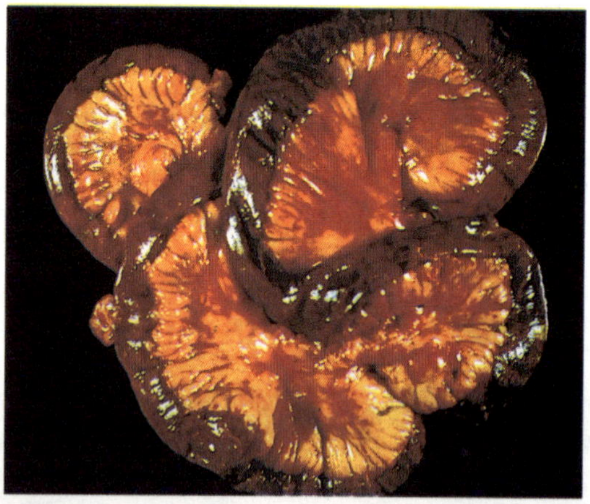

Figure 15–23

Infarcted small bowel, secondary to acute thrombotic occlusion of the superior mesenteric artery.

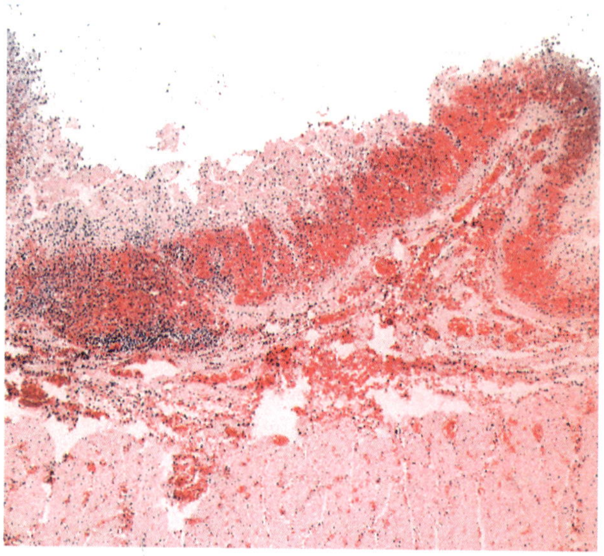

Figure 15–24

Mucosal infarction of the small bowel. The mucosa is hemorrhagic, and there is no epithelial layer. The remaining layers of the bowel are intact.

Clinical Features. Ischemic bowel injury is most common in the later years of life. With the transmural lesions, there is the sudden onset of abdominal pain, often out of proportion to the physical signs. Sometimes the pain is accompanied by bloody diarrhea. The onset of pain tends to be more sudden with mesenteric embolism than with arterial or venous thrombosis. Because this condition may progress to shock and vascular collapse within hours, the diagnosis must be made promptly, and making it requires a high index of suspicion in the appropriate context (e.g., recent major abdominal surgery, recent myocardial infarction, atrial fibrillation, or manifestations suggestive of some form of vegetative endocarditis). The mortality rate with infarction of the bowel approaches 90%, largely because the window of time between onset of symptoms and perforation caused by gangrene is so small.

By contrast, mural and mucosal ischemia may appear only as unexplained abdominal distention or gastrointestinal bleeding, sometimes accompanied by the gradual onset of abdominal pain or discomfort. Suspicion is raised if the individual has experienced conditions that favor acute hypoperfusion of the bowel, such as an episode of cardiac decompensation or shock. Mucosal and mural infarctions are not by themselves fatal, and, indeed, if the cause or causes of hypoperfusion can be corrected, the lesions may heal.

Angiodysplasia

Tortuous dilations of submucosal and mucosal blood vessels are seen most often in the cecum or right colon, usually only after the sixth decade of life. They are prone to rupture and bleed into the lumen. *Such lesions account for 20% of significant lower intestinal bleeding.* The hemorrhage may be chronic and intermittent and only cause severe anemia, but rarely it is acute and massive.

These lesions sometimes are part of a systemic disorder such as hereditary hemorrhagic telangiectasia (Osler-Weber-Rendu syndrome) or limited scleroderma, sometimes called the CREST syndrome (Chapter 5). Most often, they are isolated lesions thought to develop over decades as the result of mechanical influences operative in the colonic wall. As penetrating veins pass through the muscularis they are subject to intermittent occlusion during peristaltic contractions, but the thicker walled arteries remain patent, thus producing venous distention and ectasia.

Hemorrhoids

Hemorrhoids are variceal dilations of the anal and perianal submucosal venous plexuses. They are common after age 50 and develop in the setting of persistently elevated venous pressure within the hemorrhoidal plexus. Common predisposing conditions are straining at stool in the setting of chronic constipation and the venous stasis of pregnancy in younger women. More rarely, hemorrhoids may reflect portal hypertension, usually resulting from cirrhosis of the liver (Chapter 16).

Varicosities in the superior and middle hemorrhoidal veins appear above the anorectal line and are covered by rectal mucosa (*internal hemorrhoids*). Those that appear below the anorectal line represent dilations of the inferior hemorrhoidal plexus and are covered by anal mucosa (*external hemorrhoids*). Both are thin-walled, dilated vessels that commonly bleed, sometimes masking bleeding from far more serious proximal lesions. They may become thrombosed, particularly when subject to trauma from passage of stool. Finally, internal hemorrhoids may prolapse during straining at stool and then become trapped by the compressive anal sphincter, leading to sudden, extremely painful, edematous hemorrhagic enlargement or strangulation.

COLONIC DIVERTICULOSIS

A diverticulum is a blind pouch that communicates with the lumen of the gut. Congenital diverticula have all three layers of the bowel wall (mucosa, submucosa, and most notably the muscularis propria) and are distinctly uncommon. The prototype is *Meckel diverticulum*, described above.

Virtually all other diverticula are acquired and either lack or have an attenuated muscularis propria. *Acquired diverticula may occur anywhere in the alimentary tract, but by far the most common location is the colon*, giving rise to *diverticular disease* of the colon, also called *diverticulosis*. The colon is unique in that the outer longitudinal muscle coat is not complete but is gathered into three equidistant bands (the taeniae coli). Focal defects in the muscle wall are created where nerves and arterial vasa recta penetrate the inner circular muscle coat alongside the taeniae. The connective tissue sheaths accompanying these penetrating vessels provide potential sites for herniations.

Colonic diverticulosis is relatively infrequent in native populations of non-Western countries. Although unusual in Western adults younger than 30 years of age, in those older than the age of 60 the prevalence approaches 50%. This high prevalence is attributed to the consumption of a refined, low-fiber diet in Western societies, resulting in reduced stool bulk with increased difficulty in passage of intestinal contents. Exaggerated spastic contractions of the colon isolate segments of the colon (segmentation) in which the intraluminal pressure becomes markedly elevated, with consequent herniation of the bowel wall through the anatomic points of weakness. Thus, *two* influences are thought to be important in the genesis of diverticular protrusions: (1) *exaggerated peristaltic contractions* with abnormal elevation of intraluminal pressure and (2) *focal defects* peculiar to the normal muscular colonic wall.

Morphology

Most colonic diverticula are **small, flasklike or spherical outpouchings, usually 0.5 to 1 cm in diameter** (Fig. 15–25A). They are located in the sigmoid colon in approximately 95% of patients. Infrequently, more proximal levels and sometimes the entire colon are affected. Isolated cecal diverticula also occur. The exaggerated peristalsis often induces muscular hypertrophy in affected segments, with unusually prominent taenia coli and circular muscle bundles. Most diverticula penetrate between the bundles of circular muscle fibers adjacent to the mesenteric and lateral taeniae at sites of penetrating blood vessels. They frequently dissect into the appendices epiploicae and therefore may be inapparent on casual external inspection.

In the uninflamed state the walls are usually very thin, made up largely of mucosa and submucosa enclosed within fat or an intact peritoneal covering (Fig. 15–25B). Inflammatory changes may supervene to produce both diverticulitis and peridiverticulitis. Perforation may lead to localized peritonitis or abscess formation. When many closely adjacent diverticula become inflamed, the bowel wall may be encased by fibrous tissue, with narrowing of the lumen producing a remarkable resemblance to a cancerous stricture.

Clinical Features. In most persons, diverticular disease is asymptomatic and is discovered only at autopsy or by chance during a laparoscopy or barium enema for some other problem. In only about a fifth of the cases does intermittent cramping or sometimes continuous left-sided lower quadrant discomfort appear, with a sensation of never being able to completely empty the rectum. Super-

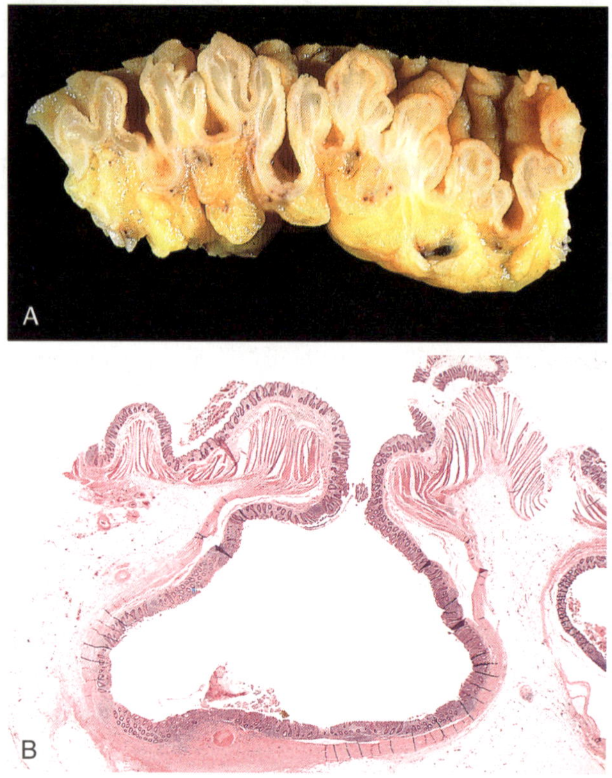

Figure 15–25

Diverticulosis. **A,** Section through the sigmoid colon showing multiple saclike diverticula protruding through the muscle wall into the mesentery. The muscularis between the diverticular protrusions is markedly thickened. **B,** Low-power micrograph of diverticulum of the colon showing protrusion of mucosa and submucosa through the muscle wall. A dilated blood vessel at the base of the diverticulum was a source of bleeding; some blood clot is present within the diverticular lumen.

imposed diverticulitis accentuates the symptoms and produces left lower quadrant tenderness and fever. Other, less common complications include minimal chronic intermittent bleeding or, rarely, brisk hemorrhage, perforation with pericolic abscess, or fistula formation.

The treatment of this condition merits brief mention, because it bears on its pathogenesis. A high-fiber diet is recommended on the theory that the increased stool bulk reduces the exaggerated peristalsis. Whether a high-fiber diet prevents disease progression or protects against superimposed diverticulitis is unclear, but the diet itself is a source of discomfort.

BOWEL OBSTRUCTION

Although any part of the gut may be involved, because of its narrow lumen, the small bowel is most commonly affected. Four entities—hernias, intestinal adhesions, intussusception, and volvulus—account for at least 80% of the cases (Table 15–6 and Fig. 15–26).

Hernias, a weakness or defect in the wall of the peritoneal cavity, may permit protrusion of a pouchlike, serosa-lined sac of peritoneum, called a *hernial sac*. The usual sites of weakness are anteriorly at the inguinal and femoral canals, at the umbilicus, and in surgical scars. Rarely, retroperitoneal hernias may occur, chiefly about the ligament of Treitz. *Hernias are of concern because segments of viscera frequently intrude and become trapped in them (external herniation)*. This is particularly true with inguinal hernias, which have narrow orifices and large sacs. The most frequent intruders are small bowel loops, but portions of omentum or large bowel also may become trapped. Pressure at the neck of the pouch may impair venous drainage of the trapped viscus. The ensuing stasis and edema increase the bulk of the herniated loop, leading to permanent trapping (*incarceration*). Further compromise of its blood supply and drainage leads to infarction of the trapped segment (*strangulation*).

Surgical procedures, infection, and even endometriosis often cause localized or general peritoneal inflammation (peritonitis). With healing, *adhesions* may develop between bowel segments or the abdominal wall and the operative site. These fibrous bridges can create closed loops through which the intestines may slide and become trapped (*internal herniation*). The sequence of events is much the same as with external hernias.

Intussusception denotes telescoping of a proximal segment of bowel into the immediately distal segment. In children, intussusception sometimes occurs without apparent anatomic basis, perhaps related to excessive peristaltic activity. In adults, such telescoping often points to an intraluminal mass (e.g., tumor) that becomes trapped by a peristaltic wave and pulls its point of attachment along with it into the distal segment. Not only does intestinal obstruction ensue, but the vascular supply may be so compromised as to cause infarction of the trapped segment.

Volvulus refers to twisting of a loop of bowel or other structure (e.g., ovary) about its base of attachment, constricting the venous outflow and sometimes the arterial supply as well. Volvulus affects the small bowel most often and rarely the redundant sigmoid. Intestinal obstruction and infarction may follow.

Table 15–6 Major Causes of Intestinal Obstruction

Mechanical Obstruction
Hernias, internal or external
Adhesions
Intussusception
Volvulus
Other Less Frequent Conditions
Tumors
Inflammatory strictures
Obstructive gallstones, fecaliths, foreign bodies
Congenital stricture, atresias
Congenital bands
Meconium in cystic fibrosis
Imperforate anus

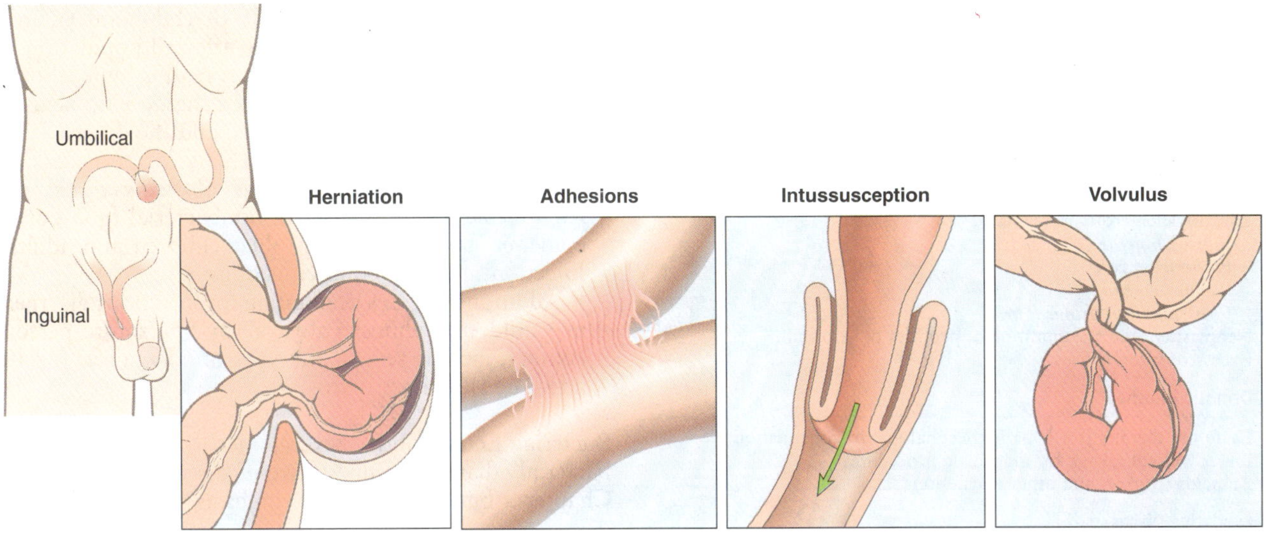

Figure 15–26

The four major causes of intestinal obstruction: (1) herniation of a segment in the umbilical or inguinal regions, (2) adhesions between intestinal loops, (3) intussusception, (4) volvulus.

ENTEROCOLITIS (DIARRHEAL DISEASES)

Diarrheal diseases of the bowel make up a veritable Augean stable of entities (as his fifth labor, Hercules cleaned the messy stables of King Augeas, which contained 3000 cattle and had not been swept for 30 years). Many are caused by microbiologic agents; others arise in the setting of malabsorptive disorders and idiopathic inflammatory bowel disease.

Although a precise definition of diarrhea is elusive, an increase in stool mass, stool frequency, or stool fluidity is perceived as diarrhea by most persons. For many individuals, this consists of daily stool production in excess of 250 gm, containing 70% to 95% water. More than 14 L/day of fluid may be lost in severe cases of diarrhea, equivalent to the circulating blood volume! Diarrhea is often accompanied by pain, urgency, perianal discomfort, and incontinence. Low-volume, painful, bloody diarrhea is known as dysentery.

We first list the major types of diarrheal diseases and then discuss infectious enterocolitis and malabsorption syndromes. Inflammatory bowel disease is presented in a subsequent section.

The major types of diarrheal diseases are:

- *Secretory diarrhea:* net intestinal fluid secretion that is isotonic with plasma and persists during fasting
- *Osmotic diarrhea:* excessive osmotic forces exerted by luminal solutes that abate with fasting
- *Exudative diarrhea:* output of purulent, bloody stools that persists on fasting; stools are frequent but may be small or large volume
- *Malabsorption diarrhea:* output of voluminous, bulky stools with increased osmolarity resulting from unabsorbed nutrients and excess fat (steatorrhea); it usually abates on fasting
- *Deranged motility diarrhea:* highly variable features regarding stool output, volume, and consistency; other forms of diarrhea must be excluded

The major causes of each of these types of diarrhea are presented in Table 15–7; selected entities are discussed here. It is important to bear in mind that several mechanisms may be operative in the same patient.

Infectious Enterocolitis

Intestinal diseases of microbial origin are marked principally by diarrhea and sometimes by ulceroinflammatory changes in the small or large intestine. *Infectious enterocolitis is a global problem of staggering proportions, causing more than 3 million deaths annually worldwide and accounting for up to one-half of deaths in children younger than 5 years of age in some countries.* Though far less prevalent in industrialized nations, infectious enterocolitis is still responsible for approximately 1.5 episodes of diarrhea per person (child and adult) per year, second only to the common cold in frequency. About 500 infants and young children die of diarrheal disease annually in the United States. Moreover, diarrhea is the most common health problem encountered by the more than 300 million people who travel internationally per year.

Among the most common offenders are rotavirus, calciviruses, and enterotoxigenic *Escherichia coli.* However, many pathogens can cause diarrhea; the major offenders vary with the age, nutrition, and immune status of the host, environment (living conditions, public health measures), and special predispositions such as foreign travel, exposure to more virulent organisms while hospitalized, and wartime dislocation. In 40% to 50% of cases, the specific agent cannot be isolated.

Table 15–7 Major Causes of Diarrheal Illnesses

Secretory Diarrhea	
Infectious: viral damage to surface epithelium	
	Rotavirus
	Norwalk virus
	Enteric adenoviruses
Infectious: enterotoxin-mediated	
	Vibrio cholerae
	Escherichia coli
	Bacillus cereus
	Clostridium perfringens
Neoplastic: tumor elaboration of peptides or serotonin	
Excessive laxative use	
Osmotic Diarrhea	
Lactulose therapy (for hepatic encephalopathy, constipation)	
Prescribed gut lavage for diagnostic procedures	
Antacids ($MgSO_4$ and other magnesium salts)	
Exudative Diseases	
Infectious: destruction of the epithelial layer	
	Shigella spp.
	Salmonella spp.
	Campylobacter spp.
	Entamoeba histolytica
Idiopathic inflammatory bowel disease	
Malabsorption	
Defective intraluminal digestion	
Defective mucosal-cell absorption	
Reduced small intestinal surface area	
Lymphatic obstruction	
Infectious: impaired mucosal-cell absorption	
	Giardia lamblia
Deranged Motility	
Decreased intestinal retention time	
	Surgical reduction of gut length
	Neural dysfunction, including irritable bowel syndrome
	Hyperthyroidism
Decreased motility (increased intestinal retention time)	
	Surgical creation of a "blind" intestinal loop
	Bacterial overgrowth in the small intestine

Worldwide, intestinal parasitic disease and protozoal infections are also major causes of chronic or recurrent infectious enterocolitis. Collectively, they affect more than one-half of the world's population, because they are endemic in less developed nations. Of the various lower alimentary tract infections, only selected examples are described here.

Viral Gastroenteritis. Viral infection of superficial epithelium in the small intestine destroys these cells and their absorptive function. Repopulation of the small intestinal villi with immature enterocytes and relative preservation of crypt secretory cells leads to net secretion of water and electrolytes, compounded by an osmotic diarrhea from incompletely absorbed nutrients.

Symptomatic disease is caused by several distinct groups of viruses:

- *Rotavirus* accounts for an estimated 130 million cases and 0.9 million deaths worldwide per year, and constitutes approximately 60% of childhood enterocolitis in the United States. The affected population is children 6 to 24 months of age; spread is by fecal-oral contamination. The prodrome for the development of diarrhea after infection is 2 days, and the disease lasts for 3 to 5 days.
- *Caliciviruses, particularly the Norwalk virus,* are responsible for most cases of nonbacterial food-borne epidemic gastroenteritis in older children and adults. Infection in young children is unusual.
- Additional viruses accounting for infectious diarrhea in children, almost always by person-to-person contact, include several subtypes of *adenovirus* (Ad40 and Ad41) and *astrovirus.*

Bacterial Enterocolitis. Several mechanisms underlying bacterial diarrheal illness were discussed briefly in Chapter 9 but are worthy of emphasis at this point:

- *Ingestion of preformed toxin,* present in contaminated food. Major offenders of food poisoning are *Staphylococcus aureus, Vibrio* spp., and *Clostridium perfringens.* One may also ingest preformed neurotoxins, exemplified by *Clostridium botulinum.*
- *Infection by toxigenic organisms,* which proliferate within the gut lumen and elaborate an enterotoxin.
- *Infection by enteroinvasive organisms,* which proliferate, invade, and destroy mucosal epithelial cells.

Infection by toxigenic or enteroinvasive organisms involves bacterial replication in the gut and depends on three key bacterial properties:

1. *The ability to adhere to mucosal epithelial cells.* To produce disease, ingested organisms must adhere to the mucosa; otherwise they are swept away by the fluid stream. Adherence is often mediated by plasmid-coded *adhesins* (rigid, wiry proteins expressed on the surface of the organism).
2. *The ability to elaborate enterotoxins.* Enterotoxigenic organisms produce polypeptides that cause diarrhea. The polypeptides may be secretagogues, which activate secretion without inducing cell damage; cholera toxin, elaborated by *Vibrio cholerae,* is the prototype toxin of this type. Alternatively, they may be cytotoxins, which cause direct epithelial cell necrosis, as exemplified by Shiga toxin. The enterotoxygenic strains of *E. coli* are the main cause of traveler's diarrhea.
3. *The capacity to invade.* Enteroinvasive organisms such as *Shigella* possess a large virulence plasmid that confers the capacity for epithelial cell invasion. This is followed by intracellular proliferation, cell lysis, and cell-to-cell spread. *S. flexneri* is the major cause of endemic bacillary dysentery in locations of poor hygiene in developing and developed countries. Other organisms such as *Salmonella typhi,* causing thyphoid fever, and *Yersinia enterocolitica* pass through mucosal epithelial cells en route to lymphatics and the bloodstream. Other species of *Salmonella,* such as *S. enteritidis* and *S. typhimurium,* cause more than half a million cases

of food poisoning in the United States, through the ingestion of contaminated eggs, chicken, and beef that have not been properly washed.

The major bacteria giving rise to *bacterial enterocolitis* are presented in Table 15–8.

Morphology

Given the multitude of bacterial pathogens, the pathologic manifestations of small intestinal and colonic bacterial disease are quite variable. **Most bacterial infections exhibit a nonspecific pattern of damage to the surface epithelium, with an increased mitotic rate in mucosal crypts and decreased maturation of surface epithelial cells. There follows hyperemia and edema of the lamina propria and variable neutrophilic infiltration into the lamina propria and epithelial layer.** In more severe infections with cytotoxin-producing or enteroinvasive bacteria, progressive destruction of the mucosa leads to erosion, ulceration, and severe submucosal inflammation. Notable features of particular infections include:

1. ***E. coli*** (a particularly versatile organism):
Enterotoxigenic strains (ETEC) affect the small intestine, with histologic features similar to *V. cholerae* (described below).
The Shiga toxin-producing strain (STEC) O157:H7 produces most severe disease in the right colon, with hemorrhage and ulceration. In children, this infection may be followed by the hemolytic uremic syndrome (Chapter 14). This is the most common strain of *E. coli* in North America.
Enteropathogenic strains (EPEC) affect the small intestine, producing villus blunting.
Enteroinvasive strains (EIEC) affect the colon, with histologic features similar to *Shigella*.
Enteroaggregative strains (EAEC) also affect the colon and show a "stacked brick" pattern of adherence in tissues.

2. ***Salmonella*** species are a major cause of common-source outbreaks of enterocolitis, producing localized mucosal disease primarily in the ileum and colon (as with *S. enteritidis, S. typhimurium,* and others). *S. typhimurium* generally causes a self-limited gastroenteritis with watery diarrhea, nausea, and fever. Life-

Table 15–8 Major Causes of Bacterial Enterocolitis

Organism	Pathogenic Mechanism	Source	Clinical Features
Escherichia coli			
ETEC	Cholera-like toxin, no invasion	Food, water	Traveler's diarrhea, including watery diarrhea
STEC	Shiga toxin, no invasion	Undercooked beef products	Hemorrhagic colitis, hemolytic-uremic syndrome (Chapter 14)
EPEC	Attachment, enterocyte effacement, no invasion	Weaning foods, water	Watery diarrhea, infants and toddlers
EIEC	Invasion, local spread	Cheese, water, person to person	Fever, pain, diarrhea, dysentery
Salmonella spp.	Invasion, translocation, lymphoid inflammation, dissemination	Milk, beef, eggs, poultry	Fever, pain, diarrhea or dysentery, bacteremia, extra-intestinal infection, common source of outbreaks
Shigella spp.	Invasion, local spread	Person to person, low inoculum	Fever, pain, diarrhea, dysentery, epidemic spread
Campylobacter	?Toxins, invasion	Milk, poultry, animal contact	Fever, pain, diarrhea, dysentery, food sources, animal reservoirs
Yersinia enterocolitica	Invasion, translocation, lymphoid inflammation, dissemination	Milk, pork	Fever, pain, diarrhea, mesenteric lymphadenitis, extra-intestinal infection, food sources
Vibrio cholerae, other *Vibrio* spp.	Enterotoxin, no invasion	Water, shellfish, person to person	Watery diarrhea, cholera, pandemic spread
Clostridium difficile	Cytotoxin, local invasion	Nosocomial environmental spread	Fever, pain, bloody diarrhea, after antibiotic use, nosocomial acquisition
Clostridium perfringens	Enterotoxin, no invasion	Meat, poultry, fish	Watery diarrhea, food sources, "pigbel"
Mycobacterium tuberculosis	Invasion, mural inflammatory foci with necrosis and scarring	Contaminated milk, swallowing of coughed-up organisms	Chronic abdominal pain, complications of malabsorption, stricture, perforation, fistulas, hemorrhage

ETEC, enterotoxigenic *E. coli;* STEC, Shiga toxin-producing *E. coli* (also called EHEC, enterohemorrhagic *E. coli*); EPEC, enteropathogenic *E. coli;* EIEC, enteroinvasive *E. coli.*

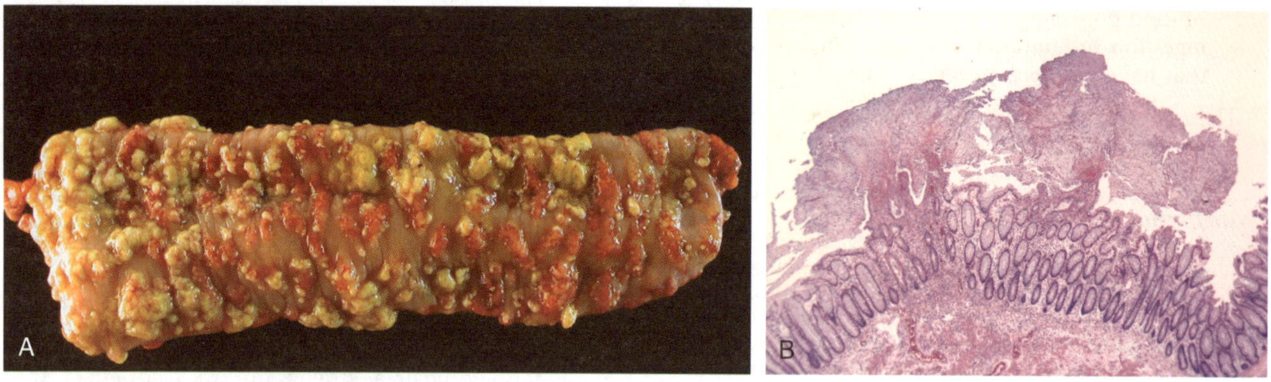

Figure 15–27

Pseudomembranous colitis from *Clostridium difficile* infection. **A,** Gross photograph showing plaques of yellow fibrin and inflammatory debris adherent to a reddened colonic mucosa. **B,** Low-power micrograph showing superficial mucosal erosion, an adherent pseudomembrane of fibrin, and inflammatory debris.

threatening systemic illness is the hallmark of *S. typhi,* whereby small intestinal invasion leads to systemic dissemination (**typhoid fever**). Typhoid fever is a protracted disease featuring **bacteremia** (first week), widespread involvement of macrophages with **splenomegaly** and **foci of necrosis in the liver** (second week), and **ulceration of Peyer's patches with intestinal bleeding and ulceration** (third week). **Gallbladder colonization** produces a chronic carrier state; chronic infection also may affect the joints, bones, meninges, and other sites.

3. ***Shigella*** affects primarily the distal colon, producing acute mucosal inflammation and erosion.

4. ***Campylobacter jejuni*** (and other species) affects the small intestine, appendix, and colon, producing many superficial ulcers, mucosal inflammation, and exudates.

5. ***Yersinia enterocolitica* and *Y. pseudotuberculosis*** affect the ileum, appendix, and colon. Peyer's patch invasion leads to mesenteric lymph node enlargement with necrotizing granulomas. Systemic spread may lead to peritonitis, pharyngitis, and pericarditis.

6. ***V. cholerae*** (cholera) affects the small intestine, especially more proximally. The mucosa is essentially intact, with only mucus-depleted crypts.

7. ***Clostridium difficile*** is a normal gut organism, but cytotoxin-producing strains may overgrow after systemic antibiotic use. A distinctive **pseudomembranous colitis** is produced, which derives its name from the plaquelike adhesion of fibrinopurulent debris and mucus to the damaged superficial mucosa (Fig. 15–27). These are not true "membranes," because the coagulum is not an epithelial layer.

8. ***C. perfringens*** shows features similar to *V. cholerae* but with some epithelial damage. Some strains produce a severe necrotizing enterocolitis with perforation.

9. Ingested ***Mycobacterium tuberculosis*** incites chronic inflammation and granuloma formation in mucosal lymphoid tissue—particularly Peyer's patches in the terminal ileum—and regional lymph nodes (Chapter 13).

Protozoal Infection. *Entamoeba histolytica* is a dysentery-causing protozoal parasite spread by fecal-oral contamination. Amebae invade the crypts of colonic glands and burrow down into the submucosa (Fig. 15–28); the organisms then fan out laterally to create a flask-shaped ulcer with a narrow neck and broad base. There may be very little inflammatory infiltrate within the ulcer. In about 40% of persons with amebic dysentery, parasites penetrate portal vessels and embolize to the liver to produce solitary, or less often numerous, discrete hepatic abscesses, some exceeding 10 cm in diameter. Some patients may present with amebic liver abscesses, without a clinical history of amebic dysentery. As with the intestinal lesions, there is a scant inflammatory reaction at the margin. Occasional amebic abscesses are encountered in the lung, heart, kidneys, and even brain. Such abscesses remain long after the acute intestinal illness has passed.

Giardia lamblia is an intestinal protozoan spread by water contaminated with feces. *Giardia* organisms attach to the small intestinal mucosa but do not appear to invade (Fig. 15–29). Small intestine morphology may range from virtually normal to marked blunting of the villi with a mixed inflammatory infiltrate in the lamina

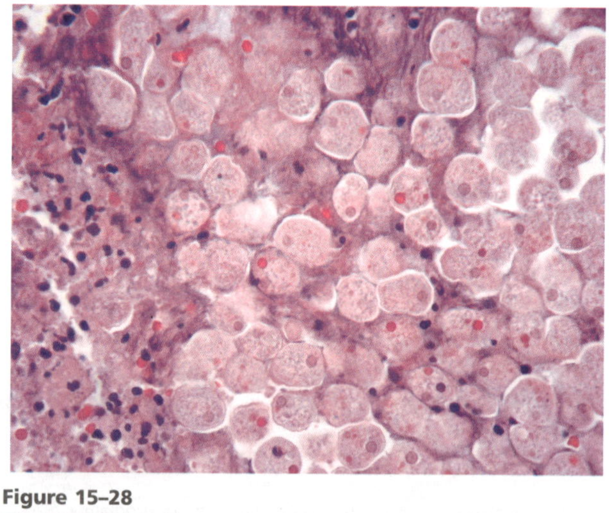

Figure 15–28

Entamoeba histolytica in the colon. Some organisms are ingesting red blood cells.

propria. A malabsorptive diarrhea seems to result from mucosal cell injury by mechanisms that are not understood.

Cryptosporidiosis has emerged as an important cause of diarrhea in animals and humans worldwide. It is the major cause of childhood diarrhea and accounts for as much as 20% of all cases of childhood diarrhea in developing countries. It is also a potentially fatal complication of AIDS. Water-borne contamination and an increased population at risk for zoonotic contamination have contributed to the increase in this disease.

Clinical Features. The clinical features of viral and protozoal infection have been briefly noted already. At the risk of oversimplification, bacterial enterocolitis takes the following forms:

- *Ingestion of preformed bacterial toxins.* Symptoms develop within a matter of hours; explosive diarrhea and acute abdominal distress herald an illness that passes within a day or so. Ingested systemic neurotoxins, as from *C. botulinum*, may produce rapid, and fatal, respiratory failure.
- *Infection with enteric pathogens.* With ingestion of enteric pathogens, an incubation period of several hours to days is followed by *diarrhea and dehydration* if the primary pathogenic mechanism is a secretory enterotoxin or *dysentery* if the primary mechanism is a cytotoxin or an enteroinvasive process. Traveler's diarrhea (e.g., Montezuma's revenge, turista) usually occurs after ingestion of feces-contaminated food or water; it begins abruptly and subsides within 2 to 3 days.
- *Insidious infection. Yersinia* and *Mycobacterium* infections may also present as subacute diarrheal illnesses mimicking Crohn disease. All enteroinvasive organisms can mimic, or even precipitate, acute onset of idiopathic inflammatory bowel disease (discussed below).

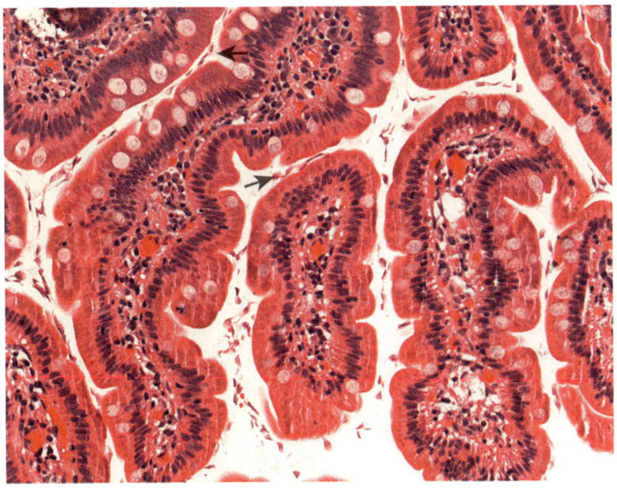

Figure 15–29

Giardia lamblia. Trophozoites (*arrows*) of the organism immediately adjacent to the duodenal surface epithelium, without mucosal invasion. (Courtesy of Drs. Melissa Upton and Paul Swanson, Department of Pathology, University of Washington, Seattle, Washington.)

In general, bacterial enterocolitis is a more severe illness than viral disease. The complications of bacterial enterocolitis result from massive fluid loss or destruction of the intestinal mucosal barrier and include dehydration, sepsis, and perforation. In the most severe cases, death ensues rapidly without quick intervention, particularly in the very young.

A distressing gastrointestinal emergency in neonates, particularly those who are premature or of low birth weight, is *necrotizing enterocolitis.* This acute, necrotizing inflammation of the small and large intestines is thought to result from a combination of functional immaturity of the neonatal gut, colonization and invasion by pathogenic organisms, and secondary ischemic injury. A small portion of terminal ileum and ascending colon may be affected, or the entire small and large intestines may be involved. The injury is initially mucosal, but in severe cases the entire bowel wall becomes hemorrhagic and gangrenous, necessitating surgical resection. In a typical case, there is abdominal distention, tenderness, ileus, and diarrhea with occult or frank blood. Onset of gangrene and perforation are immediately life-threatening.

SUMMARY

Enterocolitis (Diarrheal Diseases)

- The major types of diarrheal diseases are: secretory, osmotic, exudative, malabsorption-related, and due to deranged motility.
- Secretory diarrhea can be caused by viruses or enterotoxin-producing bacteria such as *E. coli;* in general, bacterial enterocolitis is a more serious disease than viral disease.
- *Salmonella* spp. and *Shigella* spp. cause exudative diarrhea. *Salmonella* infection is a very common cause of food poisoning. *S. typhi* can cause a systemic illness (typhoid fever).
- Bacterial enterocolitis may result from the ingestion of preformed bacterial toxins, infection with enteric pathogens, or take the form of an insidious infection that may mimic inflammatory bowel disease.
- The most common agents of enterocolitis among protozoa are *Entamoeba histolytica, Giradia lamblia* and *Cryptosporidium parvum.*

Malabsorption Syndromes

Malabsorption is characterized by defective absorption of fats, fat-soluble and other vitamins, proteins, carbohydrates, electrolytes and minerals, and water. The most common presentation is chronic diarrhea; the hallmark of malabsorption syndromes is steatorrhea (excessive fat content of the feces). At the most basic level, *malabsorption is the result of disturbance of at least one of these normal digestive functions:*

- *Intraluminal digestion*, in which proteins, carbohydrates, and fats are enzymatically broken down. The process begins in the mouth with saliva, receives a major boost from gastric peptic digestion, and continues in the small intestine, assisted by pancreatic enzyme secretion and the emulsive action of bile.

- *Mucosal absorption* in which water, electrolytes, and nutrients are absorbed and transported into the cell. Absorbed fatty acids are converted to triglycerides and are assembled with cholesterol and apoprotein B into chylomicrons. Disturbances can be caused by primary mucosal cell abnormalities or reduced small intestinal surface area. Other cases result from mucosal infections.
- *Nutrient delivery,* involving the delivery of nutrients from the intestinal cells into the lymphatics. Disturbances may be caused by congenital defects, or be secondary to tuberculosis or retroperitoneal fibrosis.

A host of disorders interrupt these three digestive functions, either directly or indirectly (Table 15–9). The malabsorptive disorders most commonly encountered in the United States are *pancreatic insufficiency, celiac disease, and Crohn disease.* Here we give some examples of the most common malabsorption syndromes caused by defects in either intraluminal digestion or mucosal absorption. Crohn disease is discussed under the heading "Inflammatory Bowel Disease."

Defects of Intraluminal Digestion. Typical features of defective intraluminal digestion are an *osmotic diarrhea* from undigested nutrients, and *steatorrhea* (excess output of undigested fat in the stool). The latter can arise either from inadequate action of pancreatic lipases or from inadequate solubilization of fat by hepatic bile secreted into the gut lumen. The most common causes are *pancreatic insufficiency* associated with chronic alcoholism, and Crohn disease, discussed below. Other causes are intestinal bacterial overgrowth, cholestatic liver disease, and surgical procedures such as extensive ileal resection and gastrojejunostomy.

Defects of Mucosal Absorption. *Lactose intolerance and abetalipoproteinemia* ares example of diseases caused by a specific defect of absorption in cells of the intestinal mucosa. *Lactose intolerance* is caused by the deficiency of disaccharidase (*lactase*). The inherited form is rare but is of great consequence, because in infants it produces milk intolerance, leading to diarrhea, weight loss, and failure to thrive. The acquired deficiency is common among adults, particularly North American blacks. Aside from the need to avoid milk products, the disorder is of minimal consequence. The intestinal mucosa is morphologically normal. Diagnosis is most readily made by measurement of breath hydrogen level, which reflects bacterial overgrowth in the presence of excess intraluminal carbohydrate.

Deficiency of apolipoprotein B (*abetalipoproteinemia*) makes the mucosal epithelial cell unable to export lipid. The protein is required for assembly of dietary lipids into chylomicrons, which are then secreted into intestinal lymphatics. In this disease, mucosal absorptive cells contain vacuolated lipid inclusions, but the mucosa is otherwise normal. This deficiency causes diarrhea and steatorrhea in infancy and significant failure to thrive. There are systemic lipid membrane abnormalities as well, readily observed in circulating erythrocytes as a characteristic burr cell transformation termed *acanthocytosis.*

Celiac disease, also known as gluten-sensitive enteropathy, is the prototype of a noninfectious cause of malabsorption resulting from a reduction in small intestinal absorptive surface area. Celiac disease is believed to be quite common, affecting 1 in 300 persons both in Europe and in the United States, and many patients have subclinical disease. The basic disorder in celiac disease is immunological sensitivity to gluten, the component of wheat and related grains (oat, barley, and rye) that contains the water-insoluble protein gliadin. Gliadin peptides are efficiently presented by antigen-presenting cells in the lamina propria of the small intestine to CD4+ T cells, thereby driving an immune response to gluten. There is hence a strong genetic susceptibility, with 95% of patients having an HLA-DQ2 haplotype and most of the remainder having HLA-DQ8. Early exposure of the immature immune system of the infant to high levels of gliadin is a prominent cofactor for manifestation of clinically overt celiac disease later in life.

The small intestinal mucosa, when exposed to gluten, accumulates intraepithelial CD8+ T cells and large numbers of lamina propria CD4+ T cells sensitized to gliadin. The CD8+ T cells that accumulate in the gut may not be specific for gliadin. Instead, these cells express the NK cell–associated NKG2D receptor, which recognizes stress-induced molecules on epithelial cells. Thus, the intestinal pathology may result from epithelial cell stress, perhaps induced by gliadin sensitivity, and CD8+ T cell-

Table 15–9 The Major Malabsorption Syndromes

Defective Intraluminal Digestion
Digestion of fats and proteins
Pancreatic insufficiency, due to pancreatitis or cystic fibrosis
Zollinger-Ellison syndrome, with inactivation of pancreatic enzymes by excess gastric acid secretion
Solubilization of fat, due to defective bile secretion
Ileal dysfunction or resection, with decreased bile salt uptake
Cessation of bile flow from obstruction, hepatic dysfunction
Nutrient preabsorption or modification by bacterial overgrowth
Distal ileal resection of bypass
Total or subtotal gastrectomy
Primary Mucosal Cell Abnormalities
Defective terminal digestion
Disaccharidase deficiency (lactose intolerance)
Bacterial overgrowth, with brush-border damage
Defective transepithelial transport
Abetalipoproteinemia
Reduced Small Intestinal Surface Area
Gluten-sensitive enteropathy (celiac disease)
Short-gut syndrome, after surgical resections
Crohn disease
Infections
Acute infectious enteritis
Parasitic infestation
Tropical sprue
Whipple disease
Lymphatic Obstruction
Lymphoma
Tuberculosis and tuberculous lymphadenitis

mediated killing of these epithelial cells. CD4+ T cells are probably also involved (based on the HLA associations), but their role and the role of antibodies remain obscure. Regardless of the precise mechanism, the effect of the immune response may be total flattening of mucosal villi (and hence loss of surface area), affecting the proximal more than the distal small intestine. In addition, lymphocytes and other inflammatory cells accumulate in the lamina propria.

The age of presentation with symptomatic diarrhea and malnutrition varies from infancy to mid-adulthood; removal of gluten from the diet is met with dramatic improvement. There is, however, a low long-term risk of malignant disease, with about a twofold increase over the usual rate. Intestinal lymphomas, especially T-cell lymphomas, are disproportionately represented; other malignancies include gastrointestinal and breast carcinomas. In some patients with celiac disease there is an associated skin disorder called dermatitis herpetiformis (Chapter 22).

Tropical sprue and *Whipple disease* are two disorders that exemplify malabsorption syndromes arising from intestinal infection. Tropical sprue resembles celiac disease in symptomatology but occurs almost exclusively in persons living in or visiting the tropics. No specific causal agent has been clearly identified, but the appearance of malabsorption within days or a few weeks of an acute diarrheal enteric infection strongly implicates an infectious process, as does prompt response to broad-spectrum antibiotic therapy. Small intestinal changes vary from near normal to a severe diffuse enteritis with villus flattening. In contrast to celiac disease, injury is seen at all levels of the small intestine.

Whipple disease is a rare systemic infection that may involve any organ of the body but principally affects the intestine, central nervous system, and joints. The hallmark of Whipple disease is a small intestinal mucosa laden with distended periodic acid-Schiff–positive macrophages in the lamina propria. The causal organism is a gram-positive and culture-resistant actinomycete, *Tropheryma whippelii*. Although *T. whippelii* is not an obligate intracellular pathogen, phagocytosed organisms and degenerated fragments thereof persist in lamina propria macrophages for years, without causing inflammation. Occurring principally in males in the fourth to fifth decades of life, Whipple disease causes a malabsorptive syndrome occasionally accompanied by lymphadenopathy, hyperpigmentation, polyarthritis, and obscure central nervous system complaints. Response to antibiotic therapy is usually prompt, but relapses are common.

Clinical Features. Clinically, the malabsorption syndromes resemble each other. The passage of abnormally bulky, frothy, greasy, yellow or gray stools is a prominent feature of malabsorption, accompanied by weight loss, anorexia, abdominal distention, borborygmi and flatus, and muscle wasting. The consequences of malabsorption affect many organ systems:

- *Hematopoietic system:* anemia from iron, pyridoxine, folate, or vitamin B_{12} deficiency (vitamin B_{12} is normally absorbed in the ileum) and bleeding from vitamin K deficiency (a fat-soluble vitamin)
- *Musculoskeletal system:* osteopenia and tetany from defective calcium, magnesium, vitamin D, and protein absorption
- *Endocrine system:* amenorrhea, impotence, and infertility from generalized malnutrition; and hyperparathyroidism from protracted calcium and vitamin D deficiency
- *Skin:* purpura and petechiae from vitamin K deficiency; edema from protein deficiency; dermatitis and hyperkeratosis from deficiencies of vitamin A (also fat soluble), zinc, essential fatty acids, and niacin; mucositis from vitamin deficiencies
- *Nervous system:* peripheral neuropathy from vitamin A and B_{12} deficiencies

INFLAMMATORY BOWEL DISEASE

Crohn disease and ulcerative colitis are chronic relapsing inflammatory disorders of unknown origin, collectively known as idiopathic inflammatory bowel disease (IBD), which share many common features. *They result from an abnormal local immune response against the normal flora of the gut, and probably against some self antigens, in genetically susceptible individuals. Crohn disease may affect any portion of the gastrointestinal tract from esophagus to anus but most often involves the ileum; about half of cases exhibit noncaseating granulomatous inflammation. Ulcerative colitis is a nongranulomatous disease limited to the colon.* Before considering these diseases separately, the pathogenesis of these two forms of IBD will be considered.

Etiology and Pathogenesis. The normal intestine is in a steady state of "physiologic" inflammation, representing a dynamic balance between (1) factors that activate the host immune system, such as luminal microbes, dietary antigens, and endogenous inflammatory stimuli; and (2) host defenses that down-regulate inflammation and maintain the integrity of the mucosa. The search for the causes of loss of this balance in Crohn disease and ulcerative colitis has revealed many parallels, but the origins of *both diseases remain unexplained* (thus their designation as *idiopathic*). The pathogenesis of IBD involves genetic susceptibility, failure of immune regulation, and triggering by microbial flora. We comment below on each of these contributors. It is important to note that Crohn disease and ulcerative colitis differ in many respects, including the natural history of the disease, pathological aspects, and in the types of therapies and responses to treatment.

Genetic Predisposition. There is little doubt that genetic factors are important in the occurrence of IBD. First-degree relatives are 3 to 20 times more likely to develop the disease, and 15% of persons with IBD have affected first-degree relatives. In keeping with an underlying immunologic dysfunction, both Crohn disease and ulcerative colitis have been linked to specific major histocompatibility complex class II alleles. Ulcerative colitis has been associated with *HLA-DRB1*, whereas *HLA-DR7* and *DQ4* alleles are associated with approximately 30% of Crohn disease cases in North American white males. Much recent interest has focused on associations of the disease with non-HLA genes. A gene called *NOD2* (or *CARD15*) is mutated in as many as 25% of Crohn disease patients in some ethnic populations. The NOD2 protein is an intracellular receptor for muramyl dipeptide, a component of the cell walls of many bacteria, and is thought to play a role in host responses to these bacteria. The protein is expressed in Paneth cells. The disease-associated mutant form may be defective in responding to the bacteria, thus allowing chronic infections to be established in the intestine and promoting inflammatory reactions by NOD2-independent pathways. Alternatively, the disease-associated form of NOD2 may promote excessive host responses to intestinal bacteria. Another gene that has recently been found to be associated with Crohn disease and ulcerative colitis is a mutant form of the *IL-23 receptor* (*IL-23R*) gene. IL-23 is a cytokine that promotes the production of IL-17 by T cells, and IL-17 has been implicated in inflammatory reactions in IBD and other chronic inflammatory diseases. It is not known if or how the mutant IL-23R influences these inflammatory reactions.

Immunologic Factors. It is not known whether the immune responses in IBD are directed against self-antigens of the intestinal epithelium or to bacterial antigens. The following general comments can be made about the immunologic responses in IBD.

- In both Crohn disease and ulcerative colitis the primary damaging agents appear to be CD4+ cells. Antineutrophil cytoplasmic antibodies and anti-tropomyosin antibodies detected in persons with ulcerative colitis do not seem to play a pathogenetic role.
- It has long been thought that Crohn disease is the result of a chronic delayed-type hypersensitivity reaction induced by interferon γ-producing T_H1 cells. However, recent results from mouse models of IBD suggest that the tissue inflammation may be the result of secretion of the cytokine IL-17 by a recently discovered subset of CD4+ T cells that is being called the "T_H17" subset.
- Although in animal models ulcerative colitis may be caused by activation of T_H2 cells, IL-4, the signature cytokine for this kind of response, has not been found, suggesting that in ulcerative colitis there may not be a predominant class of T-cell response.
- The inflammatory cytokine TNF (see Chapter 2) may play an important pathogenic role in Crohn disease. This is suggested by the effectiveness of treatment with TNF antagonists in this disorder.

Microbial Factors. The sites affected by IBD—the distal ileum and the colon—are awash in bacteria. While there is no evidence that these diseases are caused by microbes, it is quite likely that microbes provide the antigenic trigger to a fundamentally dysregulated immune system. This concept is strengthened by the observations that in murine models, IBD develops in the presence of normal gut flora but not in germ-free mice.

To summarize, IBD is a heterogeneous group of diseases characterized by an exaggerated and destructive mucosal immune response. The tissue injury in IBD is likely to be initiated by diverse genetic and immunologic pathways that are modified by environmental influences, including microbes and their products.

Inflammation is the final common pathway for the pathogenesis of IBD. Both the clinical manifestations and the morphologic changes of IBD are ultimately the result of activation of inflammatory cells—neutrophils initially and mononuclear cells later in the course. The products of these inflammatory cells cause nonspecific tissue injury. Inflammation causes (1) impaired integrity of the mucosal epithelial barrier, and (2) loss of surface epithelial cell absorptive function. The inflammation ultimately causes outright mucosal destruction, which leads to obvious loss of mucosal barrier and absorptive function. Collectively, these events give rise to the intermittent bloody diarrhea that is characteristic of these diseases. Most current therapeutic interventions act entirely or partly through nonspecific down-regulation of the immune system. Among diagnostic tests, the most useful is the detection of perinuclear antineutrophil cytoplasmic antibodies, which are present in about 75% of persons with ulcerative colitis and only 11% of individuals with Crohn disease.

Crohn Disease

This disease may affect any level of the alimentary tract, from mouth to anus, but most commonly located at the terminal ileum. When first described, the disease was thought to be limited to the ileum, and it was referred to as "terminal ileitis" or "regional enteritis." *Crohn disease must be viewed as a systemic inflammatory disease with predominant gastrointestinal involvement.* Active cases of the disease are often accompanied by extra-intestinal complications of immune origin, such as uveitis, sacroiliitis, migratory polyarthritis, erythema nodosum, bile duct inflammatory disorders, and obstructive uropathy with attendant nephrolithiasis.

When fully developed, Crohn disease is characterized by:

- Sharply limited transmural involvement of the bowel by an inflammatory process with mucosal damage
- Presence of noncaseating granulomas
- Fistula formation

Epidemiology. Worldwide in distribution, Crohn disease is much more prevalent in the United States, Great Britain, and Scandinavia than in Central Europe, and is rare in Asia and Africa. The incidence and prevalence of Crohn disease has been steadily rising in the United States and Western Europe. The annual incidence in the United States is 3 to 5 per 100,000 population, which is slightly less frequent than the incidence of ulcerative colitis. It occurs at any age, from young childhood to advanced age, but the peak incidence is between the second and third decades of life, with a minor peak in the sixth and seventh decades. Females are affected slightly more often than males. Whites appear to develop the disease two to five times more often than do nonwhites. In the United States, Crohn disease occurs three to five times more often among Jews than among non-Jews.

Morphology

In Crohn disease there is gross involvement of the small intestine alone in about 30% of cases, of small intestine and colon in 40%, and of the colon alone in about 30%. Crohn disease may involve the duodenum, stomach, esophagus, and even mouth, but these sites are distinctly uncommon. **When fully developed, Crohn disease is characterized by (1) sharply delimited and typically transmural involvement of the bowel by an inflammatory process with mucosal damage, (2) the presence of noncaseating granulomas in 40% to 60% of cases, and (3) fissuring with formation of fistulae.** In diseased segments, the serosa becomes granular and dull gray and often the mesenteric fat wraps around the bowel surface **("creeping fat"). The intestinal wall is rubbery and thick, the result of edema, inflammation, fibrosis, and hypertrophy of the muscularis propria.** As a result, the lumen is almost always narrowed; in the small intestine this is seen radiographically as the "string sign," a thin stream of barium passing through the diseased segment. Strictures may occur in the colon but are usually less severe. **A classic feature of Crohn disease is the sharp demarcation of diseased bowel segments from adjacent uninvolved bowel.** When several bowel segments are involved, the intervening bowel is essentially normal ("skip" lesions).

In the intestinal mucosa, early disease shows focal mucosal ulcers resembling canker sores (aphthous ulcers), edema, and loss of the normal mucosal texture. With progressive disease, ulcers coalesce into long, serpentine linear ulcers, which tend to be oriented along the axis of the bowel (Fig. 15–30). Because the intervening mucosa tends to be relatively spared, it acquires a coarsely textured, cobblestone appearance. **Narrow fissures develop between the folds of the mucosa,** often penetrating deeply through the bowel wall all the way to the serosa. This may lead to adhesions with adjacent loops of bowel. Further extension of fissures leads to **fistula or sinus tract formation,** to adherent viscera, to the outside skin, or into a blind cavity to form a localized abscess.

By microscopic examination, the mucosa shows several characteristic features (Fig. 15–31): (1) **inflammation,** with neutrophilic infiltration into the epithelial layer and accumulation within crypts to form **crypt abscesses**; (2) **ulceration**, which is the usual outcome of active disease; and (3) **chronic mucosal damage** in the form of architectural distortion, atrophy, and metaplasia (including rudimentary gastric metaplasia in the intestine). **Granulomas may be present anywhere in the alimentary tract, even in individuals with Crohn disease limited to one bowel segment. However, the absence of granulomas does not preclude a diagnosis of Crohn disease.** In diseased segments, the muscularis mucosae and muscularis propria are usually markedly thickened, and fibrosis affects all tissue layers. Lymphoid aggregates scattered through the various tissue layers and in the extramural fat also are characteristic.

Particularly important in persons with long-standing chronic disease are dysplastic changes appearing in the mucosal epithelial cells. These may be focal or widespread, tend to increase with time, and are thought to be related to a fivefold to sixfold increased risk of carcinoma, particularly of the colon.

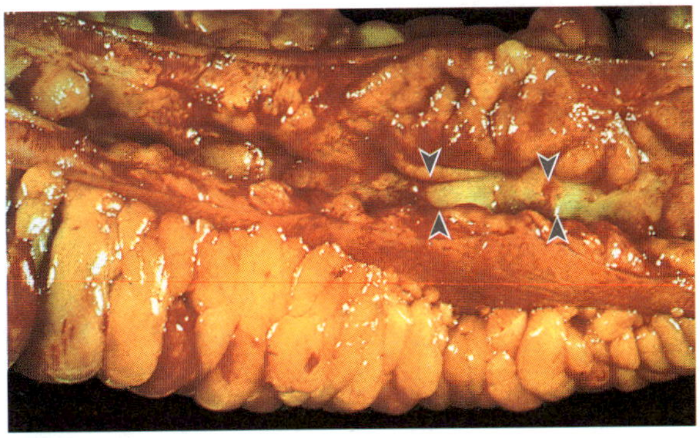

Figure 15–30

Crohn disease of the ileum showing narrowing of the lumen, bowel wall thickening, serosal extension of mesenteric fat ("creeping fat"), and linear ulceration of the mucosal surface (*arrowheads*).

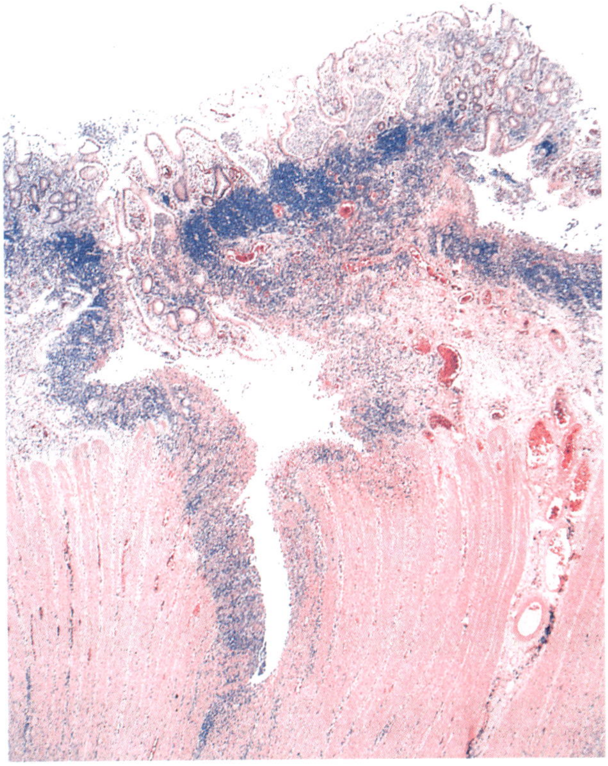

Figure 15–31

Crohn disease of the colon showing a deep fissure extending into the muscle wall, a second, shallow ulcer (upper right), and relative preservation of the intervening mucosa. Abundant lymphocyte aggregates are present, evident as dense blue patches of cells at the interface between mucosa and submucosa.

Clinical Features. The presentation of Crohn disease is highly variable and unpredictable. The dominant manifestations are recurrent episodes of diarrhea, crampy abdominal pain, and fever lasting days to weeks. These manifestations usually begin insidiously, but in some instances, particularly in young persons, the onset of the pain is so abrupt and the diarrhea so mild that abdominal exploration is performed with a diagnosis of appendicitis. Some melena is present in about 50% of cases with colon involvement; it is usually mild but sometimes massive. In most patients, after an initial attack, the manifestations remit either spontaneously or with therapy, but characteristically they are followed by relapses, and intervals between successive attacks grow shorter. In 10% to 20% of persons with Crohn disease the symptom-free interval after the initial attack may last for decades, and for a very fortunate few the first attack is the last. Alternatively, about 20% of patients experience continuously active disease following their diagnosis. For the majority, the course fluctuates between years of remission and years with clinically active disease. Superimposed on this course are the potential development of malabsorption and some of the extra-intestinal manifestations mentioned earlier.

The debilitating consequences of Crohn disease include (1) *fistula* formation to other loops of bowel, the urinary bladder, vagina, or perianal skin; (2) *abdominal abscesses* or peritonitis; and (3) *intestinal stricture* or obstruction, necessitating surgical intervention. Rare but devastating events are massive intestinal bleeding, toxic dilation of the colon, or carcinoma of the colon or small intestine. Although the increased risk for carcinoma is significant, it is substantially less than that associated with ulcerative colitis. This difference may not be intrinsic to these two conditions, but may relate to the fact that in Crohn disease the affected bowel is usually removed surgically due to obstruction, thus reducing the risk of cancer.

Ulcerative Colitis

Ulcerative colitis is an ulceroinflammatory disease affecting the colon, which is limited to the mucosa and submucosa, except in the most severe cases. Ulcerative colitis begins in the rectum and extends proximally in a continuous fashion, sometimes involving the entire colon. Like Crohn disease, ulcerative colitis is a systemic disorder associated in some persons with migratory polyarthritis, sacroiliitis, ankylosing spondylitis, uveitis, erythema nodosum, and hepatic involvement (pericholangitis and primary sclerosing cholangitis). There are several important differences between ulcerative colitis and Crohn disease (Fig. 15–32 and Table 15–10).

In ulcerative colitis:

- Well-formed granulomas are absent.
- There are no skip lesions.
- The mucosal ulcers rarely extend below the submucosa, and there is surprisingly little fibrosis.
- Mural thickening does not occur, and the serosal surface is usually completely normal.
- There appears to be a high risk of carcinoma development.

Epidemiology. Ulcerative colitis is somewhat more common than Crohn disease in the United States and Western countries, with an incidence of around 7 per 100,000 population, but it is infrequent in Asia, Africa, and South America. As with Crohn disease, the incidence of this condition has risen in recent decades. In the United States it is more common among whites than among nonwhites and exhibits no particular sex predilection. The

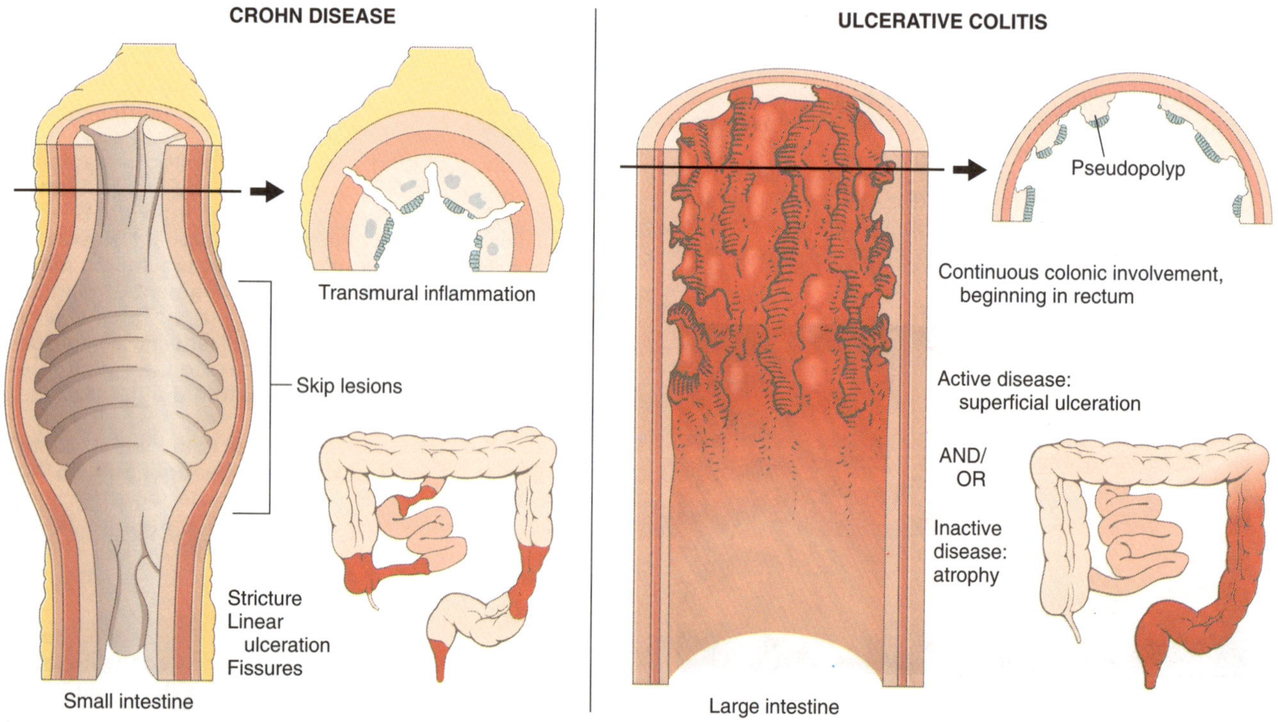

Figure 15–32

Comparison of the distribution patterns of Crohn disease and ulcerative colitis, and the different conformations of the ulcers and wall thickenings.

Table 15–10 Distinctive Features of Crohn Disease and Ulcerative Colitis*

Feature	Crohn Disease (Small intestine)	Crohn Disease (Colon)	Ulcerative Colitis
Macroscopic			
Bowel region	Ileum ± colon†	Colon ± ileum	Colon only
Distribution	Skip lesions	Skip lesions	Diffuse
Stricture	Early	Variable	Late/rare
Wall appearance	Thickened	Variable	Thin
Dilation	No	Yes	Yes
Microscopic			
Pseudopolyps	None to slight	Marked	Marked
Ulcers	Deep, linear	Deep, linear	Superficial
Lymphoid reaction	Marked	Marked	Mild
Fibrosis	Marked	Moderate	Mild
Serositis	Marked	Variable	Mild to none
Granulomas	Yes (40% to 60%)	Yes (40% to 60%)	No
Fistulas/sinuses	Yes	Yes	No
Clinical			
Fat/vitamin malabsorption	Yes	Yes, if ileum	No
Malignant potential	Yes	Yes	Yes
Response to surgery‡	Poor	Fair	Good

*Not all features present in a single case.
†Crohn disease can occur elsewhere in the small intestine as well.
‡Based on likelihood of disease recurrence after surgical removal of a diseased segment.

disease may arise at any age, with a peak incidence between ages 20 and 25 years. Ulcerative colitis has a familial association; about 20% of persons with the disorder have affected relatives. Individuals with ulcerative colitis and ankylosing spondylitis have an increased frequency of the *HLA-B27* allele, but this association is related to the spondylitis and not to ulcerative colitis.

Morphology

Ulcerative colitis involves the rectum and sigmoid and may involve the entire colon. Presentation with an even higher proximal extension (pancolitis) occurs much less frequently. Colonic involvement is continuous from the distal colon, so that skip lesions are not encountered. Active disease denotes ongoing inflammatory destruction of the mucosa, with macroscopic hyperemia, edema, and granularity with friability and easy bleeding. With severe active disease, there is extensive and broad-based ulceration of the mucosa in the distal colon or throughout its length (Fig. 15–33). Isolated islands of regenerating mucosa bulge upward to create **pseudopolyps.** Often the undermined edges of adjacent ulcers interconnect to create tunnels covered by tenuous mucosal bridges. As with Crohn disease, the ulcers of ulcerative colitis are frequently aligned along the axis of the colon, but rarely do they replicate the linear serpentine ulcers of Crohn disease. In rare cases, the muscularis propria is so compromised as to permit perforation and pericolonic abscess formation. Exposure of the muscularis propria and neural plexus to fecal material also may lead to complete shutdown of neuromuscular function. When this occurs, the colon progressively swells and becomes gangrenous (**toxic megacolon**). With indolent chronic disease or with healing of active disease, progressive mucosal atrophy leads to a flattened and attenuated mucosal surface.

The pathologic features of ulcerative colitis are those of mucosal inflammation, ulceration, and chronic mucosal damage (Fig. 15–34).

- **A diffuse, predominantly mononuclear inflammatory infiltrate in the lamina propria is almost universally present,** even at the time of clinical presentation. Neutrophilic infiltration of the epithelial layer may produce collections of neutrophils in crypt lumina (**crypt** abscesses). These are not spe-

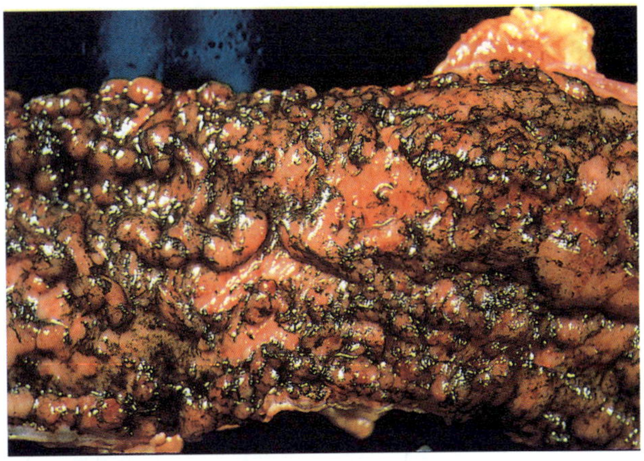

Figure 15–33

Ulcerative colitis. The pale, irregular regions comprise ulcerations that have in many instances coalesced, leaving virtual islands of residual mucosa. A tendency toward pseudopolyp formation is already evident. The darker material is adherent mucus stained by feces.

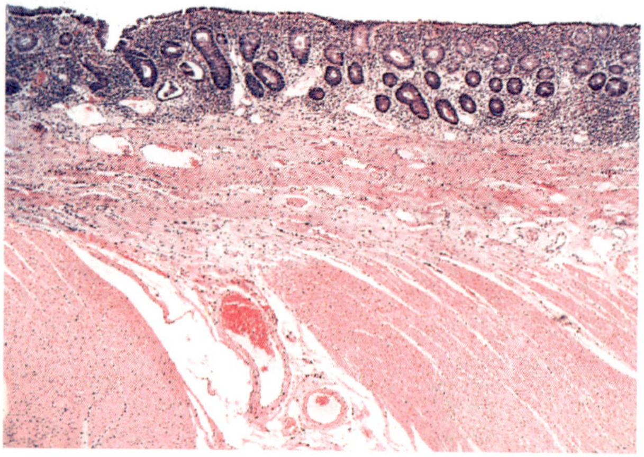

Figure 15–34

Ulcerative colitis. Low-power micrograph showing marked chronic inflammation of the mucosa with atrophy of colonic glands, moderate submucosal fibrosis, and a normal muscle wall.

cific for ulcerative colitis and may be observed in Crohn disease or any active inflammatory colitis. Unlike Crohn disease, there are no granulomas, although rupture of crypt abscesses may incite a foreign body reaction in the lamina propria.

- **Further destruction of the mucosa leads to outright** ulceration, extending into the submucosa and sometimes leaving only the raw, exposed muscularis propria.
- With remission of active disease, **granulation tissue fills in the ulcer craters**, followed by regeneration of the mucosal epithelium. **Submucosal fibrosis and mucosal architectural disarray and atrophy remain as residua of healed disease.**

The most serious complication of ulcerative colitis is the development of colon carcinoma. Two factors govern the risk: duration of the disease and its anatomic extent. It is believed that with 10 years of disease limited to the left colon the risk is minimal, and at 20 years the risk is on the order of 2%. With pancolitis, the risk of carcinoma is 10% at 20 years and 15% to 25% by 30 years. Overall, the annual incidence of colon cancer in persons with ulcerative colitis of more than 10 years' duration is 0.8% to 1%.

Clinical Features. Ulcerative colitis is a chronic relapsing disorder marked by attacks of bloody mucoid diarrhea that may persist for days, weeks, or months and then subside, only to recur after an asymptomatic interval of months to years or even decades. Presentation is usually insidious, with cramps, tenesmus, and colicky lower abdominal pain that is relieved by defecation. Some people manifest fever and weight loss. Grossly bloody stools are more common with ulcerative colitis than with Crohn disease, and the blood loss may be considerable. In the fortunate person the first attack is the last, representing about 10% of patients. At the other end of the spectrum, the explosive initial attack may lead to such serious bleeding and fluid and electrolyte imbalance as to constitute a medical emergency. For the most part, however, the vast majority of individuals with ulcerative colitis experience a relapsing course. Concurrent infections, as with enterotoxin-producing *C. difficile*, may first bring ulcerative colitis to light; they do not precipitate the disease.

Extra-intestinal manifestations, particularly migratory polyarthritis, are more common with ulcerative colitis than with Crohn disease. Uncommon but *life-threatening complications* include severe diarrhea and electrolyte derangements, massive hemorrhage, severe colonic dilation (toxic megacolon) with potential rupture, and perforation with peritonitis. Inflammatory strictures of the colorectum, while uncommon, must be differentiated from cancer.

Diagnosis can usually be made by endoscopic examination and biopsy. Specific infectious causes must always be ruled out. The most feared long-term complication of ulcerative colitis is cancer. The sequential mucosal changes from dysplasia to invasive carcinoma provide the rationale for surveillance programs of repeated colonoscopies and multiple biopsies aimed at detecting dysplasia for possible prophylactic colectomy. Since the carcinomas that develop from ulcerative colitis are frequently of an infiltrative type, early detection is of major importance. DNA damage with microsatellite instability has been detected in ulcerative colitis mucosal cells. More recently, the same type of damage was also found in nondysplastic areas of the gut of persons with ulcerative colitis, suggesting these patients may have DNA repair defects in mucosal cells throughout the intestine.

SUMMARY

Inflammatory Bowel Disease (IBD)

- Crohn disease and ulcerative colitis are idiopathic inflammatory bowel diseases believed to result from abnormal local immune responses against unknown microbes and/or self antigens in the intestine.
- *Crohn disease:*
  - Associated with HLA-DR7 and –DQ4 alleles, and with mutations in the *NOD2* gene, which encodes an intracellular sensor of microbes
  - Results from a chronic T cell-mediated inflammatory reaction involving IFN-γ-producing T_H1 cells and, perhaps, IL-17-producing T_H17 cells
  - Manifested by chronic inflammation with granulomas, ulcers, and strictures caused by fibrosis, involving the terminal ileum and colon
  - Consequences include fistula formation, abdominal abscesses, intestinal obstruction, and increased risk of carcinoma.
- *Ulcerative colitis:*
  - Associated with HLA-DRB1
  - Manifested by superficial ulcers in the colon without granulomas or extensive fibrosis; the nature of the pathologic immune response is unknown
  - The most serious complication is the increased risk of carcinoma.

TUMORS OF THE SMALL AND LARGE INTESTINES

Epithelial tumors of the intestines are a major cause of morbidity and mortality worldwide. The colon, including the rectum, is host to more primary neoplasms than any other organ in the body. Colorectal cancer ranks second only to bronchogenic carcinoma among the cancer killers in the United States. About 5% of Americans will develop colorectal cancer, and 40% of this population will die of the disease. Adenocarcinomas constitute the vast majority of colorectal cancers and represent 70% of all malignancies arising in the gastrointestinal tract. Curiously, the small intestine is an uncommon site for benign or malignant tumors despite its great length and its vast pool of dividing mucosal cells. The classification of intestinal tumors is the same for the small and large bowel (Table 15–11).

Before embarking on our discussion, several concepts pertaining to terminology must be emphasized (Fig. 15–35):

- A *polyp* is a mass that protrudes into the lumen of the gut; traction on the mass may create a stalked, or *pedunculated*, polyp. Alternatively, the polyp may be *sessile*, without a definable stalk.
- Polyps may be formed as the result of abnormal mucosal maturation, inflammation, or architecture. These polyps are *non-neoplastic* and do not have malignant potential.
- Those polyps that arise as the result of epithelial proliferation and dysplasia are termed *adenomatous polyps* or *adenomas. They are true neoplastic lesions and are precursors of carcinoma.*
- *Hyperplastic polyps* are the most common polyps of the colon and rectum. When single, they do not have malignant potential. However a lesion known as *sessile serrated adenoma*, which has some similarities with hyperplastic polyps, may have malignant potential (discussed below).

Table 15–11 Tumors of the Small and Large Intestines

Non-neoplastic Polyps
Hyperplastic polyps
Hamartomatous polyps
Juvenile polyps
Peutz-Jeghers polyps
Inflammatory polyps
Lymphoid polyps
Neoplastic Epithelial Lesions
Benign polyps
Adenomas
Malignant lesions
Adenocarcinoma
Squamous cell carcinoma of the anus
Other Tumors
Gastrointestinal stromal tumors
Carcinoid tumor
Lymphoma

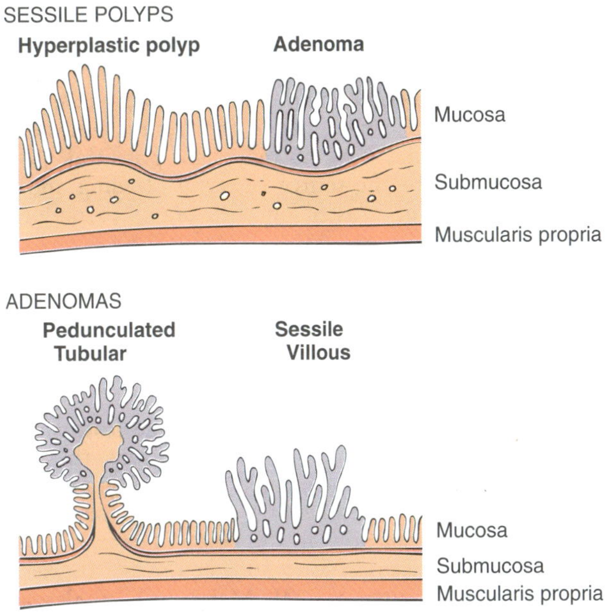

Figure 15–35

Two forms of sessile polyp (hyperplastic polyp and adenoma) and of two types of adenoma (pedunculated and sessile). There is only a loose association between the tubular architecture for pedunculated adenomas and the villous architecture for sessile polyps.

Some polypoid lesions may be caused by submucosal or mural tumors. However, as with the stomach, the term *polyp*, unless otherwise specified, refers to lesions arising from the epithelium of the mucosa.

Non-Neoplastic Polyps

The overwhelming majority of intestinal polyps occur sporadically, particularly in the colon, and increase in frequency with age. Non-neoplastic polyps represent about 90% of all epithelial polyps in the large intestine and are found in more than half of all persons age 60 years or older. Most are *hyperplastic polyps*, which are small (<5 mm in diameter), nipple-like, hemispherical, smooth protrusions of the mucosa. They may occur singly but are more often multiple. Although they may be anywhere in the colon, well over half are found in the rectosigmoid region. Histologically, they contain abundant crypts lined by well-differentiated goblet or absorptive epithelial cells, separated by a scant lamina propria. Although the vast majority of hyperplastic polyps have *no malignant potential*, it is now being recognized that some "hyperplastic polyps," the so-called sessile serrated adenomas, located on the right side of the colon, may be precursors of colorectal carcinomas. They may be solitary or multiple ("hyperplastic polyposis"). As discussed later, these polyps show microsatellite instability and can give rise to colon cancers by the mismatch repair pathway.

Juvenile polyps are essentially hamartomatous proliferations, mainly of the lamina propria, enclosing widely spaced, dilated cystic glands. They occur most frequently in children younger than 5 years old but also are found in adults of any age; in the latter group they may be called *retention polyps*. Irrespective of terminology, the lesions are usually large in children (1–3 cm in diameter) but smaller in adults; they are rounded, smooth, or slightly lobulated and sometimes have a stalk as long as 2 cm. In general, they occur singly and in the rectum, and being hamartomatous they have no malignant potential. Juvenile polyps may be the source of rectal bleeding and in some cases become twisted on their stalks to undergo painful infarction.

Polyps that develop in the Peutz-Jegher syndrome are discussed in the later section on Familial Polyposis Syndromes.

Adenomas

Adenomas are neoplastic polyps that range from small, often pedunculated, tumors to large lesions that are usually sessile. Because the incidence of adenomas in the small intestine is very low, this discussion focuses on those adenomas that arise in the colon. The prevalence of colonic adenomas is 20% to 30% before age 40, rising to 40% to 50% after age 60. Males and females are affected equally. There is a well-defined familial predisposition to sporadic adenomas, accounting for about a fourfold greater risk for adenomas among first-degree relatives, and also a fourfold greater risk of colorectal carcinoma in any person with adenomas.

All adenomatous lesions arise as the result of epithelial proliferation and dysplasia, which may range from mild to so severe as to represent transformation to carcinoma. Furthermore, there is strong evidence that most sporadic invasive colorectal adenocarcinomas arise in preexisting adenomatous lesions. Adenomatous polyps are segregated into four subtypes on the basis of the epithelial architecture:

- *Tubular adenomas*—mostly tubular glands, recapitulating mucosal topology
- *Villous adenomas*—villous projections
- *Tubulovillous adenomas*—a mixture of the above
- *Sessile serrated adenomas*—serrated epithelium lining the crypts

Tubular adenomas are by far the most common; 5% to 10% of adenomas are tubulovillous, and only 1% are villous. Most tubular adenomas are small and pedunculated; villous adenomas tend to be large and sessile. Conversely, most pedunculated polyps are tubular, and large sessile polyps usually show villous features.

The malignant risk with an adenomatous polyp is correlated with three interdependent features—polyp size, histologic architecture, and severity of epithelial dysplasia—as follows:

- Cancer is rare in tubular adenomas smaller than 1 cm in diameter.
- The likelihood of cancer is high (approaching 40%) in sessile villous adenomas larger than 4 cm in diameter.
- Severe dysplasia, when present, is often found in villous areas.
- Among these variables, *maximum diameter is the chief determinant of the risk of an adenoma's harboring carcinoma*; architecture does not provide substantive independent information.

Morphology

Tubular adenomas may arise anywhere in the colon, but about half are found in the rectosigmoid, the proportion increasing with age. In about half of the instances they occur singly, but in the remainder two or more lesions are distributed at random. The smallest adenomas are sessile; lesions 0.3 cm in size can be identified at endoscopy. Among the larger tubular adenomas up to 2.5 cm in diameter, most have slender stalks 1 to 2 cm long and raspberry-like heads (Fig. 15–36A). Histologically the stalk is covered by normal colonic mucosa, but the head is composed of neoplastic epithelium, forming branching glands lined by tall, hyperchromatic, somewhat disorderly cells, which may or may not show mucin secretion (Fig. 15–36B). In some instances there are small foci of villous architecture. In the clearly benign lesion, the branching glands are well separated by lamina propria, and the level of dysplasia or cytologic atypia is slight. However, all degrees of dysplasia may be encountered, ranging up to cancer confined to the mucosa (**intramucosal carcinoma**) or **invasive carcinoma** extending into the submucosa of the stalk. A frequent finding in any adenoma is superficial erosion of the epithelium, the result of mechanical trauma.

Villous adenomas are the larger and more ominous of the epithelial polyps. They tend to occur in older persons, most commonly in the rectum and rectosigmoid, but they may be located elsewhere. They generally are sessile, up to 10 cm in diameter, velvety or cauliflower-like masses projecting 1 to 3 cm above the surrounding normal mucosa. The histology is that of frondlike villiform extensions of the mucosa covered by dysplastic, sometimes very disorderly, sometimes piled-up, columnar epithelium (Fig. 15–37). All degrees of dysplasia may be encountered, and invasive carcinoma is found in as many as 40% of these lesions, the frequency being correlated with the size of the polyp.

Tubulovillous adenomas are composed of a broad mix of tubular and villous areas. They are intermediate between the tubular and the villous lesions in their frequency of having a stalk or being sessile, their size, the degree of dysplasia, and the risk of harboring intramucosal or invasive carcinoma.

Clinical Features. The smaller adenomas are usually asymptomatic, until such time that occult bleeding leads to clinically significant anemia. Villous adenomas are much more frequently symptomatic because of overt or occult rectal bleeding. The most distal villous adenomas may secrete sufficient amounts of mucoid material rich in protein and potassium to produce hypoproteinemia or hypokalemia. On discovery, all adenomas, regardless of their location in the alimentary tract, are to be considered potentially malignant; thus, in practical terms, prompt and adequate excision is mandated.

Familial Polyposis Syndromes

Familial polyposis syndromes are uncommon autosomal dominant disorders. Their importance lies in the propensity for malignant transformation and in the insights that such transformation has provided in unraveling the molecular basis of colorectal cancer. Individuals

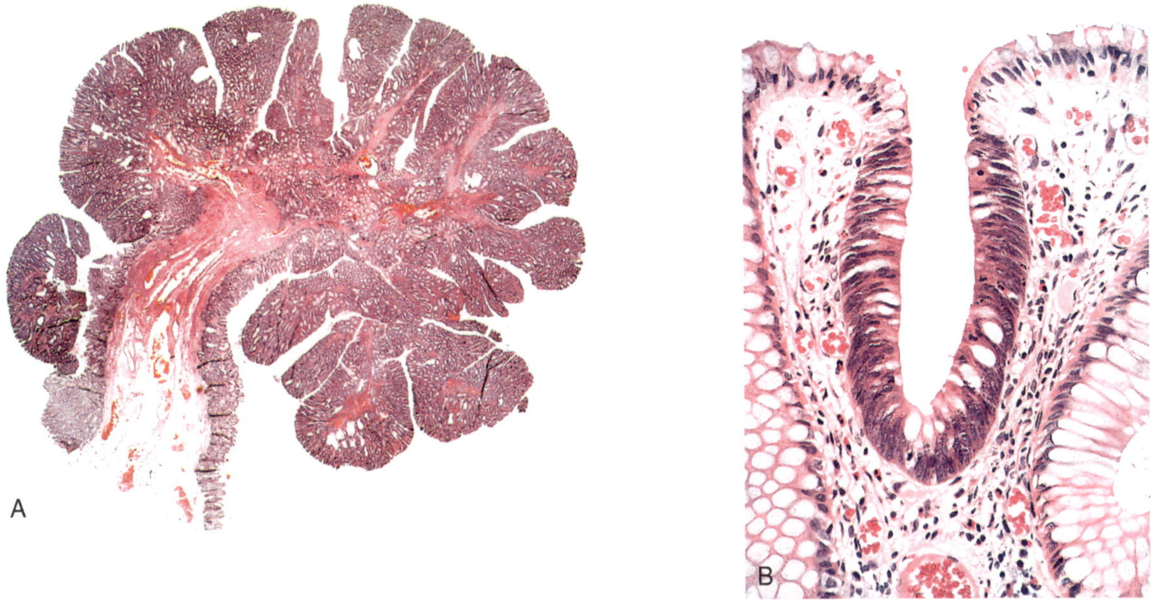

Figure 15–36

A, Pedunculated adenoma showing a fibrovascular stalk covered by normal colonic mucosa and a head that contains abundant dysplastic epithelial glands—hence the blue color. **B,** A small focus of adenomatous epithelium in an otherwise normal (mucin-secreting, clear) colonic mucosa, showing how the dysplastic columnar epithelium (deeply stained) can populate a colonic crypt ("tubular" architecture).

with *familial adenomatous polyposis* (FAP) typically develop 500 to 2500 colonic adenomas that carpet the mucosal surface (Fig. 15–38); a minimum number of 100 is required for the diagnosis. Multiple adenomas may also be present elsewhere in the alimentary tract, including almost a 100% lifetime incidence of duodenal adenomas. Most polyps are tubular adenomas; occasional polyps have villous features. Polyps usually become evident in adolescence or early adulthood. *The risk of colonic cancer is virtually 100% by midlife, unless a prophylactic colectomy is performed.* The genetic defect underlying FAP has been localized to the *APC* gene on chromosome 5q21, as discussed below; *Gardner syndrome* and the much rarer *Turcot syndrome* seem to share the same genetic defect as FAP. These syndromes differ from FAP with respect to the occurrence of extra-intestinal tumors in the latter two: osteomas, gliomas, and soft tissue tumors, to name a few.

Peutz-Jeghers polyps are uncommon hamartomatous polyps that occur as part of the rare autosomal dominant Peutz-Jeghers syndrome, characterized in addition by melanotic mucosal and cutaneous pigmentation. This syndrome is caused by germ-line mutations in the *LKB1* gene, which encodes a serine threonine kinase. *Cowden syndrome* is also characterized by hamartomatous polyps in the gastrointestinal tract and by an increased risk of neoplasms of the thyroid, breast, uterus, and skin. This syndrome is caused by germ-line mutations in the *PTEN* (phosphatase and tensin homologue) tumor suppressor gene. This gene, mutated in a large number of human cancers, encodes a phosphatase that has the ability to regulate many intracellular signaling pathways. It acts as a growth inhibitor by interrupting signals from several tyrosine kinase receptors (e.g., epidermal growth factor receptor) and by favoring apoptosis through the BAD/BCL2 pathways. Peutz-Jeghers and Cowden syndromes, like the other familial polyposis syndromes, are associated with an increased risk of both intestinal and extraintestinal malignancies.

Colorectal Carcinoma

A great majority (98%) of all cancers in the large intestine are adenocarcinomas. They represent one of the prime challenges to the medical profession, because they almost always arise in adenomatous polyps that are generally curable by resection. With an estimated 134,000 new cases per year and about 55,000 deaths, this disease accounts for nearly 15% of all cancer-related deaths in the United States.

Epidemiology. The peak incidence for colorectal cancer is 60 to 70 years of age; fewer than 20% of cases occur before the age of 50 years. Adenomas are the presumed precursor lesion for most of the tumors; the frequency with which colorectal cancer arises de novo from flat colonic mucosa remains undefined but appears to be low. Males are affected about 20% more often than females.

Both genetic and environmental influences contribute to the development of colorectal cancers. When colorectal cancer is found in a young person, preexisting ulcerative colitis or one of the polyposis syndromes must be suspected. In addition, individuals with *hereditary nonpolyposis colorectal cancer syndrome* (HNPCC, also known as Lynch syndrome), caused by germ-line mutations of DNA mismatch repair genes, are at a high risk of developing colorectal cancers. (HNPCC patients

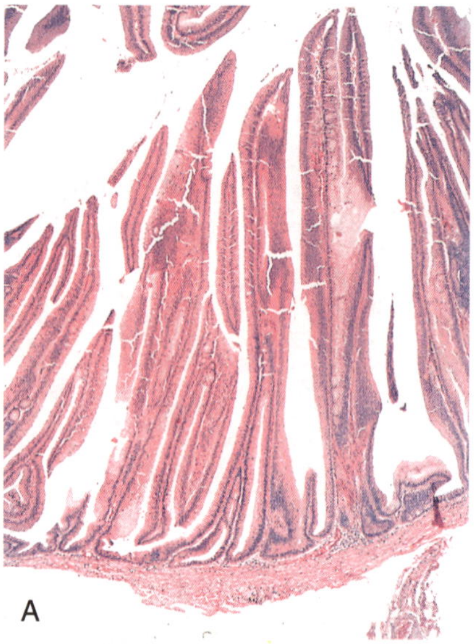

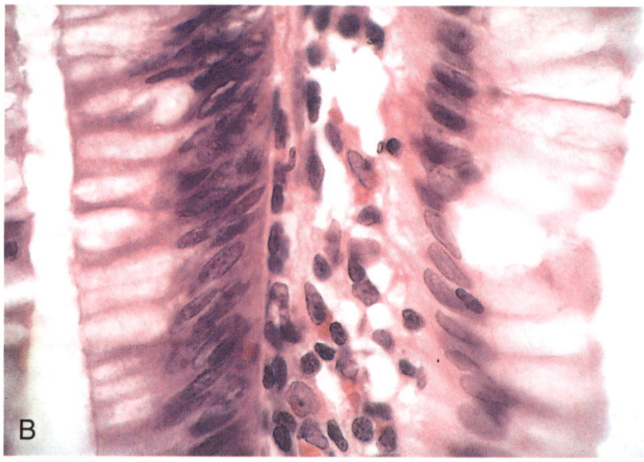

Figure 15–37

A, Sessile adenoma with villous architecture. Each frond is lined by dysplastic epithelium. **B,** Portion of a villous frond with dysplastic columnar epithelium on the left and normal colonic columnar epithelium on the right.

are also at risk of developing other tumors, such as cholangiocarcinomas.)

Colorectal carcinoma has a worldwide distribution, with the highest incidence rates in the United States, Canada, Australia, New Zealand, Denmark, Sweden, and other developed countries. Its incidence is substantially lower, up to 30-fold less, in India, South America, and Africa. The incidence in Japan, which formerly was very low, has now risen to the intermediate levels observed in the United Kingdom. Environmental influences, particularly dietary practices, are implicated in the striking geographic variation in incidence. The dietary factors receiving the most attention are (1) a low content of unabsorbable vegetable fiber, (2) a corresponding high content of refined carbohydrates, (3) a high fat content (as from meat), and (4) decreased intake of protective micronutrients such as vitamins A, C, and E. It is theorized that reduced fiber content leads to decreased stool bulk, increased fecal retention in the bowel, and an altered bacterial flora of the intestine. Potentially toxic oxidative byproducts of carbohydrate degradation by bacteria are therefore present in higher concentrations in the stool and are held in contact with the colonic mucosa for longer periods of time. Moreover, high fat intake enhances the synthesis of cholesterol and bile acids by the liver, which in turn may be converted into potential carcinogens by intestinal bacteria. Refined diets also contain less of vitamins A, C, and E, which may act as oxygen radical scavengers. Intriguing as these scenarios are, they remain unproven.

Several recent epidemiologic studies suggest that use of aspirin and other NSAIDs exerts a protective effect against colon cancer. In the Nurses' Health Study, women who used four to six tablets of aspirin per day for 10 years or more had a decreased incidence of colon cancer. It is suspected that this effect is via inhibition of cyclooxygenase-2 (COX-2). This enzyme is overexpressed in 90% of colorectal carcinoma and 40% to 90% of adenomas. How COX-2 promotes carcinogenesis is not clear. Some of its effects may be mediated by production of prostaglandin E2 (PGE_2), which seems to favor epithelial cell proliferation, inhibit apoptosis, and enhance angiogenesis. PGE_2 may promote angiogenesis by enhancing production of vascular endothelial growth factor.

The development of carcinoma from adenomatous lesions is documented by these general observations:

- Populations that have a high prevalence of adenomas have a high prevalence of colorectal cancer, and vice versa.
- The distribution of adenomas within the colorectum is more or less comparable to that of colorectal cancer.
- The peak incidence of adenomatous polyps antedates by some years the peak for colorectal cancer.
- When invasive carcinoma is identified at an early stage, surrounding adenomatous tissue is often present.
- The risk of cancer is directly related to the number of adenomas, and hence the virtual certainty of cancer in persons with familial polyposis syndromes.

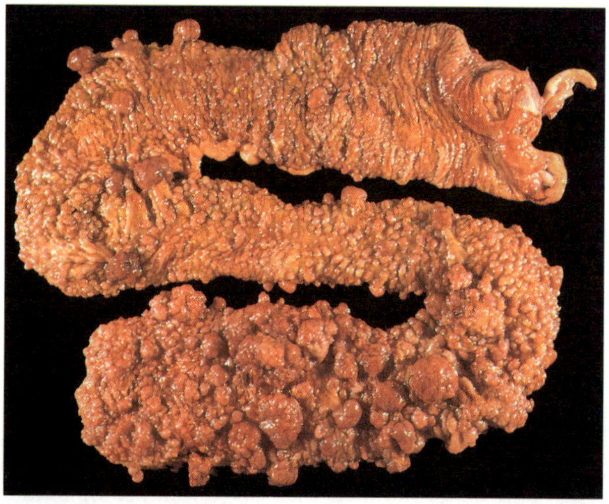

Figure 15–38

Familial adenomatous polyposis. The surface is carpeted by innumerable polypoid adenomas. (Courtesy of Dr. Tad Wieczorek, Brigham and Women's Hospital, Boston, Massachusetts.)

Table 15–12 Molecular Genetic Pathways of Colorectal Cartinogenesis

	Hereditary Colorectal Carcinoma			Sporadic Colorectal Carcinoma		
Molecular Pathway	**Clinical Phenotype**	**Histopathology**	**Genetics**	**Clinical Phenotype**	**Histopathology**	**Genetics**
Adenoma-carcinoma sequence	Familial adenomatous polyposis	Innumerable adenomatous polyps Moderately differentiated adenocarcinomas	Germ-line *APC* inactivation	Left-sided predominant cancers	Tubular, tubulovillous, and villous adenomas Moderately differentiated adenocarcinomas	Somatic inactivation or mutation of multiple genes*
Microsatellite instability	Hereditary nonpolyposis colorectal cancer	Mucinous and poorly differentiated carcinomas with lymphocytic infiltrates	Germ-line inactivation of *MLH1* or *MSH2* DNA repair genes	Right-sided predominant cancers	No precursor lesions Sessile serrated adenomas Large hyperplastic polyps Mucinous carcinomas	Somatic inactivation of *MLH1* or *MSH2* DNA repair genes

*Genes encoding APC/β-catenin, K-RAS, SMADS, p53. Adapted from Iacobuzio-Donahue CA, Montgomery EA: Gastrointestinal and Liver Pathology. Philadelphia, Elsevier, 2005.

- Programs that assiduously follow persons for the development of adenomas, and remove all that are identified, reduce the incidence of colorectal cancer.

Colorectal Carcinogenesis. Study of colorectal carcinogenesis has provided fundamental insights into the general mechanisms of cancer evolution. Many of these principles were discussed in Chapter 6. Here we will discuss concepts specifically pertinent to carcinogenesis in the colon.

It is now believed that *there are two pathogenetically distinct pathways for the development of colon cancer, the APC/β-catenin pathway (or the adenoma-carcinoma sequence), and the mismatch repair (or microsatellite instability) pathway* (Table 15–12). Both of these pathways involve the stepwise accumulation of multiple mutations, but the genes involved and the mechanisms by which the mutations accumulate are different.

The first pathway, variously called the *adenoma-carcinoma sequence, the APC/β-catenin pathway, or the chromosome instability pathway,* is characterized by chromosomal instability associated with stepwise accumulation of mutations in a number of oncogenes and tumor suppressor genes. The molecular evolution of colon cancer along this pathway occurs through a series of morphologically identifiable stages (Fig. 15–39). Ini-

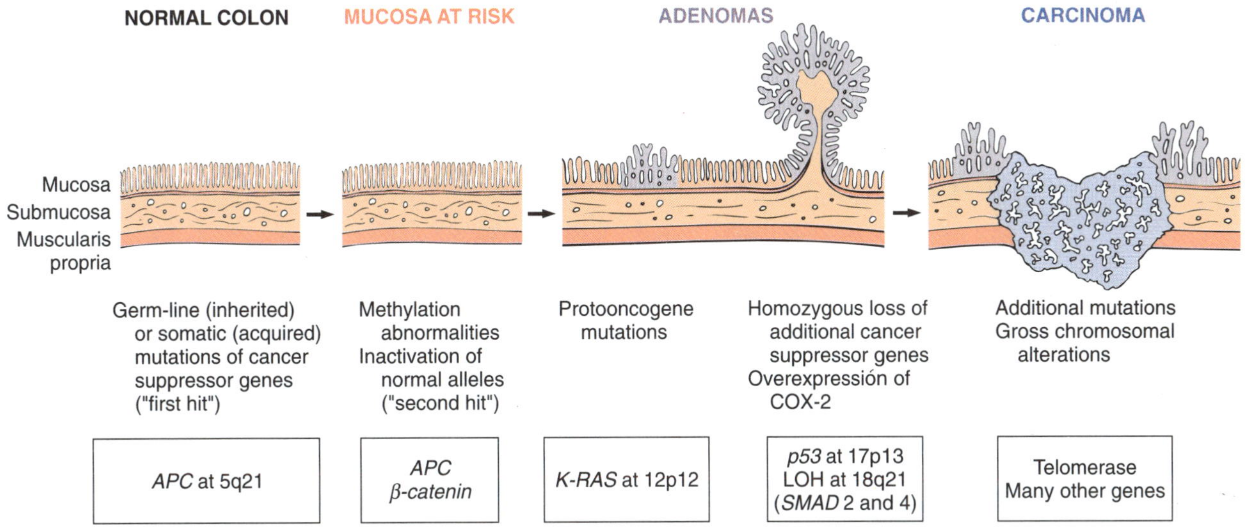

Figure 15–39

Morphologic and molecular changes in the adenoma-carcinoma sequence. It is postulated that loss of one normal copy of the tumor suppressor gene *APC* occurs early. Individuals may be born with one mutant allele, making them extremely prone to develop colon cancer, or inactivation of *APC* may occur later in life. This is the "first hit" according to Knudson's hypothesis (Chapter 6). The loss of the intact copy of *APC* follows ("second hit"). Other mutations include those on *K-RAS*, losses at 18q21 involving *SMAD2* and *SMAD4*, and the inactivation of the tumor suppressor gene *p53*, leading to the emergence of carcinoma, in which additional mutations occur. Although there seems to be a temporal sequence of changes, the accumulation of mutations, rather than their occurrence in a specific order, seems to be critical.

tially, there is localized epithelial proliferation. This is followed by the formation of small adenomas that progressively enlarge, become more dysplastic, and ultimately develop into invasive cancers. Such adenoma-carcinoma sequence, accounts for about 80% of sporadic colon tumors. The genetic correlates of this pathway are as follows:

- *Loss of the APC tumor suppressor gene.* This is believed to be the earliest event in the formation of adenomas. Recall that in the FAP and Gardner syndromes, germ-line mutations in the *APC* gene give rise to hundreds of adenomas that progress to form cancers. Both copies of the *APC* gene must be lost for adenomas to develop. As discussed in Chapter 6, the functions of the APC protein are intimately linked to β-catenin. Normal APC promotes the degradation of β-catenin; with loss of APC function, the accumulated β-catenin translocates to the nucleus and activates the transcription of several genes, such as *MYC* and cyclin D1, which promote cell proliferation. *APC* mutations are present in 60% to 80% of sporadic colon cancers.
- *Mutation of K-RAS.* The *K-RAS* gene encodes a signal transduction molecule that oscillates between an activated guanosine triphosphate–bound state and an inactive guanosine diphosphate–bound state. As discussed in Chapter 6, mutated *RAS* is trapped in an activated state that delivers mitotic signals and prevents apoptosis. *K-RAS* is mutated in fewer than 10% of adenomas less than 1 cm, in 50% of adenomas larger than 1 cm, and in 50% of carcinomas.
- *18q21 deletion.* Loss of a putative cancer suppressor gene on 18q21 has been found in 60% to 70% of colon cancers. Three genes have been mapped to this chromosome location: *DCC* (deleted in colon carcinoma), *SMAD2*, and *SMAD4*. The *SMAD* genes are considered to be the most relevant ones for colon carcinogenesis. They encode components of the transforming growth factor β (TGF-β) signaling pathway. Because TGF-β signaling normally inhibits the cell cycle, the loss of these genes may allow unrestrained cell growth.
- *Loss of p53.* Loss of this tumor suppressor gene is noted in 70% to 80% of colon cancers, yet similar losses are infrequent in adenomas, suggesting that mutations in *p53* occur late in colorectal carcinogenesis. The critical role of *p53* in cell cycle regulation was discussed in Chapter 6.

In addition to these changes, alterations in the methylation level of tumor suppressor genes occur in the development of colorectal tumors in the adenoma-carcinoma pathway.

The second pathway of colorectal carcinogenesis is characterized by genetic lesions in *DNA mismatch repair genes* (Fig. 15–40). It is involved in 10% to 15% of sporadic cases. As in the *APC*/β-catenin schema, there is accumulation of mutations, but the involved genes are different. There may be no detectable antecedent lesions, or the tumors may develop from sessile serrated adenomas. Defective DNA repair caused by inactivation of DNA mismatch repair genes is the fundamental and the most likely initiating event in colorectal cancers that follow this path. Inherited mutations in one of five DNA mismatch repair genes (*MSH2*, *MSH6*, *MLH1*, *PMS1*, and *PMS2*) give rise to the hereditary nonpolyposis colon carcinoma (HNPCC). Of these, *MLH1* and *MSH2* are the ones most commonly involved in HNPCC- derived and sporadic colon carcinomas with DNA mismatch repair gene defects. Loss of DNA mismatch repair genes leads to a hypermutable state in which simple repetitive DNA sequences, called *microsatellites*, are unstable during DNA replication, giving rise to widespread alterations in these repeats. The resulting *microsatellite instability* (MSI) is the molecular signature of defective DNA mismatch repair, and hence this pathway is often referred to as the MSI pathway. Because of the multiple mutations caused as a consequence of the defect in DNA repair, the defect is considered to lead to the establishment of a *mutator phenotype*. Most microsatellite sequences are in noncoding regions of the genes. However, some

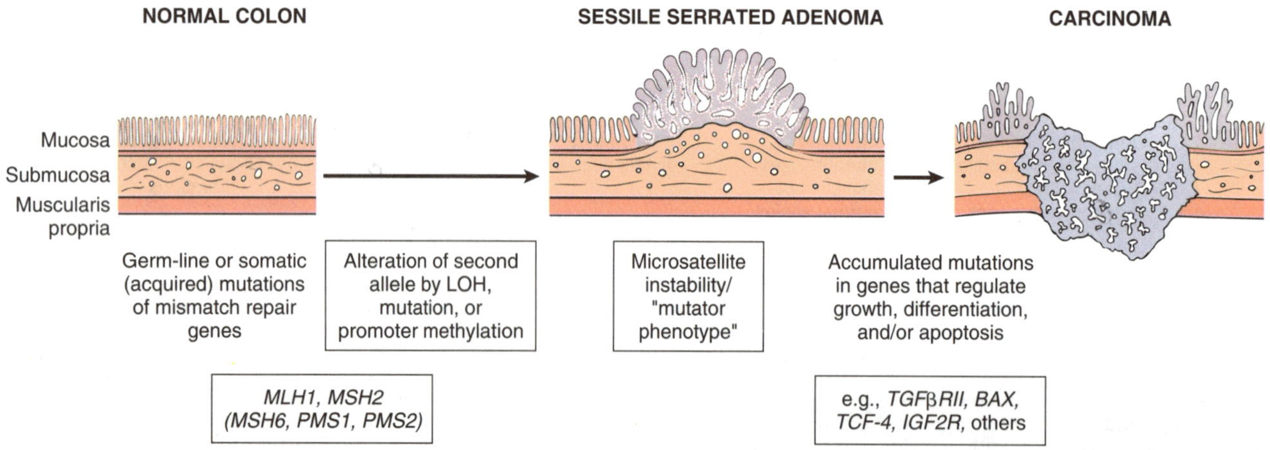

Figure 15–40

Morphologic and molecular changes in the mismatch repair pathway of colon carcinogenesis. Defects in mismatch repair genes result in microsatellite instability and permit the accumulation of mutations in numerous genes. If these mutations affect genes involved in cell survival and proliferation, cancer may develop.

microsatellite sequences are located in the coding or promoter region of genes involved in regulation of cell growth. Such genes include type II TGF-β receptor and *BAX*. TGF-β signaling inhibits the growth of colonic epithelial cells, and the *BAX* gene product causes apoptosis. Loss of mismatch repair leads to the accumulation of mutations in these and other growth-regulating genes, culminating in the emergence of colorectal carcinomas.

Although there is no readily identifiable adenoma-carcinoma sequence that typifies tumors arising from defects in mismatch repair, it has been noted that sessile serrated adenomas located on the right side of the colon display MSI and may be precancerous. Fully developed tumors that arise via the mismatch repair pathway do show some distinctive morphologic features, including proximal colonic location, mucinous histology, and infiltration by lymphocytes. In general, these tumors have a better prognosis than do stage-matched tumors that arise by the *APC*/β-catenin pathway.

A note of caution is needed in the evaluation of the molecular changes discussed in the adenoma–carcinoma sequence and the mismatch repair pathway. None of the changes listed appears universally. For instance, defects in *APC* are universal in FAP polyps but vary widely in dysplastic polyps associated with sporadic colorectal cancer. In fact, the sequence of gene alterations seen in these two pathways of hereditary colon cancer may not be as evident in sporadic tumors. Most likely, the accumulation of multiple mutations is more important than the order of their appearance.

Morphology

About 25% of colorectal carcinomas are in the cecum or ascending colon, with a similar proportion in the rectum and distal sigmoid. An additional 25% are in the descending colon and proximal sigmoid; the remainder are scattered elsewhere. Hence, a substantial portion of cancers is undetectable by digital or proctosigmoidoscopic examination. Most often carcinomas occur singly and have frequently obliterated their adenomatous origins. When multiple carcinomas are present, they are often at widely disparate sites in the colon.

Although all colorectal carcinomas begin as in situ lesions, they evolve into different morphologic patterns. **Tumors in the proximal colon tend to grow as polypoid, exophytic masses that extend along one wall of the capacious cecum and ascending colon** (Fig. 15–41). Obstruction is uncommon. **When carcinomas in the distal colon are discovered, they tend to be annular, encircling lesions that produce so-called napkin-ring constrictions of the bowel and narrowing of the lumen** (Fig. 15–42); the margins of the napkin ring are classically heaped up. Both forms of neoplasm directly penetrate the bowel wall over the course of time (probably years) and may appear as firm masses on the serosal surface.

Regardless of their gross appearance, all colon carcinomas are microscopically similar. Almost all are adenocarcinomas that range from well-differentiated (Fig. 15–43) to undifferentiated, frankly anaplastic masses. Many tumors produce mucin, which is secreted into the gland lumina or into the interstitium of the gut wall. Because these secretions dissect through the gut wall, they facilitate extension of the cancer and worsen the prognosis. Cancers of the anal zone are predominantly squamous cell in origin.

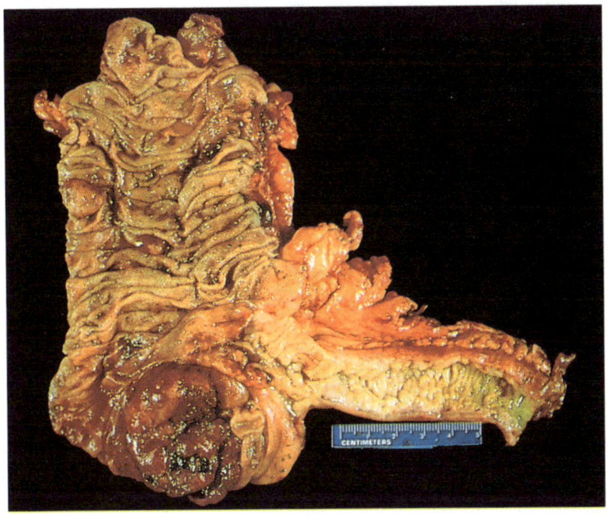

Figure 15–41

Carcinoma of the cecum. The exophytic carcinoma projects into the lumen but has not caused obstruction.

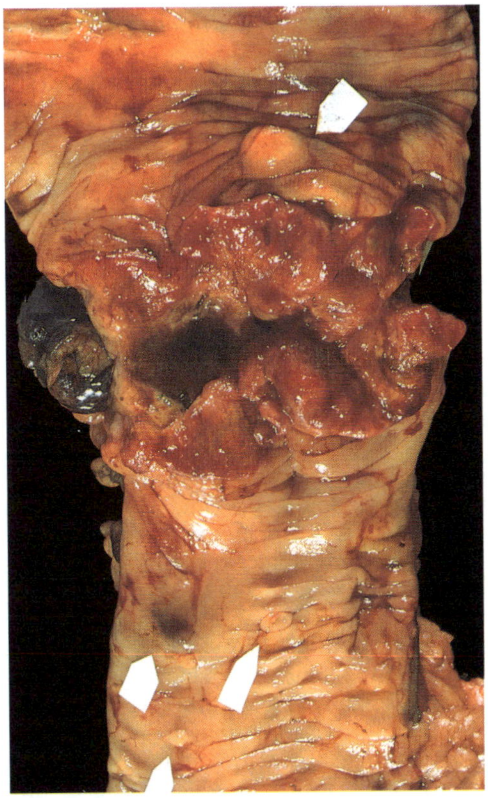

Figure 15–42

Carcinoma of the descending colon. This circumferential tumor has heaped-up edges and an ulcerated central portion. The arrows identify separate mucosal polyps.

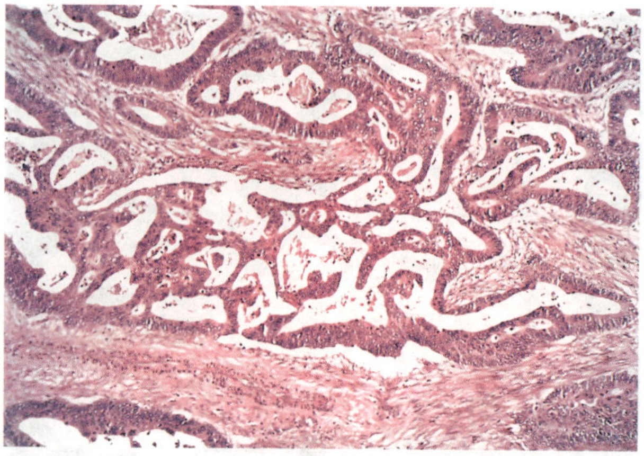

Figure 15–43

Invasive adenocarcinoma of colon showing malignant glands infiltrating the muscle wall.

Table 15–13 TNM Staging of Colon Cancers

Tumor (T)
T0 = none evident
Tis = in situ (limited to mucosa)
T1 = invasion of lamina propria or submucosa
T2 = invasion of muscularis propria
T3 = invasion through muscularis propria into subserosa or nonperitonealized perimuscular tissue
T4 = invasion of other organs or structures
Lymph Nodes (N)
0 = none evident
1 = 1 to 3 positive pericolic nodes
2 = 4 or more positive pericolic nodes
3 = any positive node along a named blood vessel
Distant Metastases (M)
0 = none evident
1 = any distant metastasis
5-Year Survival Rates
T1 = 97%
T2 = 90%
T3 = 78%
T4 = 63%
Any T; N1; M0 = 66%
Any T; N2; M0 = 37%
Any T; N3; M0 = data not available
Any M1 = 4%

Clinical Features. Colorectal cancers remain asymptomatic for years; symptoms develop insidiously and frequently have been present for months, sometimes years, before diagnosis. Cecal and right colonic cancers most often are called to clinical attention by the appearance of fatigue, weakness, and iron deficiency anemia. Left-sided lesions may produce occult bleeding, changes in bowel habit, or crampy left lower quadrant discomfort. Although anemia in females may arise from gynecologic causes, it is a clinical maxim that *iron deficiency anemia in an older man means gastrointestinal cancer until proved otherwise.*

All colorectal tumors spread by direct extension into adjacent structures and by metastasis through the lymphatics and blood vessels. In order of preference, the favored sites for metastasis are the regional lymph nodes, liver, lungs, and bones, followed by many other sites including the serosal membrane of the peritoneal cavity. In general, the disease spreads beyond the range of curative surgery in 25% to 30% of patients. Carcinomas of the anal region are locally invasive and metastasize to regional lymph nodes and distant sites. Almost 80% of malignant tumors of the anal canal are squamous cell carcinomas.

The detection and diagnosis of colorectal neoplasms rely on a variety of methods, beginning with digital rectal examination and fecal testing for occult blood loss. Barium enema, sigmoidoscopy, and colonoscopy require confirmatory biopsy for diagnosis. Computed tomography and other radiographic studies are usually used to assess metastatic spread. Serum markers for disease, such as elevated blood levels of carcinoembryonic antigen, are of little diagnostic value, because they reach significant levels only after the tumor has achieved considerable size and has very probably spread. Moreover, "positive" carcinoembryonic antigen levels may be produced by carcinomas of the lung, breast, ovary, urinary bladder, and prostate, as well as such non-neoplastic disorders as alcoholic cirrhosis, pancreatitis, and ulcerative colitis. Because *APC* mutations occur early in most colon cancers, molecular detection of *APC* mutations in epithelial cells, isolated from stools, is being evaluated as a diagnostic test. As mentioned earlier, it is not established that *APC* mutations always occur early in the development of colorectal tumors. Other tests under development involve the detection of abnormal patterns of methylation in DNA isolated from stool cells.

The single most important prognostic indicator of colorectal carcinoma is the extent (stage) of the tumor at the time of diagnosis. The American Joint Commission on Cancer uses the TNM classification (Table 15–13). The challenge is to discover these neoplasms when curative resection is possible, preferably in their "infancy" when they are still adenomatous polyps.

SUMMARY

Colorectal Carcinoma

- Common tumor in developing countries, with peak incidence at 60–70 years of age.
- Almost all are adenocarcinomas, most frequently originating from adenomatous polyps.
- There are two molecular pathways of colorectal carcinogenesis, the adenoma-carcinoma sequence and the mismatch repair (or microsatellite instability) pathway. In each pathway there is sequential accumulation of mutations in specific genes (e.g. *APC* and DNA mismatch repair genes).
- Tumors are exophytic and polypoid masses or annular lesions, composed of malignant cells forming glands and with varying degrees of differentiation.

Neoplasms of the Small Intestine

Whereas the small bowel represents 75% of the length of the alimentary tract, its tumors account for only 3% to 6% of gastrointestinal tumors, with a slight preponderance of benign tumors. The number of deaths in the United States annually is under 1000, representing only about 1% of gastrointestinal malignancies. The most frequent benign tumors in the small intestine are stromal tumors of predominantly smooth muscle origin, adenomas, and lipomas, followed by various neurogenic, vascular, and hamartomatous epithelial lesions. Small intestinal adenocarcinomas and carcinoids have a roughly equal incidence. Gastrointestinal stromal tumors (GISTs) have received much attention recently, because they have an activating mutation affecting *KIT*, a tyrosine kinase receptor that is the target of new therapeutic agents (discussed in the next section).

Adenocarcinoma of the Small Intestine. These tumors grow in a napkin-ring encircling pattern or as polypoid fungating masses, in a manner similar to colonic cancers. Most small bowel carcinomas arise in the duodenum (including the ampulla of Vater). Cramping pain, nausea, vomiting, and weight loss are the common presenting signs and symptoms, but such manifestations generally appear late in the course of these cancers. By the time of diagnosis, most have already penetrated the bowel wall, invaded the mesentery or other segments of the gut, spread to regional nodes, and sometimes metastasized to the liver and more widely. Despite these problems, wide en bloc excision of these cancers yields a 5-year survival rate of about 70%. Adenomas of the small intestine may present with anemia or rarely intussusception or obstruction. Adenomas in the immediate vicinity of the ampulla of Vater may produce biliary obstruction causing jaundice.

Other Tumors of the Gastrointestinal Tract

Gastrointestinal Stromal Tumors

In the past, these tumors were considered to be smooth muscle tumors, either benign leiomyomas or malignant leiomyosarcomas, sometimes with a spindle cell composition. However, on the basis of a molecular marker common to these tumors, they are classified as gastrointestinal stromal tumors (GISTs). With the use of immunohistochemical markers, GISTs are now subdivided into (a) tumors that show smooth muscle cell differentiation (the most common type); (b) tumors with neural differentiation (often called gastrointestinal autonomic nerve tumors; (c) tumors with smooth muscle/neural dual differentiation, and (d) tumors lacking differentiation toward these lineages. GISTs constitute the majority of nonepithelial tumors of the stomach but can be present in the small and large intestine (Fig. 15–44). An important advance in understanding the pathogenesis of these tumors, which had an immediate application in diagnosis and treatment, was the recognition that *most GISTs have a somatic mutation in the c-KIT (CD117) gene, which encodes a tyrosine kinase receptor.* Mutations in

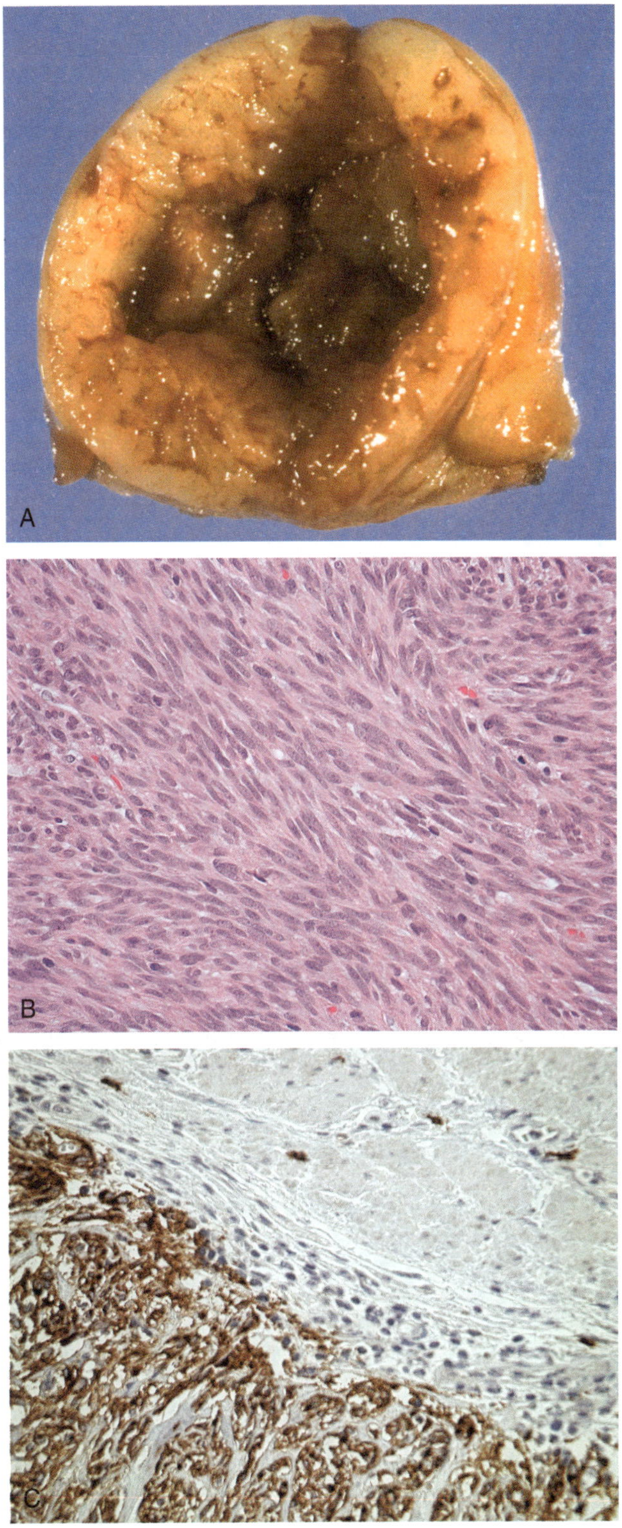

Figure 15–44

Gastrointestinal stromal tumor (GIST). **A,** GIST from the stomach wall. **B,** Histology of the tumor showing spindle cells with elongated nuclei with fine chromatin, and eosinophilic fibrillar cytoplasm. **C,** KIT stain showing strong and uniform reactivity of the tumor cells. Note KIT staining of mast cells in the adjacent normal muscle wall. (Courtesy of Dr. Brian Rubin, Department of Pathology, University of Washington, Seattle, Washington.)

this receptor (generally in exon 11) lead to consitutive signaling from the receptor, without the need for a ligand.

There seem to be no differences in the frequency of the mutation among the various histologic types of GISTs. Most GISTs occur in adults. The preferred sites for metastases of the malignant tumors are the liver, peritoneum, and lungs. Metastases can appear more than 20 years after removal of the original tumor. The recognition of the molecular defect in GISTs has led to development of drugs that are specifically targeted to the tumor cells ("targeted therapy"). The tyrosine kinase inhibitor imatinib mesylate, shown to be highly effective in the treatment of individuals with chronic myeloid leukemia, has been used very successfully in the treatment of GISTs that have a c-KIT mutation. Nevertheless, because of the development of resistance to this agent after prolonged treatment, new types of inhibitors of tyrosine kinase receptor signaling are being tested for clinical use.

Gastrointestinal Lymphoma

Any segment of the gastrointestinal tract may be involved secondarily by systemic dissemination of non-Hodgkin lymphomas. However, up to 40% of lymphomas arise in sites other than lymph nodes, and the gut is the most common extra-nodal location; 1% to 4% of all gastrointestinal malignancies are lymphomas. *By definition, primary gastrointestinal lymphomas reveal no evidence of liver, spleen, or bone marrow involvement at the time of diagnosis;* regional lymph node involvement may be present. Intestinal tract lymphomas can be of B- or T-cell origin. The most common form in Western countries is *MALT lymphoma.* This is a sporadic lymphoma that originates in B cells of the *mucosa-associated lymphoid tissue* (MALT) of the gastrointestinal tract. This type of gastrointestinal lymphoma usually affects adults, lacks a sex predilection, and may arise anywhere in the gut: stomach (55% to 60% of cases), small intestine (25% to 30%), proximal colon (10% to 15%), and distal colon (≤10%). The appendix and esophagus are only rarely involved.

Gastric MALT lymphomas arise in the setting of mucosal lymphoid activation, as a result of *Helicobacter*-associated chronic gastritis. With *H. pylori* infection, there is an intense activation of T and B cells in the mucosa. This leads to polyclonal B-cell hyperplasia and eventually to the emergence of a monoclonal B-cell neoplasm. MALT lymphoma cells are CD5 and CD10 negative, and a t(11;18) translocation is common (the translocation creates a fusion gene between the apoptosis inhibitor *BCL-2* gene in chromosome 11 and the *MLT* gene in chromosome 18).

Primary gastrointestinal lymphomas generally have a better prognosis than do those arising in other sites, because combined surgery, chemotherapy, and radiation therapy offer reasonable hopes of cure. About 50% of gastric lymphomas can regress with antibiotic treatment for *H. pylori.* Those that do not regress usually contain the t(11;18) translocation or other genetic abnormalities. Celiac disease (discussed earlier) is associated with a higher than normal risk of intestinal T-cell lymphomas.

Carcinoids

Cells generating bioactive compounds, particularly peptide and nonpeptide hormones, are normally dispersed along the length of the gastrointestinal tract mucosa and have a major role in coordinated gut function. Endocrine cells are abundant in other organs, but most of the tumors that develop from these cells arise in the gut. Tumors arising from these endocrine cells are called carcinoid tumors; they may develop in the pancreas or peripancreatic tissue, lungs, biliary tree, and even liver. The term *carcinoid* is an old reference to "carcinoma-like," which has persisted through the decades. The peak incidence of these neoplasms is in the sixth decade, but they may appear at any age. *They compose less than 2% of colorectal malignancies but almost half of small intestinal malignant tumors.*

Although all carcinoids are potentially malignant tumors, the tendency for aggressive behavior correlates with the site of origin, the depth of local penetration, and the size of the tumor. For example, *appendiceal and rectal carcinoids infrequently metastasize,* even though they may show extensive local spread. By contrast, 90% of ileal, gastric, and colonic carcinoids that have penetrated halfway through the muscle wall have spread to lymph nodes and distant sites at the time of diagnosis, especially those larger than 2 cm in diameter.

As with normal gut endocrine cells, the cells of carcinoid tumors can synthesize and secrete a variety of bioactive products and hormones. Although multiple hormones may be synthesized by a single tumor, when a tumor secretes a predominant product to cause a clinical syndrome, it may be called by that name (e.g., gastrinoma, somatostatinoma, and insulinoma).

Morphology

The appendix is the most common site of gut carcinoid tumors, followed by the small intestine (primarily ileum), rectum, stomach, and colon. In the appendix they appear as bulbous swellings of the tip, which frequently obliterate the lumen. Elsewhere in the gut, they appear as intramural or submucosal masses that create small, polypoid, or plateau-like elevations rarely larger than 3 cm in diameter (Fig. 15–45A). The overlying mucosa may be intact or ulcerated, and the tumors may permeate the bowel wall to invade the mesentery. Those that arise in the stomach and ileum are frequently multicentric, but the remainder tend to be solitary lesions. **A characteristic feature is a solid, yellow-tan appearance on transection.** The tumors are exceedingly firm because of desmoplasia; and when these fibrosing lesions penetrate the mesentery of the small bowel they may cause sufficient angulation or kinking to cause obstruction. When present, visceral metastases are usually small, dispersed nodules and rarely achieve the size seen with the primary lesions. Notably, **rectal and appendiceal carcinoids almost never metastasize.**

Histologically, the neoplastic cells may form discrete islands, trabeculae, strands, glands, or undifferentiated sheets. Whatever their organization, the tumor cells are monotonously similar, having a scant, pink granular

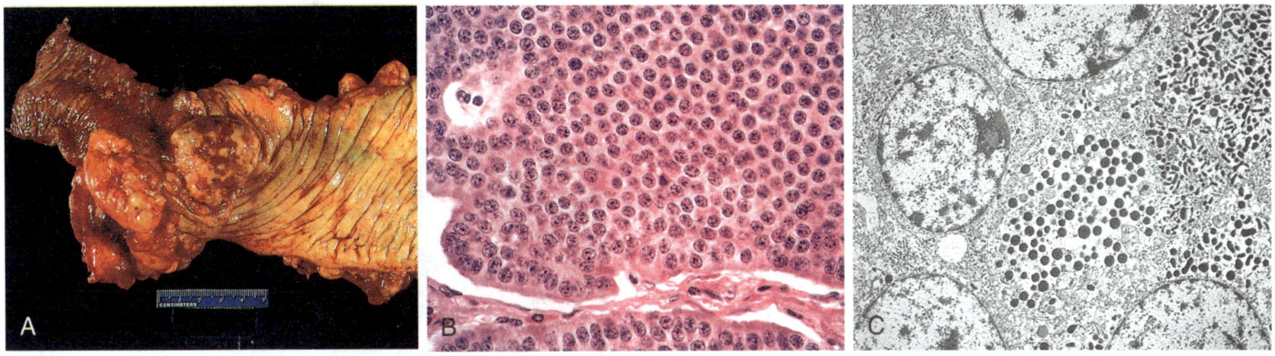

Figure 15–45

Carcinoid tumor. **A,** Multiple protruding tumors are present at the ileocecal junction. **B,** The tumor cells show a monotonous morphology, with a delicate intervening fibrovascular stroma. (H&E). **C,** Electron micrograph showing dense-core bodies in the cytoplasm.

cytoplasm and a round-to-oval stippled nucleus. In most tumors there is minimal variation in cell and nuclear size, and mitoses are infrequent or absent (Fig. 15–45B). By electron microscopy (Fig. 15–45C), the cells in most tumors contain cytoplasmic, membrane-bound secretory granules with osmophilic centers (dense-core granules). Most carcinoids can be shown to contain chromogranin A, synaptophysin, and neuron-specific enolase. Specific hormonal peptides may occasionally be identified by immunocytochemical techniques.

Clinical Features. Gastrointestinal carcinoids are frequently asymptomatic, including virtually all that arise in the appendix. Only rarely do carcinoids produce local symptoms secondary to angulation or obstruction of the small intestine. However, the secretory products of some carcinoids can produce a variety of syndromes or endocrinopathies. Gastric, peripancreatic, and pancreatic carcinoids release their products directly into the systemic circulation and can produce the Zollinger-Ellison syndrome by excess elaboration of gastrin, Cushing syndrome caused by adrenocorticotropic hormone secretion, hyperinsulinism, and others. In some instances, these tumors may be less than 1.0 cm in size and extremely difficult to find, even during surgical exploration.

Some neoplasms are associated with a distinctive *carcinoid syndrome*, detailed in Table 15–14. The syndrome occurs in about 1% of all patients with carcinoids and in 20% of those with widespread metastases. The precise basis of the carcinoid syndrome is uncertain, but most manifestations are thought to arise from elaboration of serotonin (5-hydroxytryptamine [5-HT]). Elevated levels of 5-HT and its metabolite, 5-hydroxyindoleacetic acid (5-HIAA) are present in the blood and urine of most individuals with the classic syndrome; 5-HT is degraded in the liver to functionally inactive 5-HIAA. Thus, with gastrointestinal carcinoids, hepatic dysfunction resulting from metastases must be present for the development of the syndrome. The possibility that other secretory products such as histamine, bradykinin, and prostaglandins contribute to the manifestations of this syndrome has not been excluded.

The 5-year survival rate for carcinoids (excluding appendiceal) is approximately 90%. Even with small bowel tumors that have spread to the liver, it is better than 50%. However, widespread disease usually causes death.

Table 15–14 Clinical Features of the Carcinoid Syndrome

Vasomotor disturbances
- Cutaneous flushes and apparent cyanosis (most patients)

Intestinal hypermotility
- Diarrhea, cramps, nausea, vomiting (most patients)

Asthmatic bronchoconstrictive attacks
- Cough, wheezing, dyspnea (about one-third of patients)

Hepatomegaly
- Nodular, related to hepatic metastases (some cases)

Niacin deficiency (due to shunting of niacin to serotonin synthesis)

Systemic fibrosis

Cardiac involvement
- Pulmonic and tricuspid valve thickening and stenosis
- Endocardial fibrosis, principally in right ventricle (bronchial carcinoids affect the left side)

Retroperitoneal and pelvic fibrosis

Collagenous pleural and intimal aortic plaques

APPENDIX

Diseases of the appendix loom large in surgical practice; appendicitis is the most common acute abdominal condition the surgeon is called on to treat. Despite the preeminence of this diagnostic entity, a differential diagnosis must include virtually every acute process that can occur within the abdominal cavity, as well as some emergent conditions affecting organs of the thorax. On occasion, a tumor arises in the appendix, necessitating abdominal exploration.

ACUTE APPENDICITIS

Surveys indicate that approximately 10% of persons in the United States and other Western countries develop appendicitis at some time. No age is immune, but the peak incidence is in the second and third decades, although lately a second smaller peak is appearing among elderly persons. Males are affected more often than females in a ratio of 1.5:1.

Pathogenesis. Appendiceal inflammation is associated with obstruction in 50% to 80% of cases, usually in the form of a fecalith and, less commonly, a gallstone, tumor, or ball of worms *(Oxyuriasis vermicularis)*. With continued secretion of mucinous fluid, the buildup of intraluminal pressure presumably is sufficient to cause collapse of the draining veins. Obstruction and ischemic injury then favor bacterial proliferation with additional inflammatory edema and exudation, further compromising the blood supply. Nevertheless, a significant minority of inflamed appendices have no demonstrable luminal obstruction, and the pathogenesis of the inflammation remains unknown.

Morphology

At the earliest stages, only a scant neutrophilic exudate may be found throughout the mucosa, submucosa, and muscularis propria. Subserosal vessels are congested, and often there is a modest perivascular neutrophilic infiltrate. The inflammatory reaction transforms the normal glistening serosa into a dull, granular, red membrane; this transformation signifies **early acute appendicitis** for the operating surgeon. At a later stage, a prominent neutrophilic exudate generates a fibrinopurulent reaction over the serosa (Fig. 15–46). As the inflammatory process worsens, there is abscess formation within the wall, along with ulcerations and foci of necrosis in the mucosa. This state constitutes **acute suppurative appendicitis.** Further appendiceal compromise leads to large areas of hemorrhagic green ulceration of the mucosa, and green-black gangrenous necrosis through the wall extending to the serosa, creating **acute gangrenous appendicitis** that is quickly followed by rupture and suppurative peritonitis.

The histologic criterion for the diagnosis of acute appendicitis is neutrophilic infiltration of the muscularis propria. Usually, neutrophils and ulcerations are also present within the mucosa.

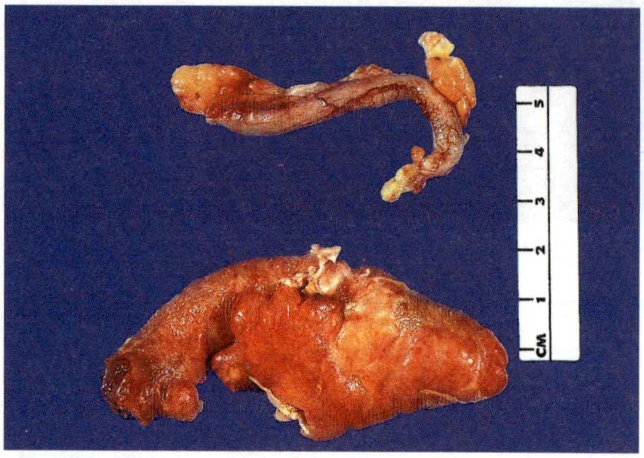

Figure 15–46

Acute appendicitis. The inflamed appendix *(bottom)* is red, swollen, and covered with a fibrinous exudate. For comparison, a normal appendix is shown *(top)*.

Clinical Features. Acute appendicitis is either the easiest or the most difficult of abdominal diagnoses. The classic case is marked by (1) mild periumbilical discomfort, followed by (2) anorexia, nausea, and vomiting, soon associated with (3) right lower quadrant tenderness, which in the course of hours is transformed into (4) a deep constant ache or pain in the right lower quadrant. Fever and leukocytosis appear early in the course. Regrettably, a large number of cases are not classic. The condition can be remarkably silent, particularly in the aged, or can fail to reveal localizing right-sided lower quadrant signs, as when the appendix is retrocecal or when there is malrotation of the colon. Moreover, the following disorders may present many of the clinical features of acute appendicitis: (1) mesenteric lymphadenitis after a viral systemic infection, (2) gastroenteritis with mesenteric adenitis, (3) pelvic inflammatory disease with tubo-ovarian involvement, (4) rupture of an ovarian follicle at the time of ovulation, (5) ectopic pregnancy, (6) Meckel diverticulitis, and other conditions as well. Thus, with conventional diagnostic techniques (starting with physical examination), an accurate diagnosis of acute appendicitis can be made only about 80% of the time. Newer preoperative imaging modalities may be increasing diagnostic accuracy to 95%. Regardless, *it is generally conceded that it is better to occasionally resect a normal appendix than to risk the morbidity and mortality (~2%) of appendiceal perforation.*

TUMORS OF THE APPENDIX

Carcinoids (discussed above) are the most common tumors in the appendix. The only other lesions worthy of mention are mucocele of the appendix and mucinous neoplasms.

Mucocele refers to dilation of the lumen of the appendix by mucinous secretion. It is caused by non-neoplastic obstruction of the lumen and is usually associated with a fecalith in the lumen, permitting the slow accumulation of sterile mucinous secretions. Eventually, the distention induces atrophy of the mucin-secreting mucosal cells and the secretions stop. This condition is usually asymptomatic; rarely, a mucocele ruptures, spilling otherwise innocuous mucin into the peritoneum.

Mucinous neoplasms range from the benign *mucinous cystadenoma*, to *mucinous cystadenocarcinoma*, which invades the wall, to a form of disseminated intraperitoneal cancer called *pseudomyxoma peritonei*. The cystadenoma is histologically identical to analogous tumors in the ovary (Chapter 19). The malignant mucin-secreting neoplasms (cystadenocarcinomas) invade the wall, allowing tumor cells to implant throughout the peritoneal cavity, which becomes filled with mucin (pseudomyxoma peritonei).

BIBLIOGRAPHY

Oral Cavity

Forastiere A, et al.: Head and neck cancer. N Engl J Med 345:1890, 2001. *[A review of molecular and clinical features of cancers of the head and neck, including the oral cavity.]*

Ha PK, Califano JA: The role of human papillomavirus in oral carcinogenesis. Crit Rev Oral Biol Med 15:188, 2004. *[Points out that the evidence that herpesviruses have a causal role in oral carcinogenesis is limited.]*

Simpson RH: Classification of salivary gland tumors—a brief histopathological review. Histol Histopathol 10:737, 1995. *[A primer on the morphologic features of salivary gland tumors.]*

Witt RL: Major salivary gland cancer. Surg Oncol Clin N Am 13:113, 2004. *[A review on diagnosis and treatment of these tumors.]*

Esophagus

Gomes L, et al.: Expression profile of malignant and non-malignant lesions of esophagus and stomach: differential activity of functional modules related to inflammation and lipid metabolism. Cancer Res 65:7127, 2005. *[An analysis of gene expression in these tumors by microarray techniques, which challenges some established views on tumor classification.]*

Mueller J, et al.: Barrett's esophagus: histopathologic definitions and diagnostic criteria. World J Surg 28:148, 2004. *[A detailed discussion of histopathologic issues regarding Barrett esophagus.]*

McCormick PA: Pathophysiology and prognosis of oesophageal varices. Scand J Gastroenterol 29 (Suppl 207):1, 1994. *[A convincing discussion of the grave nature of this disease condition.]*

Paterson WG: Etiology and pathogenesis of achalasia. Gastrointest Endosc Clin North Am 11:249, 2001.

Richter JE: Oesophageal motility disorders. Lancet 358:823, 2001.

Shaheen, NJ: Advances in Barrett's esophagus and esophageal adenocarcinoma. Gastroenterology 128:1554, 2005. *[A very good review on the diagnosis, pathogenesis, and management of these conditions.]*

Spechler SJ: Barrett's esophagus. N Engl J Med 346:836, 2002. *[An excellent discussion that touches on clinical, histologic, and prognostic issues.]*

Wild CP, Hardie, LJ: Reflux, Barrett's esophagus and adenocarcinoma: burning questions. Nat Rev Cancer 3:676, 2003. *[A discussion of the pathogenesis and molecular alterations in gastroesophageal reflux disease, Barrett esophagus, and the progression to tumor development.]*

Stomach

Atherton JC: The pathogenesis of *Helicobacter pylori*-induced gastroduodenal diseases. Ann Rev Pathol: Mech Dis 1:63, 2006.

Boussioutas A, et al.: Distinctive patterns of gene expression in premalignant gastric mucosa and gastric cancer. Cancer Res 63:2569, 2003. *[Identification of molecular signatures of premalignant lesions, and different types of gastric cancers by microarray analysis.]*

Chan FK, Leung WK: Peptic-ulcer disease. Lancet 360:933, 2002.

Dundan WG, et al.: Virulence factors of *Helicobacter pylori*. Int J Med Microbiol 290:647, 2001. *[An excellent summary of Helicobacter-elaborated toxins and enzymes.]*

Henson DE, et al.: Differential trends in the intestinal and diffuse types of gastric carcinoma in the United States, 1973–2000: increase in the signet ring cell type. Arch Pathol Lab Med 128:765, 2004. *[An analysis of incidence trends of different histological types of gastric carcinomas.]*

Lynch HT, et al.: Gastric cancer: new genetic developments. J Surg Oncol 90:114, 2005. *[A comprehensive review of the genetics and pathology of the intestinal and diffuse types of gastric carcinoma.]*

Normark S, et al.: Persistent infection with *Helicobacter pylori* and the development of gastric cancer. Adv Cancer Res 90:63, 2003. *[A review of bacterial/host relationships in the intestinal wall and the mechanisms by which H. pylori may promote tumorigenesis.]*

Peek RM Jr, Blaser MJ: *Helicobacter pylori* and gastrointestinal tract adenocarcinomas. Nat Rev Cancer 2:28, 2002. *[A review focusing on host/microbial interactions that discusses the question of susceptibility to cancer in individuals infected with H. pylori.]*

Rugge M, Genta R: Staging and grading of chronic gastritis. Hum Pathol 36:228, 2005. *[Description of a new system for staging and grading of chronic gastritis.]*

Werner M, et al.: Gastric adenocarcinoma: pathomorphology and molecular pathology. J Cancer Res Clin Oncol 124:207, 2001. *[A review of important concepts.]*

Small and Large Intestines

Bouma G, Strober W: The immunological and genetic basis of inflammatory bowel disease. Nat Rev Immunol 3:251, 2003. *[An excellent review of the immunology and molecular biology of Crohn disease and ulcerative colitis.]*

Brito GA, et al.: Pathophysiology and impact of enteric bacterial and protozoal infections: new approaches to therapy. Chemotherapy 51 (Suppl 1):23, 2005. *[An overview of the epidemiology, pathogenesis and management of infectious diarrhea.]*

Cario E: Bacterial interactions with cells of the intestinal mucosa: Toll-like receptors and NOD2. Gut 54:1182, 2005. *[A review of basic mechanisms that may involve TLR and NOD2 in the pathogenesis of inflammatory bowel disease.]*

Eckman L, Karin M: NOD2 and Crohn's disease: loss or gain of function? Immunity 22:661, 2005. *[A discussion of the role of NOD2 in the pathogenesis of Crohn disease.]*

Farrell RJ, Kelley CP: Celiac sprue. N Engl J Med 346:180, 2002. *[An excellent review of this common but under-recognized disorder.]*

Fodde R: The *APC* gene in colorectal cancer. Eur J Cancer 38:867, 2002. *[An excellent review on APC functions and its role in colorectal cancers.]*

Green PH, Jabri B: Celiac disease. Ann Rev Med 57:207, 2006. *[A comprehensive and contemporary review on celiac disease.]*

Gupta RA, Dubois R: Colorectal cancer prevention and treatment by inhibition of cyclooxygenase-2. Nature Rev Cancer 1:11, 2001. *[An excellent discussion of the clinical evidence documenting chemopreventive actions of cyclooxygenase inhibitors, and the possible molecular basis of this action.]*

Inohara N, et al.: NOD-LRR proteins: role in host-microbial interactions and inflammatory disease. Ann Rev Biochem 74:355, 2005. *[A comprehensive review of the involvement of NOD proteins in host immune responses against pathogens.]*

Isaacson PG, Du MQ: Gastrointestinal lymphoma: where morphology meets molecular biology. J Pathol 205:255, 2005. *[An excellent review on the histopathology and molecular characterization of these tumors.]*

Jass JR, et al.: Emerging concepts in colorectal neoplasia. Gastroenterology 123:862, 2002. *[An alternative view of the development of colorectal tumors.]*

Leslie A, et al.: The colorectal adenoma-carcinoma sequence. Br J Surg 89:845, 2002. *[An update on the strengths and potential limitations of the adenoma-carcinoma sequence in colorectal cancer.]*

Loeb LA, et al.: Multiple mutations and cancer. Proc Natl Acad Sci USA 199:776, 2003. *[A presentation on the current status of the mutator phenotype in cancer pathogenesis.]*

Marx J: Puzzling out the pains in the gut. Science 315:33, 2007. *[An up-to-date and brief review of newly identified mutations and immunological mediators in IBD.]*

Oldenburg WA, et al.: Acute mesenteric ischemia: a clinical review. Arch Intern Med 164:1054, 2004. *[Describes the challenges on the diagnosis and treatment of acute mesenteric ischemia.]*

Peltomäki P: Deficient DNA mismatch repair: a common etiologic factor for colon cancer. Hum Mol Genet 10:735, 2001. *[A discussion of the molecular pathways that involve mismatch repair genes and give rise to colon cancer.]*

Podolsky DK: Inflammatory bowel disease. N Engl J Med 347:417, 2002. *[An excellent summary of both Crohn disease and ulcerative colitis, highlighting the similarities and differences.]*

Sanborn RE, Blanke CD: Gastrointestinal tumors and the evolution of targeted therapy. Clin Adv Hematol Oncol 3:647, 2005. *[A review of the present status of targeted therapy for GISTs.]*

Stollman N, Raskin JB: Diverticular disease of the colon. Lancet 363:631, 2004. *[A review of pathophysiology, clinical presentation and management of diverticular disease of the colon.]*

Thielman NM, Guerrant RL: Clinical practice. Acute infectious diarrhea. N Engl J Med 350:38, 2004. *[An excellent review of the management of infectious diarrhea.]*

Weitz J, et al.: Colorectal cancer. Lancet 365:153, 2005. *[A general review of hereditary and sporadic colorectal cancer and the clinical management of the disease.]*

Wynter CV, et al.: Methylation patterns define two types of hyperplastic polyp associated with colorectal cancer. Gut 53:573, 2004. *[Identification of molecular heterogeneity among hyperplastic polyps and their malignant potential.]*

Appendix

Birnbaum BA, Wilson SR: Appendicitis at the millennium. Radiology 215:337, 2000. *[An excellent overview of pathophysiology and treatment.]*

Goede AC, et al.: Carcinoid tumor of the appendix. Br J Surg 90:1317, 2003. *[A discussion of the controversies regarding the management of these tumors.]*

Misdraji J, Graeme-Cook FM: Miscellaneous conditions of the appendix. Semin Diagn Pathol 21:151, 2004. *[A review of a variety of conditions that affect the appendix.]*

Misdraji J, Young RH: Primary epithelial neoplasms and other epithelial lesions of the appendix (excluding carcinoid tumors). Semin Diagn Pathol 21:120, 2004. *[An overview of malignant and nonmalignant tumors of the appendix.]*

Modlin IM, et al.: Current status of gastrointestinal carcinoids. Gastroenterology 128:1717, 2005. *[A comprehensive review of the pathophysiology of these tumors and their treatment.]*

Young RH: Pseudomyxoma peritonei and selected other aspects of the spread of appendiceal neoplasms. Semin Diagn Pathol 21:134, 2004. *[An excellent review of mucinous tumors of the appendix and their spread to ovaries.]*

Chapter 16

The Liver, Gallbladder, and Biliary Tract

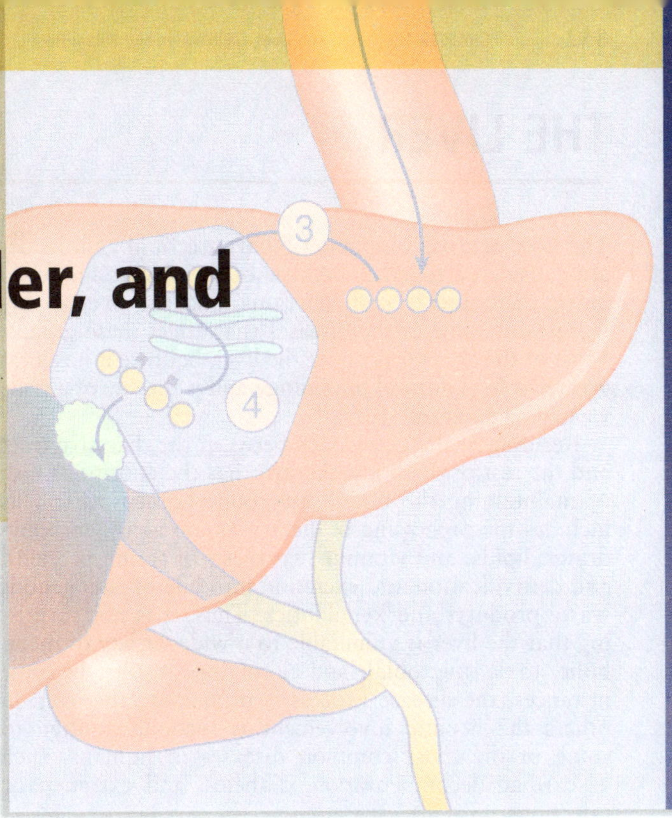

THE LIVER

The liver and its companion biliary tree and gallbladder are considered together because of their anatomic proximity, their interrelated functions, and the overlapping features of some of the diseases that affect these organs. Most of the chapter is about the liver, because it has a far greater role in normal physiology and is the site of a wide variety of diseases.

Residing at the crossroads between the digestive tract and the rest of the body, the liver has the enormous task of maintaining the body's metabolic homeostasis. This includes the processing of dietary amino acids, carbohydrates, lipids, and vitamins; synthesis of serum proteins; and detoxification and excretion into bile of endogenous waste products and xenobiotics. Thus, it is not surprising that the liver is vulnerable to a wide variety of metabolic, toxic, microbial, and circulatory insults. In some instances, the disease process is primary to the liver. In others the hepatic involvement is secondary, often to some of the most common diseases in humans, such as cardiac decompensation, diabetes, and extrahepatic infections.

The liver has enormous functional reserve, and regeneration occurs in all but the most fulminant of hepatic diseases. Surgical removal of 60% of the liver of a normal person produces minimal and transient hepatic impairment, and regeneration restores most of the liver mass within 4 to 6 weeks. In persons with massive hepatocellular necrosis that has not destroyed the hepatic reticulin framework, almost perfect restoration may occur if the individual can survive the metabolic insult of liver failure. The functional reserve and the regenerative capacity of the liver mask to some extent the clinical impact of early liver damage. However, with progression of diffuse disease or disruption of the circulation or bile flow, the consequences of deranged liver function become life-threatening.

Hepatic disorders have far-reaching consequences, given the crucial dependence of other organs on the metabolic function of the liver. Liver injury and its manifestations tend to follow characteristic morphologic and clinical patterns, regardless of cause. We first summarize the main morphologic patterns that occur in liver injury and then present a general description of the main clinical syndromes of liver disease. The remainder of the chapter describes the principal features of individual hepatic diseases.

PATTERNS OF HEPATIC INJURY

Here we describe the main patterns of morphologic liver injury and associated cellular responses. Some of these changes are localized to certain regions of the liver lobule (Fig. 16–1).

- *Degeneration and intracellular accumulation.* Moderate cell swelling caused by toxic or immunologic insults is reversible. However, more serious damage to hepatocytes may cause marked cell enlargement *(ballooning degeneration),* with irregularly clumped cytoplasm showing large, clear spaces. Substances may accumulate in viable hepatocytes, including fat, iron, copper, and retained biliary material. Accumulation of fat droplets within hepatocytes is known as *steatosis.* Multiple tiny droplets that do not displace the nucleus are known as *microvesicular steatosis* and appear in such conditions as alcoholic liver disease, Reye syndrome, and acute fatty liver of pregnancy. A single large droplet that displaces the nucleus, *macrovesicular steatosis,* may be seen in alcoholic liver disease or in the livers of obese or diabetic individuals. Retained biliary material may impart a diffuse, foamy, swollen appearance to the hepatocyte (known as feathery degeneration).

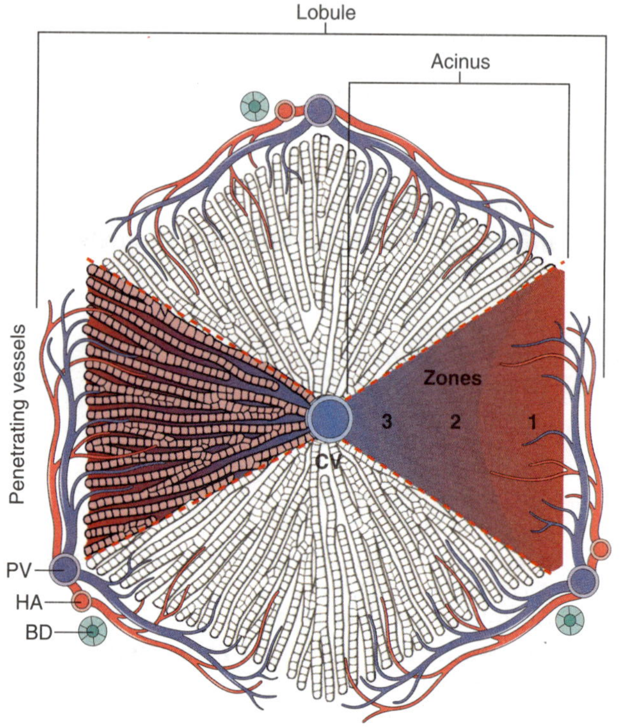

Figure 16–1

Microscopic architecture of the liver parenchyma. Both a lobule and an acinus are represented. The classic hexagonal lobule is centered around a central vein (CV), also known as terminal hepatic venule, and has portal tracts at three of its apices. The portal tracts contain branches of the portal vein (PV), hepatic artery (HA), and the bile duct (BD) system. Regions of the lobule are generally referred to as "periportal," "midzonal," and "centrilobular," according to their proximity to portal spaces and central vein. Another way of defining the architecture of the liver parenchyma is to use the blood supply as a source of reference. Using this approach, triangular acini can be recognized. Acini have at their base branches of portal vessels that penetrate the parenchyma ("penetrating vessels"). On the basis of the distance from the blood supply, the acinus is divided into zones 1 (closest to blood source), 2, and 3 (farthest from blood source).

• *Necrosis and apoptosis.* Virtually any significant insult to the liver may cause hepatocyte destruction. In coagulative necrosis, poorly stained mummified hepatocytes remain. In apoptosis, isolated hepatocytes become shrunken, pyknotic, and intensely eosinophilic (these patterns are described in Chapter 1). In the setting of ischemia and several drug and toxic reactions, hepatocyte necrosis is distributed immediately around the central vein *(centrilobular necrosis)*, extending into the midzonal area. Pure midzonal and periportal necrosis is rare. In most types of hepatic injury, a variable mixture of inflammation and hepatocyte death is encountered. Cell death may be limited to scattered cells within the hepatic parenchyma or to the interface between the periportal parenchyma and inflamed portal tracts *(interface hepatitis)*. With more severe inflammatory or toxic injury, apoptosis or necrosis of contiguous hepatocytes may span adjacent lobules in a portal-to-portal, portal-to-central, or central-to-central fashion *(bridging necrosis)*. Destruction of entire lobules *(submassive necrosis)* or most of the liver parenchyma *(massive necrosis)* is usually accompanied by hepatic failure.

• *Regeneration.* Cell death or tissue resection (such as in living-donor transplantation) triggers hepatocyte replication, to compensate for the cell or tissue loss. Hepatocyte proliferation is recognized by the presence of mitoses or by the detection of cell cycle markers by immunocytochemical staining. The cells of the canals of Hering constitute a reserve compartment of progenitor cells for hepatocytes and bile duct cells. Cells of this reserve compartment, known as *oval cells*, proliferate when hepatocytes are unable to replicate or have exhausted their replicative capacity.

• *Inflammation.* Injury to hepatocytes associated with an influx of acute or chronic inflammatory cells into the liver is termed *hepatitis*. Although hepatocyte necrosis may precede the onset of inflammation, the converse is also true. Lysis of antigen-expressing liver cells by sensitized T cells is the cause of liver damage in some forms of viral hepatitis. Inflammation may be limited to portal tracts or may spill over into the parenchyma. Foreign bodies, organisms, and a variety of drugs may incite a granulomatous reaction.

• *Fibrosis.* Fibrous tissue is formed in response to inflammation or direct toxic insult to the liver. Deposition of collagen has lasting consequences on hepatic patterns of blood flow and perfusion of hepatocytes. In the initial stages, fibrosis may develop within or around portal tracts *(portal or periportal fibrosis)* or around the central vein, or fibrous tissue may be deposited directly within the sinusoids around single or multiple hepatocytes *(pericellular fibrosis)*. With time, fibrous strands link regions of the liver (portal-to-portal, portal-to-central, central-to-central), a process called *bridging fibrosis*.

• *Cirrhosis.* With progressive parenchymal injury and fibrosis, the liver develops nodules of regenerating hepatocytes surrounded by bands of scar tissue. In this process, the normal liver architecture is destroyed, and the condition is termed cirrhosis. Depending on the size of the nodules (smaller or larger than 3 mm), cirrhosis can be classified as being micronodular or macronodular. However, this classification has little relevance for the pathogenesis or clinical course of the disease. Cirrhosis is an end-stage liver disease, and it also increases the risk of malignancy.

• *Ductular reaction.* In biliary and other forms of liver disease, the number of intrahepatic bile ducts and canals of Hering may increase. This change is known as a ductular reaction. The proliferation of biliary ductules is usually associated with fibrosis and inflammation. Ductular reaction has gained much interest recently, because some of the proliferating cells originating from the canals of Hering can function as progenitor cells for hepatocytes and bile ducts.

CLINICAL SYNDROMES

The ebb and flow of hepatic injury may be imperceptible to the individual, or hepatic function may be so impaired as to be life-threatening. The major clinical syndromes of liver disease are hepatic failure, cirrhosis, portal hypertension, and cholestasis. These conditions have characteristic clinical manifestations (Table 16–1), and a battery of laboratory tests are used to diagnose these disorders (Table 16–2). These conditions are discussed next.

Hepatic Failure

The most severe clinical consequence of liver disease is hepatic failure. It generally develops as the end point of progressive damage to the liver, either by insidious destruction of hepatocytes or by repetitive discrete waves of parenchymal damage. Less commonly, hepatic failure is the result of sudden and massive destruction of hepatic tissue. Whatever the sequence, 80% to 90% of hepatic function must be lost before hepatic failure ensues. In

Table 16–1 Clinical Consequences of Liver Disease

Characteristic Signs of Severe Hepatic Dysfunction
Jaundice and cholestasis
Hypoalbuminemia
Hyperammonemia
Hypoglycemia
Palmar erythema
Spider angiomas
Hypogonadism
Gynecomastia
Weight loss
Muscle wasting
Portal Hypertension Associated with Cirrhosis
Ascites
Splenomegaly
Esophageal varices
Hemorrhoids
Caput medusae—abdominal skin
Complications of Hepatic Failure
Coagulopathy
Hepatic encephalopathy
Hepatorenal syndrome

Table 16–2 Laboratory Evaluation of Liver Disease

Test Category	Serum Measurement*
Hepatocyte integrity	Cytosolic hepatocellular enzymes† *Serum aspartate aminotransferase* (AST) *Serum alanine aminotransferase* (ALT) Serum lactate dehydrogenase (LDH)
Biliary excretory function	Substances secreted in bile† *Serum bilirubin* *Total:* unconjugated plus conjugated *Direct:* conjugated only *Delta:* covalently linked to albumin Urine bilirubin Serum bile acids Plasma membrane enzymes† (from damage to bile canaliculus) *Serum alkaline phosphatase* Serum γ-glutamyl transpeptidase Serum 5′-nucleotidase
Hepatocyte function	Proteins secreted into the blood *Serum albumin*‡ *Prothrombin time*† (factors V, VII, X, prothrombin, fibrinogen) Hepatocyte metabolism Serum ammonia† Aminopyrine breath test (hepatic demethylation) Galactose elimination (intravenous injection)

*Most common tests are in italics.
†An elevation implicates liver disease.
‡A decrease implicates liver disease.

many cases, the balance is tipped toward decompensation by intercurrent diseases that place demands on the liver. These include systemic infections, electrolyte disturbances, stress (major surgery, heart failure), and gastrointestinal bleeding.

The alterations that cause liver failure fall into three categories:

1. *Acute liver failure with massive hepatic necrosis.* This is most often caused by *drugs* or *fulminant viral hepatitis.* Acute liver failure denotes clinical hepatic insufficiency that progresses from onset of symptoms to hepatic encephalopathy within 2 to 3 weeks. A course extending as long as 3 months is called subacute failure. *The histologic correlate of acute liver failure is massive hepatic necrosis.* It is an uncommon but life-threatening condition that often requires liver transplantation. Drug-induced acute liver failure is discussed later in this chapter.
2. *Chronic liver disease.* This is the most common route to hepatic failure and is the end point of relentless chronic liver damage ending in cirrhosis. The many causes of cirrhosis are discussed later.
3. *Hepatic dysfunction without overt necrosis.* Hepatocytes may be viable but unable to perform normal metabolic function, as in acute fatty liver of pregnancy (which can lead to acute liver failure a few days after onset), tetracycline toxicity, and Reye syndrome (a rare syndrome of fatty liver and encephalopathy in children, associated with aspirin intake and virus infection; discussed later).

Clinical Features. Regardless of cause, the clinical signs of hepatic failure occurring in individuals with chronic liver disease are much the same. *Jaundice* is an almost invariable finding. Impaired hepatic synthesis and secretion of albumin leads to *hypoalbuminemia,* which predisposes to peripheral edema. *Hyperammonemia* is attributable to defective hepatic urea cycle function. On a longer term basis, impaired estrogen metabolism and consequent hyperestrogenemia are the putative causes of *palmar erythema* (a reflection of local vasodilatation) and *spider angiomas* of the skin. Each angioma is a central, pulsating, dilated arteriole from which small vessels radiate. In the male, hyperestrogenemia also leads to *hypogonadism* and *gynecomastia.* Acute liver failure may present as jaundice or encephalopathy, but notably absent on physical examination are stigmata of chronic liver disease (e.g., gynecomastia, spider angiomas).

Hepatic failure is life-threatening for several reasons. The accumulation of toxic metabolites may have widespread effects. With severely impaired liver function, patients are highly susceptible to failure of multiple organ systems. Thus, respiratory failure with pneumonia and sepsis combines with renal failure to claim the lives of many individuals with hepatic failure. A *coagulopathy* develops, attributable to impaired hepatic synthesis of blood clotting factors. The resultant bleeding tendency may lead to massive gastrointestinal hemorrhage as well as bleeding elsewhere. Intestinal absorption of blood places a metabolic load on the liver that worsens the severity of hepatic failure. The outlook of full-blown hepatic failure is particularly grave for persons with chronic liver disease. A rapid downhill course is usual, with death occurring within weeks to a few months in about 80% of cases. About 40% of individuals with acute liver failure may recover spontaneously. The others either die without transplantation (~30%) or receive a liver transplant.

Two particular complications merit separate consideration, because they herald the most grave stages of hepatic failure: hepatic encephalopathy and hepatorenal syndrome.

Hepatic Encephalopathy

Hepatic encephalopathy is a feared complication of acute and chronic liver failure. Patients show a spectrum of disturbances in brain function, ranging from subtle behavioral abnormalities to marked confusion and stupor, to deep coma and death. These changes may progress over hours or days as, for example, in fulminant hepatic failure or, more insidiously, in someone with marginal hepatic function from chronic liver disease. Associated fluctuating neurologic signs include rigidity, hyper-reflexia, nonspecific electroencephalographic changes, and, rarely, seizures. Particularly characteristic is *asterixis* (also called flapping tremor), which is a pattern of nonrhythmic, rapid extension-flexion movements of the head and extremities, best seen when the arms are held in extension with dorsiflexed wrists.

In most instances there are only minor morphologic changes in the brain, such as edema and an astrocytic reaction. Two physiologic conditions seem to be important in the genesis of this disorder: (1) severe loss of hepatocellular function and (2) shunting of blood from portal to systemic circulation around the chronically diseased liver. The net result is exposure of the brain to an altered metabolic milieu. In the acute setting, an elevation in blood ammonia, which impairs neuronal function and promotes generalized brain edema, seems to be key. In the chronic setting, deranged neurotransmission arises from alterations in amino acid metabolism in the brain.

Hepatorenal Syndrome

The hepatorenal syndrome, which appears in individuals with severe liver disease, consists of the development of renal failure without primary abnormalities of the kidneys themselves. Excluded by this definition are concomitant damage to both liver and kidney, as may occur with exposure to carbon tetrachloride and certain mycotoxins, and the copper toxicity of Wilson disease. Also excluded are instances of advanced hepatic failure in which circulatory collapse leads to acute tubular necrosis and renal failure. Kidney function promptly improves if hepatic failure is reversed. Although the exact cause is unknown, evidence points to splanchnic vasodilatation and systemic vasoconstriction, leading to severe reduction of renal blood flow, particularly to the cortex. Onset of this syndrome is typically heralded by a drop in urine output, associated with rising blood urea nitrogen and creatinine values. *The ability to concentrate urine is retained, producing a hyperosmolar urine devoid of proteins and abnormal sediment that is surprisingly low in sodium (unlike renal tubular necrosis).* The renal failure may hasten death in the patient with acute fulminant or advanced chronic hepatic disease. Alternatively, borderline renal insufficiency (serum creatinine of 2–3 mg/dL) may persist for weeks to months, as in cirrhotic patients whose ascites is refractory to diuretic therapy.

Cirrhosis

Cirrhosis is among the top 10 causes of death in the Western world. Its major causes include alcohol abuse, chronic infections, autoimmune hepatitis, biliary disease, and iron overload. Cirrhosis is defined as a *diffuse process characterized by fibrosis and the conversion of normal liver architecture into structurally abnormal nodules.* Its three main characteristics are:

- *Bridging fibrous septa* in the form of delicate bands or broad scars around multiple adjacent lobules. Longstanding fibrosis is generally irreversible, although regression has been reported to occur in selected instances.
- *Parenchymal nodules,* varying from very small (<3 mm in diameter, micronodules) to large (several centimeters in diameter, macronodules), which are encircled by fibrotic bands. The nodules generally contain proliferating hepatocytes, although regeneration is not a required feature for the diagnosis of cirrhosis.
- *Disruption of the architecture of the entire liver.* The parenchymal cell injury and fibrosis are diffuse, extending throughout the liver; focal injury with scarring does not constitute cirrhosis.

There is no satisfactory classification of cirrhosis save for specification of the presumed underlying etiology. The most common causes of cirrhosis are chronic alcoholism and chronic hepatitis B and C, followed by biliary diseases and hemochromatosis. After all the known causes have been excluded, about 10% of cases remain, referred to as cryptogenic cirrhosis. The magnitude of the cryptogenic cirrhosis "wastebasket" speaks to the difficulty in establishing an etiologic diagnosis once cirrhosis is well established.

Pathogenesis. The major mechanisms that combine to create cirrhosis are hepatocellular death, regeneration, progressive fibrosis, and vascular changes. The many causes of hepatocellular destruction are discussed elsewhere in this chapter and include most frequently toxins and viruses. The development of cirrhosis requires that cell death occur over long periods of time and be accompanied by fibrosis. As already mentioned, regeneration is a normal compensatory response to cell death. Fibrosis is a wound-healing reaction that progresses to scar formation when the injury involves not only the parenchyma but also the supporting connective tissue. In the normal liver, extracellular matrix (ECM) consisting of interstitial collagens (fibril-forming collagens types I, III, V, and XI) is present only in the liver capsule, in portal tracts, and around central veins. The liver has no true basement membrane; instead, a delicate framework containing type IV collagen and other proteins lies in the space between sinusoidal endothelial cells and hepatocytes (the space of Disse). By contrast, in cirrhosis, types I and III collagen and other ECM components are deposited in the space of Disse (Fig. 16–2). In advanced fibrosis and cirrhosis, fibrous bands separate nodules of hepatocytes throughout the liver. Vascular changes consisting of the loss of sinusoidal endothelial cell fenestrations and the development of portal vein–hepatic vein and hepatic artery–portal vein vascular shunts contribute to defects in liver function. Collagen deposition converts sinusoids with fenestrated endothelial channels that allow free exchange of solutes between plasma and hepatocytes to higher pressure, fast-flowing vascular channels without such solute exchange. In particular, the movement of proteins (e.g., albumin, clotting factors, lipoproteins) between hepatocytes and the plasma is markedly impaired. These functional changes are aggravated by the loss of microvilli from the hepatocyte surface, which diminishes the transport capacity of the cell.

The major source of excess collagen in cirrhosis are the perisinusoidal stellate cells (formerly known as Ito cells or fat-storing cells), which lie in the space of Disse.

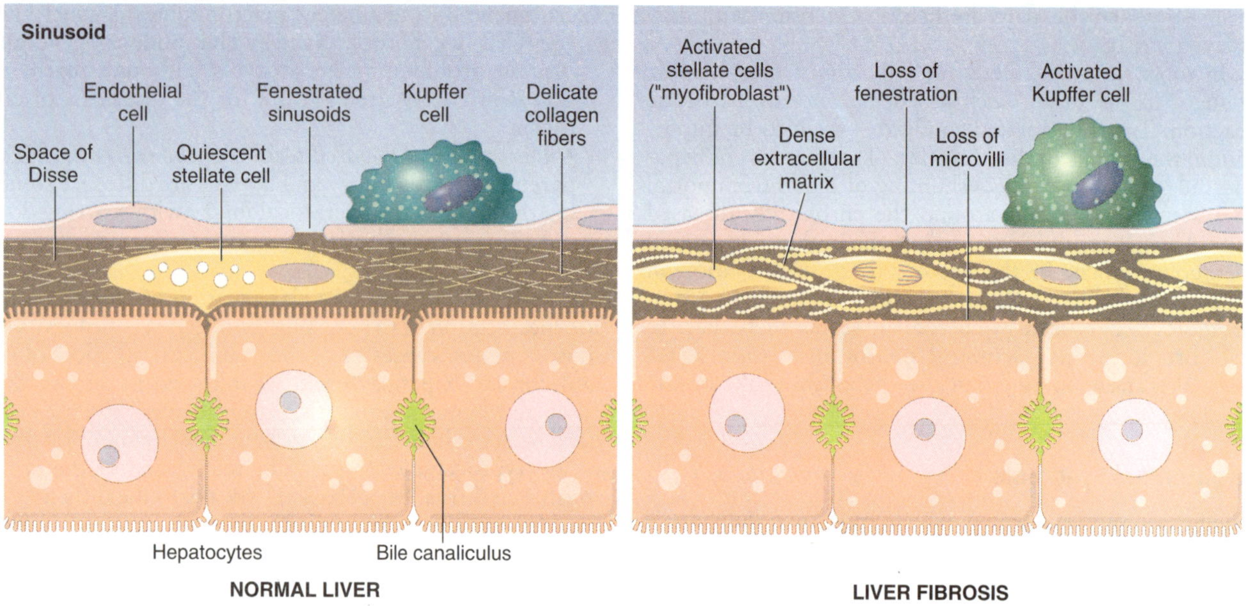

Figure 16–2

Liver fibrosis. In the normal liver, the perisinusoidal space (space of Disse) contains a delicate framework of extracellular matrix components. In liver fibrosis, stellate cells are activated to produce a dense layer of matrix material that is deposited in the perisinusoidal space. Collagen deposition blocks the endothelial fenestrations and prevents the free exchange of materials from the blood. Kupffer cells are also activated and produce cytokines that are involved in fibrosis. Note that this illustration is not to scale; the space of Disse is actually much narrower than shown.

Although they normally function as storage cells for vitamin A and fat, during the development of fibrosis they become activated, and transform into myofibroblast-like cells, which express smooth muscle α-actin and glial fibrillary acidic protein. The stimuli for the activation of stellate cells and production of collagen are believed to include reactive oxygen species (ROS), growth factors, and cytokines such as tumor necrosis factor (TNF), interleukin-1 (IL-1), and lymphotoxins, which can be produced by damaged hepatocytes or by stimulated Kupffer cells and sinusoidal endothelial cells. Activated stellate cells produce growth factors, cytokines, and chemokines that cause their further proliferation and collagen synthesis. Transforming growth factor β is the main fibrogenic agent for stellate cells. At least in its initial stages, fibrosis is a dynamic process that involves the synthesis and deposition of ECM components, activation of metalloproteinases and also of tissue inhibitors of metalloproteinases.

Clinical Features. All forms of cirrhosis may be clinically silent. When symptomatic they lead to nonspecific manifestations: anorexia, weight loss, weakness, and, in advanced disease, frank debilitation. Progression or improvement in cirrhosis depends to a large extent on the activity of the disease responsible for the cirrhosis. Incipient or overt hepatic failure may develop, usually precipitated by imposition of a metabolic load on the liver, as from systemic infection or a gastrointestinal hemorrhage. The ultimate mechanism of death in most individuals with cirrhosis is (1) progressive liver failure, (2) a complication related to portal hypertension, or (3) the development of hepatocellular carcinoma.

SUMMARY

Cirrhosis

- The three main characteristics of cirrhosis are (1) bridging fibrous septa, (2) parenchymal nodules containing replicating hepatocytes, and (3) disruption of the architecture of the entire liver.
- It is an end-stage liver disease that may have multiple causes. The most frequent are chronic hepatitis B and C and chronic alcoholism. Less frequent causes are autoimmune and biliary diseases and metabolic conditions such as hemochromatosis.
- The morphologic features of advanced cirrhosis are similar, regardless of the cause of the disease.
- Nonalcoholic fatty liver disease is a newly recognized cause of cirrhosis.
- The main complications of cirrhosis are related to decreased liver function, portal hypertension, and increased risk of hepatocellular carcinoma.

Portal Hypertension

Increased resistance to portal blood flow may develop from prehepatic, intrahepatic, and posthepatic causes (described later). *The dominant intrahepatic cause is cirrhosis, accounting for most cases of portal hypertension.* Far less frequent are schistosomiasis, massive fatty change, diffuse granulomatous diseases such as sarcoidosis and miliary tuberculosis, and diseases affecting the portal microcirculation, exemplified by nodular regenerative hyperplasia (discussed later).

Portal hypertension in cirrhosis results from increased resistance to portal flow at the level of the sinusoids and compression of central veins by perivenular fibrosis and expanded parenchymal nodules. Anastomoses between the arterial and portal systems in the fibrous bands also contribute to portal hypertension by imposing arterial pressure on the normally low-pressure portal venous system. The four major clinical consequences are (1) ascites, (2) the formation of portosystemic venous shunts, (3) congestive splenomegaly, and (4) hepatic encephalopathy (discussed earlier). The manifestations of portal hypertension in the setting of cirrhosis are described next (Fig. 16–3).

Ascites

Ascites refers to the collection of excess fluid in the peritoneal cavity. It usually becomes clinically detectable when at least 500 mL have accumulated, but many liters may collect and cause massive abdominal distention. It is generally a serous fluid having as much as 3 gm/dL of protein (largely albumin) as well as the same concentrations of solutes such as glucose, sodium, and potassium as in the blood. The fluid may contain a scant number of mesothelial cells and mononuclear leukocytes. Influx of neutrophils suggests secondary infection, whereas red cells point to possible disseminated intra-abdominal cancer. With long-standing ascites, seepage of peritoneal fluid through transdiaphragmatic lymphatics may produce hydrothorax, more often on the right side.

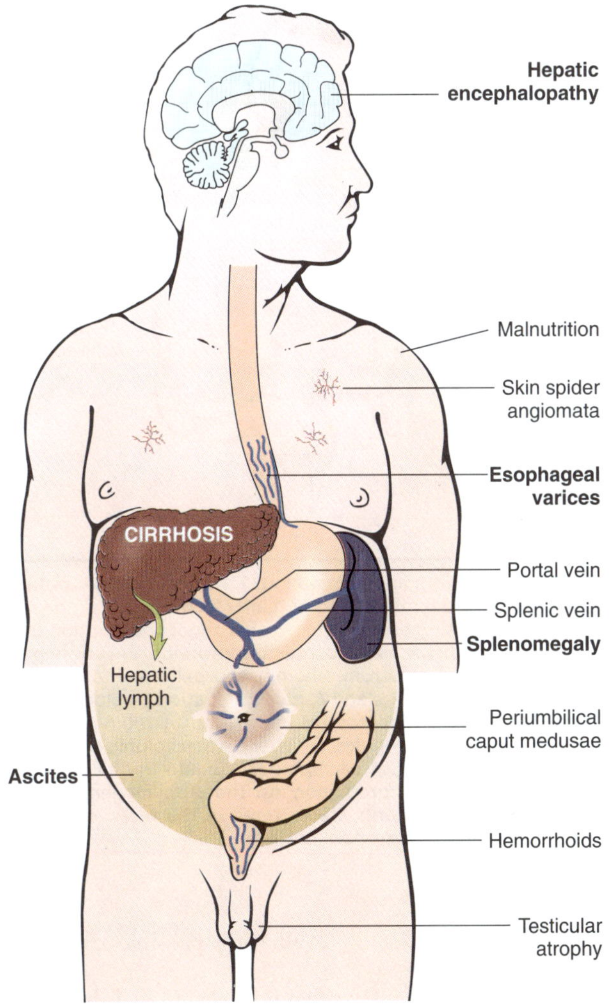

Figure 16–3

Some clinical consequences of portal hypertension in the setting of cirrhosis. The most important manifestations are in shown in **boldface** type.

The pathogenesis of ascites is complex, involving one or more of the following mechanisms:

- *Sinusoidal hypertension,* alters Starling forces and drives fluid into the space of Disse, which is then removed by hepatic lymphatics; this movement of fluid is also promoted by hypoalbuminemia.
- *Leakage of hepatic lymph* into the peritoneal cavity: normal thoracic duct lymph flow approximates 800 to 1000 mL/day. With cirrhosis, hepatic lymphatic flow may approach 20 L/day, exceeding thoracic duct capacity. Hepatic lymph is rich in proteins and low in triglycerides, as reflected in the protein-rich ascitic fluid.
- *Renal retention of sodium and water* due to secondary hyperaldosteronism (Chapter 4), despite a total body sodium value greater than normal.

Portosystemic Shunt

With the rise in portal venous pressure, bypasses develop wherever the systemic and portal circulations share capillary beds. Principal sites are veins around and within the rectum (manifest as hemorrhoids), the cardioesophageal junction (producing esophagogastric varices), the retroperitoneum, and the falciform ligament of the liver (involving periumbilical and abdominal wall collaterals). Although hemorrhoidal bleeding may occur, it is rarely massive or life threatening. Much more important are the *esophagogastric varices* that appear in about 65% of those with advanced cirrhosis of the liver and cause massive hematemesis and death in about half (Chapter 15). Abdominal wall collaterals appear as dilated subcutaneous veins extending outward from the umbilicus *(caput medusae)* and constitute an important clinical hallmark of portal hypertension.

Splenomegaly

Long-standing congestion may cause congestive splenomegaly. The degree of enlargement varies widely (usually ≤1000 gm) and is not necessarily correlated with other features of portal hypertension. Massive splenomegaly may secondarily induce a variety of hematologic abnormalities attributable to hypersplenism (Chapter 12).

Jaundice and Cholestasis

Jaundice, a common manifestation of liver disease, results from the retention of bile. Hepatic bile formation serves two major functions. Bile constitutes the primary pathway for the elimination of bilirubin, excess cholesterol, and xenobiotics that are insufficiently water soluble to be excreted into urine. Second, secreted bile salts and phospholipid molecules promote emulsification of dietary fat in the lumen of the gut. Because bile formation is one of the most sophisticated functions of the liver, it is also one of the most readily disrupted. Thus, *jaundice,* a yellow discoloration of skin and sclerae *(icterus),* occurs when systemic retention of bilirubin leads to elevated serum levels above 2.0 mg/dL (the normal in the adult is <1.2 mg/dL). *Cholestasis* is defined as systemic retention of not only bilirubin but also other solutes eliminated in bile (particularly bile salts and cholesterol).

Bilirubin and Bile Acids. Bilirubin is the end product of heme degradation (Fig. 16–4). Most of the daily production (0.2–0.3 gm) is derived from breakdown of senescent erythrocytes, with the remainder derived primarily from the turnover of hepatic hemoproteins and from premature destruction of newly formed erythrocytes in the bone marrow. The latter pathway is important in hematologic disorders associated with excessive intramedullary hemolysis of defective erythrocytes (ineffective erythropoiesis; Chapter 12). Whatever the source, heme oxygenase oxidizes heme to biliverdin, which is then reduced to bilirubin by biliverdin reductase. Bilirubin thus formed outside the liver in cells of the mononuclear phagocyte system (including the spleen) is released and bound to serum albumin. Hepatocellular processing of bilirubin involves (1) carrier-mediated uptake at the sinusoidal membrane, (2) cytosolic protein binding and delivery to the endoplasmic reticulum, (3) conjugation with one or two molecules of glucuronic acid by bilirubin uridine diphosphate-glucuronosyltransferase, and (4) excretion of the water-soluble, nontoxic bilirubin glucuronides into bile. Most bilirubin glucuronides are deconjugated by gut bacterial β-glucuronidases and degraded to colorless urobilinogens. The urobilinogens and the residue of intact pigment are largely excreted in feces. Approximately 20% of the urobilinogens are reabsorbed in the ileum and colon, returned to the liver, and promptly re-excreted into bile. Conjugated and unconjugated bile acids are also reabsorbed in the ileum and returned to the liver by *enterohepatic circulation.*

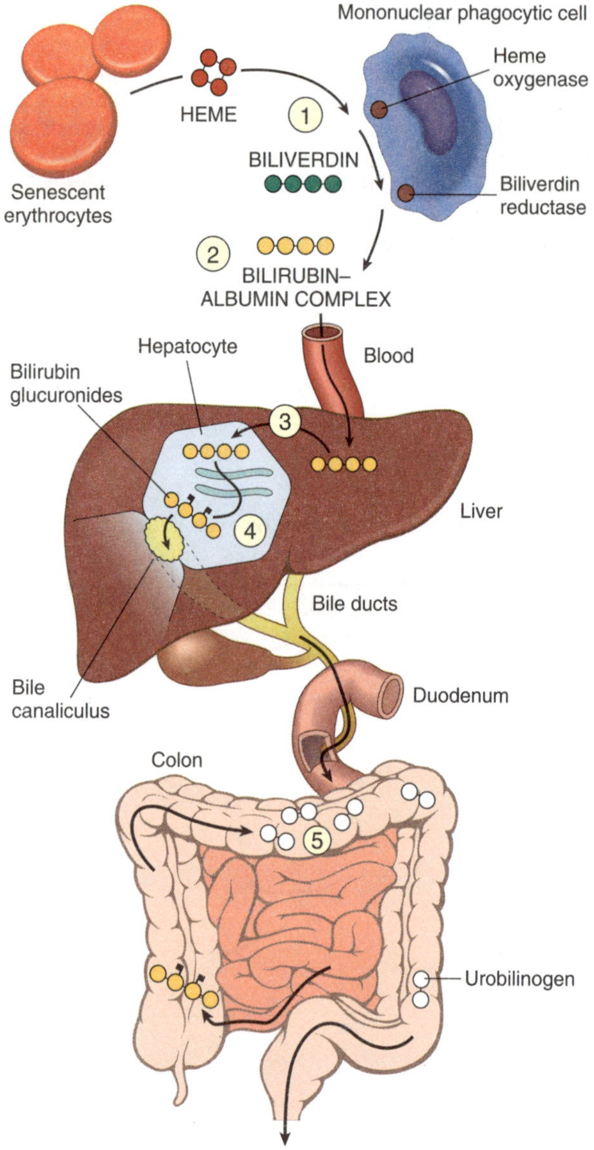

Figure 16–4

Bilirubin metabolism and elimination. **1,** Normal bilirubin production (0.2–0.3 gm/day) is derived primarily from the breakdown of senescent circulating erythrocytes, with a minor contribution from degradation of tissue heme-containing proteins. **2,** Extrahepatic bilirubin is bound to serum albumin and delivered to the liver. **3,** Hepatocellular uptake, and **4,** glucuronidation by glucuronosyltransferase in the hepatocytes generates bilirubin monoglucuronides and diglucuronides, which are water soluble and readily excreted into bile. **5,** Gut bacteria deconjugate the bilirubin and degrade it to colorless urobilinogens. The urobilinogens and the residue of intact pigments are excreted in the feces, with some reabsorption and re-excretion into bile.

Pathogenesis and Clinical Features. In the normal adult the rate of systemic bilirubin production is equal to the rates of hepatic uptake, conjugation, and biliary excretion. Jaundice occurs (bilirubin levels may reach 30–40 mg/dL in severe disease) when the equilibrium between bilirubin production and clearance is disturbed by one or more of the following mechanisms (Table 16–3): (1) excessive production of bilirubin, (2) reduced hepatic uptake, (3) impaired conjugation, (4) decreased hepatocellular excretion, and (5) impaired bile flow (both intrahepatic and extrahepatic). The first three mechanisms produce unconjugated hyperbilirubinemia, and the latter two produce predominantly conjugated hyperbilirubinemia. More than one mechanism may operate to produce jaundice, especially in hepatitis, which may produce unconjugated and conjugated hyperbilirubinemia. In general, however, one mechanism predominates, so that knowledge of the predominant form of plasma bilirubin is of value in evaluating possible causes of hyperbilirubinemia.

Of the various causes of jaundice listed in Table 16–3, the most common are hepatitis, obstruction to the flow of bile (discussed later in this chapter), and hemolytic anemia (Chapter 12). Because the hepatic machinery for conjugating and excreting bilirubin does not fully mature

Table 16–3 Main Causes of Jaundice

Predominantly Unconjugated Hyperbilirubinemia
Excess production of bilirubin
Hemolytic anemias
Resorption of blood from internal hemorrhage (e.g., alimentary tract bleeding, hematomas)
Ineffective erythropoiesis syndromes (e.g., pernicious anemia, thalassemia)
Reduced hepatic uptake
Drug interference with membrane carrier systems
Diffuse hepatocellular disease (e.g., viral or drug-induced hepatitis, cirrhosis)
Impaired bilirubin conjugation
Physiologic jaundice of the newborn
Predominantly Conjugated Hyperbilirubinemia
Decreased hepatocellular excretion
Deficiency in canalicular membrane transporters
Drug-induced canalicular membrane dysfunction (e.g., oral contraceptives, cycloporine)
Hepatocellular damage or toxicity (e.g., viral or drug-induced hepatitis, total parenteral nutrition, systemic infection)
Impaired intra- or extra-hepatic bile flow
Inflammatory destruction of intrahepatic bile ducts (e.g., primary biliary cirrhosis, primary sclerosing cholangitis, graft-versus-host disease, liver transplantation)

until about 2 weeks of age, almost every newborn develops transient and mild unconjugated hyperbilirubinemia, termed *neonatal jaundice* or physiologic jaundice of the newborn.

Jaundice may also result from inborn errors of metabolisms, including:

- *Gilbert syndrome* is a relatively common, benign, somewhat heterogeneous inherited condition presenting as mild, fluctuating unconjugated hyperbilirubinemia. The primary cause is decreased hepatic levels of glucuronosyltransferase. Although this is attributed to a mutation of the responsible gene, additional polymorphisms may play a role in the variable expression of this disorder. Affecting up to 7% of the population, the hyperbilirubinemia may go undiscovered for years and *does not have associated morbidity.*
- *Dubin-Johnson syndrome* results from an autosomal recessive defect in the transport protein responsible for hepatocellular excretion of bilirubin glucuronides across the canalicular membrane. These patients exhibit conjugated hyperbilirubinemia. Other than having a darkly pigmented liver (from polymerized epinephrine metabolites, not bilirubin) and hepatomegaly, patients are otherwise without functional problems.

Cholestasis, which results from impaired bile flow due to hepatocellular dysfunction or intrahepatic or extrahepatic biliary obstruction, may also present as jaundice. However, sometimes *pruritus* is the presenting symptom, presumably related to the elevation in plasma bile acids and their deposition in peripheral tissues, particularly skin. *Skin xanthomas* (focal accumulations of cholesterol) sometimes appear, the result of hyperlipidemia and impaired excretion of cholesterol. A *characteristic laboratory finding is elevated serum alkaline phosphatase,* an enzyme present in bile duct epithelium and in the canalicular membrane of hepatocytes. An isozyme is normally present in many other tissues such as bone, and so the increased levels must be verified as being hepatic in origin. Other manifestations of reduced bile flow relate to intestinal malabsorption, including inadequate absorption of the fat-soluble vitamins A, D, and K.

Extrahepatic biliary obstruction is frequently amenable to surgical alleviation. By contrast, cholestasis caused by diseases of the intrahepatic biliary tree or hepatocellular secretory failure (collectively termed *intrahepatic cholestasis*) cannot be benefited by surgery (short of transplantation), and the patient's condition may be worsened by an operative procedure. Thus, *there is some urgency in making a correct diagnosis of the cause of jaundice and cholestasis.*

SUMMARY

Jaundice and Cholestasis

- Jaundice occurs when retention of bilirubin leads to serum levels above 2.0 mg/dL.
- Hepatitis and intra- or extra-hepatic obstruction of bile flow are the most common causes of jaundice involving the accumulation of conjugated bilirubin.
- Hemolytic anemias are the most common causes of jaundice involving the accumulation of unconjugated bilirubin.
- Cholestasis is the impairment of bile flow resulting in the retention of bilirubin, bile acids, and cholesterol.
- Serum alkaline phosphatase is usually elevated in cholestatic conditions.

INFECTIOUS AND INFLAMMATORY DISORDERS

Chronic inflammatory disorders of the liver dominate the clinical practice of hepatology. Virtually any insult to the liver can kill hepatocytes and recruit inflammatory cells. *However, the foremost primary liver infection is viral hepatitis,* which will be discussed first. Less common is a condition called *autoimmune hepatitis,* which we will discuss later. The liver is almost always involved in blood-borne infections, whether systemic or arising within the abdomen. Those in which the hepatic lesion may be prominent include miliary tuberculosis, malaria, the salmonelloses, candidiasis, and amebiasis, which are discussed in the relevant chapters throughout this book. Only pyogenic liver abscesses will be discussed in this section, and they are presented last.

Systemic viral infections that can involve the liver include (1) infectious mononucleosis (Epstein-Barr virus), which may cause a mild hepatitis during the acute phase; (2) cytomegalovirus or herpesvirus infections, particularly in the newborn or immunosuppressed; and (3) yellow fever, which has been a major and serious cause of hepatitis in tropical countries. Infrequently, in children and the immunosuppressed, the liver is affected in the course of rubella, adenovirus, or enterovirus infections. However, unless otherwise specified, *the term viral hepatitis is reserved for infection of the liver caused by a small group of viruses having a particular affinity for the liver.* Because these viruses may cause similar patterns of disease, the histologic changes and clinical course of viral hepatitis are described together, after a presentation of the specific forms of viral hepatitis.

Viral Hepatitis

The etiologic agents of viral hepatitis (as defined above) are hepatitis viruses A (HAV), B (HBV), C (HCV), D (HDV), and E (HEV). Hepatitis G virus (HGV) is not pathogenic and will not be considered. Table 16–4 summarizes some of the features of the hepatitis viruses.

Hepatitis A Virus (HAV)

Hepatitis A (known for many years as "infectious hepatitis") is a *benign, self-limited disease* with an incubation period of 15 to 50 days (average 28 days). It is an "old" disease, having been described as a contagious jaundice in antiquity (a recommended remedy was drinking of donkey urine, according to the Babylonian Talmud), and was a major problem for the military during World War II. *HAV does not cause chronic hepatitis or a carrier state and only rarely causes fulminant hepatitis. Case fatalities from HAV occur at a very low rate, about 0.1%, and seem to be more likely to occur when patients have preexisting liver disease from other causes such as HBV or alcohol toxicity.* Nevertheless, HAV has the largest potential among the hepatitis viruses to cause epidemics. HAV occurs throughout the world and is endemic in countries with poor hygiene and sanitation, so that most natives of such countries have detectable antibodies to HAV by the age of 10 years. Clinical disease tends to be mild or asymptomatic (in children) and rare after childhood. Unfortunately, HAV infection in adults may create considerably greater morbidity than the innocuous childhood infection.

HAV is spread by ingestion of contaminated water and foods and is shed in the stool for 2 to 3 weeks before and 1 week after the onset of jaundice. HAV is not shed in any significant quantities in saliva, urine, or semen. Close personal contact with an infected individual during the period of fecal shedding, with fecal-oral contamination, accounts for most cases and explains the outbreaks in institutional settings such as schools and nurseries. *Because HAV viremia is transient, blood-borne transmission of HAV occurs only rarely; therefore, donated blood is not specifically screened for this virus.* Waterborne epidemics may occur in developing countries where people live in overcrowded, unsanitary conditions; the incidence of infectious particles in the water supply may exceed 35%, despite routine indicators of fecal pollution falling within acceptable limits. Among developed countries, sporadic infections may be contracted by the consumption of raw or steamed shellfish (oysters, mussels, clams), which concentrate the virus from seawater contaminated with human sewage. Ingestion of raw green onions contaminated with HAV caused outbreaks of the disease in the United States in 2003, involving more than 600 persons.

HAV is a small, nonenveloped, single-stranded RNA picornavirus. It reaches the liver from the intestinal tract

Table 16–4 The Hepatitis Viruses

Virus	Hepatitis A	Hepatitis B	Hepatitis C	Hepatitis D	Hepatitis E
Type of virus	ssRNA	partially dsDNA	ssRNA	Circular defective ssRNA	ssRNA
Viral family	Hepatovirus; related to picornavirus	Hepadnavirus	Flaviridae	Subviral particle in Deltaviridae family	Calicivirus
Route of transmission	Fecal-oral (contaminated food or water)	Parenteral, sexual contact, perinatal	Parenteral; intranasal cocaine use is a risk factor	Parenteral	Fecal-oral
Mean incubation period	2–4 weeks	1–4 months	7–8 weeks	Same as HBV	4–5 weeks
Frequency of chronic liver disease	Never	10%	~80%	5% (coinfection); ≤70% for superinfection	Never
Diagnosis	Detection of serum IgM antibodies	Detection of HBsAg or antibody to HBcAg	PCR for HCV RNA; 3rd-generation ELISA for antibody detection	Detection of IgM and IgG antibodies; HDV RNA serum; HDAg in liver	PCR for HEV RNA; detection of serum IgM and IgG antibodies

dsDNA, double-stranded DNA; ELISA, enzyme-linked immunosorbent assay; HBcAg, hepatitis B core antigen; HBsAg, hepatitis B surface antigen; HBV, hepatitis B virus; HCV, hepatitis C virus; HDAg, hepatitis D antigen; HDV, hepatitis D virus; HEV, hepatitis E virus; IV, intravenous; PCR, polymerase chain reaction; ssRNA, single stranded RNA.

From Washington K: Inflammatory and infectious diseases of the liver. In Iacobuzio-Donahue CA, Montgomery EA (eds): Gastrointestinal and Liver Pathology. Philadelphia, Churchill Livingstone; 2005.

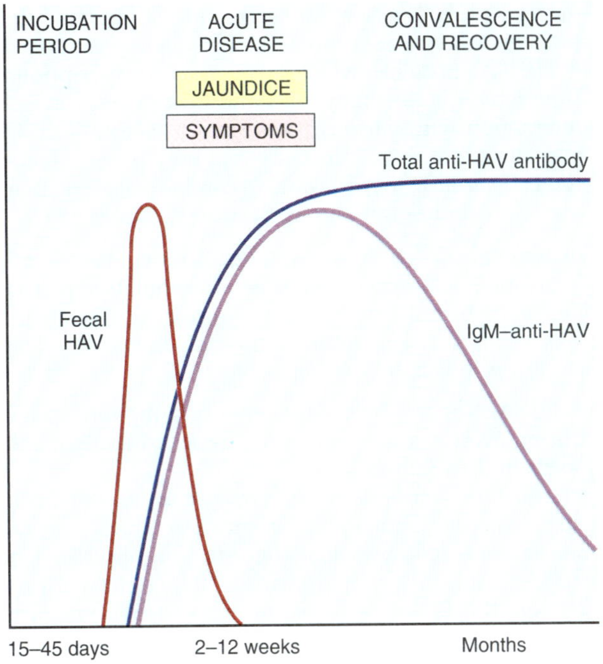

Figure 16–5

The sequence of serologic markers in acute hepatitis A infection. HAV, hepatitis A virus.

after ingestion, replicates in hepatocytes, and is shed in the bile and feces. The virus itself does not seem to be toxic to hepatocytes, and hence the liver injury seems to result from T cell–mediated damage of infected hepatocytes. As depicted in Figure 16–5, immunoglobulin M (IgM) antibodies against HAV appear in blood at the onset of symptoms. Detection of anti-HAV IgM antibody is the best diagnostic marker for the disease; IgG antibody persists beyond convalescence and is the primary defense against reinfection. However, there are no routinely available tests for IgG anti-HAV, and therefore the presence of this type of antibody is inferred from the difference between total and IgM anti-HAV. In the United States, the prevalence of seropositivity increases gradually with age, reaching 50% by age 50 years. Prevention and management of hepatitis A include (1) hygienic measures focused on the disposal of human wastes and personal hygiene, (2) passive immunization with immune serum globulin for individuals exposed to the virus or those traveling to high-exposure areas, and (3) pre-exposure prophylaxis using a virus-inactivated vaccine.

Hepatitis B Virus (HBV)

HBV can produce (1) acute hepatitis with recovery and clearance of the virus, (2) nonprogressive chronic hepatitis, (3) progressive chronic disease ending in cirrhosis, (4) fulminant hepatitis with massive liver necrosis, and (5) an asymptomatic carrier state. HBV-induced chronic liver disease is an important precursor for the development of hepatocellular carcinoma. Figure 16–6 depicts the approximate frequencies of these outcomes.

Globally, liver disease caused by HBV is an enormous problem, with an estimated worldwide carrier rate of approximately 400 million. It is estimated that HBV will infect more than 2 billion of the individuals alive today at some point in their lives. About 80% of all chronic carriers live in Asia and the Western Pacific rim, where prevalence of chronic hepatitis B is more than 10%. In the United States there are approximately 185,000 new infections per year. HBV remains in blood during the last stages of a prolonged incubation period (4–26 weeks) and during active episodes of acute and chronic hepatitis. It is also present in all physiologic and pathologic body fluids, with the exception of stool. HBV is a hardy virus and can withstand extremes of temperature and humidity. Thus, whereas blood and body fluids are the primary

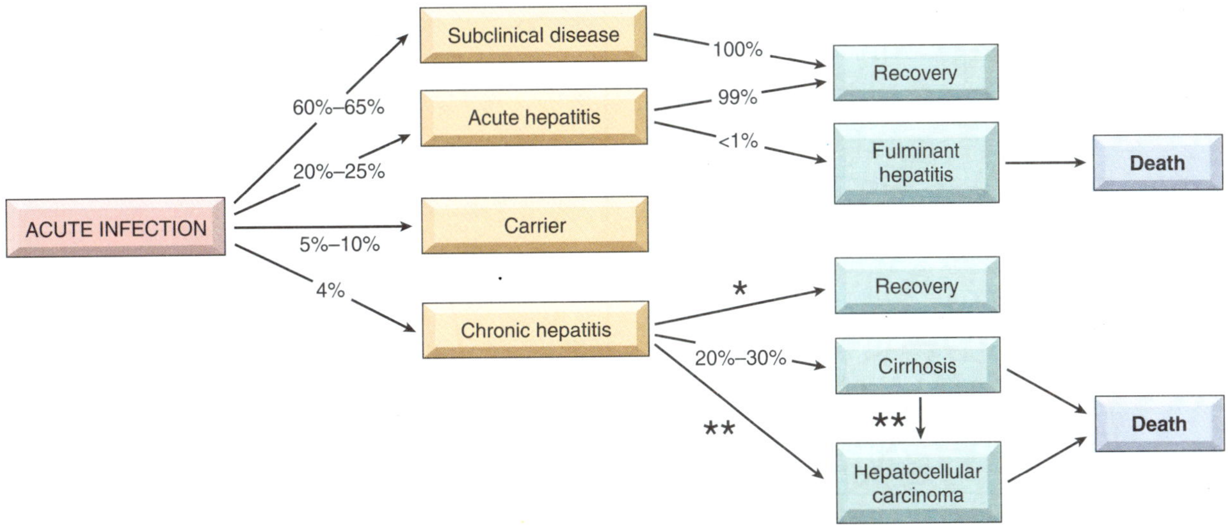

Figure 16–6

The potential outcomes of hepatitis B infection in adults, with their approximate annual frequencies in the United States.
*Estimated rate of recovery from chronic hepatitis is 0.5–1% per year; **The risk of hepatocellular carcinoma is 0.02% per year for chronic hepatitis B and 2.5% per year when cirrhosis has developed.

vehicles of transmission, virus may also be spread by contact with body secretions such as semen, saliva, sweat, tears, breast milk, and pathologic effusions. In endemic regions, vertical transmission from mother to child during birth constitutes the main mode of transmission. In areas of low prevalence, horizontal transmission via transfusion, blood products, dialysis, needle-stick accidents among health care workers, intravenous drug abuse, and sexual transmission (homosexual or heterosexual) constitute the primary mechanisms for HBV infection. In one-third of patients the source of infection is unknown. HBV infection in adults is mostly cleared, but vertical transmission produces a high rate of chronic infection.

HBV is a member of the Hepadnaviridae, a group of DNA-containing viruses that cause hepatitis in many animal species. HBV replication does not involve the integration of the virus in the DNA of the host cell, but integrated HBV is frequently found in cells. The integrated viruses generally have large deletions and rearrangements and usually become inactive. The genome of HBV is a partially double-stranded circular DNA molecule of 3200 nucleotides that encodes:

- The pre-core/core region of a nucleocapsid "core" protein (*HBcAg,* hepatitis B core antigen) and a pre-core protein designated *HBeAg* (hepatitis B "e" antigen). HBcAg is retained in the infected hepatocyte; HBeAg is secreted into blood and is essential for the establishment of persistent infection.
- Envelope glycoprotein (*HBsAg,* hepatitis B surface antigen), which may be produced and secreted into the blood in massive amounts. Blood HBsAg is immunogenic and can be visualized as spheres or tubules.
- A *DNA polymerase* with reverse transcriptase activity (genomic replication takes place through an intermediate RNA known as pregenomic RNA). In this process mutant viral genomes are frequently generated.
- *HBV-X* protein, which acts as a transcriptional transactivator for many viral and host genes, through interaction with various transcription factors. HBV-X is required for viral infectivity and may have a role in the causation of hepatocellular carcinoma by regulating p53 degradation and expression (Chapter 6).

After exposure to the virus, there is a long 45- to 160-day, (average 120 days) asymptomatic incubation period, which may be followed by acute disease lasting many weeks to months. The natural course of acute disease can be followed by serum markers (Fig. 16–7).

- HBsAg appears before the onset of symptoms, peaks during overt disease, and then declines to undetectable levels in 3 to 6 months.
- Anti-HBs antibody does not rise until the acute disease is over and is usually not detectable for a few weeks to several months after the disappearance of HBsAg. Anti-HBs may persist for life, conferring protection; this is the basis for current vaccination strategies using noninfectious HBsAg.
- HBeAg, HBV-DNA, and DNA polymerase appear in serum soon after HBsAg, and all signify active viral replication. Persistence of HBeAg is an important indicator of continued viral replication, infectivity, and probable progression to chronic hepatitis. The appearance of anti-HBe antibodies implies that an acute infection has peaked and is on the wane.
- IgM anti-HBc becomes detectable in serum shortly before the onset of symptoms, concurrent with the onset of elevated serum aminotransferase levels (indicative of hepatocyte destruction). Over a period of months the IgM anti-HBc antibody is replaced by IgG anti-HBc. As in the case of anti-HAV, there is no direct assay for IgG

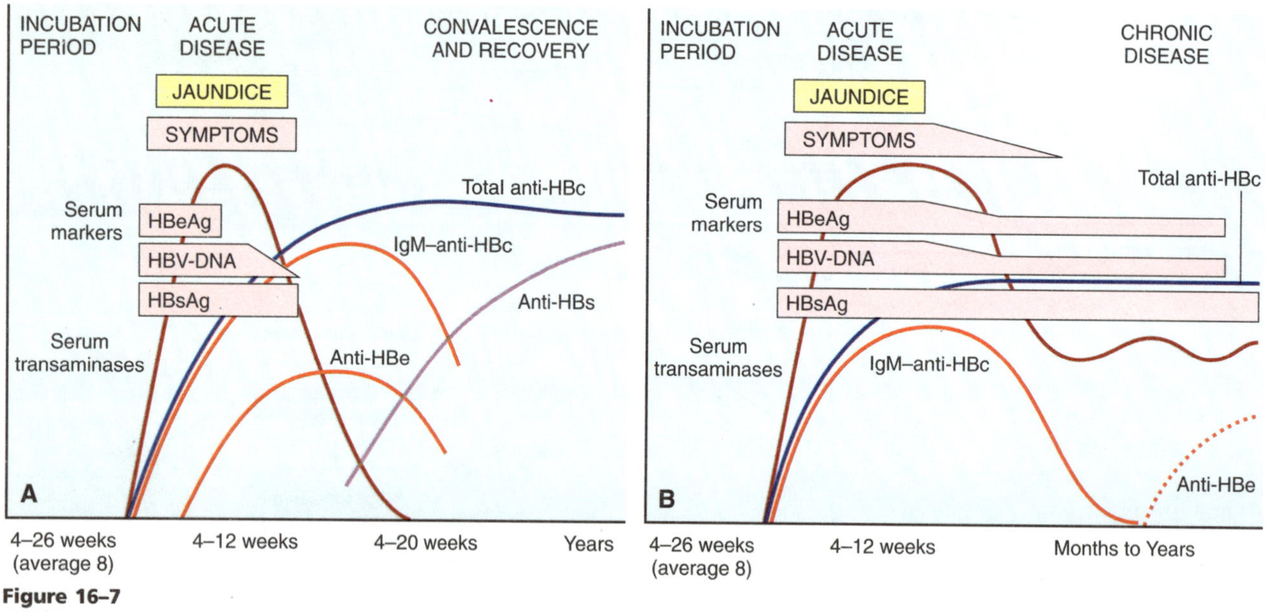

Figure 16–7

The sequence of serologic markers in acute hepatitis B infection. **A,** Resolution of active infection. **B,** Progression to chronic infection. See text for abbreviations.

anti-HBc, but its presence is inferred from decline of IgM anti-HBc in the face of rising levels of total anti-HBc.

Occasionally, mutated strains of HBV emerge that do not produce HBeAg but are replication competent and express HBcAg. In such patients, the HBeAg may be low or undetectable despite the presence of HBV viral load. A second ominous development is the appearance of vaccine-induced escape mutants, which replicate in the presence of vaccine-induced immunity. For instance, replacement of arginine at amino acid 145 of HBsAg with glycine significantly alters recognition of HBsAg by anti-HBsAg antibodies.

The host immune response to the virus is the main determinant of the outcome of the infection. The mechanisms of innate immunity protect the host during the initial phases of the infection, and a strong response by virus-specific CD4+ and CD8+ interferon γ-producing cells are associated with the resolution of acute infection. There are several reasons to believe that HBV does not cause direct hepatocyte injury. Most importantly, many chronic carriers have virions in their hepatocytes with no evidence of cell injury. Hepatocyte damage is believed to result from damage to the virus-infected cells by CD8+ cytotoxic T cells. Thus, the immune response has to be properly calibrated to clear the virus without causing widespread liver damage.

Hepatitis B can be prevented by vaccination and by the screening of donor blood, organs, and tissues. The vaccine is prepared from purified HbsAg produced in yeast. Vaccination induces a protective anti-HBs antibody response in 95% of infants, children, and adolescents. Universal vaccination has had notable success in Taiwan and Gambia, but unfortunately, it has not been adopted worldwide.

Hepatitis C Virus (HCV)

HCV is also a major cause of liver disease. The worldwide carrier rate is estimated at 175 million persons (a 3% prevalence rate, ranging widely from 0.1% to 12%, depending on the country). Persistent chronic infection exists in 3 to 4 million persons in the United States, where the number of newly acquired HCV infections per year dropped from 180,000 in the mid-1980s to about 28,000 in the mid-1990s. This welcome change resulted from the marked reduction in transfusion-associated hepatitis C (as a result of screening procedures) and a decline of infections in intravenous drug abusers (related to practices motivated by fear of human immunodeficiency virus infection). However, the death rate from HCV will continue to climb for 20 to 25 years, because of the decades-long lag time between acute infection and liver failure. *The major route of transmission is through blood inoculation, with intravenous drug use accounting for over 40% of cases in the United States.* Transmission via blood products is now fortunately rare, accounting for only 4% of all acute HCV infections. Occupational exposure among health care workers accounts for 4% of cases. The rates of sexual transmission and vertical transmission are low. Sporadic hepatitis of unknown source accounts for 40% of cases. *HCV infection has a much higher rate than HBV of progression to chronic disease and eventual cirrhosis* (Fig. 16–8). *Hepatitis C and chronic alcoholism are the main causes of chronic liver disease in the Western world,* and *hepatitis* C is the condition that most frequently requires liver transplantation in the United States.

HCV is a positive-sense single-stranded RNA virus belonging to Flaviviridae, a class of viruses that includes the HGV and the causative agents of dengue fever and yellow fever. It contains highly conserved 5′- and 3′-terminal regions that flank a single open reading frame of nearly 9500 nucleotides that encode structural and nonstructural proteins. Based on the genetic sequence, HCV is subclassified into six genotypes. Moreover, because of the poor fidelity of RNA replication, an infected person may carry many HCV variants, called quasi-species. The relationships between quasi-species development and disease progression are being investigated, but it seems that high multiplicity of quasi-species is associated with worst prognosis. In any case, this variability seriously hampers efforts to develop an HCV vaccine.

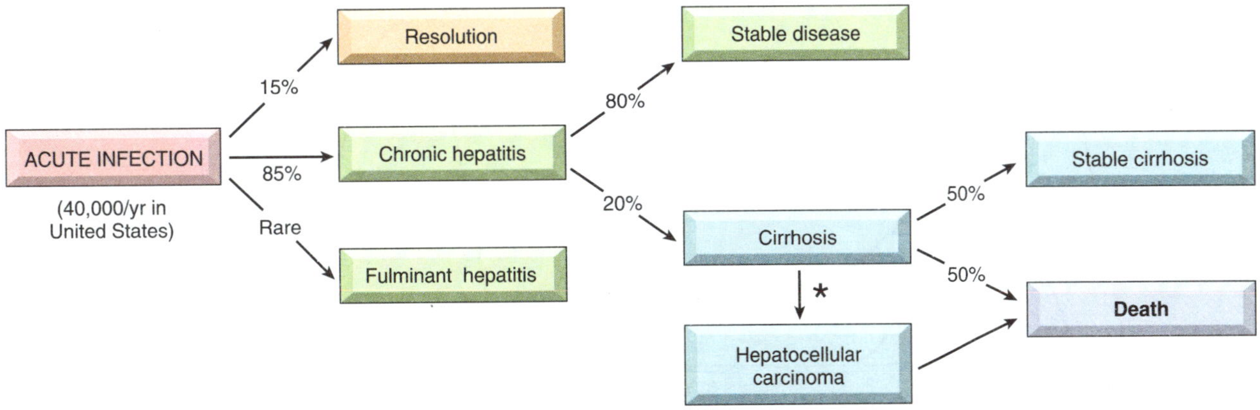

Figure 16–8

The potential outcomes of hepatitis C infection in adults, with their approximate annual frequencies in the United States. The population estimates are for newly detected infection; because of the decades-long lag time for progression from acute infection to cirrhosis, the actual annual death rate from hepatitis C is about 10,000 per year and is expected to exceed 22,000 deaths per year by 2008. *The risk of hepatocellular carcinoma is 1% to 4% per year.

The incubation period for hepatitis C ranges from 2 to 26 weeks, with a mean of 6 to 12 weeks. The clinical course of acute hepatitis C is asymptomatic in 75% of individuals and is easily missed. Thus, not much information is available for this phase of the disease. HCV RNA is detectable in blood for 1 to 3 weeks and is accompanied by elevations in serum aminotransferase. Although neutralizing anti-HCV antibodies develop within weeks to a few months, they *do not confer effective immunity* (Fig. 16–9). Strong immune responses involving CD4+ and CD8+ cells are associated with self-limited HCV infections, but it is not known why only a minority of individuals is capable of clearing HCV infection.

In persistent infection, circulating HCV-RNA is detectable, and aminotransferases show episodic elevations, or continuous elevation with fluctuating levels. In a small percentage of individuals, aminotransferase levels are persistently low even though their liver histology has not returned to normal. Increased enzyme activity may occur in the absence of clinical symptoms, presumably reflecting recurrent bouts of hepatocyte necrosis. *Persistent infection is the hallmark of HCV infection, occurring in 80% to 85% of individuals with subclinical or asymptomatic acute infection* (see Fig. 16–8). Cirrhosis develops in 20% of persistently infected individuals: it can be present at the time of diagnosis or may develop over 5 to 20 years. Alternatively, individuals may have documented chronic HCV infection for decades, without progressing to cirrhosis. Fulminant hepatitis is rare.

Hepatitis D Virus (HDV)

Also called hepatitis delta virus, HDV is a unique RNA virus that is replication defective, causing infection only when it is encapsulated by HBsAg. Thus, *though taxonomically distinct from HBV, HDV is absolutely dependent on HBV coinfection for multiplication.* Delta hepatitis arises in two settings: (1) acute coinfection after exposure to serum containing both HDV and HBV and (2) superinfection of a chronic carrier of HBV with a new inoculum of HDV. In the first case, HBV infection must become established before HBsAg is available for the development of complete HDV virions. Most coinfected individuals can clear the viruses and recover completely. The course is different in superinfected individuals. In most cases, there is an acceleration of hepatitis, progressing to more severe chronic hepatitis 4 to 7 weeks later.

Infection by HDV is worldwide, with prevalence rates ranging from 8% among HBsAg carriers in southern Italy to as high as 40% in Africa and the Middle East. Surprisingly, HDV infection is uncommon in Southeast Asia and China, areas in which HBV infection is endemic. Periodic epidemic outbreaks have occurred in subtropical areas of Peru, Colombia, and Venezuela. In the United States, HDV infection is largely restricted to drug addicts and individuals receiving multiple transfusions (e.g., hemophiliacs), who have prevalence rates of 1% to 10%.

HDV RNA and the HDV Ag are detectable in the blood and liver just before and in the early days of acute symptomatic disease. *IgM anti-HDV antibody is the most reliable indicator of recent HDV exposure,* but its appearance is transient. Nevertheless, acute coinfection by HDV and HBV is best indicated by detection of IgM against both HDV Ag and HBcAg (denoting new infection with HBV). With chronic delta hepatitis arising from HDV superinfection, HBsAg is present in serum; and anti-HDV antibodies (IgM and IgG) persist in low titer for months or longer.

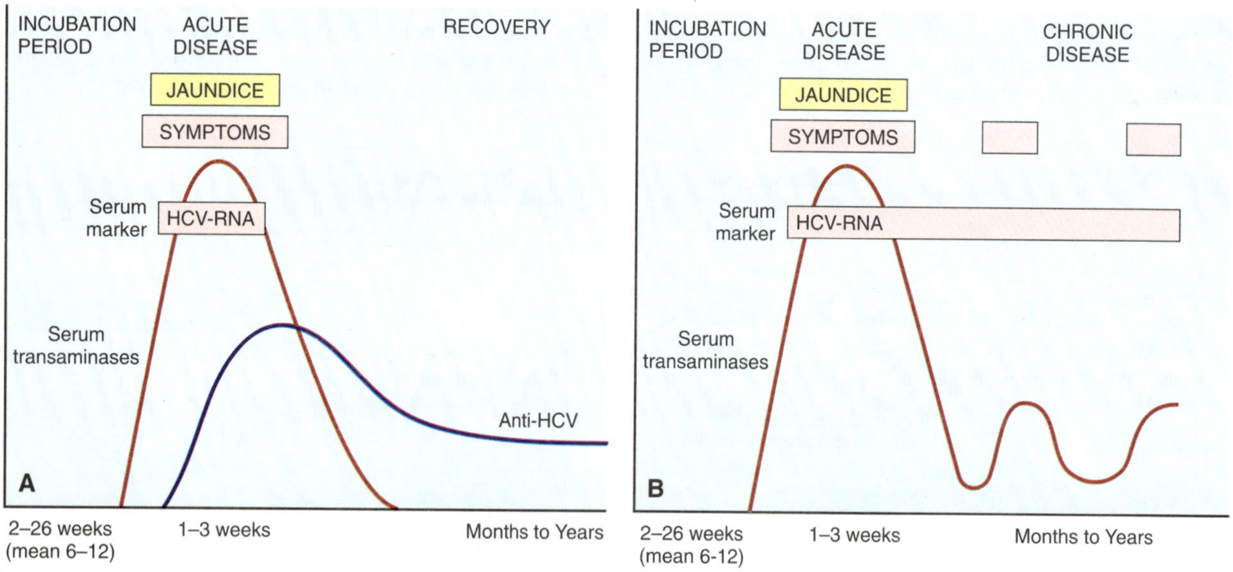

Figure 16–9

Sequence of serologic markers for hepatitis C. **A,** Acute infection with resolution. **B,** Progression to chronic infection. See text for abbreviations.

Hepatitis E Virus (HEV)

HEV hepatitis is an enterically transmitted, waterborne infection occurring primarily beyond the years of infancy. HEV is endemic in India (where it was first documented as caused by fecal contamination of drinking water). Prevalence rates of anti-HEV IgG antibodies approach 40% in the Indian population. Epidemics have been reported from Asia, sub-Saharan Africa, and Mexico. Sporadic infection seems to be uncommon; it is seen mainly in travelers and accounts for more than 50% of cases of sporadic acute viral hepatitis in India. In most cases, the disease is self-limited; HEV is not associated with chronic liver disease or persistent viremia. *A characteristic feature of the infection is the high mortality rate among pregnant women, approaching 20%.* The average incubation period after exposure is 6 weeks (range, 2–8 weeks).

HEV is a nonenveloped, single-stranded RNA virus that is best characterized as a calicivirus. A specific antigen (HEV Ag) can be identified in the cytoplasm of hepatocytes during active infection. Virus can be detected in stools, and anti-HEV IgG and IgM antibodies are detectable in serum.

Clinical Features and Outcomes of Viral Hepatitis

A number of clinical syndromes may develop after exposure to hepatitis viruses:

- Asymptomatic acute infection: serologic evidence only
- Acute hepatitis: anicteric or icteric
- Chronic hepatitis: with or without progression to cirrhosis
- Chronic carrier state: asymptomatic without apparent disease
- Fulminant hepatitis: submassive to massive hepatic necrosis with acute liver failure

Not all of the hepatotropic viruses provoke each of these clinical syndromes (see Table 16–4). With rare exceptions, HAV, HCV, and HEV do not generate a carrier state, and HAV and HEV infections do not progress to chronic hepatitis. As already mentioned, viral persistence and development of chronic disease is much more common after HCV infection than for HBV infection. Because other infectious or noninfectious causes, particularly drugs and toxins, can lead to essentially identical syndromes, serologic studies are critical for the diagnosis of viral hepatitis and identification of virus types. Here we present brief summaries of clinical outcomes of viral hepatitis.

Asymptomatic Infection. Not surprisingly, patients in this group are identified only incidentally on the basis of minimally elevated serum aminotransferases or after the fact by the presence of antiviral antibodies.

Acute Viral Hepatitis. Any one of the hepatotropic viruses can cause acute viral hepatitis. Acute infections are easily detected for HBV infections but only rarely diagnosed for HCV. Although the following description is mostly based on HBV infections, *acute hepatitis, whatever the agent, can be divided into four phases: (1) an incubation period, (2) a symptomatic preicteric phase, (3) a symptomatic icteric phase (with jaundice and scleral icterus), and (4) convalescence.* Peak infectivity, attributed to the presence of circulating infectious viral particles, occurs during the last asymptomatic days of the incubation period and the early days of acute symptoms. The preicteric phase is marked by nonspecific, constitutional symptoms. Malaise is followed in a few days by general fatigability, nausea, and loss of appetite. Weight loss, low-grade fever, headaches, muscle and joint aches, vomiting, and diarrhea are inconstant symptoms. About 10% of patients with acute hepatitis B develop a serum sickness–like syndrome consisting of fever, rash, and arthralgias, attributed to circulating immune complexes. The hepatitis-related origin of all these symptoms is suggested by elevated serum aminotransferase levels. Physical examination reveals a mildly enlarged, tender liver. In some individuals the nonspecific symptoms are more severe, with higher fever, shaking chills, and headache, sometimes accompanied by right upper quadrant pain and tender liver enlargement. Surprisingly, as jaundice appears and these patients enter the icteric phase, other symptoms begin to abate. The jaundice is caused predominantly by conjugated hyperbilirubinemia and hence is accompanied by dark-colored urine related to the presence of conjugated bilirubin. With hepatocellular damage and consequent defect in bilirubin conjugation, unconjugated hyperbilirubinemia can also occur. The stools may become light colored due to cholestasis, and the retention of bile salts may cause distressing pruritus. An icteric phase is usual in adults (but not children) infected with HAV but is absent in about half the cases involving HBV and is absent in most cases of HCV infection. In a few weeks to perhaps several months, the jaundice and most of the other systemic symptoms clear as convalescence begins.

Chronic Hepatitis is defined as symptomatic, biochemical, or serologic evidence of continuing or relapsing hepatic disease for more than 6 months, with histologically documented inflammation and necrosis. Although the hepatitis viruses are responsible for most cases, there are many causes of chronic hepatitis (described later). They include Wilson disease, α_1-antitrypsin deficiency, chronic alcoholism, drugs (isoniazid, α-methyldopa, methotrexate), and autoimmunity.

In chronic hepatitis, *etiology rather than the histologic pattern is the most important determinant of the probability of developing progressive chronic hepatitis.* In particular, HCV is notorious for causing a chronic hepatitis evolving to cirrhosis in a significant percentage of patients (see Fig. 16–8), regardless of histologic features at the time of initial evaluation.

The clinical features of chronic hepatitis are highly variable and are not predictive of outcome. In some patients, the only signs of chronic disease are persistent elevations of serum aminotransferase levels. The most common overt symptoms are fatigue and, less commonly, malaise, loss of appetite, and bouts of mild jaundice. Physical findings are few, the most common being spider angiomas, palmar erythema, mild hepatomegaly, and hepatic tenderness. Laboratory studies may reveal prolongation of the prothrombin time and, in some instances, hypergammaglobulinemia, hyperbilirubinemia, and mild elevations in alkaline phosphatase levels. Occasionally in cases of HBV and HCV, circulating antibody-antigen complexes produce immune-complex disease, in the form of vasculitis (subcutaneous or visceral, Chapter 10) and glomerulonephritis (Chapter 14). Cryoglobulinemia is found in as many as 50% of individuals with hepatitis C. The clinical course is highly variable. Persons with hepatitis C may experience spontaneous remission or may have indolent disease without progression for years. Conversely, some patients have rapidly progressive disease and develop cirrhosis within a few years. The major causes of death in patients with chronic hepatitis relate to cirrhosis, namely, liver failure, hepatic encephalopathy, massive hematemesis from esophageal varices, and hepatocellular carcinoma (see Figs. 16–6 and 16–8).

The Carrier State. A "carrier" is an individual without manifest symptoms who harbors and therefore can transmit an organism. With hepatotropic viruses, carriers are (1) those who harbor one of the viruses but are suffering little or no adverse effects, and (2) those who have nonprogressive liver damage but are essentially free of symptoms or disability. Both constitute reservoirs of infection. HBV infection early in life, particularly through vertical transmission during childbirth, produces a carrier state 90% to 95% of the time. In contrast, only 1% to 10% of HBV infections acquired in adulthood yield a carrier state. Individuals with impaired immunity are particularly likely to become carriers. The situation is less clear with HDV, although there is a well-defined low risk of posttransfusion hepatitis D, indicative of a carrier state in conjunction with HBV. HCV can clearly induce a carrier state, which is estimated to affect 0.2% to 0.6% of the general US population.

Fulminant Hepatitis. A very small proportion of patients with acute hepatitis A, B, or E may develop acute liver failure, resulting from massive hepatic necrosis. Cases with a more protracted course of several weeks or months are usually referred to as "subacute hepatic necrosis"; livers of these individuals show both massive necrosis and regenerative hyperplasia. As discussed later, drugs and chemicals can also cause massive hepatic necrosis.

Table 16–5 Main Morphologic Features of Acute and Chronic Viral Hepatitis

Acute Hepatitis

Gross: Enlarged, reddened liver; greenish if cholestatic
Parenchymal changes (microscopic)
- Hepatocyte injury: swelling (ballooning degeneration)
  - Cholestasis: canalicular bile plugs
  - HCV: mild fatty change of hepatocytes
- Hepatocyte necrosis: isolated cells or clusters
  - Cytolysis (rupture) or apoptosis (shrinkage)
  - If severe: bridging necrosis (portal-portal, central-central, portal-central)
  - Lobular disarray: loss of normal architecture
- Regenerative changes: hepatocyte proliferation
- Sinusoidal cell reactive changes
  - Accumulation of phagocytosed cellular debris in Kupffer cells
  - Influx of mononuclear cells into sinusoids
- Portal tracts
  - Inflammation: predominantly mononuclear
  - Inflammatory spillover into adjacent parenchyma, with hepatocyte necrosis

Chronic Hepatitis

Changes shared with acute hepatitis:
- Hepatocyte injury, necrosis, apoptosis, and regeneration
- Sinusoidal cell reactive changes

Portal tracts
- Inflammation:
  - Confined to portal tracts, *or*
  - Spillover into adjacent parenchyma, with necrosis of hepatocytes ("interface hepatitis"), *or*
  - Bridging inflammation and necrosis
- Fibrosis:
  - Portal deposition, *or*
  - Portal and periportal deposition, *or*
  - Formation of bridging fibrous septa

HBV: ground-glass hepatocytes (accumulation of HBsAg)
HCV: bile duct epithelial cell proliferation, lymphoid aggregate formation

Cirrhosis: the End-Stage Outcome

Morphology

The general morphologic features of acute and chronic viral hepatitis are listed in Table 16–5. Examples are presented in Figures 16–10 and 16–11. The morphologic changes in acute and chronic viral hepatitis are shared among the hepatotropic viruses and can be mimicked by drug reactions. With acute hepatitis, hepatocyte injury takes the form of diffuse swelling **(ballooning degeneration),** so that the cytoplasm looks empty and contains only scattered wisps of cytoplasmic remnants. An inconstant finding is **cholestasis,** with bile plugs in canaliculi and brown pigmentation of hepatocytes. Fatty change is mild and is unusual except with HCV infection. Whether acute or chronic, HBV infection may generate **"ground-glass"** hepatocytes (Fig. 16–12): a finely granular, eosinophilic cytoplasm shown by electron microscopy to contain massive quantities of HBsAg in the form of spheres and tubules. Other HBV-infected hepatocytes may have **"sanded" nuclei,** resulting from abundant intranuclear HBcAg.

Two patterns of **hepatocyte death** are seen. In the first, rupture of cell membranes leads to **cytolysis.** The necrotic cells appear to have "dropped out," with collapse of the sinusoidal collagen reticulin framework where the cells have disappeared; scavenger macrophage aggregates mark sites of dropout. The second pattern of cell death, **apoptosis,** is more distinctive. Apoptotic hepatocytes shrink, become intensely eosinophilic, and have fragmented nuclei; effector T cells may be present in the immediate vicinity. Apoptotic cells also are phagocytosed within hours by macrophages and hence may be difficult to find despite extensive ongoing apoptosis. In severe cases, confluent necrosis of hepatocytes may lead to **bridging necrosis** connecting portal-to-portal, central-to-central,

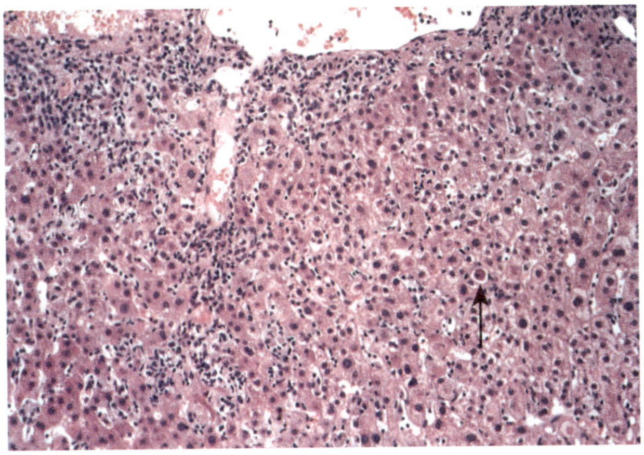

Figure 16–10

Acute viral hepatitis showing disruption of lobular architecture, inflammatory cells in sinusoids, and apoptotic cells *(arrow).*

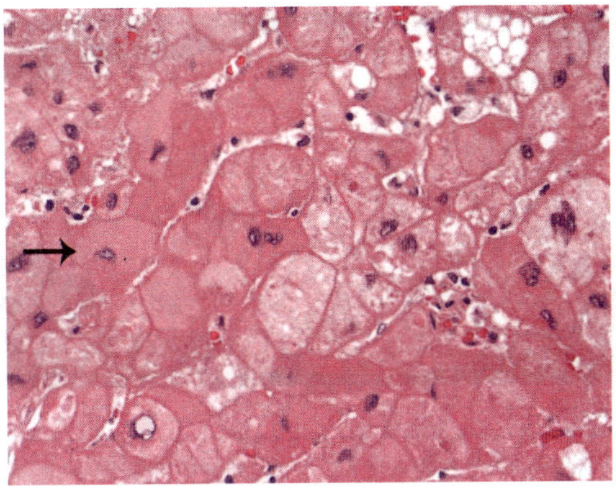

Figure 16–12

Ground-glass hepatocytes *(arrow)* in chronic hepatitis B, caused by accumulation of HBsAg in cytoplasm. (Courtesy of Dr. Matthew Yeh, University of Washington, Seattle, Washington.)

or portal-to-central regions of adjacent lobules, signifying a more severe form of acute hepatitis. Hepatocyte swelling, necrosis, and regeneration produce compression of the vascular sinusoids and loss of the normal, more or less radial array of the parenchyma (so-called **lobular disarray**).

Inflammation is a characteristic and usually prominent feature of acute hepatitis. **Kupffer cells undergo hypertrophy and hyperplasia,** and are often laden with lipofuscin pigment caused by phagocytosis of hepatocellular debris. **The portal tracts are usually infiltrated with a mixture of** inflammatory cells. The inflammatory infiltrate may spill over into the parenchyma to cause necrosis of periportal hepatocytes (**interface** hepatitis).

Finally, bile duct epithelium may become reactive and even proliferate, particularly in cases of HCV hepatitis, forming poorly defined ductular structures in the midst of the portal tract inflammation. Bile duct destruction, however, does not occur.

The histologic features of **chronic hepatitis** range from exceedingly mild to severe. Smoldering hepatocyte necrosis throughout the lobule may occur in all forms of chronic hepatitis. In the mildest forms, significant inflammation is limited to portal tracts and consists of lymphocytes, macrophages, occasional plasma cells, and rare neutrophils or eosinophils. **Lymphoid aggregates** in the portal tract are often seen in HCV infection. Liver architecture is usually well preserved. Continued **periportal necrosis** and **bridging necrosis** are harbingers of progressive liver damage. **The hallmark** of serious liver damage is the deposition of fibrous tissue. At first, only portal tracts exhibit increased fibrosis, but with time **periportal fibrosis** occurs, followed by linking of fibrous septa between lobules (**bridging fibrosis**).

Continued loss of hepatocytes and fibrosis results in cirrhosis, with fibrous septa and hepatocyte regenerative nodules. This pattern of cirrhosis is characterized by irregularly sized nodules separated by variable but mostly broad scars (Fig. 16–13). The nodules are typically greater than 0.3 cm in diameter, earning the term **macronodular cirrhosis.** While such cirrhosis is characteristic of postviral cirrhosis, it is not specific to this etiology, because hepatotoxins (carbon tetrachloride, mushroom poisoning), pharmaceutical agents (acetaminophen, α-methyldopa), and even alcohol (discussed later) may give rise to macronodular cirrhosis. Notably, in about 10% of cases an etiology for the cirrhosis cannot be identified.

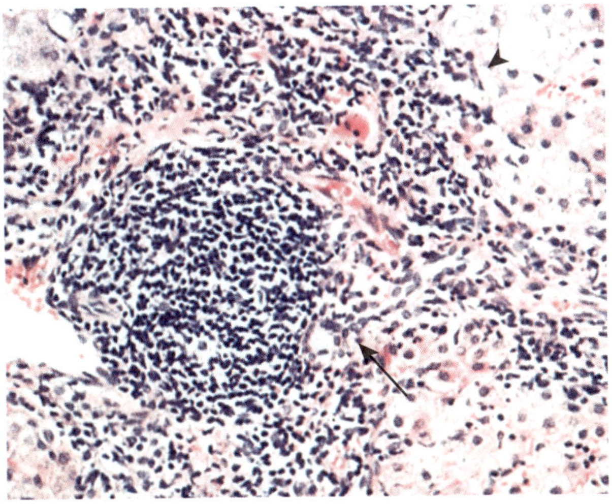

Figure 16–11

Chronic hepatitis C showing portal tract expansion with inflammatory cells and fibrous tissue (*arrow*), and interface hepatitis with spillover of inflammation into the parenchyma (*arrowhead*). A lymphoid aggregate is present in the center of the picture.

Autoimmune Hepatitis

Autoimmune hepatitis is a syndrome of chronic hepatitis in persons with a heterogeneous set of immunologic abnormalities. The histologic features are indistinguishable from chronic viral hepatitis. This disease may run an indolent or severe course and typically responds dramatically to immunosuppressive therapy. Salient features include:

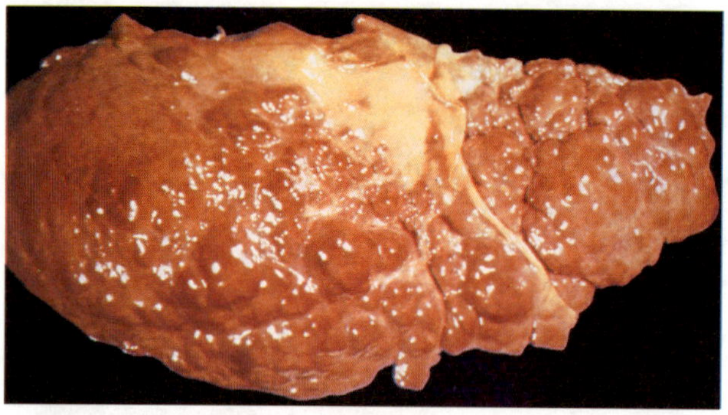

Figure 16–13

Cirrhosis resulting from chronic viral hepatitis. Note the irregular nodularity of the liver surface.

- Female predominance (70%)
- Absence of serologic markers of a viral infection
- Elevated serum IgG (>2.5 g/dL)
- High titers of autoantibodies in 80% of cases
- The presence of other forms of autoimmune diseases, seen in up to 60% of patients, including rheumatoid arthritis, thyroiditis, Sjögren syndrome, and ulcerative colitis.

Pathogenesis and Main Clinical Features. Autoimmune hepatitis can be divided into three subtypes on the basis of the autoantibodies, but the relevance of this classification to clinical management is unclear. Most patients have circulating antinuclear antibodies, anti–smooth muscle antibodies, liver kidney microsomal antibody, and anti-soluble liver/pancreas antigen. These antibodies can be detected by immunofluorescence or enzyme-linked immunosorbent assays. The best characterized among these antibodies are smooth muscle antibodies directed against cytoskeletal proteins that include actin, troponin, and tropomyosin, and liver kidney microsomal antibodies directed against components of the cytochrome P-450 system and the UDP-glucuronosyltransferases. The main effectors of cell damage in autoimmune hepatitis are believed to be CD4+ helper cells. Autoimmune hepatitis may present with mild to severe chronic hepatitis. Response to immunosuppressive therapy is usually dramatic, although a full remission of disease is unusual. The overall risk of cirrhosis, the main cause of death, is 5%.

SUMMARY

Hepatitis

- Viral hepatitis is the most common primary liver infection. Autoimmune hepatitis is much less frequent.
- HAV causes a self-limited disease that never becomes chronic; HBV can produce acute, chronic, and fulminant disease (1% or less), but the frequency of chronic disease is about 10%.
- HCV causes acute and chronic hepatitis; the acute phase is often difficult to detect and the frequency of chronic disease may reach 85%; cirrhosis develops in 20% of cases of chronic disease.
- In both acute and chronic hepatitis there is hepatocyte injury and cell death, and inflammation of portal tracts; chronic hepatitis may show bridging necrosis and fibrosis.
- Patients with longstanding HBV or HCV infections are at increased risk of developing hepatocellular carcinomas.

Pyogenic Liver Abscesses

In developing countries liver abscesses are common; most result from parasitic infections, such as amebic, echinococcal, and (less commonly) other protozoal and helminthic organisms. In developed countries parasitic liver abscesses are rare, and many occur in immigrants. In the Western world, bacterial abscesses are more common, representing a complication of an infection elsewhere. The organisms reach the liver through one of the following pathways: (1) ascending infection in the biliary tract (ascending cholangitis); (2) vascular seeding, either portal or arterial, predominantly from the gastrointestinal tract (3) direct invasion of the liver from a nearby source; or (4) a penetrating injury. Debilitating disease with immune deficiency is a common setting—for example, extreme old age, immunosuppression, or cancer chemotherapy with marrow failure.

Pyogenic (bacterial) hepatic abscesses may occur as solitary or multiple lesions, ranging from millimeters to massive lesions, many centimeters in diameter. They are generally produced by gram-negative bacteria such as *Escherichia coli* and *Klebsiella* sp. Bacteremic spread through the arterial or portal system tends to produce multiple small abscesses, whereas direct extension and trauma usually cause solitary large abscesses. Gross and microscopic features are those of any pyogenic abscess, consisting of necrotic tissue with abundant neutrophils. Occasionally, fungi or parasites rather than bacteria can be identified.

Liver abscesses are associated with fever and, in many instances, with right upper quadrant pain and tender hepatomegaly. Jaundice is often the result of extrahepatic biliary obstruction. Although antibiotic therapy may control smaller lesions, surgical drainage is often necessary. Because diagnosis is frequently delayed, particularly in persons with serious coexistent disease, the mortality rate with large liver abscesses ranges from 30% to 90%. With early recognition and management, as many as 80% of patients may survive.

ALCOHOL- AND DRUG-INDUCED LIVER DISEASE

As the major drug metabolizing and detoxifying organ in the body, the liver is subject to injury from an enormous array of therapeutic and environmental chemicals. Injury may result from direct toxicity, occur via hepatic conversion of a xenobiotic to an active toxin, or be produced by immune mechanisms, usually by the drug or a metabolite acting as a hapten to convert a cellular protein into an immunogen.

A diagnosis of drug-induced liver disease may be made on the basis of a temporal association of liver damage with drug administration and, it is hoped, recovery on removal of the drug, combined with exclusion of other potential causes. Exposure to a toxin or therapeutic agent should always be included in the differential diagnosis of any form of liver disease. By far, the most important agent that produces toxic liver injury is alcohol.

Alcoholic Liver Disease

Excessive ethanol consumption causes more than 60% of chronic liver disease in most Western countries and accounts for 40% to 50% of deaths due to cirrhosis. The following statistics attest to the magnitude of the problem in the United States:

- More than 10 million Americans are alcoholics.
- Alcohol abuse causes 100,000 to 200,000 deaths annually in the United States, the fifth leading cause of death. Of these deaths, 20,000 are attributable directly to end-stage cirrhosis; many more are the result of automobile accidents.
- From 25% to 30% of hospitalized patients have problems related to alcohol abuse.

Chronic alcohol consumption has a variety of adverse effects (Chapter 8). Of great impact, however, are the three distinctive, albeit overlapping, forms of alcoholic liver disease: *(1) hepatic steatosis (fatty liver), (2) alcoholic hepatitis, and (3) cirrhosis, collectively referred to as alcoholic liver disease* (Fig. 16–14). Ninety to 100% of heavy drinkers develop fatty liver (steatosis), and of those, 10% to 35% develop alcoholic hepatitis. However, only 8% to 20% of chronic alcoholics develop cirrhosis. Steatosis and alcoholic hepatitis may develop independently, and thus, they do not necessarily represent a continuum of changes.

Morphology

Hepatic Steatosis (Fatty Liver). After even moderate intake of alcohol, small (microvesicular) lipid droplets accumulate in hepatocytes. With chronic intake of alcohol, lipid accumulates to the point of creating large clear macrovesicular globules, compressing and displacing the nucleus to the periphery of the hepatocyte. This transformation is initially centrilobular, but in severe cases it may involve the entire lobule (Fig. 16–15). Macroscopically the fatty liver of chronic alcoholism is large (≤4–6 kg), soft, yellow, and greasy. Although there is little or no fibrosis at the outset, with continued alcohol intake fibrous tissue develops around the central veins and extends into the adjacent sinusoids. Until fibrosis appears, the fatty change is completely reversible if there is abstention from further intake of alcohol.

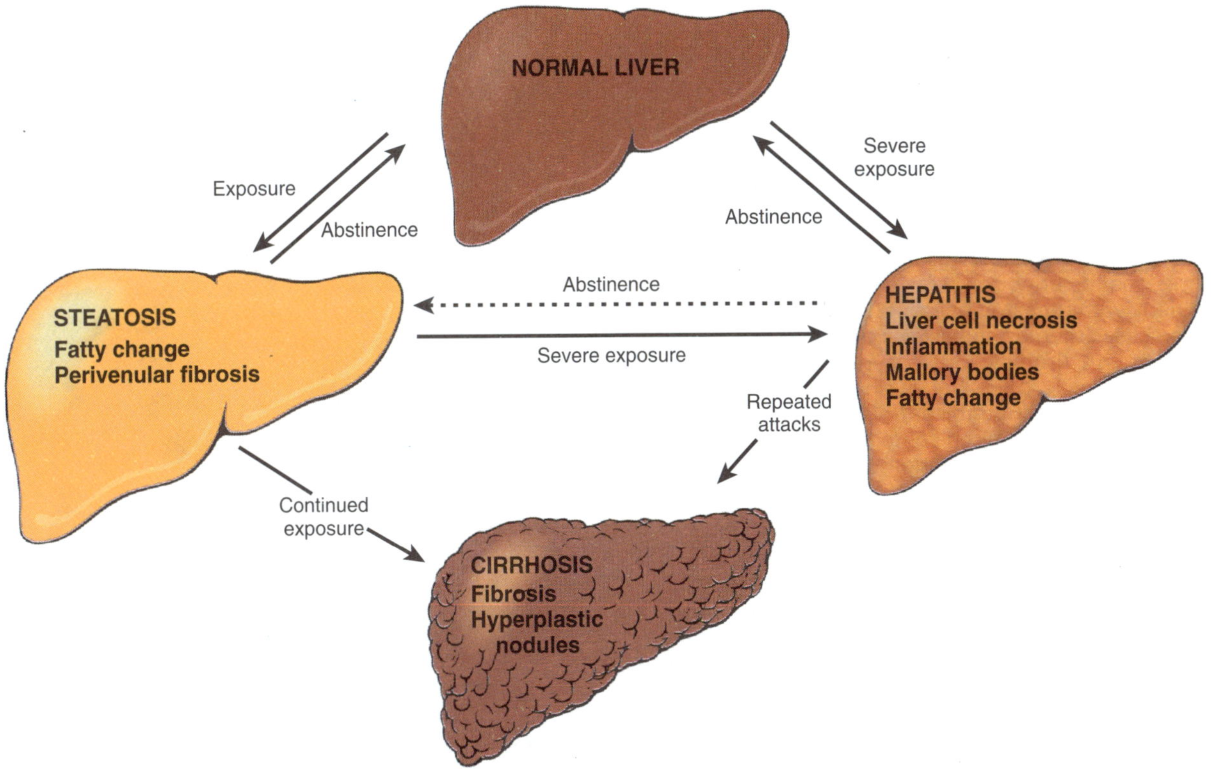

Figure 16–14

Alcoholic liver disease. The interrelationships among hepatic steatosis, hepatitis, and cirrhosis are shown, along with a depiction of key morphologic features at the microscopic level.

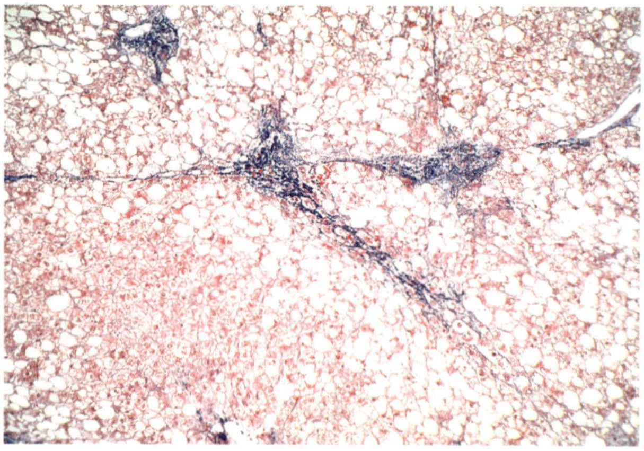

Figure 16–15

Alcoholic liver disease: macrovesicular steatosis, involving most regions of the hepatic lobule. The intracytoplasmic fat is seen as clear vacuoles. Some early fibrosis (stained *blue*) is present (Masson trichrome).

Alcoholic Hepatitis. This is characterized by the following:

Hepatocyte Swelling and Necrosis. Single or scattered foci of cells undergo swelling (ballooning) and necrosis. The swelling results from the accumulation of fat and water, as well as proteins that normally are exported.

Mallory Bodies. Scattered hepatocytes accumulate tangled skeins of intermediate filaments and other proteins, visible as eosinophilic cytoplasmic inclusions in degenerating hepatocytes (Fig. 16–16). These inclusions are a characteristic but not specific feature of alcoholic liver disease, because they are also seen in primary biliary cirrhosis, Wilson disease, chronic cholestatic syndromes, and hepatocellular tumors.

Neutrophil Infiltration. Neutrophils permeate the lobule and accumulate around degenerating hepatocytes, particularly those containing Mallory bodies. Lymphocytes and macrophages also enter portal tracts and spill into the parenchyma.

Fibrosis. Alcoholic hepatitis is almost always accompanied by a brisk sinusoidal and perivenular fibrosis; occasionally periportal fibrosis may predominate, particularly with repeated bouts of heavy alcohol intake. In some cases there is cholestasis and mild deposition of hemosiderin (iron) in hepatocytes and Kupffer cells. Macroscopically, the liver is mottled red with bile-stained areas. Although the liver may be normal or increased in size, it often contains visible nodules and fibrosis, indicative of evolution to cirrhosis.

Alcoholic Cirrhosis. The final and irreversible form of alcoholic liver disease usually evolves slowly and insidiously. At first the cirrhotic liver is yellow-tan, fatty, and enlarged, usually weighing over 2 kg. Over the span of years it is transformed into a brown, shrunken, nonfatty organ, sometimes weighing less than 1 kg. Arguably, cirrhosis may develop more rapidly in the setting of alcoholic hepatitis, within 1 to 2 years. Initially the developing fibrous septa are delicate and extend through sinusoids from central vein to portal regions as well as from portal tract to portal tract. Regenerative activity of entrapped parenchymal hepatocytes generates fairly uniformly sized nodules. Since these nodules tend to be less than 0.3 cm in diameter, this pattern of cirrhosis is termed **micronodular cirrhosis** (vs. the macronodular cirrhosis described for viral hepatitis). The nodularity eventually becomes more prominent; scattered larger nodules create a "hobnail" appearance on the surface of the liver (Fig. 16–17). As fibrous septa dissect and surround nodules, the liver becomes more fibrotic, loses fat, and shrinks progressively. Residual regenerating parenchymal islands are engulfed by ever wider bands of fibrous tissue, and the liver is converted into a mixed micronodular and macronodular pattern (Fig. 16–18). Ischemic necrosis and fibrous obliteration of nodules eventually create broad expanses of tough, pale scar tissue. Bile stasis often develops; Mallory bodies are only rarely evident at this stage. Thus, end-stage alcoholic cirrhosis eventually comes to resemble, both macroscopically and microscopically, the cirrhosis developing from viral hepatitis and other causes.

Pathogenesis. Short-term ingestion of as much as 80 gm of ethanol per day (8 beers or 7 ounces of 80-proof liquor) generally produces mild, reversible hepatic changes, such as fatty liver. Chronic intake of 50 to 60 gm/day is considered a borderline risk for severe injury. For reasons that may relate to decreased gastric metabolism of ethanol and differences in body composition,

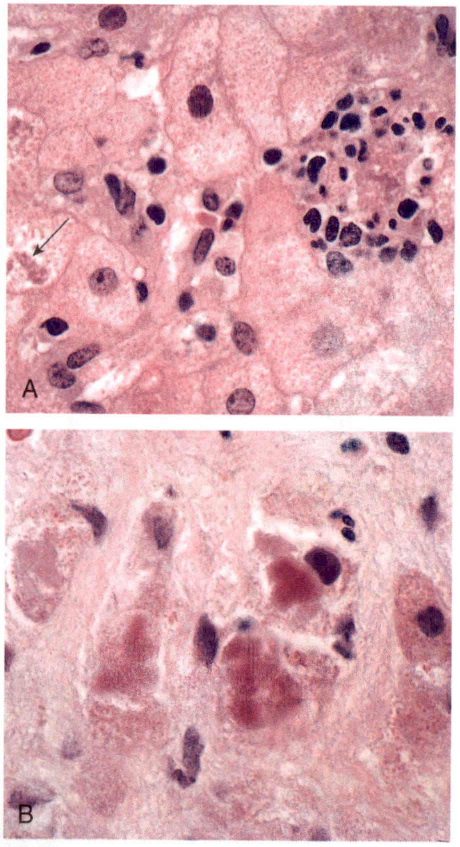

Figure 16–16

Alcoholic hepatitis. **A,** The cluster of inflammatory cells marks the site of a necrotic hepatocyte. A Mallory body is present in another hepatocyte *(arrow)*. **B,** Eosinophilic Mallory bodies are seen in hepatocytes, which are surrounded by fibrous tissue (H & E).

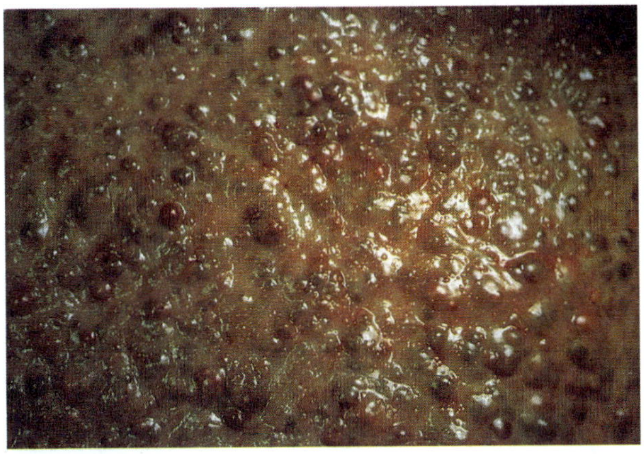

Figure 16–17

Alcoholic cirrhosis showing the characteristic diffuse nodularity of the surface induced by the underlying fibrous scarring. The average nodule size is 3 mm in this close-up view. The greenish tint is caused by bile stasis.

women seem to be more susceptible to hepatic injury than are men. It seems that what and how often one drinks may affect the risk of liver disease development; wine drinking carries less risk than beer, and binge drinking causes more liver injury (note that beer binge drinking is, unfortunately, the preferred modality of drinking in college student parties). Individual, possibly genetic, susceptibility must exist, but no reliable genetic markers of susceptibility have been identified. In addition, there is an inconstant relationship between hepatic steatosis and alcoholic hepatitis as precursors to cirrhosis, which may develop without antecedent evidence of steatosis or alcoholic hepatitis. In the absence of a clear understanding of the pathogenetic factors influencing liver damage, no "safe" upper limit for alcohol consumption can be proposed (despite the current popularity of red wines for protection against coronary vascular disease).

The metabolism of alcohol, and ethanol oxidation through the alcohol dehydrogenase and microsomal ethanol oxidizing system, were discussed in Chapter 8.

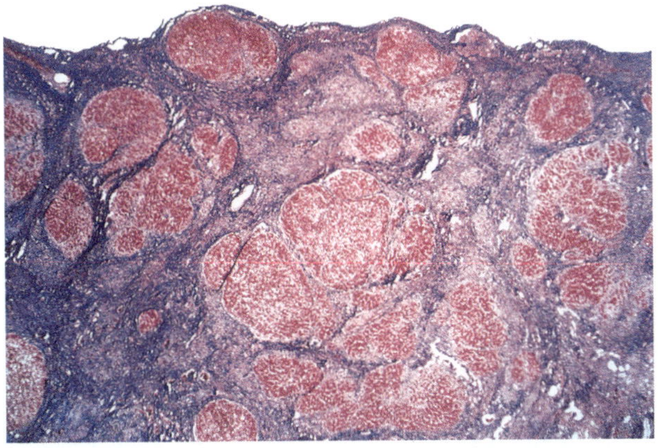

Figure 16–18

Alcoholic cirrhosis. Nodules of varying sizes are entrapped in *blue*-staining fibrous tissue (Masson trichrome stain).

As mentioned, the induction of cytochrome P-450 by alcohol leads to augmented transformation of other drugs to toxic metabolites. In particular, this can accelerate the metabolism of acetaminophen into highly toxic metabolites and increase the risk of liver injury even with therapeutic doses of this commonly used analgesic. Here we discuss the detrimental effects of alcohol and its by-products on hepatocellular function.

Hepatocellular steatosis results from (1) the shunting of normal substrates away from catabolism and toward lipid biosynthesis, because of generation of excess reduced nicotinamide-adenine dinucleotide by the two major enzymes of alcohol metabolism, alcohol dehydrogenase and acetaldehyde dehydrogenase (generating acetate); (2) impaired assembly and secretion of lipoproteins; and (3) increased peripheral catabolism of fat.

The causes of *alcoholic hepatitis* are uncertain, but the following alterations caused by alcohol are important.

- Acetaldehyde (the major intermediate metabolite of alcohol en route to acetate production) induces lipid peroxidation and acetaldehyde-protein adduct formation, which may disrupt cytoskeletal and membrane function.
- Alcohol directly affects microtubule organization (as illustrated by the detection of Mallory's hyaline), mitochondrial function, and membrane fluidity.
- Reactive oxygen species are generated during oxidation of ethanol by the microsomal ethanol oxidizing system; the free radicals react with membranes and proteins.
- Reactive oxygen species are also produced by neutrophils, which infiltrate areas of hepatocyte necrosis.

Abnormal cytokine regulation is a major feature of alcoholic hepatitis and alcoholic liver disease in general. TNF is considered to be the main effector of injury. The main stimuli for the production of cytokines in alcoholic liver disease (TNF, IL-6, IL-8, and IL-18) are the reactive oxygen species, mentioned above, and endotoxin (lipopolysaccharide) derived from gut bacteria. Because generation of acetaldehyde and free radicals is maximal in the centrilobular region of the parenchyma, this region is most susceptible to toxic injury. Pericellular fibrosis and sinusoidal fibrosis develop in this area of the lobule. Concurrent viral hepatitis, particularly hepatitis C, is a major accelerater of liver disease in alcoholics. The prevalence of hepatitis C in individuals with alcoholic disease is about 30%.

For unknown reasons, *cirrhosis* develops in only a small fraction of chronic alcoholics. Alcoholic cirrhosis includes the same features (disruption of the architecture of the entire liver, and the presence of nodules encircled by bridging fibrosis) as cirrhosis induced by viral hepatitis.

Clinical Features. *Hepatic steatosis* may give rise to hepatomegaly with mild elevation of serum bilirubin and alkaline phosphatase. Alternatively, there may be no clinical or biochemical evidence of liver disease. Severe hepatic compromise is unusual. Alcohol withdrawal and the provision of an adequate diet are sufficient treatment. For the occasional heavy drinker, mild hepatic steatosis is a common transient event.

It is estimated that 15 to 20 years of excessive drinking are necessary to develop *alcoholic hepatitis*. However, in such persons the clinical features of alcoholic hepatitis appear relatively acutely, usually after a bout of heavy drinking. Symptoms and laboratory abnormalities may be minimal or severe. Between these two extremes are the nonspecific symptoms of malaise, anorexia, weight loss, upper abdominal discomfort, tender hepatomegaly, and fever and the laboratory findings of hyperbilirubinemia, elevated alkaline phosphatase, and often a neutrophilic leukocytosis. Serum alanine aminotransferase and aspartate aminotransferase are elevated but usually remain below 500 U/mL. The outlook is unpredictable; each bout of hepatitis carries about a 10% to 20% risk of death. With repeated bouts, cirrhosis appears in about one-third of patients within a few years; alcoholic hepatitis also may be superimposed on cirrhosis. With proper nutrition and total cessation of alcohol consumption, alcoholic hepatitis may clear slowly. However, in some individuals the hepatitis persists despite abstinence and progresses to cirrhosis.

The manifestations of *alcoholic cirrhosis* are similar to other forms of cirrhosis, presented earlier. Commonly, the first signs of cirrhosis relate to complications of portal hypertension. The stigmata of cirrhosis (e.g., an abdomen grossly distended with ascites, wasted extremities, caput medusae) may be the presenting features. Alternatively, a patient may first present with life-threatening variceal hemorrhage or hepatic encephalopathy. In other cases, insidious onset of malaise, weakness, weight loss, and loss of appetite precede the appearance of jaundice, ascites, and peripheral edema. Laboratory findings reflect the developing hepatic disease, with elevated serum aminotransferase, hyperbilirubinemia, variable elevation of alkaline phosphatase, hypoproteinemia (globulins, albumin, and clotting factors), and anemia. Finally, cirrhosis may be clinically silent, discovered only at autopsy or when stress such as infection or trauma tips the balance toward hepatic insufficiency. In chronic alcoholics, alcohol may become a major caloric source in the diet, displacing other nutrients and leading to malnutrition and vitamin deficiencies (e.g., thiamine and vitamin B_{12}). This is compounded by impaired digestive function, primarily related to chronic gastric and intestinal mucosal damage, and pancreatitis.

The long-term outlook for alcoholics with liver disease is variable. The most important aspect of treatment is abstinence from alcohol. Five-year survival approaches 90% in abstainers who are free of jaundice, ascites, or hematemesis but drops to 50% to 60% in those who continue to imbibe. In the end-stage alcoholic, the immediate causes of death are (1) hepatic failure, (2) a massive gastrointestinal hemorrhage, (3) an intercurrent infection (to which these individuals are predisposed), (4) hepatorenal syndrome after a bout of alcoholic hepatitis, and (5) hepatocellular carcinoma in 3% to 6% of cases.

Drug-Induced Liver Disease

Drug-induced liver disease is a common condition that may present as a mild reaction or, much more seriously, as acute liver failure. A large number of drugs and chemicals can produce liver injury (Table 16–6). Principles of

Table 16–6 Patterns of Injury in Drug- and Toxin-Induced Hepatic Injury

Pattern of Injury	Morphologic Findings	Examples of Associated Agents
Cholestatic	Bland hepatocellular cholestasis, without inflammation	Contraceptive and anabolic steroids; estrogen replacement therapy
Cholestatic hepatitis	Cholestasis with lobular necroinflammatory activity; may show bile duct destruction	Numerous antibiotics; phenothiazines
Hepatocellular necrosis	Spotty hepatocyte necrosis Submassive necrosis, zone 3 Massive necrosis	Methyldoya, phenytoin Acetaminophen, halothane Isoniazid, phenytoin
Steatosis	Macrovesicular	Ethanol, methotrexate, corticosteroids, total parenteral nutrition
Steatohepatitis	Microvesicular, Mallory bodies	Amiodarone, ethanol
Fibrosis and cirrhosis	Periportal and pericellular fibrosis	Methotrexate, isoniazid, enalapril
Granulomas	Noncaseating epithelioid granulomas	Sulfonamides, numerous other agents
Vascular lesions	Sinusoidal obstruction syndrome (veno-occlusive disease): obliteration of central veins Budd-Chiari syndrome Sinusoidal dilatation Peliosis hepatis: blood-filled cavities, not lined by endothelial cells	High-dose chemotherapy, bush teas Oral contraceptives Oral contraceptives, numerous other agents Anabolic steroids, tamoxifen
Neoplasms	Hepatic adenoma Hepatocellular carcinoma Cholangiocarcinoma Angiosarcoma	Oral contraceptives, anabolic steroids Thorotrast Thorotrast Thorotrast, vinyl chloride

From Washington K: Metabolic and toxic conditions of the liver. In Iacobuzio-Donahue CA, Montgomery EA (eds): Gastrointestinal and Liver Pathology. Philadelphia, Churchill Livingstone; 2005.

drug and toxic injury were discussed in Chapter 8. Here it suffices to recall that drug reactions may be classified as predictable (intrinsic) reactions or unpredictable (idiosyncratic) ones. Predictable drug reactions may occur in anyone who accumulates a sufficient dose. Unpredictable reactions depend on idiosyncrasies of the host, particularly the host's propensity to mount an immune response to the antigenic stimulus, and the rate at which the host metabolizes the agent. The injury may be immediate or take weeks to months to develop. Most important, *drug-induced chronic hepatitis is clinically and histologically indistinguishable from chronic viral hepatitis or autoimmune hepatitis, and hence serologic markers of viral infection are critical for making the distinction.* Among the hepatotoxic agents, predictable drug reactions are ascribed to acetaminophen, tetracycline, antineoplastic agents, *Amanita phalloides* toxin, carbon tetrachloride, and, to a certain extent, alcohol. Examples of drugs that can cause idiosyncratic reactions include chlorpromazine (an agent that causes cholestasis in patients who are slow to metabolize it to an innocuous by-product), halothane (which can cause a fatal immune-mediated hepatitis in some persons exposed to this anesthetic on several occasions), and other drugs such as sulfonamides, α-methyldopa, and allopurinol.

The mechanism of liver injury may be direct toxic damage to hepatocytes (e.g., acetaminophen, carbon tetrachloride, and mushroom toxins) but also involves a variable combination of toxicity and inflammation with immune-mediated hepatocyte destruction (see Chapter 8). Depending on the drug, the patterns of drug-induced liver injury may include one or more of the following: hepatocellular necrosis, cholestasis, steatosis, steatohepatitis, fibrosis, and vascular lesions. These patterns of injury are similar to those that occur in other types of liver disease, requiring careful analysis to confirm the cause of the injury.

Among drugs that may cause acute liver failure are acetaminophen, halothane, antituberculosis drugs (rifampin, isoniazid), antidepressant monoamine oxidase inhibitors, industrial chemicals such as carbon tetrachloride, and mushroom poisoning *(A. phalloides)*. The most common cause (~46% of cases of acute liver failure) is acetaminophen intoxication, and about 60% of these are a consequence of accidental overdosage. Inadvertent overdosage of acetaminophen is of particular concern in children and in individuals who chronically take prescription drugs containing acetaminophen plus an opiate.

Morphology

With massive hepatic necrosis, the distribution of liver destruction is extremely capricious: **the entire liver may be involved or only random areas are affected.** With massive loss of hepatic substance, the liver may shrink to 500 to 700 gm and become transformed into a limp, red organ covered by a wrinkled, overly large capsule. On transection (Fig. 16–19), necrotic areas have a muddy red, mushy appearance with blotchy bile staining. Microscopically, complete destruction of hepatocytes in contiguous lobules leaves only a collapsed reticulin framework and preserved portal tracts. There may be surprisingly little inflammatory reaction (Fig. 16–20). Alternatively, with survival for several days there is a massive influx of inflammatory cells to begin the clean-up process.

Patient survival for more than a week permits regeneration of surviving hepatocytes. Regeneration is initially in the form of strings of ductular structures, which mature into hepatocytes. If the parenchymal framework is preserved, regeneration is orderly and native liver architecture is restored. With more massive destruction of confluent lobules, regeneration is disorderly, yielding nodular masses of liver cells. Scarring may occur in patients with a protracted course of submassive or patchy necrosis, representing a route for developing so-called macronodular cirrhosis, as noted earlier.

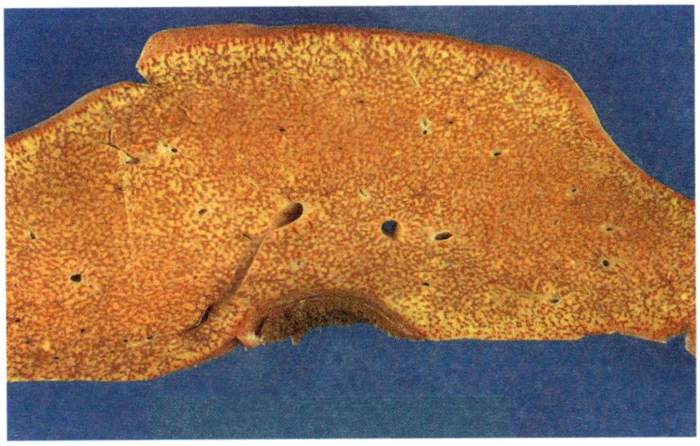

Figure 16–19

Massive necrosis, cut section of liver. The liver is small (700 gm), bile stained, soft, and congested. (Courtesy of Dr. Matthew Yeh, University of Washington, Seattle, Washington.)

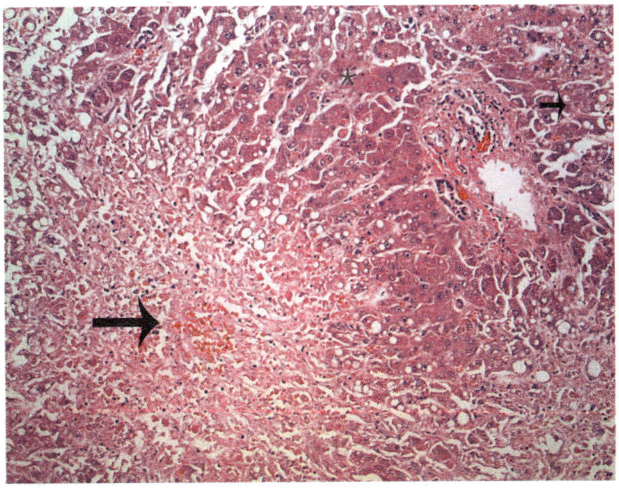

Figure 16–20

Hepatocellular necrosis caused by acetaminophen overdose. Confluent necrosis is seen in the perivenular region (zone 3; *large arrow*). There is little inflammation. The residual normal tissue is indicated by the *asterisk*. (Courtesy of Dr. Matthew Yeh, University of Washington, Seattle, Washington.)

SUMMARY

Alcohol and Drug-Induced Liver Disease

- Alcoholic liver disease has three main components: hepatic steatosis, alcoholic hepatitis, and cirrhosis; these conditions do not necessarily evolve as a continuum.
- Consumption of 50–60 gm/day of alcohol is considered to be the threshold for the development of alcoholic liver disease.
- It may take 10 to 15 years of drinking for the development of cirrhosis, which occurs only in a small proportion of chronic alcoholics; alcoholic cirrhosis has the same morphologic and clinical features as cirrhosis caused by viral hepatitis.
- The multiple pathologic effects of alcohol include changes in lipid metabolism and decreased export of lipoproteins, and cell injury caused by reactive oxygen species and cytokines.
- Drug-induced liver disease may cause multiple patterns of injury, including cholestasis, hepatitis, steatosis, necrosis and acute liver failure, sinusoidal obstruction, acute liver failure, and neoplasms.
- Drug-induced chronic hepatitis is clinically and morphologically similar to viral or autoimmune hepatitis.

METABOLIC AND INHERITED LIVER DISEASE

The most common metabolic liver disease is *nonalcoholic fatty liver disease* (NAFLD). Metabolic diseases attributable to inborn errors of metabolism include hemochromatosis, Wilson disease, and α_1-antitrypsin deficiency. These diseases may present in children or in adults. An additional set of diseases, referred to as neonatal cholestasis, appears in infancy and represents a diverse group of inherited and acquired conditions. We first consider NAFLD and then discuss inherited conditions.

Nonalcoholic Fatty Liver Disease

NAFLD is a common condition, which was first recognized in 1980. As the name denotes, NAFLD is a condition in which fatty liver and liver disease develop in individuals who do not drink alcohol. It may present as steatosis (fatty liver) or as *nonalcoholic steatohepatitis (NASH)*. The latter is similar to alcoholic hepatitis and involves hepatocyte destruction, parenchymal inflammation with neutrophils and mononuclear cells, and progressive pericellular fibrosis. NAFLD and NASH are most consistently associated with *insulin resistance*. Other key associated variables are:

- Type 2 diabetes (or family history)
- Obesity (body mass index >30 kg/m^2 in Caucasians and >25 kg/m^2 in Asians)
- Dyslipidemia (hypertriglyceridemia, low high-density lipoprotein cholesterol, high low-density lipoprotein cholesterol)

Pathogenesis and Clinical Features. The combination of insulin resistance with the conditions listed above is known as the *metabolic syndrome*. The presence of type 2 diabetes and obesity are the best predictors of severe fibrosis and disease progression. Insulin resistance results in the accumulation of triglycerides in hepatocytes by at least three mechanisms: (1) impaired oxidation of fatty acids, (2) increased synthesis and uptake of fatty acids, and (3) decrease hepatic secretion of very-low-density lipoprotein cholesterol. Fat-laden hepatocytes are highly sensitive to lipid peroxidation products generated by oxidative stress, which can damage mitochondrial and plasma membranes, causing apoptosis. Either as a consequence of oxidative stress or through release from visceral adipose tissue, levels of TNF, IL-6, and of the MCP-1 chemokine increase, contributing to liver damage and inflammation. The effects of these cytokines are opposed by adiponectin, which is produced by fat tissue.

NAFLD is the most common cause of incidental elevation of serum transaminases. Most persons with steatosis are asymptomatic; patients with NASH or more advanced NAFLD may also be asymptomatic, but some may have fatigue, malaise, right upper quadrant discomfort, or more severe symptoms of chronic liver disease. Liver biopsy is required for diagnosis. Fortunately, the frequency of progression from steatosis to NASH, and from NASH to cirrhosis, seems to be low. Nevertheless, NAFLD is considered as a significant contributor to the group of patients with "cryptogenic" cirrhosis. Present therapy of NAFLD is directed toward obesity reduction and improvement of insulin resistance. Adiponectins are being investigated as potential therapeutic agents for the treatment of persons with NASH/NAFLD.

Inherited Metabolic Diseases

Although there are a relatively large number of inherited metabolic liver diseases, in this section we discuss only some common and selected conditions. They include hemochromatosis, Wilson disease, α_1-antitrypsin deficiency, neonatal cholestasis, and Reye syndrome.

Hemochromatosis

Hereditary hemochromatosis refers to genetic disorders characterized by the excessive accumulation of body iron, most of which is deposited in the parenchymal organs such as the liver and pancreas. There are at least four genetic variants of hereditary hemochromatosis. The most common form is an autosomal recessive disease of adult onset caused by mutations in the *HFE* gene. Acquired forms of iron accumulation from known sources of excess iron are called *secondary iron overload*. Among the most important are multiple transfusions, ineffective erythropoiesis (as in β-thalassemia and sideroblastic anemia), and increased iron intake (Bantu siderosis). Chronic liver disease can also cause iron accumulation.

As discussed in Chapter 12, the total body iron pool ranges from 2 to 6 gm in normal adults; about 0.5 gm is stored in the liver, 98% of which is in hepatocytes. In hereditary hemochromatosis, iron accumulates over the lifetime of an individual from excessive intestinal absorption. Total iron accumulation may exceed 50 gm, over one-third of which accumulates in the liver. Fully developed cases show (1) cirrhosis (all patients), (2) diabetes mellitus (75% to 80% of patients), and (3) skin pigmentation (75% to 80%).

Pathogenesis. It may be recalled that the total body content of iron is tightly regulated, whereby the limited daily losses of iron are matched by gastrointestinal absorption since there is no excretory pathway for excess absorbed iron. *In hereditary hemochromatosis there is a defect in the regulation of intestinal absorption of dietary iron, leading to net iron accumulation of 0.5 to 1.0 gm/year.* The hereditary hemochromatosis gene, responsible for the most common form of this disorder, is called *HFE*. It is located on the short arm of chromosome 6 close to the human leukocyte antigen (HLA) gene complex. It encodes a protein that is similar in structure to MHC class I proteins. The role of HFE in regulating iron uptake is complex and not fully understood. It appears that HFE and the other genes involved in less common forms of hereditary hemochromatosis all regulate the levels of *hepcidin,* the iron hormone produced by the liver. Hepicidin normally down-regulates the efflux of iron from the intestines and macrophages into the plasma and inhibits iron absorption. When hepcidin levels are reduced there is increased iron absorption. Mice in whom the hepcidin gene is deleted develop iron overload resembling hemochromatosis, and mice that overexpress hepicidin develop severe iron deficiency, thus establishing the central role of hepcidin in regulating iron absorption. As might be expected, hepicidin levels are reduced in all currently known genetic forms of hemochromatosis. The interconnections between function of these various genes and hepcidin synthesis are still being elucidated.

There are two common mutations in the *HFE* gene associated with hemochromatosis. The first is a mutation at nucleotide 845 that results in a tyrosine substitution for cysteine at amino acid 282 (C282Y). The second mutation results in an aspartate substitution for histidine at amino acid 63 (H63D). In Caucasian populations of North European descent, the carrier frequency of the C282Y mutation is 1 in 70 and of homozygosity is 1 in 200. Approximately 80% of hemochromatosis patients are homozygous for the C282Y mutation and have the highest incidence of iron accumulation. Compound heterozygotes for the C282Y/H63D mutation or homozygotes for the H63D mutation make up about 10% of hereditary hemochromatosis patients. The remainder comprise variants of hereditary hemochromatosis that do not involve the *HFE* gene.

Hereditary hemochromatosis manifests typically after 20 gm of storage iron has accumulated. Regardless of source, excessive iron seems to be directly toxic to tissues by the following mechanisms: (1) lipid peroxidation by iron-catalyzed free-radical reactions, (2) stimulation of collagen formation, and (3) direct interactions of iron with DNA. Whatever the actions of iron, they may be reversible, with the exception of nonlethal DNA damage.

Morphology

The morphologic changes in hereditary hemochromatosis are characterized principally by (1) the **deposition of hemosiderin** in the following organs (in decreasing order of severity): liver, pancreas, myocardium, pituitary, adrenal, thyroid and parathyroid glands, joints, and skin; (2) **cirrhosis;** and (3) **pancreatic fibrosis.** In the liver, iron becomes evident first as golden-yellow hemosiderin granules in the cytoplasm of periportal hepatocytes, which stain blue with the Prussian blue stain (Fig. 16–21). With increasing iron load, there is progressive involvement of the rest of the lobule, along with bile duct epithelium and Kupffer cell pigmentation. Iron is a direct hepatotoxin, and inflammation is characteristically absent. At this stage the liver is typically slightly larger than normal, dense, and chocolate brown. Fibrous septa develop slowly, leading ultimately to a micronodular pattern of cirrhosis in an intensely pigmented liver.

In normal individuals the iron content of unfixed liver tissue is less than 1000 μg/gm dry weight. Adult patients with hereditary hemochromatosis exhibit over 10,000 μg/gm dry weight of iron; hepatic iron concentrations in excess of 22,000 μg/gm dry weight are associated with the development of fibrosis and cirrhosis.

The **pancreas** becomes intensely pigmented, has diffuse interstitial fibrosis, and may show some parenchymal atrophy. Hemosiderin is found in the acinar and the islet cells and sometimes in the interstitial fibrous stroma. The **heart** is often enlarged and has hemosiderin granules within the myocardial fibers. The pigmentation may induce a striking brown coloration of the myocardium. A delicate interstitial fibrosis may appear. Although **skin** pigmentation is partially attributable to hemosiderin deposition in dermal macrophages and fibroblasts, most of the coloration results from increased epidermal melanin production. The combination of these pigments renders the skin slate-gray. With hemosiderin deposition in the **joint synovial linings,** an acute synovitis may develop. There is also excessive deposition of calcium pyrophosphate, which damages the articular cartilage and sometimes produces disabling polyarthritis, referred to as pseudogout. The **testes** may be small and atrophic but are usually not discolored.

Clinical Features. Males predominate (ratio of 5 to 7:1) with slightly earlier clinical presentation, partly because physiologic iron loss (menstruation, pregnancy) retards iron accumulation in women. In the most common forms, caused by *HFE* mutations, symptoms usually first appear in the fifth to sixth decades of life. The principal manifestations include hepatomegaly, abdominal pain, skin pigmentation (particularly in sun-exposed areas), deranged glucose homeostasis or frank diabetes mellitus from destruction of pancreatic islets, cardiac dysfunction (arrhythmias, cardiomyopathy), and atypical arthritis. In some individuals the presenting complaint is amenorrhea in women and loss of libido and impotence in men. The classic clinical triad of cirrhosis with hepatomegaly, skin pigmentation, and diabetes mellitus may not develop until late in the course of the disease. Death may result from cirrhosis, hepatocellular carcinoma, or cardiac

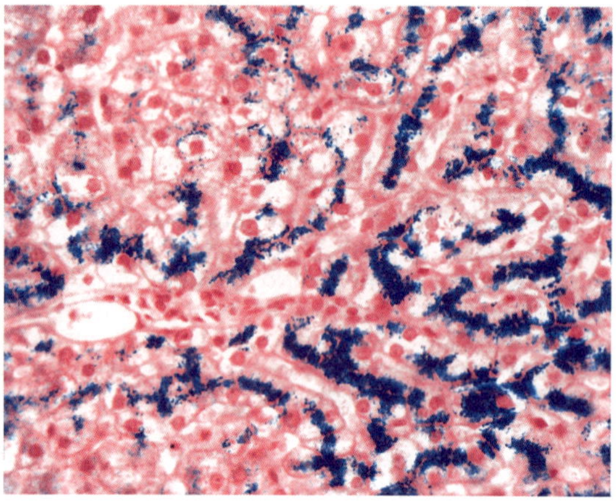

Figure 16–21

Hereditary hemochromatosis. In this Prussian blue–stained histologic section hepatocellular iron appears blue. The parenchymal architecture is normal.

disease. Treatment of iron overload does not remove the risk for development of hepatocellular carcinoma, because of the oxidative damage of DNA produced by iron. The risk of hepatocellular carcinoma development in patients with hemochromatosis is 200-fold higher than in normal populations.

Fortunately, hereditary hemochromatosis can be diagnosed long before irreversible tissue damage has occurred. Screening involves demonstration of very high levels of serum iron and ferritin, exclusion of secondary causes of iron overload, and liver biopsy if indicated. Also important is screening of family members of probands for the causative mutations. The natural course of the disease can be substantially altered by a variety of interventions, mainly phlebotomy and the use of iron chelators to drain off the excess iron. Patients diagnosed in the subclinical, precirrhotic stage and treated by regular phlebotomy have a normal life expectancy. Heterozygotes may show a mild increase in iron absorption and accumulation.

Wilson Disease

This autosomal recessive disorder of copper metabolism is characterized by the accumulation of toxic levels of copper in many tissues and organs, principally the liver, brain, and eye. The genetic defect responsible for Wilson disease is a mutation in *ATP7B*. This gene, located on chromosome 13, encodes an ATPase metal ion transporter that localizes to the Golgi region of hepatocytes. More than 80 mutations have been detected. The gene for Wilson disease has a frequency of 1:200. The incidence of this disease is approximately 1:30,000; thus, it is much less common than hereditary hemochromatosis.

Normal copper physiology involves (1) absorption of ingested copper (2–5 mg/day); (2) plasma transport in complex with albumin; (3) hepatocellular uptake, followed by incorporation into an α_2-globulin to form ceruloplasmin; (4) secretion of ceruloplasmin into plasma, where it accounts for 90% to 95% of plasma copper; and (5) hepatic uptake of desialylated, senescent ceruloplasmin from the plasma, followed by lysosomal degradation and secretion of free copper into bile. In Wilson disease, the initial steps of copper absorption and transport to the liver are normal. However, absorbed copper fails to enter the circulation in the form of ceruloplasmin, and biliary excretion of copper is markedly diminished. Defective function of *ATP7B* leads to failure to excrete copper into bile, *the primary route for copper elimination from the body.* The defect apparently also inhibits secretion of ceruloplasmin into the plasma. Copper thus accumulates progressively in the liver, apparently causing toxic liver injury by (1) promoting the formation of free radicals, (2) binding to sulfhydryl groups of cellular proteins, and (3) displacing other metals in hepatic metalloenzymes. Usually by 5 years of age, copper that is not ceruloplasmin bound spills over into the circulation, causing hemolysis and pathologic changes at other sites, such as brain, cornea, kidneys, bones, joints, and parathyroid glands. Concomitantly, urinary excretion of copper increases markedly. *The biochemical diagnosis of Wilson* disease is based on a decrease in serum ceruloplasmin, *increase in hepatic copper content, and increase in urinary excretion of copper.*

Morphology

The liver often bears the brunt of injury in Wilson disease, with hepatic changes ranging from relatively minor to massive damage. **Fatty change** may be mild to moderate, with vacuolated nuclei (glycogen or water) and occasional hepatocyte focal necrosis. An **acute hepatitis** can mimic acute viral hepatitis, save possibly for the accompanying fatty change. A **chronic hepatitis** resembles chronic hepatitis of viral, drug, or alcoholic origin but may show such distinguishing features as fatty change, vacuolated nuclei, and Mallory bodies. With progression of chronic hepatitis, **cirrhosis** develops. **Massive liver necrosis** is a rare manifestation that is indistinguishable from that caused by viruses or drugs. Excess copper deposition can often be demonstrated by special stains (e.g., rhodanine stain for copper, orcein stain for copper-associated protein). Because copper also accumulates in chronic obstructive cholestasis, and because histology cannot reliably distinguish Wilson disease from viral- and drug-induced hepatitis, demonstration of hepatic copper content in excess of 250 μg/gm dry weight is most helpful for making a diagnosis.

In the **brain,** toxic injury primarily affects the basal ganglia, particularly the putamen, which demonstrates atrophy and even cavitation. Nearly all patients with neurologic involvement develop **eye lesions** called **Kayser-Fleischer rings** (green to brown deposits of copper in Descemet membrane in the limbus of the cornea)—hence the alternative designation of this condition as hepatolenticular degeneration.

Clinical Features. The age at onset and the clinical presentation of Wilson disease are extremely variable, but the disorder rarely manifests before 6 years of age. The most common presentation is acute or chronic liver disease. Neuropsychiatric manifestations, including mild behavioral changes, frank psychosis, or a Parkinson disease–like syndrome, are the initial features in most of the remaining cases. Demonstration of Kayser-Fleischer rings or markedly elevated hepatic copper levels in a person with a low serum ceruloplasmin value strongly favor the diagnosis. Early recognition and long-term copper chelation therapy (as with D-penicillamine) have dramatically altered the usual progressive downhill course.

α_1-Antitrypsin (AAT) Deficiency

AAT deficiency is an autosomal recessive disorder marked by abnormally low serum levels of this protease inhibitor. The major function of AAT is the inhibition of proteases, particularly neutrophil elastase released at sites of inflammation. AAT deficiency leads to pulmonary emphysema, because a relative lack of this protein permits the unrestrained activity of tissue-destructive proteases (Chapter 13).

AAT is a small (394–amino acid) plasma glycoprotein synthesized predominantly by hepatocytes. The *AAT* gene, located on human chromosome 14, is very polymorphic, and at least 75 forms have been identified. Most allelic variants produce normal or mildly reduced levels of serum AAT. However, homozygotes for the Z allele (*PiZZ* genotype) have circulating AAT levels that are only 10% of normal levels. Expression of *AAT* alleles is autosomal codominant, and consequently *PiMZ* heterozygotes have intermediate plasma levels of AAT. The PiZ polypeptide contains a single amino acid substitution that results in misfolding of the nascent polypeptide in the hepatocyte endoplasmic reticulum. Because the mutant protein cannot be secreted by the hepatocyte, it accumulates in the endoplasmic reticulum and undergoes excessive lysosomal degradation. Curiously, all individuals with the *PiZZ* genotype accumulate AAT in the liver, but only 8% to 20% develop significant liver damage. This may be related to a genetic tendency that causes susceptible individuals to be less able to degrade accumulated AAT protein within hepatocytes.

Morphology

Hepatocytes in AAT deficiency contain round to oval cytoplasmic **globular inclusions** of retained AAT, which are strongly positive in a periodic acid–Schiff stain (Fig. 16–22). By electron microscopy they lie within smooth, and sometimes rough, endoplasmic reticulum. Hepatic injury associated with PiZZ homozygosity may range from marked **cholestasis** with **hepatocyte necrosis** in newborns, to **childhood cirrhosis,** or to a smoldering chronic inflammatory hepatitis or cirrhosis that becomes apparent only late in life.

Clinical Course. Among newborns with AAT deficiency, 10% to 20% show cholestasis. In older children, adolescents, and adults, presenting symptoms may be related to chronic hepatitis, cirrhosis, or pulmonary disease. The disease may remain silent until cirrhosis appears in middle to later life. Hepatocellular carcinoma develops in 2% to 3% of *PiZZ* adults, usually, but not always, in the setting of cirrhosis. The treatment and cure for the severe hepatic disease is orthotopic liver transplantation.

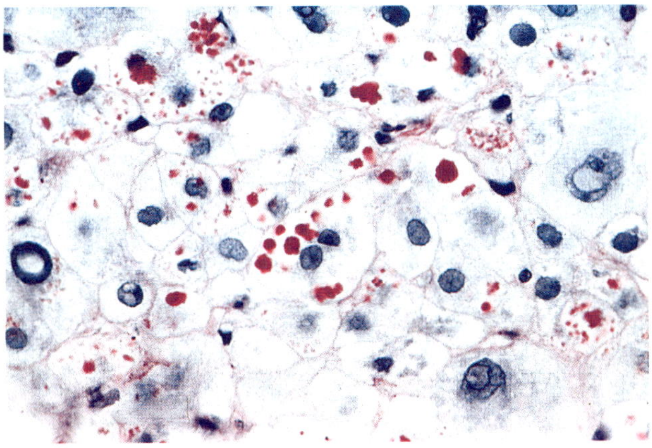

Figure 16–22

α_1-Antitrypsin deficiency. Periodic acid–Schiff stain of liver, highlighting the characteristic red cytoplasmic granules. (Courtesy of Dr. I. Wanless, Toronto General Hospital, Ontario, Canada.)

Neonatal Cholestasis

As mentioned earlier, mild transient elevations in serum unconjugated bilirubin are common in normal newborns. Prolonged conjugated hyperbilirubinemia in the newborn, termed *neonatal cholestasis,* affects approximately 1 in 2500 live births. The major causes are extrahepatic biliary atresia, discussed later, and a variety of other disorders collectively referred to as *neonatal hepatitis.* Neonatal hepatitis is not a specific entity, nor are the disorders necessarily inflammatory. Instead, the finding of "neonatal cholestasis" should evoke a diligent search for recognizable toxic, metabolic, and infectious liver diseases. *Idiopathic neonatal hepatitis* constitutes as many as 50% of cases of neonatal hepatitis.

Clinical presentation of infants with any form of neonatal cholestasis is fairly typical, with jaundice, dark urine, light or acholic stools, and hepatomegaly. Variable degrees of hepatic synthetic dysfunction, such as hypoprothrombinemia, may be present. Differentiation between the two most common causes of neonatal cholestasis (extrahepatic atresia and idiopathic hepatitis) assumes great importance, because definitive treatment of biliary atresia requires surgical intervention, whereas surgery may adversely affect the clinical course of a child with idiopathic neonatal hepatitis. Fortunately, discrimination between these diseases can be made in about 90% of cases using clinical data and liver biopsy.

Reye Syndrome

Reye syndrome is a rare disease characterized by fatty change in the liver and encephalopathy. The most severe forms are fatal. It primarily affects children younger than 4 years of age, typically developing 3 to 5 days after a viral illness. The onset is heralded by pernicious vomiting and is accompanied by irritability or lethargy and hepatomegaly. Serum bilirubin, ammonia, and aminotransferase levels are essentially normal at this time. Although most patients recover, about 25% progress to coma, accompanied by elevations in the serum levels of bilirubin, aminotransferases, and particularly ammonia.

Death occurs from progressive neurologic deterioration or liver failure. Survivors of more serious illness may be left with permanent neurologic impairments.

The pathogenesis of Reye syndrome involves a generalized loss of mitochondrial function. Reye syndrome is now recognized as the prototype of a wide variety of conditions known as *"mitochondrial hepatopathies."* Reye syndrome has been associated with aspirin administration during viral illnesses, but there is no evidence that salicylates play a causal role in this disorder. Although the case rate for classic Reye syndrome in the United States is less than 1 per million per year, this disorder and "Reye-like syndromes" must be considered in the differential diagnosis of postviral disorders in children.

Morphology

The key pathologic finding in the **liver** is microvesicular steatosis. Electron microscopy of hepatocellular mitochondria reveals pleomorphic enlargement and electron lucency of the matrices, with disruption of cristae and loss of dense bodies. In the **brain,** cerebral edema is usually present. Astrocytes are swollen and mitochondrial changes similar to those seen in the liver may develop. Inflammation is notably absent, as is any evidence of viral infection. **Skeletal muscles, kidneys,** and **heart** may also reveal microvesicular fatty change and mitochondrial alterations, though more subtle than those of the liver.

SUMMARY

Metabolic and Inherited Liver Disease

- The most common metabolic disorder is nonalcoholic fatty liver disease, which is associated with the metabolic syndrome and obesity.
- Nonalcoholic fatty liver disease may develop from steatosis that progresses to nonalcoholic steatohepatitis and finally to cirrhosis.
- The inherited and childhood metabolic diseases include hemochromatosis, Wilson disease, α_1-antitrypsin deficiency, neonatal cholestasis and Reye syndrome.
- Hemochromatosis is characterized by accumulation of iron in liver and pancreas. It is caused by a mutation in the *HFE* gene, whose product is involved in intestinal iron uptake.
- Wilson disease is the result of accumulation of copper in the liver, brain, and eyes; it is caused by a mutation in the metal ion transporter *ATP7B*.
- α_1-antitrypsin deficiency is caused by the low production of $\alpha_1$antitrypsin in individuals of *PiZZ* genotype; the main consequences are pulmonary emphysema caused by increased elastase activity, and liver injury caused by the accumulation of abnormal α_1-antitrypsin.

DISEASES OF THE INTRAHEPATIC BILIARY TRACT

Biliary tract disorders cannot be neatly divided into intrahepatic or extrahepatic, particularly because diseases may affect both intra- and extrahepatic segments, and extrahepatic biliary disorders may cause secondary changes within the liver. In addition, the biliary tree is frequently damaged as part of a more general liver disease, as in drug toxicity, viral hepatitis, and transplantation (both orthotopic liver transplantation and graft-versus-host disease after bone marrow transplantation). With these caveats, consideration will now be given to two disorders of bile ducts, primary biliary cirrhosis and primary sclerosing cholangitis, that culminate in cirrhosis (Table 16–7). Primary biliary cirrhosis is characterized by destruction of intrahepatic bile ducts, and primary sclerosing cholangitis involves extrahepatic and large intrahepatic bile ducts. Bile duct disorders initiated primarily in the extrahepatic segment are discussed in the last section of this chapter.

Primary Biliary Cirrhosis

Primary biliary cirrhosis is a chronic, progressive, and often fatal cholestatic liver disease, characterized by the destruction of intrahepatic bile ducts, portal inflammation and scarring, and the eventual development of cirrhosis and liver failure over years to decades. *The primary feature of this disease is a nonsuppurative destruction of small and medium-sized intrahepatic bile ducts;* cirrhosis appears only late in the course. In the early lesions there is a dense lymphocyte/plasma cell infiltrate around small bile ducts in portal tracts, and granulomatous lesions may also appear. Primary biliary cirrhosis is primarily a disease of middle-aged women, with an age at onset between 20 and 80 years and peak incidence between 40 and 50 years of age.

Pathogenesis and Clinical Course. More than 90% of persons with primary biliary cirrhosis have high titers of antimitochondrial antibodies. These antibodies are directed to specific domains of mitochondrial acid dehydrogenase enzymes. Despite their characterization, it is still unclear why the immune response is focused on this enzyme domain, and why intrahepatic bile ducts are the targets for these antibodies. Recent evidence suggests that exposure to certain xenobiotics may modify mitochondrial proteins leading to a decrease of immunologic tolerance to some of these proteins. Nevertheless, it is not known whether exposure to xenobiotics has a role in the pathogenesis of primary biliary cirrhosis.

The onset of primary biliary cirrhosis is insidious, usually presenting as pruritus; jaundice develops late. Over a period of two or more decades, the individuals develop hepatic decompensation, including portal hypertension with variceal bleeding, and hepatic encephalopathy. *Serum alkaline phosphatase and cholesterol levels are almost always elevated; hyperbilirubinemia is a late development and usually signifies incipient hepatic decompensation.* Associated extrahepatic conditions include the sicca complex of dry eyes and mouth (Sjögren

Table 16–7 Main Features of Primary Biliary Cirrhosis and Primary Sclerosing Cholangitis

Parameter	Primary Biliary Cirrhosis	Primary Sclerosing Cholangitis
Age	Median age 50 years (30–70)	Median age 30 years
Gender	90% female	70% male
Clinical course	Progressive	Unpredictable but progressive
Associated conditions	Sjögren syndrome (70%) Scleroderma (5%) Thyroid disease (20%)	Inflammatory bowel disease (70%) Pancreatitis (≤25%) Idiopathic fibrosing diseases (retroperitoneal fibrosis)
Serology	95% AMA positive 20% ANA positive 60% ANCA positive	0% to 5% AMA positive (low titer) 6% ANA positive 82% ANCA positive
Radiology	Normal	Strictures and beading of large bile ducts; pruning of smaller ducts
Duct lesion	Florid duct lesion; loss of small ducts	Concentric periductal fibrosis; loss of small ducts

AMA, antimitochondrial antibody; ANA, antinuclear antibody; ANCA, antineutrophil cytoplasmic antibody.

syndrome), scleroderma, thyroiditis, rheumatoid arthritis, Raynaud phenomenon, membranous glomerulonephritis, and celiac disease.

Primary Sclerosing Cholangitis

Primary sclerosing cholangitis is a chronic cholestatic disorder, characterized by progressive fibrosis and destruction of extrahepatic and large intrahepatic bile ducts. Because the changes in the ducts are patchy, retrograde cholangiography shows a characteristic "beading" of the contrast medium in the affected segments of the biliary tree. The large bile ducts show periductal fibrosis that obliterates the lumen, leaving a solid cord scar with few inflammatory cells. Primary sclerosing cholangitis is commonly seen in association with inflammatory bowel disease (Chapter 15), particularly chronic ulcerative colitis, which coexists in approximately 70% of individuals. Conversely, the prevalence of primary sclerosing cholangitis in persons with ulcerative colitis is about 4%. The disorder tends to occur in the third through fifth decades, most often after development of inflammatory bowel disease. Males are affected more often than females in a ratio of 2:1.

Pathogenesis and Clinical Course. The cause of primary sclerosing cholangitis is unknown. The association with ulcerative colitis, linkage with certain *HLA-DR* alleles, and presence of antinuclear cytoplasmic antibodies with a perinuclear localization (Chapter 10) in 80% of cases all suggest that this is an immunologically mediated disease. Antimitochondrial antibodies are present in a minority of patients. Symptoms at presentation include progressive fatigue, pruritus, and jaundice. Asymptomatic patients may come to attention only on the basis of a persistent elevation of serum alkaline phosphatase. Severely afflicted persons show symptoms associated with chronic liver disease, including weight loss, ascites, variceal bleeding, and encephalopathy. Primary sclerosing cholangitis generally has a protracted course over many years. Cholangiocarcinoma may develop in 10% to 15% of individuals with primary sclerosing cholangitis, with a median time of 5 years from diagnosis. There is no effective therapy for primary sclerosing cholangitis, and the disease has become an important indication for liver transplantation.

Morphology

In all primary biliary cirrhosis and primary sclerosing cholangitis, the end-stage liver shows extraordinary yellow-green pigmentation, associated with marked icteric discoloration of body tissues and fluids. On cut surface, the liver is hard, with a finely granular appearance (Fig. 16–23). Interlobular bile ducts are absent in the end stage of **primary biliary cirrhosis.** However, the morphology of this disease is most revealing in the precirrhotic stage. Interlobular bile ducts are destroyed by inflammation (the **florid duct lesion**), featuring intraepithelial infiltration of lymphocytes and accompanying granulomatous inflammation. There is a dense portal tract infiltrate of lymphocytes, macrophages, plasma cells, and occasional eosinophils (Fig. 16–24). The obstruction to intrahepatic bile flow leads to upstream bile ductular proliferation (Fig. 16–25), inflammation and necrosis of the adjacent periportal hepatic parenchyma, and generalized cholestasis. Over years to decades, relentless portal tract scarring and bridging fibrosis leads to cirrhosis.

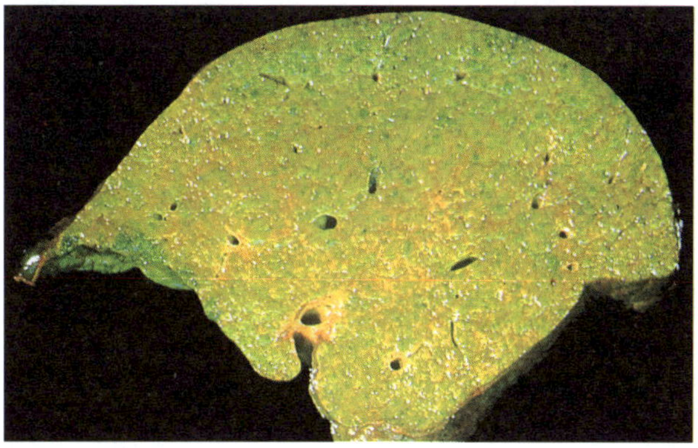

Figure 16–23

Primary biliary cirrhosis. This sagittal section through the liver demonstrates the fine nodularity and bile staining of end-stage primary biliary cirrhosis.

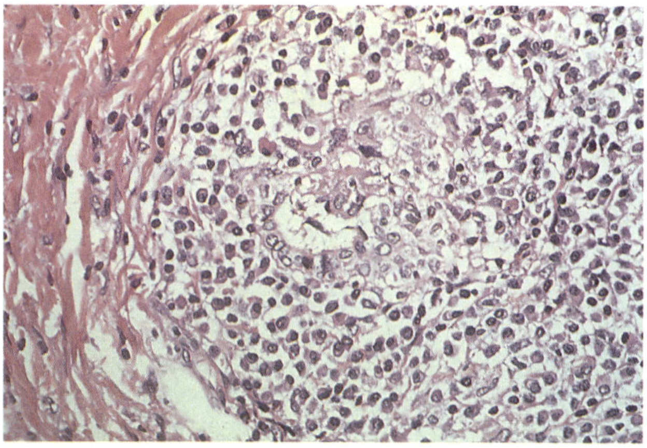

Figure 16–24

Primary biliary cirrhosis. A portal tract is markedly expanded by an infiltrate of lymphocytes and plasma cells. Note the granulomatous reaction to a bile duct undergoing destruction (florid duct lesion).

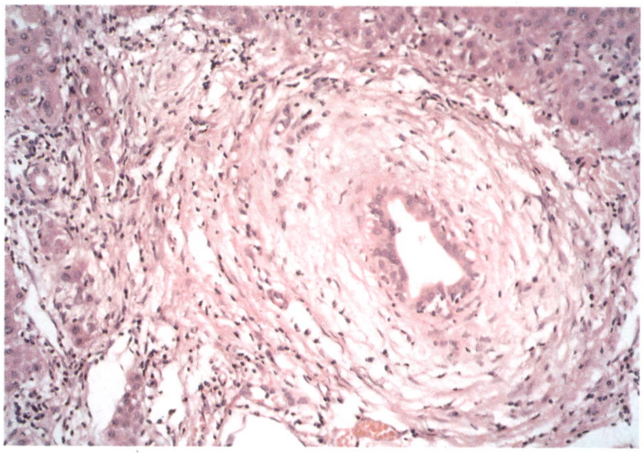

Figure 16–26

Primary sclerosing cholangitis. A bile duct undergoing degeneration is entrapped in a dense, "onion-skin" concentric scar.

The characteristic feature of **primary sclerosing cholangitis** is a fibrosing cholangitis of bile ducts. Specifically, affected portal tracts show concentric periductal onion-skin fibrosis and a modest lymphocytic infiltrate (Fig. 16–26). Progressive atrophy of the bile duct epithelium leads to obliteration of the lumen, leaving behind a solid, cordlike fibrous scar. In between areas of progressive stricture, bile ducts become ectatic and inflamed, presumably the result of down-stream obstruction. As the disease progresses over years, the entire liver becomes markedly cholestatic and fibrotic. Ultimately, biliary cirrhosis develops, much like that seen with primary and secondary biliary cirrhosis.

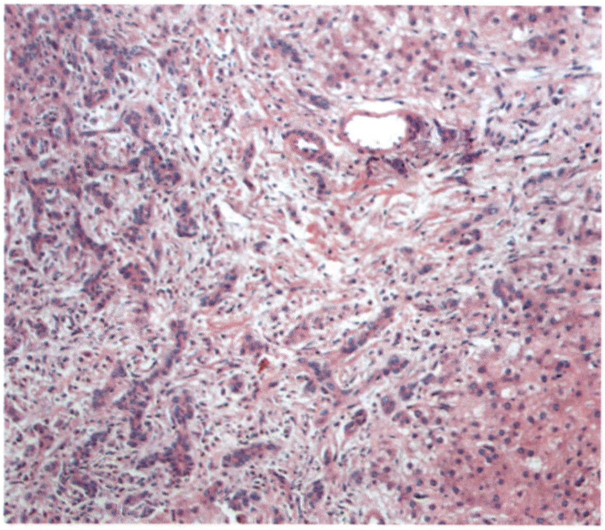

Figure 16–25

An example of ductular proliferation in a fibrotic septum. (Courtesy of Dr. Matthew Yeh, University of Washington, Seattle, Washington.)

CIRCULATORY DISORDERS

Given the enormous flow of blood through the liver, it is not surprising that circulatory disturbances have considerable impact on the liver. These disorders can be grouped according to whether blood flow into, through, or from the liver is impaired (Fig. 16–27).

Impaired Blood Flow into the Liver

Hepatic Artery Inflow

Liver infarcts are rare, thanks to the double blood supply to the liver. Interruption of the main hepatic artery does not always produce ischemic necrosis of the organ, because retrograde arterial flow through accessory vessels and the portal venous supply may sustain the liver parenchyma. The one exception is hepatic artery thrombosis in the transplanted liver, which generally leads to loss of the organ. Thrombosis or compression of an intrahepatic branch of the hepatic artery by polyarteritis nodosa (Chapter 10), embolism, neoplasia, or sepsis may result in a localized parenchymal infarct.

Portal Vein Obstruction and Thrombosis

Blockage of the portal vein may be insidious and well tolerated or may be a catastrophic and potentially lethal event; most cases fall somewhere in between. Occlusion of the portal vein or its major branches typically produces abdominal pain and, in most instances, ascites and other manifestations of portal hypertension, principally esophageal varices that are prone to rupture. The ascites, when present, is often massive and intractable. Acute impairment of visceral blood flow leads to profound congestion and bowel infarction. Extrahepatic portal vein obstruction may arise from the following:

- Peritoneal sepsis (e.g., acute diverticulitis or appendicitis leading to pylephlebitis in the splanchnic circulation)

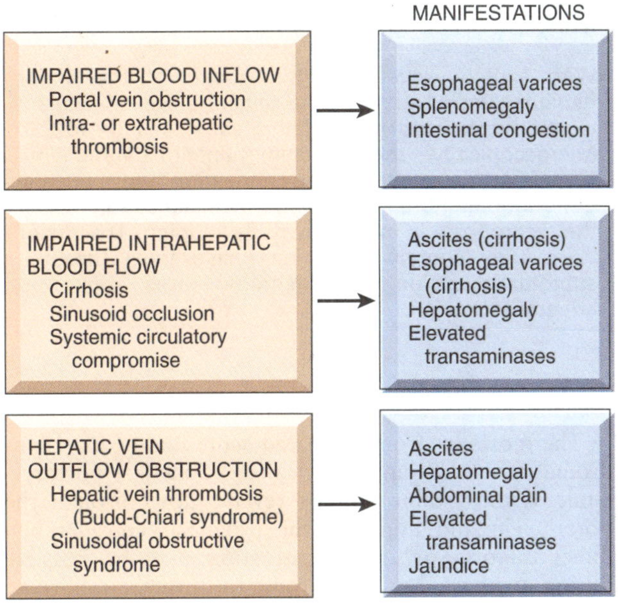

Figure 16–27

Hepatic circulatory disorders. The forms and clinical manifestations of compromised blood flow are contrasted.

- Pancreatitis that initiates splenic vein thrombosis, which propagates into the portal vein
- Thrombogenic diseases and postsurgical thromboses
- Vascular invasion by primary or secondary cancer in the liver that progressively occludes portal inflow to the liver; extensions of hepatocellular carcinoma can even occlude the main portal vein
- Banti syndrome, in which subclinical thrombosis of the portal vein (as from neonatal omphalitis or umbilical vein catheterization) produces a fibrotic, partially recanalized vascular channel presenting as splenomegaly or esophageal varices years after the occlusive event

Intrahepatic thrombosis of a portal vein radicle, when acute, does not cause ischemic infarction but instead results in a sharply demarcated area of red-blue discoloration (so-called *infarct of Zahn*). There is no necrosis, only hepatocellular atrophy and marked congestion in distended sinusoids. *Hepatoportal sclerosis* is a chronic, generally bland condition of progressive portal tract sclerosis leading to impaired portal vein inflow. In those instances in which a cause can be identified, it may be a myeloproliferative disorder with associated hypercoagulability, peritonitis, or exposure to arsenicals.

Impaired Blood Flow through the Liver

The most common intrahepatic cause of portal blood flow obstruction is cirrhosis, as was described earlier. In addition, physical occlusion of the sinusoids occurs in a small but important group of diseases. In sickle cell disease, the hepatic sinusoids may become packed with sickled erythrocytes, both free within the vascular space and erythrophagocytosed by Kupffer cells, leading to panlobular parenchymal necrosis. *Disseminated intravascular coagulation* may cause occlusion of sinusoids. This is usually inconsequential except for the periportal sinusoidal occlusion and parenchymal necrosis that may occur in the eclampsia of pregnancy. Subsequent suffusion of blood under the capsule may precipitate a fatal intra-abdominal hemorrhage.

Passive Congestion and Centrilobular Necrosis

These hepatic manifestations of systemic circulatory disorders constitute a morphologic continuum. Right-sided cardiac decompensation leads to passive congestion of the liver, and if persistent, can cause centrilobular necrosis, and perivenular fibrosis in the areas of necrosis. In most instances, the only clinical evidence of centrilobular necrosis is a small elevation of serum aminotransferase levels. The parenchymal damage may be sufficient to induce mild to moderate jaundice.

Morphology

In right-sided cardiac failure, the liver is slightly enlarged, tense, and cyanotic, with rounded edges. Microscopically, there is congestion of centrilobular sinusoids. With time, centrilobular hepatocytes become atrophic, resulting in markedly attenuated liver cell cords. An uncommon complication of sustained chronic severe congestive heart failure is so-called cardiac sclerosis. The pattern of liver fibrosis is distinctive, inasmuch as it is mostly centrilobular. The damage rarely fulfills the accepted criteria for the diagnosis of cirrhosis, but the historically sanctified term *cardiac cirrhosis* cannot easily be dislodged.

Left-sided cardiac failure or shock may lead to hepatic hypoperfusion and hypoxia. In this instance, hepatocytes in the central region of the lobule undergo ischemic necrosis. There is a sharp demarcation of viable hepatocytes in the periportal region versus necrotic hepatocytes in the centrilobular region of the parenchyma. The combination of left-sided hypoperfusion and right-sided retrograde congestion acts synergistically to generate a distinctive lesion, centrilobular hemorrhagic necrosis (Fig. 16–28). The liver takes on a variegated mottled appearance, reflecting hemorrhage and necrosis in the centrilobular regions, alternating with pale midzonal areas, known traditionally as the **"nutmeg" liver.**

Peliosis Hepatis

Sinusoidal dilation occurs in any condition in which efflux of hepatic blood is impeded. Peliosis hepatis is a rare condition in which the dilation is primary. It is most commonly associated with exposure to anabolic steroids and, rarely, oral contraceptives, and danazol. The pathogenesis is not known. Although clinical signs are generally absent even in advanced peliosis, potentially fatal intra-abdominal hemorrhage or hepatic failure may occur. Peliotic lesions usually disappear after cessation of drug treatment.

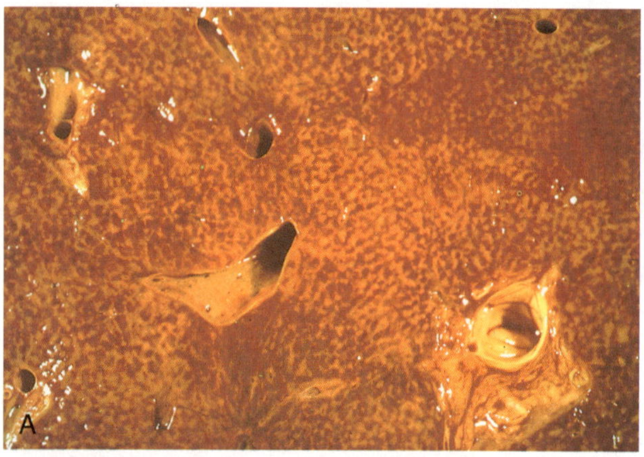

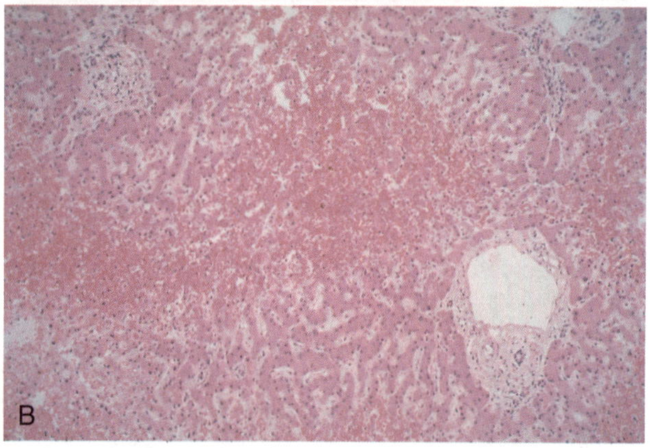

Figure 16–28

Centrilobular hemorrhagic necrosis (nutmeg liver). **A,** The cut liver section, in which major blood vessels are visible, is notable for a variegated mottled red appearance, representing hemorrhage in the centrilobular regions of the parenchyma. **B,** Microscopically, the centrilobular region is suffused with red blood cells, and hepatocytes are not readily visible. Portal tracts and the periportal parenchyma are intact.

Hepatic Vein Outflow Obstruction

Hepatic Vein Thrombosis (Budd-Chiari Syndrome)

The Budd-Chiari syndrome results from the thrombosis of two or more major hepatic veins and is characterized by hepatomegaly, weight gain, ascites, and abdominal pain. Hepatic vein thrombosis is associated with (in order of frequency) myeloproliferative disorders including polycythemia vera, pregnancy, the postpartum state, the use of oral contraceptives, paroxysmal nocturnal hemoglobinuria, and intra-abdominal cancers, particularly hepatocellular carcinoma. All these conditions produce thrombotic tendencies or, in the case of liver cancers, sluggish blood flow. Some cases are caused by mechanical obstruction to blood outflow, as by a massive intrahepatic abscess or parasitic cyst, or by obstruction of the inferior vena cava at the level of the hepatic veins by thrombus or tumor. About 10% of cases are idiopathic.

Morphology

With acutely developing thrombosis of the major hepatic veins or inferior vena cava, the liver is swollen, is red-purple, and has a tense capsule (Fig. 16–29). Microscopically, the affected hepatic parenchyma reveals severe centrilobular congestion and necrosis. Centrilobular fibrosis develops in instances in which the thrombosis is more slowly developing. The major veins may contain totally occlusive fresh thrombi, subtotal occlusion, or, in chronic cases, organized adherent thrombi.

The mortality from untreated acute Budd-Chiari syndrome is high. Prompt surgical creation of a portosystemic venous shunt permits reverse flow through the portal vein and improves the prognosis considerably; direct dilation of caval obstruction may be possible during angiography. The chronic form of the syndrome is far less grave, and more than two-thirds of the patients are alive after 5 years.

Sinusoidal Obstruction Syndrome

Originally described in Jamaican drinkers of bush-tea containing pyrrolizidine alkaloid, this condition was known as veno-occlusive disease. The new name indicates that sinusoidal obstruction syndrome is caused by toxic injury to sinusoidal endothelium. Damaged endothelial cells slough off and create emboli that block blood flow. Endothelial damage is accompanied by passage of red blood cell into the space of Disse, proliferation of stellate cells, and fibrosis of terminal branches of the hepatic vein (Fig. 16–30). Sinusoidal obstruction syndrome now occurs primarily in the first 20–30 days after bone marrow transplantation. The sinusoidal injury is believed to be caused by drugs such as cyclophosphamide, and by total body radiation, used in pre- or post-transplantation regimens. The incidence may approach 20% in recipients of allogeneic marrow transplants. The presentation of the disease varies from mild to severe. Severe sinusoidal obstruction syndrome that does not resolve after 3 months of treatment can cause death.

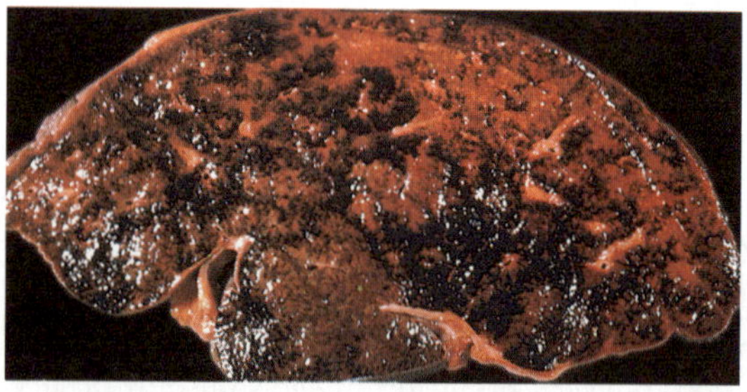

Figure 16–29

Budd-Chiari syndrome. Thrombosis of the major hepatic veins has caused extreme blood retention in the liver.

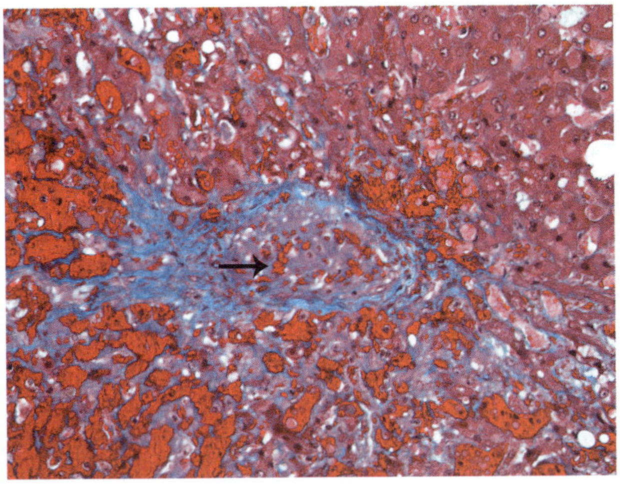

Figure 16–30

Sinusoidal obstruction syndrome (formerly known as veno-occlusive disease). A central vein is occluded by cells and newly formed collagen *(arrow)*. There is also fibrosis in the sinusoidal spaces. Fibrous tissue is stained *blue* by the Masson trichrome stain. (Courtesy of Dr. Matthew Yeh, University of Washington, Seattle, Washington.)

SUMMARY

Circulatory Disorders

- Circulatory disorders of the liver can be caused by impaired blood inflow, defects in intrahepatic blood flow, and obstruction of blood outflow.
- Portal vein obstruction by intra or extrahepatic thrombosis may cause portal hypertension, esophageal varices, and ascites.
- The most common cause of impaired intrahepatic blood flow is cirrhosis.
- Obstructions of blood outflow include hepatic vein thrombosis (Budd-Chiari syndrome) and sinusoidal obstruction syndrome, previously known as veno-occlusive disease.

TUMORS AND HEPATIC NODULES

The liver and lungs share the dubious distinction of being the visceral organs most often involved in the metastatic spread of cancers. Indeed, *the most common hepatic neoplasms are metastatic carcinomas*, with colon, lung, and breast heading the list as sites of the primary tumor. The incidence of *primary hepatic malignancies*, almost entirely constituted by *hepatocellular carcinomas* varies throughout the world, as discussed later. Two rare types of primary liver tumors are not discussed further: hepatoblastoma, a childhood hepatocellular tumor, and angiosarcoma, a tumor of blood vessels that is associated with exposure to vinylchloride and arsenic. Hepatic masses come to attention for a variety of reasons. They may generate epigastric fullness and discomfort or be detected by routine physical examination. Radiographic studies for other indications may pick up incidental liver masses. Here we discuss primary nodular and neoplastic lesions of the liver.

Hepatocellular Nodules

Solitary or multiple benign hepatocellular nodules may develop in the liver. These include lesions known as focal nodular hyperplasia, macroregenerative nodules, and dysplastic nodules.

- *Focal nodular hyperplasia* is a localized, well-demarcated but poorly encapsulated lesion, consisting of hyperplastic hepatocyte nodules with a central fibrous scar. The nodules appear in noncirrhotic livers and may reach up to many centimeters in diameter. Focal nodular hyperplasia, as the name indicates, is not a neoplasm but a nodular regeneration. It occurs in response to local vascular injury. It is usually an incidental finding, most commonly in women of reproductive age, and does not carry a risk for malignancy. In about 20% of cases, focal nodular hyperplasia coexists with hepatic cavernous hemangiomas (described below).
- *Macroregenerative* nodules appear in cirrhotic livers (Fig. 16–31). They are larger than surrounding cirrhotic nodules but do not display atypical features. Macroregenerative nodules contain more than one portal tract, have an intact reticulin framework, and do not seem to be precursors of malignant lesions.
- *Dysplastic nodules* are lesions larger than 1 mm in diameter that appear in cirrhotic livers. Hepatocytes in dysplastic nodules and in smaller lesions called dysplastic foci are highly proliferative and show atypical features such as crowding and pleomorphism. The dysplastic features can be of low or high grade. *High-grade dysplastic lesions are considered to be precursors of hepatocelluar cancers, are often monoclonal, and may contain chromosome aberrations similar to those*

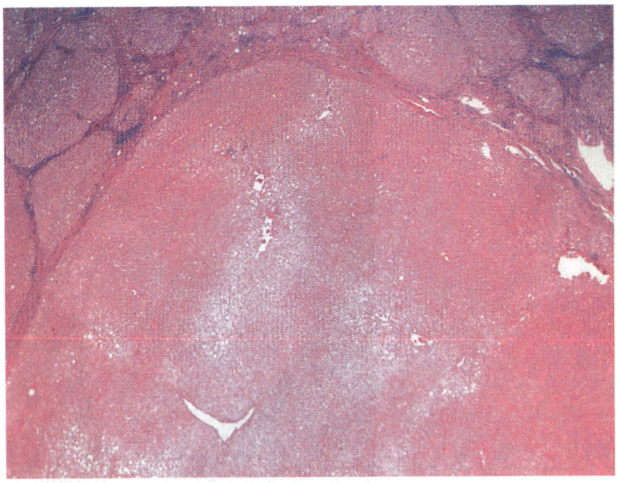

Figure 16–31

Large macroregenerative nodule in a cirrhotic liver. (Courtesy of Dr. Matthew Yeh, University of Washington, Seattle, Washington.)

present in liver cancers. Dysplastic lesions are subdivided into small-cell and large-cell dysplastic nodules or foci. Only small-cell dysplasias are precursors to cancer; large-cell dysplastic lesions contain hepatocytes that apparently have reached replicative senescence.

Benign Tumors

The most common benign lesions of the liver are *cavernous hemangiomas,* which are identical to those occurring in other parts of the body (Chapter 10). These well-circumscribed lesions consist of endothelial cell-lined vascular channels and intervening stroma. They appear as discrete red-blue, soft nodules, usually less than 2 cm in diameter, often directly beneath the capsule. Their chief clinical significance is the importance of not mistaking them for metastatic tumors; blind percutaneous needle biopsy may cause severe intra-abdominal bleeding.

Hepatic Adenoma. This benign neoplasm of hepatocytes usually occurs in women of childbearing age who have used oral contraceptive steroids, and it may regress on discontinuance of hormone use. These tumors may be pale, yellow-tan or bile-stained, well-demarcated nodules found anywhere in the hepatic substance but often beneath the capsule (Fig. 16–32). They may reach 30 cm in diameter. Histologically, liver cell adenomas are composed of sheets and cords of cells that may resemble normal hepatocytes or have some variation in cell and nuclear size. Portal tracts are absent; instead, prominent arterial vessels and draining veins are distributed through the substance of the tumor. Liver cell adenomas are significant for three reasons: (1) when they present as an intrahepatic mass, they may be mistaken for the more ominous hepatocellular carcinoma; (2) subcapsular adenomas are at risk for rupture, particularly during pregnancy (under estrogenic stimulation), causing life-threatening intra-abdominal hemorrhage; and (3) although adenomas are not considered precursors of hepatocellular carcinoma, adenomas carrying β-catenin mutations carry a risk of developing into cancers.

Hepatocellular Carcinomas (HCC)

Epidemiology. Worldwide, HCC (also known as liver cell carcinoma or, erroneously, hepatoma) constitutes approximately 5.4% of all cancers, but the incidence varies widely in different areas of the world. More than 85% of cases occur in countries with high rates of chronic HBV infection. Highest incidences are found in Asian countries (Southeast China, Korea, Taiwan) and African countries such as Mozambique, in which HBV is transmitted vertically, and, as already discussed, the carrier state starts in infancy. Moreover, many of these populations are exposed to aflatoxin, which, combined with HBV infection, increases the risk of HCC development by more than 200-fold over noninfected, nonexposed populations. The peak incidence of HCC in these areas is between 20 and 40 years of age, and in almost 50% of cases, HCC may appear in the absence of cirrhosis. In Western countries HCC incidence is rapidly increasing. It tripled in the United States during the last 25 years, but it is still much lower (8- to 30-fold) than the incidence in some Asian countries. In Western populations HCC is rarely present before age 60, and in almost 90% of cases tumors develop in persons with cirrhosis.

There is a pronounced male preponderance of HCC throughout the world, about 3:1 in low-incidence areas and as high as 8:1 in high-incidence areas. These differences may be related to the greater prevalence of HBV infection, alcoholism, and chronic liver disease among males.

Pathogenesis. Several general factors relevant to the pathogenesis of HCC were discussed in Chapter 6. Only a few points deserve emphasis at this time.

- Three major etiologic associations have been established: infection with HBV or HCV, chronic alcoholism, and aflatoxin exposure. Other conditions include hemochromatosis and tyrosinemia.
- Many variables, including age, gender, chemicals, viruses, hormones, alcohol, and nutrition, interact in

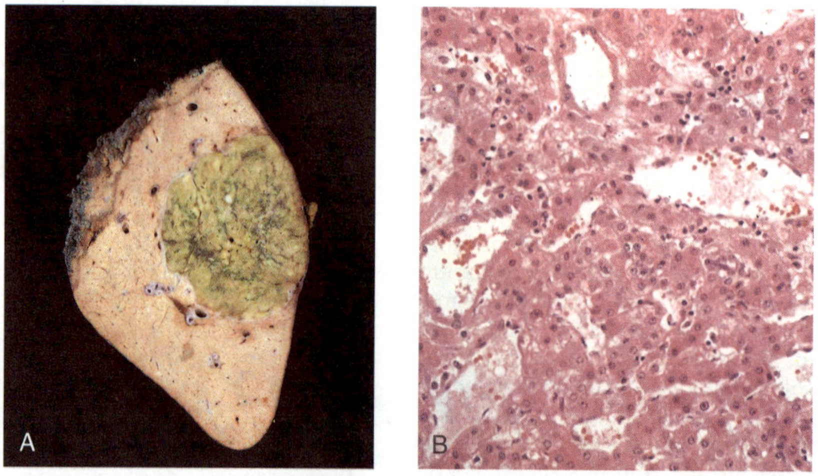

Figure 16–32

Hepatic adenoma. **A,** Surgically resected specimen showing a discrete mass underneath the liver capsule. **B,** Photomicrograph showing adenoma, with cords of hepatocytes.

the development of HCC. For example, the disease most likely to give rise to HCC is, in fact, the extremely rare hereditary tyrosinemia, in which almost 40% of patients develop this tumor despite adequate dietary control.

- The development of cirrhosis seems to be an important, but not requisite, contributor to the emergence of HCC. Carcinogenesis is greatly enhanced in the presence of cell injury and replication, as occurs in chronic viral hepatitis.
- In many parts of the world, including Japan and Central Europe, chronic HCV infection is the greatest risk factor in the development of liver cancer. HCC in patients with hepatitis C occurs almost exclusively in the setting of cirrhosis.
- In certain regions of the world, such as China and South Africa, where HBV is endemic, there is also high exposure to dietary aflatoxins derived from the fungus *Aspergillus flavus*. These carcinogenic toxins are found in "moldy" grains and peanuts. Aflatoxin can bind covalently with cellular DNA and cause a mutation in *p53*.

Despite the detailed knowledge about the etiologic agents of HCC, the pathogenesis of the tumor is still uncertain. *In most cases, it develops from small-cell, high-grade dysplastic nodules in cirrhotic livers.* As already discussed, these nodules may be monoclonal and may contain chromosomal aberrations similar to those seen in HCCs. The cell of origin of HCC has been the subject of considerable debate. It seems that *the tumors may arise from both mature hepatocytes and progenitor cells (known as ductular cells or oval cells)*. Distinguishing high-grade dysplastic nodules from early HCC is difficult even in biopsies, because there are no molecular markers specific for these stages. An important criterion is nodule vascularization, visualized by imaging, which is almost always a clear indication of malignancy.

An almost universal feature of HCC is the presence of structural and numeric chromosomal abnormalities. The precise origin of HCC genetic instability is not known, but some entities seem to be most important:

- Cell death, hepatocyte replication, and inflammation, seen in all forms of chronic hepatitis, are believed to be main contributors to DNA damage.
- Poor regulation of hepatocyte replication can occur by point mutations or overexpression of specific cellular genes (such as *β-catenin*), mutations or loss of heterozygosity of tumor suppressor genes (such as *p53*), methylation changes, and constitutive expression of growth factors.
- Defects in DNA repair, particularly those in repair systems for double-stranded DNA breaks, perpetuate DNA damage and may cause chromosome defects.

Neither HBV nor HCV contains oncogenes. The already mentioned *HBV-X* gene may have some oncogenic potential (Chapter 6). The tumorigenic capacity of these viruses probably relates primarily to their capacity to cause continuing cell death, chronic inflammation, and regeneration.

Morphology

Primary liver carcinomas, of which almost all are HCC, may appear grossly as (1) a **unifocal,** usually massive tumor (Fig. 16–33); (2) a **multifocal tumor** made of nodules of variable size; or (3) a **diffusely infiltrative** cancer, permeating widely and sometimes involving the entire liver, blending imperceptibly into the cirrhotic liver background. Particularly in the latter two patterns, it may be difficult to distinguish regenerative nodules of cirrhotic liver from nodules of neoplasm of similar size. Discrete tumor masses are usually yellow-white, punctuated sometimes by bile staining and areas of hemorrhage or necrosis. **All patterns of HCC have a strong propensity for invasion of vascular channels.** Extensive intrahepatic metastases ensue, and occasionally snakelike masses of tumor invade the portal vein (with occlusion of the portal circulation) or inferior vena cava, extending even into the right side of the heart.

Histologically, HCCs range from well-differentiated lesions that reproduce hepatocytes arranged in cords, trabeculae or glandular patterns (Fig. 16–34), to poorly differentiated lesions, often composed of large multinucleate anaplastic tumor giant cells. **In the better differentiated variants, globules of bile may be found within the cytoplasm of cells and in pseudocanaliculi** between cells. Acidophilic hyaline inclusions within the cytoplasm may be present, resembling Mallory bodies. There is surprisingly scant stroma in most HCCs, explaining the soft consistency of these tumors.

A distinctive clinicopathologic variant of HCC is the **fibrolamellar carcinoma,** which occurs in young male and female adults (20–40 years of age) with equal incidence, has no association with cirrhosis or other risk factors (Fig. 16–35). It usually consists of a single large, hard "scirrhous" tumor with fibrous bands coursing through it, vaguely resembling focal nodular hyperplasia. Histologically it is composed of well-differentiated polygonal cells growing in nests or cords and separated by parallel lamellae of dense collagen bundles.

Clinical Features. Although primary carcinomas in the liver may present with silent hepatomegaly, they are often encountered in individuals with cirrhosis of the liver who already have symptoms of the underlying disorder. In these persons, *rapid increase in liver size, sudden wors-*

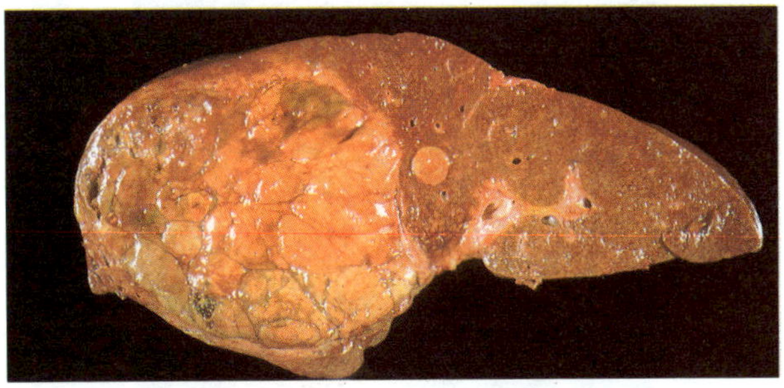

Figure 16–33

Hepatocellular carcinoma, unifocal, massive type. A large neoplasm with extensive areas of necrosis has replaced most of the right hepatic lobe in this noncirrhotic liver. A satellite tumor nodule is directly adjacent.

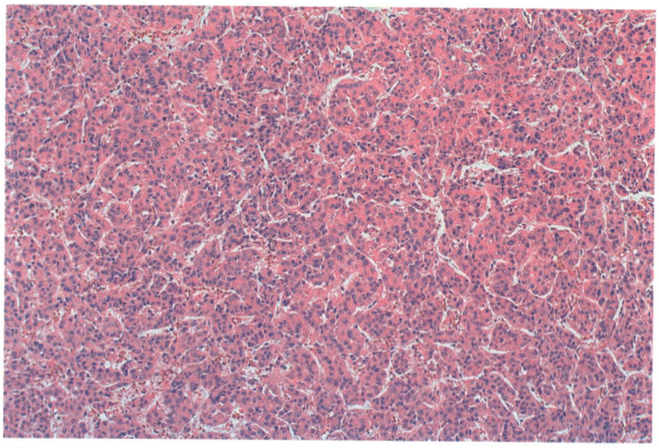

Figure 16–34

Hepatocellular carcinoma Carcinoma cells forming trabecular, pseudoacinar, and pseudoglandular architecture. (Courtesy of Dr. Matthew Yeh, University of Washington, Seattle, Washington.)

ening of ascites, or the appearance of bloody ascites, fever, and pain call attention to the development of a tumor. Laboratory studies are helpful but not diagnostic. Approximately 50% of patients have elevated serum α-fetoprotein. However, this tumor "marker" lacks specificity, because modest elevations are also encountered in other conditions, such as cirrhosis, massive liver necrosis, chronic hepatitis, normal pregnancy, fetal distress or death, fetal neural tube defects such as anencephaly and spina bifida (Chapter 23), and gonadal germ cell tumors (Chapter 18). *Very high levels (>1000 ng/mL), however, are rarely encountered except in HCC.*

The overall prognosis of HCC is grim, but it is significantly better for individuals who have a single tumor less than 2 cm in diameter and good liver function. The median survival is 7 months, with death from (1) profound cachexia, (2) gastrointestinal or esophageal variceal bleeding, (3) liver failure with hepatic coma, or (4) rarely, rupture of the tumor with fatal hemorrhage. Early detection of the tumors is critical for successful treatment. The most effective therapies are surgical resection of smaller tumors detected by ultrasound screening of persons with chronic liver disease, and liver transplantation for patients with small tumors and good liver function. Nevertheless, the tumor recurrence rate is greater than 60% at 5 years. The best hope for preventing HCC in regions endemic for HBV infection is a comprehensive anti-HBV immunization program.

Summary

Liver Tumors

- The liver is the most common site of metastatic cancers from primary tumors of the colon, lung, and breast.
- The main primary tumors are hepatocellular carcinomas and cholangiocarcinomas; hepatocellular carcinomas are by far the most common.
- HCC is a common tumor in regions of Asia and Africa, and its incidence is increasing in the United States.
- The main etiologic agents for hepatocellular carcinoma are hepatitis B and C, alcoholic cirrhosis, hemochromatosis, and more rarely, tyrosinemia. In the Western population about 90% of hepatocellular carcinomas develop in cirrhotic livers; in Asia almost 50% of cases develop in noncirrhotic livers.
- The chronic inflammation and cellular regeneration associated with viral hepatitis may be predisposing factors for the development of carcinomas.
- Hepatocellular carcinomas may be unifocal or multifocal, tend to invade blood vessels, and recapitulate normal liver architecture to varying degrees.

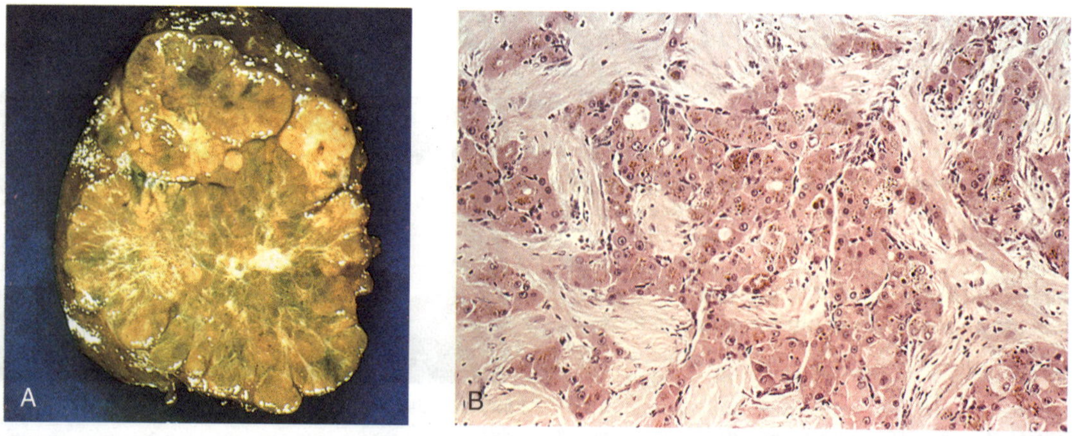

Figure 16–35

Fibrolamellar carcinoma. **A,** Resected specimen with an outer rim of normal liver. **B,** Nests and cords of tumor cells separated by dense bundles of collagen.

DISORDERS OF THE GALLBLADDER AND THE EXTRAHEPATIC BILIARY TRACT

Disorders of the gallbladder and biliary tract affect a large proportion of the world's population. *Cholelithiasis (gallstones)* accounts for more than 95% of these diseases. It is estimated that about 2% of the United States federal health budget is spent on cholelithiasis and its complications. Moreover, the burden of gallstones in the US population is calculated to weigh 25 to 50 tons, distributed among more than 20 million persons! In this section we first discuss gallbladder diseases (cholelithiasis and cholecystitis) and then examine some disorders of the extrahepatic bile ducts. It should be kept in mind that lesions of the extrahepatic biliary tract may extend to intrahepatic bile ducts and that tumors of the biliary tract (cholangiocarcinomas, described later) may have intra- or extrahepatic locations.

GALLBLADDER DISEASES

Cholelithiasis (Gallstones)

Gallstones afflict 10% to 20% of adult populations in northern hemisphere Western countries. Adult prevalence rates are higher in Latin American countries (20% to 40%) and are low in Asian countries (3% to 4%). In the United States there are about 1 million new cases of gallstones diagnosed annually, and two-thirds of these individuals undergo surgery.

There are two main types of gallstones. *In the West about 80% are cholesterol stones, containing crystalline cholesterol monohydrate.* The remainder are composed predominantly of bilirubin calcium salts and are designated *pigment stones.*

Pathogenesis and Risk Factors. Bile is the only significant pathway for elimination of excess cholesterol from the body, either as free cholesterol or as bile salts. Cholesterol is water insoluble and is rendered water soluble by aggregation with bile salts and lecithins secreted into bile. When cholesterol concentrations exceed the solubilizing capacity of bile (supersaturation), cholesterol can no longer remain dispersed and nucleates into solid cholesterol monohydrate crystals. Cholesterol gallstone formation involves four simultaneously occurring conditions:

- Supersaturation of the bile with cholesterol
- Establishment of nucleation sites by microprecipitates of calcium salts
- Hypomobility of the gallbladder (stasis), which promotes nucleation
- Mucus hypersecretion to trap the crystals, enhancing their aggregation into stones.

The pathogenesis of pigment stones is also complex. It is clear, however, that the presence of unconjugated bilirubin in the biliary tree increases the likelihood of pigment stone formation, as occurs in hemolytic anemias and infections of the biliary tract. The precipitates are primarily insoluble calcium bilirubinate salts.

The major risk factors for gallstones are listed in Table 16–8. However, 80% of individuals with gallstones have no identifying risk factors other than age and gender. Here we comment about some of these risk factors:

- *Age and gender.* The prevalence of gallstones increases throughout life. In the United States, less than 5% to 6% of the population younger than age 40 has stones, in contrast to 25% to 30% of those older than 80 years. The prevalence in white women is about twice as high as in men.
- *Ethnic and geographic.* Cholesterol gallstone prevalence approaches 75% in Native American populations—the Pima, Hopi, and Navajos—whereas pigment stones are rare; the prevalence seems to be related to biliary cholesterol hypersecretion. Gallstones are more prevalent in Western industrialized societies and uncommon in developing societies.
- *Heredity.* In addition to ethnicity, family history alone imparts increased risk, as do a variety of inborn errors of metabolism such as those associated with impaired bile salt synthesis and secretion.
- *Environment.* Estrogenic influences, including oral contraceptives and pregnancy, increase hepatic cholesterol uptake and synthesis, leading to excess biliary secretion of cholesterol. Obesity, rapid weight loss, and treatment with the hypocholesterolemic agent clofibrate are also strongly associated with increased biliary cholesterol secretion.
- *Acquired disorders.* Any condition in which gallbladder motility is reduced predisposes to gallstones,

Table 16–8 Risk Factors for Gallstones

Cholesterol Stones
Demography: Northern Europeans, North and South Americans, Native Americans, Mexican Americans.
Advancing age
Female sex hormones
Female gender
Oral contraceptives
Pregnancy
Obesity
Rapid weight reduction
Gallbladder stasis
Inborn disorders of bile acid metabolism
Hyperlipidemia syndromes
Pigment Stones
Demography: Asian more than Western, rural more than urban
Chronic hemolytic syndromes
Biliary infection
Gastrointestinal disorders: ileal disease (e.g., Crohn disease), ileal resection or bypass, cystic fibrosis with pancreatic insufficiency

such as pregnancy, rapid weight loss, and spinal cord injury. In most cases, however, gallbladder hypomotility is present without obvious cause.

Morphology

Cholesterol stones arise exclusively in the gallbladder and consist of 50% to 100% cholesterol. **Pure cholesterol stones** are pale yellow; increasing proportions of calcium carbonate, phosphates, and bilirubin impart gray-white to black discoloration (Fig. 16–36). They are ovoid and firm; they can occur singly but most often there are several, with faceted surfaces resulting from apposition to one another. **Most cholesterol stones are radiolucent, although as many as 20% may have sufficient calcium carbonate to render them radiopaque.**

Pigment stones may arise anywhere in the biliary tree and are trivially classified as black and as brown. In general, black pigment stones are found in sterile gallbladder bile, while brown stones are found in infected intrahepatic or extrahepatic ducts. The stones contain calcium salts of unconjugated bilirubin and lesser amounts of other calcium salts, mucin glycoproteins, and cholesterol. Black stones are usually small and present in large quantities (Fig. 16–37) and crumble easily. Brown stones tend to be single or few in number and are soft with a greasy, soaplike consistency that results from the presence of retained fatty acid salts released by the action of bacterial phospholipases on biliary lecithins. Because of calcium carbonates and phosphates, **50% to 75% of black stones are radiopaque.** Brown stones, which contain calcium soaps, are radiolucent.

Clinical Features. Among persons with gallstones, 70% to 80% remain asymptomatic throughout life, while the remainder become symptomatic at the rate of 1% to 3% per year. The risk for the appearance of symptoms diminishes with time. The symptoms are striking: pain tends to be excruciating, either constant or "colicky" (spasmodic)

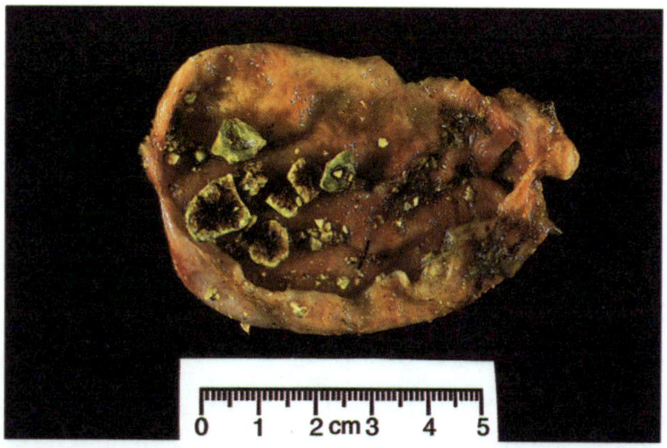

Figure 16–36

Cholesterol gallstones. Mechanical manipulation during laparoscopic cholecystectomy has caused fragmentation of several cholesterol gallstones, revealing interiors that are pigmented because of entrapped bile pigments. The gallbladder mucosa is reddened and irregular as a result of coexistent acute and chronic cholecystitis.

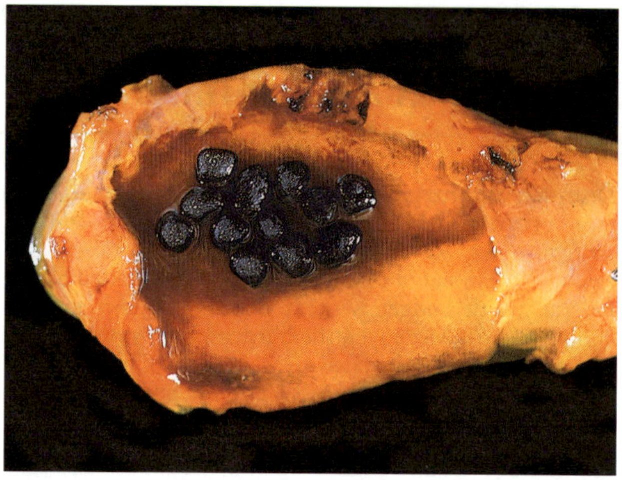

Figure 16–37

Pigmented gallstones. Several faceted black gallstones are present in this otherwise unremarkable gallbladder from a person with a mechanical mitral valve prosthesis, leading to chronic intravascular hemolysis.

from an obstructed gallbladder or when small gallstones move down-stream and lodge in the biliary tree. Inflammation of the gallbladder, in association with stones, also generates pain. More severe complications include empyema, perforation, fistulae, inflammation of the biliary tree, and obstructive cholestasis or pancreatitis. The larger the calculi, the less likely they are to enter the cystic or common ducts to produce obstruction; it is the very small stones, or "gravel," that are more dangerous. Occasionally a large stone may erode directly into an adjacent loop of small bowel, generating intestinal obstruction ("gallstone ileus").

Cholecystitis

Inflammation of the gallbladder may be acute, chronic, or acute superimposed on chronic, and almost always occurs in association with gallstones. In the United States, cholecystitis is one of the most common indications for abdominal surgery. Its epidemiologic distribution closely parallels that of gallstones.

Morphology

In **acute cholecystitis** the gallbladder is usually enlarged (twofold to threefold) and tense, and it assumes a bright red or blotchy, violaceous to green-black discoloration, imparted by subserosal hemorrhages. The serosal covering is frequently layered by fibrin and, in severe cases, by a suppurative exudate. In 90% of cases stones are present, often obstructing the neck of the gallbladder or the cystic duct. The gallbladder lumen is filled with a cloudy or turbid bile that may contain fibrin, blood, and frank pus. When the contained exudate is virtually pure pus, the condition is referred to as **empyema of the gallbladder.** In mild cases the gallbladder wall is thickened, edematous, and hyperemic. In more severe cases the gallbladder is transformed into a green-black necrotic organ, termed **gangrenous cholecystitis.** Histologically the inflammatory reactions are not distinctive and consist of the usual patterns of acute inflammation (i.e., edema, leukocytic infiltration, vascular congestion, frank abscess formation, or gangrenous necrosis).

The morphologic changes in **chronic cholecystitis** are extremely variable and sometimes minimal. The mere presence of stones within the gallbladder, even in the absence of acute inflammation, is often taken as sufficient justification for the diagnosis. The gallbladder may be contracted, of normal size, or enlarged. Mucosal ulcerations are infrequent; the submucosa and subserosa are often thickened from fibrosis. In the absence of superimposed acute cholecystitis, mural lymphocytes are the only sentinels of inflammation.

Acute Calculous Cholecystitis

Acute inflammation of a gallbladder that contains stones is termed *acute calculous cholecystitis* and is precipitated by obstruction of the gallbladder neck or cystic duct. *It is the most common major complication of gallstones and the most common reason for emergency cholecystectomy.* Symptoms may appear with remarkable suddenness and constitute an acute surgical emergency. On the other hand, symptoms may be mild and resolve without medical intervention.

Acute calculous cholecystitis is initially the result of chemical irritation and inflammation of the gallbladder wall in the setting of obstruction to bile outflow. The action of phospholipases derived from the mucosa hydrolyzes biliary lecithin to lysolecithin, which is toxic to the mucosa. The normally protective glycoprotein mucous layer is disrupted, exposing the mucosal epithelium to the direct detergent action of bile salts. Prostaglandins released within the wall of the distended gallbladder contribute to mucosal and mural inflammation. Distention and increased intraluminal pressure may also compromise blood flow to the mucosa. These events occur in the absence of bacterial infection; only later may bacterial contamination develop.

Acute Non-Calculous Cholecystitis

Between 5% and 12% of gallbladders removed for acute cholecystitis contain no gallstones. Most of these cases occur in seriously ill patients: (1) the postoperative state after major, nonbiliary surgery; (2) severe trauma (e.g., motor vehicle accidents); (3) severe burns; and (4) sepsis. Many events are thought to contribute to acute acalculous (non-calculous) cholecystitis, including dehydration, gallbladder stasis and sludging, vascular compromise, and, ultimately, bacterial contamination.

Chronic Cholecystitis

Chronic cholecystitis may be the sequel to repeated bouts of acute cholecystitis, but in most instances it develops without any history of acute attacks. Like acute cholecystitis it is almost always associated with gallstones. However, gallstones do not seem to have a direct role in the initiation of inflammation or the development of pain, because chronic acalculous cholecystitis causes symptoms and morphologic alterations similar to those seen in the calculous form. Rather, supersaturation of bile predisposes to both chronic inflammation and, in most instances, stone formation. Microorganisms, usually *Escherichia coli* and enterococci, can be cultured from the bile in only about one-third of cases. Unlike acute calculous cholecystitis, stone obstruction of gallbladder outflow in chronic cholecystitis is not a requisite. Nevertheless, the symptoms of chronic cholecystitis are similar to those of the acute form and range from biliary colic to indolent right upper quadrant pain and epigastric distress. Because most gallbladders removed at elective surgery for gallstones show features of chronic cholecystitis, one must conclude that biliary symptoms emerge after long-term coexistence of gallstones and low-grade inflammation.

Clinical Features. *Acute calculous cholecystitis* may barely achieve notice or may announce itself acutely, with severe, steady upper abdominal pain often radiating to the right shoulder. Sometimes, when stones are present in the gallbladder neck or in ducts, the pain is colicky. Fever, nausea, leukocytosis, and prostration are classic; the presence of conjugated hyperbilirubinemia suggests obstruction of the common bile duct. The right subcostal region is markedly tender and rigid as a result of spasm of the abdominal muscles; occasionally a tender, distended gallbladder can be palpated. Mild attacks usually subside spontaneously over 1 to 10 days; however, recurrence is common. Approximately 25% of symptomatic patients are sufficiently ill to require surgical intervention.

Symptoms arising from *acute acalculous cholecystitis* are usually obscured by the generally severe clinical condition of the patient. Diagnosis therefore rests on keeping this possibility in mind.

Chronic cholecystitis does not have the striking manifestations of the acute forms and is usually characterized by recurrent attacks of either steady or colicky epigastric or right upper quadrant pain. Nausea, vomiting, and intolerance for fatty foods are frequent accompaniments.

The diagnosis of both acute and chronic cholecystitis usually rests on the detection of gallstones or dilatation of the bile ducts by ultrasonography, typically accompanied by evidence of a thickened gallbladder wall. Attention to this disorder is important, because of the following complications:

- Bacterial superinfection with cholangitis or sepsis
- Gallbladder perforation and local abscess formation
- Gallbladder rupture with diffuse peritonitis
- Biliary enteric (cholecystenteric) fistula, with drainage of bile into adjacent organs, entry of air and bacteria into the biliary tree, and potentially gallstone-induced intestinal obstruction (ileus)
- Aggravation of preexisting medical illness, with cardiac, pulmonary, renal, or liver decompensation

DISORDERS OF EXTRAHEPATIC BILE DUCTS

Choledocholithiasis and Cholangitis

These conditions are considered together because they frequently go hand in hand. *Choledocholithiasis* is the presence of stones within the biliary tree. In Western nations, almost all stones are derived from the gallbladder; in Asia, there is a much higher incidence of primary ductal and intrahepatic, usually pigmented, stone formation. Choledocholithiasis may not immediately obstruct major bile ducts; asymptomatic stones are found in about 10% of patients at the time of surgical cholecystectomy. Symptoms may develop because of (1) biliary obstruction, (2) pancreatitis, (3) cholangitis, (4) hepatic abscess, (5) chronic liver disease with secondary biliary cirrhosis, or (6) acute calculous cholecystitis.

Cholangitis is the term used for acute inflammation of the wall of bile ducts, almost always caused by bacterial infection of the normally sterile lumen. It can result from any lesion obstructing bile flow, most commonly choledocholithiasis, and also from surgical reconstruction of the biliary tree. Uncommon causes include tumors, indwelling stents or catheters, acute pancreatitis, and benign strictures. Bacteria most likely enter the biliary tract through the sphincter of Oddi, rather than by the hematogenous route. *Ascending cholangitis* refers to the propensity of bacteria, once within the biliary tree, to infect intrahepatic biliary ducts. The usual pathogens are *E. coli, Klebsiella, Clostridium, Bacteroides,* or *Enterobacter;* group D streptococci are also common, and two or more organisms are found in half of the cases. In some world populations, parasitic cholangitis is a significant problem: *Fasciola hepatica* or schistosomiasis in Latin America and the Near East, *Clonorchis sinensis* or *Opisthorchis viverrini* in the Far East, and cryptosporidiosis in individuals with acquired immunodeficiency syndrome.

Bacterial cholangitis usually produces fever, chills, abdominal pain, and jaundice. The most severe form of cholangitis is suppurative cholangitis, in which purulent bile fills and distends bile ducts, with an attendant risk of liver abscess formation. Because sepsis rather than cholestasis is the dominant risk in cholangitic patients, prompt diagnosis and intervention are imperative.

Secondary Biliary Cirrhosis

Prolonged obstruction of the extrahepatic biliary tree results in profound damage to the liver itself. The most common cause of obstruction is extrahepatic cholelithiasis. Other obstructive conditions include biliary atresia (discussed below), malignancies of the biliary tree and head of the pancreas, and strictures resulting from previous surgical procedures. The initial morphologic features of cholestasis were described earlier and are entirely reversible with correction of the obstruction. However, secondary inflammation resulting from biliary obstruction initiates periportal fibrogenesis, which eventually leads to scarring and nodule formation, generating secondary biliary cirrhosis. Subtotal obstruction may promote secondary bacterial infection of the biliary tree (ascending cholangitis), which further contributes to the damage. Enteric organisms such as coliforms and enterococci are common culprits.

Biliary Atresia

The infant presenting with neonatal cholestasis was discussed previously in the context of neonatal hepatitis. A major contributor to neonatal cholestasis is biliary atresia, accounting for one-third of infants with neonatal cholestasis and occurring in approximately 1 in 10,000 live births. Biliary atresia *is defined as a complete obstruction of bile flow caused by destruction or absence of all or part of the extrahepatic bile ducts.* It is the most frequent cause of death from liver disease in early childhood and accounts for more than half of the children referred for liver transplantation.

The salient features of biliary atresia include (1) inflammation and fibrosing stricture of the hepatic or common bile ducts; (2) inflammation of major intrahepatic bile ducts, with progressive destruction of the intrahepatic biliary tree; (3) florid features of biliary obstruction on liver biopsy (i.e., marked bile ductular proliferation, portal tract edema and fibrosis, and parenchymal cholestasis); and (4) periportal fibrosis and cirrhosis within 3 to 6 months of birth.

Clinical Course. Infants with biliary atresia present with neonatal cholestasis, as discussed earlier; there is a slight female preponderance. They have normal birth weights and postnatal weight gain. Stools change from initially normal to acholic as the disease evolves. Laboratory findings do not distinguish between biliary atresia and intrahepatic cholestasis, but a liver biopsy provides evidence of bile duct obstruction in 90% of cases of biliary atresia. Liver transplantation remains the definitive treatment. Without surgical intervention, death usually occurs within 2 years of birth.

SUMMARY

Diseases of the Gallbladder and Extrahepatic Bile Ducts

- Gallbladder diseases include cholelithiasis and acute and chronic cholecystitis.
- Gallstone formation is a common condition in Western countries. The great majority of the gallstones are cholesterol stones. Pigmented stones containing bilirubin and calcium are most common in Asian countries.
- Risk factors for the development of cholesterol stones are advancing age, female gender, estrogen use, obesity, and heredity.
- Cholecystitis almost always occurs in association with cholelithiasis, although in about 10% of cases it occurs in the absence of gallstones.
- Acute calculous cholecystitis is the most common reason for emergency cholecystectomy.

TUMORS

Carcinoma of the Gallbladder

Carcinoma of the gallbladder, which develops from the epithelial lining of the organ, is the most frequent malignant tumor of the biliary tract. It is slightly more common in women and occurs most frequently in the seventh decade of life. For unknown reasons carcinoma of the gallbladder is more frequent in Mexico and Chile. In the United States the incidence is highest in Hispanics and Native Americans. Only rarely is it discovered at a resectable stage, and the mean 5-year survival has remained at a dismal 5% rate. Gallstones are present in 60% to 90% of cases. However, in Asia, where pyogenic and parasitic diseases of the biliary tree are more common, gallstones are less important. Presumably, gallbladders containing stones or infectious agents develop cancer as a result of recurrent trauma and chronic inflammation. The role of carcinogenic derivatives of bile acids is unclear, but the presence of a abnormal choledochopancreatic duct junction is considered to be a risk factor.

Morphology

Cancers of the gallbladder assume either **exophytic** or **infiltrating** patterns of growth. The infiltrating pattern is more common and usually appears as a poorly defined area of diffuse thickening and induration of the gallbladder wall that may cover several square centimeters or involve the entire gallbladder. These tumors are scirrhous and very firm. The exophytic pattern grows into the lumen as an irregular, cauliflower mass, but at the same time it invades the underlying wall (Fig. 16–38). **Most carcinomas of the gallbladder are adenocarcinomas.** They may be papillary, poorly differentiated, or undifferentiated infiltrating tumors (Fig. 16–39). About 5% are squamous cell carcinomas or have adenosquamous differentiation. A minority are carcinoid tumors. By the time gallbladder cancers are discovered, **most have invaded the liver directly** and many have extended to the cystic duct and adjacent bile ducts and portal hepatic lymph nodes. The peritoneum, gastrointestinal tract, and lungs are less common sites of seeding.

Clinical Features. Preoperative diagnosis of carcinoma of the gallbladder is the exception, occurring in fewer than 20% of patients. Presenting symptoms are insidious and typically indistinguishable from those associated with cholelithiasis: abdominal pain, jaundice, anorexia, and nausea and vomiting. The fortunate person develops early obstruction and acute cholecystitis before extension of the tumor into adjacent structures or undergoes cholecystectomy for coexistent symptomatic gallstones. Preoperative diagnosis rests largely on detection of gallstones along with abnormalities in the gallbladder wall documented by imaging studies.

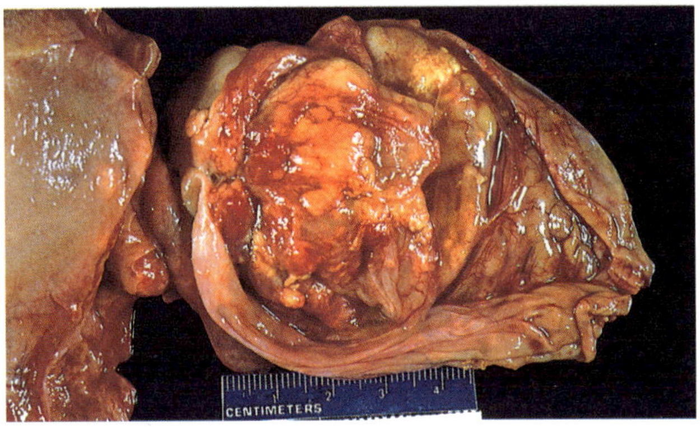

Figure 16–38

Adenocarcinoma of the gallbladder. The opened gallbladder contains a large, exophytic tumor that virtually fills the lumen.

Cholangiocarcinomas

Cholangiocarcinomas are adenocarcinomas with biliary differentiation arising from cholangiocytes in ducts within and outside of the liver. Extrahepatic cholangiocarcinomas, constituting approximately two-thirds of these tumors, may develop at the hilum (known as Klatskin tumors) or more distally in the biliary tree, as far as the peripancreatic portion of the distal common bile duct. Cholangiocarcinomas occur mostly in individuals of 50 to 70 years of age. Because both intra- and extrahepatic cholangiocarcinomas are generally asymptomatic until they reach an advanced stage, the prognosis is poor and most patients have unresectable tumors. Risk factors include primary sclerosing cholangitis (already described), fibrocystic diseases of the biliary tree, and exposure to Thorotrast (which is no longer used in radiography of the biliary tree). The incidence of intrahepatic cholangiocarcinomas is increasing worldwide, while that of extrahepatic tumors has decreased. The causes for these changes in incidence are unknown, but suggest that intra- and extrahepatic cholangiocarcinomas may have different pathogenesis.

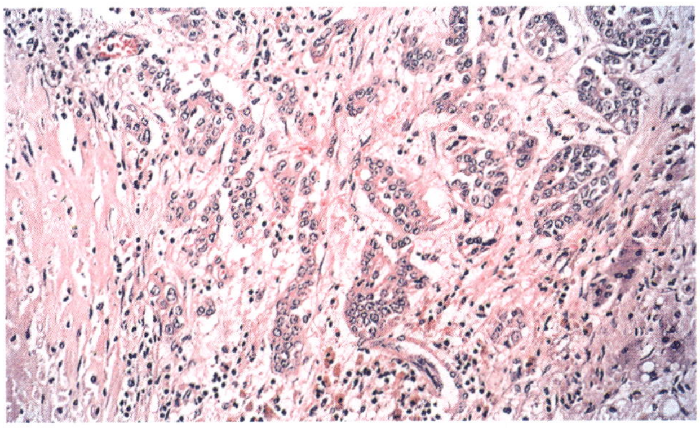

Figure 16–39

Adenocarcinoma of the gallbladder. Malignant glandular structures are present within the gallbladder wall, which is fibrotic.

Morphology

Cholangiocarcinomas appear as more or less well-differentiated adenocarcinomas, typically with an abundant fibrous stroma (desmoplasia) explaining their firm, gritty consistency (Fig. 16–40). Most exhibit clearly defined glandular and tubular structures lined by somewhat anaplastic cuboidal to low columnar epithelial cells. Bile pigment and hyaline inclusions are not found within the cells.

Because partial or complete obstruction of bile ducts rapidly leads to jaundice, extrahepatic biliary tumors tend to be relatively small at the time of diagnosis. Most appear as firm, gray nodules within the bile duct wall; some may be diffusely infiltrative lesions, creating ill-defined thickening of the wall; others are papillary, polypoid lesions. Uncommonly, squamous features are present. For the most part, an abundant fibrous stroma accompanies the epithelial proliferation. Cholangiocarcinomas may spread to extrahepatic sites such as regional lymph nodes, lungs, bones, and adrenal glands. Cholangiocarcinoma has a greater propensity for extrahepatic spread than hepatocellular carcinomas.

Pathogenesis and Clinical Features. The feature common to the risk factors for cholangiocarcinomas is that they all cause chronic cholestasis and inflammation. Recent studies of the pathogenesis of cholangiocarcinomas in humans and experimental animals have demonstrated several consistent changes, including overexpression of the tyrosine kinase receptors ErbB-2 and c-met, up-regulation of cyclooxygenase-2 (COX-2), and a high frequency of abnormalities in the *p16* tumor suppressor gene. ErbB-2 and COX-2 inhibitors are being investigated for potential use as therapeutic agents.

Intrahepatic cholangiocarcinoma is detected by the presence of a liver mass and unspecific symptoms such as weight loss, pain, anorexia, and ascites. Symptoms arising from extrahepatic cholangiocarcinomas (jaundice, decolorization of the stools, nausea and vomiting, and weight loss) result from biliary obstruction. Associated changes are elevated levels of serum alkaline phosphatase and aminotransferases, bile-stained urine, and prolonged prothrombin time. Surgical resection is the only treatment available, but the results are variable. Mean survival times range from 6 to 18 months, regardless of whether aggressive resection or palliative surgery is performed.

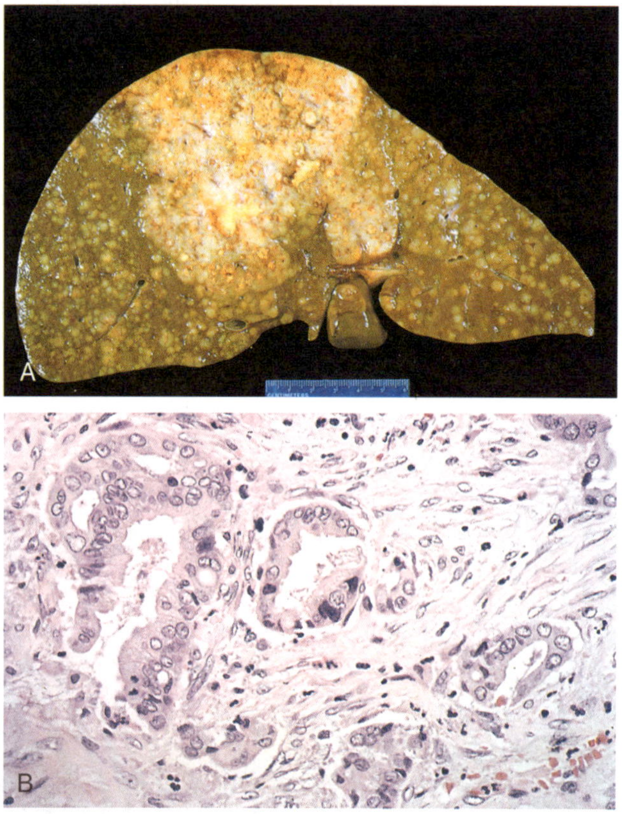

Figure 16–40

Cholangiocarcinoma. **A,** Massive neoplasm in the right lobe and multiple metastases throughout the liver. **B,** Tumor cells forming glandular structures surrounded by dense sclerotic stroma.

BIBLIOGRAPHY

Bataller R, Brenner DA: Liver fibrosis. J Clin Invest 115:209, 2005. *[A current review.]*

Bruix J, et al.: Focus on hepatocellular carcinoma. Cancer Cell 5:215, 2004. *[Excellent discussion on the clinical features of hepatocellular carcinomas and the development of strategies for detection and treatment.]*

Clark JM, et al.: Nonalcoholic fatty liver disease. Gastroenterology 122:1649, 2002. *[An excellent overview.]*

Cortez-Pinto H, Camilo ME: Nonalcoholic fatty liver disease/nonalcoholic steatohepatitis (NAFLD/NASH): diagnosis and clinical course. Best Pract Res Clin Gastro 18:1089, 2004. *[An excellent discussion of the spectrum of NAFLD.]*

Deleve LD, et al.: Toxic injury to hepatic sinusoids: sinusoidal obstruction syndrome (venocclusive disease). Semin Liver Dis 22:27, 2002. *[A presentation of the modern concepts of the disease.]*

El-Serag HB, et al.: The continuing increase in the incidence of hepatocellular carcinoma in the United States. Ann Intern Med 139:817, 2003. *[Data showing the trends in the incidence of hepatocellular carcinoma, with a good discussion about the causes of the increased incidence.]*

Ferrell L: Liver pathology: cirrhosis, hepatitis, and primary liver tumors: update and diagnostic problems. Mod Pathol 13:679, 2000. *[An excellent guide to pathologic evaluation of liver disease.]*

Friedman SL: Stellate cells: a moving target in hepatic fibrogenesis. Hepatology 40:1041, 2004. *[A short editorial discussing new results and ideas about the function of stellate cells.]*

Ganem D, Prince AM: Hepatitis B virus infection—natural history and clinical consequences. N Engl J Med 350:1118, 2004. *[Very good concise review of the topics.]*

Garg R, et al.: Insulin resistance as a pro-inflammatory state: mechanisms mediators, and therapeutic interventions. Curr Drug Targets 4:487, 2003. *[An interesting paper on the pro-inflammatory state mediated by insulin resistance, which is important for the development of nonalcoholic fatty liver disease.]*

Gershwin ME, et al.: Primary biliary cirrhosis: an orchestrated immune response against epithelial cells. Immunol Rev 174:210, 2000. *[A thorough discussion of potential mechanisms for autoimmune destruction of the biliary tree.]*

Gunawan B, Kaplowitz N: Clinical perspectives on xenobiotic-induced hepatotoxicity. Drug Metab Rev 36:301, 2004. *[A comprehensive and current review.]*

Hui AY, Friedman SL: Molecular basis of hepatic fibrosis. Exp Rev Mol Med 5:1, 2003. *[A very well done analysis of the cellular and molecular pathogenesis of fibrosis.]*

Kaplowitz N: Idiosyncratic drug hepatotoxicity. Nat Rev Drug Discov 4:489, 2005. *[Current review of a complex subject.]*

Kleiner DE: The liver biopsy in chronic hepatitis C: a view from the other side of the microscope. Semin Liver Dis 25:52, 2005. *[An excellent review of diagnostic issues.]*

LaRusso NF, et al: Primary sclerosing cholangitis: summary of a workshop. Hepatology 44:746, 2006. *[A comprehensive review of all aspects of this disease.]*

Lazaridis KN, Gores GJ: Cholangiocarcinoma. Gastroenterology128:1655, 2005. *[An excellent review on the epidemiology, pathology, pathogenesis, and treatment of cholangiocarcinomas.]*

Lee WM: Acetaminophen and the U.S. acute liver failure study group: Lowering the risks of hepatic failure. Hepatology 40:6, 2004. *[A discussion of acetaminophen as the leading cause of acute liver failure.]*

Lok A, McMahon BJ: Chronic hepatitis B. Hepatology 34:1225, 2001. *[Excellent overview.]*

Mandayam S, et al.: Epidemiology of alcoholic liver disease. Semin Liver Dis 24:217, 2004. *[An overview of the epidemiology of alcoholic liver disease.]*

Marchesini G, et al.: Nonalcoholic fatty liver, steatohepatitis and the metabolic syndrome. Hepatology 37:917, 2003. *[Very good overview of the association between nonalcoholic fatty liver disease and components of the metabolic syndrome.]*

Pietrangelo A: hereditary hemochromatosis—a new look at an old disease. N Engl J Med 350:2383, 2004. *[A modern approach to the pathogenesis of hemochromatosis.]*

Pietrangelo A: Hereditary hemochromatosis. Biochim et Biophys Acta 1763:700, 2006. *[A unifying hypothesis of inherited disorders of iron overload.]*

Poulson J, Lee WM: The management of acute liver failure. Hepatology 41:1179, 2005. *[A very comprehensive position paper from the American Association for the Study of Liver Disease.]*

Rehermann B, Nascimbeni M: Immunology of hepatitis B virus and hepatitis C virus infection. Nat Rev Immunol 5:215, 2005. *[Current review of critical issues in hepatitis B and C virus-induced liver disease.]*

Roskams TA, et al.: Nomenclature of the finer branches of the biliary tree: canals, ductules, and ductular reactions in human livers. Hepatology 39:1739, 2004. *[A consensus paper about the identification of the branches of the biliary tree, which is of importance for liver disease and stem cell research.]*

Sirica AE: Cholangiocarcinoma: molecular targeting strategies for chemoprevention and therapy. Hepatology 41:5, 2005. *[Excellent review on newly identified molecular markers and their potential as therapeutic targets.]*

Schilsky ML, Oikonomou I: Inherited metabolic liver disease. Curr Opin Gastroenterol 21:275, 2005. *[An update on hemochromatosis, Wilson disease, and α_1-antitrypsin deficiency.]*

Vaquero J, et al.: Pathogenesis of hepatic encephalopathy in acute liver failure. Semin Liver Dis 23:259, 2003. *[An excellent discussion of the mechanisms of encephalopathy.]*

Worman HJ, Courvalin JC: Antinuclear antibodies specific for primary biliary cirrhosis. Autoimmun Rev 2:211, 2003. *[A review of a very complex issue.]*

Chapter 17

The Pancreas*

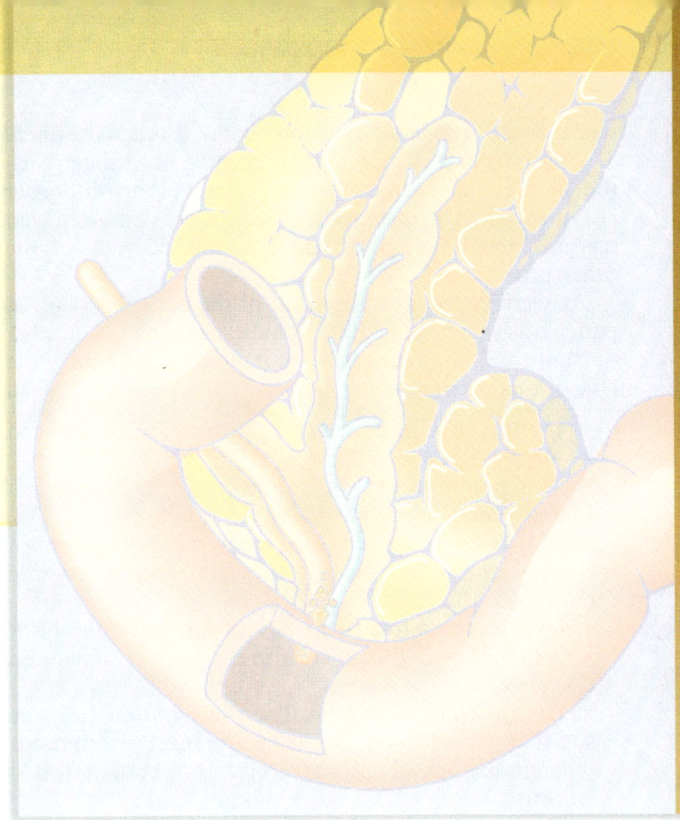

The pancreas has critical endocrine functions, and the exocrine portion of the pancreas is a major source of extremely potent digestive enzymes. Consequently, diseases affecting the pancreas can wreak major havoc and can be the source of significant morbidity and mortality. A general truism from the practice of surgery is particularly apt: "You don't mess around with the pancreas." Unfortunately, despite its physiologic importance, the retroperitoneal location of the pancreas and the generally vague signs and symptoms associated with its injury allow many pancreatic diseases to progress undiagnosed for extended periods of time; recognition of disease often requires a high degree of suspicion.

The adult pancreas is a transversely oriented retroperitoneal organ extending from the "C" loop of the duodenum to the hilum of the spleen. Although the pancreas does not have well-defined anatomic subdivisions, adjacent vessels and ligaments can demarcate the organ into a head, body, and tail.

The pancreas gets its name from the Greek *pankreas,* meaning "all flesh." It is, however, a complex lobulated organ with distinct endocrine and exocrine elements. The endocrine portion constitutes only 1% to 2% of the pancreas and is composed of about 1 million cell clusters, the islets of Langerhans; these cells secrete insulin, glucagon, and somatostatin. The most significant disorders of the *endocrine* pancreas include diabetes mellitus and neoplasms; these are described in detail in Chapter 20 and will not be discussed further here.

The *exocrine pancreas* is composed of *acinar cells* that produce the digestive enzymes, and the ductules and ducts that convey them to the duodenum. The acinar cells produce mostly proenzyme forms of digestive enzymes and store them in membrane-bound *zymogen granules.* When acinar cells are stimulated to secrete, the granules fuse with the apical plasma membrane and release their contents into the central acinar lumen.

These secretions are transported to the duodenum through a series of anastomosing ducts. The epithelial cells lining the ducts are also active participants in pancreatic secretion: cuboidal epithelial cells lining the smaller ductules secrete bicarbonate-rich fluid, while the columnar epithelial cells lining the larger ducts produce mucin. The epithelial cells of the larger pancreatic ducts express the *cystic fibrosis transmembrane conductance regulator (CFTR);* aberrant expression of this membrane protein affects the viscosity of the pancreatic secretions and has a fundamental role in the pathophysiology of pancreatic disease in persons with cystic fibrosis (Chapter 7).

In general, the exocrine products of the pancreas are secreted as enzymatically inert proenzymes (e.g. trypsinogen); amylase and lipase are exceptions and are secreted in an active form. The strategy of producing most pancreatic enzymes in an inactive zymogen form is largely to prevent self-digestion; it also focuses the eventual

*The authors acknowledge Drs. Michael J. Clare-Salzer, James M. Crawford, Ralph M. Hruban, and Robb E. Wilentz and thank them for their previous contributions to many aspects of this chapter.

work of the activated enzymes to the duodenal lumen. The proenzymes remain largely inactive until they reach the duodenum; there, enteropeptidase (a brush-border enzyme) cleaves trypsinogen into active trypsin. Activated trypsin then functions to catalyze the cleavage of the other proenzymes.

As we will see, autodigestion of the pancreas (e.g., in pancreatitis) can be a catastrophic event. Thus, a number of "fail-safe" mechanisms have evolved to minimize the risk of this occurring:

- The majority of pancreatic enzymes are synthesized as inactive proenzymes.
- The proenzymes are sequestered in membrane-bound zymogen granules.
- Activation of proenzymes requires conversion of trypsinogen to trypsin by duodenal enteropeptidase (enterokinase).
- Trypsin inhibitors (e.g., serine protease inhibitor Kazal type l or SPINK1) are also secreted by acinar and ductal cells.
- Trypsin contains a critical self-recognition cleavage site that allows trypsin to inactivate itself in situations wherein there is a high local concentration of activated enzyme.
- Most of the secreted enzymes have acidic pH optima and are relatively inactive in the bicarbonate-rich pancreatic fluid.
- Enzymes within lysosomes can degrade zymogen granules if normal acinar secretion is blocked.
- Acinar cells are remarkably resistant to the action of activated enzymes such as trypsin, chymotrypsin, and phospholipase A_2.

Diseases of the exocrine pancreas include cystic fibrosis, congenital anomalies, acute and chronic pancreatitis, and neoplasms. Cystic fibrosis is discussed in detail in Chapter 7; the remainder of this chapter will discuss the other pathologic processes.

CONGENITAL ANOMALIES

Pancreatic development is a complex process involving fusion of dorsal and ventral primordia; subtle deviations in this process frequently give rise to congenital variations in pancreatic anatomy. While most of these do not cause disease per se, variants (especially in ductal anatomy) can present unique challenges to the endoscopist and surgeon. For example, failure to recognize idiosyncratic anatomy could conceivably result in inadvertent severing of a pancreatic duct during surgery, resulting in pancreatitis.

Agenesis. Very rarely, the pancreas may be totally absent, a condition usually (but not invariably) associated with additional severe malformations that are incompatible with life. IPF1 is a homeodomain transcription factor critical for normal pancreas development, and *IPF1* gene mutations on chromosome 13q12.1 have been associated with pancreatic agenesis.

Pancreas divisum is the most common clinically significant congenital pancreatic anomaly, with an incidence of 3% to 10%. It occurs when the fetal duct systems of the pancreatic primordia fail to fuse. As a result, the main pancreatic duct (Wirsung) is very short and drains only a small portion of the head of the gland, while the bulk of the pancreas (from the dorsal pancreatic primordium) drains through the minor sphincter. The relative stenosis caused by the bulk of the pancreatic secretions passing through the minor sphincter predisposes such individuals to chronic pancreatitis.

Annular pancreas is a relatively uncommon variant on pancreatic fusion; the outcome is a ring of pancreatic tissue that completely encircles the duodenum. It can present with signs and symptoms of duodenal obstruction such as gastric distention and vomiting.

Ectopic Pancreas. Aberrantly situated, or *ectopic,* pancreatic tissue occurs in about 2% of the population; favored sites are the stomach and duodenum, followed by the jejunum, Meckel diverticulum, and ileum. These embryologic rests are typically small (millimeters to centimeters in diameter) and are located in the submucosa; they are composed of normal pancreatic acini with occasional islets. Though usually incidental and asymptomatic, ectopic pancreas can cause pain from localized inflammation, or—rarely—can cause mucosal bleeding. Approximately 2% of islet cell tumors arise in ectopic pancreatic tissue.

Congenital cysts probably result from anomalous ductal development. In *polycystic disease,* kidney, liver, and pancreas can all contain cysts (see Chapter 14). Pancreatic cysts range from microscopic to 5 cm in diameter. They are lined by duct-type cuboidal epithelium or can lack a cell lining altogether, and are enclosed in a thin, fibrous capsule. In general, unilocular cysts tend to be benign, while multilocular cysts are more often neoplastic and possibly malignant (see below).

PANCREATITIS

Inflammation of the pancreas can have clinical manifestations ranging from mild, self-limited disease to a life-threatening acutely destructive process; durations can vary from transient to irreversible loss of function. By definition, in *acute pancreatitis* the organ can return to normal if the underlying cause of inflammation is removed. In contrast, *chronic pancreatitis* is defined by the presence of irreversible destruction of exocrine pancreatic parenchyma.

Acute Pancreatitis

Acute pancreatitis is a group of reversible lesions characterized by inflammation; severity can range from focal edema and fat necrosis to widespread parenchymal necrosis with severe hemorrhage. Acute pancreatitis is relatively common, with an annual incidence in industrialized countries of 10 to 20 per 100,000 people. Approximately 80% of cases are attributable to either biliary tract disease or alcoholism (Table 17–1). Roughly 5% of patients with gallstones develop acute pancreatitis, and gallstones are implicated in 35% to 60% of cases overall. Excessive alcohol intake as a cause of acute pancreatitis varies from 65% of cases in the United States to 5% or less in the United Kingdom.

Table 17–1 Etiologic Factors in Acute Pancreatitis

Metabolic	
	Alcoholism
	Hyperlipoproteinemia
	Hypercalcemia
	Drugs (e.g., thiazide diuretics)
	Genetic
Mechanical	
	Trauma
	Gallstones
	Iatrogenic injury
	Perioperative injury
	Endoscopic procedures with dye injection
Vascular	
	Shock
	Atheroembolism
	Polyarteritis nodosa
Infectious	
	Mumps
	Coxsackievirus
	Mycoplasma pneumoniae

Other causes of acute pancreatitis include:

- Non-gallstone obstruction of the pancreatic ducts (e.g., due to periampullary tumors, pancreas divisum, biliary "sludge," and parasites—generally *Ascaris lumbricoides*)
- Medications including thiazide diuretics, azathioprine, estrogens, sulfonamides, furosemide, methyldopa, pentamidine, and procainamide
- Infections with mumps, coxsackievirus, or *Mycoplasma pneumoniae*
- Metabolic disorders, including hypertriglyceridemia, hyperparathyroidism, and other hypercalcemic states
- Ischemia due to vascular thrombosis, embolism, vasculitis, or shock
- Trauma, both blunt force and iatrogenic during surgery or endoscopy
- Inherited mutations in genes encoding pancreatic enzymes or their inhibitors (e.g., *SPINK1*). For example, *hereditary pancreatitis* is an autosomal dominant disease with an 80% penetrance characterized by recurrent attacks of severe pancreatitis usually beginning in childhood. It is caused by mutations in the *PRSS1* gene that affect a site on the trypsinogen molecule that is essential for the cleavage (inactivation) of trypsin by trypsin itself. When this site is mutated, trypsinogen and trypsin become resistant to inactivation, leading to ongoing activation of other digestive proenzymes, and eventually the development of pancreatitis.

Notably, 10% to 20% of patients with acute pancreatitis have no identifiable cause *(idiopathic pancreatitis)*, although a growing body of evidence suggests that many may have an underlying genetic basis.

Morphology

The morphology of acute pancreatitis ranges from trivial inflammation and edema to extensive necrosis and hemorrhage. The basic alterations are **(1) microvascular leakage causing edema, (2) necrosis of fat by lipases, (3) an acute inflammatory reaction, (4) proteolytic destruction of pancreatic parenchyma, and (5) destruction of blood vessels with hemorrhage.**

In milder forms, histologic alterations include interstitial edema and focal areas of fat necrosis in the pancreatic substance and peripancreatic fat (Fig. 17–1A). Fat necrosis results from enzymatic destruction of fat cells; the released fatty acids combine with calcium to form insoluble salts that precipitate in situ.

In more severe forms, such as **acute necrotizing pancreatitis,** necrosis of pancreatic tissue affects acinar and ductal tissues as well as the islets of Langerhans; vascular damage causes hemorrhage into the parenchyma of the pancreas. Macroscopically, the pancreas exhibits red-black hemorrhage interspersed with foci of yellow-white, chalky fat necrosis (Fig. 17–1B). Fat necrosis can also occur in extra-pancreatic fat, including the omentum and bowel mesentery, and even outside the abdominal cavity (e.g., in subcutaneous fat). In most

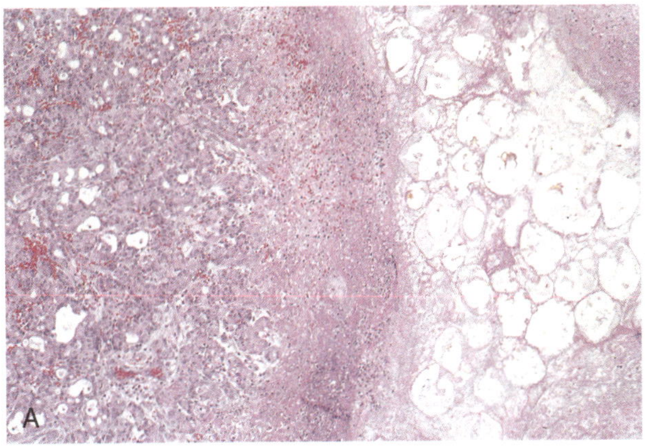

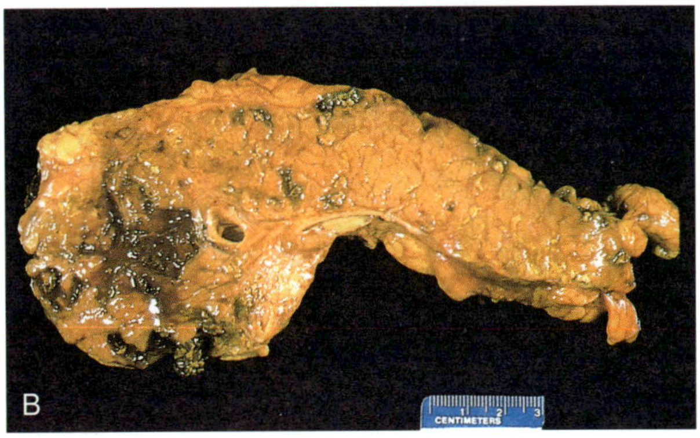

Figure 17–1

Acute pancreatitis. **A,** The microscopic field shows a region of fat necrosis *(right)*, and focal pancreatic parenchymal necrosis *(center)*. **B,** The pancreas has been sectioned longitudinally to reveal dark areas of hemorrhage in the pancreatic substance and a focal area of pale fat necrosis in the peripancreatic fat *(upper left)*.

cases the peritoneum contains a serous, slightly turbid, brown-tinged fluid with globules of fat (derived from enzymatically digested adipose tissue). In the most severe form, **hemorrhagic pancreatitis,** extensive parenchymal necrosis is accompanied by diffuse hemorrhage.

Pathogenesis. The histologic changes seen in acute pancreatitis strongly suggest *autodigestion of the pancreatic substance by inappropriately activated pancreatic enzymes.* Recall that the zymogen forms of pancreatic enzymes must be enzymatically cleaved to be activated; trypsin is central in this process and *activation of trypsin is thus a critical triggering event in acute pancreatitis.* If trypsin is inappropriately generated from its proenzyme trypsinogen, it can activate other proenzymes (e.g., phospholipases and elastases) that can then take part in the process of autodigestion. Trypsin also converts prekallikrein to its activated form, thus sparking the kinin system and, by activation of factor XII (Hageman factor), also sets in motion the clotting and complement systems (Chapter 4). Three possible pathways can incite the initial enzyme activation that may lead to acute pancreatitis (Fig. 17–2):

• *Pancreatic duct obstruction.* Impaction of a gallstone or biliary sludge, or extrinsic compression of the ductal system by a mass blocks ductal flow, increases intraductal pressure, and allows accumulation of an enzyme-rich interstitial fluid. Since lipase is secreted in an active form, this can cause local fat necrosis. Injured tissues, periacinar myofibroblasts, and leukocytes then release pro-inflammatory cytokines that promote local inflammation, and interstitial edema through a leaky microvasculature. Edema further compromises local blood flow, causing vascular insufficiency and ischemic injury to acinar cells.

• *Primary acinar cell injury.* This pathogenic mechanism comes into play in acute pancreatitis caused by ischemia, viruses (e.g., mumps), drugs, and direct trauma to the pancreas.

• *Defective intracellular transport of proenzymes within acinar cells.* In normal acinar cells, digestive enzymes intended for zymogen granules (and eventually extracellular release) and hydrolytic enzymes destined for lysosomes are transported in discrete pathways after synthesis in the ER. However, at least in some animal models of metabolic injury, pancreatic proenzymes and lysosomal hydrolases become packaged together. This

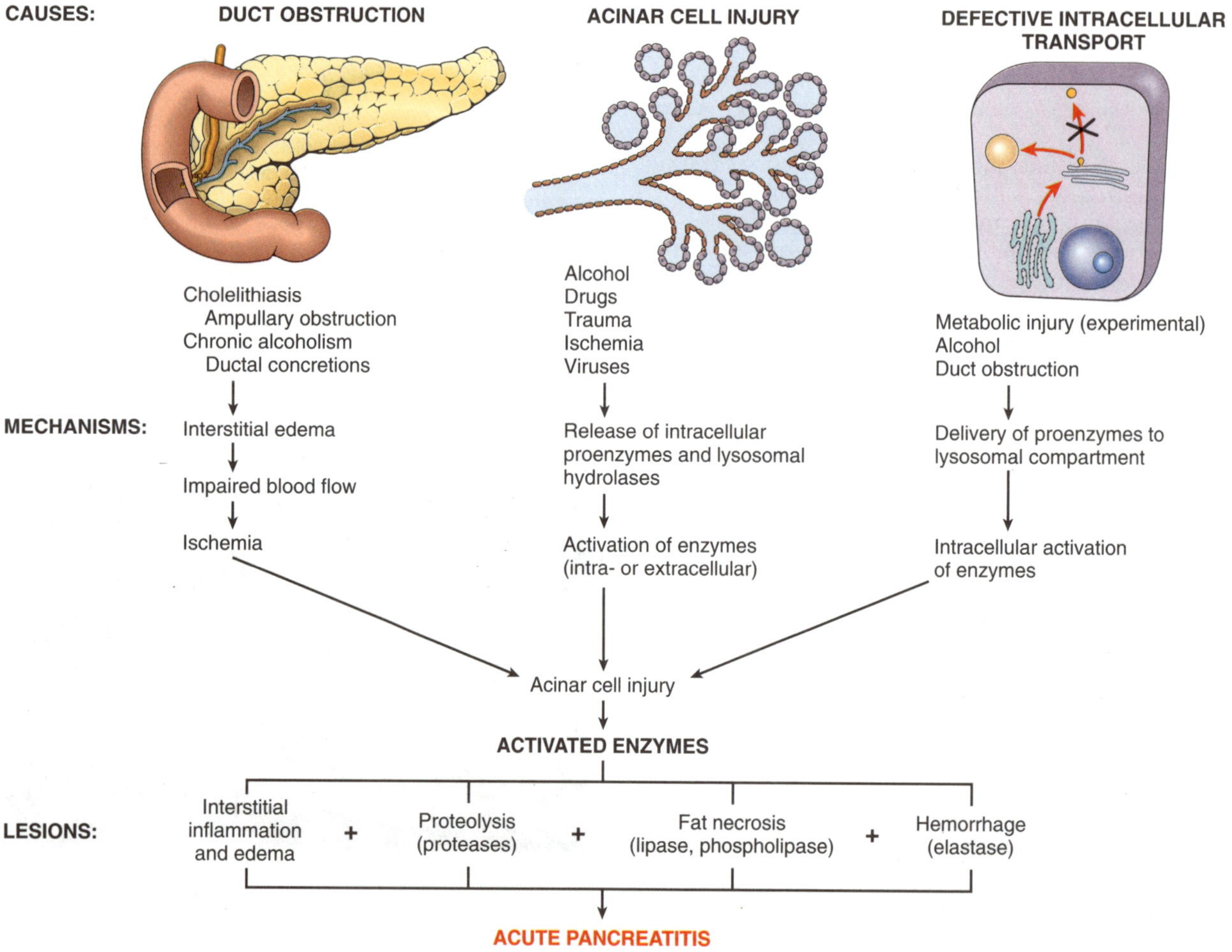

Figure 17–2

Proposed pathogenesis of acute pancreatitis.

results in proenzyme activation, lysosomal rupture (action of phospholipases), and local release of activated enzymes. It is not clear how extensive a role such a mechanism has in human pancreatitis, although aberrant acinar cell packaging of digestive enzymes has been demonstrated after pancreatic duct obstruction.

The manner by which alcohol causes pancreatitis is unknown, although abnormal proenzyme trafficking (described above) has been implicated. Other proposed mechanisms include contraction of the sphincter of Oddi (the muscle regulating the tone at the ampulla of Vater) and direct toxic effects on acinar cells. Alcohol ingestion also causes increased secretion of protein-rich pancreatic fluid, potentially leading to deposition of inspissated protein plugs and obstruction of small pancreatic ducts, followed by the sequence of events described above.

Clinical Features. *Abdominal pain* is the cardinal manifestation of acute pancreatitis. Its severity varies from mild and uncomfortable to severe and incapacitating. Suspected acute pancreatitis is primarily diagnosed by the presence of elevated plasma levels of amylase and lipase and the exclusion of other causes of abdominal pain.

Full-blown acute pancreatitis is a medical emergency of the first magnitude. Such individuals usually have the sudden calamitous onset of an "acute abdomen" with a painful, rigid abdomen and the ominous absence of bowel sounds. Characteristically, the pain is constant and intense and is often referred to the upper back; it must be differentiated from other causes such as ruptured acute appendicitis, perforated peptic ulcer, acute cholecystitis with rupture, and occlusion of mesenteric vessels with infarction of the bowel.

The manifestations of severe acute pancreatitis are attributable to systemic release of digestive enzymes and explosive activation of the inflammatory response. Patients show increased vascular permeability, leukocytosis, disseminated intravascular coagulation, acute respiratory distress syndrome (due to alveolar capillary injury), and diffuse fat necrosis. *Peripheral vascular collapse (shock) can rapidly ensue* as a result of electrolyte disturbances and loss of blood volume, compounded by endotoxemia (from breakdown of the barriers between gastrointestinal flora and the bloodstream), and a massive release of cytokines and vasoactive agents.

Laboratory findings include markedly elevated serum amylase during the first 24 hours, followed (within 72–96 hours) by rising serum lipase levels. Hypocalcemia can result from precipitation of calcium in the extensive areas of fat necrosis; if persistent, it is a poor prognostic sign. The enlarged inflamed pancreas can be visualized by computed tomography (CT) or magnetic resonance imaging.

The crux of the management of acute pancreatitis is supportive therapy (e.g., maintaining blood pressure and alleviating pain), and "resting" the pancreas by total restriction of food and fluids. In 40% to 60% of cases of acute necrotizing pancreatitis, the necrotic debris become infected, usually by gram-negative organisms from the alimentary tract, further complicating the clinical course. Although most individuals with acute pancreatitis eventually recover, some 5% die from shock during the first week of illness; acute respiratory distress syndrome and acute renal failure are ominous complications. In surviving patients, sequelae include sterile *pancreatic abscesses* or *pancreatic pseudocysts* (see below).

Pancreatic Pseudocysts

A common sequela of acute pancreatitis is a *pancreatic pseudocyst.* Liquefied areas of necrotic pancreatic tissue become walled off by fibrous tissue to form a cystic space, lacking an epithelial lining (hence the prefix "pseudo"). Drainage of pancreatic secretions into this space over months to years (from damaged pancreatic ducts) can cause massive enlargement of the cyst. Such collections account for approximately 75% of all pancreatic cysts. While many pseudocysts spontaneously resolve, they can become secondarily infected, and larger pseudocysts can compress or even perforate into adjacent structures.

Morphology

Pseudocysts are usually solitary; they are commonly attached to the surface of the gland and involve peripancreatic tissues such as the lesser omental sac or the retroperitoneum between the stomach and transverse colon or liver (Fig. 17–3A). They can range from 2 to 30 cm in diameter. Since pseudocysts form by walling off areas of hemorrhagic fat necrosis, they are typically composed of necrotic debris encased by fibrous walls of granulation tissue lacking an epithelial lining (Fig. 17–3B).

Chronic Pancreatitis

Chronic pancreatitis is characterized by longstanding inflammation and fibrosis of the pancreas with destruction of the exocrine pancreas; in its late stages, the endocrine parenchyma is also lost. Although chronic pancreatitis can result from recurrent bouts of acute pancreatitis, *the chief distinction between acute and chronic pancreatitis is the irreversible impairment in pancreatic function in the latter.* The prevalence of chronic pancreatitis is difficult to determine but probably ranges between 0.04% and 5% of the population. By far *the most common cause of chronic pancreatitis is long-term alcohol abuse;* middle-aged males constitute the bulk of this group. Less common causes of chronic pancreatitis include:

- Long-standing pancreatic duct *obstruction* (e.g., by pseudocysts, calculi, neoplasms, or pancreas divisum)
- *Tropical pancreatitis,* a poorly characterized disorder seen in Africa and Asia, attributed to malnutrition
- *Hereditary pancreatitis* due to *PRSS1* mutations (see above), or mutations in the *SPINK1* gene encoding trypsin inhibitor.
- *Chronic pancreatitis associated with CFTR mutations.* As discussed in detail in Chapter 7, cystic fibrosis is caused by mutations in the *CFTR* gene. Recall that the CFTR protein is also expressed in pancreatic ductal epithelium, and *CFTR* mutations decrease bicarbonate secretion, thereby promoting protein plugging.

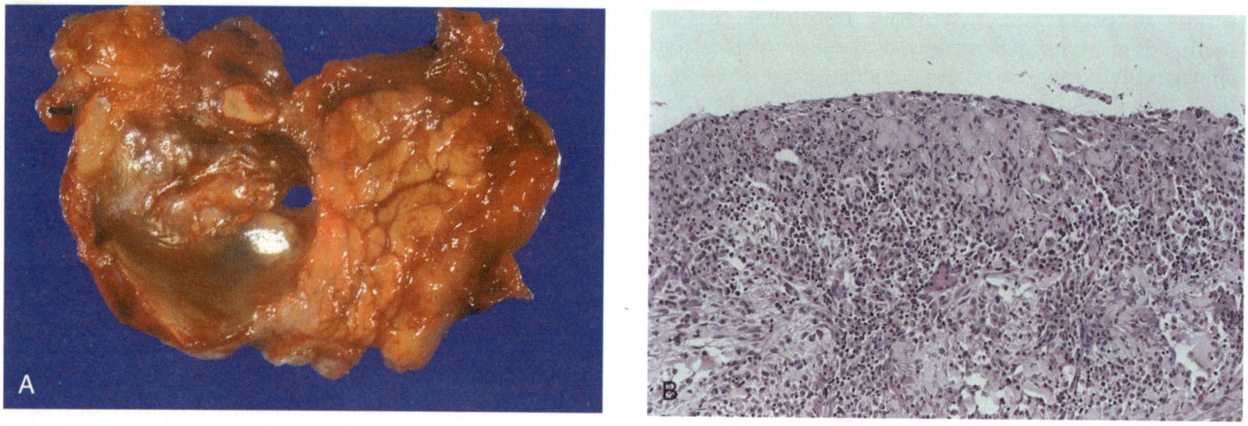

Figure 17–3

Pancreatic pseudocyst. **A,** Cross-section revealing a poorly defined cyst with a necrotic brownish wall. **B,** Histologically the cyst lacks a true epithelial lining and instead is lined by fibrin, granulation tissue, and chronic inflammation.

In typical cystic fibrosis (with Δ 508 mutation, Chapter 7) the secretory defects in the pancreatic ducts are quite severe, giving rise to pancreatic atrophy early in the course of the disease, rather than progressing to chronic pancreatitis. A subset of individuals with certain *CFTR* mutations develop chronic pancreatitis; interestingly, *the other clinical features of cystic fibrosis are typically absent, and the sweat chloride level is normal.* The mutations of the *CFTR* gene in such persons are distinct from those associated with cystic fibrosis. Alternatively, CFTR-related pancreatitis can also be seen in individuals who inherit two distinct *CFTR* gene mutations (compound heterozygotes).

As many as 40% of individuals with chronic pancreatitis have no recognizable predisposing factors. However, as with acute pancreatitis, a growing number of these "idiopathic" cases are associated with inherited mutations in genes important for normal pancreatic exocrine function.

Morphology

Chronic pancreatitis is characterized by **parenchymal fibrosis,** reduced number and size of acini, and variable **dilation of the pancreatic ducts;** there is a relative sparing of the islets of Langerhans (Fig. 17–4A). **Acinar loss** is a constant feature, usually with a chronic inflammatory infiltrate around remaining lobules and ducts. The ductal epithelium may be atrophied, hyperplastic, or exhibit squamous metaplasia, and ductal concretions can occur (Fig. 17–4B). The remaining islets of Langerhans become embedded in the sclerotic tissue and may fuse and appear enlarged; eventually they also disappear. Grossly, the gland is hard, sometimes with extremely dilated ducts and visible calcified concretions.

Pathogenesis. Although the pathogenesis of chronic pancreatitis is not well defined, several hypotheses are proposed:

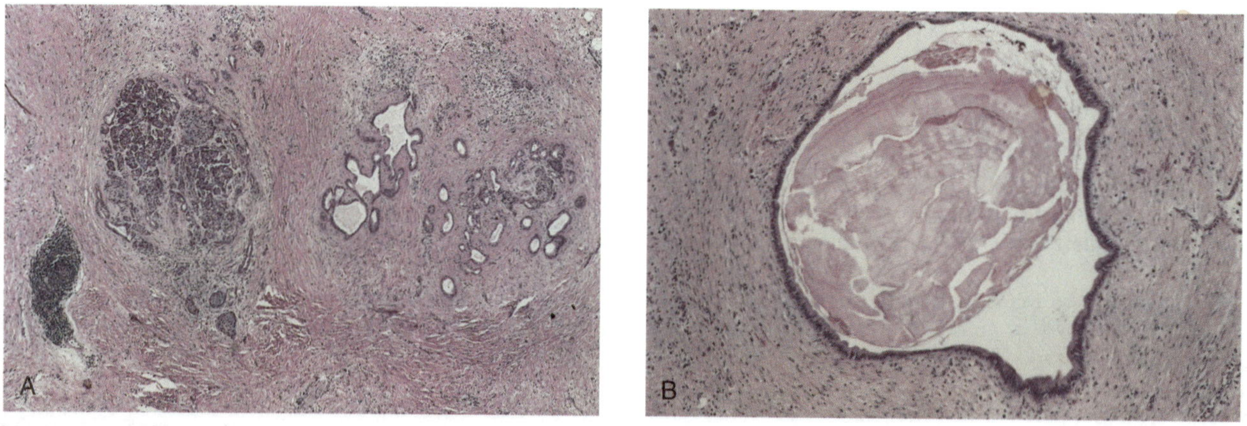

Figure 17–4

Chronic pancreatitis. **A,** Extensive fibrosis and atrophy has left only residual islets *(left)* and ducts *(right),* with a sprinkling of chronic inflammatory cells and acinar tissue. **B,** A higher power view demonstrating dilated ducts with inspissated eosinophilic concretions in a patient with alcoholic chronic pancreatitis.

- *Ductal obstruction by concretions.* Many of the inciting agents in chronic pancreatitis (e.g., alcohol) increase the protein concentration of pancreatic secretions, and these proteins can form ductal plugs.
- *Toxic-metabolic.* Toxins, including alcohol and its metabolites, can exert a direct toxic effect on acinar cells, leading to lipid accumulation, acinar cell loss, and eventually parenchymal fibrosis.
- *Oxidative stress.* Alcohol-induced oxidative stress may generate free radicals in acinar cells, leading to membrane lipid oxidation and subsequent chemokine expression that recruits mononuclear inflammatory cells. Oxidative stress also promotes the fusion of lysosomes and zymogen granules with resulting acinar cell necrosis, inflammation, and fibrosis.
- *Necrosis-fibrosis.* Acute pancreatitis can cause local perilobular fibrosis, duct distortion, and altered pancreatic secretions. Over time and with multiple episodes, this can lead to loss of pancreatic parenchyma and fibrosis.

Clinical Features. Chronic pancreatitis can present in several different ways. It may announce itself with repeated bouts of jaundice or vague indigestion, persistent or recurrent abdominal and back pain, or it may be entirely silent until pancreatic insufficiency and diabetes mellitus develop (the latter due to islet destruction). Attacks can be precipitated by alcohol abuse, overeating (increases demand on pancreatic secretions), or opiates or other drugs that increase the muscle tone of the sphincter of Oddi.

The diagnosis of chronic pancreatitis requires a high degree of suspicion. During an attack of abdominal pain, there may be mild fever and modest elevations of serum amylase. In end-stage disease, however, acinar destruction may preclude such a diagnostic laboratory clue. Gallstone-induced obstruction may present as jaundice or elevations in serum levels of alkaline phosphatase. A very helpful finding is visualization of calcifications within the pancreas by CT or ultrasonography. Weight loss and hypoalbuminemic edema from malabsorption caused by pancreatic exocrine insufficiency can also point toward the disease.

Although chronic pancreatitis is usually not acutely life-threatening, the long-term outlook for individuals with chronic pancreatitis is poor, with a 50% mortality rate over 20 to 25 years. Severe *pancreatic exocrine insufficiency* and chronic malabsorption may develop, as can *diabetes mellitus.* In other patients, *severe chronic pain* may dominate. *Pancreatic pseudocysts* (described above) develop in about 10% of patients. Individuals with hereditary pancreatitis have a 40% lifetime risk of developing pancreatic cancer. The degree to which other forms of chronic pancreatitis contribute to cancer development is unclear.

SUMMARY

Pancreatitis

- *Acute pancreatitis* is characterized by inflammation and reversible parenchymal damage with lesions ranging from focal edema and fat necrosis to widespread parenchymal necrosis and hemorrhage; clinical manifestations vary from mild abdominal pain to a rapidly fatal vascular collapse.
- *Chronic pancreatitis* is characterized by irreversible parenchymal damage and scar formation; clinical manifestations include chronic malabsorption (due to pancreatic exocrine insufficiency) and diabetes mellitus (due to islet cell loss).
- Both entities share similar pathogenic mechanism, and indeed recurrent acute pancreatitis can result in chronic pancreatitis. Ductal obstruction and alcohol are the most common causes of both forms. Inappropriate activation of pancreatic digestive enzymes (due to mutations in genes encoding trypsinogen or trypsin inhibitors) and primary acinar injury (due to toxins, infections, ischemia, or trauma) also cause pancreatitis.

PANCREATIC NEOPLASMS

Pancreatic exocrine neoplasms can be cystic or solid; some are benign, while others are among the most lethal of all malignancies.

Cystic Neoplasms

Roughly 5% to 15% of all pancreatic cysts are neoplastic; these constitute less than 5% of all pancreatic neoplasms. Some of these are entirely benign (e.g., serous cystadenoma); others, such as mucinous cystic neoplasms, can be benign but frequently have malignant potential.

Serous Cystadenomas

Serous cystadenomas account for about a quarter of all pancreatic cystic neoplasms; they are composed of glycogen-rich cuboidal cells surrounding small cysts containing clear, straw-colored fluid (Fig. 17–5). The tumors typically present in the seventh decade of life with nonspecific symptoms such as abdominal pain; the female-to-male ratio is 2:1. These tumors are almost uniformly benign, and surgical resection is curative in the vast majority of patients.

Mucinous Cystic Neoplasms

Mucinous cystic neoplasms almost always arise in women, usually in the body or tail of the pancreas, and present as painless, slow-growing masses. The cystic spaces are filled with thick, tenacious mucin, and the cysts are lined by a columnar mucinous epithelium with an associated densely cellular stroma (Fig. 17–6). These tumors can be benign, borderline malignant, or malignant. Benign mucinous cystadenomas lack significant cytologic or architectural atypia, while borderline mucinous cystic neoplasms show significant cytologic and architectural atypia but no tissue invasion. Malignant mucinous cystadenocarcinomas are invasive.

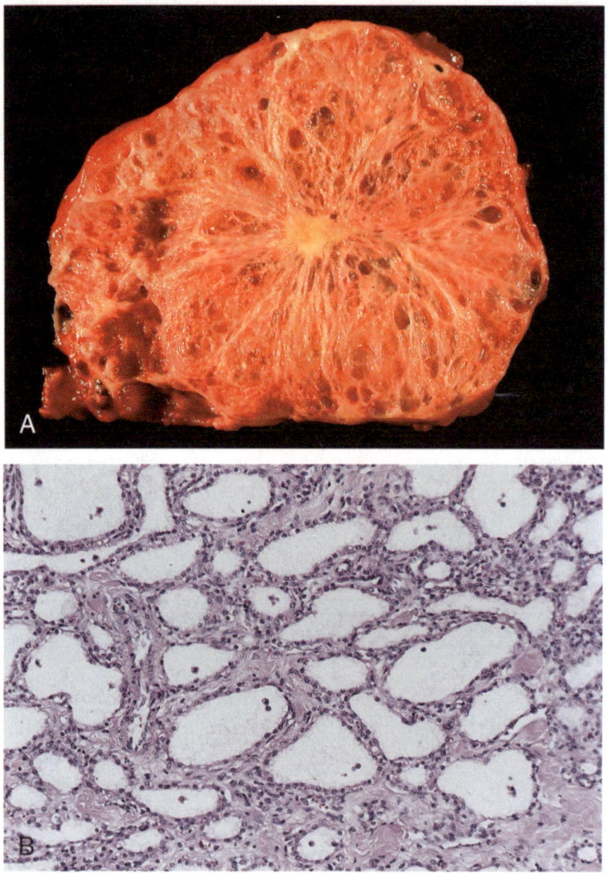

Figure 17–5

Serous cystadenoma. **A,** Cross-section through a serous cystadenoma. Only a thin rim of normal pancreatic parenchyma remains. The cysts are relatively small and contain clear, straw-colored fluid. **B,** The cysts are lined by cuboidal epithelium without atypia.

Intraductal Papillary Mucinous Neoplasms

Intraductal papillary mucinous neoplasms (IPMNs) also produce cysts containing mucin, and can be benign, borderline malignant, or malignant. In contrast to mucinous cystic neoplasms, IPMNs arise more frequently in men than in women and more frequently involve the head of the pancreas. IPMNs arise in the main pancreatic ducts and lack the cellular stroma seen in mucinous cystic neoplasms (Fig. 17–7).

Pancreatic Carcinoma

Pancreatic carcinoma is the fourth leading cause of cancer death in the United States, preceded only by lung, colon, and breast cancers. Although it is substantially less common than the other three malignancies, pancreatic carcinoma is near the top of the list among lethal cancers because it has one of the highest mortality rates. Nearly 30,000 Americans are diagnosed with pancreatic cancer annually, and virtually all will die of it; the 5-year survival rate is dismal—less than 5%.

Pathogenesis. Like all cancers, pancreatic cancer is fundamentally a genetic disease arising as a consequence of inherited and acquired mutations in cancer-associated genes. In a pattern analogous to that seen in colon cancer (Chapter 6), there is a progressive accumulation of genetic changes in pancreatic epithelium as it proceeds from non-neoplastic, to noninvasive lesions in small ducts and ductules, to invasive carcinoma (Fig. 17–8). Antecedent lesions are called "pancreatic intraepithelial neoplasias" (PanINs). Evidence in favor of their precursor relationship to frank malignancy includes the fact that they are often found adjacent to infiltrating carcinomas and share a number of the same genetic mutations. Moreover, the epithelial cells in PanINs show dramatic telomere shortening, potentially predisposing these lesions to accumulating additional chromosomal abnormalities on their way to becoming invasive carcinoma. The more common molecular alterations in pancreatic carcinogenesis affect *K-RAS, p16, SMAD4,* and *p53:*

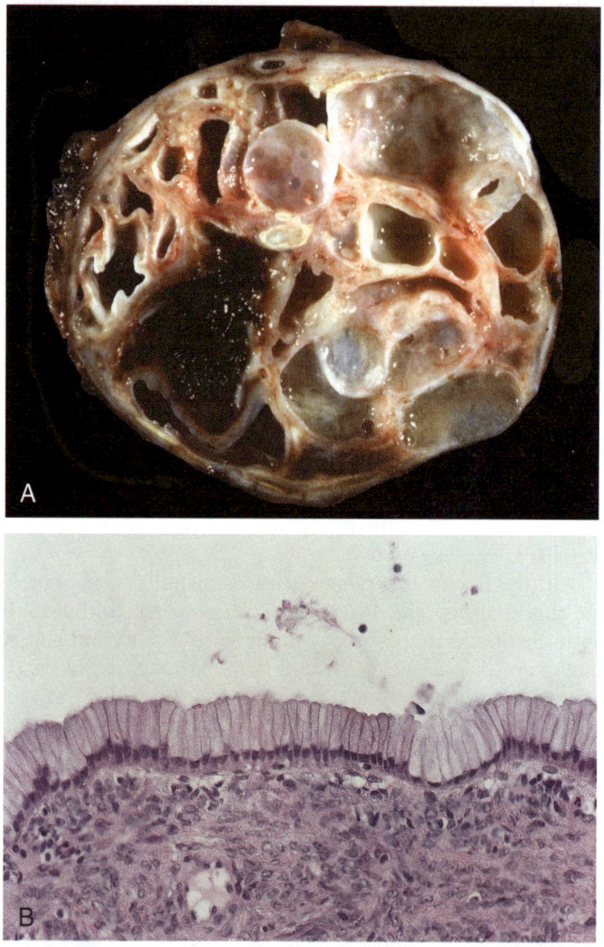

Figure 17–6

Pancreatic mucinous cystadenoma. **A,** Cross-section through a mucinous multiloculated cyst in the tail of the pancreas. The cysts are large and filled with tenacious mucin. **B,** The cysts are lined by columnar mucinous epithelium, with a densely cellular accompanying stroma.

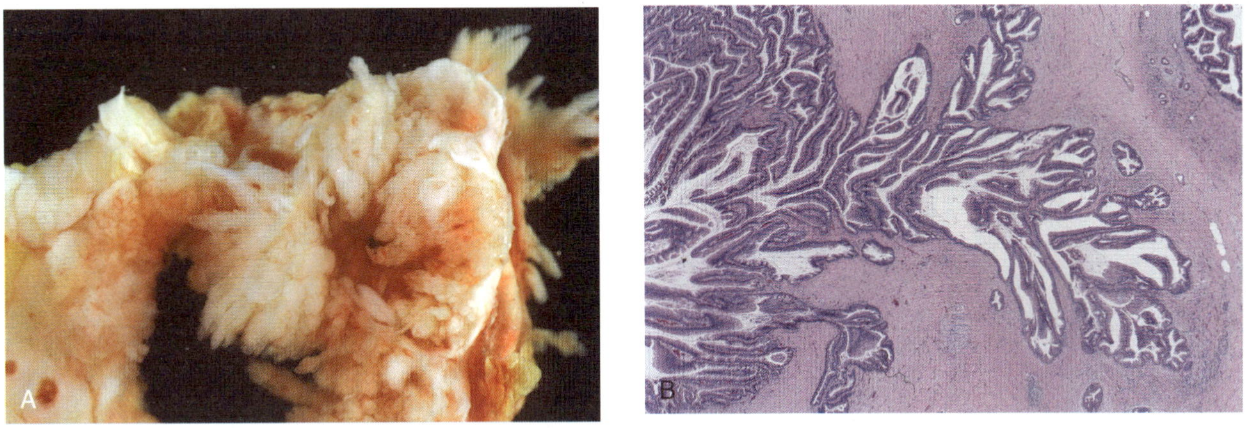

Figure 17–7

Intraductal papillary mucinous neoplasm. **A,** Cross-section through the head of the pancreas showing a prominent papillary neoplasm distending the main pancreatic duct. **B,** The papillary mucinous neoplasm involved the main pancreatic duct *(left)* and is extending down into the smaller ducts and ductules *(right).*

- The *K-RAS* gene is the most frequently altered oncogene in pancreatic cancer; it is activated by point mutation in 80% to 90% of cases. These mutations impair the intrinsic GTPase activity of the K-RAS protein so that it is constitutively active. In turn, K-RAS activates several intracellular signal transduction pathways culminating in the activation of FOS and JUN transcription factors.
- The *p16 (CDKN2A)* gene is the most frequently inactivated tumor suppressor gene in pancreatic cancer, being turned off in 95% of cases. The p16 protein has a critical role in cell cycle control; inactivation removes an important checkpoint.
- The *SMAD4* tumor suppressor gene is inactivated in 55% of pancreatic cancers; it codes for a protein that plays an important role in signal transduction downstream of the transforming growth factor-β receptor. Its normal function is most likely to suppress growth and promote apoptosis.
- Inactivation of the *p53* tumor suppressor gene occurs in 50% to 70% of pancreatic cancers. The *p53* gene product acts both as a cell cycle checkpoint and as an inducer of apoptosis (Chapter 6).

What causes these molecular changes is unknown. It is primarily a disease of the elderly, with 80% of cases occurring between the ages of 60 and 80. Carcincoma of the pancreas is more common in blacks than in whites. The strongest environmental influence is smoking, which doubles the risk. Chronic pancreatitis and diabetes mellitus are also both associated with an increased risk of pancreatic cancer. It is difficult to sort out whether chronic pancreatitis is the cause of pancreatic cancer or an effect of the disease, since small pancreatic cancers can block the pancreatic duct and thereby produce chronic pancreatitis. A similar argument applies to the association of diabetes mellitus with pancreatic cancer, since diabetes can occur as a consequence of pancreatic cancer.

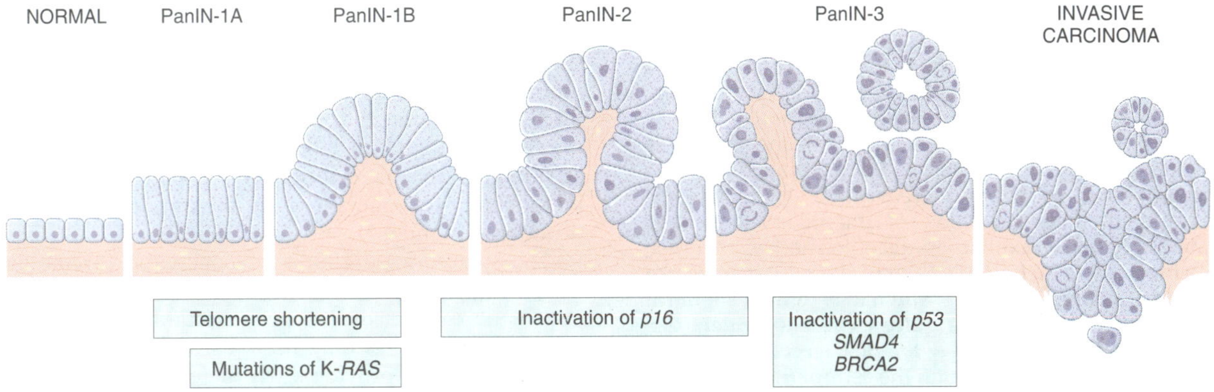

Figure 17–8

Model for the development of pancreatic cancer. It is postulated that telomere shortening, and mutations of the oncogene *K-RAS* occur at early stages, inactivation of the *p16* tumor suppressor gene occurs at intermediate stages, and the inactivation of the *p53, SMAD4,* and *BRCA2* tumor suppressor genes occurs at late stages. Note that while there is a general temporal sequence of changes, the accumulation of multiple mutations is more important than their occurrence in a specific order. (Adapted from Wilentz RE, et al.: Loss of expression of Dpc4 in pancreatic intraepithelial neoplasia: evidence that *DPC4* inactivation occurs late in neoplastic progression. Cancer Res 60:2002, 2000.)

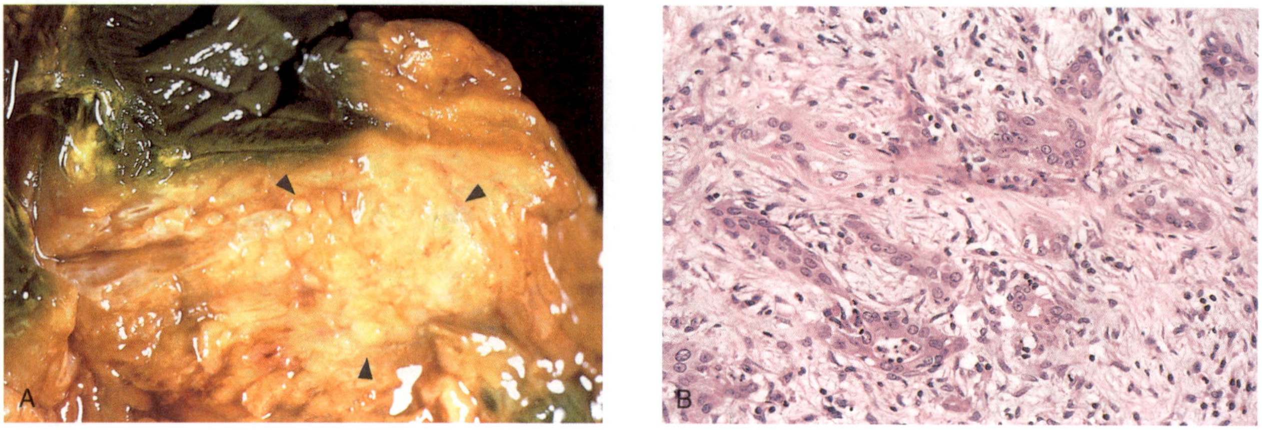

Figure 17–9

Carcinoma of the pancreas. **A,** A cross-section through the head of the pancreas and adjacent common bile duct showing both an ill-defined mass in the pancreatic substance *(arrowheads)* and the green discoloration of the duct resulting from total obstruction of bile flow. **B,** Poorly formed glands are present in a densely fibrotic (desmoplastic) stroma within the pancreatic substance.

Familial clustering of pancreatic cancer has been reported, and a growing number of inherited syndromes are now recognized that increase pancreatic cancer risk. In particular, familial pancreatitis (related to mutations in the *PRSS1* trypsinogen gene; see above) incurs a 50- to 80-fold increased risk of pancreatic malignancy.

Morphology

Approximately 60% of pancreatic cancers arise in the head of the gland, 15% in the body, and 5% in the tail; in 20%, the neoplasm diffusely involves the entire organ. Carcinomas of the pancreas are usually hard, stellate, gray-white, poorly defined masses (Fig. 17–9A).

The vast majority of carcinomas are **ductal adenocarcinomas** recapitulating to some degree the normal duct epithelium by forming glands and secreting mucin. Two features are characteristic of pancreatic cancer: it is highly invasive (even "early" invasive pancreatic cancers invade peripancreatic tissues extensively), and it elicits an intense non-neoplastic host reaction composed of fibroblasts, lymphocytes, and extracellular matrix **(desmoplastic response).**

Most carcinomas of the head of the pancreas obstruct the distal common bile duct as it courses through the head of the pancreas. In 50% of such cases, there is marked distention of the biliary tree, and patients typically exhibit jaundice. In marked contrast, **carcinomas of the body and tail of the pancreas do not impinge on the biliary tract and hence remain silent for some time. They may be quite large and widely disseminated by the time they are discovered.** Pancreatic cancers often extend through the retroperitoneal space, entrapping adjacent nerves, and occasionally invade the spleen, adrenals, vertebral column, transverse colon, and stomach. Peripancreatic, gastric, mesenteric, omental, and portahepatic lymph nodes are frequently involved, and the liver is often enlarged because of metastatic deposits. Distant metastases occur, principally to the lungs and bones.

Microscopically, pancreatic carcinoma is usually a **moderately to poorly differentiated adenocarcinoma forming abortive tubular structures or cell clusters and exhibiting an aggressive, deeply infiltrative growth pattern** (Fig. 17–9B). Dense stromal fibrosis accompanies tumor invasion, and there is a proclivity for perineural invasion within and beyond the organ. Lymphatic invasion is also commonly seen.

Less common variants of pancreatic cancer include: **acinar cell carcinomas** showing prominent acinar cell differentiation with zymogen granules and exocrine enzyme production; **adenosquamous carcinomas** with focal squamous differentiation in addition to glandular differentiation; **undifferentiated carcinomas with osteoclast-like giant cells.**

Clinical Features. *Carcinomas of the pancreas typically remain silent until their extension impinges on some other structure.* Pain is usually the first symptom, but by that point these cancers are usually beyond cure. *Obstructive jaundice* can be associated with carcinoma in the head of the pancreas, but it rarely draws attention to the cancer soon enough. Weight loss, anorexia, and generalized malaise and weakness are signs of advanced disease. *Migratory thrombophlebitis (Trousseau syndrome)* occurs in about 10% of patients and is attributable to the elaboration of platelet-aggregating factors and procoagulants from the tumor or its necrotic products (Chapter 4).

The symptomatic course of pancreatic carcinoma is distressingly brief and progressive. Fewer than 20% of pancreatic cancers overall are resectable at the time of diagnosis. There has long been a search for biochemical tests that could provide early detection of pancreatic cancers. Indeed, serum levels of many enzymes and antigens (e.g., carcinoembryonic and CA19-9 antigens) are elevated, but these markers are neither specific nor sensitive enough to be used as screening tests. Several imaging techniques, such as endoscopic ultrasonography and CT, are helpful in diagnosis and performing percutaneous needle biopsy but are not useful as screening tests.

SUMMARY

Pancreatic Neoplasms

- Pancreatic cancer probably arises from precursor lesions (PanINs), developing by a progressive accumulation of characteristic mutations of oncogenes (e.g., *K-RAS*) and tumor suppressor genes (e.g., *p16, p53,* and *SMAD4*).
- Typically, they are ductal adenocarcinomas with a dense stroma.
- Pancreatic cancer is usually only diagnosed after it is deeply invasive; it is an aggressive malignancy with a high mortality rate.
- Obstructive jaundice is a feature of the carcinoma of the head of the pancreas.

BIBLIOGRAPHY

DiMagno MJ, DiMagno EP: Chronic pancreatitis. Curr Opin Gastroenterol 21:544, 2005. *[An excellent general review on the topic.]*

Furukawa T, et al.: Molecular mechanisms of pancreatic carcinogenesis. Cancer Sci 97:1, 2006 *[A good, current discussion of the pathways in pancreatic carcinogenesis.]*

Gullo L, et al.: Alcoholic pancreatitis: new insights into an old disease. Curr Gastroenterol Rep 7:96, 2005. *[A good discussion of the potential mechanisms linking alcohol and pancreatitis.]*

Maitra A, Kern SE, Hruban RH: Molecular pathogenesis of pancreatic cancer. Best Pract Res Clin Gastroent 20:211, 2006. *[An excellent review of molecular alterations in pancreatic cancer.]*

Mayerle J, et al.: Current management of acute pancreatitis. Nat Clin Pract Gastroenterol Hepatol 2:473, 2005. *[Good overview of the diagnosis and clinical management of the disease.]*

Pandol SJ: Acute pancreatitis. Curr Opin Gastroenterol 21:538, 2005. *[An excellent general review on the topic.]*

Paju A, Stenman UH: Biochemistry and clinical role of trypsinogens and pancreatic secretory trypsin inhibitor. Crit Rev Clin Lab Sci 43:103, 2006. *[An extremely thorough and complete review of the biochemistry of trypsinogens and their inhibitors, correlating with diagnosis and clinical diseases.]*

Sakorafas GH, Sarr MG: Cystic neoplasms of the pancreas; what a clinician should know. Cancer Treat Rev 31:507, 2005. *[A complete clinically oriented overview of pancreatic cystic neoplasms.]*

Whitcomb DC: Mechanisms of disease: advances in understanding the mechanisms leading to chronic pancreatitis. Nat Clin Pract Gastroenterol Hepatol 1:46, 2004. *[A nice summary of the advances in our understanding of the genetic and immunologic contributions to chronic pancreatitis.]*

Chapter 18

The Male Genital System*

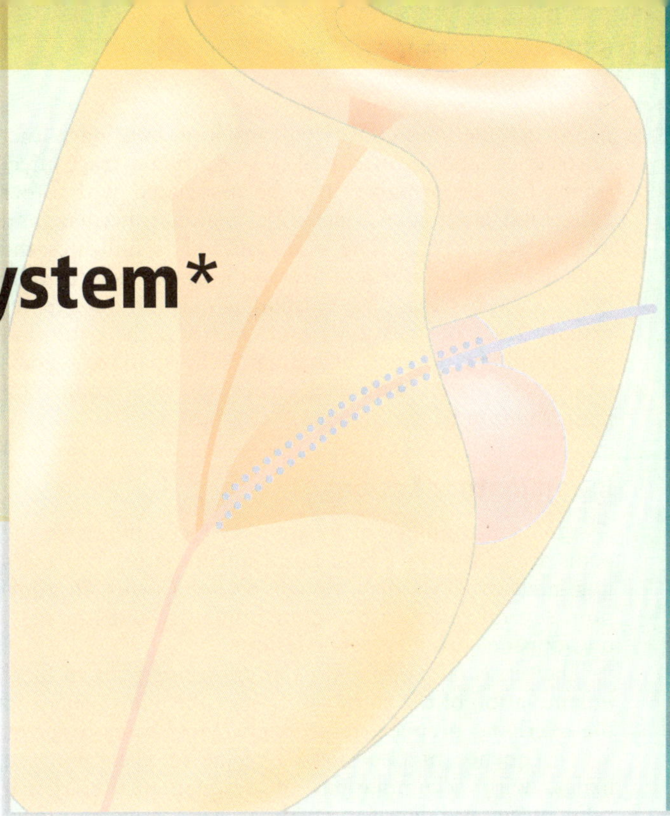

Disorders of the male genital system include a variety of malformations, inflammatory conditions, and neoplasms involving the penis and scrotum, prostate, and testes. In this chapter the major anatomic subdivisions of the male genital system are considered individually, because many of the diseases discussed tend to involve the various organs in a fairly selective fashion. The major exception to this anatomic grouping is the discussion of sexually transmitted diseases (STDs), which are described separately because of their frequent multisystem involvement. Because of many similarities in their presentations in both sexes, the manifestations of selected STDs in females are also considered in this chapter.

*The contributions of Dr. Dennis Burns to this chapter in previous editions of this book and Dr. Tamara Lotan's contributions to this chapter are gratefully acknowledged.

PENIS

The penis may be affected by many congenital and acquired disorders. Only the most common malformations, inflammatory conditions, and neoplasms are considered here. Of the inflammatory disorders affecting the penis, a significant number represent STDs, which are discussed later in the chapter.

Malformations

The most common malformations of the penis include abnormalities in the location of the distal urethral orifice, termed *hypospadias* and *epispadias*. *Hypospadias,* the more common of the two lesions, occurs in 1 in 250 live male births and designates an abnormal opening of the urethra along the ventral aspect of the penis. The urethral orifice, which may lie anywhere along the shaft of the penis, is sometimes constricted, resulting in urinary tract obstruction and an increased risk of urinary tract infections. The abnormality may be associated with other congenital anomalies, including inguinal hernias and undescended testes. The term *epispadias* indicates the presence of the urethral orifice on the dorsal aspect of the penis. Like hypospadias, epispadias may produce lower urinary tract obstruction; in other cases, the condition may result in urinary incontinence. Epispadias is commonly associated with *bladder extrophy,* a congenital malformation of the bladder.

Inflammatory Lesions

A significant number of inflammatory conditions of the penis are caused by STDs. Local inflammatory processes unrelated to STDs may also involve the penis. In addition, several other systemic inflammatory diseases may, on occasion, produce penile lesions.

The terms *balanitis* and *balanoposthitis* refer to local inflammation of the glans penis, or of the glans penis and the overlying prepuce, respectively. Most cases occur as a consequence of poor local hygiene in uncircumcised males, with accumulations of desquamated epithelial cells, sweat, and debris, termed *smegma,* acting as a local irritant. In such cases, the distal penis is typically red, swollen, and tender; a purulent discharge may be present. *Phimosis* represents a condition in which the prepuce cannot be retracted easily over the glans penis. Although phimosis may occur as a congenital anomaly, most cases are acquired from scarring of the prepuce secondary to previous episodes of balanoposthitis. Regardless of its origin, most cases of phimosis are accompanied by evidence of ongoing distal penile inflammation. When a stenotic prepuce is forcibly retracted over the glans penis, the circulation to the glans may be compromised, with resultant congestion, swelling, and pain of the distal penis, a condition known as *paraphimosis.* Urinary retention may develop in severe cases.

Fungi may infect the skin of the penis and scrotum, because growth of fungi is favored by warm, moist conditions at this site and poor local hygiene. *Genital candidiasis* may occur in otherwise normal individuals, but it is particularly common in patients with diabetes mellitus. Candidiasis typically presents as an erosive, painful, intensely pruritic lesion involving the glans penis, scrotum, and adjacent intertriginous areas. Scrapings or biopsy specimens of the lesions reveal characteristic budding yeast forms and pseudohyphae within the superficial epidermis.

Neoplasms

More than 95% of penile neoplasms originate from squamous epithelium. In the United States, squamous cell carcinomas of the penis are relatively uncommon, accounting for about 0.4% of all cancers in males. In developing countries, however, penile carcinoma occurs at much higher rates. Most cases occur in uncircumcised patients older than 40 years of age. Several factors have been implicated in the pathogenesis of squamous cell carcinoma of the penis, including poor hygiene (with resultant exposure to potential carcinogens in smegma), smoking, and infection with human papillomavirus (HPV), particularly types 16 and 18.

As with squamous cell carcinomas at other sites, carcinomas of the penis are generally preceded by the appearance of malignant cells confined to the epidermis, termed *intraepithelial neoplasia* or *carcinoma in situ.* Three clinical variants of carcinoma in situ, all strongly associated with HPV infection, occur on the penis. *Bowen disease* occurs in older uncircumcised males and appears grossly as a solitary, plaquelike lesion on the shaft of the penis. Histologic examination reveals morphologically malignant cells throughout the epidermis with no invasion of the underlying stroma (Fig. 18–1). Bowen disease is not unique to the penis but may also occur elsewhere on the skin and on mucosal surfaces, including the vulva and oral mucosa. Its major clinical importance lies in the potential for progression to invasive squamous cell carcinoma, a complication estimated to occur in as many as 33% of cases involving the penis. When Bowen disease presents as an erythematous patch on the glans penis, it is called *erythroplasia of Queyrat.* Bowenoid papulosis occurs in young, sexually active males and is histologically identical to Bowen disease. Clinically, however, it presents with multiple reddish brown papules on the glans and is most often transient, with only rare progression to carcinoma in immunocompetent patients.

Squamous cell carcinoma of the penis appears as a gray, crusted, papular lesion, most commonly on the glans penis or prepuce. In many cases, the carcinoma infiltrates the underlying connective tissue to produce an indurated, ulcerated lesion with irregular margins (Fig. 18–2). The histologic appearance is usually that of a keratinizing squamous cell carcinoma with infiltrating margins, indistinguishable from squamous carcinomas in other sites. *Verrucous carcinoma* is a variant of squamous

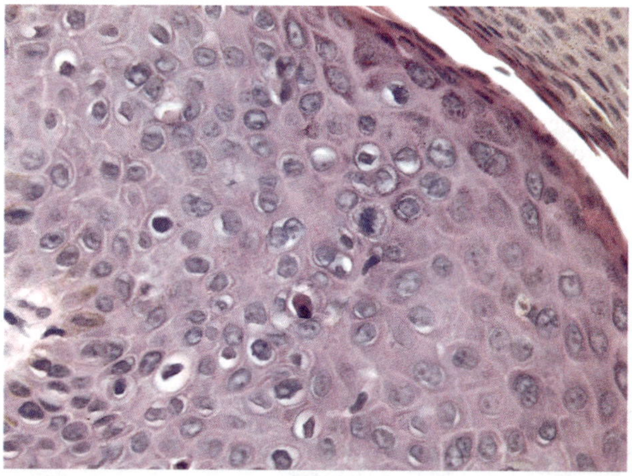

Figure 18–1

Bowen disease (carcinoma in situ) of the penis. The epithelium above the intact basement membrane (not seen in this picture) shows hyperchromatic, dysplastic, dyskeratotic epithelial cells with scattered mitoses above the basal layer.

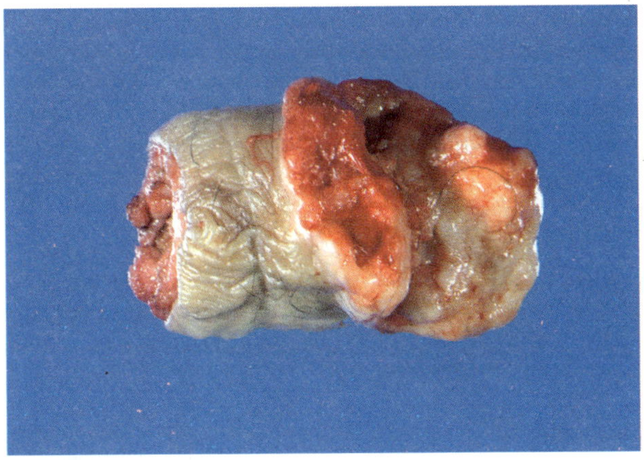

Figure 18–2

Carcinoma of the penis. The glans penis is deformed by a firm, ulcerated, infiltrative mass.

cell carcinoma characterized by a papillary architecture, less striking cytologic atypia, and rounded, pushing deep margins. Most cases of squamous cell carcinoma of the penis are indolent, locally infiltrative lesions. Regional metastases are present in the inguinal lymph nodes in approximately 25% of patients at the time of diagnosis. Distant metastases are relatively uncommon. The overall 5-year survival rate averages 70%.

SUMMARY

Neoplasms of the Penis

- Squamous cell carcinoma and its precursor lesions are the most important penile lesions. All are associated with HPV infection.
- Carcinoma in situ of the penis occurs in three forms: Bowen disease, Bowenoid papulosis, and erythroplasia of Queyrat. Histologically they are similar but have distinctive clinical presentations.
- Squamous cell carcinoma occurs on the glans or shaft of the penis as an ulcerated infiltrative lesion that may spread to inguinal nodes and infrequently to distant sites. Most cases occur in uncircumcised males who are smokers.

SCROTUM, TESTIS, AND EPIDIDYMIS

The skin of the scrotum may be affected by several inflammatory processes, including local fungal infections and systemic dermatoses. Neoplasms of the scrotal sac are unusual. *Squamous cell carcinoma,* the most common of these, is of historical interest in that it represents the first human malignancy associated with environmental influences, dating from Sir Percival Pott's observation of a high incidence of the disease in chimney sweeps. Several disorders unrelated to the testes and epididymis may also present as scrotal enlargement. *Hydrocele,* the most common cause of scrotal enlargement, is an accumulation of serous fluid within the tunica vaginalis. It may arise in response to neighboring infections or tumors, or it may be idiopathic. Accumulations of blood or lymphatic fluid within the tunica vaginalis, termed *hematoceles* and *chyloceles,* respectively, may also cause testicular enlargement. In extreme cases of lymphatic obstruction, caused, for example, by filariasis, the scrotum and the lower extremities may enlarge to grotesque proportions, a condition termed *elephantiasis.*

The more important disorders of the scrotum involve the testes and their adnexal structures. Testicular diseases may be congenital, inflammatory, or neoplastic. They may manifest themselves in a variety of ways, including infertility, atrophy, enlargement, and local pain. Distinguishing among many of these conditions, particularly those associated with testicular enlargement, on the basis of physical examination alone can be exceedingly difficult.

Cryptorchidism and Testicular Atrophy

Cryptorchidism represents *failure of testicular descent* into the scrotum. Normally, the testes descend from the coelomic cavity into the pelvis by the third month of gestation and then through the inguinal canals into the scrotum during the last 2 months of intrauterine life. The diagnosis of cryptorchidism is difficult to establish with certainty before 1 year of age, particularly in premature infants, because complete testicular descent into the scrotum is not invariably present at birth. By 1 year of age, cryptorchidism is present in 1% of the male population. Approximately 10% of these cases are bilateral. Several influences, including hormonal abnormalities, intrinsic testicular abnormalities, and mechanical problems (e.g., obstruction of the inguinal canal), may interfere with normal testicular descent, resulting in malpositioning of the gonad anywhere along its migration pathway. Additionally, cryptorchidism is a common feature of several congenital syndromes, such as the Prader-Willi syndrome (Chapter 7). In the vast majority of cases, however, the cause of the cryptorchidism is unknown. Not surprisingly, bilateral cryptorchidism causes sterility. Unilateral cryptorchidism may be associated with atrophy of the contralateral descended gonad and therefore may also lead to sterility. In addition to infertility, failure of descent is also associated with a 3- to 5-fold increased risk of *testicular malignancy.* Individuals with unilateral cryptorchidism are also at increased risk for the development of cancer in the contralateral, normally descended testis, suggesting that some intrinsic abnormality, rather than simple failure of descent, may be responsible for the increased cancer risk. Surgical placement of the undescended testis into the scrotum (orchiopexy) before puberty decreases the likelihood of testicular atrophy and reduces, but does not eliminate, the risk of cancer and infertility.

Morphology

Cryptorchidism involves the right testis somewhat more commonly than the left. In approximately 10% of cases, the condition is bilateral. The cryptorchid testis may be of normal size early in life, although some degree of atrophy is usually present by the time of puberty. Microscopic evidence of tubular atrophy is evident by 5 to 6 years of age, and hyalinization is present by the time of puberty. Loss of tubules is usually accompanied by hyperplasia of Leydig cells. Foci of **intratubular germ cell neoplasia** (discussed later) may be present in cryptorchid testes and may be the source of subsequent tumors developing in these organs. Atrophic changes similar to those seen in cryptorchid testes may be caused by several other conditions, including chronic ischemia, trauma, radiation, antineoplastic chemotherapy, and conditions associated with chronic elevation in estrogen levels (e.g., cirrhosis). Intratubular germ cell neoplasia is not a feature of these latter conditions, however.

SUMMARY

Cryptorchidism

- Cryptorchidism refers to incomplete descent of the testis from the abdomen to the scrotum and is present in about 1% of 1-year-old males.
- Bilateral or, in some cases, unilateral cryptorchidism is associated with tubular atrophy and sterility.
- The cryptorchid testis has a 3- to 5-fold higher risk of testicular cancer arising in foci of intratubular germ cell neoplasia within the atrophic tubules. Orchiopexy reduces the risk of sterility and cancer.

Inflammatory Lesions

Inflammatory lesions of the testis are more common in the epididymis than in the testis proper. Some of the more important inflammatory diseases of the testis are associated with venereal disease and are discussed later in this chapter. Other causes of testicular inflammation include nonspecific epididymitis and orchitis, mumps, and tuberculosis. *Nonspecific epididymitis* and *orchitis* usually begin as a primary urinary tract infection with secondary ascending infection of the testis through the vas deferens or lymphatics of the spermatic cord. The involved testis is typically swollen and tender and contains a predominantly neutrophilic inflammatory infiltrate. Orchitis complicates *mumps infection* in roughly 20% of infected adult males but rarely occurs in children. The affected testis is edematous and congested and contains a predominantly lymphoplasmacytic inflammatory infiltrate. Severe cases may be associated with considerable loss of seminiferous epithelium with resultant tubular atrophy, fibrosis, and sterility. Several conditions, including infections and autoimmune injury, may elicit a granulomatous inflammatory reaction in the testis. Of these, *tuberculosis* is the most common. Testicular tuberculosis generally begins as an epididymitis, with secondary involvement of the testis. The histologic changes include granulomatous inflammation and caseous necrosis, identical to that seen in active tuberculosis in other sites.

Testicular Neoplasms

Testicular neoplasms are the most important cause of firm, painless enlargement of the testis. Such neoplasms occur in roughly 5 per 100,000 males, with a peak incidence between the ages of 20 and 34 years. Tumors of the testis represent a heterogeneous group of neoplasms composed of germ cell tumors and sex cord/stromal tumors. In adults, 95% of testicular tumors arise from germ cells, and all are malignant. Neoplasms derived from Sertoli or Leydig cells (sex cord/stromal tumors) are uncommon and, in contrast to tumors of germ cell origin, usually pursue a benign clinical course. The remainder of this section will focus on testicular germ cell tumors.

The cause of testicular neoplasms remains unknown. As noted previously, *cryptorchidism is associated with a 3- to 5-fold increase in the risk of cancer* in the undescended testis, as well as an increased risk of cancer in the contralateral descended testis. A history of cryptorchidism is present in approximately 10% of cases of testicular cancer. Intersex syndromes, including androgen insensitivity syndrome and gonadal dysgenesis, are also associated with an increased frequency of testicular cancer. Cytogenetic studies show a wide range of abnormalities in testicular germ cell neoplasms, the most common of which is an isochromosome of the short arm of chromosome 12. However, the role of these chromosomal aberrations in the pathogenesis of testicular neoplasms remains unclear. The risk of neoplasia is increased in siblings of males with testicular cancers, although no consistent hereditary genetic abnormalities have been identified to account for this increased risk. The development of cancer in one testis is associated with a markedly increased risk of neoplasia in the contralateral testis. Testicular tumors are more common in whites than in blacks, and the incidence has increased in Caucasian populations over recent decades.

Classification and Histogenesis. Several different classification schemes have been proposed for testicular neoplasms, based on the histologic features of the tumors and on differing theories about their histogenesis. The World Health Organization classification is the most widely used in the United States (Table 18–1). In this schema, germ cell tumors of the testis are divided into two broad categories, based on whether they contain a single histologic pattern (60% of cases) or multiple histologic patterns (40% of cases). This classification is based on the view that germ cell tumors of the testis arise from primitive cells that may either differentiate along gonadal lines to produce *seminomas* or transform into a totipotential cell population, giving rise to *nonseminomatous germ cell tumors.* Such totipotential cells may remain largely undifferentiated to form *embryonal carcinomas,* may differentiate along extra-embryonic lines to form *yolk sac tumors* and *choriocarcinomas,* or may differentiate along

Table 18–1 Simplified Classification of Testicular Germ Cell Tumors

Tumors with One Histologic Pattern
Seminoma
*Embryonal carcinoma
*Yolk sac tumor
*Choriocarcinoma
*Teratomas Mature Immature With malignant transformation of somatic elements
Tumors with More Than One Histologic Pattern

*Together grouped as non-seminomatous tumors.

somatic cell lines to produce *teratomas*. This proposed histogenesis is supported by the high frequency of mixed histologic patterns among nonseminomatous germ cell tumors. The morphology of the more common forms is presented below, along with a discussion of some of their more salient clinical features.

It is now widely believed that most testicular tumors arise from in situ lesions characterized as *intratubular germ cell neoplasia*. This lesion is present in conditions associated with a high risk of developing germ cell tumors (e.g., cryptorchidism, dysgenetic testes). Furthermore, foci of such in situ lesions are seen in testicular tissue adjacent to a testicular germ cell tumor in virtually all cases.

Morphology

Seminomas, sometimes referred to as "classic" seminomas to distinguish them from the less common spermatocytic seminoma discussed below, account for about 50% of testicular germ cell neoplasms. They are histologically identical to ovarian dysgerminomas and to germinomas occurring in the central nervous system and other extra-gonadal sites. Seminomas are large, soft, well-demarcated, usually homogeneous, gray-white tumors that bulge from the cut surface of the affected testis (Fig. 18–3). The neoplasms are typically confined to the testis by an intact tunica albuginea. Large tumors may contain foci of coagulation necrosis, usually without hemorrhage. The presence of hemorrhage should prompt careful scrutiny for an associated nonseminomatous germ cell component to the tumor. Microscopically, seminomas are composed of **large, uniform cells with distinct cell borders, clear, glycogen-rich cytoplasm, and round nuclei with conspicuous nucleoli** (Fig. 18–4). The cells are often arrayed in small lobules with intervening fibrous septa. A lymphocytic infiltrate is usually present and may, on occasion, overshadow the neoplastic cells. A granulomatous inflammatory reaction may also be present. In as many as 25% of cases, cells staining positively for human chorionic gonadotropin (hCG) can be seen. Some of these hCG-expressing cells are morphologically similar to syncytiotrophoblasts, and they are presumably the source of the elevated serum hCG concentrations that may be encountered in some males with pure seminoma.

Another, less common, morphologic variant of seminoma is the so-called **spermatocytic seminoma.** These tumors, which tend to occur in older patients than do classic seminomas, contain a mixture of medium-sized cells, large uninucleate or multinucleate tumor cells, and small cells with round nuclei that are reminiscent of secondary spermatocytes. There is no association with intratubular germ cell neoplasia, and metastases are exceedingly rare, in contrast to the behavior of classic seminoma.

Embryonal carcinomas are ill-defined, invasive masses containing foci of hemorrhage and necrosis (Fig. 18–5). The primary lesions may be small, even in patients with systemic metastases. Larger lesions may invade the epididymis and spermatic cord. The constituent cells are **large and primitive looking, with basophilic cytoplasm, indistinct cell borders, and large nuclei with prominent nucleoli.** The neoplastic cells may be arrayed in undifferentiated, solid sheets or may contain glandular structures and irregular papillae (Fig. 18–6). In most cases, other patterns of germ cell neoplasia (e.g., yolk sac carcinoma, teratoma, choriocarci-

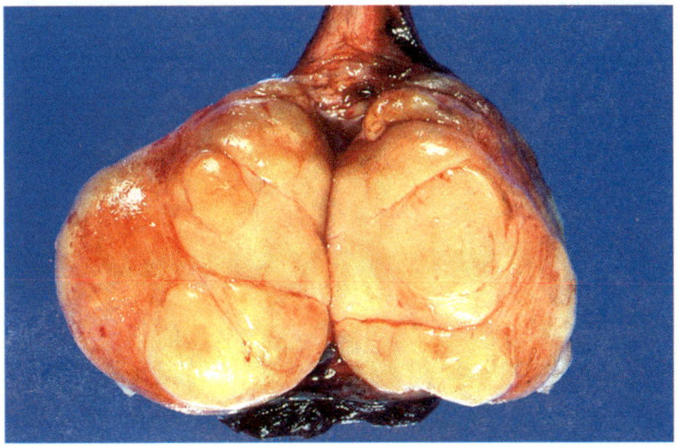

Figure 18–3

Seminoma of the testis appears as a fairly well circumscribed, pale, fleshy, homogeneous mass.

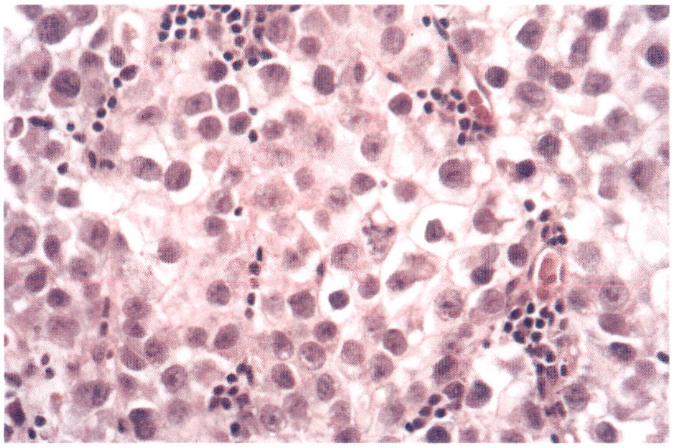

Figure 18–4

Seminoma of the testis. Microscopic examination reveals large cells with distinct cell borders, pale nuclei, prominent nucleoli, and a sparse lymphocytic infiltrate.

noma) are admixed with the embryonal areas. Pure embryonal carcinomas comprise 2% to 3% of all testicular germ cell tumors. As with other germ cell tumors of the testes, foci of intratubular germ cell neoplasia are frequently present in the adjacent seminiferous tubules.

Yolk sac tumors, also termed **endodermal sinus tumors,** are the most common primary testicular neoplasm in children younger than 3 years of age. In adults, yolk sac tumors are most often seen admixed with embryonal carcinoma. In the histogenetic scheme noted previously, yolk sac tumors represent **endodermal sinus** differentiation of totipotential neoplastic cells. Grossly, these tumors are often large and may be well demarcated. Histologic examination discloses low cuboidal to columnar epithelial cells forming microcysts, sheets, glands, and papillae, often associated with eosinophilic hyaline globules (Fig. 18–7). A distinctive feature is the presence of structures resembling primitive glomeruli, the so-called **Schiller-Duvall** bodies. α-fetoprotein (AFP) can be demonstrated within the cytoplasm of the neoplastic cells by immunohistochemical techniques.

Choriocarcinomas represent differentiation of pluripotential neoplastic germ cells along **trophoblastic** lines. Grossly, the primary tumors are often small, nonpalpable lesions, even with extensive systemic metastases. Microscopically, choriocarcinomas are composed of sheets of small cuboidal cells irregularly intermingled with or capped by large, eosinophilic syncytial cells containing multiple dark, pleomorphic nuclei; these represent **cytotrophoblastic** and **syncytiotrophoblastic** differentiation, respectively (Fig. 18–8). Well-formed placental villi are not seen. The hormone hCG can be identified with appropriate immunohistochemical staining, particularly within the cytoplasm of the syncytiotrophoblastic elements.

Teratomas represent differentiation of neoplastic germ cells along **somatic** cell lines. These tumors form firm masses that on cut surface often contain cysts and recognizable areas of cartilage. Histologically, three major variants of pure teratoma are recognized. **Mature teratomas** contain fully differentiated tissues from one or more germ cell layers (e.g., neural tissue, cartilage, adipose tissue, bone, epithelium) in a haphazard array (Fig. 18–9). **Immature teratomas,** in contrast, contain immature somatic elements reminiscent of those in developing fetal tissue. **Teratomas with somatic-type malignancies** are characterized by the development of frank malignancy in preexisting teratomatous elements, usually in the form of a squamous cell carcinoma or adenocarcinoma. Pure teratomas in prepubertal males are usually benign. In adults, teratomas metastasize in as many as 37% of cases. As with other germ cell tumors, testicular teratomas in adults often contain other malignant germ cell elements and therefore should be generally regarded as malignant neoplasms.

Mixed germ cell tumors, as noted, account for approximately 40% of all testicular germ cell neoplasms. Combinations of any of the described patterns may occur in mixed tumors, the most common of which is a combination of teratoma, embryonal carcinoma, and yolk sac tumors.

Clinical Features. Clinically, it is best to consider testicular germ cell tumors under two broad categories: Seminomas and non-seminomatous tumors. As will be evident from the discussion that follows, these two groups of tumors have somewhat distinctive clinical presentation and natural history.

Individuals with testicular germ cell neoplasms present most frequently with *painless enlargement of the testis.* However, some tumors, especially nonseminomatous germ cell neoplasms, may have widespread metastases at diagnosis, in the absence of a palpable testicular lesion.

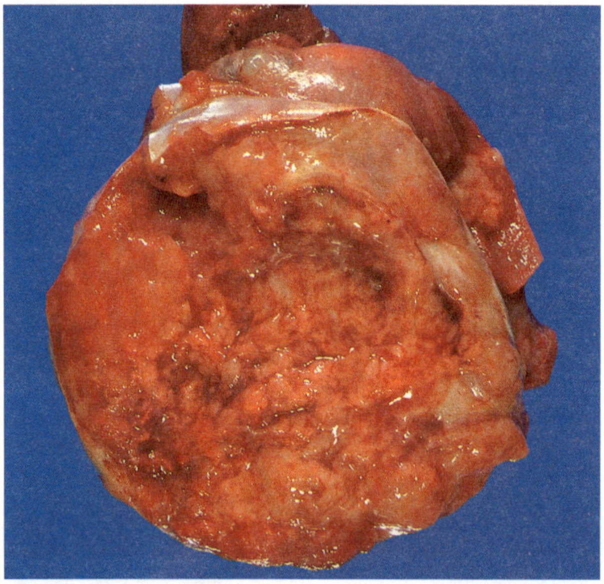

Figure 18–5

Embryonal carcinoma. In contrast to the seminoma illustrated in Figure 18–3, the embryonal carcinoma is a hemorrhagic mass.

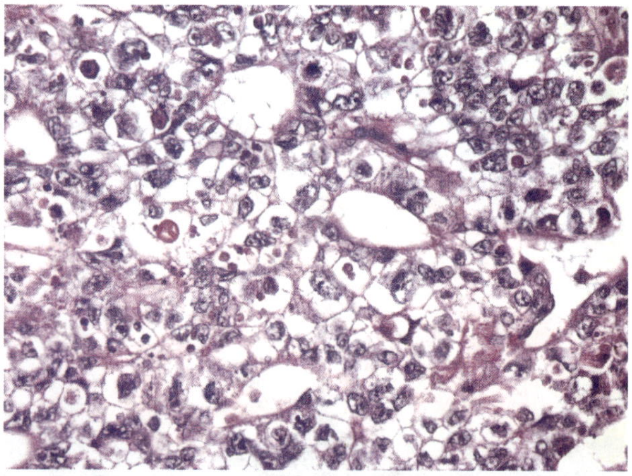

Figure 18–6

Embryonal carcinoma shows sheets of undifferentiated cells as well as primitive glandular differentiation. The nuclei are large and hyperchromatic.

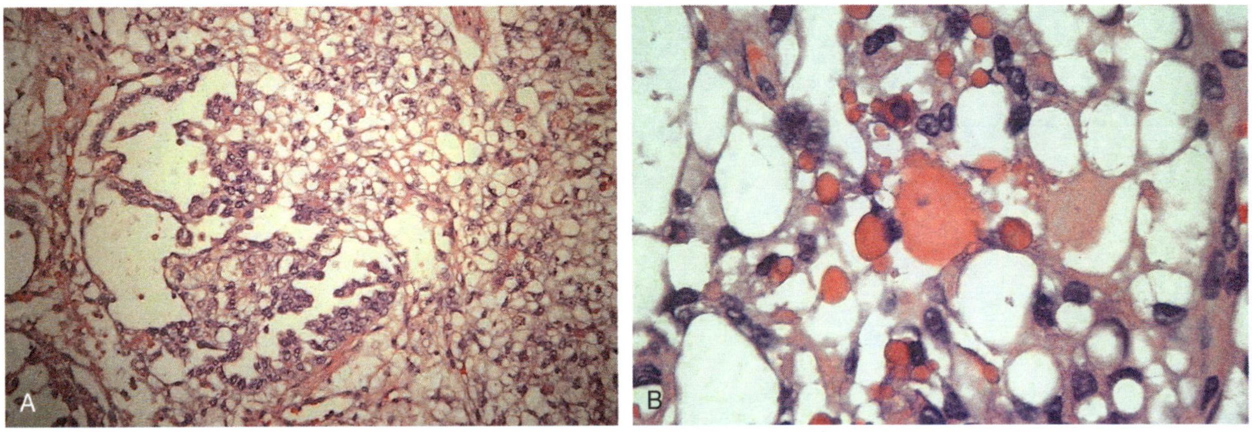

Figure 18–7

Yolk sac carcinoma. **A,** Low-power photomicrograph demonstrating areas of loosely textured, microcystic tissue and a papillary structure resembling a developing glomerulus. **B,** Higher power photomicrograph demonstrating characteristic hyaline droplets within the microcystic areas of the tumor. α-fetoprotein is present within the droplets.

Seminomas often remain confined to the testis for prolonged intervals and may reach considerable size before diagnosis. Metastases are most commonly encountered in the iliac and para-aortic lymph nodes, particularly in the upper lumbar region. Hematogenous metastases occur later. In contrast, *nonseminomatous germ cell neoplasms tend to metastasize earlier,* by both lymphatic and hematogenous routes. Hematogenous metastases are most common in the liver and lungs. Metastatic lesions are typically histologically identical to the primary testicular tumor; rarely they may contain other germ cell elements. Testicular germ cell neoplasms are staged as follows:

Stage I: Tumor confined to the testis
Stage II: Regional lymph node metastases only
Stage III: Nonregional lymph node and/or distant organ metastases

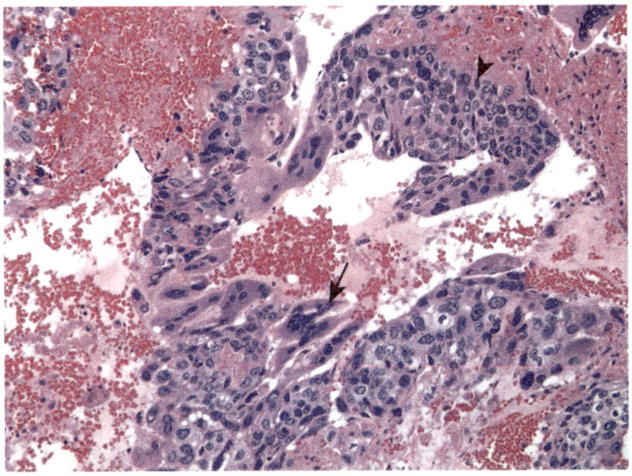

Figure 18–8

Choriocarcinoma shows cytotrophoblastic cells with central nuclei (*arrowhead,* upper right) and syncytiotrophoblastic cells with multiple dark nuclei embedded in eosinophilic cytoplasm (*arrow,* middle). Hemorrhage and necrosis are prominent.

Assay of *tumor markers* secreted by tumor cells is important in the clinical evaluation and staging of germ cell neoplasms (Table 18–2). hCG, produced by neoplastic syncytiotrophoblastic cells, is always elevated in patients with choriocarcinoma. As noted, other germ cell tumors, including seminoma, may also contain syncytiotrophoblastic cells without cytotrophoblastic elements and hence may elaborate hCG. Approximately 10% to 25% of seminomas elaborate hCG. AFP is a glycoprotein normally synthesized by the fetal yolk sac and several other fetal tissues. Nonseminomatous germ cell tumors containing elements of yolk sac (endodermal sinus) often produce AFP; in contrast to hCG, the presence of AFP is a reliable indicator of the presence of a nonseminomatous component to the germ cell neoplasm, because yolk sac elements are not found in pure seminomas. Because mixed patterns are common, most nonseminomatous tumors have elevations of both hCG and AFP. In addition to their role in the primary diagnosis and staging of testicular germ cell tumors, serial determinations of hCG and AFP are useful for monitoring patients for persistent or recurrent tumor after therapy. It should be noted, however, that AFP is also elevated in hepatocellular carcinoma (Chapter 16).

The treatment of testicular germ cell neoplasms is considered a success story of chemotherapy. Although roughly 8000 new cases of testicular cancer occur in the United States yearly, fewer than 400 men are expected to die of the disease. In fact, after being treated for testicular cancer, Lance Armstrong won the Tour de France bicycle race a record seven times! The treatment is determined by both the histologic pattern of the tumor and the stage of disease at the time of diagnosis. Seminomas are exquisitely radiosensitive, and they also respond well to chemotherapy. The prognosis of many nonseminomatous germ cell tumors has improved dramatically with the introduction of platinum-based chemotherapy regimens.

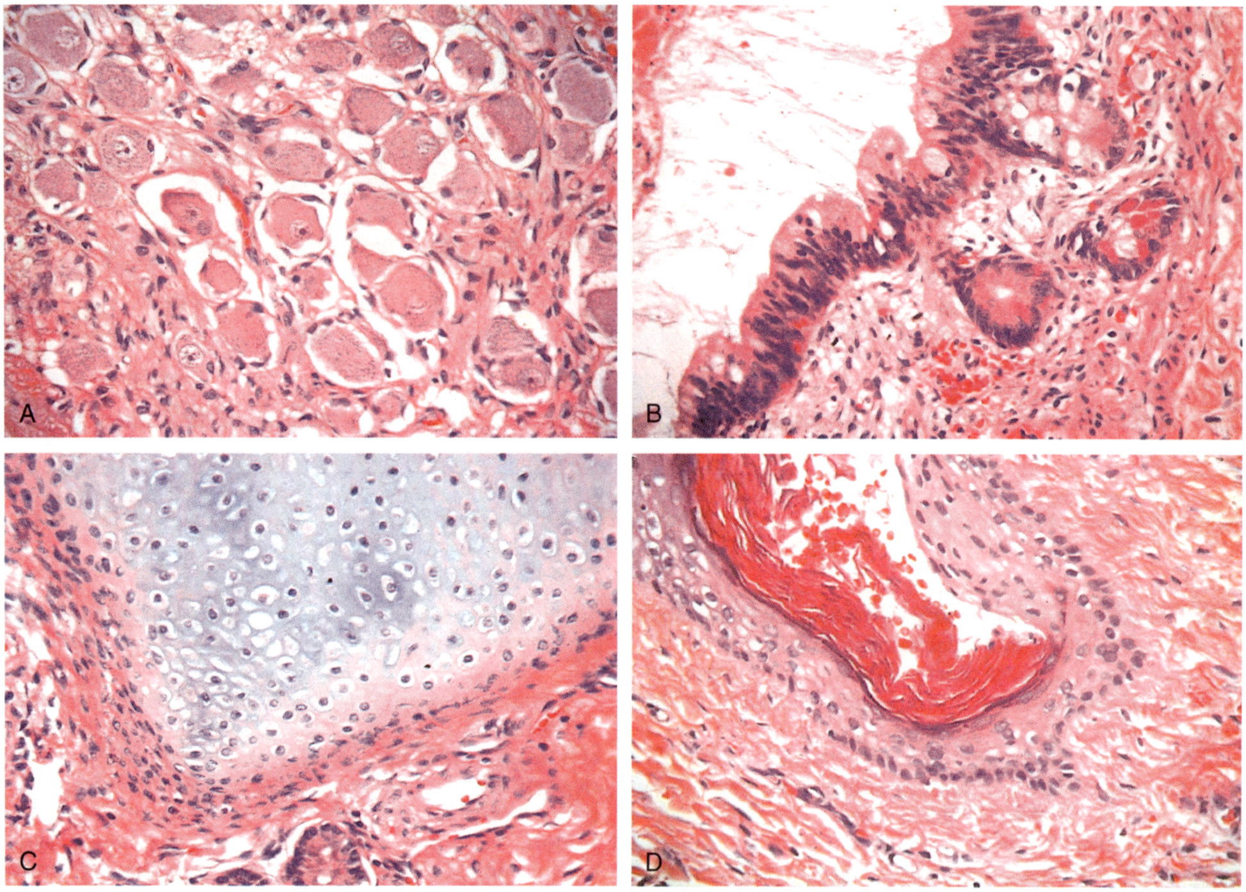

Figure 18–9

Teratoma. Testicular teratomas contain mature cells from endodermal, mesodermal, and ectodermal lines. Pictured here are four different fields from the same tumor containing **(A)** neural (ectodermal), **(B)** glandular (endodermal), **(C)** cartilaginous (mesodermal), and **(D)** squamous epithelial elements.

Table 18–2 Summary of Testicular Tumors

Tumor	Peak Age (yr)	Morphology	Tumor Markers
Seminoma	40–50	Sheets of uniform polygonal cells with cleared cytoplasm; lymphocytes in the stroma	10% have elevated hCG
Embryonal carcinoma	20–30	Poorly differentiated, pleomorphic cells in cords, sheets, or papillary formation; most contain some yolk sac and choriocarcinoma cells	90% have elevated hCG or AFP or both
Yolk sac tumor	3	Poorly differentiated endothelium-like, cuboidal, or columnar cells	90% have elevated AFP
Choriocarcinoma (pure)	20–30	Cytotrophoblast and syncytiotrophoblast without villus formation	100% have elevated hCG
Teratoma	All ages	Tissues from all three germ-cell layers with varying degrees of differentiation	50% have elevated hCG or AFP or both
Mixed tumor	15–30	Variable, depending on mixture; commonly teratoma and embryonal carcinoma	90% have elevated hCG and AFP

AFP, α-fetoprotein; hCG, human chorionic gonadatropin.

SUMMARY

Testicular Tumors

- Testicular tumors are the most common cause of painless testicular enlargement. They occur with increased frequency in undescended testis and in males with gonadal dysgenesis.
- Germ cells are the source of 95% of testicular tumors, and the remainder arise from Sertoli or Leydig cells. Germ cell tumors may be composed of one histologic pattern (60% of cases) or mixed patterns (40%).They are often preceded by in situ lesions.
- The most common single histologic patterns of testicular tumors are seminoma, embryonal carcinoma, yolk sac tumors, choriocarcinoma, and teratoma. Mixed tumors conatain more than one element, most commonly embryonal carcinoma, teratoma, and yolk sac tumors.
- Clinically testicular tumors can be divided into two groups: seminomas and nonseminomatous tumors. Seminomas remain confined to the testis for a long time and spread mainly to para-aortic nodes—rarely to distant sites. Nonseminomatous tumors tend to spread earlier both by lymphatics and blood vessels.
- hCG is produced by syncytiotrophoblasts and is always elevated in choriocarcinomas and in those seminomas that have syncytiotrophoblasts. AFP is made by yolk sac cells and is elevated in yolk sac tumors. Most nonseminomatous tumors have mixed patterns and hence elevation of both hCG and AFP.

PROSTATE

The most important categories of prostatic disease are inflammatory lesions (prostatitis), nodular hyperplasia, and carcinoma.

Prostatitis

Prostatitis may be acute or chronic. The classification of prostatitis is based on a combination of clinical features, microscopic examination, and, in selected cases, culture of fractionated urine specimens obtained before and after prostatic massage. *Acute bacterial prostatitis* is caused by the same organisms associated with other acute urinary tract infections, particularly *Escherichia coli* and other gram-negative rods. Most patients with acute prostatitis have concomitant infection of the urethra and urinary bladder (acute urethrocystitis). In these cases, organisms may reach the prostate by direct extension from the urethra or urinary bladder or by vascular channels from more distant sites. *Chronic prostatitis* may follow clinical episodes of acute prostatitis, or may develop insidiously, without previous episodes of acute infection. In some cases of chronic prostatitis, bacteria similar to those responsible for acute bacterial prostatitis can be isolated. Such cases are designated as *chronic bacterial prostatitis.* In other instances the presence of an increased number of leukocytes in prostatic secretions attests to prostatic inflammation, but bacteriologic findings are negative. Such cases, termed *chronic abacterial prostatitis,* account for most cases of chronic prostatitis. Several nonbacterial agents implicated in the pathogenesis of nongonococcal urethritis, including *Chlamydia trachomatis* and *Ureaplasma urealyticum,* can also cause chronic abacterial prostatitis.

Morphology

Acute prostatitis is characterized by the presence of an acute, neutrophilic inflammatory infiltrate, congestion, and stromal edema. Neutrophils are initially most conspicuous within the prostatic glands. As the infection progresses, the inflammatory infiltrate destroys glandular epithelium and extends into the surrounding stroma, resulting in the formation of microabscesses. Grossly visible abscesses are uncommon but can develop with extensive tissue destruction, e.g. in diabetic patients.

The histologic features of **chronic prostatitis** are nonspecific in most cases and include a variable amount of lymphoid infiltrate, evidence of glandular injury, and, frequently, concomitant acute inflammatory changes. Evidence of tissue destruction and fibroblastic proliferation, along with the presence of other inflammatory cells, such as neutrophils, is required for a histologic diagnosis of chronic prostatitis.

A morphologic variant of chronic prostatitis, **granulomatous prostatitis,** deserves special mention. Granulomatous prostatitis is not a single disease but is instead a morphologic reaction to a variety of different insults. Granulomatous inflammation may be encountered with systemic inflammatory processes (e.g., disseminated tuberculosis, sarcoidosis, fungal infections, Wegener granulomatosis). It may also occur as a nonspecific reaction to inspissated prostatic secretions and after transurethral resection of prostatic tissue. The morphologic features of granulomatous prostatitis include multinucleate giant cells and variable numbers of foamy histiocytes, sometimes accompanied by eosinophils. Caseous necrosis is only seen in the setting of tuberculous prostatitis. It is not seen in other forms of granulomatous prostatitis.

Clinical Features. The clinical manifestations of prostatitis include *dysuria, urinary frequency, lower back pain,* and *poorly localized suprapubic or pelvic pain.* The prostate may be enlarged and tender, particularly in acute prostatitis, in which local symptoms are often accompanied by fever and leukocytosis. Chronic prostatitis, even if asymptomatic, may serve as a reservoir for organisms capable of causing urinary tract infections. Chronic bacterial prostatitis, therefore, is one of the most important causes of recurrent urinary tract infection in men.

SUMMARY

Prostatitis

- Prostatitis may be acute or chronic and the latter may be bacterial or abacterial. Acute bacterial prostatitis is caused by *E. coli* and other gram-negative rods that cause urinary tract infections. Chronic bacterial prostatitis is caused by the same organisms and may follow acute infection or arise insidiously. Chronic abacterial prostatitis is caused by *C. trachomatis* and *U. urealyticum*.
- Clinically, acute prostatitis causes dysuria, frequency, and low back pain. Chronic prostatitis may be symptomatic or silent. It is an important cause of recurrent urinary tract infection in males.

Nodular Hyperplasia of the Prostate

The normal prostate consists of glandular and stromal elements surrounding the urethra. The prostatic parenchyma can be divided into several biologically distinct regions, the most important of which are the peripheral, central, transitional, and periurethral zones (Fig. 18–10). The types of proliferative lesions are different in each region. For example, most *hyperplastic* lesions arise in the inner transitional and central zones of the prostate, while most *carcinomas* (70% to 80%) arise in the peripheral zones.

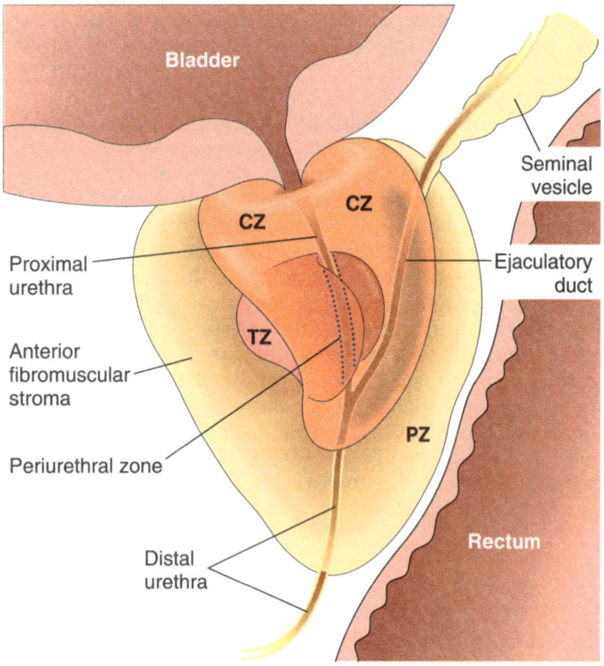

Figure 18–10

Adult prostate. The normal prostate contains several distinct regions, including a central zone (CZ), a peripheral zone (PZ), a transitional zone (TZ), and a periurethral zone. Most carcinomas arise from the peripheral glands of the organ and are often palpable during digital examination of the rectum. Nodular hyperplasia, in contrast, arises from more centrally situated glands and is more likely to produce urinary obstruction early in its course than is carcinoma.

Nodular hyperplasia, also termed *glandular* and *stromal hyperplasia,* is an extremely common abnormality of the prostate. It is present in a significant number of men by the age of 40, and its frequency rises progressively with age, reaching 90% by the eighth decade. Prostatic hyperplasia is characterized by proliferation of both stromal and epithelial elements, with resultant enlargement of the gland and, in some cases, urinary obstruction. "Benign prostatic hypertrophy" (BPH), a time-honored synonym for nodular hyperplasia of the prostate, is both redundant and a misnomer, because all hypertrophies are benign and the fundamental lesion is a hyperplasia rather than a hypertrophy.

Although the cause of nodular hyperplasia remains incompletely understood, it is clear that *androgens have a central role in its development.* Nodular hyperplasia does not occur in males castrated before the onset of puberty nor in men with genetic diseases that block androgen activity. Dihydrotestosterone (DHT), an androgen derived from testosterone through the action of 5α-reductase, and its metabolite, 3α-androstanediol, seem to be major hormonal stimuli for stromal and glandular proliferation in men with nodular hyperplasia. DHT binds to nuclear androgen receptors and, in turn, stimulates synthesis of DNA, RNA, growth factors, and other cytoplasmic proteins, leading to hyperplasia. This forms the basis for the current use of 5α-reductase inhibitors in the treatment of symptomatic nodular hyperplasia. Because no study has shown a conclusive association between circulating androgen levels and the development of nodular hyperplasia, it follows that local, intraprostatic concentrations of androgens and androgen receptors contribute to the pathogenesis of this condition. Experimental work has also identified age-related increases in estrogen levels that may increase the expression of DHT receptors on prostatic parenchymal cells, thereby functioning in the pathogenesis of nodular hyperplasia.

Morphology

As noted, nodular hyperplasia arises most commonly in the inner, periurethral glands of the prostate, particularly from those that lie above the verumontanum. The affected prostate is enlarged, with weights in excess of 300 gm reported in severe cases. The cut surface contains many fairly well-circumscribed nodules that bulge from the cut surface (Fig. 18–11). This nodularity may be present throughout the prostate, but it is **usually most pronounced in the inner (central and transitional) region.** The nodules may have a solid appearance or may contain cystic spaces, the latter corresponding to dilated glandular elements seen in histologic sections. The urethra is usually compressed by the hyperplastic nodules, often to a slitlike orifice. In some cases, hyperplastic glandular and stromal elements lying just under the epithelium of the proximal prostatic urethra may project into the bladder lumen as a pedunculated mass, resulting in a ball-valve type of urethral obstruction.

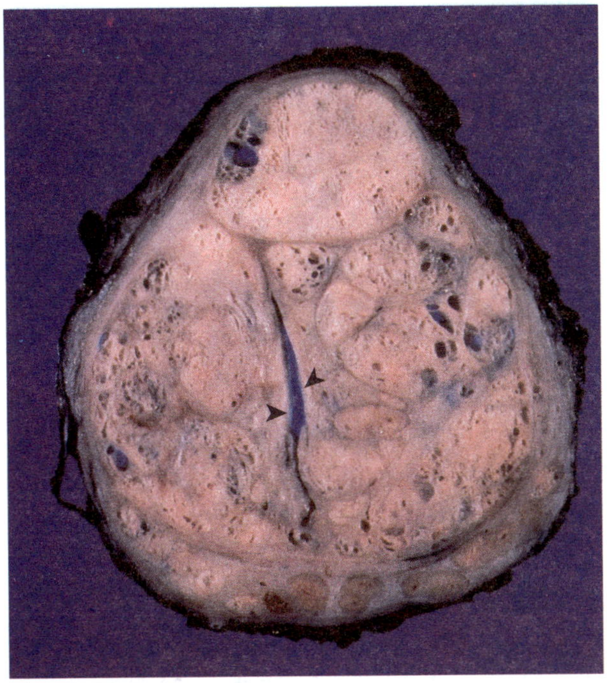

Figure 18–11

Nodular prostatic hyperplasia. Well-defined nodules compress the urethra (*arrowheads*) into a slitlike lumen.

Microscopically the hyperplastic nodules are composed of varying proportions of proliferating glandular elements and fibromuscular stroma. The hyperplastic glands are lined by tall, columnar epithelial cells and a peripheral layer of flattened basal cells; crowding of the proliferating epithelium results in the formation of papillary projections in some glands (Fig. 18–12). The glandular lumina often contain inspissated, proteinaceous secretory material, termed **corpora amylacea.** The glands are surrounded by proliferating stromal elements. Other nodules are composed predominantly of spindle-shaped stromal cells and connective tissue. Areas of infarction are fairly common in advanced cases of nodular hyperplasia and are frequently accompanied by foci of squamous metaplasia in adjacent glands.

Clinical Features. Clinical manifestations of prostatic hyperplasia occur in only about 10% of men with the disease. Because nodular hyperplasia preferentially involves the inner portions of the prostate, its most common manifestations are those of *lower urinary tract obstruction.* These include difficulty in starting the stream of urine (hesitancy) and intermittent interruption of the urinary stream while voiding. Some men may develop complete urinary obstruction, with resultant painful distention of the bladder and, if neglected, hydronephrosis (Chapter 14). Symptoms of obstruction are frequently accompanied by urinary urgency, frequency, and nocturia, all indicative of bladder irritation. The combination of residual urine in the bladder and chronic obstruction increases the risk of urinary tract infections.

SUMMARY

Nodular Hyperplasia of the Prostate

- Nodular hyperplasia of prostate is characterized by benign proliferation of stromal and glandular elements. DHT, an androgen derived from testosterone, is the major hormonal stimulus for proliferation.
- Nodular hyperplasia most commonly affects the inner periuretheral zone of the prostate, and the nodules compress the prostatic urethra. Microscopically the nodules have variable proportions of

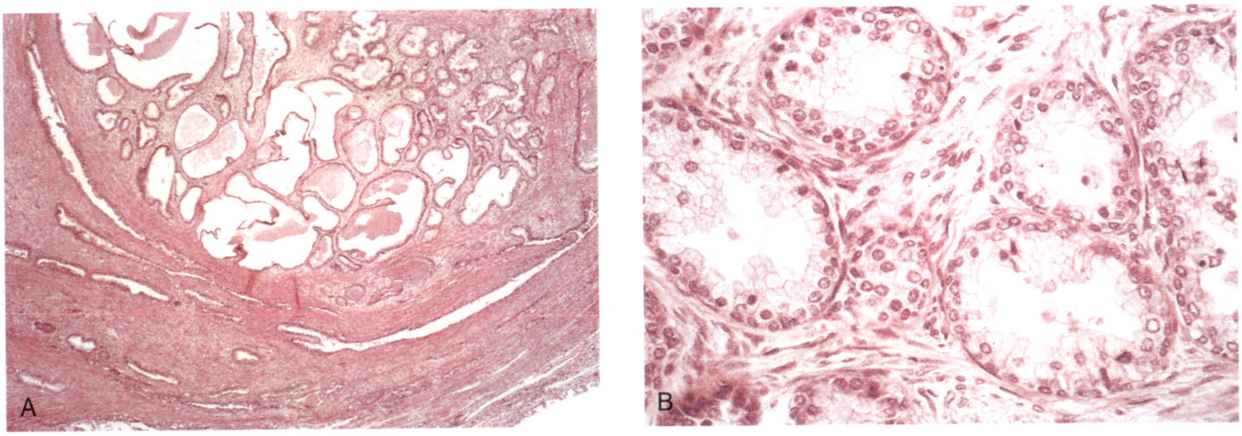

Figure 18–12

Nodular hyperplasia. **A,** Low-power photomicrograph demonstrates a well-demarcated nodule at the top of the field, populated by hyperplastic glands. In other cases of nodular hyperplasia, the nodularity is caused predominantly by stromal, rather than glandular, proliferation. **B,** Higher power photomicrograph demonstrates the morphology of the hyperplastic glands, with the characteristic dual cell population: the inner columnar secretory cells, and the outer flattened basal cell layer.

stroma and glands. Hyperplastic glands are lined by two cell layers: an inner columnar layer and an outer layer composed of flattened basal cells.
- Clinical symptoms are seen in 10% of affected patients and include hesitancy, urgency, nocturia, and poor urinary stream. Chronic obstruction predisposes to recurrent urinary tract infections. Acute urinary obstruction may occur.

Carcinoma of the Prostate

Carcinoma of the prostate is the most common visceral cancer in males, ranking as the second most common cause of cancer-related deaths in men older than 50 years of age, after carcinoma of the lung. It is predominantly a disease of older males, with a peak incidence between the ages of 65 and 75 years. Latent cancers of the prostate are even more common than those that are clinically apparent, with an overall frequency of more than 50% in men older than 80 years of age.

Although the cause of carcinoma of the prostate remains unknown, clinical and experimental observations suggest that hormones, genes, and environment all have a role in its pathogenesis. Cancer of the prostate does not develop in males castrated before puberty, indicating that *androgens* probably contribute to its development. A hormonal influence is further suggested by the observation that the growth of many carcinomas of the prostate can be inhibited by orchiectomy or by the administration of estrogens such as diethylstilbestrol. As in the case of nodular hyperplasia of the prostate, however, the function of hormones in the pathogenesis of carcinoma of the prostate is not fully understood.

Hereditary contributions have also been implicated in light of the increased risk of disease among first-degree relatives of patients with prostate cancer. Symptomatic carcinoma of the prostate is more common and occurs at an earlier age in American blacks than in whites, Asians, or Hispanics. Whether such racial differences occur as a consequence of genetic influences, environmental factors, or some combination of the two remains unknown. However, the frequency of *incidental* prostatic cancers is comparable in all races, suggesting that race figures more importantly in the growth of established lesions than in the initial development of carcinoma. Much effort is focused on finding prostate cancer genes, but no definitive data are available. In studies of familial cases, several susceptibility loci on chromosome 1 have been identified. In sporadic cases, hypermethylation of glutathione *S*-transferase p1 *(GSTP1)*, a genome caretaker gene on chromosome 11, and telomere shortening are relatively common genetic alterations. Recent studies implicate overexpression of two ETS family transcription factors in the pathogenesis of prostate cancer. Recall that these transcription factors are also involved in Ewing sarcoma. Interestingly, racial variations in the number of CAG repeats in the androgen receptor gene seem to be linked to the higher incidence of prostate cancer in African Americans. Perhaps these polymorphisms influence the action of androgens on prostatic epithelium.

A possible role for *environmental influences* is suggested by the increased frequency of prostatic carcinoma in certain industrial settings and by significant geographic differences in the incidence of the disease. Carcinoma of the prostate is particularly common in Scandinavian countries and relatively uncommon in Japan and certain other Asian countries. Males emigrating from low-risk to high-risk areas maintain a lower risk of prostate cancer; the risk of disease is intermediate in subsequent generations, in keeping with an environmental influence on the development of this disease. Among environmental influences, a diet high in animal fat has been suggested as a risk factor.

Morphology

Seventy to eighty percent of prostate cancers arise in the outer (peripheral) glands and hence may be palpable as irregular hard nodules by rectal digital examination. Because of the peripheral location, prostate cancer is less likely to cause urethral obstruction in its initial stages than is nodular hyperplasia. Early lesions typically appear as ill-defined masses just beneath the capsule of the prostate. On cut surface, foci of carcinoma appear as firm, gray-white to yellow lesions that infiltrate the adjacent gland with ill-defined margins (Fig. 18–13). Metastases to regional pelvic lymph nodes may occur early. Locally advanced cancers often infiltrate the seminal vesicles and periurethral zones of the prostate and may invade the adjacent soft tissues and the wall of the urinary bladder. Denonvilliers fascia, the connective tissue layer separating the lower genitourinary structures from the rectum, usually prevents growth of the tumor posteriorly. Invasion of the rectum therefore is less common than is invasion of other contiguous structures.

Microscopically, most prostatic carcinomas are **adenocarcinomas** exhibiting variable degrees of differentiation. The better differentiated lesions are composed of small glands that infiltrate the adjacent stroma

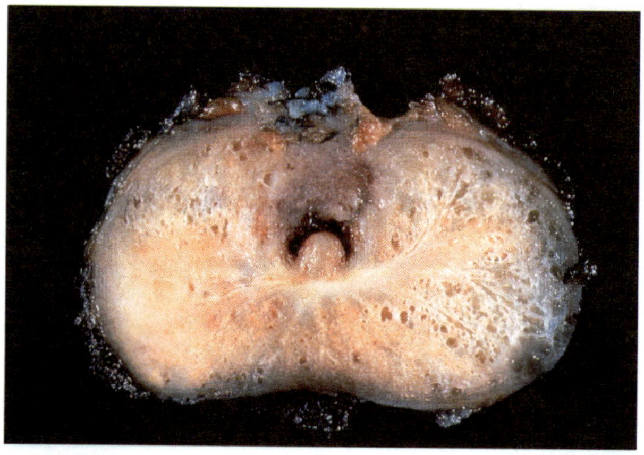

Figure 18–13

Adenocarcinoma of the prostate. Carcinomatous tissue is seen on the posterior aspect *(lower left)*. Note the solid whiter tissue of cancer in contrast to the spongy appearance of the benign peripheral zone on the contralateral side.

in an irregular, haphazard fashion. In contrast to normal and hyperplastic prostate, the glands in carcinomas lie "back to back" and appear to dissect sharply though the native stroma (Fig. 18–14). The neoplastic glands are lined by a single layer of cuboidal cells with conspicuous nucleoli; the basal cell layer seen in normal or hyperplastic glands is absent. With increasing degrees of anaplasia, irregular, ragged glandular structures, papillary or cribriform epithelial structures, and, in extreme cases, sheets of poorly differentiated cells are present. Glands adjacent to areas of invasive carcinoma of the prostate often contain foci of epithelial atypia, or **prostatic intraepithelial neoplasia (PIN)**. Because of its frequent coexistence with infiltrating carcinoma, PIN has been suggested as a probable precursor to carcinoma of the prostate. PIN has been subdivided into high-grade and low-grade patterns, depending on the degree of atypia. Importantly, high-grade PIN shares molecular changes with invasive carcinoma, lending support to the argument that PIN is an intermediate between normal and frankly malignant tissue.

A number of histologic grading schemes have been proposed for carcinoma of the prostate. They are based on features such as the degree of glandular differentiation, the architecture of the neoplastic glands, nuclear anaplasia, and mitotic activity. A commonly used method for grading is the **Gleason system.** Despite the potential difficulties associated with incomplete sampling in biopsy material and the subjectivity inherent in histologic evaluation, Gleason grade has proved to correlate reasonably well with both the anatomic stage of prostatic carcinoma (discussed later) and the prognosis.

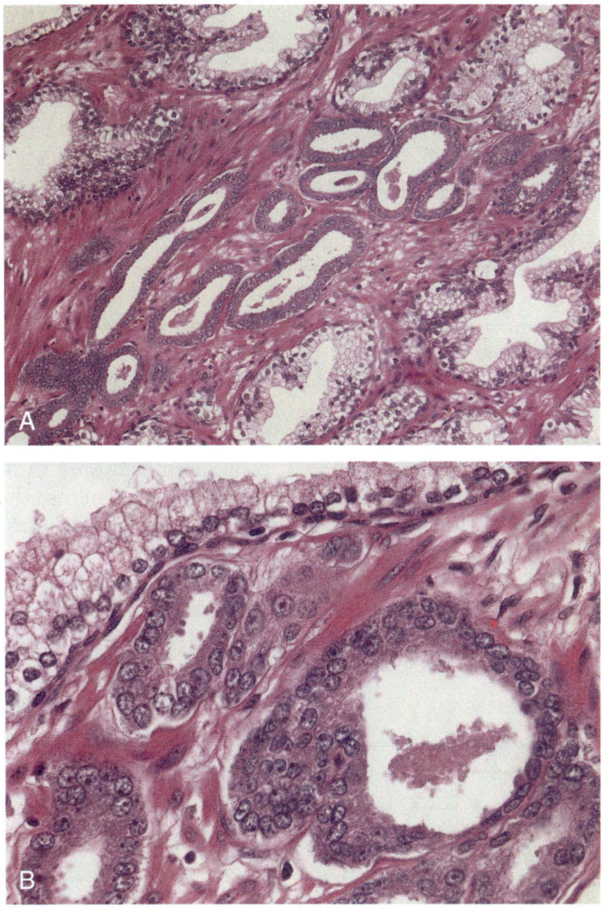

Figure 18–14

A, Photomicrograph of a small focus of adenocarcinoma of the prostate demonstrating small glands crowded in between larger benign glands. **B,** Higher magnification shows several small malignant glands with enlarged nuclei, prominent nucleoli, and dark cytoplasm, as compared with the larger benign gland *(top).*

Clinical Features. Carcinomas of the prostate are often clinically silent, particularly during their early stages. Approximately 10% of localized carcinomas are discovered unexpectedly, during histologic examination of prostate tissue removed for nodular hyperplasia. In autopsy studies, the incidence approaches 30% in men between 30 and 40 years of age. Because most cancers begin in the peripheral regions of the prostate, they may be discovered during routine digital rectal examination. More extensive disease may produce signs and symptoms of "prostatism," including local discomfort and evidence of lower urinary tract obstruction similar to that encountered in patients with nodular hyperplasia. Physical examination in such cases typically reveals evidence of locally advanced disease, in the form of a hard, fixed prostate. More aggressive carcinomas of the prostate may first come to clinical attention because of the presence of metastases. Regrettably, this is not an uncommon mode of presentation. Bone metastases, particularly to the axial skeleton, are common and may cause either osteolytic (destructive) or, more commonly, osteoblastic (bone-producing) lesions. *The presence of osteoblastic metastases in an older male is strongly suggestive of advanced prostatic carcinoma.*

Assay of serum levels of *prostate-specific antigen* (PSA) has gained widespread use in the diagnosis of early carcinomas. PSA is a 33-kD proteolytic enzyme produced by both normal and neoplastic prostatic epithelium. PSA is secreted in high concentrations into prostatic acini and thence into seminal fluid, where it increases sperm motility by maintaining seminal secretions in a liquid state. Traditionally, a serum PSA level of 4.0 ng/L has been used as the upper limit of normal. Cancer cells produce more PSA, but any condition that disrupts the normal architecture of the prostate, including adenocarcinoma, nodular hyperplasia, and prostatitis, may also cause an elevation in serum levels of PSA. Although serum PSA levels tend to be higher in men with carcinomas than in those with nodular hyperplasia, considerable overlap in serum levels exists between the two conditions. Moreover, in a minority of cases of cancer of the prostate, especially those confined to the prostate, serum PSA is not elevated. Because of these problems with both specificity and sensitivity, PSA is of limited value when used as an isolated screening test for cancer of the prostate. Its diagnostic value is enhanced considerably, however, when it is used in conjunction with other procedures, such as digital rectal examination, transrectal sonography, and needle biopsy. In contrast to its limitations as a diagnostic screening test, serum PSA concentration is of great value in monitoring patients after treatment for prostate cancer, with rising levels after ablative therapy indicative of recurrence and/or the development of metastases. Several refinements in the testing of PSA values may further enhance its diagnostic utility. These include rate of change of PSA values with time (PSA velocity), determination of the ratio between the serum PSA value and volume of the prostate gland (PSA density), and the measurement of free versus bound forms of circulating PSA. Free PSA levels greater than 25% indicate a lower risk for cancer, whereas levels below 10% are worrisome. Such refinements are likely to be most useful when PSA levels are between 4 and 10 ng/mL, the "gray zone."

Anatomic staging of the extent of disease has an important role in the evaluation and treatment of prostatic carcinoma (Table 18–3). Prostate cancer is staged by clinical examination, surgical exploration, radiographic imaging techniques, and, in some systems, the histologic grade of the tumor and levels of tumor markers. The anatomic extent of disease and the histologic grade influence the therapy for prostate cancer and correlate well with prognosis. Carcinoma of the prostate is treated with various combinations of surgery, radiation therapy, and hormonal manipulations. Localized disease is usually treated with surgery, external-beam, or internal (radioactive seeds) radiation therapy. Hormonal therapy has a central role in the treatment of advanced carcinomas. Specifically, most prostate cancers are androgen sensitive and are inhibited to some degree by androgen ablation. Surgical or pharmacologic castration, estrogens, and androgen receptor-blocking agents have all been used to control the growth of disseminated lesions. Serial evaluation of serum levels of PSA, as noted, is useful to monitor patients for recurrent or progressive disease. The prognosis for patients with limited-stage disease is favorable: more than 90% of patients with stage T1 or T2 lesions survive 10 years or longer. The outlook for patients with disseminated disease remains poor, with 10-year survival rates in this group ranging from 10% to 40%.

Table 18–3 Staging of Prostatic Adenocarcinoma Using the TNM System

TNM Designation	Anatomic Findings
Extent of Primary Tumor (T)	
T1	CLINICALLY INAPPARENT LESION (BY PALPATION/IMAGING STUDIES)
T1a	Involvement of ≤5% of resected tissue
T1b	Involvement of >5% of resected tissue
T1c	Carcinoma present on needle biopsy (following elevated PSA)
T2	PALPABLE OR VISIBLE CANCER CONFINED TO PROSTATE
T2a	Involvement of ≤50% of one lobe
T2b	Involvement of >50% of one lobe, but unilateral
T2c	Involvement of both lobes
T3	LOCAL EXTRAPROSTATIC EXTENSION
T3a	Extracapsular extension
T3b	Seminal vesical invasion
T4	INVASION OF CONTIGUOUS ORGANS AND/OR SUPPORTING STRUCTURES INCLUDING BLADDER NECK, RECTUM, EXTERNAL SPHINCTER, LEVATOR MUSCLES, OR PELVIC FLOOR
Status of Regional Lymph Nodes (N)	
N0	NO REGIONAL NODAL METASTASES
N1	METASTASIS IN REGIONAL LYMPH NODES
Distant Metastases (M)	
M0	NO DISTANT METASTASES
M1	DISTANT METASTASES PRESENT
M1a	Metastases to distant lymph nodes
M1b	Bone metastases
M1c	Other distant sites

PSA, prostate-specific antigen.

SUMMARY

Carcinoma of the Prostate

- Carcinoma of the prostate is a common cancer of older men between 65 and 75 years of age. It is more common in American blacks than in Caucasians.
- Carcinomas of the prostate arise most commonly in the outer, peripheral glands and may be palpable by rectal exam. Microscopically, they are adenocarcinomas with variable differentiation and anaplasia. Neoplastic glands are lined by a single layer of cells. Grading of prostate cancer by the Gleason system correlates with anatomic stage and prognosis.
- Most localized cancers are clinically silent and are detected by routine monitoring of PSA concentrations in older men. Advanced cancers present with metastases, frequently to the bones.
- Serum PSA concentrations under 4 ng/mL are considered normal, and values over 10 ng/mL are suggestive of prostate cancer. PSA levels may also be elevated above 4 ng/mL in non-neoplastic conditions such as nodular hyperplasia and prostatitis, hence biopsy is required for diagnosis. Evaluation of PSA concentrations after treatment has great value in monitoring progressive or recurrent disease.

SEXUALLY TRANSMITTED DISEASES (STDs)

STDs have complicated human existence for centuries and continue to do so at the present time. Globally, approximately 15 million new cases of STD occur every year, and of these, 4 million affect 15- to 19-year-olds and 6 million affect 20- to 24-year-olds. Of the 10 leading infectious diseases that require notification of the Centers for Disease Control in the United States, five are STDs (Table 18–4). These include chlamydia, gonorrhea,

Table 18–4 Classification of Important Sexually Transmitted Diseases

	Disease or Syndrome and Population Principally Affected		
Pathogens	**Males**	**Both**	**Females**
Viruses			
Herpes simplex virus		Primary and recurrent herpes, neonatal herpes	
Hepatitis B virus		Hepatitis	
Human papillomavirus	Cancer of penis (some cases)	Condyloma acuminatum	Cervical dysplasia and cancer, vulvar cancer
Human immunodeficiency virus		Acquired immunodeficiency syndrome	
Chlamydiae			
Chlamydia trachomatis	Urethritis, epididymitis, proctitis	Lymphogranuloma venereum	Urethral syndrome, cervicitis, bartholinitis, salpingitis, and sequelae
Mycoplasmas			
Ureaplasma urealyticum	Urethritis		Cervicitis
Bacteria			
Neisseria gonorrhoeae	Epididymitis, prostatitis, urethral stricture	Urethritis, proctitis, pharyngitis, disseminated gonococcal infection	Cervicitis, endometritis, bartholinitis, salpingitis and sequelae (infertility, ectopic pregnancy, recurrent salpingitis)
Treponema pallidum		Syphilis	
Haemophilus ducreyi		Chancroid	
Calymmatobacterium granulomatis		Granuloma inguinale (donovanosis)	
Shigella sp.	Enterocolitis*		
Campylobacter sp.	Enterocolitis*		
Protozoa			
Trichomonas vaginalis	Urethritis, balanitis	Vaginitis	
Entamoeba histolytica	Amebiasis*		
Giardia lamblia	Giardiasis*		

*Most important in homosexual populations.
Modified and updated from Krieger JN: Biology of sexually transmitted diseases. Urol Clin North Am 11:15, 1984.

acquired immunodeficiency syndrome (AIDS), syphilis, and hepatitis B. In the United States, the two most common STDs are genital herpes and genital HPV infection, but these do not require notification. Several of these entities, such as human immunodeficiency virus (HIV) infection, HPV, hepatitis B, and infection with *E. histolytica,* are discussed in other chapters. Our comments here focus on some of the more important of these entities that are not conveniently addressed in other areas of this book.

Syphilis

Syphilis, or lues, is a chronic venereal infection caused by the spirochete *Treponema pallidum*. First recognized in epidemic form in sixteenth-century Europe as the Great Pox, syphilis has remained an endemic infection in all parts of the world. In the United States, approximately 6000 cases are reported every year, and this number has been on an upward trajectory since 2000. There is a strong racial disparity, with African Americans affected 30 times more often than whites.

T. pallidum is a fastidious spirochete whose only natural hosts are humans. The usual source of infection is an active cutaneous or mucosal lesion in a sexual partner in the early (primary or secondary) stages of syphilis. The organism is transmitted from such lesions during sexual intercourse across minute breaks in the skin or mucous membranes of the uninfected partner. In cases of congenital syphilis, *T. pallidum* is transmitted across the placenta from mother to fetus, particularly during the early stages of maternal infection. Once introduced into the body, the organisms are rapidly disseminated to distant sites by lymphatics and the bloodstream, even before the appearance of lesions at the primary inoculation site. Between 9 and 90 days (a mean of 21 days) after the initial infection, a primary lesion, termed a *chancre,* appears at the point of entry. Systemic dissemination of organisms continues during this period, while the host mounts an immune response. Two types of antibodies are formed: nontreponemal antibodies and antibodies to specific treponemal antigens. As discussed in detail later, detection of these antibodies plays an important part in the diagnosis of syphilis. This acquired immunity, however, fails to eradicate spirochetes introduced during the primary inoculation.

The chancre of primary syphilis resolves spontaneously over a period of 4 to 6 weeks and is followed in approximately 25% of untreated patients by the development of *secondary syphilis*. The manifestations of secondary syphilis, discussed in more detail later, include generalized lymphadenopathy and variable mucocutaneous lesions and reflect the presence of organisms disseminated throughout the body during the primary phase of the disease. *The mucocutaneous lesions of both primary and secondary syphilis are teeming with spirochetes and are highly infectious.* Like the chancre, the lesions of secondary syphilis resolve without any specific antimicrobial therapy, at which point patients are said to be in *early latent phase syphilis*. Mucocutaneous lesions may recur during this phase of the disease. The US Public Health Service has restricted the definition of early latent syphilis to the period 1 year after infection.

Patients with untreated syphilis then enter into an asymptomatic, *late latent* phase of the illness. In about one-third of cases, subsequent symptomatic lesions may develop over the next 5 to 20 years. This late symptomatic phase, or *tertiary syphilis*, is marked by the development of lesions in the cardiovascular system, central nervous system, or, less frequently, other organs. Spirochetes are much more difficult to demonstrate during the later stages of disease, and patients with late latent or tertiary syphilis are much less likely to be infectious than are those in the primary or secondary stages of disease.

Syphilis is common in HIV-infected patients. Like all other ulcerative genital diseases, syphilis promotes the transmission of HIV, and HIV stimulates progression of syphilis.

Morphology

The macroscopic lesions of syphilis vary with the stage of disease and are discussed later. The fundamental microscopic lesion of syphilis is a **proliferative endarteritis** and an accompanying **inflammatory infiltrate rich in plasma cells.** The treponemes cause endothelial hypertrophy and proliferation, followed by intimal fibrosis and narrowing of the vessel lumen. Local ischemia caused by the vascular changes undoubtedly accounts for some of the local cell death and fibrosis seen in syphilis, although other factors, including delayed hypersensitivity, also appear to contribute to parenchymal injury. Spirochetes are readily demonstrable in histologic sections of early lesions with the use of standard silver stains (e.g., Warthin-Starry stains). There is no evidence that the organisms cause direct toxic injury to the host tissues. Large areas of parenchymal damage in tertiary syphilis result in the formation of a **gumma,** an irregular, firm mass of necrotic tissue surrounded by resilient connective tissue. Microscopically the gumma contains a central zone of coagulation necrosis surrounded by a mixed inflammatory infiltrate composed of lymphocytes, plasma cells, activated macrophages (epithelioid cells), occasional giant cells, and a peripheral zone of dense fibrous tissue.

Primary Syphilis

This stage is characterized by the presence of a chancre at the site of initial inoculation. The chancre of syphilis is characteristically indurated and has been referred to in the past as a "hard chancre" to distinguish it from the "soft chancre" of chancroid caused by *Haemophilus ducreyi;* (discussed later). The primary chancre in males is usually on the penis. In females, multiple chancres may be present, usually in the vagina or on the uterine cervix. The chancre begins as a small, firm papule, which gradually enlarges to produce a painless ulcer with well-defined, indurated margins and a "clean," moist base (Fig. 18–15). Spirochetes are readily demonstrable in material scraped from the ulcer base using dark-field and immunofluorescence microscopy (Fig. 18–16). Regional lymph nodes are often slightly enlarged and firm, but painless. Histologic examination of the ulcer reveals the usual lymphocytic and plasmacytic inflammatory infiltrate and proliferative vascular changes as described before. Even without therapy, the primary chancre resolves over a period of several weeks to form a subtle scar. *Serologic tests for syphilis are often negative during the early stages of primary syphilis* and therefore should be complemented by dark-field microscopy or direct fluorescent antibody testing if primary syphilis is suspected.

Secondary Syphilis

Within approximately 2 months of resolution of the chancre, the lesions of secondary syphilis occur. The manifestations of secondary syphilis are varied but typically include a combination of *generalized lymph node enlargement* and a variety of *mucocutaneous lesions*. Skin lesions are usually symmetrically distributed and may be maculopapular, scaly, or pustular. *Involvement of the palms of the hands and soles of the feet is common.* In moist skin areas, such as the anogenital region, inner thighs, and axillae, broad-based, elevated lesions termed *condylomata lata* may occur. Superficial mucosal lesions resembling condylomata lata can occur anywhere, but they are particularly common in the oral cavity, pharynx, and external genitalia. Histologic examination of mucocutaneous lesions during the secondary phase of the disease reveals the characteristic *proliferative endarteritis,* accompanied by a *lymphoplasmacytic inflammatory infiltrate.* Spirochetes are present and easily demonstrable within the mucocutaneous lesions; they are therefore contagious. Lymph node enlargement is most common in the neck and inguinal areas. Biopsy of enlarged nodes reveals nonspecific hyperplasia of germinal centers accompanied by increased numbers of plasma cells or, less commonly, granulomas or neutrophils. Less common manifestations of secondary syphilis include hepatitis, renal disease, eye disease (iritis), and gastrointestinal abnormalities. The mucocutaneous lesions of secondary syphilis resolve over a period of several weeks, at which point the patient enters the early latent phase of the disease, which lasts approximately 1 year. Lesions may recur at any time during the early latent phase, during which the disease may still be spread. *Both nontrepone-*

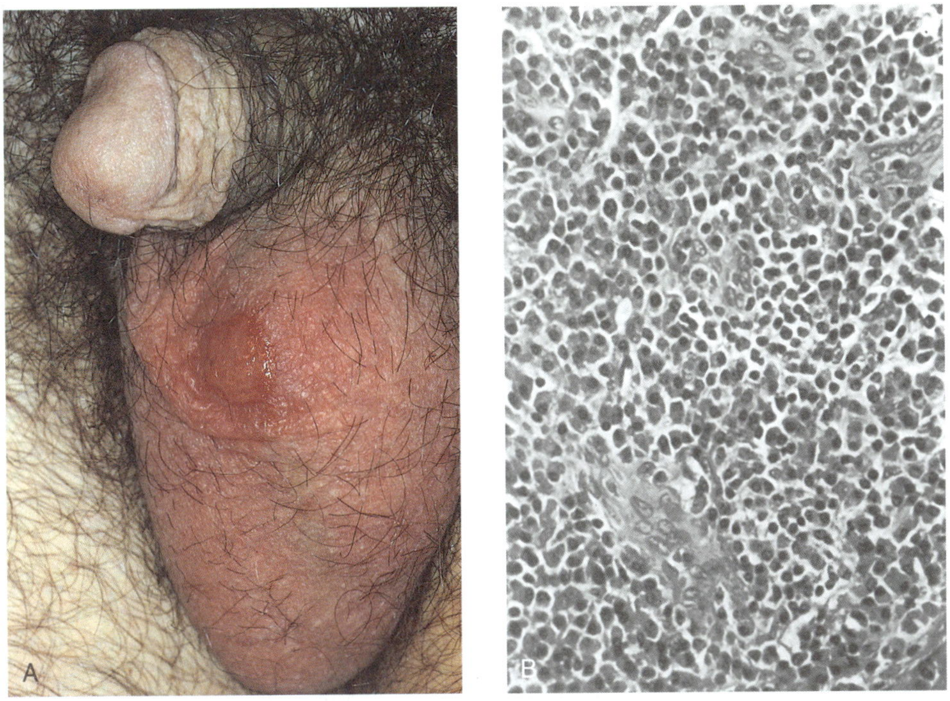

Figure 18–15

A, Syphilitic chancre of the scrotum. Such lesions are typically painless despite the presence of ulceration, and they heal spontaneously. **B,** Histology of chancre with diffuse plasmacytic infiltrate and endothelial proliferation. (Courtesy of Dr. Richard Johnson, New England Deaconess Hospital, Boston, Massachusetts.)

mal and antitreponemal antibody tests are strongly positive in virtually all cases of secondary syphilis.

Tertiary Syphilis

Tertiary syphilis develops in approximately one-third of untreated patients, usually after a latent period of 5 years or more. This phase of syphilis is divided into three major categories: cardiovascular syphilis, neurosyphilis, and so-called benign tertiary syphilis. The various forms may occur singly or in combination in a given patient. *Nontreponemal antibody tests may revert to negative during the tertiary phase, although antitreponemal antibody tests remain positive.*

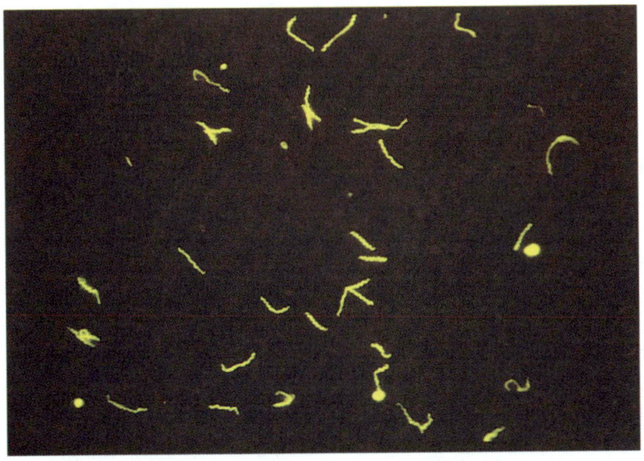

Figure 18–16

Treponema pallidum (dark-field microscopy) showing several spirochetes in scrapings from the base of the chancre. (Courtesy of Dr. Paul Southern, Department of Pathology, University of Texas Southwestern Medical School, Dallas, Texas.)

Cardiovascular syphilis, in the form of *syphilitic aortitis,* accounts for more than 80% of cases of tertiary disease; it is much more common in men than in women. Briefly, the disease is fundamentally an endarteritis of the vasa vasorum of the proximal aorta. Occlusion of the vasa vasorum results in scarring of the media of the proximal aortic wall, with consequent loss of elasticity. The aortic disease is characterized by slowly progressive dilation of the aortic root and arch, with resultant aortic insufficiency and aneurysms of the proximal aorta. In some cases there is narrowing of the coronary artery ostia caused by subintimal scarring with secondary myocardial ischemia. The morphologic and clinical features of syphilitic aortitis are discussed in greater detail with diseases of the blood vessels (Chapter 10).

Neurosyphilis accounts for only about 10% of cases of tertiary syphilis. Variants of neurosyphilis include chronic meningovascular disease, tabes dorsalis, and a generalized brain parenchymal disease termed *general paresis.* They are discussed in detail in Chapter 23. An increased frequency of neurosyphilis has been noted in patients with concomitant HIV infection.

A third, relatively uncommon, form of tertiary syphilis is the so-called benign tertiary syphilis, characterized by the development of gummas in various sites. These lesions are probably related to the development of delayed hypersensitivity. *Gummas occur most commonly in bone, skin, and the mucous membranes of the upper airway and mouth,* although any organ may be affected. Skeletal involvement characteristically causes local pain, tenderness, swelling, and, sometimes, pathologic fractures. Involvement of skin and mucous membranes may produce nodular lesions, or, in exceptional cases, destructive, ulcerative lesions that mimic malignant neoplasms. *Spirochetes are rarely demonstrable within the lesions.* Once common, gummas have become exceedingly rare thanks to the development of effective antibiotics such as penicillin. They are reported now mostly in patients with AIDS.

Congenital Syphilis

T. pallidum may be transmitted across the placenta from an infected mother to the fetus at any time during pregnancy. The likelihood of maternal transmission is greatest during the early (primary and secondary) stages of disease, when spirochetes are most numerous. Because the manifestations of maternal disease may be subtle, routine serologic testing for syphilis is mandatory in all pregnancies. The stigmata of congenital syphilis typically do not develop until after the fourth month of pregnancy. In the absence of treatment, as many as 40% of infected infants die in utero, typically after the fourth month.

Manifestations of *congenital syphilis* include stillbirth, infantile syphilis, and late (tardive) congenital syphilis. Among infants who are stillborn, the most common manifestations are *hepatomegaly, bone abnormalities, pancreatic fibrosis,* and *pneumonitis.* Liver shows extramedullary hematopoiesis and portal tract inflammation. Changes in the bones include inflammation and disruption of the osteochondral junction in long bones and, on occasion, bone resorption and fibrosis of the flat bones of the skull. The lungs may be firm and pale as a result of the presence of inflammatory cells and fibrosis in the alveolar septa (pneumonia alba). Spirochetes are readily demonstrable in tissue sections.

Infantile syphilis refers to congenital syphilis in liveborn infants that is clinically manifest at birth or within the first few months of life. Affected infants present with chronic rhinitis (snuffles) and mucocutaneous lesions similar to those seen in secondary syphilis in adults. Visceral and skeletal changes resembling those seen in stillborn infants may also be present.

Late, or tardive, congenital syphilis refers to cases of untreated congenital syphilis of more than 2 years' duration. Classic manifestations include the Hutchinson triad: notched central incisors, interstitial keratitis with blindness, and deafness from eighth cranial nerve injury. Other changes include a saber shin deformity caused by chronic inflammation of the periosteum of the tibia, deformed molar teeth ("mulberry" molars), chronic meningitis, chorioretinitis, and gummas of the nasal bone and cartilage with a resultant "saddle-nose" deformity.

In cases of congenital syphilis, the placenta is enlarged, pale, and edematous. Microscopy reveals proliferative endarteritis involving the fetal vessels, a mononuclear inflammatory reaction (villitis), and villous immaturity.

Serologic Tests for Syphilis

Although polymerase chain reaction (PCR)–based testing for syphilis has been developed, serology remains the mainstay of diagnosis. Serologic tests for syphilis include nontreponemal antibody tests and antitreponemal antibody tests. Nontreponemal tests measure antibody to cardiolipin, an antigen that is present in both host tissues and the treponemal cell wall. These antibodies are detected by the rapid plasma reagin (RPR) and Venereal Disease Research Laboratory (VDRL) tests. Nontreponemal antibody tests begin to become positive after 1 to 2 weeks of infection and are usually positive by 4 to 6 weeks. Titers of these antibodies usually fall after successful treatment. The VDRL and RPR, widely used as screening tests for syphilis, are also used to monitor the results of therapy. They may be negative, however, in the late latent or tertiary phases of the disease. Nontreponemal antibodies may persist in some patients even after successful treatment. Two additional points about nontreponemal antibody tests deserve emphasis:

- *Nontreponemal antibody tests are often negative during the early stages of disease,* even in the presence of a primary chancre. Hence, during this period, direct visualization of the spirochetes by dark-field or immunofluorescence may be the only way to confirm the diagnosis. However, this requires rapid transit of specimens to the laboratory. Thus, despite its value, direct visualization is not commonly performed, and treatment is based on clinical impressions.
- As many as 15% of positive VDRL tests represent *biologic false-positive results.* These false-positive tests, which may be acute (transient) or chronic (persistent), increase in frequency with age. Conditions associated with false-positive VDRL results include certain acute infections, collagen vascular diseases (e.g., systemic lupus erythematosus), drug addiction, pregnancy, hypergammaglobulinemia of any cause, and lepromatous leprosy.

Treponemal antibody tests include the fluorescent treponemal antibody absorption test and the microhemagglutination assay for *Treponema pallidum* antibodies. These tests also become positive within 4 to 6 weeks after an infection, but, unlike nontreponemal antibody tests, they remain positive indefinitely, even after successful treatment. They are not recommended as primary screening tests, because they remain positive after treatment, and as many as 2% of the general population have false-positive test results.

Serologic response may be delayed, exaggerated (false-positive results), or even absent in some patients with syphilis and coexistent HIV infection. However, in most cases, these tests remain extremely useful in the diagnosis and management of syphilis in patients with AIDS.

SUMMARY

Syphilis

- Syphilis is an STD caused by *T. pallidum*, and has three stages. In primary syphilis a painless lesion called chancre develops on the external genitalia along with regional lymph node enlargement. Secondary syphilis presents with generalized lymphadenopathy and mucocutaneous lesions that may be maculopapular or take the form of flat raised lesions called condyloma lata. Tertiary syphilis causes proximal aortitis with aortic insufficiency, and involvement of the brain, meninges, and the spinal cord, or focal granulomatous lesions called gummas in multiple organs.
- Maternal transmission of the spirochetes, mostly during primary and secondary stages, causes congenital syphilis. This may cause stillbirth or widespread tissue injury in liver, spleen, lung, bones, and pancreas.
- Histologically, most syphilitic lesions demonstrate proliferative endarteritis and a plasma cell–rich inflammatory infiltrate. Gummas have a central area of necrosis surrounded by lymphoplasmacytic infiltrate and epitheloid cells.
- Syphilis is diagnosed by direct demonstration of bacteria within the lesions in primary and secondary stages or by serologic tests (all stages). Nontreponemal antibody tests (VDRL and RPR) are directed against treponemal cell wall and cross-react with host tissues. They are the first tests to become positive and are useful for screening, but they may be negative in advanced disease. False-positive nontreponemal test may occur in SLE, in drug addicts, and during pregnancy. Treponeme-specific antibody tests become positive later but remain positive indefinitely.

Gonorrhea

Gonorrhea is a sexually transmitted infection of the lower genitourinary tract caused by *Neisseria gonorrhoeae*. With the exception of chlamydial infection of the genitourinary tract, discussed later, gonorrhea is the most common reportable communicable disease in the United States. With an estimated 650,000 cases each year in the United States it remains a major public health problem. The gravity of gonococcal infections is increased by the emergence of strains of *N. gonorrhoeae* that are resistant to multiple antibiotics.

Humans are the only natural reservoir for *N. gonorrhoeae*. The organism is highly fastidious, and spread of infection requires direct contact with the mucosa of an infected person, usually during sexual intercourse. There is no evidence that gonorrhea is transmitted by contact with toilet seats or other fomites. The bacteria initially attach to mucosal epithelium, particularly of the columnar or transitional type, using a variety of membrane-associated adhesion molecules and structures termed *pili* (Chapter 9). Such attachment prevents the organism from being unceremoniously flushed by body fluids such as urine or endocervical mucus. The organism then penetrates through the epithelial cells and invades the deeper tissues of the host.

Morphology

N. gonorrhoeae provokes an intense, suppurative inflammatory reaction. In males this is manifested most often as a **purulent urethral discharge,** associated with an edematous, congested urethral meatus. Gram-negative diplococci, many within the cytoplasm of neutrophils, are readily identified in Gram stains of the purulent exudate (Fig. 18–17). Ascending infection may result in the development of **acute prostatitis, epididymitis** (Fig. 18–18), and **orchitis.** Abscesses may complicate severe cases. Urethral and endocervical exudates tend to be less conspicuous in females, although acute inflammation of adjacent structures, such as the Bartholin glands, is fairly common. Ascending infection involving the uterus, fallopian tubes, and ovaries results in **acute salpingitis,** sometimes complicated by tubo-ovarian abscesses. The acute inflammatory process is followed by the development of granulation tissue and scarring, with resultant strictures and other permanent deformities of the involved structures, giving rise to **pelvic inflammatory disease.**

Clinical Features. In most infected males, gonorrhea is manifested by the presence of *dysuria, urinary frequency, and a mucopurulent urethral exudate* within 2 to 7 days of the time of initial infection. Treatment with appropriate antimicrobial therapy results in eradication of the organism and prompt resolution of symptoms. Untreated infections may ascend to involve the prostate, seminal vesicles, epididymis, and testis. Neglected cases may be

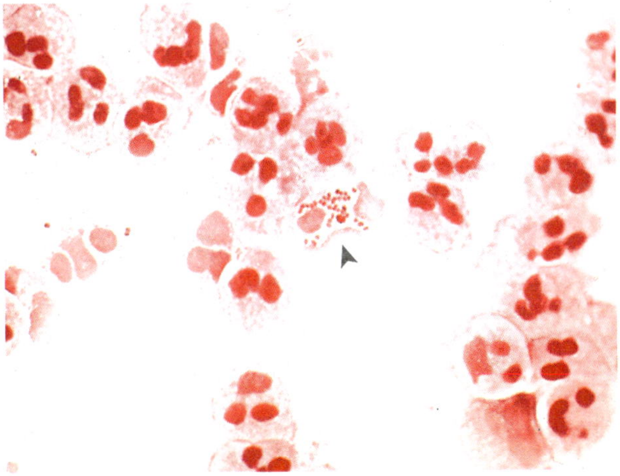

Figure 18–17

Neisseria gonorrhoeae. Gram stain of urethral discharge, demonstrating characteristic gram-negative, intracellular diplococci (*arrowhead*). (Courtesy of Dr. Rita Gander, Department of Pathology, University of Texas Southwestern Medical School, Dallas, Texas.)

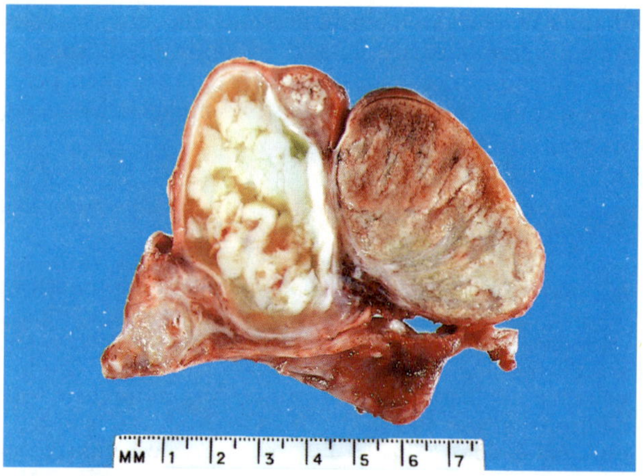

Figure 18–18

Acute epididymitis caused by gonococcal infection. The epididymis is replaced by an abscess. Normal testis is seen on the right.

SUMMARY

Gonorrhea

- Gonorrhea is a common STD affecting the genitourinary tract that can become disseminated in individuals with deficiency of complement.
- In males there is a severe, symptomatic uretheritis that can spread to the prostate, epididymis, and testis. In females the initial lesions on the cervix and urethera are less prominent than in males, but ascending infection to fallopian tubes and ovaries can cause scarring and deformity with resultant sterility.
- Pregnant females can transmit gonorrhea to newborns during passage through the birth canal.
- Diagnosis can be made by culture of the exudates as well as by nucleic acid amplification techniques.

complicated by chronic urethral stricture and, in more advanced cases, by permanent sterility. Untreated men may also become chronic carriers of *N. gonorrhoeae.*

Among female patients, initial infection may be asymptomatic or associated with *dysuria, lower pelvic pain, and vaginal discharge.* Untreated cases may be complicated by ascending infection, leading to acute inflammation of the fallopian tubes (salpingitis) and ovaries. Chronic scarring of the fallopian tubes may occur, with resultant infertility and an increased risk of ectopic pregnancy. Gonococcal infection of the upper genital tract may spread to the peritoneal cavity, where the exudate may extend up the right paracolic gutter to the dome of the liver, resulting in gonococcal perihepatitis.

Other sites of primary infection, more commonly encountered in male homosexuals than in heterosexuals, include the oropharynx and the anorectal area, with resultant acute pharyngitis and proctitis, respectively.

Disseminated infection is much less common than local infection, occurring in 0.5% to 3% of cases of gonorrhea. It is more common in females than males. Manifestations include, most commonly, tenosynovitis, arthritis, and pustular or hemorrhagic skin lesions. Endocarditis and meningitis are rare manifestations. Strains that cause disseminated infection are usually resistant to the lytic action of complement.

Gonococcal infection may be transmitted to infants during passage through the birth canal. The affected neonate may develop purulent infection of the eyes (ophthalmia neonatorum), an important cause of blindness in the past. The routine administration of antibiotic ointment to the eyes of newborns has resulted in a marked reduction in the incidence of this disorder.

Both culture and nucleic acid amplification techniques can be used for diagnosis of gonococcal infections. The advantages of culture are that it can be done on nongenital sources such as eye and rectum, and antibiotic sensitivity can be determined. Nucleic acid amplification methods can usually be done on urine and urethral samples. They are somewhat more sensitive than culture. Overall, molecular methods are being used increasingly.

Nongonococcal Urethritis and Cervicitis

Nongonococcal urethritis (NGU) and cervicitis are the most common forms of STDs today. A variety of organisms has been implicated in the pathogenesis of NGU and cervicitis, including *C. trachomatis, Trichomonas vaginalis, U. urealyticum,* and *Mycoplasma genitalium. Most cases are apparently caused by C. trachomatis, and this organism is believed to be the most common bacterial cause of STD in the United States. U. urealyticum* is the next most common cause of NGU.

C. trachomatis is a small gram-negative bacterium that is an obligate intracellular parasite. It exists in two forms. The infectious form, the so-called elementary body, is capable of at least limited survival in the extracellular environment. The elementary body is taken up by host cells, primarily via a process of receptor-mediated endocytosis. Once inside the cell, the elementary body differentiates into a metabolically active form, termed the *reticulate body.* Using energy sources from the host cell, the reticulate body replicates and ultimately forms new elementary bodies capable of infecting additional cells. They preferentially infect columnar epithelial cells.

C. trachomatis infections may be associated with a spectrum of clinical features that are virtually indistinguishable from those caused by *N. gonorrhoeae.* Thus, patients may develop epididymitis, prostatitis, pelvic inflammatory disease, pharyngitis, conjunctivitis, perihepatic inflammation, and, among persons engaging in anal intercourse, proctitis. *C. trachomatis* also causes lymphogranuloma venereum, discussed in the next section.

The morphologic and clinical features of chlamydial infection, with the exception of lymphogranuloma venereum, are virtually identical to those of gonorrhea. The primary infection is characterized by a *mucopurulent discharge containing a predominance of neutrophils.* Organisms are not visible in gram-stained sections. In contrast to the gonococcus, *C. trachomatis* cannot be isolated with the use of conventional culture media. The diagnosis is best made by nucleic acid amplification tests on voided urine. Although culture can be done from genital swabs, it is not possible from urine. Molecular tests are also more sensitive than culture. Other manifestations of chlamydial infection include a reactive arthritis, predominantly in patients who are HLA-B27 positive. This condition, designated Reiter syndrome, typically presents as a combination of urethritis, conjunctivitis, arthritis, and generalized mucocutaneous lesions.

SUMMARY

Nongonococcal Urethritis and Cervicitis

- NGU and cervicitis are the most common STDs. The majority are caused by *C. trachomatis* and the rest by *T. vaginalis, U. urealyticum,* and *M. genitalium.*
- *C. trachomatis* is a gram-negative intracellular bacterium that causes a disease that is clinically indistinguishable from gonorrhea in both men and in women. Diagnosis requires detection of the bacteria by molecular methods. Culture from genital swabs is possible but requires special methods.
- In patients who are HLA-B27 positive, *C. trachomatis* infection can cause reactive arthritis along with conjunctivitis, and generalized mucocutaneous lesions, together called Reiter syndrome.

Lymphogranuloma Venereum

Lymphogranuloma venereum (LGV) is a chronic, ulcerative disease caused by certain strains of *C. trachomatis,* which are distinct from those causing the more common NGU or cervicitis discussed before. It is a sporadic disease in the United States and Western Europe, but is endemic in parts of Asia, Africa, the Caribbean region, and South America. As in the case of granuloma inguinale (discussed later), sporadic cases of LGV are associated most often with sexual promiscuity.

Morphology

The patient with LGV may present with nonspecific urethritis, papular or ulcerative lesions involving the lower genitalia, regional adenopathy, or an anorectal syndrome. The lesions contain a **mixed granulomatous and neutrophilic inflammatory response,** with a variable number of chlamydial inclusions in the cytoplasm of epithelial cells or inflammatory cells. Regional lymphadenopathy is common, usually occurring within 30 days of the time of infection. Lymph node involvement is characterized by a granulomatous inflammatory reaction associated with irregularly shaped foci of necrosis and neutrophilic infiltration (**stellate abscesses**). With time, the inflammatory reaction gives rise to extensive fibrosis that can cause local lymphatic obstruction with **lymphedema** and strictures. Rectal strictures are particularly common in women. In active lesions, the diagnosis of LGV may be made by demonstration of the organism in biopsy sections or smears of exudate. In more chronic cases, the diagnosis rests on the demonstration of antibodies to the appropriate chlamydial serotypes in the patient's serum. Nucleic acid amplification tests have also been developed.

Chancroid (Soft Chancre)

Chancroid, sometimes called the "third" venereal disease (after syphilis and gonorrhea), is an acute, ulcerative infection caused by *Haemophilus ducreyi,* a small, gram-negative coccobacillus. The disease is most common in tropical and subtropical areas and is more prevalent in lower socioeconomic groups, particularly among men who have regular contact with prostitutes. *Chancroid is one of the most common causes of genital ulcers in Africa and southeast Asia,* where it serves as an important cofactor in the transmission of HIV-1 infection. Chancroid is probably underdiagnosed in the United States, because most STD clinics do not have facilities for isolating *H. ducreyi,* and PCR-based tests are not widely available.

Morphology

Four to seven days after inoculation, the person with chancroid develops a tender, **erythematous papule** involving the external genitalia. In males the primary lesion is usually on the penis; in females most lesions occur in the vagina or periurethral area. Over the course of several days the surface of the primary lesion erodes to produce an **irregular ulcer,** which is more likely to be painful in males than in females. In contrast to the primary chancre of syphilis, the ulcer of chancroid is not indurated, and multiple lesions may be present. The base of the ulcer is covered by shaggy, yellow-gray exudate. The regional **lymph nodes,** particularly in the inguinal region, become enlarged and tender in about 50% of cases within 1 to 2 weeks of the primary inoculation. In untreated cases, the inflamed and enlarged nodes (buboes) may erode the overlying skin to produce chronic, draining ulcers.

Microscopically, the ulcer of chancroid contains a superficial zone of neutrophilic debris and fibrin, with an underlying zone of granulation tissue containing areas of necrosis and thrombosed vessels. A dense, lymphoplasmacytic inflammatory infiltrate is present beneath the layer of granulation tissue. Coccobacillary organisms are sometimes demonstrable in Gram or silver stains, but they are often obscured by the mixed bacterial growth frequently present at the ulcer base. In the majority of cases, *H. ducreyi* can be cultured from the ulcer when appropriate media are used.

Granuloma Inguinale

Granuloma inguinale is a chronic inflammatory disease caused by *Calymmatobacterium granulomatis,* a minute, encapsulated coccobacillus related to the *Klebsiella* genus. This disease is uncommon in the United States and Western Europe but is endemic in rural areas in certain tropical and subtropical regions. When it occurs in urban settings, transmission of *C. granulomatis* is typically associated with sexual promiscuity. Untreated cases are characterized by extensive scarring, often associated with lymphatic obstruction and lymphedema (elephantiasis) of the external genitalia. Culture of the organism is difficult, and PCR-based assays are not widely available.

Morphology

Granuloma inguinale begins as a raised, papular lesion involving the moist, stratified squamous epithelium of the genitalia. The lesion eventually undergoes ulceration, accompanied by the development of abundant granulation tissue, which is manifested grossly as a protuberant, soft, painless mass. As the lesion enlarges, its borders become raised and indurated. Disfiguring scars may develop in untreated cases and are sometimes associated with urethral, vulvar, or anal strictures. Regional lymph nodes typically are spared or show only nonspecific reactive changes, in contrast to chancroid.

Microscopic examination of active lesions reveals marked epithelial hyperplasia at the borders of the ulcer, sometimes mimicking carcinoma **(pseudoepitheliomatous hyperplasia).** A mixture of neutrophils and mononuclear inflammatory cells is present at the base of the ulcer and beneath the surrounding epithelium. The organisms are demonstrable in Giemsa-stained smears of the exudate as minute coccobacilli within vacuoles in macrophages (Donovan bodies). Silver stains (e.g., the Warthin-Starry stain) may also be used to demonstrate the organism.

SUMMARY

Lymphogranuloma Venereum, Chancroid, and Granuloma Inguinale

- LGV is caused by *C. trachomatis* serotypes that are distinct from those that cause NGU. LGV is associated with urethritis, ulcerative genital lesions, lymphadenopathy, and involvement of the rectum. The lesions show both acute and chronic inflammation; they progress to fibrosis causing lymphedema and rectal strictures.
- *H. ducreyi* infection causes an acute painful ulcerative genital infection called *chancroid*. Inguinal node involvement occurs in many cases and leads to their enlargement and ulceration. Ulcers show a superficial area of acute inflammation and necrosis, with an underlying zone of granulation tissue and mononuclear infiltrate. Diagnosis is possible by culture of the organism.
- *Granuloma inguinale* is a chronic fibrosing STD caused by *C. granulomatis*. The initial papular lesion on the genitalia expands, ulcerates, and may cause urethral, vulvar, or anal strictures. Microscopically there is granulation tissue and intense epithelial hyperplasia that can mimic a squamous cell carcinoma. Organisms are visible as small intracellular coccobacilli within vacuolated macrophages (Donovan bodies).

Trichomoniasis

T. vaginalis is a sexually transmitted protozoan that is a frequent cause of vaginitis. The trophozoite form adheres to, and causes superficial lesions of, the mucosa. In females, *T. vaginalis* infection is often associated with loss of acid-producing Döderlein bacilli. It may be asymptomatic, but frequently it causes itching and a profuse, frothy, yellow vaginal discharge. Urethral colonization may cause urinary frequency and dysuria. *T. vaginalis* infection is usually asymptomatic in males but in some cases may present as nongonococcal urethritis. The organism is usually demonstrable in smears of vaginal scrapings.

Genital Herpes Simplex

Genital herpes infection, or herpes genitalis, is a common STD that affects an estimated 50 million people in the United States. Although both herpes simplex virus 1 (HSV-1) and HSV-2 can cause genital or oral infections, most cases of genital herpes are caused by HSV-2. Current studies reveal that an increasing number of genital infections are being caused by HSV-1, in part due to the increasing practice of oral sex. Genital HSV infection may occur in any sexually active population. As with other STDs, the risk of infection is directly related to the number of sexual contacts. HSV is transmitted when the virus comes into contact with a mucosal surface or broken skin of a susceptible host. Such transmission requires direct contact with an infected person, because the virus is readily inactivated at room temperature, particularly if dried.

Morphology

The initial lesions of genital HSV infection are **painful, erythematous vesicles** on the mucosa or skin of the lower genitalia and adjacent extra-genital sites. The anorectal area is a particularly common site of primary infection among homosexual males. Histologic changes include the presence of **intraepithelial vesicles** accompanied by necrotic cellular debris, neutrophils, and cells harboring characteristic intranuclear viral inclusions. The classic **Cowdry type A inclusion** appears as a light purple, homogeneous intranuclear structure surrounded by a clear halo. Infected cells commonly fuse to form multinucleated syncytia. The inclusions readily stain with antibodies to HSV, permitting a rapid, specific diagnosis of HSV infection in histologic sections or smears.

As mentioned earlier, both HSV-1 and HSV-2 can cause genital or oral infection, and both can produce primary or recurrent mucocutaneous lesions that are clinically indistinguishable. The manifestations of HSV infection vary considerably, depending on whether the infection is primary or recurrent. Primary infection is often mildly symptomatic with HSV-2. Among persons experiencing their first episode, locally painful vesicular lesions are often accompanied by dysuria, urethral discharge, local lymph node enlargement and tenderness, and systemic manifestations, such as fever, muscle aches, and headache. HSV is actively shed during this period, and it continues to be shed until the mucosal lesions have completely healed. Signs and symptoms may last for several weeks during the primary phase of disease. Recurrences are much more common with HSV-1 than HSV-2 and are typically milder and of shorter duration than the primary episode. As with primary infection, HSV is shed while active lesions are present.

Among immunocompetent adults, herpes genitalis is generally not life-threatening. However, HSV does pose a major threat to immunosuppressed patients, in whom fatal, disseminated disease may develop. *Neonatal herpes infection* occurs in about half of infants delivered vaginally of mothers suffering from either primary or recurrent genital HSV infection. The viral infection is acquired during passage through the birth canal. Its incidence has risen in parallel with the rise in genital HSV infection. The manifestations of neonatal herpes, which typically develop during the second week of life, include rash, encephalitis, pneumonitis, and hepatic necrosis. Approximately 60% of affected infants die of the disease, with significant morbidity occurring in about half of the survivors. The laboratory diagnosis of genital herpes relies on viral culture. Molecular diagnostic tests are also available but they are used mostly in extragenital herpes, particularly in central nervous system infections.

Human Papillomavirus Infection

HPV is the cause of a number of squamous proliferations in the genital tract, including condylomata acuminata, some precancerous lesions, and some carcinomas (Chapter 19). *Condylomata acuminata,* also known as venereal warts, are caused by HPV types 6 and 11. They occur on the penis as well as on the female genitalia. They should not be confused with the condylomata lata seen in secondary syphilis. Genital HPV infection may be transmitted to neonates during vaginal delivery. These infants may subsequently develop recurrent and potentially life-threatening papillomas of the upper respiratory tract.

Morphology

In males, condylomata acuminata usually occur on the coronal sulcus or inner surface of the prepuce, where they range from small, sessile lesions to large, papillary proliferations measuring several centimeters in diameter. In females, they commonly occur on the vulva (see Fig. 19–2; Chapter 19). The microscopic appearance is that of an exuberant proliferation of stratified squamous epithelium supported by fibrovascular papillae. The more superficial epithelial cells contain irregular, hyperchromatic nuclei surrounded by a characteristic clear perinuclear halo, a change referred to as **koilocytosis** (see Fig. 19–3; Chapter 19).

SUMMARY

Herpes Simplex Virus and Human Papillomavirus

- HSV-2, and less commonly HSV-1, can cause genital infections. Initial (primary) infection causes painful, erythematous, intraepithelial vesicles on the mucosa and skin of external genitalia along with regional lymph node enlargement. Recurrent lesions are more common with HSV-1 than HSV-2 and they are milder.
- Histologically, the vesicles contain necrotic cells and fused multinucleated giant cells containing purple, intranuclear inclusions (Cowdry's type A) that stain with antibodies to HSV.
- Neonatal herpes can be life threatening and occurs in children born to mothers with genital herpes. Affected infants have generalized herpes including encephalitis and consequent high mortality.
- HPV causes many proliferative lesions of the genital mucosa including condyloma acuminata, carcinoma in situ, and frank cancers. Condylomas are papillary proliferations in which the superficial cells show koilocytic changes.

BIBLIOGRAPHY

Andriole G, et al.: Dihydrotestosterone and the prostate: the scientific rationale for 5α-reductase inhibitors in the treatment of benign prostatic hyperplasia. J Urol 172:1399, 2004. *[Review of the role of DHT in the etiology and therapy of prostatic nodular hypertrophy.]*

Barry MJ: Prostate-specific-antigen: testing for early diagnosis of prostate cancer. N Engl J Med 344:1373, 2001. *[An excellent summary of clinical use of PSA.]*

Blanchard TJ, Maybe DC: Chlamydial infections. Br J Clin Pract 48:201, 1994. *[A review of the clinical spectrum of chlamydial infections, including their role as sexually transmitted pathogens.]*

Chapple CR: Pharmacological therapy of benign prostatic hyperplasia/lower urinary tract symptoms: an overview for the practicing clinician. BJU Int 9:738, 2004. *[Review of current clinical guidelines for therapy of symptomatic prostatic nodular hyperplasia.]*

Clyne B, Jerrard DA: Syphilis testing. J Emerg Med 18:361, 2000. *[A readable, current review of laboratory methods used in the diagnosis of syphilis.]*

Donovan B: Sexually transmitted infections other than HIV. Lancet 363:545, 2004. *[A clinical review of STDs.]*

Frankel S, et al.: Screening for prostate cancer. Lancet 361:1122, 2003. *[Review of the usefulness of early cancer screening and PSA.]*

Fredlund H, et al.: Molecular genetic methods for diagnosis and characterization of *C. trachomatis* and *N. gonorrhoeae:* impact on epidemiologic surveillance and interventions. APMIS 112:771, 2004. *[A detailed discussion of molecular tests and their applications.]*

Gah BT: Syphilis in adults. Sex Transm Infect 81:448, 2005. *[A good overview of syphilis.]*

Gori S, et al.: Germ cell tumours of the testis. Crit Rev Oncol Hematol 53:141, 2005. *[An informative review of the predisposing factors, clinical features, and treatment of testicular neoplasms.]*

Han M, et al.: Prostate-specific antigen and screening for prostate cancer. Med Clin North Am 88:245, 2004. *[Review of the physiology, diagnostic utility, and measurement of serum PSA.]*

Ishihara S, et al.: *Mycoplasma genitalium* uretheritis in men. Int J Antimicrob Agents 245:523, 2004. *[A discussion of M. genitalium infection as a cause of NGU.]*

Lee KL, Peehl DM: Molecular and cellular pathogenesis of benign prostatic hyperplasia. J Urol 172:1784, 2004. *[Review of current understanding of the etiology of prostatic nodular hyperplasia.]*

Lipsky BA: Prostatitis and urinary tract infection in men: what's new; what's true? Am J Med 106:327, 1999. *[A recent summary of clinical features and treatment of acute and chronic prostatitis.]*

Misra S, et al.: Penile carcinoma: a challenge for the developing world. Lancet Oncol. 5:240, 2004. *[An excellent summary of the epidemiology, pathophysiology, staging and therapy of penile carcinoma.]*

Nelson WG, et al.: Prostate cancer. N Engl J Med 349(4):366, 2003. *[Excellent review of current understanding of the molecular mechanisms of prostate carcinogenesis.]*

Nickel JC, Moon T: Chronic bacterial prostatitis: an evolving clinical enigma. Urology 66:2, 2005. *[Review of the etiology and treatment of chronic prostatitis.]*

Reuter VE: Origins and molecular biology of testicular germ cell tumors. Mod Pathol 18 (Suppl 2):S51, 2005. *[A review of recent developments in the pathobiology of germ cell tumors.]*

Sesterhenn IA, Davis CJ Jr: Pathology of germ cell tumors of the testis. Cancer Control 11:374, 2004. *[A concise summary of histologic classification of testicular neoplasms, including discussions of the roles of immunohistochemistry and serum markers in their diagnosis.]*

Sulak PJ: Sexually transmitted diseases. Semin Reprod Med 21:399, 2003. *[An exhaustive review of STDs.]*

Chapter 19

The Female Genital System and Breast

ANTHONY MONTAG, MD*
VINAY KUMAR, MD

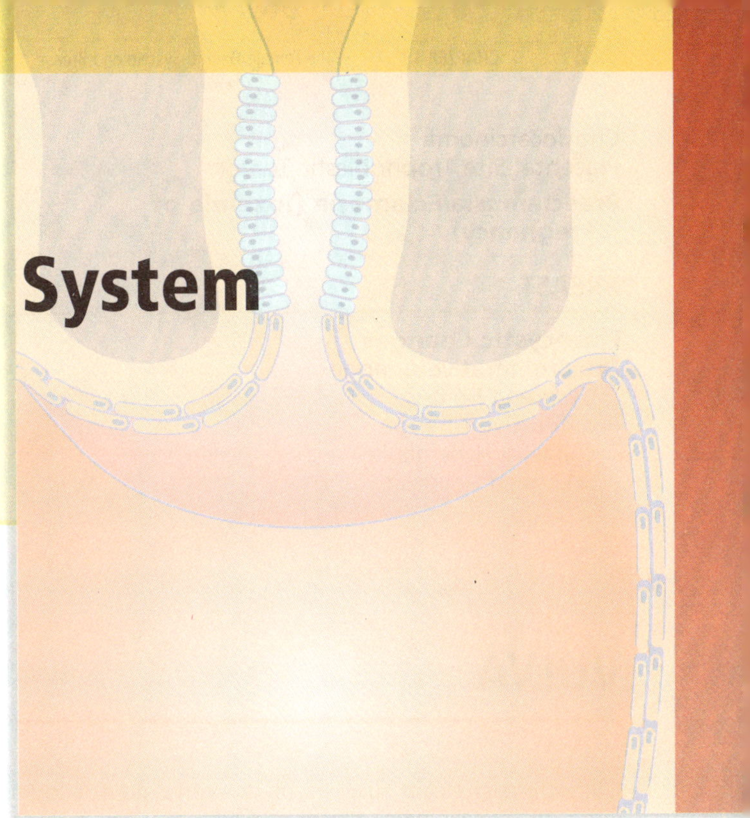

* Dr. Christopher Crum and Susan Laster made valuable contributions to this chapter in the previous edition. Dr. Suzanne Conzen and Pedram Argani were extremely helpful in the revision of the section on breast diseases in this edition. Their help is gratefully acknowledged.

VULVA

Clinically significant diseases of the vulva do not loom large in gynecologic practice. Only the uncommon carcinomas are life threatening. Far more frequent are the inflammatory disorders (vulvitis), which are more uncomfortable than serious. Only a few other conditions bear mentioning here: non-neoplastic epithelial disorders (discussed later); the painful Bartholin cysts caused by obstruction of the excretory ducts of the glands; and imperforate hymen in children, impeding secretions and menstrual flow later in life.

VULVITIS

The moist hair-bearing skin and delicate membrane of the vulva are vulnerable to many nonspecific microbe-induced inflammations and dermatologic disorders. Intense itching (pruritus) and subsequent scratching often exacerbate the primary condition. There are also many specific forms of vulvar infection related to sexually transmitted diseases. Most are discussed in Chapter 18. The five most important of these infectious agents in North America are human papillomavirus (HPV), producing condylomata acuminata and vulvar intraepithelial neoplasia (both discussed in some detail later); herpes genitalis (herpes simplex virus [HSV 1 or 2]), causing a vesicular eruption; gonococcal suppurative infection of the vulvovaginal glands; syphilis, with its primary chancre at the site of inoculation; and candidal vulvitis.

Contact Dermatitis

One of the most common causes of vulvar pruritus is a reactive inflammation to an exogenous stimulus, whether an irritant (contact irritant dermatitis) or an allergen (contact allergic dermatitis). Irritant dermatitis presents as well-defined erythematous weeping and crusting papules and plaques and may be a reaction to urine, soaps, detergents, antiseptics, deodorants, or alcohol. Allergic dermatitis has a similar gross appearance and may result from allergy to perfumes and other additives in creams, lotions, and soaps, chemical treatments on clothing, and other antigens. Both forms of contact dermatitis may present as an acute spongiotic dermatitis or as a subacute dermatitis with epithelial hyperplasia or subacute dermatitis (see Chapter 22).

NON-NEOPLASTIC EPITHELIAL DISORDERS

The epithelium of the vulvar mucosa may undergo atrophic thinning or hyperplastic thickening. For want of a better term, these alterations were previously referred to as "dystrophies" but are now simply referred to as non-neoplastic epithelial disorders to differentiate them from the premalignant lesions discussed later. There are two forms of non-neoplastic epithelial disorders: lichen sclerosus and lichen simplex chronicus. Both may coexist in different areas in the same person, and both may appear macroscopically as depigmented white lesions, referred to as *leukoplakia.* Similar white patches or plaques are also seen with (1) vitiligo (loss of pigment) of the skin, (2) a variety of benign dermatoses such as psoriasis and lichen planus (Chapter 22), (3) carcinoma in situ, (4) Paget disease (described later), and (5) invasive carcinoma. Thus, leukoplakia is merely a descriptive term that gives no indication of its underlying nature. Only biopsy and microscopic examinations can differentiate among these similar-looking lesions.

Lichen Sclerosus

This lesion is characterized by thinning of the epidermis and disappearance of rete pegs, hydropic degeneration of the basal cells, superficial hyperkeratosis, and dermal fibrosis with a scant perivascular, mononuclear inflammatory cell infiltrate (Fig. 19–1). The lesions appear clin-

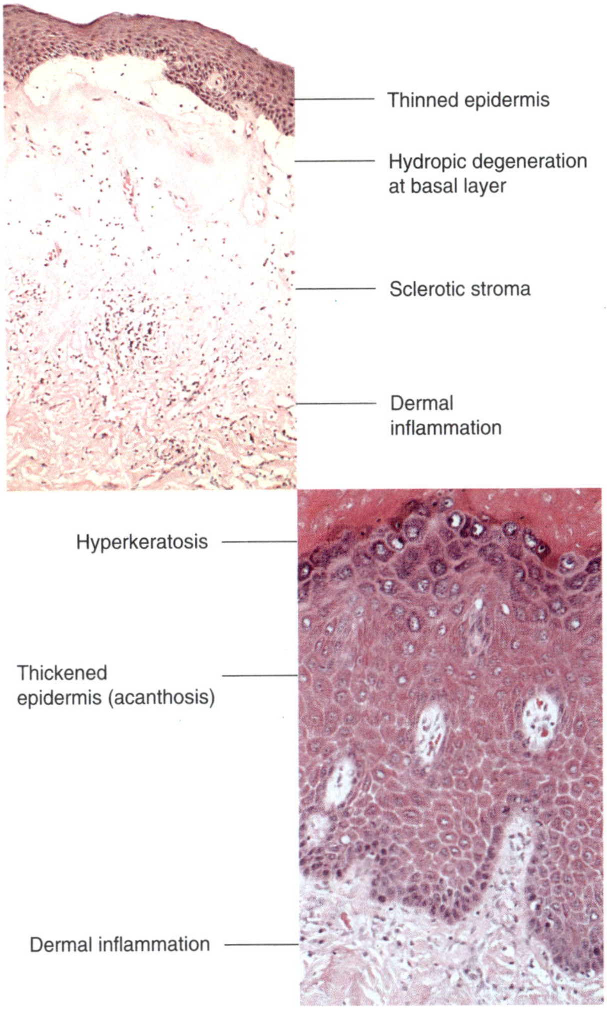

Figure 19–1

Inflammatory vulvar disorders. Lichen sclerosus (*upper panel*). Lichen simplex chronicus (*lower panel*). The main features of the lesions are indicated in the figures.

ically as smooth, white plaques or papules that in time may extend and coalesce. The surface is smoothed out and sometimes resembles parchment. When the entire vulva is affected, the labia become somewhat atrophic and stiffened, and the vaginal orifice is constricted. It occurs in all age groups but is most common in postmenopausal women. It may also be encountered elsewhere on the skin. The pathogenesis is uncertain, but the presence of activated T cells in the subepithelial inflammatory infiltrate and the increased frequency of autoimmune disorders in these women suggests an autoimmune reaction may be involved. Although the lesion in lichen sclerosus is not pre-malignant by itself, women with symptomatic lichen sclerosus have approximately a 15% chance of developing squamous cell carcinoma in their lifetime.

Lichen Simplex Chronicus

Previously called "hyperplastic dystrophy," this disorder is the end stage of many inflammatory dermatoses and is marked by epithelial thickening, expansion of the stratum granulosum, and significant surface hyperkeratosis. It appears clinically as an area of leukoplakia. The epithelium may show increased mitotic activity in both the stratum basalis and spinosum. Leukocytic infiltration of the dermis is sometimes pronounced. The hyperplastic epithelial changes show no atypia (see Fig. 19–1). There is generally no increased predisposition to cancer, but suspiciously, lichen simplex chronicus is often present at the margins of established cancer of the vulva.

SUMMARY

Non-neoplastic Epithelial Disorders

- Lichen sclerosus is characterized by atrophic epithelium, usually with dermal fibrosis.
- Lichen sclerosus carries an increased risk of developing squamous cell carcinoma.
- Lichen simplex chronicus is characterized by thickened epithelium, usually with an inflammatory infiltrate.

TUMORS

Condylomas and Low-Grade Vulvar Intraepithelial Neoplasia (VIN)

Condylomas are essentially anogenital warts, but in the moist environment of the vulva they tend to be large. Most fall into two distinctive biologic forms, but rarer types also exist. *Condylomata lata,* not commonly seen today, are flat, moist, minimally elevated lesions that occur in secondary syphilis (Chapter 18). The more common *condylomata acuminata* may be papillary and distinctly elevated or somewhat flat and rugose. They occur anywhere on the anogenital surface, sometimes singly but more often in multiple sites. On the vulva they range from a few millimeters to many centimeters in diameter and are red-pink to pink-brown (Fig. 19–2). The histologic appearance of these lesions was described earlier (Chapter 18), but particularly significant is the characteristic cellular morphology, namely, perinuclear cytoplasmic vacuolization with nuclear angular pleomorphism and koilocytosis (Fig. 19–3). Such cells are considered to be hallmarks of HPV infection. Indeed, there is a strong association with HPV 6 and HPV 11. The HPV can be transmitted venereally and identical lesions occur in men on the penis and around the anus. Vulvar condylomas are not precancerous but may coexist with foci of intraepithelial neoplasia in the vulva (VIN grade I) and cervix. Indeed, according to some authorities, VIN I and condylomas, both caused by HPV of low malignant potential, should be segregated from VIN II and VIN III, discussed later. The types of HPV isolated from the cancers differ from those most often found in condylomas.

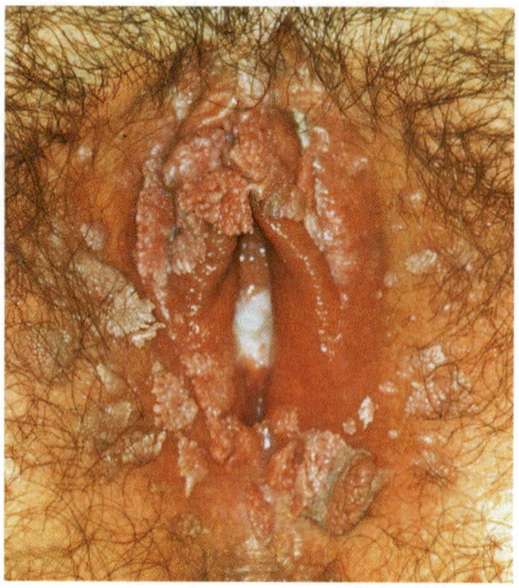

Figure 19–2

Numerous condylomas of the vulva. (Courtesy of Dr. Alex Ferenczy, McGill University, Montreal, Quebec, Canada.)

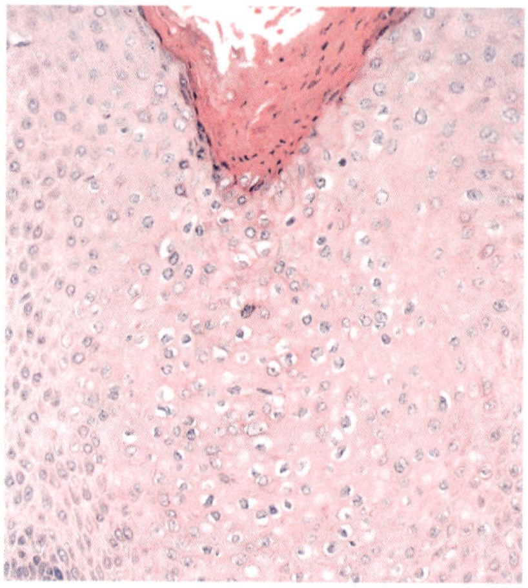

Figure 19–3

Histopathology of condyloma acuminatum showing acanthosis, hyperkeratosis, and cytoplasmic vacuolation (koilocytosis, *center*).

High-Grade Vulvar Intraepithelial Neoplasia and Carcinoma of the Vulva

Carcinoma of the vulva represents about 3% of all genital tract cancers in women, occurring mostly in women older than age 60 years. However, there has been an increase in the frequency of high grade VIN in the past few decades, principally among younger women (40–60 years of age). In all age groups, approximately 90% of carcinomas are squamous cell carcinomas; the remainder are adenocarcinomas, melanomas, or basal cell carcinomas.

Many findings suggest that there are two biologic forms of vulvar carcinoma. The most common is seen in relatively younger patients, particularly in cigarette smokers. HPV, especially type 16 and less frequently other types, is present in 75% to 90% of cases; in many cases there is coexisting vaginal or cervical carcinoma, carcinoma in situ, or condylomata acuminata, suggesting a common causal agent, probably HPV. Often in these women, in situ cancerous changes (i.e. VIN) confined to the epithelium precede the development of the overt cancer. The VIN may be graded VIN II, or VIN III (carcinoma in situ). It may be found in multiple, apparently separate foci, or it may coexist with an invasive lesion. Whether VIN is always destined to become an invasive cancer remains unclear, but there is good evidence that, at least in some individuals, the VIN has been present for many years, perhaps decades. Whether genetic, immunologic, or environmental influences (e.g., cigarette smoking or superinfection with new strains of HPV) determine the course is unclear.

The other subgroup of vulvar carcinoma occurs in older women. It is not associated with HPV but is often preceded by years of non-neoplastic epithelial changes, principally lichen sclerosus and, rarely, lichen simplex chronicus. Frequently the overlying epithelium lacks the typical cytologic changes of VIN, but it may display dyskeratotic cells, angular budding, and basal keratinization. Occasionally epithelial changes of VIN precede the appearance of the overt neoplasm. Tumors tend to be well differentiated and highly keratinizing.

Morphology

VIN and early vulvar carcinomas appear as areas of **leukoplakia** caused by epithelial thickening involving any region of the vulva or adjacent skin. In about one-fourth of cases the lesions are pigmented with melanin. In the course of time, these areas are transformed into overt **exophytic** or ulcerative **endophytic tumors.** HPV-positive tumors are more often multifocal and appear warty or condylomatous.

Histologically, HPV-positive neoplasms tend to be poorly differentiated **squamous cell carcinoma,** whereas the HPV-negative lesions, which are usually unifocal, tend to show well-differentiated keratinizing squamous cells. Although all patterns tend to remain confined to their site of origin for a few years, ultimately, direct invasion with involvement of regional nodes and lymphohematogenous spread occurs. The risk of such spread is correlated with the size of the tumor and the depth of invasion.

Women with a tumor less than 2 cm in diameter have about a 75% 5-year survival after radical excision, whereas only 10% of those with larger lesions survive 10 years.

Extramammary Paget Disease

Paget disease of the vulva, like that of the breast, is essentially a form of intraepithelial carcinoma. Unlike the breast, where Paget disease is virtually always associated with an underlying carcinoma, the majority of cases of vulvar Paget disease have no demonstrable underlying carcinoma. Occasionally there is an accompanying subepithelial or submucosal tumor arising in an adnexal structure, typically sweat glands. In cases without an underlying primary, the tumor likely arises from aberrant differentiation of epithelial progenitor cells in the epidermis.

Vulvar Paget disease presents as a red, scaly, crusted plaque and may appear as an inflammatory dermatosis. Histologically large epithelioid cells infiltrate the epithelium, singly and in groups, with abundant granular cytoplasm and occasional cytoplasmic vacuoles (Fig. 19–4) containing mucin that stains positive for periodic acid–Schiff. When the Paget cells are confined to the epithelium, the lesion may persist for years or even decades without evidence of invasion. However, in some instances, particularly when there is an associated appendageal tumor, the Paget cells extend into the skin appendages, invade locally, and ultimately metastasize more widely to distant sites, usually within the first 2 to 5 years.

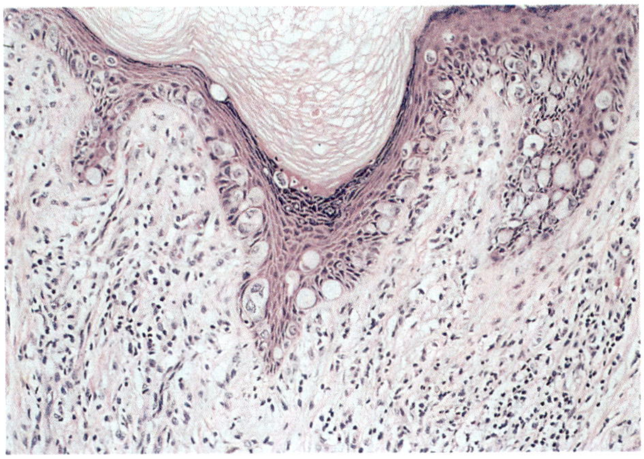

Figure 19–4

Paget disease of the vulva, with scattered large, clear tumor cells within the squamous epithelium.

SUMMARY

Squamous Carcinoma of the Vulva

- As many as 90% of vulvar squamous cell carcinomas are HPV related, usually presenting as poorly differentiated lesions, sometimes multifocal. They often evolve from vulvar intraepithelial neoplasia.
- Non-HPV-related vulvar squamous cell carcinoma occurs in older individuals, is usually well differentiated and unifocal, and is associated with lichen sclerosus or other inflammatory conditions.

Paget Disease of the Vulva

- Red, scaly plaque, microscopically characterized by the spread of malignant cells within the epithelium, occasionally with invasion of underlying dermis
- In a minority of cases there is an underlying carcinoma of a vulvar or perineal gland

VAGINA

The vagina in adults is seldom the site of primary disease. More often it is secondarily involved in the spread of cancer or infections arising in close proximity (e.g., cervix, vulva, bladder, rectum). The only primary disorders discussed here are a few congenital anomalies, vaginitis, and primary tumors.

Congenital anomalies of the vagina are fortunately uncommon and include entities such as total absence of the vagina, a septate or double vagina (usually associated with a septate cervix and, sometimes, uterus), and congenital small lateral Gartner duct cysts arising from persistent embryonic remnants.

VAGINITIS

Vaginitis is a relatively common clinical problem that is usually transient and not serious. It produces a vaginal discharge (leukorrhea). A large variety of organisms have been implicated, including bacteria, fungi, and parasites. Many represent normal commensals that become pathogenic in conditions such as diabetes, systemic antibiotic therapy that disrupts the normal microbial flora, after abortion or pregnancy, or in elderly persons with compromised immune function, and in patients with the acquired immunodeficiency syndrome. In adults, primary gonorrheal infection of the vagina is uncommon. However, it may occur in a newborn born to an infected mother. The only other organisms worthy of specific mention, because they are frequent offenders, are *Candida albicans* and *Trichomonas vaginalis.* Candidal (monilial) vaginitis produces a curdy white discharge. This organism is present in about 5% of normal adults, and so the appearance of symptomatic infection almost always involves predisposing influences or sexual transmission of a new, more aggressive strain. Biopsy specimens, which are rarely obtained, reveal only superficial, nonspecific submucosal inflammation. *T. vaginalis,* also a frequent offender, produces a watery, copious gray-green discharge in which parasites can also be identified microscopically. However, *Trichomonas* can also be identified in about 10% of asymptomatic women, and so active infection usually represents a sexually transmitted new strain (Chapter 18). The inflammatory reaction is confined to the superficial squamous mucosa without invasion of the underlying tissue.

Nonspecific atrophic vaginitis may be encountered in postmenopausal women with preexisting atrophy and thinning of the squamous vaginal mucosa.

VAGINAL INTRAEPITHELIAL NEOPLASIA AND SQUAMOUS CELL CARCINOMA

Extremely uncommon, these lesions usually occur in women older than age 60 years, with risk factors similar to those for carcinoma of the cervix, discussed below. A preexisting or concurrent cervical intraepithelial neoplasia or carcinoma of the cervix is frequently present. Vaginal intraepithelial neoplasia is a precursor lesion associated with HPV infection in nearly all cases. Invasive squamous cell carcinoma of the vagina is associated with the presence of HPV DNA in more than half of cases.

Of particular interest is vaginal clear cell adenocarcinoma, usually encountered in young women in their late teens to early 20s whose mothers took diethylstilbestrol during pregnancy. Sometimes these cancers do not appear until the third or fourth decade of life. The overall risk is less than 1 per 1000 of those exposed in utero. In about one-third of instances these cancers arise in the cervix. Much more frequently, perhaps in one-third of the population at risk, small glandular or microcystic inclusions appear in the vaginal mucosa. These benign lesions, called *vaginal adenosis,* appear as red granular foci and are lined by mucus-secreting or ciliated columnar cells. It is from such inclusions that the rare clear cell adenocarcinoma arises.

SARCOMA BOTRYOIDES

Sarcoma botryoides (embryonal rhabdomyosarcoma), producing soft polypoid masses, is another, fortunately rare, form of primary vaginal cancer. It is usually encountered in infants and children younger than the age of 5 years. It may occur in other sites, such as the urinary bladder and bile ducts. These lesions are described in more detail in Chapter 21.

CERVIX

The cervix must serve as a barrier to the ingress of air and the microflora of the normal vaginal tract, yet it must permit the escape of menstrual flow and be capable of dilating to accommodate childbirth. No small wonder it is often the seat of disease. Fortunately, most cervical lesions are relatively banal inflammations (cervicitis), but this is also the site of one of the most common cancers in women; squamous cell carcinoma.

CERVICITIS

During development, the columnar mucus-secreting epithelium of the endocervix meets the squamous epithelial covering of the exocervix at the external os; thus, the entire "exposed" cervix is covered by squamous epithelium. The endocervical columnar epithelium is not visible to the naked eye or colposcopically. In time, in most young women, there is distal growth of the columnar epithelium that extends beyond the exocervical os, a condition called ectropion; thus, the squamocolumnar junction comes to lie visibly on the exocervix. This "exposed" mucus-secreting columnar epithelium may appear reddened and moist and has mistakenly been called cervical "erosion," but in fact it is the result of normal changes in adult women. Remodeling occurs continuously with regeneration of both squamous and columnar epithelium. The region in which this takes place is known as the *transformation zone* (Fig. 19–5). Frequently, overgrowth of the regenerating squamous epithelium blocks the orifices of endocervical glands in the transformation zone to produce small *nabothian cysts* lined by columnar mucus-secreting epithelium. In the transformation zone, there may be a mild inflammatory infiltrate resulting, possibly, from changes in the vaginal pH or the ever-present microflora of the vagina.

Inflammations of the cervix are extremely common and are associated with a mucopurulent to purulent vaginal discharge. Cytologic examination of the discharge reveals white cells and inflammatory atypia of shed epithelial cells, as well as possible microorganisms. These inflammations have been variously subdivided into noninfectious and infectious cervicitis. Because microorganisms are invariably present in the vagina, with or without associated inflammatory changes on cytologic examination, it is difficult to differentiate noninfectious from infectious cervicitis. Often present are indigenous and, for the most part, incidental vaginal aerobes and anaerobes, streptococci, staphylococci, enterococci, and *Escherichia coli.* Much more important are *Chlamydia trachomatis, Ureaplasma urealyticum, T. vaginalis, Candida* spp., *Neisseria gonorrhoeae,* herpes simplex II (genitalis), and one or more types of HPV. Many of these microorganisms are transmitted sexually, and so the cervicitis may represent a sexually transmitted disease. Among these pathogens, *C. trachomatis* is by far the most common and accounts for as many as 40% of cases of cervicitis encountered in sexually transmitted disease

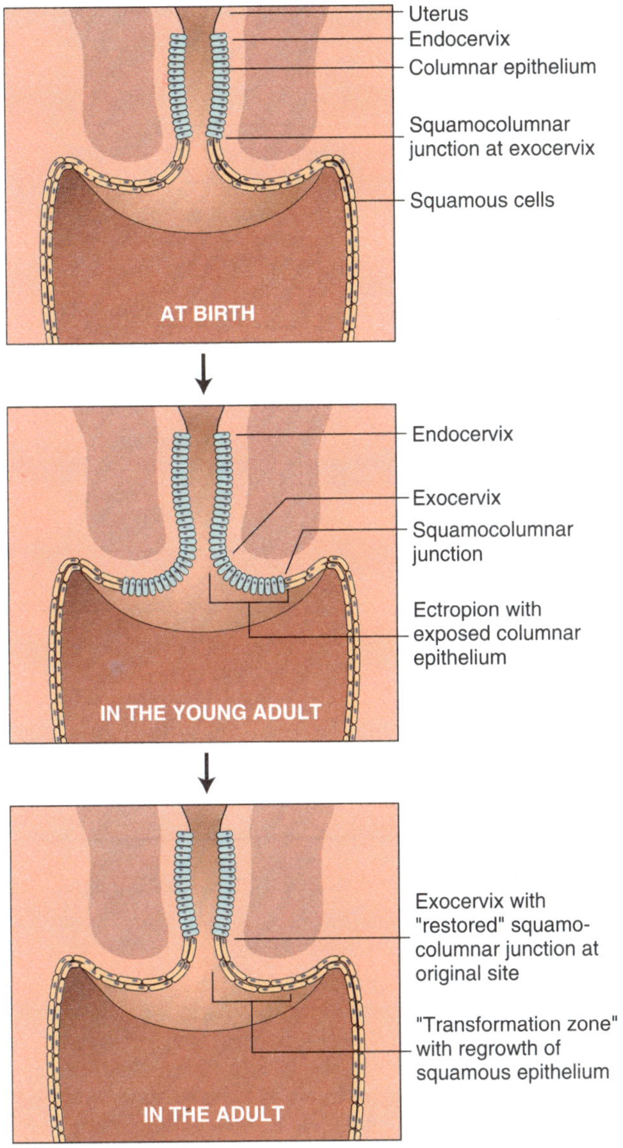

Figure 19–5

Development of the cervical transformation zone.

clinics, thus being far more common than gonorrhea. Herpetic infections of the cervix are noteworthy, because this organism may be transmitted to the infant during passage through the birth canal, sometimes resulting in a serious, sometimes fatal, systemic herpetic infection (Chapter 7).

Morphology

Nonspecific cervicitis may be either **acute** or **chronic.** Excluding gonococcal infection, which causes a specific form of acute disease, the relatively uncommon **acute nonspecific form** is limited to postpartum women and is usually caused by staphylococci or streptococci. The chronic form is a nearly ubiquitous entity usually referred to as **nonspecific cervicitis.**

Specific forms include herpesvirus ulcerative lesions and changes caused by *C. trachomatis.* Chronic cervicitis is not easily defined, but it consists of inflammation and epithelial regeneration common in all women of reproductive age. The cervical epithelium may show hyperplasia and reactive changes. These changes may occur in both squamous and columnar mucosa. Eventually, columnar epithelium undergoes squamous metaplasia or transformation into a stratified squamous epithelium.

Cervicitis commonly comes to attention on routine examination or because of marked leukorrhea. Culture of the discharge must be interpreted cautiously, because commensal organisms are virtually always present. Only the identification of known pathogens is helpful. When the lesion is severe, inflammatory changes can make differentiation from carcinoma difficult on cytologic preparations and even with colposcopy. Differentiation of inflammatory changes from premalignant dysplasia may also be difficult on cervical biopsy specimen.

TUMORS OF THE CERVIX

Despite dramatic improvements in early diagnosis and treatment, cervical carcinoma continues to be one of the major causes of cancer-related deaths in women, particularly in the developing world. The only other "tumor" meriting mention is the endocervical polyp.

Cervical Intraepithelial Neoplasia (CIN) and Squamous Cell Carcinoma

Cervical carcinoma was once the most frequent form of cancer in women around the world. Since the introduction of the Papanicolaou (Pap) smear 50 years ago, the incidence of cervical cancer has plummeted. The Pap smear remains the most successful cancer screening test ever developed. In populations that are screened regularly, cervical cancer mortality is reduced by as much as 99%. In the United States, Pap screening has dramatically lowered the incidence of invasive cervical tumors to about 10,500 new cases annually and the mortality to about 3900 cases per year, ranking it 13th in cancer deaths for women. Many of the cases of cervical carcinoma now occur in women who have not had regular screening. Over the same period the incidence of precursor CIN has increased (this being in part attributable to better case finding) to its present level of more than 50,000 cases annually. This growing divergence is a testament to detection of precursor lesions by the Pap smear at an early stage, permitting discovery of these lesions when curative treatment is possible.

It is important to emphasize here that nearly all invasive cervical squamous cell carcinomas arise from precursor epithelial changes referred to as CIN. However, not all cases of CIN progress to invasive cancer, and indeed many persist without change or even regress, as will be pointed out.

Cervical Intraepithelial Neoplasia

Cytologic examination can detect CIN long before any abnormality can be seen grossly. The follow-up of such women has revealed that precancerous epithelial changes (CIN) may precede the development of an overt cancer by many years, or in some cases even decades. However, as noted earlier, only a fraction of cases of CIN progress to invasive carcinoma. The precancerous changes referred to as CIN may begin as low-grade CIN and progress to higher grade CIN, or they may begin at the outset as high-grade CIN, depending on the location of the HPV infection in the transformation zone, the type of HPV infection (high versus low risk), and other contributing host factors. On the basis of histology, precancerous changes are graded as follows:

CIN I: Mild dysplasia
CIN II: Moderate dysplasia
CIN III: Severe dysplasia and carcinoma in situ

However, in cytologic smears, the current Bethesda system separates the precancerous lesions into only two groups: low-grade and high-grade squamous intraepithelial lesions (SIL). The low-grade lesions correspond to CIN I or flat condylomas (described later) and the high-grade lesions to CIN II or III. Progression from a lower grade to a higher grade is not inevitable. Although studies vary, with CIN I the likelihood of regression is 50% to 60%, that of persistence is 30%, and that of progression to CIN III, is 20%. With progression, only 1% to 5% become invasive. With CIN III the likelihood of regression is only 33% and of progression 60% to 74% (in various studies). It is evident that the higher the grade of CIN, the greater the likelihood of progression, but it should be noted that in many cases even the higher grade lesions do not progress to cancer.

Epidemiology and Pathogenesis. The peak age incidence of CIN is about 30 years, whereas that of invasive carcinoma is about 45 years. Although invasive tumors are occasionally seen in women in their early 20s, precancerous changes usually take many years, perhaps decades, to evolve into overt carcinomas.

Important risk factors for the development of CIN and invasive carcinoma are:

- Early age at first intercourse
- Multiple sexual partners
- A male partner with multiple previous sexual partners
- Persistent infection by "high-risk" papillomaviruses.

Many other risk factors can be related to these four, including the higher incidence in lower socioeconomic groups, the rarity among virgins, and the association with multiple pregnancies. They point to the likelihood of sexual transmission of a causative agent, in this case HPV. Indeed, HPV can be detected by molecular methods in nearly all precancerous lesions and invasive neoplasms. More specifically, certain high-risk HPV types, including 16, 18, 45, and 31, account for the majority of cervical carcinomas, with smaller contributions by HPV 33, 35, 39, 45, 52, 56, 58, and 59. By contrast, condylomas, which are benign lesions, are associated with infection by

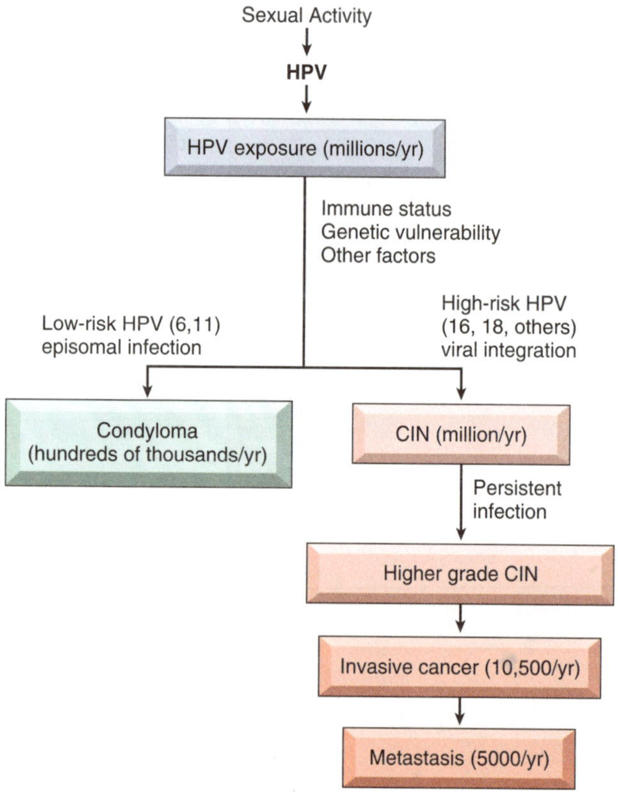

Figure 19–6

An attempt to depict the sequence of events that may follow human papillomavirus (HPV) infection. CIN, cervical intraepithelial neoplasia.

low-risk HPV types (i.e., 6, 11, 42, and 44; Fig. 19–6). In these benign lesions the viral DNA does not integrate into the host genome, remaining in the free episomal form. By contrast, HPV types 16 and 18 usually integrate into the host genome and express large amounts of E6 and E7 proteins, which block or inactivate tumor suppressor genes *p53* and *RB*, respectively (Chapter 6). The result is a transformed cell phenotype, capable of autonomous growth and susceptible to the acquisition of further mutations. The recently introduced HPV vaccine is very effective in preventing HPV infections and hence cervical cancers.

Although many women harbor these viruses, only a few develop cancer, suggesting other influences on cancer risk. Among the other well-defined risk factors are cigarette smoking and exogenous or endogenous immunodeficiency. For example, the incidence of carcinoma in situ is increased approximately fivefold in women infected with human immunodeficiency virus when compared with controls.

Morphology

The cervical epithelial changes included within the term **CIN** begin with mild dysplasia, called **CIN I** or **flat condyloma.** This lesion is characterized by koilocytotic changes mostly in the superficial layers of the epithelium. **Koilocytosis,** as you will recall from the earlier discussion of condylomata acuminata, is composed of nuclear hyperchromasia and angulation with perinuclear vacuolization produced by cytopathic effect of HPV. In CIN II the dysplasia is more severe, with maturation of keratinocytes delayed into the middle third of the epithelium. It is associated with some variation in cell and nuclear size, heterogeneity of nuclear chromatin and mitoses above the basal layer, extending in to the middle third of the epithelium. The superficial layer of cells shows some differentiation, and in some cases it shows the koilocytotic changes described. The next level of dysplasia, not always distinct from CIN II, is CIN III, marked by even greater variation in cell and nuclear size, marked chromatin heterogeneity, disorderly orientation of the cells, and normal or abnormal mitoses; these changes affect virtually all layers of the epithelium and are characterized by loss of maturation. Differentiation of surface cells and koilocytotic changes have usually disappeared (Figs. 19–7 and 19–8). CIN II and III may begin as CIN I or arise de novo, depending in part on the associated HPV type. In time, dysplastic changes become more atypical and may extend into the endocervical glands, but **the alterations are confined to the epithelial layer and its glands.** These changes constitute **carcinoma in situ.** The next stage, if it is to appear, is invasive cancer. However, as previously emphasized, there is no inevitability to this progression.

Cervical precancers produce cytologic abnormalities that often (but not always) reflect the severity of CIN. Interestingly, the majority (>70%) of CINs of all grades are associated with "high-risk" HPVs. Moreover, as many as one-half of "nondiagnostic" Pap smear abnormalities (e.g., atypical squamous cells of undetermined significance) may be associated with high-risk HPVs, yet less than 25% of these changes will be followed by a biopsy-proven CIN II or CIN III. Among women with cytologically normal smears, 10% to 15% harbor high-risk HPVs. Of these, approximately 10% will eventually develop a high-grade CIN.

Although HPV testing can identify the pool of women at risk for cervical cancer, most sexually active women will contract cervical HPV infections at some point in their lifetime. This limits the usefulness of HPV testing as a screening tool for cervical cancer. Thus, cervical cytology and cervical examinations (colposcopy) remain the mainstays of cervical cancer prevention. Nevertheless, women who test HPV negative with the use of molecular probes for HPV DNA are *at extremely low risk for harboring a CIN,* and guidelines for frequency of future screening for this group are being formulated.

Invasive Carcinoma of the Cervix

The importance of cervical cancer as a cause of morbidity and mortality around the world, particularly in developing countries, has already been emphasized. The most common cervical carcinomas are squamous cell carcinomas (75%), followed by adenocarcinomas and adenosquamous carcinomas (20%), and small-cell neuroendocrine carcinomas (<5%). The squamous cell lesions are increasingly appearing in younger women, now with a peak incidence at about 45 years, some 10 to 15 years after detection of their precursors. In some individuals with particularly aggressive intraepithelial changes, the time interval may be considerably shorter, whereas in other women CIN precursors may persist for life. Many variables, both constitutional and acquired, modify the course. The only reliable way to monitor the course of the disease is with careful follow-up and repeat biopsies. The relative proportion of adenocarcinoma has been increasing in recent decades; glandular lesions are not detected well by Pap smear and other screening techniques, and invasive squamous carcinoma is becoming less frequent.

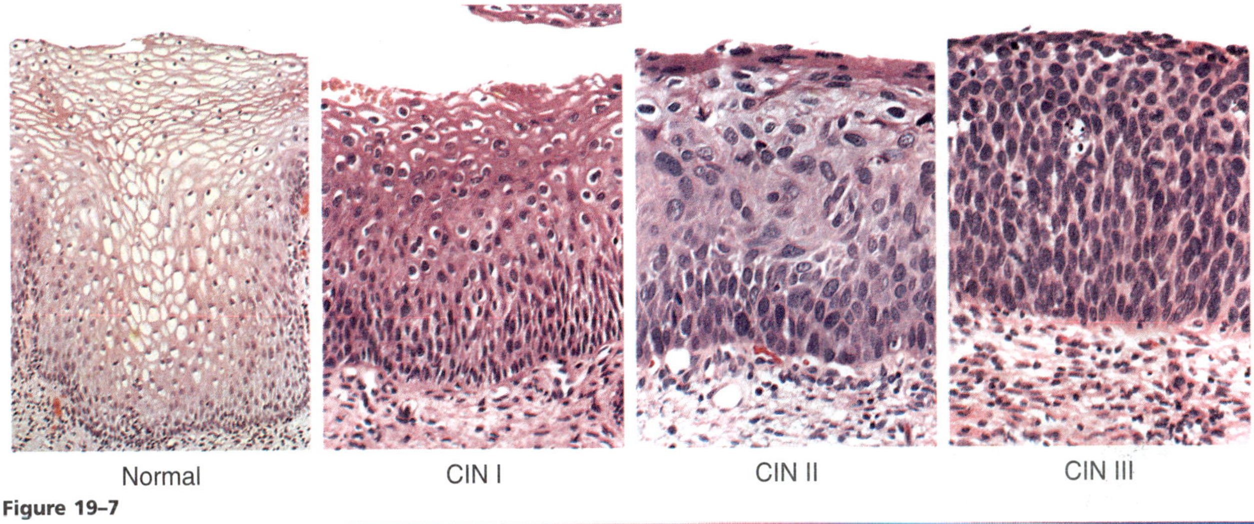

Figure 19–7

Spectrum of CIN: normal squamous epithelium for comparison; CIN I with koilocytotic atypia; CIN II with progressive atypia in all layers of the epithelium; CIN III (carcinoma in situ) with diffuse atypia and loss of maturation.

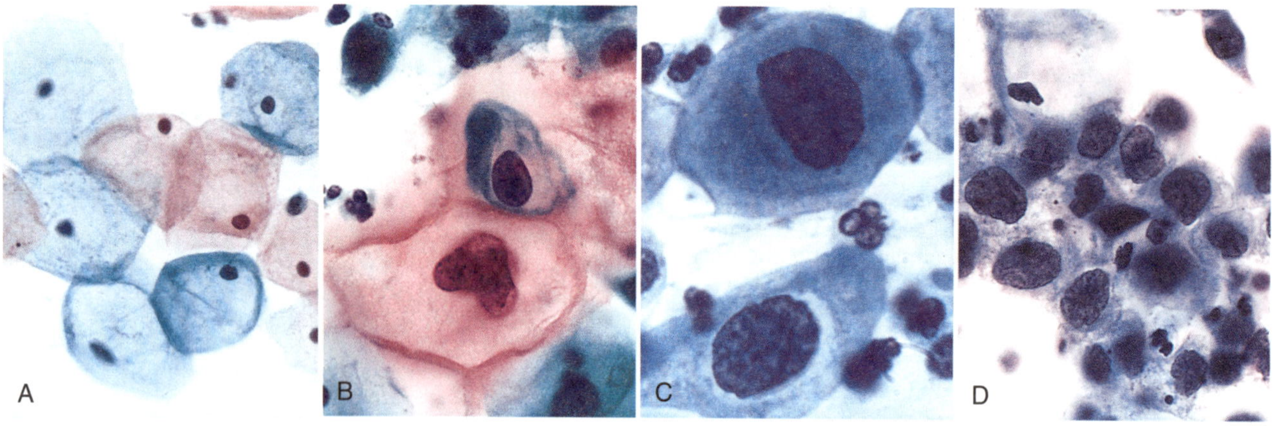

Figure 19–8

The cytology of CIN as seen on the Papanicolaou smear. **A–B,** Cytoplasmic staining in superficial cells may be either red or blue. **A,** Normal exfoliated superficial squamous epithelial cells. **B,** CIN I. **C,** CIN II. **D,** CIN III. Note the reduction in cytoplasm and the increase in the nucleus-to-cytoplasm ratio as the grade of the lesion increases. This reflects the progressive loss of cellular differentiation on the surface of the cervical lesions from which these cells are exfoliated (see Figure 19–7). (Courtesy of Dr. Edmund S. Cibas, Brigham and Women's Hospital, Boston, Massachusetts.)

Morphology

Invasive carcinomas of the cervix develop in the region of the transformation zone and range from microscopic foci of early stromal invasion to grossly conspicuous tumors encircling the os (Fig. 19–9). Thus, the tumors may be invisible or exophytic. Tumors encircling the cervix and penetrating into the underlying stroma produce a "barrel cervix," which can be identified by direct palpation. Extension into the parametrial soft tissues can fix the uterus to the pelvic structures. Spread to pelvic lymph nodes is determined by tumor depth and the presence of capillary-lymphatic invasion, ranging from less than 1% for tumors under 3 mm in depth to over 10% once invasion exceeds 5 mm. Distant metastases, including para-aortic nodal involvement, remote organ involvement, or invasion of adjacent structures such as bladder or rectum, occur late in the course of disease. With the exception of neuroendocrine tumors, which are uniformly aggressive in their behavior, cervical carcinomas are graded from 1 to 3 based on cellular differentiation and staged from 1 to 4 depending on clinical spread.

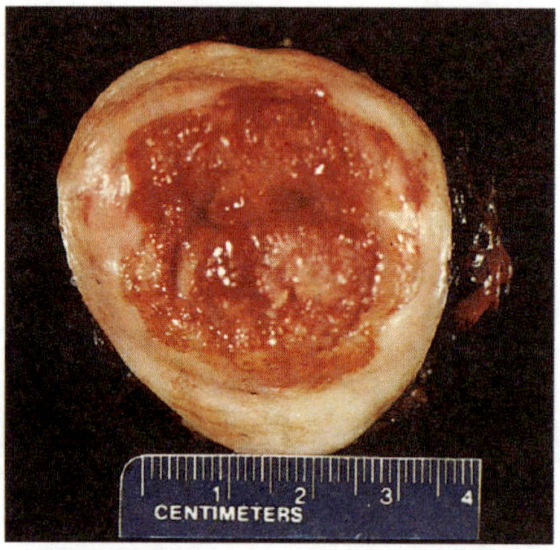

Figure 19–9

Carcinoma of the cervix, well advanced.

Clinical Course. With the advent of the Pap smear, an increasing proportion of cervical carcinomas are diagnosed early in their course (stage 1). The vast majority of cervical neoplasms are diagnosed in the preinvasive phase and appear as white areas on colposcopic examination after application of dilute acetic acid. More advanced cases of cervical cancer are invariably seen in women who either have never had a Pap smear or have waited many years since the prior smear. Such tumors may be symptomatic, called to attention by unexpected vaginal bleeding, leukorrhea, painful coitus (dyspareunia), and dysuria. Mortality is most strongly related to tumor extent and in some cases (as in neuroendocrine tumors) to cell type. Detection of precursors by cytologic examination and their eradication by laser vaporization or cone biopsy is the most effective method of cancer prevention. However, once cancer develops, the outlook hinges on stage, with 5-year survivals as follows: stage 0 (preinvasive), 100%; stage 1, 90%; stage 2, 82%; stage 3, 35%; and stage 4, 10%. Because tumor spread is gradual, 5-year survival of women even with positive pelvic nodes approaches 50%. Chemotherapy may improve survival in advanced cases.

SUMMARY

Cervical Neoplasia

- Risk factors for cervical carcinoma include early age at first intercourse, multiple sexual partners, cigarette smoking, immunodeficiency, and infection by "high-risk" papillomaviruses.

- Nearly all cervical carcinoma is HPV related, particularly certain HPV subtypes (16, 18, 45, 31, and others). HPV vaccine can prevent the occurrence of cervical cancer.
- HPV virus E6 and E7 proteins cause inactivation of *p53* and *RB* genes, respectively, resulting in increased cell proliferation and suppression of apoptosis.
- High-grade cervical dysplasias (CIN II and III) contain HPV incorporated into the cell genome, and cytologically have increased chromatin abnormality and an increased nuclear-to-cytoplasmic ratio.
- Not all HPV infections progress to CIN III or invasive carcinoma. The time course from infection to invasive disease may be 10 years or more.
- The Pap smear is a highly effective screening tool in the detection of cervical dysplasia and carcinoma, and has reduced the incidence of cervical carcinoma.

Endocervical Polyp

Although these lesions may protrude as polypoid masses (sometimes through the exocervix), they may in reality be inflammatory in origin. They can be as large as a few centimeters, are soft and yielding to palpation, and have a smooth, glistening surface with underlying cystically dilated spaces filled with mucinous secretion. The surface epithelium and lining of the underlying cysts are composed of the same mucus-secreting columnar cells that line the endocervical canal. The stroma is edematous and may contain scattered mononuclear cells. Superimposed chronic inflammation may lead to squamous metaplasia of the covering epithelium and ulcerations. These lesions may bleed and thus cause some concern, but they have no malignant potential.

BODY OF UTERUS

The uterine corpus with its lining endometrium is the principal seat of female reproductive tract disease. Many disorders of this organ are common, often chronic and recurrent, and sometimes disastrous. Only the more frequent and significant ones are considered here.

ENDOMETRITIS

Inflammation of the endometrium is seen as part of the wider spectrum of pelvic inflammatory disease, a condition with consequences for the integrity of the fallopian tubes and subsequent fertility, as discussed below. Endometritis may be associated with retained products of conception subsequent to miscarriage or delivery, or a foreign body such as an intrauterine device. Retained tissue or foreign bodies act as a nidus for infection, frequently by flora ascending from the vaginal and intestinal tract, and removal of the offending tissue or foreign body typically results in resolution.

Endometritis is classified as acute or chronic based on whether there is a predominant neutrophilic or lymphoplasmacytic response; however, components of both may be present in a given uterus. Generally the diagnosis of chronic endometritis requires the presence of plasma cells. Acute endometritis is frequently due to *N. gonorrhoeae* or *C. trachomatis*. Histologically, neutrophilic infiltrate in the superficial endometrium and glands coexists with a stromal lymphoplasmacytic infiltrate. Prominent lymphoid follicles are more commonly seen in chlamydial infection. By contrast, *Mycoplasma* infection has a subtle lymphocytic stromal infiltrate. All forms of endometritis may present with fever, abdominal pain, menstrual abnormalities, infertility and ectopic pregnancy due to damage to the fallopian tubes (see below).

Occasionally tuberculosis may present with a granulomatous endometritis, frequently with tuberculous salpingitis and peritonitis. Although seen in the United States mainly in immunocompromised individuals, it is common in other countries where tuberculosis is endemic and should receive consideration in the differential diagnosis of pelvic inflammatory disease in women who have recently emigrated from endemic areas.

ADENOMYOSIS

Adenomyosis refers to the growth of the basal layer of the endometrium down into the myometrium. Nests of endometrial stroma, glands, or both, are found well down in the myometrium between the muscle bundles. In the fortuitous microscopic section, continuity between these nests and the overlying endometrium can be established. The uterine wall often becomes thickened and the uterus is enlarged and globular as a result of the presence of endometrial tissue and a reactive hypertrophy of the myometrium. Because these glands derive from the stratum basalis of the endometrium, they do not undergo cyclical bleeding. Nevertheless, marked adenomyosis may produce menorrhagia, dysmenorrhea, and pelvic pain before the onset of menstruation.

ENDOMETRIOSIS

Endometriosis is characterized by endometrial glands and stroma in a location outside the endomyometrium. It occurs in as many as 10% of women in their reproductive years and in nearly half of women with infertility. It is a common cause of dysmenorrhea, and pelvic pain, and may present as a pelvic mass filled with degenerating blood (chocolate cyst). It is frequently multifocal and may involve tissue in the pelvis (ovaries, pouch of Douglas, uterine ligaments, tubes, and rectovaginal septum), less frequently in more remote sites of the peritoneal cavity and about the umbilicus and uncommonly lymph nodes, lungs, and even heart, skeletal muscle, or bone.

Three possibilities (not mutually exclusive) have been invoked to explain the origin of these dispersed lesions (Fig. 19–10). First, the *regurgitation theory,* currently the most accepted, proposes menstrual backflow through the fallopian tubes with subsequent implantation. Indeed, menstrual endometrium is viable and survives when injected into the anterior abdominal wall; however, this theory cannot explain lesions in the lymph nodes, skeletal muscle, or lungs. Second, the *metaplastic theory* proposes endometrial differentiation of coelomic epithelium, which is the origin of the endometrium itself. This theory, too, cannot explain endometriotic lesions in the lungs or lymph nodes. Third, the *vascular* or *lymphatic dissemination theory* has been invoked to explain extrapelvic or intranodal implants. Conceivably, all pathways are valid in individual instances.

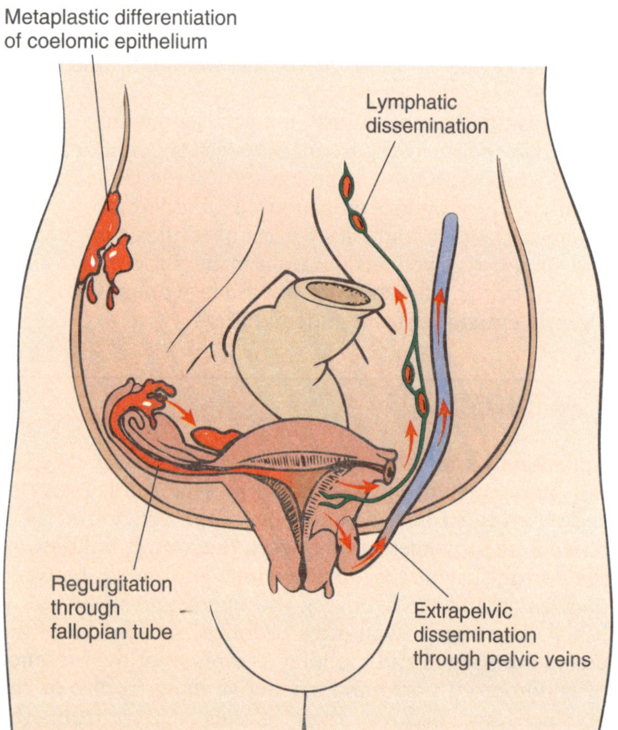

Figure 19–10

The potential origins of endometrial implants.

Morphology

In contrast to adenomyosis, **endometriosis** almost always contains **functioning endometrium,** which undergoes cyclic bleeding. Because blood collects in these aberrant foci, they usually appear grossly as red-blue to yellow-brown nodules or implants. They vary in size from microscopic to 1 to 2 cm in diameter and lie on or just under the affected serosal surface. Often individual lesions coalesce to form larger masses. When the ovaries are involved, the lesions may form large, blood-filled cysts that are transformed into so-called **chocolate cysts** as the blood ages (Fig. 19–11). Seepage and organization of the blood leads to widespread fibrosis, adherence of pelvic structures, sealing of the tubal fimbriated ends, and distortion of the oviducts and ovaries. The histologic diagnosis at all sites depends on finding two of the following three features within the lesions: endometrial glands, stroma, or hemosiderin pigment.

The clinical manifestations of endometriosis depend on the distribution of the lesions. Extensive scarring of the oviducts and ovaries often produces discomfort in the lower abdominal quadrants and eventually causes sterility. Pain on defecation reflects rectal wall involvement, and dyspareunia (painful intercourse) and dysuria reflect involvement of the uterine and bladder serosa, respectively. In almost all cases, there is severe dysmenorrhea and pelvic pain as a result of intrapelvic bleeding and periuterine adhesions.

DYSFUNCTIONAL UTERINE BLEEDING AND ENDOMETRIAL HYPERPLASIA

By far the most common problem for which women seek medical attention is some disturbance in menstrual function: *menorrhagia* (profuse or prolonged bleeding at the time of the period), *metrorrhagia* (irregular bleeding between the periods), *ovulatory* (intermenstrual) or *postmenopausal* bleeding. Common causes include polyps, leiomyomas, endometrial carcinoma, endometrial hyperplasia, and endometritis. Vaginal bleeding may also

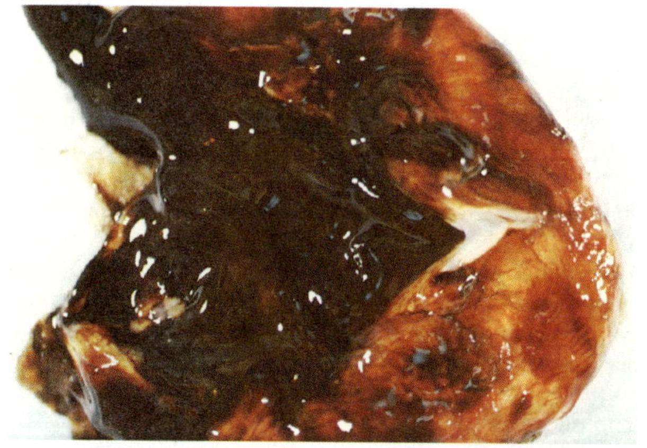

Figure 19–11

This ovary has been sectioned to reveal a large endometriotic cyst with degenerated blood ("chocolate" cyst).

be due to lesions of the cervix and vagina, such as polyps, cervicitis, or carcinoma.

Dysfunctional Uterine Bleeding

Abnormal bleeding in the absence of a well-defined organic lesion in the uterus is called dysfunctional uterine bleeding. The probable cause of abnormal uterine bleeding, dysfunctional or organic (related to a well-defined lesion), depends somewhat on the age of the woman (Table 19–1).

The various causes of dysfunctional bleeding can be segregated into four groups:

- *Failure of ovulation.* Anovulatory cycles are very common at both ends of reproductive life; with any dysfunction of the hypothalamic-pituitary axis, adrenal, or thyroid; with a functioning ovarian lesion producing an excess of estrogen; with malnutrition, obesity, or debilitating disease; and with severe physical or emotional stress. Regardless of the basis for the failure of ovulation, it leads to an excess of estrogen relative to progesterone. Thus, the endometrium goes through a proliferative phase that is not followed by the normal secretory phase. The endometrial glands may develop mild cystic changes or in other places may appear disorderly with a relative scarcity of stroma, which requires progesterone for its support. The poorly supported endometrium partially collapses, with rupture of spiral arteries, accounting for the bleeding.
- *Inadequate luteal phase.* The corpus luteum may fail to mature normally or may regress prematurely, leading to a relative lack of progesterone. The endometrium under these circumstances reveals delay in the development of the secretory changes expected at the date of biopsy.
- *Contraceptive-induced bleeding.* Older oral contraceptives containing synthetic estrogens and progestin induced a variety of endometrial responses—for example, a lush, decidua-like stroma and inactive, nonsecretory glands. The pills in current use have corrected these abnormalities.
- *Endomyometrial disorders,* including chronic endometritis, endometrial polyps, and submucosal leiomyomas.

Table 19–1 Causes of Abnormal Uterine Bleeding by Age Group

Age Group	Cause(s)
Prepuberty	Precocious puberty (hypothalamic, pituitary, or ovarian origin)
Adolescence	Anovulatory cycle
Reproductive age	Complications of pregnancy (abortion, trophoblastic disease, ectopic pregnancy) Organic lesions (leiomyoma, adenomyosis, polyps, endometrial hyperplasia, carcinoma) Anovulatory cycle Ovulatory dysfunctional bleeding (e.g., inadequate luteal phase)
Perimenopause	Anovulatory cycle Irregular shedding Organic lesions (carcinoma, hyperplasia, polyps)
Postmenopause	Organic lesions (carcinoma, hyperplasia, polyps) Endometrial atrophy

Endometrial Hyperplasia

An excess of estrogen relative to progestin, if sufficiently prolonged or marked, will induce exaggerated endometrial proliferation (hyperplasia), which can be preneoplastic. The severity of hyperplasia is classified based on architectural crowding and cytologic atypia, ranging from simple hyperplasia to complex hyperplasia, and finally atypical hyperplasia (Fig. 19–12). These three categories represent a continuum based on the level and duration of the estrogen excess. Not surprisingly, in time the hyperplasia may become autonomously proliferating, no longer needing estrogenic influence, eventually giving rise to carcinoma. The risk of developing carcinoma is dependent on the severity of the hyperplastic changes and associated cellular atypia. Simple hyperplasia carries a negligible risk, while a person with atypical hyperplasia with cellular atypia has a 20% risk of developing endometrial carcinoma. Any estrogen excess may lead to hyperplasia. Potential contributors include failure of ovulation, such as is seen around the menopause; prolonged administration of estrogenic steroids without counterbalancing progestin; estrogen-producing ovarian lesions such as polycystic ovaries (including Stein-Leventhal syndrome); cortical stromal hyperplasia; and granulosa-theca cell tumors of the ovary. A common risk factor is obesity, because adipose tissue processes steroid precursors into estrogens. When atypical hyperplasia is discovered, it must be carefully evaluated for the presence of cancer and must be monitored by repeated endometrial biopsy.

SUMMARY

Non-neoplastic Disorders of Endometrium

- Endometriosis refers to location of endometrial glands and stroma outside the uterus and may involve the pelvic or abdominal peritoneum, and sometimes distant sites like lymph nodes and lungs.
- The ectopic endometrium in endometriosis undergoes cyclincal bleeding and is a common cause of dysmenorrhea and pelvic pain.
- Adenomyosis refers to growth of endometrium into the myometrium with uterine enlargement. Unlike endometriosis there is no cyclical bleeding.
- Endometrial hyperplasia results from an excess of estrogen, whether endogenous or exogenous.
- Risk factors for developing hyperplasia include anovulatory cycles, polycystic ovary syndrome, estrogen-producing ovarian tumor, obesity, and hormone intake.
- The severity of hyperplasia is graded by architectural and cytologic criteria. Complex architecture associated with cytologic atypia has a 20% risk of developing carcinoma.

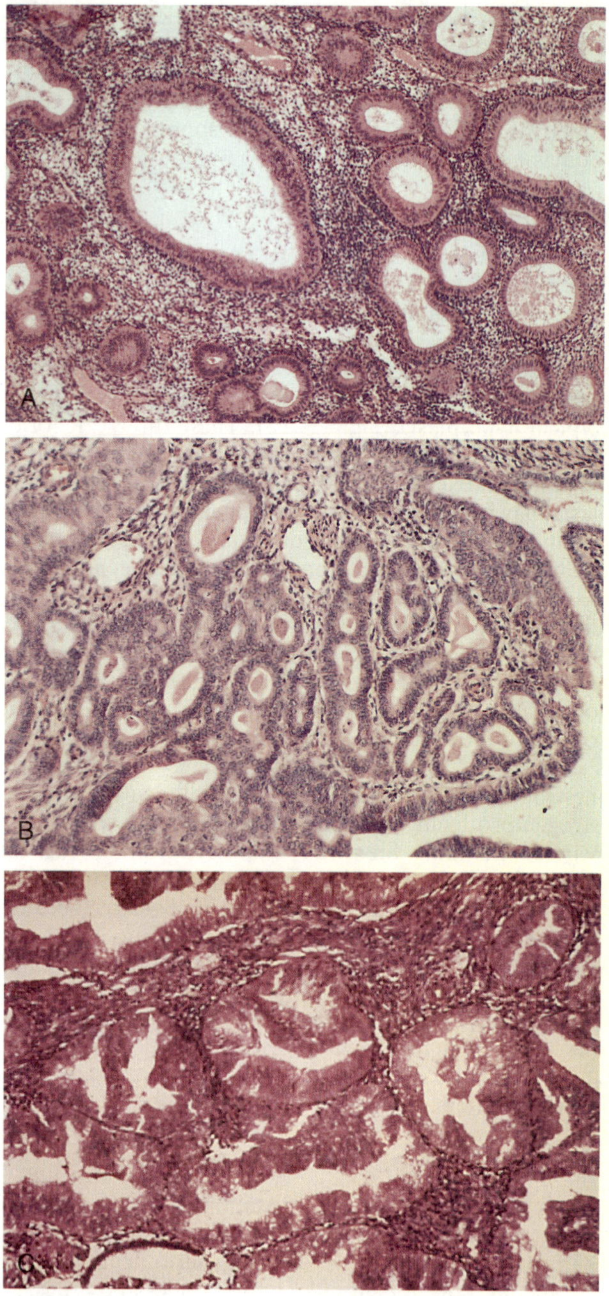

Figure 19–12

A, Anovulatory or "disordered" endometrium with dilatation of glands. **B,** Complex hyperplasia displaying a nest of closely packed glands. **C,** Atypical endometrial hyperplasia with crowding of glands, unfolding of tall columnar cells, and some loss of polarity.

TUMORS OF THE ENDOMETRIUM AND MYOMETRIUM

The most common neoplasms of the body of the uterus are endometrial polyps, smooth muscle tumors, and endometrial carcinomas. All tend to produce bleeding from the uterus as the earliest manifestation.

Endometrial Polyps

These are sessile, usually hemispheric (rarely pedunculated) lesions that are 0.5 to 3 cm in diameter. Larger polyps may project from the endometrial mucosa into the uterine cavity. Histologically they are composed of endometrium resembling the basalis, frequently with small muscular arteries. Some have an essentially normal endometrial architecture, but more often they have cystically dilated glands. The stromal cells in most endometrial polyps are monoclonal and have a cytogenetic rearrangement at 6p21, making it clear that they are the neoplastic component of the polyp.

Although endometrial polyps may occur at any age, they develop more commonly at the time of menopause. Their clinical significance lies in the production of abnormal uterine bleeding and, more important, the risk (however rare) of giving rise to a cancer.

Leiomyoma and Leiomyosarcoma

Benign tumors that arise from the smooth muscle cells in the myometrium are properly termed *leiomyomas.* However, because they are firm, they are more often referred to as *fibroids.* They are the most common benign tumor in females and are found in 30% to 50% of women during reproductive life. Some genetic influence may be involved; these tumors are considerably more frequent in blacks than in whites. Estrogens and possibly oral contraceptives stimulate their growth; conversely, they shrink postmenopausally. These tumors are clearly monoclonal, and nonrandom chromosomal abnormalities have been found in about 40% of tumors.

Morphology

Macroscopically leiomyomas are typically **sharply circumscribed,** firm gray-white masses with a characteristic **whorled cut surface.** They may occur singly, but most often multiple tumors are scattered within the uterus, ranging in size from small seedlings to massive neoplasms that dwarf the size of the uterus (Fig. 19–13). Some are embedded within the myometrium (intramural), whereas others may lie directly beneath the endometrium (submucosal) or directly beneath the serosa (subserosal). The latter may develop attenuated stalks and even become attached to surrounding organs, from which they develop a blood supply and then free themselves from the uterus to become "parasitic" leiomyomas. Larger neoplasms may develop foci of ischemic necrosis with areas of hemorrhage and cystic softening, and after menopause they may become densely collagenous and even calcified. Histologically, the tumors are characterized by **whorling bundles of smooth muscle cells** duplicating the histology of the normal myometrium. Foci of fibrosis, calcification, ischemic necrosis, cystic degeneration, and hemorrhage may be present.

Leiomyomas of the uterus may be entirely asymptomatic and be discovered only on routine pelvic or post mortem examination. The most frequent manifestation, when present, is menorrhagia, with or without metror-

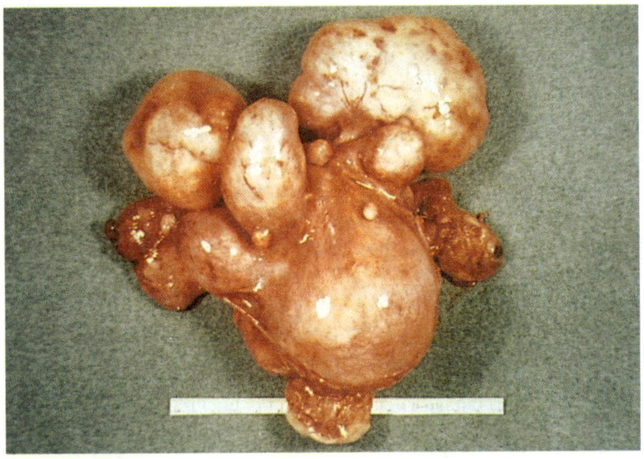

Figure 19–13

Multiple leiomyomas of the uterus. Several large, almost pedunculated tumors protrude from the dome of the fundus. The lower uterine segment and cervix are below *(on top of white bar)*. (Courtesy of Dr. Kyle Molberg, Department of Pathology, University of Texas Southwestern Medical School, Dallas, Texas.)

rhagia. Large masses in the pelvic region may become palpable to the woman or may produce a dragging sensation. Benign leiomyomas rarely transform into sarcomas, and the presence of multiple lesions does not increase the risk of harboring a malignancy.

Leiomyosarcomas typically arise de novo from the mesenchymal cells of the myometrium, not from preexisting leiomyomas. They are almost always solitary tumors, in contradistinction to the frequently multiple leiomyomas.

Morphology

Grossly, leiomyosarcomas develop in several distinct patterns: as bulky masses infiltrating the uterine wall, as polypoid lesions projecting into the uterine cavity, or as deceptively discrete tumors that masquerade as large, benign leiomyomas. They are frequently soft, hemorrhagic, and necrotic. Histologically, they present a wide range of differentiation, from those that closely resemble leiomyoma to wildly anaplastic tumors. With this range in morphology, it is understandable that some well-differentiated tumors lie at the interface between benign and malignant, and sometimes these are designated as smooth muscle tumors of uncertain malignant potential. The diagnostic features of leiomyosarcoma include tumor necrosis, which is distinct from the degenerative necrosis frequently seen in leiomyomas, cytologic atypia, and mitotic activity. Since increased mitotic activity alone is sometimes seen in benign smooth muscle tumors in young women, an assessment of all three features is necessary to make a diagnosis of malignancy.

Recurrence after removal is common with these cancers, and many metastasize, typically to the lungs, yielding a 5-year survival rate of about 40%. Understandably, the more anaplastic tumors have a poorer outlook than the better differentiated lesions.

SUMMARY

Uterine Smooth Muscle Neoplasms

- Benign smooth muscle tumors, called leiomyomas, are common and frequently multiple; they may present as menorrhagia, as a pelvic mass, or as a cause of infertility.
- Malignant smooth muscle tumors, called leiomyosarcomas, seem to arise de novo; multiple benign smooth muscle tumors do not increase the risk of malignancy.
- Criteria of malignancy include necrosis, cytologic atypia, and mitotic activity.

Endometrial Carcinoma

In the United States and many other Western countries, endometrial carcinoma is the most frequent cancer occurring in the female genital tract. Some years ago, it was much less common than cervical cancer. However, early detection of CIN by periodic cytologic examinations and its appropriate treatment have dramatically reduced the incidence of invasive cervical cancer.

Epidemiology and Pathogenesis. Endometrial cancer appears most frequently between the ages of 55 and 65 years and is distinctly uncommon in women younger than 40 years of age. There are two clinical settings in which endometrial carcinomas arise: in perimenopausal women with estrogen excess and in older women with endometrial atrophy. These scenarios are correlated with differences in histology: *endometrioid* and *serous carcinoma* of the endometrium, respectively.

There is a constellation of well-defined risk factors for endometrioid carcinoma:

- Obesity: increased synthesis of estrogens in fat depots and from adrenal and ovarian precursors
- Diabetes
- Hypertension
- Infertility: women tend to be nulliparous, often with nonovulatory cycles.

These risk factors point to *increased estrogen stimulation*, and indeed it is well recognized that prolonged estrogen replacement therapy and estrogen-secreting ovarian tumors increase the risk of this form of cancer. The great preponderance of endometrial carcinomas arise in the setting just described. Many of these risk factors are the same as those for endometrial hyperplasia, and *endometrial carcinoma frequently arises on a background of endometrial hyperplasia*. These tumors are termed *endometrioid* because of their similarity to normal endometrial glands. Breast carcinoma occurs in women with endometrial cancer (and vice versa) more frequently than by chance alone.

Dissecting the pathogenesis of endometrioid carcinoma is aided by analysis of two familial cancer syndromes that have an increased risk of the endometrioid type of endometrial carcinoma:

- Endometrial carcinoma is the second most common cancer associated with *hereditary nonpolyposis colon cancer syndrome,* an inherited genetic defect in a DNA mismatch repair gene. Sporadic cases of endometrioid-type endometrial carcinoma also have a high frequency of inactivation of these genes by methylation of the promoter, and as a consequence have relatively unstable genomes (microsatellite instability).
- Persons with *Cowden's syndrome,* a multiple hamartoma syndrome that carries an increased risk of carcinoma of the breast, thyroid, and endometrium, have mutations in *PTEN,* a tumor suppressor gene. Sporadic cases of endometrioid carcinoma also harbor mutations in *PTEN.* In fact, both mismatch repair gene and *PTEN* mutations are early events in endometrial carcinogenesis, occurring in the progression from abnormal proliferation to atypical hyperplasia.

Serous carcinoma of the endometrium is pathophysiologically distinct. It typically arises in a background of atrophy, sometimes in the setting of an endometrial polyp. Mutations in DNA mismatch repair genes and *PTEN* are rare in serous carcinoma; however, nearly all cases have mutations in the *p53* tumor suppressor gene.

Morphology

Endometrioid carcinomas closely resemble normal endometrium and may be exophytic or infiltrative (Fig. 19–14A, B). They frequently show a range of patterns, including mucinous, tubal (ciliated), and squamous (occasionally adenosquamous) differentiation. Tumors originate in the mucosa and may infiltrate the myometrium and enter vascular spaces, with metastases to regional lymph nodes. For this group of tumors, grading (grades I–III) and staging closely parallel outcome: stage I, confined to the corpus; stage II, involvement of the cervix; stage III, beyond the uterus but within the true pelvis; stage IV, distant metastases or involvement of other viscera. One exception is synchronous endometrioid tumors arising in the uterus and ovary. This scenario often signifies two separate primary neoplasms rather than stage III disease and has a favorable prognosis. **Serous carcinoma** forms small tufts and papillae rather than the glands seen in endometrioid carcinoma, and has much greater cytologic atypia. They behave as poorly differentiated cancers are not graded, and are particularly aggressive (Fig. 19–14C, D).

Clinical Course. The first clinical indication of all endometrial carcinomas is marked leukorrhea and irregular bleeding. This is cause for concern in a postmenopausal

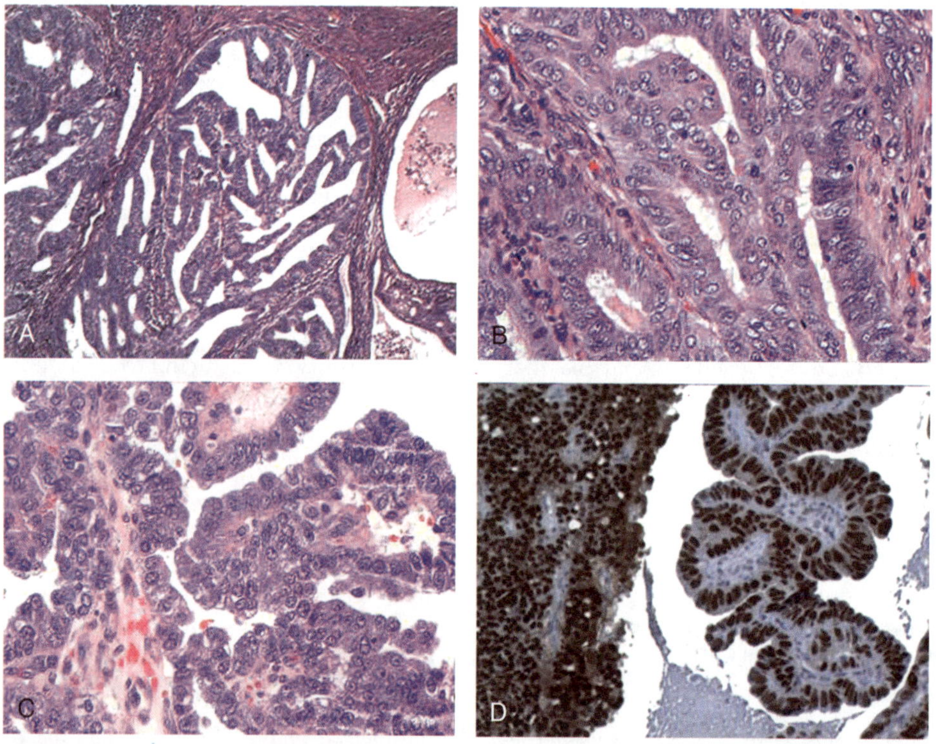

Figure 19–14

Endometrial carcinoma: **A,** Endometrioid type, infiltrating myometrium and displaying cribriform architecture. **B,** Higher magnification reveals loss of polarity and nuclear atypia. **C,** Serous carcinoma of the endometrium displaying formation of papillae and marked cytologic atypia. **D,** Immunohistochemical stain for *p53* reveals accumulation of mutant *p53* in serous carcinoma.

woman, since it reflects erosion and ulceration of the endometrial surface. With progression, the uterus may be palpably enlarged, and in time it becomes fixed to surrounding structures by extension of the cancer beyond the uterus. Fortunately, these are usually late-metastasizing neoplasms, but dissemination eventually occurs, with involvement of regional nodes and more distant sites. With therapy, stage I carcinoma is associated with a 5-year survival rate of 90%; this rate drops to 30% to 50% in stage II and to less than 20% in stages III and IV. The prognosis for papillary serous carcinomas is strongly dependent on the extent of tumor, as determined by operative staging with peritoneal cytology. This is critical, since very small or superficial serous tumors may nonetheless spread via the fallopian tube to the peritoneal cavity.

SUMMARY

Endometrial Carcinoma

- Clinically and molecularly there are two major types of endometrial carcinoma.
- *Endometrioid carcinoma* is associated with estrogen excess and endometrial hyperplasia. Early molecular changes include inactivation of DNA mismatch repair genes and the *PTEN* gene.
- *Serous carcinoma* of the endometrium arises in older women, usually associated with endometrial atrophy. Mutations in the *p53* gene are an early event.
- Stage is the major determinant of survival. Serous tumors tend to present more frequently with extrauterine extension and are therefore frequently of more advanced stage.

FALLOPIAN TUBES

The most common disease of the fallopian tubes is inflammation (salpingitis), almost always as a component of pelvic inflammatory disease. Less common are ectopic (tubal) pregnancy, followed in order of frequency by endometriosis and the rare primary tumors. Only a few comments on salpingitis and tumors follow.

Inflammations of the tube are almost always microbial in origin. With the declining incidence of gonorrhea, nongonococcal organisms, such as *Chlamydia, Mycoplasma hominis,* coliforms, and (in the postpartum setting) streptococci and staphylococci, are now the major offenders. The morphologic changes produced by gonococci conform to those already described (Chapter 18). Nongonococcal infections differ in that they are more invasive, penetrating the wall of the tubes and thus tend more often to give rise to blood-borne infections and seeding of the meninges, joint spaces, and sometimes the heart valves. Tuberculous salpingitis is far less common and is encountered almost always in combination with tuberculosis of the endometrium. All forms of salpingitis may produce fever, lower abdominal or pelvic pain, and pelvic masses when the tubes become distended with either exudate or, later, burned-out inflammatory debris and secretions (Fig. 19–15). Adherence of the tube to the ovary and adjacent ligamentous tissues results in a *tubo-ovarian abscess,* or when infection subsides, a tubo-ovarian complex. Even more serious is the potential for adhesions of the tubal plicae, creating luminal culs-de-sac

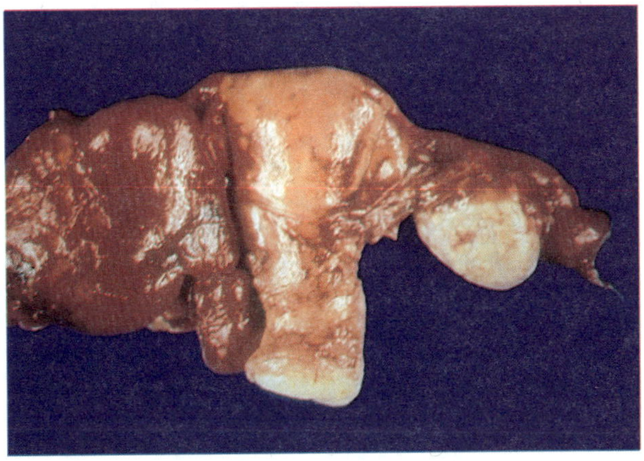

Figure 19–15

Pelvic inflammatory disease, asymmetric albeit bilateral. The left side has a large inflammatory mass totally obscuring the tube and ovary. The right is less involved, but the tube is widely adherent to the still recognizable ovary.

and increasing the risk of tubal ectopic pregnancy (discussed below). Damage or obstruction of the tubal lumina may produce permanent sterility.

Primary adenocarcinomas of the fallopian tubes may be of papillary serous or endometrioid histology. Although less common than ovarian tumors, fallopian tube carcinomas seem to be increased in women with *BRCA* mutations. In studies of prophylactic oophorectomies from such women, 10% had occult foci of malignancy, equally divided between the ovary and fallopian tube, where it usually occurred in the fimbria. Because the lumen and fimbria of the fallopian tube have access to the peritoneal cavity, fallopian tube carcinomas frequently involve the omentum and peritoneal cavity at presentation.

SUMMARY

Fallopian Tube Disease

- Salpingitis may be acute and clinically evident, as with gonorrhea, or chronic and subclinical, as with *Mycoplasma* or *Chlamydia*.
- Salpingitis results in scarring of the fallopian tube lining, increasing the risk of tubal ectopic pregnancy. Extension beyond the fallopian tube gives rise to pelvic inflammatory disease.
- Fallopian tube carcinomas usually present at an advanced stage, with involvement of the peritoneal cavity.

OVARIES

The ovaries are affected by physiologic changes involving the menstrual cycle, changes associated with aging, as well as a variety of tumors from its component tissues. In the U.S., carcinomas of the ovaries account for more deaths than do cancers of the cervix and uterine corpus together. It is less the frequency of the carcinomas than their lethality (because of their silent growth) that makes them so dangerous. Ovarian cysts are commonplace and can be broadly divided into those arising from the ovarian follicle and those with an epithelial lining.

FOLLICLE AND LUTEAL CYSTS

Follicle and luteal cysts in the ovaries are so commonplace as almost to constitute physiologic variants. These innocuous lesions originate in unruptured graafian follicles or in follicles that have ruptured and immediately sealed. Such cysts are often multiple and develop immediately subjacent to the serosal covering of the ovary. Usually, they are small (1–1.5 cm in diameter) and are filled with clear serous fluid. Occasionally, they achieve diameters of 4 to 5 cm and may thus become palpable masses and produce pelvic pain. When small they are lined by granulosa lining cells or luteal cells, but as the fluid accumulates, pressure may cause atrophy of these cells. Sometimes these cysts rupture, producing intraperitoneal bleeding and acute abdominal symptoms.

POLYCYSTIC OVARIES

Oligomenorrhea, hirsutism, infertility, and sometimes obesity may appear in young women (usually in girls after menarche) secondary to excessive production of estrogens and androgens (mostly the latter) by multiple cystic follicles in the ovaries. This condition is called *polycystic ovaries,* or *Stein-Leventhal syndrome.*

The ovaries are usually twice normal in size, are gray-white with a smooth outer cortex, and are studded with subcortical cysts 0.5 to 1.5 cm in diameter. Histologically, there is a thickened, fibrotic outer tunica, overlying innumerable cysts lined by granulosa cells with a hypertrophic and hyperplastic luteinized theca interna. There is a conspicuous absence of corpora lutea.

The principal biochemical abnormalities in most patients are excessive production of androgens, high concentrations of luteinizing hormone, and low concentrations of follicle-stimulating hormone. The origins of these changes are poorly understood, but it is proposed that the ovaries in this condition elaborate excess androgens, which are converted in peripheral fatty depots to estrone, and these, through the hypothalamus, inhibit the secretion of follicle-stimulating hormone by the pituitary. The basis of excess ovarian androgen secretion is mysterious.

TUMORS OF THE OVARY

With more than 23,000 new cases diagnosed annually, ovarian cancer is the fifth most common cancer in US women. It is also the fifth leading cause of cancer death in women, with close to 14,000 deaths estimated in 2006. Tumors of the ovary are amazingly diverse pathologic entities. This diversity is attributable to the three cell types that make up the normal ovary: the multipotential surface (coelomic) covering epithelium, the totipotential germ cells, and the multipotential sex cord/stromal cells. Each of these cell types gives rise to a variety of tumors (Fig. 19–16).

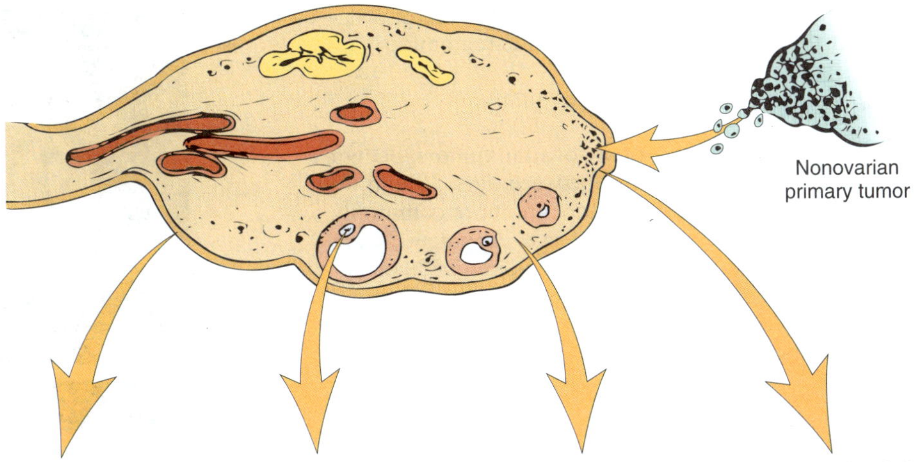

ORIGIN	SURFACE EPITHELIAL CELLS (Surface epithelial–stromal cell tumors)	GERM CELL	SEX CORD–STROMA	METASTASIS TO OVARIES
Overall frequency	65%–70%	15%–20%	5%–10%	5%
Proportion of malignant ovarian tumors	90%	3%–5%	2%–3%	5%
Age group affected	20+ years	0–25+ years	All ages	Variable
Types	• Serous tumor • Mucinous tumor • Endometrioid tumor • Clear cell tumor • Brenner tumor • Cystadenofibroma	• Teratoma • Dysgerminoma • Endodermal sinus tumor • Choriocarcinoma	• Fibroma • Granulosa-theca cell tumor • Sertoli-Leydig cell tumor	

Figure 19–16

Derivation of various ovarian neoplasms and some data on their frequency and age distribution.

Neoplasms of surface epithelial origin account for the great majority of primary ovarian tumors, and in their malignant forms account for almost 90% of ovarian cancers. Germ-cell and sex cord/stromal cell tumors are much less frequent and, although they constitute 20% to 30% of ovarian tumors, are collectively responsible for fewer than 10% of malignant tumors of the ovary.

Pathogenesis. Several risk factors for epithelial ovarian cancers have been recognized. Two of the most important are nulliparity and family history. There is a higher incidence of carcinoma in unmarried women and married women with low parity. Interestingly, prolonged use of oral contraceptives reduces the risk somewhat. Although only 5% to 10% of ovarian cancers are familial, much is being learned about the molecular pathogenesis of these cancers by identifying the culprit genes in these cases. A majority of hereditary ovarian cancers seem to be caused by mutations in the *BRCA* genes, *BRCA1* and *BRCA2*. These, as will be discussed later, are also associated with hereditary breast cancer. Indeed, with mutations in these genes there is increased risk for both ovarian and breast cancers. The average lifetime risk for ovarian cancer approximates 30% in *BRCA1* carriers, with figures varying from 16% to 44% in different studies. The risk in *BRCA2* carriers is somewhat lower. Although mutations in *BRCA* genes are present in the majority of the familial cases of ovarian cancer, such mutations are seen in only 8% to 10% of sporadic ovarian cancers. Thus, there must be other molecular pathways to ovarian neoplasms. For example, the protein HER2/NEU is overexpressed in 35% of ovarian cancers, and is associated with a poor prognosis. K-RAS protein is overexpressed in up to 30% of tumors, mostly mucinous cystadenocarcinomas. As with other cancers, *p53* is mutated in about 50% of all ovarian cancers.

SURFACE EPITHELIAL-STROMAL TUMORS

These neoplasms are derived from the coelomic mesothelium that covers the surface of the ovary. With repeated ovulation and scarring the surface epithelium is pulled into the cortex of the ovary, forming small epithelial cysts. These can undergo metaplasia and neoplastic transformation into epithelial tumors of the various histologic types. Benign lesions are usually cystic (cystadenoma) or can have an accompanying stromal component (cystadenofibroma). Malignant tumors may also be cystic (cystadenocarcinoma) or solid (carcinoma). The surface epithelial tumors also have an intermediate, borderline category currently referred to as *tumors of low malignant potential.* These seem to be low-grade cancers with limited invasive potential. Thus, they have a better prognosis than the fully malignant ovarian carcinomas.

Serous Tumors

These are the most frequent of the ovarian tumors. Benign lesions are usually encountered between ages 30 and 40 years, and malignant serous tumors are more commonly seen between 45 and 65 years of age. About 60% are benign, 15% of low malignant potential, and 25% malignant. Combined, borderline and malignant serous tumors are the most common malignant ovarian tumors and account for about 60% of all ovarian cancers.

Morphology

Grossly, serous tumors may be small (5–10 cm) in diameter, but most are large, spherical to ovoid, cystic structures, as large as 30 to 40 cm in diameter. **About 25% of the benign forms are bilateral.** In the benign form, the serosal covering is smooth and glistening. In contrast, the surface of the cystadenocarcinoma shows nodular irregularities, which represent penetration of the tumor to or through the serosa. On transection, the small cystic tumor may reveal a single cavity, but larger ones are usually divided by multiple septa into a multiloculated mass (Fig. 19–17). The cystic spaces are usually filled with a clear serous fluid, although a considerable amount of mucus may also be present. Jutting into the cystic cavities are polypoid or papillary projections, which become more marked in malignant tumors (see Fig. 19–17).

Histologically, the benign tumors are characterized by a single layer of **tall columnar epithelium** that lines the cyst or cysts. The cells are in part ciliated and in part dome-shaped secretory cells. **Psammoma bodies** (concentrically laminated calcified concretions) are common in the tips of papillae. When frank carcinoma develops, anaplasia of the lining cells appears, as does invasion of the stroma. Papillary formations are complex and multilayered, with invasion of the axial fibrous tissue by nests or totally undifferentiated sheets of malignant cells. Between these clearly benign and obviously malignant forms are the **tumors of low malignant potential,** with milder cytologic atypia and typically, little or no stromal invasion. Tumors of low malignant potential may seed the peritoneum, but typically the implants of tumor are "noninvasive." Occasionally, tumors of low malignant potential may present with "invasive" peritoneal implants that behave as carcinoma. Retrospective histologic studies of these tumors often reveal a greater degree of tumor complexity and cellular anaplasia. A micropapillary variant of serous low malignant potential tumor has been described that seems to have a worse prognosis and seems to evolve from a conventional serous low malignant potential tumor. Mutations in *BRAF* and *K-RAS* are common in tumors in this sequence. High-grade serous carcinomas, by contrast, have mutations in *p53* and *BRCA1,* and typically lack mutations in *K-RAS* and *BRAF.*

In general, malignant serous tumors spread to regional lymph nodes, including periaortic lymph nodes, but distant lymphatic and hematogenous metastases are infrequent.

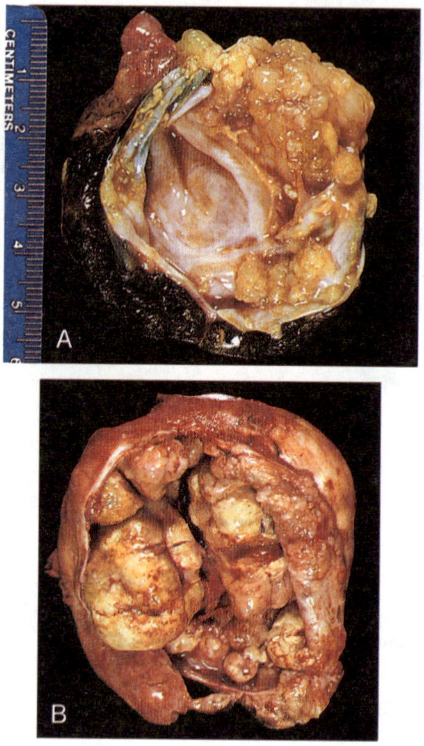

Figure 19–17

A, Borderline serous cystadenoma opened to display a cyst cavity lined by delicate papillary tumor growths. **B,** Cystadenocarcinoma. The cyst is opened to reveal a large, bulky tumor mass. (Courtesy of Dr. Christopher Crum, Brigham and Women's Hospital, Boston, Massachusetts.)

The prognosis for the individual with clearly invasive serous cystadenocarcinoma after surgery, radiation, and chemotherapy, is poor and depends heavily on the stage of the disease at the time of diagnosis. If the tumor appears to be confined to the ovary, the frankly carcinomatous lesions yield a 5-year survival of about 70%, whereas tumors of low malignant potential demonstrate about 100% survival. With cancers that have penetrated the capsule, the 10-year survival rate is only 13%. The 5-year survival for stage I serous low malignant potential tumor is nearly 100%, and even with peritoneal metastases it is nearly 75%, although almost 40% of such women eventually die of their tumors.

Mucinous Tumors

Mucinous tumors are in most respects analogous to the serous tumors, differing essentially in that the epithelium consists of mucin-secreting cells similar to those of the endocervical mucosa. These tumors occur in women in the same age range as those with serous tumors, but mucinous lesions are considerably less likely to be malignant, accounting for about 10% of all ovarian cancers. Only 10% of mucinous tumors are malignant *(cystadenocarcinomas),* while 10% are of low malignant potential, and 80% are benign.

Morphology

Only about 5% of benign and 20% of malignant mucinous tumors are bilateral, a much lower incidence than for their serous counterparts. Bilateral mucinous tumors of the ovary must be differentiated from metastatic adenocarcinomas of the gastrointestinal tract, which may present as ovarian masses.

On gross examination they may be indistinguishable from serous tumors except by the mucinous nature of the cystic contents. However, **they are more likely to be larger and multilocular, and papillary formations are less common (Fig. 19–18A). (Unlike in their serous counterparts, psammoma bodies are not found within the tips of the papillae.) Prominent papillation, serosal penetration, and solidified areas point to malignancy.**

Histologically, mucinous tumors are classified according to the character of the mucin-producing epithelial cells. Essentially three types may be identified. The first two, which are not always distinguishable, include tumors with endocervical and intestinal-type epithelia (Fig. 19–18B). The latter is almost always present in mucinous tumors with low malignant potential, and mucinous carcinomas. The third type is the müllerian mucinous cystadenoma, which is typically associated with an endometriotic cyst. This tumor probably represents an endometrial tumor with mucinous differentiation.

Rupture of mucinous tumors may result in mucinous deposits in the peritoneum; however, these typically do not result in long-term growth of tumor in the peritoneum. Implantation of mucinous tumor cells in the peritoneum with production of copious amounts of mucin is called **pseudomyxoma peritonei**. The vast majority if not all cases of pseudomyxoma peritonei are caused by metastasis from the gastrointestinal tract, primarily the appendix (Chapter 15). Metastasis of mucinous tumor of the gastrointestinal tract to the ovaries (the so-called **Krukenberg tumor**) may also mimic an ovarian primary tumor. Clues to metastatic spread of a gastrointestinal tumor include bilateral ovarian involvement, infiltration of the stroma by small glands and individual cells, and "dirty" necrosis of the tumor (necrosis associated with cellular debris)

The prognosis of mucinous cystadenocarcinoma is somewhat better than that for the serous counterpart, but the stage rather than the histologic type is the major determinant of treatment success.

Endometrioid Tumors

These tumors may be solid or cystic, but sometimes they develop as a mass projecting from the wall of an endometriotic cyst filled with chocolate-colored fluid. Microscopically they are distinguished by the formation of tubular glands, similar to those of the endometrium, within the linings of cystic spaces. Although benign and borderline forms exist, endometrioid tumors are usually malignant. They are bilateral in about 30% of cases, and 15% to 30% of women with these ovarian tumors have a concomitant endometrial carcinoma. Similar to endometrial cancer, endometrioid carcinomas have mutations in the *PTEN* suppressor gene.

Brenner Tumor

The Brenner tumor is an uncommon, solid, usually unilateral ovarian tumor consisting of an abundant stroma containing nests of transitional-like epithelium resembling that of the urinary tract. Occasionally, the nests are cystic and are lined by columnar mucus-secreting cells. Brenner tumors are generally smoothly encapsulated and gray-white on transection and range from a few centimeters to 20 cm in diameter. These tumors may arise from the surface epithelium or from urogenital epithe-

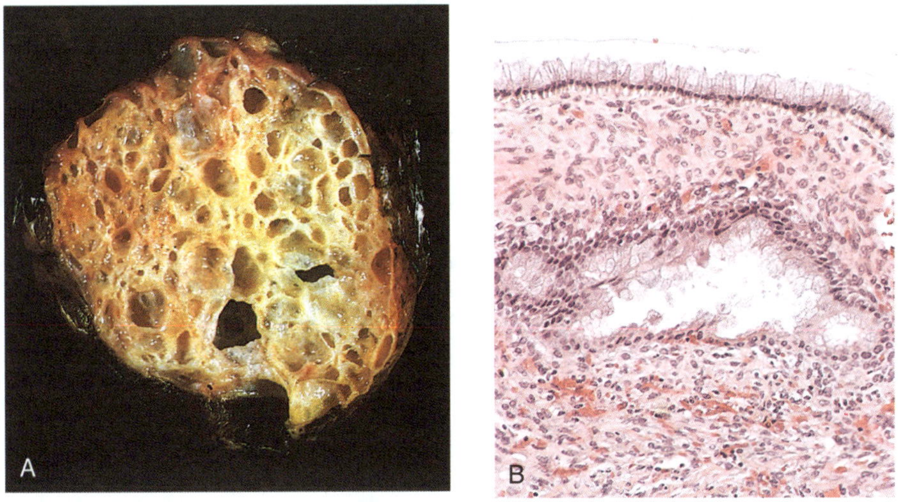

Figure 19–18

A, A mucinous cystadenoma with its multicystic appearance and delicate septa. Note the presence of glistening mucin within the cysts. **B,** Columnar cell lining of mucinous cystadenoma.

lium trapped within the germinal ridge. Rarely, they are formed as nodules within the wall of a mucinous cystadenoma. Although most are benign, both malignant and borderline tumors have been described.

OTHER OVARIAN TUMORS

Many other types of tumors of germ-cell or sex cord/stromal origin also arise in the ovary, but only the teratomas of germ-cell origin are sufficiently common to be described here. Table 19–2 presents some salient features of a few other neoplasms of germ-cell and sex cord origin. Interestingly, the testis, essentially an identical gonad in the early embryo until sex determination, has a completely inverted pattern of tumor formation. Epithelial tumors are vanishingly rare in the testis, benign cystic teratomas are never seen, and malignant germ-cell tumors are the most common.

Teratomas

These neoplasms of germ-cell origin constitute 15% to 20% of ovarian tumors. They display the distressing behavior of arising in the first two decades of life, and the younger the person, the greater is the likelihood of

Table 19–2 Selected Ovarian Neoplasms

	Peak Incidence	Usual Location	Morphologic Features	Behavior
Germ-Cell Origin				
Dysgerminoma	Second to third decades Occur with gonadal dysgenesis	80% to 90% unilateral	Counterpart of testicular seminoma. Solid large to small gray masses. Sheets or cords of large cleared cells separated by scant fibrous strands. Stroma may contain lymphocytes and occasional granuloma.	All malignant but only one-third aggressive and spread; all radiosensitive with 80% cure.
Choriocarcinoma	First three decades of life	Unilateral	Identical to placental tumor. Often small, hemorrhagic focus with two types of epithelium; cytotrophoblast and syncytiotrophoblast.	Metastasizes early and widely. Primary focus may disintegrate, leaving only "mets." In contrast to placental tumors, ovarian primaries are resistant to chemotherapy.
Sex Cord Tumors				
Granulosa-thecal cell	Most postmenopausal but at any age	Unilateral	May be tiny or large, gray to yellow (with cystic spaces). Composed of mixture of cuboidal granulosa cells in cords, sheets, or strands and spindled or plump lipid-laden thecal cells. Granulosal elements may recapitulate ovarian follicle as Call-Exner bodies.	May elaborate large amounts of estrogen (from thecal elements) and so may promote endometrial or breast carcinoma. Granulosal element may be malignant (5% to 25%).
Thecoma-fibroma	Any age	Unilateral	Solid gray fibrous cells to yellow (lipid-laden) plump thecal cells.	Most hormonally inactive. Few elaborate estrogens. About 40%, for obscure reasons, produce ascites and hydrothorax (Meigs syndrome). Rarely malignant.
Sertoli-Leydig cell	All ages	Unilateral	Usually small, gray to yellow-brown, and solid. Recaps development of testis with tubules, or cords and plump pink Sertoli cells.	Many masculinizing or defeminizing. Rarely malignant.
Metastases to Ovary				
	Older ages	Mostly bilateral	Usually solid gray-white masses as large as 20 cm in diameter. Anaplastic tumor cells, cords, glands, dispersed through fibrous background. Cells may be "signet-ring" mucin-secreting.	Primaries are gastrointestinal tract (Krukenberg tumors), breast, and lung.

malignancy. However, more than 90% of these germ-cell neoplasms are benign mature cystic teratomas. The immature malignant variant is rare.

Benign (Mature) Cystic Teratomas

Almost all of these neoplasms are marked by differentiation of totipotential germ cells into mature tissues representing all three germ cell layers: ectoderm, endoderm, and mesoderm. Usually there is the formation of a cyst lined by recognizable epidermis replete with adnexal appendages—hence the common designation *dermoid cysts*. Most are discovered in young women as ovarian masses or are found incidentally on abdominal radiographs or scans because they contain foci of calcification produced by contained teeth. About 90% are unilateral, more often on the right. Rarely do these cystic masses exceed 10 cm in diameter. On transection, they are often filled with sebaceous secretion and matted hair that, when removed, reveal a hair-bearing epidermal lining (Fig. 19–19). Sometimes there is a nodular projection from which teeth protrude. Occasionally, foci of bone and cartilage, nests of bronchial or gastrointestinal epithelium, and other recognizable lines of development are also present.

For unknown reasons these neoplasms sometimes produce infertility. In about 1% of cases there is malignant transformation of one of the tissue elements, usually taking the form of a squamous cell carcinoma. Also, for unknown reasons, these tumors are prone to undergo torsion (10% to 15% of cases), producing an acute surgical emergency.

Immature Malignant Teratomas

These neoplasms are found early in life, the mean age being 18 years. They differ strikingly from benign mature teratomas insofar as they are often bulky, are predominantly solid or near-solid on transection, and are punctuated here and there by areas of necrosis; uncommonly, one of the cystic foci may contain sebaceous secretion, hair, and other features similar to those in the mature teratoma. Microscopically, the distinguishing feature is a variety of immature or barely recognizable areas of differentiation toward cartilage, bone, muscle, nerve, and other structures. Particularly ominous are foci of neuroepithelial differentiation, because most such lesions are aggressive and metastasize widely. Immature teratomas are both graded and staged in an effort to predict their future. Those of grade I, stage I can often be cured with appropriate therapy, whereas the opposite end of the spectrum carries a much graver outlook.

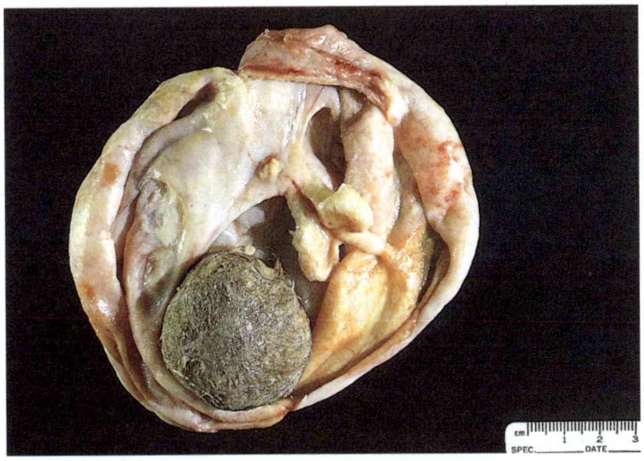

Figure 19–19

Opened mature cystic teratoma (dermoid cyst) of the ovary. A ball of hair *(bottom)* and a mixture of tissues are evident. (Courtesy of Dr. Christopher Crum, Brigham and Women's Hospital, Boston, Massachusetts.)

Specialized Teratomas

These curiosities are mentioned only because they tend to evoke "I don't believe it" reactions. Struma ovarii is composed entirely of mature thyroid tissue that, interestingly, may hyperfunction and produce hyperthyroidism. These tumors appear as small, solid, unilateral brown ovarian masses. Equally incongruous is the ovarian carcinoid, which in rare instances has produced the carcinoid syndrome! If you practice medicine long enough, you may come across a combined struma ovarii and carcinoid in the same ovary. More ominously, one of these elements may become malignant.

Clinical Correlations for All Ovarian Tumors

All ovarian neoplasms pose formidable clinical challenges, because they produce no symptoms or signs until they are well advanced. The clinical presentation of all ovarian tumors is remarkably similar despite their great morphologic diversity, except for the functioning neoplasms that have hormonal effects. Ovarian tumors of surface cell origin are usually asymptomatic until they become large enough to cause local pressure symptoms (e.g., pain, gastrointestinal complaints, urinary frequency). Indeed, about 30% of all ovarian neoplasms are discovered incidentally on routine gynecologic examination. Larger masses, notably the common epithelial tumors, may cause an increase in abdominal girth. Smaller masses, particularly dermoid cysts, sometimes become twisted on their pedicles (torsion), producing severe abdominal pain mimicking an "acute abdomen." Fibromas and malignant serous tumors often cause ascites, the latter resulting from metastatic seeding of the peritoneal cavity, so that tumor cells can be identified in the ascitic fluid. Functioning ovarian tumors often come to attention because of the endocrinopathies they induce.

Unfortunately, treatment of ovarian tumors remains unsatisfactory, as proved by the only modest increase of survival that has been achieved since the mid-1970s. Screening detection methods are being developed, but to this point they are of limited value in discovering ovarian cancers while they are still curable. Among the many markers that have been explored, elevations of the protein CA-125 have been reported in 75% to 90% of women with epithelial ovarian cancer. However, this protein is undetectable in as many as 50% of women with cancer limited to the ovary and, moreover, it is present in high concentrations in a variety of benign conditions, as well as nonovarian cancers. It is useful as a screening test in asymptomatic postmenopausal women because of the low incidence of confounding variables. However, as with carcinoembryonic antigen in colon cancer (Chapter 15), CA-125 measurements are of greatest value in monitoring response to therapy.

SUMMARY

Ovarian Tumors

- Tumors may arise from any of the major components of the ovary: surface epithelium, ovarian stromal and follicle lining granulosa cells, or germ cells.
- Epithelial tumors are the most common malignant ovarian tumors and are more common in women older than 40 years of age.
- The major types of epithelial tumors are serous, endometrioid, and mucinous. Each has a benign, malignant, and a low malignant potential (borderline) counterpart.
- Germ-cell tumors (mostly cystic teratomas) are the most common ovarian tumor in young women; the majority are benign.
- Germ-cell tumors may differentiate toward oogonia (dysgerminoma), primitive embryonal tissue (embryonal), yolk sac (endodermal sinus tumor), placental tissue (choriocarcinoma), or multiple fetal tissues (teratoma).
- Sex cord stromal tumors may display differentiation toward granulosa, Sertoli, Leydig, or ovarian stromal cell. Depending on differentiation, they may produce estrogens or androgens.

DISEASES OF PREGNANCY

Diseases of pregnancy and pathologic conditions of the placenta are important causes of intrauterine or perinatal death, premature birth, congenital malformations, intrauterine growth retardation, maternal death, and a great deal of morbidity for both mother and child. Here we discuss only a limited number of disorders in which knowledge of the morphologic lesions contributes to an understanding of the clinical problem.

PLACENTAL INFLAMMATIONS AND INFECTIONS

Infections reach the placenta by two pathways: (1) ascending infection through the birth canal and (2) hematogenous (transplacental) infection.

Ascending infections are by far the most common; in most instances, they are bacterial and are associated with premature birth and premature rupture of the membranes. The chorioamnion shows polymorphonuclear leukocytic infiltration with edema and congestion of the vessels (acute chorioamnionitis). When the infection extends beyond the membranes, it may involve the umbilical cord and placental villi and cause acute vasculitis of the cord. Ascending infections are caused by mycoplasmas, *Candida,* and the numerous bacteria of the vaginal flora. Uncommonly, placental infections may arise by the *hematogenous spread* of bacteria and other organisms; histologically, the villi are most often affected (villitis). Syphilis, tuberculosis, listeriosis, toxoplasmosis, and various viruses (rubella, cytomegalovirus, herpes simplex) can all cause placental villitis. Transplacental infections can affect the fetus and give rise to the so-called TORCH complex (Chapter 7).

ECTOPIC PREGNANCY

Ectopic pregnancy is implantation of the fertilized ovum in any site other than the normal uterine location. The condition occurs in as many as 1% of pregnancies. In more than 90% of these cases, implantation is in the oviducts (tubal pregnancy); other sites include the ovaries, the abdominal cavity, and the intrauterine portion of the oviducts (interstitial pregnancy). Any factor that retards passage of the ovum along its course through the oviducts to the uterus predisposes to an ectopic pregnancy. In about half of the cases, such obstruction is based on chronic inflammatory changes in the oviduct, although intrauterine tumors and endometriosis may also hamper passage of the ovum. In approximately 50% of tubal pregnancies, no anatomic cause can be demonstrated. Ovarian pregnancies probably result from those rare instances where the ovum is fertilized within its follicle just at the time of rupture. Gestation within the abdominal cavity occurs when the fertilized egg drops out of the fimbriated end of the oviduct and implants on the peritoneum.

Morphology

In all sites, ectopic pregnancies are characterized by fairly normal early development of the embryo, with the formation of placental tissue, the amniotic sac, and decidual changes. An abdominal pregnancy is occasionally carried to term. With tubal pregnancies, however, the invading placenta eventually burrows through the wall of the oviduct, causing **intratubal hematoma (hematosalpinx), intraperitoneal hemor-**

rhage, or both. The tube is usually locally distended as much as 3 to 4 cm by a contained mass of freshly clotted blood in which may be seen bits of gray placental tissue and fetal parts. The histologic diagnosis depends on the visualization of placental villi or, rarely, of the embryo. Less commonly, poor attachment of the placenta to the tubal wall results in death of the embryo, with spontaneous proteolysis and absorption of the products of conception.

Until rupture occurs, an ectopic pregnancy may be indistinguishable from a normal one, with cessation of menstruation and elevation of serum and urinary placental hormones. Under the influence of these hormones, the endometrium (in ~50% of cases) undergoes the characteristic hypersecretory and decidual changes. However, the absence of elevated gonadotropin levels does not exclude this diagnosis, because poor attachment with necrosis of the placenta is common. Rupture of an ectopic pregnancy may be catastrophic, with the sudden onset of intense abdominal pain and signs of an acute abdomen, often followed by shock. Prompt surgical intervention is necessary.

SUMMARY

Ectopic Pregnancy

- Any implantation outside the uterine corpus is ectopic; the most common site is a fallopian tube.
- Chronic salpingitis with scarring is a major risk factor for tubal ectopic pregnancy.
- Approximately 1% of pregnancies implant ectopically. Rupture of an ectopic pregnancy is a medical emergency that may result in exsanguination and death.

GESTATIONAL TROPHOBLASTIC DISEASE

Traditionally, the gestational trophoblastic tumors have been divided into three overlapping morphologic categories: *hydatidiform mole, invasive mole,* and *choriocarcinoma.* They range in level of aggressiveness from the hydatidiform moles, most of which are benign, to the highly malignant choriocarcinomas. All elaborate human chorionic gonadotropin (hCG), which can be detected in the circulating blood and urine at titers considerably higher than those found during normal pregnancy; the titers progressively rising from hydatidiform mole to invasive mole to choriocarcinoma. In addition to aiding diagnosis, the fall or (alternatively) rise in the level of the hormone in the blood or urine can be used to monitor the effectiveness of treatment. Clinicians therefore prefer the term *gestational trophoblastic disease,* because the response to therapy as judged by the hormone titers is significantly more important than any arbitrary anatomic segregation of one lesion from another. Nonetheless, it is necessary to understand their individual characteristics to appreciate the spectrum of lesions.

Hydatidiform Mole: Complete and Partial

The typical hydatidiform mole is a voluminous mass of swollen, sometimes cystically dilated, chorionic villi, appearing grossly as grapelike structures. The swollen villi are covered by varying amounts of normal to highly atypical chorionic epithelium. Two distinctive subtypes of moles have been characterized: *complete* and *partial* moles. The complete hydatidiform mole does not permit embryogenesis and therefore never contains fetal parts. All of the chorionic villi are abnormal, and the chorionic epithelial cells are diploid (46,XX or, uncommonly, 46,XY). The partial hydatidiform mole is compatible with early embryo formation and therefore contains fetal parts, has some normal chorionic villi, and is almost always triploid (e.g., 69,XXY; Table 19–3). The two patterns result from abnormal fertilization; in a complete mole an empty egg is fertilized by two spermatozoa (or a diploid sperm), yielding a diploid karyotype composed of entirely paternal genes, while in a partial mole a normal egg is fertilized by two spermatozoa (or a diploid sperm), resulting in a triploid karyotype with a preponderance of paternal genes.

The incidence of complete hydatidiform moles is about 1 to 1.5 per 2000 pregnancies in the United States and other Western countries. For unknown reasons there is a much higher incidence in Asian countries. Moles are most common before age 20 years and after age 40 years, and a history of the condition increases the risk in subsequent pregnancies. Although traditionally discovered at 12 to 14 weeks of pregnancy because of a gestation that was "too large for dates," early monitoring of pregnancies by ultrasound has lowered the gestational age of detection, leading to the more frequent diagnosis of "early complete hydatidiform mole." In either instance, elevations of hCG in the maternal blood and absence of fetal parts or fetal heart sounds are typical.

Table 19–3 Features of Complete and Partial Hydatidiform Mole

Feature	Complete Mole	Partial Mole
Karyotype	46,XX (46,XY)	Triploid (69,XXY)
Villous edema	All villi	Some villi
Trophoblast proliferation	Diffuse; circumferential	Focal; slight
Atypia	Often present	Absent
Serum hCG	Elevated	Less elevated
hCG in tissue	++++	+
Behavior	2% choriocarcinoma	Rare choriocarcinoma

hCG, human chorionic gonadotropin.

Morphology

The uterus may be normal in size (as in early moles), but in fully developed cases the uterine cavity is filled with a delicate, friable mass of thin-walled, translucent cystic structures (Fig. 19–20). Fetal parts are rarely seen in complete moles but are common in partial moles. Microscopically, the **complete mole** shows hydropic swelling of chorionic villi and virtual absence of vascularization of villi. The central substance of the villi is a loose, myxomatous, edematous stroma. The chorionic epithelium almost always shows some degree of proliferation of both cytotrophoblast and syncytiotrophoblast (Fig. 19–21). The proliferation may be mild, but in many cases there is striking circumferential hyperplasia. Histologic grading to predict the clinical outcome of moles has been supplanted by careful following of hCG levels. In **partial moles** the villous edema involves only some of the villi and the trophoblastic proliferation is focal and slight. The villi of partial moles have a characteristic irregular scalloped margin. In most cases of partial mole there is evidence of an embryo or fetus. This may be in the form of fetal red blood cells in placental villi or, in some cases, a fully formed fetus that, despite a triploid karyotype, is morphologically nearly normal in appearance.

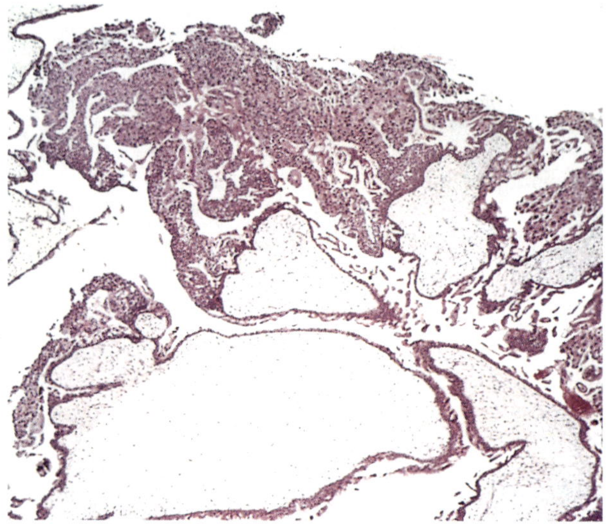

Figure 19–21

A microscopic image of a complete mole showing distended hydropic villi *(below)* and proliferation of the chorionic epithelium *(above).* (Courtesy of Dr. Kyle Molberg, Department of Pathology, University of Texas Southwestern Medical School, Dallas, Texas.)

Overall, 80% to 90% of moles do not recur after thorough curettage; 10% of complete moles are invasive, but not more than 2% to 3% give rise to choriocarcinoma. Partial moles rarely give rise to choriocarcinomas. With complete moles, monitoring the post-curettage blood and urinary hCG concentrations, particularly the more definitive β-subunit of the hormone, permits detection of incomplete removal or a more ominous complication and leads to the institution of appropriate therapy, including in some cases chemotherapy, which is almost always curative.

Invasive Mole

Invasive moles are complete moles that are more invasive locally but do not have the aggressive metastatic potential of a choriocarcinoma.

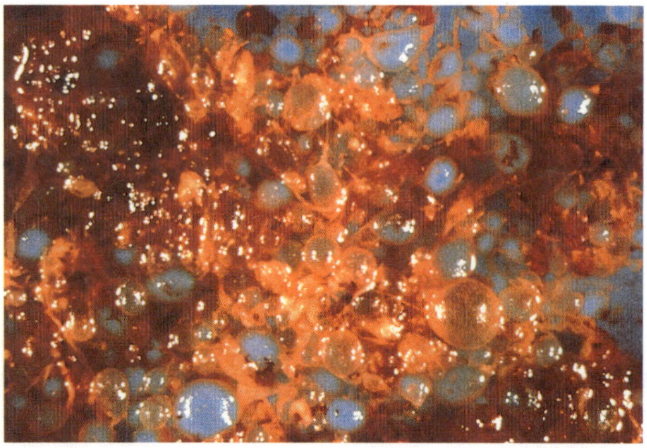

Figure 19–20

Complete hydatidiform mole suspended in saline showing numerous swollen (hydropic) villi.

An invasive mole retains hydropic villi, which penetrate the uterine wall deeply, possibly causing rupture and sometimes life-threatening hemorrhage. Local spread to the broad ligament and vagina may also occur. Microscopically, the epithelium of the villi is marked by hyperplastic and atypical changes, with proliferation of both cuboidal and syncytial components.

Although the marked invasiveness of this lesion makes removal technically difficult, metastases do not occur. Hydropic villi may embolize to distant organs, such as lungs or brain, but these emboli do not constitute true metastases and may actually regress spontaneously. Because of the greater depth of invasion into the myometrium, an invasive mole is difficult to remove completely by curettage, and therefore serum hCG may remain elevated. This alerts the clinician to the need for further treatment. Fortunately, in most cases cure is possible through chemotherapy.

Choriocarcinoma

This very aggressive malignant tumor arises either from gestational chorionic epithelium or, less frequently, from totipotential cells within the gonads or elsewhere. Choriocarcinomas are rare in the Western hemisphere, and in the United States they occur in about 1 in 30,000 pregnancies. They are much more common in Asian and African countries, reaching a frequency of 1 in 2000 pregnancies. The risk is somewhat greater before age 20 and is significantly elevated after age 40. Approximately 50% of choriocarcinomas arise in complete hyaditidiform moles; about 25% arise after an abortion, and most of the remainder occur during what had been a normal pregnancy. Stated in another way, the more abnormal the conception, the greater is the risk of developing gestational choriocarcinoma. Most cases are discovered by the appearance of a bloody, brownish discharge accompanied by a rising titer of hCG, particularly the β-subunit, in blood and urine, and the absence of marked uterine enlargement, such as would be anticipated with a mole. In general, the titers are much higher than those associated with a mole. In those instances that follow abortion or pregnancy, the positive correlation between increasing maternal age and increasing frequency of this neoplasm suggests an origin from an abnormal ovum rather than from retained chorionic epithelium.

Morphology

Choriocarcinomas usually appear as very hemorrhagic, necrotic masses within the uterus. Sometimes the necrosis is so complete that anatomic diagnosis is difficult. Indeed, the primary lesion may self-destruct, and only the metastases tell the story. Very early, the tumor insinuates itself into the myometrium and into vessels. **In contrast to the case with hydatidiform moles and invasive moles, chorionic villi are not formed; instead, the tumor is purely epithelial, composed of anaplastic cuboidal cytotrophoblast and syncytiotrophoblast (Fig. 19–22).**

By the time most choriocarcinomas are discovered, there is usually widespread dissemination via the blood, most often to the lungs (50%), vagina (30% to 40%), brain, liver, and kidneys. Lymphatic invasion is uncommon.

Despite the extreme aggressiveness of these neoplasms, which made them nearly uniformly fatal in the past, present-day chemotherapy has achieved remarkable results. Nearly 100% of cases can be cured, even with neoplasms that have spread beyond the pelvis and vagina and into the lungs. Equally remarkable are reports of healthy infants born later to these survivors. By contrast, there is relatively poor response to chemotherapy in choriocarcinomas that arise in the gonads (ovary or testis). This striking difference in prognosis may be related to the presence of paternal antigens on placental choriocarcinomas but not on gonadal lesions. Conceivably, a maternal immune response against the foreign (paternal) antigens helps by acting as an adjunct to chemotherapy.

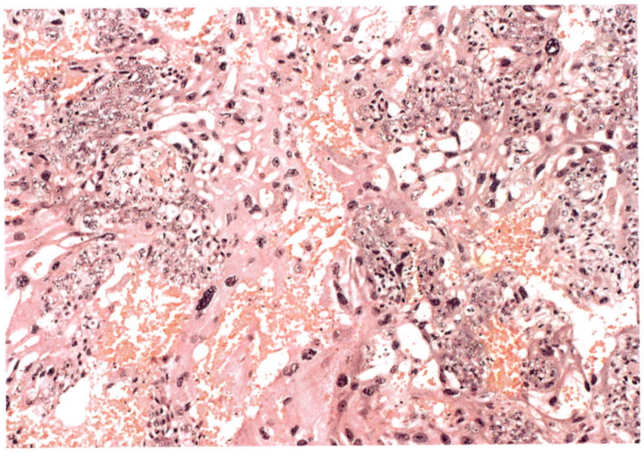

Figure 19–22

Photomicrograph of choriocarcinoma illustrating both neoplastic cytotrophoblast and syncytiotrophoblast. (Courtesy of Dr. David R. Genest, Brigham and Women's Hospital, Boston, Massachusetts.)

Placental Site Trophoblastic Tumor

These uncommon tumors are diploid, are often XX in karyotype, and are derived from the placental site or intermediate trophoblast. They typically arise a few months after a pregnancy. Because intermediate trophoblasts do not produce hCG in large amounts, hCG concentrations are elevated, but only slightly. More typically these tumors produce human placental lactogen. These tumors are indolent and generally have a favorable outcome if confined to the endomyometrium. However, they are not as sensitive to chemotherapy as other trophoblastic tumors, and the prognosis is poor when spread has occurred beyond the uterus.

SUMMARY

Gestational Trophoblastic Disease

- Molar disease is due to an abnormal contribution of paternal chromosomes in the gestation.
- Partial moles are triploid and have two sets of paternal chromosomes. They are typically accompanied by a triploid embryo or fetus. There is a low rate of persistent disease.
- Complete moles are diploid or near diploid, and all chromosomes are paternal. No embryonic or fetal tissues are associated with complete mole.
- Among complete moles, 10% to 15% have persistent disease, usually invasive mole. Only 2% of complete moles subsequently develop choriocarcinoma.
- Gestational choriocarcinoma is a highly invasive and frequently metastatic tumor that, in contrast to ovarian choriocarcinoma, is highly responsive to chemotherapy and curable in most cases.
- Placental site trophoblastic tumor is an indolent and usually early-stage tumor of intermediate trophoblast that produces human placental lactogen and does not respond well to chemotherapy.

PREECLAMPSIA/ECLAMPSIA (TOXEMIA OF PREGNANCY)

The development of hypertension, accompanied by proteinuria and edema in the third trimester of pregnancy, is referred to as *preeclampsia.* This syndrome occurs in 5% to 10% of pregnancies, particularly with first pregnancies in women older than age 35 years. In those severely affected, convulsive seizures may appear, and the symptom complex is then termed *eclampsia.* By long historical precedent, preeclampsia and eclampsia have been referred to as *toxemia of pregnancy.* No blood-borne toxin has ever been identified, however, and so the historically sanctified term (still in use) is clearly a misnomer. Full-blown eclampsia may lead to disseminated intravascular coagulation, with all of its attendant widespread ischemic organ injuries, and so eclampsia is potentially fatal. However, recognition and early treatment of preeclampsia has now made eclampsia and, particularly, fatal eclampsia rare.

The triggering events initiating these syndromes are unknown, but a *basic feature underlying all cases is inadequate maternal blood flow to the placenta secondary to inadequate development of the spiral arteries* of the uteroplacental bed. In the third trimester of normal pregnancy, the musculoelastic walls of the spiral arteries are replaced by a fibrinous material, permitting them to dilate into wide vascular sinusoids. In preeclampsia and eclampsia, the musculoelastic walls are retained and the channels remain narrow. Recent studies suggest that an imbalance between proangiogenic and antiangiogenic factors predates the onset of preeclampsia. Increases in the antiangiogenic factor sFlt1 and reduction in the level of the proangiogenic factor VEGF have been noted. While the exact basis of vascular abnormalities remains unknown, several consequences ensue:

- Placental hypoperfusion with an increased predisposition to the development of infarcts
- Reduced elaboration by the trophoblast of the vasodilators prostacyclin, prostaglandin E_2, and nitric oxide, which in normal pregnancies oppose the effects of renin-angiotensin—hence the hypertension of preeclampsia and eclampsia
- Production by the ischemic placenta of thromboplastic substances such as tissue factor and thromboxane, which probably account for the development of disseminated intravascular coagulation.

Morphology

The morphologic changes of preeclampsia/ eclampsia are variable and depend somewhat on the severity of the toxemic state.

Placental changes are most consistent. They include the following:

- **Infarcts,** which are a feature of normal pregnancy, are much more numerous in about one-third of women with severe preeclampsia/eclampsia. They may, however, be absent.
- **Retroplacental hemorrhages** occur in as many as 15% of patients.
- Placental villi reveal the changes of **premature aging** with villous edema, hypovascularity, and increased production of syncytial epithelial knots.
- Prominent in well-advanced eclampsia is **acute atherosis** in the spiral arteries, characterized by thickening and fibrinoid necrosis of the vessel wall with focal accumulations of lipid-containing macrophages. Necrosis of these cells releases lipid, which is followed by the accumulation of lymphocytes and macrophages within and about the vessels. Such lesions accentuate the placental ischemia.

Multiorgan changes may be present, reflecting the development of disseminated intravascular coagulation, which is discussed more fully in Chapter 12. Only major findings are considered here. The kidneys are variably affected, depending on the severity of the disseminated intravascular coagulation. Basically, the changes consist of fibrin thrombi within the glomerular capillaries, accompanied by endothelial swelling and possibly mesangial hyperplasia. Focal glomerulitis may ensue. When numerous glomeruli are affected, blood flow to the cortex is reduced, possibly resulting in renal cortical necrosis that may be bilateral and fatal. Microvascular thrombi are also found in the brain, pituitary, heart, and elsewhere. They have the potential of producing focal ischemic lesions accompanied by microhemorrhages.

Clinical Features. Preeclampsia appears insidiously in the 24th to 25th weeks of gestation, with the development of edema, proteinuria, and rising blood pressure. Should the condition evolve into eclampsia, renal function is impaired, the blood pressure mounts, and convulsions may occur. Prompt therapy early in the course aborts the organ changes, with clearance of all abnormalities promptly after delivery or cesarean section.

SUMMARY

Preeclampsia/Eclampsia

- Preeclampsia is characterized by edema, proteinuria, and hypertension in the second to third trimesters of pregnancy.
- Eclampsia is characterized, in addition, by seizures, and it can be fatal when accompanied by disseminated intravascular coagulation and multiple organ failure.
- Eclampsia is due to abnormalities in the maternal/placental blood flow, with resultant placental ischemia and infarction and abnormalities in production of vasodilators.

BREAST

Lesions of the female breast are much more common than lesions of the male breast, which is remarkably seldom affected. These lesions usually take the form of palpable, sometimes painful, nodules or masses. Fortunately, most are innocent, but as is well known, breast cancer was the foremost cause of cancer deaths in women in the United States until 1986, when it was supplanted by carcinoma of the lung. The conditions to be described should be considered in terms of their possible confusion clinically with malignancy. This problem is most acute with fibrocystic change, because it is the most common cause of breast "lumps" and because of the continuing controversy about the association of particular variants with breast carcinoma. However, a significant proportion of women have sufficient irregularity of the "normal" breast tissue to cause them to seek clinical attention (Fig. 19–23).

Before we turn to the extremely common fibrocystic change, several relatively minor lesions should be mentioned. *Supernumerary nipples or breasts* may be found along the embryonic ridge (milk line). Besides being curiosities, these congenital anomalies are subject to the same diseases that affect the definitive breasts. *Congenital inversion of the nipple* is of significance because similar changes may be produced by an underlying cancer. *Galactocele* is a cystic dilation of an obstructed duct that arises during lactation. Besides being painful "lumps," the cysts may rupture to incite a local inflammatory reaction, which may yield a persistent focus of induration that may arouse suspicion of malignancy.

FIBROCYSTIC CHANGES

This designation is applied to a miscellany of changes in the female breast that range from those that are innocuous to patterns associated with an increased risk of breast carcinoma. Some of these alterations (stromal fibrosis and microcysts or macrocysts) produce palpable "lumps." It is widely accepted that this range of changes is the consequence of an *exaggeration and distortion of the cyclic breast changes that occur normally in the menstrual cycle.* Estrogenic therapy and oral contraceptives do not seem to increase the incidence of these alterations; indeed, oral contraceptives may *decrease* the risk.

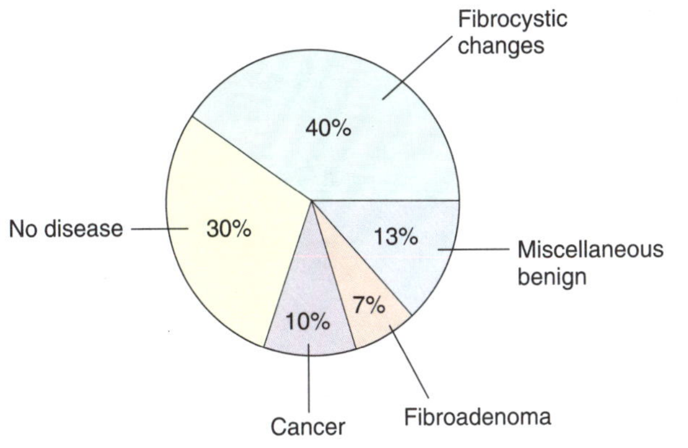

Figure 19–23

Representation of the findings in a series of women seeking evaluation of apparent breast "lumps."

Traditionally, these breast alterations have been called *fibrocystic disease;* however, physicians have expressed much dissatisfaction with this term. Most of the changes encompassed within the diagnosis of fibrocystic disease have little clinical significance except that they cause nodularity; only a small minority represent forms of epithelial hyperplasia that are clinically important. Thus, the term *fibrocystic changes* is preferred, since it does not stigmatize the subject with "a disease." Regardless of such semantic issues, the "lumps" produced by the various patterns of fibrocystic change must be distinguished from cancer, and the distinction between the trivial variants and the not-so-trivial ones can be made by examination of fine-needle aspiration material or more definitively by biopsy and histologic evaluation. In a somewhat arbitrary manner, the alterations are here subdivided into nonproliferative and proliferative patterns. The nonproliferative lesions include cysts and/or fibrosis *without* epithelial cell hyperplasia, known as *simple fibrocystic change.* The proliferative lesions include a range of innocuous to atypical duct or ductular epithelial cell hyperplasias and *sclerosing adenosis.* All tend to arise during reproductive period of life but may persist after menopause. The various changes, particularly the nonproliferative ones, are so common, being found at autopsy in 60% to 80% of women, that they almost constitute physiologic variants.

Nonproliferative Change

Cysts and Fibrosis

Nonproliferative change is the most common type of alteration, characterized by an increase in fibrous stroma associated with dilation of ducts and formation of cysts of various sizes.

Morphology

Grossly, a single large cyst may form within one breast, but the disorder is usually multifocal and often bilateral. The involved areas show ill-defined, diffusely increased density and discrete nodularities. The cysts vary from smaller than 1 cm to 5 cm in diameter. Unopened, they are brown to blue **(blue dome cysts)** and are filled with serous, turbid fluid (Fig. 19–24). The secretory products within the cysts may calcify to appear as microcalcifications in mammograms. Histologically, in smaller cysts, the epithelium is more cuboidal to columnar and is sometimes multilayered in focal areas. In larger cysts it may be flattened or even totally atrophic (Fig. 19–25). Occasionally, mild epithelial proliferation leads to piled-up masses or small pap-

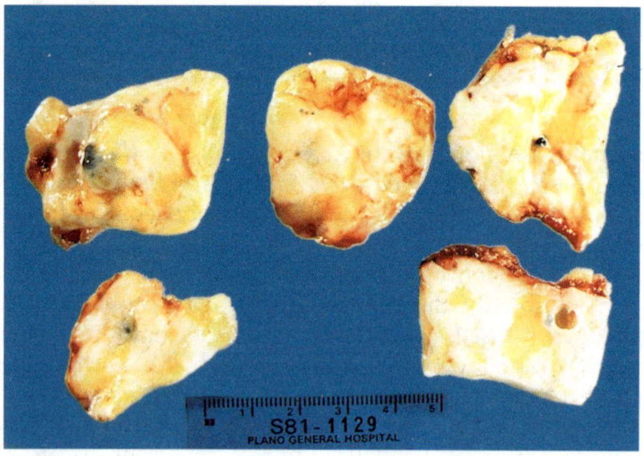

Figure 19–24

Several biopsy specimens showing fibrocystic change of the breast. The scattered, poorly demarcated white areas represent foci of fibrosis. The biopsy specimen at the *lower right* reveals a transected empty cyst; those on the left have unopened blue dome cysts. (Courtesy of Dr. Kyle Molberg, Department of Pathology, University of Texas Southwestern Medical School, Dallas, Texas.)

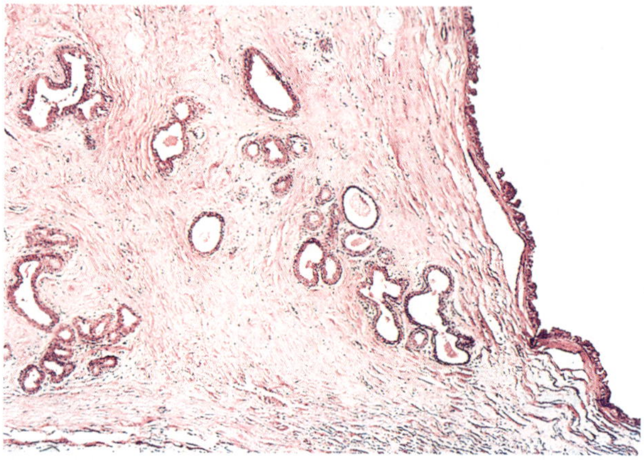

Figure 19–25

Microscopic detail of fibrocystic change of the breast revealing dilation of ducts producing microcysts and, at right, the wall of a large cyst with visible lining epithelial cells. (Courtesy of Dr. Kyle Molberg, Department of Pathology, University of Texas Southwestern Medical School, Dallas, Texas.)

illary excrescences. Frequently, cysts are lined by large polygonal cells that have an abundant granular, eosinophilic cytoplasm, with small, round, deeply chromatic nuclei, called **apocrine metaplasia;** this is virtually always benign.

The stroma surrounding all forms of cysts is usually compressed fibrous tissue, having lost its normal delicate, myxomatous appearance. A stromal lymphocytic infiltrate is common in this and all other variants of fibrocystic change.

Proliferative Change

Epithelial Hyperplasia

The terms *epithelial hyperplasia* and *proliferative fibrocystic change* encompass a range of proliferative lesions within the ductules, the terminal ducts, and sometimes the lobules of the breast. Some of the epithelial hyperplasias are mild and orderly, and carry little risk of carcinoma, but at the other end of the spectrum are the more florid atypical hyperplasias that carry a significantly greater risk, commensurate with the severity and atypicality of the changes. The epithelial hyperplasias are often accompanied by other histologic variants of fibrocystic change.

Morphology

The gross appearance of epithelial hyperplasia is not distinctive and is dominated by coexisting fibrous or cystic changes. Histologically, there is an almost infinite spectrum of proliferative alterations. The ducts, ductules, or lobules may be filled with orderly cuboidal cells, within which small gland patterns can be discerned (called **fenestrations**) (Fig. 19–26). Sometimes the proliferating epithelium projects in multiple small papillary excrescences into the ductal lumen **(ductal papillomatosis).** The degree of hyperplasia, manifested in part by the number of layers of intraductal epithelial proliferation, can be mild, moderate, or severe.

In some instances the hyperplastic cells become monomorphic with complex architectural patterns. In short, they have changes approaching those of ductal carcinoma in situ (described later). Such hyperplasia is called **atypical.** The line separating the epithelial hyperplasias without atypia from atypical hyperplasia is difficult to define, just as it is difficult to clearly distinguish between atypical hyperplasia and carcinoma in situ. However, these distinctions are important, as will soon become clear.

Atypical lobular hyperplasia is the term used to describe hyperplasias that cytologically resemble lobular carcinoma in situ, but the cells do not fill or distend more than 50% of the acini within a lobule. Atypical lobular hyperplasia is associated with an increased risk of invasive carcinoma.

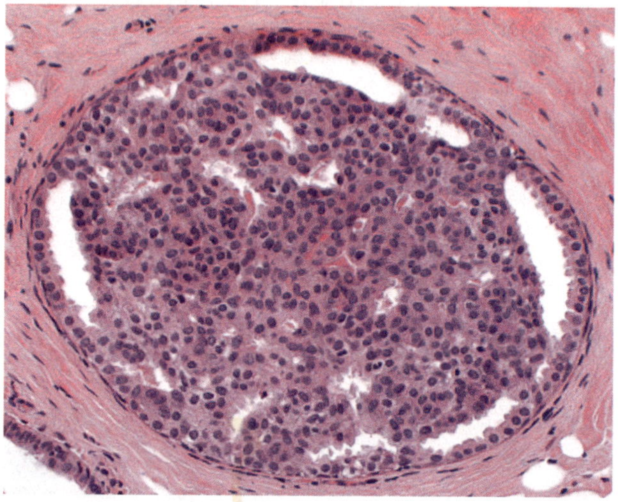

Figure 19–26

Epithelial hyperplasia. The lumen is filled with a heterogeneous population of cells of different morphologies. Irregular slit-like fenestrations are prominent at the periphery.

Epithelial hyperplasia per se does not often produce a clinically discrete breast mass. Occasionally, it produces microcalcifications on mammography, raising fears about cancer. Such nodularity as may be present usually relates to other concurrent variants of fibrocystic change; however, florid papillomatosis may be associated with a serous or serosanguineous nipple discharge.

Sclerosing Adenosis

This variant is less common than cysts and hyperplasia, but it is significant because its clinical and morphologic features may be deceptively similar to those of carcinoma. These lesions contain marked intralobular fibrosis and proliferation of small ductules and acini.

Morphology

Grossly, the lesion has a hard, rubbery consistency, similar to that of breast cancer. Histologically, sclerosing adenosis is characterized by proliferation of lining epithelial cells and myoepithelial cells in small ducts and ductules, yielding masses of small gland patterns within a fibrous stroma (Fig. 19–27). Aggregated glands or proliferating ductules may be virtually back to back, with single or multiple layers of cells in contact with one another **(adenosis)**. Marked stromal fibrosis, which may compress and distort the proliferating epithelium, is always associated with the adenosis; hence, the designation **sclerosing adenosis. This overgrowth of fibrous tissue may completely compress the lumina of the acini and ducts, so that they appear as solid cords of cells.** This pattern may then be difficult to distinguish histologically from an invasive scirrhous carcinoma. The presence of double layers of epithelium and the identification of myoepithelial elements are helpful in suggesting a benign diagnosis.

Although sclerosing adenosis is sometimes difficult to differentiate clinically and histologically from carcinoma, it is associated with only a minimally increased risk of progression to carcinoma.

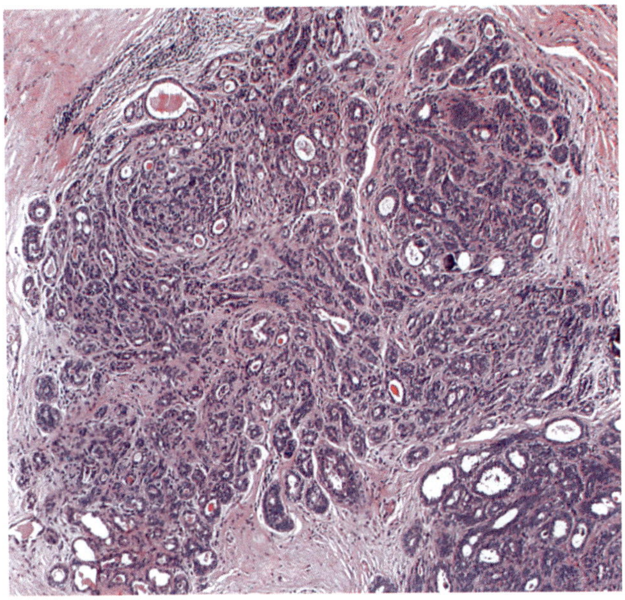

Figure 19–27

Sclerosing adenosis. The involved terminal duct lobular unit is enlarged, and the acini are compressed and distorted by the surrounding dense stroma. Calcifications are often present within the lumens. Although this lesion is frequently mistaken for an invasive carcinoma, unlike carcinomas, the acini are arranged in a swirling pattern, and the outer border is usually well circumscribed.

Relationship of Fibrocystic Changes to Breast Carcinoma

The relationship of fibrocystic changes to breast carcinoma is controversial. Only some reasonably supportable summary statements are possible. Clinically, although certain features of fibrocystic change tend to distinguish it from cancer, the only certain way of making this distinction is through biopsy and histologic examination. With respect to the relationship of the various patterns of fibrocystic change to cancer, the statements below currently represent the best-informed opinion:

- *Minimal or no increased risk of breast carcinoma:* fibrosis, cystic changes (microscopic or macroscopic), apocrine metaplasia, mild hyperplasia, fibroadenoma.
- *Slightly increased risk (1.5–2 times):* moderate to florid hyperplasia (without atypia), ductal papillomatosis, sclerosing adenosis.
- *Significantly increased risk (5 times):* atypical hyperplasia, ductular or lobular (seen in 15% of biopsies).
- Proliferative lesions may be multifocal, and the risk of subsequent carcinoma extends to both breasts.
- *A family history of breast cancer may increase the risk in all categories* (e.g., to ~10-fold with atypical hyperplasia).

Fortunately, most women who have lumps related to fibrocystic change can be reassured that there is little or no increased predisposition to cancer. The need to differentiate among the many variants and the grounds for dissatisfaction with the unqualified terms *fibrocystic changes* or, even worse, *fibrocystic disease* are apparent.

SUMMARY

Fibrocystic Changes

- Classified as nonproliferative cystic lesions or proliferative lesions
- Proliferative lesions include epithelial proliferations of ducts and lobules, with or without features of atypia, and adenosis, the proliferation of terminal ducts, sometimes associated with fibrosis (sclerosing adenosis).
- Atypical hyperplasia of ductular or lobular epithelium is associated with a five-fold increase in the risk of developing carcinoma; when associated with a family history of breast carcinoma, the risk is 10-fold.

INFLAMMATIONS

Inflammations of the breast are uncommon and during the acute stages usually cause pain and tenderness in the involved areas. Included in this category are several forms of mastitis and traumatic fat necrosis, none of which are associated with increased risk of cancer.

Acute mastitis develops when bacteria gain access to the breast tissue through the ducts; when there is inspissation of secretions; through fissures in the nipples, which usually develop during the early weeks of nursing; or from various forms of dermatitis involving the nipple.

Morphology

Staphylococcal infections induce single or multiple abscesses accompanied by the typical clinical acute inflammatory changes. They are usually small, but when sufficiently large they may heal with residual foci of scarring that are palpable as localized areas of induration. Streptococcal infections generally spread throughout the entire breast, causing pain, marked swelling, and breast tenderness. Resolution of these infections rarely leaves residual areas of induration.

Mammary duct ectasia (periductal or plasma cell mastitis) is a nonbacterial chronic inflammation of the breast associated with inspissation of breast secretions in the main excretory ducts. Ductal dilation with ductal rupture leads to reactive changes in the surrounding breast substance. It is an uncommon condition, usually encountered in women in their 40s and 50s who have borne children.

Morphology

Usually the inflammatory changes are confined to an area drained by one or several of the major excretory ducts of the nipple. There is increased firmness of the tissue, and on cross-section dilated ropelike ducts are apparent from which thick, cheesy secretions can be extruded. Histologically, the ducts are filled by granular debris, sometimes containing leukocytes, principally lipid-laden macrophages. The lining epithelium is generally destroyed. **The most distinguishing features are the prominence of a lymphocytic and plasma cell infiltration and occasional granulomas in the periductal stroma.**

Mammary duct ectasia is of principal importance because it leads to induration of the breast substance and, more significantly, to retraction of the skin or nipple, mimicking the changes caused by some carcinomas.

Traumatic fat necrosis is an uncommon and innocuous lesion that is significant only because it produces a mass. Most, but not all, women with this condition report some antecedent trauma to the breast.

Morphology

During the early stage of traumatic fat necrosis, the lesion is small, often tender, rarely more than 2 cm in diameter, and sharply localized. It consists of a central focus of necrotic fat cells surrounded by neutrophils and lipid-filled macrophages, which is later enclosed by fibrous tissue and mononuclear leukocytes. Eventually the focus is replaced by scar tissue, or the debris becomes encysted within the scar. Calcifications may develop in either the scar or cyst wall.

TUMORS OF THE BREAST

Tumors are the most important lesions of the female breast. Although they may arise from either connective tissue or epithelial structures, it is the latter that give rise to the common breast neoplasms. Here we will describe fibroadenoma, phyllodes tumor, papilloma and papillary carcinoma, and carcinoma of the breast.

Fibroadenoma

Fibroadenoma is by far the most common benign neoplasm of the female breast. An absolute or relative increase in estrogen activity is thought to contribute to its development, and indeed similar lesions may appear with fibrocystic changes (fibroadenomatoid changes). Fibroadenomas usually appear in young women; the peak incidence is in the third decade of life.

Morphology

The fibroadenoma occurs as a discrete, usually solitary, freely movable nodule, 1 to 10 cm in diameter. Rarely, multiple tumors are encountered and, equally rarely, they may exceed 10 cm in diameter **(giant fibroadenoma)**. Whatever their size, they are usually easily "shelled out." Grossly, all are firm, with a uniform tan-white color on cut section, punctuated by softer yellow-pink specks representing the glandular areas (Fig. 19–28). Histologically there is a loose fibroblastic stroma containing ductlike, epithelium-lined spaces of various forms and sizes. These ductlike or glandular spaces are lined with single or multiple layers of cells that are regular and have a well-defined, intact basement membrane. Although in some lesions the ductal spaces are open, round to oval, and fairly regular **(pericanalicular fibroadenoma),** others are compressed by extensive proliferation of the stroma, so that on cross-section they appear as slits or irregular, star-shaped structures **(intracanalicular fibroadenoma)** (Fig. 19–29).

Clinical Features. Clinically, fibroadenomas usually present as solitary, discrete, movable masses. They may enlarge late in the menstrual cycle and during pregnancy. After menopause they may regress and calcify. Cytogenetic studies reveal that the stromal cells are monoclonal and so represent the neoplastic element of these tumors. The basis of ductal proliferation is not clear; perhaps the

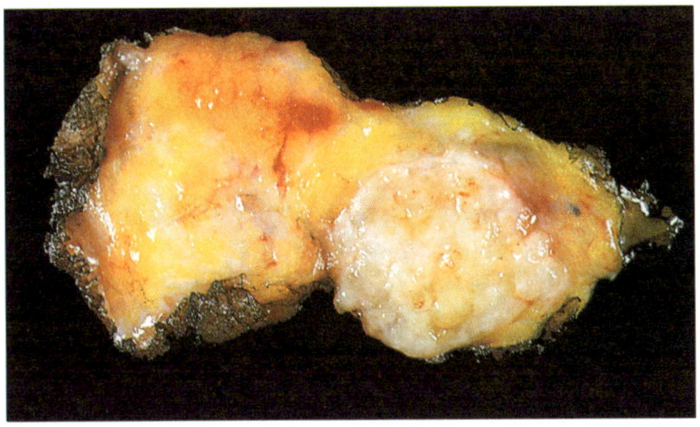

Figure 19–28

Fibroadenoma. A rubbery, white, well-circumscribed mass is clearly demarcated from the surrounding yellow adipose tissue. The fibroadenoma does not contain adipose tissue and therefore appears denser than the surrounding normal tissue on mammogram.

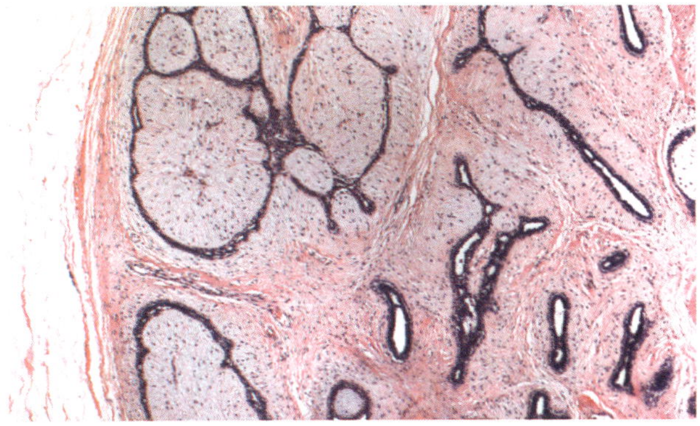

Figure 19–29

Fibroadenoma. The lesion consists of a proliferation of intralobular stroma surrounding and often pushing and distorting the associated epithelium. The border is sharply delimited from the surrounding tissue.

neoplastic stromal cells secrete growth factors that induce proliferation of epithelial cells. Fibroadenomas almost never become malignant.

Phyllodes Tumor

These tumors are much less common than fibroadenomas and are thought to arise from the periductal stroma and not from preexisting fibroadenomas. They may be small (3–4 cm in diameter), but most grow to large, possibly massive size, distending the breast. Some become lobulated and cystic; because on gross section they exhibit leaflike clefts and slits, they have been designated phyllodes (Greek for "leaflike") tumors. In the past they had the tongue-tangling name *cystosarcoma phyllodes*, an unfortunate term because these tumors are usually benign. The most ominous change is the appearance of increased stromal cellularity with anaplasia and high mitotic activity, accompanied by rapid increase in size, usually with invasion of adjacent breast tissue by malignant stroma. Most of these tumors remain localized and are cured by excision; malignant lesions may recur, but they also tend to remain localized. Only the most malignant, about 15% of cases, metastasize to distant sites.

Intraductal Papilloma

This is a neoplastic papillary growth within a duct. Most lesions are solitary, found within the principal lactiferous ducts or sinuses. They present clinically as a result of (1) the appearance of serous or bloody nipple discharge, (2) the presence of a small subareolar tumor a few millimeters in diameter, or (3) rarely, nipple retraction.

Morphology

The tumors are usually solitary and less than 1 cm in diameter, consisting of delicate, branching growths within a dilated duct or cyst. Histologically, they are composed of multiple papillae, each having a connective tissue axis covered by cuboidal or cylindrical epithelial cells that are frequently double layered, with the outer epithelial layer overlying a myoepithelial layer.

In some cases there are multiple papillomas in several ducts or *intraductal papillomatosis*. These lesions sometimes become malignant, whereas the solitary papilloma almost always remains benign. Papillary carcinoma must also be excluded; it often lacks a myoepithelial component and shows either severe cytologic atypia or monotonous ductal epithelium.

Carcinoma

No cancer is more feared by women than carcinoma of the breast, and for good reason. In the United States it is estimated by the American Cancer Society that 212,920 new invasive breast cancers will be discovered in women in 2006, and there will be 40,940 deaths, making this scourge second only to lung cancer as a cause of cancer death in women. The data make clear that despite advances in diagnosis and treatment, almost one-fourth of women who develop these neoplasms will die of the disease. However, it is also important to emphasize that although the lifetime risk is one in eight for women in the United States, 75% of women with breast cancer are older than age 50. Only 5% are younger than the age of 40. For unknown reasons (possibly related in some part to earlier detection via mammography), there has been an increase in the incidence of breast cancer throughout the world. In the United States the increase was holding steady at about 1% a year, when it started to climb in 1980 to 3% to 4% a year. Fortunately, the rate has now plateaued at about 111 cases per 100,000 women. Understandably, then, there has been intense study of the possible origins of this form of cancer and of means to diagnose it early enough to permit cure.

Epidemiology and Risk Factors. A large number of risk factors have been identified that modify a woman's likelihood of developing this form of cancer. Table 19–4 divides the risk factors into well-established and less well-established groups and indicates, where possible, the relative risk imposed by each. Comments about some of the more important risk factors follow.

Table 19–4 Breast Cancer Risk Factors

Factor	Relative Risk
Well-Established Influences	
Geographic factors	Varies in different areas
Age	Increases after age 30 yr
Family history	
First-degree relative with breast cancer	1.2–3.0
Premenopausal	3.1
Premenopausal and bilateral	8.5–9.0
Postmenopausal	1.5
Postmenopausal and bilateral	4.0–5.4
Menstrual history	
Age at menarche <12 yr	1.3
Age at menopause >55 yr	1.5–2.0
Pregnancy	
First live birth from ages 25 to 29 yr	1.5
First live birth after age 30 yr	1.9
First live birth after age 35 yr	2.0–3.0
Nulliparous	3.0
Benign breast disease	
Proliferative disease without atypia	1.6
Proliferative disease with atypical hyperplasia	>2.0
Lobular carcinoma in situ	6.9–12.0
Less Well-Established Influences	
Exogenous estrogens	
Oral contraceptives	
Obesity	
High-fat diet	
Alcohol consumption	
Cigarette smoking	

Extensively modified from Bilimoria MM, Morrow M: The women at increased risk for breast cancer: evaluation and management strategies. CA Cancer J Clin 46:263, 1995.

Geographic Variations. There are surprising differences among countries in the incidence and mortality rates of breast cancer. The risk for this form of neoplasia is significantly higher in North America and northern Europe than in Asia and Africa. For example, the incidence and mortality rates are five times higher in the United States than in Japan. These differences seem to be environmental rather than genetic in origin, because migrants from low-incidence locales to high-incidence areas tend to acquire the rates of their adoptive countries, and vice versa. Diet, reproductive patterns, and nursing habits are thought to be involved.

Age. Breast cancer is uncommon in women younger than age 30. Thereafter, the risk steadily increases throughout life, but after menopause the upward slope of the curve almost plateaus.

Genetics and Family History. About 5% to 10% of breast cancers are related to specific inherited mutations. Women are more likely to carry a breast cancer susceptibility gene if they develop breast cancer before menopause, have bilateral cancer, have other associated cancers (e.g., ovarian cancer), have a significant family history (i.e., multiple relatives affected before menopause), or belong to certain ethnic groups. About half of women with hereditary breast cancer have mutations in gene *BRCA1* (on chromosome 17q21.3), and an additional one-third have mutations in *BRCA2* (on chromosome 13q12-13). These are large, complex genes that do not exhibit close homology to each other, nor to other known genes. Although their exact role in carcinogenesis and their relative specificity for breast cancer are still being elucidated, both of these genes are thought to function in DNA repair (Chapter 6). They act as tumor suppressor genes, since cancer arises when both alleles are inactive or defective—one caused by a germ-line mutation and the second by a subsequent somatic mutation. Genetic testing is available, but it is complicated by the hundreds of different mutant alleles, only some of which confer cancer susceptibility. The degree of penetrance, the age at cancer onset, and the association with susceptibility to other types of cancers can vary with the type of mutation. However, most carriers will develop breast cancer by the age of 70 years, as compared with only 7% of women who do not carry a mutation. The role of these genes in nonhereditary sporadic breast cancer is less clear, because mutations affecting *BRCA1* and *BRCA2* are infrequent in these tumors. It is possible that other mechanisms, such as methylation of regulatory regions, act to inactivate the genes in sporadic cancer. Less common genetic diseases associated with breast cancer are the Li-Fraumeni syndrome (caused by germ-line mutations in *p53;* Chapter 6), Cowden disease (caused by germ-line mutations in *PTEN;* discussed earlier and in Chapter 15), and carriers of the ataxia-telangiectasia gene (Chapter 6).

Other Risk Factors. *Prolonged exposure to exogenous estrogens* postmenopausally, known as hormone replacement therapy, prevents or at least delays the onset of osteoporosis. However, according to recent studies, relatively short-term use of combined estrogen plus progestin hormone therapy is associated with an increased risk of breast cancer, diagnosis at a more advanced stage of breast cancer, and more abnormal mammograms. Because the 2002 Women's Health Initiative report suggested greater harm than benefit of combined estrogen plus a progestin, there has been a precipitous decline in estrogen and progestin use and a serious reevaluation of menopausal hormone therapy.

Oral contraceptives have also been suspected of increasing the risk of breast cancer. Once again the evidence is contradictory, and the newer formulations of balanced low doses of combined estrogens and progestins seem to be safe. A large, well-designed study provides solid evidence that birth control pills do not increase the risk of breast cancer even in women who have taken the pill for a long time and in women with a family history of breast cancer.

Ionizing radiation to the chest increases the risk of breast cancer. The magnitude of the risk depends on the radiation dose, the time since exposure, and age. Only women irradiated before age 30, during breast development, seem to be affected. For example, 20% to 30% of women irradiated for Hodgkin lymphoma in their teens and 20s develop breast cancer, but the risk for women treated later in life is not elevated. The low doses of radiation associated with mammographic screening have little, if any, effect on the incidence of breast cancer. Any possible effect is compensated for by the demonstrated benefits of earlier detection of breast cancer.

Many other less well-established risk factors, such as obesity, alcohol consumption, and a diet high in fat, have been implicated in the development of breast cancer on the basis of population studies. Obesity is a recognized risk factor in postmenopausal women.

Pathogenesis. As is the case with all cancers, the cause of breast cancer remains unknown. However, three sets of influences seem to be important: (1) genetic changes, (2) hormonal influences, and (3) environmental variables.

Genetic Changes. In addition to those producing the well-established familial syndromes mentioned earlier, genetic changes have also been implicated in the genesis of sporadic breast cancer. As with most other cancers, mutations affecting proto-oncogenes and tumor suppressor genes in breast epithelium contribute to the oncogenic transformation process. Among the best characterized is overexpression of the *HER2/NEU* proto-oncogene, which has been found to be amplified in up to 30% of invasive breast cancers. This gene is a member of the epidermal growth factor receptor family, and its overexpression is associated with a poor prognosis. Analogously, amplification of *RAS* and *MYC* genes has also been reported in some human breast cancers. Mutations of the well-known tumor suppressor genes *RB* and *p53* may also be present. A large number of genes including the estrogen receptor may be inactivated by promoter hypermethylation. Most likely, multiple acquired genetic alterations are involved in the sequential transformation of a normal epithelial cell into a cancerous cell. An important concept resulting from genetic analyses of breast cancers is that it is heterogeneous at the molecular level. Gene expression profiling can stratify breast cancer into five subtypes: luminal A (estrogen receptor positive), luminal B (estrogen receptor positive), *HER2/NEU* overexpressing (estrogen receptor negative), basal-like (estrogen receptor and *HER2/NEU* negative), and normal breast like. These subtypes are reproducible and are associated with different outcomes.

Hormonal Influences. Endogenous estrogen excess, or more accurately, hormonal imbalance, clearly has a significant role. Many of the risk factors mentioned (long duration of reproductive life, nulliparity, and late age at birth of first child) imply increased exposure to estrogen peaks during the menstrual cycle (see Table 19–4). Functioning ovarian tumors that elaborate estrogens are associated with breast cancer in postmenopausal women. Estrogens stimulate the production of growth factors by normal breast epithelial cells and by cancer cells. It is hypothesized that the estrogen and progesterone receptors normally present in breast epithelium, and often present in breast cancer cells, may interact with growth promoters, such as transforming growth factor α, platelet-derived growth factor, and fibroblast growth factor elaborated by human breast cancer cells, to create an autocrine mechanism of tumor development.

Environmental Variables. Environmental influences are suggested by the variable incidence of breast cancer in genetically homogeneous groups and the geographic differences in prevalence, as discussed earlier. Other important environmental variables include irradiation and exogenous estrogens, described earlier.

Morphology

Cancer of the breast affects the left breast slightly more often than the right. About 4% of women with breast cancer have bilateral primary tumors or sequential lesions in the same breast. The locations of the tumors within the breast are:

Upper outer quadrant	50%
Central portion	20%
Lower outer quadrant	10%
Upper inner quadrant	10%
Lower inner quadrant	10%

Breast cancers are classified into those that have not penetrated the limiting basement membrane (noninvasive) and those that have (invasive). The chief forms of carcinoma of the breast are classified as follows:

A. Noninvasive
   1. Ductal carcinoma in situ (DCIS; intraductal carcinoma)
   2. Lobular carcinoma in situ (LCIS)

B. Invasive (infiltrating)
   1. Invasive ductal carcinoma ("not otherwise specified")
   2. Invasive lobular carcinoma
   3. Medullary carcinoma
   4. Colloid carcinoma (mucinous carcinoma)
   5. Tubular carcinoma
   6. Other types

Of these, invasive ductal carcinoma is by far the most common. Because it usually has an abundant fibrous stroma, it is also referred to as **scirrhous carcinoma.**

Noninvasive (in Situ) Carcinoma (including Paget Disease). There are two types of noninvasive breast carcinoma: DCIS and LCIS. Morphologic studies have shown that both usually arise from the terminal duct lobular unit. DCIS tends to fill, distort, and unfold involved lobules and thus appears to involve ductlike spaces. In contrast, LCIS usually expands but does not alter the underlying lobular architecture. Both are confined by a basement membrane and do not invade into stroma or lymphovascular channels.

DCIS has a wide variety of histologic appearances. Architectural patterns are often mixed and include solid, comedo, cribriform, papillary, micropapillary, and clinging types. Necrosis may be present in any of these types. Nuclear appearance tends to be uniform in a given case, and ranges from bland and monotonous (low nuclear grade) to pleomorphic (high nuclear grade). The **comedo** subtype is distinctive and is characterized by cells with high-grade nuclei distending spaces with extensive central necrosis (Fig. 19–30). The name derives from the toothpaste-like necrotic tissue that can be extruded from transected ducts with gentle pressure. Calcifications are frequently associated with DCIS, as a result of either calcified necrotic debris or secretory material. The incidence of DCIS markedly increases from less than 5% of breast cancers in unscreened populations up to 40% of those screened by mammography, primarily because of the detection of calcifications. Currently, DCIS only rarely presents as a palpable or radiologically detectable mass. If detection is delayed, a palpable mass or nipple discharge may develop. The cells in the better differentiated tumors express estrogen and, less often, progesterone receptors. The prognosis for DCIS is excellent, with

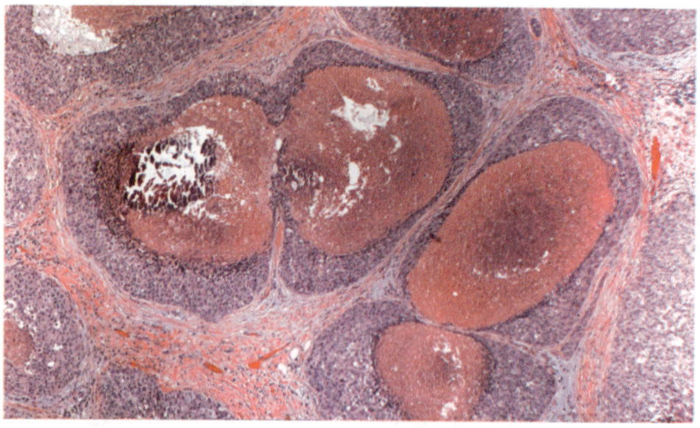

Figure 19–30

Comedo DCIS fills several adjacent ducts and is characterized by large central zones of necrosis with calcified debris. This type of DCIS is most frequently detected as radiologic calcifications.

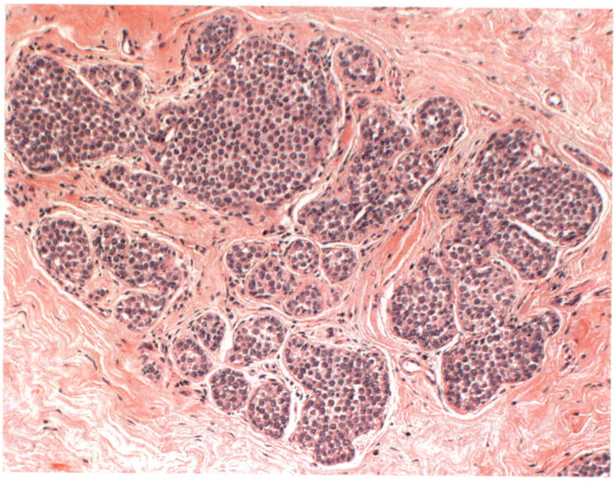

Figure 19–31

Lobular carcinoma in situ. A monomorphic population of small, rounded, loosely cohesive cells fills and expands the acini of a lobule. The underlying lobular architecture can still be recognized.

over 97% long-term survival after simple mastectomy. Some women develop distant metastases without local recurrence; such cases usually have extensive high-nuclear-grade DCIS and probably had undetected small areas of invasion. At least one-third of women with small areas of untreated low-nuclear-grade DCIS will eventually develop invasive carcinoma. When invasive cancer does develop, it is usually in the same breast and quadrant as the earlier DCIS. Current treatment strategies attempt to eradicate the DCIS by surgery and radiation. Treatment with the anti-estrogenic tamoxifen may also decrease the risk of recurrence. Treatment with aromatase inhibitors for postmenopausal women is being examined.

Paget disease of the nipple is caused by the extension of DCIS up to the lactiferous ducts and into the contiguous skin of the nipple. The malignant cells disrupt the normal epidermal barrier, which allows extracellular fluid to be extruded onto the surface. The clinical appearance is usually of a unilateral crusting exudate over the nipple and areolar skin. In about half of cases, an underlying invasive carcinoma will also be present. Prognosis is based on the underlying carcinoma and is not worsened by the presence of Paget disease.

LCIS, like the low-nuclear-grade DCIS and unlike high-nuclear-grade DCIS, has a uniform appearance. The cells are monomorphic with bland, round nuclei and occur in loosely cohesive clusters in ducts and lobules (Fig. 19–31). Intracellular mucin vacuoles (signet ring cells) are common. LCIS is virtually always an incidental finding, and, unlike DCIS, it does not form masses and is only rarely associated with calcifications. Therefore, the incidence of LCIS is almost unchanged in mammographically screened populations. Approximately one-third of women with LCIS will eventually develop invasive carcinoma. Unlike DCIS, **subsequent invasive carcinomas arise in either breast at significant frequency.** About one-third of these cancers will be of lobular type (as compared with ~10% of cancers in women who develop de novo lobular carcinoma), but most are of no special type. Thus, **LCIS is both a marker of increased risk of developing breast cancer in either breast and a direct precursor of some cancers.** Current treatment requires either close clinical and radiologic follow-up of both breasts or bilateral prophylactic mastectomy.

Invasive (Infiltrating) Carcinoma. The morphology of the subtypes of invasive carcinoma is presented first, followed by the clinical features of all.

Invasive ductal carcinoma is a term used for all carcinomas that cannot be subclassified into one of the specialized types described below and does not indicate that this tumor specifically arises from the ductal system. **Carcinomas of "no special type" or "not otherwise specified" are synonyms for ductal carcinomas.** The majority (70% to 80%) of cancers fall into this group. This type of cancer is usually associated with DCIS, but rarely LCIS is present. Most ductal carcinomas produce a desmoplastic response, which replaces normal breast fat (resulting in a mammographic density) and forms a hard, palpable mass (Figs. 19–32 and 19–33). The microscopic appearance is quite heterogeneous, ranging from tumors with well-developed

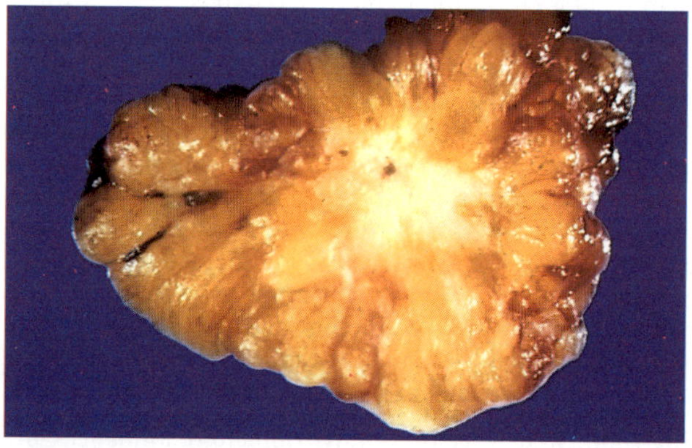

Figure 19–32

A cut section of an invasive ductal carcinoma of the breast. The lesion is retracted, infiltrating the surrounding breast substance, and would be stony hard on palpation.

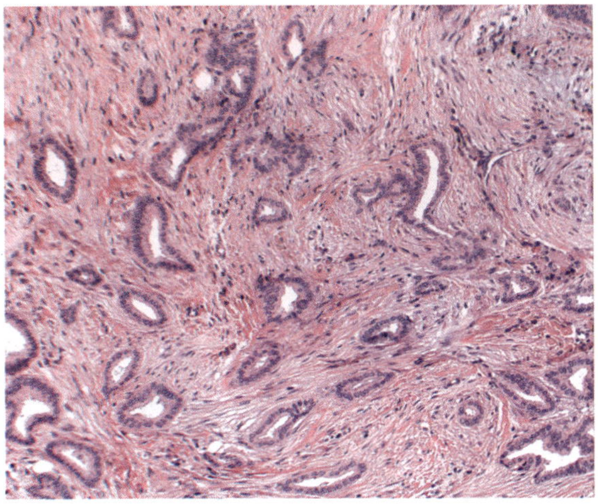

Figure 19–33

Well-differentiated invasive carcinoma of no special type. Well-formed tubules and nests of cells with small monomorphic nuclei invade into the stroma with a surrounding desmoplastic response.

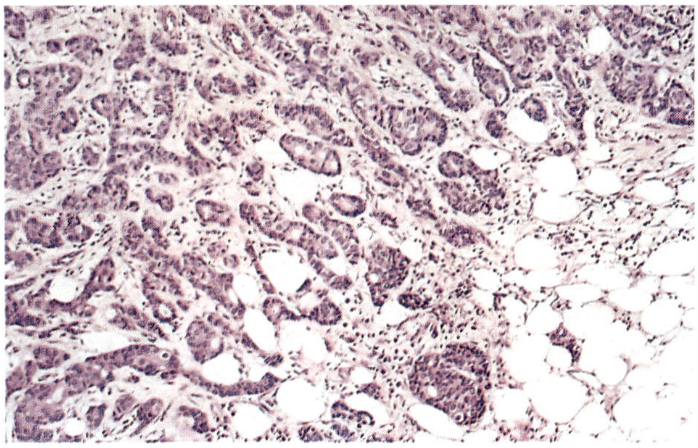

Figure 19–34

The margin of a cancer of the breast revealing tumorous infiltration of the adjacent fatty tissue *(right).*

tubule formation and low-grade nuclei to tumors consisting of sheets of anaplastic cells. The tumor margins are usually irregular (Fig. 19–34) but are occasionally pushing and circumscribed. Invasion of lymphovascular spaces or along nerves may be seen. Advanced cancers may cause dimpling of the skin, retraction of the nipple, or fixation to the chest wall. About two-thirds express estrogen or progestagen receptors, and about one-third overexpress HER2/NEU.

Inflammatory carcinoma is defined by the clinical presentation of an enlarged, swollen, erythematous breast, usually without a palpable mass. The underlying carcinoma is generally poorly differentiated and diffusely invades the breast parenchyma. The blockage of numerous dermal lymphatic spaces by carcinoma results in the clinical appearance. True inflammation is minimal or absent. Most of these tumors have distant metastases, and the prognosis is extremely poor.

Invasive lobular carcinoma consists of cells morphologically identical to the cells of LCIS. Two-thirds of the cases are associated with adjacent LCIS. The cells invade individually into stroma and are often aligned in strands or chains. Occasionally they surround cancerous or normal-appearing acini or ducts, creating a so-called bull's-eye pattern. Although most present as palpable masses or mammographic densities, a significant subgroup may have a diffusely invasive pattern without a desmoplastic response and may be clinically occult. Lobular carcinomas, more frequently than ductal carcinomas, metastasize to cerebrospinal fluid, serosal surfaces, gastrointestinal tract, ovary and uterus, and bone marrow. Lobular carcinomas are also more frequently multicentric and bilateral (10% to 20%). Almost all of these carcinomas express hormone receptors, but HER2/NEU overexpression is very rare or absent. These tumors comprise fewer than 20% of all breast carcinomas.

Medullary carcinoma is a rare subtype of carcinoma constituting fewer than 1% of cases. These cancers consist of sheets of large anaplastic cells with pushing, well-circumscribed borders (Fig. 19–35). Clinically, they can be mistaken for fibroadenomas. There is invariably a pronounced lymphoplasmacytic infiltrate. DCIS is usually absent or minimal. Medullary carcinomas, or medullary-like carcinomas, occur with increased frequency in women with *BRCA1* mutations, although most women with medullary carcinoma are not carriers. These carcinomas uniformly lack hormone receptors and do not overexpress HER2/NEU.

Colloid (mucinous) carcinoma is also a rare subtype. The tumor cells produce abundant quantities of extracellular mucin that dissects into the surrounding stroma (Fig. 19–36). Like medullary carcinomas, they often present as well-circumscribed masses and can be mistaken for fibroadenomas. Grossly the tumors are usually soft and gelatinous. Most express hormone receptors, and rare examples may overexpress HER2/NEU.

Tubular carcinomas rarely present as palpable masses but account for 10% of invasive carcinomas smaller than 1 cm found with mammographic screening. They usually present as irregular mammographic densities. Microscopically, the carcinomas consist of well-formed tubules with low-grade nuclei. Lymph node metastases are rare, and prognosis is excellent. Virtually all tubular carcinomas express hormone receptors, but overexpression of HER2/NEU is highly unusual.

Features Common to All Invasive Cancers. In all the forms of breast cancer discussed previously, progression of the disease leads to certain local morphologic features. These include a tendency to become adherent to the pectoral muscles or deep fascia of the chest wall, with consequent fixation of the lesion, as well as adherence to the overlying skin, with retraction or dimpling of the skin or nipple. The latter is an important sign, because it may be the first indication of a lesion, observed by the woman herself during self-examination. Involvement of the lymphatic pathways may cause localized lymphedema. In these cases the skin becomes thickened around exaggerated hair follicles, a change known as peau d'orange (orange peel).

Spread of Breast Cancer. Spread eventually occurs through lymphatic and hematogenous channels. Lymph node metastases are present in about 40% of cancers presenting as palpable masses but in fewer than 15% of cases found by mammography. Outer quadrant and centrally located lesions typically spread first to the axillary nodes.

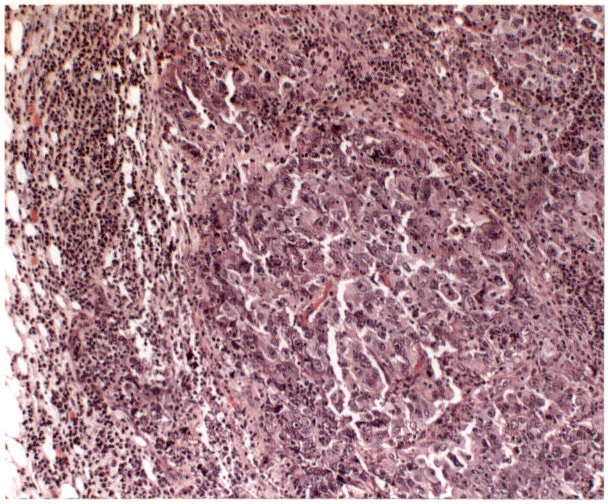

Figure 19–35

Medullary carcinoma. The cells are highly pleomorphic with frequent mitoses and grow as sheets of cohesive cells. A lymphoplasmacytic infiltrate is prominent.

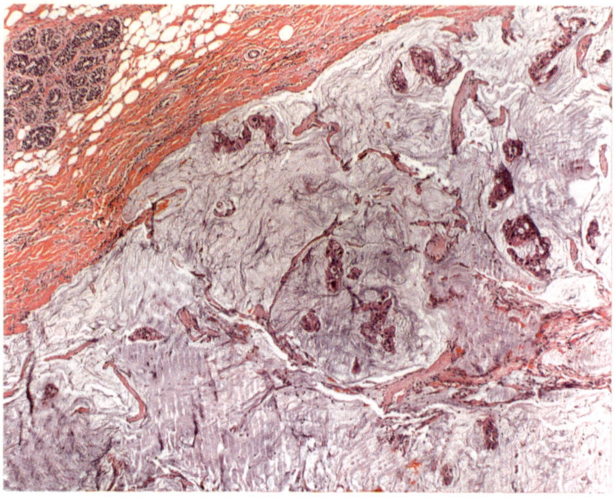

Figure 19–36

Mucinous (colloid) carcinoma. The tumor cells arer present as small clusters within large pools of mucin. The borders are typically well circumscribed, and these cancers often mimic benign masses.

Those in the inner quadrants often involve the lymph node along the internal mammary arteries. The supraclavicular nodes are sometimes the primary site of spread, but they may become involved only after the axillary and internal mammary nodes are affected. More distant dissemination eventually ensues, with metastatic involvement of almost any organ or tissue in the body. Favored locations are the lungs, skeleton, liver, and adrenals and (less commonly) the brain, spleen, and pituitary. However, no site is exempt. *Metastases may appear many years after apparent therapeutic control of the primary lesion, sometimes 15 years later.* Nevertheless, with each passing year the scene brightens.

Clinical Course. Breast cancer is often discovered by the woman or her physician as a deceptively discrete, solitary, painless, and movable mass. At this time, the carcinoma is typically 2 to 3 cm in size, and involvement of the regional lymph nodes (most often axillary) is already present in about half of patients. With mammographic screening, carcinomas are frequently detected before they become palpable. The average invasive carcinoma found by screening is around 1 cm in size, and only 15% of these have nodal metastases. In addition, in many women DCIS is detected before the development of invasive carcinoma. As women age, fibrous breast tissue is replaced by fat and screening becomes more sensitive, as a result of the increased radiolucency of the breast and the increased incidence of malignancy. The current controversy over the best time to begin mammographic screening must take into account the benefit to some women balanced against the morbidity of the majority of women who will be proved to have benign changes. Magnetic resonance imaging is being studied in high-risk, young patients with dense breasts that are difficult to image by mammography as adjunct to mammographic screening.

Prognosis is influenced by the following variables (note that the first three are components of tumor stage):

1. *The size of the primary carcinoma.* Invasive carcinomas smaller than 1 cm have an excellent prognosis in the absence of lymph node metastases and may not require systemic therapy.
2. *Lymph node involvement and the number of lymph nodes involved by metastases.* With no axillary node involvement, the 5-year survival rate is close to 90%. The survival rate decreases with each involved lymph node and is less than 50% with 16 or more involved nodes. Sentinel node biopsy has been introduced as an alternative, less morbid, procedure to replace a full axillary dissection. The first one or two draining lymph nodes are identified by using a dye or a radioactive tracer, or both. A negative sentinel lymph node is highly predictive of the absence of metastatic carcinoma in the remaining lymph nodes. The sentinel lymph node can be examined by more extensive procedures, such as serial sectioning or immunohistochemical studies for cytokeratin-positive cells. However, the clinical significance of the finding of micrometastases (defined as metastatic deposits measuring less than 0.2 cm) is still unknown.
3. *Distant metastases.* Patients who develop hematogenous spread are rarely curable, although chemotherapy may prolong survival.
4. *The grade of the carcinoma.* The most common grading system for breast cancer evaluates tubule formation, nuclear grade, and mitotic rate to divide carcinomas into three groups. Well-differentiated carcinomas have a significantly better prognosis as compared with poorly differentiated carcinomas. Moderately differentiated carcinomas initially have a better prognosis, but survival at 20 years approaches that of poorly differentiated carcinomas.
5. *The histologic type of carcinoma.* All specialized types of breast carcinoma (tubular, medullary,

cribriform, adenoid cystic, and mucinous) have a somewhat better prognosis than carcinomas of no special type ("ductal carcinomas").

6. *The presence or absence of estrogen or progesterone receptors.* The presence of hormone receptors confers a slightly better prognosis. However, the reason for determining their presence is to predict the response to therapy. The highest rate of response (~80%) to anti-estrogen therapy (oophorectomy or tamoxifen) is seen in women whose tumors have both estrogen and progesterone receptors. Lower rates of response (25% to 45%) are seen if only one of the receptors is present. If both are absent, very few patients (<10%) respond.
7. *The proliferative rate of the cancer.* Proliferation can be measured by mitotic counts, flow cytometry, or immunohistochemical markers for cell cycle proteins. Mitotic counts are included as part of the grading system. The optimal method for evaluating proliferation has not been determined. High proliferative rates are associated with a poorer prognosis.
8. *Aneuploidy.* Carcinomas with an abnormal DNA content (aneuploidy) have a slightly worse prognosis as compared with carcinomas with a DNA content similar to normal cells.
9. *Overexpression of HER2/NEU.* Overexpression of this membrane-bound protein is almost always caused by amplification of the gene. Therefore, overexpression can be determined by immunohistochemistry (which detects the protein in tissue sections) or by fluorescence in situ hybridization (which detects the number of gene copies). Overexpression is associated with a poorer prognosis. However, the importance of evaluating HER2/NEU is to predict response to a monoclonal antibody ("Herceptin") to the gene product. This is one of the first examples whereby an antitumor antibody therapy has been developed on the basis of a specific gene abnormality present in the tumor.

The major prognostic factors are used by the American Joint Committee on Cancer to divide breast carcinomas into clinical stages as follows:

- Stage 0. DCIS or LCIS (5-year survival rate: 92%).
- Stage I. Invasive carcinoma 2 cm or less in diameter (including carcinoma in situ with microinvasion) without nodal involvement (or only metastases < 0.02 cm in diameter) (5-year survival rate: 87%).
- Stage II. Invasive carcinoma 5 cm or less in diameter with up to three involved axillary nodes or invasive carcinoma greater than 5 cm without nodal involvement (5-year survival rate: 75%).
- Stage III. Invasive carcinoma 5 cm or less in diameter with four or more involved axillary nodes; invasive carcinoma greater than 5 cm in diameter with nodal involvement; invasive carcinoma with 10 or more involved axillary nodes; invasive carcinoma with involvement of the ipsilateral internal mammary lymph nodes; or invasive carcinoma with skin involvement (edema, ulceration, or satellite skin nodules), chest wall fixation, or clinical inflammatory carcinoma (5-year survival rate: 46%).
- Stage IV. Any breast cancer with distant metastases (5-year survival rate: 13%).

Why some cancers recur following postoperative therapy whereas others do not remains a mystery. Clearly, similar-looking tumors have subtle genetic differences that cannot at present be detected. As mentioned earlier, gene chip technology (microarray analysis) allows comparison of expression of thousands of genes within individual tumors (Chapter 6), and such analysis has revealed differences in breast tumors. This may allow the development of therapy that is specifically targeted to the genetic abnormalities in a given tumor. The first commercial test to predict chemotherapy response using mRNA levels of several genes (using paraffin sections) has been approved in the United States. Clinical trials are ongoing worldwide to determine whether or not microarray gene expression patterns can predict benefit from chemotherapy.

SUMMARY

Breast Carcinoma

- The lifetime risk of developing breast cancer for an American woman is 1 in 8.
- The majority (75%) of breast cancer occurs after the age of 50.
- Risk factors include delayed child bearing, long duration between menarche and menopause, atypical proliferative lesions, and family history of breast cancer in a first-degree relative, particularly if the disease was multifocal or premenopausal.
- Only 5% to 10% of all breast cancers are related to inherited mutations; the majority are in the *BRCA1* and *BRCA2* genes, less commonly in *p53*, *PTEN* or *ATM* genes.
- Ductal carcinoma in situ (DCIS) is a precursor to invasive ductal carcinoma and is typically found on mammographic examination as calcifications or as a mass. When carcinoma develops in a woman with a previous diagnosis of DCIS, it is usually in the same breast and of ductal histology.
- Lobular carcinoma in situ (LCIS) is frequently an incidental finding and does not tend to produce a mass lesion. When carcinoma develops in a woman with a previous diagnosis of LCIS, it occurs in the affected or unaffected breast with the same frequency and may be lobular or ductal carcinoma.
- The natural history of breast carcinoma is long, with metastases sometimes appearing decades after the initial diagnosis.
- Prognosis is dependent on tumor size, lymph node involvement, distant metastasis at presentation, tumor grade and histologic type, proliferation rate, estrogen receptor status, aneuploidy, and overexpression of *HER2/NEU*.

MALE BREAST

The rudimentary male breast is relatively free of pathologic involvement. Only two disorders occur with sufficient frequency to be considered here: *gynecomastia* and *carcinoma.*

Gynecomastia

As in females, male breasts are subject to hormonal influences, but they are considerably less sensitive than are female breasts. Nonetheless, enlargement of the male breast, or gynecomastia, may occur in response to absolute or relative estrogen excesses. Gynecomastia, then, is the male analogue of fibrocystic change in the female. The most important cause of such hyperestrinism in the male is cirrhosis of the liver, with consequent inability of the liver to metabolize estrogens. Other causes include Klinefelter syndrome, estrogen-secreting tumors, estrogen therapy, and, occasionally, digitalis therapy. Physiologic gynecomastia often occurs in puberty and in extreme old age.

The morphologic features of gynecomastia are similar to those of intraductal hyperplasia. Grossly, a button-like, subareolar swelling develops, usually in both breasts but occasionally in only one.

Carcinoma

This is a rare occurrence, with a frequency ratio to breast cancer in the female of 1:125. It occurs in advanced age. Because of the scant amount of breast substance in the male, the tumor rapidly infiltrates the overlying skin and underlying thoracic wall. Both morphologically and biologically, these tumors resemble invasive carcinomas in the female. Unfortunately, almost half have spread to regional nodes and more distant sites by the time they are discovered.

BIBLIOGRAPHY

Bell DA: Origins and molecular pathology of ovarian cancer. Mod Pathol 18 (Suppl 2):S19, 2005. *[Current summary of ovarian carcinogenesis, a topic that is controversial.]*

Burstein HJ, et al.: Ductal carcinoma in situ of the breast. N Engl J Med 350:1430, 2004. *[An excellent clinical pathologic and molecular discussion.]*

Cannistra S: Cancer of ovary. N Engl J Med 351:2519, 2004. *[A comprehensive review.]*

Crum CP: Contemporary theories of cervical carcinogenesis: the virus, the host and the stem cell. Mod Pathol 13:243, 2000. *[A review of current opinion on cervical carcinogenesis.]*

DiCristofano A, Ellenson LH: Endometrial carcinoma. Annual Review of Pathology: Mechanisms of Disease, Vol. 2:57, 2007. *[A comprehensive discussion of pathogenesis.]*

Ehrmann DA: Polycystic ovary syndrome. N Engl J Med 352:1223, 2004. *[A detailed review.]*

Holschneider CH, Berek JS: Ovarian cancer: epidemiology, biology, and prognostic factors. Semin Surg Oncol 19:3, 2000. *[An excellent review of the pathogenesis of ovarian cancers.]*

Hui P, et al.: Gestational trophoblastic diseases: recent advances in histopathologic diagnosis and related genetic aspects. Adv Anat Pathol 12:116, 2005. *[Discussion of moles and choriocarcinoma, with review of genetics.]*

Lazo PA: The molecular genetics of cervical carcinoma. Br J Cancer 80:208, 1999. *[A review of molecular cervical carcinogenesis.]*

Matias-Guiu X, et al.: Molecular pathology of endometrial hyperplasia and carcinoma. Hum Pathol 32:569, 2001. *[A comprehensive review of the molecular pathways in endometrial carcinogenesis.]*

Santen RJ, Mansel R: Benign breast disorders. N Engl J Med 353:275, 2005. *[A good review of benign breast lesions and risk of cancer.]*

Sherman ME: Theories of endometrial carcinogenesis: a multidisciplinary approach. Mod Pathol 13:295, 2000. *[A review of the molecular basis of endometrial cancers.]*

Wells M: Recent advances in endometriosis with emphasis on pathogenesis, molecular pathology, and neoplastic transformation. Int J Gynecol Pathol 23:316, 2004. *[A good review of current theories on endometriosis.]*

Wilkinson N, Rollason TP: Recent advances in the pathology of smooth muscle tumours of the uterus. Histopathology 39:331, 2001. *[A good introduction to smooth muscle tumors.]*

Wooster R, Weber BL: Breast and ovarian cancer. N Engl J Med 348:2339, 2003. *[Discussion of genetics of breast and ovarian cancer.]*

Yager JD, Davidson NE: Estrogen carcinogenesis in breast cancer. N Engl J Med 354:273, 2006. *[Role of estrogens including those used in hormonal replacement therapy in breast cancer.]*

Chapter 20

The Endocrine System

ANIRBAN MAITRA, MBBS

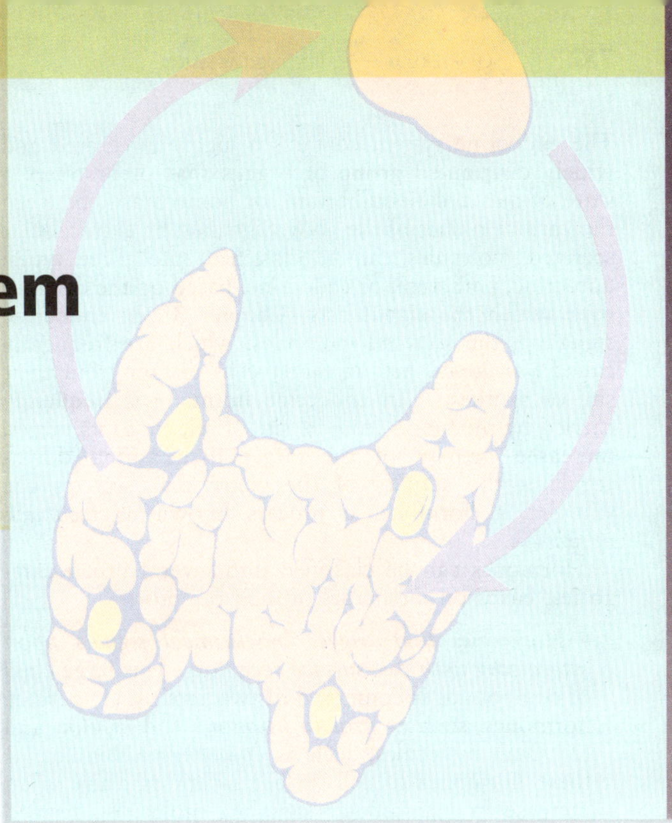

The endocrine system contains a highly integrated and widely distributed group of organs that orchestrates a state of metabolic equilibrium, or homeostasis, between the various tissues of the body. Signaling by extracellular secreted molecules can be classified into three types: autocrine, paracrine, or endocrine, based on the distance over which the signal acts (Chapter 3). In endocrine signaling, the secreted molecules, which are frequently called *hormones,* act on target cells distant from their site of synthesis. An endocrine hormone is frequently carried by the blood from its site of release to its target. Increased activity of the target tissue often down-regulates the activity of the gland that secretes the stimulating hormone, a process known as *feedback inhibition.*

Hormones can be classified into several broad categories, based on the nature of their receptors:

- *Hormones that trigger biochemical signals upon interacting with cell-surface receptors:* This large class of compounds is composed of two groups: (1) peptide hormones, such as *growth hormone* and *insulin,* and (2) small molecules, such as *epinephrine.* Binding of these hormones to cell surface receptors leads to an increase in intracellular signaling molecules, termed *second messengers,* such as cyclic adenosine monophosphate (cAMP); production of mediators from membrane phospholipids (e.g., inositol 1,4,5-trisphosphate); and shifts in the intracellular levels of ionized calcium. The elevated levels of one or more of these can control proliferation, differentiation, survival, and functional activity of cells, mainly by regulating the expression of specific genes.
- *Hormones that diffuse across the plasma membrane and interact with intracellular receptors:* Many lipid-soluble hormones diffuse across the plasma membrane and interact with receptors in the cytosol or the nucleus. The resulting hormone-receptor complexes bind specifically to promoter and enhancer elements in DNA, thereby affecting the expression of specific target genes. Hormones of this type include the *steroids* (e.g., estrogen, progesterone, and glucocorticoids) and *thyroxine.*

Several processes may disturb the normal activity of the endocrine system, including impaired synthesis or release of hormones, abnormal interactions between hormones and their target tissues, and abnormal responses of target organs to their hormones. Endocrine diseases can be generally classified as (1) diseases of *underproduction or overproduction* of hormones and their resulting biochemical and clinical consequences, and (2) diseases associated with the development of *mass lesions,* which may be nonfunctional or may be associated with overproduction or underproduction of hormones. The study of endocrine diseases requires integration of morphologic findings with biochemical measurements of the levels of hormones, their regulators, and other metabolites.

PITUITARY

The pituitary gland is a small, bean-shaped structure that lies at the base of the brain within the confines of the sella turcica. It is intimately related to the hypothalamus, with which it is connected by both a "stalk," composed of axons extending from the hypothalamus, and a rich venous plexus constituting a portal circulation. Along with the hypothalamus, the pituitary has a central role in the regulation of most of the other endocrine glands. The pituitary is composed of two morphologically and functionally distinct components: the anterior lobe (adenohypophysis) and the posterior lobe (neurohypophysis). Diseases of the pituitary, accordingly, can be divided into those that primarily affect the anterior lobe and those that primarily affect the posterior lobe.

The *anterior pituitary,* or *adenohypophysis,* is composed of epithelial cells derived embryologically from the developing oral cavity. In routine histologic sections, a colorful array of cells containing basophilic cytoplasm, eosinophilic cytoplasm, or poorly staining ("chromophobic") cytoplasm is present (Fig. 20–1). Detailed studies using electron microscopy and immunocytochemistry have demonstrated that the staining properties of these cells are related to the presence of various trophic hormones within their cytoplasm. The release of trophic hormones is in turn under the control of factors produced in the hypothalamus; while most hypothalamic factors are stimulatory and promote pituitary hormone release, others (e.g., somatostatin and dopamine) are inhibitory in their effects (Fig. 20–2). Rarely, symptoms of pituitary disease may be caused by an excess or lack of the hypothalamic factors rather than a primary pituitary abnormality.

Symptoms of pituitary disease can be divided into the following:

- *Hyperpituitarism:* This disorder arises from excessive secretion of trophic hormones. It most often results from an *anterior pituitary adenoma,* but may also be caused by other pituitary and extra-pituitary lesions that are described below. The symptoms of hyperpituitarism are discussed in the context of individual tumors later in this chapter.
- *Hypopituitarism:* This is caused by deficiency of trophic hormones and results from a variety of destructive processes, including *ischemic injury, surgery or radiation,* and *inflammatory reactions.* In addition, *nonfunctional pituitary adenomas* may encroach upon and destroy adjacent native anterior pituitary parenchyma and cause hypopituitarism.
- *Local mass effects:* Among the earliest changes referable to mass effect are *radiographic abnormalities of the sella turcica,* including sellar expansion, bony

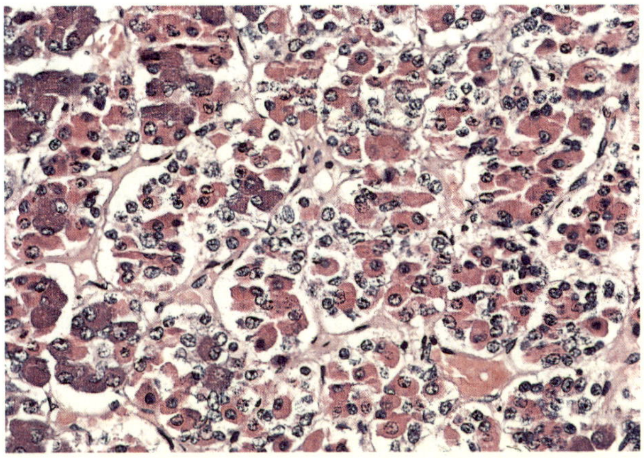

Figure 20–1

Photomicrograph of normal anterior pituitary. The gland is populated by several distinct cell populations containing a variety of stimulating (trophic) hormones. Each of the hormones has different staining characteristics, resulting in a mixture of cell types in routine histologic preparations.

erosion, and disruption of the diaphragma sellae. Because of the close proximity of the optic nerves and chiasm to the sella, expanding pituitary lesions often compress decussating fibers in the optic chiasm. This gives rise to *visual field abnormalities,* classically in the form of defects in the lateral (temporal) visual fields—a so-called *bitemporal hemianopsia.* In addition, a variety of other visual field abnormalities may be caused by asymmetric growth of many tumors. As in the case of any expanding intracranial mass, pituitary adenomas may produce signs and symptoms of *elevated intracranial pressure,* including headache, nausea, and vomiting. Pituitary adenomas that extend beyond the sella turcica into the base of the brain (invasive pituitary adenoma) produce *seizures* or *obstructive hydrocephalus;* involvement of cranial nerves can result in *cranial nerve palsy.* On occasion, acute hemorrhage into an adenoma is associated with clinical evidence of rapid enlargement of the lesion and depression of consciousness, a situation appropriately termed *pituitary apoplexy.* Acute pituitary apoplexy is a neurosurgical emergency, because it may cause sudden death.

HYPERPITUITARISM AND PITUITARY ADENOMAS

The most common cause of hyperpituitarism is an adenoma arising in the anterior lobe. Other, less common causes include hyperplasia and carcinomas of the anterior pituitary, secretion of hormones by some extrapituitary tumors, and certain hypothalamic disorders. *Pituitary adenomas are classified on the basis of hormone(s) produced by the neoplastic cells, which are detected by immunohistochemical stains performed on tissue sections* (Table 20–1); rarely, ultrastructural examination may be required to determine the specific lineage of the neoplastic cell. Pituitary adenomas can be *functional* (i.e., associated with hormone excess and clinical manifestations thereof) or *silent* (i.e., immunohistochemical and/or ultrastructural demonstration of hormone production at the tissue level only, without clinical manifestations of hormone excess). Both functional and silent pituitary adenomas are usually composed of a single cell type and produce a single predominant hormone, although exceptions are known to occur. Some pituitary adenomas can secrete two hormones (growth hormone and prolactin being the most common combination); rarely, pituitary adenomas are plurihormonal. Pituitary adenomas may also be *hormone negative,* based on absence of immunohistochemical reactivity and ultrastructural demonstration of lineage-specific differentiation.

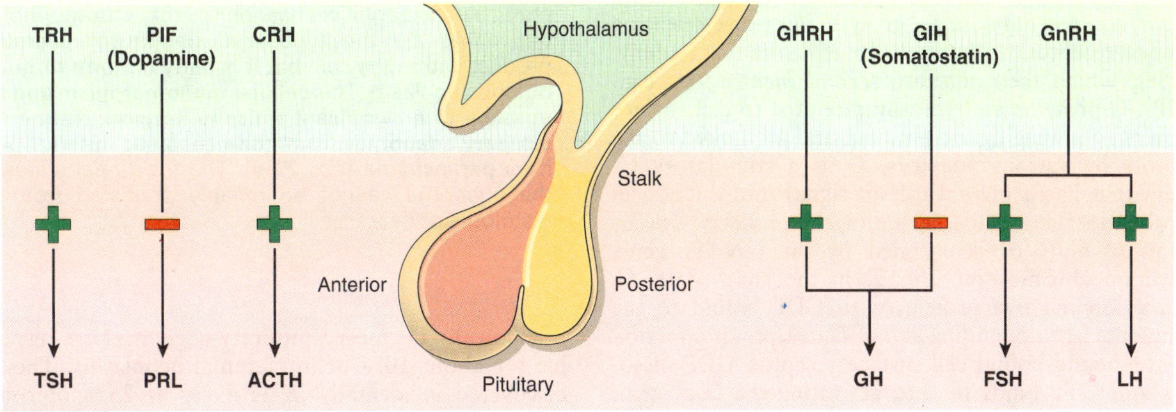

Figure 20–2

The adenohypophysis (anterior pituitary) releases six hormones that are, in turn, under the control of various stimulatory and inhibitory hypothalamic releasing factors: ACTH, adrenocorticotropic hormone (corticotropin); FSH, follicle-stimulating hormone; GH, growth hormone (somatotropin); LH, luteinizing hormone; PRL, prolactin; and TSH, thyroid-stimulating hormone (thyrotropin). The stimulatory releasing factors are CRH (corticotropin-releasing hormone), GHRH (growth hormone-releasing hormone), GnRH (gonadotropin-releasing hormone), and TRH (thyrotropin-releasing hormone). The inhibitory hypothalamic factors are growth hormone inhibitory hormone (GIH, or somatostatin) and PIF (prolactin inhibitory factor, or dopamine).

Table 20–1 Classification of Pituitary Adenomas*

Prolactin cell (lactotroph) adenoma
Growth hormone cell (somatotroph) adenoma
Thyroid-stimulating hormone cell (thyrotroph) adenomas
ACTH cell (corticotroph) adenomas
Gonadotroph cell adenomas Silent gonadotroph adenomas includes most so-called null cell adenomas
Mixed (plurihormonal) adenomas Growth hormone-prolactin mixed adenomas most common
Hormone-negative adenomas

ACTH, adrenocorticotropic hormone.
*For each of the pituitary cell types, the adenoma may be *functional* (producing symptoms of hormone excess) or *silent*. The heterogeneous category of "nonfunctional" adenomas includes silent pituitary adenomas and true hormone-negative adenomas (rare).

Most pituitary adenomas occur as isolated lesions. In about 3% of cases, however, adenomas are associated with *multiple endocrine neoplasia type 1* (MEN-1, discussed later). Pituitary adenomas are designated, somewhat arbitrarily, *microadenomas* if less than 1 cm in diameter and *macroademomas* if they exceed 1 cm in diameter. Silent and hormone-negative adenomas are likely to come to clinical attention at a later stage than those associated with endocrine abnormalities and are therefore more likely to be macroadenomas; in addition, these adenomas may cause *hypo*pituitarism as they encroach on and destroy adjacent anterior pituitary parenchyma.

Pathogenesis. There have been several advances in understanding the molecular pathogenesis of pituitary adenomas. Guanine nucleotide–binding protein (G-protein) mutations are the best-characterized molecular abnormalities in these neoplasms. G-proteins have a critical role in signal transduction, transmitting signals from *cell surface receptors* (e.g., growth hormone–releasing hormone receptor) to *intracellular effectors* (e.g., adenyl cyclase), which then generate *second messengers* (e.g., cAMP). G-proteins are typically recruited to cell surface receptors following ligand binding, and are linked to the receptors by various adaptors. G_s is a stimulatory G-protein that has a pivotal role in signal transduction in several endocrine organs, including the pituitary. The α-subunit of G_s ($G_s\alpha$) is encoded by the *GNAS1* gene, located on chromosome 20q13. In the basal state, G_s exists as an inactive protein, with GDP bound to the guanine nucleotide-binding site of $G_s\alpha$. Upon interaction with the ligand-bound cell surface receptor, GDP dissociates and GTP binds to $G_s\alpha$, activating the G-protein. GTP-bound $G_s\alpha$ directly interacts with and activates its effectors (such as adenyl cyclase), with a resultant increase in intracellular cAMP. cAMP acts as a potent mitogenic stimulus for a variety of endocrine cell types, promoting cellular proliferation and hormone synthesis and secretion. The activation of $G_s\alpha$, and the resultant generation of cAMP, are *transient* because of an intrinsic GTPase activity in the α-subunit, which hydrolyzes GTP into GDP. *A mutation in the α-subunit that interferes with its intrinsic GTPase activity therefore results in constitutive activation of $G_s\alpha$, persistent generation of cAMP, and unchecked cellular proliferation.* Approximately 40% of growth hormone–secreting somatotroph cell adenomas and a minority of adrenocorticotrophic hormone (ACTH)–secreting corticotroph cell adenomas bear *GNAS1* mutations. Pituitary adenomas that arise in the context of familial MEN-1 syndrome harbor, by definition, mutations in the *MEN-1 (menin)* gene (discussed later). Additional molecular abnormalities present in *aggressive or advanced pituitary adenomas* include activating mutations of the *RAS* oncogene, overexpression of the *C-MYC* oncogene, and inactivation of the metastasis suppressor gene *NM23,* suggesting that these genetic events are linked to disease progression.

Morphology

The usual pituitary adenoma is a well-circumscribed, soft lesion that may, in the case of smaller tumors, be confined by the sella turcica. Larger lesions typically extend superiorly through the sellar diaphragm into the suprasellar region, where they often compress the optic chiasm and adjacent structures (Fig. 20–3). As these adenomas expand, they frequently erode the sella turcica and anterior clinoid processes. They may also extend locally into the cavernous and sphenoidal sinuses. In as many as 30% of cases the adenomas are grossly nonencapsulated and infiltrate adjacent bone, dura, and (uncommonly) brain. Such lesions are designated **invasive adenomas.** Foci of hemorrhage and/or necrosis are common in larger adenomas.

Microscopically, pituitary adenomas are composed of relatively uniform, polygonal cells arrayed in sheets, cords, or papillae. Supporting connective tissue, or reticulin, is sparse, accounting for the soft, gelatinous consistency of many lesions. The nuclei of the neoplastic cells may be uniform or pleomorphic. Mitotic activity is usually scanty. The cytoplasm of the constituent cells may be acidophilic, basophilic, or chromophobic, depending on the type and amount of secretory product within the cell, but it is fairly uniform throughout the neoplasm. **This cellular monomorphism and the absence of a significant reticulin network distinguish pituitary adenomas from non-neoplastic anterior pituitary parenchyma** (Fig. 20–4). The functional status of the adenoma cannot be reliably predicted from its histologic appearance.

Clinically diagnosed pituitary adenomas are responsible for about 10% of intracranial neoplasms. They are discovered incidentally in as many as 25% of routine autopsies. In fact, the most recent data using high-resolution computed tomography or magnetic resonance imaging suggest that approximately 20% of "normal" adult pituitary glands harbor an incidental lesion measuring 3 mm or more in diameter, usually a silent adenoma. Pituitary adenomas are usually found in adults, with a peak incidence from the 30s to the 50s.

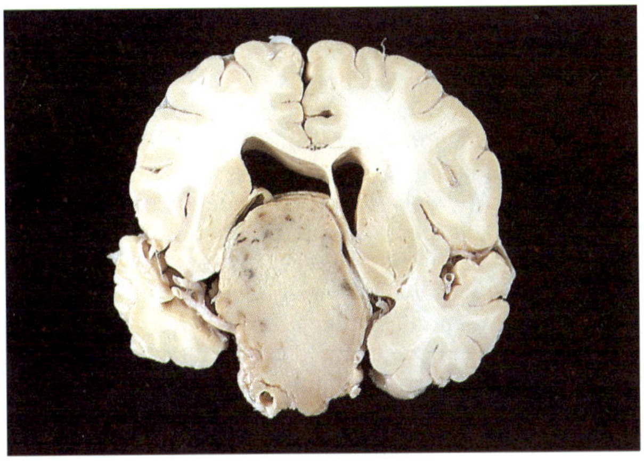

Figure 20–3

Gross view of a pituitary adenoma. This massive, nonfunctional adenoma has grown far beyond the confines of the sella turcica and has distorted the overlying brain. Nonfunctional adenomas tend to be larger at the time of diagnosis than those that secrete a hormone.

SUMMARY

Hyperpituitarism

- The most common cause of hyperpituitarism is an anterior lobe pituitary adenoma.
- Pituitary adenomas can be macroadenomas (>1 cm) or microadenomas (<1 cm), and clinically, they can be functional or silent.
- Most adenomas consist of one cell type and produce one hormone, although there are exceptions.
- Mutation of the *GNAS1* gene, which results in constitutive activation of a stimulatory G-protein, is one of the more common genetic alterations.
- The two distinctive morphologic features of most adenomas are their cellular monomorphism and absence of a reticulin network.

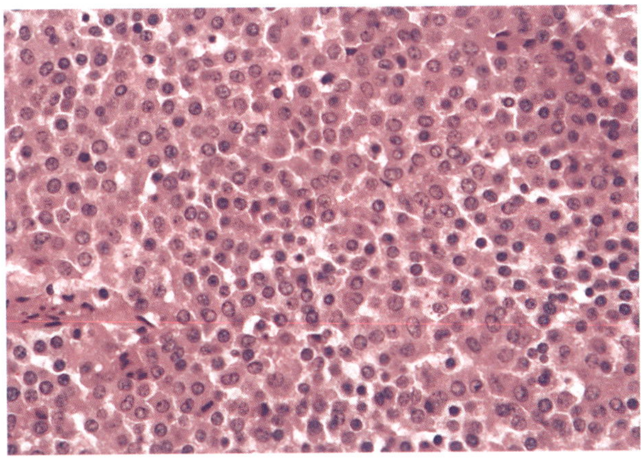

Figure 20–4

Photomicrograph of pituitary adenoma. The monomorphism of these cells contrasts markedly to the mixture of cells seen in the normal anterior pituitary in Figure 20–1. Note also the absence of reticulin network.

Prolactinomas

Prolactinomas are the most common type of hyperfunctioning pituitary adenoma. They range from small microadenomas to large, expansile tumors associated with considerable mass effect. Prolactin is demonstrable within the cytoplasm of the neoplastic cells by immunohistochemical techniques.

Hyperprolactinemia causes amenorrhea, galactorrhea, loss of libido, and infertility. Because many of the manifestations of hyperprolactinemia (e.g., amenorrhea) are more obvious in premenopausal females than in males or postmenopausal females, prolactinomas are usually diagnosed at an earlier stage in females of reproductive age than in other individuals. In contrast, hormonal manifestations may be quite subtle in men and older women, in whom the tumors may reach considerable size before coming to clinical attention. Hyperprolactinemia may be caused by conditions other than prolactin-secreting pituitary adenomas, including pregnancy, high-dose estrogen therapy, renal failure, hypothyroidism, hypothalamic lesions, and dopamine-inhibiting drugs (e.g., reserpine). In addition, any mass in the suprasellar compartment may disturb the normal inhibitory influence of hypothalamus on prolactin secretion, resulting in hyperprolactinemia, known as the *stalk effect*. It should be kept in mind, therefore, that *mild* elevations of serum prolactin (<200 μg/L) in an individual with a pituitary adenoma do not necessarily indicate a prolactin-secreting neoplasm.

Growth Hormone–Producing Adenomas

Growth hormone–producing (somatotroph cell) neoplasms, including those that produce a mixture of growth hormone and other hormones (e.g., prolactin), are the second most common type of functional pituitary adenoma. Because the clinical manifestations of excessive growth hormone may be subtle, somatotroph cell adenomas may be quite large by the time they come to clinical attention. Microscopically, growth hormone–producing adenomas are composed of densely or sparsely granulated cells, and immunohistochemical stains demonstrate growth hormone within the cytoplasm of the neoplastic cells. Small amounts of immunoreactive prolactin are often present as well.

Persistent hypersecretion of growth hormone stimulates the hepatic secretion of insulin-like growth factor I (somatomedin C), which causes many of the clinical manifestations. If a growth hormone–secreting adenoma occurs before the epiphyses close, as is the case in prepubertal children, excessive levels of growth hormone result in *gigantism*. This is characterized by a generalized increase in body size, with disproportionately long arms and legs. If elevated levels of growth hormone persist, or present after closure of the epiphyses, individuals develop *acromegaly*, in which growth is most conspicuous in soft tissues, skin, and viscera and in the bones of the face, hands, and feet. Enlargement of the jaw results in its protrusion (prognathism), with broadening of the lower face and separation of the teeth. The hands and feet are enlarged, with broad, sausage-like fingers. In practice, most cases of gigantism are also accompanied by evidence of acromegaly. Growth hormone excess is also associated with a number of other disturbances, including abnormal glucose tolerance and diabetes mellitus, generalized muscle weakness, hypertension, arthritis, osteoporosis, and congestive heart failure. Prolactin is demonstrable in a number of growth hormone–producing adenomas and in some cases may be released in sufficient quantities to produce signs and symptoms of hyperprolactinemia.

Corticotroph Cell Adenomas

Most corticotroph cell adenomas are small (microadenomas) at the time of diagnosis, although some tumors may be quite large. These adenomas stain positively with periodic acid–Schiff (PAS) stains, as a result of the accumulation of glycosylated ACTH protein. As in the case of other pituitary hormones, the secretory granules can be detected by immunohistochemical methods. By electron microscopy they appear as membrane-bound, electron-dense granules averaging 300 nm in diameter.

Corticotroph cell adenomas may be clinically silent or may cause *hypercortisolism* (also known as *Cushing syndrome*) because of the stimulatory effect of ACTH on the adrenal cortex. Cushing syndrome, discussed in more detail later with diseases of the adrenal gland, may be caused by a wide variety of conditions in addition to ACTH-producing pituitary neoplasms. When the hypercortisolism is caused by excessive production of ACTH by the pituitary, the process is designated *Cushing disease,* because it is the pattern of hypercortisolism originally described by Dr. Harvey Cushing. Large, clinically aggressive corticotroph adenomas may develop after surgical removal of the adrenal glands for treatment of Cushing syndrome. This condition, known as *Nelson syndrome,* occurs in most cases because of a loss of the inhibitory effect of adrenal corticosteroids on a preexisting corticotroph microadenoma. Because the adrenals are absent in individuals with Nelson syndrome, hypercortisolism does not develop. Instead, patients present with the mass effects of the pituitary tumor. In addition, because ACTH is synthesized as part of a larger prohormone that includes melanocyte-stimulating hormone (MSH), there may also be hyperpigmentation.

Other Anterior Pituitary Neoplasms

- *Gonadotroph (luteinizing hormone [LH]–producing and follicle-stimulating hormone [FSH]–producing)* adenomas can be difficult to recognize, because they secrete hormones inefficiently and variably, and the secretory products usually do not cause a recognizable clinical syndrome. Gonadotroph adenomas are most frequently found in middle-aged men and women when the tumors have become large enough to cause neurologic symptoms, such as impaired vision, headaches, diplopia, or pituitary apoplexy. The neoplastic cells usually demonstrate immunoreactivity for the common gonadotropin α-subunit and the specific β-FSH and β-LH subunits; FSH is usually the predominant secreted hormone. The availability of reliable immunoassays for the gonadotropin β-subunit and the recognition of gonadotroph-specific transcription factors have led to the reclassification of many previously described hormone-negative adenomas *("null cell adenomas")* as silent gonadotroph adenomas.
- *Thyrotroph (thyroid-stimulating hormone [TSH]–producing) adenomas* account for about 1% of all pituitary adenomas and are a rare cause of hyperthyroidism.
- *Nonfunctioning pituitary adenomas* comprise both clinically silent counterparts of the functioning adenomas described above (for example, a *silent gonadotroph adenoma*) and true *hormone-negative* (null cell) adenomas; the latter are quite infrequent and, as stated above, many have been reclassified using improved diagnostic techniques. Nonfunctioning adenomas constitute approximately 25% of all pituitary tumors. Not surprisingly, the typical presentation of nonfunctioning adenomas is mass effects. These lesions may also compromise the residual anterior pituitary sufficiently to produce hypopituitarism.
- *Pituitary carcinomas are exceedingly rare.* In addition to local extension beyond the sella turcica, these tumors virtually always have distant metastases.

SUMMARY

Clinical Manifestations of Pituitary Adenomas

- *Prolactinomas:* amenorrhea, galactorrhea, loss of libido, and infertility
- *Growth hormone (somatotroph cell) adenomas:* gigantism (children), acromegaly (adults), impaired glucose tolerance, and diabetes mellitus
- *Corticotroph cell adenomas:* Cushing syndrome, hyperpigmentation
- All pituitary adenomas, particularly nonfunctioning adenomas, may be associated with mass effects and hypopituitarism.

HYPOPITUITARISM

Hypofunction of the anterior pituitary may occur with loss or absence of 75% or more of the anterior pituitary parenchyma. This may be *congenital* (exceedingly rare) or may result from a wide range of *acquired* abnormalities that are intrinsic to the pituitary. Less frequently, disorders that interfere with the delivery of pituitary hormone–releasing factors from the hypothalamus, such as hypothalamic tumors, may also cause hypofunction of the anterior pituitary. *Hypopituitarism accompanied by evidence of posterior pituitary dysfunction in the form of diabetes insipidus* (see later) *is almost always of hypothalamic origin.* Most cases of anterior pituitary hypofunction are caused by the following:

- Nonfunctioning pituitary adenomas (see above)
- Ischemic necrosis of the anterior pituitary is an important cause of pituitary insufficiency. In general, the anterior pituitary tolerates ischemic insults fairly

well; loss of as much as half of the anterior pituitary parenchyma causes no clinical consequences. However, with destruction of larger amounts of the anterior pituitary (≥75%), signs and symptoms of hypopituitarism develop. *Sheehan syndrome,* or postpartum necrosis of the anterior pituitary, is the most common form of clinically significant ischemic necrosis of the anterior pituitary. During pregnancy the anterior pituitary enlarges considerably, largely because of an increase in the size and number of prolactin-secreting cells. However, this physiologic enlargement of the gland is not accompanied by an increase in blood supply from the low-pressure portal venous system. The enlarged gland is thus vulnerable to ischemic injury, especially in women who develop significant hemorrhage and hypotension during the peripartum period. The posterior pituitary, because it receives its blood directly from arterial branches, is much less susceptible to ischemic injury in this setting and is therefore usually not affected. Clinically significant pituitary necrosis may also be encountered in conditions other than pregnancy, including disseminated intravascular coagulation, sickle cell anemia, elevated intracranial pressure, traumatic injury, and shock of any origin. The residual gland is shrunken and scarred.

- Ablation of the pituitary by surgery or radiation
- Other, less common causes of anterior pituitary hypofunction include inflammatory lesions such as sarcoidosis or tuberculosis, trauma, and metastatic neoplasms involving the pituitary. Rarely, mutations affecting the pituitary transcription factor Pit-1 can cause multihormonal deficiency.

The clinical manifestations of anterior pituitary hypofunction depend on the specific hormone(s) that are lacking. Children can develop growth failure *(pituitary dwarfism)* as a result of growth hormone deficiency. Gonadotropin or gonadotropin-releasing hormone (GnRH) deficiency leads to amenorrhea and infertility in women and decreased libido, impotence, and loss of pubic and axillary hair in men. TSH and ACTH deficiencies result in symptoms of hypothyroidism and hypoadrenalism, respectively, and are discussed later in the chapter. Prolactin deficiency results in failure of postpartum lactation. The anterior pituitary is also a rich source of MSH, synthesized from the same precursor molecule that produces ACTH; therefore, one of the manifestations of hypopituitarism is pallor from loss of stimulatory effects of MSH on melanocytes.

POSTERIOR PITUITARY SYNDROMES

The posterior pituitary, or neurohypophysis, is composed of modified glial cells (termed *pituicytes*) and axonal processes extending from nerve cell bodies in the supraoptic and paraventricular nuclei of the hypothalamus. The hypothalamic neurons produce two peptides: antidiuretic hormone (ADH) and oxytocin. They are stored in axon terminals in the neurohypophysis and released into the circulation in response to appropriate stimuli. Oxytocin stimulates the contraction of smooth muscle in the pregnant uterus and those surrounding the lactiferous ducts of the mammary glands. Abnormal oxytocin synthesis and release has not been associated with significant clinical abnormalities. The clinically important posterior pituitary syndromes involve ADH production. They include *diabetes insipidus* and *secretion of inappropriately high levels of ADH.*

ADH is a nonapeptide hormone synthesized predominantly in the supraoptic nucleus. In response to several different stimuli, including increased plasma oncotic pressure, left atrial distention, exercise, and certain emotional states, ADH is released from axon terminals in the neurohypophysis into the general circulation. The hormone acts on the collecting tubules of the kidney to promote the resorption of free water. ADH deficiency causes *diabetes insipidus,* a condition characterized by excessive urination (polyuria) caused by an inability of the kidney to properly resorb water from the urine. Diabetes insipidus can result from several causes, including head trauma, neoplasms, and inflammatory disorders of the hypothalamus and pituitary, and from surgical procedures involving the hypothalamus or pituitary. The condition sometimes arises spontaneously ("idiopathic") in the absence of an underlying disorder. Diabetes insipidus from ADH deficiency is designated as *central,* to differentiate it from *nephrogenic* diabetes insipidus as a result of renal tubular unresponsiveness to circulating ADH. The clinical manifestations of both diseases are similar and include the excretion of large volumes of dilute urine with an inappropriately low specific gravity. Serum sodium and osmolality are increased as a result of excessive renal loss of free water, resulting in thirst and polydipsia. Patients who can drink water can generally compensate for urinary losses; patients who are obtunded, bedridden, or otherwise limited in their ability to obtain water may develop life-threatening dehydration.

In the *syndrome of inappropriate ADH (SIADH)* secretion, ADH excess is caused by several extracranial and intracranial disorders. It causes resorption of excessive amounts of free water, with resultant hyponatremia. The most common causes of SIADH include the secretion of ectopic ADH by malignant neoplasms (particularly small-cell carcinomas of the lung), non-neoplastic diseases of the lung, and local injury to the hypothalamus and/or neurohypophysis. The clinical manifestations of SIADH are dominated by hyponatremia, cerebral edema, and resultant neurologic dysfunction. Although total body water is increased, blood volume remains normal and peripheral edema does not develop.

THYROID

The thyroid gland consists of two bulky lateral lobes connected by a relatively thin isthmus, usually located below and anterior to the larynx. The thyroid gland develops embryologically from an evagination of the developing pharyngeal epithelium that descends from the foramen cecum at the base of the tongue to its normal position in the anterior neck. This pattern of descent explains the occasional presence of *ectopic thyroid tissue,* most commonly located at the base of the tongue *(lingual thyroid)* or at other sites abnormally high in the neck.

The thyroid is divided into lobules, each composed of about 20 to 40 evenly dispersed follicles. The follicles range from uniform to variable in size and are lined by cuboidal to low columnar epithelium, which is filled with thyroglobulin, the iodinated precursor protein of active thyroid hormone. In response to trophic factors from the hypothalamus, TSH *(thyrotropin)* is released by thyrotrophs in the anterior pituitary into the circulation. The binding of TSH to its receptor on the thyroid follicular epithelium results in activation and conformational change in the receptor, allowing it to associate with a stimulatory G-protein (Fig. 20–5). Activation of the G-protein eventually results in an increase in intracellular cAMP levels, which stimulates thyroid hormone synthesis and release via cAMP-dependent protein kinases. Thyroid follicular epithelial cells convert thyroglobulin into *thyroxine* (T_4) and lesser amounts of *triiodothyronine* (T_3). T_4 and T_3 are released into the systemic circulation, where most of these peptides are reversibly bound to circulating plasma proteins, such as T_4-binding globulin, for transport to peripheral tissues. The binding proteins serve to maintain the serum unbound ("free") T_3 and T_4 concentrations within narrow limits while ensuring that the hormones are readily available to the tissues. In the periphery the majority of free T_4 is de-iodinated to T_3; the latter binds to thyroid hormone nuclear receptors in target cells with 10-fold greater affinity than T_4, and has proportionately greater activity. *The interaction of thyroid hormone with its nuclear thyroid hormone receptor (TR) results in the formation of a hormone-receptor complex that binds to thyroid hormone response elements (TREs) in target genes, regulating their transcription.* Thyroid hormone has diverse cellular effects, including up-regulation of carbohydrate and lipid catabolism and stimulation of protein synthesis in a wide range of cells. The net result of these processes is an increase in the basal metabolic rate.

It is important to recognize diseases of the thyroid, because most are amenable to medical or surgical management. These diseases include conditions associated with excessive release of thyroid hormones (hyperthyroidism), those associated with thyroid hormone deficiency (hypothyroidism), and mass lesions of the thyroid. We first consider the clinical consequences of disturbed thyroid function, then focus on the disorders that generate these problems.

HYPERTHYROIDISM

Thyrotoxicosis is a hypermetabolic state caused by elevated circulating levels of free T_3 and T_4. Because it is caused most commonly by hyperfunction of the thyroid gland, it is often referred to as hyperthyroidism. However, in certain conditions the oversupply is related either to excessive release of preformed thyroid hormone (e.g., in thyroiditis) or to an extra-thyroidal source, rather than to hyperfunction of the gland (Table 20–2). *Thus, strictly speaking, hyperthyroidism is only one (albeit*

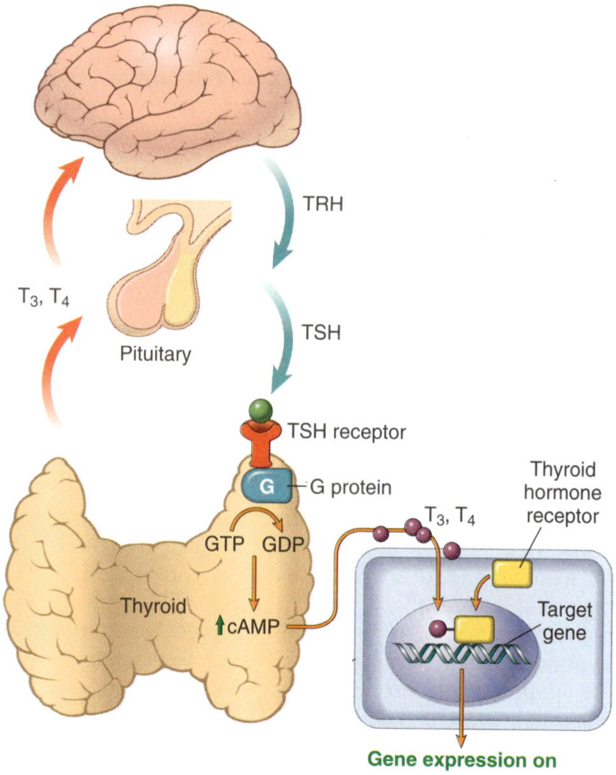

Figure 20–5

Homeostasis in the hypothalamus-pituitary-thyroid axis and mechanism of action of thyroid hormones. Secretion of thyroid hormones (T_3 and T_4) is controlled by trophic factors secreted by both the hypothalamus and the anterior pituitary. Decreased levels of T_3 and T_4 stimulate the release of thyrotropin-releasing hormone (TRH) from the hypothalamus and thyroid-stimulating hormone (TSH) from the anterior pituitary, causing T_3 and T_4 levels to rise. Elevated T_3 and T_4 levels, in turn, suppress the secretion of both TRH and TSH. This relationship is termed a *negative-feedback loop.* TSH binds to the TSH receptor on the thyroid follicular epithelium, which causes activation of G-proteins, release of cyclic AMP (cAMP), and cAMP-mediated synthesis and release of thyroid hormones (T_3 and T_4). In the periphery, T_3 and T_4 interact with the thyroid hormone receptor (TR) to form a hormone-receptor complex that translocates to the nucleus and binds to so-called thyroid response elements (TREs) on target genes initiating transcription.

Table 20–2 Cause of Thyrotoxicosis

Associated with Hyperthyroidism	
PRIMARY	
Diffuse toxic hyperplasia (Graves disease)	
Hyperfunctioning ("toxic") multinodular goiter	
Hyperfunctioning ("toxic") adenoma	
SECONDARY	
TSH-secreting pituitary adenoma (rare)*	
Not Associated with Hyperthyroidism	
Subacute granulomatous thyroiditis (*painful*)	
Subacute lymphocytic thyroiditis (*painless*)	
Struma ovarii (ovarian teratoma with thyroid)	
Factitious thyrotoxicosis (exogenous thyroxine intake)	

TSH, Thyroid-stimulating hormone.
*Associated with increased TSH; *all other causes of thyrotoxicosis associated with decreased TSH.*

the most common) category of thyrotoxicosis. With this disclaimer, we will follow the common practice of using the terms *thyrotoxicosis* and *hyperthyroidism* interchangeably.

The clinical manifestations of thyrotoxicosis are truly protean and include changes referable to the *hypermetabolic state* induced by excessive amounts of thyroid hormone as well as those related to *overactivity of the sympathetic nervous system:*

- *Constitutional symptoms:* The skin of thyrotoxic individuals tends to be soft, warm, and flushed; *heat intolerance* and excessive sweating are common. Increased sympathetic activity and hypermetabolism result in *weight loss despite increased appetite.*
- *Gastrointestinal:* Stimulation of the gut results in hypermotility, malabsorption, and diarrhea.
- *Cardiac:* Palpitations and tachycardia are common; elderly patients may develop congestive heart failure due to aggravation of preexisting heart disease.
- *Neuromuscular:* Patients frequently experience nervousness, tremor, and irritability. Nearly 50% develop proximal muscle weakness *(thyroid myopathy).*
- *Ocular manifestations:* a wide, staring gaze and lid lag are present because of sympathetic overstimulation of the levator palpebrae superioris (Fig. 20–6). However, true *thyroid ophthalmopathy* associated with proptosis is a feature seen only in Graves disease.
- *Thyroid storm* is used to designate the abrupt onset of severe hyperthyroidism. This condition occurs most commonly in individuals with underlying Graves disease (discussed later), probably resulting from an acute elevation in catecholamine levels, as might be encountered during stress. Thyroid storm is a medical emergency: a significant number of untreated patients die of cardiac arrhythmias.
- *Apathetic hyperthyroidism* refers to thyrotoxicosis occurring in the elderly, in whom old age and various co-morbidities may blunt the typical features of thyroid hormone excess seen in younger patients. The diagnosis of thyrotoxicosis in these individuals is often made during laboratory work-up for unexplained weight loss or worsening cardiovascular disease.

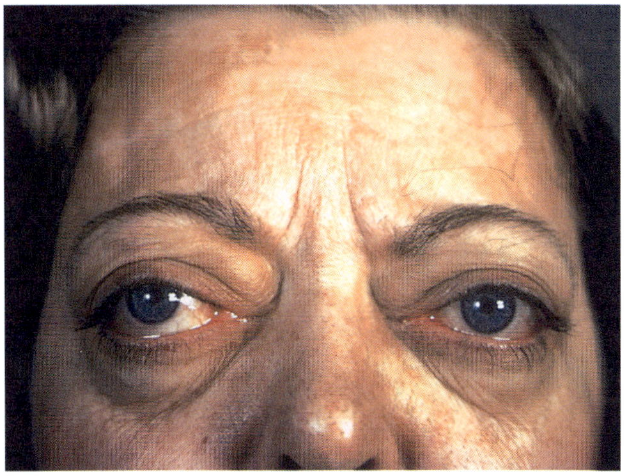

Figure 20–6

Patient with hyperthyroidism. A wide-eyed, staring gaze, caused by overactivity of the sympathetic nervous system, is one of the features of this disorder. In Graves disease, one of the most important causes of hyperthyroidism, accumulation of loose connective tissue behind the orbits also adds to the protuberant appearance of the eyes.

The diagnosis of hyperthyroidism is based on clinical features and laboratory data. The measurement of serum TSH concentration using sensitive assays provides the most useful single screening test for hyperthyroidism, because TSH levels are decreased even at the earliest stages, when the disease may still be subclinical. In rare cases of pituitary- or hypothalamus-associated (secondary) hyperthyroidism, TSH levels are either normal or raised. A low TSH value is usually associated with increased levels of free T_4. In an occasional person, hyperthyroidism results predominantly from increased circulating levels of T_3 (T_3 toxicosis). In these cases free T_4 levels may be decreased, and direct measurement of serum T_3 may be useful. Once the diagnosis of thyrotoxicosis has been confirmed by a combination of TSH and free thyroid hormone assays, measurement of radioactive iodine uptake by the thyroid gland is often valuable in determining the etiology. For example, there may be diffusely increased uptake in the whole gland (Graves disease), increased uptake in a solitary nodule (toxic adenoma), or decreased uptake (thyroiditis).

HYPOTHYROIDISM

Hypothyroidism is caused by any structural or functional derangement that interferes with the production of adequate levels of thyroid hormone. As in the case of hyperthyroidism, this disorder is sometimes divided into primary and secondary categories, depending on whether the hypothyroidism arises from an intrinsic abnormality in the thyroid or results from hypothalamic or pituitary disease (Table 20–3).

The clinical manifestations of hypothyroidism include cretinism and myxedema. *Cretinism* refers to hypothyroidism developing in infancy or early childhood. This

Table 20-3 Causes of Hypothyroidism

Primary
Postablative: surgery, radioiodine therapy, or external radiation
Hashimoto thyroiditis*
Iodine deficiency*
Congenital biosynthetic defect (dyshormonogenetic goiter)*
Drugs (lithium, iodides, *p*-aminosalicylic acid)*
Rare developmental abnormalities of the thyroid (thyroid dysgenesis)
Secondary
Pituitary or hypothalamic failure (uncommon)

*Associated with enlargement of thyroid ("goitrous hypothyroidism"). Hashimoto thyroiditis and postablative hypothyroidism account for the vast majority of cases of hypothyroidism, particularly in regions with adequate dietary iodine.

disorder was formerly fairly common in areas of the world where dietary iodine deficiency is endemic, including the Himalayas, inland China, Africa, and other mountainous areas. It has now become much less frequent because of the widespread supplementation of foods with iodine. On rare occasions cretinism may also result from inborn errors in metabolism (e.g., enzyme deficiencies) that interfere with the biosynthesis of normal levels of thyroid hormone (sporadic cretinism). Clinical features of cretinism include impaired development of the skeletal system and central nervous system, with severe mental retardation, short stature, coarse facial features, a protruding tongue, and umbilical hernia. The severity of the mental impairment in cretinism seems to be directly influenced by the time at which thyroid deficiency occurs in utero. Normally, maternal hormones that are critical to fetal brain development, including T_3 and T_4, cross the placenta. If there is maternal thyroid deficiency before the development of the fetal thyroid gland, mental retardation is severe. In contrast, reduction in maternal thyroid hormones later in pregnancy, after the fetal thyroid has developed, allows normal brain development.

Hypothyroidism developing in older children and adults results in a condition known as *myxedema.* Myxedema, or Gull disease, was first linked with thyroid dysfunction in 1873 by Sir William Gull in a paper addressing the development of a "cretinoid state" in adults. Manifestations of myxedema include generalized apathy and mental sluggishness that in the early stages of disease may mimic depression. Individuals with myxedema are listless, cold intolerant, and often obese. Mucopolysaccharide-rich edema accumulates in skin, subcutaneous tissue, and a number of visceral sites, with resultant broadening and coarsening of facial features, enlargement of the tongue, and deepening of the voice. Bowel motility is decreased, resulting in constipation. Pericardial effusions are common; in later stages the heart is enlarged, and heart failure may supervene.

Laboratory evaluation has a vital role in the diagnosis of suspected hypothyroidism because of the nonspecific nature of symptoms. *Measurement of the serum TSH is the most sensitive screening test for this disorder.* The serum TSH is increased in primary hypothyroidism because of a loss of feedback inhibition of thyrotropin-releasing hormone (TRH) and TSH production by the hypothalamus and pituitary, respectively. The TSH concentration is not increased in persons with hypothyroidism caused by primary hypothalamic or pituitary disease. Serum T_4 is decreased in individuals with hypothyroidism of any origin.

THYROIDITIS

Thyroiditis, or inflammation of the thyroid gland, encompasses a diverse group of disorders characterized by some form of thyroid inflammation. These diseases include conditions that result in acute illness with severe thyroid pain (e.g., infectious thyroiditis, subacute granulomatous thyroiditis) and disorders in which there is relatively little inflammation and the illness is manifested primarily by thyroid dysfunction (subacute lymphocytic [painless] thyroiditis and fibrous [Reidel] thyroiditis). This section focuses on the more common and clinically significant types of thyroiditis: (1) Hashimoto thyroiditis (or chronic lymphocytic thyroiditis), (2) subacute granulomatous thyroiditis, and (3) subacute lymphocytic thyroiditis.

Chronic Lymphocytic (Hashimoto) Thyroiditis

Hashimoto thyroiditis is the most common cause of hypothyroidism in areas of the world where iodine levels are sufficient. It is characterized by gradual thyroid failure because of autoimmune destruction of the thyroid gland. This disorder is most prevalent between 45 and 65 years of age and is more common in women than in men, with a female predominance of 10:1 to 20:1. Although it is primarily a disease of older women, it can occur in children and is a major cause of nonendemic goiter in children.

Pathogenesis. Hashimoto thyroiditis is an autoimmune disease in which the overriding feature is progressive depletion of thyroid epithelial cells (thyrocytes), which are gradually replaced by mononuclear cell infiltration and fibrosis. Multiple immunologic mechanisms may contribute to the death of thyrocytes (Fig. 20–7), although sensitization of autoreactive CD4+ T-helper cells to thyroid antigens seems to be the initiating event. The effector mechanisms for thyrocyte death include:

- The possible reaction of CD4+ T cells to thyroid antigens, thus producing cytokines—notably interferon γ (IFN-γ)—which promote inflammation and activate macrophages, as in delayed-type hypersensitivity reactions. Injury to the thyroid results from the toxic products of inflammatory cells.
- CD8+ cytotoxic T-cell-mediated cell death: CD8+ cytotoxic T cells may recognize antigens on thyroid cells and kill these cells.
- Binding of antithyroid antibodies followed by antibody-dependent cell-mediated cytotoxicity mediated by natural killer (NK) cells has been invoked as another mechanism of thyrocyte death, on the basis of the

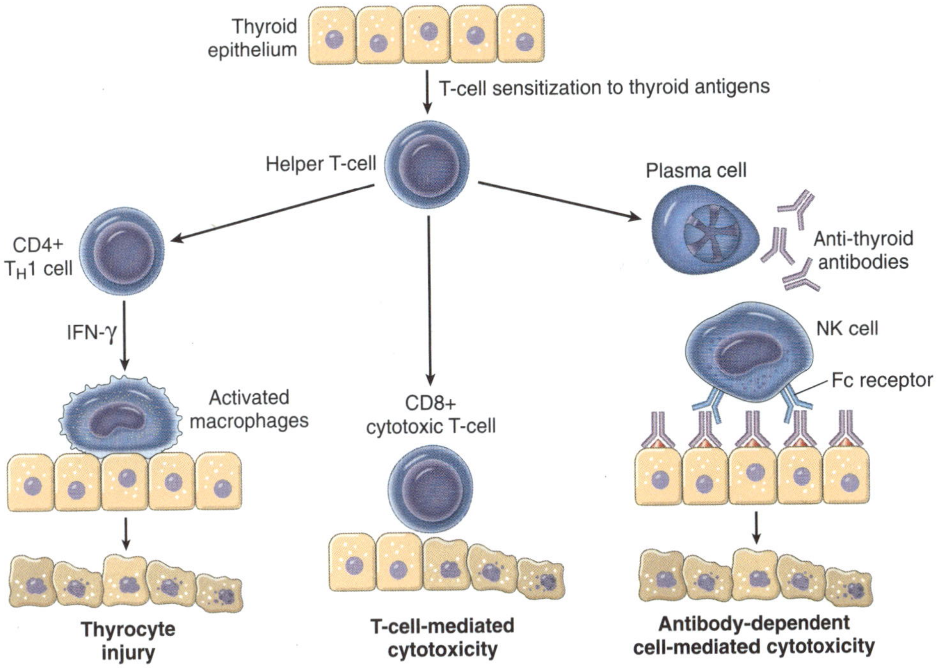

Figure 20–7

Pathogenesis of Hashimoto thyroiditis. Sensitization of autoreactive CD4+ helper T cells to thyroid antigens seems to be the initiating event for all proposed mechanisms of thyroid cell death. Sensitized CD4+ helper T cells then either differentiate into T_H1 cells with resulting delayed-type hypersensitivity reaction, or stimulate cytotoxic T-cell responses and help B cells (not shown) to develop into antibody-secreting plasma cells.

finding of NK cells in the cellular infiltrates. However, the importance of this mechanism is not proved.

There is a significant *genetic component* to disease pathogenesis. Hashimoto thyroiditis occurs with increased frequency in first-degree relatives, and unaffected family members often have circulating thyroid autoantibodies. Association studies have reported linkage between *HLA-DR3* and *HLA-DR5* alleles and Hashimoto thyroiditis, but the associations are generally weak. Several non-HLA genes are also linked to autoimmune thyroid disease, including genes encoding the T-cell inhibitory receptor CTLA-4, but again the associations are weak and of uncertain significance.

Morphology

Grossly, the thyroid is usually diffusely and symmetrically enlarged, although more localized enlargement may be seen in some cases. The capsule is intact, and the gland is well demarcated from adjacent structures. The cut surface is pale, gray-tan, firm, and somewhat friable. Microscopic examination reveals widespread infiltration of the parenchyma by a **mononuclear inflammatory infiltrate** containing small lymphocytes, plasma cells, and well-developed **germinal centers** (Fig. 20–8). The thyroid follicles are atrophic and are lined in many areas by epithelial cells distinguished by the presence of abundant eosinophilic, granular cytoplasm, termed **Hürthle,** or **oxyphil, cells.** This is a metaplastic response of the normally low cuboidal follicular epithelium to ongoing injury; ultrastructurally the Hürthle cells are characterized by numerous prominent mitochondria. Interstitial connective tissue is increased and may be abundant. Less commonly, the thyroid is small and atrophic as a result of more extensive fibrosis (**fibrosing variant**). Unlike in Reidel thyroiditis, the fibrosis does not extend beyond the capsule of the gland.

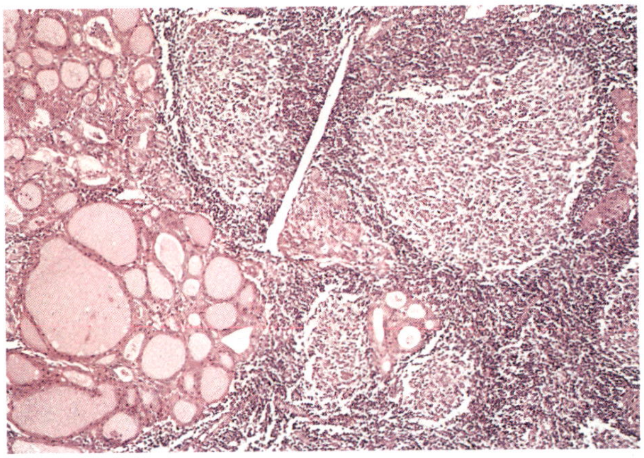

Figure 20–8

Photomicrograph of Hashimoto thyroiditis. The thyroid parenchyma contains a dense lymphocytic infiltrate with germinal centers. Residual thyroid follicles lined by deeply eosinophilic Hürthle cells are also seen.

Clinical Features. Hashimoto thyroiditis comes to clinical attention as *painless enlargement of the thyroid, usually associated with some degree of hypothyroidism,* in a middle-aged woman. The enlargement of the gland is usually symmetric and diffuse, but in some cases it may be sufficiently localized to raise a suspicion of neoplasm. In the usual clinical course, hypothyroidism develops gradually. In some cases, however, it *may be preceded by transient thyrotoxicosis* caused by disruption of thyroid follicles, with secondary release of thyroid hormones ("hashitoxicosis"). During this phase, free T_4 and T_3 concentrations are elevated, TSH is diminished, and radioactive iodine uptake is decreased. As hypothyroidism supervenes, T_4 and T_3 levels progressively fall, accompanied by a compensatory increase in TSH. Patients with Hashimoto thyroiditis often have *other autoimmune diseases* and are at *increased risk for the development of B-cell non-Hodgkin lymphomas.* However, there is no established risk for developing thyroid epithelial neoplasms.

Subacute Granulomatous (de Quervain) Thyroiditis

Subacute granulomatous thyroiditis, also known as de Quervain thyroiditis, is much less common than is Hashimoto disease. de Quervain thyroiditis is most common between the ages of 30 and 50 and, like other forms of thyroiditis, occurs more frequently in women than in men. Subacute thyroiditis is believed to be caused by a *viral infection* or a postviral inflammatory process. The majority of patients have a history of an upper respiratory infection just before the onset of thyroiditis. In contrast to autoimmune thyroid disease, the immune response is not self-perpetuating, so the process is limited.

Morphology

The gland is firm, with an intact capsule, and may be unilaterally or bilaterally enlarged. Histologically, there is disruption of thyroid follicles, with extravasation of colloid leading to a polymorphonuclear infiltrate, which is replaced over time by lymphocytes, plasma cells, and macrophages. The extravasated colloid provokes a granulomatous reaction, with exuberant giant cells, some containing fragments of colloid. Healing occurs by resolution of inflammation and fibrosis.

Clinical Features. The onset of this form of thyroiditis is often acute, characterized by *pain* in the neck (particularly when swallowing), fever, malaise, and variable enlargement of the thyroid. Transient hyperthyroidism may occur, as in other cases of thyroiditis, as a result of disruption of thyroid follicles and release of excessive thyroid hormone. Thyroid function tests are similar to those encountered in thyrotoxicosis associated with other forms of thyroiditis. The leukocyte count and erythrocyte sedimentation rates are increased. With progression of disease and gland destruction, a transient hypothyroid phase may ensue. The condition is typically self-limited, with most patients returning to a euthyroid state within 6 to 8 weeks.

Subacute Lymphocytic Thyroiditis

Subacute lymphocytic thyroiditis is also known as "silent" or "painless" thyroiditis; in a subset of patients the onset of disease follows pregnancy *(postpartum thyroiditis).* This disease is most likely autoimmune in etiology, because circulating antithyroid antibodies are found in the majority of patients. It mostly affects middle-aged women, who present with a *painless* neck mass or features of thyroid hormone excess. There is an initial phase of thyrotoxicosis (likely to be secondary to thyroid tissue damage), followed by return to a euthyroid state within a few months. Patients with one episode of postpartum thyroiditis are at an increased risk of recurrence after subsequent pregnancies. In a minority of affected individuals the condition eventually progresses to hypothyroidism. Except for possible mild symmetric enlargement, the thyroid appears normal on gross inspection. The histologic features consist of lymphocytic infiltration and hyperplastic germinal centers within the thyroid parenchyma; unlike Hashimoto thyroiditis, follicular atrophy or Hürthle cell metaplasia are not commonly seen.

Other Forms of Thyroiditis

Two uncommon variants are described here:

- *Riedel thyroiditis,* a rare disorder of unknown etiology, is characterized by extensive fibrosis involving the thyroid and contiguous neck structures. The presence of a hard and fixed thyroid mass clinically simulates a thyroid neoplasm. It may be associated with idiopathic fibrosis in other sites in the body, such as the retroperitoneum. The presence of circulating antithyroid antibodies in most patients suggests an autoimmune etiology.
- *Palpation thyroiditis,* caused by vigorous clinical palpation of the thyroid gland, results in multifocal follicular disruption associated with chronic inflammatory cells and occasional giant-cell formation. Unlike de Quervain thyroiditis, abnormalities of thyroid function are not present, and palpation thyroiditis is usually an incidental finding in specimens resected for other reasons.

SUMMARY

Thyroiditis

- Chronic lymphocytic (Hashimoto) thyroiditis is the most common cause of hypothyroidism in regions where dietary iodine levels are sufficient.
- Hashimoto thyroiditis is an autoimmune disease, characterized by progressive destruction of thyroid parenchyma, "Hürthle cell" change, and mononuclear (lymphoplasmacytic) infiltrates, with or without extensive fibrosis.
- Multiple autoimmune mechanisms account for Hashimoto disease, including cytotoxicity mediated by CD8+ T cells, cytokines (IFN-γ), and antithyroid antibodies.
- Subacute granulomatous (de Quervain) thyroiditis is a self-limited disease, probably secondary to

a viral infection, and is characterized by pain and the presence of a granulomatous inflammation in the thyroid.
• Subacute lymphocytic thyroiditis often occurs following a pregnancy (postpartum thyroiditis), is typically painless, and is characterized by lymphocytic inflammation in the thyroid.

GRAVES DISEASE

In 1835 Robert Graves reported on his observations of a disease characterized by "violent and long continued palpitations in females" associated with enlargement of the thyroid gland. *Graves disease is the most common cause of endogenous hyperthyroidism.* It is characterized by a triad of manifestations:

• *Thyrotoxicosis,* caused by a diffusely enlarged, hyperfunctional thyroid, is present in all cases.
• An infiltrative *ophthalmopathy* with resultant exophthalmos is noted in as many as 40% of patients.
• A localized, infiltrative *dermopathy* (sometimes designated *pretibial myxedema*) is seen in a minority of cases.

Graves disease has a peak incidence between the ages of 20 and 40, with *women being affected as much as seven times more commonly than men.* This is a very common disorder that is said to be present in 1.5% to 2.0% of women in the United States. Genetic factors are important in the causation of Graves disease. An increased incidence of Graves disease occurs among family members of affected patients, and the concordance rate in monozygotic twins is as high as 60%. As is a recurring theme with other autoimmune disorders, there is a genetic susceptibility to Graves disease associated with the presence of certain HLA haplotypes, specifically HLA-B8 and -DR3, and allelic variants (polymorphisms) in genes encoding the inhibitory T-cell receptor CTLA-4 and the tyrosine phosphatase PTPN22.

Pathogenesis. *Graves disease is an autoimmune disorder* in which a variety of antibodies may be present in the serum, including antibodies to the TSH receptor, thyroid peroxisomes, and thyroglobulin. Of these, *autoantibodies to the TSH receptor are central to disease pathogenesis,* and include:

• *Thyroid-stimulating immunoglobulin:* An IgG antibody that binds to the TSH receptor and mimics the action of TSH, stimulating adenyl cyclase, with resultant increased release of thyroid hormones. Almost all persons with Graves disease have detectable amounts of this autoantibody to the TSH receptor. This antibody is relatively specific for Graves disease, in contrast to thyroglobulin and thyroid peroxidase antibodies.
• *Thyroid growth-stimulating immunoglobulins (TGIs):* Also directed against the TSH receptor, TGIs have been implicated in the proliferation of thyroid follicular epithelium.
• *TSH-binding inhibitor immunoglobulins (TBII):* These anti-TSH receptor antibodies prevent TSH from binding normally to its receptor on thyroid epithelial cells. In so doing, some forms of TBIIs mimic the action of TSH, resulting in the stimulation of thyroid epithelial cell activity, whereas other forms may actually *inhibit* thyroid cell function. It is not unusual to find the coexistence of stimulating *and* inhibiting immunoglobulins in the serum of the same patient, a finding that may explain why some patients with Graves disease spontaneously develop episodes of hypothyroidism.

The trigger for the initiation of the autoimmune reaction in Graves disease remains uncertain, although the underlying mechanism is likely to be breakdown in helper T-cell tolerance, resulting in the production of anti-TSH autoantibodies. A T-cell–mediated autoimmune phenomenon is also involved in the development of the *infiltrative ophthalmopathy* characteristic of Graves disease. In Graves ophthalmopathy the volume of the retro-orbital connective tissues and extra-ocular muscles is increased as a result of several causes, including: (1) marked infiltration of the retro-orbital space by mononuclear cells, predominantly T cells; (2) inflammatory edema and swelling of extra-ocular muscles; (3) accumulation of extracellular matrix components, specifically hydrophilic glycosaminoglycans such as hyaluronic acid and chondroitin sulfate; and (4) increased numbers of adipocytes (fatty infiltration). These changes displace the eyeball forward and can interfere with the function of the extraocular muscles.

Autoimmune disorders of the thyroid thus span a continuum in which Graves disease, characterized by hyperfunction of the thyroid, lies at one extreme and Hashimoto disease, manifesting as hypothyroidism, occupies the other end. Sometimes hyperthyroidism may supervene on preexisting Hashimoto thyroiditis *(hashitoxicosis),* while at other times individuals with Graves disease may spontaneously develop thyroid hypofunction; occasionally, families may experience coexistence of Hashimoto and Graves disease within the affected kindred. Not surprisingly, there is also an element of histologic overlap between the autoimmune thyroid disorders (most characteristically, prominent intra-thyroidal lymphoid cell infiltrates with germinal center formation). In both disorders the frequency of other autoimmune diseases, such as systemic lupus erythematosus, pernicious anemia, type 1 diabetes, and Addison disease, is increased.

Morphology

In the typical case of Graves disease, the thyroid gland is diffusely enlarged because of the presence of **diffuse hypertrophy and hyperplasia** of thyroid follicular epithelial cells. The gland is usually smooth and soft, and its capsule is intact. Microscopically, the follicular epithelial cells in untreated cases are tall, columnar, and more crowded than usual. This crowding often results in the formation of small papillae, which project into the follicular lumen (Fig. 20–9). Such papillae lack

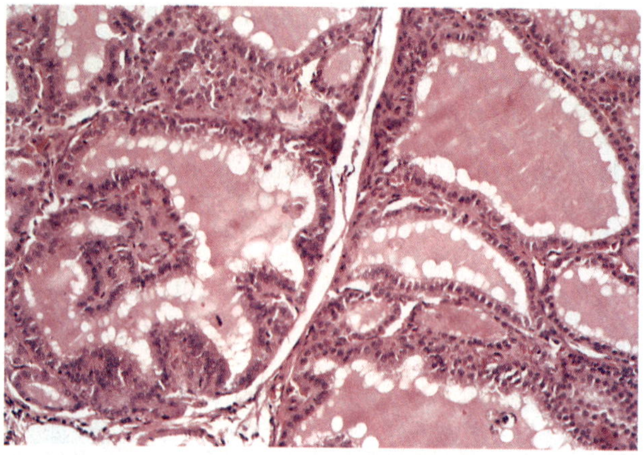

Figure 20–9

Photomicrograph of a diffusely hyperplastic gland in a case of Graves disease. The follicles are lined by tall columnar epithelial cells that project into the lumens of the follicles. These cells actively resorb the colloid in the centers of the follicles, resulting in the "scalloped" appearance of the edges of the colloid.

fibrovascular cores, in contrast to those of papillary carcinoma. The colloid within the follicular lumen is pale, with scalloped margins. Lymphoid infiltrates, consisting predominantly of T cells, with fewer B cells and mature plasma cells, are present throughout the interstitium; germinal centers are common. Preoperative therapy alters the morphology of the thyroid in Graves disease. For example, preoperative administration of iodine causes involution of the epithelium and the accumulation of colloid by blocking thyroglobulin secretion; with continued administration, fibrosis of the gland results.

Changes in extra-thyroidal tissues include generalized lymphoid hyperplasia. In individuals with ophthalmopathy, the tissues of the orbit are edematous, because of the presence of hydrophilic glycosaminoglycans. In addition, there is infiltration by lymphocytes, mostly T cells. Orbital muscles are edematous initially but may undergo fibrosis late in the course of the disease. The dermopathy, if present, is characterized by thickening of the dermis, as a result of deposition of glycosaminoglycans and lymphocyte infiltration.

Clinical Features. The clinical manifestations of Graves disease include those common to all forms of thyrotoxicosis (discussed earlier), as well as those associated uniquely with Graves disease: *diffuse hyperplasia of the thyroid, ophthalmopathy, and dermopathy.* The degree of thyrotoxicosis varies from case to case and may sometimes be less conspicuous than other manifestations of the disease. Diffuse enlargement of the thyroid is present in all cases of Graves disease. The thyroid enlargement is usually smooth and symmetric, but it may be asymmetric. Increased flow of blood through the hyperactive gland often produces an audible bruit. Sympathetic overactivity produces a characteristic wide, staring gaze and lid lag. The ophthalmopathy of Graves disease results in abnormal protrusion of the eyeball (exophthalmos). The extra-ocular muscles are often weak. The exophthalmos may persist or progress despite successful treatment of the thyrotoxicosis, sometimes resulting in corneal injury. The infiltrative dermopathy, or pretibial myxedema, is most common in the skin overlying the shins, where it presents as scaly thickening and induration of the skin. The skin lesions may be slightly pigmented papules or nodules and often have an orange-peel texture. Laboratory findings in Graves disease include elevated serum free T_4 and T_3 and depressed serum TSH. Because of ongoing stimulation of the thyroid follicles by thyroid-stimulating immunoglobulins, radioactive iodine uptake is increased and radioiodine scans show a *diffuse uptake* of iodine.

SUMMARY

Graves disease

- Graves disease, the most common cause of endogenous hyperthyroidism, is characterized by the triad of thyrotoxicosis, ophthalmopathy, and dermopathy.
- Graves disease is an autoimmune disorder caused by activation of thyroid epithelial cells by autoantibodies to the TSH receptor that mimic TSH action.
- The thyroid in Graves disease is characterized by diffuse hypertrophy and hyperplasia of follicles and lymphoid infiltrates; glycosaminoglycan deposition and lymphoid infiltrates characterize the ophthalmopathy and dermopathy.
- Laboratory features include elevations in serum free T_3 and T_4, and decreased serum TSH.

DIFFUSE AND MULTINODULAR GOITER

Enlargement of the thyroid, or *goiter,* is the most common manifestation of thyroid disease. *Diffuse and multinodular goiters reflect impaired synthesis of thyroid hormone,* most often caused by dietary iodine deficiency. Impairment of thyroid hormone synthesis leads to a compensatory rise in the serum TSH, which, in turn, causes hypertrophy and hyperplasia of thyroid follicular cells and, ultimately, gross enlargement of the thyroid gland. The compensatory increase in functional mass of the gland is able to overcome the hormone deficiency, ensuring a *euthyroid* metabolic state in the vast majority of individuals. If the underlying disorder is sufficiently severe (e.g., a congenital biosynthetic defect), the compensatory responses may be inadequate to overcome the impairment in hormone synthesis, resulting in *goitrous hypothyroidism.* The degree of thyroid enlargement is proportional to the level and duration of thyroid hormone deficiency. Goiters arise in both an endemic and a sporadic distribution.

Endemic goiter occurs in geographic areas where the soil, water, and food supply contain little iodine. The term *endemic* is used when goiters are present in more than 10% of the population in a given region. Such conditions are particularly common in mountainous areas of the world, including the Himalayas and the Andes. With increasing availability of dietary iodine supplementation, the frequency and severity of endemic goiter have declined significantly. *Sporadic goiter* occurs less commonly than endemic goiter. The condition is more common in females than in males, with a peak incidence in puberty or young adult life, when there is an increased physiologic demand for T_4. Sporadic goiter may be caused by several conditions, including the ingestion of substances that interfere with thyroid hormone synthesis at some level, such as excessive calcium and vegetables belonging to the Brassicaceae (Cruciferae) family (e.g., cabbage, cauliflower, Brussels sprouts, and turnips). In other instances, goiter may result from hereditary enzymatic defects that interfere with thyroid hormone synthesis *(dyshormonogenetic goiter)*. In most cases, however, the cause of sporadic goiter is not apparent.

Morphology

In most cases, TSH-induced hypertrophy and hyperplasia of thyroid follicular cells results initially in diffuse, symmetric enlargement of the gland **(diffuse goiter)**. The follicles are lined by crowded columnar cells, which may pile up and form projections similar to those seen in Graves disease. If dietary iodine subsequently increases, or if the demands for thyroid hormone decrease, the stimulated follicular epithelium involutes to form an enlarged, colloid-rich gland **(colloid goiter)**. The cut surface of the thyroid in such cases is usually brown, somewhat glassy, and translucent. Microscopically, the follicular epithelium may be hyperplastic in the early stages of disease or flattened and cuboidal during periods of involution. Colloid is abundant during the latter periods. With time, recurrent episodes of hyperplasia and involution combine to produce a more irregular enlargement of the thyroid, termed **multinodular goiter**. Virtually all long-standing simple goiters convert into multinodular goiters. They may be nontoxic or may induce thyrotoxicosis **(toxic multinodular goiter)**. The pathogenesis of nodules in multinodular goiters has many similarities to the molecular events involved in the formation of benign neoplasm of the thyroid (i.e., follicular adenomas). Because normal thyroid cells are heterogeneous in their response to TSH and their ability to replicate, the development of nodules may reflect clonal evolution and subsequent emergence of a clone of cells having a proliferative advantage. Consistent with this model, both polyclonal and monoclonal nodules coexist within the same multinodular goiter, with the latter presumably having arisen as a result of the acquisition of a genetic abnormality favoring growth. Multinodular goiters are multilobulated, asymmetrically enlarged glands, which may reach massive size. On the cut surface, irregular nodules containing variable amounts of brown, gelatinous colloid are present (Fig. 20–10). Regressive changes are quite common, particularly in older lesions, and include areas of fibrosis, hemorrhage, calcification, and cystic change. The microscopic appearance includes colloid-rich follicles lined by flattened, inactive epithelium and areas of follicular epithelial hypertrophy and hyperplasia, accompanied by the regressive changes noted above.

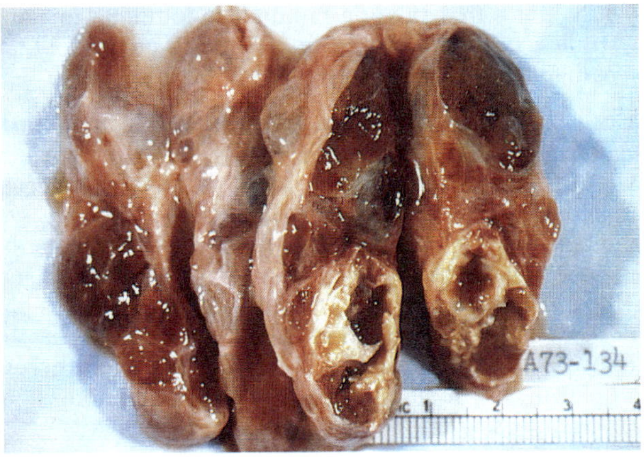

Figure 20–10

Multinodular goiter. The gland is coarsely nodular and contains areas of fibrosis and cystic change. Note the brown gelatinous colloid characteristic of this condition ("colloid goiter").

Clinical Features. The dominant clinical features of goiter are those caused by the *mass effects* of the enlarged gland. In addition to the obvious cosmetic problem of a large neck mass, goiters may also cause airway obstruction, dysphagia, and compression of large vessels in the neck and upper thorax. In a minority of patients, a hyperfunctioning ("toxic") nodule may develop within a long-standing goiter, resulting in *hyperthyroidism.* This condition, known as *Plummer syndrome,* is not accompanied by the infiltrative ophthalmopathy and dermopathy of Graves disease. Less commonly, goiter may be associated with clinical evidence of *hypothyroidism.* Goiters are also clinically significant because of their ability to mask or to mimic neoplastic diseases arising in the thyroid.

NEOPLASMS OF THE THYROID

The thyroid gland gives rise to a variety of neoplasms, ranging from circumscribed, benign adenomas to highly aggressive, anaplastic carcinomas. From a clinical standpoint, the possibility of neoplastic disease is of major concern in individuals who present with *thyroid nodules.* Fortunately, the overwhelming majority of solitary nodules of the thyroid prove to be benign lesions, either follicular adenomas or localized, non-neoplastic conditions (e.g., nodular hyperplasia, simple cysts, or foci of thyroiditis). Carcinomas of the thyroid, in contrast, are uncommon, accounting for much less than 1% of solitary thyroid nodules. Several clinical criteria provide a clue to the nature of a given thyroid nodule:

- *Solitary nodules,* in general, are more likely to be neoplastic than are multiple nodules.
- *Nodules in younger patients* are more likely to be neoplastic than are those in older patients.
- *Nodules in males* are more likely to be neoplastic than are those in females.
- A history of *radiation* treatment to the head and neck region is associated with an increased incidence of thyroid malignancy.

- Nodules that take up radioactive iodine in imaging studies (*hot nodules*) are more likely to be benign than malignant.

Such statistics and general trends, however, are of little significance in the evaluation of a given individual, in whom the timely recognition of a malignancy, however uncommon, can be life-saving. Ultimately, it is the morphologic evaluation of a given thyroid nodule, done by fine-needle aspiration biopsy and histologic study of surgically resected thyroid parenchyma, that provides the most definitive information about its nature. In the following sections, we will consider the major thyroid neoplasms, including adenomas and carcinomas of various types.

Adenomas

Adenomas of the thyroid are benign neoplasms derived from follicular epithelium. As in the case of all thyroid neoplasms, follicular adenomas are usually solitary. Clinically and morphologically, they may be difficult to distinguish, on the one hand, from hyperplastic nodules or, on the other hand, from the less common follicular carcinomas. Although the vast majority of adenomas are nonfunctional, a small proportion produces thyroid hormones ("toxic adenomas") and causes clinically apparent thyrotoxicosis.

Pathogenesis. The *TSH receptor signaling pathway* plays an important role in the pathogenesis of toxic adenomas. *Activating ("gain of function") somatic mutations in one of two components of this signaling system*—most often the TSH receptor itself and, less commonly, the α-subunit of G_s—cause chronic overproduction of cAMP, generating cells that acquire a growth advantage. This results in clonal expansion of epithelial cells within the follicular adenoma, which can autonomously produce thyroid hormone and cause symptoms of thyroid excess. About 20% of follicular adenomas have point mutations in the *RAS* family of oncogenes, which have also been identified in approximately half of follicular carcinomas. This finding has raised the possibility that some adenomas may progress to carcinomas.

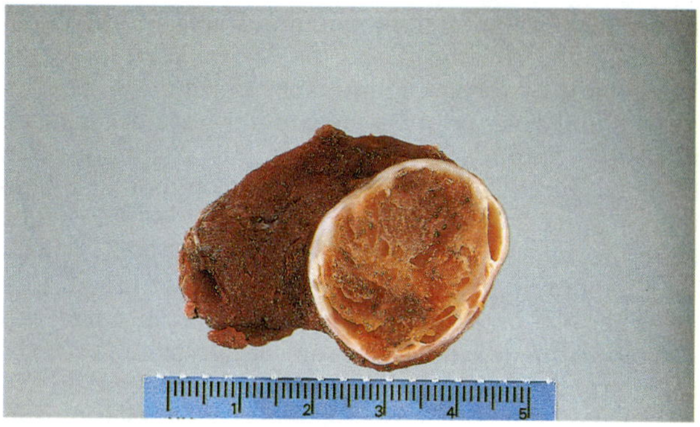

Figure 20–11

Follicular adenoma of the thyroid. A solitary, well-circumscribed nodule is seen.

Morphology

The typical thyroid adenoma is a **solitary,** spherical lesion that compresses the adjacent non-neoplastic thyroid. The neoplastic cells are demarcated from the adjacent parenchyma by a **well-defined, intact capsule** (Fig. 20-11). **These features are important in making the distinction from multinodular goiters,** which contain multiple nodules on their cut surface (even though the patient may present clinically with a solitary dominant nodule), do not demonstrate compression of the adjacent thyroid parenchyma, and lack a well-formed capsule. Microscopically, the constituent cells are arranged in uniform follicles that contain colloid (Fig. 20–12). The follicular growth pattern within the adenoma is usually quite distinct from the adjacent non-neoplastic thyroid, and this is another distinguishing feature from multinodular goiters, in which nodular and uninvolved thyroid parenchyma demonstrate comparable growth patterns. Papillary change is not a typical feature of adenomas and, if present, should raise the suspicion of an encapsulated papillary carcinoma (discussed later). The neoplastic cells are uniform, with well-defined cell borders. Occasionally, the neoplastic cells acquire brightly eosinophilic granular cytoplasm (oxyphil or Hürthle cell change) (Fig. 20–13); the clinical presentation and behavior of a **Hürthle cell adenoma** are no different from those of a conventional adenoma. Similar to endocrine tumors at other anatomic sites, even benign follicular adenomas may, on occasion, exhibit focal nuclear pleomorphism, atypia, and prominent nucleoli **(endocrine atypia);** by itself this does not constitute a feature of malignancy. The hallmark of all follicular adenomas is the presence of an intact well-formed capsule encircling the tumor. **Careful evaluation of the integrity of the capsule is therefore critical in the distinction of follicular adenomas from follicular carcinomas,** which demonstrate capsular and/or vascular invasion (see below).

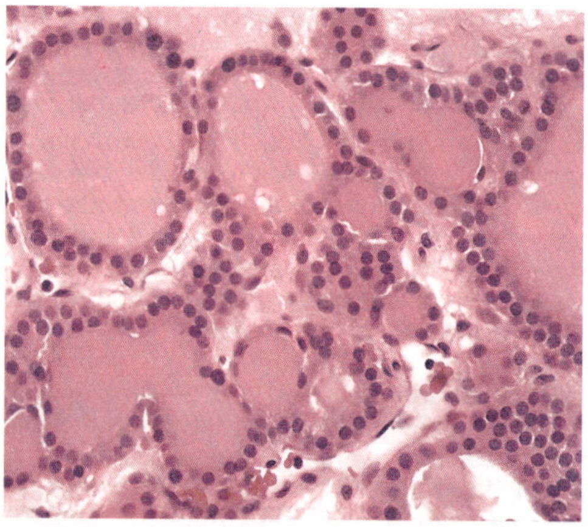

Figure 20–12

Photomicrograph of follicular adenoma. Well-differentiated follicles resemble normal thyroid parenchyma.

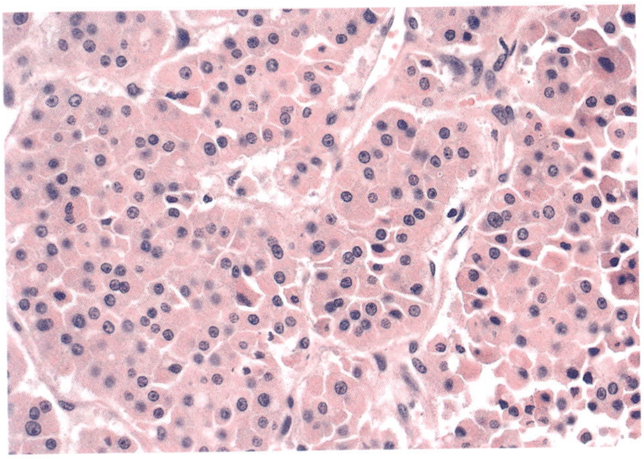

Figure 20–13

Hürthle cell adenoma. A high-power view showing that the tumor is composed of cells with abundant eosinophilic cytoplasm and small regular nuclei. (Courtesy of Dr. Mary Sunday, Brigham and Women's Hospital, Boston, Massachusetts.)

Clinical Features. Most adenomas of the thyroid present as painless nodules, often discovered during a routine physical examination. Larger masses may produce local symptoms such as difficulty in swallowing. As previously stated, persons with toxic adenomas can present with features of thyrotoxicosis. After injection of radioactive iodine, most adenomas take up iodine less avidly than does normal thyroid parenchyma. On radionuclide scanning, therefore, adenomas appear as "cold" nodules relative to the adjacent normal thyroid gland. Toxic adenomas, however, will appear as "warm" or "hot" nodules in the scan. As many as 10% of "cold" nodules eventually prove to be malignant. By contrast, malignancy is virtually nonexistent in "hot" nodules. Additional techniques used in the preoperative evaluation of suspected adenomas are ultrasonography and fine-needle aspiration biopsy. Because of the need for evaluating capsular integrity, *the definitive diagnosis of thyroid adenoma can only be made after careful histologic examination of the resected specimen.* Suspected adenomas of the thyroid are therefore removed surgically to exclude malignancy. Thyroid adenomas have an excellent prognosis and do not recur or metastasize.

Carcinomas

Clinically significant carcinomas of the thyroid are relatively uncommon in the United States, being responsible for less than 1% of cancer-related deaths; in contrast, it is not unusual to detect a microscopic (clinically silent) tumor as an incidental finding at autopsy. Most cases of thyroid carcinoma occur in adults, although some forms, particularly papillary carcinomas, may present in childhood. A female predominance has been noted among persons developing thyroid carcinoma in the early and middle adult years, probably related to the expression of estrogen receptors on neoplastic thyroid epithelium. In contrast, cases presenting in childhood and late adult life are distributed equally among males and females, largely related to exogenous influences (see later). The major subtypes of thyroid carcinoma and their relative frequencies are as follows:

- Papillary carcinoma (75% to 85% of cases)
- Follicular carcinoma (10% to 20% of cases)
- Medullary carcinoma (5% of cases)
- Anaplastic carcinomas (<5% of cases)

Most thyroid carcinomas are derived from the follicular epithelium, except for medullary carcinomas; the latter are derived from the parafollicular, or C, cells. Because of the unique clinical and biologic features associated with each variant of thyroid carcinoma, these subtypes will be described separately, after discussion of pathogenesis.

Pathogenesis. Both genetic and environmental variables are implicated in the pathogenesis of thyroid cancers.

Genetic Variables. Genetic influences are implicated in both familial and nonfamilial ("sporadic") forms of thyroid cancer. Familial medullary thyroid cancers account for most inherited cases of thyroid cancer, while familial papillary and follicular cancers are very rare. Distinct genes are involved in the pathogenesis of individual histologic variants.

- *Papillary thyroid carcinomas:* Two major types of genetic alterations—chromosomal rearrangements and point mutations—are involved in the pathogenesis of papillary thyroid carcinomas. Notably, these alterations lead to activation of similar tumorigenic pathways—the mitogen-activating protein (MAP) kinase signaling pathway—and therefore occur in nonoverlapping subsets of tumors. Chromosomal rearrangements involving the tyrosine kinase receptor gene *RET* (located on chromosome 10q11) occur in approximately a fifth of papillary thyroid carcinomas. Such rearrangements result in the formation of novel fusion genes, known as *ret/PTC* (ret/papillary thyroid carcinoma), which constitutively activate *RET* and the downstream MAP kinase signaling pathway. The frequency of *ret/PTC* rearrangements is significantly higher in papillary cancers arising in children and in the backdrop of radiation exposure. The RET protein is a receptor tyrosine kinase that plays essential roles in the development of neuroendocrine cells. The *NTRK1* gene (neurotrophic tyrosine kinase receptor 1, located on chromosome 1q) is similarly rearranged in approximately 5% to 10% of papillary carcinomas. In contrast to these chromosomal rearrangements, approximately a third to a half of papillary thyroid carcinomas harbor point mutations in the *BRAF* oncogene, which also activate the MAP kinase signaling pathway.
- *Follicular thyroid carcinomas:* Approximately one-half of follicular thyroid carcinomas harbor mutations in the *RAS* family of oncogenes (*HRAS, NRAS,* and *KRAS*). Recently, a unique translocation has been described between *PAX-8,* a paired homeobox gene important in thyroid development, and the gene encoding peroxisome proliferator-activated receptor γ1 *(PPARγ1),* a nuclear hormone receptor implicated in terminal differentiation of cells. The *PAX8-PPARγ1* fusion is present in approximately one-third of follicular thyroid carcinomas, specifically those cancers with a

t(2;3)(q13;p25) translocation, which permits juxtaposition of portions of both genes. Follicular carcinomas seem to arise by two distinct and virtually nonoverlapping molecular pathways: tumors carry either a *RAS* mutation or a *PAX8-PPARγ1* fusion; rarely are both genetic abnormalities present in the same case.

- *Medullary thyroid carcinomas:* Medullary carcinomas arise from the parafollicular C cells in the thyroid. Familial medullary thyroid carcinomas occur in multiple endocrine neoplasia type 2 (see below), and are associated with germ-line *RET* proto-oncogene mutations leading to constitutive activation of the receptor. *RET* mutations are also seen in nonfamilial (sporadic) medullary thyroid cancers. Chromosomal rearrangements such as *ret/PTC* translocations, reported in papillary cancers, are not seen in medullary carcinomas.
- *Anaplastic carcinomas:* These highly aggressive and lethal tumors can arise de novo or by "dedifferentiation" of a well-differentiated papillary or follicular carcinoma. Inactivating point mutations in the *p53* tumor suppressor gene are rare in well-differentiated thyroid carcinomas but common in anaplastic tumors.

Environmental Variables. Exposure to ionizing radiation, particularly during the first 2 decades of life, has emerged as one of the most important influences predisposing to the development of thyroid cancer. In the past, radiation therapy was liberally used in the treatment of several head and neck lesions in infants and children, including reactive tonsillar enlargement, acne, and tinea capitis. As many as 9% of people receiving such treatment during childhood subsequently developed thyroid malignancies, usually several decades after exposure. The incidence of carcinoma of the thyroid is substantially higher, in addition, among atomic bomb survivors in Japan and in those exposed to ionizing radiation after the Chernobyl nuclear plant disaster. *The overwhelming majority of cancers arising in this setting are papillary thyroid cancers, and most have RET gene rearrangements.* Long-standing multinodular goiter has been suggested as a predisposing factor in some cases, since areas with iodine deficiency-related endemic goiter have a higher prevalence of follicular carcinomas.

Papillary Carcinoma

As mentioned above, papillary carcinomas represent the most common form of thyroid cancer. They may occur at any age, and they account for the vast majority of thyroid carcinomas associated with previous exposure to ionizing radiation.

Morphology

Papillary carcinomas may present as solitary or multifocal lesions within the thyroid. In some cases, they may be well circumscribed and even encapsulated; in other instances, they infiltrate the adjacent parenchyma with ill-defined margins. The lesions may contain areas of fibrosis and calcification and are often cystic. On the cut surface, they may appear granular and may sometimes contain grossly discernible papillary foci (Fig. 20–14A). The definitive diagnosis of papillary carcinoma can be made only after microscopic examination. As currently used, **the diagnosis of papillary carcinoma is based on nuclear features** even in the absence of a papillary architecture. The nuclei of papillary carcinoma cells contain very finely dispersed chromatin, which imparts an **optically clear** appearance, giving rise to the designation "ground-glass" or "Orphan Annie eye" nuclei (Fig. 20–14C, D). In addition, invaginations of the cytoplasm may give the appearance of intranuclear inclusions (hence the term **pseudo-inclusions**) in cross-sections. A **papillary architecture** is present in many cases (Fig. 20–14B), although some tumors are composed predominantly or exclusively of follicles; these **follicular variants** still behave biologically as papillary carcinomas if they have the nuclear features described. When present, the papillae of papillary carcinoma differ from those seen in areas of hyperplasia. Unlike hyperplastic papillary lesions, the neoplastic papillae have dense fibrovascular cores. Concentrically calcified structures termed **psammoma bodies** are often present within the papillae. Foci of lymphatic permeation by tumor are often present, but invasion of blood vessels is relatively uncommon, particularly in smaller lesions. Metastases to adjacent cervical lymph nodes are estimated to occur in about half of cases.

Clinical Features. Papillary carcinomas are nonfunctional tumors, and thus they present most often as a painless mass in the neck, either within the thyroid or as metastasis in a cervical lymph node. The presence of isolated cervical nodal metastases, interestingly, does not seem to have a significant influence on the generally good prognosis of these lesions. In a minority of patients, hematogenous metastases are present at the time of diagnosis, most commonly to the lung. Papillary carcinomas are indolent lesions, with 10-year survival rates in excess of 95%. In general, the prognosis is less favorable among elderly persons and in patients with invasion of extra-thyroidal tissues or distant metastases.

Follicular Carcinoma

Follicular carcinomas are the second most common form of thyroid cancer. They usually present at an older age than do papillary carcinomas, with a peak incidence in the middle adult years. The incidence of follicular carcinoma is increased in areas of dietary iodine deficiency, suggesting that, in some cases, nodular goiter may predispose to the development of the neoplasm. The high frequency of *RAS* mutations in follicular adenomas and carcinomas suggests that they may be related tumors.

Morphology

Microscopically, most follicular carcinomas are composed of fairly uniform cells forming small follicles, reminiscent of normal thyroid (Fig. 20–15); in other cases, follicular differentiation may be less apparent. Similar to follicular adenomas, Hürthle cell variants of follicular carcinomas may be seen. Follicular carcinomas may be grossly infiltrative or minimally invasive. The latter are sharply demarcated lesions that may be impossible to distinguish from follicular adenomas on gross examination. **This distinction requires extensive**

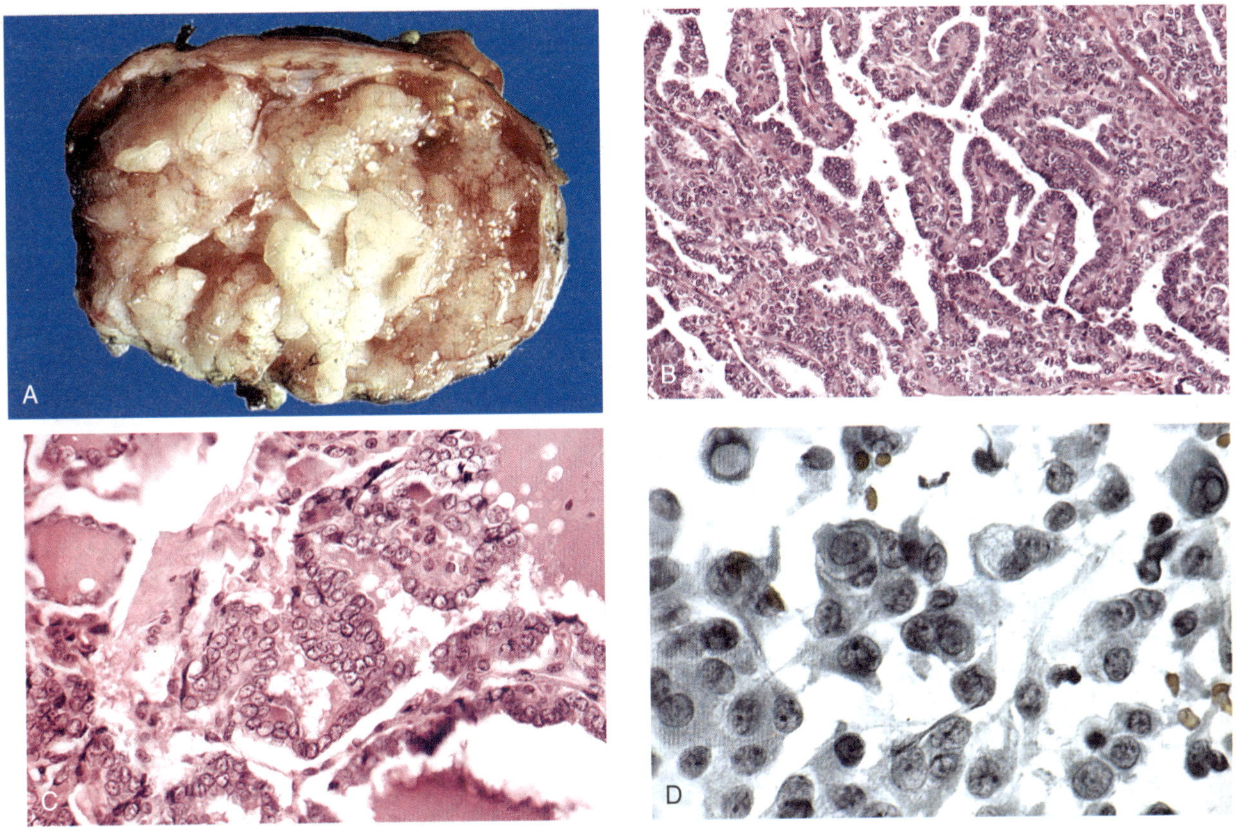

Figure 20–14

Papillary carcinoma of the thyroid. **A,** A papillary carcinoma with grossly discernible papillary structures. This particular example contained well-formed papillae (**B**), lined by cells with characteristic empty-appearing nuclei, sometimes termed "Orphan Annie eye" nuclei (**C**). **D,** Cells obtained by fine-needle aspiration of a papillary carcinoma. Characteristic intranuclear inclusions are visible in some of the aspirated cells. (Courtesy of Dr. S. Gokasalan, Department of Pathology, University of Texas Southwestern Medical School, Dallas, Texas.)

histologic sampling of the tumor-capsule-thyroid interface, to exclude capsular and/or vascular invasion (Fig. 20–16). Extensive invasion of adjacent thyroid parenchyma makes the diagnosis of carcinoma obvious in some cases. As mentioned earlier, follicular lesions in which the nuclear features are typical of papillary carcinomas should be regarded as papillary cancers.

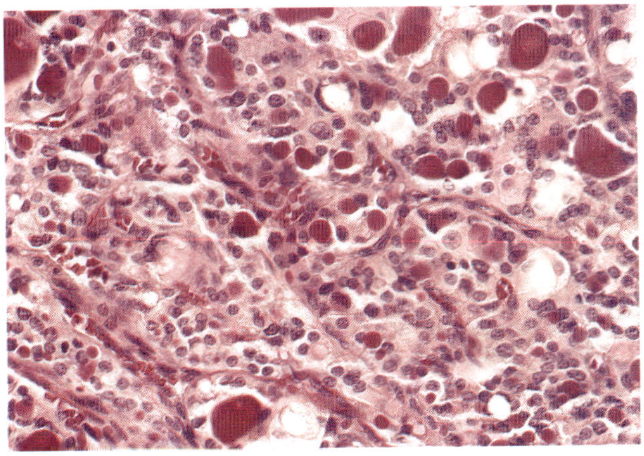

Figure 20–15

Follicular carcinoma of the thyroid. A few of the glandular lumens contain recognizable colloid.

Clinical Features. Follicular carcinomas present most frequently as solitary "cold" thyroid nodules. In rare cases, they may be hyperfunctional. These neoplasms tend to metastasize through the bloodstream to the lungs, bone, and liver. Regional nodal metastases are uncommon, in contrast to papillary carcinomas. Follicular carcinomas are treated with surgical excision. Well-differentiated metastases may take up radioactive iodine, which can be used to identify, and ablate, such lesions. Because better differentiated lesions may be stimulated by TSH, patients are usually treated with thyroid hormone after surgery to suppress endogenous TSH.

Medullary Carcinoma

Medullary carcinomas of the thyroid are neuroendocrine neoplasms derived from the parafollicular cells, or C cells, of the thyroid. Like normal C cells, medullary carcinomas secrete calcitonin, the measurement of which plays an important role in the diagnosis and postoperative follow-up of patients. In some cases, the tumor cells elaborate other polypeptide hormones such as somatostatin, serotonin, and vasoactive intestinal peptide (VIP). Medullary carcinomas arise *sporadically* in about 80% of cases. The remaining 20% are *familial* cases occurring in the setting of MEN syndromes 2A or 2B, or familial medullary thyroid carcinoma (FMTC) without an asso-

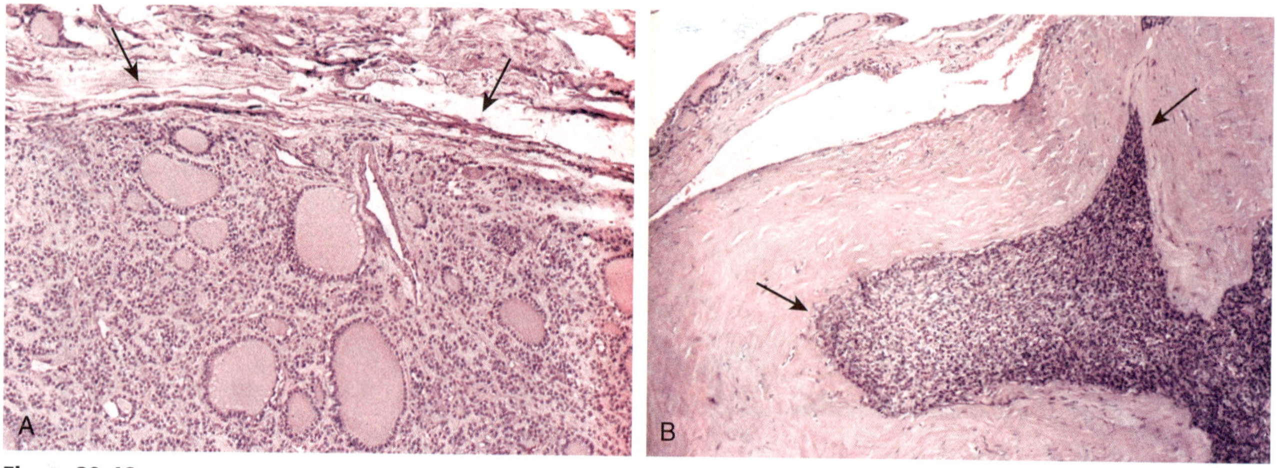

Figure 20–16

Capsular invasion in follicular carcinoma. Evaluating the integrity of the capsule is critical in distinguishing follicular adenomas from follicular carcinomas. In adenomas **(A),** a fibrous capsule, usually thin but occasionally more prominent, surrounds the neoplastic follicles and no capsular invasion is seen *(arrows);* compressed normal thyroid parenchyma is usually present external to the capsule *(top).* **B,** In contrast, follicular carcinomas demonstrate capsular invasion *(arrows)* that may be minimal, as in this case, or widespread with extension into local structures of the neck.

ciated MEN syndrome, as discussed later. Recall that both familial and sporadic medullary forms demonstrate activating *RET* mutations. Sporadic medullary carcinomas, as well as FMTC, occur in adults, with a peak incidence in the fifth to sixth decades. Cases associated with MEN-2A or MEN-2B, in contrast, occur in younger patients and may even arise in children.

Morphology

Medullary carcinomas may arise as a solitary nodule or may present as multiple lesions involving both lobes of the thyroid. **Multicentricity** is particularly common in familial cases. Larger lesions often contain areas of necrosis and hemorrhage and may extend through the capsule of the thyroid. Microscopically, medullary carcinomas are composed of polygonal to spindle-shaped cells, which may form nests, trabeculae, and even follicles. Acellular **amyloid deposits,** derived from altered calcitonin molecules, are present in the adjacent stroma in many cases (Fig. 20–17) and are a distinctive feature of these tumors. Calcitonin is readily demonstrable both within the cytoplasm of the tumor cells and in the stromal amyloid by immunohistochemical methods. Electron microscopy reveals variable numbers of intracytoplasmic membrane-bound electron-dense granules (Fig. 20–18). One of the peculiar features of familial medullary carcinomas is the presence of **multicentric C-cell hyperplasia** in the surrounding thyroid parenchyma, a feature usually absent in sporadic lesions. While the precise criteria for defining what constitutes hyperplasia are variable, the presence of multiple prominent clusters of C cells scattered throughout the parenchyma should raise the specter of a familial tumor, even if that history is not available. Foci of C-cell hyperplasia are believed to represent the precursor lesions from which medullary carcinomas arise.

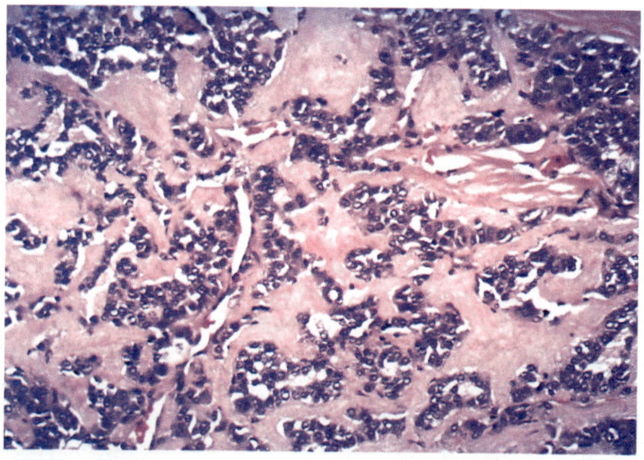

Figure 20–17

Medullary carcinoma of the thyroid. These tumors typically contain amyloid, visible here as homogeneous extracellular material, derived from calcitonin molecules secreted by the neoplastic cells.

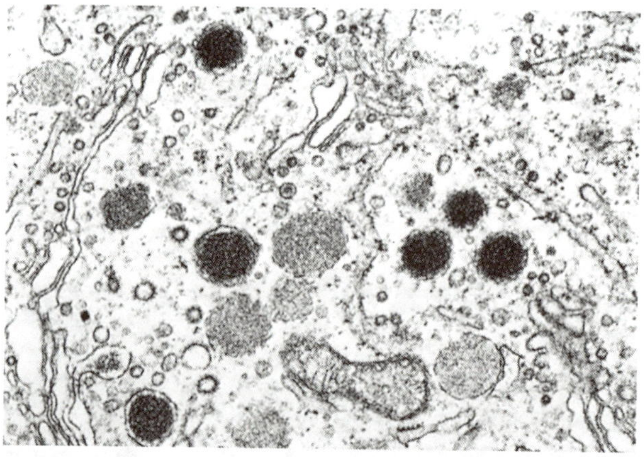

Figure 20–18

Electron micrograph of medullary thyroid carcinoma. These cells contain membrane-bound secretory granules that are the sites of storage of calcitonin and other peptides (original magnification ×30,000).

Clinical Features. Sporadic cases of medullary carcinoma present most often as a mass in the neck, sometimes associated with compression effects such as dysphagia or hoarseness. In some instances the initial manifestations are caused by the secretion of a peptide hormone (e.g., diarrhea caused by the secretion of VIP). Notably, hypocalcemia is not a feature, despite the presence of raised calcitonin levels. Screening of relatives for elevated calcitonin levels or *RET* mutations permits early detection of tumors in familial cases. As discussed at the end of this chapter, all MEN-2 kindred carrying *RET* mutations are offered prophylactic thyroidectomies to preempt the development of medullary carcinomas; often, the only histologic finding in the resected thyroid of these asymptomatic carriers is the presence of C-cell hyperplasia or small (<1 cm) "micromedullary" carcinomas. Recent studies have shown that specific *RET* mutations correlate with an aggressive behavior in medullary carcinomas.

Anaplastic Carcinoma

Anaplastic carcinomas of the thyroid are among the most aggressive human neoplasms, with a near-uniform mortality rate. Individuals with anaplastic carcinoma are older than those with other types of thyroid cancer, with a mean age of 65 years. About half of the patients have a history of multinodular goiter, whereas 20% of the patients with these tumors have a history of differentiated carcinoma; another 20% to 30% have a concurrent differentiated thyroid tumor, frequently a papillary carcinoma. These findings have led to speculation that anaplastic carcinoma develops by "dedifferentiation" from more differentiated tumors as a result of one or more genetic changes, including loss of function of the *p53* tumor suppressor gene.

Morphology

Anaplastic carcinomas present as bulky masses that typically grow rapidly beyond the thyroid capsule into adjacent neck structures. Microscopically, these neoplasms are composed of highly anaplastic cells, which may take on several histologic patterns, including (1) large, pleomorphic **giant cells;** (2) **spindle cells** with a sarcomatous appearance; (3) **mixed** spindle and giant-cell lesions; and (4) **small cells,** resembling those seen in small-cell carcinomas at other sites. It is unlikely that a true small-cell carcinoma exists in the thyroid, and most of the "anaplastic small-cell" tumors ultimately proved to be medullary carcinomas or malignant lymphomas. Foci of papillary or follicular differentiation may be present in some tumors, suggesting origin from a better differentiated carcinoma.

Clinical Features. Anaplastic carcinomas grow with wild abandon despite therapy. Metastases to distant sites are common, but in most cases death occurs in less than 1 year as a result of aggressive local growth and compromise of vital structures in the neck.

SUMMARY

Thyroid Neoplasms

- Most thyroid neoplasms present as solitary thyroid nodules; only 1% of all thyroid nodules are neoplastic.
- Follicular adenomas are the most common benign neoplasms, while papillary carcinoma is the most common malignancy.
- Multiple genetic pathways are involved in thyroid carcinogenesis. Some of the genetic abnormalities that are fairly unique to thyroid cancers include PAX8-PPARγ1 fusion (in follicular carcinoma), chromosomal rearrangements involving the *RET* oncogene (papillary cancers), and mutations of *RET* (medullary carcinomas).
- *Follicular adenomas and carcinomas* are both composed of well-differentiated follicular epithelial cells, and are distinguished by evidence of capsular and/or vascular invasion in the latter.
- *Papillary carcinomas* are recognized based on nuclear features (ground-glass nuclei, pseudo-inclusions) even in the absence of papillae. Psammoma bodies are a characteristic feature of papillary cancers; these neoplasms typically metastasize via lymphatics but their prognosis is excellent.
- *Medullary cancers* are nonepithelial neoplasms arising from the parafollicular C cells and can occur in either sporadic (80%) or familial (20%) settings. Multicentricity and C-cell hyperplasia are features of familial cases. Amyloid deposits are a characteristic histologic finding.
- *Anaplastic carcinomas* are thought to arise by dedifferentiation of more differentiated neoplasms. They are highly aggressive, uniformly lethal cancers.

PARATHYROID GLANDS

The parathyroid glands are derived from the developing pharyngeal pouches that also give rise to the thymus. They normally lie in close proximity to the upper and lower poles of each thyroid lobe, but they may be found anywhere along the pathway of descent of the pharyngeal pouches, including the carotid sheath and the thymus and elsewhere in the anterior mediastinum. Most of the gland is composed of *chief cells*. The chief cells vary from light to dark pink with H&E stains, depending on their glycogen content. They contain secretory granules of *parathyroid hormone (PTH). Oxyphil cells* are found throughout the normal parathyroid either singly or in small clusters. They are slightly larger than the chief cells, have acidophilic cytoplasm, and are tightly packed with mitochondria. *The activity of the parathyroids is controlled by the level of free (ionized) calcium in the bloodstream rather than by trophic hormones secreted by the hypothalamus and pituitary.* Normally, decreased levels of free calcium stimulate the synthesis and secretion of PTH, which in turn:

- Activates osteoclasts, thereby mobilizing calcium from bone
- Increases the renal tubular reabsorption of calcium
- Increases the conversion of vitamin D to its active dihydroxy form in the kidneys
- Increases urinary phosphate excretion
- Augments gastrointestinal calcium absorption.

The net result of these activities is an increase in the level of free calcium, which inhibits further PTH secretion. Abnormalities of the parathyroids include both hyperfunction and hypofunction. *Tumors of the parathyroid glands, unlike thyroid tumors, usually come to attention because of excessive secretion of PTH rather than mass effects.*

HYPERPARATHYROIDISM

Hyperparathyroidism occurs in two major forms, *primary* and *secondary,* and, less commonly, as *tertiary* hyperparathyroidism. The first condition represents an autonomous, spontaneous overproduction of PTH, while the latter two conditions typically occur as secondary phenomena in individuals with chronic renal insufficiency.

Primary Hyperparathyroidism

Primary hyperparathyroidism is one of the most common endocrine disorders, and it is an important cause of *hypercalcemia.* There has been a dramatic increase in the detection of cases beginning in the latter half of the last century, mainly as a result of the greater availability and use of advanced analyzers for detecting serum electrolytes. The frequency of occurrence of the various parathyroid lesions underlying the hyperfunction is as follows:

- Adenoma—75% to 80%
- Primary hyperplasia (diffuse or nodular)—10% to 15%
- Parathyroid carcinoma—less than 5%

In more than 95% of cases, primary hyperparathyroidism is caused by sporadic parathyroid adenomas or sporadic hyperplasia. The genetic defects identified in familial primary hyperparathyroidism include multiple endocrine neoplasia syndromes, specifically MEN-1 and MEN-2A (see below). Familial hypocalciuric hypercalcemia is a rare cause of hyperparathyroidism, caused by inactivating mutations in the calcium-sensing receptor *(CASR)* gene on parathyroid cells, leading to constitutive PTH secretion.

Molecular Pathogenesis of Parathyroid Tumors. Although the detailed discussion of genetic alterations in parathyroid tumors is beyond the scope of this book, two genes whose abnormalities are commonly associated with these tumors will be mentioned. The first of these, called *PRAD1* (for *parathyroid adenomatosis gene 1*), is located on chromosome 11q. The protein product of *PRAD1* belongs to a family of cell-cycle regulators known as cyclins (hence the protein is named cyclin D1). Overexpression of cyclin D1 is common in parathyroid tumors (adenomas and carcinomas) as well as in hyperplasia, and presumably contributes to abnormal growth. In 10% to 20% of adenomas, activation of the cyclin D1 gene occurs by a pericentromeric inversion of chromosome 11 that juxtaposes *PRAD1* with the 5′-regulatory region of the parathyroid hormone gene, thus directing overexpression of cyclin D1 in the parathyroid gland. The second common abnormality involves the tumor suppressor gene *MEN1* on chromosome 11q13, germ-line mutations of which are responsible for the MEN-1 syndrome. Approximately 20% to 30% of parathyroid tumors not associated with the MEN-1 syndrome also demonstrate mutations of the *MEN1* gene.

Morphology

The morphologic changes seen in primary hyperparathyroidism include those in the parathyroid glands as well as those in other organs affected by elevated levels of calcium. In 75% to 80% of cases, one of the parathyroids harbors a solitary **adenoma,** which, like the normal parathyroids, may lie in close proximity to the thyroid gland or in an ectopic site (e.g., the mediastinum). The typical parathyroid adenoma is a well-circumscribed, soft, tan nodule, invested by a delicate capsule. **By definition, parathyroid adenomas are almost invariably confined to single glands** (Fig. 20–19), and the remaining glands are normal in size or somewhat shrunken, as a result of feedback inhibition by elevations in serum calcium. Most parathyroid adenomas weigh between 0.5 and 5 gm. Microscopically, parathyroid adenomas are composed predominantly of chief

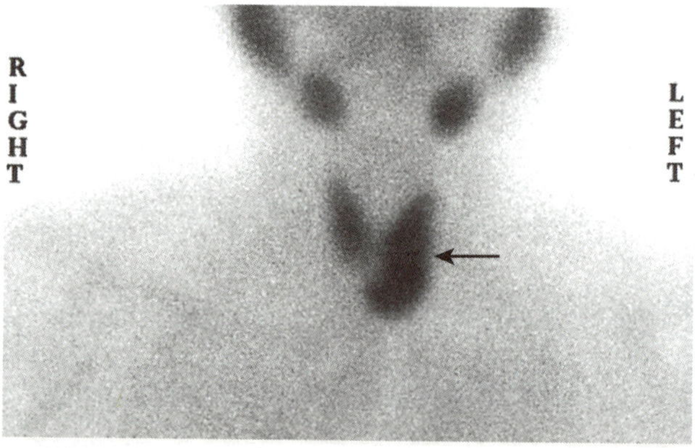

Figure 20–19

Technetium-99m–sestamibi radionuclide scan demonstrates an area of increased uptake corresponding to the left inferior parathyroid gland *(arrow).* This patient had a parathyroid adenoma. Preoperative scintigraphy is useful in localizing and distinguishing adenomas from parathyroid hyperplasia, where more than one gland would demonstrate increased uptake.

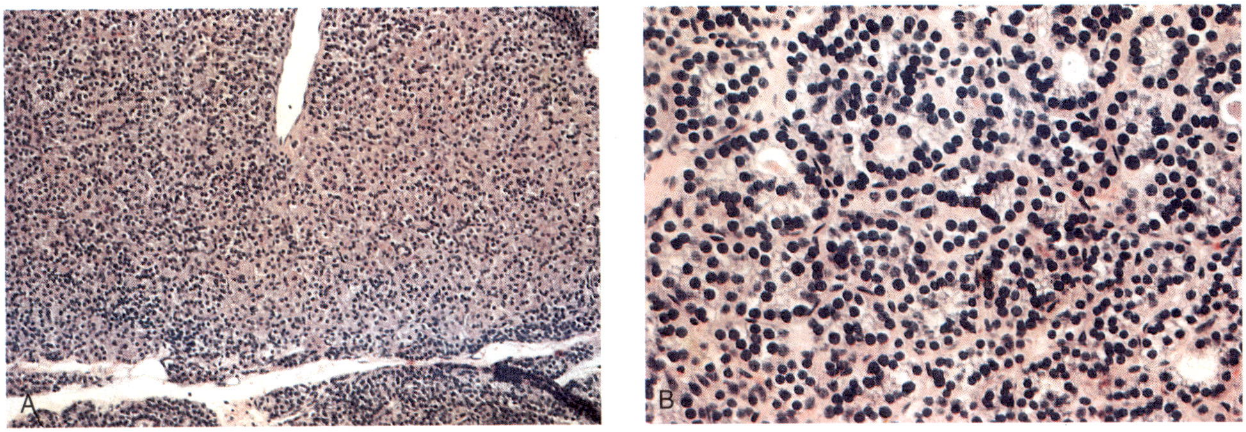

Figure 20–20

A, Solitary chief-cell parathyroid adenoma *(low-power view)* revealing clear delineation from the residual gland below. **B,** High-power detail of chief-cell parathyroid adenoma. There is slight variation in nuclear size and tendency to follicular formation but no anaplasia.

cells (Fig. 20–20). In most cases, at least a few nests of larger oxyphil cells are also present. A rim of compressed, non-neoplastic parathyroid tissue, generally separated by a fibrous capsule, is often visible at the edge of the adenoma. This constitutes a helpful internal control, since the chief cells of the adenoma are larger and show greater nuclear size variability than the normal chief cells. It is not uncommon to find bizarre and pleomorphic nuclei even within adenomas (so-called endocrine atypia), and this should not be used as a criterion for malignancy. Mitotic figures are rare. In contrast to the normal parathyroid parenchyma, adipose tissue is inconspicuous within the adenoma.

Parathyroid hyperplasia is characteristically a multiglandular process. In some cases, however, enlargement may be grossly apparent in only one or two glands, complicating the distinction between hyperplasia and adenoma. The combined weight of all glands may exceed 1 gm but is often less. Microscopically, the most common pattern seen is that of chief-cell hyperplasia, which may involve the glands in a diffuse or multinodular pattern. Less commonly, the constituent cells contain abundant clear cytoplasm due to accumulation of glycogen, a condition designated as water-clear cell hyperplasia. As in the case of adenomas, stromal fat is inconspicuous within foci of hyperplasia.

Parathyroid carcinomas are usually firm or hard tumors, adhering to the surrounding tissue as a result of fibrosis or infiltrative growth (intraoperatively, a fibrous and adherent parathyroid is often a clue that the surgeon is dealing with a carcinoma rather than an adenoma). Parathyroid carcinomas are larger than adenomas, almost always more than 5 gm and sometimes exceeding 10 gm. Like their adenomatous counterparts, parathyroid carcinomas are typically single-gland disorders, and chief cells tend to predominate in most cases. The cytologic features and mitotic activity can be quite variable, showing considerable overlap with those in adenomas; therefore, neither can be reliably used to diagnose parathyroid carcinomas. The only two valid criteria for malignancy are (1) invasion of surrounding tissues and (2) metastatic dissemination.

Morphologic changes in other organs deserving special mention are found in the skeleton and kidneys. **Skeletal changes** include prominence of osteoclasts, which in turn erode bone matrix and mobilize calcium salts, particularly in the metaphyses of long tubular bones. Bone resorption is accompanied by increased osteoblastic activity and the formation of new bone trabeculae. In many cases the resultant bone contains widely spaced, delicate trabeculae reminiscent of those seen in osteoporosis. In more severe cases the cortex is grossly thinned and the marrow contains increased amounts of fibrous tissue accompanied by foci of hemorrhage and cyst formation **(osteitis fibrosa cystica)**. Aggregates of osteoclasts, reactive giant cells, and hemorrhagic debris occasionally form masses that may be mistaken for neoplasms (**brown tumors** of hyperparathyroidism). PTH-induced hypercalcemia favors the formation of urinary tract stones (nephrolithiasis) as well as calcification of the renal interstitium and tubules (nephrocalcinosis). Metastatic calcification secondary to hypercalcemia may also be seen in other sites, including the stomach, lungs, myocardium, and blood vessels.

Clinical Features. Primary hyperparathyroidism is usually a disease of adults and is more common in women than in men by a ratio of nearly 3:1. *The most common manifestation of primary hyperparathyroidism is an increase in serum ionized calcium.* In fact, primary hyperparathyroidism is the most common cause of *clinically silent hypercalcemia*. It should be noted that other conditions also produce hypercalcemia (Table 20–4). *Malignancy,* in particular, is the most common cause of *clinically apparent hypercalcemia* in adults (Chapter 6). The prognosis for individuals with malignancy-associated hypercalcemia is poor, in that it more frequently occurs in individuals with advanced cancers. In persons with hypercalcemia caused by parathyroid hyperfunction, serum PTH is inappropriately elevated, whereas serum PTH is low to undetectable in hypercalcemia caused by nonparathyroid diseases, including malignancy. Other laboratory alterations referable to PTH excess include hypophosphatemia and increased urinary excretion of both calcium and phosphate.

Primary hyperparathyroidism has been traditionally associated with a constellation of symptoms that included "painful bones, renal stones, abdominal groans, and psychic moans". Pain, secondary to fractures of bones

Table 20–4 Causes of Hypercalcemia

Raised PTH	Decreased PTH
Hyperparathyroidism	Hypercalcemia of malignancy
Primary (adenoma > hyperplasia)*	Osteolytic metastases
Secondary†	PTH-rP mediated
Tertiary†	Vitamin D toxicity
Familial hypocalciuric hypercalcemia	Immobilization
	Drugs (thiazide diuretics)
	Granulomatous diseases (sarcoidosis)

PTH, parathyroid hormone; PTH-rP, PTH-related protein.
*Primary hyperparathyroidism is the most common cause of hypercalcemia overall. Malignancy is the most common cause of *symptomatic* hypercalcemia. Primary hyperparathyroidism and malignancy account for nearly 90% of cases of hypercalcemia.
†Secondary and tertiary hyperparathyroidism are most commonly associated with progressive renal failure.

weakened by osteoporosis or osteitis fibrosa cystica and resulting from renal stones, with obstructive uropathy, was at one time a prominent manifestation of primary hyperparathyroidism. Because serum calcium is now routinely assessed in the work-up of most patients who need blood tests for unrelated conditions, clinically silent hyperparathyroidism is detected early. Hence, many of the classic clinical manifestations, particularly those referable to bone and renal disease, are seen much less frequently. Additional signs and symptoms that may be encountered in hyperparathyroidism include the following:

- *Gastrointestinal disturbances,* including constipation, nausea, peptic ulcers, pancreatitis, and gallstones
- *Central nervous system alterations,* including depression, lethargy, and seizures
- *Neuromuscular abnormalities,* including weakness and hypotonia
- *Polyuria* and secondary polydipsia

Although some of these alterations, for example, polyuria and muscle weakness, are clearly related to hypercalcemia, the pathogenesis of many of the other manifestations of the disorder remains poorly understood.

Secondary Hyperparathyroidism

Secondary hyperparathyroidism is caused by any condition associated with a chronic depression in the serum calcium level, because low serum calcium leads to compensatory overactivity of the parathyroids. *Renal failure is by far the most common cause of secondary hyperparathyroidism.* The mechanisms by which chronic renal failure induces secondary hyperparathyroidism are complex and not fully understood. Chronic renal insufficiency is associated with decreased phosphate excretion, which in turn results in hyperphosphatemia. The elevated serum phosphate levels directly depress serum calcium levels and thereby stimulate parathyroid gland activity. In addition, loss of renal substances reduces the availability of α_1-hydroxylase necessary for the synthesis of the active form of vitamin D, which in turn reduces intestinal absorption of calcium (Chapter 8).

Morphology

The parathyroid glands in secondary hyperparathyroidism are hyperplastic. As in the case of primary hyperplasia, the degree of glandular enlargement is not necessarily symmetric. Microscopically, the hyperplastic glands contain an increased number of chief cells, or cells with more abundant, clear cytoplasm **(water-clear cells),** in a diffuse or multinodular distribution. Fat cells are decreased in number. **Bone changes** similar to those seen in primary hyperparathyroidism may also be present. **Metastatic calcification** may be seen in many tissues, including lungs, heart, stomach, and blood vessels.

Clinical Features. The clinical manifestations of secondary hyperparathyroidism are usually dominated by those related to chronic renal failure. Bone abnormalities *(renal osteodystrophy)* and other changes associated with PTH excess are, in general, less severe than those seen in primary hyperparathyroidism. Serum calcium remains near normal because the compensatory increase in PTH levels sustains serum calcium. The metastatic calcification of blood vessels (secondary to hyperphosphatemia) may occasionally result in significant ischemic damage to skin and other organs, a process sometimes referred to as *calciphylaxis.* In a minority of patients, parathyroid activity may become autonomous and excessive, with resultant hypercalcemia, a process sometimes termed *tertiary hyperparathyroidism.* Parathyroidectomy may be necessary to control the hyperparathyroidism in such patients.

SUMMARY

Hyperparathyroidism

- Primary hyperparathyroidism is the most common cause of asymptomatic hypercalcemia.
- In the majority of cases, primary hyperparathyroidism is caused by a sporadic parathyroid adenoma, and, less commonly, by parathyroid hyperplasia.
- Parathyroid adenomas are solitary, while hyperplasia is typically a multiglandular process.
- Skeletal manifestations of hyperparathyroidism include bone resorption, *osteitis fibrosa cystica,* and "brown tumors." Renal changes include nephrolithiasis (stones) and nephrocalcinosis.
- The clinical manifestations of hyperparathyroidism can be summarized as "painful bones, renal stones, abdominal groans, and psychic moans."
- Secondary hyperparathyroidism is most often caused by renal failure, and the parathyroid glands are hyperplastic.
- Malignancies are the most important cause of symptomatic hypercalcemia, which results from osteolytic metastases or release of PTH-related protein from non-parathyroid tumors.

HYPOPARATHYROIDISM

Hypoparathyroidism is far less common than is hyperparathyroidism. The major causes of hypoparathyroidism include the following:

- *Surgical ablation:* inadvertent removal of parathyroids during thyroidectomy.
- *Congenital absence:* usually occurs in conjunction with thymic aplasia and cardiac defects in DiGeorge syndrome (Chapters 5 and 7)
- *Autoimmune hypoparathyroidism:* a hereditary polyglandular deficiency syndrome arising from autoantibodies to multiple endocrine organs (parathyroid, thyroid, adrenals, and pancreas). Chronic fungal infections involving the skin and mucous membranes (mucocutaneous candidiasis) are sometimes encountered in these individuals, suggesting an underlying defect in T-cell function. This condition is discussed more extensively in the context of autoimmune adrenalitis.

The major clinical manifestations of hypoparathyroidism are referable to hypocalcemia and include *increased neuromuscular irritability (tingling, muscle spasms, facial grimacing, and sustained carpopedal spasm or tetany)*, cardiac arrhythmias, and, on occasion, *increased intracranial pressures* and *seizures*. Morphologic changes are generally inconspicuous but may include cataracts, calcification of the cerebral basal ganglia, and dental abnormalities.

ENDOCRINE PANCREAS

The endocrine pancreas consists of about 1 million microscopic clusters of cells, the islets of Langerhans, which contain four major cell types—β, α, δ, and PP (pancreatic polypeptide) cells. The cells can be differentiated morphologically by their staining properties, by the ultrastructural structure of their granules, and by their hormone content. *The β cell produces insulin,* which is the most potent anabolic hormone known, with multiple synthetic and growth-promoting effects; *the α cell secretes glucagon,* inducing hyperglycemia by its glycogenolytic activity in the liver; *δ cells contain somatostatin,* which suppresses both insulin and glucagon release; and *PP cells contain a unique pancreatic polypeptide* (vasoactive intestinal peptide, VIP) that exerts several gastrointestinal effects, such as stimulation of secretion of gastric and intestinal enzymes and inhibition of intestinal motility.

DIABETES MELLITUS

Diabetes mellitus is not a single disease entity but rather a *group of metabolic disorders sharing the common underlying feature of hyperglycemia.* Hyperglycemia in diabetes results from defects in insulin secretion, insulin action, or, most commonly, both. The chronic hyperglycemia and attendant metabolic dysregulation of diabetes mellitus may be associated with secondary damage in multiple organ systems, especially the kidneys, eyes, nerves, and blood vessels. Diabetes affects an estimated 21 million people in the United States (or nearly 7% of the population), as many as a third of whom are undiagnosed. Diabetes is a leading cause of end-stage renal disease, adult-onset blindness, and nontraumatic lower extremity amputations in the United States, underscoring the impact of this disease on the burden of health care costs. It also greatly increases the risk of developing coronary artery disease and cerebrovascular disease. In concert with great technologic advances, there have been pronounced changes in human behavior, with increasingly sedentary life styles and poor eating habits. This has contributed to the simultaneous escalation of diabetes and obesity worldwide, which some have termed the "diabesity" epidemic.

Diagnosis

Blood glucose levels are normally maintained in a very narrow range, usually 70 to 120 mg/dL. The diagnosis of diabetes is established by elevation of blood glucose by any one of three criteria:

1. A random blood glucose concentration of 200 mg/dL or higher, with classical signs and symptoms (discussed below)
2. A fasting glucose concentration of 126 mg/dL or higher on more than one occasion, or
3. An abnormal oral glucose tolerance test (OGTT), in which the glucose concentration is 200 mg/dL or higher 2 hours after a standard carbohydrate load (75 gm of glucose).

Derangements in carbohydrate metabolism proceed along a continuum. Individuals with serum fasting glucose values less than 110 mg/dL, or less than 140 mg/dL following an OGTT, are considered to be euglycemic. However, those with serum fasting glucose greater than 110 but less than 126 mg/dL, or OGTT values of greater than 140 but less than 200 mg/dL, are considered to have *impaired glucose tolerance.* Individuals with impaired glucose tolerance have a significant risk of progressing to overt diabetes over time, with as many as 5% to 10% advancing to full-fledged diabetes mellitus per year. In addition, those with impaired glucose tolerance are at *risk for cardiovascular disease,* due to abnormal carbohydrate metabolism and the coexistence of other risk factors (see Chapter 10).

Classification

Although all forms of diabetes mellitus share hyperglycemia as a common feature, the underlying causes of hyperglycemia vary widely. *The vast majority of cases of diabetes fall into one of two broad classes:*

- *Type 1 diabetes* is characterized by an absolute deficiency of insulin secretion caused by pancreatic β-cell destruction, usually resulting from an autoimmune attack. Type 1 diabetes accounts for approximately 10% of all cases.
- *Type 2 diabetes* is caused by a combination of peripheral resistance to insulin action and an inadequate compensatory response of insulin secretion by the pancreatic β cells ("relative insulin deficiency"). Approximately 80% to 90% of patients have type 2 diabetes.

A variety of monogenic and secondary causes make up the remaining cases of diabetes (Table 20–5). It should be stressed that while the major types of diabetes have different pathogenic mechanisms, *the long-term complications in kidneys, eyes, nerves, and blood vessels are the same and are the principal causes of morbidity and death.*

Normal Insulin Physiology and Glucose Homeostasis

Before discussing the pathogenesis of the two major types of diabetes, we briefly review normal insulin physiology and glucose metabolism. *Normal glucose homeostasis is tightly regulated by three interrelated processes:* (1) glucose production in the liver, (2) glucose uptake and utilization by peripheral tissues, chiefly skeletal muscle, and, (3) actions of insulin and counter-regulatory hormones (e.g., glucagon). *The principal metabolic function of insulin is to increase the rate of glucose transport into certain cells in the body* (Fig. 20–21). These are the *striated muscle cells* (including myocardial cells) and, to a lesser extent, *adipocytes,* representing collectively about two-thirds of the entire body weight. Glucose uptake in other peripheral tissues, most notably the brain, is insulin independent. In muscle cells, glucose is then either stored as glycogen or oxidized to generate adenosine triphosphate (ATP). In adipose tissue, glucose is primarily stored as lipid. Besides promoting lipid synthesis (lipogenesis), insulin also inhibits lipid degradation (lipolysis) in adipocytes. Similarly, insulin promotes amino acid uptake and protein synthesis while inhibiting protein degradation. *Thus, the metabolic effects of insulin can be summarized as anabolic, with increased synthesis and reduced degradation of glycogen, lipid, and protein.* In addition to these metabolic effects, insulin has several *mitogenic* functions, including initiation of DNA synthesis in certain cells and stimulation of their growth and differentiation.

Insulin reduces the production of glucose from the liver. Insulin and glucagon have opposing regulatory effects on glucose homeostasis. During *fasting* states, low insulin and high glucagon levels facilitate hepatic gluconeogenesis and glycogenolysis (glycogen breakdown) while decreasing glycogen synthesis, thereby preventing hypoglycemia. Thus, *fasting* plasma glucose levels are determined primarily by hepatic glucose output. Following a meal, insulin levels rise and glucagon levels fall in response to the large glucose load. *The most important stimulus that triggers insulin release is glucose itself, which initiates insulin synthesis in the pancreatic β cells.* Other agents, including intestinal hormones and certain amino acids (leucine and arginine), stimulate insulin

Table 20–5 Etiologic Classification of Diabetes Mellitus

1. Type 1 Diabetes
β-cell destruction, leads to absolute insulin deficiency
2. Type 2 Diabetes
Insulin resistance with relative insulin deficiency
3. Genetic Defects of β-Cell Function
MODY, caused by mutations in: HNF-4α (MODY1) Glucokinase (MODY2) HNF-1α (MODY3) IPF-1 (MODY4) HNF-1β (MODY5) Neuro D1 (MODY6) Mitochondrial DNA mutations
4. Genetic Defects in Insulin Processing or Insulin Action
Defects in proinsulin conversion Insulin gene mutations Insulin receptor mutations
5. Exocrine Pancreatic Defects
Chronic pancreatitis Pancreatectomy Neoplasia Cystic fibrosis Hemochromatosis Fibrocalculous pancreatopathy
6. Endocrinopathies
Growth hormone excess (acromegaly) Cushing syndrome Hyperthyroidism Pheochromocytoma Glucagonoma
7. Infections
Cytomegalovirus Coxsackievirus B
8. Drugs
Glucocorticoids Thyroid hormone β-adrenergic agonists
9. Genetic Syndromes Associated with Diabetes
Down syndrome Kleinfelter syndrome Turner syndrome
10. Gestational Diabetes Mellitus

HNF, hepatocyte nuclear factor; IPF-1, insulin promoter factor 1; MODY, maturity-onset diabetes of the young; Neuro D1, neurogenic differentiation factor 1.

Adapted from the Report of the American Diabetes Association (ADA) Expert Committee on the Diagnosis and Classification of Diabetes Mellitus. *Diabetic Care* 25 (Suppl.1):S5-S20, 2002.

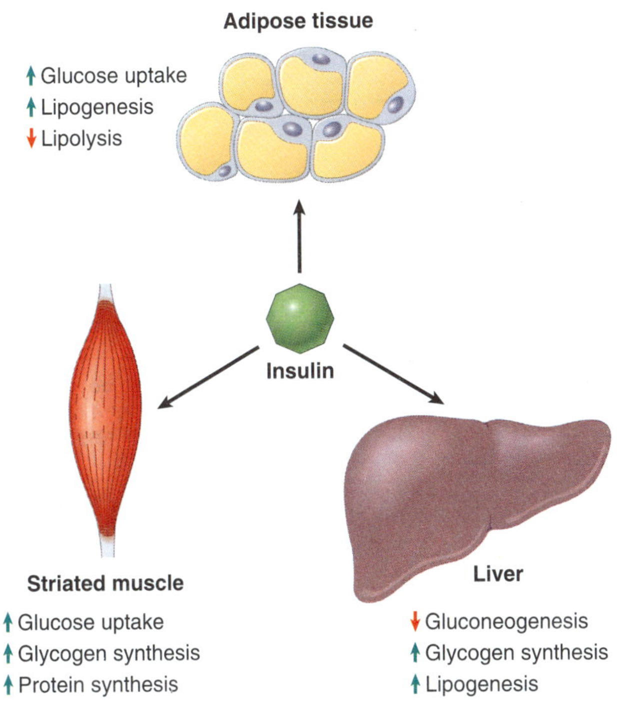

Figure 20–21

Metabolic actions of insulin in striated muscle, adipose tissue, and liver.

release but not its synthesis. In peripheral tissues (skeletal muscle and adipose tissue), secreted insulin binds to the *insulin receptor,* triggering a number of intracellular responses that promote glucose uptake and post-prandial glucose utilization, thereby maintaining glucose homeostasis. Abnormalities at various points along this complex signaling cascade, from synthesis and release of insulin by β cells to insulin receptor interactions in peripheral tissues, can result in the diabetic phenotype.

Pathogenesis of Type 1 Diabetes Mellitus

Type 1 diabetes is an *autoimmune disease* in which islet destruction is caused primarily by T lymphocytes reacting against as yet poorly defined β-cell antigens, resulting in a reduction in β-cell mass. Recent studies have implicated immunologic epitopes on insulin hormone itself as a target antigen for autoimmune injury, but it remains to be convincingly established whether this is a universal phenomenon in all cases of type 1 diabetes or in only a subset. What is also unclear is how immunologic tolerance breaks down in the setting of type 1 diabetes. As in all autoimmune diseases, genetic susceptibility and environmental influences play important roles in the pathogenesis. Type 1 diabetes most commonly develops in childhood, becomes manifest at puberty, and is progressive with age. Most individuals with type 1 diabetes depend on exogenous insulin supplementation for survival, and without insulin, they develop serious metabolic complications such as acute ketoacidosis and coma.

Although the clinical onset of type 1 diabetes is abrupt, this disease in fact results from a chronic autoimmune attack on β cells that usually starts many years before the disease becomes evident (Fig. 20–22). The classic manifestations of the disease (hyperglycemia and ketosis) occur late in its course, after more than 90% of the β cells have been destroyed. *Several mechanisms contribute to β-cell destruction, and it is likely that many of these immune mechanisms work together to produce progressive loss of β cells,* resulting in clinical diabetes:

- *T lymphocytes* react against β-cell antigens and cause cell damage. These T cells include CD4+ T cells of the T_H1 subset, which cause tissue injury by activating macrophages, and CD8+ cytotoxic T lymphocytes, which directly kill β cells and also secrete cytokines that activate macrophages. In the rare cases in which the pancreatic lesions have been examined at the early active stages of the disease, the islets show cellular necrosis and lymphocytic infiltration. This lesion is called *insulitis.*
- Locally produced *cytokines* damage β cells. Among the cytokines implicated in the cell injury are IFN-γ, produced by T cells, and tumor necrosis factor and interleukin-1, produced by macrophages that are activated during the immune reaction.
- *Autoantibodies* against a variety of β-cell antigens, including insulin and glutamic acid decarboxylase, are also detected in the blood of 70% to 80% of patients and may contribute to islet damage.

Type 1 diabetes has a *complex pattern of genetic association,* and putative susceptibility genes have been

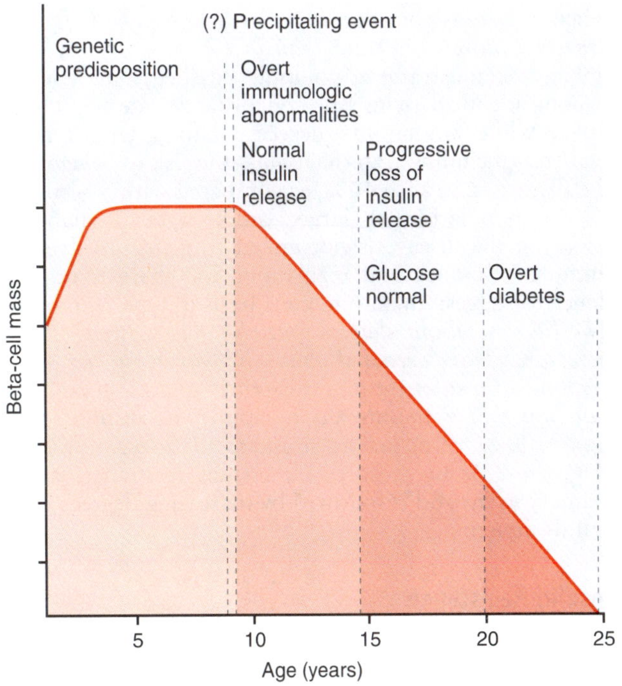

Figure 20–22

Stages in the development of type 1 diabetes mellitus. The stages are listed from left to right, and hypothetical β-cell mass is plotted against age. (From Eisenbarth GE: Type 1 diabetes—a chronic autoimmune disease. N Engl J Med 314:1360, 1986.)

mapped to at least 20 chromosomal regions. Of these, *the principal susceptibility locus for type 1 diabetes resides in the region that encodes the class II MHC molecules on chromosome 6p21 (HLA-D)*. Between 90% and 95% of Caucasians with type 1 diabetes have *HLA-DR3*, or *DR4*, or both, in contrast to about 40% of normal subjects, and 40% to 50% of patients are *DR3/DR4* heterozygotes, in contrast to 5% of normal subjects. Despite the high relative risk of type 1 diabetes in individuals with particular class II alleles, most persons who inherit these alleles do not develop the disease. Another gene shown to be weakly associated with the disease encodes the T-cell inhibitory receptor CTLA-4. Individuals with type 1 diabetes show increased frequency of a splice variant that may abrogate the normal ability of this receptor to keep self-reactive T lymphocytes under control. As mentioned above, we do not know the actual genes in the many other susceptibility loci. There is also evidence to suggest that *environmental factors*, especially infections, may be involved in type 1 diabetes as in other autoimmune diseases. It has been proposed that viruses may be an initiating trigger, perhaps because some viral antigens are antigenically similar to β cell antigens (molecular minicry), but this idea is unproved. The controversy is compounded by recent evidence indicating that infections are actually protective.

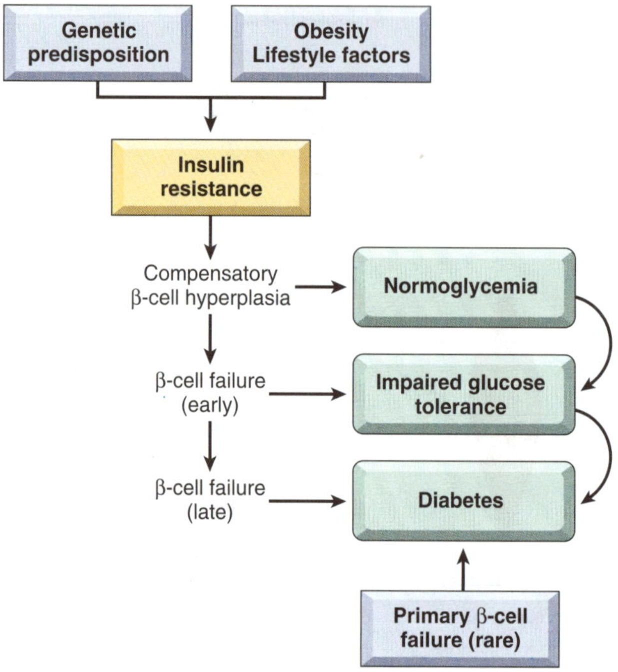

Figure 20–23

Pathogenesis of type 2 diabetes mellitus. Genetic predisposition and environmental influences converge to cause insulin resistance. Compensatory β-cell hyperplasia can maintain normoglycemia, but eventually β-cell secretory dysfunction sets in, leading to impaired glucose tolerance and eventually frank diabetes. Rare instances of primary β-cell failure can directly lead to type 2 diabetes without a state of insulin resistance.

Pathogenesis of Type 2 Diabetes Mellitus

While much has been learned in recent years, the pathogenesis of type 2 diabetes remains enigmatic. Environmental influences, such as a sedentary life style and dietary habits, clearly have a role, as will become evident when obesity is considered. Nevertheless, *genetic factors are even more important than in type 1 diabetes,* with linkage demonstrable to multiple "diabetogenic" genes. Among identical twins, the concordance rate is 50% to 90%, while among first-degree relatives with type 2 diabetes (including fraternal twins) the risk of developing the disease is 20% to 40%, as compared with 5% to 7% in the population at large. Unlike type 1 diabetes, however, the disease is not linked to genes involved in immune tolerance and regulation, and there is no evidence to suggest an autoimmune basis to type 2 diabetes. *The two metabolic defects that characterize type 2 diabetes are (1) a decreased ability of peripheral tissues to respond to insulin (insulin resistance) and (2) β-cell dysfunction that is manifested as inadequate insulin secretion in the face of insulin resistance and hyperglycemia* (Fig. 20–23). In most cases, insulin resistance is the primary event and is followed by increasing degrees of β-cell dysfunction.

Insulin Resistance

Insulin resistance is defined as resistance to the effects of insulin on glucose uptake, metabolism, or storage. Insulin resistance is a characteristic feature of most individuals with type 2 diabetes and is an almost universal finding in diabetic individuals who are obese. The evidence that insulin resistance has a major role in the pathogenesis of type 2 diabetes can be gauged from the findings that (1) insulin resistance is often detected 10 to 20 years before the onset of diabetes in predisposed individuals (e.g., offspring of type 2 diabetics), and (2) in prospective studies, insulin resistance is the best predictor for subsequent progression to diabetes. *It is recognized that insulin resistance is a complex phenomenon, influenced by a variety of genetic and environmental factors.*

Genetic Defects of the Insulin Receptor and Insulin Signaling Pathway. Loss-of-function abnormalities of either the insulin receptor or its down-stream signaling molecules are obvious candidates for mediating insulin resistance in type 2 diabetes. Much of the role of genetic defects in the insulin signaling pathway has been elucidated from targeted disruption of these genes in knockout mouse models of diabetes. Unfortunately, the extrapolation of these single-gene knockout models to human disease has been less than gratifying, underscoring the *multifactorial etiology of insulin resistance in humans.* Point mutations of the insulin receptor are relatively rare, accounting for no more than 1% to 5% of patients with insulin resistance (see "Monogenic Forms of Diabetes"). The vast majority of individuals with conventional type 2 diabetes, however, do *not* harbor inactivating mutations in either the insulin receptor or other components of the insulin-signaling pathway.

Obesity and Insulin Resistance. The association of obesity with type 2 diabetes has been recognized for decades, with visceral obesity being common in the majority of type 2 diabetics. Insulin resistance is *the link between obesity and diabetes* (Fig. 20–24). The risk for diabetes increases as the body mass index (a measure of body fat content) increases, suggesting a dose-response relationship between body fat and insulin resistance. Although many details of the "adipo-insulin axis" remain to be elucidated, there has been a substantial increase in our recognition of some of the putative pathways leading to insulin resistance:

- *Role of free fatty acids (FFAs):* Cross-sectional studies have demonstrated an inverse correlation between fasting plasma FFAs and insulin sensitivity. The level of intracellular triglycerides is often markedly increased in muscle and liver tissues in obese individuals, presumably because excess circulating FFAs are deposited in these organs. Intracellular triglycerides and products of fatty acid metabolism are potent inhibitors of insulin signaling and result in an acquired insulin resistance state. These "lipotoxic" effects of FFAs are most likely mediated through a decrease in activity of key insulin-signaling proteins.
- *Role of adipocytokines in insulin resistance:* Adipose tissue is not merely a passive storage depot for fat; it can operate as a functional endocrine organ, releasing hormones in response to extracellular stimuli or changes in the metabolic status. *A variety of proteins released into the systemic circulation by adipose tissue have been identified, and these are collectively termed adipocytokines.* Among these are *leptin, adiponectin,* and *resistin;* changes in their levels are associated with insulin resistance. For example, adiponectin levels are *reduced* in states of obesity and insulin resistance, suggesting that, under physiologic conditions, this cytokine contributes to insulin sensitivity in peripheral tissues. Conversely, levels of resistin are increased in obesity, and this cytokine contributes to insulin resistance.
- *Role of the PPARγ and thiazolidinediones (TZD):* TZDs are a class of antidiabetic compounds that were first developed in the early 1980s as antioxidants. The target receptor for TZDs has been identified as PPARγ, a nuclear receptor and transcription factor. *PPARγ is most highly expressed in adipose tissue, and its activation by TZDs results in modulation of gene expression in adipocytes,* eventually leading to reduction of insulin resistance. The targets of PPARγ activation include several of the adipocytokines discussed above. PPARγ activation also decreases concentrations of FFAs, which you will recall as another element contributing to insulin resistance in obesity.
- A family of proteins called *sirtuins,* which were identified as being involved in aging, have also been implicated in diabetes. The best-studied mammalian sirtuin, called Sirt-1, has been shown to improve glucose tolerance, enhance β cell insulin secretion, and increase production of adiponectin. It remains to be seen if sirtuin abnormalities are involved in the pathogenesis of type 2 diabetes.

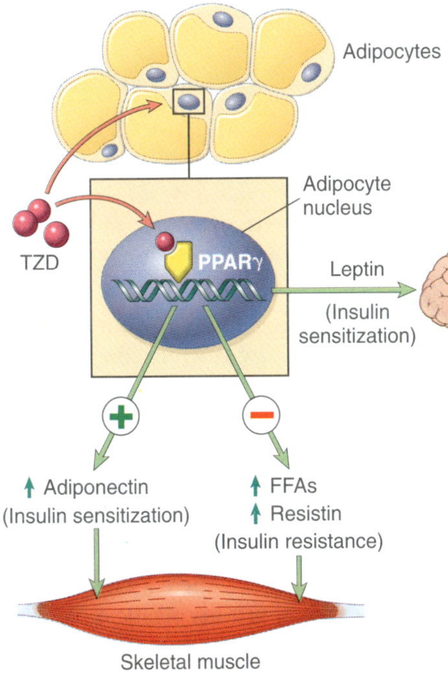

Figure 20–24

Obesity and insulin resistance: the missing links? Adipocytes release a variety of factors (free fatty acids [FFAs] and adipocytokines) that may have a role in modulating insulin resistance in peripheral tissues (illustrated here is striated muscle). Excess FFAs and resistin are associated with insulin resistance; in contrast, adiponectin, whose levels are decreased in obesity, is an insulin-sensitizing adipocytokine. Leptin is also an insulin-sensitizing agent but acts via central receptors (in the hypothalamus). The peroxisome proliferator-activated receptor γ (PPARγ) is a adipocyte nuclear receptor that is activated by a class of insulin-sensitizing drugs called thiazolidinediones (TZDs). The mechanism of action of TZDs may eventually be mediated through modulation of adipocytokine and FFA levels that favor a state of insulin sensitivity.

To summarize, insulin resistance in type 2 diabetes is a complex and multifactorial phenomenon. Genetic defects in the insulin signaling pathway are not common, and when present, they are more likely to be subtle variations in function of multiple components in this pathway rather than a single profound inactivating mutation. Insulin resistance is present in the overwhelming majority of individuals, and obesity is central to this phenomenon (see Fig. 20–24). Several possible links between obesity and insulin resistance have been suggested, including excessive amounts of FFAs and a variety of adipocyte-specific products (adipocytokines). TZDs are insulin-sensitizing drugs that act via the PPARγ receptor, and represent one of the many major advances achieved in ameliorating insulin resistance in diabetes.

β-Cell Dysfunction

β-cell dysfunction in type 2 diabetes reflects the inability of these cells to adapt themselves to the long-term demands of peripheral insulin resistance and increased insulin secretion. In states of insulin resistance, insulin secretion is initially higher for each level of glucose than in controls. This hyperinsulinemic state is a compensation for peripheral resistance and can often maintain normal plasma glucose for years. Although the data in humans are scant, studies from animal models of diabetes support the aforementioned sequence of events wherein β-cell hyperplasia in the pre-diabetic state is followed by decrease in β-cell mass that coincides with clinical progression to diabetes. Eventually, however, β-cell compensation becomes inadequate, and there is progression to overt diabetes. The underlying bases for failure of β-cell adaptation is not known, although it is postulated that several mechanisms, including adverse effects of high circulating FFAs ("lipotoxicity") or chronic hyperglycemia ("glucotoxicity"), may have a role. *β-cell dysfunction in type 2 diabetes encompasses both qualitative and quantitative aspects.*

- Qualitative β-cell dysfunction is initially manifest as subtle abnormalities, such as loss in the normal pulsatile, oscillating pattern of insulin secretion, and attenuation of the rapid first phase of insulin secretion triggered by elevation in plasma glucose. Over time, the secretory defect progresses to encompass all phases of insulin secretion, and even though some basal insulin secretion persists in type 2 diabetes, it is inadequate for overcoming insulin resistance.
- Quantitative β-cell dysfunction is manifest as a *decrease in β-cell mass, islet degeneration, and deposition of islet amyloid.* Islet amyloid protein (amylin) is a characteristic finding in individuals with type 2 diabetes, and it is present in more than 90% of diabetic islets examined. Islet amyloidosis is associated with a decrease in β-cell mass, although it is uncertain whether the amyloid is a cause or consequence of cell damage in type 2 diabetes. In this context, it is important to note that even a "normal" β-cell mass in diabetic individuals may, in fact, indicate a relative reduction as compared with the expected hyperplasia needed to compensate for insulin resistance.

Monogenic Forms of Diabetes

Types 1 and 2 diabetes are genetically complex, and despite the associations with multiple susceptibility loci, no single gene defect (mutation) can account for predisposition to these entities. In contrast, monogenic forms of diabetes (Table 20–5) are uncommon examples of the *diabetic phenotype occurring secondary to loss-of-function mutations within a single gene.* Monogenic causes of diabetes result from either a primary defect in β-cell function or a defect in insulin–insulin receptor signaling.

Pathogenesis of the Complications of Diabetes

Most of the available experimental and clinical evidence suggests that the complications of diabetes are a consequence of the metabolic derangements, mainly hyperglycemia. At least three distinct metabolic pathways seem to be involved in the pathogenesis of long-term diabetic complications, although the primacy of any one has not been established. These pathways include:

1. *Non-enzymatic glycosylation.* This is the process by which glucose chemically attaches to free amino groups of proteins without the aid of enzymes. The degree of nonenzymatic glycosylation is directly related to blood glucose level; indeed, the measurement of glycosylated hemoglobin levels in blood is useful in the management of diabetes mellitus, because it provides an index of the average blood glucose levels over the 120-day life span of erythrocytes. The early glycosylation products of collagen and other long-lived proteins in interstitial tissues and blood vessel walls undergo a slow series of chemical rearrangements to form irreversible *advanced glycosylation end products* (AGEs), which accumulate over the lifetime of the vessel wall. AGEs have a number of chemical and biologic properties that are pathogenic to extracellular matrix components and to the target cells of diabetic complications:

- AGE formation on proteins such as collagen causes cross-links between polypetides; this in turn may trap nonglycosylated plasma and interstitial proteins. In large vessels, trapping low-density lipoprotein, for example, retards its efflux from the vessel wall and enhances the deposition of cholesterol in the intima, thus accelerating atherogenesis. In capillaries, including those of renal glomeruli, plasma proteins such as albumin bind to the glycated basement membrane, accounting in part for the basement membrane thickening characteristic of diabetic glomerulopathy.
- Circulating plasma proteins are modified by the addition of AGE residues; these proteins, in turn, bind to AGE receptors on several cell types (endothelial cells, mesangial cells, macrophages). The biologic effects of AGE-receptor signaling include (1) release of cytokines and growth factors from macrophages and mesangial cells; (2) increased endothelial permeability; (3) increased procoagulant activity on endothelial cells and macrophages; and (4) enhanced proliferation and synthesis of extracellular matrix by fibroblasts and smooth muscle cells. All these effects can potentially contribute to diabetic complications.

2. *Activation of protein kinase C.* Activation of intracellular protein kinase C (PKC) by calcium ions and the second messenger diacylglycerol (DAG) is an important signal transduction pathway in many cellular systems. Intracellular hyperglycemia can stimulate the de novo synthesis of DAG from glycolytic intermediates and hence cause activation of PKC. The down-stream effects of PKC activation are numerous and include production of *pro-angiogenic molecules* such as vascular endothelial growth factor, implicated in the neovascularization seen in diabetic retinopathy, and pro-fibrogenic molecules like transforming growth factor β, leading to increased deposition of extracellular matrix and basement membrane material.

3. *Intracellular hyperglycemia with disturbances in polyol pathways.* In some tissues that do not require insulin for glucose transport (e.g., nerves, lens, kidneys, blood vessels), hyperglycemia leads to an increase in intracellular glucose that is then metabolized by the enzyme *aldose reductase* to sorbitol, a polyol, and eventually to fructose. While accumulated sorbitol and fructose have traditionally been implicated in causing cell injury via increased intracellular osmolarity and water influx, accumulating evidence suggests that the deleterious consequences of the aldose reductase pathway arise primarily by an increase in cellular susceptibility to

oxidative stress. This is because intracellular antioxidant reserves are diminished in the course of sorbitol metabolism. The importance of this pathway in human diabetes is not clear because clinical trials using an aldose reductase inhibitor fail to significantly ameliorate the development of diabetic neuropathy.

SUMMARY

Pathogenesis of Diabetes Mellitus and Its Long-Term Complications

- Type 1 diabetes is an autoimmune disease characterized by progressive destruction of islet β cells, leading to absolute insulin deficiency. Several immune mechanisms probably contribute to β-cell damage, including T cells, cytokines, and autoantibodies.
- Type 2 diabetes has no autoimmune basis; instead, features central to its pathogenesis are insulin resistance and β-cell dysfunction, resulting in relative insulin deficiency.
- Obesity has an important relationship with insulin resistance (and hence, type 2 diabetes), probably mediated by cytokines released from adipose tissues (adipocytokines). Other players in the "adipo-insulin axis" include free fatty acids (which may cause "lipotoxicity") and the PPARγ receptor, which modulates adipocytokine levels.
- Monogenic forms of diabetes are uncommon and are caused by single-gene defects that result in primary β-cell dysfunction (e.g., *glucokinase* mutation) or lead to abnormalities of insulin–insulin receptor signaling (e.g., insulin receptor gene mutations).
- The long-term complications of diabetes are similar in both types and involve three underlying mechanisms: formation of AGEs through nonenzymatic glycosylation, activation of PKC, and accumulation of intracellular sorbitol.

Morphology of Diabetes and Its Late Complications

Pathologic findings in the pancreas are variable and not necessarily dramatic. The important morphologic changes are related to the many late systemic complications of diabetes. There is extreme variability among patients in the time of onset of these complications, their severity, and the particular organ or organs involved. In individuals with tight control of diabetes the onset may be delayed. In most patients, however, morphologic changes are likely to be found in arteries **(macrovascular disease)**, basement membranes of small vessels **(microangiopathy)**, kidneys **(diabetic nephropathy)**, retina **(retinopathy)**, nerves **(neuropathy)**, and other tissues. These changes are seen in both type 1 and type 2 diabetes (Fig. 20–25).

Pancreas. Lesions in the pancreas are inconstant and rarely of diagnostic value. Distinctive changes are more commonly associated with type 1 than with type 2 diabetes. One or more of the following alterations may be present.

- **Reduction in the number and size of islets.** This is most often seen in type 1 diabetes, particularly with rapidly advancing disease. Most of the islets are small, inconspicuous, and not easily detected.
- **Leukocytic infiltration of the islets** (insulitis) principally composed of T lymphocytes similar to that in animal models of autoimmune diabetes (Fig. 20–26A). This may be seen in type 1 diabetics at the time of clinical presentation. The distribution of insulitis may be strikingly uneven. Eosinophilic infiltrates may also be found, particularly in diabetic infants who fail to survive the immediate postnatal period.
- **In type 2 diabetes there may be a subtle reduction in islet cell mass,** demonstrated only by special morphometric studies.
- **Amyloid replacement of islets in long-standing type 2 diabetes** appears as deposition of pink, amorphous material beginning in and around capillaries and between cells. At advanced stages the islets may be virtually obliterated (Fig. 20–26B); fibrosis may also be observed. This change is often seen in long-standing cases of type 2 diabetes. Similar lesions may be found in elderly nondiabetics, apparently as part of normal aging.
- **An increase in the number and size of islets is especially characteristic of nondiabetic newborns of diabetic mothers.** Presumably, fetal islets undergo hyperplasia in response to the maternal hyperglycemia.

Diabetic Macrovascular Disease. Diabetes exacts a heavy toll on the vascular system. The hallmark of diabetic macrovascular disease is accelerated atherosclerosis affecting the aorta and large and medium-sized arteries. Except for its greater severity and earlier age of onset, atherosclerosis in diabetics is indistinguishable from that in nondiabetics (Chapter 10). Myocardial infarction, caused by atherosclerosis of the coronary arteries, is the most common cause of death in diabetics. Significantly, it is almost as common in diabetic women as in diabetic men. In contrast, myocardial infarction is uncommon in nondiabetic women of reproductive age. Gangrene of the lower extremities, as a result of advanced vascular disease, is about 100 times more common in diabetics than in the general population. The larger renal arteries are also subject to severe atherosclerosis, but the most damaging effect of diabetes on the kidneys is exerted at the level of the glomeruli and the microcirculation. This is discussed later.

Hyaline arteriolosclerosis, the vascular lesion associated with hypertension (Chapters 10 and 14), is both more prevalent and more severe in diabetics than in nondiabetics, but it is not specific for diabetes and may be seen in elderly nondiabetics without hypertension. It takes the form of an amorphous, hyaline thickening of the wall of the arterioles, which causes narrowing of the lumen (Fig. 20–27). Not surprisingly, in diabetics it is related not only to the duration of the disease but also to the level of blood pressure.

Diabetic Microangiopathy. One of the most consistent morphologic features of diabetes is **diffuse thickening of basement membranes.** The thickening is most

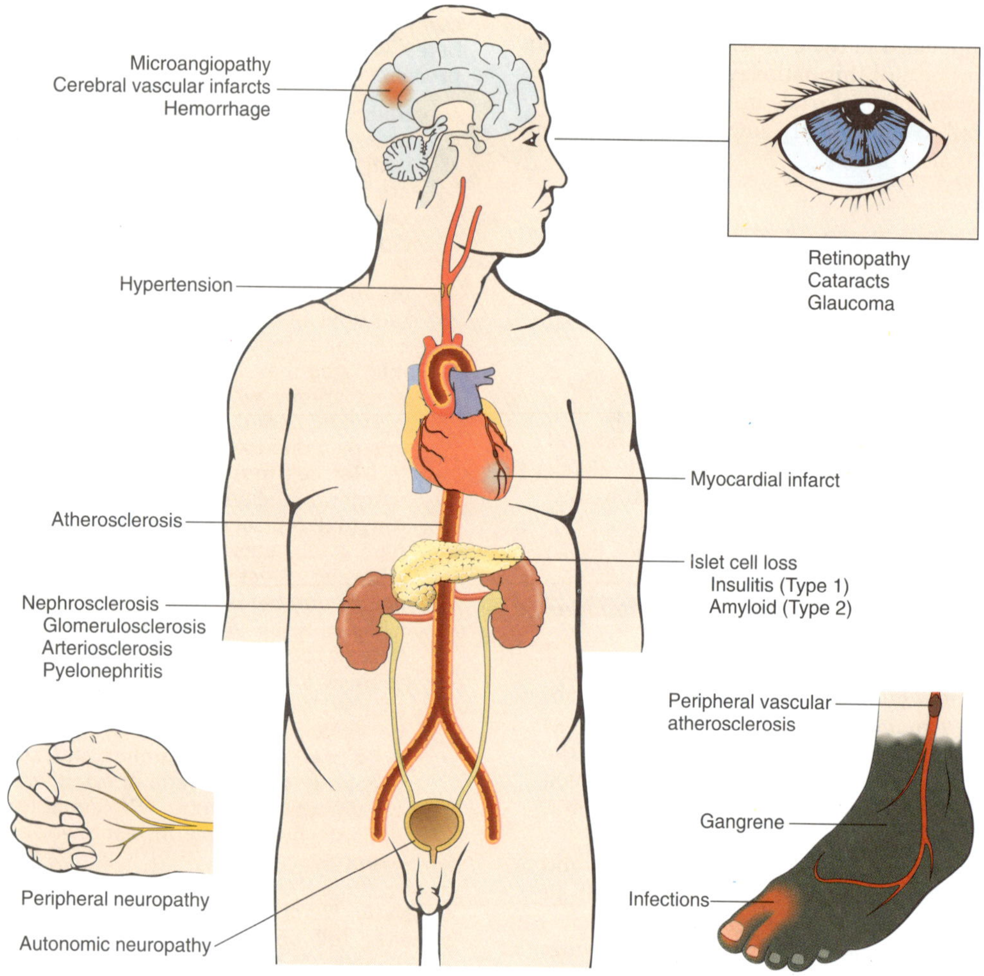

Figure 20–25

Long-term complications of diabetes.

evident in the capillaries of the skin, skeletal muscle, retina, renal glomeruli, and renal medulla. However, it may also be seen in such nonvascular structures as renal tubules, the Bowman capsule, peripheral nerves, and placenta. By both light and electron microscopy, the basal lamina separating parenchymal or endothelial cells from the surrounding tissue is markedly thickened by concentric layers of hyaline material composed

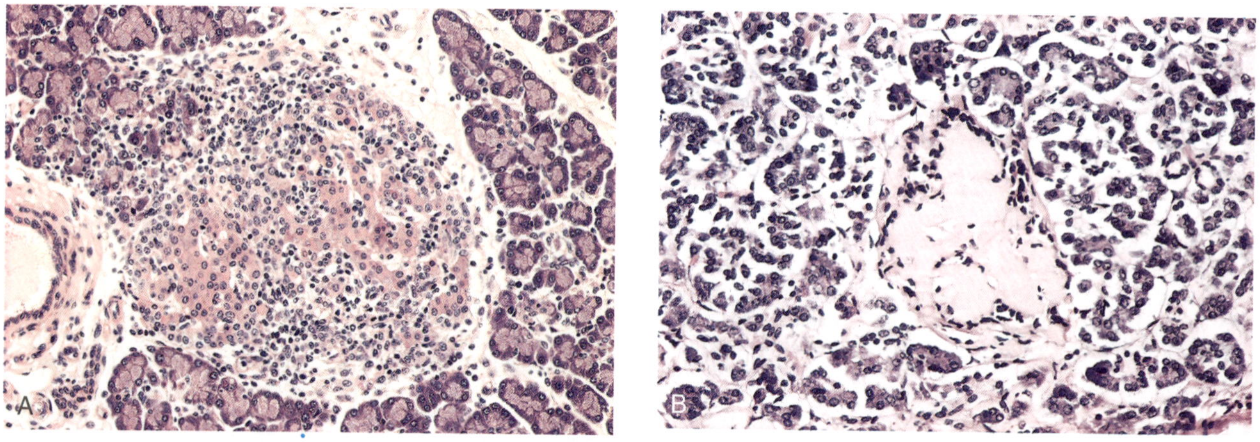

Figure 20–26

A, Insulitis, shown here from a rat (BB) model of autoimmune diabetes, and seen in type 1 human diabetes. **B,** Amyloidosis of a pancreatic islet in type 2 diabetes. (**A,** Courtesy of Dr. Arthur Like, University of Massachusetts, Worchester, Massachusetts.)

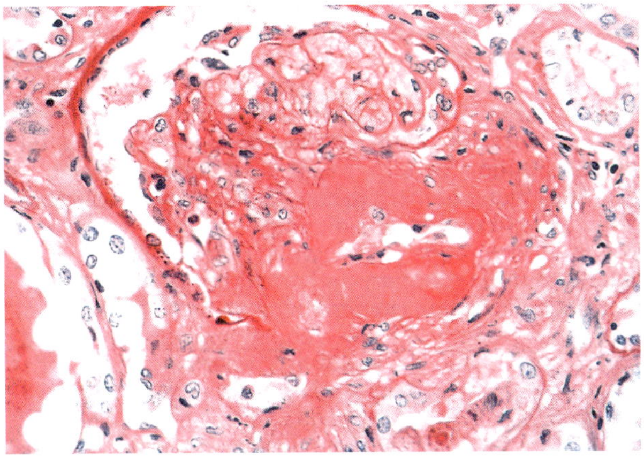

Figure 20–27

Severe renal hyaline arteriolosclerosis. Note a markedly thickened, tortuous afferent arteriole. The amorphous nature of the thickened vascular wall is evident. (PAS stain; courtesy of Dr. M.A. Venkatachalam, Department of Pathology, University of Texas Health Science Center at San Antonio.)

predominantly of type IV collagen (Fig. 20–28). It should be noted that **despite the increase in the thickness of basement membranes, diabetic capillaries are more leaky than normal to plasma proteins. The microangiopathy underlies the development of diabetic nephropathy, retinopathy, and some forms of neuropathy.** An indistinguishable microangiopathy can be found in aged nondiabetic patients, but rarely to the extent seen in individuals with long-standing diabetes.

Diabetic Nephropathy. The kidneys are prime targets of diabetes (see also Chapter 14). Renal failure is second only to myocardial infarction as a cause of death from this disease. Three lesions are encountered: (1) glomerular lesions; (2) renal vascular lesions, principally arteriolosclerosis; and (3) pyelonephritis, including necrotizing papillitis.

The most important glomerular lesions are capillary basement membrane thickening, diffuse mesangial sclerosis, and nodular glomerulosclerosis. The glomerular capillary basement membranes are thick-

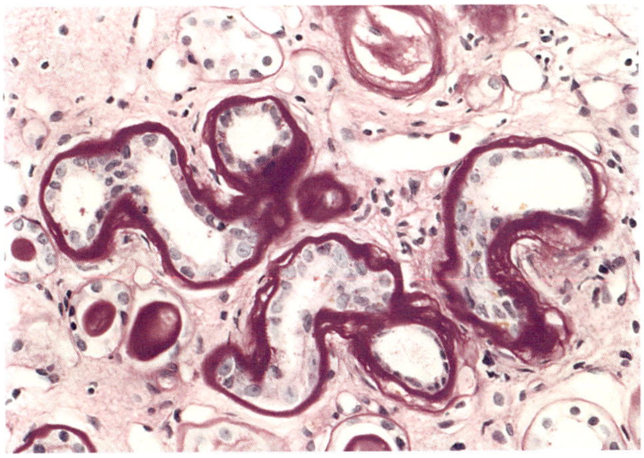

Figure 20–28

Renal cortex showing thickening of tubular basement membranes in a diabetic patient (PAS stain).

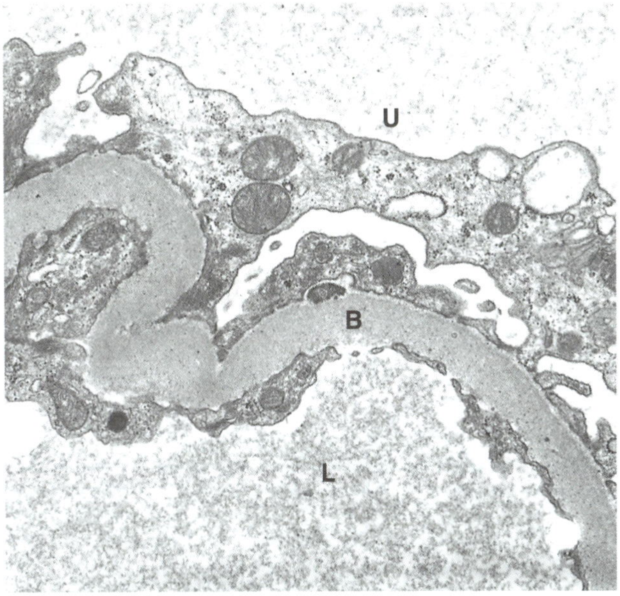

Figure 20–29

Renal glomerulus showing markedly thickened glomerular basement membrane (B) in a diabetic. L, glomerular capillary lumen; U, urinary space. (Courtesy of Dr. Michael Kashgarian, Department of Pathology, Yale University School of Medicine, New Haven, Connecticut.)

ened throughout their entire length. This change can be detected by electron microscopy within a few years of the onset of diabetes, sometimes without any associated change in renal function (Fig. 20–29).

Diffuse mesangial sclerosis consists of a diffuse increase in mesangial matrix along with mesangial cell proliferation and is always associated with basement membrane thickening. It is found in most individuals with disease of more than 10 years' duration. When glomerulosclerosis becomes marked, patients manifest the nephrotic syndrome, characterized by proteinuria, hypoalbuminemia, and edema (Chapter 14).

Nodular glomerulosclerosis describes a glomerular lesion made distinctive by ball-like deposits of a laminated matrix situated in the periphery of the glomerulus (Fig. 20–30). These nodules are PAS positive and usually contain trapped mesangial cells. This distinctive change has been called the Kimmelstiel-Wilson lesion, after the pathologists who described it. Nodular glomerulosclerosis is encountered in approximately 15% to 30% of long-term diabetics and is a major cause of morbidity and mortality. Diffuse mesangial sclerosis may also be seen in association with old age and hypertension; on the contrary, the nodular form of glomerulosclerosis, once certain unusual forms of nephropathies have been excluded (see Chapter 14), is essentially pathogonomic of diabetes. Both the diffuse and the nodular forms of glomerulosclerosis induce sufficient ischemia to cause scarring of the kidneys, manifested by a finely granular cortical surface (Fig. 20–31).

Renal atherosclerosis and arteriolosclerosis constitute part of the macrovascular disease in diabetics. The kidney is one of the most frequently and severely affected organs; however, the changes in the arteries and arterioles are similar to those found throughout the body. **Hyaline arteriolosclerosis affects not only the**

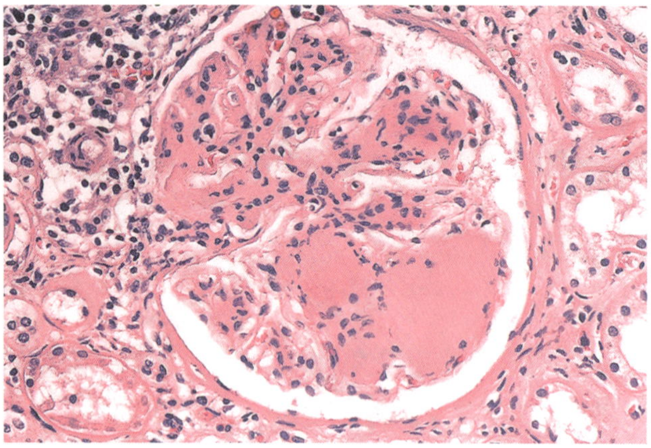

Figure 20–30

Nodular glomerulosclerosis in a person with long-standing diabetes. (Courtesy of Dr. Lisa Yerian, Department of Pathology, University of Chicago, Chicago, Illinois.)

afferent but also the efferent arterioles. Such efferent arteriolosclerosis is rarely if ever encountered in persons who do not have diabetes.

Pyelonephritis is an acute or chronic inflammation of the kidneys that usually begins in the interstitial tissue and then spreads to affect the tubules. Both the acute and chronic forms of this disease occur in nondiabetics as well as in diabetics but are more common in diabetics than in the general population, and once affected, diabetics tend to have more severe involvement. One special pattern of acute pyelonephritis, **necrotizing papillitis** (or papillary necrosis), is much more prevalent in diabetics than in nondiabetics.

Ocular Complications of Diabetes. Visual impairment, sometimes even total blindness, is one of the more feared consequences of long-standing diabetes. **The ocular involvement may take the form of retinopathy, cataract formation, or glaucoma.** Retinopathy, the most common pattern, consists of a constellation of changes that together are considered by many ophthalmologists to be virtually diagnostic of the disease. **The lesion in the retina takes two forms: nonproliferative (background) retinopaty and proliferative retinopathy.**

Nonproliferative retinopathy includes intraretinal or preretinal hemorrhages, retinal exudates, microaneurysms, venous dilations, edema, and, most importantly, thickening of the retinal capillaries (microangiopathy). The retinal exudates can be either "soft" (microinfarcts) or "hard" (deposits of plasma proteins and lipids) (Fig. 20–32). The microaneurysms are discrete saccular dilations of retinal choroidal capillaries that appear through the ophthalmoscope as small red dots. Dilations tend to occur at focal points of weakening, resulting from loss of pericytes. Retinal edema presumably results from excessive capillary permeability. Underlying all of these changes is the microangiopathy, which is thought to lead to loss of capillary pericytes and hence to focal weakening of capillary structure.

The so-called proliferative retinopathy is a process of neovascularization and fibrosis. This lesion leads to serious consequences, including blindness, especially if it involves the macula. Vitreous hemorrhages can result from rupture of newly formed capillaries; the resultant organization of the hemorrhage can pull the retina off its substratum (retinal detachment).

Diabetic Neuropathy. The central and peripheral nervous systems are not spared by diabetes. The most frequent pattern of involvement is a peripheral, symmetric neuropathy of the lower extremities that affects

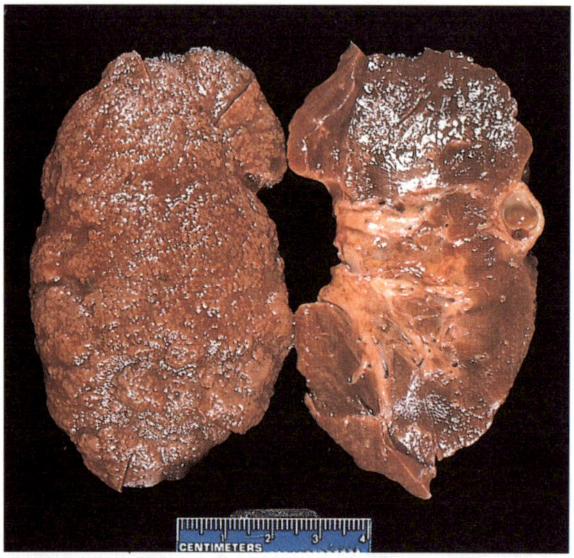

Figure 20–31

Nephrosclerosis in a person with long-standing diabetes. The kidney has been bisected to demonstrate both diffuse granular transformation of the surface *(left)* and marked thinning of the cortical tissue *(right).* Additional features include some irregular depressions, the result of pyelonephritis, and an incidental cortical cyst *(far right).*

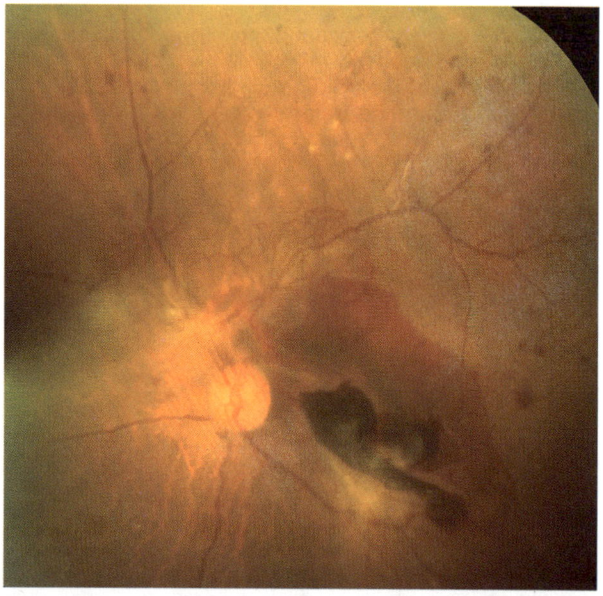

Figure 20–32

Diabetic retinopathy, demonstrating advanced proliferative retinopathy with retinal hemorrhages, exudates, neovascularization, and tractional retinal detachment in the lower right corner. (Courtesy of Dr. Rajendra Apte, Washington University School of Medicine, St. Louis, Missouri.)

both motor and sensory function but particularly the latter. Other forms include peripheral neuropathy, which produces disturbances in bowel and bladder function and sometimes sexual impotence, and diabetic mononeuropathy, which may manifest as sudden footdrop, wristdrop, or isolated cranial nerve palsies. The neurologic changes may be caused by microangiopathy and increased permeability of the capillaries that supply the nerves as well as direct axonal damage due to alterations in sorbitol metabolism (as discussed).

Clinical Features. It is difficult to sketch with brevity the diverse clinical presentations of diabetes mellitus. Only a few characteristic patterns will be presented (Table 20–6). In the initial 1 or 2 years following manifestation of overt *type 1 diabetes,* the exogenous insulin requirements may be minimal to none secondary to ongoing endogenous insulin secretion (referred to as the "*honeymoon period*"), but shortly thereafter any residual β-cell reserve is exhausted and insulin requirements increase dramatically. Although β-cell destruction is a gradual process, the transition from impaired glucose tolerance to overt diabetes may be abrupt, heralded by an event with increased insulin requirements such as infection. The onset is marked by polyuria, polydipsia, polyphagia, and in severe cases, ketoacidosis, all resulting from metabolic derangements (Fig. 20–33). Since insulin is a major anabolic hormone in the body, *deficiency of insulin results in a catabolic state that affects not only glucose metabolism but also fat and protein metabolism.* The assimilation of glucose into muscle and adipose tissue is sharply diminished or abolished. Not only does storage of glycogen in liver and muscle cease, but also reserves are depleted by glycogenolysis. The resultant hyperglycemia exceeds the renal threshold for reabsorption, and glycosuria ensues. The glycosuria induces an osmotic diuresis and thus *polyuria,* causing a profound loss of water and electrolytes. The obligatory renal water loss combined with the hyperosmolarity resulting from the increased levels of glucose in the blood tends to deplete intracellular water, triggering the osmoreceptors of the thirst centers of the brain. In this manner, intense thirst *(polydipsia)* appears. With a deficiency of insulin, the scales swing from insulin-promoted anabolism to catabolism of proteins and fats. Proteolysis follows, and the gluconeogenic amino acids are removed by the liver and used as building blocks for glucose. The catabolism of proteins and fats tends to induce a negative energy balance, which in turn leads to increasing appetite *(polyphagia),* thus completing the classic triad of diabetes: *polyuria, polydipsia,* and *polyphagia.* Despite the increased appetite, catabolic effects prevail, resulting in weight loss and muscle weakness. The combination of polyphagia and weight loss is paradoxical and should always raise the suspicion of diabetes.

In individuals with type 1 diabetes, deviations from normal dietary intake, unusual physical activity, infection, or any other forms of stress may rapidly influence the treacherously fragile metabolic balance, predisposing one to *diabetic ketoacidosis.* The plasma glucose is usually in the range of 500 to 700 mg/dL as a result of absolute insulin deficiency and unopposed effects of counter-regulatory hormones (epinephrine, glucagon). The marked hyperglycemia causes an osmotic diuresis and dehydration characteristic of the ketoacidotic state. The second major effect is activation of the ketogenic machinery. Insulin deficiency leads to activation of lipoprotein lipase, with resultant excessive breakdown of adipose stores, giving rise to increased levels of FFAs, oxidation of which by the liver produces *ketone bodies.* Ketogenesis is an adaptive phenomenon in times of starvation, gen-

Table 20–6 Type 1 versus Type 2 Diabetes Mellitus

Parameter	Type 1	Type 2
Clinical		
	Onset <20 years Normal weight Markedly decreased blood insulin Antibodies to islet cells Ketoacidosis common	Onset >30 years Obesity Increased blood insulin (early); normal to moderate decreased insulin (late) No antibodies to islet cells Ketoacidosis rare; nonketotic hyperosmolar coma
Genetics		
	30% to 70% concordance in twins Linkage to MHC class II HLA genes	50% to 90% concordance in twins No HLA linkage Linkage to candidate "diabetogenic" genes
Pathogenesis		
	Autoimmune destruction of β-cells mediated by T cells and humoral mediators Absolute insulin deficiency	Insulin resistance in skeletal muscle, adipose tissue, and liver β-cell dysfunction and relative insulin deficiency
Islet cells		
	Insulitis early Marked atrophy and fibrosis β-cell depletion	No insulitis Focal atrophy and amyloid deposition Mild β-cell depletion

HLA, human leukocyte antigen; MHC, major histocompatibility complex.

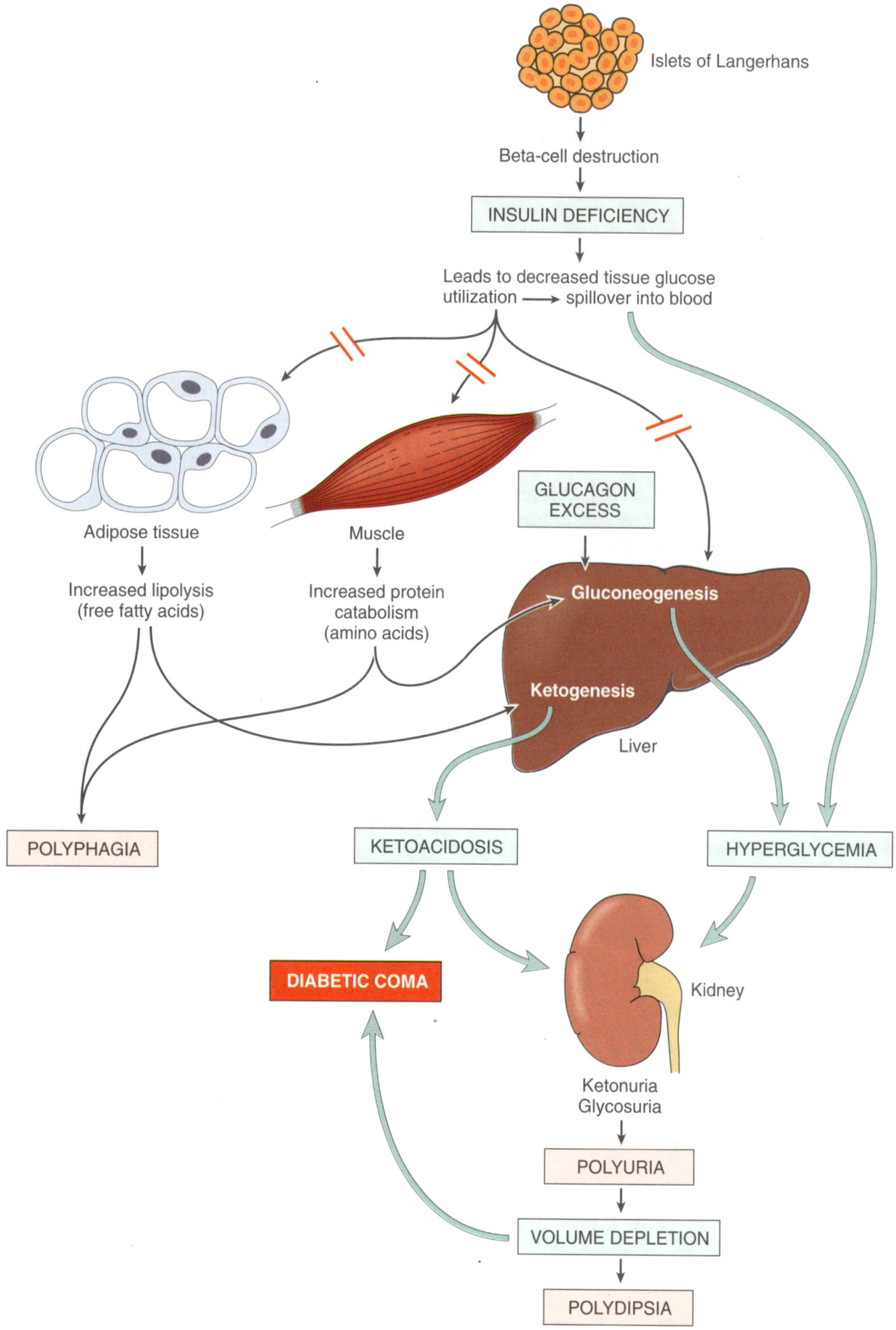

Figure 20–33

Sequence of metabolic derangements leading to diabetic coma in type 1 diabetes mellitus. An absolute insulin deficiency leads to a catabolic state, eventuating in ketoacidosis and severe volume depletion. These bring about sufficient central nervous system compromise to cause coma, and eventual death if left untreated.

erating ketones as a source of energy for consumption by vital organs (e.g., brain). The rate at which ketone bodies are formed may exceed the rate at which they can be used by peripheral tissues, leading to *ketonemia* and *ketonuria*. If the urinary excretion of ketones is compromised by dehydration, the plasma hydrogen ion concentration increases, resulting in metabolic ketoacidosis.

Type 2 diabetes mellitus may also present with polyuria and polydipsia, but unlike type 1 diabetes, patients are often older (>40 years) and frequently obese. However, with the increase in obesity and sedentary life style in our society, type 2 diabetes is now seen in children and adolescents with increasing frequency. In some cases medical attention is sought because of unexplained weakness or weight loss. *Most frequently, however, the diagnosis is made after routine blood or urine testing in asymptomatic persons.*

In the decompensated state, individuals with type 2 diabetes may develop *hyperosmolar nonketotic coma*, a syndrome engendered by the severe dehydration resulting from sustained osmotic diuresis in patients who do not drink enough water to compensate for urinary losses from chronic hyperglycemia. Typically, the person is an elderly diabetic who is disabled by a stroke or an infection and is unable to maintain adequate water intake. Furthermore, the absence of ketoacidosis and its symptoms (nausea, vomiting, respiratory difficulties) delays the seeking of medical attention in these patients until severe dehydration and coma occur.

As previously discussed, it is the long-term effects of diabetes, more than the acute metabolic complications, that are responsible for the overwhelming proportion of morbidity and mortality attributable to this disease. In most instances, these complications appear approximately 15 to 20 years after the onset of hyperglycemia.

- *In both forms of long-standing diabetes, cardiovascular events such as myocardial infarction, renal vascular insufficiency, and cerebrovascular accidents are the most common causes of mortality.* The impact of cardiovascular disease can be gauged by its involvement in as many as 80% of deaths of type 2 diabetics; in fact, diabetics have a 3 to 7.5 times greater incidence of death from cardiovascular causes than nondiabetic populations. The hallmark of cardiovascular disease is *accelerated atherosclerosis* of the large and medium-sized arteries (i.e., macrovascular disease). The importance of *obesity* in the pathogenesis of insulin resistance has already been discussed, but it is also an independent risk factor for development of atherosclerosis.
- *Diabetic nephropathy* is a leading cause of end-stage renal disease in the United States. The earliest manifestation of diabetic nephropathy is the appearance of small amounts of albumin in the urine (>30 mg/day, but <300 mg/day; i.e., *microalbuminuria*). Without specific interventions, approximately 80% of type 1 diabetics and 20% to 40% of type 2 diabetics will develop *overt nephropathy with macroalbuminuria* (>300 mg/day) over the next 10 to 15 years, usually accompanied by the appearance of hypertension. The progression from overt nephropathy to *end-stage renal disease* can be highly variable and is evidenced by a progressive drop in glomerular filtration rate. By 20 years after diagnosis, more than 75% of type 1 diabetics and about 20% of type 2 diabetics with overt nephropathy will develop end-stage renal disease, requiring dialysis or renal transplantation.
- *Visual impairment*, sometimes even total blindness, is one of the more feared consequences of long-standing diabetes. This disease is currently the fourth leading cause of acquired blindness in the United States. Approximately 60% to 80% of patients develop some form of *diabetic retinopathy* approximately 15 to 20 years after diagnosis. In addition to retinopathy, diabetics also have an increased propensity for *glaucoma* and *cataract formation*, both of which contribute to visual impairment in diabetes.
- *Diabetic neuropathy* typically presents with decreased sensation in the distal extremities with less evident motor abnormalities (sensorimotor neuropathy). The loss of pain sensation can result in the development of ulcers that heal poorly and are a major cause of morbidity. As many as 20% to 40% of diabetics also develop autonomic dysfunction over time, as manifested by impediments in bowel and bladder control.
- *Diabetics are plagued by an enhanced susceptibility to infections of the skin, as well as to tuberculosis, pneumonia, and pyelonephritis.* Such infections cause the deaths of about 5% of diabetics. In an individual with diabetic neuropathy, a trivial infection in a toe may be the first event in a long succession of complications (gangrene, bacteremia, pneumonia) that may ultimately lead to death.

PANCREATIC ENDOCRINE NEOPLASMS

Pancreatic endocrine neoplasms, also known as "islet cell tumors," are rare in comparison with tumors of the exocrine pancreas, accounting for only 2% of all pancreatic neoplasms. They are most common in adults, may be single or multiple, and benign or malignant, the latter metastasizing to lymph nodes and liver. Pancreatic endocrine neoplasms have a propensity to elaborate pancreatic hormones, but some may be totally nonfunctional. Like any other endocrine neoplasms, it is difficult to predict the biologic behavior of a pancreatic endocrine neoplasm purely on the basis of light microscopic criteria. In general, tumors less than 2 cm in size tend to behave in an indolent manner, but there are significant exceptions to this rule. The functional status of the tumor may have some import on prognosis, since approximately 90% of insulinomas are benign, while 60% to 90% of other functioning and nonfunctioning pancreatic endocrine neoplasms tend to be malignant. Fortunately, insulinomas are also the most common subtype of pancreatic endocrine noplasms.

Insulinomas

β-cell tumors (insulinomas) are the most common of pancreatic endocrine neoplasms and may be responsible for the elaboration of sufficient insulin to induce clinically significant hypoglycemia. There is a characteristic clinical triad resulting from these pancreatic lesions: (1) attacks of hypoglycemia occur with blood glucose amounts below 50 mg/dL of serum; (2) the attacks consist principally of such central nervous system manifestations as confusion, stupor, and loss of consciousness; and (3) the attacks are precipitated by fasting or exercise and are promptly relieved by feeding or parenteral administration of glucose.

Morphology

Insulinomas are most often found within the pancreas and are generally benign. Most are solitary lesions, although multiple tumors or tumors ectopic to the pancreas may be encountered. Bona fide carcinomas, making up only about 10% of cases, are diagnosed on the basis of criteria for malignancy listed above. Solitary tumors are usually small (often <2 cm in diameter) and are encapsulated, pale to red-brown nodules located anywhere in the pancreas. Histologically, these benign tumors look remarkably like giant islets, with preservation of the regular cords of monotonous cells and their orientation to the vasculature. Not even the malignant lesions present much evidence of anaplasia (Fig. 20–34A), and they may be deceptively encapsulated. By immunocytochemistry, insulin can be localized in the tumor cells (Fig. 20–34B). Under the electron microscope, neoplastic β cells, like their normal counterparts, display distinctive round granules that contain polygonal or rectangular dense crystals separated from the enclosing membrane by a distinct halo. It should be cautioned that granules may be present in the absence of clinically significant hormone activity.

While as many as 80% of islet cell tumors may demonstrate excessive insulin secretion, hypoglycemia is mild in all but 20%, and many cases never become clinically symptomatic. The critical laboratory findings in insulinomas are high circulating levels of insulin and a high insulin-to-glucose ratio. Surgical removal of the tumor is usually followed by prompt reversal of the hypoglycemia. It is important to note that *there are many other causes of hypoglycemia besides insulinomas.* These include diffuse liver disease, secretion of insulin-like growth factor-2 (IGF-2) by some fibrosarcomas, and self-injection of insulin.

Gastrinomas

Marked hypersecretion of gastrin usually has its origin in gastrin-producing tumors *(gastrinomas),* which are just as likely to arise in the duodenum and peripancreatic soft tissues as in the pancreas (so-called "gastrinoma triangle"). Zollinger and Ellison first called attention to the *association of pancreatic islet cell lesions with hypersecretion of gastric acid and severe peptic ulceration,* which are present in 90% to 95% of patients (Zollinger-Ellison syndrome).

Morphology

Gastrinomas may arise in the pancreas, the peripancreatic region, or the wall of the duodenum. **Over half of gastrin-producing tumors are locally invasive or have already metastasized at the time of diagnosis.** In approximately 25% of patients, gastrinomas arise in conjunction with other endocrine tumors, thus conforming to the MEN-1 syndrome (see below); MEN-1–associated gastrinomas are frequently multifocal, while sporadic gastrinomas are usually single. As with insulin-secreting tumors of the pancreas, gastrin-producing tumors are histologically bland and rarely exhibit marked anaplasia.

In Zollinger-Ellison syndrome, hypergastrinemia from a pancreatic or duodenal tumor stimulates extreme gastric acid secretion, which in turn causes *peptic ulceration.* The duodenal and gastric ulcers are often *multiple;* although they are identical to those found in the general population, they are often *intractable* to usual modalities

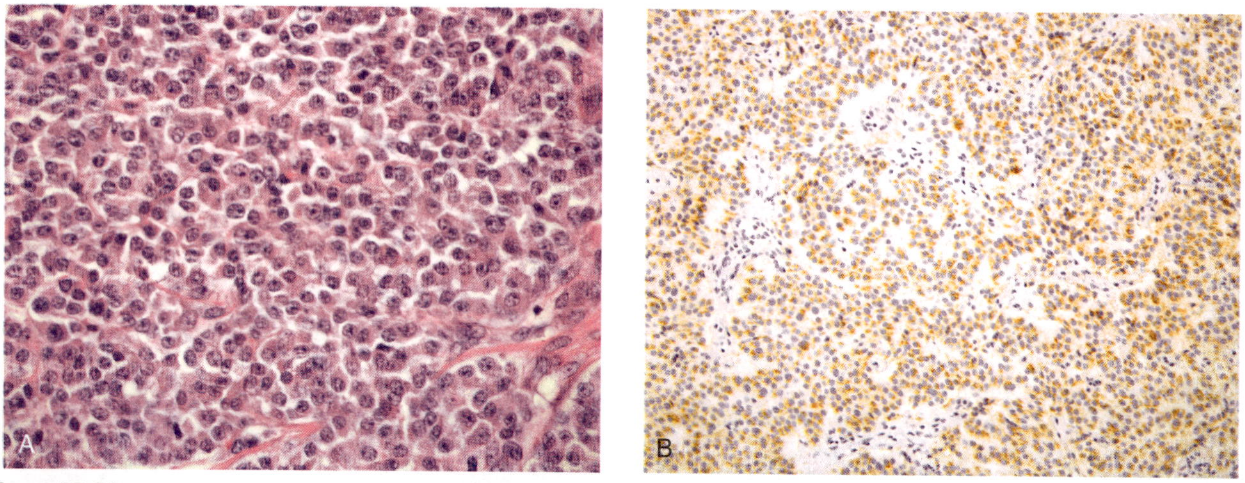

Figure 20–34

Pancreatic endocrine tumor ("islet cell tumor"). **A,** The neoplastic cells are monotonous and demonstrate minimal pleomorphism or mitotic activity (H&E stain). **B,** Immunoreactivity for insulin confirms the neoplasm is an insulinoma. Clinically, the patient had episodic hypoglycemia.

of therapy. In addition, ulcers may also occur in *unusual locations* such as the jejunum; when intractable jejunal ulcers are found, Zollinger-Ellison syndrome should be considered. More than 50% of the patients have diarrhea; in 30% it is the presenting symptom.

Other Rare Pancreatic Endocrine Neoplasms

- *α-Cell tumors (glucagonomas)* are associated with increased serum glucagon and a syndrome consisting of mild diabetes mellitus, a characteristic skin rash *(necrolytic migratory erythema),* and anemia. They occur most frequently in peri- and postmenopausal women and are characterized by extremely high plasma glucagon levels.
- *δ-Cell tumors (somatostatinomas)* are associated with diabetes mellitus, cholelithiasis, steatorrhea, and hypochlorhydria. They are exceedingly difficult to localize preoperatively. High plasma somatostatin levels are required for diagnosis.
- *VIPoma (watery diarrhea, hypokalemia, achlorhydria or WDHA syndrome)* is an endocrine tumor that induces the eponymous characteristic syndrome, caused by release of vasoactive intestinal peptide (VIP) from the tumor. Some of these tumors are locally invasive and metastatic.

ADRENAL CORTEX

The *adrenal glands* are paired endocrine organs consisting of both cortex and medulla, which differ in their development, structure, and function. The *cortex* consists of three layers of distinct cell types. Beneath the capsule of the adrenal is the narrow layer of zona glomerulosa. An equally narrow zona reticularis abuts the medulla. Intervening is the broad zona fasciculata, which makes up about 75% of the total cortex. The adrenal cortex synthesizes three different types of steroids: (1) *glucocorticoids* (principally cortisol), which are synthesized primarily in the zona fasciculata with a small contribution from the zona reticularis; (2) *mineralocorticoids,* the most important being aldosterone, which is generated in the zona glomerulosa; and (3) *sex steroids* (estrogens and androgens), which are produced largely in the zona reticularis. The *adrenal medulla* is composed of chromaffin cells, which synthesize and secrete *catecholamines,* mainly epinephrine. This section deals first with disorders of the adrenal cortex and then of the medulla. Diseases of the adrenal cortex can be conveniently divided into those associated with cortical hyperfunction and those characterized by cortical hypofunction.

ADRENOCORTICAL HYPERFUNCTION (HYPERADRENALISM)

Just as there are three basic types of corticosteroids elaborated by the adrenal cortex (glucocorticoids, mineralocorticoids, and sex steroids), so there are three distinctive hyperadrenal clinical syndromes: (1) *Cushing syndrome,* characterized by an excess of cortisol; (2) *hyperaldosteronism;* and (3) *adrenogenital* or virilizing syndromes, caused by an excess of androgens. The clinical features of some of these syndromes overlap somewhat because of the overlapping functions of some of the adrenal steroids.

Hypercortisolism (Cushing Syndrome)

This disorder is caused by any condition that produces an elevation in glucocorticoid levels. *In clinical practice, most cases of Cushing syndrome are caused by the administration of exogenous glucocorticoids.* The remaining cases are endogenous and caused by one of the following (Fig. 20–35):

- Primary hypothalamic-pituitary diseases associated with hypersecretion of ACTH
- Primary adrenocortical hyperplasia or neoplasia
- The secretion of ectopic ACTH by nonendocrine neoplasms

Primary hypothalamic-pituitary disease associated with oversecretion of ACTH, also known as *Cushing disease,* accounts for more than half of the cases of spontaneous, endogenous Cushing syndrome. The disorder affects women about five times more frequently than men, and it occurs most frequently during the 20s and 30s. In the vast majority of cases, the *pituitary gland contains an ACTH-producing microadenoma* that does not produce mass effects in the brain; some corticotroph tumors qualify as macroadenomas (>10 mm). In the remaining patients, the anterior pituitary contains areas of *corticotroph cell hyperplasia* without a discrete adenoma. Corticotroph cell hyperplasia may be primary, or arise secondarily from excessive stimulation of ACTH release by a hypothalamic corticotropin-releasing hormone–producing tumor. The adrenal glands in patients with Cushing disease are characterized by variable degrees of bilateral nodular cortical hyperplasia (discussed later), caused by elevated levels of ACTH. The cortical hyperplasia, in turn, is responsible for the hypercortisolism.

Primary adrenal neoplasms, such as adrenal adenoma and carcinoma, and *primary cortical hyperplasia,* are responsible for about 10% to 20% of cases of endogenous Cushing syndrome. This form of Cushing syndrome is also designated *ACTH-independent Cushing syndrome* or adrenal Cushing syndrome because the adrenals function autonomously. The biochemical sine qua non of adrenal Cushing syndrome is elevated levels of cortisol with low serum levels of ACTH. In most cases, adrenal Cushing syndrome is caused by a unilateral adrenocorti-

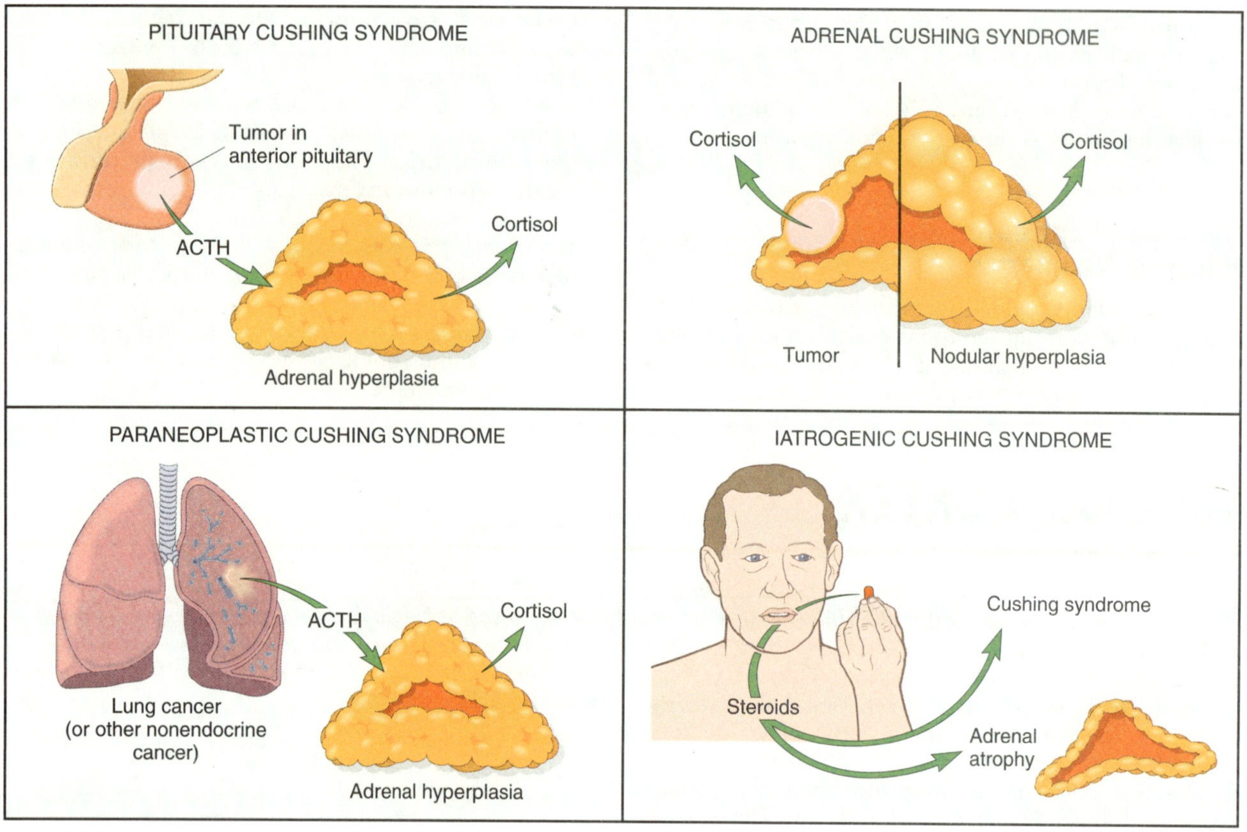

Figure 20–35

Schematic representation of the various forms of Cushing syndrome, illustrating the three endogenous forms, as well as the more common exogenous (iatrogenic) form. ACTH, adrenocorticotropic hormone.

cal neoplasm, which may be either benign (adenoma) or malignant (carcinoma). Primary bilateral hyperplasia of the adrenal cortices is a rare cause of Cushing syndrome. There are two variants of this entity; the first presents as macronodules (<3 mm) and the second as micronodules (>3 mm) that are often pigmented ("primary pigmented nodular adrenocortical disease"). The micronodular variant is a familial disease, usually associated with features of overactivity in other endocrine organs such as the pituitary, thyroid, and gonads.

Secretion of ectopic ACTH by nonendocrine tumors accounts for most of the remaining cases of endogenous Cushing syndrome. Commonly, the responsible tumor is a *small-cell carcinoma of the lung,* although other neoplasms, including *carcinoid tumors, medullary carcinomas of the thyroid, and islet cell tumors of the pancreas,* have also been associated with the syndrome. In addition to tumors that elaborate ectopic ACTH, an occasional neoplasm produces ectopic corticotropin-releasing hormone, which in turn causes ACTH secretion and hypercortisolism. As with Cushing syndrome associated with hypothalamic-pituitary disease, nodular cortical hyperplasia is present in the adrenals.

Morphology

The main lesions of Cushing syndrome are found in the pituitary and adrenal glands. The **pituitary** in Cushing syndrome shows changes regardless of the cause. The most common alteration, resulting from high levels of endogenous or exogenous glucocorticoids, is termed **Crooke hyaline change.** In this condition, the normal granular, basophilic cytoplasm of the ACTH-producing cells in the anterior pituitary is replaced by homogeneous, lightly basophilic material. This alteration is the result of the accumulation of intermediate keratin filaments in the cytoplasm.

The morphology of the **adrenal glands** depends on the cause of the hypercortisolism. The adrenals have one of the following abnormalities: (1) cortical atrophy; (2) diffuse hyperplasia; (3) nodular hyperplasia; and (4) an adenoma, rarely a carcinoma. In patients in whom the syndrome results from exogenous glucocorticoids, suppression of endogenous ACTH results in bilateral **cortical atrophy,** due to a lack of stimulation of the zonae fasciculata and reticularis by ACTH. The zona glomerulosa is of normal thickness in such cases, because this portion of the cortex functions independently of ACTH. In cases of endogenous hypercortisolism, in contrast, the adrenals either are hyperplastic or contain a cortical neoplasm. **Diffuse hyperplasia** is found in 60% to 70% of cases of endogenous Cushing syndrome. The adrenal cortex is diffusely thickened and yellow, as a result of an increase in the size and number of lipid-rich cells in the zonae fasciculata and reticularis. Some degree of nodularity is common but is pronounced in **nodular hyperplasia** (Fig. 20–36). This takes the form of bilateral, 0.5- to 2.0-cm, yellow

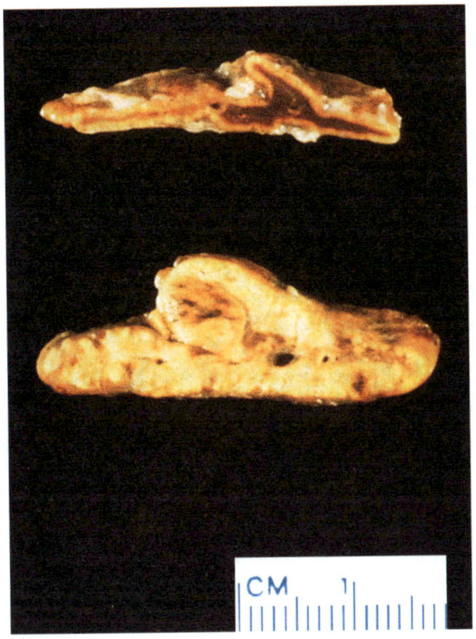

Figure 20–36

Adrenocortical hyperplasia. The adrenal cortex (bottom) is yellow, thickened, and multinodular as a result of hypertrophy and hyperplasia of the lipid-rich zonae fasciculata and reticularis. The top shows a normal adrenal for comparison.

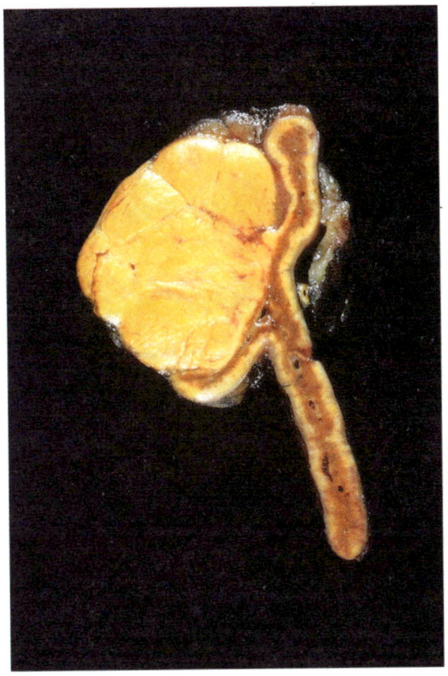

Figure 20–37

Adrenocortical adenoma. The adenoma is distinguished from nodular hyperplasia by its solitary, circumscribed nature. The functional status of an adrenocortical adenoma cannot be predicted from its gross or microscopic appearance.

nodules scattered throughout the cortex, separated by intervening areas of widened cortex. The combined adrenals may weigh as much as 30 to 50 gm. This macronodularity appears to be an extension of the diffuse hyperplasia, because the cortex between the nodules exactly resembles that found in the diffuse form of this condition. **Primary adrenocortical neoplasms** causing Cushing syndrome may be malignant or benign. The adrenocortical **adenomas** are yellow tumors surrounded by thin or well-developed capsules, and most weigh less than 30 gm (Fig. 20–37). Their morphology is identical to that of nonfunctional adenomas and of adenomas associated with hyperaldosteronism (see below). Microscopically, they are composed of cells that are similar to those encountered in the normal zona fasciculata. The **carcinomas** associated with Cushing syndrome, by contrast, tend to be larger than the adenomas. These tumors are unencapsulated masses frequently exceeding 200 to 300 gm in weight, having all of the anaplastic characteristics of cancer, as detailed later. With both functioning benign and malignant tumors, the adjacent adrenal cortex and that of the contralateral adrenal gland are atrophic because of suppression of endogenous ACTH by high cortisol levels.

Clinical Features. The signs and symptoms of Cushing syndrome are an exaggeration of the known actions of glucocorticoids. Cushing syndrome usually develops gradually and, like many other endocrine abnormalities, may be quite subtle in its early stages. A major exception to this insidious onset is Cushing syndrome associated with small-cell carcinomas of the lung, where the rapid course of the underlying disease precludes development of many of the characteristic features. Early manifestations of Cushing syndrome include hypertension and weight gain. With time, the more characteristic centripetal distribution of adipose tissue becomes apparent, with resultant truncal obesity, "moon" facies, and accumulation of fat in the posterior neck and back ("buffalo hump"). Hypercortisolism causes selective atrophy of fast-twitch (type II) myofibers, with resultant decreased muscle mass and proximal limb weakness. Glucocorticoids induce gluconeogenesis and inhibit the uptake of glucose by cells, with resultant *hyperglycemia, glucosuria,* and *polydipsia,* mimicking diabetes mellitus. The catabolic effects on proteins cause loss of collagen and resorption of bone. Thus, the skin is thin, fragile, and easily bruised; *cutaneous striae* are particularly common in the abdominal area. Bone resorption results in the development of *osteoporosis,* with consequent increased susceptibility to fractures. Because glucocorticoids suppress the immune response, patients with Cushing syndrome are also at increased risk for a variety of infections. Additional manifestations include *hirsutism* and *menstrual abnormalities,* as well as a number of *mental disturbances,* including mood swings, depression, and frank psychosis. Extra-adrenal Cushing syndrome caused by pituitary or ectopic ACTH secretion is usually associated with increased skin pigmentation, because of melanocyte-stimulating activity in the ACTH precursor molecule.

SUMMARY

Hypercortisolism (Cushing syndrome)

- The most common cause of hypercortisolism is exogenous administration of steroids.
- Endogenous hypercortisolism is most often secondary to an ACTH-producing pituitary micro-

adenoma ("Cushing disease"), followed by primary adrenal neoplasms ("ACTH-independent" hypercortisolism), and paraneoplastic ACTH production by tumors (e.g., small-cell lung cancer).
• The morphologic features in the adrenal include bilateral cortical atrophy (in exogenous steroid-induced disease), bilateral diffuse or nodular hyperplasia (most common finding in endogenous Cushing syndrome), or an adrenocortical neoplasm.

Hyperaldosteronism

Excessive levels of aldosterone cause *sodium retention and potassium excretion, with resultant hypertension and hypokalemia.* Hyperaldosteronism may be primary, or it may be secondary to an extra-adrenal cause. In *secondary hyperaldosteronism,* aldosterone release occurs in response to activation of the renin-angiotensin system. It is characterized by *increased levels of plasma renin* and is encountered in conditions associated with:

- Decreased renal perfusion (arteriolar nephrosclerosis, renal artery stenosis)
- Arterial hypovolemia and edema (congestive heart failure, cirrhosis, nephrotic syndrome)
- Pregnancy (caused by estrogen-induced increases in plasma renin substrate)

Primary hyperaldosteronism, in contrast, indicates a primary, autonomous overproduction of aldosterone, with resultant suppression of the renin-angiotensin system and *decreased plasma renin activity.* Primary hyperaldosteronism is caused either by an aldosterone-producing adrenocortical neoplasm, usually an adenoma, or by primary adrenocortical hyperplasia. Some cases are idiopathic; these may be caused by overactivity of the aldosterone synthase gene, *CYP11B2.*

Morphology

In roughly 80% of cases, primary hyperaldosteronism is caused by an **aldosterone-secreting adenoma** in one adrenal gland, a condition referred to as **Conn syndrome.** In most cases, the adenomas are solitary, small (<2cm in diameter), encapsulated lesions, although multiple adenomas may be present in an occasional patient; carcinomas resulting in hyperaldosteronism are rare. In contrast to cortical adenomas associated with Cushing syndrome, those associated with hyperaldosteronism do not usually suppress ACTH secretion. Therefore, the adjacent adrenal cortex and that of the contralateral gland are not atrophic. They are bright yellow on cut section and, surprisingly, are composed of lipid-laden cortical cells more closely resembling fasciculata cells than glomerulosa cells (the normal source of aldosterone). In general, the cells tend to be uniform in size and shape; occasionally there is some nuclear and cellular pleomorphism (Fig. 20–38). A characteristic feature of aldesterone-producing adenomas is the presence of eosinophilic, laminated cytoplasmic inclusions, known as **spironolactone bodies.** These are typically found after treatment with the anti-hypertensive drug spironolactone, which is the drug of choice in primary hyperaldosteronism. In about 15% of cases, primary hyperaldosteronism is caused by bilateral **primary adrenocortical hyperplasia,** characterized by bilateral nodular hyperplasia of the adrenal glands, highly reminiscent of those found in the nodular hyperplasia of Cushing syndrome.

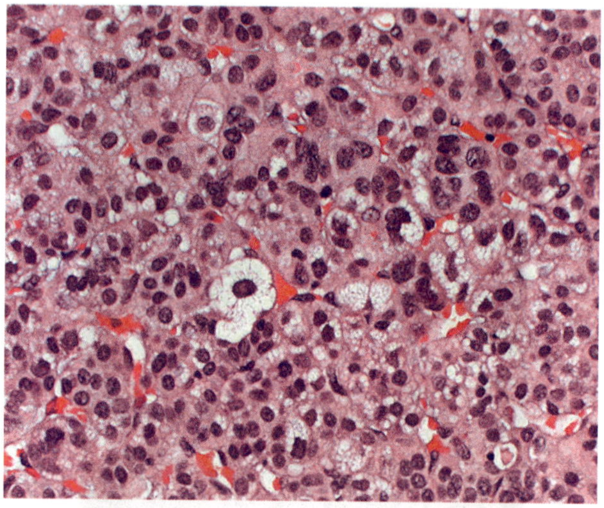

Figure 20–38

Histologic features of an adrenal cortical adenoma. The neoplastic cells are vacuolated because of the presence of intracytoplasmic lipid. There is mild nuclear pleomorphism. Mitotic activity and necrosis are not seen.

Clinical Features. The clinical manifestations of primary hyperaldosteronism are those of hypertension and hypokalemia. Serum renin levels, as mentioned earlier, are low. Conn syndrome occurs most frequently in middle adult life and is more common in females than in males (2:1). Although aldosterone-producing adenomas account for less than 1% of cases of hypertension, it is important to recognize them, because they cause a surgically correctable form of hypertension. Primary adrenal hyperplasia associated with hyperaldosteronism occurs more often in children and young adults than in older adults; surgical intervention is not very beneficial in these patients, and this condition is best managed with medical therapy with an aldosterone antagonist such as spironolactone. The treatment of secondary hyperaldosteronism rests on correcting the underlying cause of the stimulation of the renin-angiotensin system.

Adrenogenital Syndromes

Excess of androgens may be caused by a number of diseases, including primary gonadal disorders and several primary adrenal disorders. The adrenal cortex secretes two compounds—dehydroepiandrosterone and androstenedione—which require conversion to testosterone in peripheral tissues for their androgenic effects. Unlike gonadal androgens, adrenal androgen formation is regulated by ACTH; thus, excessive secretion can occur either as a "pure" syndrome or as a component of

Cushing disease. The adrenal causes of androgen excess include *adrenocortical neoplasms* and an uncommon group of disorders collectively designated *congenital adrenal hyperplasia (CAH)*. Adrenocortical neoplasms associated with symptoms of androgen excess *(virilization)* are more likely to be carcinomas than adenomas. They are morphologically identical to other functional or nonfunctional cortical neoplasms.

CAHs represent a group of autosomal recessive disorders, each characterized by a hereditary defect in an enzyme involved in adrenal steroid biosynthesis, particularly cortisol. In these conditions, decreased cortisol production results in a compensatory increase in ACTH secretion due to absence of feedback inhibition. The resultant adrenal hyperplasia causes increased production of cortisol precursor steroids, which are then channeled into synthesis of androgens with virilizing activity. Certain enzyme defects may also impair aldosterone secretion, adding salt loss to the virilizing syndrome. The most common enzymatic defect in CAH is 21-hydroxylase deficiency, which accounts for more than 90% of cases. 21-Hydroxylase deficiency may range from a total lack to a mild loss, depending on the nature of the underlying mutation involving the *CYP21B* gene, which encodes this enzyme.

Morphology

In all cases of CAH, the adrenals are **hyperplastic bilaterally,** sometimes expanding to 10 to 15 times their normal weights, because of the sustained elevation in ACTH. The adrenal cortex is thickened and nodular, and on cut section, the widened cortex appears brown as a result of depletion of all lipid. The proliferating cells are mostly compact, eosinophilic, lipid-depleted cells, intermixed with lipid-laden clear cells. In addition to cortical abnormalities, **adrenomedullary dysplasia** has also been recently reported in patients with the salt-losing 21-hydroxylase deficiency. The medullary dysplasia is characterized by incomplete migration of the chromaffin cells to the center of the gland, with pronounced intermingling of nests of chromaffin and cortical cells in the periphery. Hyperplasia of corticotroph (ACTH-producing) cells is present in the anterior pituitary in most patients.

Clinical Features. The clinical manifestations of CAH are determined by the specific enzyme deficiency and include abnormalities related to androgen metabolism, sodium homeostasis, and (in severe cases) glucocorticoid deficiency. Depending on the nature and severity of the enzymatic defect, the onset of clinical symptoms may occur in the perinatal period, later childhood, or (less commonly) adulthood.

In 21-hydroxylase deficiency, *excessive androgenic activity* causes signs of masculinization in females, ranging from clitoral hypertrophy and pseudo-hermaphroditism in infants to oligomenorrhea, hirsutism, and acne in postpubertal females. In males, androgen excess is associated with enlargement of the external genitalia and other evidence of precocious puberty in prepubertal patients and with oligospermia in older individuals. In some forms of CAH (e.g., 11β-hydroxylase deficiency), the accumulated intermediary steroids have mineralocorticoid activity, with resultant *sodium retention* and *hypertension*. In other cases, however, including about one-third of persons with 21-hydroxylase deficiency, the enzymatic defect is severe enough to produce mineralocorticoid deficiency, with resultant *salt (sodium) wasting*. Cortisol deficiency places individuals with CAH at risk for *acute adrenal insufficiency* (discussed later).

CAH should be suspected in any neonate with ambiguous genitalia; severe enzyme deficiency in infancy can be a life-threatening condition, with vomiting, dehydration, and salt wasting. In the milder variants, women may present with delayed menarche, oligomenorrhea, or hirsutism. In all such cases, an androgen-producing ovarian neoplasm must be excluded. Individuals with congenital adrenal hyperplasia are treated with exogenous glucocorticoids, which, in addition to providing adequate levels of glucocorticoids, also suppress ACTH levels and thus decrease the excessive synthesis of the steroid hormones responsible for many of the clinical abnormalities.

SUMMARY

Adrenogenital Syndromes

- The adrenal cortex can secrete excess androgens in two settings: adrenocortical neoplasms (usually "virilizing" carcinomas) or congenital adrenal hyperplasia (CAH).
- CAH is a group of autosomal recessive disorders characterized by defects in steroid biosynthesis, usually cortisol; the common subtype is caused by deficiency of the enzyme 21-hydroxylase.
- Reduction in cortisol production causes a compensatory increase in ACTH secretion, which in turn stimulates androgen production. Androgens have virilizing effects, including masculinization in females (ambiguous genitalia, oligomenorrhea, hirsutism), precocious puberty in males, and in some instances, salt (sodium) wasting and hypotension.
- There is bilateral hyperplasia of the adrenal cortex, and a subset of 21-hydroxylase-deficient patients also demonstrates "adrenomedullary dysplasia."

ADRENAL INSUFFICIENCY

Adrenocortical insufficiency, or hypofunction, may be caused by either primary adrenal disease (primary hypoadrenalism) or decreased stimulation of the adrenals resulting from a deficiency of ACTH (secondary hypoadrenalism). The patterns of adrenocortical insufficiency can be considered under the following headings: (1) primary *acute* adrenocortical insufficiency (adrenal crisis), (2) primary *chronic* adrenocortical insufficiency *(Addison disease)*, and (3) secondary adrenocortical insufficiency.

Acute Adrenocortical Insufficiency

Acute adrenocortical insufficiency occurs most commonly in the clinical settings listed in Table 20–7. Individuals with chronic adrenocortical insufficiency may develop an acute crisis after any stress that taxes their limited physiologic reserves. In patients maintained on exogenous corticosteroids, rapid withdrawal of steroids or failure to increase steroid doses in response to an acute stress may precipitate a similar adrenal crisis, because of the inability of the atrophic adrenals to produce glucocorticoid hormones. *Massive adrenal hemorrhage* may destroy the adrenal cortex sufficiently to cause acute adrenocortical insufficiency. This condition may occur in patients maintained on anticoagulant therapy, in postoperative patients who develop disseminated intravascular coagulation, during pregnancy, and in patients suffering from overwhelming sepsis (Waterhouse-Friderichsen syndrome) (Fig. 20–39). This catastrophic syndrome is classically associated with *Neisseria meningitidis* septicemia but can also be caused by other organisms, including *Pseudomonas* species, pneumococci, and *Haemophilus influenzae*. The pathogenesis of the Waterhouse-Friderichsen syndrome remains unclear, but it probably involves endotoxin-induced vascular injury with associated disseminated intravascular coagulation (Chapter 12).

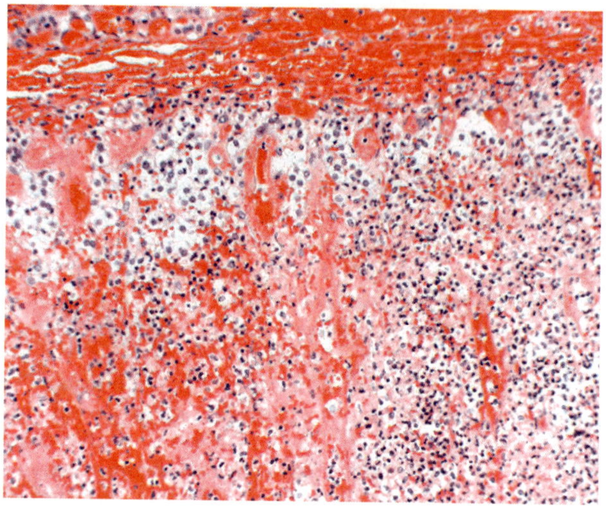

Figure 20–39

Acute adrenal insufficiency caused by severe bilateral adrenal hemorrhage in an infant with overwhelming sepsis (Waterhouse-Friderichsen syndrome). At autopsy the adrenals were grossly hemorrhagic and shrunken; microscopically, little residual cortical architecture is discernible.

Chronic Adrenocortical Insufficiency (Addison Disease)

Addison disease, or chronic adrenocortical insufficiency, is an uncommon disorder resulting from progressive destruction of the adrenal cortex. More than 90% of all cases are attributable to one of four disorders: *autoimmune adrenalitis, tuberculosis, the acquired immune deficiency syndrome (AIDS) or metastatic cancers* (Table 20–7).

- *Autoimmune adrenalitis* accounts for 60% to 70% of cases and is by far the most common cause of primary adrenal insufficiency in developed countries. As the name implies, there is autoimmune destruction of steroid-producing cells, and autoantibodies to several key steroidogenic enzymes have been detected in these patients. In about half of the patients the autoimmune disease is apparently restricted to the adrenal glands *(isolated autoimmune Addison disease);* in the remaining patients, other autoimmune diseases, such as Hashimoto disease, pernicious anemia, type I diabetes mellitus, and idiopathic hypoparathyroidism, coexist *(autoimmune polyendocrinopathy syndrome)*. A subset of autoimmune polyendocrinopathy syndrome is associated with mutations in the autoimmune regulator 1 *(AIRE1)* gene on chromosome 21q22.
- *Infections,* particularly tuberculosis and those produced by fungi, may also cause primary chronic adrenocortical insufficiency. Tuberculous adrenalitis, which once accounted for as many as 90% of cases of Addison disease, has become less common with the advent of antituberculous therapy. However, with the resurgence of tuberculosis in many urban centers, this cause of adrenal deficiency must be borne in mind. When present, tuberculous adrenalitis is usually associated with active infection in other sites, particularly the lungs and genitourinary tract. Among fungi, disseminated infections caused by *Histoplasma capsulatum* and *Coccidioides immitis* may also result in chronic adrenocortical insufficiency. Patients with AIDS are at risk for developing adrenal insufficiency from several infectious (cytomegalovirus, *Mycobacterium avium-intracellulare*) and noninfectious (Kaposi sarcoma) complications of their disease.
- *Metastatic neoplasms* involving the adrenals are another potential cause of adrenal insufficiency. The adrenals are a fairly common site for metastases in persons with disseminated carcinomas. Although adrenal function is preserved in most such patients, the metastatic growths sometimes destroy sufficient adrenal cortex to produce a degree of adrenal insufficiency. Carcinomas of the lung and breast are the source of a majority of metastases in the adrenals, although many other neoplasms, including gastrointestinal carcinomas, malignant melanomas, and hematopoietic neoplasms, may also metastasize to the organ.

Table 20–7 Causes of Adrenal Insufficiency

Causes of Adrenal Insufficiency
Acute
Waterhouse-Friderichsen syndrome
Sudden withdrawal of long-term corticosteroid therapy
Stress in patients with underlying chronic adrenal insufficiency
Chronic
MAJOR CONTRIBUTORS
Autoimmune adrenalitis
Tuberculosis
Acquired immunodeficiency syndrome
Metastatic disease
MINOR CONTRIBUTORS
Systemic amyloidosis
Fungal infections
Hemochromatosis
Sarcoidosis

Secondary Adrenocortical Insufficiency

Any disorder of the hypothalamus and pituitary, such as metastatic cancer, infection, infarction, or irradiation, that reduces the output of ACTH leads to a syndrome of hypoadrenalism having many similarities to Addison disease. With secondary disease, the hyperpigmentation of primary Addison disease is lacking because melanotropic hormone levels are low. ACTH deficiency may occur alone, but in some instances, it is only one part of panhypopituitarism, associated with multiple tropic hormone deficiencies. In patients with primary disease, serum ACTH levels may be normal, but the destruction of the adrenal cortex does not permit a response to exogenously administered ACTH in the form of increased plasma levels of cortisol. By contrast, secondary adrenocortical insufficiency is characterized by low serum ACTH and a prompt rise in plasma cortisol levels in response to ACTH administration.

Morphology

The appearance of the adrenal glands varies with the cause of the adrenocortical insufficiency. In **secondary hypoadrenalism** the adrenals are reduced to small, flattened structures that usually retain their yellow color because of a small amount of residual lipid. A uniform, thin rim of atrophic yellow cortex surrounds a central, intact medulla. Histologically, there is atrophy of cortical cells with loss of cytoplasmic lipid, particularly in the zonae fasciculata and reticularis. **Primary** autoimmune adrenalitis is characterized by irregularly shrunken glands, which may be exceedingly difficult to identify within the suprarenal adipose tissue. Histologically, the cortex contains only scattered residual cortical cells in a collapsed network of connective tissue. A variable lymphoid infiltrate is present in the cortex and may extend into the subjacent medulla (Fig. 20–40). The medulla is otherwise preserved. In cases of **tuberculosis or fungal diseases** the adrenal architecture is effaced by a granulomatous inflammatory reaction identical to that encountered in other sites of infection. Demonstration of the responsible organism may require the use of special stains. When hypoadrenalism is caused by **metastatic carcinoma,** the adrenals are enlarged and their normal architecture is obscured by the infiltrating neoplasm.

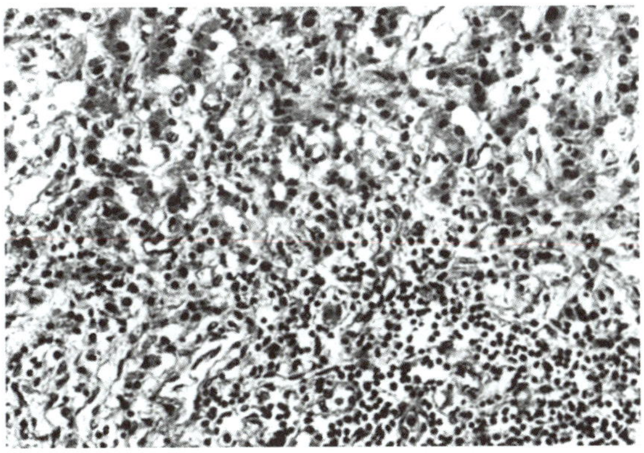

Figure 20–40

Autoimmune adrenalitis. In addition to loss of all but a subcapsular rim of cortical cells, there is an extensive mononuclear cell infiltrate.

Clinical Features. In general, clinical manifestations of adrenocortical insufficiency do not appear until at least 90% of the adrenal cortex has been compromised. The initial manifestations often include progressive weakness and easy fatigability, which may be dismissed as nonspecific complaints. *Gastrointestinal disturbances* are common and include anorexia, nausea, vomiting, weight loss, and diarrhea. In individuals with primary adrenal disease, increased levels of ACTH precursor hormone stimulate melanocytes, with resultant *hyperpigmentation* of the skin and mucosal surfaces. The face, axillae, nipples, areolae, and perineum are particularly common sites of hyperpigmentation. By contrast, hyperpigmentation is not seen in individuals with secondary adrenocortical insufficiency. Decreased mineralocorticoid (aldosterone) activity in patients with primary adrenal insufficiency results in potassium retention and sodium loss, with consequent *hyperkalemia, hyponatremia, volume depletion,* and *hypotension;* in contrast, secondary hypoadrenalism is characterized by deficient cortisol and androgen output but normal or near-normal aldosterone synthesis. Hypoglycemia may occasionally occur as a result of glucocorticoid deficiency and impaired gluconeogenesis. Stresses such as infections, trauma, or surgical procedures in such patients may precipitate an acute adrenal crisis, manifested by intractable vomiting, abdominal pain, hypotension, coma, and vascular collapse. Death follows rapidly unless corticosteroids are replaced immediately.

SUMMARY

Adrenocortical Insufficiency (Hypoadrenalism)

- Primary adrenocortical insufficiency can be acute (Waterhouse-Friderichsen syndrome) or chronic (Addison disease)
- Chronic adrenal insufficiency in the developed world is most often secondary to autoimmune adrenalitis, which can be an isolated lesion, or part of an autoimmune polyglandular syndrome.
- Tuberculosis and opportunistic pathogens associated with the human immunodeficiency virus, and tumors metastatic to the adrenals, are the other important causes of chronic hypoadrenalism.
- Patients typically present with fatigue, weakness, and gastrointestinal disturbances. Primary adrenocortical insufficiency is also characterized by high ACTH levels with associated skin pigmentation.

ADRENOCORTICAL NEOPLASMS

It should be evident from the discussion of adrenocortical hyperfunction that functional adrenal neoplasms may be responsible for any of the various forms of hypera-

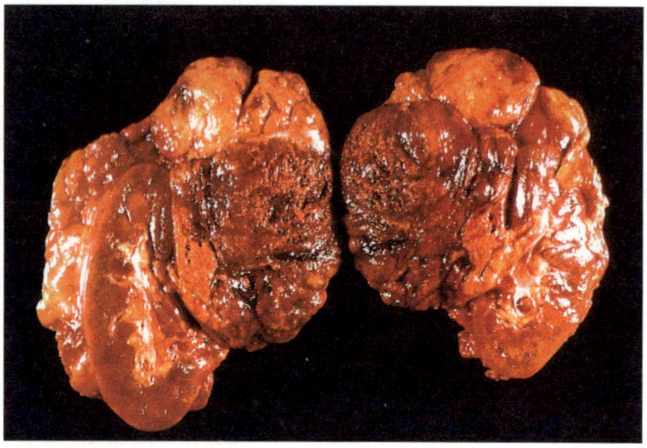

Figure 20–41

Adrenal carcinoma. The bright yellow tumor dwarfs the kidney and compresses the upper pole. It is largely hemorrhagic and necrotic.

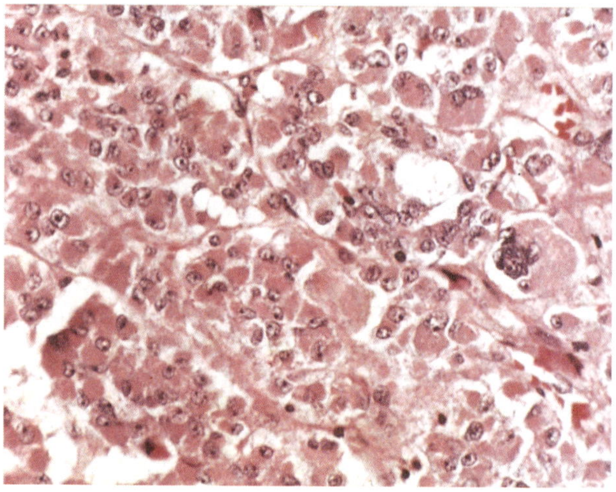

Figure 20–42

Adrenal carcinoma with marked anaplasia.

drenalism. While functional adenomas are most commonly associated with hyperaldosteronism and with Cushing syndrome, a virilizing neoplasm is more likely to be a carcinoma. However, not all adrenocortical neoplasms elaborate steroid hormones. Determination of whether a cortical neoplasm is functional or not is based on clinical evaluation and measurement of the hormone or its metabolites in the laboratory. In other words, *functional and nonfunctional adrenocortical neoplasms cannot be distinguished on the basis of morphologic features.*

Morphology

Adrenocortical adenomas were described in the earlier discussions of Cushing syndrome and hyperaldosteronism. Most cortical adenomas do not cause hyperfunction and are usually encountered as incidental findings at the time of autopsy or during abdominal imaging for an unrelated cause. In fact, the half-facetious appellation of **"adrenal incidentaloma"** has crept into the medical lexicon to describe these incidentally discovered tumors. On cut surface, adenomas are usually yellow to yellow-brown, owing to the presence of lipid within the neoplastic cells (see Fig. 20–37). As a general rule they are small, averaging 1 to 2 cm in diameter. Microscopically, adenomas are composed of cells similar to those populating the normal adrenal cortex. The nuclei tend to be small, although some degree of pleomorphism may be encountered even in benign lesions ("endocrine atypia") (see Fig. 20–38). The cytoplasm of the neoplastic cells ranges from eosinophilic to vacuolated, depending on their lipid content; mitotic activity is generally inconspicuous.

Adrenocortical carcinomas are rare neoplasms that may occur at any age, including in childhood. Two rare inherited causes of adrenal cortical carcinomas include the Li-Fraumeni syndrome (Chapter 6) and the Beckwith-Wiedemann syndrome (Chapter 7). In most cases, adrenocortical carcinomas are large, invasive lesions that efface the native adrenal gland. On cut surface, adrenocortical carcinomas are typically variegated, poorly demarcated lesions containing areas of necrosis, hemorrhage, and cystic change (Fig. 20–41). Microscopically, adrenocortical carcinomas may be composed of well-differentiated cells resembling those seen in cortical adenomas or bizarre, pleomorphic cells, which may be difficult to distinguish from those of an undifferentiated carcinoma metastatic to the adrenal (Fig. 20–42). Adrenal cancers have a strong tendency to invade the adrenal vein, vena cava, and lymphatics. Metastases to regional and periaortic nodes are common, as are distant hematogenous spread to the lungs and other viscera. Bone metastases are unusual. The median patient survival is about 2 years.

ADRENAL MEDULLA

The adrenal medulla is embryologically, functionally, and structurally distinct from the adrenal cortex. It is populated by cells derived from the neural crest (*chromaffin* cells) and their supporting (sustentacular) cells. The chromaffin cells, so named because of their brown-black color after exposure to potassium dichromate, synthesize and secrete catecholamines in response to signals from preganglionic nerve fibers in the sympathetic nervous system. Similar collections of cells are distributed throughout the body in the extra-adrenal paraganglion system. The most important diseases of the adrenal medulla are neoplasms, which include both neuronal neoplasms (including neuroblastomas and more mature ganglion cell tumors) and neoplasms composed of chromaffin cells (pheochromocytomas).

PHEOCHROMOCYTOMA

Pheochromocytomas are neoplasms composed of chromaffin cells, which, like their non-neoplastic counterparts, synthesize and release catecholamines and, in some cases, other peptide hormones. These tumors are of special importance because, although uncommon, they (like aldosterone-secreting adenomas) give rise to a surgically correctable form of hypertension.

Pheochromocytomas usually subscribe to a convenient "rule of 10s":

- *10% of pheochromocytomas arise in association with one of several familial syndromes.* These include the MEN-2A and MEN-2B syndromes (described later), type 1 neurofibromatosis (Chapter 23), von Hippel-Lindau disease (Chapters 14 and 23), and Sturge-Weber syndrome (Chapter 23).
- *10% of pheochromocytomas are extra-adrenal,* occurring in sites such as the organ of Zuckerkandl and the carotid body, where they are usually called *paragangliomas* rather than pheochromocytomas.
- *10% of adrenal pheochromocytomas are bilateral;* this figure may rise to 50% in cases that are associated with familial syndromes.
- *10% of adrenal pheochromocytomas are biologically malignant,* although the associated hypertension represents a serious and potentially lethal complication of even "benign" tumors. Frank malignancy is somewhat more common in tumors arising in extra-adrenal sites.

Morphology

Pheochromocytomas range from small, circumscribed lesions confined to the adrenal to large, hemorrhagic masses weighing several kilograms. On cut surface, smaller pheochromocytomas are yellow-tan, well-defined lesions that compress the adjacent adrenal (Fig. 20–43). Larger lesions tend to be hemorrhagic, necrotic, and cystic and typically efface the adrenal gland. Incubation of the fresh tissue with potassium dichromate solutions turns the tumor a dark brown color, as noted previously.

Microscopically, pheochromocytomas are composed of polygonal to spindle-shaped chromaffin cells and their supporting cells, compartmentalized into small nests, or "Zellballen," by a rich vascular network (Fig. 20–44). The cytoplasm of the neoplastic cells often has a finely granular appearance, highlighted by a variety of silver stains, because of the presence of granules containing catecholamines. Electron microscopy reveals variable numbers of membrane-bound, electron-dense granules, representing catecholamines and sometimes other peptides. The nuclei of the neoplastic cells are often quite pleomorphic. Both capsular and vascular invasion may be encountered in benign lesions, and the presence of mitotic figures per se does not imply malignancy. **Therefore, the definitive diagnosis of malignancy in pheochromocytomas is based exclusively on the presence of metastases.** These may involve regional lymph nodes as well as more distant sites, including liver, lung, and bone.

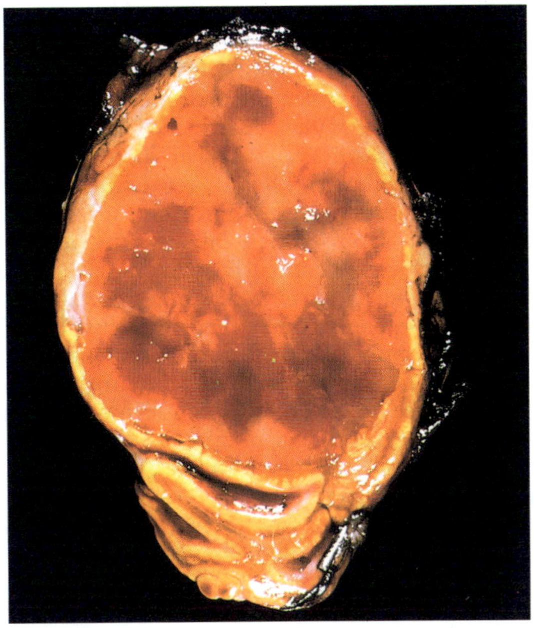

Figure 20–43

Pheochromocytoma. The tumor is enclosed within an attenuated cortex and demonstrates areas of hemorrhage. The comma-shaped residual adrenal is seen below.

Clinical Features. The dominant clinical manifestation of pheochromocytoma is *hypertension.* Classically, this is described as an abrupt, precipitous elevation in blood pressure, associated with tachycardia, palpitations, headache, sweating, tremor, and a sense of apprehension. Such episodes may also be associated with pain in the abdomen or chest, nausea, and vomiting. In practice, *isolated, paroxysmal episodes of hypertension occur in*

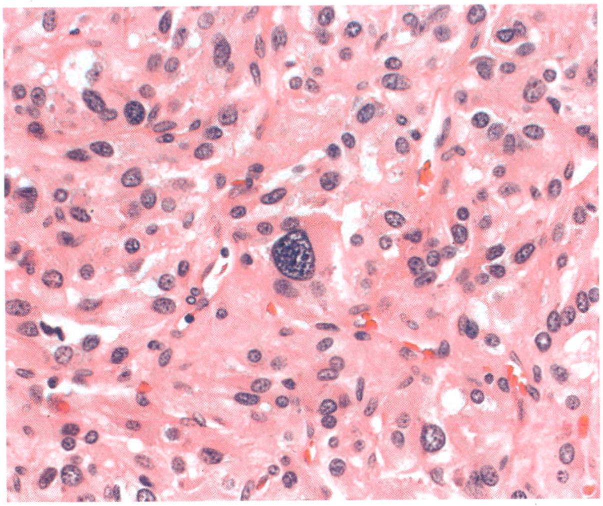

Figure 20–44

Photomicrograph of pheochromocytoma, demonstrating characteristic nests of cells ("Zellballen") with abundant cytoplasm. Granules containing catecholamine are not visible in this preparation. It is not uncommon to find bizarre cells even in pheochromocytomas that are biologically benign, and this criterion by itself should not be used to diagnose malignancy.

fewer than half of individuals with pheochromocytoma. In about two-thirds of patients the hypertension occurs in the form of a chronic, sustained elevation in blood pressure, although an element of labile hypertension is often present as well. Whether sustained or episodic, the hypertension is associated with an increased risk of myocardial ischemia, heart failure, renal injury, and cerebrovascular accidents. Sudden cardiac death may occur, probably secondary to catecholamine-induced myocardial irritability and ventricular arrhythmias. In some cases, pheochromocytomas secrete other hormones such as ACTH and somatostatin and may therefore be associated with clinical features related to the secretion of these and other peptide hormones. The laboratory diagnosis of pheochromocytoma is based on demonstration of increased urinary excretion of free catecholamines and their metabolites, such as vanillylmandelic acid and metanephrines. Isolated benign pheochromocytomas are treated with surgical excision, after pre- and intraoperative medication of patients with adrenergic-blocking agents. Multifocal lesions may require long-term medical treatment for hypertension.

NEUROBLASTOMA AND OTHER NEURONAL NEOPLASMS

Neuroblastoma is the most common extra-cranial solid tumor of childhood. These neoplasms occur most commonly during the first 5 years of life and may arise during infancy. Neuroblastomas may occur anywhere in the sympathetic nervous system and occasionally within the brain, but they are most common in the abdomen; most cases arise in either the adrenal medulla or the retroperitoneal sympathetic ganglia. Most neuroblastomas are sporadic, although familial cases also occur. These tumors are discussed in Chapter 7, along with other pediatric neoplasms.

MULTIPLE ENDOCRINE NEOPLASIA SYNDROMES

The MEN syndromes are a group of inherited diseases resulting in proliferative lesions (hyperplasias, adenomas, and carcinomas) of multiple endocrine organs. Like other inherited cancer disorders (Chapter 6), endocrine tumors arising in the context of MEN syndromes have certain distinctive features that contrast with their sporadic counterparts:

- These tumors occur at a *younger age* than sporadic cancers.
- They arise in *multiple endocrine organs,* either *synchronously* or *metachronously.*
- Even in one organ, the tumors are often *multifocal.*
- The tumors are usually preceded by an *asymptomatic stage of endocrine hyperplasia* involving the cell of origin of the tumor (for example, patients with MEN-1 syndrome develop varying degrees of islet cell hyperplasia, some of which progress to pancreatic tumors).
- These tumors are usually *more aggressive* and *recur* in a higher proportion of cases than similar endocrine tumors that occur sporadically.

Unraveling the genetic basis of the MEN syndromes and applying the knowledge to therapeutic decision making has been one of the success stories of translational research. The salient features of the MEN syndromes are discussed below.

MULTIPLE ENDOCRINE NEOPLASIA TYPE 1

MEN type 1 is inherited in an autosomal dominant pattern. The gene *(MEN1)* is located at 11q13 and is a tumor suppressor gene; thus, inactivation of both alleles of the gene is believed to be the basis of tumorigenesis. Organs commonly involved include the parathyroid (95%), pancreas (~40%), and pituitary (~30%)—the "3 Ps."

- *Parathyroid:* Primary hyperparathyroidism, arising from multiglandular parathyroid hyperplasia, is the most consistent feature of MEN-1.
- *Pancreas:* Endocrine tumors of the pancreas are the leading cause of death in MEN-1. These tumors are usually aggressive and present with metastatic disease or multifocality. Pancreatic endocrine tumors are often functional (i.e., they secrete hormones). Zollinger-Ellison syndrome, associated with gastrinomas, and hypoglycemia, related to insulinomas, are common endocrine manifestations.
- *Pituitary:* The most frequent pituitary tumor in MEN-1 patients is a prolactin-secreting macroadenoma. Some individuals develop acromegaly from somatotrophin-secreting tumors.

MULTIPLE ENDOCRINE NEOPLASIA TYPE 2

MEN type 2 is actually two distinct groups of disorders that are unified by the occurrence of activating mutations of the *RET* protooncogene. There is a strong *genotype-phenotype correlation* within the MEN-2 syndrome, and differences in mutation patterns possibly account for the variable features in the two subtypes. MEN-2 is inherited in an autosomal dominant pattern. The *RET* protooncogene is located at 10q11.2.

Multiple Endocrine Neoplasia, Type 2A

Organs commonly involved include:

- *Thyroid:* Medullary carcinoma of the thyroid develops in virtually all untreated cases, and the tumors usually occur in the first 2 decades of life. The tumors are commonly multifocal, and foci of C-cell hyperplasia can be found in the adjacent thyroid.
- *Adrenal medulla:* 50% of patients develop adrenal pheochromocytomas; fortunately, no more than 10% are malignant.
- *Parathyroid:* Approximately a third of patients develop parathyroid gland hyperplasia with primary hyperparathyroidism.

Multiple Endocrine Neoplasia, Type 2B

Organs commonly involved include the thyroid and adrenal medulla. The spectrum of thyroid and adrenal medullary disease is similar to that in MEN-2A. *However, unlike MEN-2A, patients with MEN-2B:*

- Do not develop primary hyperparathyroidism
- *Develop extraendocrine manifestations:* ganglioneuromas of mucosal sites (gastrointestinal tract, lips, tongue) and marfanoid habitus

Before the advent of genetic testing, family members of individuals with the MEN-2 syndrome were screened with annual biochemical tests, which often lacked sensitivity. Now, routine genetic testing identifies *RET* mutation carriers earlier and more reliably in MEN-2 kindreds; *all persons carrying germ-line RET mutations are advised to have prophylactic thyroidectomy to prevent the inevitable development of medullary carcinomas.* Surgical intervention based on the results of a single genetic test represents a new paradigm in the practice of "molecular medicine."

BIBLIOGRAPHY

Arighi E, et al.: RET tyrosine kinase signaling in development and cancer. Cytokine Growth Factor Rev 16:441; 2005. *[A review on the role of RET tyrosine kinase dysfunction in human disease, both loss-of-function mutations as observed in certain forms of Hirschsprung disease, and gain-of-function mutations as seen in endocrine neoplasia.]*

Bartalena L, et al.: Graves ophthalmopathy: state of the art and perspective. J Endocrinol Invest 27:295; 2004. *[A review on the pathophysiology of Graves ophthalmopathy, including orbital cell types involved in the disease process, and potential therapies.]*

Biddinger SB, Kahn CR: From mice to men: insights into insulin resistance syndromes. Annu Rev Physiol doi:10.1146/annurev.physiol.68.040104.124723 (2005). *[A seminal review summarizing how animal models have provided insights into mechanisms of insulin resistance and type 2 diabetes.]*

Falchetti A, et al.: Lessons from genes mutated in multiple endocrine neoplasia syndromes. Ann Endocrinol (Paris) 66:195, 2005. *[A review of the genetics of MEN syndromes, including the current state of knowledge on MEN1 and RET.]*

Farnebo LO: Primary hyperparathyroidism. Scand J Surg 93:282; 2005. *[A clinically oriented review on this subject.]*

Findling JW, Raff H: Screening and diagnosis of Cushing syndrome. Endocrinol Metab Clin North Am 34:385, 2005. *[This review covers some of the more intricate aspects on differential diagnosis of Cushing syndrome, including pertinent laboratory tests, that were not specifically covered in the current chapter.]*

Gumbs AA, et al.: Review of the clinical, histological, and molecular aspects of pancreatic endocrine neoplasms. J Surg Oncol 81:45, 2002. *[A review on the pathology and genetics of pancreatic endocrine neoplasms, including a molecular classification that has prognostic importance.]*

Heaney AP, Melmed S: Molecular targets in pituitary tumors. Nat Rev Cancer 4:285, 2004. *[A review on the molecular genetics of pituitary neoplasms with a focus on identification of therapeutic targets.]*

Kasuga M: Insulin resistance and pancreatic beta cell failure. J Clin Invest 7:1756–1760, 2006. *[A scholarly review of the pathophysiology of type 2 diabetes.]*

Kent SC, et al.: Expanded T cells from pancreatic lymph nodes of type 1 diabetic subjects recognize an insulin epitope. Nature 435:151, 2005. *[A research article detailing the identification of T-cell subsets that recognize an insulin epitope, in patients with long-standing type 1 diabetes; not listed is a companion paper in the same issue describing the importance of similar insulin epitopes in mouse models of diabetes.]*

Koerner A, et al.: Adipocytokines: leptin—the classical, resistin—the controversial, adiponectin—the promising, and more to come. Best Pract Res Clin Endocrinol Metab 19:525, 2005. *[A comprehensive review on adipocytokines, which are increasingly being implicated in the pathogenesis of type 2 diabetes in the setting of obesity.]*

Kroll TG: Molecular events in follicular thyroid tumors. Cancer Treat Res 122:85, 2004. *[A scholarly article on the genetics of thyroid carcinomas, emphasizing the parallels between thyroid tumors and hematologic malignancies, with an eye on potential therapeutic targets.]*

Marzotti S, Falorni A: Addison's disease. Autoimmunity 37:333, 2004. *[A review on the pathogenesis of adrenal insufficiency, particularly autoimmune adrenalitis.]*

Merke DP, Bornstein SR: Congenital adrenal hyperplasia. Lancet 365:2125, 2005. *[This article reviews the epidemiology, genetics, pathophysiology, diagnosis, and management of CAH, and provides an overview of clinical challenges and future therapies.]*

Reid JR, Wheeler SF: Hyperthyroidism: diagnosis and management. Am Fam Physician 623, 2005. *[A clinically oriented review on hyperthyroidism, with a diagnostic algorithm for identifying the causative etiology.]*

Report of the Expert Committee on the Diagnosis and Classification of Diabetes Mellitus. Diabetes Care 25 (Suppl 1):S5, 2002. *[A consensus statement from the American Diabetes Association on the new "etiology-based" classification of diabetes.]*

Schott M, et al.: Thyrotropin receptor autoantibodies in Graves disease. Trends Endocrinol Metab 16:243, 2005. *[A review on the role of anti-TSHR autoantibodies in Graves disease, and methods for detecting these antibodies.]*

Stassi G, DeMaria R: Autoimmune thyroid disease: new models of cell death in autoimmunity. Nat Rev Immunol 2:195, 2002. *[A review on autoimmune thyroid disorders, particularly the pathogenesis of Hashimoto and other thyroiditis.]*

Stumvoll M, et al.: Type 2 diabetes: principles of pathogenesis and therapy. Lancet 365:1333, 2005. *[An outstanding and state-of-the-art review on a complicated subject, summarizing current knowledge on obesity and insulin resistance, β-cell dysfunction, and genetics of diabetes. Strongly recommended.]*

Vaugh ED Jr: Diseases of the adrenal gland. Med Clin North Am 88:443, 2004. *[A one-stop shop summarizing major adrenal diseases, mostly from a clinical perspective.]*

Waki H, Tontonoz P: Endocrine functions of adipose tissue. Annual Review of Pathology: Mechanisms of Disease, Vol. 2:31, 2007. *[A timely review on adipokines.]*

Wolford JK, et al.: Genetic basis of type 2 diabetes mellitus: implications for therapy. Treat Endocrinol 3:257, 2004. *[Another review on genetics of type 2 diabetes, this one from the potential for therapy and primary prevention.]*

Xing M: *BRAF* mutation in thyroid cancer. Endocr Relat Cancer 12:245, 2005. *[A review on the role of BRAF point mutations as an oncogenic event in papillary thyroid cancers, and its diagnostic utility.]*

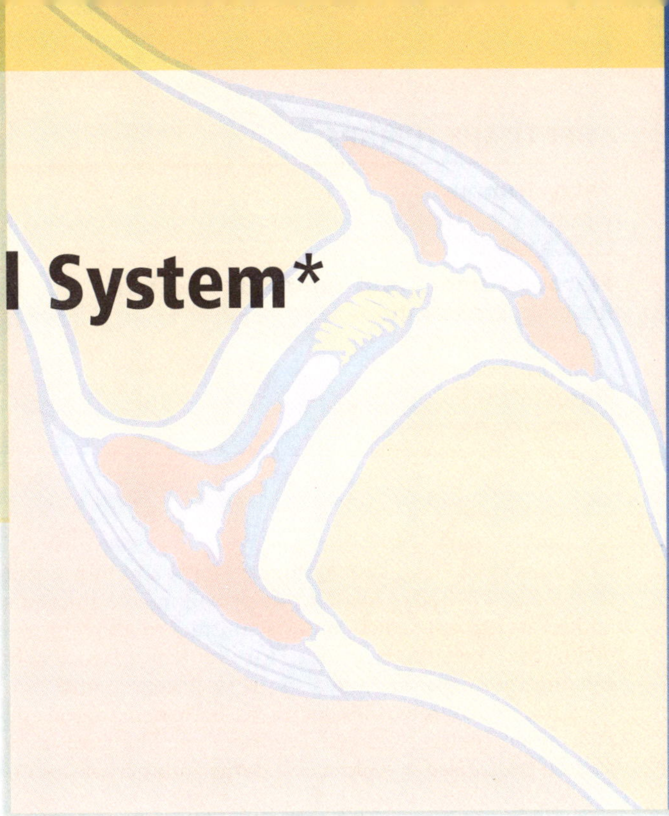

Chapter 21

The Musculoskeletal System*

*The authors acknowledge the contributions of Dr. Dennis K. Burns to previous editions of this book.

SOFT TISSUE TUMORS

Fatty Tumors
Lipoma
Liposarcoma

Fibrous Tumors and Tumor-Like Lesions
Reactive Proliferations
- Nodular Fasciitis
- Myositis Ossificans

Fibromatoses
Fibrosarcoma

Fibrohistiocytic Tumors
Benign Fibrous Histiocytoma (Dermatofibroma)
Malignant Fibrous Histiocytoma

Smooth Muscle Tumors
Leiomyoma
Leiomyosarcoma

Synovial Sarcoma

The musculoskeletal system imparts form and movement to the human body. Aside from providing the fulcrums and levers against which muscles contract to allow movement, the skeleton is critical for mineral (particularly calcium) homeostasis, and also protects viscera and supplies an environment conducive to both hematopoiectic and mesenchymal stem cell development. The term *musculoskeletal disease* embraces a large number of conditions ranging from localized, benign lesions of the bone such as the osteochondroma to generalized disorders such as osteoporosis, osteogenesis imperfecta, and muscular dystrophy. In this chapter we will first consider some of the more common conditions affecting the bones and joints, then discuss selected diseases of skeletal muscle, concluding with a brief commentary about tumors arising in the various soft tissues of the body.

BONES

CONGENITAL DISEASES OF BONE

Congenital diseases of bone range from localized malformations to hereditary disorders associated with abnormalities affecting the entire skeletal system. Developmental anomalies resulting from localized problems in the migration of mesenchymal cells and the formation of condensations are called *dysostoses*. They are usually limited to defined embryologic structures and can result from mutations in specific homeobox genes. Some of the more common lesions include *aplasia* (e.g., congenital absence of a digit or rib), the formation of extra bones (e.g., supernumerary digits or ribs), and abnormal fusion of bones (e.g., premature closure of the cranial sutures or congenital fusion of the ribs). Such malformations may occur as isolated, sporadic lesions or as components of a more complex syndrome. Mutations that interfere with bone or cartilage growth and/or maintenance of normal matrix components (e.g. those affecting growth factors or their receptors) have more diffuse effects; such disorders are called *dysplasias*. The number of such disorders (well over 200) renders the discussion of all but the most common impossible in the limited space here. In addition, a number of hereditary metabolic disorders not usually thought of as primary skeletal diseases (e.g., mucopolysaccharidoses like Hurler syndrome) can also affect the bone matrix; such conditions are discussed briefly with other genetic disorders in Chapter 7.

Osteogenesis Imperfecta

Osteogenesis imperfecta (OI), also known as "brittle bone disease", is actually a group of hereditary disorders caused by defective synthesis of type I collagen. Because type I collagen is a major component of extracellular matrix in other parts of the body, there are also numerous extraskeletal manifestations (affecting e.g., skin, joints, and eyes). The molecular pathology underlying OI characteristically involves gene mutations in the coding sequences for α_1 or α_2 chains of type I collagen. Because successful collagen synthesis and extracellular export require formation of a complete and intact triple helix, any primary defect in a collagen chain tends to disrupt the entire structure and results in its premature degradation (an example of a *dominant negative mutation*; see Chapter 7). As a consequence, most defects manifest as autosomal dominant disorders and can have a disastrous phenotype. There is, however, a broad spectrum of severity, and mutations that result in qualitatively normal collagen but at only reduced levels generally have milder manifestations.

The fundamental abnormality in all forms of OI is too little bone, resulting in extreme skeletal fragility. There are four major subtypes, with an extremely broad range of clinical outcomes. Thus, the type II variant is uniformly fatal pre- or immediately post-partum due to multiple fractures that occur *in utero*. In contrast, patients with type I OI have a normal lifespan, with only a modestly increased proclivity to fractures during childhood (decreasing in frequency after puberty). The classic finding of *blue sclerae* in type I OI is attributable to decreased scleral collagen content; this causes a relative transparency that allows the underlying choroid to be seen. *Hearing loss* can be related to conduction defects in the middle and inner ear bones, and *small misshapen teeth* are a result of dentin deficiency.

Achrondroplasia

Achondroplasia is a major cause of dwarfism. The underlying etiology is a point mutation in the fibroblast growth factor receptor 3 (FGFR3) that results in its constitutive activation. Unfortunately, activated FGFR3 *inhibits* chondrocyte proliferation; as a result, the normal epiphyseal growth plate expansion is suppressed and long bone growth is severely stunted. Because the most common mutation leads to ligand-independent FGFR3 activation, the disorder is typically autosomal dominant. The affected individuals are typically heterozygotes, since homozygosity leads to abnormalities in chest development and death from respiratory failure soon after birth. Interestingly, four of five cases represent new spontaneous mutations.

Achondroplasia affects all bones that form from a cartilaginous framework. The most conspicuous changes include marked, disproportionate shortening of the proximal extremities, bowing of the legs, and a lordotic (sway-backed) posture. The cartilage growth plates are disorganized and hypoplastic, in contrast to the expanded, orderly columns normally seen at the epiphyses.

Thanatophoric dwarfism is a lethal variant of dwarfism, affecting 1 in every 20,000 live births (*thanatophoric* means "death loving"). This disease is also caused by FGFR3 mutations, but involves missense or point mutations in different domains of the receptors, distinct from those in achondroplasia. Affected heterozygotes have extreme shortening of the limbs, frontal bossing of the skull, and an extremely small thorax, which is the cause of fatal respiratory failure in the perinatal period.

Osteopetrosis

Osteopetrosis is a group of rare genetic disorders characterized by reduced osteoclast-mediated bone resorption and therefore defective bone remodelling. Osteopetrosis (literally "stone bone") is a seemingly apt name, since the affected bone is grossly dense and stone-like. Paradoxically, the bone is architecturally unsound and fractures as readily as a piece of chalk. There are four variants distinguished on the basis of clinical findings and modes of inheritance.

Bone resorption occurs through osteoclast-driven enzymatic degradation of the proteinaceous bone matrix. However, before the matrix can be digested, it must first be decalcified. This is achieved by osteoclasts tightly applying themselves to the bony surface (at sites called *Howship lacunae*) and sealing their edges to prevent leaks. This is important because the extracellular space between osteoclast and bone becomes functionally analogous to a secondary lysosome. The space is acidified by a proton pump, and the inorganic hydroxyapatite matrix is dissolved. The osteoclast also releases a number of matrix degrading enzymes; as part of the degradative process, mediators that were previously deposited in the matrix (largely by osteoblasts) are also released and become active.

The precise nature of the osteoclast dysfunction is unknown in most cases. Nevertheless, there is a variant associated with *carbonic anhydrase II deficiency* that makes excellent pathogenic sense because this enzyme is required for the osteoclast hydrogen ion excretion and, therefore, for acidification of the site of bone resorbtion. Thus, defective bone remodeling in these patients is directly attributable to reduced bone demineralization.

Besides fractures, patients with osteopetrosis frequently have cranial nerve problems (due to compression from surrouding bone), and recurrent infections. The latter is attributable to diminished hematopoiesis resulting from reduced marrow space. Indeed, osteopetrotic patients often develop impressive hepatosplenomegaly due to expansive extramedullary hematopoiesis.

Because osteoclasts are derived from marrow monocyte precursors, bone marrow transplants hold the promise of re-populating recipients with progenitors capable of differentiating into fully functional osteoclasts. Indeed, many of the skeletal abnormalities appear to be reversible once normal precursor cells are provided.

SUMMARY

Congenital Diseases of Bone

- Congenital malformations are called *dysostoses* and can result in the absence of bones, supernumerary bones, or inappropriately fused bones; these are typically due to mutations in homeobox genes affecting localized migration and condensation of primitive mesenchymal cells.
- Abnormalities in bone organogenesis are called *dysplasias;* these can be caused by mutations in a variety of signal transduction pathways or in components of the extracellular matrix:
  - Achondroplasia (dwarfism) occurs as a consequence of constitutive FGFR3 activation resulting in defective cartilage synthesis at growth plates.
  - Osteogenesis imperfecta (brittle bone disease) is a group of disorders related to abnormal type I collagen synthesis with resultant bone fragility and susceptibility to fractures.
  - Osteopetrosis results in a dense but architecturally unsound bone due to defective osteoclast-induced bone remodeling.

ACQUIRED DISEASES OF BONE DEVELOPMENT

Many nutritional, endocrine, and systemic disorders affect the skeletal system. Nutritional deficiencies causing bone disease include deficiencies of vitamin C (involved in collagen cross-linking; deficiency causes *scurvy*) and vitamin D (involved in calcium uptake; deficiency causes *rickets* and *osteomalacia*). Both of these are discussed in greater detail with other nutritional diseases in Chapter 8. Primary and secondary hyperparathyroidism (discussed in Chapter 20) also cause significant skeletal changes, which will be briefly reviewed in this section. The major focus of the discussion here will be *osteoporosis,* resulting from a loss of bone mass, and *Paget disease,* a disease associated with the loss of osteoclast function.

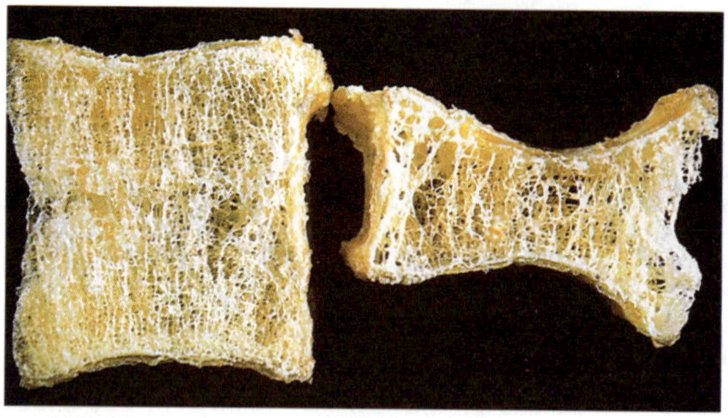

Figure 21–1

Osteoporotic vertebral body *(right)* shortened by compression fractures, compared with a normal vertebral body. Note that the osteoporotic vertebra has a characteristic loss of horizontal trabeculae and thickened vertical trabeculae.

Osteoporosis

Osteoporosis is a disease characterized by increased porosity of the skeleton resulting from reduced bone mass. It is associated with an increase in bone fragility and susceptibility to fractures. The disorder may be localized to a certain bone or region, as in *disuse osteoporosis of a limb,* or may involve the entire skeleton, as a manifestation of a *metabolic bone disease.* Generalized osteoporosis may be primary, or secondary to a large variety of conditions (Table 21–1).

The most common forms of osteoporosis are *senile* and *postmenopausal* osteoporosis; senile osteoporosis affects all aging individuals, while postmenopausal osteoporosis obviously affects only women after menopause. Peak bone mass is achieved during young adulthood, but beginning in the third or fourth decade in both sexes, bone resorption begins to outpace bone deposition; this age-related bone loss—averaging 0.7% per year—is a normal biological phenomenon. Such losses generally occur in areas containing abundant cancelloues (trabecular) bone and are therefore more pronounced in the spine and femoral neck. Hence these sites are more prone to fractures in individuals with osteoporosis. Clearly, if one begins with a greater bone mass, the effects of gradual bone loss are delayed. However, the rate of loss with each cycle of remodeling can be accelerated by the postmenopausal state. Hence females are more vulnerable to osteoporosis and its complications. Regardless of the underlying cause, the progressive loss of bone mass is clinically significant because of the resultant increase in the risk of fractures. Roughly a million Americans each year experience a significant osteoporosis-related fracture; when the morbidity and mortality associated with osteoporosis-related fractures are taken into account, the annual cost of osteoporosis in the United States exceeds $14 billion.

Table 21–1 Categories of Generalized Osteoporosis

Primary	
Postmenopausal Senile	
Secondary	
ENDOCRINE DISORDERS	DISEASE DRUGS
Hyperparathyroidism Hypo or hyperthyroidism Hypogonadism Pituitary tumors Diabetes, type 1 Addison disease	Anticoagulants Chemotherapy Corticosteroids Anticonvulsants Alcohol
NEOPLASIA	MISCELLANEOUS
Multiple myeloma Carcinomatosis	Osteogenesis imperfecta Immobilization Pulmonary disease Homocystinuria Anemia
GASTROINTESTINAL DISORDERS	
Malnutrition Malabsorption Hepatic insufficiency Vitamin C, D deficiencies Idiopathic	

Morphology

The hallmark of osteoporosis is a loss of bone, which tends to be **most conspicuous in parts of the skeleton containing abundant trabecular bone.** The bony trabeculae are thinner and more widely separated than usual, resulting in an increased susceptibility to fractures (Fig. 21–1). In postmenopausal osteoporosis, the bone loss is often particularly severe in the vertebral bodies, which may fracture and collapse. Similar bone loss is common in other weight-bearing bones, such as the femoral necks, another common site for fractures. The major microscopic changes are thinning of the trabeculae and widening of Haversian canals. Osteoclastic activity is present but is not dramatically increased. The mineral content of the remaining bone is normal, and thus there is no alteration in the ratio of minerals to protein matrix.

Pathogenesis. In adults there is a dynamic equilibrium between bone formation by osteoblasts (Fig. 21–2A), maintenance by osteocytes, and resorption by osteoclasts (Fig. 21–2B). Osteoporosis occurs when the balance tilts in favor of resorption.

Although a complete understanding of the underlying control mechanisms of bone remodeling is not yet

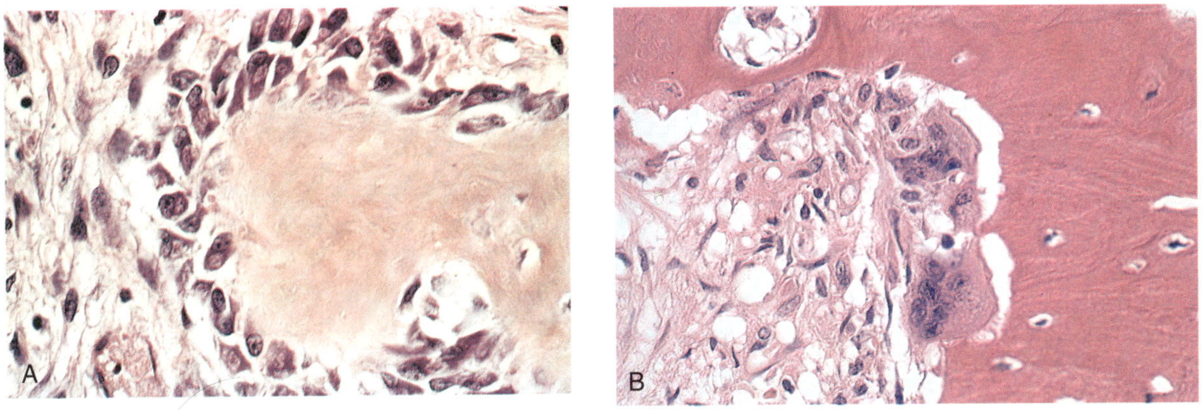

Figure 21–2

Cells of bone. **A,** Active osteoblasts synthesizing bone matrix proteins. The surrounding spindle cells represent osteoprogenitor cells. **B,** Two osteoclasts resorbing bone. The smaller blue nuclei surrounded by a halo of clearing in the dense pink lamellar bone are osteocytes in their individual lacunae.

known, there are a number of exciting new insights. Central to these is the recognition that novel members of the tumor necrosis factor (TNF) receptor family influence osteoclast function (Fig. 21–3). The story begins with RANK, which stands for *r*eceptor *a*ctivator for *n*uclear factor κB. This name derives from the ability of the receptor to activate the NFκB transcriptional pathway on cells that bear RANK; such RANK-expressing cells include macrophages (and thus, osteoclasts). RANK is activated by interaction with RANK ligand (a cell surface TNF family member) that is synthesized and expressed by bone stromal cells and osteoblasts. Stromal cells and osteoblasts also produce a cytokine called macrophage colony-stimulating factor (M-CSF) that attaches to a distinct macrophage cell surface receptor. Together, RANK ligand and M-CSF conspire to convert macrophages into bone-crunching osteoclasts. RANK activation is therefore a major stimulus for bone resorption. The resorptive activity induced by the RANK–RANK ligand pathway is regulated by a molecule called *osteoprotegerin (OPG)*, also secreted by osteoblasts and stromal cells. OPG is a "decoy receptor" that can bind RANK ligand and thus short-circuit its interaction with RANK. Binding of RANK ligand to OPG instead of RANK curtails osteoclast formation and bone-resorbing activity. Dysregulation of RANK, RANK ligand, and OPG interactions is likely a major contributor in the pathogenesis of osteoporosis. Such dysregulation can occur for a variety of reasons, including aging, changes in cytokine environment, and estrogen deficiency (Fig. 21–4 and see below). Regardless of the upstream influences, the final common pathway in osteoporosis involves an imbalance of osteoblast bone formation, osteoclast bone resorption, *and* osteoblast (and stromal cell) regulation of osteoclast activation.

- *Age-related changes.* With increasing age, osteoblasts replicate and synthesize matrix with progressively diminished gusto. The various growth factors deposited in the ECM also tend to become less potent with time. Unfortunately, while new bone synthesis

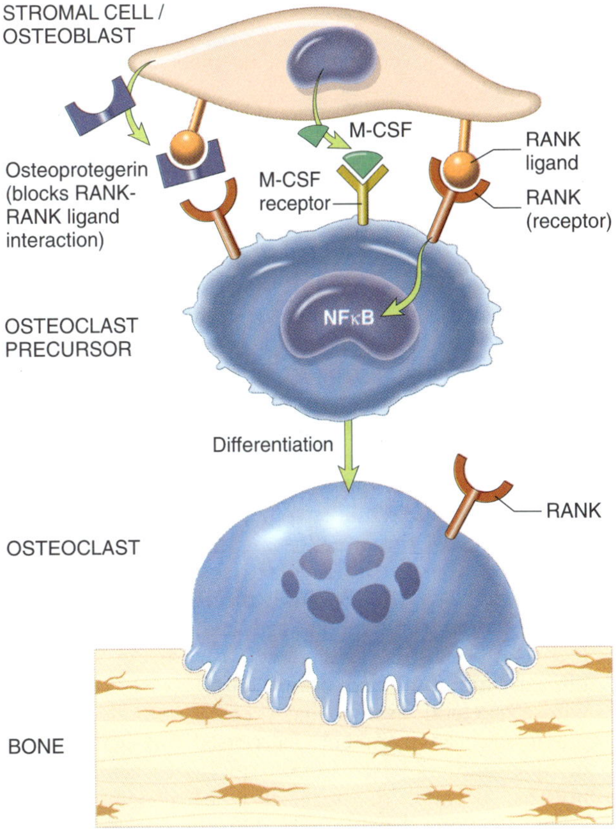

Figure 21–3

Paracrine mechanisms regulating osteoclast formation and function. Osteoclasts are derived from the same stem cells that produce macrophages. RANK (receptor activator for nuclear factor-κB) receptors on osteoclast precursors bind RANK ligand (RANKL) expressed by osteoblasts and marrow stromal cells. Along with macrophage colony-stimulating factor (M-CSF), the RANK-RANKL interaction drives the differentiation of functional osteoclasts. Stromal cells also secrete osteoprotegerin (OPG) that acts as a decoy receptor for RANKL, preventing it from binding the RANK receptor on osteoclast precursors. Consequently OPG prevents bone resorption by inhibiting osteoclast differentiation.

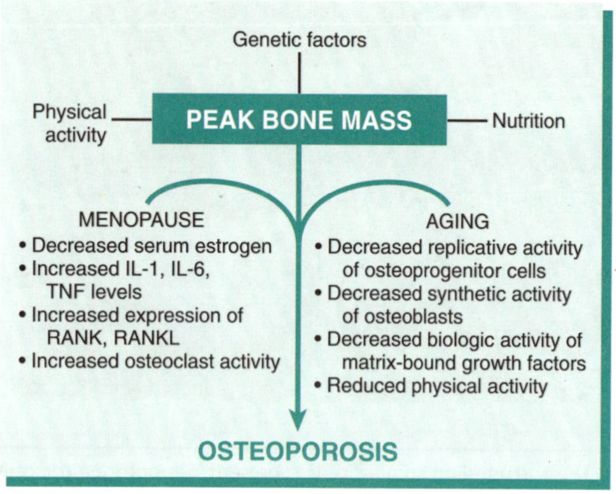

Figure 21–4

Pathophysiology of postmenopausal and senile osteoporosis (see text).

wanes with advancing age, osteoclasts retain their youthful vigor (Fig. 21–4).

• *Hormonal influences.* The decline in estrogen levels associated with menopause correlates with an annual decline of as much as 2% of cortical bone and 9% of cancellous bone. This can add up to 35% of cortical bone and 50% of trabecular bone within 30–40 years! It is therefore not surprising that roughly half of postmenopausal women will suffer an osteoporotic fracture (compared to 2–3% of men of comparable age). *The hypoestrogenic effects are attributable in part to augmented cytokine production* (especially interleukin-1 and TNF). These translate into increased RANK–RANK ligand activity and diminished OPG (see Fig. 21–4). Despite some compensatory osteoblastic activity, it is inadequate to keep pace with the osteoclast bone resorption. While estrogen replacement can ameliorate some of the bone loss, it is increasingly associated with other cardiovascular risks (see Chapter 10).

• *Physical activity.* Because mechanical forces stimulate bone remodeling, reduced physical activity increases bone loss. This effect is obvious in an immobilized limb, but also occurs diffusely in astronauts whose skeletal system has been "unloaded" in a gravity-free environment. Decreased physical activity in older individuals also contributes to senile osteoporosis. Because the magnitude of skeletal loading influences bone density more than the number of load cycles, the type of physical activity is important. Thus, resistance exercises such as weight training increase bone mass more effectively than endurance activities such as jogging.

• *Genetic factors.* Vitamin D receptor polymorphisms account for approximately 75% of the maximal peak bone mass achieved in any given individual. Additional genetic variables can influence calcium uptake, or PTH synthesis and responses.

• *Calcium nutritional state.* The majority of adolescent girls (but not boys) have insufficient dietary intake. Unfortunately, this calcium deficiency occurs during a period of rapid bone growth. As a result, they do not achieve the maximal peak bone that could be otherwise expected, and are therefore likely to develop clinically significant osteoporosis at an earlier age.

• *Secondary causes of osteoporosis.* These include prolonged glucocorticoid therapy (increases bone resorption and reduces bone synthesis.)

Clinical Course. The clinical outcome of osteoporosis depends on which bones are involved. Thoracic and lumbar vertebral fractures are extremely common, and produce loss of height and various deformities, including kyphoscoliosis that can compromise respiratory function. Pulmonary embolism and pneumonia are common complications of fractures of the femoral neck, pelvis, or spine, and result in as many as 50,000 deaths annually.

Osteoporosis is difficult to diagnose because it remains asymptomatic until skeletal fragility is announced with a fracture. Moreover, it cannot be reliably detected in plain radiographs until 30%–40% of bone mass has already disappeared; serum levels of calcium, phosphorus, and alkaline phosphatase are notoriously insensitive. The current state of the art for bone loss estimation involves specialized radiographic techniques to assess density, e.g., dual-energy absorptiometry and quantitative computed tomography.

Osteoporosis prevention and treatment begins with adequate dietary calcium intake, vitamin D supplementation, and a regular exercise regimen—starting before the age of 30—to increase the peak bone density. Calcium and vitamin D supplements later in life can also modestly reduce bone loss. Bisphosphonate administration is an important part of the therapeutic strategy in osteoporosis due to its ability to decrease bone resorption. Selective estrogen receptor agonists are another class of drugs that act by increasing bone mass (similar to endogenous estrogens) but without the side effects associated with estrogen use. Parathyroid hormone administration is yet another approach, and may be especially applicable for patients who cannot tolerate estrogen therapy.

Paget Disease (Osteitis Deformans)

This unique skeletal disease is characterized by repetitive episodes of frenzied, regional osteoclastic activity and bone resorption *(osteolytic stage),* followed by exuberant bone formation *(mixed osteoclastic-osteoblastic stage),* and finally by an apparent exhaustion of cellular activity *(osteosclerotic stage).* The net effect of this process is a *gain in bone mass;* however, the newly formed bone is disordered and lacks strength.

Paget disease usually does not occur until mid-adulthood but becomes progressively more common thereafter. There is marked variation in prevalence in different populations; it is rare in the native populations of Scandinavia, China, Japan, and Africa, but is relatively common in whites in much of Europe, Australia, New Zealand, and the United States, affecting up to 10% of the adult populations.

Morphology

Paget disease may present as a solitary lesion (monostotic) or may occur at multiple sites in the skeleton (polyostotic) with marked variation at each location. In the initial **lytic phase,** osteoclasts (and their associated Howship lacunae) are numerous and abnormally large. Osteoclasts persist in the **mixed phase,** but the bone surfaces become lined by prominent osteoblasts. The marrow is replaced by loose connective tissue containing osteoprogenitor cells, as well as numerous blood vessels needed to meet the increased metabolic demands of the tissue. The newly formed bone may be woven or lamellar, but eventually all of it is remodeled into a heightened caricature of lamellar bone. The pathognomonic histologic feature is a **mosaic pattern** of lamellar bone (likened to a jigsaw puzzle) due to prominent cement lines that haphazardly anneal units of lamellar bone (Fig. 21–5). As the osteoblastic activity burns out, the periosseous fibrovascular tissue recedes and is replaced by normal marrow. Although thickened, the resulting cortex is softened and prone to deformation and fracture under stress.

Pathogenesis. When he first described the disease, Sir James Paget attributed the skeletal changes to an inflammatory process, and assigned the moniker *osteitis deformans.* Ironically, after many years and multiple alternative theories, he may ultimately be correct. Current evidence suggests that a *paramyxovirus* infection ultimately underlies Paget disease. Paramyxovirus antigens and particles resembling paramyxovirus can be demonstrated in osteoclasts. The causal connection is that paramyxoviruses can induce IL-1 secretion from infected cells, and this cytokine—as well as M-CSF—is produced in large amounts in pagetic bone. As noted above, these potently activate osteoclasts. Nevertheless, as intriguing as these observations are, no infectious virus has been isolated from affected tissue. Other pathogenic mechanisms are suggested by the observations that osteoclasts in Paget disease appear to be intrinsically hyperresponsive to activating agents such as vitamin D and RANK ligand.

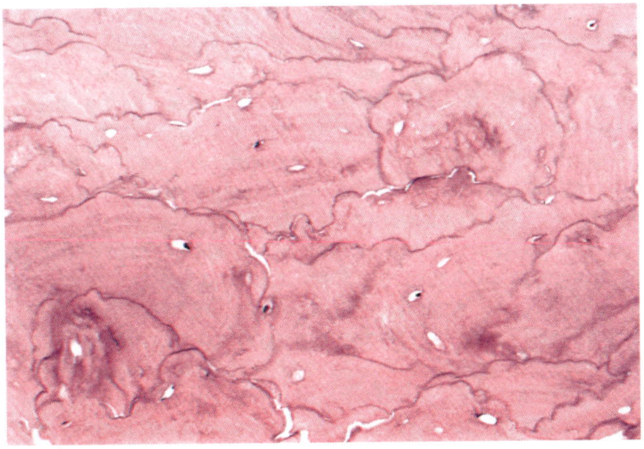

Figure 21–5

Mosaic pattern of lamellar bone pathognomonic of Paget disease.

Clinical Course. The clinical findings depend on the extent and site of the disease. Paget disease is *monostotic* (tibia, ilium, femur, skull, vertebra, and humerus) in about 15% of cases and *polyostotic* (pelvis, spine, and skull) in the remainder; the axial skeleton or proximal femur is involved in as many as 80% of cases. Involvement of the ribs, fibula, and small bones of the hands and feet is unusual. Although Paget disease can produce a plethora of skeletal, neuromuscular, and cardiovascular complications, most cases are mild and are discovered only as incidental radiographic findings. Elevations in serum alkaline phosphatase and increased urinary excretion of hydroxyproline reflect exuberant bone turnover.

In some patients, the early hypervascular bone lesions cause warmth of the overlying skin and subcutaneous tissue. In patients with extensive polyostotic disease, hypervascularity can result in high-output congestive heart failure. In the proliferative phase of the disease involving the skull, common symptoms, attributable to nerve impingement, include headache and visual and auditory disturbances. All these are caused by deformities of the bones of the skull and impingement on cranial nerves. Back pain is common with vertebral lesions and may be associated with disabling fractures and nerve root compression. Affected long bones in the legs are often deformed due to the inability of pagetoid bone to appropriately remodel in response to the stress of weight-bearing. Brittle long bones in particular are subject to *chalkstick fractures.*

The development of a sarcoma in association with osteoblastic lesions is a dreaded but fortunately rare complication of Paget disease, occurring in only an estimated 1% of patients. The sarcomas are usually osteogenic, although other histologic variants can occur. Their distribution generally parallels that of the Paget lesions, with the exception of vertebral bodies, which rarely harbor malignancy. The prognosis of patients who develop secondary sarcomas is exceedingly poor, but in the absence of malignant transformation, Paget disease usually follows a relatively benign course. Most patients have mild symptoms that are readily controlled by calcitonin or bisphosphonates.

Rickets and Osteomalacia

Both rickets and osteomalacia are manifestations of vitamin D deficiency or its abnormal metabolism (and are detailed in Chapter 8). The fundamental change is defective bone mineralization resulting in overabundant nonmineralized osteoid. This contrasts with osteoporosis, where the mineral content of the remaining bone is normal, but the total bone mass is decreased. *Rickets* refers to a childhood disorder in which deranged bone growth produces distinctive skeletal deformities. *Osteomalacia* is the adult counterpart; bone that forms during the remodeling process is undermineralized, resulting in osteopenia and predisposition to fractures.

Hyperparathyroidism

As discussed in Chapter 20, parathyroid hormone (PTH) plays a central role in calcium homeostasis via its effects on:

- Osteoclast activation, increasing bone resorption and calcium mobilization. This effect is mediated indirectly by increased RANKL production by osteoblasts.
- Increased resorption of calcium by the renal tubules
- Increased urinary excretion of phosphates
- Increased synthesis of active vitamin D, $1,25(OH)_2$-D, by the kidneys, which in turn enhances calcium absorption from the gut and mobilizes bone calcium by inducing RANKL

The net result is an elevation in serum calcium, which, under normal circumstances, inhibits further PTH production. However, excessive or inappropriate levels of PTH can result from autonomous parathyroid secretion *(primary hyperparathyroidism)* or can occur in the setting of underlying renal disease (*secondary hyperparathyroidism;* see also Chapter 20).

In either setting, *hyperparathyroidism leads to significant skeletal changes related to unabated osteoclast activity.* The entire skeleton is affected, although some sites can be more severely affected than others. PTH is directly responsible for the bone changes seen in primary hyperparathyroidism, but additional influences contribute to the development of bone disease in secondary hyperparathyroidism. In chronic renal insufficiency there is inadequate $1,25\text{-}(OH)_2$-D synthesis that ultimately affects gastrointestinal calcium absorption. The hyperphosphatemia of renal failure also suppresses renal α_1-hydroxylase, further impairing vitamin D synthesis; additional influences include metabolic acidosis and aluminum deposition in bone.

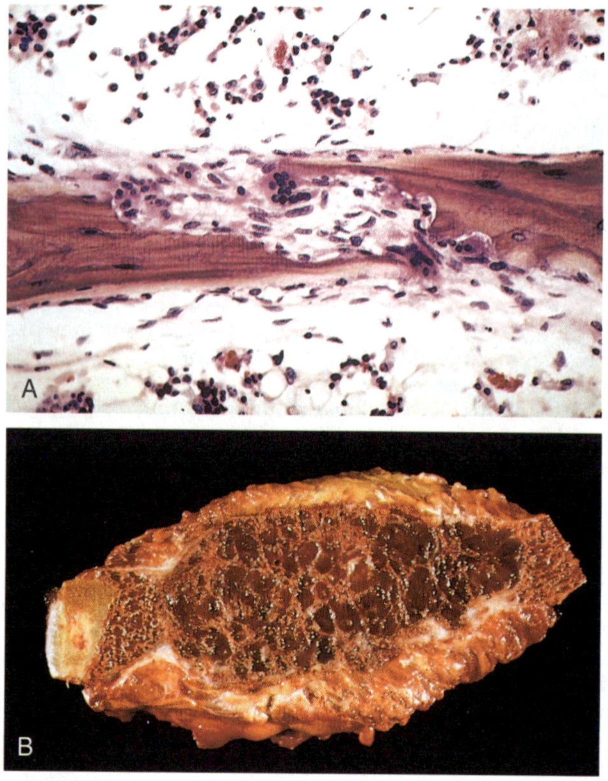

Figure 21–6

Bony manifestations of hyperparathyroidism. **A,** Osteoclasts gnawing into and disrupting lamellar bone. **B,** Resected rib, with expansile cystic mass ("brown tumor").

Morphology

The hallmark of PTH excess is **increased osteoclastic activity, with bone resorption.** Cortical and trabecular bone are lost and replaced by loose connective tissue. Bone resorption is especially pronounced in the subperiosteal regions and produces characteristic radiographic changes, best seen along the radial aspect of the middle phalanges of the second and third fingers. Microscopically, excessive resorptive activity is manifested by the presence of **increased numbers of osteoclasts and accompanying erosion of bone surfaces** (Fig. 21–6A). The marrow space contains increased amounts of loose fibrovascular tissue. Hemosiderin deposits are present, reflecting episodes of hemorrhage resulting from fractures of the weakened bone. In some instances, collections of osteoclasts, reactive giant cells, and hemorrhagic debris form a distinct mass, termed a **brown tumor of hyperparathyroidism** (Fig. 21–6B). Cystic change is common in such lesions (hence the name **osteitis fibrosa cystica**), and they can be confused with primary bone neoplasms.

As bone mass decreases, affected patients are increasingly susceptible to fractures, bone deformation, and joint pathology. Fortunately, reduction of PTH level can result in complete lesion regression.

SUMMARY

Acquired Diseases of Bone Development

- Nutritional deficiencies can affect bone integrity by altering the quality of the protein matrix (e.g., vitamin C is involved in collagen cross-linking) or by influencing bone mineralization (e.g., vitamin D is involved in calcium uptake).
- Osteoporosis results from decreased bone mass and is clinically significant because it predisposes bone to fracture. Although osteoporosis is multifactorial, the two most common forms are *senile osteoporosis* due to aging-related losses of osteoblast function, and *postmenopausal osteoporosis* due to increased osteoclastic activity caused by the relative absence of estrogen.
- Paget disease may result from a paramyxovirus infection and is caused by aberrant and excessive osteoclast activity, followed by exuberant–but structurally unsound–osteoblast deposition of bone.
- Primary or secondary (due to renal failure) overproduction of PTH *(hyperparathyroidism)* results in increased osteoclast activity and bone resorption, leading to fractures and deformities.

FRACTURES

Fractures rank among the most common bone pathologies. They are classified as:

- *complete* or *incomplete*
- *closed* when the overlying tissue is intact, or *compound* when the fracture extends into the overlying skin
- *comminuted* when the bone is splintered
- *displaced,* when the fractured bone is not aligned

If the break occurs at the site of previous disease (e.g., a bone cyst, a malignant tumor, or a brown tumor associated with elevated PTH), the result is a *pathologic fracture.* A *stress fracture* develops slowly over time as a collection of micro-fractures associated with increased physical activity, especially with repetitive weight on bone (as in military boot camps).

In all cases, the repair of a fracture is a highly regulated process that involves overlapping stages:

- The trauma of the bone fracture ruptures associated blood vessels; the resulting blood coagulum creates a fibrin mesh scaffold to recruit inflammatory cells, fibroblasts, and endothelium. Degranulated platelets and marauding inflammatory cells subsequently release a host of cytokines (e.g., platelet-derived growth factor and FGF) that activate bone progenitor cells, and within a week, the involved tissue is primed for new matrix synthesis. This *soft tissue callus* is able to hold the ends of the fractured bone in apposition, but it is non-calcified and cannot support weight bearing.
- Bone progenitors in the medullary cavity deposit new foci of woven bone, and activated mesenchymal cells at the fracture site differentiate into cartilage-synthesizing chondroblasts. In uncomplicated fractures, this early repair process peaks within 2–3 weeks. The newly formed cartilage acts as a nidus for *endochondral ossification,* recapitulating the process of bone formation in epiphyseal growth plates. This connects the trabeculae in adjacent bone. With ossification, the fractured ends are bridged by a *bony callus.*
- Although excess fibrous tissue, cartilage, and bone are produced in the early callus, subsequent weight-bearing leads to resorption of the callus from non-stressed sites; at the same time there is fortification of regions that support greater loads. This callus remodeling restores the original size and shape of the bone, including the spongy cancellous architecture of the medullary cavity.

The healing of a fracture can be disrupted by many factors:

- Displaced and comminuted fractures frequently result in some deformity; devitalized fragments of splintered bone require resorption, which delays healing, enlarges the callus, and requires inordinately long periods of remodeling that may never completely normalize.
- Inadequate immobilization permits constant movement at the fracture site so that the normal constituents of callus do not form. In this case, the healing site is composed mainly of fibrous tissue and cartilage, perpetuating the instability and resulting in delayed union and nonunion.
- Too much motion along the fracture gap (as in nonunion), causes the central portion of the callus to undergo cystic degeneration; the luminal surface can actually become lined by synovial-like cells, creating a false joint, or *pseudoarthrosis.* In the setting of a nonunion or pseudoarthrosis, normal healing can only be achieved if the interposed soft tissues are removed and the fracture site stabilized.
- *Infection* (a risk in comminuted and open fractures) is a serious obstacle to fracture healing. The infection must be eradicated before successful bone reunion and remodeling can occur.
- Bone repair will obviously be impaired by inadequate levels of calcium or phosphorus, vitamin deficiencies, systemic infection, diabetes, and vascular insufficiency.

Generally, with uncomplicated fractures in children and young adults, practically perfect reconstitution is the norm. In older age groups, or for fractures occurring with an underlying disease (e.g. osteoporosis), repair is frequently less than optimal and typically requires orthopedic intervention to achieve the best result.

OSTEONECROSIS (AVASCULAR NECROSIS)

Ischemic necrosis with resultant bone infarction occurs relatively frequently. Mechanisms contributing to bone ischemia include:

- vascular compression or disruption (e.g., following a fracture)
- steroid administration
- thromboembolic disease (e.g., nitrogen bubbles in caisson disease; see Chapter 4)
- primary vessel disease (e.g., vasculitis)

Most cases of bone necrosis are due to fracture or occur after corticosteroid use.

Morphology

The pathologic features of bone necrosis are the same regardless of cause. Dead bone with empty lacunae is interspersed with areas of fat necrosis and insoluble calcium soaps. The cortex is usually not affected because of collateral blood supply; in subchondral infarcts, the overlying articular cartilage also remains viable because the synovial fluid can provide nutritive support. With time, osteoclasts can resorb many of the necrotic bony trabeculae; any dead bone fragments that remain act as scaffolds for new bone formation, a process called **creeping substitution.**

Clinical Course. Symptoms depend on the size and location of injury. *Subchondral infarcts* initially declare with pain during physical activity, becoming more persistent with time. *Medullary infarcts* are usually clinically silent except for large ones (e.g., with Gaucher disease, caisson disease, or sickle cell disease). Medullary infarcts are usually stable; subchondral infarcts, however, often collapse and can lead to severe osteoarthritis. Roughly 50,000 joint replacements are performed each year in the United States specifically to treat the consequences of osteonecrosis.

OSTEOMYELITIS

The term *osteomyelitis* formally designates inflammation of the bone and marrow cavity; as commonly used, however, it almost always implies infection. Osteomyelitis can be a complication of systemic infection but more frequently occurs as an isolated focus of disease; it can be an acute process or a chronic, debilitating illness. Although any microorganism can cause osteomyelitis, the most common etiologic agents are pyogenic bacteria and *Mycobacterium tuberculosis.*

Pyogenic Osteomyelitis

Most cases of acute osteomyelitis are caused by bacteria. The offending organisms reach the bone by one of three routes: (1) hematogenous dissemination (most common); (2) extension from an infection in adjacent joint or soft tissue; or (3) traumatic implantation after compound fractures or orthopedic procedures. Overall, *Staphylococcus aureus* is the most frequent causal organism; its propensity to infect bone may be related to the expression of surface proteins that allow adhesion to bone matrix. *Escherichia coli* and group B streptococci are important causes of acute osteomyelitis in neonates, whereas *Salmonella* is an especially common pathogen in individuals with sickle cell disease. Mixed bacterial infections, including anaerobes, are typically responsible for osteomyelitis developing after bone trauma. In as many as 50% of cases, no organisms can be isolated.

Morphology

The morphologic changes in osteomyelitis depend on the stage (acute, subacute, or chronic) and location of the infection. Causal bacteria proliferate, induce an acute inflammatory reaction, and cause cell death. Entrapped bone undergoes early necrosis; the dead bone in infected sites is called a **sequestrum.** Bacteria and inflammation can percolate throughout the Haversian systems to reach the periosteum. In children, the periosteum is loosely attached to the cortex; therefore, sizable **subperiosteal** abscesses can form and extend for long distances along the bone surface. Lifting of the periosteum further impairs the blood supply to the affected region, and both suppurative and ischemic injury can cause segmental bone necrosis. Rupture of the periosteum can lead to an abscess in the surrounding soft tissue and formation of a **draining sinus.** Sometimes the sequestrum crumbles and forms free foreign bodies that pass through the sinus tract.

In infants (uncommonly in adults), epiphyseal infection can spread into the adjoining joint to produce suppurative arthritis, sometimes with extensive destruction of the articular cartilage and permanent disability. An analogous process can involve vertebrae, with an infection destroying intervertebral discs and spreading into adjacent vertebrae.

After the first week of infection chronic inflammatory cells become more numerous. Leukocyte cytokine release stimulates osteoclastic bone resorption, fibrous tissue ingrowth, and bone formation in the periphery. Reactive woven or lamellar bone can be deposited; when it forms a shell of living tissue around a segment of devitalized bone it is called an **involucrum** (Fig. 21–7). Viable organisms can persist in the sequestrum for years after the original infection.

Clinical Features. Osteomyelitis classically manifests as an acute systemic illness with malaise, fever, leukocytosis, and throbbing pain over the affected region. Symptoms can also be subtle with only unexplained fever, particularly in infants, or only localized pain in the adult. Diagnosis is suggested by characteristic radiologic findings: a destructive lytic focus surrounded by a sclerotic rim. In many untreated cases, blood cultures are positive, but biopsy and bone cultures are usually required to identify the pathogen. A combination of antibiotics and surgical drainage is usually curative, but up to a quarter of cases do not resolve and persist as chronic infections. Chronicity may develop when there is delay in diagnosis, extensive bone necrosis, abbreviated antibiotic therapy, inadequate surgical debridement, and/or weakened host defenses. Besides occasional acute flare-ups, chronic osteomyelitis is also complicated by pathologic fracture, secondary amyloidosis, endocarditis, sepsis, development of squamous cell carcinoma in the sinus tract, and rarely osteosarcoma.

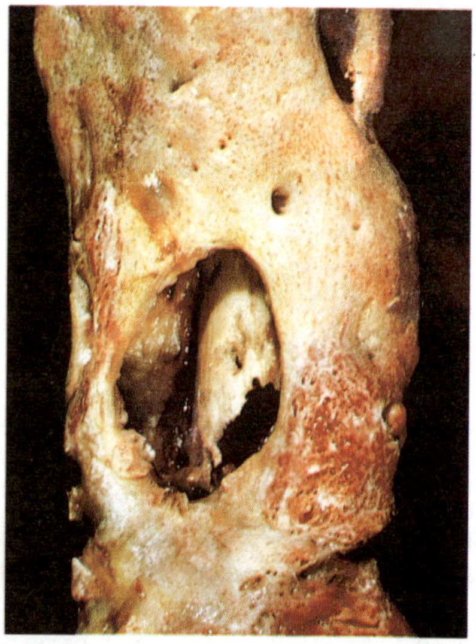

Figure 21–7

Resected femur from a person with chronic osteomyelitis. Necrotic bone (the sequestrum) visible in the center of a draining sinus tract is surrounded by a rim of new bone (the involucrum).

Tuberculous Osteomyelitis

Mycobacterial infection of bone has long been a problem in developing countries; with the resurgence of tuberculosis (due to immigration patterns and increasing numbers of immunocompromised hosts) it is becoming an important disease in other countries as well. Bone infection complicates an estimated 1% to 3% of cases of pulmonary tuberculosis. The organisms usually reach the bone through the bloodstream, although direct spread from a contiguous focus of infection (e.g., from mediastinal nodes to the vertebrae) can also occur. With hematogenous spread, *long bones and vertebrae are favored sites*. The lesions are often solitary but can be multicentric, particularly in patients with an underlying immunodeficiency. Because the tubercle bacillus is microaerophilic, the synovium, with its higher oxygen pressures, is a common site of initial infection. The infection then spreads to the adjacent epiphysis, where it causes a typical granulomatous inflammation with caseous necrosis and extensive bone destruction. *Tuberculosis of the vertebral bodies, or Pott disease, is an important form of osteomyelitis.* Infection at this site causes vertebral deformity and collapse, with secondary neurologic deficits. Extension of the infection to the adjacent soft tissues with the development of psoas muscle abscesses is fairly common in Pott disease.

BONE TUMORS

Primary bone tumors are considerably less common than are bone metastases from other primary sites; metastatic disease will be discussed at the end of this section.

Primary bone tumors exhibit great morphologic diversity and clinical behaviors—from benign to aggressively malignant. Most are classified according to the normal cell of origin and apparent pattern of differentiation; Table 21–2 lists the salient features of the most common primary bone neoplasms, excluding multiple myeloma and other hematopoietic tumors. Overall, matrix-producing and fibrous tumors are the most common, and among the benign tumors, osteochondroma and fibrous cortical defect occur most frequently. Osteosarcoma is the most common primary bone cancer, followed by chondrosarcoma and Ewing sarcoma. Benign tumors markedly outnumber their malignant counterparts, particularly before age 40; bone tumors in the elderly are much more likely to be malignant.

Most bone tumors develop during the first several decades of life and have a propensity to originate in the long bones of the extremities. Nevertheless, specific tumor types target certain age groups and anatomic sites; such clinical information is often critical for the appropriate diagnosis. For instance, most osteosarcomas occur

Table 21–2 Tumors of Bone

Tumor Type	Common Locations	Age (yr)	Morphology
Bone-Forming			
BENIGN			
Osteoma	Facial bones, skull	40–50	Exophytic growths attached to bone surface; histologically resemble normal bone
Osteoid osteoma	Metaphysis of femur and tibia	10–20	Cortical tumors, characterized by pain; histologically interlacing trabeculae of woven bone
Osteoblastoma	Vertebral column	10–20	Arise in vertebral transverse and spinous processes; histologically similar to osteoid osteoma
MALIGNANT			
Primary osteosarcoma	Metaphysis of distal femur, proximal tibia, and humerus	10–20	Grow outward, lifting periosteum, and inward to the medullary cavity; microscopically malignant cells form osteoid; cartilage may also be present
Secondary osteosarcoma	Femur, humerus, pelvis	>40	Complications of polyostotic Paget disease; histologically similar to primary osteosarcoma
Cartilaginous			
BENIGN			
Osteochondroma	Metaphysis of long tubular bones	10–30	Bony excrescences with a cartilaginous cap; may be solitary or multiple and hereditary
Chondroma	Small bones of hands and feet	30–50	Well-circumscribed single tumors resembling normal cartilage; arise with medullary cavity of bone; uncommonly multiple and hereditary
MALIGNANT			
Chondrosarcoma	Bones of shoulder, pelvis, proximal femur, and ribs	40–60	Arise within medullary cavity and erode cortex; microscopically well differentiated cartilage-like or anaplastic
Miscellaneous			
Giant-cell tumor (usually benign)	Epiphysis of long bone	20–40	Lytic lesions that erode cortex; microscopically, contain osteoclast-like giant cells and round to spindle-shaped mononuclear cells; majority are benign
Ewing tumor (malignant)	Diaphysis and metaphysis	10–20	Arise in medullary cavity; microscopically, sheets of small round cells that contain glycogen; aggressive neoplasm

during adolescence, with half arising around the knee, either in the distal femur or proximal tibia. In contrast, chondrosarcomas tend to develop during mid- to late adulthood and involve the trunk, limb girdles, and proximal long bones.

Most bone tumors arise without any prior known cause. Nevertheless, genetic syndromes (e.g., Li-Fraumeni and retinoblastoma syndromes; see Chapter 6) are associated with osteosarcomas, as are (rarely) bone infarcts, chronic osteomyelitis, Paget disease, radiation, and metal orthopedic devices.

In terms of clinical presentations, benign lesions are frequently asymptomatic and are detected as incidental findings. Others produce pain or a slowly growing mass. Occasionally, a sudden pathologic fracture is the first manifestation. Radiologic imaging is critical in the evaluation of bone tumors; however, biopsy and histologic study are necessary for the final diagnosis.

Bone-Forming Tumors

The tumor cells in the following neoplasms all produce bone that is usually woven and variably mineralized.

Osteoma

Osteomas are benign lesions of bone that in many cases represent developmental aberrations or reactive growths rather than true neoplasms. They are most commonly encountered in the head and neck, including the paranasal sinuses, but can occur elsewhere as well; they are typically seen in middle age. Osteomas are usually solitary and present as localized, slowly growing, hard, exophytic masses on the bone surface. Multiple lesions are a feature of Gardner syndrome, a hereditary condition discussed further below. Histologically, osteomas are a bland mixture of woven and lamellar bone. Although they may cause local mechanical problems (e.g., obstruction of a sinus cavity) and cosmetic deformities, they are not invasive and do not undergo malignant transformation.

Osteoid Osteoma and Osteoblastoma

Osteoid osteomas and *osteoblastomas* are benign neoplasms with very similar histologic features. Both lesions typically arise during the teenage years and 20s, with a male predilection (2 : 1 in osteoid osteomas). They are distinguished primarily by their size, site of origin, and their radiographic appearance as well-circumscribed lesions, usually involving the cortex and rarely the medullary cavity. The central area of the tumor, termed the *nidus*, is characteristically radiolucent but may become mineralized and sclerotic. *Osteoid osteomas* arise most often in the proximal femur and tibia, and are by definition less than 2 cm, whereas osteoblastomas are larger. Localized pain is an almost universal complaint with osteoid osteomas, and is usually relieved by aspirin. *Osteoblastomas* arise most often in the vertebral column; they also cause pain, although it is often more difficult to localize and is not responsive to aspirin. Local excision is the treatment of choice; incompletely resected lesions can recur. Malignant transformation is rare *unless* the lesion is treated with radiation.

Morphology

Grossly, both lesions are round-to-oval masses of hemorrhagic gritty tan tissue. A rim of sclerotic bone is present at the edge of both types of tumors; however, it is much more conspicuous in osteoid osteomas. Microscopically, both neoplasms are composed of interlacing trabeculae of woven bone surrounded by osteoblasts (Fig. 21–8). The intervening stroma is loose, vascular connective tissue containing variable numbers of giant cells.

Osteosarcoma

Osteosarcoma is a bone-producing malignant mesenchymal tumor. Outside of myeloma and lymphoma, osteosarcoma is the most common primary malignant tumor of bone, accounting for approximately 20% of primary bone cancers; a little over 2000 cases are diagnosed annually in the United States. Osteosarcomas occur in all age groups but some 75% of patients are younger than age 20, with a second peak occuring in the elderly, usually with other conditions, including Paget disease, bone infarcts, and prior irradiation. Men are more commonly affected than women (1.6 : 1). Although any bone can be involved, most tumors arise in the metaphyseal region of the long bones of the extremities, with almost 60% occurring about the knee, 15% around the hip, 10% at the shoulder, and 8% in the jaw. Several subtypes of osteosarcoma are recognized on the basis of the site of involvement within the bone (e.g., medullary vs cortical), degree of differentiation, solitary vs multicentric, presence of underlying disease, and histologic variants; the most common type of osteosarcoma is primary, solitary, intramedullary, and poorly differentiated, producing a predominantly bony matrix.

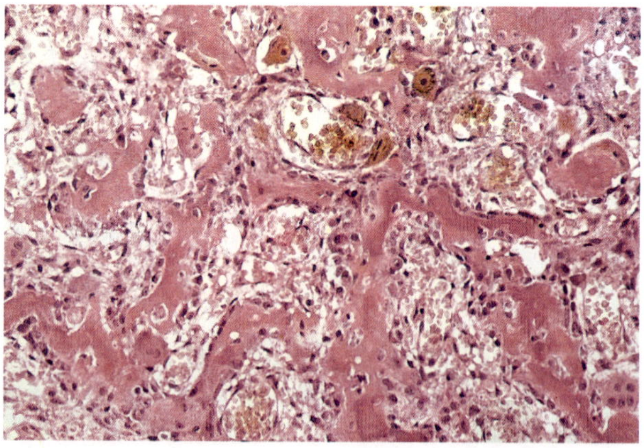

Figure 21–8

Osteoid osteoma showing randomly oriented trabeculae of woven bone rimmed by prominent osteoblasts. The intertrabecular spaces are filled by vascular loose connective tissue.

Morphology

Grossly, osteosarcomas are gritty, gray-white tumors, often exhibiting hemorrhage and cystic degeneration. Tumors frequently destroy the surrounding cortices and produce soft tissue masses (Fig. 21–9A). They spread extensively in the medullary canal, infiltrating and replacing the marrow, but only infrequently penetrating the epiphyseal plate or entering the joint space. Tumor cells vary in size and shape, and frequently have large hyperchromatic nuclei; bizarre tumor giant cells are common, as are mitoses. **The production of mineralized or unmineralized bone (osteoid) by malignant cells is essential for diagnosis of osteosarcoma.** (Fig. 21–9B). The neoplastic bone is typically coarse and ragged but can also be deposited in broad sheets. Cartilage and fibrous tissue can also be present in varying amounts. When malignant cartilage is abundant, the tumor is called a **chondroblastic osteosarcoma**. Vascular invasion is common, as is spontaneous tumor necrosis.

Pathogenesis. Several genetic mutations are closely associated with the development of osteosarcoma. In particular, *RB* gene mutations occur in 60% to 70% of sporadic tumors, and individuals with hereditary retinoblastomas (due to germ-line mutations in the *RB* gene) have a thousandfold greater risk of developing osteosarcoma. Spontaneous osteosarcomas also frequently exhibit mutations in genes that regulate the cell cycle including *p53,* cyclins, cyclin-dependent kinases, and kinase inhibitors. Many osteosarcomas develop at sites of greatest bone growth.

Clinical Features. Osteosarcomas typically present as painful enlarging masses, although a pathologic fracture can be the first symptom. Radiographs usually show a large, destructive, mixed lytic and blastic mass with indistinct infiltrating margins. The tumor frequently breaks through the cortex and lifts the periosteum, resulting in reactive periosteal bone formation. A triangular shadow on x-ray between the cortex and raised periosteum (*Codman triangle*) is characteristic of osteosarcomas. Osteosarcomas typically spread hematogenously; at the time of diagnosis, approximately 10% to 20% of patients have demonstrable pulmonary metastases.

Despite aggressive behavior, standard treatment with chemotherapy and limb-salvage therapy currently yields long-term survivals of 60% to 70%.

Secondary osteosarcomas occur in an older age group than do primary osteosarcomas. They most commonly develop in the setting of Paget disease or previous radiation exposure. Secondary osteosarcomas are highly aggressive tumors that do not respond well to therapy.

Cartilage-Forming Tumors

These neoplasms produce hyaline or myxoid cartilage; fibrocartilage and elastic cartilage are rare components. Like the bone-forming tumors, cartilaginous tumors comprise a spectrum from benign, self-limited growths to highly aggressive malignancies; again, benign cartilage tumors are much more common than malignant ones. Only the more common types are discussed here.

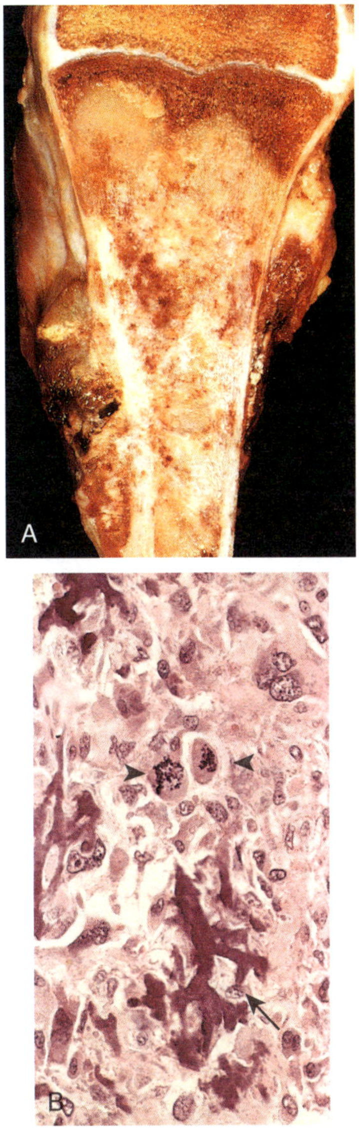

Figure 21–9

Osteosarcoma. **A,** Mass involving the upper end of the tibia. The tan-white tumor fills most of the medullary cavity of the metaphysis and proximal diaphysis. It has infiltrated through the cortex, lifted the periosteum, and formed soft tissue masses on both sides of the bone. **B,** Histologic appearance, with coarse, lacelike pattern of neoplastic bone (*arrow*) produced by anaplastic tumor cells. Note the wildly aberrant mitotic figures (*arrowheads*).

Osteochondroma

Osteochondromas are also called *exostoses;* they are relatively common benign cartilage-capped outgrowths attached by a bony stalk to the underlying skeleton. Solitary osteochondromas are usually first diagnosed in late adolescence and early adulthood (male-to-female ratio of 3:1); multiple osteochondromas become apparent during childhood, occurring as *multiple hereditary exostosis,* an autosomal dominant disorder. Inactivation of both copies of the *EXT* gene in chondrocytes is implicated in both sporadic and hereditary osteochondromas. This tumor suppressor gene encodes glycosyltransferases essential for polymerization of heparin sulfate, an important component of cartilage. This finding and other molecular genetic studies support the concept that osteochondromas are true neoplasms and not simple malformations.

Osteochondromas develop only in bones of endochondral origin arising at the metaphysis near the growth plate of long tubular bones, especially about the knee; they tend to stop growing once the normal growth of the skeleton is completed (Fig. 21–10). Occasionally they develop from bones of the pelvis, scapula, and ribs, and in these sites are frequently sessile. Rarely, exostoses involve the short tubular bones of hands and feet.

Morphology

Osteochondromas vary from 1–20 cm in size. The cap is benign hyaline cartilage, resembling disorganized growth plate undergoing endochondral ossification. Newly formed bone forms the inner portion of the head and stalk, with the stalk cortex merging with the cortex of the host bone.

Clinical Features. Osteochondromas are slow-growing masses that are painful when they impinge on a nerve or if the stalk is fractured. In many cases, they are detected only incidentally. In multiple hereditary exostosis, deformity of the underlying bone suggests an associated disturbance in epiphyseal growth. Osteochondromas rarely progress to chondrosarcoma or other sarcoma, although patients with the hereditary syndrome are at increased risk of malignant transformation.

Chondroma

Chondromas are benign tumors of hyaline cartilage. When they arise within the medulla, they are termed *enchondromas;* when on the bone surface they are called *juxtacortical chondromas.* Enchondromas are usually diagnosed in persons between ages 20 and 50; they are typically solitary and located in the metaphyseal region of tubular bones, the favored sites being the short tubular bones of the hands and feet. *Ollier disease* is characterized by *multiple chondromas* preferentially involving one side of the body, and *Maffucci syndrome* is characterized by *multiple chondromas associated with benign soft tissue angiomas.* Chondromas probably develop from slowly proliferating rests of growth plate cartilage.

Morphology

Enchondromas are gray-blue, translucent nodules usually smaller than 3 cm. Microscopically, there is well-circumscribed hyaline matrix and cytologically benign chondrocytes. At the periphery, there is endochondral ossification, while the center frequently calcifies and dies. In the hereditary multiple chondromatoses, the islands of cartilage exhibit greater cellularity and atypia, making them difficult to distinguish from chondrosarcoma.

Clinical Features. Most enchondromas are detected as incidental findings; occasionally they are painful or cause pathologic fractures. On x-ray, the unmineralized nodules of cartilage produce well-circumscribed oval lucencies surrounded by thin rims of radiodense bone *(O-ring sign).* Calcified matrix exhibits irregular opacities. The growth potential of chondromas is limited, and most remain stable, although they can recur if incompletely excised. Solitary chondromas rarely undergo malignant transformation, but those associated with enchondromatoses are at increased risk. Maffucci syndrome is associated with an increased risk of developing other types of malignancies, including ovarian carcinomas and brain gliomas.

Chondrosarcoma

Chondrosarcomas comprise a variety of tumors sharing the ability to produce neoplastic cartilage; they are subclassified according to site (e.g., *intramedullary* vs *juxtacortical*), and histologic variants (see below). Chondrosarcomas occur roughly half as frequently as osteosarcomas; most patients are age 40 or older, with men affected twice as frequently as women.

Morphology

Conventional chondrosarcomas arise within the medullary cavity of the bone to form an expansile glistening mass that often erodes the cortex (Fig. 21–11A).

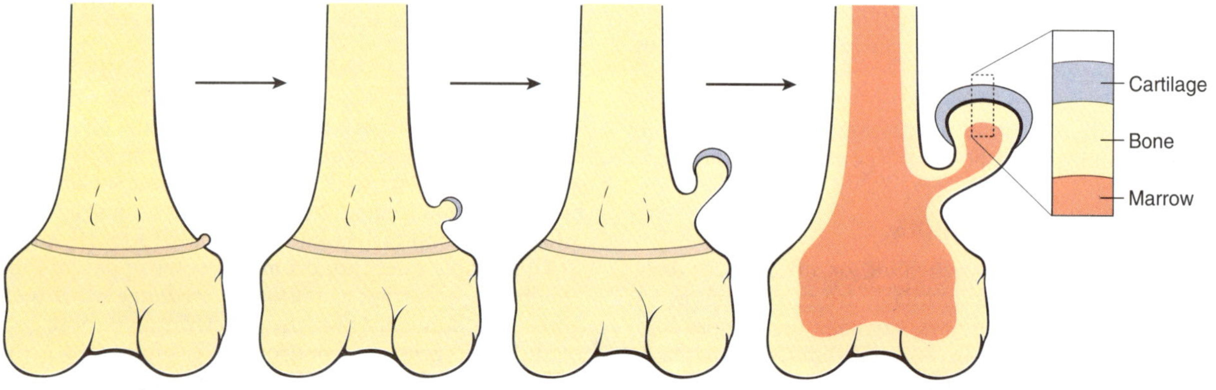

Figure 21–10

The development of an osteochondroma, beginning with an outgrowth from the epiphyseal cartilage.

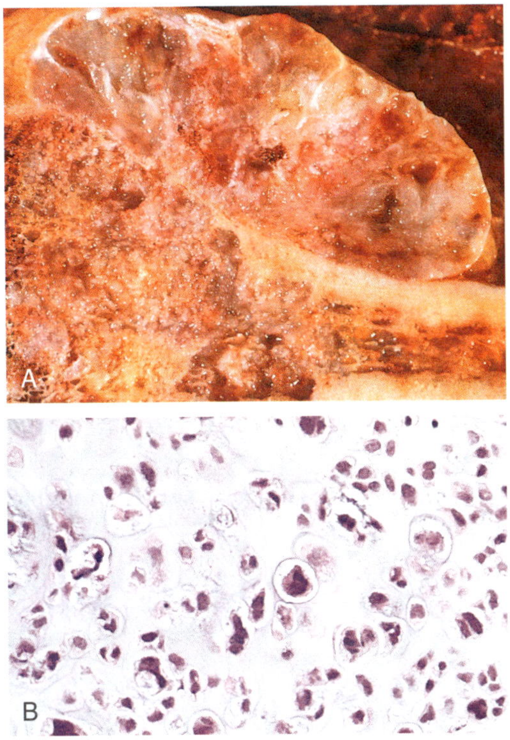

Figure 21–11

Chondrosarcoma. **A,** Islands of hyaline and myxoid cartilage expand the medullary cavity and grow through the cortex to form a sessile paracortical mass. **B,** Anaplastic chondrocytes within a chondroid matrix.

They exhibit malignant hyaline and myxoid cartilage. In **myxoid chondrosarcomas,** the tumors are viscous and gelatinous, and the matrix oozes from the cut surface. Spotty calcifications are typically present, and central necrosis can create cystic spaces. The adjacent cortex is thickened or eroded, and the tumor grows with broad pushing fronts into marrow spaces and the surrounding soft tissue. Tumor grade is determined by cellularity, cytologic atypia, and mitotic activity (Fig. 21–11B). Low-grade tumors resemble normal cartilage. Higher grade lesions contain pleomorphic chondrocytes with frequent mitotic figures. Multinucleate cells are present with lacunae containing two or more chondrocytes.

Approximately 10% of patients with conventional low-grade chondrosarcomas have a second high-grade poorly differentiated component (**dedifferentiated chondrosarcomas**) that include foci of fibro- or osteosarcomas. Other histologic variants include **clear-cell** and **mesenchymal chondrosarcomas.**

Clinical Features. Chondrosarcomas commonly arise in the pelvis, shoulder, and ribs; in contrast to enchondromas, chondrosarcomas rarely involve the distal extremities. They typically present as painful, progressively enlarging masses. A slowly growing low-grade tumor causes reactive thickening of the cortex, whereas a more aggressive high-grade neoplasm destroys the cortex and forms a soft tissue mass; consequently, the more radiolucent the tumor the greater the likelihood that it is high grade. There is also a direct correlation between grade and biologic behavior of the tumor. Fortunately, most conventional chondrosarcomas are indolent and low-grade, with a 5-year survival rate of 80% to 90% (vs 43% for grade 3 tumors); grade 1 tumors rarely metastasize, whereas 70% of the grade 3 tumors disseminate. Size is another prognostic feature, with tumors larger than 10 cm being significantly more aggressive than smaller tumors. Chondrosarcomas metastasize hematogenously, preferentially to the lungs and skeleton. Conventional chondrosarcomas are treated with wide surgical excision; chemotherapy is added for the mesenchymal and dedifferentiated variants because of their aggressive clinical course.

Fibrous and Fibro-Osseous Tumors

Fibrous tumors of the skeleton are extremely common and comprise a wide diversity of morphologic variants.

Fibrous Cortical Defect and Nonossifying Fibroma

Fibrous cortical defects occur in 30% to 50% of all children older than age 2; they are probably developmental defects rather than true neoplasms. The vast majority are smaller than 0.5 cm and arise in the metaphysis of the distal femur or proximal tibia; almost 50% are bilateral or multiple. Larger lesions (5–6 cm) develop into *nonossifying fibromas.*

Morphology

Fibrous cortical defects and nonossifying fibromas both present as sharply demarcated radiolucencies surrounded by a thin zone of sclerosis. Grossly, they are gray to yellow-brown, and microscopically are cellular lesions composed of cytologically benign fibroblasts and activated macrophages, including multinucleated forms. The fibroblasts classically exhibit a storiform (pinwheel) pattern (Fig. 21–12).

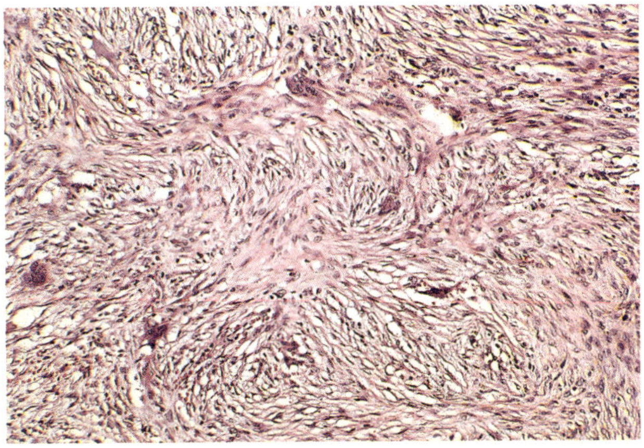

Figure 21–12

Fibrous cortical defect or nonossifying fibroma. Characteristic storiform pattern of spindle cells interspersed with scattered osteoclast-type giant cells.

Clinical Features. Fibrous cortical defects are asymptomatic and are usually only detected as incidental radiographic lesions. Most undergo spontaneous differentiation into normal cortical bone within a few years and do not require a biopsy. The few that enlarge into nonossifying fibromas can present with pathologic fracture; in such cases biopsy is necessary to rule out other tumors.

Fibrous Dysplasia

Fibrous dysplasia is a benign tumor that is probably more appropriately labeled a localized developmental arrest; all components of normal bone are present, but they fail to differentiate into mature structures. Fibrous dysplasia occurs as one of three clinical patterns: (1) involvement of a single bone (monostotic); (2) involvement of multiple bones (polyostotic); and (3) polyostotic disease, associated with café au lait skin pigmentations and endocrine abnormalities, especially precocious puberty *(McCune-Albright syndrome)*. In the latter the skeletal, skin, and endocrine lesions result from a somatic (not hereditary) embryonic mutation yielding a G-protein that constitutively activates adenyl cyclase with resultant cyclic adenosine monophosphate overproduction and cellular hyperfunctioning.

Monostotic fibrous dysplasia accounts for 70% of cases. It usually begins in early adolescence, and ceases with epiphyseal closure; there is no gender predilection. In descending order of frequency, ribs, femur, tibia, jawbones, calvaria, and humerus are most commonly affected. Lesions are asymptomatic and usually discovered incidentally. However, fibrous dysplasia can cause marked enlargement and distortion of bone, so that if the face or skull is involved, disfigurement can occur.

Polyostotic fibrous dysplasia without endocrine dysfunction accounts for the majority of the remaining cases. It presents at a slightly earlier age than the monostotic type and can progress into adulthood. In descending order of frequency, femur, skull, tibia, and humerus are most commonly involved. Craniofacial involvement is present in 50% of patients with moderate skeletal involvement, and in 100% of patients with extensive skeletal disease. Polyostotic disease tends to involve the shoulder and pelvic girdles, resulting in severe deformities and spontaneous fractures.

McCune-Albright syndrome accounts for 3% of all cases. The associated endocrinopathies include sexual precocity (girls more often than boys), hyperthyroidism, growth hormone-secreting pituitary adenomas, and primary adrenal hyperplasia. The severity of manifestations depends on the number and cell types that harbor the G-protein mutation. The bone lesions are often unilateral, and the skin pigmentation is usually limited to the same side of the body. The cutaneous macules are classically large, dark to light brown (*café au lait*), and irregular.

Morphology

Grossly, fibrous dysplasia is characterized by well-circumscribed, intramedullary lesions of varying sizes; large masses expand and distort the bone. Lesional tissue is tan-white and gritty; microscopically, it exhibits curved trabeculae of woven bone (mimicking Chinese characters), without osteoblastic rimming, and surrounded by a moderately cellular fibroblastic proliferation (Fig. 21–13).

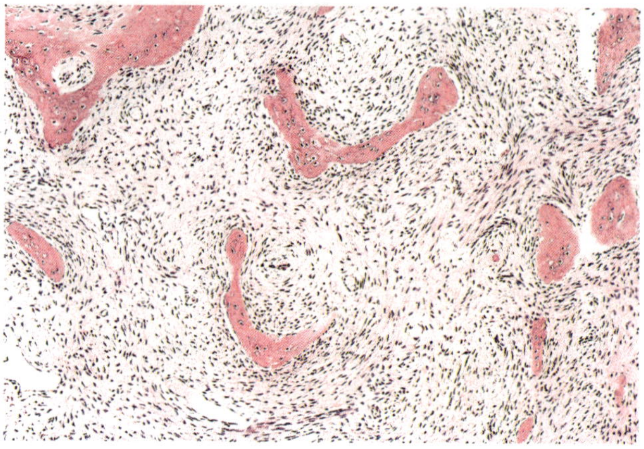

Figure 21–13

Fibrous dysplasia. Curved trabeculae of woven bone arising in a fibrous tissue. Note the absence of osteoblasts rimming the bones.

Clinical Course. The natural history depends on the extent of skeletal involvement; individuals with monostotic disease usually have minimal symptoms. By x-ray, lesions exhibit a characteristic ground-glass appearance with well-defined margins. Symptomatic lesions are readily cured by conservative surgery. Polyostotic involvement is frequently associated with progressive disease, and more severe skeletal complications (e.g., fractures, long bone deformities, and craniofacial distortion). Rarely, polyostotic disease can transform into osteosarcoma, *especially following radiotherapy.*

Miscellaneous Bone Tumors

Ewing Sarcoma and Primitive Neuroectodermal Tumor

Ewing sarcoma and primitive neuroectodermal tumors (PNETs) are primary malignant small round-cell tumors of bone and soft tissue. Because they share an identical chromosome translocation, they should be viewed as the same tumor, differing only in degree of differentiation. PNETs demonstrate neural differentiation whereas Ewing sarcomas are undifferentiated by traditional marker analysis.

These two malignancies account for 6% to 10% of primary malignant bone tumors. After osteosarcomas, they are the second most common pediatric bone sarcomas. Most patients are 10 to 15 years old, and 80% are younger than age 20. Boys are affected slightly more frequently than girls, and there is a striking racial predilection; blacks are rarely afflicted. The common chromosomal abnormality is a translocation that causes fusion of the *EWS* gene on 22q12 with a member of the *ETS* family of transcription factors. The most common fusion partners are the *FL1* gene on 11q24, and the *ERG* gene on 21q22. The resulting chimeric protein functions as a constitutively active transcription factor to stimulate cell proliferation. At a practical level, these translocations are of diagnostic importance. Thus, approximately 95% of patients with Ewing tumor have t(11;22) (q24;q12) or t(21;22) (q22;q12).

Morphology

Ewing sarcoma and PNETs arise in the medullary cavity and invade the cortex and periosteum to produce a soft tissue mass. The tumor is tan-white, frequently with hemorrhage and necrosis. It is composed of sheets of uniform small, round cells that are slightly larger than lymphocytes with few mitoses and little intervening stroma (Fig. 21–14). The cells have scant glycogen-rich cytoplasm. The presence of **Homer-Wright rosettes** (tumor cells circled about a central fibrillary space) indicates neural differentiation.

Clinical Features. Ewing sarcoma and PNETs typically present as painful enlarging masses in the diaphyses of long tubular bones (especially the femur) and the pelvic flat bones. Some patients have systemic signs and symptoms, including fever, elevated erythrocyte sedimentation rate, anemia, and leukocytosis that can mimic infection. X-rays show a destructive lytic tumor with infiltrative margins and extension into surrounding soft tissues. There is a characteristic periosteal reaction depositing bone in an onionskin fashion.

Treatment includes chemotherapy and surgical excision with or without radiation. The 5-year survival is currently 75%, with 50% achieving long-term durable remissions.

Giant-Cell Tumor of Bone

Giant-cell tumors (GCTs) are dominated by multinucleated osteoclast-type giant cells, hence the synonym *osteoclastoma*. GCT is relatively uncommon; it is benign but locally aggressive, usually arising in individuals in their 20s to 40s. Current opinion suggests that the giant cell component is likely a reactive macrophage population and the mononuclear cells are neoplastic. The latter show complex cytogenetic abnormalities.

Morphology

Tumors are large and red-brown with frequent cystic degeneration. They are composed of uniform oval mononuclear cells with frequent mitoses, with scattered osteoclast-type giant cells containing 100 or more nuclei (Fig. 21–15). Necrosis, hemorrhage, and reactive bone formation are also commonly present.

Clinical Course. Although almost any bone can be involved, the majority of GCTs arise in the epiphysis of long bones around the knee (distal femur and proximal tibia), frequently causing arthritis-like symptoms. Occasionally, GCTs present as pathologic fractures. Most are solitary. Radiographically, GCTs are large, purely lytic, and eccentric; the overlying cortex is frequently destroyed, producing a bulging soft tissue mass with a thin shell of reactive bone. Although GCTs are histologically benign, roughly half recur after simple curettage, and as many as 4% metastasize to the lungs.

Metastatic Disease

Metastatic tumors are the most common malignant tumor of bone. Pathways of spread include (1) direct extension, (2) lymphatic or hematogenous dissemination, and (3) intraspinal seeding. Any cancer can spread to bone, but certain tumors exhibit a distinct skeletal predilection. In adults more than 75% of skeletal metastases originate from cancers of the prostate, breast, kidney, and lung. In children, neuroblastoma, Wilms' tumor,

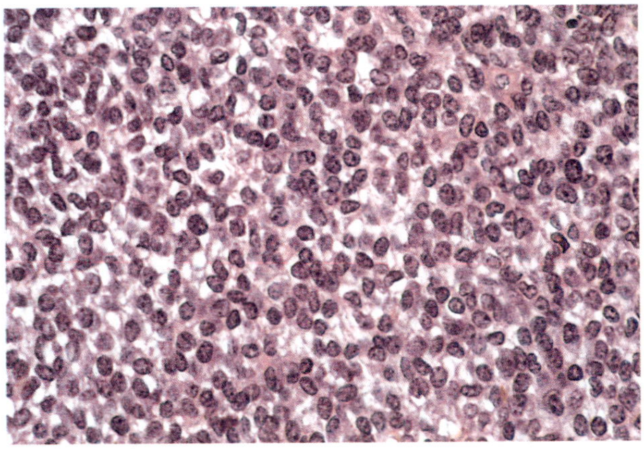

Figure 21–14

Ewing sarcoma. Sheets of small round cells with scant, cleared cytoplasm.

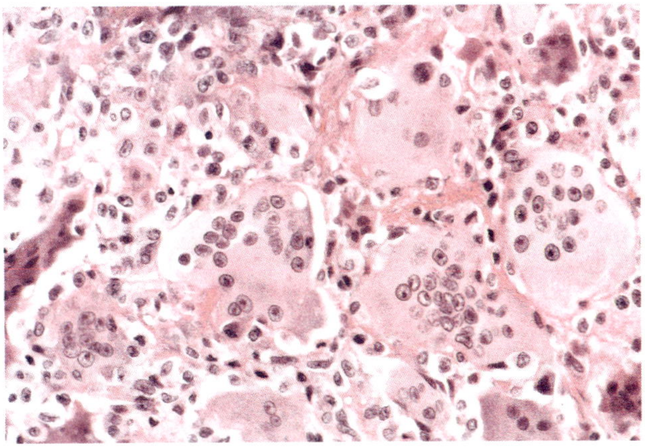

Figure 21–15

Benign giant-cell tumor showing abundant multinucleated giant cells and a background of mononuclear cells.

osteosarcoma, Ewing sarcoma, and rhabdomyosarcoma are the common sources of bony metastases.

Most metastases involve the axial skeleton (vertebral column, pelvis, ribs, skull, sternum), proximal femur, and humerus, in descending order. Presumably the red marrow in these areas, with its rich capillary network, slow blood flow, and nutrient environment, facilitates tumor cell implantation and growth.

The radiologic appearance of metastases can be purely lytic, purely blastic, or both. In lytic lesions (e.g., kidney, lung, and melanoma), the metastatic cells secrete substances such as prostaglandins, interleukins, and PTHRp that stimulate osteoclastic bone resorption; the tumor cells themselves do not directly resorb bone. Similarly, metastases that elicit a sclerotic response (e.g., prostate adenocarcinoma) do so by stimulating osteoblastic bone formation. Most metastases induce a mixed lytic and blastic reaction.

SUMMARY

Bone Tumors

- Bone tumors of non-hematopoietic origin have diverse gross and microscopic appearances, with clinical behaviors ranging from completely benign to rapidly fatal. Diagnosis rests on a combination of clinical presentation (age, gender, and symptoms), site of the lesion, radiologic appearance, and histologic features.
- Most bone tumors are categorized according to the nature of the matrix they produce; chondroid and bony matrices are roughly equally represented. Benign lesions far outnumber malignant tumors. Metastatic tumors are the most common form of skeletal malignancy.
- Major tumor types can be subdivided into:
  - Abnormal development
    - Fibrous cortical defects—common developmental defects composed of cytologically benign fibroblasts
    - Fibrous dysplasias—failure of normal bone elements to differentiate into mature structures
    - Osteoma—developmental bony aberrations, primarily of the head and neck
  - Benign neoplasms
    - Osteoid osteoma—islands of woven bone, typically of the proximal femur or tibia
    - Osteochondroma—cartilage-capped outgrowths at epiphyseal growth plates
  - Malignant neoplasms
    - Osteosarcoma—malignant mesenchymal tumor forming bone; 20% of primary bone tumors
    - Chondrosarcoma—malignant mesenchymal tumor forming cartilage
    - Ewing tumor—aggressive neural crest-derived neoplasm of adolescents
  - Neoplasms of uncertain potential
    - Giant cell tumor—occasionally (4%) malignant tumor composed of a mixture of neoplastic mononuclear cells and reactive osteoclast-like giant cells, typically occupying long bone epiphyses

JOINTS

The joints are subject to a wide variety of disorders, including degeneration, infections, immune-mediated injury, metabolic derangements, and neoplasms. In this section we will confine our comments to some of the most common forms of arthritis, namely, degenerative joint disease (*osteoarthritis*), gout, and infectious arthritis, as well as the two most common benign joint tumors. Rheumatoid arthritis (RA), another important and potentially devastating joint disease, is discussed in detail in Chapter 5.

ARTHRITIS

Osteoarthritis

Osteoarthritis, or *degenerative joint disease,* is the most common joint disorder. It is a frequent, if not inevitable, part of aging and is an important cause of physical disability in individuals over the age of 65. *The fundamental feature of osteoarthritis is degeneration of the articular cartilage;* any structural changes in the underlying bone are secondary. Although the term *osteoarthritis* implies an inflammatory disease, and inflammatory cells can be present, osteoarthritis is primarily a degenerative disorder of articular cartilage.

In most cases, osteoarthritis appears insidiously with age and without apparent initiating cause *(primary osteoarthritis).* In such cases the disease is usually *oligoarticular* (i.e., affecting only a few joints). In the unusual circumstance (less than 5% of cases) when osteoarthritis strikes in youth, there is typically some predisposing condition, such as previous traumatic injury, developmental deformity, or underlying systemic disease such as diabetes, ochronosis, hemochromatosis, or marked obesity. In these settings the disease is called *secondary osteoarthritis* and often involves one or several predisposed joints. Gender has some influence; knees and hands are more commonly affected in women, whereas hips are more commonly affected in men. It is estimated that the economic toll of osteoarthritis in the United States is more than $33 billion annually.

Morphology

The earliest structural changes in osteoarthritis include enlargement, proliferation, and disorganization of the chondrocytes in the superficial part of the articular cartilage. This process is accompanied by increasing water content of the matrix with decreasing concentration of the proteoglycans (the proteoglycan component conveys turgor and elasticity). Subsequently, vertical and horizontal **fibrillation and cracking of the matrix** occur as the superficial layers of the cartilage are degraded (Fig. 21–16A). Gross examination at this stage reveals a soft granular articular cartilage surface. Eventually, full-thickness portions of the cartilage are lost, and the subchondral bone plate is exposed. Friction smooths and burnishes the exposed bone, giving it the appearance of polished ivory **(bone eburnation)** (Fig. 21–16B). The underlying cancellous bone becomes sclerotic and thickened. Small fractures can dislodge pieces of cartilage and subchondral bone into the joint, forming loose bodies **(joint mice)**. The fracture gaps allow synovial fluid to be forced into the subchondral regions to form fibrous walled cysts. Mushroom-shaped **osteophytes** (bony outgrowths) develop at the margins of the articular surface. In severe disease, a fibrous synovial **pannus** covers the peripheral portions of the articular surface.

Pathogenesis. *Articular cartilage bears the brunt of the degenerative changes in osteoarthritis.* Normal articular cartilage performs two functions: (1) along with the synovial fluid, it provides virtually friction-free movement within the joint; and (2) in weight-bearing joints, it spreads the load across the joint surface in a manner that allows the underlying bones to absorb shock and weight. These functions require the cartilage to be elastic (i.e., to regain normal architecture after compression) and to have high tensile strength. These attributes are provided by proteoglycans and type II collagen, respectively, both produced by chondrocytes. As with adult bone, articular cartilage constantly undergoes matrix degradation and replacement. Normal chondrocyte function is critical to maintain cartilage synthesis and degradation; any imbalance can lead to osteoarthritis.

Chondrocyte function can be affected by a variety of influences. Although osteoarthritis is not exclusively a wear-and-tear phenomenon, mechanical stresses and aging nevertheless figure prominently. *Genetic factors* also seem to contribute to osteoarthritis susceptibility, particularly in the hands and hips, but the responsible genes are not known. The risk of osteoarthritis is also increased with increasing bone density, as well as sustained high estrogen levels.

Regardless of the inciting stimulus, early osteoarthritis is marked by degenerating cartilage containing more water and less proteoglycan. The collagen network is also diminished, presumably as a result of decreased local synthesis and increased breakdown; chondrocyte apoptosis is increased. Overall, cartilage tensile strength and resilience are compromised. In response to these degenerative changes, chondrocytes in the deeper layers proliferate and attempt to "repair" the damage by synthesizing new collagen and proteoglycans. Although these reparative changes are initially able to keep pace, matrix changes and chondrocyte loss eventually predominate.

Clinical Course. Osteoarthritis is an insidious disease, predominantly affecting patients beginning in their 50s and 60s. Characteristic symptoms include deep, aching pain exacerbated by use, morning stiffness, crepitus (grating or popping sensation in the joint), and limited range of movement. Osteophyte impingement on spinal foramina can cause nerve root compression with radicular pain, muscle spasms, muscle atrophy, and neurologic deficits. Hips, knees, lower lumbar and cervical vertebrae, proximal and distal interphalangeal joints of the fingers,

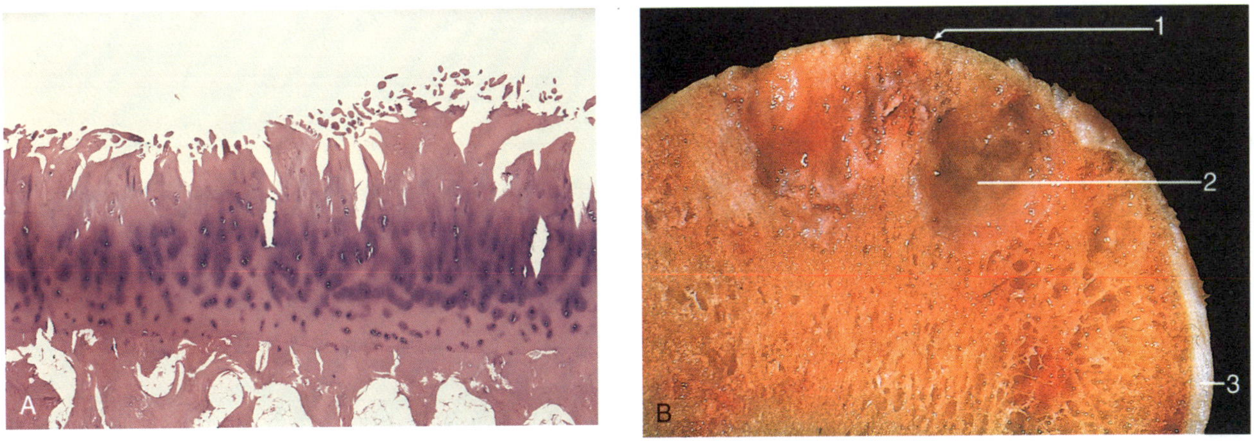

Figure 21–16

Osteoarthritis. **A,** Histologic demonstration of the characteristic fibrillation of the articular cartilage. **B,** Severe osteoarthritis with 1, Eburnated articular surface exposing subchondral bone. 2, Subchondral cyst. 3, Residual articular cartilage.

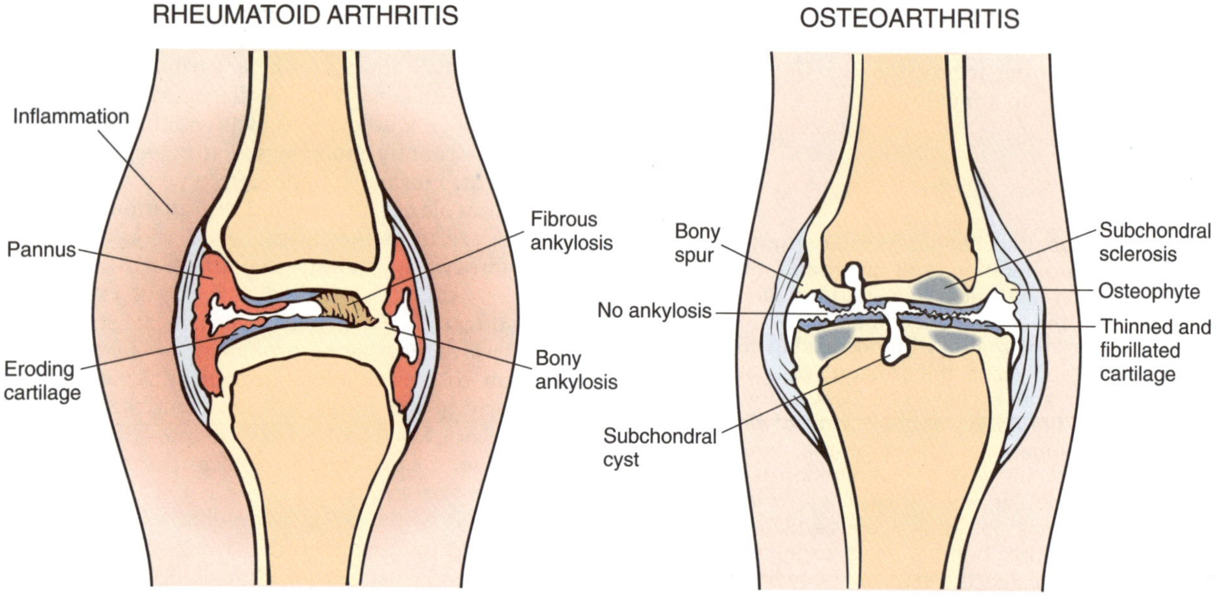

Figure 21–17

Comparison of the morphologic features of RA and osteoarthritis (also see Chapter 5 for a more detailed discussion of RA).

first carpometacarpal joints, and first tarsometatarsal joints of the feet are commonly involved. *Heberden nodes* in the fingers, representing prominent osteophytes at the distal interphalangeal joints, are characteristic in women. Aside from complete inactivity, there is no predicted way to prevent or halt the progression of primary osteoarthritis; it can stabilize for years but is generally slowly progressive. With time, significant joint deformity can occur, but unlike rheumatoid arthritis (Chapter 5), fusion does not take place. A comparison of the important morphologic features of these two disorders is shown in Figure 21–17.

Gout

Gout is a disorder caused by the tissue accumulation of excessive amounts of *uric acid, an end product of purine metabolism*. It is marked by recurrent episodes of acute arthritis, sometimes accompanied by the formation of large crystalline aggregates called *tophi*, and chronic joint deformity. All of these result from precipitation of monosodium urate crystals from supersaturated body fluids. Although an elevated level of uric acid is an essential component of gout, not all such individuals develop gout, indicating that influences besides hyperuricemia contribute to the pathogenesis. Gout is traditionally divided into primary and secondary forms, accounting for about 90% and 10% of cases, respectively (see Table 21–3). *Primary gout* designates cases wherein the basic cause is unknown or (less commonly) when it is due to an inborn metabolic defect that causes hyperuricemia. In *secondary gout* the cause of the hyperuricemia is known, but gout is not necessarily the main or even dominant clinical disorder.

Table 21–3 Classification of Gout

Clinical Category	Metabolic Defect
Primary Gout (90% of cases)	
Enzyme defects unknown (85% to 90% of primary gout)	• Overproduction of uric acid Normal excretion (majority) Increased excretion (minority) Underexcretion of uric acid with normal production
Known enzyme defects—e.g., partial HGPRT deficiency (rare)	• Overproduction of uric acid
Secondary Gout (10% of cases)	
Associated with increased nucleic acid turnover—e.g., leukemias	• Overproduction of uric acid with increased urinary excretion
Chronic renal disease	• Reduced excretion of uric acid with normal production
Inborn errors of metabolism	• Overproduction of uric acid with increased urinary excretion e.g., complete HGPRT deficiency (Lesch-Nyhan syndrome)

HGPRT, hypoxanthine guanine phosphoribosyl transferase.

Morphology

The major morphologic manifestations of gout are acute arthritis, chronic tophaceous arthritis, tophi in various sites, and gouty nephropathy.

Acute arthritis is characterized by a dense neutrophilic infiltrate permeating the synovium and synovial fluid. Long, slender, needle-shaped **monosodium urate crystals** are frequently found in the cytoplasm of the neutrophils as well as in small clusters in the synovium. The synovium is edematous and congested, and contains scattered mononuclear inflammatory cells. When the episode of crystallization abates and the crystals resolubilize, the attack remits.

Chronic tophaceous arthritis evolves from repetitive precipitation of urate crystals during acute attacks. The urates can heavily encrust the articular surfaces and form visible deposits in the synovium (Fig. 21–18A). The synovium becomes hyperplastic, fibrotic, and thickened by inflammatory cells, forming a pannus that destroys the underlying cartilage, and leading to juxta-articular bone erosions. In severe cases, fibrous or bony ankylosis ensues, resulting in loss of joint function.

Tophi are the pathognomonic hallmarks of gout. They are formed by large aggregations of urate crystals surrounded by an intense inflammatory reaction of lymphocytes, macrophages, and foreign-body giant cells, attempting to engulf the masses of crystals (Fig. 21–18B). Tophi can appear in the articular cartilage of joints and in the periarticular ligaments, tendons, and soft tissues, including the ear lobes, nasal cartilages, and skin of the fingertips. Superficial tophi can lead to large ulcerations of the overlying skin.

Gouty nephropathy refers to multiple different renal complications associated with urate deposition, variously forming medullary tophi, intratubular precipitations, or free uric acid crystals and renal calculi. Secondary complications such as pyelonephritis can occur, especially when there is urinary obstruction.

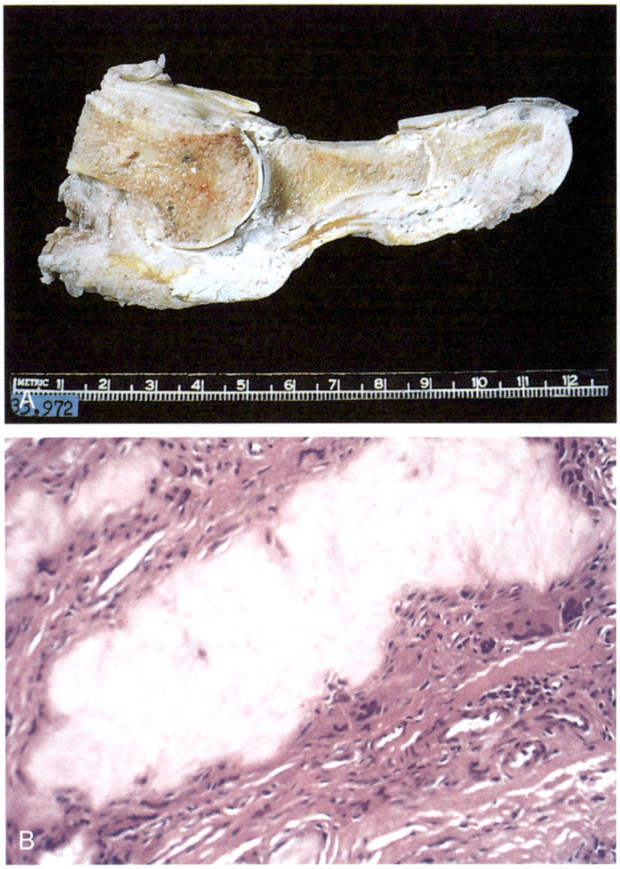

Figure 21–18

Gout. **A,** Amputated great toe with white tophi involving the joint and soft tissues. **B,** Photomicrograph of a gouty tophus. An aggregate of dissolved urate crystals is surrounded by reactive fibroblasts, mononuclear inflammatory cells, and giant cells.

Pathogenesis. Elevated uric acid levels can result from overproduction of uric acid, reduced excretion, or both (see Table 21–3). Most cases of gout are characterized by a primary overproduction of uric acid. Less commonly, uric acid is produced at normal rates, and hyperuricemia occurs because of decreased renal excretion of urate. To understand these influences, a brief review of normal uric acid synthesis and excretion is warranted.

- *Uric acid synthesis.* Uric acid is the end product of purine catabolism; consequently increased urate synthesis typically reflects some abnormality in purine nucleotide production. The synthesis of purine nucleotides involves two different but interlinked pathways: the *de novo* and *salvage pathways* (Fig. 21–19).
- *The de novo pathway* is involved in the synthesis of purine nucleotides from nonpurine precursors. The starting substrate is ribose-5-phosphate, which is ultimately converted into inosinic acid, guanylic acid, and adenylic acid. Particularly important in the context of gout are (1) the negative feedback regulation of amidophosphoribosyltransferase (amido-PRT) and 5-phosphoribosyl-1-pyrophosphate (PRPP) synthetase by the purine nucleotide end products and (2) the activation of amido-PRT by its PRPP substrate.
- *The salvage pathway* is involved in the synthesis of purine nucleotides from free purine bases, derived from dietary intake and by catabolizing nucleic acids and purine nucleotides. In this pathway purine nucleotides are formed in a single-step condensation between PRPP and hypoxanthine, guanine, or adenine. These reactions are catalyzed by two transferases: hypoxanthine guanine phosphoribosyltransferase (HGPRT) and adenine phosphoribosyltransferase (APRT).
- *Uric acid excretion.* Circulating uric acid is freely filtered by the glomerulus and virtually completely resorbed in the proximal tubules of the kidney. A small fraction of the resorbed urate is subsequently secreted by the distal nephron and excreted in the urine.

Although the cause of excessive uric acid biosynthesis in *primary gout* is unknown in most cases, rare patients have identifiable enzymatic defects. For example, complete lack of HGPRT gives rise to the *Lesch-Nyhan syndrome*. This X-linked genetic condition is characterized by excessive excretion of uric acid, severe neurologic disease with mental retardation, and self-mutilation (but

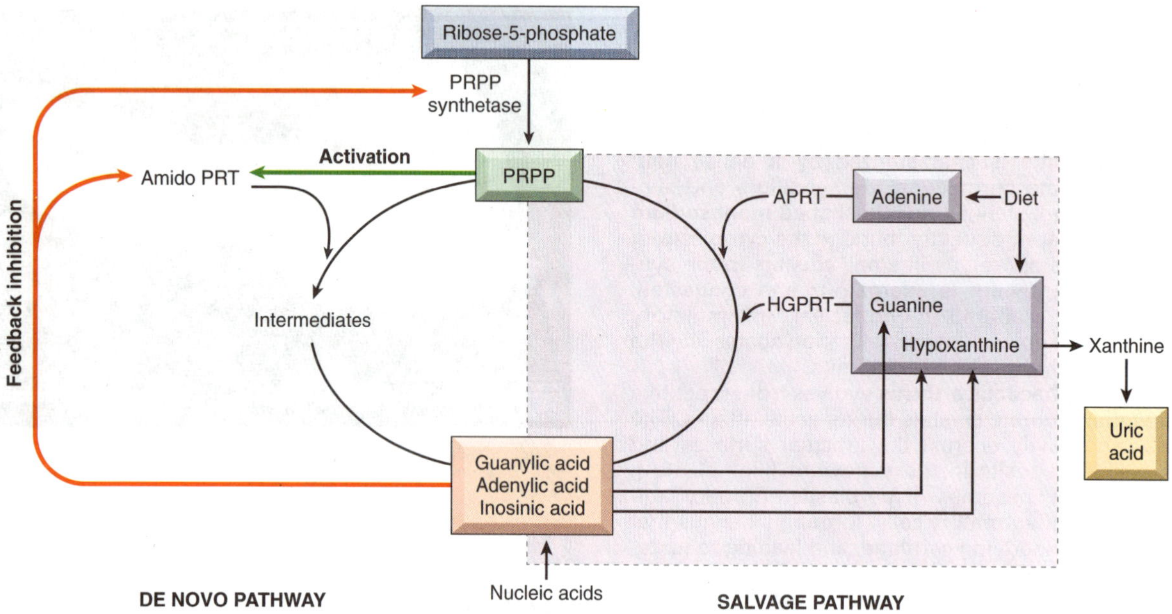

Figure 21–19

Purine metabolism. The conversion of PRPP to purine nucleotides is catalyzed by amido-PRT in the de novo pathway and by APRT and HGPRT in the salvage pathway. APRT, adenosine phosphoribosyltransferase; HGPRT, hypoxanthine-guanine phosphoribosyltransferase; PRPP, phosphoribosyl pyrophosphate; PRT, phosphoribosyltransferase.

interestingly, little in the way of gout!). Because of the almost complete absence of HGPRT, purine nucleotide synthesis via the salvage pathway is blocked. This has two effects: an accumulation of PRPP, a key substrate for the de novo pathway, and increased activity of amido-PRT (due to elevated PRPP and reduced feedback inhibition from purine nucleotides). As a consequence, de novo pathway purine biosynthesis is augmented, resulting eventually in excess production of the uric acid end product. Less severe deficiencies of HGPRT (*partial deficiency;* see Table 21–3) cause clinically severe gouty arthritis, occasionally associated with mild neurologic disease.

In *secondary gout,* hyperuricemia can be caused by increased urate production (e.g., rapid cell lysis during chemotherapy for lymphoma or leukemia) or decreased excretion (chronic renal insufficiency), or both. Reduced renal excretion may also be caused by drugs such as thiazide diuretics, presumably because of effects on uric acid tubular transport.

Whatever the cause, increased levels of uric acid in the blood and other body fluids (e.g., synovium) lead to the precipitation of monosodium urate crystals. This, in turn, triggers a chain of events that culminate in joint injury (Fig. 21–20). The precipitated crystals are directly chemotactic, and can also activate complement to generate chemotactic C3a and C5a fragments. This leads to a local accumulation of neutrophils and macrophages in the joints and synovial membranes; in attempting to phagocytize the crystals, these cells become activated, leading to the release a host of additional mediators including chemokines, toxic free radicals, and leukotrienes–particularly leukotriene B_4. The activated neutrophils also liberate destructive lysosomal enzymes. Macrophages participate in joint injury by secreting a variety of proinflammatory mediators such as IL-1, IL-6, and TNF. While intensifying the inflammatory response, these cytokines can also directly activate synovial cells and cartilage cells to release proteases (e.g., collagenase) that cause tissue injury. The resulting acute arthritis typically remits in days to weeks, even if untreated. Repeated bouts, however, can lead to the permanent damage seen in chronic tophaceous arthritis.

Clinical Features. Gout is more common in men than in women; it does not usually cause symptoms before the age of 30. Four stages are classically described: (1) asymptomatic hyperuricemia, (2) acute gouty arthritis, (3) "intercritical" gout, and (4) chronic tophaceous gout. *Asymptomatic hyperuricemia* appears around puberty in males and after menopause in women. After a long interval of years, *acute arthritis* appears in the form of sudden onset of excruciating joint pain associated with localized erythema and warmth; constitutional symptoms are uncommon, except possibly mild fever. The vast majority of first attacks are monarticular; 50% occur in the first metatarsophalangeal joint (great toe), and 90% in the instep, ankle, heal, or wrist. Untreated, acute gouty arthritis may last for hours to weeks, but it gradually completely resolves and the patient enters an *asymptomatic intercritical period.* Although some individuals never have another attack, most experience a second episode within months to a few years. In the absence of appropriate therapy, the attacks recur at shorter intervals and frequently become polyarticular. Eventually, after a

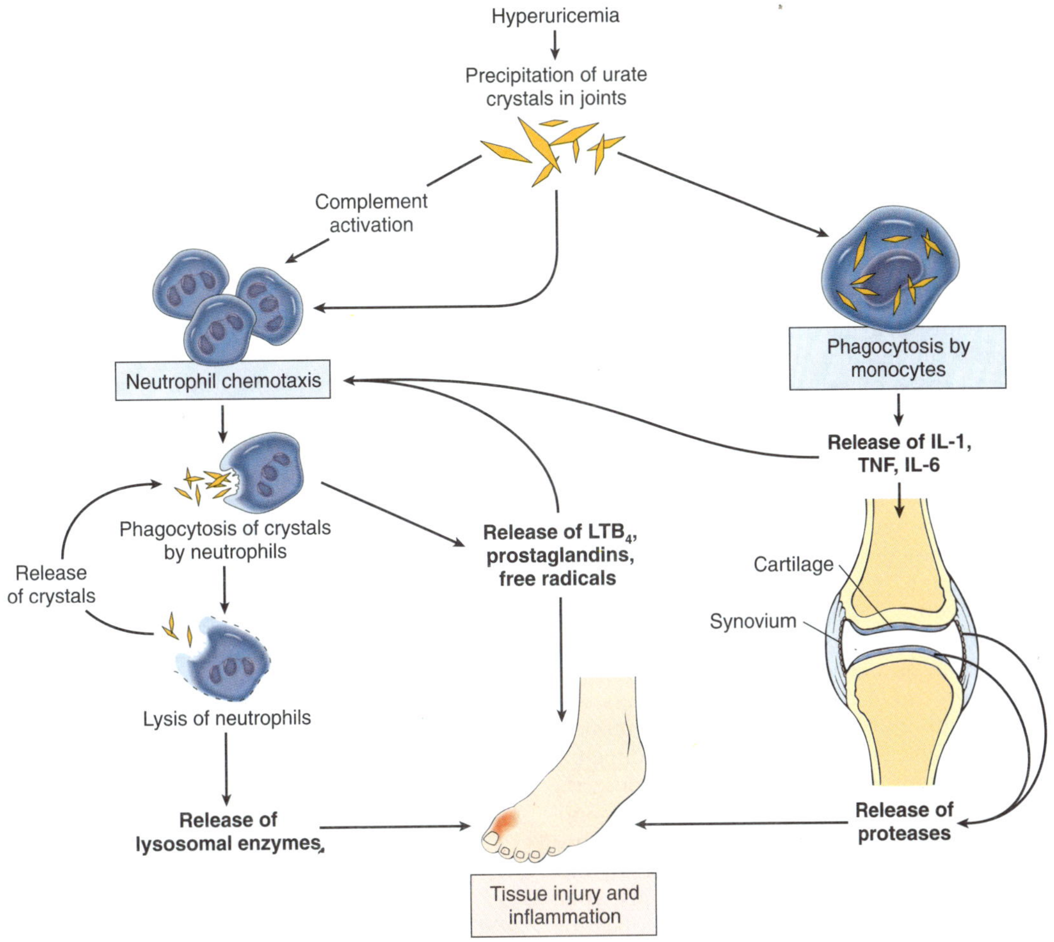

Figure 21–20

Pathogenesis of acute gouty arthritis. IL, interleukin; LTB_4, leukotriene B_4; TNF, tumor necrosis factor.

decade or so, symptoms fail to resolve completely after each attack, and the disease progresses to *chronic tophaceous gout.* At this stage, radiographs show characteristic juxta-articular bone erosion caused by the crystal deposits and loss of the joint space. Progression leads to severe crippling disease.

Renal manifestations of gout can appear as renal colic associated with the passage of gravel and stones, and can evolve into chronic gouty nephropathy. About 20% of individuals with chronic gout die of renal failure.

Numerous drugs are available to abort or prevent acute attacks of arthritis and mobilize tophaceous deposits. Their use is important because many aspects of gout are related to the duration and severity of hyperuricemia. Generally, gout does not materially shorten the life span, but it can certainly impair quality of life.

Pseudogout

Pseudogout is also known as *chondrocalcinosis* or–more formally–calcium pyrophosphate crystal deposition disease. Pseudogout typically first occurs in those age 50 or older, becoming more common with increasing age, and eventually reaching a prevalence of 30% to 60% in those age 85 or older. There is no gender or race predilection.

Although not all pathways that can lead to crystal formation are known, most probably they involve enzymes that produce or degrade pyrophosphate, resulting in its accumulation and eventual crystallization with calcium. In a hereditary variant with a mutation in a transmembrane pyrophosphate transport channel, crystals develop relatively early in life and there is severe osteoarthritis.

Much of the subsequent joint pathology in pseudogout involves the recruitment and activation of inflammatory cells, and is reminiscent of gout (see above). Joint involvement can last from several days to weeks and may be monoarticular or polyarticular; the knees, followed by the wrists, elbows, shoulders, and ankles, are most commonly affected. Ultimately, approximately 50% of patients experience significant joint damage. Therapy is supportive; no known treatment prevents or retards crystal formation.

Infectious Arthritis

Microorganisms of any type can lodge in joints during hematogenous dissemination. Articular structures can also become infected by direct inoculation or by contiguous spread from osteomyelitis or a soft tissue abscess. Infectious arthritis is serious because it can cause rapid joint destruction and permanent deformities.

Suppurative Arthritis

Bacteria can seed joints during episodes of bacteremia; joint infection with such microorganisms almost uniformly results in a suppurative arthritis. Although virtually any bacteria can be causal, *Haemophilus influenzae* predominates in children under age 2 years, *S. aureus* is the main causative agent in older children and adults, and *gonococcus* is prevalent during late adolescence and young adulthood. Individuals with sickle cell disease are prone to infection with *Salmonella* at any age. Both genders are affected equally, except for gonococcal arthritis, which occurs mainly in sexually active women. Those with deficiency of certain complement proteins (C5, C6, and C7) are particularly susceptible to disseminated gonococcal infections and hence arthritis.

Classically, there is sudden onset of pain, redness, and swelling of the joint with restricted range of motion. Fever, leukocytosis, and elevated erythrocyte sedimentation rate are common. In gonococcal infections, the course tends to be more subacute. In 90% of nongonococcal suppurative arthritis, the infection involves only a single joint—usually the knee—followed in order by hip, shoulder, elbow, wrist, and sternoclavicular joints. Joint aspiration is typically purulent, and allows identification of the causal agent.

Lyme Arthritis

Lyme disease is caused by infection with the spirochete *Borrelia burgdorferi,* transmitted by deer ticks of the *Ixodes ricinus* complex; it is named for the Connecticut town where the disease was first recognized in the 1970s. With more than 20,000 cases reported annually, it is the leading arthropod-borne disease in the United States. As in another major spirochetal disease, syphilis, clinical disease caused by Lyme spirochetes involves multiple organ systems and is usually divided into three stages. In *stage 1 Borrelia* spirochetes multiply at the site of the tick bite and cause an expanding area of redness, often with an indurated or pale center. This skin lesion, called *erythema chronicum migrans,* may be accompanied by fever and lymphadenopathy but usually disappears in a few weeks' time. In *stage 2,* the *early disseminated stage,* spirochetes spread hematogenously and cause secondary annular skin lesions, lymphadenopathy, migratory joint and muscle pain, cardiac arrhythmias, and meningitis, often with cranial nerve involvement. If the disease is not treated, antibodies develop that are useful for serodiagnosis of *Borrelia* infection. Some spirochetes, however, escape host antibody and T-cell responses by sequestering themselves in the central nervous system or as intracellular forms within endothelial cells. In *stage 3,* the *late disseminated stage,* which occurs 2 or 3 years after the initial bite, Lyme *Borrelia* organisms cause a chronic arthritis, sometimes with severe damage to large joints, and an encephalitis that varies from mild to debilitating.

Lyme arthritis develops in roughly 60% to 80% of untreated patients and is the dominant feature of late disease. The arthritis may be caused by immune responses against *Borrelia* antigens that cross-react with proteins in the joints, although surprisingly little is concretely understood about the pathogenesis of Lyme arthritis. The disease tends to be remitting and migratory, primarily involving large joints, especially the knees, shoulders, elbows, and ankles, in descending order of frequency. Histologically, there is a chronic papillary synovitis with synoviocyte hyperplasia, fibrin deposition, mononuclear cell infiltrates, and onionskin thickening of arterial walls; in severe cases, the morphology closely resembles rheumatoid arthritis. In only 25% of cases do silver stains reveal a sprinkling of organisms, and formal diagnosis of Lyme arthritis may depend on the clinical story and/or appropriate serologic studies. Chronic arthritis with pannus formation and permanent deformities develops in roughly one of ten patients.

SUMMARY

Arthritis

- *Osteoarthritis* (degenerative joint disease) is by far the most common form of joint pathology; it represents a primary degenerative disorder of articular cartilage with matrix breakdown exceeding synthesis. Inflammation is secondary.
- The vast majority of cases occur without apparent precipitating cause except increasing age. Local production of pro-inflammatory cytokines and other mediators (IL-1, TNF, nitric oxide), increased bone density, and sustained high estrogen levels are also associated with osteoarthritis.
- *Gout and pseudogout.* Increased circulating levels of uric acid (due to variations in urate metabolism, decreased renal excretion, or to increased cell turnover; *gout*) or calcium pyrophosphate *(pseudogout)* can lead to crystal deposition in the joint space. Resulting inflammatory cell recruitment and activation leads to joint injury by degrading cartilage and inciting local fibrosis.
- Either direct infection of a joint space *(suppurative arthritis)* or cross-reactive immune responses to systemic infections (e.g., in some cases of *Lyme arthritis*) can lead to joint inflammation and injury.

JOINT TUMORS AND TUMOR-LIKE LESIONS

Primary neoplasms of joints are unusual; in general, they reflect the cells and tissue types (synovial membrane, vessels, fibrous tissue, and cartilage) native to the joints. Benign tumors are much more frequent than their malignant counterparts. The rare malignant neoplasms of these structures are discussed below with the soft tissue tumors.

In comparison, reactive *tumor-like lesions such as ganglions and synovial cysts* are much more common than neoplasms; these typically result from trauma or degenerative processes.

Ganglion and Synovial Cysts

A *ganglion* is a small (<1.5 cm) cyst located near a joint capsule or tendon sheath; the wrist is an especially common site. Lesions manifest as firm to fluctuant pea-sized nodules. These are grossly translucent and microscopically lack a true cell lining, because they arise by cystic degeneration of connective tissue. Lesions can be multilocular through coalescence of adjacent areas of myxoid change. The cyst fluid is similar to synovial fluid, although there is no communication with the joint space. Ganglions are usually completely asymptomatic. Classically, these can be treated by "Bible therapy"; whacking them with a large tome is usually sufficient to rupture the cyst, and re-accumulation is uncommon.

Herniation of synovium through a joint capsule or massive enlargement of a bursa can produce a *synovial cyst*. A good example is the *Baker cyst* that occurs in the popliteal fossa.

Pigmented Villonodular Tenosynovitis and Giant-Cell Tumor of Tendon Sheath

Villonodular synovitis is a catch-all term for several closely related benign neoplasms of synovium. Although these were previously considered reactive proliferations (hence the designation *synovitis*), cytogenetic studies show consistent chromosomal changes that prove they are neoplastic, clonal proliferations. Classic examples include *pigmented villonodular synovitis* (PVNS, involving joint synovium), and *giant-cell tumor of tendon sheath* (GCT). Whereas PVNS tends to involve joints diffusely, GCT usually occurs as a single tendon sheath nodule. Both PVNS and GCT typically arise in people in their 20s to 40s without gender predilection.

Morphology

Grossly, PVNS and GCT are red-brown to orange-yellow. In PVNS the joint synovium becomes a contorted mass of red-brown folds, finger-like projections, and nodules (Fig. 21–21A). In contrast, GCT is well circumscribed and contained. Tumor cells in both lesions resemble synoviocytes (Fig. 21–21B). In PVNS they spread along the surface and infiltrate the subsynovial compartment. In GCT the cells grow in a solid nodular aggregate. Other typical findings include hemosiderin deposits, foamy macrophages, multinucleated giant cells, and zones of scarring.

PVNS usually presents as a monoarticular arthritis; it affects the knee in 80% of cases, followed by the hip and ankle. Patients typically complain of pain, locking, and recurrent swelling. Tumor progression limits the range of movement of the joint. Aggressive lesions erode into adjacent bones and soft tissues, causing confusion with other tumors. In contrast, GCT manifests as a solitary, slowly growing, painless mass frequently involving wrist and finger tendon sheaths; it is the most common soft tissue tumor of the hand. Cortical erosion of adjacent bone occurs in approximately 15% of cases. Both lesions are amenable to surgical resection, although both tend to recur locally.

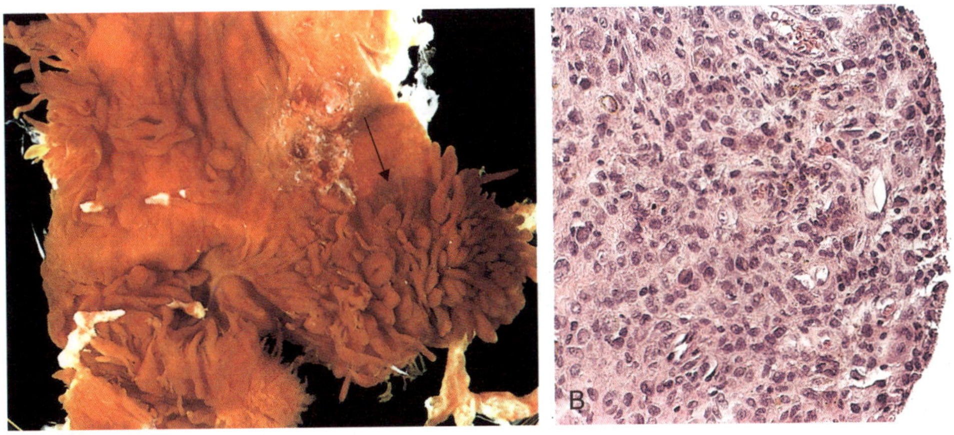

Figure 21–21

Pigmented villonodular synovitis (PVNS). **A,** Excised synovium with fronds and nodules typical of PVNS *(arrow)*. **B,** Sheets of proliferating cells in PVNS bulging the synovial lining.

SKELETAL MUSCLE

Normal skeletal muscle development and function critically depend on a tight integration with the central and peripheral nervous systems (Chapter 23). The principal element of this integrated system is called the *motor unit.* It is comprised of a motor neuron in the brain or spinal cord, its associated peripheral axon and distal neuromuscular junction, and finally, the skeletal muscle fibers that are innervated. Depending on the nature of the nerve fiber doing the enervation, the associated skeletal muscle develops into one of two major subpopulations; *type I "slow twitch"* or *type II "fast twitch"* fibers. The different fibers are distinguishable by unique metabolic and biochemical attributes, and can be identified using specific staining techniques. A single "type I" or "type II" neuron will innervate multiple muscle fibers and these fibers are usually randomly scattered in a "checkerboard pattern" within a circumscribed area within the larger muscle (Fig. 21–22A). A helpful mnemonic for type I fibers is "one slow fat red ox" referring to type I fibers being *slow*-twitch and more dependent on *fat* catabolism for energy through mitochondrial *ox*idative phosphorylation; the *red* refers to this being the dark (red) meat on birds where fiber type grouping in different muscles (e.g., thigh *vs.* breast meat) is quite pronounced. The counter-mnemonic for type II fibers ("two fast glycogen white anaerobes") is not nearly so memorable.

Diseases that affect skeletal muscle can involve any portion of the motor unit; these include primary disorders of the motor neuron or axon, abnormalities of the neuromuscular junction, and a wide variety of disorders primarily affecting the skeletal muscle itself (*myopathies*). For purposes of the following discussion, we will divide skeletal muscle disease into 1) disorders characterized by neurogenic changes or myofiber atrophy, 2) the more common muscular dystrophies, 3) selected congenital, toxic, and infectious myopathies (*inflammatory* myopathies such as *dermatomyositis* are discussed in Chapter 5), and 4) disorders of the neuromuscular junction. At the end of this section we will also briefly touch on primary skeletal muscle tumors.

MUSCLE ATROPHY

Muscle atrophy is a non-specific response in a variety of muscle disorders. It is characterized by abnormally small myofibers; the type of fibers affected by the atrophy, their distribution in the muscle, and their specific morphology help identify the etiology of the atrophic changes.

Clearly loss of muscle innervation causes atrophy of the associated fibers. As discussed in detail below, neurogenic atrophy is characterized by involvement of both fiber types and by clustering of myofiers into small groups. Simple disuse (e.g., prolonged bed rest, immobilization to allow healing of a bone fracture, etc.) can also cause profound atrophy. Exogenous glucocorticoids or endogenous hypercortisolism (e.g., in Cushing syndrome) are another cause of muscle atrophy, typically involving proximal muscle groups more than distal ones. Disuse- and steroid-induced atrophy primarily affects the type II fibers and causes a random distribution of the atrophic myofibers. Finally, atrophic myofibers are also found in myopathies. As discussed later, the finding of additional morphologic changes like myofiber degeneration and regeneration, chronic remodeling of the tissue or inflammatory infiltrates are features that suggest a myopathic etiology.

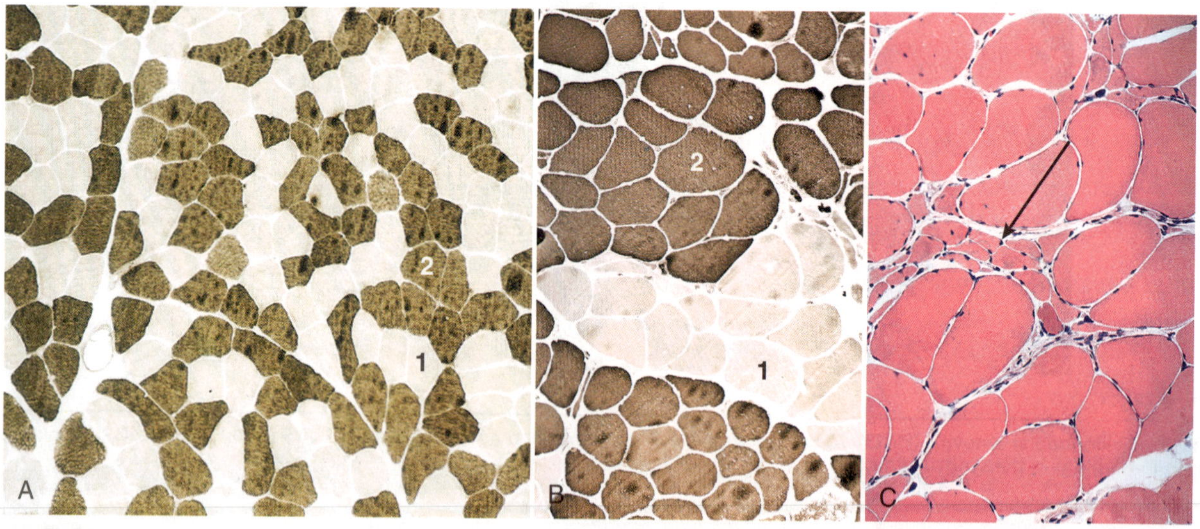

Figure 21–22

A, ATPase histochemical staining, at pH 9.4, of normal muscle showing checkerboard distribution of intermingled type 1 (*light*) and type 2 (*dark*) fibers. **B,** in contrast, fibers of either histochemical type are grouped together after reinnervation of muscle. **C,** A cluster of atrophic fibers (group atrophy) in the center (*arrow*).

Neurogenic Atrophy

Deprived of their normal enervation, skeletal fibers undergo progressive atrophy. It is important to recall that loss of a single neuron will affect all muscle fibers in a motor unit, so that the atrophy tends to be scattered over the field. However, following re-enervation, adjacent intact neurons send out sprouts to engage the neuromuscular junction of the previously de-enervated fibers. Once the new connection is established these fibers assume the type of the innervating neuron. In this manner, whole groups of fibers can eventually fall under the influence of the same neuron, and become the same fiber type (*fiber type grouping*) (Fig. 21–22B). In that setting, if the relevant enervating neuron now becomes injured, rather large coalescent groups of fibers are cut off from the trophic stimulation and wither away (*grouped atrophy*, Fig. 21–22C), a hallmark of recurrent neurogenic atrophy.

MUSCULAR DYSTROPHY

The muscular dystrophies are a heterogeneous group of inherited disorders, often presenting in childhood, that are characterized by progressive degeneration of muscle fibers leading to muscle weakness and wasting. Histologically, in advanced cases muscle fibers are replaced by fibrofatty tissue. This histologic feature distinguishes dystrophies from myopathies (described later), which also present with muscle weakness.

X-Linked Muscular Dystrophy (Duchenne and Becker Muscular Dystrophy)

The two most common forms of muscular dystrophy are X-linked: *Duchenne muscular dystrophy* (DMD) and *Becker muscular dystrophy* (BMD). DMD is the most severe and the most common form of muscular dystrophy, with an incidence of about 1 per 3500 live male births. DMD becomes clinically evident by age 5, with progressive weakness leading to wheelchair dependence by age 10 to 12 years, and death by the early 20s. Although the same gene is involved in both BMD and DMD, BMD is less common and much less severe.

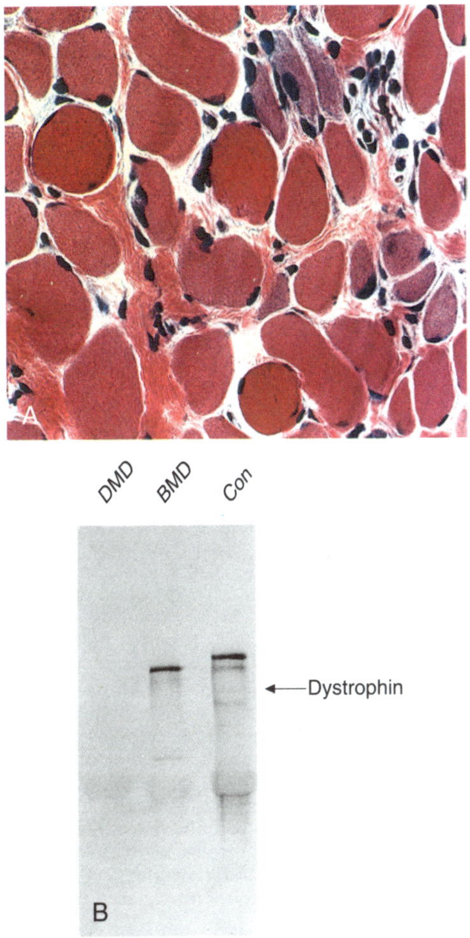

Figure 21–23

A, Duchenne muscular dystrophy (DMD) showing variation in muscle fiber size, increased endomysial connective tissue, and regenerating fibers *(blue hue).* **B,** Western blot showing absence of dystrophin in DMD and altered dystrophin size in Becker muscular dystrophy (BMD) compared with control (Con) (Courtesy of Dr. L. Kunkel, Children's Hospital, Boston, Massachusetts).

Morphology

The histologic features of DMD and BMD are similar and include **marked variation in muscle fiber size,** caused by concomitant myofiber hypertrophy and atrophy. Many of the residual muscle fibers show a range of **degenerative changes,** including fiber splitting and necrosis, whereas other fibers show evidence of **regeneration,** including sarcoplasmic basophilia, nuclear enlargement, and nucleolar prominence. **Connective tissue is increased** throughout the muscle (Fig. 21–23A). The definitive diagnosis is based on the demonstration of **abnormal staining for dystrophin** in immunohistochemical preparations or by western blot analysis of skeletal muscle. In the late stages of the disease, extensive fiber loss and adipose tissue infiltration are present in most muscle groups. Changes in cardiac muscle in either DMD or BMD include variable degrees of fiber hypertrophy and interstitial fibrosis.

Pathogenesis. DMD and BMD are caused by abnormalities in the dystrophin gene located on the short arm of the X chromosome (Xp21). Dystrophin is a large protein (427 kD) that is expressed in a wide variety of tissues, including muscles of all types, brain, and peripheral nerves. As shown schematically in Figure 21–24, dystrophin attaches portions of the sarcomere to the cell membrane, maintaining the structural and functional integrity of skeletal and cardiac myocytes. The role of dystrophin in transferring the force of contraction to connective tissue has been proposed as the basis for the

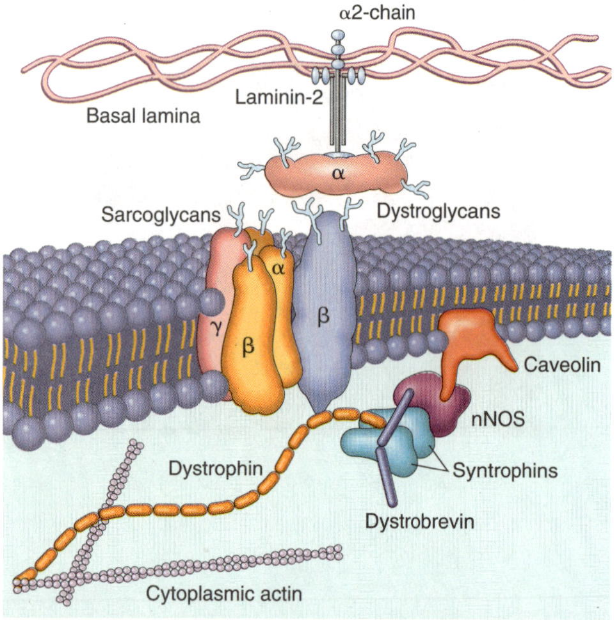

Figure 21–24

The relationship between the cell membrane (sarcolemma) and the sarcolemmal associated proteins. Dystrophin, an intracellular protein, forms an interface between the cytoskeletal proteins and a group of transmembrane proteins, the dystroglycans and the sarcoglycans. These transmembrane proteins interact with the ECM, including the laminin proteins. Mutations in dystrophin are associated with the X-linked muscular dystrophies, mutations in caveolin and the sarcoglycan proteins with the autosomal limb girdle muscular dystrophies, and mutations in the α_2-laminin (merosin) with a form of congenital muscular dystrophy.

myocyte degeneration that occurs with dystrophin defects, or with changes in other proteins that interact with dystrophin (Fig. 21–24, and see later). Muscle biopsy specimens from *individuals with DMD show virtually no dystrophin by either immunohistochemical staining or western blot analysis, explaining the greater severity of their presentation* (see Fig. 21–23B). In comparison, *individuals with BMD show diminished amounts of an abnormal molecular weight dystrophin,* reflecting mutations that apparently permit limited synthesis of a defective (but still partially active) protein.

The dystrophin gene spans roughly 2400 kilobases (~1% of the total X chromosome), making it one of the largest in the human genome; its enormous size is a probable explanation for its particular vulnerability to mutation. Deletions appear to represent a large proportion of the genetic abnormalities, with frameshift and point mutations accounting for the rest. Approximately two-thirds of the cases are familial, with the remainder representing new mutations. In affected families, females are carriers; they are clinically asymptomatic but often have elevated serum creatine kinase and can show mild histologic abnormalities on muscle biopsy. Female carriers, however, are at risk for developing dilated cardiomyopathy.

Clinical Features. Boys with DMD are normal at birth, and early motor milestones are met on time. Walking, however, is often delayed, and the first indications of muscle weakness are clumsiness and inability to keep up with peers. Weakness begins in the pelvic girdle muscles and then extends to the shoulder girdle. Enlargement of the calf muscles associated with weakness, a phenomenon termed *pseudohypertrophy,* is an important clinical finding. The increased muscle bulk is caused initially by an increase in the size of the muscle fibers and then, as the muscle atrophies, by an increase in fat and connective tissue. Pathologic changes are also found in the heart, and patients may develop heart failure or arrhythmias. Although there are no well-established structural abnormalities of the central nervous system, cognitive impairment seems to be a component of the disease and is severe enough in some patients to be considered mental retardation. Serum creatine kinase is elevated during the first decade of life but returns to normal in the later stages of the disease, as muscle mass decreases. Death results from respiratory insufficiency, pulmonary infection, and cardiac decompensation.

Boys with BMD develop symptoms at a later age than those with DMD. The onset occurs in later childhood or in adolescence, and it is accompanied by a generally slower and more variable rate of progression. Although cardiac disease is frequently seen in these patients, many have a nearly normal life span.

Autosomal Muscular Dystrophies

Other forms of muscular dystrophy share many features of DMD and BMD but have distinct clinical and pathologic characteristics. Some of these muscular dystrophies affect specific muscle groups, and the formal diagnosis is based largely on the clinical pattern of muscle weakness. Several autosomal muscular dystrophies affect the proximal musculature of the trunk and limbs (similar to the X-linked muscular dystrophies), and are termed *limb girdle muscular dystrophies.* Limb girdle muscular dystrophies can be inherited either as autosomal dominant or autosomal recessive disorders; six dominant subtypes and ten recessive subtypes have been identified. Mutations of the *sarcoglycan complex of proteins* cause four of the recessive forms of these dystrophies (see Fig. 21–24), with other forms being associated with other cytoskeletal proteins or caveolin.

Myotonic Dystrophy

Myotonia is a sustained involuntary contraction of a group of muscles; it is the cardinal neuromuscular symptom in myotonic dystrophy. Patients often complain of "stiffness" and have difficulty in releasing their grip, for instance, after a handshake. Myotonia can often be elicited by percussion of the thenar eminence.

Myotonic dystrophy is inherited as an autosomal dominant trait; it is associated with a CTG trinucleotide repeat expansion on chromosome 19 that affects the mRNA for the dystrophila myotonia-protein kinase. In normal subjects, fewer than 30 CTG repeats are present;

disease develops with expansion of this repeat, and in severely affected individuals several thousand repeats may be present. Expansion of the trinucleotide repeat influences the eventual concentration of the protein product. Like other "trinucleotide repeat disorders" (e.g., fragile X syndrome, Huntington disease; see Chapter 7), myotonic dystrophy tends to increase in severity and appear at a younger age in succeeding generations, a phenomenon termed *anticipation*. With each new generation there is expansion of the CTG repeats during gametogenesis, and this seems to correspond to the clinical feature of anticipation.

The disease often presents in late childhood with gait abnormalities attributable to weakness of foot dorsiflexors; it progresses to weakness of the intrinsic muscles of the hands and wrist extensors; atrophy of facial muscles with ptosis ensues.

SUMMARY

Muscular Dystrophy

- Muscular dystrophies are inherited disorders usually manifesting in childhood as skeletal muscular weakness and wasting; cardiac muscle can also be affected with congestive heart failure.
- The most common muscular dystrophies are X-linked and related to defective synthesis (Duchenne muscular dystrophy) or mutated forms (Becker muscular dystrophy) of *dystrophin*. Other forms of muscular dystrophy can involve other proteins of the sarcoglycan complex; specific diagnoses strongly depend on the patterns of clinical presentation.
- Myotonic dystrophy presents with muscle weakness as well as myotonia; the most common form is a trinucleotide repeat disorder affecting the synthesis of an intracellular protein kinase.

MYOPATHY

The term *myopathy* encompasses a heterogeneous group of disorders, both morphologically and clinically. For purposes of this discussion, we will segregate these into congenital and toxic (i.e., acquired) forms. Although a complete review is beyond the scope of this text, recognition of these disorders is important for genetic counseling or appropriate treatment of acquired disease.

Congenital Myopathies

Important subcategories include disorders caused by *inherited mutations of ion channels (channelopathies)*, *inborn errors of metabolism* (exemplified by glycogen and lipid storage diseases), and *mitochondrial abnormalities*.

- *Ion channel myopathies* are a group of familial diseases characterized clinically by myotonia, relapsing episodes of hypotonic paralysis (associated with variably abnormal serum potassium concentrations), or both. As their name indicates, these diseases are caused by mutations in genes that encode ion channels. Thus, *hyperkalemic periodic paralysis* results from mutations in the gene for the skeletal muscle sodium channel protein SCN4A, which regulates sodium entry during contraction. *Malignant hyperthermia* is a rare clinical syndrome characterized by a dramatic hypermetabolic state (tachycardia, tachypnea, muscle spasms, and later hyperpyrexia) triggered by anesthesia, usually involving halogenated inhalational agents and succinylcholine; mutations have been identified in genes encoding calcium channels.
- *Myopathies due to inborn errors of metabolism* include disorders of glycogen synthesis and degradation (see Chapter 7), and abnormalities in lipid handling. Specifically, abnormalities of the carnitine transport system or deficiencies of the mitochondrial dehydrogenase enzyme systems can lead to significant lipid accumulation within myocytes *(lipid myopathies)*.
- *Mitochondrial myopathies* can involve mutations in either mitochondrial or nuclear DNA that encodes mitochondrial constituents. The mitochondrial genome (mtDNA) encodes one-fifth of the proteins involved in mitochondrial oxidative phosphorylation, as well as 22 mitochondrial-specific tRNAs and 2 rRNA species. Diseases that involve mtDNA show maternal inheritance, because only the oocyte contributes mitochondria to the embryo. Mitochondrial myopathies typically present in young adulthood with proximal muscle weakness, and sometimes with severe involvement of the ocular musculature *(external ophthalmoplegia)*. There can also be neurologic symptoms, lactic acidosis, and cardiomyopathy. The most consistent pathologic findings in skeletal muscle are irregular muscle fibers and aggregates of abnormal mitochondria; the latter impart a blotchy red appearance to the muscle fiber on the modified Gomori trichrome stain, hence the term *ragged red fibers* (Fig. 21–25A). The electron microscopic appearance is also often distinctive: there are increased numbers of, and abnormalities in, the shape and size of mitochondria, some of which contain paracrystalline *parking lot inclusions* or alterations in the structure of cristae (Fig. 21–25B).

Toxic Myopathies

Important subcategories include disorders caused by *intrinsic* exposures (e.g. thyroxine) versus *extrinsic* exposures (e.g., alcohol, therapeutic drugs).

- *Thyrotoxic myopathy* can present as either acute or chronic proximal muscle weakness, and can precede the onset of other signs of thyroid dysfunction. Find-

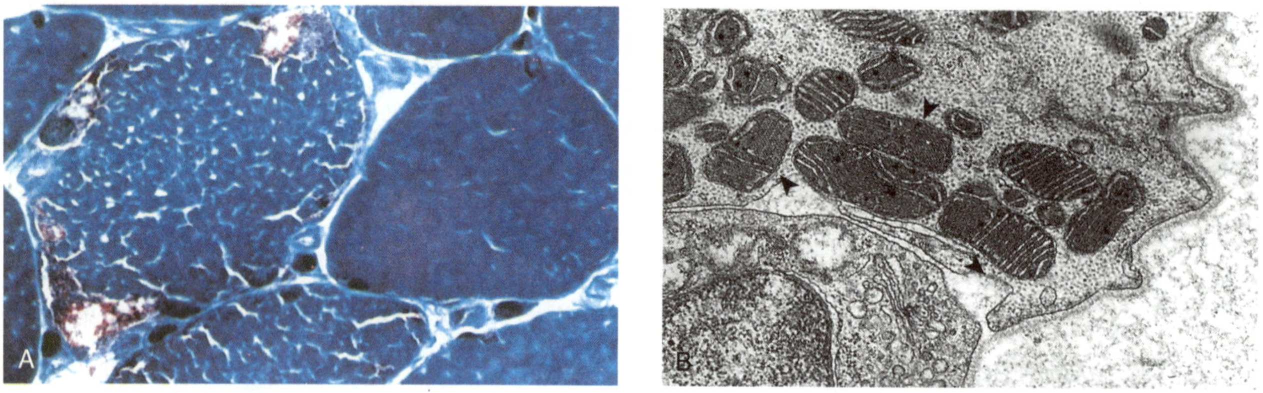

Figure 21–25

A, Mitochondrial myopathy showing an irregular fiber with subsarcolemmal collections of mitochondria that stain red with the modified Gomori trichrome stain *(ragged red fiber).* **B,** Electron micrograph of mitochondria from biopsy specimen in **A** showing "parking lot" inclusions (*arrowheads*).

ings include myofiber necrosis, regeneration, and interstitial lymphocytes.

- *Ethanol myopathy* can occur with binge drinking, where there is an acute toxic rhabdomyolysis with accompanying myoglobinuria that can cause renal failure. Clinically, the patient may acutely develop pain that is either generalized or confined to a single muscle group. On histology, there is myocyte swelling and necrosis, myophagocytosis, and regeneration.
- *Chloroquine* can also produce a proximal myopathy in humans. The most prominent finding is myocyte vacuolization, and with progression, myocyte necrosis.

DISEASES OF THE NEUROMUSCULAR JUNCTION

Myasthenia Gravis

Myasthenia gravis is an autoimmune disorder of the neuromuscular junction characterized by muscle weakness. The disease affects roughly 3 in 100,000 persons; it can present at any age and has a predilection for women. Thymic hyperplasia is found in 65% and a thymoma in 15% of patients. Circulating antibodies to the skeletal muscle acetylcholine receptors (AChRs) are present in nearly all patients, associated with a decrease in the number of AChRs. The disease can be transferred to animals with serum from affected patients, demonstrating the causal role of the anti-AChR antibodies.

Pathogenesis. In most cases, the autoantibodies against the AChR lead to loss of functional AChRs at the neuromuscular junction either by (1) increasing the internalization and degradation of the receptors, and/or (2) blocking the binding of acetylcholine (ACh) to its receptor. Notably, the autoantibodies do not appear to cause disease by inducing muscle destruction. Despite the evidence that anti-AChR antibodies function critically in the pathogenesis of the disease, antibody levels and neurologic deficit are not always correlated. The link between autoimmunity to AChRs and the thymic abnormalities is also unclear. Nevertheless, most patients show improvement after thymectomy.

Clinical Features. Typically, weakness is first noticed in the extraocular muscles; drooping eyelids *(ptosis)* and double vision *(diplopia)* cause the patient to seek medical attention. The generalized muscle weakness can fluctuate dramatically, with alterations occurring over the course of days, hours, or even minutes. Repetitive electrophysiologic stimulation typically elicits diminishing muscle strength, and patients show marked improvement after administration of anticholinesterase agents—the latter presumably by increasing the levels of ACh in the neuromuscular synapse; both maneuvers are diagnostically useful. Sensory and autonomic functions are not affected in myasthenia gravis. Respiratory compromise was a major cause of mortality in the past; 95% of patients now survive more than 5 years after diagnosis because of improved treatment (anticholinesterase drugs, prednisone, plasmapheresis, and thymic resection), as well as ventilatory support.

Lambert-Eaton Myasthenic Syndrome

The *Lambert-Eaton myasthenic syndrome* characteristically develops as a paraneoplastic process (see Chapter 6), most commonly in the setting of small-cell lung carcinoma (60% of cases); it can also occur in the absence of malignancy. Although individuals with Lambert-Eaton syndrome also present with muscle weakness, the syndrome is distinct from myasthenia gravis in several ways: (1) anticholinesterase administration does not improve symptoms; (2) autonomic function is affected; and (3) electrophysiologic studies demonstrate that repeated stimulation elicits *increasing* muscle strength. In these patients, the content of ACh is normal in neuromuscular junction synaptic vesicles, and the postsynaptic membrane is normally responsive to ACh, but fewer vesicles than normal are released in response to each presynaptic action potential. This is attributed to antibodies that recognize presynaptic calcium channels; a similar disease can be transferred to animals with these antibodies.

SKELETAL MUSCLE TUMORS

Skeletal muscle neoplasms are almost all malignant. The benign rhabdomyoma is rare and will not be covered here. *Cardiac rhabdomyomas* are examples of hamartomas.

Rhabdomyosarcoma

Rhabdomyosarcoma is the most common soft tissue sarcoma of childhood and adolescence, usually appearing before age 20. Interestingly, they occur most commonly in the head and neck or genitourinary tract, usually at sites where there is little, if any, skeletal muscle as a normal constituent.

Chromosomal translocations are found in most cases; the more common t(2;13) translocation fuses the *PAX3* gene on chromosome 2 with the *FKHR* gene on chromosome 13. *PAX3* functions upstream of genes that control skeletal muscle differentiation, and tumor development probably involves dysregulation of muscle differentiation by the chimeric PAX3-FKHR protein.

Morphology

The gross appearance of rhabdomyosarcomas is variable. Some tumors, particularly those arising near the mucosal surfaces of the bladder or vagina, can present as soft, gelatinous, grapelike masses, designated **sarcoma botryoides.** In other cases they are poorly defined, infiltrating masses. Rhabdomyosarcoma is histologically subclassified into the **embryonal, alveolar,** and **pleomorphic** variants. The **rhabdomyoblast** is the diagnostic cell in all types; it exhibits granular eosinophilic cytoplasm rich in thick and thin filaments. The rhabdomyoblasts may be round or elongated; the latter are known as **tadpole or strap cells** (Fig. 21–26) and may contain cross-striations visible by light microscopy. The diagnosis of rhabdomyosarcoma is based on the demonstration of skeletal muscle differentiation, either in the form of sarcomeres under the electron microscope or by immunohistochemical demonstration of muscle-associated antigens such as desmin and muscle-specific actin.

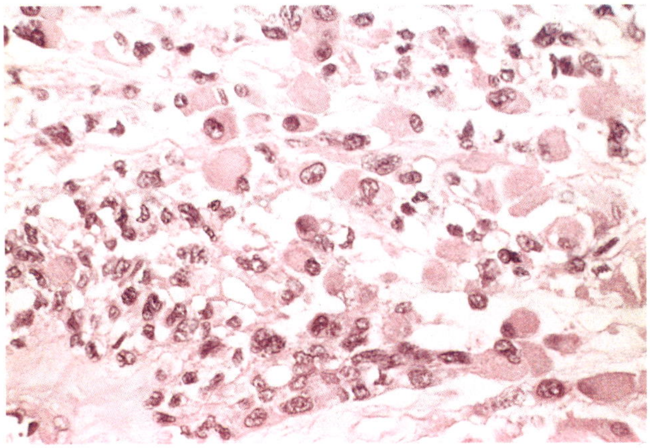

Figure 21–26

Rhabdomyosarcoma. The rhabdomyoblasts are large and round and have abundant eosinophilic cytoplasm; no cross-striations are evident here.

Rhabdomyosarcomas are aggressive neoplasms treated with a combination of surgery, chemotherapy, and radiation. Location and the histologic variant of the tumor influence survival; embryonal, pleomorphic, and alveolar variants have progressively worsening prognoses. The malignancy is curable in almost two-thirds of children, but adults do much more poorly.

SOFT TISSUE TUMORS

By convention, the term *soft tissue* describes any nonepithelial tissue other than bone, cartilage, CNS, hematopoietic, and lymphoid tissues. Soft tissue tumors are classified according to the tissue type they recapitulate, including fat, fibrous tissue, and neurovascular tissue (Table 21–4). In some soft tissue neoplasms, however, no corresponding normal counterpart is known. With the exception of skeletal muscle neoplasms (see above), benign soft tissue tumors outnumber their malignant counterparts by at least 100:1. In the United States, approximately 8000 soft tissue sarcomas are diagnosed annually, representing less than 1% of all invasive malignancies. Nevertheless, they cause 2% of all cancer deaths, reflecting their lethal nature.

Most soft tissue tumors arise without antecedent causes, although rarely radiation, burn injury, or toxin exposure are implicated. Kaposi sarcoma (Chapter 11) is associated with the human herpesvirus 8, but viruses are probably not important in the pathogenesis of most sarcomas. A small minority of sarcomas are associated with genetic syndromes, most notably neurofibromatosis type 1 (neurofibroma, malignant schwannoma), Gardner syndrome (fibromatosis), Li-Fraumeni syndrome (soft tissue sarcoma), and Osler-Weber-Rendu syndrome (telangiectasia). Specific chromosomal abnormalities and genetic derangements in these syndromes provide important clues about the genesis of the neoplasms. Even in sporadic soft tissue sarcomas, characteristic chromosomal abnormalities can be detected. These provide insight into pathogenesis, as well as diagnostic markers. Some tumors, such as Ewing sarcoma and synovial sarcoma, are eventually defined by their translocation.

Soft tissue tumors can arise in any location, although approximately 40% occur in the lower extremities, especially the thigh. The incidence generally increases with age, although 15% arise in children. Certain sarcomas

Table 21–4 Soft Tissue Tumors

• Tumors of Adipose Tissue
Lipomas
Liposarcoma
• Tumors and Tumor-like Lesions of Fibrous Tissue
Nodular fasciitis
Fibromatoses
Superficial fibromatoses
Deep fibromatoses
Fibrosarcoma
• Fibrohistiocytic Tumors
Fibrous histiocytoma
Dermatofibrosarcoma protuberans
Malignant fibrous histiocytoma
• Tumors of Skeletal Muscle
Rhabdomyoma
Rhabdomyosarcoma
• Tumors of Smooth Muscle
Leiomyoma
Smooth muscle tumors of uncertain malignant potential
Leiomyosarcoma
• Vascular Tumors
Hemangioma
Lymphangioma
Hemangioendothelioma
Hemangiopericytoma
Angiosarcoma
• Peripheral Nerve Tumors
Neurofibroma
Schwannoma
Malignant peripheral nerve sheath tumors
• Tumors of Uncertain Histogenesis
Synovial sarcoma
Alveolar soft part sarcoma
Epithelioid sarcoma
Granular cell tumor

tend to appear in certain age groups, e.g., rhabdomyosarcoma in children, synovial sarcoma in young adulthood, and liposarcoma and malignant fibrous histiocytoma in later adult life.

Several features of soft tissue tumors influence prognosis:

- *Accurate histologic classification is critical.* Although cell morphology and architectural arrangement are important, these features are often inadequate to distinguish different sarcomas, particularly if they are poorly differentiated. Consequently, immunohistochemistry, electron microscopy, cytogenetics, and molecular genetics are indispensable in assigning the correct diagnosis in some cases.
- *Sarcoma grade is important for predicting behavior.* Grading, usually I to III, is based on the degree of differentiation, the average number of mitoses per high-power field, cellularity, pleomorphism, and an estimate of the extent of necrosis (presumably a reflection of rate of growth). Mitotic counts and necrosis are the most important predictors.
- *Staging helps determine the prognosis.* With tumors larger than 20 cm, metastases develop in 80% of cases; in contrast, for tumors 5 cm or smaller, metastases occur in only 30% of cases.
- In general, tumors arising in superficial locations (e.g., skin) have a better prognosis than deep-seated lesions; overall, the 10-year survival rate for sarcomas is approximately 40%.

With this brief background, we now turn to the individual tumors and tumor-like lesions; only the more common will be covered. Some of the soft tissue tumors are presented elsewhere; we have already discussed some of the joint and skeletal muscle tumors above. Tumors of peripheral nerve are briefly covered in Chapter 23, and tumors of vascular origin, including Kaposi sarcoma, are highlighted in Chapter 11.

FATTY TUMORS

Lipoma

Lipomas are benign tumors of fat, and are the most common soft tissue tumors of adulthood. Most lipomas are solitary lesions; multiple lipomas usually suggest the presence of rare autosomal dominant syndromes. Lipomas can be subclassified based on their histologic features (e.g., conventional, myolipoma, spindle cell, myelolipoma, pleomorphic, angiolipoma), and/or characteristic chromosomal rearrangements. Most lipomas are mobile, slowly enlarging, painless masses (angiolipomas can present with local pain); complete excision is usually curative.

Morphology

Conventional lipomas (the most common subtype) are soft, yellow, well-encapsulated masses of mature adipocytes; they can vary considerably in size. Histologically, they consist of mature white fat cells with no pleomorphism.

Liposarcoma

Liposarcomas are malignant neoplasms of adipocytes. They occur most commonly in the fifth and sixth decades. Most liposarcomas arise in the deep soft tissues or in visceral sites. The prognosis of liposarcomas is greatly influenced by the histologic subtype; well-differentiated and myxoid variants tend to grow in a fairly indolent fashion and have a more favorable outlook than do the more aggressive round cell and pleomorphic variants, which tend to recur after excision and metastasize to lungs. Amplification of a region of 12q is common in well-differentiated liposarcomas; this region contains the *MDM2* gene whose product binds to and inactivates p53 protein. A t(12;16) chromosomal translocation is associated with myxoid liposarcomas and with some cases of round cell liposarcoma; the rearrangement affects a transcription factor that plays a role in normal adipocyte differentiation.

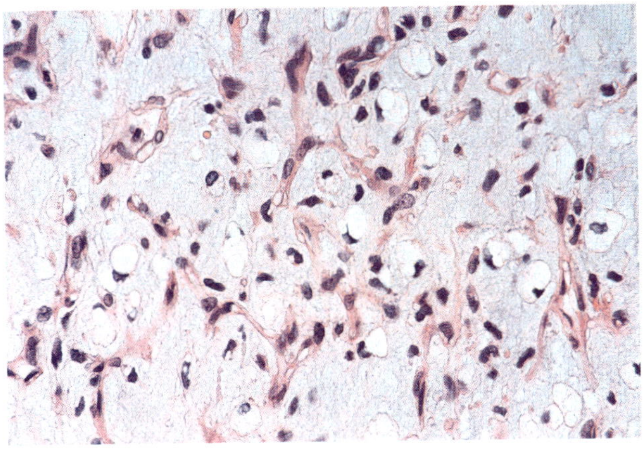

Figure 21–27

Myxoid liposarcoma. Adult-appearing fat cells and more primitive cells, with lipid vacuoles *(lipoblasts)* are scattered in abundant myxoid matrix.

Morphology

Liposarcomas usually present as relatively well-circumscribed lesions. Several different histologic subtypes are recognized, including two low-grade variants, the **well-differentiated liposarcoma** and the **myxoid liposarcoma,** the latter characterized by abundant, mucoid extracellular matrix. Some well-differentiated lesions can be difficult to distinguish histologically from lipomas, whereas very poorly differentiated tumors can resemble various other high-grade malignancies. In most cases, cells indicative of fatty differentiation are present. Such cells are known as **lipoblasts;** they recapitulate fetal fat cells with cytoplasmic lipid vacuoles that scallop the nucleus (Fig. 21–27).

FIBROUS TUMORS AND TUMOR-LIKE LESIONS

Fibrous tissue proliferations are a heterogeneous group of lesions. At one end of the spectrum, *nodular fasciitis* is not a true tumor but rather a reactive, self-limited proliferation. At the other end, *fibrosarcomas* are highly malignant neoplasms that tend to recur locally and can metastasize. *Fibromatoses* fall somewhere in the middle; these are characterized as benign lesions that nevertheless exhibit persistent local growth and can defy adequate surgical excision. Distinguishing the various lesions requires considerable skill and experience on the part of the pathologist.

Reactive Proliferations

Nodular Fasciitis

Nodular fasciitis is a self-limited, reactive fibroblastic proliferation that typically occurs in adults on the volar aspect of the forearm, followed in frequency by the chest and back. Patients characteristically present with a several-week history of a solitary, rapidly growing, and occasionally painful mass. Preceding trauma is noted in 10% to 15% of cases. Lesions of nodular fasciitis rarely recur after excision.

Morphology

Characteristically, the lesion is several centimeters in greatest dimension and nodular with poorly defined margins. Histologically, it is richly cellular and consists of plump, randomly arranged, immature-appearing fibroblasts in an abundant myxoid stroma (Fig. 21–28). The cells vary in size and shape (spindle to stellate) and have conspicuous nucleoli and numerous mitoses.

Myositis Ossificans

Myositis ossificans is distinguished from other fibroblastic proliferations by the presence of *metaplastic bone.* It usually develops in the proximal muscles of the extremities in athletic adolescents and young adults after trauma. The involved area is initially swollen and painful, eventually evolving into a painless, hard, well-demarcated mass. It is critical to distinguish the lesion from extraskeletal osteosarcoma. Simple excision of myositis ossificans is usually curative.

Fibromatoses

The fibromatoses are a group of fibroblastic proliferations distinguished by their tendency to grow in an infiltrative fashion and, in many cases, to recur after surgical removal. Although some lesions are *locally aggressive, they do not metastasize.* The fibromatoses are divided into two major clinicopathologic groups: superficial and deep.

- The *superficial fibromatoses* arise in the superficial fascia and include such entities as palmar fibromatosis *(Dupuytren contracture)* and penile fibromatosis *(Peyronie disease).* Superficial lesions are genetically distinct from their deep-seated cousins and are generally more innocuous (they can be associated with trisomy 3 and 8); they also come to clinical attention earlier, because they cause deformity of the involved structure.

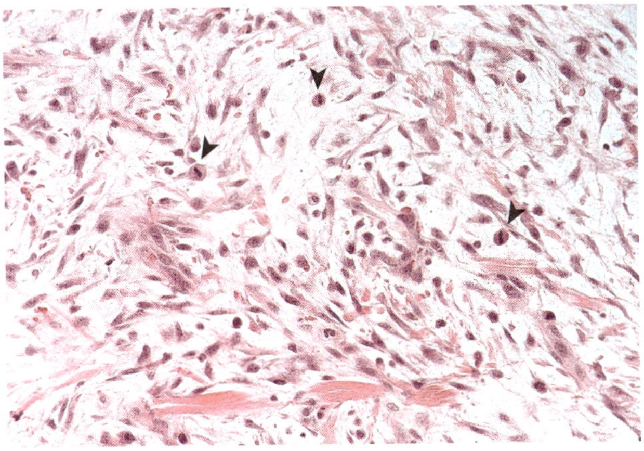

Figure 21–28

Nodular fasciitis. A highly cellular lesion composed of plump, randomly oriented spindle cells surrounded by myxoid stroma. Note the prominent mitotic activity *(arrowheads).*

• The *deep fibromatoses* include the so-called *desmoid tumors* that arise in the abdominal wall and muscles of the trunk and extremities, and within the abdomen (mesentery and pelvic walls). They can be isolated lesions, or a component of *Gardner syndrome,* an autosomal dominant disorder including colonic adenomatous polyps and osteomas. Mutations in the *APC* or β-catenin genes are present in the majority of these tumors. Deep fibromatoses tend to grow in a locally aggressive manner and recur after excision.

Morphology

These tumors are gray-white, firm to rubbery, poorly demarcated, infiltrative masses 1 to 15 cm in greatest dimension. Histologically, fibromatoses are composed of plump cells arranged in broad sweeping fascicles that penetrate the adjacent tissue; mitoses are infrequent. Immunohistochemical and ultrastructural studies show that these cells are probably **myofibroblasts.** Some lesions may be quite cellular, particularly early in their evolution, whereas others, especially the superficial fibromatoses, contain abundant dense collagen.

In addition to being disfiguring or disabling, fibromatoses are occasionally painful. Although curable by adequate excision, they frequently recur when incompletely removed. Some tumors respond to tamoxifen, and in other cases chemotherapy or irradiation are effective. Rare reports of metastases likely represent misdiagnosis of an original fibrosarcoma.

Fibrosarcoma

Fibrosarcomas are malignant neoplasms composed of fibroblasts. Most occur in adults, typically in the deep tissues of the thigh, knee, and retroperitoneal area. They tend to grow slowly, and have usually been present for several years at the time of diagnosis. As with other sarcomas, fibrosarcomas often recur locally after excision (>50% of cases) and can metastasize hematogenously (>25% of cases), usually to the lungs.

Morphology

Fibrosarcomas are soft unencapsulated, infiltrative masses frequently with areas of hemorrhage and necrosis. Better differentiated lesions can appear deceptively encapsulated. Histologic examination discloses all degrees of differentiation, from tumors that closely resemble fibromatosis, to densely packed lesions with spindled cells growing in a herringbone fashion (Fig. 21–29), to highly cellular neoplasms exhibiting architectural disarray, pleomorphism, frequent mitoses, and necrosis.

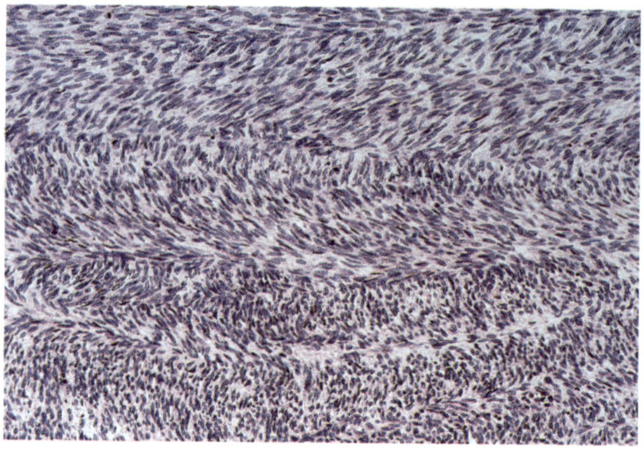

Figure 21–29

Fibrosarcoma. Malignant spindle cells here are arranged in a herringbone pattern.

FIBROHISTIOCYTIC TUMORS

Fibrohistiocytic tumors are composed of a mixture of fibroblasts and phagocytic, lipid-laden cells resembling activated macrophages. The neoplastic cells in many cases are most likely fibroblasts. Nevertheless, detailed immunohistochemical analyses demonstrate that a significant number of such tumors actually derive from other cell types. Consequently, the term *fibrohistiocytic,* especially in regard to the malignant variants, should be considered descriptive and not necessarily connoting a specific cellular origin. These tumors span a broad range of histologic patterns and biologic behavior, from self-limited benign lesions to high-grade sarcomas.

Benign Fibrous Histiocytoma (Dermatofibroma)

Dermatofibromas are relatively common benign lesions in adults presenting as circumscribed, small (<1 cm) mobile nodules in the dermis or subcutaneous tissue. Histologically, these typically consist of bland, interlacing spindle cells admixed with foamy, lipid-rich histiocyte-like cells. The borders of the lesions tend to be infiltrative, but extensive local invasion does not occur. They are cured by simple excision. The pathogenesis of these lesions is uncertain.

Malignant Fibrous Histiocytoma

Malignant fibrous histiocytoma (MFH) is a term rather loosely applied to a variety of soft tissue sarcomas characterized by considerable cytologic pleomorphism, the presence of bizarre multinucleate cells, and storiform architecture (Fig. 21–30). Despite the name, the phenotype of many such tumors is fibroblastic and not histiocytic. Nevertheless, it is also important to note that several tumors diagnosed as MFH actually exhibit markers for cells of other origin (e.g., smooth muscle cells, adipocytes, skeletal muscle cells) and are therefore more appropriately classified as leiomyosarcomas, liposarcomas, and the like. Alternatively, some tumors designated as MFH are so poorly differentiated that they do not express any discernible precursor phenotype. Consequently, any discussion of "typical" behaviors or characteristics is

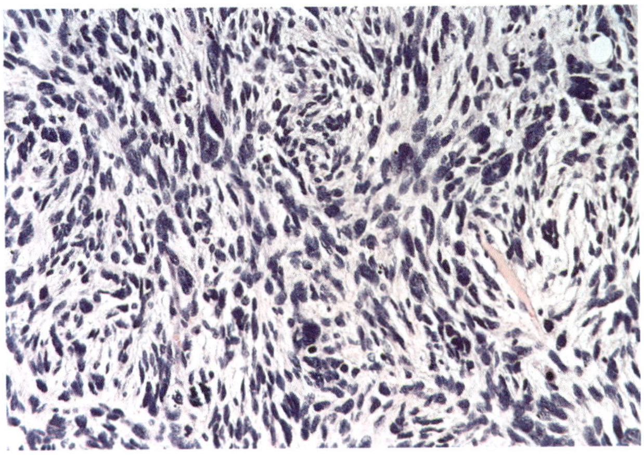

Figure 21–30

Malignant fibrous histiocytoma. There are fascicles of plump spindle cells in a swirling (storiform) pattern. (Courtesy of Dr. J. Corson, Brigham and Women's Hospital, Boston, Massachusetts.)

confounded by the extremely heterogeneous collection of tumors that have this same general histologic appearance. Indeed, if a cell of origin *can* be established, the tumors tend to behave like others of that same class. Having said that, MFH exhibiting fibroblastic differentiation are usually large (5–20 cm), gray-white unencapsulated masses that often appear deceptively circumscribed. They usually arise in the musculature of the proximal extremities or in the retroperitoneum. Most of these tumors are extremely aggressive, recur unless widely excised, and have a metastatic rate of 30% to 50%.

SMOOTH MUSCLE TUMORS

Leiomyoma

Benign smooth muscle tumors, or *leiomyomas,* are common, well-circumscribed neoplasms that can arise from smooth muscle cells anywhere in the body, but are encountered most commonly in the uterus (see Chapter 19).

Leiomyosarcoma

Leiomyosarcomas comprise 10% to 20% of soft tissue sarcomas. They occur in adults, more commonly females. Skin and deep soft tissues of the extremities and retroperitoneum are common sites. They commonly present as firm, painless masses; retroperitoneal tumors can be large and bulky and cause abdominal symptoms. Histologically, they show spindle cells with cigar-shaped nuclei arranged in interweaving fascicles. Treatment depends on the size, location, and grade of the tumor. Superficial or cutaneous leiomyosarcomas are usually small and have a good prognosis, whereas retroperitoneal tumors are large, cannot be entirely excised, and cause death by both local extension and metastatic spread.

SYNOVIAL SARCOMA

Synovial sarcoma was originally believed to recapitulate synovium; however, the cell of origin is unclear and is most certainly *not* a synoviocyte. Reflecting a non-joint origin, less than 10% of synovial sarcomas are intra-articular. Synovial sarcomas account for approximately 10% of all soft tissue sarcomas, typically occurring in individuals in their 20s to 40s. Most develop in deep soft tissues around the large joints of the extremities, with 60% to 70% occurring around the knee; many have been present for several years at the time of presentation. Most synovial sarcomas show a characteristic t(X;18) translocation that produces a fusion product combining the *SYT* gene (encoding a transcription factor) with either *SSX1* or *SSX2* genes (encoding transcription inhibitors). The specific type of translocation relates to prognosis.

Morphology

Histologically, synovial sarcomas may be biphasic or monophasic. Classic **biphasic** synovial sarcoma exhibits differentiation of tumor cells into both epithelial-like cells and spindle cells. The epithelial cells are cuboidal to columnar and form glands or grow in solid cords or aggregates. The spindle cells are arranged in densely cellular fascicles that surround the epithelial cells (Fig. 21–31). Many synovial sarcomas are **monophasic,** that is, composed of spindled cells or, rarely, epithelial cells only. Lesions composed solely of spindled cells are easily mistaken for fibrosarcomas or malignant peripheral nerve sheath tumors. Immunohistochemistry is helpful, because the tumor cells are positive for keratin and epithelial membrane antigen, differentiating them from most other sarcomas.

Synovial sarcomas are treated aggressively with limb-sparing surgery and chemotherapy. Common metastatic sites are lung, bone, and regional lymph nodes. The 5-year survival rate varies from 25% to 62%, and only 10% to 30% live for more than 10 years.

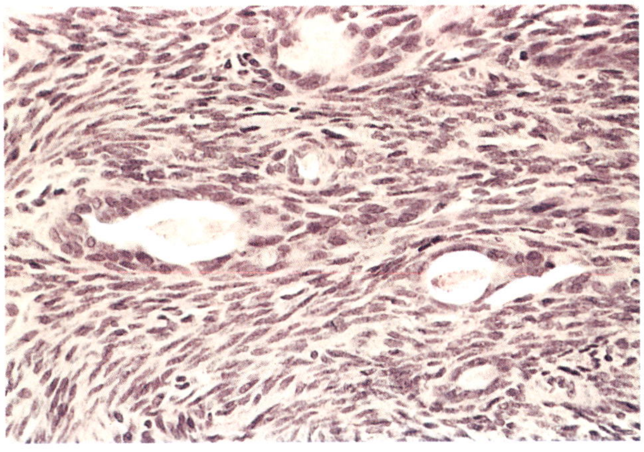

Figure 21–31

Synovial sarcoma exhibiting a classic biphasic spindle cell and gland-like histologic appearance.

BIBLIOGRAPHY

Chakkalakal JV, et al: Molecular, cellular, and pharmacological therapies for Duchenne/Becker muscular dystrophies. FASEB J 19:880, 2005. *[Extensive overview and assessment of the potential therapies for these disorders.]*

Chitnis T, Khoury SJ: Immunologic neuromuscular disorders. J Allergy Clin Immunol 111:S659, 2003. *[Excellent review of the pathogenesis, diagnosis, and therapies of multiple autoimmune neuromuscular disorders, including the myasthenic syndromes.]*

DiCaprio MR, Enneking WF: Fibrous dysplasia. Pathophysiology, evaluation, and treatment. J Bone Joint Surg Am 87:1848, 2005. *[Recent overview of monostotic and polyostotic fibrous dysplasia, including pathogenesis.]*

DiMauro S, Gurgel-Giannetti J: The expanding phenotype of mitochondrial myopathy. Curr Opin Neurol 18:538, 2005. *[Nice overview of the new developments in our understanding of mitochondrial myopathies.]*

Dos Santos NR, et al: Molecular mechanisms underlying human synovial sarcoma development. Genes Chromosomes Cancer 30:1, 2001. *[An informative review of the molecular aberrations associated with the synovial sarcoma-associated t(X;18) chromosomal translocation and their relationship to histologic patterns and clinical behavior.]*

Ellman MH, Becker MA: Crystal-induced arthropathies: recent investigative advances. Curr Opin Rheumatol 18:249, 2006. *[Excellent summary of the recent developments in the understanding of the molecular and cellular biology underlying gout and pseudogout.]*

Felson DT: Risk factors for osteoarthritis: understanding joint vulnerability. Clin Orthop Relat Res 427(Suppl):S16, 2004. *[Summary of the epidemiology of osteoarthritis and the roles played by hormonal status, genetic factors, nutrition, and mechanical factors in its development.]*

Fletcher JA: Molecular biology and cytogenetics of soft-tissue sarcomas: relevance for targeted therapies. Cancer Treat Res 120:99, 2004. *[A good overview of soft tissue tumors.]*

Gatchel JR, Zoghbi HY: Diseases of unstable repeat expansion: mechanisms and common principles. Nat Rev Genet 6:743, 2005. *[Comprehensive review of all of these diseases, including myotonic dystrophy.]*

Janknecht R: EWS-ETS oncoproteins: the linchpins of Ewing tumors. Gene 363:1, 2005. *[Excellent summary of the molecular basis of Ewing sarcoma.]*

Lane NE: Epidemiology, etiology, and diagnosis of osteoporosis. Am J Obstet Gynecol 194:S3, 2006. *[A current, comprehensive review of many of the clinical aspects of postmenopausal osteoporosis.]*

Luyten FP: Mesenchymal stem cells in osteoarthritis. Curr Opin Rheumatol 16:599, 2004. *[A succinct and thought-provoking review of the role of mesenchymal stem cells in osteoarthritis pathogenesis and therapy.]*

Mankin HJ, Hornicek FJ: Diagnosis, classification, and management of soft tissue sarcomas. Cancer Control 12:5, 2005. *[An overview of a massive topic; entire textbooks are devoted to these relatively uncommon tumors.]*

McNally EM, Pytel P: Muscle diseases: The muscular dystrophies. Annual Review of Pathology: Mechanisms of Disease, Vol. 2:87, 2007.

Millington-Ward S, et al: Emerging therapeutic approaches for osteogenesis imperfecta. Trends Mol Med 11:299, 2005. *[An exciting overview of new genetic therapies for osteogenesis imperfecta.]*

Mondry A, et al: Bone and the kidney: a systems biology approach to the molecular mechanisms of renal osteodystrophy. Curr Mol Med 5:489, 2005. *[A well-written discussion about the interplay of kidney and bone in metabolic bone disease.]*

Potts JT: Parathyroid hormone: past and present. J Endocrinol 187:311, 2005. *[Excellent review of parathyroid hormone and its role in bone resorption and potential for treating osteoporosis.]*

Roodman GD, Windle JJ: Paget disease of bone. J Clin Invest 115:200, 2005. *[Terrific review about the viral and/or inflammatory pathogenic pathways in Paget disease.]*

Sandberg AA: Cytogenetics and molecular genetics of bone and soft-tissue tumors. Am J Med Genet 115:189, 2002. *[Succinct summary of the cytogenetic alterations in a variety of soft tissue tumors.]*

Sandberg AA: Genetics of chondrosarcoma and related tumors. Curr Opin Oncol 16:342, 2004. *[A good review of the known genetic abnormalities in these tumors.]*

Steere AC, Glickstein L: Elucidation of Lyme arthritis. Nat Rev Immunol 4:143, 2004. *[An update on the arthritis component of the disease by the person who originally described Lyme disease.]*

Tolar J, et al: Osteopetrosis. N Engl J Med 351:2839, 2004. *[Imminently readable review of the disorder.]*

Uitterlinden AG, et al: Genetics and biology of vitamin D receptor polymorphisms. Gene 338:143, 2004. *[Scholarly review of the vitamin D polymorphisms and their effect on bone metabolism.]*

Ulrich-Vinther M, et al: Articular cartilage biology. J Am Acad Orthop Surg 11:421, 2003. *[Clinically-oriented review discussing the general biology of articular cartilage and approaches to therapy in osteoarthritis.]*

Wada T, et al: RANKL-RANK signaling in osteoclastogenesis and bone disease. Trends Mol Med 12:17, 2006. *[Good review of the mechanisms of activating osteoclasts, and the role of these pathways in disease.]*

Wang LL: Biology of osteogenic sarcoma. Cancer J 11:294, 2005. *[Current overview of the underlying genetic and pathologic basis for osteosarcoma.]*

Xia SJ, et al: Molecular pathogenesis of rhabdomyosarcoma. Cancer Biol Ther 1:97, 2002. *[Scholarly discussion of the PAX3-FKHR genetic translocation in rhabdomyosarcomas.]*

Chapter 22

The Skin

ALEXANDER J.F. LAZAR, MD, PhD*

Cutaneous disorders are extremely common and range from irritating acne to life-threatening melanoma. Many cutaneous disorders are intrinsic to the skin, but some are manifestations of systemic disease. Among this latter group are systemic lupus erythematosus, acquired immunodeficiency syndrome (e.g., Kaposi sarcoma), and genetic syndromes such as neurofibromatosis and Muir-Torre syndrome. Thus, skin provides a uniquely accessible window for the recognition of numerous and varied disorders.

Skin is not merely a passive, protective mantle, but rather a complex organthe largest of the bodywith regulated cellular and molecular events that govern interactions with the external environment. Skin is constantly bathed with microbial and nonmicrobial antigens that are processed by bone marrow–derived dendritic Langerhans cells, which in turn communicate with the immune system by migrating to regional lymph nodes. Squamous cells (keratinocytes) help maintain skin homeostasis by secreting a plethora of cytokines that not only regulate interactions among the epidermal cells but also diffuse into and influence the dermal microenvironment. The dermis contains both CD4+ helper and CD8+ cytotoxic T lymphocytes; some of these T cells home selectively to the skin by virtue of homing receptors called the cutaneous lymphocyte antigen (CLA). The epidermis contains intraepithelial lymphocytes, including γ/δ T cells. All these cells are rich sources of cytokines. The local tissue response involving these T cells and cytokines accounts for the microscopic patterns and clinical expressions of cutaneous inflammatory and infectious disease. These patterns can be recognized and interpreted through the microscope by the experienced observer.

This chapter focuses on diseases of the skin that are common and/or illustrative. The practice of der-

*The author thanks Professors Ronald Rapini and Robert Jordan and the Department of Dermatology at The University of Texas Medical School at Houston for many of the clinical photographs in this chapter. The contributions of Dr. George Murphy to this chapter in previous editions are gratefully acknowledged.

matopathology is unique in its close interaction with clinicians (particularly dermatologists, who spend considerable time studying skin pathology in their training) and reliance on clinical presentation and history to render a diagnosis. In effect, the clinical assessment of the condition involving the patient's skin is the gross examination that is subsequently correlated with the microscopic findings to make a diagnosis. Diseases of the skin can be perplexing, because dermatologists and dermatopathologists have a large and unique lexicon not commonly used in describing lesions in other tissues. Because knowledge of dermatologic terms and disease forms the basis of clear understanding and communication, some of these are defined below.

Macroscopic Terms

Macule: Flat, circumscribed area of any size distinguished from surrounding skin by coloration
Papule: Elevated solid area 5 mm or less in diameter
Nodule: Elevated solid area more than 5 mm in diameter
Plaque: Elevated flat-topped area, usually more than 5 mm in diameter
Vesicle: Fluid-filled raised area 5 mm or less in diameter
Bulla: Fluid-filled raised area more than 5 mm in diameter; a large vesicle
Blister: Common term used for vesicle or bulla
Pustule: Discrete, pus-filled raised area
Scale: Dry, horny, platelike excrescence; usually the result of imperfect cornification
Lichenification: Thickened and rough skin characterized by prominent skin markings; usually the result of repeated rubbing in susceptible persons (see "Lichen Simplex Chronicus")
Excoriation: A traumatic lesion characterized by breakage of the epidermis, causing a raw linear area usually due to scratching.

Microscopic Terms

Hyperkeratosis: Hyperplasia of the stratum corneum, often associated with a qualitative abnormality of the keratin
Parakeratosis: Mode(s) of keratinization characterized by retention of the nuclei in the stratum corneum; on mucosal membranes, parakeratosis is normal.
Acanthosis: Epidermal hyperplasia preferentially involving the stratum spinosum
Dyskeratosis: Abnormal keratinization occurring prematurely within individual cells or groups of cells below the stratum granulosum
Acantholysis: Loss of intercellular connections resulting in lack of cohesion between keratinocytes
Papillomatosis: Hyperplasia of the papillary dermis with elongation and/or widening of the dermal papillae
Lentiginous: Refers to a linear pattern of melanocyte proliferation within the epidermal basal cell layer; lentiginous melanocytic hyperplasia can occur as a reactive change or as part of a neoplasm of melanocytes
Spongiosis: Intercellular edema of the epidermis

ACUTE INFLAMMATORY DERMATOSES

Literally thousands of specific inflammatory dermatoses exist, hence the clinical variants and nomenclature are challenging to master at any stage of training. In general, acute lesions last from days to weeks and are characterized by inflammation (unlike other tissues, these are often marked by mononuclear cells rather than neutrophils and defined as acute because of the limited course of their natural history), edema, and sometimes epidermal, vascular, or subcutaneous injury. Some acute lesions may persist, resulting in transition to a chronic phase, while others are characteristically self-limited and never progress.

Urticaria

Urticaria (hives) is a common disorder mediated by *localized mast cell degranulation resulting in dermal microvascular hyperpermeability.* This gives rise to erythematous, edematous, and pruritic plaques termed *wheals.*

Pathogenesis. In most cases, urticaria results from antigen-induced release of vasoactive mediators from mast cell granules via sensitization with specific immunoglobulin E (IgE) antibodies (type I hypersensitivity; Chapter 5). This IgE-dependent degranulation can follow exposure to a number of antigens including pollens, foods, drugs, and insect venom. IgE-independent urticaria may result from substances that directly incite mast cell degranulation, such as opiates and certain antibiotics. In the vast majority of cases, no clinical cause is discovered despite extensive searching. Hereditary angioneurotic edema results from inherited deficiency of C1 esterase inhibitor, yielding uncontrolled activation of the early components of the complement system (Chapter 2). The resulting urticaria affects the lips, throat, eyelids, genitals, and distal extremities. When the larynx is affected it can be dangerous since airway patency may be compromised.

Morphology

The histologic features of urticaria are often subtle with very sparse superficial perivenular infiltrate of mononuclear cells and rare admixed neutrophils. Scattered eosinophils may be present. Superficial dermal edema results in more widely spaced collagen bundles. Degranulation of mast cells, that normally reside around superficial dermal venules, is often not prominent in routine H & E stains, but these can sometimes be highlighted using a Giemsa stain.

Clinical Features. Urticaria generally occurs between the ages of 20 and 40 years. Individual lesions develop and fade within hours (usually <24 hours), but episodes may persist for days or even months. Persistent lesions are sometimes due to urticarial vasculitis associated with temporary vascular damage. Lesions vary from small, pruritic papules to large edematous plaques with erythema resulting from superficial vascular dilation. Increased vascular permeability leads to localized dermal edema. Sites include any area exposed to pressure, such as the trunk, distal extremities, and ears. In general, this condition is more irritating and embarrassing than life-threatening and is managed with antihistamines or steroids in more severe cases.

Acute Eczematous Dermatitis

Eczema is a clinical term that embraces a number of conditions with different underlying etiologies. All are characterized by red, *papulovesicular, oozing, and crusted lesions* at an early stage. The degree of these changes varies with clinical subtype. With persistence, these lesions develop into raised, *scaling plaques*. Clinical differences permit classification of eczematous dermatitis into: (1) allergic contact, (2) atopic, (3) drug-related eczematous, (4) photoeczematous, and (5) primary irritant forms. Most of these forms resolve completely when the offending stimulus is removed or exposure to it is limited, thus stressing the importance of investigating the underlying cause. Only the most common form, contact dermatitis, will be discussed here.

Pathogenesis. After initial exposure to an environmental contact sensitizing agent, such as poison ivy, self-proteins modified by the agent are processed by epidermal Langerhans cells that then migrate to draining lymph nodes and present the antigen to naive T cells. This sensitization event leads to acquisition of immunologic memory; on re-exposure to the antigen, the now-educated CD4+ T lymphocytes migrate to the affected skin sites. Here they release cytokines that recruit additional inflammatory cells and also mediate the epidermal damage as in any delayed-type hypersensitivity reaction (Chapter 5).

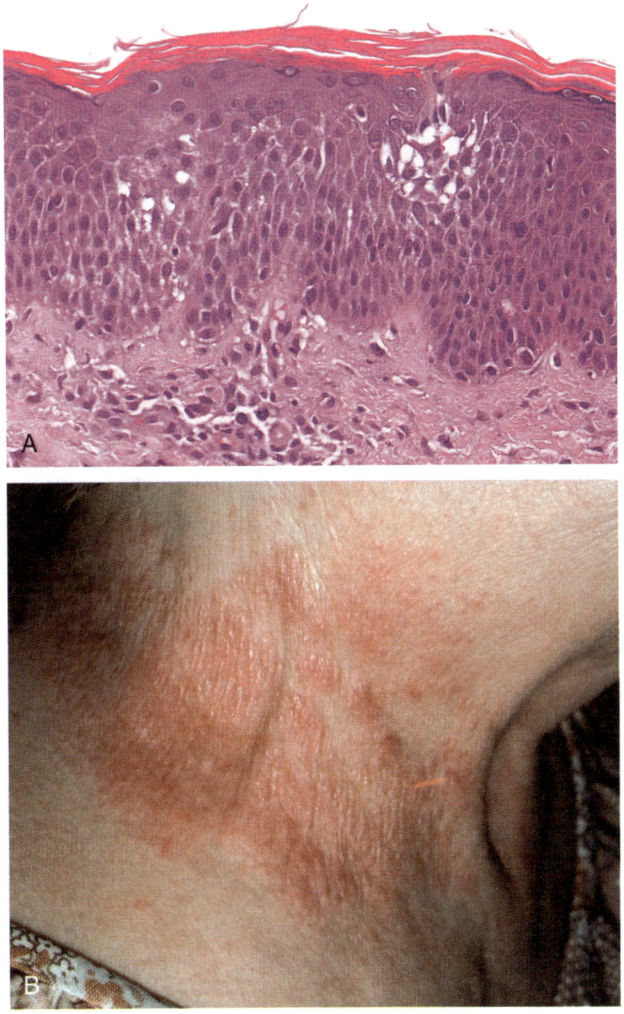

Figure 22–1

Eczematous dermatitis. **A,** Fluid accumulation between epidermal cells results in spongiosis that can proceed to small vesicles if intercellular connections are stretched until broken—thus the term spongiotic dermatitis. **B,** Note the patterned erythema and scale associated with nickel contact dermatitis resulting from this woman's necklace.

Morphology

Spongiosis—the accumulation of edema fluid within the epidermis—characterizes all forms of acute eczematous dermatitis—hence the synonym **"spongiotic dermatitis."** Edema seeps into the intercellular spaces of the epidermis, splaying apart keratinocytes. Intercellular bridges are stretched and become more prominent visually, giving a "spongy" appearance (Fig. 22–1A). This is accompanied by a superficial perivascular lymphocytic infiltrate, papillary dermal edema, and mast cell degranulation. Eosinophils may be present and especially prominent in spongiotic eruptions provoked by drugs, but in general there are no specific features for differentiating the various causes of eczema and careful clinical correlation is needed.

Clinical Features. Lesions of acute eczematous dermatitis are pruritic (itchy), edematous, oozing plaques, often containing vesicles and bullae. With persistent antigen stimulation, lesions may become progressively scaly (hyperkeratotic) as the epidermis thickens (acanthosis) and can become chronic. Some of these changes also result from scratching or rubbing of the lesion (see "Lichen Simplex Chronicus"). The clinical causes of eczema are sometimes divided into "inside" and "outside" jobs—disease resulting from external application of antigen (such as poison ivy) or reaction to an internal circulating antigen (such as ingested food or drug).

Susceptibility to atopic dermatitis is often inherited and this form can be more chronic, although it sometimes improves with age. Atopic individuals often suffer from asthma as well (Chapter 5), perhaps another expression of an irritable and overactive immune system.

Erythema Multiforme

Erythema multiforme is an uncommon, usually self-limited disorder that seems to be a *hypersensitivity response to certain infections and drugs.* Among antecedent infections are those caused by herpes simplex, mycoplasmas, and fungi such as *Histoplasma Capsulatum,* and *Coccidiodes imitis.* The implicated drugs include sulfonamides, penicillin, salicylates, hydantoins, and antimalarials. Patients present with an array of *"multiform" lesions, including macules, papules, vesicles, and bullae, as well as the characteristic targetoid lesion consisting of a red macule or papule with a pale vesicular or eroded center* (Fig. 22–2A).

Pathogenesis. The lesions of erythema multiforme result from the action of CLA positive, skin-homing cytotoxic T cells that are concentrated in the central portion of the lesions, while CD4+ helper and Langerhan cells are more prominent in the raised, erythematous periphery. The cytotoxic cells directed against an inciting drug or microbe presumably respond to cross-reactive antigens of the basal cell layer of skin and mucosae and damage these tissues.

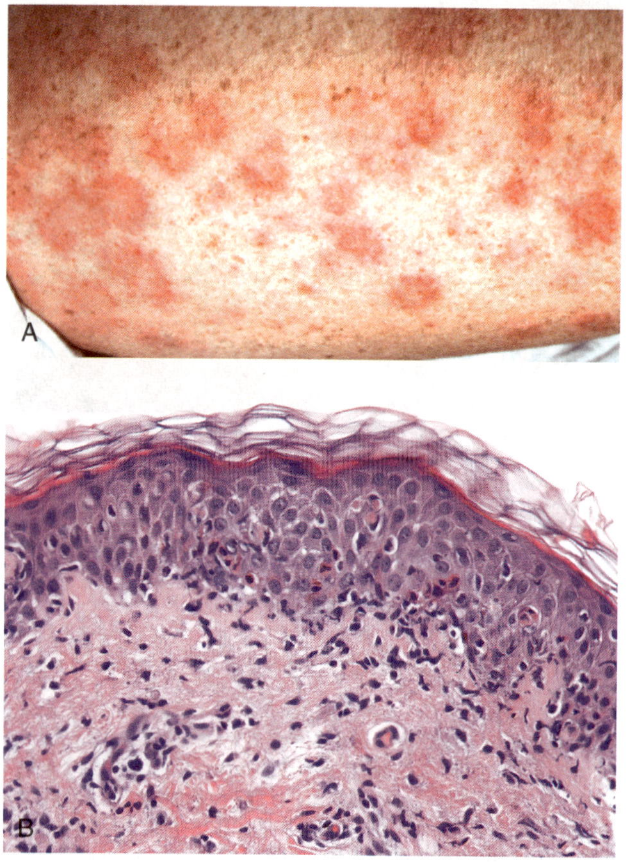

Figure 22–2

Erythema multiforme. **A,** Lesions show a central zone of dusky pink-gray discoloration that correlates with epidermal necrosis or early blister formation, surrounded by a pink-red rim, producing the characteristic target-like appearance of erythema multiforme minor. **B,** Early lesions show alignment of lymphocytes along the dermoepidermal junction with injury to basal epidermal cells as a result of the cytotoxic assault. This is an interface dermatitis (there is destruction of cells at the epidermal-dermal interface), but it lacks the chronic features seen in lichen planus, discussed below.

Morphology

Early lesions show a superficial perivascular, lymphocytic infiltrate associated with dermal edema and margination of lymphocytes along the dermoepidermal junction in intimate association with degenerating keratinocytes (Fig. 22–2B). With time, discrete, confluent zones of basal epidermal necrosis occur, with concomitant blister formation. In the more rare and severe form of this disease, toxic epidermal necrosis, the necrosis extends through the full thickness of the epidermis.

Clinical Features. Erythema multiforme manifests with a broad range of severity. The forms associated with infection, most often herpesvirus, are sometimes termed erythema multiforme minor because of their less severe clinical presentation. More severe forms of this disease are termed erythema multiforme major, Stevens-Johnson syndrome, and toxic epidermal necrolysis. These latter clinical forms of this disease continuum can be life-threatening because they can cause sloughing of large portions of the epidermis and loss of moisture and infectious barriers. They are most often seen as idiopathic reactions to drugs such as antibiotics or nonsteroidal anti-inflammatory agents.

CHRONIC INFLAMMATORY DERMATOSES

This category focuses on the persistent inflammatory dermatoses that exhibit their most characteristic features over many months to years, although they may begin with an acute stage. The skin surface in some chronic inflammatory dermatoses is roughened as a result of excessive or abnormal scale formation and shedding (desquamation).

Psoriasis

Psoriasis is a common chronic inflammatory dermatosis affecting 1% to 2% of people in the United States. In rare cases it is associated with arthritis, myopathy, enteropathy, and spondylitic heart disease.

Pathogenesis. Psoriasis is an immunologic disease with contributions from genetic susceptibility and environmental factors. It is not known if the inciting antigens are self or environmental. Sensitized populations of T cells enter the skin, including dermal CD4+ T_H1 cells and CD8+ T cells that accumulate in the epidermis. T cells homing to the skin secrete cytokines and growth factors that induce keratinocyte hyper-proliferation, resulting in the characteristic lesions. Psoriatic lesions can be induced in susceptible individuals by local trauma, a process known as the *Koebner phenomenon.* The trauma may induce a local inflammatory response that promotes lesion development. While reserved for use in severe psoriatic arthritis, recent therapeutics exploit advances in our understanding of T-cell biology. Various clinically useful agents block (1) T-cell activation and proliferation; (2) T cell trafficking and keratinocyte interaction with T cells; and (3) binding of tumor necrosis factor to its receptor thus inhibiting T cell functions.

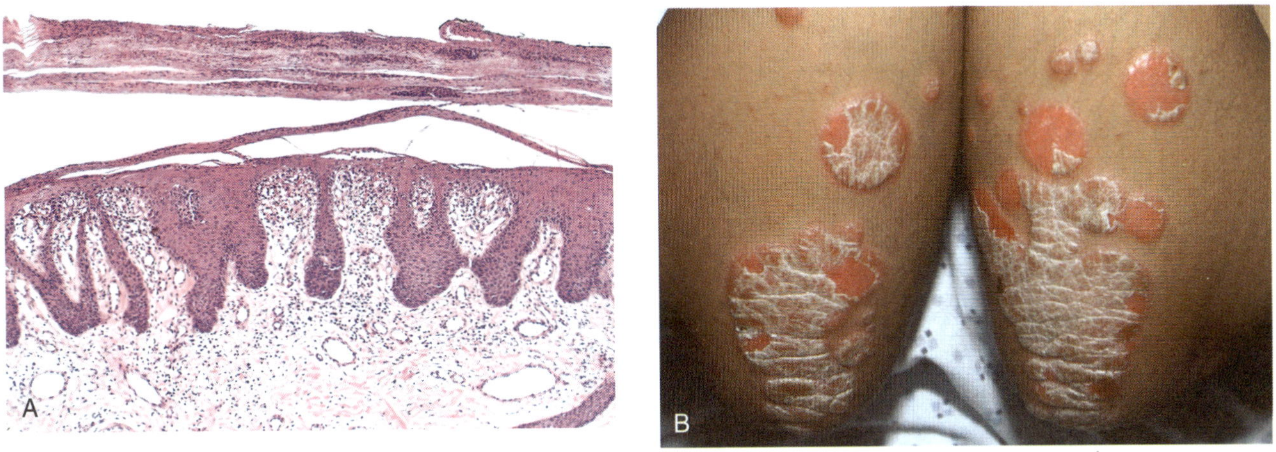

Figure 22–3

Psoriasis. **A,** Established plaques show marked epidermal hyperplasia with uniform downward extension of rete ridges (psoriasiform hyperplasia) as well as prominent parakeratotic scale focally infiltrated by neutrophils. Superficial fungal infections can show a strikingly similar epidermal pattern, and thus infection should be excluded using special stains. **B,** Chronic plaques of psoriasis show silvery-white scale on the surface of erythematous plaques.

Morphology

There is marked epidermal thickening (**acanthosis**), with regular downward elongation of the rete ridges (Fig. 22–3A). This downward growth has been likened to "test tubes in a rack." Increased epidermal cell turnover and lack of maturation results in **loss of the stratum granulosum with extensive overlying parakeratotic scale.** There is thinning of the epidermal cell layer overlying the tips of dermal papillae (suprapapillary plates) and blood vessels within the papillae are dilated and tortuous. These vessels bleed readily when the scale is removed, giving rise to multiple punctate bleeding points (**Auspitz sign**). Neutrophils form small aggregates within both the spongiotic superficial epidermis (**pustules of Kogoj**) and the parakeratotic stratum corneum (**Munro microabscesses**). Similar changes can be seen in superficial fungal infections, and it is important to exclude this possibility with special stains in new diagnoses of psoriasis.

Clinical Features. Psoriasis most frequently affects the skin of the elbows, knees, scalp, lumbosacral areas, intergluteal cleft, and glans penis. *The most typical lesion is a well-demarcated, pink to salmon-colored plaque covered by loosely adherent silver-white scale* (Fig. 22–3B). Nail changes occur in 30% of cases of psoriasis and consist of yellow-brown discoloration, with pitting, thickening, and crumbling and separation of the nail plate from the underlying bed (onycholysis). In most cases, psoriasis is limited in distribution, but it can be widespread and severe on occasion. There are a variety of clinical subtypes of this disease, defined by the severity and pattern of involvement.

Lichen Planus

"Pruritic, purple, polygonal, planar papules, and plaques" are the tongue-twisting traditional "*p*'s" of this disorder of skin and mucosa. Lichen planus is self-limited and usually resolves spontaneously 1 to 2 years after onset. Oral lesions may persist for years.

Pathogenesis. The pathogenesis is not known. Expression of altered antigens at the level of the basal cell layer and the dermoepidermal junction may elicit a CD8+ T cell-mediated cytotoxic immune response. The altered antigens could be due to viral infection or perhaps drug treatment.

Morphology

Lichen planus, the prototypic **interface dermatitis,** is characterized by a dense, continuous infiltrate of lymphocytes along the dermoepidermal junction (Fig. 22–4A). The lymphocytes are intimately associated with basal keratinocytes that show degeneration and necrosis. Thus the changes are at the interface of the squamous epithelium and papillary dermis. Perhaps as a response to damage, the basal cells show a resemblance in size and contour to more mature cells of the stratum spinosum (squamatization). This pattern of inflammation causes the dermoepidermal interface to assume an angulated, zigzag contour ("sawtoothing"). Anucleate, necrotic basal cells are seen in the inflamed papillary dermis and are referred to as colloid bodies or **Civatte bodies.** Although these changes bear some similarities to those in erythema multiforme (discussed earlier), lichen planus shows well-developed changes of chronicity: epidermal hyperplasia, hypergranulosis, and hyperkeratosis.

Clinical Features. Cutaneous lesions consist of *pruritic, violaceous, flat-topped papules, which may coalesce focally to form plaques* (Fig. 22–4B). These papules are often highlighted by white dots or lines, called *Wickham's striae.* Hyperpigmentation may result from melanin loss into the dermis from the damaged basal cell layer. Multiple lesions are symmetrically distributed, particularly on the extremities, often about the wrists and elbows, and

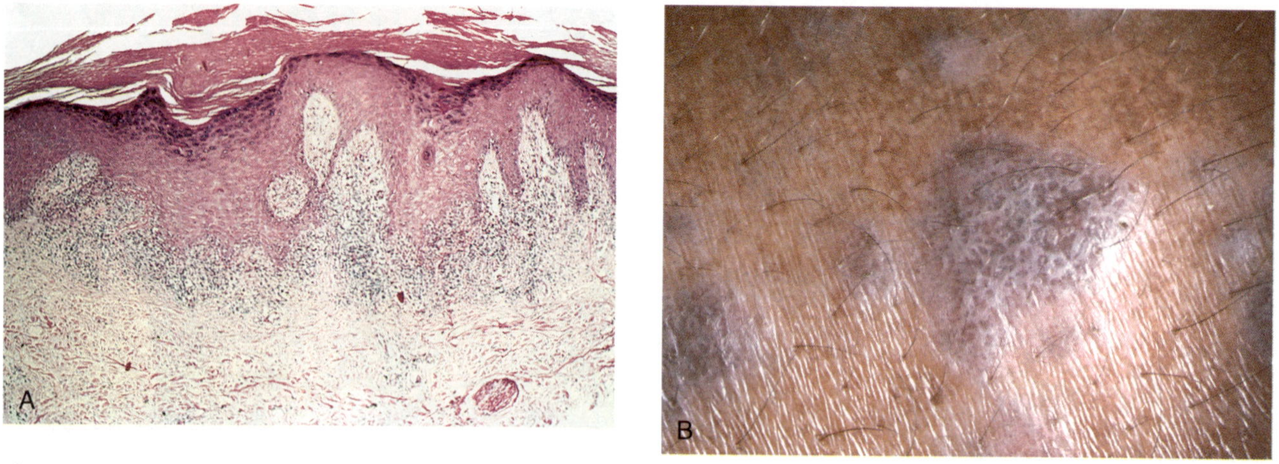

Figure 22–4

Lichen planus. **A,** There is a band of lymphocytes along the dermoepidermal junction, and the rete ridges have acquired a pointed, or "saw-tooth," architecture. This is also an interface dermatitis, but the infiltrate is more bandlike (lichenoid) than is seen in erythema multiforme, and hyperkeratosis and hypergranulosis are definite signs of chronicity. **B,** Multiple flat-topped papules with white, lacey or netlike markings (Wickham striae) are characteristic.

on the glans penis. In 70% of cases, oral lesions are present as white, reticulated, or netlike areas involving the mucosa.

Lichen Simplex Chronicus

Lichen simplex chronicus presents as roughening of the skin that takes on an appearance reminiscent of lichen on a tree. It is a response to local repetitive trauma such as continual rubbing or scratching. When this condition is localized to nodules, it is termed *prurigo nodularis.*

Pathogenesis. The pathogenesis of lichen simplex chronicus is not understood, but it is probable that repetitive trauma induces epithelial hyperplasia with eventual dermal scarring.

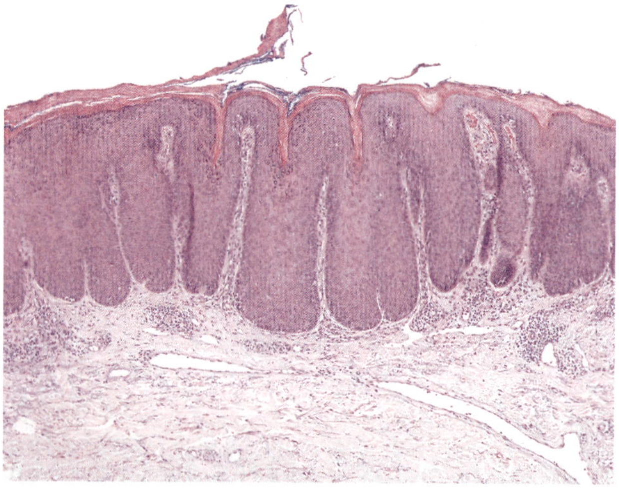

Figure 22–5

Lichen simplex chronicus. Acanthosis with hyperkeratosis and hypergranulosis are distinctive. Superficial dermal fibrosis with vascular ectasia is also common. There is no overt cytologic atypia thus distinguishing this from squamous cell carcinoma.

Morphology

Lichen simplex chronicus is characterized by **acanthosis** with **hyperkeratosis** and **hypergranulosis.** There is elongation of the rete ridges and fibrosis of the papillary dermis with a chronic inflammatory infiltrate (Fig. 22–5). Interestingly, these lesions are similar to normal volar (palms and soles) skin, another area conditioned by constant "trauma," but at these sites the changes appear to represent an adaptive response to such stimuli.

Clinical Features. The lesions are often raised and erythematous, with increased scale and can be mistaken for keratinocytic neoplasms. Often lichen simplex chronicus is superimposed upon, and masks another (often pruritic) dermatosis. It is therefore important to rule out an underlying cause, but keep in mind that the lesion can be entirely self-inflicted.

SUMMARY

Inflammatory Dermatoses

- There are many specific inflammatory dermatoses; they may be mediated by IgE antibodies (urticaria), antigen-specific T cells (eczema, erythema multiforme, and psoriasis), and trauma (lichen simplex chronicus).
- The histologic features can be grouped into patterns of inflammation such as interface dermatitis (e.g. lichen planus and erythema multiforme), superficial perivascular dermatitis, and panniculitis (inflammation in subcutaneous fat) that provide insight into the mechanism and the ability to organize the diseases into pathogenic categories.
- Careful clinical correlation is needed to diagnose specific skin diseases, since the features overlap within histologic pattern groups.

INFECTIOUS DERMATOSES

Bacterial Infection

Numerous bacterial infections occur in skin. These range from superficial infections caused by *Staphylococcus* and *Streptococcus* spp., known as *impetigo,* to deeper dermal abscesses caused by anaerobes like *Pseudomonas aeruginosa,* associated with puncture wounds. The pathogensis is similar to that of similar microbial infections elsewhere (Chapter 19).

Morphology

Skin biopsy typically shows spongiotic epidermis with a neutrophilic infiltrate. Bacterial cocci can be demonstrated using Gram stain in the superficial epidermis. Microbiologic culture with assessment of sensitivities to various antibiotics can be useful.

Clinical Features. One of the most common skin bacterial infections is *impetigo;* it is primarily seen in children but can sometimes affect adults. The disease involves direct contact, usually with *Staphylococcus aureus,* or less commonly *Streptococcus pyogenes.* The disease often begins as a single small macule that rapidly evolves into a larger lesion with a "honey-colored crust" (dried serum or scab). The areas most often involved are the extremities, nose, and mouth (Fig. 22–6). Individuals colonized by *S. aureus* or *S. pyogenes* (usually nasal or anal) are more likely to suffer from this disease. A less common bullous form of impetigo that can mimic an autoimmune blistering disorder may occur in children.

Fungal Infection

Fungal infections are varied and range from superficial infections with *Candida* species to life-threatening infections of immunosuppressed individuals with *Aspergillus* species. In general, a fungal infection can be very superficial (stratum corneum, hair, and nails), deep, involving the dermis or subcutis, or systemic involving skin by hematogenous spread (often in an immunocompromised host).

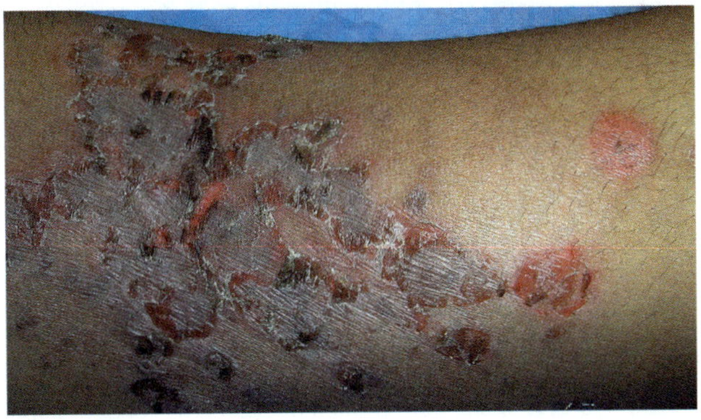

Figure 22–6

Microbial infections. This child's arm is involved by impetigo resulting from a superficial bacterial infection. (Courtesy of Dr. Angela Wyatt, New York, New York.)

Pathogenesis. Superficial infections are often associated with a neutrophilic infiltrate in the epidermis. While dermal infections by bacteria induce neutrophil-rich abscesses, dermal fungal infections often elicit a granulomatous response, perhaps indicating that different signals from the immune system are driving the responses. The deeper infections are usually more destructive; in particular, *Aspergillus* can be angioinvasive.

Morphology

Superficial *Candida* infections often induce a clinical response that can mimic psoriasis. While psoriasis is not caused by fungal infection, such infections can mimic psoriasis so closely that it is essential to perform a fungal stain to exclude infection in a new diagnosis of psoriasis. This indicates that psoriasiform hyperplasia is a generalized response of skin to stimulation by the immune system. Deeper fungal infections produce greater tissue damage, probably induced by both the microbes themselves and the vigorous host immune response to their presence.

Clinical Features. Superficial infections such as those seen with *Candida* usually show erythematous macules with superficial scale that can be pruritic, while deeper infections such as those seen with *Aspergillus* species in immunocompromised hosts are erythematous, often nodular, and sometimes show evidence of local hemorrhage.

Verrucae (Warts)

Verrucae are common lesions of children and adolescents, although they may be encountered at any age. They are caused by human papillomavirus (HPV). Transmission usually involves direct contact between individuals or autoinoculation. Verrucae are generally self-limited, most often regressing spontaneously within 6 months to 2 years.

Pathogenesis. As mentioned earlier, verrucae are caused by HPV. Some members of the HPV family are associated with preneoplastic and invasive cancers of the anogenital region (Chapters 18 and 19). However, in contrast to HPV-associated carcinomas, most warts are caused by distinct low-risk HPV types that lack potential for causing malignant transformation. Mechanistically, the virus subverts cell cycle control to allow increased proliferation of epithelial cells and production of new virus. Normal immune response usually limits the growth of these tumors, but immunodeficiency can be associated with increased numbers and size of verrucae.

Morphology

Histologic features common to verrucae include **epidermal hyperplasia** that is often undulant in character (so-called verrucous or papillomatous epidermal hyperplasia; Fig. 22–7A, *top*) and cytoplasmic vacuolization (**koilocytosis**) that preferentially involves the more superficial epidermal layers, producing halos of pallor surrounding infected nuclei. Infected cells may also demonstrate prominent keratohyaline granules and jagged eosinophilic intracytoplasmic protein aggregates as a result of impaired maturation (Fig. 22–7A, bottom).

Clinical Features. Warts can be classified into several types on the basis of their morphology and location. In addition, each type of wart is generally caused by a distinct HPV type. *Verruca vulgaris* is the most common type of wart. These lesions occur anywhere but are found most frequently on the hands, particularly on the dorsal surfaces and periungual areas, where they appear as gray-white to tan, flat to convex, 0.1- to 1-cm papules with a rough, pebble-like surface (Fig. 22–7B). *Verruca plana,* or *flat wart,* is common on the face or dorsal surfaces of the hands. These warts are flat, smooth, tan macules. *Verruca plantaris* and *verruca palmaris* occur on the soles and palms, respectively. These rough, scaly lesions may reach 1 to 2 cm in diameter, coalesce, and be confused with ordinary calluses. *Condyloma acuminatum (venereal wart)* occurs on the penis, female genitalia, urethra, and perianal areas (Chapters 18 and 19).

BLISTERING (BULLOUS) DISORDERS

Although vesicles and bullae (blisters) occur as a secondary phenomenon in several unrelated conditions (e.g., herpesvirus infection, spongiotic dermatitis), there is a group of disorders in which blisters are the primary and most distinctive features. Blisters can occur at multiple levels within the skin, and assessment of their location within the skin is essential for an accurate histologic diagnosis (Fig. 22–8).

Pemphigus (Vulgaris and Foliaceus)

Pemphigus is a rare autoimmune blistering disorder resulting from loss of integrity of normal intercellular attachments within the epidermis and mucosal epithelium. Most individuals who develop pemphigus are middle-aged and older. There are three major variants: (1) pemphigus vulgaris, (2) pemphigus foliaceus, and (3) paraneoplastic pemphigus. The latter is associated

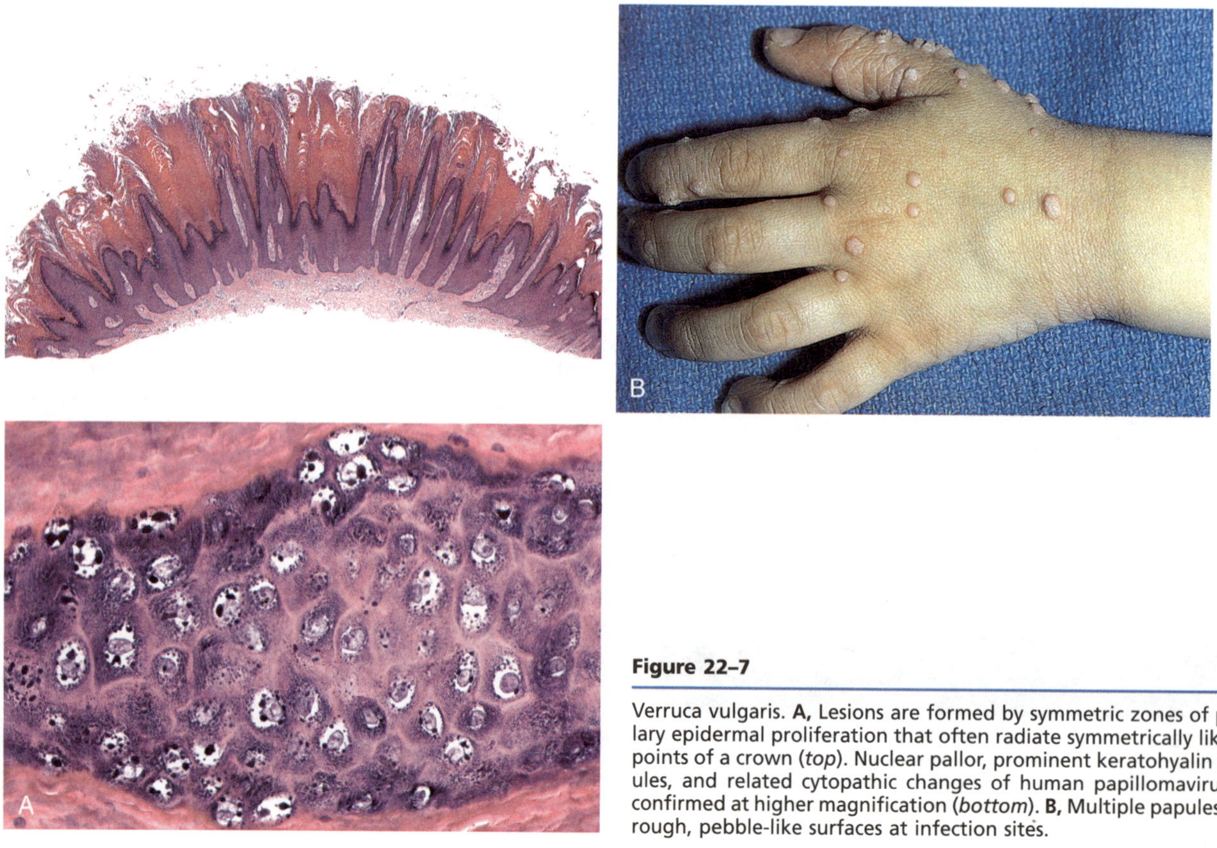

Figure 22–7

Verruca vulgaris. **A,** Lesions are formed by symmetric zones of papillary epidermal proliferation that often radiate symmetrically like the points of a crown (*top*). Nuclear pallor, prominent keratohyalin granules, and related cytopathic changes of human papillomavirus are confirmed at higher magnification (*bottom*). **B,** Multiple papules with rough, pebble-like surfaces at infection sites.

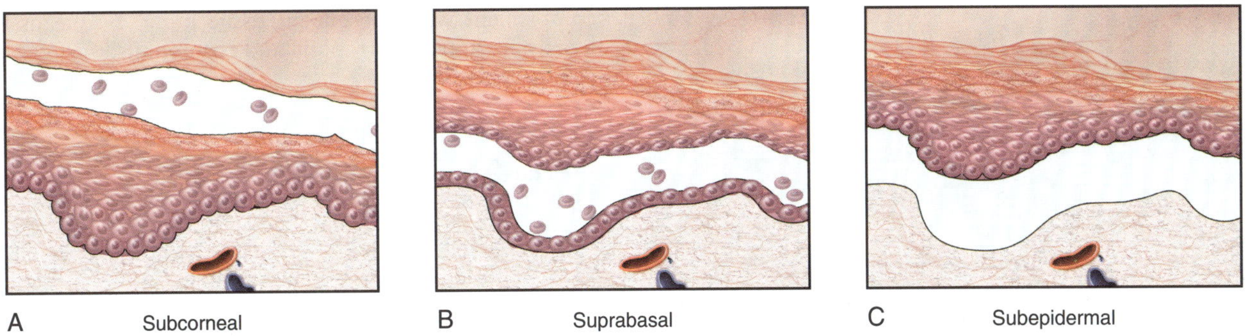

Figure 22–8

Levels of blister formation. **A,** Subcorneal (as in pemphigus foliaceus). **B,** Suprabasal (as in pemphigus vulgaris). **C,** Subepidermal (as in bullous pemphigoid or dermatitis herpetiformis). Assessment of the levels of epidermal separation forms the basis of the initial differential diagnosis of these lesions.

with internal malignancy and will not be discussed here.

Pathogenesis. Both pemphigus vulgaris and pemphigus foliaceus are caused by a type II hypersensitivity reaction (antibody directed against a fixed tissue antigen; Chapter 5) and show linkage to specific HLA types. Patient sera contain pathogenic IgG antibodies to intercellular desmosomal proteins (desmoglein types 1 and 3) of skin and mucous membranes. The distribution of these proteins within the epidermis determines the location of the lesions. By direct immunofluorescence, lesional sites show a characteristic netlike pattern of intercellular IgG deposits (Fig. 22–9). The antibodies seem to function primarily by disrupting the intercellular adhesive function of the desmosomes and may activate intercellular proteases as well.

Morphology

The common histologic denominator in all forms of pemphigus is **acantholysis** (lysis of the intercellular adhesion sites) within a squamous epithelial surface. Detached from their moorings, acantholytic cells become rounded. In pemphigus vulgaris, acantholysis selectively involves the layer of cells immediately above the basal cell layer, giving rise to a **suprabasal acantholytic blister** (Fig. 22–10B). In pemphigus foliaceus, acantholysis selectively involves the superficial epidermis at the level of the stratum granulosum (Fig. 22–11B). Variable superficial dermal infiltration by lymphocytes, histiocytes, and eosinophils accompanies all forms of pemphigus.

Clinical Features. *Pemphigus vulgaris,* by far the most common type, involves mucosa and skin, especially on the scalp, face, axillae, groin, trunk, and points of pressure. The primary lesions are superficial vesicles and bullae that rupture easily, leaving erosions covered with serum crust (Fig. 22–10A). *Pemphigus foliaceus,* a more rare and benign form of pemphigus, results in bullae confined to skin, with infrequent involvement of mucous membranes. The blisters are so superficial that only zones of erythema and crusting sites of previous blister rupture are detected (Fig. 22–11A). An epidemic form occurs in

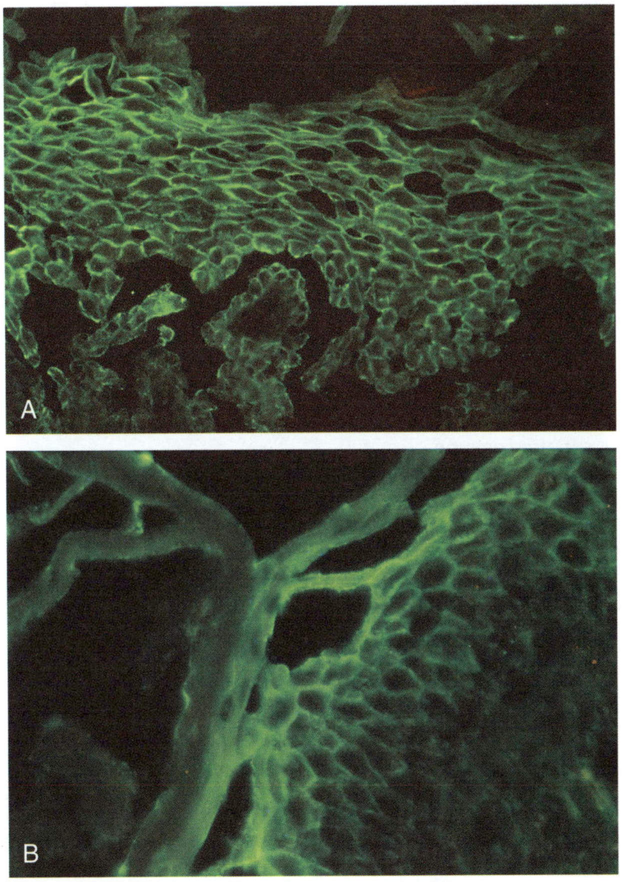

Figure 22–9

A, Pemphigus vulgaris. There is uniform deposition of immunoglobulin and complement (*green*) along the cell membranes of keratinocytes, producing a characteristic "fishnet" appearance. **B,** The immunoglobulin deposits are more superficial in pemphigus foliaceus.

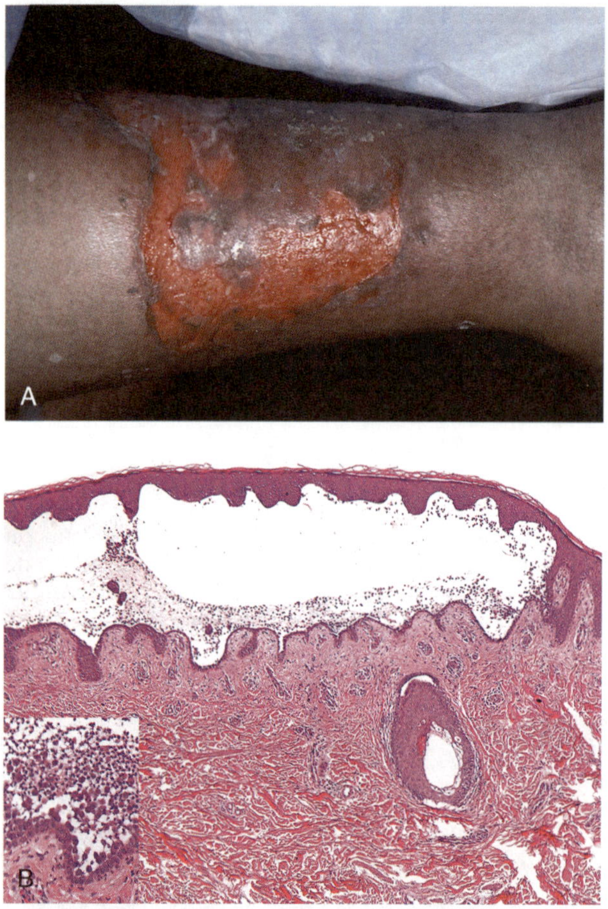

Figure 22–10

Pemphigus vulgaris. **A,** This eroded area on the leg represents confluent blisters with loss of their roofs. **B,** Suprabasal acantholysis results in an intraepidermal blister containing rounded keratinocytes that are separating from their neighbors. Initially, a single row of basal cells is present on the floor of the blister (suprabasal split), but these cells can divide and repopulate this area with keratinocytes, as seen in this case (inset). This is an early part of the healing response. Follicular involvement by acantholysis is also common.

South America (*fogo selvagem*), putatively associated with a specific infectious agent.

Bullous Pemphigoid

Generally affecting elderly individuals, bullous pemphigoid shows a wide range of clinical presentations, typically with generalized cutaneous lesions and involvement of mucosal surfaces.

Pathogenesis. Bullous pemphigoid is an autoimmune disease in which the characteristic finding is linear deposition of IgG antibodies and complement in the basement membrane zone (Fig. 22–12A). Reactivity also occurs in the basal cell–basement membrane attachment plaques (hemidesmosomes), where most of the bullous pemphigoid antigen (BPAG) is located. This protein is involved normally in dermoepidermal bonding. IgG autoantibodies to hemidesmosome components fixes complement with subsequent tissue injury by means of locally recruited neutrophils and eosinophils.

Morphology

Bullous pemphigoid is characterized by a **subepidermal, nonacantholytic** blister. Early lesions show a perivascular infiltrate of lymphocytes and variable numbers of eosinophils, occasional neutrophils, superficial dermal edema, and associated basal cell layer vacuolization. The vacuolated basal cell layer eventually gives rise to a fluid-filled blister (Fig. 22–12B). Because the blister roof involves full-thickness epidermis, it is more resistant to rupture than blisters in pemphigus.

Clinical Features. Clinically, *lesions are tense bullae, filled with clear fluid, on normal or erythematous skin* (Fig. 22–12C). The bullae do not rupture as readily as in pemphigus and, if uncomplicated by infection, heal without

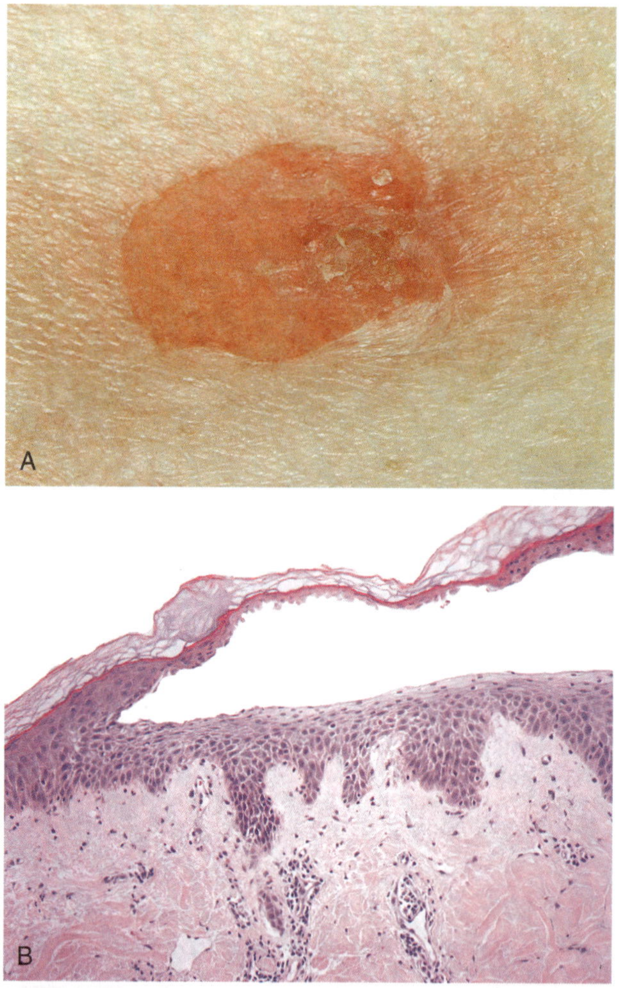

Figure 22–11

Pemphigus foliaceus. **A,** Blisters are much less erosive than those seen in pemphigus vulgaris, since the level of the blisters is more superficial (subcorneal). **B,** Subcorneal separation of the epithelium is seen.

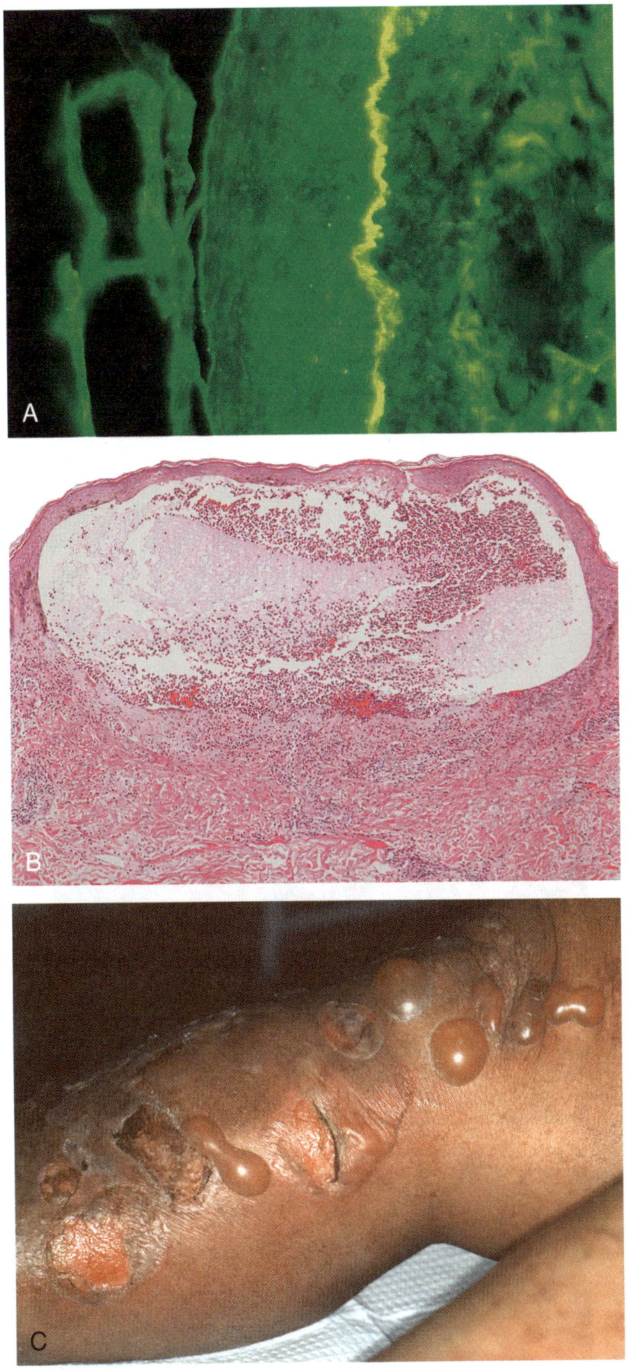

Figure 22–12

Bullous pemphigoid. **A,** In bullous pemphigoid, both IgG antibody and complement can be detected by direct immunofluorescence as a linear band outlining the subepidermal basement membrane zone (epidermis is on the left side of the fluorescent band). **B,** The subepidermal vesicle has an inflammatory infiltrate rich in eosinophils. **C,** Tense, fluid-filled blisters result from vacuolization of the basal layer, producing subepidermal blisters. (**B,** Courtesy of Dr. Victor G. Prieto, Houston, Texas.)

scarring. Sites of occurrence include the inner aspects of the thighs, flexor surfaces of the forearms, axillae, groin, and lower abdomen. Oral involvement is present in as many as one-third of patients. Gestational pemphigoid (also known as *herpes gestationis,* a misnomer, since there is no viral etiology) occurs late in the second or third trimester of pregnancy and resolves after childbirth.

Dermatitis Herpetiformis

Dermatitis herpetiformis is a rare disorder characterized by *urticaria and grouped vesicles.* The disease affects predominantly males, often in the third and fourth decades. In some cases it occurs in association with intestinal celiac disease and responds to a gluten-free diet (Chapter 15).

Pathogenesis. The association of dermatitis herpetiformis with celiac disease provides a clue to its pathogenesis. Genetically predisposed individuals develop IgA antibodies to dietary gluten (derived from the wheat protein gliadin). The antibodies cross-react with reticulin, a component of the anchoring fibrils that tether the epidermal basement membrane to the superficial dermis. The resultant injury and inflammation produce a subepidermal blister. Some people with dermatitis herpetiformis and gluten-sensitive enteropathy respond to a gluten-free diet.

Morphology

As an early event, fibrin and neutrophils accumulate selectively at the **tips of dermal papillae,** forming small microabscesses (Fig. 22–13A). The basal cells overlying these microabscesses show vacuolization and focal dermoepidermal separation that ultimately coalesce to form a true **subepidermal blister.** By direct immunofluorescence, dermatitis herpetiformis shows discontinuous, **granular deposits of IgA** selectively localized in the tips of dermal papillae (Fig. 22–13B).

Clinical Features. The urticarial plaques and vesicles of dermatitis herpetiformis are extremely *pruritic.* The lesions are bilateral, symmetric, and grouped involving preferentially the extensor surfaces, elbows, knees, upper back, and buttocks (Fig. 22–13C).

SUMMARY

Blistering Disorders

- Blistering disorders are traditionally classified according to the epidermal layer where the separation occurs.
- This group of diseases is often caused by autoreactive antibodies to constituents of the epithelium or basement membrane.
- Pemphigus is associated with formation of IgG auto-antibodies to intercellular desmogleins with resulting acantholysis in the epidermis. This gives rise to bullae that are subcorneal (superficial) in pemphigus foliaceus and suprabasal (deeper) in pemphigus vulgaris.

- Bullous pemphigoid shows deposition of IgG auto-antibodies to basement membrane proteins and produces a subepidermal blister.
- Dermatitis herpetiformis is associated with deposition of IgA auto-antibodies to fibrils that bind epidermal basement membrane to dermis, thus producing subepidermal blisters. This disease may be associated with celiac disease.

TUMORS

Benign and Premalignant Epithelial Lesions

Benign epithelial neoplasms are common and usually biologically inconsequential. These tumors are probably derived from stem cells that reside in the epidermis and hair follicles, that tend to differentiate toward cells and structures in the epidermis and adenexa. The overwhelming majority of these tumors show limited growth and do not undergo malignant transformation.

Seborrheic Keratosis

These common epidermal tumors occur most frequently in middle-aged or older individuals. They arise spontaneously and may become particularly numerous on the trunk, although the extremities, head, and neck may also be involved.

Pathogenesis. Recent work has demonstrated that a significant fraction of these tumors harbor activating mutations in *fibroblast growth factor (FGF) receptor 3*. The explosive onset of hundreds of lesions may occur as a *paraneoplastic syndrome* (sign of Lesser-Trelat) in rare cases. Patients with this presentation may harbor internal malignancies that produce growth factors that stimulate epidermal proliferation.

Morphology

These neoplasms are exophytic and composed of sheets of small cells that most resemble monotonous basal cells of the normal epidermis (Fig. 22–14A). Variable melanin pigmentation is present within these basaloid cells, accounting for the brown coloration seen clinically. Hyperkeratosis occurs at the surface and the presence of small keratin-filled cysts (horn cysts) and down-growths of keratin into the main tumor mass (pseudo-horn cysts) are characteristic features.

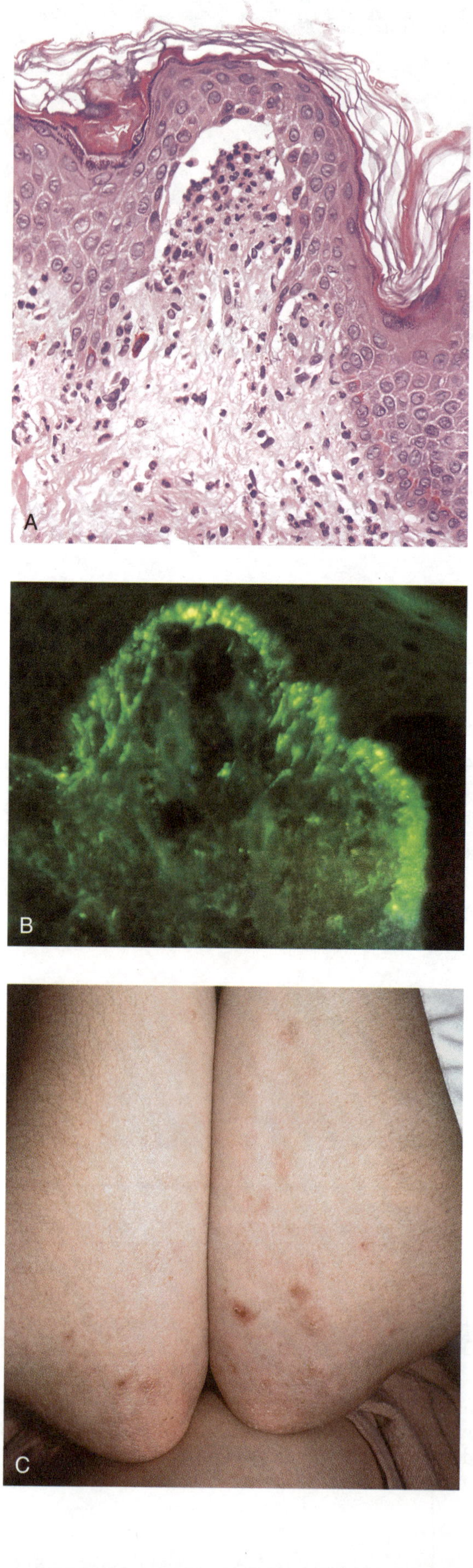

Figure 22–13

Dermatitis herpetiformis. **A,** The blisters are associated with basal cell layer injury initially caused by accumulation of neutrophils (microabscesses) at the tips of dermal papillae. **B,** Selective deposition of IgA autoantibody at the tips of dermal papillae is characteristic. **C,** Lesions consist of intact and eroded (usually scratched) erythematous blisters, often grouped (seen here on elbows and arms). (**B,** Courtesy of Dr. Victor G. Prieto, Houston, Texas.)

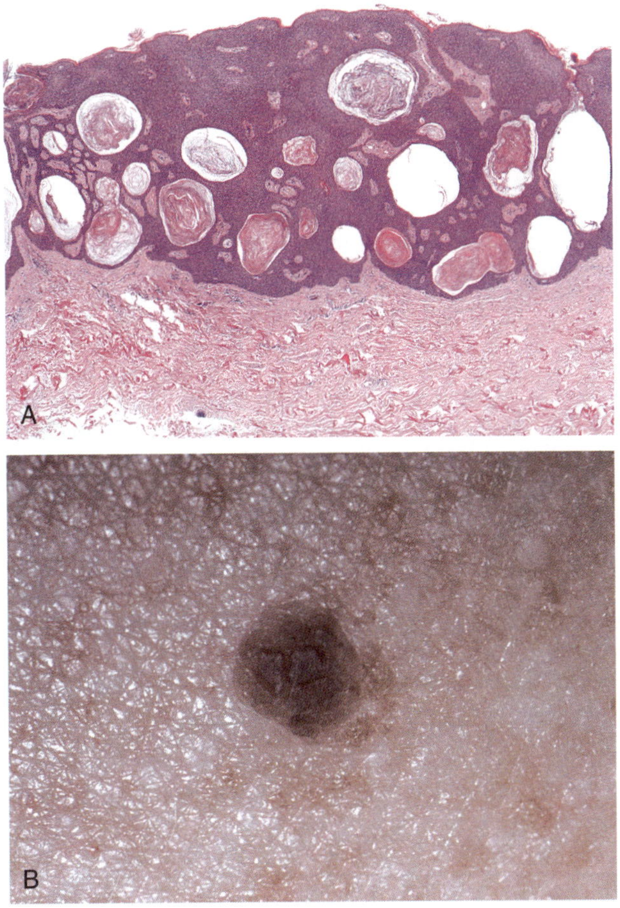

Figure 22–14

Seborrheic keratosis. **A,** The lesions consist of an orderly proliferation of uniform, benign basaloid keratinocytes with a tendency to form keratin microcysts (horn cysts). **B,** This roughened, brown, waxy lesion almost appears to be "stuck on" the skin.

Clinical Features. Clinically, seborrheic keratoses appear as *round, flat, coin-like plaques that vary in diameter from millimeters to centimeters* (Fig. 22–14B). They are tan to dark brown and usually show a velvety to granular surface. Occasionally, they become inflamed or mimic melanoma because of their pigmentation, warranting their removal.

Sebaceous Adenoma

Sebaceous adenomas are rare tumors that primarily occur in the head and neck region of older individuals. They usually present as flesh-colored papules and can be a marker for an internal malignancy. Knowledge of this association can save a life.

Pathogenesis. Much has been learned about the pathogenesis of these tumors by their association with the Muir-Torre syndrome. In this condition, the tumors may be multiple or be distributed outside of the head and neck region. In addition there may be internal malignancy, most often colon carcinoma. These cases are a subset of the hereditary nonpolyposis colorectal carcinoma syndrome (Chapters 6 and 15). This syndrome is associated with microsatellite instability due to loss of a DNA mismatch repair protein, either MLH1 or MSH2 (Fig. 22–15A).

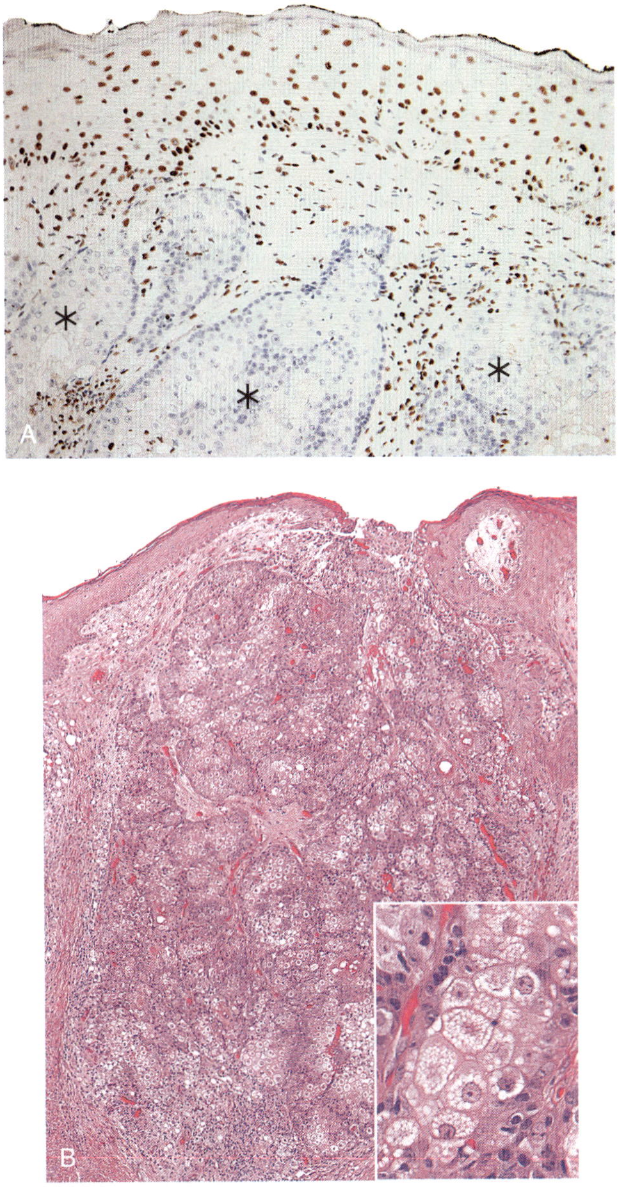

Figure 22–15

Sebaceous adenoma. **A,** Immunohistochemistry reveals loss of nuclear expression of the DNA mismatch repair protein MSH2 (*asterisks*), but retention in normal epidermis and lymphocytes, indicating probable association with the Muir-Torre syndrome. **B,** This lesion shows a lobular proliferation of sebocytes with increased peripheral basaloid cells and more mature sebocytes in the central portion. Vacuolated cytoplasm is characteristic of mature sebocytes (inset, lower right corner).

Morphology

Sebaceous adenomas show a lobular proliferation of sebocytes that maintain an organoid appearance (Fig. 22–15B). The basal cell layer is normally two cells thick, but this is variably expanded in adenomas with maturation to mature sebocytes in the center of the lesion. These cells have clear cytoplasm vacuolated by vesicles filled with sebum. The tumors lack the severe cytologic atypia and infiltrative border characteristic of carcinoma.

Clinical Features. Sebaceous adenomas are benign, and their growth is usually self-limited. They tend to occur in areas such as the face, where numerous prominent sebaceous glands are normally present. Clinically these can be separated from the much more common sebaceous hyperplasia, which has an umbilicated (dimpled) center and consists of hypertrophic sebaceous glands surrounding a central hair follicle.

Actinic Keratosis

Before the development of overt malignancy of the epidermis, a series of progressively dysplastic changes occurs. Because such skin dysplasia is usually the result of chronic exposure to sunlight and is associated with hyperkeratosis, these lesions are called actinic (sun-related) keratoses.

Pathogenesis. Whether all actinic keratoses would result in carcinoma with time is conjectural. Many lesions regress or remain stable. However, enough do become malignant to warrant local eradication. Mutation of *p53* is often an early event with molecular changes suggestive of ultraviolet light injury.

Morphology

Lower portions of the epidermis show **cytologic atypia,** often with hyperplasia of basal cells (Fig. 22–16A) or with early atrophy that results in diffuse thinning of the epidermal surface of the lesion. The dermis contains thickened, blue-gray elastic fibers (solar elastosis), the result of chronic sun damage. The stratum corneum is thickened with retained nuclei (parakeratosis). Some but not all lesions progress to full-thickness atypia amounting to squamous cell carcinoma in situ (Fig. 22–16C). A useful acronym for remembering the histologic features is SPAIN—a sun-soaked country perfect for acquiring such lesions—solar elastosis (dermal sun damage), parakeratosis, atypia (keratinocytic), inflammation (lymphocytes in the superficial dermis), and not full thickness (atypia). (Acronym courtesy of Dr. Zeina Tannous, Massachusetts General Hospital, Boston, Massachusetts.)

Clinical Features. Lesions of actinic keratosis, very common in fair-skinned individuals, are usually *less than 1 cm in diameter; tan-brown, red, or skin colored; and have a rough, sandpaper-like consistency* (Fig. 22–16B). As would be expected, there is a predilection for sun-exposed areas (face, arms, dorsum of the hands), and the lesions accumulate with age and degree of sun exposure. The lesions can be treated with local cryotherapy (superficial freezing) or topical chemotherapeutic and other agents.

SUMMARY

Benign and Premalignant Tumors

- *Seborrheic Keratosis:* Round, flat plaques made up of proliferating monotonous basal cells of epi-

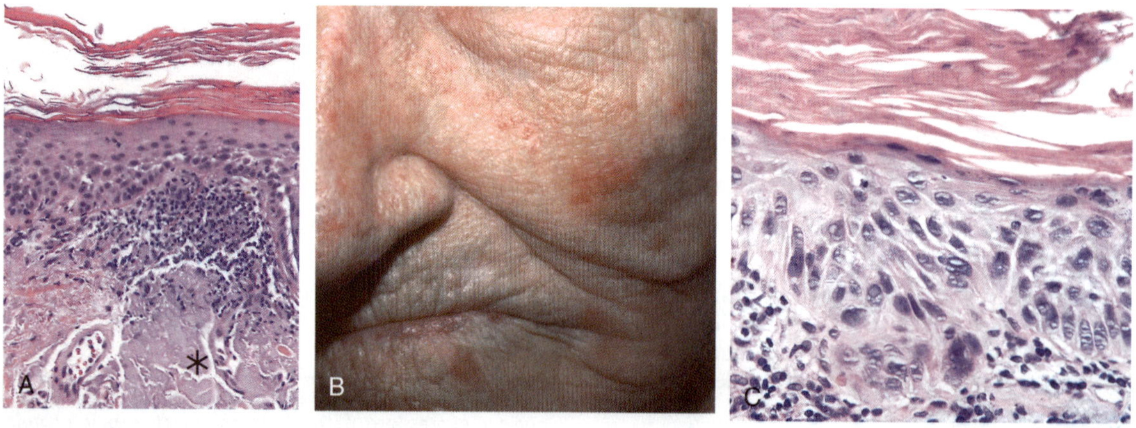

Figure 22–16

Actinic keratosis. **A,** Basal cell layer atypia (dysplasia) is associated with marked hyperkeratosis, parakeratosis, and dermal solar elastosis (*asterisk*). **B,** Most lesions form subtle zones of redness or sandpaper-like keratinization as seen in the lesions on the cheek, nose, and chin of this woman. **C,** More advanced lesions show full-thickness atypia, qualifying as carcinoma in situ.

dermis containing melanin. Hyperkeratosis with keratin-filled cysts characteristic.

- *Sebaceous Adenoma:* Multiple flesh colored nodules in head and neck region arising from sebaceous glands. May be a marker of internal malignancy with loss of DNA mismatch repair genes.
- *Actinic Keratosis:* Present on sun-exposed skin, they show cytologic atypia in lower parts of epidemis, that can infrequently progress to carcinoma *in situ.*

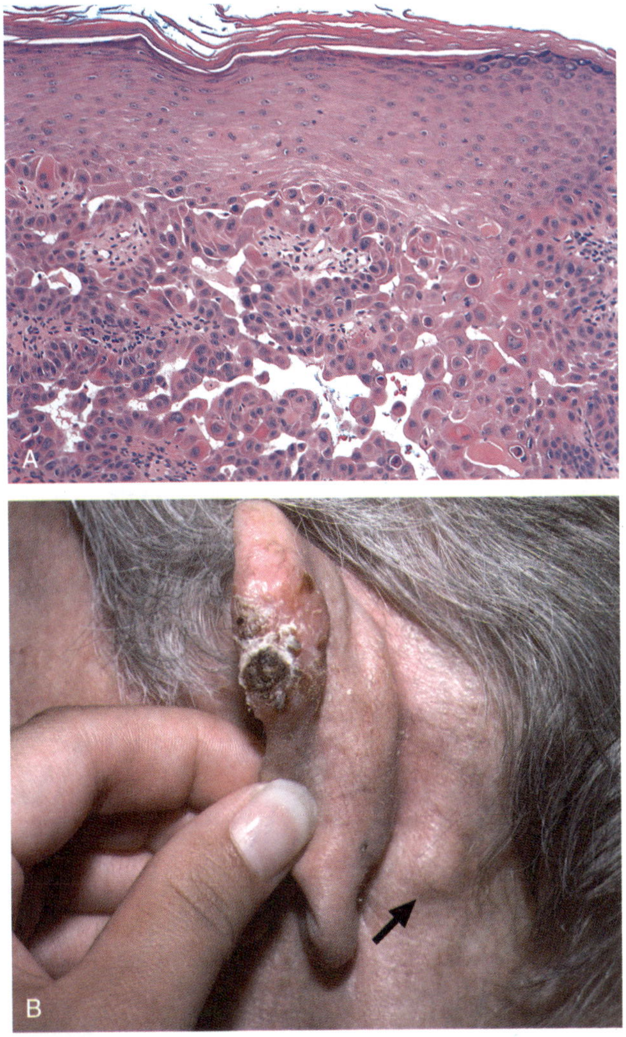

Figure 22–17

Invasive squamous cell carcinoma. **A,** The carcinoma invades the dermis as irregular projections of atypical squamous epithelium; this particular case is acantholytic (i.e., the squamous cells are poorly cohesive). **B,** A nodular and hyperkeratotic lesion occurring on the ear, unfortunately with early metastasis to a prominent postauricular lymph node (*arrow*).

Malignant Epidermal Tumors

Squamous Cell Carcinoma

Squamous cell carcinoma is *a common tumor arising on sun-exposed sites in older people.* Except for lesions on the lower legs, these tumors have a higher incidence in men than in women. In addition to sunlight, predisposing factors include industrial carcinogens (tars and oils), chronic ulcers, old burn scars, ingestion of arsenicals, and ionizing radiation.

Pathogenesis. The most common exogenous cause of cutaneous squamous cell carcinoma is UV light exposure, with subsequent unrepaired DNA damage (Chapter 6). Individuals who are immunosuppressed as a result of chemotherapy or organ transplantation, or who have *xeroderma pigmentosum,* are at increased risk. In addition to inducing mutations, UV light (UVB in particular) may have a transient immunosuppressive effect on skin by impairing antigen presentation by Langerhans cells. This may contribute to tumorigenesis by weakening immunosurveillance. Immunosuppressed patients, particularly organ transplant recipients, are likely to be associated with high-risk HPV types. *p53* mutations with associated UV mutation signatures are common, as are activating mutations in *RAS.* As with squamous cell carcinomas at other sites, those in the skin may be preceded by *in situ* lesions.

Morphology

Squamous cell carcinoma in situ is characterized by highly atypical cells at **all levels** of the epidermis, with nuclear crowding and disorganization. The squamous dyplasia is broad and occupies the full thickness of the epithelium. When these cells break through the basement membrane, the process has become invasive (Fig. 22–17A). Invasive squamous cell carcinomas exhibit variable differentiation, ranging from tumors formed by atypical squamous cells arranged in orderly lobules showing large zones of keratinization to neoplasms formed by highly anaplastic, rounded cells with foci of necrosis and only abortive, single-cell keratinization (dyskeratosis). While morphologic variation is wide, all squamous cell carcinomas share the feature of keratinization.

Clinical Features. Squamous cell carcinomas *in situ* appear as sharply defined, red, scaling plaques; many arise from prior actinic keratoses. More advanced, invasive lesions are nodular, show variable scale, and may ulcerate (Fig. 22–17B). The likelihood of metastasis is related to the thickness of the lesion and degree of invasion into the subcutis. Tumors arising in the context of actinic keratoses may behave in a less aggressive fashion, while those arising in burn scars, ulcers, and skin not exposed to the sun tend to behave less predictably.

Invasive squamous cell carcinomas of the skin are often discovered while small and resectable; less than 5% have metastases to regional nodes at diagnosis. Mucosal squamous cell carcinomas (oral, pulmonary, esophageal, etc.) are generally a much more aggressive.

Basal Cell Carcinoma

Basal cell carcinoma, the most common human cancer, is a *slow-growing tumor that rarely metastasizes.* It tends to occur at sites subject to chronic sun exposure and in lightly pigmented people. As with squamous cell carcinoma, the incidence of basal cell carcinoma increases with immunosuppression (though not as dramatically as that of squamous cell carcinoma) and in individuals with inherited defects in DNA repair.

Pathogenesis. Basal cell carcinoma has been associated with dysregulation of the sonic hedgehog, or *PTCH,* pathway. Inherited defects in the *PTCH* gene with subsequent loss of heterozygosity in the numerous individual tumor foci cause the familial basal cell carcinoma syndrome, Gorlin syndrome. Thus, *PTCH* functions as a classic tumor suppressor. Since the *PTCH* pathway is also important in embryonic development, subtle developmental anomalies are also noted in these individuals. Some component of the *PTCH* pathway is also mutated in the great majority of sporadic basal cell carcinomas; mutations in *p53* are also common.

Morphology

Tumor cells resemble the normal epidermal basal cell layer from which they are derived. Because they arise from the epidermis or sometimes follicular epithelium, they are not encountered on mucosal surfaces. Two common patterns are seen: either **multifocal growths** originating from the epidermis (superficial type), or **nodular lesions** growing downward into the dermis as cords and islands of variably basophilic cells with hyperchromatic nuclei, embedded in a fibrotic to mucinous matrix (Fig. 22–18A). Peripheral tumor cell nuclei align in the outermost layer (palisading) with separation from the stroma, creating a cleft or separation artifact (Fig. 22–18B).

Clinical Features. Clinically, these tumors present as *pearly papules, often containing prominent, dilated subepidermal blood vessels (telangiectasia)* (Fig. 22–18C). Some tumors contain melanin pigment and thus appear similar to melanocytic nevi or melanomas. Advanced lesions may ulcerate, and extensive local invasion of bone or facial sinuses may occur after many years of neglect. These tumors are usually treated with complete local excision, although immunomodulatory therapies that direct the innate immune response against the tumor are currently being tested as well.

SUMMARY

Malignant Epidermal Tumors

- The incidence of both basal cell and squamous cell carcinoma is strongly correlated with increasing lifetime sun exposure.

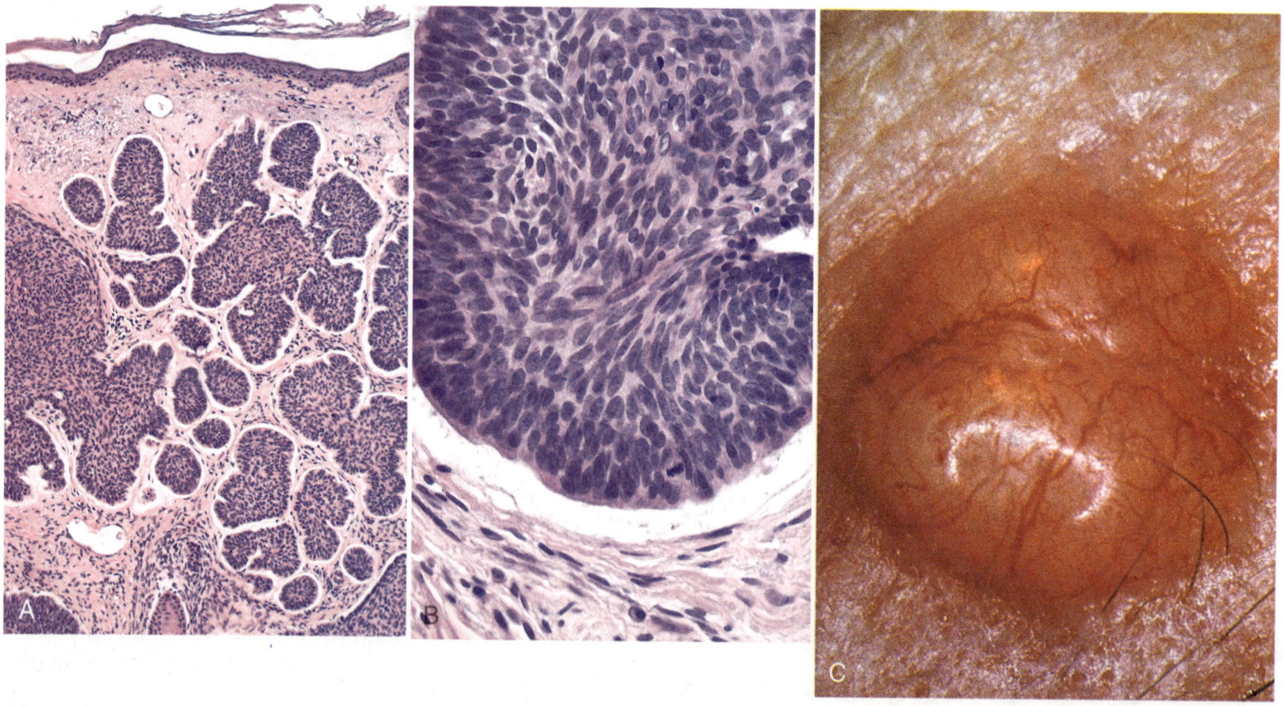

Figure 22–18

Basal cell carcinoma. **A,** The lesion is formed by multiple nodules of basaloid cells infiltrating a fibrotic stroma. **B,** The cells have scant cytoplasm, small hyperchromatic nuclei, and a peripheral palisade with clefting from the stroma. Note the similarity of these cells to the basal cells of normal epithelium. **C,** This lesion is a prototypical pearly, smooth-surfaced papule with associated telangiectatic vessels.

- Basal cell carcinoma, the most common malignant tumor world-wide, is a locally aggressive tumor associated with mutations in the PTCH pathway. Metastasis is exquisitely rare.
- Cutaneous squamous cell carcinoma can progress from actinic keratoses but most arise from chemical exposure, at thermal burn sites, or in association with HPV infection in the setting of immunosuppression.
- Cutaneous squamous cell carcinoma has potential for metastasis, but is much less aggressive than squamous cell carcinoma at mucosal sites.

Tumors and Tumor-Like Lesions of Melanocytes

Melanocytic Nevi

Strictly speaking, the term *nevus* denotes any congenital lesion of the skin. *Melanocytic* nevus, however, refers to any benign congenital or acquired neoplasm of melanocytes.

Common Nevus

Pathogenesis. Melanocytic nevi are derived from the transformation of highly dendritic melanocytes that are normally interspersed among basal keratinocytes. Progressive growth of nevus cells from the dermoepidermal junction into the underlying dermis is accompanied by *maturation.* Superficial nevus cells are larger and less mature, tend to produce melanin pigment, and grow in nests; deeper nevus cells are smaller and more mature, produce little or no pigment, and grow in cords. This sequence of maturation of individual nevus cells is of diagnostic importance, since melanomas usually show little or no maturation. The majority of benign nevi have been shown to harbor an activating mutation in BRAF (a protein downstream from RAS in the extracellular receptor kinase pathway) or less commonly in *RAS* itself. These two mutations are mutually exclusive; the growth of melanocytic nevi is self-limited.

Morphology

Melanocytic nevi are initially composed of round-to-oval cells that grow in "nests" along the dermoepidermal junction. Nuclei are uniform and round, and contain inconspicuous nucleoli with little or no mitotic activity. Such lesions, believed to represent an early developmental stage, are called **junctional nevi.** Eventually, most junctional nevi grow into the underlying dermis as nests or cords of cells (**compound nevi**), and in older lesions the epidermal nests may be lost entirely to leave pure **dermal nevi** (Fig. 22–19A). Clinically, compound and dermal nevi are often more elevated than are junctional nevi.

Clinical Features. Common melanocytic nevi are tan-to-brown, uniformly pigmented, small (usually ≤5 mm across), solid regions of elevated skin (papules) with well-defined, rounded borders (Fig. 22–19B). There are numerous types of melanocytic nevi, with varied clinical appearance. Although usually these lesions are of cosmetic interest only (sometimes even referred to as "beauty spots" and prominently displayed on some celebrated faces), they can become irritating or mimic melanoma and thus may be surgically removed.

Dysplastic Nevus

Dysplastic nevi may occur *sporadically or in a familial form.* The latter are inherited in an autosomal dominant fashion and are considered precursors of melanoma. In the sporadic form, the risk of malignant transformation seems very low.

Pathogenesis. A subset of dysplastic nevi are precursors of melanoma. In individuals with a family history of melanoma, the melanomas occur only in individuals who first develop dysplastic nevi. In these cases, the lifetime risk of developing melanoma is close to 100%. The number of dysplastic nevi correlates with the risk of developing melanoma and transition from dysplastic nevus to early melanoma has been documented both clinically and histologically. Despite such documented

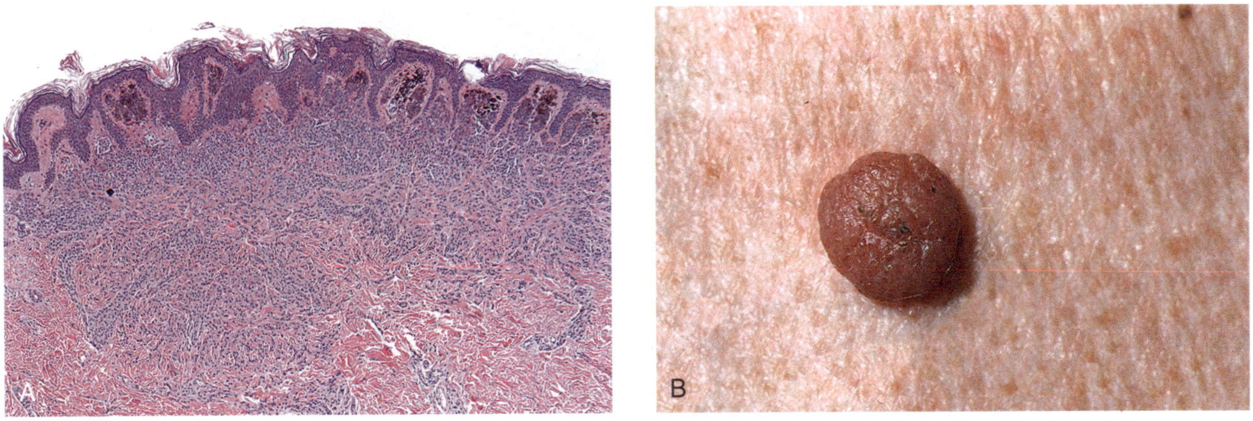

Figure 22–19

Melanocytic nevus. **A,** This dermal nevus shows rounded melanocytes extending into the dermis with loss of pigmentation and cells becoming smaller and more separated with depth—all reassuring signs of appropriate maturation. **B,** Melanocytic nevi are relatively small, symmetric, and uniformly pigmented.

evolution from dysplastic nevi to melanoma, most melanomas arise de novo and not from a preexisting nevus. Thus, the likelihood that any particular individual nevus, dysplastic or otherwise, would develop into melanoma is exceedingly low. Consequently, these lesions should be viewed as markers of melanoma risk. Activating *RAS* or *BRAF* mutations are encountered in dysplastic as well as in melanocytic nevi; additional complementing mutations occur in melanoma.

Morphology

Dysplastic nevi consist mainly of compound nevi with both architectural and cytologic evidence of abnormal growth. In this sense they have some histologic and clinical properties that are reminiscent of both benign nevi and melanoma. **Nevus cell nests within the epidermis may be enlarged and exhibit abnormal fusion or coalescence with adjacent nests. As part of this process, single nevus cells begin to replace the normal basal cell layer along the dermoepidermal junction, producing so-called lentiginous hyperplasia** (see Fig. 22–22B). Cytologic atypia consisting of irregular, often angulated, nuclear contours and hyperchromasia is frequently observed (Fig. 22–20A, B). Associated alterations also occur in the superficial dermis. These consist of a sparse lymphocytic infiltrate, loss of melanin pigment with phagocytosis by dermal macrophages (melanin pigment incontinence), and linear fibrosis surrounding epidermal nests of melanocytes. These are all elements of the host response to these lesions.

Clinical Features. *Dysplastic nevi are usually larger than most acquired nevi* (often >5 mm across) and may occur as hundreds of lesions on the body surface (Fig. 22–20C). They are flat macules to slightly raised plaques, with a "pebbly" surface. They usually show variable pigmentation (variegation) and irregular borders (Fig. 22–20C, inset). Unlike ordinary nevi, *dysplastic nevi have a tendency to occur on body surfaces not exposed to the sun* as well as on sun-exposed body surfaces. Dysplastic nevi have been documented in multiple members of families prone to the development of malignant melanoma (the "familial melanoma syndrome").

Melanoma

Melanoma is less common but much more deadly than basal or squamous cell carcinoma. Today, as a result of increased public awareness of the earliest signs of skin melanomas, most melanomas are cured surgically. Nonetheless, the incidence of these lesions has increased dramatically over the last several decades, at least in part a result of increasing sun exposure, necessitating vigorous surveillance.

Pathogenesis. As with other cutaneous malignancies, sunlight plays an important role in the development of melanoma. The incidence is highest in sun-exposed skin and in geographic locales such as New Zealand and Australia where sun exposure is high and the protective mantle of melanin is sparse. Intense intermittent exposure at an early age is particularly harmful. Sunlight, however, does not seem to be the only predisposing factor; the presence of preexisting nevi and hereditary predisposition also play a role.

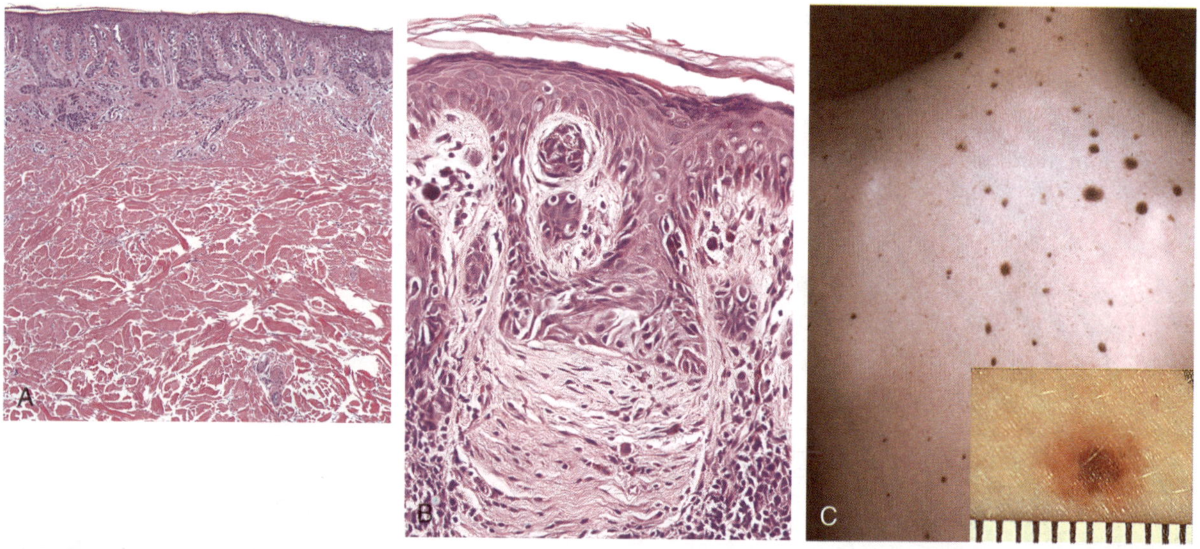

Figure 22–20

Dysplastic nevus. **A,** Compound dysplastic nevi feature a central dermal component with an asymmetric "shoulder" of exclusively junctional melanocytes (*left*). The former correlates with the more pigmented and raised central zone (see **C,** inset), and the latter with the less pigmented flat peripheral rim. **B,** An important feature is the presence of cytologic atypia (irregular, dark-staining nuclei) at high magnification. The dermis shows peculiar but characteristic parallel bands of fibrosis often encountered in dysplastic nevi—part of the host response to these lesions. **C,** Numerous irregular nevi on the back of this individual suggest the dysplastic nevus syndrome; the clinical features are intermediate to those of benign nevi and melanoma. The lesions are usually greater than 5 mm in diameter with irregular borders and variable pigmentation (inset).

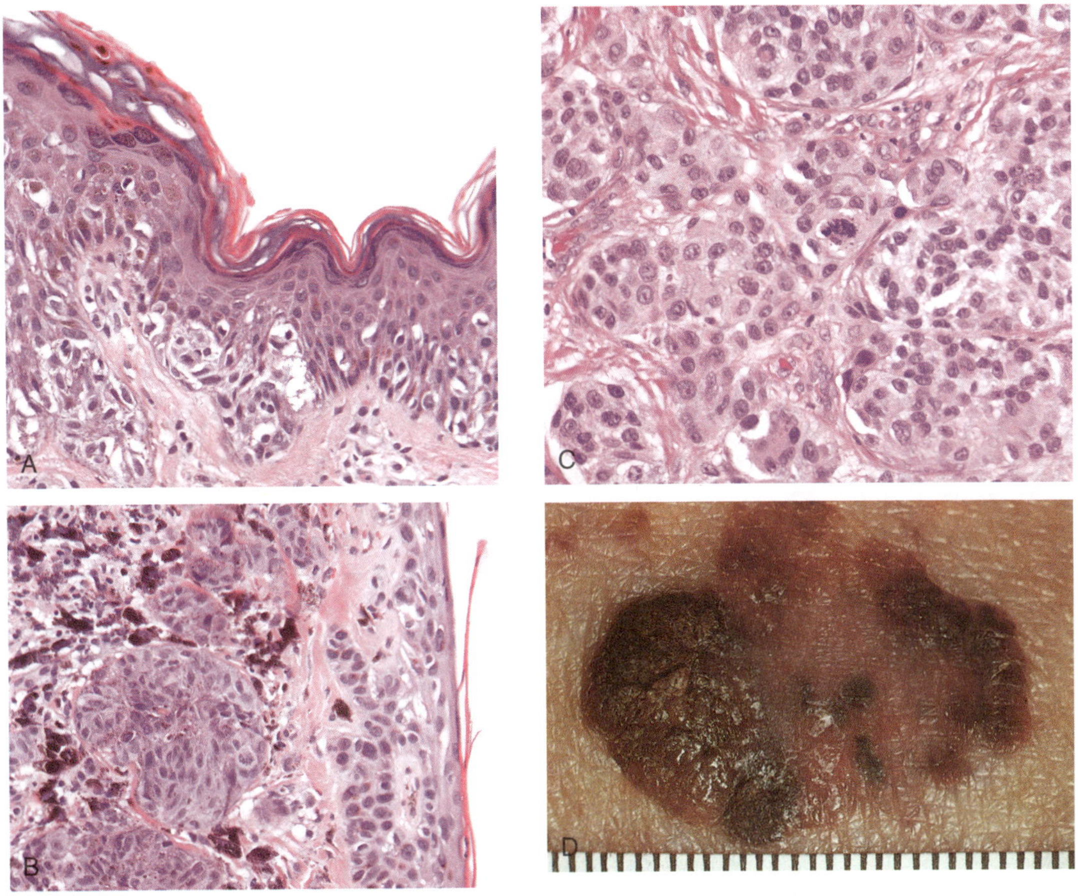

Figure 22–21

Melanoma. **A,** Radial growth, showing irregular nested and single-cell spread of melanoma cells in the epidermis. **B,** Vertical growth showing nodular aggregates of malignant cells extending deeply within the dermis (epidermis is on the right). **C,** Melanoma cells have hyperchromatic nuclei of irregular size and shape with prominent nucleoli. Mitoses, including atypical forms such as seen in the center of this field, are often encountered. **D,** Lesions clinically tend to be larger than nevi, with irregular contours and pigmentation. Macular areas are early superficial (radial) growth, while elevated areas often indicate dermal invasion (vertical growth).

Central to an understanding of the complicated histology of melanoma is the concept of radial and vertical growth. Simply stated, *radial growth* indicates the initial tendency of a melanoma to grow horizontally within the epidermis (in situ) and superficial dermal layers, often for a prolonged period (Fig. 22–21A). During this stage of growth, melanoma cells do not have the capacity to metastasize, and there is no evidence of angiogenesis. With time, the pattern of growth assumes a *vertical component,* and the melanoma now grows downward into the deeper dermal layers as an expansile mass lacking cellular maturation (Figs. 22–21B and 22–22E). This event is often heralded clinically by the development of a nodule in the relatively flat radial growth phase and correlates with the emergence of a clone of cells with metastatic potential. The probability of metastasis is predicted by measuring the depth of invasion in millimeters of this vertical growth phase nodule below the top of the granular cell layer of the overlying epidermis (Breslow thickness). Other indicators of metastatic potential are lymphatic density, mitotic rate, and overlying ulceration. *Metastases involve not only regional lymph nodes but also liver, lungs, brain, and virtually any other site that can be seeded by the hematogenous route.* Sentinel lymph node biopsy (first draining node(s) of a primary melanoma) at the time of surgery provides additional information on biological aggressiveness. In some cases, metastases may appear for the first time many years after complete surgical excision of the primary tumor, suggesting a long phase of dormancy.

Most melanomas occur sporadically, but a few are hereditary (<5% to 10 %). Molecular genetic analysis of such familial as well as sporadic cases has provided important insights into the pathogenesis of melanoma. Germ-line mutations in the *CDKN2A* gene (located on 9p21) are found in as many as 40% of the rare individuals with familial melanoma. This gene encodes $p16^{INK4A}$, a cyclin-dependent kinase inhibitor that regulates the G1-S transition of the cell cycle in a retinoblastoma protein (pRB)-dependent fashion (Chapter 6). The *CDNK2A* gene can also be silenced by methylation. Sporadic activating mutations in either *NRAS* or *BRAF* are also seen in a high portion of melanomas but are generally mutually exclusive since *BRAF* functions downstream of *RAS.*

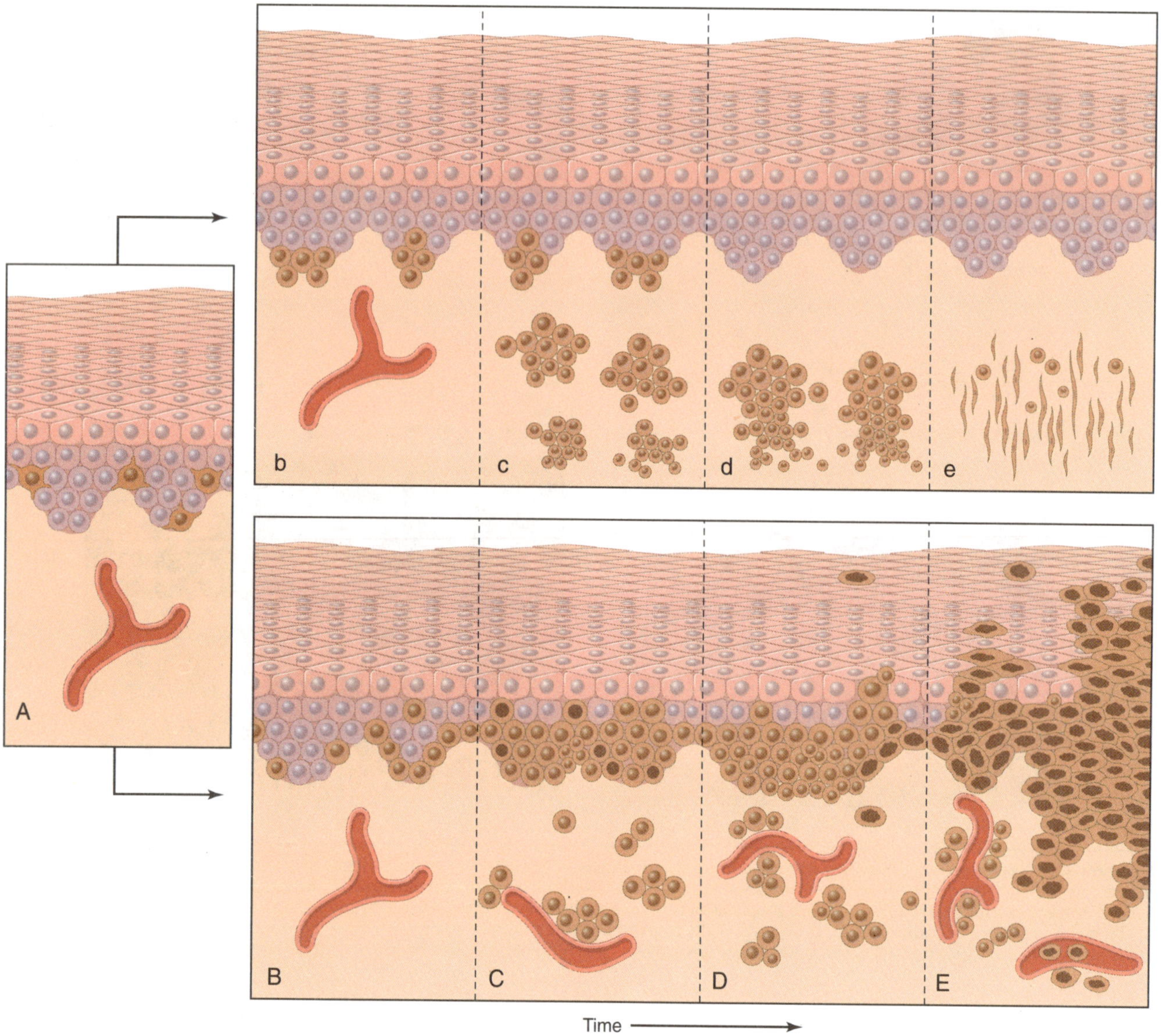

Figure 22–22

Possible steps in development of melanocytic nevi and melanoma. **A,** Normal skin shows only scattered melanocytes. *Top row:* **b,** Junctional nevus. **c,** Compound nevus. **d,** Intradermal nevus. **e,** Intradermal nevus with neurotization (extreme maturation). *Bottom row:* **B,** Lentiginous melanocytic hyperplasia. **C,** Lentiginous compound nevus with abnormal architecture and cytologic features (dysplastic nevus). **D,** Early or radial growth-phase melanoma (large dark cells in epidermis) arising in a nevus. **E,** Melanoma in vertical growth phase with metastatic potential. Note that no melanocytic nevus precursor is identified in most cases of melanoma. They are believed to arise de novo, perhaps using the same pathway.

Suppression of the *PTEN* gene on 10q23.3 is also seen in primary melanomas, allowing activation of the *AKT* pathway that promotes cell proliferation. Surprisingly, unlike most malignancies, deletion of *p53* is quite uncommon, perhaps because of overlapping cell cycle control functions of *CDNK2A* and *p53*. Polymorphisms in the melanocortin-1-receptor (*MC1R*) locus, associated with red hair, fair skin, and easy freckling, are also markers of melanoma susceptibility. As with other tumors, malignant transformation of melanocytes is a multistep process with activating mutations in proto-oncogenes and loss of tumor suppressor genes. The prevalence of these mutations varies in individual cases and types of melanoma, and much current research is directed toward finding agents that can target specific defects in these tumors.

Morphology

Individual melanoma cells are usually considerably larger than nevus cells. They contain large nuclei with irregular contours having chromatin characteristically clumped at the periphery of the nuclear membrane and prominent eosinophilic nucleoli often described as "cherry red" (Fig. 22–21D). Malignant cells grow as poorly formed nests or individual cells at all levels of the epidermis and as dermal expansile, balloon-like nodules; these constitute the radial and vertical growth phases, respectively (see Figs. 22–21A, B and 22–22D and E).

The nature and extent of the vertical growth phase determine the biologic behavior of melanomas, and thus it is important to observe and record these parameters and mitotic rate. By using these and other variables in aggregate, accurate predictive statements regarding prognosis are possible.

Clinical Features. Although most of these lesions arise in the skin, other less common sites of origin include the *oral* and *anogenital mucosal surfaces,* the *esophagus,* the *meninges,* and notably the *eye.* The following comments apply to cutaneous melanomas.

Clinically, melanoma of the skin is usually asymptomatic, although itching may be an early manifestation. *The most important clinical sign of the disease is a change in the color or size of a pigmented lesion.* Unlike benign nevi, melanomas exhibit striking variations in pigmentation, appearing in shades of black, brown, red, dark blue, and gray (Fig. 22–21D). The borders of melanomas are irregular and often "notched." The main clinical warning signs of melanoma are (1) enlargement of a preexisting mole, (2) itching or pain in a preexisting mole, (3) development of a new pigmented lesion during adult life, (4) irregularity of the borders of a pigmented lesion, and (5) variegation of color within a pigmented lesion. These principles are expressed in the so-called ABCs of melanoma: *a*symmetry, *b*order, *c*olor, *d*iameter, and *e*volution (change of an existing nevus). It is vitally important to recognize and intervene in melanoma as rapidly as possible. The vast majority of superficial lesions are cured surgically, while melanomas that become metastatic have a virtually uniformly poor prognosis, with no effective therapy in most cases.

SUMMARY

Melanocytic Lesions, Benign and Malignant

- Most *melanocytic nevi* tend to show activating mutations in just one gene, usually BRAF or less often NRAS, but the vast majority of nevi never undergo malignant transformation.
- Most *dysplastic nevi* are best regarded as markers of melanoma risk rather than premalignant lesions. They are compound nevi with cytologic atypia.
- *Melanoma* is a highly aggressive malignancy; tumors only a few millimeters in thickness can give rise to metastasis and ultimately the death of the patient.
- In most cases, melanoma progresses from an intraepithelial (in situ) to invasive (dermal) form. Characteristics of the dermal tumor such as thickness and mitotic activity correlate strongly with overall survival.

BIBLIOGRAPHY

Curtin JA, et al.: Distinct sets of genetic alterations in melanoma. N Engl J Med 353:2135, 2005. *[A modified classification of melanoma based on both clinical and genetic features of the tumors is presented. Molecular classification schemes such as this will be critical for progress in targeted therapy for cancer.]*

Elder DE: Precursors of melanoma and their mimics: nevi of special sites. Mod Pathol 19(Suppl 2):S4, 2006. *[The histology and pathogenesis of nevi and their relationship to melanoma is discussed in a balanced fashion.]*

Haluska FG, et al.: Genetic alterations in signaling pathways in melanoma. Clin Cancer Res 12(Pt 2): 2301s, 2006. *[The genetic pathways relevant to melanoma are reviewed with suggestions of possible future therapeutic development.]*

Kupper TS, Fuhlbrigge RC: Immune surveillance in the skin: Mechanisms and clinical consequences. Nat Rev 4:211, 2004. *[Lymphocytic subtypes and targeting is reviewed with the relationship of these to cutaneous inflammatory diseases providing insight into common pathogenic features of this class of skin disease.]*

Nousari HC, Anhalt GJ: Pemphigus and bullous pemphigoid. Lancet 354:667, 1999. *[The clinical and pathogenic features, including immunologic findings, of bullous disorders and their clinical management is reviewed.]*

Ridky TW, Khavari PA: Pathways sufficient to induce epidermal carcinogenesis. Cell Cycle 3:621, 2004. *[This work discusses models of human epidermal carcinogenesis and indicates that multiple mutations in multiple specific pathways are required for malignant transformation.]*

Rubin AI, Chen EH, Ratner D: Basal cell carcinoma. N Engl J Med 353:2262, 2005. *[The epidemiology, clinical presentation and treatment options for basal cell carcinoma are succinctly reviewed.]*

Schon MP, Boehncke WH: Psoriasis. N Engl J Med 352:1899, 2005. *[The pathogenesis, clinical features and treatment options are discussed.]*

Tsai KY, Tsao H: The genetics of skin cancer. Am J Med Genet 131C:82, 2004. *[The genetic bases for skin malignancies are presented along with their associations with the human genetic syndromes that predispose to their occurrence and provide insight into their pathogenesis.]*

Chapter 23

The Nervous System*

MATTHEW P. FROSCH, MD, PhD

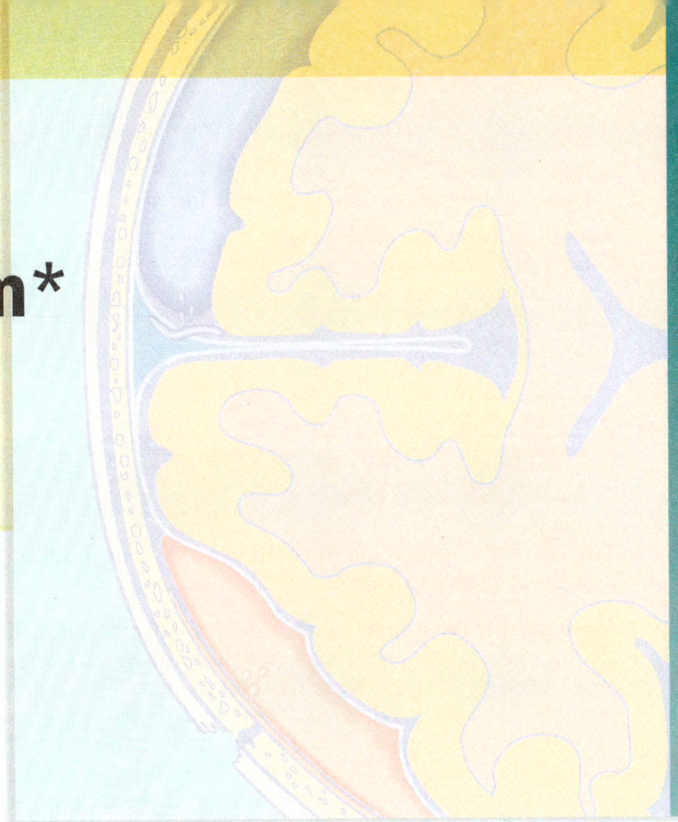

*The author is greatly appreciative of the contributions to this chapter from Drs. D. Burns and V. Kumar (Basic Pathology, 7th edition) and Drs. U. De Girolami and D. Anthony (from co-authored chapters in Robbins and Cotran: Pathologic Basis of Disease, 7th edition).

PATTERNS OF INJURY IN THE NERVOUS SYSTEM

The cellular constituents of the nervous system respond in different ways to various forms of injury.

Markers of Neuronal Injury. In response to injury, changes can be observed in neurons and their processes (axons and dendrites). Within 12 hours of an irreversible hypoxic/ischemic insult, *acute neuronal injury* becomes evident even on routine hematoxylin and eosin (H & E) staining (Fig. 23–1A). There is shrinkage of the cell body, pyknosis of the nucleus, disappearance of the nucleolus, and loss of Nissl substance, with intense eosinophilia of the cytoplasm *("red neurons")*. Often, the nucleus assumes the angulated shape of the shrunken cell body. Areas of cerebral ischemia may progress to coagulative necrosis. Injured axons undergo swelling and show disruption of axonal transport. The swellings (*spheroids*) can be recognized on H & E stains (Fig. 23–1B) and can be highlighted by silver staining or immunohistochemistry for axonally transported proteins such as amyloid precursor protein. Axonal injury also leads to cell body enlargement and rounding, peripheral displacement of the nucleus, enlargement of the nucleolus, and dispersion of Nissl substance (from the center of the cell to the periphery, so-called *central chromatolysis;* Fig. 23–1C).

Many neurodegenerative diseases are associated with specific intracellular inclusions that help in diagnosing the disease (e.g., Lewy bodies in Parkinson disease and tangles in Alzheimer disease). In some neurodegenerative diseases, neuronal processes also become thickened and tortuous; these can be seen as *dystrophic neurites.*

Viral infections can form inclusions in neurons, just as they do in other cells of the body. With age, neurons also accumulate complex lipids in their cytoplasm and lysosomes (*lipofuscin*).

Astrocytes in Injury and Repair. Astrocytes are the principal cells responsible for repair and scar formation in the brain, a process termed *gliosis.* In response to injury, astrocytes undergo both hypertrophy and hyperplasia. The nucleus enlarges and becomes vesicular, and the nucleolus is prominent. The previously scant cytoplasm expands to a bright pink, somewhat irregular swath around an eccentric nucleus, from which emerge numerous stout, ramifying processes (*gemistocytic astrocyte*). There is minimal extracellular matrix deposition. Unlike the repair after injury elsewhere in the body, fibroblasts participate in healing after brain injury only to a limited extent (usually after penetrating brain trauma or around abscesses). In settings of long-standing gliosis, astrocytes have less distinct cytoplasm and appear more fibrillar *(fibrillary astrocytes). Rosenthal fibers* are thick, elongated, brightly eosinophilic protein aggregates that can be found in astrocytic processes in chronic gliosis and in some low-grade gliomas.

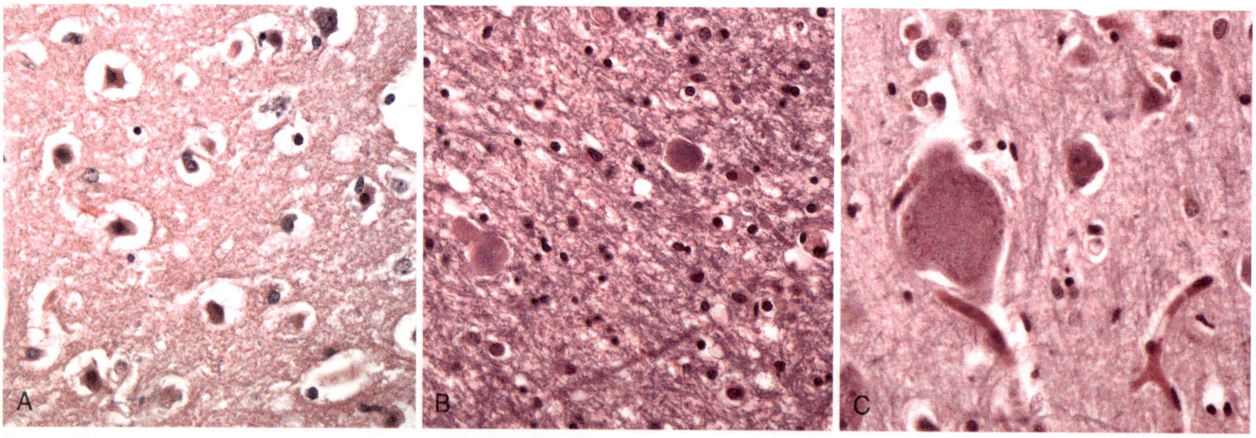

Figure 23–1

Patterns of neuronal injury. **A,** Acute hypoxic/ischemic injury in cerebral cortex, where the individual cell bodies are shrunken, along with the nuclei. They also are prominently stained by eosin, leading to the term "red neurons." **B,** Axonal spheroids are visible as bulbous swellings at points of disruption or altered axonal transport (H&E). **C,** With axonal injury there can be swelling of the cell body and peripheral dispersal of the Nissl substance, termed chromatolysis (H&E).

Corpora amylacea represent a degenerative change in astrocytes and occur in increasing numbers with advancing age. These are round, faintly basophilic, periodic acid–Schiff (PAS)-positive, concentrically lamellated aggregates of polyglucosans that range between 5 and 50 µm, and are located wherever there are astrocytic end processes, especially in the subpial and perivascular zones.

Other Cells. *Oligodendrocytes,* which produce myelin, have a limited repertoire of morphologic changes, apart from cell death or damage to myelin, as in multiple sclerosis. In progressive multifocal leukoencephalopathy, viral inclusions can be seen in oligodendrocytes, with a smudgy, homogeneous-appearing enlarged nucleus.

Ependymal cells line the ventricular system and are located in the region of the obliterated central canal of the spinal cord. Disruption of ependymal cells is often associated with a local proliferation of subependymal astrocytes to produce small irregularities on the ventricular surfaces termed *ependymal granulations.* Certain infectious agents, particularly cytomegalovirus (CMV), can produce extensive ependymal injury, and viral inclusions may be seen in them.

Choroid plexus is responsible for the secretion of CSF and is in continuity with the ependyma, extending into the ventricular cavities. It has a specialized epithelial covering with a fibrovascular stroma that may contain meningothelial cells.

Microglia are bone marrow–derived cells that function as the phagocytes of the CNS. When activated after tissue injury, infection, or trauma, they proliferate and become more evident. They may be recognizable as activated macrophages in areas of demyelination, organizing infarct, or hemorrhage, or they develop elongated nuclei (*rod cells*) in neurosyphilis or other infections. When these elongated microglia form aggregates at sites of tissue injury, they are termed *microglial nodules.* Similar collections can be found congregating around portions of dying neurons, termed *neuronophagia.*

EDEMA, HERNIATION, AND HYDROCEPHALUS

The brain and spinal cord exist within a rigid compartment defined by the skull and spinal canal, and lined by dura. Nerves and blood vessels pass through this structure via specific foramina, but the brain is confined to the cranial vault. The advantage of housing the delicate CNS within such a protective environment is obvious, yet these rigid confines provide little room for brain parenchymal expansion in disease states. Disorders that upset this delicate balance include generalized cerebral edema, hydrocephalus, and focally expanding mass lesions.

Cerebral Edema

Cerebral edema is the accumulation of excess fluid within the brain parenchyma. This term should be distinguished from hydrocephalus, an increase in CSF volume within all or part of the ventricular system. There are two underlying mechanisms for the development of cerebral edema that often occur together particularly when there is generalized injury.

- *Vasogenic edema* occurs when the integrity of the normal blood-brain barrier is disrupted. With increased vascular permeability, fluid shifts from the vascular compartment into the intercellular spaces of the brain. Vasogenic edema can be either localized—because of abnormal permeability of vessels adjacent to inflammation or tumors~~or~~ generalized.
- *Cytotoxic edema* implies an increase in intracellular fluid secondary to neuronal, glial, or endothelial cell membrane injury, as might be encountered in an individual with a generalized hypoxic/ischemic insult or with exposure to some toxins.

Morphology

The edematous brain is softer than normal and often appears to "overfill" the cranial vault. In generalized edema the gyri are flattened, the intervening sulci are narrowed, and the ventricular cavities are compressed (Fig. 23–2).

Hydrocephalus

After being produced by the choroid plexus within the ventricles, cerebrospinal fluid (CSF) circulates through the ventricular system and exits through the foramina of Luschka and Magendie. CSF fills the subarachnoid space around the brain and spinal cord, contributing to the cushioning of the nervous system within its bony confines. The arachnoid granulations are responsible for the resorption of CSF. The balance between CSF generation and resorption keeps the volume of this fluid stable. *Hydrocephalus* refers to the accumulation of excessive CSF within the ventricular system. Most cases occur as a consequence of impaired flow or impaired resorption of CSF; in rare instances (e.g., tumors of the choroid

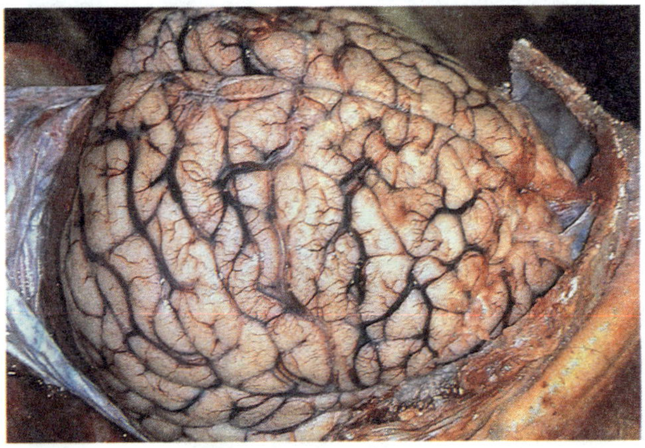

Figure 23–2

Cerebral edema. The surfaces of the gyri are flattened as a result of compression of the expanding brain by the dura mater and inner surface of the skull. Such changes are associated with a dangerous increase in intracranial pressure.

plexus), overproduction of CSF may be responsible. When hydrocephalus develops in infancy before closure of the cranial sutures, there is enlargement of the head. Hydrocephalus developing after fusion of the sutures, in contrast, is associated with expansion of the ventricles and increased intracranial pressure, without a change in head circumference (Fig. 23–3).

If there is an obstacle to the flow of CSF within the ventricular system, then a portion of the ventricles enlarges while the remainder does not. This pattern is referred to as *noncommunicating hydrocephalus* and is most commonly seen with masses at the formamen of Monro or aqueduct of Sylvius. In *communicating hydrocephalus* all of the ventricular system is enlarged; here the cause is most often reduced resorption of CSF.

The term *hydrocephalus ex vacuo* refers to dilation of the ventricular system with a compensatory increase in CSF volume secondary to a loss of brain parenchyma, as may occur after infarcts or with a degenerative disease.

Herniation

When the volume of brain tissue increases beyond the limit permitted by compression of veins and displacement of CSF, intracranial pressure may rise. Because the cranial vault is subdivided by rigid dural folds (falx and tentorium), a focal expansion of the brain causes it to be displaced in relation to these partitions. If the expansion is sufficiently severe, herniation will occur (Fig. 23–4). Herniations are named by either the part of the brain that is displaced or the structure across which it moves. The usual consequence of such displacement is compromise of the blood supply to the "pushed" tissue, resulting in infarction. This often leads to another round of swelling and further herniation.

Subfalcine (cingulate) herniation occurs when unilateral or asymmetric expansion of a cerebral hemisphere displaces the cingulate gyrus under the edge of falx. This may be associated with compression of branches of the anterior cerebral artery.

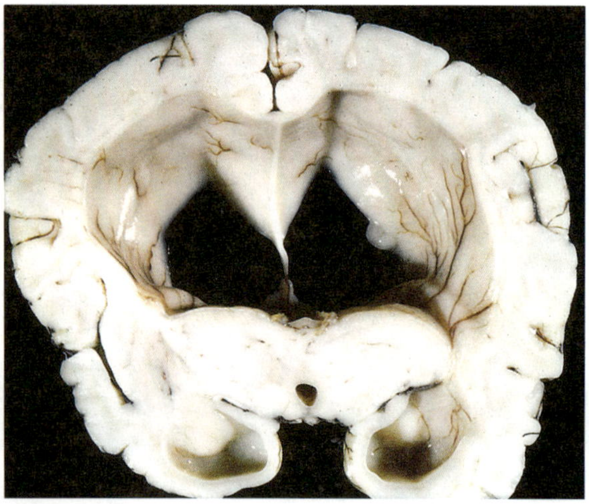

Figure 23–3

Hydrocephalus. Dilated lateral ventricles seen in a coronal section through the midthalamus.

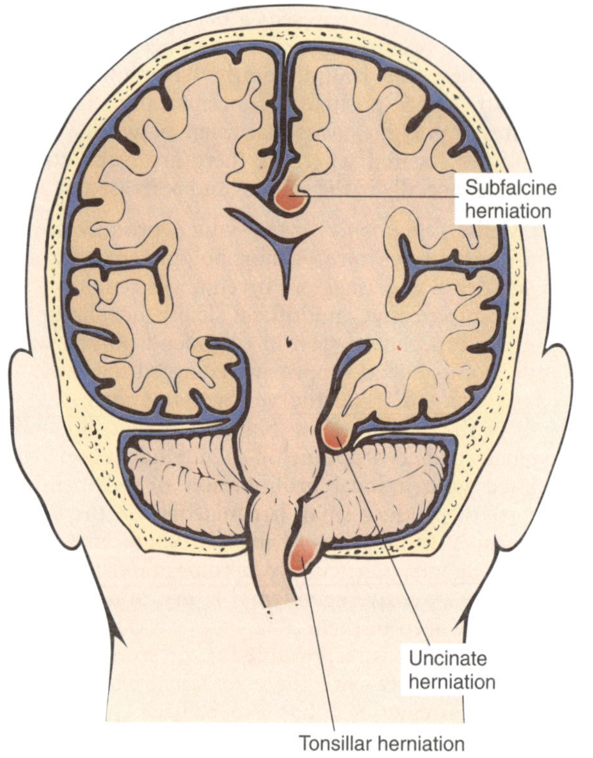

Figure 23–4

Patterns of brain herniation: subfalcine (cingulate), transtentorial (uncinate, mesial temporal), and tonsillar. (Adapted from Fishman RA: Brain edema. N Engl J Med 293:706, 1975.)

Transtentorial (uncinate) herniation occurs when the medial aspect of the temporal lobe is compressed against the free margin of the tentorium. As the temporal lobe is displaced, the third cranial nerve is compromised, resulting in pupillary dilation and impairment of ocular movements on the side of the lesion ("blown pupil"). The posterior cerebral artery may also be compressed, resulting in ischemic injury to the territory supplied by that vessel, including the primary visual cortex. When the extent of herniation is large enough the contralateral cerebral peduncle may be compressed, resulting in hemiparesis ipsilateral to the side of the herniation. Because hemispheric lesions typically cause contralateral weakness, this ipsilateral hemiparesis can be a false localizing sign that would suggest to the examiner that the patient has a lesion in the opposite, unaffected hemisphere. The changes in the peduncle in this setting are known as Kernohan's notch. Progression of transtentorial herniation is often accompanied by hemorrhagic lesions in the midbrain and pons, termed *Duret hemorrhages* (Fig. 23–5). These linear or flame-shaped lesions usually occur in the midline and paramedian regions, and are believed to be due to tearing of penetrating veins and arteries supplying the upper brain stem. The presence of Duret hemorrhages implies a grim prognosis.

Tonsillar herniation refers to displacement of the cerebellar tonsils through the foramen magnum. This pattern of herniation is life-threatening, because it causes brain stem compression and compromises vital respiratory and cardiac centers in the medulla.

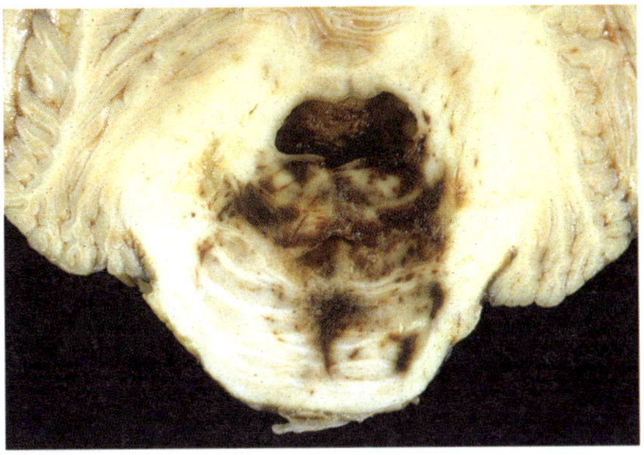

Figure 23–5

Duret hemorrhage. As mass effect displaces the brain downwards, there is disruption of the vessels that enter the pons along the midline, leading to hemorrhage.

SUMMARY

Edema, Herniation, and Hydrocephalus

•C erebral edema is the accumulation of excess fluid within the brain parenchyma. Hydrocephalus is an increase in CSF volume within all or part of the ventricular system.

• Increases in tissue volume of the brain (as a result of increased CSF volume, edema, or hemorrhage) increase the pressure inside the fixed capacity of the skull.

• Increases in pressure can damage the brain either by decreasing perfusion or by displacing tissue across dural barriers inside the skull or through openings in the skull (herniations).

CEREBROVASCULAR DISEASES

Cerebrovascular disease is the third leading cause of death (after heart disease and cancer) in the United States; it is also the most prevalent neurologic disorder in terms of both morbidity and mortality. The term *cerebrovascular disease* denotes any abnormality of the brain caused by a pathologic process involving blood vessels. The three basic processes are (1) thrombotic occlusion of vessels, (2) embolic occlusion of vessels, and (3) vascular rupture. The first two share many characteristics, because their effect on the brain is the sameloss of oxygen and metabolic substrates resulting in brain infarction. Thrombosis and embolism cause ischemic injury or infarction of specific regions of the brain, depending on the vessel involved. A similar pattern of injury occurs diffusely when there is complete loss of perfusion (or delivery of oxygen and metabolic substrate). Hemorrhage accompanies rupture of vessels, leading to direct tissue damage as well as secondary ischemic injury. "Stroke" is the clinical designation that applies to all these conditions, particularly when symptoms begin acutely.

Hypoxia, Ischemia, and Infarction

The brain requires a constant delivery of glucose and oxygen from the blood. Although the brain accounts for only 1% to 2% of body weight, it receives 15% of the resting cardiac output and accounts for 20% of the total body oxygen consumption. Cerebral blood flow remains constant over a wide range of blood pressure and intracranial pressure because of autoregulation of vascular resistance. The brain is a highly aerobic tissue, with oxygen being the limiting substance. The brain may be deprived of oxygen by any of several mechanisms: *functional hypoxia* in a setting of a low partial pressure of oxygen; impaired oxygen-carrying capacity; inhibition of oxygen use by tissue; or *ischemia,* either *transient* or *permanent,* after interruption of the normal circulatory flow. Cessation of blood flow can result from a reduction in perfusion pressure, as in hypotension, or secondary to vascular obstruction, or both.

Global Cerebral Ischemia

This pattern of widespread ischemic/hypoxic injury occurs when there is a generalized reduction of cerebral perfusion, usually below systolic pressures of less than 50 mm Hg, such as in cardiac arrest, shock, and severe hypotension. The clinical outcome varies with the severity of the insult. When mild, there may be only a transient postischemic confusional state, with eventual complete recovery. Irreversible damage of CNS tissue does occur in some individuals who suffer mild or transient global ischemic insults. Neurons are much more sensitive to hypoxia than are glial cells. There is also variability in the susceptibility of different populations of neurons in different regions of the CNS; pyramidal cells of the Sommer sector (CA1) of the hippocampus, Purkinje cells of the cerebellum, and pyramidal neurons in the neocortex are the most susceptible to ischemia of short duration. In severe global cerebral ischemia, widespread neuronal death, irrespective of regional vulnerability, occurs. Individuals who survive in this state often remain severely impaired neurologically and deeply comatose (persistent vegetative state). Other patients meet the clinical criteria for "brain death," including evidence of diffuse cortical injury (isoelectric, or "flat," electroencephalogram) and brain stem damage, including absent reflexes and respiratory drive. When patients with this pervasive form of injury are maintained on mechanical ventilation, the brain gradually undergoes an autolytic process, resulting in the so-called "respirator brain."

Morphology

In the setting of global ischemia, the brain is swollen, with wide gyri and narrowed sulci. The cut surface shows poor demarcation between gray and white matter. The histopathologic changes that attend irreversible ischemic injury (infarction) are grouped into three categories. **Early changes,** occurring 12 to 24 hours after the insult, include acute neuronal cell change (red neurons; see Fig. 23–1A) characterized initially by microvacuolization, followed by cytoplasmic eosinophilia, and later nuclear pyknosis and karyorrhexis. Similar changes occur somewhat later in astrocytes and oligodendroglia. After this, the reaction to tissue damage begins with infiltration by neutrophils (Fig. 23–6A). **Subacute changes,** occurring at 24 hours to 2 weeks, include necrosis of tissue, influx of macrophages, vascular proliferation, and reactive gliosis (Fig. 23–6B). **Repair,** seen after 2 weeks, is characterized by removal of all necrotic tissue, loss of organized CNS structure, and gliosis (Fig. 23–6C). In the cerebral cortex the neuronal loss and gliosis produce an uneven destruction of the neocortex, with preservation of some layers and involvement of others—a pattern termed pseudolaminar necrosis.

Border zone ("watershed") infarcts are wedge-shaped areas of infarction that occur in those regions of the brain and spinal cord that lie at the most distal fields of arterial perfusion. In the cerebral hemispheres, the border zone between the anterior and the middle cerebral artery distributions is at greatest risk. Damage to this region produces a band of necrosis over the cerebral convexity a few centimeters lateral to the interhemispheric fissure. Border zone infarcts are usually seen after hypotensive episodes.

Focal Cerebral Ischemia

Cerebral arterial occlusion leads to focal ischemia and~~if~~ sustained~~to~~ infarction of CNS tissue in the distribution of the compromised vessel. The size, location, and shape of the infarct and the extent of tissue damage that results are determined by modifying variables, most importantly the adequacy of collateral flow. The major source of collateral flow is the circle of Willis. Partial collateralization is also provided over the surface of the brain through cortical-leptomeningeal anastomoses. In contrast, there is little if any collateral flow for the deep penetrating vessels supplying structures such as the thalamus, basal ganglia, and deep white matter.

Occlusive vascular disease of severity sufficient to lead to cerebral infarction may be due to *in situ thrombosis* or *embolization* from a distant source. Overall, embolic infarctions are more common. Cardiac mural thrombi are a frequent source; myocardial infarct, valvular disease, and atrial fibrillation are important predisposing factors. Thromboemboli also arise in arteries, most often from atheromatous plaques within the carotid arteries. Other

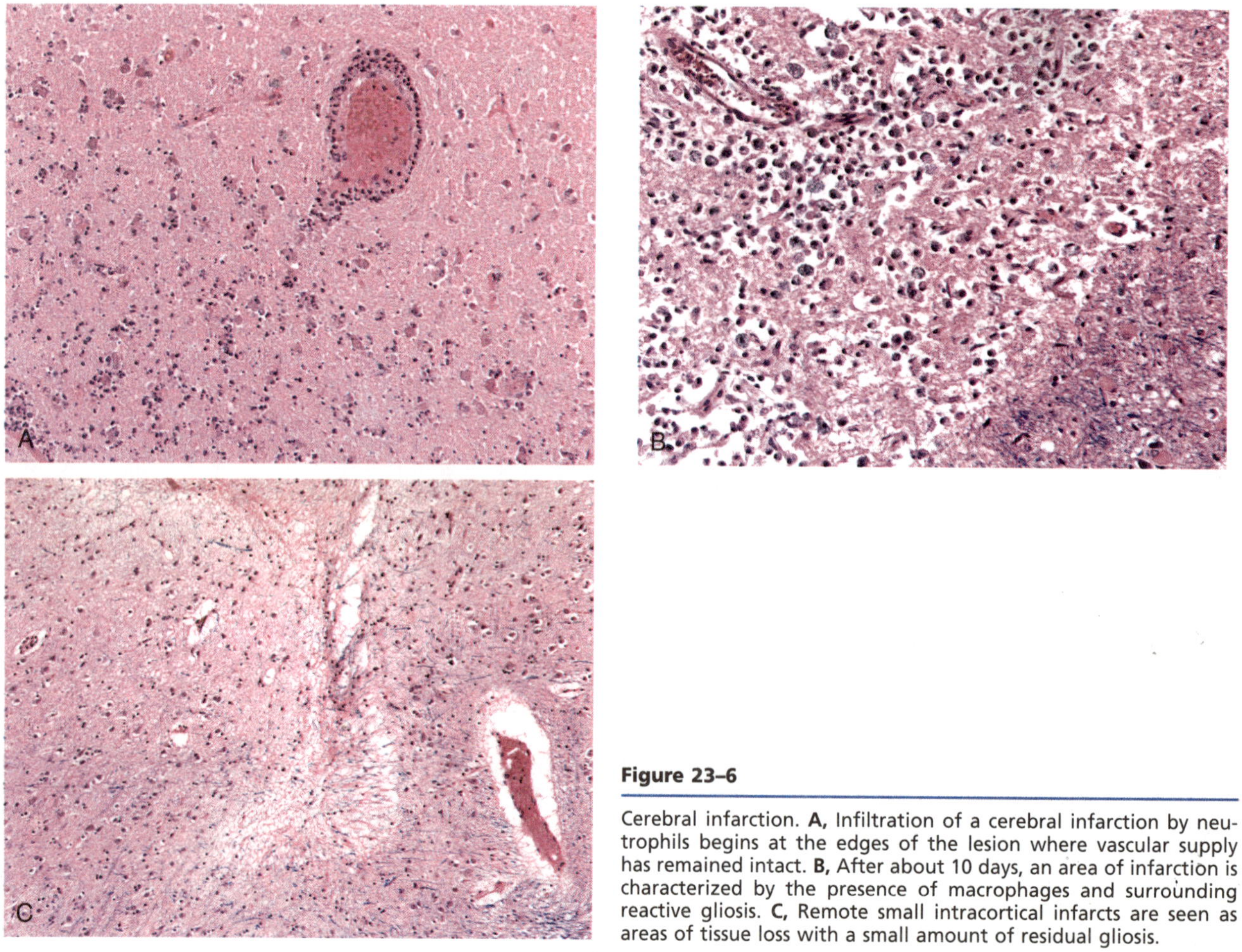

Figure 23–6

Cerebral infarction. **A,** Infiltration of a cerebral infarction by neutrophils begins at the edges of the lesion where vascular supply has remained intact. **B,** After about 10 days, an area of infarction is characterized by the presence of macrophages and surrounding reactive gliosis. **C,** Remote small intracortical infarcts are seen as areas of tissue loss with a small amount of residual gliosis.

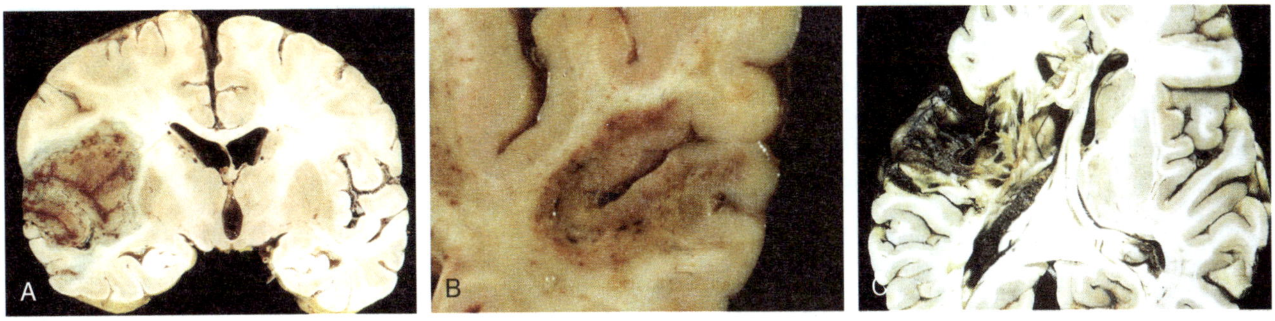

Figure 23–7

Cerebral infarction. **A,** Section of the brain showing a large, discolored, focally hemorrhagic region in the left middle cerebral artery distribution (hemorrhagic, or red, infarction). **B,** An infarct with punctate hemorrhages, consistent with ischemia-reperfusion injury, is present in the temporal lobe. **C,** Old cystic infarct shows destruction of cortex and surrounding gliosis.

sources of emboli include paradoxical emboli, particularly in children with cardiac anomalies; emboli associated with cardiac surgery; and emboli of other material (tumor, fat, or air). The territory of distribution of the middle cerebral artery~~the~~ direct extension of the internal carotid artery~~is~~ most frequently affected by embolic infarction; emboli tend to lodge where vessels branch or in areas of preexisting luminal stenosis.

The majority of thrombotic occlusions causing cerebral infarctions are due to *atherosclerosis;* the most common sites of primary thrombosis are the carotid bifurcation, the origin of the middle cerebral artery, and at either end of the basilar artery. Atherosclerotic stenoses can develop superimposed thrombosis, accompanied by anterograde extension, fragmentation, and distal embolization.

Infarcts can be divided into two broad groups based on their macroscopic and corresponding radiologic appearance (Fig. 23–7). *Nonhemorrhagic infarcts* can be treated with thrombolytic therapies, if identified shortly after presentation. This approach is contraindicated when lesions are *hemorrhagic,* with multiple, sometimes confluent, petechial hemorrhages (Fig. 23–7A, B). The hemorrhage occurs secondary to reperfusion of ischemic tissue, either through collaterals or after dissolution of intravascular occlusions.

Morphology

The macroscopic appearance of a **nonhemorrhagic infarct** changes in time. During the first 6 hours of irreversible injury, little can be observed. By 48 hours the tissue becomes pale, soft, and swollen, and the corticomedullary junction becomes indistinct. From 2 to 10 days the brain becomes gelatinous and friable, and the previously ill-defined boundary between normal and abnormal tissue becomes more distinct as edema resolves in the adjacent tissue that has survived. From 10 days to 3 weeks, the tissue liquefies, eventually leaving a fluid-filled cavity lined by dark gray tissue, which gradually expands as dead tissue is removed (Fig. 23–7C).

Microscopically, the tissue reaction follows a characteristic sequence: **After the first 12 hours** ischemic neuronal change (red neurons; see Fig. 23–1A) and both cytotoxic and vasogenic edema predominate. There is loss of the usual tinctorial characteristics of white and gray matter structures. Endothelial and glial cells, mainly astrocytes, swell, and myelinated fibers begin to disintegrate. **Until 48 hours,** there is some neutrophilic emigration followed by mononuclear phagocytic cells in the ensuing **2 to 3 weeks.** Macrophages containing myelin breakdown products or blood may persist in the lesion for months to years. As the process of phagocytosis and liquefaction proceeds, astrocytes at the edges of the lesion progressively enlarge, divide, and develop a prominent network of protoplasmic extensions.

After several months the striking astrocytic nuclear and cytoplasmic enlargement recedes. In the wall of the cavity, astrocyte processes form a dense feltwork of glial fibers admixed with new capillaries and a few perivascular connective tissue fibers. In the cerebral cortex the cavity is delimited from the meninges and subarachnoid space by a gliotic layer of tissue, derived from the molecular layer of cortex. The pia and arachnoid are not affected and do not contribute to the healing process.

The microscopic picture and evolution of **hemorrhagic infarction** parallel ischemic infarction, with the addition of blood extravasation and resorption. In persons receiving anticoagulant treatment, hemorrhagic infarcts may be associated with extensive intracerebral hematomas.

Intracranial Hemorrhage

Hemorrhage within the skull can occur in a variety of locations, and each location is associated with a set of underlying causes. Hemorrhages within the brain itself can occur secondary to hypertension or other forms of vascular wall injury. Alternatively, they can arise in a specific lesion like an arteriovenous malformation, a cavernous malformation, or an intraparenchymal tumor. Subarachnoid hemorrhages are most commonly seen with aneurysms but occur also with other vascular malformations. Hemorrhages associated with the dura (in either subdural or epidural spaces) make up a pattern associated with trauma.

Primary Brain Parenchymal Hemorrhage

Spontaneous (nontraumatic) intraparenchymal hemorrhages occur most commonly in mid to late adult life, with a peak incidence at about 60 years of age. Most are caused by rupture of a small intraparenchymal vessel. Hypertension is the most common underlying cause, and brain hemorrhage accounts for roughly 15% of deaths among individuals with chronic hypertension. Hypertensive intraparenchymal hemorrhages typically occur in the basal ganglia, thalamus, pons, and cerebellum (Fig. 23–8).

Intracerebral hemorrhage can be clinically devastating when it affects large portions of the brain and extends into the ventricular system; alternatively, it can affect small regions and be clinically silent. Over weeks or months there is a gradual resolution of the hematoma, sometimes with considerable clinical improvement. Again, the location and size of the bleed will determine the clinical manifestations.

Morphology

Acute hemorrhages are characterized by extravasation of blood with compression of the adjacent parenchyma. Old hemorrhages show an area of cavitary destruction of brain with a rim of brownish discoloration. On microscopic examination, the early lesion consists of a central core of clotted blood surrounded by a rim of brain tissue showing anoxic neuronal and glial changes as well as edema. Eventually the edema resolves, pigment- and lipid-laden macrophages appear, and proliferation of reactive astrocytes become visible at the periphery of the lesion. The cellular events then follow the same time course observed after cerebral infarction.

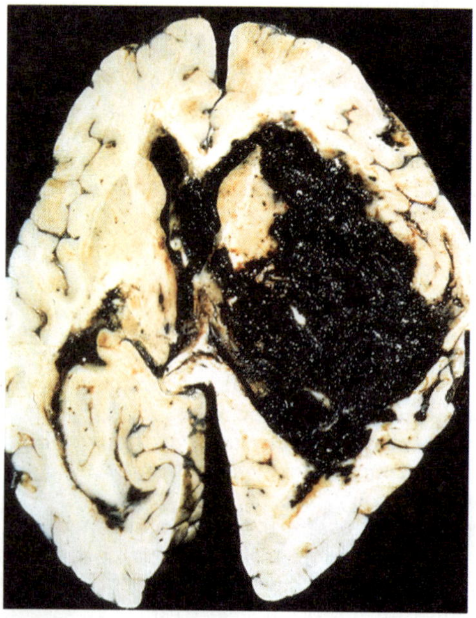

Figure 23–8

Cerebral hemorrhage. Massive hypertensive hemorrhage rupturing into a lateral ventricle.

Cerebral Amyloid Angiopathy

Cerebral amyloid angiopathy (CAA) is a disease in which amyloidogenic peptides~~ty~~pically the same ones found in Alzheimer disease (see below)~~de~~posit in the walls of medium- and small-caliber meningeal and cortical vessels. This deposition results in weakening of the vessel wall and increases the risk of hemorrhage. Since CAA is limited to leptomeningeal and cortical vessels with sparing of the vasculature of white matter and deep gray structures, hemorrhages associated with CAA have a distribution that is different from that of hypertensive intraparenchymal hemorrhages. CAA-associated hemorrhages are often referred to as *lobar hemorrhages* because of the involvement of the cerebral cortex. As in other locations, amyloid in the vessel walls can be identified by Congo Red stains. The affected vessels are rigid, with a pipe-like appearance.

Subarachnoid Hemorrhage and Saccular Aneurysms

The most frequent cause of clinically significant subarachnoid hemorrhage is rupture of a *saccular (berry) aneurysm*. Hemorrhage into the subarachnoid space may also result from vascular malformation, trauma (in which case it is usually associated with other signs of the injury), rupture of an intracerebral hemorrhage into the ventricular system, hematologic disturbances, and tumors.

Rupture can occur at any time, but in about one-third of cases it is associated with acute increases in intracranial pressure, such as with straining at stool or sexual orgasm. Blood under arterial pressure is forced into the subarachnoid space, and individuals are stricken with sudden, excruciating headache (classically described as "the worst headache I've ever had") and rapidly lose consciousness. Between 25% and 50% of individuals die with the first rupture, although those who survive typically improve and recover consciousness in minutes. Recurring bleeding is common in survivors; it is currently not possible to predict which individuals will have recurrences of bleeding. The prognosis worsens with each episode of bleeding.

About 90% of saccular aneurysms occur in the anterior circulation near major arterial branch points (Fig. 23–9); multiple aneurysms exist in 20% to 30% of cases. Although they are sometimes referred to as *congenital,* they are not present at birth but develop over time because of underlying defects in the vessel media. Besides an association with disorders of extracellular matrix proteins, there is an increased risk of aneurysms in individuals with autosomal dominant polycystic kidney disease.

Overall, aneurysms have a roughly 1.3% per year rate of bleeding. However, the probability of rupture increases with the size of the lesion, such that aneurysms greater than 10 mm have a roughly 50% risk of bleeding per year. In the early period after a subarachnoid hemorrhage, there is a risk of additional ischemic injury from vasospasm involving other vessels. In the healing phase of subarachnoid hemorrhage, meningeal fibrosis and scarring occur, sometimes leading to obstruction of CSF flow as well as interruption of the normal pathways of CSF resorption.

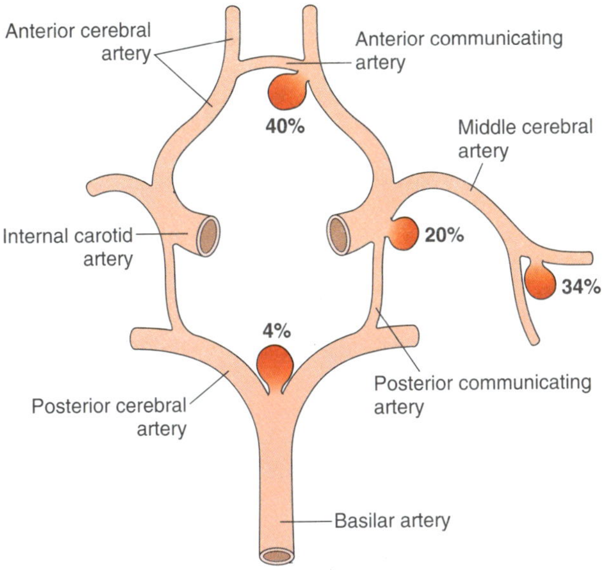

Figure 23–9

Relative frequency of common sites of saccular (berry) aneurysms in the circle of Willis.

Morphology

An unruptured saccular aneurysm is a thin-walled outpouching of an artery. At the neck of the aneurysm, the muscular wall and intimal elastic lamina stop short and are absent from the aneurysm sac itself; the sac is made up of thickened hyalinized intima. The adventitia covering the sac is continuous with that of the parent artery (Fig. 23–10). Rupture usually occurs at the apex of the sac with extravasation of blood into the subarachnoid space, the substance of the brain, or both.

While saccular aneurysms are the most common type of intracranial aneurysm, other types include atherosclerotic (fusiform, mostly of the basilar artery), mycotic, traumatic, and dissecting aneurysms. These latter three, as with saccular aneurysms, are most often found in the anterior circulation. They usually present with cerebral infarction from vascular occlusion instead of subarachnoid hemorrhage.

Vascular Malformations

Vascular malformations of the brain are classified into four principal types based on the nature of the abnormal vessels: *arteriovenous malformations (AVM)*, the most common), *cavernous angiomas, capillary telangiectasias, and venous angiomas*. AVMs affect males twice as frequently as females; the lesion is most often recognized clinically between the ages of 10 and 30 years, presenting as a seizure disorder, an intracerebral hemorrhage, or a subarachnoid hemorrhage. Large AVMs occurring in the newborn period can lead to high-output congestive heart failure because of blood shunting directly from arteries to veins. The risk of bleeding makes AVM the most dangerous type of vascular malformation.

Morphology

AVMs involve vessels in the subarachnoid space extending into brain parenchyma or they may occur exclusively within the brain. In macroscopic appearance, they resemble a tangled network of wormlike vascular channels (Fig. 23–11). Microscopically, they are enlarged blood vessels separated by gliotic tissue, often with evidence of prior hemorrhage. Some vessels can be recognized as arteries with duplicated and fragmented internal elastic lamina, while others show

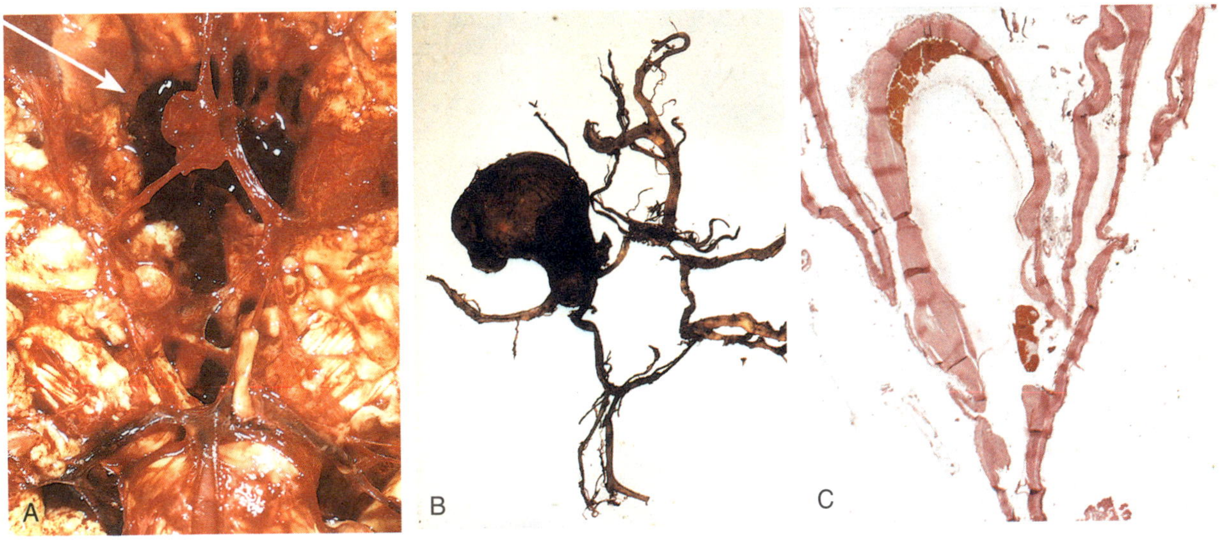

Figure 23–10

Saccular aneurysms. **A,** View of the base of the brain, dissected to show the circle of Willis with an aneurysm of the anterior cerebral artery (*arrow*). **B,** Dissected circle of Willis to show large aneurysm. **C,** Section through a saccular aneurysm showing the hyalinized fibrous vessel wall (H&E).

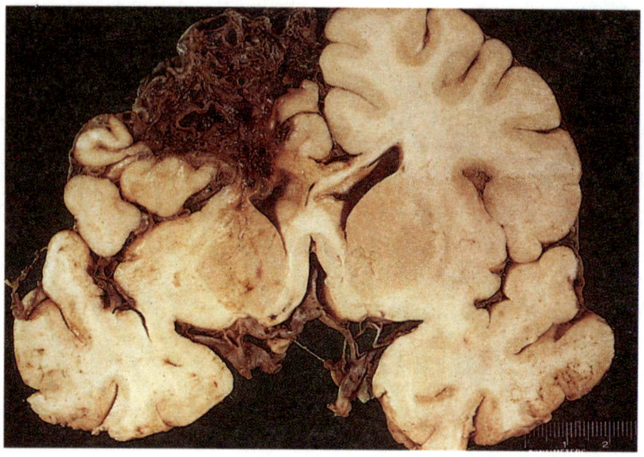

Figure 23–11

Arteriovenous malformation.

marked thickening or partial replacement of the media by hyalinized connective tissue.

Cavernous hemangiomas consist of distended, loosely organized vascular channels with thin collagenized walls; they are devoid of intervening nervous tissue (thus distinguishing them from capillary telangiectasias). They occur most often in the cerebellum, pons, and subcortical regions, and have a low flow without arteriovenous shunting. Foci of old hemorrhage, infarction, and calcification frequently surround the abnormal vessels.

Capillary telangiectasias are microscopic foci of dilated, thin-walled vascular channels separated by relatively normal brain parenchyma and occurring most frequently in the pons. **Venous angiomas** (varices) consist of aggregates of ectatic venous channels. These latter two types of vascular malformation are unlikely to bleed or cause symptoms, and are most commonly discovered as incidental lesions.

Other Vascular Diseases

Hypertensive Cerebrovascular Disease

The most important effects of hypertension on the brain include massive hypertensive intracerebral hemorrhage (discussed earlier), lacunar infarcts, slit hemorrhages, and hypertensive encephalopathy. Over the past few decades there has been a decreasing threshold for treatment of hypertension and more extensive screening for early disease, both of which have contributed to an overall decline in the incidence of these complications. Nevertheless, these continue to be important diseases because of poor patient compliance or inadequate access to health care.

Hypertension affects the deep penetrating arteries and arterioles that supply the basal ganglia and hemispheric white matter as well as the brain stem. Hypertension causes several changes, including hyaline arteriolar sclerosis in arterioles. Arteriolar walls affected by hyaline change are weaker than are normal vessels and are more vulnerable to rupture. In some instances, chronic hypertension is associated with the development of minute aneurysms in vessels that are less than 300 μm in diameter. These *Charcot-Bouchard microaneurysms* can rupture.

An important clinical and pathologic outcome of arteriolar sclerosis is the development of *lacunes* or *lacunar infarcts*. These small cavitary infarcts are just a few millimeters wide (<15 mm as an arbitrary definition). They are found most commonly in deep gray matter (basal ganglia and thalamus), internal capsule, deep white matter, and pons, and they consist of cavities of tissue loss with scattered lipid-laden macrophages and surrounding gliosis. Depending on their location in the CNS, lacunes can either be clinically silent or cause significant neurologic impairment.

Hypertension also gives rise to rupture of the small-caliber penetrating vessels and the development of small hemorrhages. In time, these hemorrhages resorb, leaving behind a slitlike cavity (*slit hemorrhage*) surrounded by brownish discoloration.

Acute hypertensive encephalopathy is a clinicopathologic syndrome characterized by diffuse cerebral dysfunction, including headaches, confusion, vomiting, and convulsions, sometimes leading to coma. Rapid therapeutic intervention to reduce the accompanying increased intracranial pressure is required, since the syndrome does not usually remit spontaneously. Patients coming to postmortem examination may show an edematous brain, with or without transtentorial or tonsillar herniation. Petechiae and fibrinoid necrosis of arterioles in the gray and white matter may be seen microscopically.

Vasculitis

A variety of inflammatory processes that involve blood vessels may lead to luminal compromise and cerebral infarcts. Infectious arteritis of small and large vessels was previously seen in association with syphilis and tuberculosis, but now more commonly occurs in the setting of immunosuppression and opportunistic infection (such as toxoplasmosis, aspergillosis, and CMV encephalitis). Some of the systemic forms of vasculitis, such as polyarteritis nodosa, may involve cerebral vessels and cause single or multiple infarcts throughout the brain. *Primary angiitis of the CNS* is an inflammatory disorder that involves multiple small to medium-sized parenchymal and subarachnoid vessels and is characterized by chronic inflammation, multinucleated giant cells (with or without granuloma formation), and destruction of the vessel wall. Affected individuals manifest a diffuse encephalopathic clinical picture, often with cognitive dysfunction; improvement occurs with steroid and immunosuppressive treatment.

SUMMARY

Cerebrovascular Diseases

- Stroke is the clinical term for a disease with acute onset of a neurologic deficit as the result of vascular lesions, either hemorrhage or loss of blood supply.

- Cerebral infarction follows loss of blood supply and can be widespread, focal, or affect regions with the least robust vascular supply ("watershed" infarcts).
- Focal cerebral infarcts are most commonly embolic; if there is subsequent fragmentation of an embolism, a nonhemorrhagic infarct can become hemorrhagic.
- Primary intraparenchymal hemorrhages are typically due to either hypertension (most commonly in white matter, deep gray matter, or posterior fossa contents) or cerebral amyloid angiopathy.
- Spontaneous subarachnoid hemorrhage is usually caused by a structural vascular abnormality, such as an aneurysm or arteriovenous malformation.

CENTRAL NERVOUS SYSTEM TRAUMA

Trauma to the brain and spinal cord is a significant cause of death and disability. Severity and site of injury affect the outcome: injury of several cubic centimeters of brain parenchyma may be clinically silent (if in the frontal lobe), severely disabling (spinal cord), or fatal (involving the brain stem).

The magnitude and distribution of traumatic brain lesions depend on the shape of the object causing the trauma, the force of impact, and whether the head is in motion at the time of injury. A blow to the head may be *penetrating* or *blunt;* it may cause an *open* or a *closed injury.* Severe brain damage can occur in the absence of external signs of head injury, and conversely, severe lacerations and even skull fractures do not necessarily indicate damage to the underlying brain. In addition to skull or spinal fractures, trauma can cause parenchymal injury and vascular injury; combinations are common.

Traumatic Parenchymal Injuries

When there is impact of an object with the head, injury may occur from collision of the brain with the skull at the site of impact (a *coup* injury) or on the opposite side (*contrecoup*). Both coup and contrecoup lesions are *contusions,* with comparable gross and microscopic appearances. A contusion is caused by rapid tissue displacement, disruption of vascular channels, and subsequent hemorrhage, tissue injury, and edema. Since they are the points of impact, crests of gyri are most susceptible, whereas cerebral cortex along the sulci is less vulnerable. The most common locations where contusions occur correspond to the most frequent sites of direct impact and to regions of the brain that overlie a rough and irregular inner skull surface, such as the frontal lobes along the orbital gyri and the temporal lobes. If there is penetration of the brain, either by a projectile such as a bullet or a skull fragment from a fracture, a *laceration* occurs, with tissue tearing, vascular disruption, hemorrhage, and injury along a linear path.

Morphology

Contusions, when seen on cross-section, are wedge shaped, with the broad base spanning the surface and centered on the point of impact (Fig. 23–12A). The histologic appearance of contusions is independent of the type of trauma. In the earliest stages there is edema and hemorrhage. During the next few hours, blood extravasates throughout the involved tissue, across the width of the cerebral cortex, and into the white matter and subarachnoid spaces. Although functional effects are seen earlier, morphologic evidence of injury in the neuronal cell body (pyknosis of nucleus, eosinophilia of the cytoplasm, disintegration of cell) takes about 24 hours to appear. The inflammatory response to the injured tissue follows its usual course, with neutrophils preceding the appearance of macrophages. In contrast to ischemic lesions in which the superficial layer of cortex may be preserved and gliotic, trauma affects the superficial layers most severely.

Old traumatic lesions have a characteristic macroscopic appearance: they are depressed, retracted, yellowish brown patches involving the crests of gyri (Fig. 23–12B). More extensive hemorrhagic regions of brain trauma give rise to larger cavitated lesions, which can resemble remote infarcts. In sites of old contusions, gliosis and residual hemosiderin-laden macrophages predominate.

Although injury to the surface of the brain is often the most dramatic, widespread injury to axons within the brain (called *diffuse axonal injury*) can be even more devastating. The movement of one region of brain relative to another is thought to lead to the disruption of axonal integrity and function. Angular acceleration alone, in the absence of impact, may cause axonal injury as well as hemorrhage. As many as 50% of patients who develop coma shortly after trauma, even without cerebral contusions, are believed to have white matter damage and diffuse axonal injury. Although these changes may be widespread, lesions are most commonly found near the angles of the lateral ventricles and in the brain stem.

Diffuse axonal injury is characterized by the wide but often asymmetric distribution of axonal swellings that appears within hours of the injury and may persist for much longer. These are best demonstrated with silver stains or by immunohistochemistry for proteins within axons.

Concussion describes reversible altered consciousness from head injury in the absence of contusion. The characteristic transient neurologic dysfunction includes loss of consciousness, temporary respiratory arrest, and loss of reflexes. Although neurologic recovery is complete, amnesia for the event persists. The pathogenesis of the sudden disruption of nervous activity is unknown.

Traumatic Vascular Injury

Vascular injury is a frequent component of CNS trauma and results from direct trauma and disruption of the

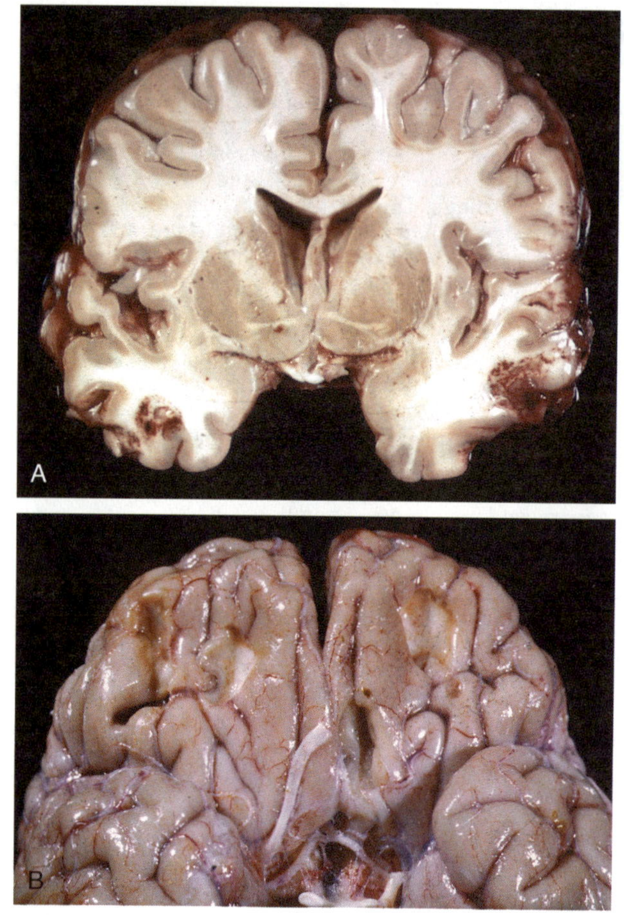

Figure 23–12

Cerebral trauma. **A,** Acute contusions are present in both temporal lobes, with areas of hemorrhage and tissue disruption. **B,** Remote contusions are present on the inferior frontal surface of this brain, with a yellow color (associated with the term *plaque jaune*).

vessel wall, leading to hemorrhage. Depending on which vessels rupture, hemorrhage may occur in any of several compartments (sometimes in combination): *epidural, subdural, subarachnoid,* and *intraparenchymal* (Fig. 23–13A). Subarachnoid and intraparenchymal hemorrhages most often occur at sites of contusions and lacerations.

Epidural Hematoma

The dura is normally tightly applied to the inside of the skull, fused with the periosteum. Vessels that run in the dura, most importantly the middle meningeal artery, are vulnerable to injury, particularly with skull fractures. In children, in whom the skull is deformable, a temporary displacement of the skull bones may tear a vessel in the absence of a skull fracture. Once a vessel has been torn, the accumulation of blood under arterial pressure can cause separation of the dura from the inner surface of the skull (Fig. 23–13B). The expanding hematoma has a smooth inner contour that compresses the brain surface. *Clinically, patients can be lucid for several hours between the moment of trauma and the development of neurologic signs.* An epidural hematoma may expand rapidly and is a neurosurgical emergency requiring prompt drainage.

Subdural Hematoma

The rapid movement of the brain that occurs in trauma can tear the bridging veins that extend from the cerebral hemispheres through the subarachnoid and subdural space to empty into dural sinuses. These vessels are particularly prone to tearing, and their disruption leads to bleeding into the subdural space. In elderly patients with brain atrophy the bridging veins are stretched out and the brain has additional space for movement, accounting for the higher rate of subdural hematomas in these patients, even after relatively minor head trauma. Infants are also susceptible to subdural hematomas because their bridging veins are thin-walled.

Subdural hematomas most often become manifest within the first 48 hours after injury. They are most common over the lateral aspects of the cerebral hemispheres and are bilateral in about 10% of cases. Neurologic signs are attributable to the pressure exerted on the adjacent brain. These may be focal, but often the clinical manifestations are nonlocalizing and include headache or confusion. In time there may be slowly progressive neurologic deterioration, rarely with acute decompensation.

Morphology

On macroscopic examination the acute subdural hematoma appears as a collection of freshly clotted blood apposed along the contour of the brain surface, without extension into the depths of sulci (Fig. 23–13C). The underlying brain is flattened, and the subarachnoid space is often clear. Typically, venous bleeding is self-limited; breakdown and organization of the hematoma take place over time. Subdural hematomas organize by lysis of the clot (about 1 week), growth of fibroblasts from the dural surface into the hematoma (2 weeks), and early development of hyalinized connective tissue (1–3 months). Organized hematomas are attached to the inner surface of the dura and are not adherent to the underlying arachnoid. The lesion can eventually retract as the granulation tissue matures, until there is only a thin layer of reactive connective tissue ("subdural membranes"). Subdural hematomas commonly rebleed (**chronic subdural hematomas**), presumably from the thin-walled vessels of the granulation tissue, leading to microscopic findings consistent with a variety of ages. The treatment of symptomatic subdural hematomas is to remove the organized blood and associated organizing tissue.

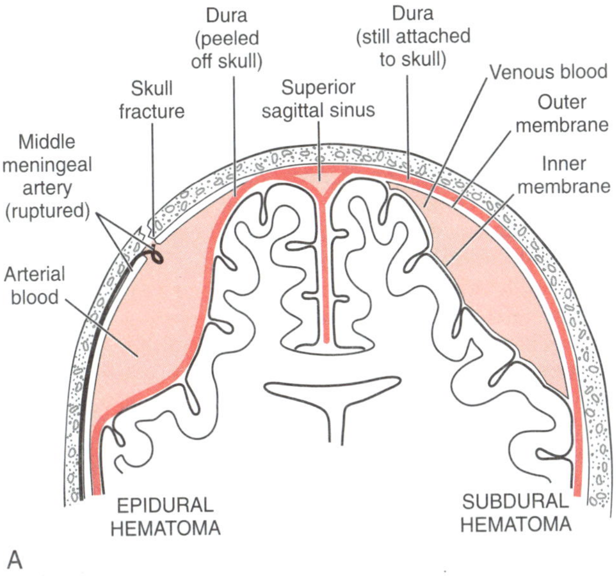

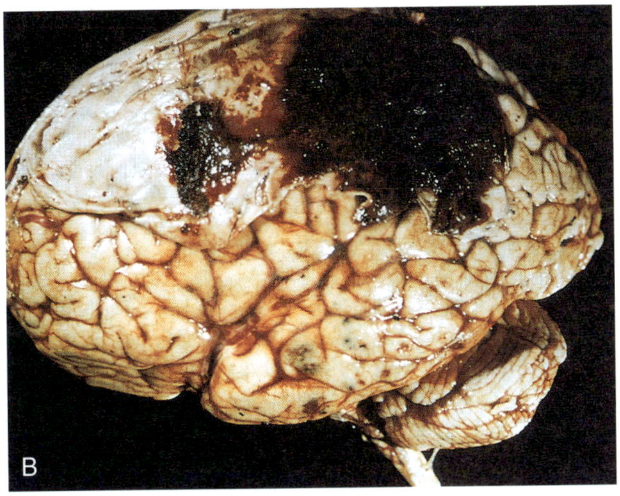

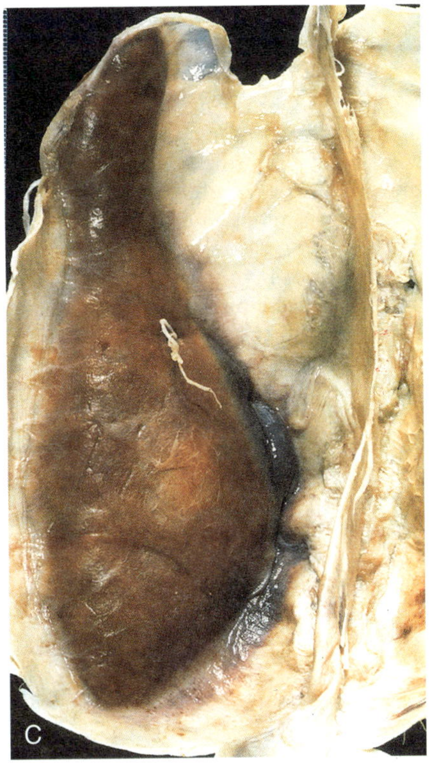

Figure 23–13

Traumatic intracranial hemorrhages. **A,** Epidural hematoma (*left*) in which rupture of a meningeal artery, usually associated with a skull fracture, leads to accumulation of arterial blood between the dura and the skull. In a subdural hematoma (*right*), damage to bridging veins between the brain and the superior sagittal sinus leads to the accumulation of blood between the dura and the arachnoid. **B,** Epidural hematoma covering a portion of the dura. **C,** Large organizing subdural hematoma attached to the dura. (**B,** Courtesy of Dr. Raymond D. Adams, Massachusetts General Hospital, Boston, Massachusetts.)

SUMMARY

Traumatic Parenchymal Injury

- Physical injury to the brain can occur when the inside of the skull comes into forceful contact with the brain.
- If the head is able to move there may be contact between the skull and brain, both at the original point of contact (coup injury) and the opposite side where the brain eventually hits the skull as it moves within it (contrecoup injury).
- Rapid displacement of the head and brain can lead to tearing of axons (diffuse axonal injury), which often causes immediate onset of severe and minimally reversible neurologic deficits.
- T earing of blood vessels associated with trauma can lead to accumulation of blood in any of three spaces: epidural hematoma, subdural hematoma, or subarachnoid hemorrhage.

CONGENITAL MALFORMATIONS AND PERINATAL BRAIN INJURY

The incidence of CNS malformations, giving rise to mental retardation, cerebral palsy, or neural tube defects, is estimated at 1% to 2%. Malformations of the brain are more common in the setting of multiple birth defects. Prenatal or perinatal insults may either cause failure of normal CNS development or result in tissue destruction. Because different parts of the brain develop at different times during gestation (and afterwards), the timing of an injury will be reflected in the pattern of malformation. Although the pathogenesis and etiology of many malformations remain unknown, both genetic and environmental factors are clearly at play. Mutations affecting molecules in pathways of neuronal and glial development, migration, and connection can cause CNS malformation. Additionally, some toxic compounds and infectious agents are known to have teratogenic effects.

Malformations

Neural Tube Defects

Among the earliest stages in brain development is the formation of the neural tube, the inside of which will become the ventricular system and the wall of which will become the brain and spinal cord. Failure of a portion of the neural tube to close, or reopening after successful closure, may lead to one of several malformations. All are characterized by abnormalities involving some combination of neural tissue, menginges, and overlying bone or soft tissues. Collectively, neural tube defects are the most frequent CNS malformations.

Folate deficiency during the initial weeks of gestation is a risk factor; prenatal vitamins are aimed, in part, at reducing this risk. The combination of ultrasound and maternal screening for elevated α-fetoprotein has increased the early detection of neural tube defects. The overall recurrence risk in subsequent pregnancies is 4% to 5%.

The most common neural tube defects involve the spinal cord. These can range from asymptomatic bony defect (spina bifida occulta) to a severe malformation with a flattened, disorganized segment of spinal cord, associated with an overlying meningeal outpouching.

Myelomeningocele is an extension of CNS tissue through a defect in the vertebral column (Fig. 23–14). They occur most commonly in the lumbosacral region; patients have motor and sensory deficits in the lower extremities and problems with bowel and bladder control. The symptoms derive from the abnormal spinal cord in this region, and are often compounded by infections extending from thin or ulcerated overlying skin.

At the other end of the developing brain, *anencephaly* is a malformation of the anterior end of the neural tube, with absence of the brain and top of skull. An *encephalocele* is a diverticulum of malformed CNS tissue extending through a defect in the cranium. It most often involves the occipital region or the posterior fossa. When it occurs anteriorly, brain tissue can extend into the sinuses.

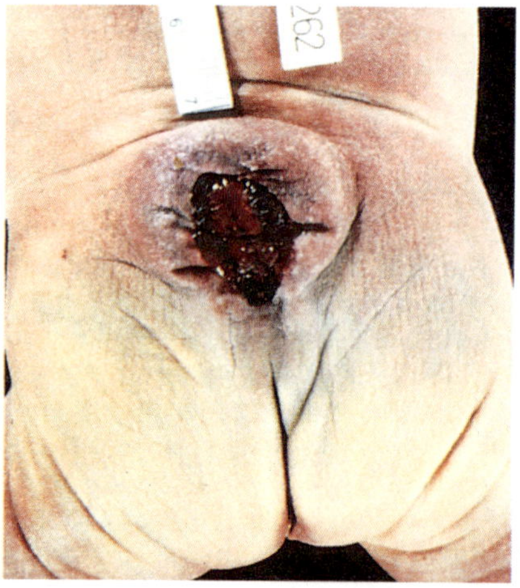

Figure 23–14

Myelomeningocele. These defects occur because the caudal neural tube fails to close properly. In meningomyelocele, both the meninges and spinal cord parenchyma are included in the cystlike structure visible just above the buttocks. Because such lesions expose the CNS to the outside environment, infection is a common complication.

Forebrain Malformations

The volume of brain may be abnormally large (*megalencephaly*) or small (*microencephaly*). Microencephaly, by far the more common of the two, is usually associated with a small head as well (microcephaly). It can occur in a wide range of clinical settings, including chromosome abnormalities, fetal alcohol syndrome, and human immunodeficiency virus 1 (HIV-1) infection acquired in utero. All causes are associated with a decreased number of neurons destined for the cerebral cortex. Disruption of normal neuronal migration and differentiation during development can lead to a disruption of the normal gyration and six-layered neocortical architecture. *Lissencephaly* (*agyria*) or, in case of more patchy involvement, *pachygyria* is characterized by an absence of normal gyration and a smooth-surfaced brain. The cortex is abnormally thickened and is usually only four-layered. Single-gene defects have been identified in some cases of lissencephaly. *Polymicrogyria* is characterized by an increased number of irregularly formed gyri that result in an irregular bumpy or cobblestone-like surface. These changes can be focal or widespread. The normal cortical architecture can be altered in different ways and adjacent gyri often show fusion of the superficial molecular layer. *Holoprosencephaly* is characterized by a disruption of the normal midline patterning. Mild forms may just show absence of the olfactory bulbs and related structures (arrhinencephaly). In severe forms the brain is not divided into hemispheres or lobes. The severe forms may be associated with facial midline defects like cyclopia. Holoprosencephaly as well as polymicrogyria can be the result of acquired or genetically determined disruption of normal development. Several single-gene defects including mutations in sonic hedgehog have been linked to holoprosencephaly.

Posterior Fossa Anomalies

The most common malformations in this region of the brain result in either misplaced or absent cerebellum. Typically, these are associated with hydrocephalus.

The *Arnold-Chiari malformation* (Chiari type II malformation) consists of a small posterior fossa and a misshapen midline cerebellum with downward extension of *vermis* through the foramen magnum; hydrocephalus and a lumbar myelomeningocele are typically also present. In the *Chiari I malformation,* low-lying cerebellar tonsils extend through the foramen magnum at the base of the skull. This can lead to obstruction of CSF flow and compression of the medulla, resulting in symptoms of headache or cranial nerve deficits. Increasing the space for the tissue through neurosurgery can alleviate the symptoms.

Unlike Chiari malformation, the *Dandy-Walker malformation* is characterized by an enlarged posterior fossa. The cerebellar vermis is absent, or present only in rudimentary form in its anterior portion. In its place is a large midline cyst that is lined by ependyma and is contiguous with leptomeninges on its outer surface. Dysplasias of brainstem nuclei are commonly found in association with Dandy-Walker malformation.

Spinal Cord Abnormalities

In addition to neural tube defects, structural alterations inside the spinal cord (and not associated with abnormalities of the bony spine or overlying skin) can occur. These lesions are characterized by a discontinuous or confluent expansion of the ependyma-lined central canal of the cord (*hydromyelia*) or by formation of a fluid-filled cleft-like cavity in the inner portion of the cord (*syringomyelia, syrinx*). A syrinx may also develop as an acquired lesion during life secondary to alterations in CSF flow by tumor or trauma. These lesions are associated with destruction of the adjacent gray and white matter and are surrounded by a dense feltwork of reactive gliosis. The cervical spinal cord is most often affected.

Perinatal Brain Injury

A variety of exogenous factors can injure the developing brain. Injuries that occur early in gestation may destroy brain tissue without evoking the usual "reactive" changes in the parenchyma and therefore may be difficult to distinguish from malformations. Brain injury occurring in the perinatal period is an important cause of childhood neurologic disability. *Cerebral palsy* is a term for nonprogressive neurologic motor deficits characterized by spasticity, dystonia, ataxia/athetosis, and paresis attributable to injury occurring during the prenatal and perinatal periods. Signs and symptoms may not be apparent at birth and declare themselves only later as development proceeds.

Two major types of injury occur in the perinatal period: hemorrhages and/or infarcts. These are different from the otherwise similar lesions in adults because of their locations and the types of reaction in the surrounding tissue. In premature infants there is an increased risk of *intraparenchymal hemorrhage* within the germinal matrix, near the junction between the thalamus and the caudate nucleus. Hemorrhages may extend into the ventricular system and thence to the subarachnoid space, sometimes leading to hydrocephalus. Infarcts may occur in the supratentorial periventricular white matter (*periventricular leukomalacia*), especially in premature babies. The residua of these infarcts are chalky yellow plaques consisting of discrete regions of white matter necrosis and mineralization (Fig. 23–15). When severe enough to involve the gray and white matter, large cystic lesions can develop throughout the hemispheres; this condition is termed *multicystic encephalopathy.*

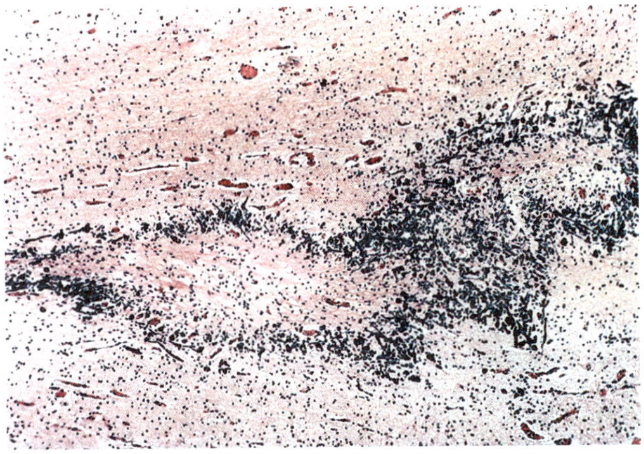

Figure 23–15

Perinatal brain injury. Periventricular leukomalacia: central focus of white matter necrosis with a peripheral rim of mineralized axonal processes (staining *blue*).

- Perinatal brain injury mostly takes one of two forms: either hemorrhage, often in the region of the germinal matrix with the risk of extension into the ventricular system, or ischemic lesions, leading to periventricular leukomalacia.

SUMMARY

Congenital Malformations and Perinatal Brain Injury

- Malformations of the brain can occur because of genetic factors or external insults.
- The timing of the injury will determine the pattern of the injury, based on the type of developmental processes occurring at the point of injury.
- Patterns of malformation include alterations in the closure of the neural tube, proper formation of the separate portions of the neural tissue, and migration of neurons to the appropriate locations.

INFECTIONS OF THE NERVOUS SYSTEM

The brain and its coverings, as with all other parts of the body, can be affected by infections. Some infectious agents have a relative or absolute predilection for the nervous system (such as rabies), while others can affect many other organs as well as the brain (such as *Staphylococcus aureus* and other bacteria). Damage to nervous tissue may be the consequence of direct injury of neurons or glia by the infectious agent, or it may occur indirectly through the elaboration of microbial toxins, the destructive effects of the inflammatory response, or the influence of immune-mediated mechanisms.

An infectious agent must use one of several different possible routes of entry to cause disease in the nervous system.

- *Hematogenous spread* via the arterial blood supply is the most common means of entry. There can also be retrograde venous spread, through the anastomoses between veins of the face and the venous sinuses of the skull.
- *Direct implantation* of microorganisms is almost invariably post-traumatic, with introduction of foreign material. It can, in rare cases, be iatrogenic, as when microbes are introduced with a lumbar puncture needle.
- *Local extension* from an established infection in the skull or spine can occur. The infection may originate in an air sinus, most often the mastoid or frontal; from an infected tooth; from a surgical site in the cranium

or spine causing osteomyelitis, bone erosion, and propagation of the infection into the CNS; or from a congenital malformation, such as meningomyelocele.

• *Peripheral nerves* can also serve as the path of entry of a few pathogens, in particular certain viruses, such as rabies and herpes zoster.

Epidural and Subdural Infections

These spaces can be involved with bacterial or fungal infections, usually as a consequence of direct local spread. Epidural abscess, commonly associated with osteomyelitis, arises from an adjacent focus of infection, such as sinusitis or a surgical procedure. When the process occurs in the spinal epidural space, it may cause spinal cord compression and constitute a neurosurgical emergency. Infections of the skull or air sinuses may also spread to the subdural space, producing subdural empyema. The underlying arachnoid and subarachnoid spaces are usually unaffected, but a large subdural empyema may produce a mass effect. In addition, thrombophlebitis may develop in the bridging veins that cross the subdural space, resulting in venous occlusion and infarction of the brain. Symptoms include those referable to the source of the infection. Most patients are febrile, with headache and neck stiffness, and if untreated may develop focal neurologic signs, lethargy, and coma. With treatment, including surgical drainage, resolution of the empyema occurs from the dural side; if resolution is complete, a thickened dura may be the only residual finding. With prompt treatment, complete recovery is usual.

Meningitis

Meningitis is an inflammatory process of the leptomeninges and CSF within the subarachnoid space. Meningoencephalitis develops with spread of the infection from the meninges into the underlying brain. Meningitis is usually caused by an infection, but *chemical meningitis* may also occur in response to a nonbacterial irritant introduced into the subarachnoid space. Infectious meningitis is broadly classified into *acute pyogenic* (usually bacterial), *aseptic* (usually viral), and *chronic* (usually tuberculous, spirochetal, or cryptococcal) on the basis of the characteristics of inflammatory exudate on CSF examination and the clinical evolution of the illness.

Acute Pyogenic Meningitis (Bacterial Meningitis)

While a wide range of bacteria can cause acute pyogenic meningitis, there is a relationship between the age of a patient and the most likely organisms. In neonates, common organisms are *Escherichia coli* and the group B streptococci; at the other extreme of life, *Streptococcus pneumoniae* and *Listeria monocytogenes* are more common. Among adolescents and in young adults, *Neisseria meningitides* is the most common pathogen, with occasional clusters of cases representing public health concerns. Regardless of the organism, patients typically show systemic signs of infection superimposed on clinical evidence of meningeal irritation and neurologic impairmentincluding headache, photophobia, irritability, clouding of consciousness, and neck stiffness. Lumbar puncture reveals an increased pressure, abundant neurophils, elevated protein, and reduced glucose. Bacteria may be seen on a smear or can be cultured, sometimes a few hours before the neutrophils appear. If untreated, pyogenic meningitis can be fatal; however, effective antimicrobial agents have markedly reduced the mortality.

Morphology

In acute meningitis, an exudate is evident within the leptomeninges over the surface of the brain (Fig. 23–16A). The meningeal vessels are engorged and prominent. From the areas of greatest accumulation, tracts of pus can be followed along blood vessels on the brain surface. When the meningitis is fulminant, the inflammatory cells infiltrate the walls of the leptomeningeal veins and may spread into the substance of the brain (focal cerebritis), or the inflammation may extend to the ventricles, producing ventriculitis. On microscopic examination, neutrophils fill the entire subarachnoid space in severely affected areas or may be found predominantly around the leptomeningeal blood vessels in less severe cases. In untreated meningitis, Gram stain reveals varying numbers of the causative organism. Bacterial meningitis may be associated with abscesses in the brain (Fig. 23–16B), discussed later. Phlebitis may also lead to venous occlusion and hemorrhagic infarction of the underlying brain. If treated early, there may be little evidence of the infection after it resolves.

Aseptic Meningitis (Viral Meningitis)

Aseptic meningitis is a misnomer; it is a clinical term for an illness comprising meningeal irritation, fever, and alterations of consciousness of relatively acute onset without recognizable organisms. The clinical course is less fulminant than in pyogenic meningitis, is usually self-limiting, and most often is treated symptomatically. The CSF shows an increased number of lymphocytes (pleiocytosis), the protein elevation is only moderate, and glucose content is nearly always normal. In approximately 70% of cases, a pathogen can eventually be identified, most commonly an enterovirus. There are no distinctive macroscopic characteristics except for brain swelling, seen in only some instances. On microscopic examination, there is either no recognizable abnormality or a mild to moderate infiltration of the leptomeninges with lymphocytes.

Chronic Meningitis

Several pathogens, including mycobacteria and some spirochetes, are associated with chronic meningitis; for these organisms there may also be a parenchymal component of the disease.

Tuberculous Meningitis

Tuberculous meningitis usually presents with generalized symptoms of headache, malaise, mental confusion, and vomiting. There is only a moderate increase in cellularity

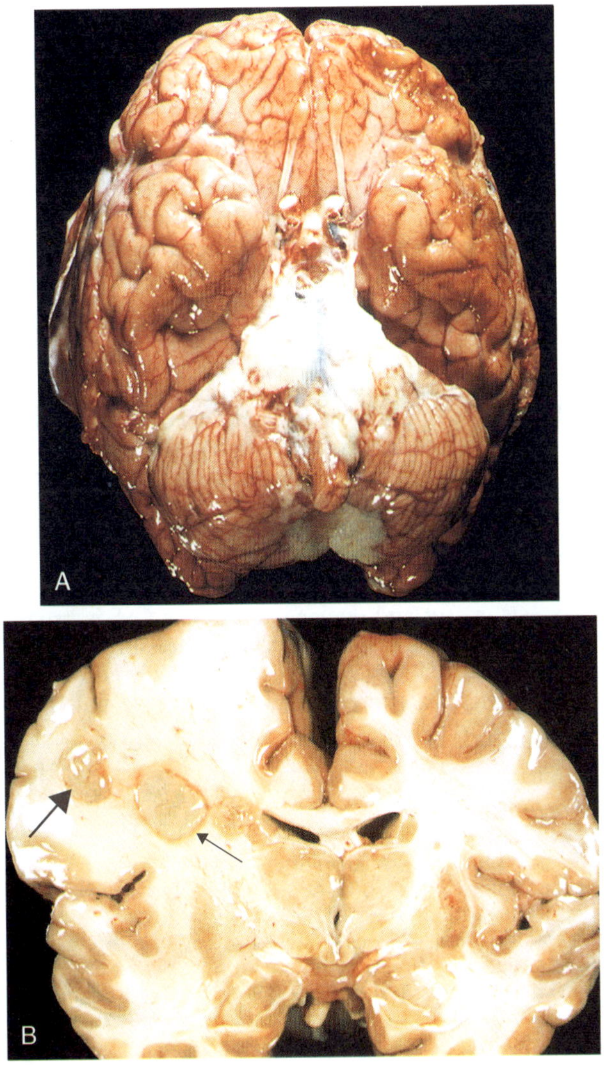

Figure 23–16

Bacterial infections. **A,** Pyogenic meningitis. A thick layer of suppurative exudate covers the brain stem and cerebellum, and thickens the leptomeninges. **B,** Cerebral abscesses in the frontal white matter (*arrows*). (**A,** From Golden JA, Louis DN: Images in clinical medicine: acute bacterial meningitis. N Engl J Med 333:364, 1994. Copyright © 1994 Massachusetts Medical Society. All rights reserved.)

of the CSF (pleiocytosis) made up of mononuclear cells, or a mixture of polymorphonuclear and mononuclear cells; the protein level is elevated, often strikingly so, and the glucose content typically is moderately reduced or normal. Infection with *Mycobacterium tuberculosis* may also result in a well-circumscribed intraparenchymal mass (*tuberculoma*), which may be associated with meningitis. Chronic tuberculous meningitis is a cause of arachnoid fibrosis, which may produce hydrocephalus.

Morphology

The subarachnoid space contains a gelatinous or fibrinous exudate, most often at the base of the brain, obliterating the cisterns and encasing cranial nerves. There may be discrete white granules scattered over the leptomeninges. Arteries running through the subarachnoid space may show **obliterative endarteritis** with inflammatory infiltrates in their walls and marked intimal thickening. The infection may spread through the CSF to the choroid plexuses and ependymal surface. On microscopic examination there are mixtures of lymphocytes, plasma cells, and macrophages. Florid cases show well-formed granulomas, often with caseous necrosis and giant cells, similar to the lesions of tuberculosis elsewhere in the body. Similar findings are observed in tuberculomas within the brain.

Neurosyphilis

Neurosyphilis is a tertiary stage of syphilis and occurs in only about 10% of individuals with untreated infection. One of the major manifestations is meningeal, called meningovascular neurosyphilis. As with other chronic infections, there can be parenchymal disease as well. *Paretic neurosyphilis* is caused by invasion of the brain by *Treponema pallidum* and manifests as insidious but progressive loss of mental and physical functions with mood alterations (including delusions of grandeur), terminating in severe dementia. *Tabes dorsalis* is another form of neurosyphilis, resulting from damage to the sensory nerves in the dorsal roots producing impaired joint position sense and resultant ataxia (locomotor ataxia); loss of pain sensation, leading to skin and joint damage (Charcot joints); other sensory disturbances, particularly characteristic "lightning pains"; and absence of deep tendon reflexes. Individuals with HIV infection are at increased risk for neurosyphilis, and the rate of progression and severity of the disease seem to be accelerated. These individuals may have asymptomatic infection, acute syphilitic meningitis, or meningovascular syphilis; direct parenchymal invasion of the brain is much less common.

Morphology

Meningovascular neurosyphilis is a chronic meningitis usually involving the base of the brain and sometimes the cerebral convexities and the spinal leptomeninges. As with tuberculous meningitis, there may be an associated obliterative endarteritis, but in this situation it has a distinctive perivascular inflammatory reaction rich in plasma cells and lymphocytes. **Cerebral gummas** (mass lesions rich in plasma cells) may also occur in relation to meninges and extend into the brain. When **paretic neurosyphilis** is present there is parenchymal damage particularly in the frontal lobe, characterized by loss of neurons with proliferation of microglia (rod cells) and gliosis. The spirochetes can rarely be demonstrated in tissue sections. The findings in **tabes dorsalis** consist of loss of both axons and myelin in the dorsal roots, with pallor and atrophy in the dorsal columns of the spinal cord.

Neuroborreliosis represents involvement of the nervous system by the spirochete *Borrelia burgdorferi,* the pathogen of Lyme disease. Neurologic symptoms are highly variable and include aseptic meningitis, facial nerve palsies, mild encephalopathy, and polyneuropathies.

Parenchymal Infections

The entire gamut of microbial organisms (virus to parasites) can potentially infect the brain. The different types of pathogens have different patterns of involvement, although the distinctions are not absolute. In general, viral infections produce the most diffuse involvement, bacteria (when not associated with meningitis) produce the most localized, and other organisms give more mixed patterns. In patients with underlying immunosuppression, more widespread involvement with any agent is typical.

Brain Abscesses

Brain abscesses are nearly always caused by bacterial infections; these can arise by direct implantation of organisms, local extension from adjacent foci (mastoiditis, paranasal sinusitis), or hematogenous spread (usually from a primary site in the heart, lungs, or distal bones or after tooth extraction). Predisposing conditions include acute bacterial endocarditis, which tends to produce multiple abscesses; cyanotic congenital heart disease, in which there is a right-to-left shunt and loss of pulmonary filtration of organisms; and chronic pulmonary sepsis, as in bronchiectasis.

Abscesses are destructive lesions, and patients almost invariably present clinically with progressive focal deficits in addition to the general signs of raised intracranial pressure. The CSF white cell count and protein level are raised, but the glucose content is normal. A systemic or local source of infection may be apparent, or a small systemic focus may have ceased to be symptomatic. The increased intracranial pressure and progressive herniation can be fatal, and abscess rupture can lead to ventriculitis, meningitis, and venous sinus thrombosis. With surgery and antibiotics, the otherwise high mortality rate can be reduced, with earlier intervention leading to better outcomes.

Morphology

Abscesses are discrete lesions with central liquefactive necrosis and a surrounding fibrous capsule (Fig. 23–16B). On microscopic examination, there is exuberant neovascularization around the necrosis that is responsible for the marked edema and formation of granulation tissue. Outside the fibrous capsule is a zone of reactive gliosis.

Viral Encephalitis

Viral encephalitis is a parenchymal infection of the brain that is almost invariably associated with meningeal inflammation (and therefore is better termed *meningoencephalitis*). While different viruses may show varying patterns of injury, the most characteristic histologic features are perivascular and parenchymal mononuclear cell infiltrates, microglial nodules, and neuronophagia (Fig. 23–17A, B). Certain viruses may form inclusion bodies.

The nervous system is particularly susceptible to viruses such as rabies and polio. Some viruses infect specific CNS cell types, while others preferentially involve particular areas of the brain (such as medial temporal lobes, limbic system) because of their routes of entry. In addition to direct infection of the nervous system, the CNS can also be injured by immune mechanisms after systemic viral infections. Intrauterine viral infection may cause *congenital malformations,* as occurs with rubella.

Arboviruses

Arboviruses (arthropod-borne viruses) are an important cause of epidemic encephalitis, especially in tropical regions of the world, and are capable of causing serious morbidity and high mortality. Among the more commonly encountered types are Eastern and Western equine encephalitis and West Nile virus. Animal hosts act as disease reservoirs for the arboviruses, which are mostly transmitted by mosquitoes. Patients develop generalized neurologic symptoms, such as seizures, confusion, delirium, and stupor or coma, as well as focal signs, such as reflex asymmetry and ocular palsies. The CSF is usually colorless but with a slightly elevated pressure and, initially, a neutrophilic pleiocytosis that rapidly converts to lymphocytes; the protein level is elevated, but sugar content is normal.

Morphology

Although the various arbovirus encephalitides differ in epidemiology and prognosis, their histopathologic picture is similar albeit of differing severity and extent. Characteristically, there is a lymphocytic meningoencephalitis (sometimes with neutrophils) with a typically perivascular distribution (Fig. 23–17A). Multifocal gray and white matter necrosis is seen; there is evidence of individual neuronal necrosis with phagocytosis of the debris, termed neuronophagia; localized collections of microglia, termed microglial nodules, are often present (Fig. 23–17B). In severe cases there may be a necrotizing vasculitis with associated focal hemorrhages.

Herpes Simplex Virus Type 1

Herpes simplex virus (HSV) type 1 produces an encephalitis that occurs in any age group but is most common in children and young adults. Only some patients have prior oral herpetic lesions. The most common presenting symptoms are alterations in mood, memory, and behavior, reflecting the involvement of frontal and temporal lobes.

Morphology

Herpes encephalitis starts in, and most severely involves, the inferior and medial regions of the temporal lobes and the orbital gyri of the frontal lobes (Fig. 23–17C). The infection is necrotizing and often hemorrhagic in the most severely affected regions. Perivascular inflammatory infiltrates are usually present, and Cowdry type A intranuclear viral inclusion bodies can be found in both neurons and glia.

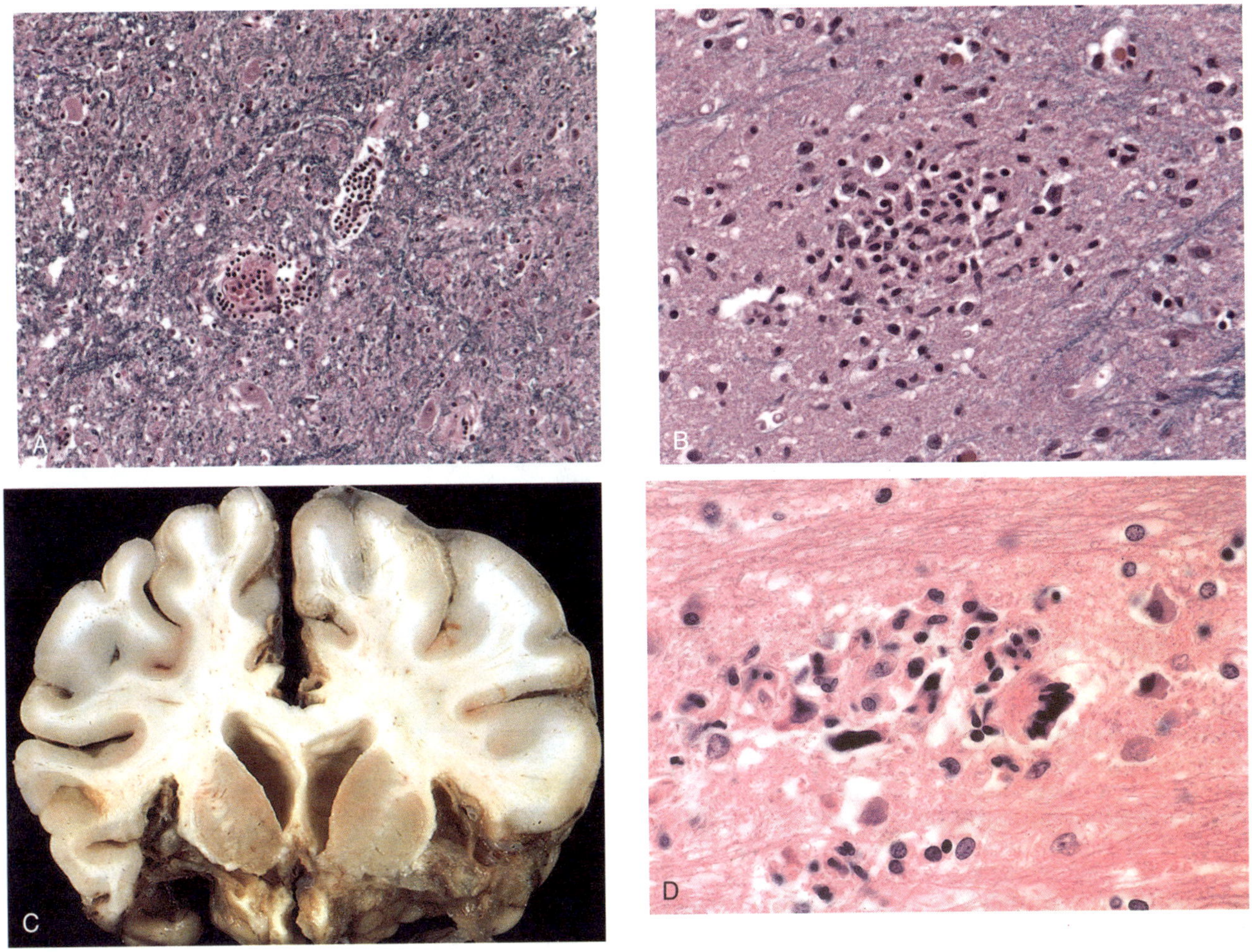

Figure 23–17

Viral infections. Characteristic findings of viral meningitis include perivascular cuffs of lymphocytes (**A**) and microglial nodules (**B**). **C**, Herpes encephalitis showing extensive destruction of inferior frontal and anterior temporal lobes. **D**, HIV encephalitis. Note the microglial nodule and multinucleated giant cell. (**C**, Courtesy of Dr. T.W. Smith, University of Massachusetts Medical School, Worcester.)

Herpes Simplex Virus Type 2

HSV-2 also affects the nervous system and usually manifests in adults as a meningitis. Disseminated severe encephalitis occurs in many neonates born by vaginal delivery to women with active primary HSV genital infections. The dependence on route of delivery indicates that the infection is acquired during passage through the birth canal rather than transplacentally.

Varicella-Zoster Virus (Herpes Zoster)

Varicella-zoster virus (VZV) causes chickenpox during its primary infection, usually without any evidence of neurologic involvement. The virus establishes latent infection in neurons of dorsal root ganglia. Reactivation in adults manifests as a painful, vesicular skin eruption in the distribution of one or a few dermatomes (*shingles*). This is usually a self-limited process, but there may be a persistent pain syndrome in the affected region (*post-herpetic neuralgia*).

VZV may cause a granulomatous arteritis, which may cause infarcts. In immunosuppressed patients, acute herpes zoster encephalitis can occur. Inclusion bodies can be found in glia and neurons.

Cytomegalovirus

CMV infects the nervous system in fetuses and immunosuppressed individuals. The outcome of infection in utero is periventricular necrosis that produces severe brain destruction followed later by microcephaly with periventricular calcification. CMV is a common opportunistic viral pathogen in individuals with acquired immunodeficiency syndrome (AIDS).

Morphology

The most common pattern of involvement in the immunosuppressed patient is that of a subacute encephalitis, associated with CMV inclusion-bearing cells. Although any type of cell within the CNS (neurons, glia, ependyma, endothelium) can be infected by CMV, there is a tendency for the virus to localize in the paraventricular subependymal regions of the brain. This results in a severe hemorrhagic necrotizing ventriculoencephalitis and choroid plexitis.

Poliovirus

Poliovirus is an enterovirus that causes paralytic poliomyelitis. Although it has been eradicated by immunization in many parts of the world, there are still many regions where it remains a problem. Infection with poliovirus most often causes a subclinical or mild gastroenteritis; in a small fraction of cases it secondarily invades the nervous system and damages motor neurons in the spinal cord and brain stem. With loss of motor neurons, it produces a flaccid paralysis with muscle wasting and hyporeflexia in the corresponding region of the body. In the acute disease, death can occur from paralysis of respiratory muscles. *Post-polio syndrome* is a poorly understood progressive weakness associated with decreased muscle bulk and pain, typically developing 25 to 35 years after the resolution of the initial illness.

Rabies

Rabies is a severe encephalitis transmitted to humans by the bite of a rabid animal; various animals are the natural reservoir for the virus. Exposure to some species of bat, even without a bite, is also a risk factor for developing infection. Virus enters the CNS by ascending along the peripheral nerves from the wound site, so the incubation period depends on the distance between the wound and the brain, usually taking a few months. The disease manifests initially with nonspecific symptoms of malaise, headache, and fever. As the infection advances, the patient shows extraordinary CNS excitability; the slightest touch is painful, with violent motor responses progressing to convulsions. Contracture of the pharyngeal musculature may create an aversion to swallowing even water (hydrophobia). Periods of alternating mania and stupor progress to coma and death from respiratory center failure.

Human Immunodeficiency Virus

HIV can have direct effects on the nervous system as well as setting the stage for opportunistic infections or tumors that can involve the nervous system (Table 23–1). As many as 60% of individuals with AIDS develop neurologic dysfunction during the course of their illness; in some, it dominates the clinical picture. Patterns of direct injury to the brain include:

- *Aseptic HIV-1 meningitis* occurring within 1 to 2 weeks of seroconversion in about 10% of patients. This is associated with a mild lymphocytic meningitis, perivascular inflammation, and some myelin loss in the hemispheres.
- *HIV-1 meningoencephalitis (subacute encephalitis)* causing AIDS-dementia complex. This dementia begins insidiously with mental slowing, memory loss, and mood disturbances, such as apathy and depression. The brains of individuals with HIV-1 encephalitis show chronic inflammatory reaction with widely distributed infiltrates of microglial nodules containing macrophage-derived multinucleated giant cells (Fig. 23–17D). It is thought that neuronal injury follows the secretion of cytokines and chemokines from HIV-infected cells of the macrophage lineage.

Table 23–1 Primary HIV-Associated Neurologic Disorders

Central Nervous System
Primary HIV encephalopathies
Multinucleate giant-cell encephalitis (HIV encephalitis)
HIV-associated white matter disease (HIV leukoencephalopathy)
Neocortical/gray matter disease (HIV poliodystrophy)
Mixed patterns
Vacuolar myelopathy
Lymphocytic meningitis
Acute, monophasic meningitis
Chronic aseptic meningitis
Cerebral vasculitis
Peripheral Nervous System
Distal symmetric polyneuropathy
Inflammatory demyelinating neuropathies
Spinal and cranial radiculitis
Vasculitic neuropathy
Skeletal Muscle
Inflammatory myopathy (polymyositis)
Mitochondrial myopathy
Nemaline myopathy

HIV, human immunodeficiency virus.

- *Vacuolar myelopathy* involving the tracts of the spinal cord can resemble subacute combined degeneration, although serum levels of vitamin B_{12} are normal. The pathogenesis of the lesion is unknown; it does not appear to be caused directly by HIV-1, and virus is not present within the lesions.

Progressive Multifocal Leukoencephalopathy (PML)

PML is caused by JC virus, a polyomavirus. The virus preferentially infects oligodendrocytes, so demyelination is its principal pathologic effect. The disease occurs almost invariably in immunosuppressed individuals in various clinical settings, including chronic lymphoproliferative or myeloproliferative illnesses, immunosuppressive therapy, and AIDS. Most people show serologic evidence of exposure to JC virus during childhood, and it is believed that PML results from virus reactivation because of immunosuppression. Patients develop focal and relentlessly progressive neurologic symptoms and signs, and imaging studies show extensive, often multifocal, ring-enhancing lesions in the hemispheric or cerebellar white matter.

Morphology

The lesions consist of patches of irregular, ill-defined destruction of the white matter that enlarge as the disease progresses (Fig. 23–18). Each lesion is an area of demyelination, in the center of which are scattered lipid-laden macrophages and a reduced number of axons. At the edge of the lesion are greatly enlarged oligodendrocyte nuclei whose chromatin is replaced by glassy amphophilic viral inclusion. The virus also infects astrocytes, leading to bizarre giant forms with irregular, hyperchromatic, sometimes multiple nuclei that can be mistaken for tumor.

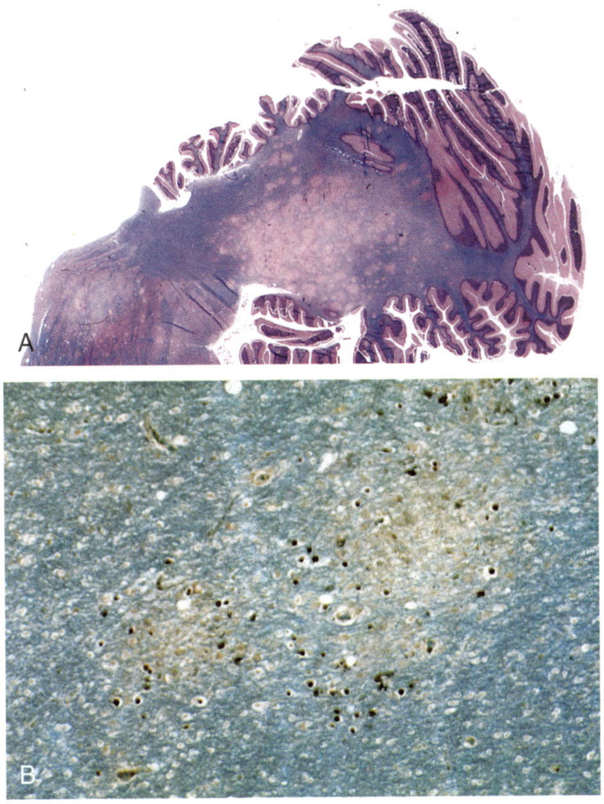

Figure 23–18

Progressive multifocal leukoencephalopathy. **A,** Section stained for myelin showing irregular, poorly defined areas of demyelination, which become confluent in places. **B,** Enlarged oligodendrocyte nuclei stained for viral antigens surround an area of early myelin loss.

Fungal Encephalitis

Candida albicans, Mucor, Aspergillus fumigatus, and *Cryptococcus neoformans* are the most common fungi that can cause encephalitis, but in endemic areas, *Histoplasma capsulatum, Coccidioides immitis,* and *Blastomyces dermatitidis* can also infect the CNS, especially in the setting of immunosuppression.

Parenchymal invasion, usually in the form of granulomas or abscesses, can occur with most of the fungi and often coexists with a meningitis. *Candida* usually produces multiple microabscesses, with or without granuloma formation. Although most fungi invade the brain by hematogenous dissemination, direct extension may also occur, particularly with *Mucor,* most commonly in diabetics with ketoacidosis. *Aspergillus* tends to cause a distinctive pattern of widespread septic hemorrhagic infarctions because of its marked predilection for invasion of blood vessel walls and subsequent thrombosis.

Cryptococcal meningitis and meningoencephalitis is observed often in association with AIDS. It can be fulminant and fatal in as little as 2 weeks, or indolent, or it can evolve over months or years. The CSF may have few cells but a high level of protein. The mucoid encapsulated yeasts can be visualized in the CSF by India ink preparations and in tissue sections by PAS and mucicarmine as well as silver stains (Fig. 23–19).

Other Meningoencephalitides

While a wide range of other organisms can infect the nervous system and its covering, only three will be considered here.

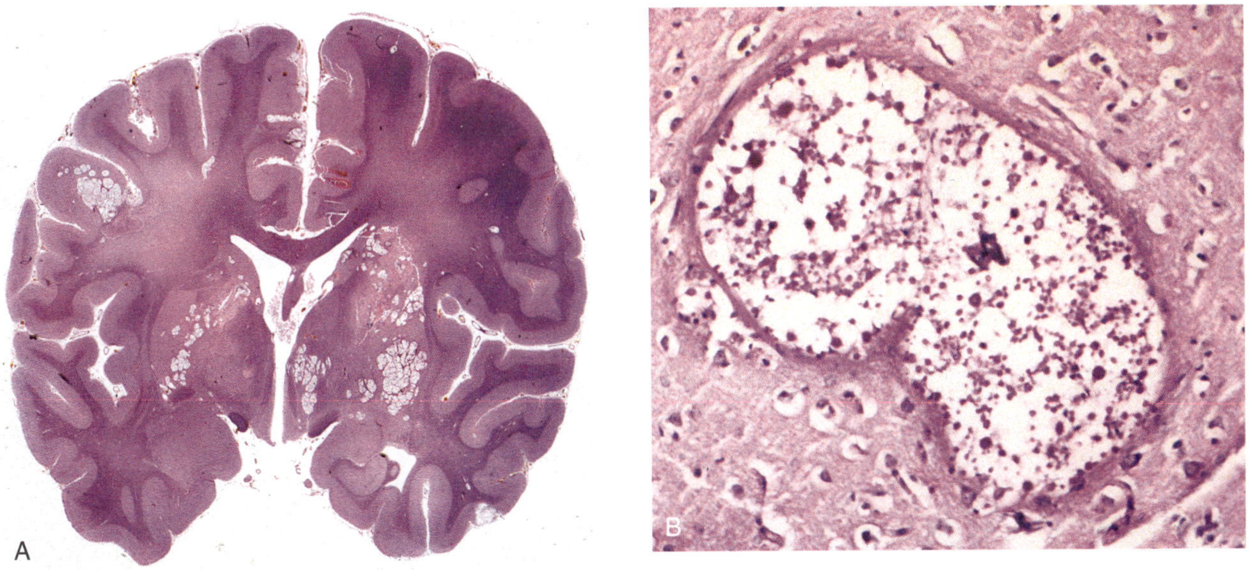

Figure 23–19

Cryptococcal infection. **A,** Whole-brain section showing the numerous areas of tissue destruction associated with the spread of organisms in the perivascular spaces. **B,** At higher magnification it is possible to see the cryptococci in the lesions.

Cerebral Toxoplasmosis

Cerebral toxoplasmosis—infection with the protozoan *Toxoplasma gondii*—is one of the most common causes of neurologic symptoms and morbidity in persons with AIDS. The clinical symptoms are subacute, evolving during a 1- or 2-week period, and may be both focal and diffuse. Computed tomography and magnetic resonance imaging studies can show multiple ring-enhancing lesions; however, this radiographic appearance is not pathognomonic.

Morphology

The brain shows abscesses, frequently multiple, most often involving the cerebral cortex (near the gray-white junction) and deep gray nuclei. Acute lesions consist of central foci of necrosis with variable petechiae surrounded by acute and chronic inflammation, macrophage infiltration, and vascular proliferation. Both free tachyzoites and encysted bradyzoites may be found at the periphery of the necrotic foci.

Cysticercosis

Cysticercosis is the consequence of an end-stage infection by the tapeworm *Tenia solium*. Because humans are an accidental (and inappropriate) host, larvae that inadvertently infect humans will encyst. These cysts can be found throughout the body, although they are common within the brain and subarachnoid space. They typically present as a mass lesion and can cause seizures. Symptoms can intensify when the organism dies within the cyst, as happens after therapy.

Morphology

The organism is encysted within a smooth lining; around the cyst, there is often a marked degree of gliosis. The body wall and hooklets from mouth parts are most commonly recognized. If the organism within the cyst has died, there can be an intense inflammatory infiltrate that will often contain eosinophils.

Amebic meningoencephalitis has different patterns of disease with different species of the parasite. *Naegleria* species, associated with swimming in nonflowing warm fresh water, causes a rapidly fatal necrotizing encephalitis. In contrast, *Acanthamoeba* causes a chronic granulomatous meningoencephalitis.

Prion Diseases

This group of diseases includes sporadic, familial, iatrogenic and variant forms of Creutzfeldt-Jakob disease (CJD). Several animal diseases from this group are also known, including scrapie in sheep and goats and bovine spongiform encephalopathy in cattle ("mad cow" disease). All these disorders are associated with abnormal forms of a normal cellular protein, termed prion protein (PrP^c). The abnormal form of this protein can act as an infectious agent, since it propagates itself and injures the cells in which it is present. Most cases of prion disease are either sporadic or associated with mutations in the gene that encodes PrP^c.

The unique pathogenesis of prion diseases is related to changes in the conformation of PrP from its native PrP^c form to an abnormal configuration called either PrP^{sc} (for scrapie) or PrP^{res} (for protease *res*istant) (Fig. 23–20). In the abnormal conformation, the prion protein becomes resistant to protease digestion. Once formed, PrP^{sc} can then initiate comparable transformation of other PrP^c molecules. The infectious nature of PrP^{sc} protein comes from this ability to propagate the pathologic conformational change. The conformational change can occur spontaneously at an extremely low rate and accounts for sporadic cases of prion disease. If there is a mutation in the gene encoding PrP^c, then the change can occur at a higher rate; this results in familial forms of prion disease.

Accumulation of PrP^{sc} in neural tissue seems to be the cause of cell injury, but how this material leads to the development of cytoplasmic vacuoles and eventual neuronal death is still unknown.

Creutzfeldt-Jakob Disease

CJD is a rare but well-characterized prion disease that manifests clinically as a rapidly progressive dementia. It is sporadic in about 85% of cases, with a worldwide annual incidence of about 1 per million; familial forms also exist. The disease has a peak incidence in the seventh decade. There are well-established cases of iatrogenic transmission by deep implantation electrodes and contaminated preparations of human growth hormone. The clinical presentation begins with subtle changes in memory and behavior that rapidly progress to dementia. The disease is uniformly fatal, with an average duration of only 7 months.

Morphology

The progression of the dementia in CJD is usually so rapid that there is little, if any, macroscopic evidence of brain atrophy. On microscopic examination, the pathognomonic finding is a **spongiform transformation of the cerebral cortex and deep gray matter structures** (caudate, putamen); this consists of a multifocal process that results in the uneven formation of small, apparently empty, microscopic vacuoles of varying sizes within the neuropil and sometimes in the perikaryon of neurons (Fig. 23–20A). In advanced cases, there is severe neuronal loss, reactive gliosis, and sometimes expansion of the vacuolated areas into cyst-like spaces ("status spongiosus"). No inflammatory infiltrate is present. In all forms of prion disease, immunohistochemical staining demonstrates the presence of proteinase K-resistant PrP^{sc} in tissue. Western blotting of tissue extracts after partial protease digestion allows detection of diagnostic PrP^{sc}.

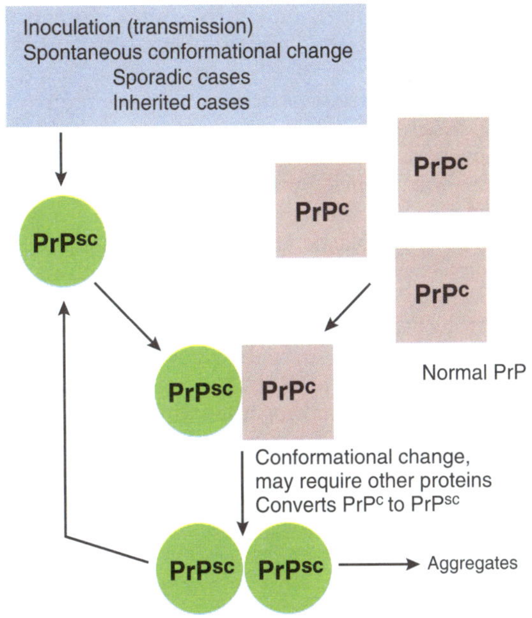

Figure 23–20

Proposed mechanism for the conversion of PrP^c through protein–protein interactions. The initiating molecules of PrP^{sc} may arise through inoculation (as in directly transmitted cases) or through an extremely low-rate spontaneous conformational change. The effect of the mutations in PrP^c is to increase the rate of the conformational change once PrP^{sc} is able to recruit and convert other molecules of PrP^c into the abnormal form of the protein. Although the model is drawn with no other proteins involved, it is possible that other proteins play critical roles in the conversion of Prp^c to PrP^{sc}.

Variant Creutzfeldt-Jakob Disease

Starting in 1995, a series of cases with a CJD-like illness appeared in the United Kingdom. They differed from typical CJD in several important respects: the disease affected young adults, behavioral disorders figured prominently in the early stages of the disease, and the neurologic syndrome progressed more slowly than in individuals with other forms of CJD. The neuropathologic findings and molecular features of these new cases were similar to those of CJD, suggesting a close relationship between the two illnesses. Multiple lines of evidence indicate that this new disease is a consequence of exposure to the prion disease of cattle, bovine spongiform encephalopathy. vCJD has a similar pathologic appearance, in general, to other forms of CJD, with spongiform change and absence of inflammation. In vCJD, however, there are abundant cortical amyloid plaques, surrounded by spongiform change (Fig. 23–21B).

SUMMARY

Infections of the Nervous System

- Pathogens from viruses through parasites can infect the brain; in addition, prion disease represents a form of protein-induced transmissible disease that is unique to the nervous system.
- Different pathogens may use distinct routes to reach the brain, and will cause different patterns of disease.
- Bacterial infections may cause meningitis, cerebral abscesses, or a chronic meningoencephalitis.
- V iral infections can cause meningitis or meningoencephalitis.
- HIV can affect the brain directly with a meningoencephalitis or by increasing the risk of other opportunistic infections (toxoplasmosis, CMV) or CNS lymphoma.
- Prion diseases are transmitted by an altered form of a normal cellular protein. They can be sporadic, transmitted, or inherited.

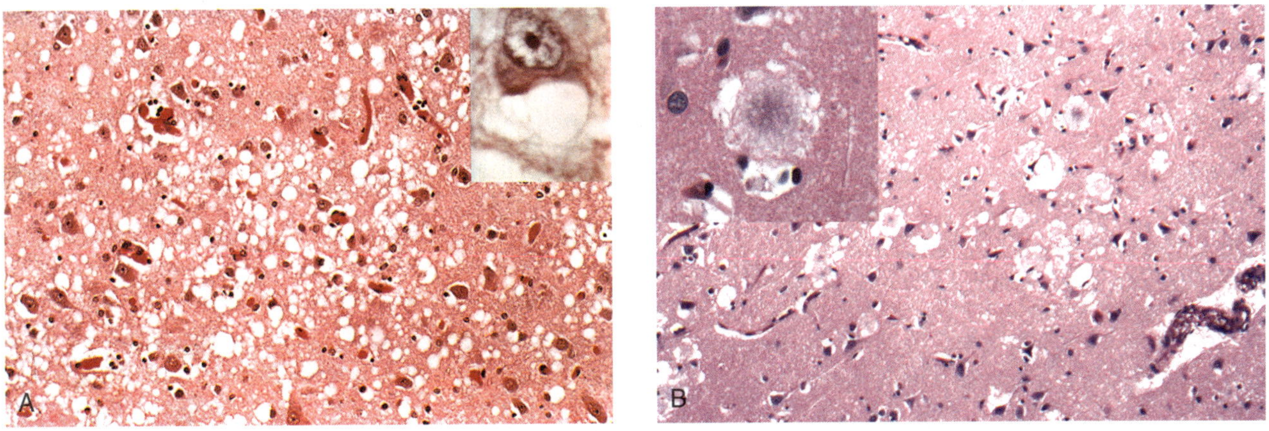

Figure 23–21

Prion disease. **A,** Histology of CJD showing spongiform change in the cerebral cortex. *Inset,* High magnification of neuron with vacuoles. **B,** Variant CJD (vCJD) is characterized by amyloid plaques (see *inset*) that sit in the regions of greatest spongiform change.

TUMORS

The annual incidence of tumors of the CNS ranges from 10 to 17 per 100,000 persons for intracranial tumors and 1 to 2 per 100,000 persons for intraspinal tumors; about half to three-quarters are primary tumors, and the rest are metastatic. Tumors of the CNS are a larger proportion of cancers of childhood, accounting for as many of 20% of all tumors. CNS tumors in childhood differ from those in adults both in histologic subtype and location. In childhood, tumors are likely to arise in the posterior fossa, while in adults they are mostly supratentorial.

Tumors of the nervous system have unique characteristics that set them apart from neoplastic processes elsewhere in the body.

- Histologic distinction between benign and malignant lesions may be more subtle in the CNS than in other organs.
- The pattern of growth of low-grade lesions (low mitotic rate, cellular uniformity, and slow growth) may still include infiltration of large regions of the brain, thereby leading to serious clinical deficits and poor prognosis.
- The anatomic site of the neoplasm can have lethal consequences irrespective of histologic classification; for example, a benign meningioma, by compressing the medulla, can cause cardiorespiratory arrest. Moreover, the ability to resect a lesion may be limited because of its location.
- The pattern of spread of primary CNS neoplasms differs from that of other tumors. Although even the most highly malignant gliomas rarely metastasize outside the CNS, the subarachnoid space does provide a pathway for spread so that seeding along the brain and spinal cord can occur.

Gliomas

Gliomas are tumors of the brain parenchyma that histologically resemble different types of glial cells. The major types of tumor in this category are *astrocytomas, oligodendrogliomas,* and *ependymomas.*

Astrocytoma

Several different categories of astrocytic tumors are recognized, the most common being fibrillary and pilocytic astrocytomas. Astrocytomas have characteristic histologic features, distribution within the brain, age groups typically affected, and clinical course.

Fibrillary Astrocytoma

Fibrillary astrocytomas account for about 80% of adult primary brain tumors. They are most frequent in the fourth through sixth decades. They are usually found in the cerebral hemispheres. The most common presenting signs and symptoms are seizures, headaches, and focal neurologic deficits related to the anatomic site of involvement. Fibrillary astrocytomas show a spectrum of histologic differentiation that correlates well with clinical course and outcome. Based on the degree of differentiation, they are classified into three groups: astrocytoma, anaplastic astrocytoma, and glioblastoma multiforme, the least differentiated of all.

For well-differentiated astrocytomas, symptoms can be static or progress only slowly during a number of years with a mean survival of more than 5 years. Eventually, however, patients usually enter a period of more rapid clinical deterioration that is generally correlated with the appearance of anaplastic features and more rapid growth of the tumor. Many patients present with glioblastoma from the start, rather than having their tumor evolve from a lower grade lesion. Independent of the initial lesion, the prognosis for patients with glioblastoma is very poor. Current state-of-the-art treatment, comprising resection (when feasible) together with radiotherapy and chemotherapy, yields a mean survival of only 8 to 10 months; fewer than 10% of patients are alive after 2 years.

Morphology

The macroscopic appearance of fibrillary astrocytoma is that of a poorly defined, gray, infiltrative tumor that expands and distorts the invaded brain (Fig. 23–22A). Infiltration beyond the grossly evident margins is always present. The cut surface of the tumor is either firm, or soft and gelatinous; cystic degeneration may be seen. In glioblastoma, variation in the gross appearance of the tumor from region to region is characteristic (Fig. 23–22B). Some areas are firm and white, others are soft and yellow (the result of tissue necrosis), and yet others show regions of cystic degeneration and hemorrhage.

Well-differentiated fibrillary astrocytomas are characterized by a mild to moderate increase in the number of glial cell nuclei, somewhat variable nuclear pleomorphism, and an intervening feltwork of fine, GFAP-positive astrocytic cell processes that give the background a fibrillary appearance. The transition between neoplastic and normal tissue is indistinct, and tumor cells can be seen infiltrating normal tissue at some distance from the main lesion. Anaplastic astrocytomas show regions that are more densely cellular and have greater nuclear pleomorphism; increased mitoses are often observed. The highest grade tumor, known as glioblastoma, has a histologic appearance similar to anaplastic astrocytoma with the additional features of **necrosis and vascular or endothelial cell proliferation and pseudo-palisading nuclei** (Fig. 23–22C). High-grade astrocytomas have abnormal vessels that are "leaky" and will show contrast enhancement with imaging studies.

Pilocytic Astrocytoma

Pilocytic astrocytomas are relatively benign tumors, often cystic, that typically occur in children and young adults and are usually located in the cerebellum but may also appear in the floor and walls of the third ventricle, the optic nerves, and occasionally the cerebral hemispheres. Symptomatic recurrence from incompletely resected lesions is often associated with cyst enlargement rather

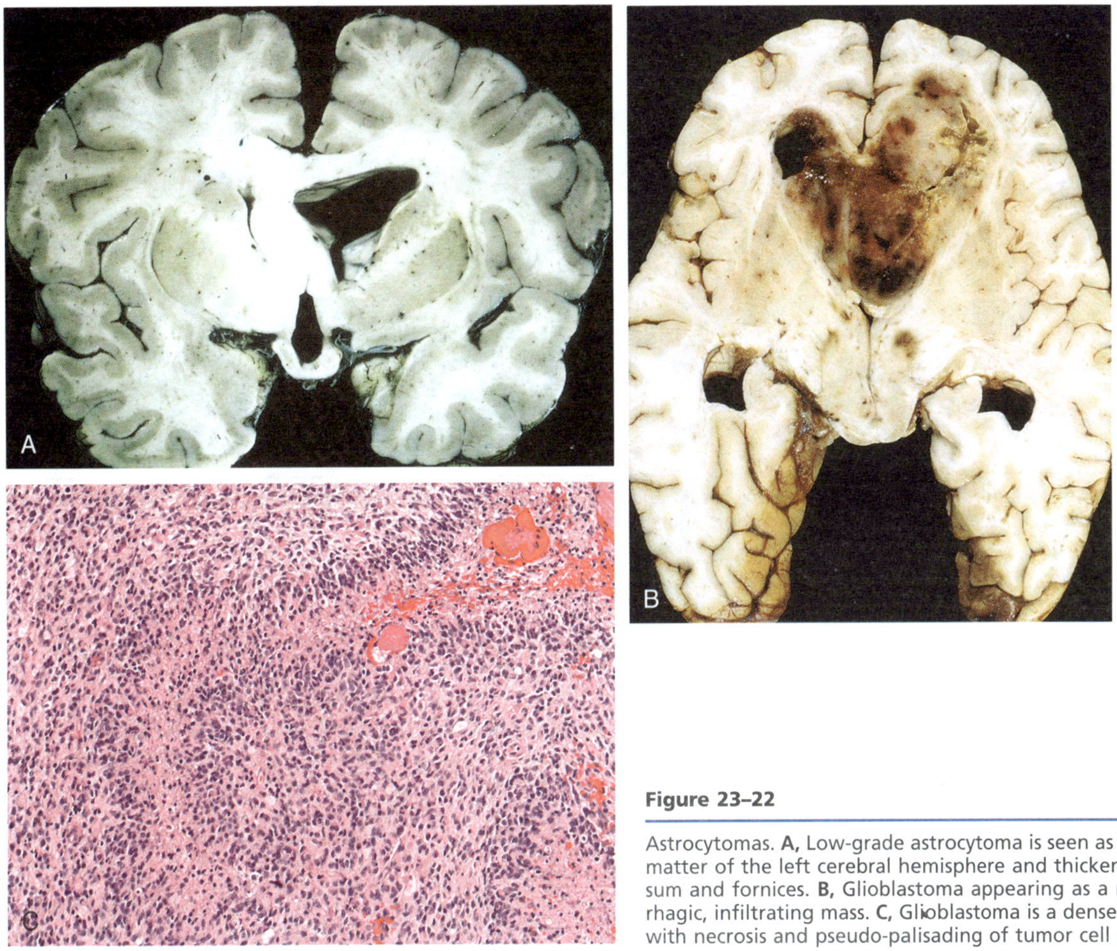

Figure 23–22

Astrocytomas. **A,** Low-grade astrocytoma is seen as expanded white matter of the left cerebral hemisphere and thickened corpus callosum and fornices. **B,** Glioblastoma appearing as a necrotic, hemorrhagic, infiltrating mass. **C,** Glioblastoma is a densely cellular tumor with necrosis and pseudo-palisading of tumor cell nuclei.

than growth of the solid component. Tumors that extend into the hypothalamic region from the optic tract can have a more difficult clinical course because of location.

Morphology

A pilocytic astrocytoma is often cystic, with a mural nodule in the wall of the cyst; if solid, it is usually well circumscribed. The tumor is composed of areas with bipolar cells with long, thin "hairlike" processes that are GFAP positive; Rosenthal fibers, eosinophilic granular bodies, and microcysts are often present. Necrosis and mitoses are absent.

Oligodendroglioma

These tumors constitute about 5% to 15% of gliomas and are most common in the fourth and fifth decades. Patients may have had several years of neurologic complaints, often including seizures. The lesions are found mostly in the cerebral hemispheres, with a predilection for white matter.

Patients with oligodendrogliomas have a better prognosis than do patients with astrocytomas. Current treatment with surgery, chemotherapy, and radiotherapy yields an average survival of 5 to 10 years. Patients with anaplastic oligodendroglioma have a worse prognosis. The most common genetic findings are loss of heterozygosity for chromosomes 1p and 19q; tumors with just those specific changes have a consistent and long-lasting response to chemotherapy and radiation.

Morphology

Oligodendrogliomas are infiltrative tumors that form gelatinous, gray masses, and may show cysts, focal hemorrhage, and calcification. On microscopic examination, the tumor is composed of sheets of regular cells with spherical nuclei containing finely granular chromatin (similar to normal oligodendrocytes) surrounded by a clear halo of cytoplasm (Fig. 23–23A). The tumor typically contains a delicate network of anastomosing capillaries. Calcification, present in as many as 90% of these tumors, ranges from microscopic foci to massive depositions. Mitotic activity is usually very difficult to detect. With increasing cell density, nuclear anaplasia, increased mitotic activity and necrosis, the tumor becomes higher grade (anaplastic oligodendroglioma).

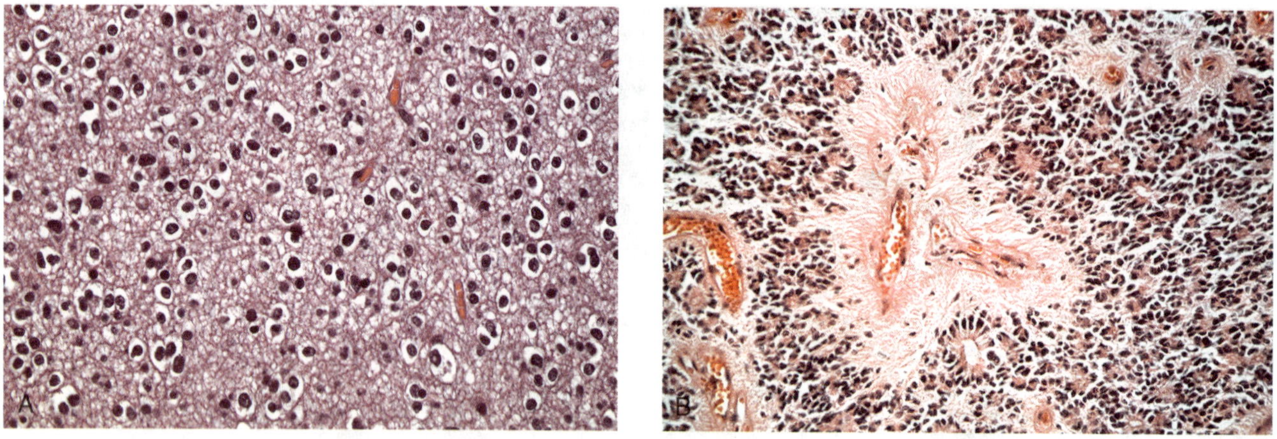

Figure 23–23

Other gliomas. **A,** In oligodendroglioma tumor cells have round nuclei, often with a cytoplasmic halo. Blood vessels in the background are thin and can form an interlacing pattern. **B,** Microscopic appearance of ependymoma.

Ependymoma

Ependymomas most often arise next to the ependyma-lined ventricular system, including the central canal of the spinal cord. In the first two decades of life, they typically occur near the fourth ventricle and constitute 5% to 10% of the primary brain tumors in this age group. In adults, the spinal cord is their most common location; tumors in this site are particularly frequent in the setting of neurofibromatosis type 2 (see below). Because ependymomas usually grow within the ventricles, CSF dissemination is a common occurrence. The clinical outcome for completely resected supratentorial and spinal ependymomas is better than for those in the posterior fossa.

Morphology

In the fourth ventricle, ependymomas are typically solid or papillary masses extending from the floor of the ventricle. These tumors are composed of cells with regular, round to oval nuclei with abundant granular chromatin. Between the nuclei there is a variably dense fibrillary background. Tumor cells may form round or elongated structures (**rosettes,** canals) that resemble the embryologic ependymal canal, with long, delicate processes extending into a lumen (Fig. 23–23B); more frequently present are **perivascular pseudo-rosettes** in which tumor cells are arranged around vessels with an intervening zone consisting of thin ependymal processes directed toward the wall of the vessel. Anaplastic ependymomas show increased cell density, high mitotic rates, necrosis. and less evident ependymal differentiation.

Neuronal Tumors

Central neurocytoma is a low-grade neuronal neoplasm found within and adjacent to the ventricular system (most commonly the lateral or third ventricles), characterized by evenly spaced, round, uniform nuclei and often islands of neuropil.

Gangliogliomas are tumors with a mixture of glial elements (looking like a low-grade astrocytoma) and mature-appearing neurons. Most of these tumors are slow growing, but the glial component occasionally becomes frankly anaplastic, and the disease then progresses rapidly. These lesions often present with seizures.

Dysembryoplastic neuroepithelial tumor is a distinctive, low-grade tumor of childhood, showing slow growth and a relatively good prognosis after resection; it often presents as a seizure disorder. These lesions are typically located in the superficial temporal lobe and consist of small round cells with features of neurons arranged in columns and around central cores of processes. These typically form multiple discrete intracortical nodules that have a myxoid background. There are well-differentiated "floating neurons" that sit in the pools of mucopolysaccharide-rich fluid of the myxoid background.

Poorly Differentiated Neoplasms

Some tumors, though of neuroectodermal origin, express few if any of the phenotypic markers of mature cells of the nervous system. The most common is the *medulloblastoma,* accounting for 20% of pediatric brain tumors.

Medulloblastoma

This tumor occurs predominantly in children and exclusively in the cerebellum. Neuronal and glial markers may be expressed, but the tumor is often largely undifferentiated. The tumor is highly malignant, and the prognosis for untreated patients is dismal; however, it is exquisitely radiosensitive. With total excision and radiation, the 5-year survival rate may be as high as 75%. Tumors of similar histology and poor degree of differentiation can be found elsewhere in the nervous system (called CNS primitive neuroectodermal tumor, or CNS PNET).

Morphology

In children, medulloblastomas are located in the midline of the cerebellum; lateral tumors occur more often in adults. The tumor is often well circumscribed, gray, and friable, and may be seen extending to the surface of the cerebellar folia and involving the leptomeninges (Fig. 23–24A). Medulloblastomas are extremely cellular, with sheets of anaplastic ("small blue") cells (Fig. 23–24B). Individual tumor cells are small, with little cytoplasm and hyperchromatic nuclei; mitoses are abundant.

Other Parenchymal Tumors

Primary Central Nervous System Lymphoma

Primary CNS lymphoma accounts for 2% of extranodal lymphomas and 1% of intracranial tumors. It is the most common CNS neoplasm in immunosuppressed individuals (including transplant recipients and persons with AIDS); under these circumstances the CNS lymphomas are nearly all driven by Epstein-Barr virus. In nonimmunosuppressed populations the age spectrum is relatively wide, with the incidence increasing after 60 years of age; most of these tumors are diffuse large B-cell lymphomas. Regardless of the clinical context, primary brain lymphoma is an aggressive disease with relatively poor response to chemotherapy as compared with peripheral lymphomas.

Individuals with primary brain lymphoma often have multiple sites of tumor within the brain parenchyma; nodal, bone marrow, or extranodal involvement outside of the CNS is a rare and late complication. Conversely, lymphoma arising outside the CNS rarely involves the brain parenchyma; when it does occur, there is usually tumor within the CSF and around intradural nerve roots.

Morphology

Lesions often involve deep gray structures, as well as white matter and cortex. Periventricular spread is common. The tumors are relatively well defined as compared with glial neoplasms but are not as discrete as metastases. They often show extensive areas of central necrosis. The tumors are nearly always high grade, most commonly large-cell lymphomas, although other histologic types can be observed (Chapter 12). Within lesions, malignant cells infiltrate the parenchyma of the brain and accumulate around blood vessels.

Germ-Cell Tumors

Primary brain germ-cell tumors occur along the midline, most commonly in the pineal and the suprasellar regions. They account for 0.2% to 1% of brain tumors in people of European descent but as many as 10% of brain tumors in Japanese. They are a tumor of the young, with 90% occurring during the first two decades. Germ-cell tumors in the pineal region show a strong male predominance.

Germ-cell tumors in the brain share many of the features of their counterparts in the gonads. The histologic classification of brain germ-cell tumors is similar to that used in the testis (Chapter 18), although the CNS tumor that is the counterpart to the testicular seminoma is called a germinoma. CNS involvement by a gonadal germ-cell tumor is not uncommon.

Meningiomas

Meningiomas are predominantly benign tumors of adults, usually attached to the dura, and arising from the meningothelial cell of the arachnoid. Meningiomas may be found along any of the external surfaces of the brain as well as within the ventricular system, where they arise from the stromal arachnoid cells of the choroid plexus. They usually come to attention because of vague nonlocalizing symptoms, or with focal findings referable to

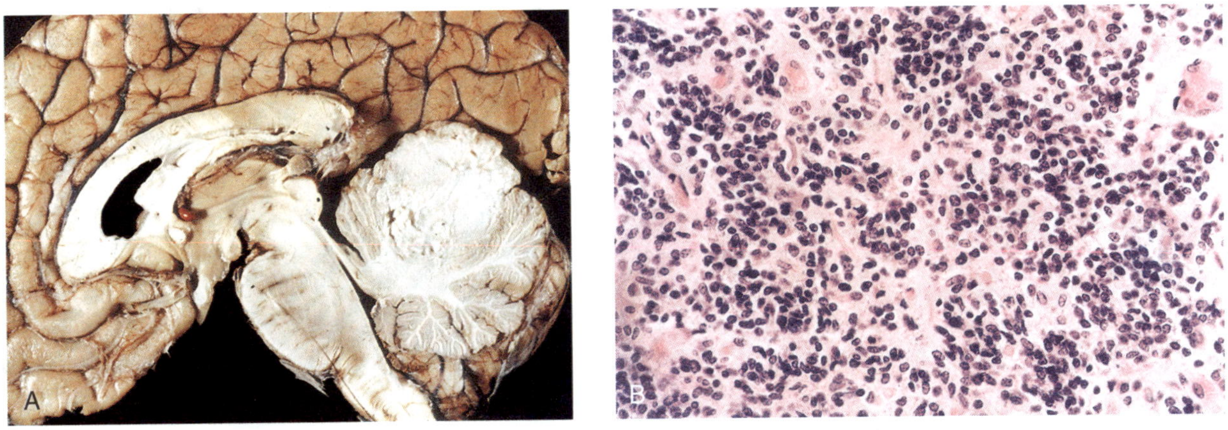

Figure 23–24

Medulloblastoma. **A,** Sagittal section of brain showing medulloblastoma destroying the superior midline cerebellum. **B,** Microscopic appearance of medulloblastoma.

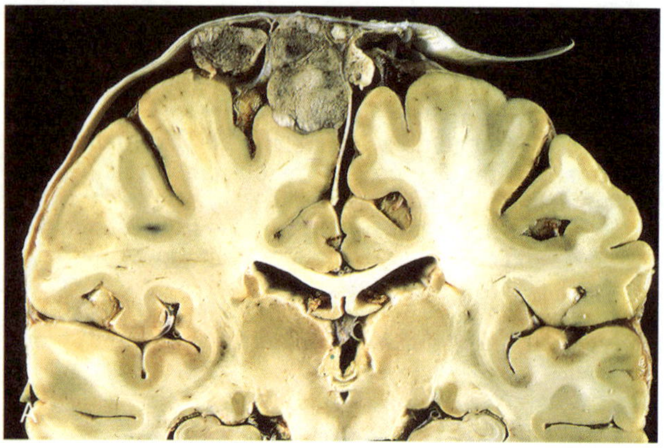

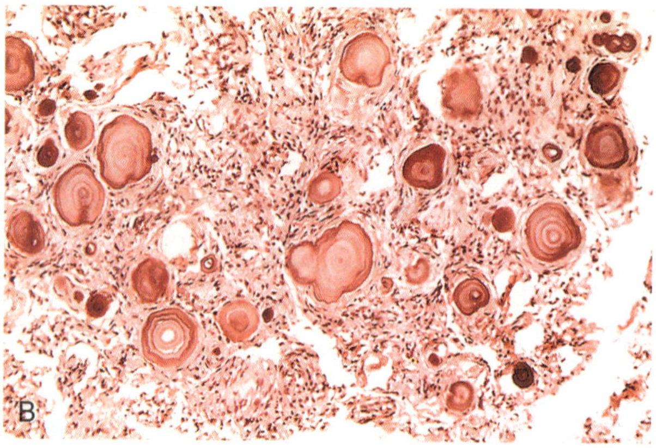

Figure 23–25

Meningioma. **A,** Parasagittal multilobular meningioma attached to the dura with compression of underlying brain. **B,** Meningioma with a whorled pattern of cell growth and psammoma bodies.

compression of underlying brain. When a person has multiple meningiomas, especially in association with eighth nerve schwannomas or glial tumors, a possible diagnosis of neurofibromatosis type 2 (NF2) should be considered (see below). About half of meningiomas not associated with NF2 still have mutations in the *NF2* gene on the long arm of chromosome 22 (22q).

Morphology

Meningiomas grow as well-defined dural-based masses that compress underlying brain but are easily separated from it (Fig. 23–25A). Extension into the overlying bone may be present. There are many different histologic patterns found in meningiomas, including: **syncytial,** named for the whorled clusters of cells that sit in tight groups without visible cell membranes; **fibroblastic,** with elongated cells and abundant collagen deposition between them; **transitional,** which shares features of the syncytial and fibroblastic types; **psammomatous,** with numerous psammoma bodies (Fig. 23–25B); **secretory,** with PAS-positive intracytoplasmic droplets and intracellular lumina by electron microscopy; and **microcystic,** with a loose, spongy appearance.

Atypical meningiomas—lesions with a higher rate of recurrence, more aggressive local growth, and a possible need for therapy in addition to surgery—are recognized by several histologic features including a higher mitotic rate.

Anaplastic (malignant) meningiomas are highly aggressive tumors that resemble a high-grade sarcoma, although there is usually some histologic evidence that indicates a meningothelial cell origin.

Although most meningiomas are easily separable from underlying brain, some tumors infiltrate the brain. The presence of brain invasion is associated with increased risk of recurrence.

The overall prognosis of meningiomas is influenced by the size and location of the lesion, surgical accessibility, and histologic grade.

Metastatic Tumors

Metastatic lesions, mostly carcinomas, account for approximately a quarter to half of intracranial tumors in hospital patients. The five most common primary sites are lung, breast, skin (melanoma), kidney, and gastrointestinal tract, accounting for about 80% of all metastases. The meninges are also a frequent site of involvement by metastatic disease. In the brain, metastases form sharply demarcated masses, often at the gray matter–white matter junction, usually surrounded by a zone of edema (Fig. 23–26). The boundary between tumor and brain parenchyma is well defined microscopically as well, with surrounding reactive gliosis.

In addition to the direct and localized effects produced by metastases, *paraneoplastic syndromes* may involve the peripheral and central nervous systems, sometimes even preceding the clinical recognition of the malignant neoplasm. These syndromes are most commonly associated

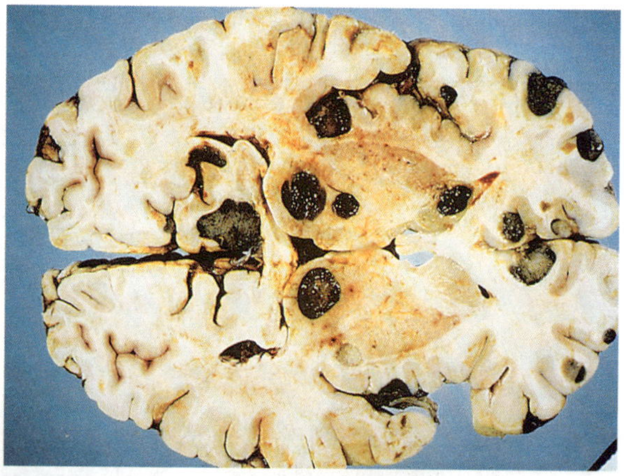

Figure 23–26

Metastatic melanoma. Metastatic lesions are distinguished grossly from most primary CNS tumors by their multicentricity and well-demarcated margins. The dark pigment in the tumor nodules in this case is characteristic of most malignant melanomas.

with small-cell carcinoma of the lung. Many, but not all, individuals with paraneoplastic syndromes have antibodies against tumor antigens. There are several manifestations of paraneoplastic syndromes; some characteristic patterns include:

- *Subacute cerebellar degeneration* resulting in ataxia, with destruction of Purkinje cells, gliosis, and a mild inflammatory infiltrate
- *Limbic encephalitis* causing a subacute dementia, with perivascular inflammatory cuffs, microglial nodules, some neuronal loss, and gliosis, all centered in the medial temporal lobe
- *Subacute sensory neuropathy* leading to altered pain sensation, with loss of sensory neurons from dorsal root ganglia, in association with inflammation.

SUMMARY

Tumors

- Tumors of the nervous system may arise from the cells of the coverings (meningiomas), from cells intrinsic to the brain (gliomas, neuronal tumors, choroid plexus tumors), or other cell populations within the skull (primary CNS lymphoma, germ-cell tumors), or they may spread from elsewhere in the body (metastases).
- Even low-grade or benign tumors can have a poor clinical outcome depending on where in the brain they occur.
- Glial tumors are broadly classified into astrocytomas, oligodendrogliomas, and ependymomas. Increasing tumor malignancy is associated with more cytologic anaplasia, increased cell density, necrosis, and mitotic activity. The most aggressive and poorly differentiated glial tumor is glioblastoma; it contains anaplastic astrocytes and shows striking vascular abnormalities.
- Metastatic spread of brain tumors to other regions of the body is rare, but the brain is not comparably protected against spread of tumors from elsewhere. Carcinomas are more commonly metastatic to the nervous system than lymphoid malignancies; sarcomas infrequently metastasize to the brain.

PRIMARY DISEASES OF MYELIN

Within the CNS, axons are tightly ensheathed by myelin, which serves as an electrical insulator to allow rapid propagation of impulses. Myelin consists of multiple layers of the specialized plasma membrane of oligodendrocytes, with most of the cytoplasm excluded. These portions of the oligodenrocyte membrane contain specialized proteins and lipids that contribute to the orderly packing of the layers. An oligodendrocyte extends processes toward many different axons and wraps a segment of roughly a few hundred microns of axon. Each of these segments is called an *internode,* and the gaps between internodes are known as *nodes of Ranvier.* Although myelinated axons are present in all areas of the brain, they are the dominant component in the white matter; therefore, most diseases of myelin are primarily white matter disorders.

The myelin in peripheral nerves is similar to the myelin in the CNS but has several important differences: Peripheral myelin is made by Schwann cells, not oligodendrocytes; each cell in the peripheral nerve contributes to only one internode, while in the CNS, many internodes comes from a single oligodendrocyte; and the specialized proteins and lipids are also different. Therefore, most diseases of CNS myelin do not significantly involve the peripheral nerves, and vice versa.

If the myelin along a set of axons is disrupted, there are changes in the ability of these axons to transmit signals. The symptoms of diseases of myelin are related to this disruption of neuronal communication; the exact nature of the symptoms depends on the site (or sites, since most disease of myelin affect many regions of the brain at the same time) where myelin disruption occurs. The natural history of demyelinating diseases is determined, in part, by the limited capacity of the CNS to regenerate normal myelin and by the degree of secondary damage to axons that occurs as the disease runs its course.

In general, diseases involving myelin are separated into two broad groups. *Demyelinating diseases* of the CNS are acquired conditions characterized by preferential damage to previously normal myelin. The most common diseases in this group result from immune-mediated injury, such as multiple sclerosis (MS) and related disorders. Other processes that can cause this type of disease include viral infection of oligodendrocytes as in progressive multifocal leukoencephalopathy (see above), and injury caused by drugs and other toxic agents.

In contrast, when myelin is not formed properly or has abnormal turnover kinetics, the resulting diseases are referred to as *dysmyelinating.* As would be expected, dysmyelinating diseases are associated with mutations affecting the proteins required for formation of normal myelin or in mutations that affect the synthesis or degradation of myelin lipids. The other general term for these diseases is *leukodystrophy.*

Multiple Sclerosis

MS is an autoimmune demyelinating disorder characterized by *distinct episodes of neurologic deficits, separated in time, attributable to white matter lesions that are separated in space.* It is the most common of the demyelinating disorders, having a prevalence of approximately 1 per 1000 persons in most of the United States and Europe. The disease becomes clinically apparent at any age, although onset in childhood or after age 50 years is relatively rare. Women are affected twice as often as men. In most individuals with MS the illness shows relapsing and remitting episodes of neurologic deficits. The frequency of relapses tends to decrease during the course of the illness, but there is a steady neurologic deterioration in a subset of patients.

It is believed that MS, like other autoimmune diseases, is caused by a combination of environmental and genetic factors that result in a loss of tolerance to self proteins (in this case, myelin antigens). A transmissible agent has been proposed, but none has ever been conclusively identified. The risk of developing MS is 15-fold higher when the disease is present in a first-degree relative. The concordance rate for monozygotic twins is approximately 25%, with a much lower rate for dizygotic twins; this indicates a strong, but not causative, role for genes. Genetic linkage of MS susceptibility to the HLA-DR2 extended haplotype is also well established.

Given the prominence of chronic inflammatory cells within and around MS plaques, immune mechanisms that may cause myelin destruction have been the focus of much investigation. Experimental allergic encephalomyelitis is an animal model of MS in which demyelination and inflammation occur after immunization with myelin, myelin proteins, or certain peptides from myelin proteins. In this model, the lesions are caused by a T cell-mediated delayed type hypersensitivity reaction to myelin proteins, and the same immune mechanism is thought to be central to the pathogenesis of MS. While MS is characterized by the presence of demyelination out of proportion to axonal loss, some injury to axons does occur. Toxic effects of lymphocytes, macrophages, and their secreted molecules have been implicated in initiating the process of axonal injury, sometimes even leading to neuronal death.

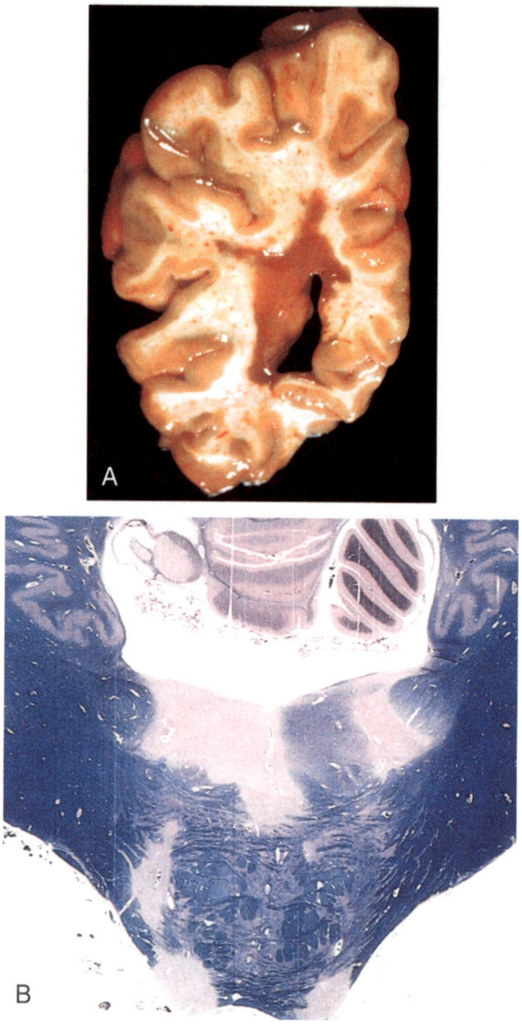

Figure 23–27

Multiple sclerosis. **A,** Section of fresh brain showing a plaque around occipital horn of the lateral ventricle. **B,** Unstained regions of demyelination (MS plaques) around the fourth ventricle. (Luxol fast blue–PAS stain for myelin.)

Morphology

MS is a white matter disease; abnormalities on the surface of the brain are usually restricted to those regions where myelinated fiber tracts course superficially (brain stem and spinal cord). Affected areas show multiple, well-circumscribed, slightly depressed, glassy, gray-tan, irregularly shaped lesions, termed **plaques** (Fig. 23–27A). These commonly occur beside the ventricles. They are also frequent in the optic nerves and chiasm, brain stem, ascending and descending fiber tracts, cerebellum, and spinal cord. The lesions have sharply defined borders at the microscopic level (Fig. 23–27B). In an **active plaque** there is evidence of ongoing myelin breakdown with abundant macrophages containing myelin debris. Lymphocytes and monocytes are present, mostly as perivascular cuffs. Small active lesions are often centered on small veins. Axons are relatively preserved, although they may be reduced in number. When plaques become quiescent (**inactive plaques**), the inflammation mostly disappears, leaving behind little to no myelin. Instead, astrocytic proliferation and gliosis are prominent. There can also be **shadow plaques,** where the border between normal and affected white matter is not sharply circumscribed. Here, thinned-out myelin sheaths can be demonstrated, especially at the outer edges, suggesting that this border region represents either incomplete myelin loss or partial remyelination.

Clinical Features. The course of MS is variable, but commonly there are multiple episodes of new symptoms (*relapses*) followed by episodes of recovery (*remissions*); typically, the recovery is not complete. The consequence of this pattern of relapsing-remitting disease is the gradual, often stepwise, accumulation of increasing neurologic deficits. Although MS lesions can occur anywhere in the CNS and, as a consequence, may induce a wide range of clinical manifestations, certain patterns of neurologic symptoms and signs are commonly observed. Unilateral visual impairment occurring over the course of a few days is a frequent initial manifestation of MS; it is due to involvement of the optic nerve (*optic neuritis, retrobulbar neuritis*). When this occurs as the first event, only a minority (10% to 50%) go on to develop full-blown MS. Involvement of the brain stem produces cranial nerve signs and ataxia, and can disrupt conjugate eye movements.

Spinal cord lesions give rise to motor and sensory impairment of trunk and limbs, spasticity, and difficulties with the voluntary control of bladder function. Changes in cognitive function can be present, but are often much milder than the other findings. In any individual patient it is hard to predict when the next relapse will occur; most current treatments aim at decreasing the rate and severity of relapses rather than recovering lost function.

The CSF in MS patients shows a mildly elevated protein level with an increased proportion of γ-globulin; in one-third of cases there is moderate pleiocytosis. When the immunoglobulin is examined further, most MS patients show *oligoclonal bands,* representing antibodies directed against a variety of antigenic targets. Although these antibodies constitute a marker for disease activity, it is not clear if they are a critical part of the disease mechanism.

Magnetic resonance imaging has greatly added to the understanding of MS, since it can show the distribution of lesions across the nervous system during active disease. From this work it has become clear that there are often more lesions in the brains of MS patients than might be expected by clinical examination, and that lesions can come and go much more often than was previously suspected.

Other Acquired Demyelinating Diseases

Immune-mediated demyelination can be found after a number of systemic infectious illnesses, including relatively mild viral diseases. These are not thought to be related to direct spread of the infectious agents to the nervous system. It is believed that the immune response to pathogen-associated antigens cross-reacts with myelin antigens, and that this results in myelin damage.

There are two general patterns of post-infectious pathology involving autoimmune reaction to myelin; unlike MS, they are monophasic illnesses with relatively abrupt onset. With *acute disseminated encephalomyelitis,* symptoms typically develop a week or two after the antecedent infection and suggest diffuse brain involvement with headache, lethargy, and coma rather than the focal findings typical of MS. Symptoms progress rapidly, with a fatal outcome in as many as 20% of cases; in the remaining patients there is complete recovery. *Acute necrotizing hemorrhagic encephalomyelitis* is a more devastating related disorder, which typically affects young adults and children.

Central pontine myelinolysis is a nonimmune process characterized by loss of myelin involving the center of the pons, most often after rapid correction of hyponatremia. It occurs in a variety of clinical settings including alcoholism and severe electrolyte or osmolar imbalance. Although the most characteristic lesion occurs in the pons, similar lesions can be found elsewhere in the brain. Because of the involvement of fibers in the pons carrying signals to motor neurons in the spinal cord, patients often present with rapidly evolving quadriplegia.

As discussed earlier, progressive multifocal leukoencephalopathy is a demyelinating disease that occurs following reactivation of JC virus in immunosuppressed patients.

Leukodystrophies

Leukodystrophies are inherited dysmyelinating diseases in which the clinical symptoms derive from either abnormal myelin synthesis or turnover. Some of these disorders involve lysosomal enzymes, while others involve peroxisomal enzymes; a few are associated with mutations in myelin proteins. Most are autosomal recessive, although X-linked diseases occur (Table 23–2).

Morphology

Much of the pathology of leukodystrophies is found in the white matter, which is diffusely abnormal in color (gray and translucent) and volume (decreased). Some diseases may show patchy involvement early, while others have a predilection for occipital lobe involvement as they begin. In the end, though, nearly all of the white matter is usually affected. With the loss of white matter, the brain becomes atrophic, the ventricles enlarge, and secondary changes can be found in the gray matter. Myelin loss is common across the leukodystrophies, often with macrophages stuffed with lipid. Some of the diseases also show specific inclusions, related to the accumulation of particular lipids.

Clinical Features. Each of the various leukodystrophies has a characteristic clinical presentation, and most can be diagnosed by genetic or biochemical methods. Despite differences in underlying mechanisms, the leukodystrophies share many features because of the common myelin target. Affected children are normal at birth but begin to miss developmental milestones during infancy and childhood. Diffuse involvement of white matter leads to deterioration in motor skills, spasticity, hypotonia, or ataxia. In general, the earlier the age at onset, the more severe the deficiency and clinical course.

Table 23–2 Selected Leukodystrophies

Metabolic Disorder	Inheritance	Abnormality
Metachromatic leukodystrophy	AR	Arylsulfatase A deficiency
Krabbe disease	AR	Galactocerebroside β-galactosidase deficiency
Adrenoleukodystrophy	AR, X	Peroxisomal defects; elevated very long chain fatty acids
Canavan disease	AR	Aspartoacylase deficieny
Pelizaeus-Merzbacher disease	X	Mutations in proteolipid protein
Vanishing white matter disease	AR	Translation initiation factor; link to myelin unclear
Alexander disease	AR	Mutations in glial fibrillary acidic protein

AR, autosomal recessive inheritance; X, X-linked inheritance.

SUMMARY

Primary Diseases of Myelin

- Because of the critical role of myelin in nerve conduction, diseases of myelin can lead to widespread and severe neurologic deficits.
- Diseases of myelin can be grouped into *demyelinating diseases* (in which normal myelin is broken down for inappropriate reasons~~often~~ by inflammatory processes), and *dysmyelinating diseases* (which are metabolic disorders that include the leukodystrophies in which the underlying structure of the myelin is abnormal or its turnover is abnormal).
- M ultiple sclerosis, an autoimmune demyelinating disease, is the most common disorder of myelin, affecting young adults often with a relapsing-remitting course with eventual progressive accumulation of neurologic deficits.
- O ther less common forms of immune-mediated demyelination often follow infections and are more acute illnesses.

ACQUIRED METABOLIC AND TOXIC DISTURBANCES

Toxic and acquired metabolic diseases are relatively common causes of neurologic illnesses. Because of the metabolic demands of the brain, it is particularly vulnerable to nutritional diseases and alterations in metabolic state. Surprisingly, even though we might expect metabolic alterations to affect the entire brain uniformly, there can be very distinct clinical presentations because of unique features or requirements of different anatomic regions. In the next section, only a few of the more common types of injury will be discussed.

Nutritional Diseases

Thiamine Deficiency. In addition to the systemic effects of thiamine deficiency (*beriberi*), there may also be abrupt development of confusion, abnormalities in eye movement and ataxia, a syndrome termed *Wernicke encephalopathy.* The acute stages, if unrecognized and untreated, may be followed by a prolonged and largely irreversible condition, *Korsakoff syndrome,* associated with profound memory disturbances. Because the two syndromes are closely linked, the term Wernicke-Korsakoff syndrome is often applied.

The syndrome is particularly common in the setting of chronic alcoholism but may also be encountered in patients with thiamine deficiency resulting from gastric disorders, including carcinoma, chronic gastritis, or persistent vomiting. Treatment with thiamine can reverse the manifestations of Wernicke syndrome.

Morphology

Wernicke encephalopathy is characterized by foci of hemorrhage and necrosis, particularly in the mammillary bodies but also adjacent to the ventricle, especially the third and fourth ventricles. Despite the presence of necrosis, there is relative preservation of many of the neurons in these structures. Early lesions show dilated capillaries with prominent endothelial cells. Subsequently, the capillaries leak red cells into the interstitium, producing hemorrhage. As the lesions resolve, there is infiltration of macrophages and development of a cystic space with hemosiderin-laden macrophages as a permanent sign of the process. Lesions in the medial dorsal nucleus of the thalamus seem to be the best correlate of the memory disturbance in Korsakoff syndrome.

Vitamin B_{12} Deficiency. In addition to pernicious anemia, deficiency of vitamin B_{12} may lead to devastating neurologic deficits associated with changes in the spinal cord. This disorder involves both ascending and descending fiber bundles in the spinal cord and is responsible for its name, *subacute combined degeneration of the spinal cord.* Symptoms develop over weeks, initially with slight ataxia and numbness and tingling in the lower extremities, but can progress rapidly to include spastic weakness of the lower extremities. Complete paraplegia can also occur. With prompt vitamin replacement therapy, clinical improvement occurs; however, if complete paraplegia has developed, recovery is poor.

Acquired Metabolic Disorders

Individuals with several systemic derangements may develop evidence of CNS dysfunction; only those associated with glucose levels and liver dysfunction will be considered here.

Hypoglycemia. Since the brain requires glucose as a substrate for its energy production, the cellular effects of diminished glucose resemble those of oxygen deprivation (hypoxia). The pattern of injury resembles global hypoxia, with injury particularly evident in the CA1 area of the hippocampus. One important difference, however, is that the Purkinje cells of the cerebellum are relatively spared in hypoglycemia. As with anoxia, if the level and duration of hypoglycemia are of sufficient severity, there may be widespread injury to many areas of the brain.

Hyperglycemia. Hyperglycemia is most commonly found in the setting of inadequately controlled diabetes mellitus and can be associated with either ketoacidosis or hyperosmolar coma. Systemically there is dehydration; however, patients develop confusion, stupor, and eventually coma because of the mass action transport of glucose (insulin-independent) into neurons associated with osmotic accumulation of water. The hyperglycemia must be corrected gradually; otherwise, severe cerebral edema may follow.

Hepatic encephalopathy. Individuals with decreased hepatic function develop depressed levels of consciousness leading to coma. In the early stages patients have a characteristic "flapping" tremor (asterixis) when extending their arms with palms facing the observer. Since the liver fails to clear ammonia through the urea cycle, it is thought that this metabolic product causes the changes in brain function, although the absolute levels of ammonia in symptomatic patients vary widely. Potential mechanisms are diverse but include alterations in synaptic transmission as well as metabolic alterations in astrocytes as they attempt to detoxify the ammonia. The cellular response in the CNS is predominantly glial, with astrocytes in the cortex and basal ganglia developing swollen pale nuclei (called *Alzheimer type II cells*).

Toxic Disorders

The list of toxins with effects on the brain is extremely long. Among the major categories of neurotoxic substances are *metals,* including lead (often causing a diffuse encephalopathy), as well as arsenic and mercury; *industrial chemicals,* including organophosphates as in pesticides and methanol (causing blindness from retinal damage); and *environmental pollutants* such as carbon monoxide (combining hypoxia with selective injury to the globus pallidus).

Ethanol is a drug with several different types of effects on the brain. While the acute intoxication effects of ethanol are reversible, excessive intake can result in profound metabolic disturbances, including brain swelling and death. Chronic alcohol exposure leads to cerebellar dysfunction in about 1% cases, with truncal ataxia, unsteady gait, and nystagmus. This is associated with atrophy in the anterior vermis of the cerebellum. The brain can also be affected by exposure to alcohol during development (fetal alcohol syndrome; Chapter 7).

Neurotoxic side effects have also been associated with the administration of chemotherapeutic agents for the treatment of tumors. *Methotrexate,* an important antineoplastic agent, may cause CNS injury, particularly in persons receiving intrathecal or high-dose systemic therapy in conjunction with radiation therapy. The morphologic changes associated with methotrexate toxicity are most prominent in white matter and consist of necrosis, demyelination, gliosis, and calcification.

Ionizing radiation can cause rapidly evolving symptoms of an intracranial mass, including headaches, nausea, vomiting, and papilledema, even after months to years after irradiation. The pathologic findings consist of large areas of coagulative necrosis in white matter with adjacent edema. Adjacent to the area of coagulative necrosis, blood vessels exhibit thickened walls with intramural fibrin-like material.

DEGENERATIVE DISEASES AND DEMENTIAS

Dementia, defined as the development of memory impairment and other cognitive deficits with preservation of a normal level of consciousness, is emerging as one of the most important public health issues in the industrialized world. There are many causes of dementia (Table 23–3); regardless of etiology, dementia is not part of normal aging and always represents a pathologic process.

Table 23–3 Major Causes of Dementia

Primary Neurodegenerative Disorders
Alzheimer disease
Pick disease and other frontotemporal degenerations
Parkinson disease and diffuse Lewy body disease
Progressive supranuclear palsy
Huntington disease
Motor neuron disease
Infections
Prion-associated disorders (Creutzfeldt-Jakob disease, fatal familial insomnia, others)
HIV encephalopathy (AIDS dementia complex)
Progressive multifocal leukoencephalopathy
Miscellaneous forms of viral encephalitis
Neurosyphilis
Chronic meningitis
Vascular and Traumatic Diseases
Multi-infarct dementia and other chronic vascular disorders
Global hypoxic-ischemic brain injury
Chronic subdural hematomas
Metabolic and Nutritional Diseases
Thiamine deficiency (Wernicke-Korsakoff syndrome)
Vitamin B_{12} deficiency
Niacin deficiency (pellagra)
Endocrine diseases
Miscellaneous
Brain tumors
Neuronal storage diseases
Toxic injury (including mercury, lead, manganese, bromides)

AIDS, acquired immunodeficiency syndrome; HIV, human immunodeficiency virus.

While the diseases to be discussed in this section are considered as “degenerative”~~that~~ is, reflecting an underlying cellular degeneration of neurons in the brain~~not~~ all forms of dementia are degenerative.

Vascular disorders are an important cause of dementia. Patients who suffer multiple, bilateral, gray and white matter (centrum semiovale) infarcts during the course of months or years develop dementia, called *vascular (multi-infarct) dementia.* When the pattern of injury preferentially involves large areas of the subcortical white matter with myelin and axon loss, the disorder is referred to as *Binswanger disease.*

In this section, we will discuss the main causes of dementia, including Alzheimer, Parkinson, and Huntington diseases and a few other selected disorders.

Alzheimer Disease

Alzheimer disease is the most common cause of dementia in the elderly. The disease usually becomes clinically apparent as insidious impairment of higher intellectual function, with alterations in mood and behavior. Later, progressive disorientation, memory loss, and aphasia indicate severe cortical dysfunction, and over the next 5 to 10 years, the patient becomes profoundly disabled, mute, and immobile. Death usually occurs from intercurrent pneumonia or other infections. When considered by age groups, the incidence of Alzheimer disease is 3%

for individuals 65 to 74 years old, 19% for 75 to 84 years, and 47% for 85 years or more. This increasing incidence with age has given rise to major medical, social, and economic problems in countries with a growing number of elderly. Although pathologic examination of brain tissue remains necessary for the definitive diagnosis of Alzheimer disease, the combination of clinical assessment and modern radiologic methods allows accurate diagnosis in 80% to 90% of cases.

Most cases are sporadic, although at least 5% to 10% are familial. In general, patients rarely become symptomatic before 50 years of age, but early onset can be seen with some of the heritable forms. Evidence from familial forms of the disease indicates that the accumulation of a peptide (β amyloid, or Aβ) in the brain initiates a chain of events that result in the morphologic changes of Alzheimer disease and dementia. This peptide is derived from a larger membrane protein known as amyloid precursor protein (APP), which is processed in either of two ways (Fig. 23–28). It can be cleaved by two enzymes, α-secretase and γ-secretase, in a process that prevents formation of Aβ, or it can be cut by β-site APP-cleaving enzyme and γ-secretase to generate Aβ. Generation and accumulation of Aβ occur slowly with advancing age. Mutations in APP or in components of γ-secretase (presenilin-1 or presenilin-2) lead to early onset familial Alzheimer disease by increasing the rate at which Aβ accumulates. Alzheimer disease occurs in almost all patients with trisomy 21 (Down syndrome)where the gene encoding APP is locatedwho survive beyond 45 years (due to APP gene dosage effects).

The search for genes associated with typical, sporadic Alzheimer disease is beginning to identify genetic associations that may provide new clues about the pathogenesis of the disease. An allele of apolipoprotein, called ε4 (ApoE4), is associated with as many as 30% of cases, and is thought to both increase the risk and lower the age of onset of the disease. ApoE4 may contribute to the deposition of Aβ, but how it does so is not known. Another gene, called *SORL1,* has recently been found to also be associated with late-onset Alzheimer disease. Deficiency of the SORL1 protein may alter the intracellular trafficking of APP, shuttling it to a compartment where the Aβ peptide is generated by enzymatic cleavage, the net result being increased generation of this pathogenic peptide.

Accumulation of Aβ has several effects on neurons and neuronal function. Small aggregates of Aβ can alter neurotransmission, and the aggregates can be toxic to neurons and synaptic endings. Larger deposits, in the form of plaques, also lead to neuronal death, elicit a local inflammatory response that can result in further cell injury, and may cause altered region-to-region communi-

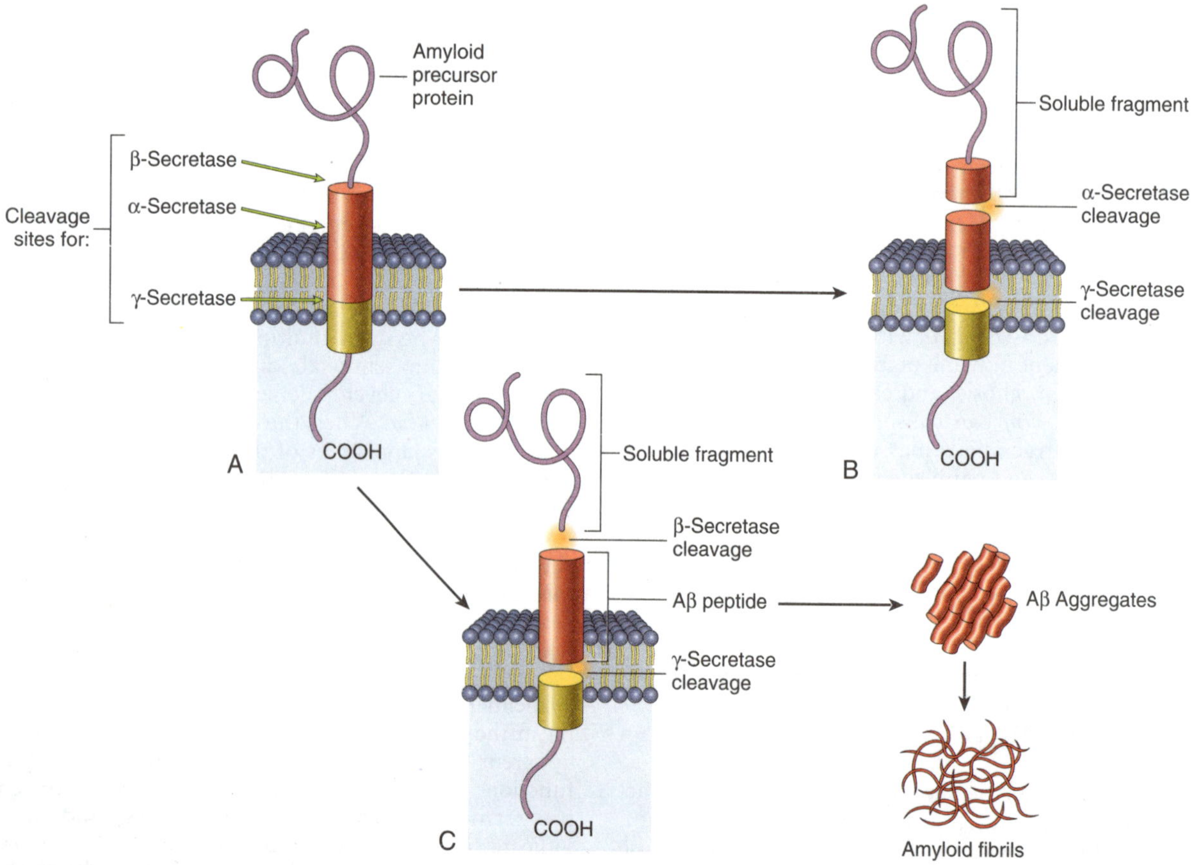

Figure 23–28

Amyloid precursor protein (APP) is a transmembrane protein. **A,** Cellular trafficking of APP involves synthesis and maturation of APP through the endoplasmic reticulum and Golgi apparatus, with eventual expression in the cell surface. **B,** Surface APP can be processed to generate soluble secreted APPs through α-secretase cleavage or can be reinternalized into an endosomal compartment. **C,** Generation of Aβ by β- and γ-secretases may occur in the endosomal and other compartments. Aβ fragments form amyloid fibrils.

cation through mechanical effects on axons and dendrites. The presence of Aβ also leads neurons to hyperphosphorylate the microtubule binding protein tau. With this increased level of phosphorylation, tau redistributes within the neuron from the axon into dendrites and cell body and aggregates into tangles. This process also results in neuronal dysfunction and cell death. The anatomic distribution of these changes, which occur roughly in parallel, are responsible for the clinical signs and symptoms; they appear to develop well in advance of clinical presentation.

Morphology

Macroscopic examination of the brain shows a variable degree of cortical atrophy with widening of the cerebral sulci that is most pronounced in the frontal, temporal, and parietal lobes. With significant atrophy, there is compensatory ventricular enlargement (hydrocephalus ex vacuo). At the microscopic level, Alzheimer disease is diagnosed by the presence of **plaques** (a type of extracellular lesion); and **neurofibrillary tangles** (a type of intracellular lesion) (Fig. 23–29). Because these may also be present to a lesser extent in the brains of elderly nondemented individuals, the current criteria for a diagnosis of Alzheimer disease are based on a combination of clinical and pathologic features. There is a fairly constant pattern of progression of involvement of brain regions: pathologic changes (specifically plaques, tangles, and the associated neuronal loss and glial reaction) are evident earliest in the entorhinal cortex, then spread through the hippocampal formation and isocortex, and then extend into the neocortex. Silver staining methods or immunohistochemistry are extremely helpful in assessing the true burden of these changes in a brain.

Neuritic plaques are focal, spherical collections of dilated, tortuous, silver-staining neuritic processes (dystrophic neurites), often around a central amyloid core (Fig. 23–29). Neuritic plaques range in size from 20 to 200 μm in diameter; microglial cells and reactive astrocytes are present at their periphery. Plaques can be found in the hippocampus and amygdala as well as in the neocortex, although there is usually relative sparing of primary motor and sensory cortices until late in the course of the disease. The amyloid core contains Aβ (Fig. 23–29B). Aβ deposits can also be found that lack any surrounding neuritic reaction, termed *diffuse plaques;* these are typically found in superficial portions of cerebral cortex as well as in basal ganglia and cerebellar cortex and may represent an early stage of plaque development.

Neurofibrillary tangles are bundles of paired helical filaments visible as basophilic fibrillary structures in the cytoplasm of the neurons that displace or encircle the nucleus (Fig. 23–29C); tangles can remain after neurons die, then becoming a form of extracellular pathology. They are commonly found in cortical neurons, especially in the entorhinal cortex, as well as in other sites such as pyramidal cells of the hippocampus, the amygdala, the basal forebrain, and the raphe nuclei. A major component of paired helical filaments is abnormally hyperphosphorylated forms of the protein **tau** (Fig. 23–29C). Tangles are not specific to Alzheimer disease, being found in other degenerative diseases as well.

Frontotemporal Dementia

Another major category of disease that results in dementia is called *frontotemporal dementias*; these disorders share clinical features (progressive deterioration of language and changes in personality) corresponding to degeneration and atrophy of temporal and frontal lobes. The symptoms often occur before memory disturbance, and this difference in presentation can assist in their separation from cases of Alzheimer disease on clinical grounds. Some of these dementias are caused by mutations in the gene encoding tau, the protein found in tangles. The basic gross finding is atrophy affecting predominantly the frontal and temporal lobes. Different subgroups are characterized by specific inclusions. In some cases the disease defining inclusions consist of abnormal accumulations of tau.

Parkinsonism

Parkinsonism is a clinical syndrome characterized by diminished facial expression (masked facies), stooped posture, slowness of voluntary movement, festinating gait

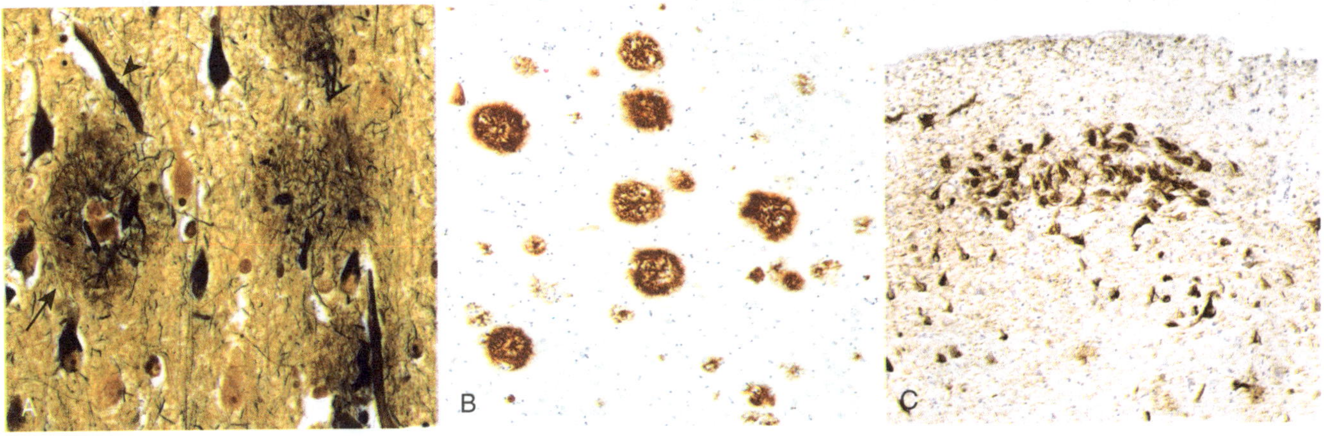

Figure 23–29

Alzheimer disease. **A,** Plaques (*arrow*) contain a central core of amyloid and a surrounding region of dystrophic neurites and tangles are filamentous intracellular inclusions (Bielschowsky stain). **B,** Immunohistochemistry against Aβ shows that the peptide is present in the core of the plaques as well as in the surrounding region. **C,** Neurons containing tangles are stained by immunohistochemistry for tau.

(progressively shortened, accelerated steps), rigidity, and a "pill-rolling" tremor. This type of motor disturbance is seen in a number of conditions that share damage to dopaminergic neurons of the substantia nigra or to their projection to the striatum. Parkinsonism can be induced by drugs that affect these neurons, particularly dopamine antagonists and toxins; one toxin, MPTP has now become an important tool in animal models to develop and test new therapies. Other diseases in which parkinsonism may be present include post-encephalitic parkinsonism (associated with the influenza pandemic), multiple system atrophy, progressive supranuclear palsy, corticobasal degeneration, and some cases of Huntington disease.

Idiopathic Parkinson disease is the most common neurodegenerative disease associated with parkinsonism; the diagnosis is made in patients with progressive parkinsonism in the absence of a toxic or other known underlying etiology and if they show clinical response to L-dihydroxyphenylalanine (L-DOPA) treatment (see below). Parkinson disease has been targeted for many novel therapeutic approaches, including transplantation, gene therapy, and stem cell injection. Currently used neurosurgical approaches to Parkinson disease include the placement of lesions in the extrapyramidal system to compensate for the loss of nigrostriatal function (pallidotomy) or placement of stimulating electrodes (deep brain stimulation).

While most Parkinson disease is sporadic, there are both autosomal dominant and recessive forms of the disease. Genetic analysis has identified specific causal mutations. For example α-synuclein mutations cause autosomal dominant Parkinson disease, as can gene duplications and triplications. Even in cases of Parkinson disease not caused by mutations in this gene, the diagnostic feature of the disease~~the~~ Lewy body~~is~~ an inclusion containing α-synuclein. This is a widely expressed neuronal protein that is involved in synaptic transmission and other cellular processes. How the alterations in sequence or protein levels result in disease is unclear, but the presence of α-synuclein in the Lewy bodies has suggested that defective degradation of the protein in the proteasome might play a role. This is supported by the identification of two other genetic loci for Parkinson disease, which involve genes encoding parkin (an E3 ubiquitin ligase) and UCHL-1 (an enzyme involved in recovery of ubiquitin from proteins targeted to the proteasome).

Morphology

On pathologic examination, the typical macroscopic findings are pallor of the substantia nigra (Fig. 23–30A, B) and locus ceruleus. On microscopic examination there is loss of the pigmented, catecholaminergic neurons in these regions associated with gliosis; **Lewy bodies** (Fig. 23–30C) may be found in some of the remaining neurons. These are single or multiple, intracytoplasmic, eosinophilic, round to elongated inclusions that often have a dense core surrounded by a pale halo. Ultrastructurally, Lewy bodies are composed of fine filaments, densely packed in the core but loose at the rim. These filaments are composed of α-synuclein, along with other proteins including neurofilament and ubiquitin. Lewy bodies may also be found in the cholinergic cells of the basal nucleus of Meynert, as well as in other brain-stem nuclei. Similar but less distinct inclusions are also found in cerebral cortical neurons, especially in the cingulate gyrus and the parahippocampal gyrus. The presence of Lewy bodies in limbic and neocortical structures is associated with cognitive impairment—the disorder recognized as dementia with Lewy bodies, discussed below.

Clinical Features. L-DOPA therapy is often extremely effective in symptomatic treatment, but it does not significantly alter the progressive nature of the disease. Over time, L-DOPA becomes less effective at providing the patient with symptomatic relief and begins to cause fluctuations in motor function on its own. The disease usually progresses over 10 to 15 years, with eventual severe motor slowing to the point of near immobility. Death is usually the result of intercurrent infection or trauma from frequent falls caused by postural instability.

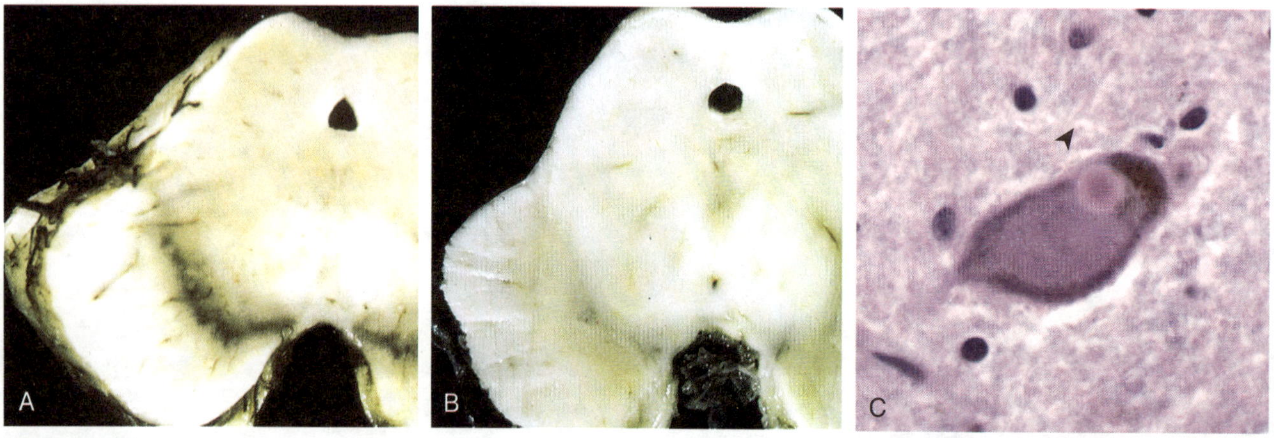

Figure 23–30

Parkinson disease. **A,** Normal substantia nigra. **B,** Depigmented substantia nigra in idiopathic Parkinson disease. **C,** Lewy body in a neuron from the substantia nigra stains pink (*arrowhead*).

About 10% to 15% of individuals with Parkinson disease develop dementia, with the incidence increasing with advancing age. Characteristic features of this disorder include a fluctuating course and hallucinations. While many affected individuals also have pathologic evidence of Alzheimer disease, the dementia in other Parkinson disease patients is attributed to widely disseminated Lewy bodies in the cerebral cortex.

Huntington Disease

Huntington disease (HD) is an inherited autosomal dominant disease characterized clinically by progressive movement disorders and dementia, with degeneration of the striatum (caudate and putamen). The movement disorder consists of jerky, hyperkinetic, sometimes dystonic movements (chorea) affecting all parts of the body; patients may develop parkinsonism with bradykinesia and rigidity. The disease is relentlessly progressive, resulting in death after an average course of about 15 years.

All individuals with *HD have the same type of mutation—a trinucleotide repeat expansion* in a gene located on 4p16.3 that encodes a large protein (huntingtin). There is a polymorphic CAG trinucleotide repeat in the gene, encoding a polyglutamine tract in the protein. Normal alleles contain 11 to 34 copies of the repeat; in disease-causing alleles the number of repeats is increased, sometimes into the hundreds. There is strong genotype-phenotype correlation in the sense that the larger the number of repeats, the earlier the onset of the disease. Once the symptoms begin, however, the course of the illness is not significantly dependent on repeat length.

Repeat expansions occur during spermatogenesis, and paternal transmission is associated with early onset in the next generation. Newly occurring mutations are uncommon, and most apparently "sporadic" cases can be related to errors in paternal identification or the death of a parent before expression of the disease. Some unaffected fathers have expanded repeats that are further expanded during transmission to their children. The identification of individuals in the presymptomatic phase of their disease obviously carries with it an immense ethical burden and should not be undertaken in the absence of appropriate counseling.

It remains unclear how the huntingtin protein with an expanded polyglutamine tract causes disease. One hypothesis is that the mutant huntingtin with expanded polyglutamine stretches binds to and sequesters various transcription factors and thus reduces synthesis of critical proteins. An alternative, and not exclusive, possibility is that the mutant huntingtin causes functional abnormalities in mitochondria, which lead to neurodegeneration. Some of these functional abnormalities may, in fact, result from decreased transcription and synthesis of proteins involved in mitochondrial electron transport and anti-oxidant proteins. The protein is widely expressed throughout the body, so it is also unclear why there is such restricted involvement of brain areas. Abnormal huntingtin is able to aggregate, and protein aggregates can be observed in tissue. It is possible that the abnormal protein fails to fold properly, and accumulation of misfolded protein triggers apoptosis in some neurons. However, this mechanism of pathogenesis has not been formally proved.

Morphology

On gross examination, the brain is small and shows striking atrophy of the caudate nucleus and, sometimes less dramatically, the putamen (Fig. 23–31). Pathologic changes develop over the course of the illness in a medial to lateral direction in the caudate and from dorsal to ventral in the putamen. The globus pallidus may be atrophied secondarily, and the lateral and third ventricles are dilated. Atrophy is frequently also seen in the frontal lobe, less often in the parietal lobe, and occasionally in the entire cortex.

On microscopic examination there is severe loss of neurons from these regions of the striatum. Loss of the small neurons generally precedes that of the larger. The medium-sized, spiny neurons that use γ-aminobutyric acid as their neurotransmitter, along with enkephalin, dynorphin, and substance P, are especially affected. There is also fibrillary gliosis that is more extensive than in the usual reaction to neuronal loss. There is a direct relationship between the degree of degeneration in the striatum and the severity of motor symptoms; a similar but less strong relationship exists between cortical neuronal loss and dementia. In remaining striatal neurons and in the cortex, there are intranuclear inclusions that contain aggregates of ubiquitinated huntingtin protein.

Clinical Features. The age at onset is most commonly in the fourth and fifth decades and is related to the length of the CAG repeat. When repeat lengths exceed 70 copies, the disease can present in adolescence or even earlier, so-called juvenile HD. Motor symptoms often precede the cognitive impairment. The movement disorder of HD is choreiform, with increased and involuntary jerky movements of all parts of the body; writhing movements of the extremities are typical. Early symptoms of higher cortical dysfunction include forgetfulness and thought and affective disorders, and there may be pro-

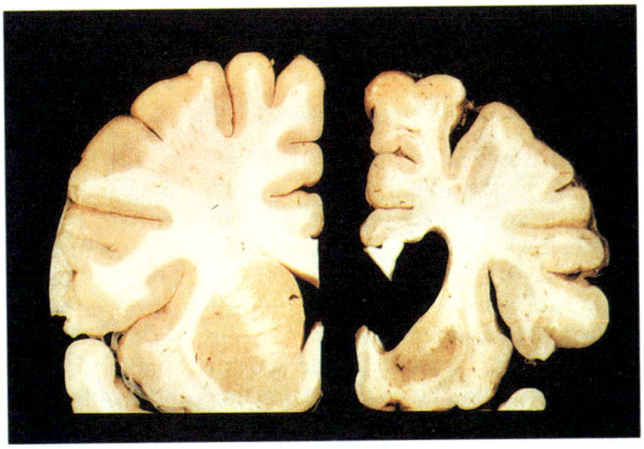

Figure 23–31

Huntington disease. Normal hemisphere on the left compared with the hemisphere with Huntington disease on the right showing atrophy of the striatum and ventricular dilation. (Courtesy of Dr. J.P. Vonsattel, Columbia University, New York, New York.)

gression to a severe dementia. HD patients have an increased risk of suicide, with intercurrent infection being the most common natural cause of death.

Spinocerebellar Degenerations

This is a clinically heterogeneous group of illnesses that include several distinct diseases; these can be distinguished on the basis of their patterns of inheritance, age at onset, and constellation of signs and symptoms. This group of diseases affects, to a variable extent, the cerebellar cortex, spinal cord, other brain regions, and peripheral nerves. Because of this pattern of involvement, clinical findings may include a combination of cerebellar and sensory ataxia, spasticity, and sensorimotor peripheral neuropathy. Degeneration of neurons, without distinctive histopathologic changes, occurs in the affected areas and is associated with mild gliosis.

Among the many forms of spinocerebellar ataxias (known in general as SCAs), there are several (SCA1–3, 6, 7, 17) that are caused by expansion of a CAG repeat encoding a polyglutamine tract similar to Huntington disease. In these forms of SCA, neuronal intranuclear inclusions containing the abnormal protein can be found, and there is a correlation between the degree of repeat expansion and age of onset. Other SCAs are caused by nucleotide repeat expansions in untranslated regions.

Friedreich ataxia is an autosomal recessive progressive illness, generally beginning in the first decade of life with gait ataxia, followed by hand clumsiness and dysarthria. Deep tendon reflexes are depressed or absent, and an extensor plantar reflex (Babinski sign) is typically present. Joint position and vibratory sense are impaired, and there is sometimes loss of pain and temperature sensation and light touch. Most patients develop pes cavus and kyphoscoliosis. There is a high incidence of cardiac disease and diabetes. Most patients become wheelchair bound within 5 years of onset; the cause of death is intercurrent pulmonary infections and cardiac disease. In most cases there is a GAA trinucleotide repeat expansion in a gene for a protein that is involved in determining iron levels in cells. This expansion does not cause a change in the structure of the protein but rather leads to extremely low levels of the protein.

Diseases of Motor Neurons

These are a series of diseases that affect the lower motor neurons in the spinal cord and brain stem, and upper motor neurons (Betz cells) in the motor cortex. Loss of lower motor neurons results in denervation of muscular targets with symptoms of muscular atrophy, weakness, and fasciculations. Loss of the projection of upper motor neurons onto the lower motor neurons results in paresis, hyperreflexia, spasticity, and positive Babinski sign. Sensory systems and cognitive functions are usually unaffected, but types with dementia do occur.

Amyotrophic Lateral Sclerosis (Motor Neuron Disease; Lou Gehrig's Disease)

This is the most common form of neurodegeneration affecting the motor system. It is characterized by muscle atrophy ("amyotrophy") and hyper-reflexia due to loss of both upper and lower motor neurons. The "lateral sclerosis" refers to the degeneration of the corticospinal tracts in the lateral portion of the spinal cord, as a result of loss of upper motor neurons.

The disease affects men slightly more frequently than women and becomes clinically manifest in the fifth decade or later. While most cases are sporadic, 5% to 10% are familial, mostly with autosomal dominant inheritance. The best understood locus for the disease is on chromosome 21, involving the gene encoding a form of superoxide dismutase, SOD1. Mutations in this gene cause approximately half of the familial cases of amyotrophic lateral sclerosis. A wide variety of missense mutations have been identified that seem to generate an adverse gain-of-function phenotype. As with huntingtin, the mutation may cause misfolding of the protein, leading to apoptosis.

Morphology

Grossly, the most evident changes are found in anterior roots of the spinal cord, which are thin and gray (rather than white). In especially severe cases, the precentral gyrus (motor cortex) may be somewhat atrophic. Microscopic examination demonstrates a reduction in the number of anterior horn cell neurons throughout the length of the spinal cord associated with reactive gliosis and loss of anterior root myelinated fibers. Similar findings are found with involvement of motor cranial nerve nuclei, nearly always sparing those of the extraocular muscles. Death of upper motor neurons—a finding that may be hard to demonstrate by microscopic examination—results in degeneration of the descending corticospinal tracts. This is usually easily seen in the spinal cord. With the loss of innervation from the death of anterior horn cells, skeletal muscles show neurogenic atrophy.

Clinical Features. Early symptoms include asymmetric weakness of the hands, manifested by dropping objects and difficulty performing fine motor tasks, and cramping and spasticity of the arms and legs. As the disease progresses, muscle strength and bulk diminish and involuntary contractions of individual motor units, termed *fasciculations,* occur. The disease eventually involves the respiratory muscles, leading to recurrent bouts of pulmonary infection, which are the usual cause of death. The severity of involvement of the upper and lower motor neurons is variable, although most patients have involvement at both levels. Familial cases develop symptoms earlier than most sporadic cases do, but the clinical course is comparable with roughly a 50% 5-year survival. In some patients, degeneration of the lower brain stem cranial motor nuclei occurs early and progresses rapidly, a pattern of disease referred to as *bulbar amyotrophic lateral sclerosis*. In these individuals, abnormalities of swallowing and speaking dominate.

Bulbospinal Atrophy (Kennedy Disease)

This X-linked adult-onset disease affecting lower motor neurons is characterized by distal limb amyotrophy and bulbar signs such as dysphagia and atrophy and fasciculations of the tongue. Affected individuals manifest androgen insensitivity with gynecomastia, testicular atrophy, and oligospermia. This is a trinucleotide-repeat disorder, similar to Huntington disease; in this case, the polyglutamine repeat is in the androgen receptor.

Spinal Muscular Atrophy

These are a distinctive group of autosomal recessive motor neuron diseases that begin in childhood or adolescence. There is loss of lower motor neurons and weakness associated with muscle fiber atrophy that often involves entire fascicles (panfascicular atrophy). The most common form of spinal muscular atrophy, SMA1 (Werdnig-Hoffmann disease), has its onset at birth or within the first 4 months of life and usually leads to death within the first 3 years of life. All forms of the disease are associated with mutations in the same gene (*SMN*) on chromosome 5.

SUMMARY

Degenerative Diseases

- Neurodegenerative diseases cause symptoms that depend on the pattern of involvement of the brain.
- Diseases that affect cerebral cortex primarily (e.g., Alzheimer disease) are more likely to cause cognitive change, alterations in personality, and memory disturbance. Accumulation of the Aβ petide, derived from amyloid precursor protein, is central to the pathogenesis of Alzheimer disease.
- Diseases that affect basal ganglia (e.g., Huntington or Parkinson disease) have motor symptoms as prominent clinical features. Parkinson disease is caused by loss of dopaminergic neurons, and Huntington disease is caused by trinucleotide repeat expansions in the gene encoding huntingtin, resulting in disease-causing gain of function.
- Diseases that affect the cerebellum (e.g., SCA) manifest as ataxia, along with other symptoms.
- Diseases that affect upper and lower motor neurons (e.g., amyotrophic lateral sclerosis) will present with weakness as the dominant feature.
- Many of these diseases are associated with abnormal aggregation of proteins, which may lead to loss of function or may trigger apoptosis. Familal forms of these diseases are associated with mutations in the genes encoding these proteins.

DISEASES OF THE PERIPHERAL NERVOUS SYSTEM

The peripheral nervous system begins a few millimeters from the pial surface of the brain and spinal cord, where Schwann cell processes replace oligodendroglial processes as the source of myelin. In the peripheral nervous system myelin shares some structural similarities with CNS myelin but also contains several proteins that are unique to the periphery. Abnormalities in some of these structural proteins have been implicated in the development of certain hereditary peripheral nerve disorders. Myelinated axons in the peripheral nerves are invested by concentric laminations of Schwann cell cytoplasm. The myelin sheath contributed by each Schwann cell is termed a *myelin internode,* and the space between adjacent internodes is termed the *node of Ranvier*. Each myelin internode is formed by a single, dedicated Schwann cell. The normal peripheral nerve also contains many smaller-diameter unmyelinated axons, which lie in small groups within the cytoplasm of a single Schwann cell. Groups of myelinated and unmyelinated axons, in turn, are compartmentalized into discrete fascicles by concentrically arrayed *perineurial cells.* Axons are insulated from the interstitial fluids of the body by a "blood-nerve" barrier, somewhat analogous to the blood-brain barrier, formed by tight junctions between endothelial cells in small peripheral nerve vessels and tight junctions between adjacent perineurial cells. Disorders of the peripheral nervous system include peripheral neuropathies and neoplasms arising from Schwann cells and other nerve sheath elements.

Patterns of Nerve Injury

A variety of disease processes can affect nerves (Table 23–4). In general, there are two main patterns of response of peripheral nerve to injury based on the target of the insult: either the Schwann cell or the axon. Diseases that affect primarily the Schwann cell lead to a loss of myelin, referred to as *segmental demyelination.* In contrast, primary involvement of the neuron and its axon leads to axonal degeneration. In some diseases, axonal degeneration may be followed by *axonal regeneration.*

Segmental Demyelination

Segmental demyelination occurs when there is dysfunction or death of the Schwann cell or damage to the myelin sheath; there is no primary abnormality of the axon. The process affects some Schwann cells, and their corresponding internodes, while sparing others (Fig. 23–32). The disintegrating myelin is engulfed initially by Schwann cells and later by macrophages. The denuded axon provides a stimulus for remyelination, with a population of cells within the endoneurium differentiating to replace injured Schwann cells. These cells proliferate and encircle the axon and, in time, remyelinate the denuded portion. Remyelinated internodes, however, are shorter than normal, and several are required to bridge the demyelinated region (see Fig. 23–32). In addition to being shortened, remyelinated internodes have thinner myelin in proportion to the diameter of the axon than normal internodes.

With repetitive cycles of demyelination and remyelination, there is an accumulation of tiers of Schwann cell processes that, on transverse section, appear as concentric layers of Schwann cell cytoplasm and redundant basement membrane that surround a thinly myelinated axon (*onion bulbs*) (Fig. 23–33). In time, many chronic demyelinating neuropathies give way to axonal injury.

Table 23–4 Causes and Types of Peripheral Neuropathies

Nutritional and Metabolic Neuropathies
Diabetes, thiamine deficiency, phyridoxine deficiency, alcoholism, renal failure
Toxic Neuropathies
Lead, arsenic, cisplatin, vincristine, organic solvents
Inflammatory Neuropathies
Guillain-Barré syndrome, chronic inflammatory demyelinating neuropathy, vasculitic neuropathy, leprosy, sarcoidosis
Hereditary Neuropathies
Hereditary motor and sensory neuropathies (Charcot-Marie-Tooth disease, Refsum disease, Dejerine-Sottas disease), hereditary sensory neuropathies, leukodystrophies
Miscellaneous
Amyloid neuropathy, paraneoplastic neuropathies, neuropathies associated with immunoglobulin abnormalities

Axonal Degeneration

Axonal degeneration is the result of primary destruction of the axon, with secondary disintegration of its myelin sheath. Damage to the axon may be due either to a focal event occurring at some point along the length of the nerve (such as trauma or ischemia) or to a more generalized abnormality affecting the neuron cell body (*neuronopathy*) or its axon (*axonopathy*). When axonal injury occurs as the result of a focal lesion, such as traumatic transection of a nerve, the distal portion of the fiber undergoes *Wallerian degeneration* (see Fig. 23–32). Within a day, the axon breaks down, and Schwann cells begin to degrade the myelin and then engulf axon fragments, forming small oval compartments (*myelin ovoids*). Macrophages are recruited into the area and participate in the phagocytosis of axonal and myelin-derived debris. In the slowly evolving neuronopathies or axonopathies, evidence of myelin breakdown is scant because only a few fibers are degenerating at any given time. The stump of the proximal portion of the severed nerve shows degenerative changes involving only the most distal two or three internodes and then undergoes regenerative activity.

The proximal stumps of degenerated axons can develop new growth cones as the axon regrows. These growth cones will use the Schwann cells vacated by the degenerated axons to guide them, if properly aligned with the distal nerve segment. The presence of multiple closely aggregated thinly myelinated small-caliber axons is evidence of regeneration (*regenerating cluster*). Regrowth of axons is a slow process, on the order of 1 to 2 mm per day, apparently limited by the rate of the slow component of axonal transport, the movement of tubulin, actin, and intermediate filaments. Despite its slow pace, axonal regeneration accounts for some of the potential for functional recovery following peripheral axonal injury.

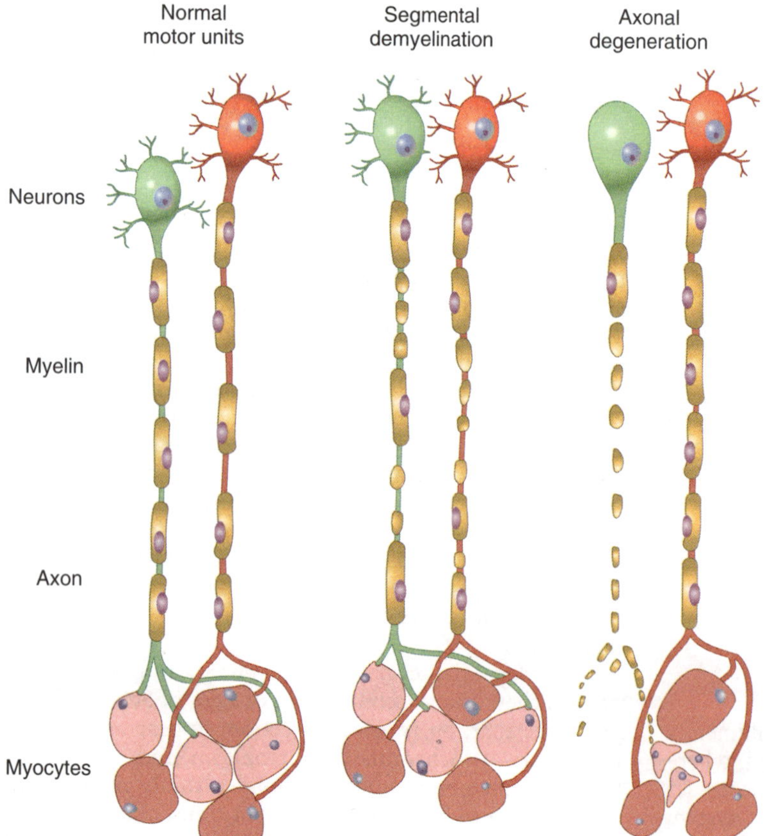

Figure 23–32

Normal and abnormal motor units. *Normal motor units:* Two adjacent motor units are shown. *Segmental demyelination:* Random internodes of myelin are injured and are remyelinated by multiple Schwann cells, while the axon and myocytes remain intact. *Axonal degeneration:* The axon and its myelin sheath undergo anterograde degeneration (shown for the *green* neuron), with resulting denervation atrophy of the myocytes within its motor unit.

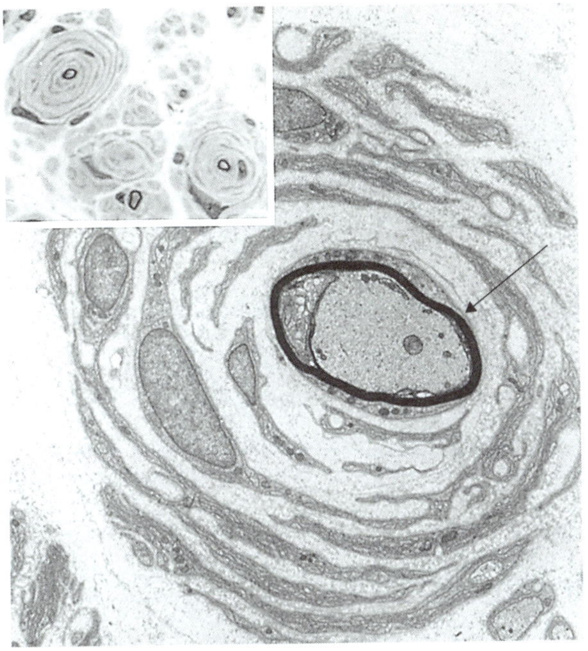

Figure 23–33

Electron micrograph of a single, thinly myelinated axon (*arrow*) surrounded by concentrically arranged Schwann cells, forming an onion bulb. *Inset,* Light microscopic appearance of an onion bulb neuropathy, characterized by "onion bulbs" surrounding axons. (From Dickersin DR: Diagnostic Electron Microscopy: A Text-Atlas. New York, Igaku-Shoin Medical Publishers, 2000, p. 984.)

Guillain-Barré Syndrome

This is one of the most common life-threatening diseases of the peripheral nervous system. It may develop spontaneously or after a systemic infection (usually viral) or other stress. Patients with Guillain-Barré syndrome present with rapidly progressive, ascending motor weakness that may lead to death from failure of respiratory muscles. Sensory involvement is usually much less striking than is motor dysfunction. The dominant histopathologic findings are segmental demyelination along with scant infiltration of peripheral nerves by macrophages and reactive lymphocytes. The CSF usually contains increased levels of protein but only a minimal cellular reaction. Because of those cases with infectious antecedents, an immunologic basis is considered most likely; treatments include plasmapheresis or intravenous immunoglobulin, which can shorten the course of the disease. With supportive care, most affected individuals recover over time.

Neoplasms of the Peripheral Nervous System

These tumors arise from cells of the peripheral nerve, including Schwann cells, perineurial cells, and fibroblasts. Many express Schwann cell characteristics, including the presence of S-100 antigen as well as the potential for melanocytic differentiation. As nerves exit the brain and spinal cord, there is a transition between myelination by oligodendrocytes and myelination by Schwann cells. This occurs within several millimeters of the substance of the brain; thus, in addition to arising along the peripheral course of nerve, these tumors can arise within the confines of the dura. When they do this, they may cause changes in adjacent brain or spinal cord.

Schwannoma

These are benign tumors arising from Schwann cells. Symptoms are referable to local compression of the involved nerve, or to compression of adjacent structures (such as brain stem or spinal cord). They are often encountered within the cranial vault, in the cerebellopontine angle, where they are attached to the vestibular branch of the eighth nerve (Fig. 23–34A). These patients often present with tinnitus and hearing loss, and the tumor is often referred to as an acoustic neuroma, although it is more accurately called a vestibular schwannoma. Elsewhere within the dura, sensory nerves are preferentially involved, including branches of the trigeminal nerve and dorsal roots. When extradural, schwannomas are most commonly found in association with large nerve trunks, where motor and sensory modalities are intermixed. Sporadic schwannomas are associated with mutations in the *NF2* gene on chromosome 22 (see below).

Morphology

Schwannomas are well-circumscribed encapsulated masses that are attached to the nerve but can be separated from it. Tumors form firm, gray masses but may also have areas of cystic and xanthomatous change. On microscopic examination, tumors show a mixture of two growth patterns (Fig. 23–34B). In the Antoni A pattern of growth, elongated cells with cytoplasmic processes are arranged in fascicles in areas of moderate to high cellularity with little stromal matrix; the "nuclear-free zones" of processes that lie between the regions of nuclear palisading are termed Verocay bodies. In the Antoni B pattern of growth, the tumor is less densely cellular with a loose meshwork of cells along with microcysts and myxoid changes. In both areas, the cytology of the individual cells is similar, with elongated cell cytoplasm and regular oval nuclei. Because the lesion displaces the nerve of origin as it grows, axons are largely excluded from the tumor. These tumors are usually uniformly immunoreactive for S-100 protein.

Neurofibroma

The most common form of neurofibroma occurs in the skin (*cutaneous neurofibroma*) or in peripheral nerve (*solitary neurofibroma*). These arise sporadically or in association with type 1 neurofibromatosis (NF1; see below). The skin lesions are evident as nodules, sometimes with overlying hyperpigmentation; they may grow to be large and become pedunculated. The risk of malignant transformation from these tumors is extremely small, and cosmetic concerns are their major morbidity.

The second type is the *plexiform neurofibroma,* mostly arising in individuals with NF1. Of major concern in the

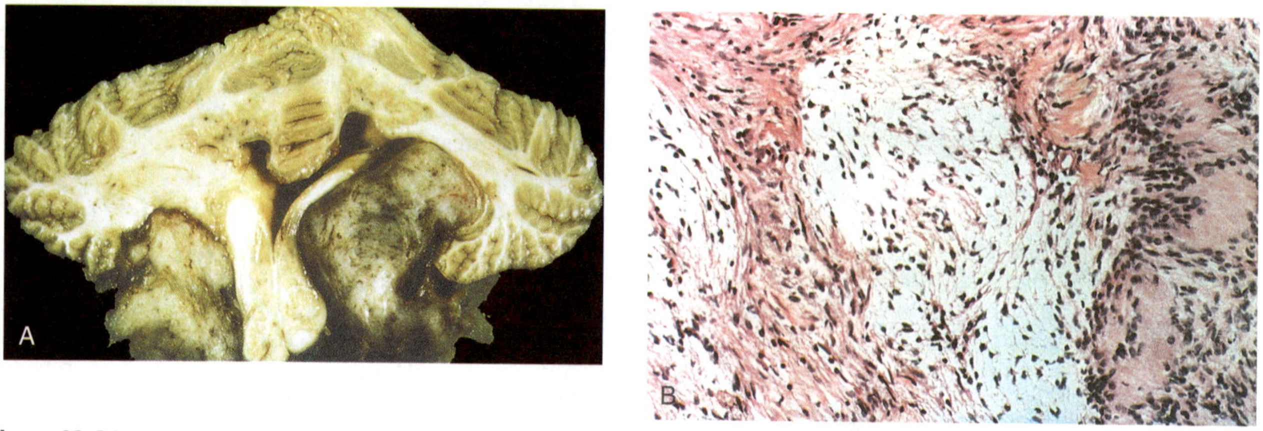

Figure 23–34

Schwannoma. **A,** Bilateral eighth-nerve schwannomas. **B,** Tumor showing cellular areas (Antoni A), including Verocay bodies (*far right*), as well as looser, myxoid regions (Antoni B areas, *center*). (**A,** Courtesy of Dr. K.M. Earle.)

care of these individuals is the difficulty in surgical removal of these plexiform tumors when they involve major nerve trunks and their potential for malignant transformation.

Morphology

Cutaneous neurofibroma. Present in the dermis and subcutaneous fat, these well-delineated but unencapsulated masses are composed of spindle cells. Although they are not invasive, the adnexal structures are sometimes enwrapped by the edges of the lesion. The stroma of these tumors is highly collagenized and contains little myxoid material. Lesions within peripheral nerves are of identical histologic appearance.

Plexiform neurofibroma. These tumors may arise anywhere along a nerve, although large nerve trunks are the most common site. They are frequently multiple. At the site of each lesion, the host nerve is irregularly expanded, as each of its fascicles is infiltrated by the neoplasm. Unlike the case with schwannomas, it is not possible to separate the lesion from the nerve. The proximal and distal extremes of the tumor may have poorly defined margins, as fingers of tumor and individual cells insert themselves between the nerve fibers. On microscopic examination, the lesion has a loose, myxoid background with a low cellularity. A number of cell types are present, including Schwann cells with typical elongated nuclei and extensions of pink cytoplasm, larger multipolar fibroblastic cells, and a sprinkling of inflammatory cells, often including mast cells.

Malignant Peripheral Nerve Sheath Tumor

These are highly malignant sarcomas that are locally invasive, frequently leading to multiple recurrences and eventual metastatic spread. Despite their name, these tumors do not arise from malignant transformation of schwannomas. Instead, they arise de novo or from transformation of a plexiform neurofibroma. These tumors can also occur after radiation therapy.

Morphology

The lesions are poorly defined tumor masses with frequent infiltration along the axis of the parent nerve as well as invasion of adjacent soft tissues. Necrosis is commonly present. A wide range of histologic findings may be encountered; often, the tumor cells resemble Schwann cells, with elongated nuclei and prominent bipolar processes. Fascicle formation may be present. Mitoses, necrosis, and extreme nuclear anaplasia are common. Some but not all malignant peripheral nerve sheath tumors are immunoreactive for S-100 protein.

FAMILIAL TUMOR SYNDROMES

Several inherited syndromes are associated with an increased risk of particular types of tumors. Those discussed here are inherited diseases characterized by the development of hamartomas and neoplasms throughout the body with particular involvement of the nervous system. Because of the combination of cutaneous manifestations and nervous system involvement, these disorders have been grouped in the past under the term "neurophakomatoses." Most of these syndromes are linked to loss of tumor suppressor genes. Symptoms are referable in part to the location of hamartomas or neoplasms; developmental delay and seizure disorders may contribute to disability in some affected individuals.

Type 1 Neurofibromatosis

This autosomal dominant disorder is characterized by neurofibromas (plexiform and solitary), gliomas of the optic nerve, pigmented nodules of the iris (*Lisch nodules*), and cutaneous hyperpigmented macules (*café au lait spots*). It is one of the more common genetic disorders, having a frequency of 1 in 3000. Individuals with NF1 have a propensity for the neurofibromas to undergo malignant transformation at a higher rate than that observed for comparable tumors in the general population. This is especially true for plexiform neurofibromas. The *NF1* gene is a tumor suppressor gene. The product of the gene is believed to be involved in G-protein–dependent signal transduction pathways (Chapter 6), but how *NF1* mutations lead to tumor development is unknown. The course of the disease is highly variable and independent of the particular mutation, with some individuals carrying a mutated gene and having no symptoms, while others develop progressive disease with spinal deformities, disfiguring lesions, and compression of vital structures, including the spinal cord.

Type 2 Neurofibromatosis

This is an autosomal dominant disorder in which patients develop a range of tumors, most commonly bilateral vestibular (acoustic) schwannomas and multiple meningiomas. Gliomas, typically ependymomas of the spinal cord, also occur in these patients. Individuals with NF2 may also have non-neoplastic lesions within the nervous system where Schwann cells or glial cells are present in small collections in inappropriate places.

This disorder is much less common than NF1, having a frequency of 1 in 40,000 to 50,000. Unlike NF1, in NF2 there is some correlation between the type of mutation and clinical symptoms, with nonsense mutations usually causing a more severe phenotype than missense mutations. As mentioned previously, the *NF2* gene is commonly mutated in sporadic meningiomas and schwannomas as well.

Tuberous Sclerosis

Tuberous sclerosis is an autosomal dominant syndrome characterized by the development of hamartomas and benign neoplasms involving the brain and other tissues. Hamartomas within the CNS occur as cortical tubers and subependymal hamartomas. Seizures, which can be difficult to control with antiepileptic drugs, are associated with the cortical lesion. Extracerebral lesions include renal angiomyolipomas, retinal glial hamartomas, and pulmonary lesions and cardiac rhabdomyomas. Cysts may be found at various sites, including the liver, kidneys, and pancreas. Cutaneous lesions include angiofibromas, leathery thickenings in localized patches (shagreen patches), hypopigmented areas (ash-leaf patches), and subungual fibromas. Tuberous sclerosis results from disruption of the tumor suppressor genes *TSC1*, which encodes hamartin, or *TSC2*, which encodes tuberin. These two proteins form dimers that regulate signaling pathways involved in protein synthesis and cell proliferation. Abnormalities of the proteins may alter neuronal proliferation, differentiation, and migration.

Morphology

Cortical hamartomas of tuberous sclerosis are firm areas of the cortex that, in contrast to the softer adjacent cortex, have been likened to potatoes, hence the appellation "tubers." These hamartomas are composed of haphazardly arranged neurons that lack the normal laminar organization of the cortex. These large cells may express a mixture of glial and neuronal features, having large vesicular nuclei with nucleoli, resembling neurons, and abundant eosinophilic cytoplasm like gemistocytic astrocytes. Similar hamartomatous features are present in the subependymal nodules, where the large astrocyte-like cells cluster beneath the ventricular surface.

von Hippel–Lindau Disease

This is an autosomal dominant inherited disease in which affected individuals develop hemangioblastomas within the cerebellar hemispheres, retina, and less commonly the brain stem and spinal cord. Patients may also have cysts involving the pancreas, liver, and kidneys and have a high propensity to develop renal cell carcinoma of the kidney. The disease frequency is 1 in 30,000 to 40,000. Therapy is directed at the symptomatic neoplasms, including resection of the cerebellar hemangioblastomas and laser therapy for retinal hemangioblastomas. Missense mutations in the tumor-suppressor gene *VHL* result in adrenal pheochromocytoma as well as hemangioblastoma. The VHL protein controls angiogenesis, especially in response to hypoxia (Chapter 6).

Morphology

The cerebellar capillary hemangioblastoma, the principal neurologic manifestation of the disease, is a highly vascular neoplasm that occurs as a mural nodule associated with a large, fluid-filled cyst. On microscopic examination, the lesion consists of variable proportions of capillary-size or somewhat larger thin-walled vessels with intervening stromal cells, with vacuolated, lightly PAS-positive, lipid-rich cytoplasm.

SUMMARY

Neoplasms of the Peripheral Nervous System and Familial Tumor Syndromes

- Neoplasms of the peripheral nervous system may originate from Schwann cells, perineurial cells and fibroblasts. They include schwannoma, neurofibroma, and malignant peripheral nerve sheat tumor.
- Familial tumor syndromes include neurofibromatosis, tuberous sclerosis, and von Hippel-Lindau disease.
- Genetic defects have been identified for each of these syndromes: *NF1* and *NF2* genes in neurofibromatosis, *TSC1* and *TSC2* genes in tuberosclerosis, and defects in the *VHL* gene in von-Hippel Lindau disease.

BIBLIOGRAPHY

Standard Textbooks of Neuropathology

Burger PC, et al: Surgical Pathology of the Nervous System and its Coverings. New York, Churchill Livingstone, 2002.

Ellison D, Love S: Neuropathology: A Reference Text of CNS Pathology. London, Mosby, 1998.

Graham DI, Lantos PL: Greenfield's Neuropathology, 7th edition. London, Arnold Press, 2002.

Vascular Disease

Kalimo H: Pathology & Genetics. Cerebrovascular Diseases. Basel, ISN Neuropath Press, 2005.

Traumatic Injury

McArthur DL, et al.: Moderate and severe traumatic brain injury: epidemiologic, imaging and neuropathologic perspectives. Brain Pathol 14:185, 2004.

Congenital and Perinatal Diseases

du Plessis AJ, Volpe JJ: Perinatal brain injury in the preterm and term newborn. Curr Opin Neurol 15:151, 2002.

Golden JA, Harding BN: Pathology & Genetics. Developmental Neuropathology. Basel, ISN Neuropath Press, 2004.

Emsley JG, et al: Adult neurogenesis and repair of the adult CNS with neural progenitors, precursors, and stem cells. Prog Neurobiol 75:321, 2005.

Mochida GH, Walsh CA: Genetic basis of developmental malformations of the cerebral cortex. Arch Neurol 61:637, 2004.

Infectious Diseases

Collinge J: Molecular neurology of prion disease. J Neurol Neurosurg Psychiatry 76:906, 2005.

Gray F, Keohane C: The neuropathology of HIV infection in the era of highly active antiretroviral therapy (HAART). Brain Pathol 13:79, 2003.

Neoplasms

Ironside JW, et al: Diagnostic Pathology of Nervous System Tumours. London, Churchill Livingstone, 2002.

Kleihues P, Cavanee WK: Pathology & Genetics. Tumors of the Nervous System. Basel, IARC Press, 2000.

Louis DN: Molecular pathology of malignant gliomas. Annu Rev Pathol: Mech Dis 1:97, 2006.

Disease of Myelin

Morales Y, et al: The pathology of multiple sclerosis: evidence for heterogeneity. Adv Neurol 98:27, 2006.

Weiner HL: Multiple sclerosis is an inflammatory T-cell-mediated autoimmune disease. Arch Neurol 61:1613, 2004.

Metabolic Disorders.

Horster F, et al: Disorders of intermediary metabolism: toxic leukoencephalopathies. J Inherit Metab Dis 28:345, 2005.

Neurodegenerative Diseases

Dickson DW: Neurodegeneration: The Molecular Pathology of Dementia and Movement Disorders. Basel, ISN Neuropath Press, 2003.

Gandhi S, Wood NW: Molecular pathogenesis of Parkinson's disease. Hum Mol Genet 14:2749, 2005.

Goedert M, Spillantini MG: A century of Alzheimer's disease. Science 314:777, 2006.

Golde TE: The Aβ hypothesis: leading us to rationally-designed therapeutic strategies for the treatment or prevention of Alzheimer disease. Brain Pathol 15:84, 2005.

Greenamyre JT: Huntington's diseasemaking connections. N Engl J Med 356:518, 2007.

Hersch SM, Ferrante RJ: Translating therapies for Huntington's disease from genetic animal models to clinical trials. NeuroRx 1:298, 2004.

Selkoe DJ: Defining molecular targets to prevent Alzheimer disease. Arch Neurol 62:192, 2005.

Selkoe DJ: Cell biology of protein misfolding: the examples of Alzheimer's and Parkinson's diseases. Nat Cell Biol 6:1054, 2004.

Shovronsky DM, Lee VM-Y, Trojanowski JQ: Neurodegenerative diseases: new concepts of pathogenesis and their therapeutic implications. Annu Rev Pathol: Mech Dis 1:151, 2006.

Peripheral Nervous System

Dyck PJ, Thomas PK: Peripheral Neuropathy, 4th edition. Philadelphia, Saunders, 2005.

Engel AG: Myology, 3rd edition. McGraw-Hill, 2004.

Karpati G: Structural Basis of Skeletal Muscle Diseases. Basel, ISN Neuropath Press, 2002.

Familial Tumor Syndromes

Grino PB, Nathanson KL, Henske EP: The tuberous sclerosis complex. N Engl J Med 355:1345, 2006.

Kaelin WG, Jr.: von Hippel-Lindau disease. Annual Review of Pathology: Mechanisms of Disease, Vol. 2:145, 2007.

McClatchey AI: Neurofibromatosis. Annual Review of Pathology: Mechanisms of Disease, Vol. 2:191, 2007.

Yohay KH: The genetic and molecular pathogenesis of NF1 and NF2. Semin Pediatr Neurol 13:21, 2006.

Index

Note: Page numbers followed by f indicate figures; those followed by t indicate tables.

F

W